To Paul Preissler M.D.

with appreciation for teaching
Dartmouth medical students.

Geo Buchbad MD

March 1981.

HEART DISEASE
IN INFANCY AND CHILDHOOD

JOHN D. KEITH

M.D., F.R.C.P.(C), F.A.C.C.

Professor Emeritus of Paediatrics,
University of Toronto Faculty of Medicine;
Physician-in-Charge (1938–1973), Cardiac Clinic and Department,
The Hospital for Sick Children, Toronto, Ontario, Canada

RICHARD D. ROWE

M.D., Ch.B.(N.Z.), F.R.C.P.(Ed.), F.R.C.P.(C)

Professor of Paediatrics,
University of Toronto Faculty of Medicine;
Director, Division of Cardiology, Department of Paediatrics,
The Hospital for Sick Children, Toronto, Ontario, Canada

PETER VLAD

M.D.

Professor of Pediatrics,
State University of New York at Buffalo, School of Medicine;
Chief, Division of Cardiology, Department of Pediatrics, and Director, Edward C. Lambert
Department of Cardiology,
Children's Hospital of Buffalo, Buffalo, New York, U.S.A.

HEART DISEASE
IN INFANCY AND CHILDHOOD
THIRD EDITION

MACMILLAN PUBLISHING CO., INC.

NEW YORK

COLLIER MACMILLAN CANADA, LTD.

TORONTO

BAILLIÈRE TINDALL

LONDON

MACMILLAN PUBLISHING CO., INC.
866 Third Avenue, New York, New York 10022

COLLIER MACMILLAN CANADA, Ltd.

BAILLIÈRE TINDALL · London

Library of Congress Cataloging in Publication Data

Main entry under title:

Heart disease in infancy and childhood.

   Previous editions written by J. D. Keith, R. D. Rowe, and P. Vlad.
   Includes bibliographies and index.
   1. Pediatric cardiology. I. Keith, John D.
II. Rowe, Richard Desmond, (date)   III. Vlad, Peter.
IV. Keith, John D. Heart disease in infancy and childhood. [DNLM: 1. Heart diseases—In infancy and childhood. WS290 K28h]
RJ421.K4   1978   618.9'21'2   76-54304
ISBN 0-02-36220-2
Baillière Tindall SBN 07020 06 254

Printing: 1 2 3 4 5 6 7 8   Year: 8 9 0 1 2 3 4

PREFACE TO THE THIRD EDITION

THE WORLD medical literature has become increasingly voluminous. The *Index Medicus* now reviews 2250 journals regularly and records the titles and origins of the pertinent articles, many relating to the cardiovascular field. From time to time excellent summary papers appear covering current knowledge on a particular segment of the discipline. The modern textbook, therefore, is a series of adequate summaries in the form of chapters, and because of the immensity of the world literature the need for such reviews is more urgent than ever before. In this third edition of *Heart Disease in Infancy and Childhood* the authors have done their best to assimilate the currently available data and to present them under suitable headings.

As was pointed out by Dr. Clement Smith, when Dr. Thomas Morgan Roch published the first textbook of pediatrics in 1896 only 7 of the 1100 pages were devoted to congenital diseases of the heart. Knowledge in this field was slow in evolving until cardiac catheterization, angio-cardiography, and modern cardiac surgery shed new light on the subject and led to the current literature, which each year represents the harvest of new articles published on a multiplicity of facets. There have been many pioneers in the field, discovering and rediscovering noteworthy features of heart anomalies or other aspects of cardiovascular disease in the young. A major review of the harvest achieved by cardiac catheterization and angiocardiography, and their impact on modern cardiac surgery, has been made in this third edition.

Perhaps the first important approach in the sphere of children's heart disease was made by Dr. Maude Abbott, whose initial efforts were encouraged by Sir William Osler and whose contributions began at the turn of the century and proceeded over the next 40 or 50 years until her death in 1943. As a result of her extensive study she established a working classification of congenital heart disease and thereby helped to focus clinical attention on individual anomalies.

In past years the energetic clinical and research activities have led to many subdivisions and have broadened the concept of cardiovascular disease in the young, so that an increasing number of subspecialties are now involved in the total picture. Initially, the clinician, the pathologist, the physiologist, the radiologist, and the bacteriologist were caught up in the stream of events. Now many other specialties and subspecialties have demonstrated the value of their investigative approaches so today there are many partners in the field of pediatric cardiology. Current converts have been added in these categories of the third edition.

The history of various forms of heart disease in the early decades of life has been changing visibly with the passage of time. Modern diagnosis and therapy have had a major impact on this process. In the past, the pace was slower, with a gradual control of certain specific diseases such as diphtheria, rheumatic fever, pneumonia, and so forth. In recent years, particularly in the last two to three decades, the pace has quickened and the natural history information is evolving steadily in relation to many advances, medical and surgical, in the field of pediatric cardiology. The assessment of this natural history process has been a major project of The Hospital for Sick Children in Toronto, and, therefore, a major concern of the authors of this book. A data-processing file was established many years ago and now covers a period of 25 to 30 years and constitutes one of the largest pools of data available in any one medical center. This valuable material had been a major contribution to each chapter of this third edition. Approximately 25,000 infants and children are now recorded in the files of the hospital, most covered by repeated visits, and many clinical, surgical, and investigative items are included. To handle this data adequately has involved modern, sophisticated computer techniques. These allow a ready source of information to study individual lesions or groups of lesions in infancy and childhood. Overall appraisal of a problem can be made in a much shorter time. Segments of the problem can be studied by pulling selected individual records. A combination of the two approaches has proved most valuable.

The progress made in the field of atherosclerosis in adult life has encouraged the pediatric cardiologist to explore the early stages of this pathologic process. From early childhood to early adult life offers such a time interval and ultimately should prove rewarding in any attempt to identify the significance of various factors in the atherosclerotic picture. The authors have brought much of this material together, based on personal experience as well as the investigations of others.

When one of us (J.D.K.) began the practice of pediatric cardiology in 1938 at The Hospital for Sick Children, Toronto, the hospital beds were crowded with rheumatic fever patients (the majority with heart involvement), usually occupying 40 beds at any one time. Since then this disease has subsided most dramatically, until today only an occasional child with rheumatic fever with or without heart disease is seen on the wards of the hospital.

However, the pattern of care of the rheumatic fever patient is one of repeated visits to the doctor's office and prolonged followup. This approach has proved most useful in the field of congenital heart disease and has resulted in the accumulation of important information regarding the natural history of the defects and the influence of medical and surgical therapy on them.

It has long been recognized that the age group that one is most likely to encounter in congenital heart anomalies is the first year of life. The majority of cases are identified first in this period, but it is only recently that persistent efforts have been made to correct the more difficult and complicated anomalies in the early months of life and most particularly in the neonate. This has led to advances in early diagnosis, surgical techniques, anesthesia, technology of the heart-lung pump machine, and intensive care support. This third edition of our book attempts to summarize the important aspects of the current progress in each of these fields of endeavor.

In our data file we have 747 cases in which transposition of the great arteries was the prime diagnosis. This group, which includes a wide spectrum of anatomic variations, has proved most useful to us in thoroughly understanding the multiple problems presented by this anomaly and has led to medical and surgical management that has steadily lowered the mortality.

Since Dr. Mustard introduced his technique for surgical correction of transposed great arteries at The Hospital for Sick Children, Toronto, we have had special interest in following the cases that were successfully corrected. Two hundred and fifty have had the Mustard procedure. The data available in this followup are recorded in the chapter on transposed great vessels (Chapter 33), which includes the early and late complications that may be identified.

Several areas in the field of pediatric cardiology have assumed increasing importance in recent years and have been emphasized in the 62 chapters of the present edition. The value of the *noninvasive* method of investigation has been enhanced by hemodynamic correlation. Echocardiography has been of special benefit for children with heart disease because of its ability to assess chamber dimension and ventricular function as well as identify great-vessel position and valve movement. Exercise physiology, because of added methodology, is rapidly assuming a new role in the evaluation of the child both before and after cardiac surgery. Nuclide techniques are similarly expanding so that myocardial imaging, as well as shunt detection and ventricular function, is being applied even to the newly born.

The expanded role of cardiology in the *first month of life* has been permitted by better support methods. The new neonatology has allowed more sophisticated hemodynamic explorations and new pharmacologic approaches to be tested. Obvious benefits are visible with new techniques for opening or closing the ductus arteriosus at this age.

With the improved results of cardiac surgery in the past decade two new populations of patients are beginning to form. One is that of children with complex cardiac malformation who have successfully been treated by palliative operations and for whom newer techniques of repair of more lasting nature are currently being considered. The other is that of patients who have had a definitive surgical repair. Better appreciation of the late consequences of congenital heart disease is leading to a more appropriate structuring of followup for the latter group of patients. Staged evaluations now include—in addition to the classic ones—echocardiography, nuclide studies, exercise testing, electrocardiographic monitoring, and cardiac catheterization and angio-cardiography. For most such patients lifelong surveillance is being recommended. The psychologic effects of living with congenital heart disease for both parent and child is gradually being revealed.

There are other issues and problems. For example, can techniques involving radiation be replaced by harmless physical methods? Are the results of early repair better than those with early palliation followed by later repair? What is the long-range fate of the child carrying prosthetic devices required by some surgical methods? What is the long-range effect, if any, of circulatory arrest employed in the execution of certain corrective operations? Are there genetic consequences on the offspring of the congenital cardiac restored to reproductive age? What are the ethics of diagnostic and surgical interventions offered to individuals with incorrectable heart defects or with multiple and intractable extracardiac malformations? And, at this time of fiscal stress, what should be the order of priority of the complex malformation in the competition for the health dollar? The third edition touches on some of these matters, but does not provide answers to any. These questions remain to challenge pediatric cardiologists in the years ahead.

J. D. K.

R. D. R.

P. V.

ACKNOWLEDGMENTS

WE ACKNOWLEDGE with gratitude our debt to the Ontario Heart Foundation for the continued support of our cardiovascular research over many years. By funding fellowships, technical assistance, equipment, and supplies this organization has facilitated our studies and helped immeasurably in solving problems and assembling data that have been set down in this volume. The work of the Foundation has been greatly advanced by the continuing efforts of the late president, Mr. John Schultz, and his Board of Directors.

We are indebted to a number of friends and colleagues in the preparation of this third edition. We would like to record our gratitude to Professor Emeritus of Paediatrics, Harry Bain, who has been Professor of Paediatrics at the University of Toronto and the Chief Physician at The Hospital for Sick Children during the past decade. His long, hard-working day has not infrequently included problems relating to the Cardiac Department. As the hospital and the Department of Paediatrics has grown steadily in the past 10 years so has the Cardiac Department. It is a pleasure to acknowledge the value of his advice, comments, and criticism as the occasion demanded.

Dr. Langford Kidd is now Harriet Lane Home Professor and Director of the Division of Cardiology in the Pediatric Department at Johns Hopkins Hospital, Baltimore. While he was at The Hospital for Sick Children in Toronto, he played a major part in collecting the data that appear in many chapters, particularly those relating to cardiac catheterization and angiocardiography.

Our cardiac surgeons—Dr. William Mustard, Dr. George Trusler, and Dr. William Williams—have permitted us to use much of their case material and illustrations of surgical procedures. They have developed cardiac surgery at The Hospital for Sick Children to a very high level. The decisions in relation to cardiac surgery and postoperative management result from the continuous close cooperation with weekly meetings with them. The integration of the two departments has led to a very happy relationship over the years. We especially acknowledged this to Dr. Mustard in 1977, at the beginning of his retirement.

Dr. Peter Fleming has given us expert advice on bacteriology when needed, and his help has been especially appreciated in the chapter on bacterial endocarditis.

The Perinatal Division of The Hospital for Sick Children, headed by Dr. P. R. Swyer with his associates Dr. G. W. Chance, Dr. M. H. Bryan, Dr. M. J. O'Brien, and Dr. P. Fitzhardinge, has given us a long and valued collaboration over the many difficult cardiorespiratory problems in that area.

We have tried whenever possible to include in each chapter the experiences gathered at The Hospital for Sick Children. In the process of collecting such data we have been dependent on a team effort that has involved the assistance and cooperation of cardiac research fellows, nurses, secretaries, and colleagues of the hospital staff.

Mrs. Mirzda Janiss, who supervised the cardiac catheterization laboratories for many years and now manages the electrocardiographic section, has played a major role in our unit over the years. Her ability to create a smooth operation and a pleasant atmosphere was as much related to her ability with people as to her technical competence. She has been ably assisted by the following nurses: Mrs. B. Carver, Mrs. J. Griffiths, Mrs. M. Toole, Mrs. G. Lamont, Mrs. I. Hecht, Miss C. Williams, Miss G. Robinson, Mrs. E. Grady, Mrs. P. Grande, Mrs. K. Hunter, Mrs. S. Balcone, Mrs. D. Evans, Mrs. A. Lewandowsky, and Mrs. H. McKim.

Since the publication of the second edition of this book, a number of cardiac fellows have been attached to the Cardiac Department of The Hospital for Sick Children for varying periods of time, and all have contributed directly or indirectly to the material used in presenting our experience with the numerous types of heart disease encountered in the pediatric age group. The following fellows have contributed in assembling the data referred to in this third edition:

Dr. Simón Muñoz Armas   Caracas, Venezuela

Dr. Robert Arnold   Liverpool, England

Dr. Pierre Auger   Levis, Quebec, Canada

Dr. Kalim Aziz   Chicago, Illinois, USA

Dr. Hugh Bain   Newcastle, England

Dr. Donald S. Beanlands   Ottawa, Ontario, Canada

Dr. Margherita Bini   Padova, Italy

Dr. Bjorn Bjarke   Stockholm, Sweden

Dr. Iain F. S. Black   Philadelphia, Pennsylvania, USA

Dr. Andrew Blackwood   Melbourne, Australia

Dr. Felipe Constancio Bolaños   Buenos Aires, Argentina

Dr. Michael Braudo   Toronto, Ontario, Canada

Dr. Samuel Brew-Graves   Nigeria

Dr. A. Louise Calder   Auckland, New Zealand

Dr. A. G. M. Campbell   Aberdeen, Scotland

Dr. Joan Coggin   Loma Linda, California, USA

Dr. Su-Chiung Chen   St. Louis, Missouri, USA

Dr. Athanasios Chrysohou   Salonika, Greece

Dr. Malcolm Clarke   Stoke-on-Trent, England

Dr. T. Emmett Cleary   Toronto, Ontario, Canada

Dr. George F. Collins   Montreal, Quebec, Canada

Dr. John F. Collins   St. John's, Newfoundland, Canada

Dr. Maria Colombi   Browns Mills, New Jersey, USA

Dr. Georges Delisle   Quebec City, Quebec, Canada

Dr. Fiza Durrani   Chichester, England

Dr. R. N. Easthope, Wellington, New Zealand

Dr. Bachoo Edibam   Nagpur, India

Dr. George Emmanouilides   Los Angeles, California, USA

Dr. John R. Evans   Toronto, Ontario, Canada

Dr. Harvest Fadahunsi   Nigeria

Dr. Joel Fagan   Calgary, Alberta, Canada

Dr. John Fay   Kingston, Ontario, Canada

Dr. Ian Findlay   Melbourne, Australia

Dr. Eugene Fischmann   Washington, D.C., USA

Dr. Peter Forbath   Toronto, Ontario, Canada

Dr. Constance Forsyth   Dundee, Scotland

Dr. Rodney S. Fowler   Toronto, Ontario, Canada

Dr. Beat Friedli   Geneva, Switzerland

Dr. Hiroshi Fukuda   Fukuoka City, Japan

Dr. Irving H. Glass   Deceased, 1976

Dr. Michael J. Godman   Edinburgh, Scotland

Dr. Katherine Hallidie-Smith   London, England

Dr. Richard Hawker   Australia

Dr. Edison Hobson   Brantford, Ontario, Canada

Dr. Ronald Hope   Miami, Florida, USA

Dr. Dyanand Jagdeo   Toronto, Ontario, Canada

Dr. Hirohisa Kato   Kurume-Shi, Japan

Dr. George Khoury   Morgantown, West Virginia, USA

Dr. Luis Lasso-Avalos   Mexico City, Mexico

Dr. Ronald M. Lauer   Iowa City, Iowa, USA

Dr. Mok Dock Li   London, Ontario, Canada

Dr. Sahat M. Manoeroeng   Medan, Indonesia

Dr. Keith McKenzie   Kingston, Jamaica

Dr. Yves Marquis   Quebec City, Quebec, Canada

Dr. Colin Miller   Kingston, Jamaica

Dr. Shiela Mitchell   Bethesda, Maryland, USA

Dr. H. Conner Mulholland   Belfast, Northern Ireland

Dr. David Mymin   St. Boniface, Manitoba, Canada

Dr. Maurice Nanton   Halifax, Nova Scotia, Canada

Dr. Catherine Neill   Baltimore, Maryland, USA

Dr. Ralph Nimchan   Laredo, Texas, USA

Dr. Aron Nordenberg   Harrisburg, Pennsylvania, USA

Dr. J. H. O'Hanley   Charlottetown, Prince Edward Island, Canada

Dr. Peter M. Olley   Toronto, Ontario, Canada

Dr. K. Ross Parker   Hamilton, Ontario, Canada

Dr. Andre Pasternac   Montreal, Quebec, Canada

Dr. Richard G. Pearse   London, England

Dr. Gerald B. Peckham St. John's, Newfoundland, Canada

Dr. Akos Pereszlenyi Toronto, Ontario, Canada

Dr. Antonio Peschiera Kalamazoo, Michigan, USA

Dr. Douglas Pickering Oxford, England

Dr. Dennis Pittaway Durban, South Africa

Dr. Dorothy Radford Brisbane, Australia

Dr. L. K. Rathi Laxmikant, USA

Dr. Nigel Roberts Los Angeles, California, USA

Dr. Lydia Rodriquez Mexico City, Mexico

Dr. Richard D. Rowe Toronto, Ontario, Canada

Dr. Michael Scott Lurgan, Northern Ireland

Dr. William Sears USA

Dr. Frank Sellers Ottawa, Ontario, Canada

Dr. Pravin Shah Rochester, New York, USA

Dr. Reda Shaher Albany, New York, USA

Dr. Ali Shams Toronto, Ontario, Canada

Dr. John Stone Toronto, Ontario, Canada

Dr. Walter Singh Bramalea Ontario, Canada

Dr. Robert Sommerville Calgary, Alberta, Canada

Dr. Henry M. Sondheimer Syracuse, New York, USA

Dr. J. Richardo Suarez-Arana San Salvador, El Salvador

Dr. Paul R. Swyer Toronto, Ontario, Canada

Dr. Otto Teixeira Ottawa, Ontario, Canada

Dr. Michael Tyrrell Saskatoon, Saskatchewan, Canada

Dr. Richard Van Praagh Boston, Massachusetts, USA

Dr. Stella Van Praagh Boston, Massachusetts, USA

Dr. Preecha Vichitbandha Bangkok, Thailand

Dr. Dennis J. Vince Vancouver, British Columbia, Canada

Dr. Shyama Virmani St John's, Newfoundland, Canada

Dr. Nino Vitarelli Rome, Italy

Dr. Alfredo Vizcaino Mexico City, Mexico

Dr. Peter Vlad Buffalo, New York, USA

Dr. David Watson Jackson, Mississippi, USA

Dr. Geoffrey Watson Manchester, England

Dr. Stephen Weyman St. John, New Brunswick, Canada

Dr. Warren S. Whelan London, Ontario, Canada

Dr. Gordon Williams Leeds, England

Dr. Tadeusz Zakrzewski Temple, Arizona, USA

Dr. Vera Rose is responsible for the cardiac records system at The Hospital for Sick Children, which involves filing of all clinical, physiologic, and pathologic data on each patient as well as preparing a punch card for subsequent analysis. This has facilitated the ease with which information can be studied. We are indebted to her and to her staff for the careful work that has been involved in the handling of this material. In the past two years, Mr. David Cook has played a major role in this department and has made the data more readily retrievable. The hospital librarians, Mrs. I. Jeryn and Mrs. M. Northgrave, as always, have made our literature searches the lighter.

The atmosphere at the hospital is apparent to those who work in it or visit it frequently. This aspect of The Hospital for Sick Children has always been unique, partly because it is a children's hospital and partly because it has become, in its 100 years, a landmark institution known for its striving for excellence. The desired standards are difficult to maintain at an ideal level, but continuous efforts are made in this direction by our Chairman of the Board, Mr. Duncan Gordon, who has had a long interest in the hospital and who, with the assistance of his able Board, has made many wise decisions over the years. Perhaps one of the most important decisions the Board has had to make from time to time is the appointment of a Director to the Hospital. In recent years, we have been blessed with two very able directors: Mr. John Law, formerly Vice-President of the Board, and Mr. Douglas Snedden, the present Executive Director to the Hospital. In any modern medical institution the administrative staff plays an extremely important part in developing a successful program. Investigators are universally aware of their presence in the background of all new or expanding activities. The difficult and delicate art of encouraging research and at the same time of keeping costs within bounds has been developed to a high degree by these partners in our work at The Hospital for Sick Children. The ability to judge the opinion of experts, to make them clarify their views before a project is supported, and to present financial restrictions with graciousness when such is necessary requires the hard-working tact of a diplomat and the patience of Job.

We are indebted to numerous secretaries but especially to Miss Elaine Smith and Mrs Dianne Zandona, who typed and retyped numerous chapters with speed and accuracy; both of these young ladies are remarkable, each in her own way. Dr. Kenneth Bloom has generously reviewed all sections on echocardiography in chapters other than his own.

It is a pleasure to draw attention to the continued cooperation we have received from Ms. Joan C. Zulch, Medical Editor of the Macmillan Publishing Co., Inc. She has helped us understand the production aspects of book publishing more fully. Her cooperation, patience, and tactful nudging, coupled with her obvious competence and humor, have allowed us to weather a third edition together.

CONTRIBUTORS

Bloom, Kenneth R., M.B., B.Ch., F.C.P.(S.A.) Assistant Professor of Paediatrics, University of Toronto Faculty of Medicine, Toronto, Ontario, Canada.

Char, Florence, M.D. Professor of Pediatrics, University of Arkansas for Medical Sciences, Little Rock, Arkansas, U.S.A.

Culham, J. A. Gordon, M.D., F.R.C.P.(C) Lecturer in Radiology, University of Toronto Faculty of Medicine; Radiologist, The Hospital for Sick Children, Toronto, Ontario, Canada.

Dische, M. Renate, M.D., Ph.D. Associate Professor of Pathology, University of Toronto Faculty of Medicine, Toronto, Ontario, Canada.

Duckworth, John W. A., M.B., Ch.B., M.D. Professor of Anatomy, University of Toronto Faculty of Medicine; Consultant in Anatomy and Embryology, Department of Pathology, The Hospital for Sick Children, Toronto, Ontario, Canada.

Fowler, Rodney S., M.D., F.R.C.P.(C), F.A.A.P. Associate Professor of Paediatrics, University of Toronto Faculty of Medicine; Staff Physician, The Hospital for Sick Children, Toronto, Ontario, Canada.

Freedom, Robert M., M.D., F.R.C.P.(C), F.A.C.C. Associate Professor of Paediatrics and Cardiovascular Pathology, University of Toronto Faculty of Medicine; Cardiologist and Co-Director of the Cardiovascular Pathology Registry, The Hospital for Sick Children, Toronto, Ontario, Canada.

Friedli, Beat, M.D., M.S.C. Pediatric Cardiologist, Clinique Universitaire de Pédiatrie, Geneva, Switzerland.

Gilday, David L., B.Eng., M.D. Assistant Professor of Radiology, University of Toronto Faculty of Medicine, Toronto, Ontario, Canada.

Gingell, Robert L., M.D. Assistant Professor of Pediatrics, State University of New York at Buffalo, School of Medicine; Cardiologist, Children's Hospital of Buffalo, Buffalo, New York, U.S.A.

Godman, Michael J., M.B., M.R.C.P. Senior Lecturer, Department of Child Life and Health, University of Edinburgh; Consultant Cardiologist, Royal Hospital for Sick Children, Edinburgh, Scotland.

Izukawa, Teruo, M.D. Associate Professor of Paediatrics, University of Toronto Faculty of Medicine; Staff Physician, The Hospital for Sick Children, Toronto, Ontario, Canada.

Keith, John D., M.D., F.R.C.P.(C), F.A.C.C. Professor Emeritus of Paediatrics, University of Toronto Faculty of Medicine; Physician-in-Charge (1938–1973), Cardiac Clinic and Department, The Hospital for Sick Children, Toronto, Ontario, Canada.

Kidd, B. S. Langford, M.D., F.R.C.P.(Ed.), F.R.C.P.(C) Harriet Lane Home Professor of Pediatric Cardiology and Director, Helen B. Taussig Children's Cardiac Center, Johns Hopkins University School of Medicine, Baltimore, Maryland, U.S.A.

Lowden, J. Alexander, M.D., Ph.D. Associate Professor of Paediatrics, University of Toronto Faculty of Medicine; Associate Director, Research Institute, The Hospital for Sick Children, Toronto, Ontario, Canada.

McClure, Peter D., M.D., C.M., F.R.C.P.(C) Associate Professor of Paediatrics, University of Toronto Faculty of Medicine, Toronto, Ontario, Canada.

McGreal, Douglas A., M.D., F.R.C.P., D.C.H. Associate Professor of Paediatrics, University of Toronto Faculty of Medicine; Neurologist, The Hospital for Sick Children, Toronto, Ontario, Canada.

Manning, James, A., M.D.   Professor of Pediatrics, University of Rochester School of Medicine and Dentistry; Director, Pediatric Cardiology Section, Strong Memorial Hospital, Rochester, New York, U.S.A.

Moës, C. A. F., M.D.   Associate Professor of Radiology, University of Toronto Faculty of Medicine, Toronto, Ontario, Canada.

Olley, Peter M., M.B., F.R.C.P.(C), M.R.C.P., F.A.C.C.   Associate Professor of Paediatrics, University of Toronto Faculty of Medicine; Physician-in-Charge, Cardiac Catheterization Laboratories, The Hospital for Sick Children, Toronto, Ontario, Canada.

Pearse, Richard G., M.A., M.B., B.Chir.(Cantab.), M.R.C.P.   Lecturer in Paediatrics, St. Thomas' Hospital, London, England.

Rose, Vera, M.D., B.Sc., M.B., B.S., F.R.C.P.(C)   Assistant Professor of Paediatrics, University of Toronto Faculty of Medicine; Staff Physician and Associate Special Consultant, The Hospital for Sick Children, Toronto, Ontario, Canada.

Rowe, Richard D., M.D., Ch.B.(N. Z.), F.R.C.P.(Ed.), F.R.C.P.(C)   Professor of Paediatrics, University of Toronto Faculty of Medicine; Director, Division of Cardiology, Department of Paediatrics, The Hospital for Sick Children, Toronto, Ontario, Canada.

Sass-Kortsak, Andrew, M.D.   Professor of Paediatrics, University of Toronto Faculty of Medicine; Chief, Genetic-Metabolic Division, Research Institute, The Hospital for Sick Children, Toronto, Ontario, Canada.

Sondheimer, Henry M., M.D.   Assistant Professor of Pediatrics, State University of New York, Upstate Medical Center, College of Medicine, Syracuse, New York, U.S.A.

Uchida, Irene A., Ph.D.   Professor of Pediatrics and Director, Regional Cytogenetics Laboratory, McMaster University School of Medicine, Hamilton, Ontario, Canada.

Van Praagh, Richard, M.D.   Professor of Pathology, Children's Hospital Medical Center, Harvard Medical School; Director, Cardiac Pathology and Embryology, and Research Associate in Cardiology, Children's Hospital Medical Center, Boston, Massachusetts, U.S.A.

Vlad, Peter, M.D.   Professor of Pediatrics, State University of New York at Buffalo, School of Medicine; Chief, Division of Cardiology, Children's Hospital of Buffalo, Buffalo, New York, U.S.A.

CONTENTS

UNIT III
SPECIFIC MALFORMATIONS

SECTION A
Shunts

SECTION B
Conotruncal Malpositions

SECTION C
Obstructions, Regurgitations, and Other Malformations

1

Prevalence, Incidence, and Epidemiology

John D. Keith

AN ACCURATE appraisal of the incidence of heart disease in infancy and childhood is difficult to achieve, although a gradual accumulation of new data over recent years now permits a better understanding of the breadth of the problem. Congenital heart disease is the most common cardiac condition in childhood, with rheumatic heart disease a diminishing second. The remaining groups occur under the headings of myocarditis, pericarditis, and many other etiologic factors. A comparison of the relative frequency of various forms of heart disease in childhood as recorded at The Hospital for Sick Children, Toronto, over a 20-year period appears in Table 1–1.

Table 1–1. **RELATIVE FREQUENCY OF VARIOUS FORMS OF CARDIOVASCULAR DISEASE IN CHILDHOOD, THE HOSPITAL FOR SICK CHILDREN, 1950–1970**

Congenital heart disease	10,535
Rheumatic heart disease	714
Myocarditis	91
Pericarditis (nonrheumatic)	52
Marfan's disease	39
Anemia with cardiac involvement	27
Friedrich's ataxia with cardiac involvement	13
Rheumatoid arthritis with pericarditis	8
Glycogen storage disease of heart	5
Tumor of heart—primary	11
—secondary	10

PREVALENCE OF CONGENITAL HEART DISEASE

IN the past, estimates of the incidence of congenital heart anomalies have varied from 0.5 per thousand to 21.0 per thousand (Malpas, 1937; DePorte and Parkhurst, 1945; Gardiner and Keith, 1951; Dodge et al., 1958; Carlgren, 1959; Muir, 1960). More recent studies have revealed several sources of error in such statistics and indicate that the figures given frequently fall far short of the true total. There are minor and, at times, major differences from one medical center to another. This is inevitable, since the diagnostic criteria and methods of diagnosis, completeness of follow-up, the presence or absence of specific epidemics, as well as the age of the child when first seen, all may affect the analysis.

A rubella epidemic may produce more cases of patent ductus arteriosus in some specific region of the world. Drugs such as thalidomide, hormone preparations, and other as-yet-unidentified substances may increase the prevalence of congenital heart disease. Autopsy material available in children's hospitals increases the accuracy of diagnosis; however, unless a wide cross-section of the live population, as seen in practice or any outpatient department, is included, a biased impression would be obtained.

An adequate follow-up of apparently normal children is necessary since many showing no evidence of congenital heart disease early in life may do so later on. This is particularly true for such lesions as the atrial septal defect, bicuspid aortic valve, anomalies of the aortic arch, and, at times, coarctation of the aorta.

A cardiac anomaly, such as the ventricular septal defect, may close spontaneously early in life before the child is adequately examined or investigated to confirm the presence of this lesion. It is important to know whether an investigator has excluded stillbirths or not, since the incidence of congenital heart disease in such infants is higher than in the general population.

The recognition and diagnosis of congenital heart disease is most likely to occur among infants and children living in or near a large modern city where a special interest is taken in the problem and complete diagnostic facilities are available. Furthermore, children with certain congenital heart defects may be

Table 1–2.   INCIDENCE OF CONGENITAL HEART DISEASE IN LIVE BIRTHS

INVESTIGATOR	NO. OF LIVE BIRTHS	PERCENT WITH C.H.D.
Richards et al. (New York City), 1946–1953	5628	0.76
Neel (Japan), 1948–1954	64,569	0.70
Carlgren (Sweden), 1941–1967	58,103	0.77
Landtman (Finland), 1945–1950	1,745,419	0.8 (approx.)
Kerebijn (Holland), 1958	1817	0.82
Yerushalmy (California), 1970	19,000	1.17
Mitchell et al. (U.S.A.), 1971	56,109	0.76
Rose (Canada), 1971	28,698	0.75

referred to such medical centers because they are blue or in heart failure, or because they may have an operable defect, thus concentrating the cases in that area. The types of defects seen in any large hospital may not be truly representative of the general population.

The approach most likely to lead to reliable incidence figures is that followed by Yerushalmy (1970), Mitchell and associates (1971), and Rose (1971). These studies are based on a large number of births in the communities concerned, and the incidence data on congenital heart defects are related to base population data. However, even this information has its sources of error since it depends on the completeness and frequency of examinations, the length of follow-up, the presence or absence of epidemics, and whether or not stillbirths are excluded.

Selected studies in various countries that have attempted to relate the prevalence of congenital heart disease to live births are shown in Table 1–2.

Richards and coworkers (1955) found that if stillbirths are included, the incidence of congenital malformations of the heart works out at 0.83 percent. If stillbirths are excluded, the figure falls to 0.70 percent. Mitchell and colleagues (1971) record similar findings, i.e., 0.81 percent if stillbirths are included, 0.76 percent if related only to live births.

Richards and associates (1955) found the incidence of congenital heart disease to be 1.73 percent in prematures, whereas it was 0.49 percent in full-term infants. A three- to fourfold increase in prevalence of ventricular septal defect has been described in premature infants compared with full-term (Hoffman and Rudolph, 1965; Mitchell et al., 1971). Hoffman points out that whether prematurity is diagnosed by birth weight or gestational age, it is a significant factor in assessing the incidence of congenital heart disease as a whole or of the ventricular septal defect in particular.

Thus, review of the data that have accumulated over the past 10 to 20 years suggests now that the incidence of congenital heart disease is approximately 1 percent of live births. It is now clear, however, that this is not the final answer, because the aortic bicuspid valve is unaccounted for and may account for an additional 1 percent, making the total 2 percent.

Individual Congenital Heart Defects

Some anomalies are found with much greater frequency than others. On the basis of the material available at The Hospital for Sick Children, Toronto, over a 24-year period, an approximation of the incidence of the various defects in relation to each other has been worked out, as shown in Table 1–3.

Table 1–3.   INCIDENCE OF VARIOUS CONGENITAL HEART DEFECTS

Hospital for Sick Children, 1950–1973 (15,104 cases) Listed by Primary Diagnosis

DEFECT	NUMBER	PERCENT	APPROXIMATE FREQUENCY PER LIVE BIRTH
Bicuspid aortic valve			1 in 78
Ventricular septal defect	4245	28.3	1 in 532
Isolated	3460		
With associated defects	785		
Atrial septal defect	1565	10.3	1 in 1548
Ostium secundum	1053		
Ostium primum	207		
AV canal defect	305		

Table 1–3. INCIDENCE OF VARIOUS CONGENITAL HEART DEFECTS (Cont.)

Hospital for Sick Children, 1950–1973 (15,104 cases) Listed by Primary Diagnosis

DEFECT	NUMBER	PERCENT	APPROXIMATE FREQUENCY PER LIVE BIRTH
Pulmonary stenosis	1471	9.9	1 in 1620
Isolated with intact septum	1380		
Infundibular	40		
Infundibular and valvular	51		
Patent ductus arteriosus	1466	9.8	1 in 1340
Tetralogy of Fallot	1426	9.7	1 in 1834
Isolated	947		
With associated defects	479		
Aortic stenosis	1058	7.1	1 in 2787
Valvular	735		
Discrete subvalve	27		
Subaortic muscular	103		
Supravalvular	19		
With associated defects	174		
Coarctation of the aorta	762	5.1	1 in 2323
Isolated	359		
With associated defects	403		
Transposition of the great arteries	747	4.9	1 in 3319
D-TGA	666		
With intact septum and	326		
pulmonary stenosis	29		
With VSD	214		
With VSD and pulmonary stenosis	97		
L-TGA	81		
Dextrocardia	255	1.65	
Isolated	70		
With other defects incl. D- and L-TGA or any other anomaly that may occur with dextrocardia	185		
Common ventricle	222	1.5	
With normally related great vessels	83		
With D-TGA	85		
With L-TGA	54		
Mitral and aortic atresia incl.			
Hypoplastic left heart syndrome	221	1.5	1 in 4978
Partial anomalous pulmonary venous drainage	208	1.38	
Isolated	31		
With ASD	154		
With other associated defect	23		
Total anomalous pulmonary venous drainage	203	1.35	1 in 11616
Vascular ring anomalies	187	1.21	
Tricuspid atresia	176	1.20	1 in 9956
Isolated	65		
With associated defects	111		
Endocardial fibroelastosis	140	0.94	1 in 6336
Pulmonary atresia with normal aortic root	108	0.71	
Isolated	19		
With associated defects	89		
Truncus arteriosus	102	0.7	1 in 11616
Type I	19		
Types II and III	4		
Unspecified	79		

Table 1–3. INCIDENCE OF VARIOUS CONGENITAL HEART DEFECTS (Cont.)

Hospital for Sick Children, 1950–1973 (15,104 cases) Listed by Primary Diagnosis

DEFECT	NUMBER	PERCENT	APPROXIMATE FREQUENCY PER LIVE BIRTH
Congenital aortic regurgitation		91	0.6
Isolated	49		
With other defects	42		
Double-outlet right ventricle		74	0.48
PA anterior to aorta	21		
Aorta anterior to PA	6		
Side by side	7		
Unspecified relationship of GA	40		
Ebstein's anomaly		48	0.32
Isolated	28		
With other defects	20		
Coronary artery anomalies		45	0.31
Unspecified	5		
Origin from PA	24		
Coronary AV fistula	11		
Aneurysm	5		
Congenital mitral stenosis		30	0.20
Isolated	12		
With other defects	18		
Interrupted aortic arch		26	0.175
Primary pulmonary hypertension		23	0.171
Aortopulmonary window		22	0.171
Isolated lesion	14		
With PDA	5		
With VSD	4		
Common atrium		21	0.17
Tumor of the heart		13	0.086
Cor triatriatum		9	0.06
Ectopia cordis		2	0.013
Total	15,104	100.00	

The most common lesions are the first nine listed. These include bicuspid aortic valve, ventricular septal defect, tetralogy of Fallot, patent ductus arteriosus, atrial septal defect, aortic stenosis, pulmonary stenosis, transposition of the great arteries, and coarctation of the aorta.

These nine types of defects comprise 85 percent of our total experience of congenital heart disease.

When comparing the relative frequencies of defects in our hospital series, which represent the type of lesion encountered by the practicing pediatric cardiologist and cardiac surgeon, the relative incidence of these defects in the population is similar in three recent studies—Yerushalmy (1970), Mitchell (1971), and Rose (1971). Some exceptions, however, deserve comment.

Bicuspid Aortic Valve as an Isolated Defect. The high incidence of bicuspid aortic valve has been recognized since 1886 when Osler reported 1.2 percent of 800 routine autopsies revealed this anomaly. This figure excluded eight cases of infective endocarditis. Such exclusion appears legitimate since infective endocarditis was a common event at that time and when it occurred the patient usually died in the hospital after a lengthy illness, thus increasing the ratio in routine autopsies.

Roberts (1970) reports finding 13 aortic bicuspid valves in 1440 postmortems on adults (0.9 percent). All had thickened but functioning cusps. More recently Silver (1973) examined 1057 adult hearts at consecutive autopsies and found ten with bicuspid aortic valves (1 percent). In addition, there were three with infective endocarditis and two with associated congenital defects of the heart (coarctation of the aorta).

Izukawa and Keith found seven bicuspid aortic valves as an isolated cardiac anomaly in 550 consecutive autopsies on infants and children, giving an incidence of 1.3 percent (see Table 1–4).

Table 1–4. INCIDENCE OF ISOLATED BICUSPID VALVES

	NO. OF AUTOPSIES	NO. OF BICUSPID AORTIC VALVES	PERCENT
Osler (1886)	800	10	1.2
Roberts (1970)	1440	13	0.9
Silver (1973)	1057	10	1.0
Izukawa and Keith (1973)	550	7	1.3

Bicuspid Aortic Valve in Association with Other Congenital Heart Defects. Bicuspid aortic valve shows the following incidence with other defects: coarctation of aorta, 29 percent; interrupted aortic arch, 27.2 percent; aortic stenosis, 19 percent; primary endocardial fibroelastosis, 18 percent; ventricular septal defect (isolated), 13.3 percent; and endocardial cushion defect, 8.1 per cent.

The association with coarctation of the aorta accounts for 45 percent of all the bicuspid aortic valves in our autopsy series among 1785 congenital heart defects. The ventricular septal defect is second with 30 percent; aortic stenosis is third with 11 percent; endocardial fibroelastosis is fourth with 10 percent; endocardial cushion defect is fifth with 8 percent. Thus, these five defects account for 74 percent of the total.

They are followed by a variety of other congenital heart diseases with an incidence of bicuspid aortic valve at, or only slightly above, that of normal children. For example, in 123 children with tetralogy of Fallot only one had a bicuspid aortic valve, an incidence of 0.8 percent.

Endocardial fibroelastosis is well recognized as a secondary phenomenon in several congenital heart defects—particularly severe aortic stenosis in early life, aortic atresia or mitral stenosis, coarctation of the aorta, and congenital mitral regurgitation. As a primary phenomenon it has been considered by some as a myocardiopathy or a late stage of myocarditis. This is discussed elsewhere (see Chapter 52). However, the finding of an incidence of 18 percent of aortic bicuspid valves among 50 primary cases contributes additional evidence that endocardial fibroelastosis is a congenital abnormality of the heart.

The incidence of 13.3 percent with bicuspid aortic valve among the uncomplicated cases of ventricular septal defect coming to autopsy suggests that if this is present in the usual patient seen in office practice with classic signs of the septal opening, he or she may eventually develop one or more of the complications that revolve around a bicuspid aortic valve.

Other Exceptions. At The Hospital for Sick Children, Toronto, the relative frequency of tetralogy of Fallot is approximately two times and that of transposition of the great arteries about three times that found in the prospective population studies. This difference can be explained by the fact that a referral center such as The Hospital for Sick Children, Toronto, where diagnostic laboratory and surgical expertise has been established for some time in the community encourages physicians to refer patients in the above two categories, especially when the diagnosis is recognized or even suspected. In this way the Johns Hopkins Hospital, Baltimore, will probably have a greater number of cases with tetralogy of Fallot in their series, due to their great interest in this particular lesion dating back nearly 30 years. Transposition of the great arteries will obviously rate high in the experience of the Great Ormond Street Hospital for Sick Children in London, England, because of their success in both diagnosis and treatment, which has been outstanding.

Aortic stenosis is the type of lesion that in our series is approximately twice that reported from the prospective studies (Yerushalmy, 1970; Mitchell et al., 1971). Aortic stenosis is a type of lesion that many times presents with a murmur suggestive of ventricular septal defect or pulmonary stenosis in the first few years of life, and only with the passage of time is this impression corrected. The left-heart catheterization studies often required to confirm the diagnosis of aortic stenosis are usually not performed until the child is five or six years of age. The length of follow-up in the prospective series of Yerushalmy (1970) and Mitchell and coworkers (1971), which averaged three to five years, and the number of cardiac catheterizations done suggest that a significant number of cases may yet prove to have aortic stenosis at a later time.

MORTALITY IN CONGENITAL HEART DISEASE

If all the children born with congenital heart disease remained alive, a very large population of children with cardiac anomalies would soon accumulate. However, it is widely recognized that many die in the first few weeks of life and that a further number succumb before the end of the first year. The incidence of death in different age groups in congenital heart disease in The Hospital for Sick Children population is shown in Table 1–5.

Among the 10,535 cases of congenital heart disease seen in the 20-year period from 1950 to 1970, 2870 or 27.2 percent died during our period of observation, which may have lasted for a few days or for many years. The age at death is indicated in Table 1–5.

Table 1–5. AGE AT DEATH AMONG 2870 INFANTS AND CHILDREN WITH CONGENITAL HEART DISEASE, THE HOSPITAL FOR SICK CHILDREN

	CASES	PERCENT
In first month of life	980	34.14
One month to one year	1047	36.48
One year to five years	449	15.64
Five years and over	394	13.72
Total	2870	100.00

A glance at Table 1–5 shows that approximately one-third of these children died in the first month of life. An equal number died between one month and 12 months, and another third died after one year of age. The deaths include the severe anomalies of the heart that cannot be controlled medically or successfully treated by surgery. They also include children who have died with multiple defects causing death, in which the heart is a contributor. There are a few cases in which the heart defect was simply an incidental finding.

The first month of life is a particularly lethal time for the child with malformations of the heart. Approximately the same number die in the first four weeks as die in the next 48 weeks. Twice as many die in the first month as die after one year of age from this cause.

It is in the first few weeks of life, therefore, that the pediatrician or pediatric cardiologist is most often involved in problems relating to the heart. It is clearly important to know which defects cause death in this period since the more severe lesions are brought to the attention of the physician first.

There has been some change in the order of importance in this regard during recent years that deserves comment. The trends in neonatal mortality are shown in Table 1–6 for Toronto, Baltimore, Boston, and Buffalo. These figures are taken from postmortem data.

Mitral and aortic atresia (or severe stenosis) are frequently grouped with coarctation of the aorta when they appear with heart failure in infancy and are referred to as the hypoplastic left-heart syndrome. These two groups of defects now comprise 41 percent of our neonatal deaths with congenital heart disease.

Deaths from transposition of the great arteries have diminished somewhat, probably due to improved medical and surgical techniques. The other figures show little change in recent years apart from pulmonary atresia or stenosis. Such cases may be found more frequently since the medical profession is now fully aware of the success of modern management and therapy.

Among the leading causes of death in infancy and childhood the Toronto Department of Public Health rates congenital cardiac deaths fifth in order of statistical significance (Table 1–7).

It is difficult to evaluate congenital heart disease as a cause of death precisely since in some cases it is the

Table 1–6. TYPES OF CONGENITAL HEART MALFORMATION IN FIRST MONTH OF LIFE BY AUTOPSY DATA

TYPE OF CARDIAC ANOMALY	TORONTO 111 Cases 1968–1970	BALTIMORE 83 Cases 1969–1971	BOSTON 350 Cases 1960–1969	BUFFALO 165 Cases 1949–1964
	(Percent)			
Mitral atresia Mitral stenosis Aortic atresia Aortic stenosis	24.3	10	15	22
Coarctation of the aorta	17.1	13	14	13
TGAD and L	11.7	28	19	15
Pulmonary atresia	3.6	3	11	6
Pulmonary stenosis	3.6	2		
Atrial septal defect	1.8	6	0	0
AV canal	3.6	1.4	0	4
Tetralogy of Fallot	4.5	4	0.3	7
VSD	4.5	12	0.6	2
Dextrocardia or levocardia	3.6	0	0	0
TAPVD	1.8	1	4.9	0.6
Truncus arteriosus	5.4	2	3	4
EFE	2.7	0	0	0
PDA*	0.9	2	0.6	2
Miscellaneous	16.2	19	0	0

* There were other patients who died with a PDA, but the cause of death was usually respiratory distress syndrome, prematurity, or pneumonia.

Table 1–7. CAUSES OF DEATH—BIRTH TO 14 YEARS TORONTO, 1969*

CAUSE OF DEATH	NO. OF DEATHS	PERCENT OF TOTAL GROUP
Anoxic and hypoxic conditions	63	21.9
Malformations—all types other than congenital heart disease	44	15.3
Accidental causes	43	14.9
Immaturity, unqualified	31	10.8
Congenital cardiac deaths and circulatory system	22	7.6
Pneumonia, all forms	13	4.5
Birth injury and difficult labor	10	3.5
Malignant neoplasms	10	3.5
Conditions of placenta and cord	9	3.1
Gastroenteritis	6	2.1
Epilepsy	3	1.0
Hemolytic disease of newborn	2	0.7
Simple meningitis	1	0.3
All other causes	31	10.8
Total	288	100.0

* From Department of Public Health, Statistical Services, Toronto.

primary cause and in others of secondary importance and yet crucial. In a third group the cardiac lesion is simply an incidental finding at postmortem (e.g., bicuspid aortic valve).

A very significant appraisal relating cardiac malformation deaths to population is available in the data provided by Mitchell and coworkers (1971). They report that of 420 cases of congenital heart disease (occurring among 56,000 births) 35.2 percent died during three-to four-year follow-up of all cases;

18.6 percent (of the 420) died in the first month of life, 11.9 percent between one month and one year, and 4.7 percent after one year. Many of these cases died from causes other than the heart. However, the heart defect was considered to be the cause of death in only half of these cases, or 18 percent of the 420; 6.6 percent of the 420 died of congenital heart disease when under one month, 8.1 percent between one month and one year, and 3.3 percent one year and over.

INCIDENCE OF CONGENITAL HEART DISEASE IN FAMILIES

WHEN a baby with congenital heart disease is born, the parents eventually ask the doctor whether they are likely to have another child with similar anomaly. The publications of McKeown and associates (1953), Anderson (1954), and Polani and Campbell (1955) indicate that after one case of congenital heart disease has appeared in a family, there is approximately a 2 percent chance of a similar event in subsequent pregnancies (see Chapter 9).

We have seen in Table 1–2 that congenital heart disease occurs in at least 1/100 live births. A chance of a recurrence in other sibs is as indicated above, 1/50. This is still not a very serious risk.

Nora and associates (1970) have carried this a step further, demonstrating that the risk of a recurrence of a congenital heart defect in another child in a family varies with the frequency the lesion is found in the general population and the type of lesion in the first affected child. This is demonstrated in Table 1–8.

Thus, if a child has a ventricular septal defect, the chance of his brothers or sisters having some form of congenital heart disease is approximately 4.4 percent or 1 in 22. On the other hand, pulmonary atresia,

which is a less commonly encountered lesion, carries a much lower risk of 1.3 percent or 1 in 77. (See also Chapter 9.)

Table 1–8. OBSERVED RECURRENCE RISK IN SIBS OF 1405 CHILDREN WITH CONGENITAL HEART LESIONS

ORIGINAL ANOMALY IDENTIFIED	AFFECTED SIBS WITH SOME FORM OF CONGENITAL HEART DISEASE (Percent)
Ventricular septal defect	4.4
Patent ductus arteriosus	3.4
Tetralogy	2.7
Atrial septal defect	3.2
Pulmonary stenosis	2.9
Aortic stenosis	2.2
Coarctation	1.8
Transposition	1.9
Tricuspid atresia	1.0
Ebstein's anomaly	1.1
Truncus	1.2
Pulmonary atresia	1.3

HEREDITARY DISORDERS AND SYNDROMES IN CONGENITAL HEART DISEASE

THE studies of McKusick and the experience of pediatricians and cardiologists have added to our knowledge of congenital heart disease as part of distinct clinical syndromes. These can be grouped in the following manner: (1) hereditary disorders with normal chromosomes in which congenital heart disease is common but is only one of many abnormalities present and (2) syndromes with abnormal chromosomes in which congenital heart disease is common but is only one of many abnormalities present.

The types of cardiac defects that may be encountered in (1) and (2) are summarized as follows:

1. Aortic regurgitation and/or mitral regurgitation, which may be found in any of the following syndromes:
   Marfan's
   Hurler (mucopolysaccharidoses)
   Hunter
   Morquio Ulrich
   Scheie
   Maroteauz-Lamy
   Osteogenesis imperfecta
   Forney
2. Atrial septal defect, which may be found at times in the following syndromes:
   Holt Oram
   Focal dermal hypoplasia
   Smith-Lemli-Opitz
   Radial aplasia thrombocytopenia
   Ellis van Crefeld
3. Patent ductus arteriosus, which may be found in the following syndromes:
   Acrocephalosyndactyly
   Cerebrohepatorenal (Zellweger)
   Fanconi pancytopenia

   Lissencephaly
   Incontinentia pigmenti (Block-Sulzberger)
4. Tetralogy of Fallot:
   Oculoauriculovertebral dysplasia (Goldenhar)
   Radial aplasia thrombocytopenia
   Smith-Lemli-Opitz
5. Ventricular septal defect:
   Apert
   de Lange
   Klippel-Feil
6. Cardiomyopathy:
   Tuberous sclerosis
   Glycogen storage disease
7. Pulmonary artery stenosis:
   Cutis laxa
   Leopard (lentigines)
   Neurofibromatosis
8. Pulmonary valve stenosis:
   Noonan's
9. Supravalvular aortic stenosis:
   Hypercalcemia, idiopathic
10. Aneurysms:
    Marfan's
    Ehler's Danlos
11. Aortic stenosis:
    Alkaptonuria
12. Dextrocardia:
    Kartageners
13. Pulmonary AV fistula:
    Osler Reudu Weber
14. Systemic hypertension:
    Riley Day
15. Conduction abnormalities:
    Refsum
    Surdo-cardiac

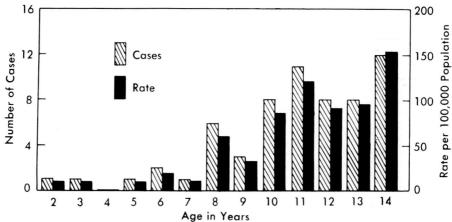

Figure 1-1. Incidence of rheumatic heart disease in the different age groups in the child population (city of Toronto in the year 1962).

PREVALENCE OF RHEUMATIC HEART DISEASE

THE prevalence of rheumatic heart disease has been estimated in the school population in many studies in the past. These have been summarized by several authors (see Table 1–9). The incidence in these references varied from 0.08 to 0.5 per thousand school population. The incidence varied somewhat with the location, chiefly in relation to time of reporting. Rheumatic fever was much more common in the 1920s and 1930s in schoolchildren in North America than it has been in the 1950s and 1960s. In Toronto, Gardiner and Keith in 1951, reporting through the Toronto Heart Registry, found the figure to be 1.6 per thousand schoolchildren. Rose, Boyd, and Ashton from the Toronto Registry, in 1964, found it to be 0.8 per thousand (0.08 percent).

As will be indicated in the discussion on rheumatic fever in Chapter 13, there has been a marked decline in the mortality from rheumatic heart disease in childhood over the past 25 years. It has fallen from being the second leading cause of death from disease in childhood to one of relative insignificance in the pediatric age group.

As one might expect, the incidence of rheumatic heart disease in different age groups in childhood gradually rises as one approaches adolescence (Figure 1-1). At six years of age, there are approximately 4 cases per thousand population, but by 12 years of age the incidence has risen to 12 per thousand. Now, as in the past, the type of valve involved in childhood rheumatic fever is the mitral valve, with varying degrees of mitral regurgitation. Mitral stenosis, which used to be seen with regularity in Canada and the United States in the teen-age group, has now become a rarity and is much more common in India and Pakistan (Chapter 9).

It is difficult to prove what factors are responsible, but overcrowding, poor living conditions, diet, epidemics, and streptococcal virulence all may play a part. The decline has been greatest where antibiotics have been used widely.

Table 1–9. INCIDENCE OF RHEUMATIC CARDITIS IN SCHOOL SURVEYS IN NORTH AMERICA

		AGE IN YEARS	RATE (PERCENT)	REFERENCES
New York	1920	6–17	0.4	Halsey, R. H., 1921
Boston	1926	6–17	0.4	Robey, W. A., 1927
Philadelphia	1934	6–18	0.5	Cahan, J. M., 1937
Toronto	1948–9	5–15	0.1	Gardiner and Keith, 1951
Buffalo	1949–52	5–18	0.1	Mattison et al., 1953
Chicago	1959–60	6–13	0.1	Miller, R. A., 1962
New York	1961	5–18	0.1	Brownell et al., 1963
Denver	1962–64	10–13	0.1	Morton et al., 1967
Colorado (rural)	1965	10–13	0.3	Morton et al., 1970
Toronto	1965	10–13	0.08	Boyd and Rose, 1969

REFERENCES

Abbott, M. E.: *Nelson's Loose-leaf Living Medicine*, **4**:207, 1927. Thomas Nelson & Sons, New York.

Adams, F. H.: Heart disease in the infant under 2 years of age. From Good, R. A., and Platou, E. S. (eds.): *Essays on Pediatrics in Honor of Dr. Irvine McQuarrie.* Lancet Publications, Inc., Mineapolis, 1955.

Alimurung, M. M.; Herrera, F., Jr.; Guytingco, A.; et al.: Heart disease in the Philippines. A seven-year (1947–53) postwar survey of four Manila general hospitals. *Am. Heart J.*, **50**:293, 1955.

American Heart Association; Editorial: The congenital bicuspid aortic valve. *Circulation*, **4**:485, 1961.

Anderson, R. C.: Causative factors underlying congenital heart malformations. *Pediatrics*, **14**:143, 1954.

Antia, A. U., and Williams, A. O.: Congenital heart disease in Nigeria. Necropsy study of 47 cases. *Br. Heart J.*, **33**:133, 1971.

Apley, J., and Perry, C. B.: A six-year survey of the cases seen at a school cardiac clinic. *Arch. Dis. Child.*, **29**:317, 1954.

Arey, J. B.: Pathologic findings in the neonatal period. *J. Pediatr.* **34**:144, 1949.

Bacon, A. P. C., and Matthews, M. B.: Congenital bicuspid aortic valves and the etiology of isolated valvular stenosis. *Q. J. Med.*, **28**:545, 1959.

Baker, C., and Somerville, J.: Results of surgical treatment of aortic stenosis. *Br. Med. J.*, **1**:197, 1964.

Birnbaum, R.: *A Clinical Manual of the Malformations and Congenital Disease of the Foetus* (translated by G. Blacker). J. & A. Churchill, Ltd., London, 1912, p. 3.

Boesen, I., and Vendel, S.: Post mortem diagnoses in 1145 children under age of 4 years with congenital heart disease. VIII International Pediatrics Congress, Copenhagen. Scientific Exhibitions, 1956, p. 17.

Brown, J. W.: *Congenital Heart Disease.* John Bale, London, 1939.

Campbell, M.: The frequency of different types of congenital heart disease. *Br. Heart J.* **15**:462, 1953.

———: The natural history of congenital aortic stenosis. *Br. Heart J.*, **30**:514, 1968.

———: Calcific aortic stenosis and congenital bicuspid aortic valves. *Br. Heart J.*, **30**:606, 1968.

Campbell, M., and Kauntz, R.: Congenital aortic valvular stenosis. *Br. Heart J.*, **15**:179, 1953.

Carlgren, L. E.: The incidence of congenital heart disease in children born in Gothenburg, 1941–1950. *Br. Heart J.*, **21**:40, 1959.

———: The incidence of congenital heart disease in Gothenburg. *Proc. Ass. Eur. Paediatr. Cardiol.*, **5**:2, 1969.

Cho, K. H.; Nahn, C. C.; Lee, D. Y.; and Cho, C. B.: Heart disease in Korea; five-year survey of heart disease in Seoul. *Proceedings III Asian-Pacific Congress of Cardiology*, **1**:190, 1964.

City of Toronto, Department of Public Health: *Annual Statements*, 1959–1969.

Clawson, B. J.: Types of congenital heart diseases in 15,597 autopsies. *Lancet*, **64**:134, 1944.

Coleman, E. N.: Progress report on infants with serious cardiac malformations. *Br. Heart J.*, **31**:441, 1969.

DePorte, J. V., and Parkhurst, E.: Congenital malformations and birth injuries among children born in New York State, in 1940–1942. *N. Y. State J. Med.*, **45**:1097, 1945.

Dodge, H. J.; Maresh, G. J.; and Morris, N. M.: Prevalence of heart disease in relation to some population characteristics of Colorado school children. *Am. J. Public Health;* **48**:62, 1958.

Dogramaci, I., and Green, H.: Factors in the etiology of congenital heart anomalies. *J. Pediatr.,* **30**:295, 1947.

Edwards, J. E.: The congenital bicuspid aortic valve. *Circulation,* **23**:485, 1961.

Fowler, R. S.: Sudden death in aortic stenosis in childhood. Presented at the 6th World Congress of Cardiology, Sept. 1970, London.

Furuta, S.: The phonocardiogram in congenital heart disease; a structural and functional consideration. *Jap. Circ. J.,* **25**:8, 1961.

Gardiner, J. H., and Keith, J. D.: Prevalence of heart disease in Toronto children: 1948–1949 cardiac registry. *Pediatrics,* **7**:713, 1951.

Gelfman, R., and Levine, S.: The incidence of acute and subacute bacterial endocarditis in congenital heart disease. *Am. J. Med. Sci.,* **204**:324, 1942.

Gibson, S., and Clifton, W. M.: Congenital heart disease: A clinical and post mortem study of one hundred and five cases. *Am. J. Dis. Child.,* **55**:761, 1938.

Gore, I.: Dissecting aneurysms of the aorta in persons under forty years of age. *Arch. Path.,* **55**:1, 1953.

Grant, R. T.; Wood, J. E.; and Jones, T. D.: Heart valve irregularities in relation to subacute bacterial endocarditis. *Heart,* **14**:247, 1928.

Harris, L. E., and Steinberg, A. G.: Abnormalities observed during the first days of life in 8,716 live-born infants. *Pediatrics,* **14**:314, 1954.

Henikoff, L. M.; Stevens, W. A., Jr.; and Perry, L. W.: Detection of heart disease in children. *Circulation,* **38**:375, 1968.

Hoffman, J. I. E.: Natural history of congenital heart disease. *Circulation,* **37**:97, 1968.

Hoffman, J. I. E., and Rudolph, A. M.: The natural history of ventricular septal defects in infancy. *Am. J. Cardiol.,* **16**:634, 1965.

————: The natural history of isolated ventricular septal defect. *Adv. Pediatr.,* **17**:57, 1970.

Hohn, A. R.; Tingelstad, J. B.; Israel, R.; et al.: Intrapulmonary shunts in congestive heart disease. *Am. J. Dis. Child.,* **115**:202, 1968.

Hoh, A. R.; Van Praagh, S.; Moore, A. A. D.; Vlad, P.; and Lambert, E. C.: Aortic stenosis. *Circulation,* **32**:4, 1965.

Hutcheson, J. M.; Heitmancik, M. R.; and Herrmann, G. R.: Changes in the incidence and types of heart disease. *Am. Heart J.,* **46**:565, 1953.

Hutchins, G. M., et al: Development of endocardial valvuloids with valvular insufficiency. *Arch. Pathol.,* **93**:401, 1972.

Hutchins, G. M., and Vie, S. A.: The progression of interstitial myocarditis to idiopathic endocardial fibroelastosis. *Am. J. Pathol.,* **66**:483, 1972.

Imperial, E. S., and Felarca, A.: Autopsy study of heart disease in the Philippines General Hospital; based on a review of 6,000 consecutive cases. *Am. Heart J.,* **66**:470, 1963.

Izukawa, T., and Keith, J. D.: Personal communication, 1973.

Jones, H. W.: Vital capacity on heart disease. *Br. Med. J.,* **1**:795, 1928.

Jones, T. D., and Bland, E. F.: Rheumatic fever and heart disease: completed ten-year observations on 1,000 patients. *Trans. Assoc. Am. Physicians,* **57**:265, 1942.

Kennedy, W. P.: Epidemiologic Aspects of the Problem of Congenital Malformations. The National Foundation. III, 1967.

Kerrebijn, K. F.: Incidence in infants and mortality from congenital malformations of the circulatory system. *Acta Paediatr. Scand.,* **55**:316, 1966.

Lambert, E. C.; Canent, R. V.; and Hohn, A. R.: Congenital cardiac anomalies in the newborn. *Pediatrics,* **37**:343, 1966.

Landtman, B.: Clinical and morphological studies in congenital heart disease. A review of 777 cases. *Acta Paediatr. Scand.,* Suppl. **213**:1, 1971.

Lewis, D. S.; Beattie, W. W.; and Abbott, M. E.: Differential study of case of pulmonary stenosis of inflammatory origin. *Am. J. Med. Sci.,* **165**:636, 1923.

Lewis, T., and Grant, R. T.: Observations relating to subacute infective endocarditis; notes on normal structure of aortic valve, bicuspid aortic valves of congenital origin; bicuspid aortic valves in subacute infective endocarditis. *Heart,* **10**:20, 1923.

McIntosh, R.; Merritt, K. K.; Richards, M. R.; Samuels, M. H.; and Bellows, M. T.: The incidence of congenital malformations: a study of 5,964 pregnancies. *Pediatrics,* **14**:505, 1954.

McKeown, T.; MacMahon, B.; and Parsons, C. G.: The familial incidence of congenital malformation of the heart. *Brit. Heart J.,* **15**:273, 1953.

McKusick, V. A.: Chronic constrictive pericarditis. Some clinical and laboratory observations. *Bull. Johns Hopkins Hosp.,* **90**:3, 1952.

MacMahon, B.: Association of congenital malformation of the heart with birth rank and maternal age. *Br. J. Soc. Med.,* **6**:178, 1952.

MacMahon, B.; McKeown, T.; and Record, R. G.: The incidence and life expectation of children with congenital heart disease. *Br. Heart J.,* **15**:121, 1953.

Mall, F.: On the frequency of localized anomalies in human embryos and infants at birth. *Am. J. Anat.,* **22**:49, 1917.

Malpas, P.: The incidence of human malformations and the significance of changes in the maternal environment in their causation. *J. Obstet. Gynaecol. Br. Emp,* **44**:434, 1937.

Mark, H., and Young, D.: Congenital heart disease in the adult. *Am. J. Cardiol.* **15**:293, 1965.

Mehrizi, A.; Hirsch, M. S.; and Taussig, H. B.: Congenital heart disease in the neonatal period. *J. Pediatr.* **65**:721, 1964.

Miller, H. C.: Analysis of fetal and neo-natal deaths in 4,117 consecutive births. *Pediatrics,* **5**:184, 1950.

Miller, R. A.; Stamler, J.; Smith, J. M.; Milne, W. S.; Paul, M. H.; Abrams, I.; Hastreiter, A. R.; Restivo, R. M.; and DeBoer, L.: The detection of heart disease in children. Results of mass trials with use of tape recorded heart sounds. II. The Michigan City study. *Circulation,* **32**:956, 1965.

Mitchell, S. C.: Incidence of congenital heart disease. Personal communication, 1963.

Mitchell, S. C.; Korones, S. B.; and Berendes, H. W.: Congenital heart disease in 56,109 births. *Circulation,* **43**:323, 1971.

Morton, W. E.; Huhn, L. A.; and Lichty, J. A.: Rheumatic heart disease epidemiology. *JAMA,* **199**:879, 1967.

Muir, C. S.: Incidence of congenital heart disease in Singapore. *Br. Heart J.,* **22**:243, 1960.

Murphy, D. P.: *Congenital Malformations: A Study of Parental Characteristics, with Special Reference to the Reproductive Process,* 2nd ed J. B. Lippincott Company, Philadelphia, 1947.

Neel, J. V.: A study of major congenital defects in Japanese infants. *Am. J. Hum. Genet.,* **10**:398, 1958.

Nora, J. J.: Multifactorial inheritance hypothesis for the etiology of congenital heart diseases. *Circulation,* **38**:604, 1968.

Nora, J. J.; Trygstad, C. W.; Mangos, J. A.; et al.; Peritoneal dialysis in the treatment and intractable congestive heart failure of infancy and childhood. *J. Pediatr.* **68**:693, 1966.

Nora, J. J.; Vargo, T. A.; Nora, A. H.; et al.: Dexamphetamine: a possible environmental trigger in cardiovascular malformations. *Lancet,* **1**:1290, 1970.

Ober, W. B., and Moore, T. E., Jr.: Congenital cardiac malformations in the neonatal period: an autopsy study. *N. Engl. J. Med.,* **253**:271, 1955.

Osler, W.: The bicuspid condition of the aortic valves. *Trans. Assoc. Am. Physicians,* **2**:185, 1886.

Paget, J.: On obstructions of the branches of the pulmonary artery. *Trans. R. Med. Chir. Soc., Lond.,* **27**:162, 1844.

Peacock, T. B.: *On Malformations of the Human Heart,* 2nd ed. J. Churchill & Sons, London, 1866.

Perinatal Problems. The second report of the British Perinatal Mortality Survey (1958). Ed. Neville R. Butler (E. & S. Livingstone Ltd. 1969).

Polani, P. E., and Campbell, M.: An aetiological study of congenital heart disease. *Ann. Hum. Genet.,* **19**:209, 1955.

Pomerance, A.: Ageing changes in human heart valves. *Br. Heart J.,* **29**:22, 1967.

Rauh, L. W.: The incidence of organic heart disease in Cincinnati school children. *Am. Heart J.,* **18**:705, 1939.

Report by the National Heart Foundation of Australia: Cardiac surgery, 1970.

Report by National Heart Foundation of Australia: Cardiac surgery, 1971.

Reynolds, J. L.: Heart disease screening of preschool children. *Am. J. Dis. Child.,* **119**:488, 1970.

Richards, M. R.; Merritt, K. K.; Samuels, M. H.; and Langmann, A. G.: Congenital malformations of the cardiovascular system in a series of 6,053 infants. *Pediatrics*, **15**:12, 1955.

Roberts, W. C.: Anomalous left ventricular band. An unemphasized cause of a precordial musical murmur. *Am. J. Cardiol.*, **23**:735, 1969.

————: Anatomically isolated aortic valvular disease: The case against its being of rheumatic etiology. *Am. J. Med.*, **49**:151, 1970.

————: The congenital bicuspid aortic valve: A study of 85 autopsy patients. *Am. J. Cardiol.*, **26**:72, 1970.

————: The structure of the aortic valve in clinically isolated aortic stenosis. An autopsy study of 162 patients over 15 years of age. *Circulation*, **42**:91, 1970.

Roberts, W. C., and Elliott, L. P.: Lesions complicating a congenitally bicuspid aortic valve. Anatomic and radiographic features. *Radiol. Clin. N. Am.*, **6**:409, 1968.

Roberts, W. C.; Friesinger, C. C.; Cohen, L. S.; et al.: Acquired pulmonic atresia. Total obstruction of right ventricular outflow after systemic to pulmonary arterial anastomoses for cyanotic congenital cardiac disease. *Am. J. Cardiol.*, **24**:335, 1969.

Robinson, S.; Aggeler, D. M.; and Daniloff, G. T.: Heart disease in San Francisco school children. *J. Pediatr.* **33**:49, 1948.

Rose, V.; Boyd, A. R.; and Ashton, T.: Incidence of heart disease in children in the City of Toronto. *Can. Med. Assoc. J.*, **91**:95, 1964.

Rose, V.: Live births, City of Toronto. Personal communication, 1971.

Rowe, R. D., and Cleary, T. E.; Congenital cardiac malformation in the newborn period; frequency in a children's hospital. *Can. Med. Assoc. J.*, **83**:299, 1960.

Schrire, V.: Experience with congenital heart disease at Groote Schuur Hospital, Cape Town; an analysis of 1,439 patients studied over an eleven-year period. *S. Afr. Med. J.*, **37**:1175, 1963.

Shann, M. K. M.: Congenital heart disease in Taiwan, Republic of China. *Circulation*, **39**:251, 1969.

Silver, M.: Bicuspid aortic valve as an isolated defect. Personal communication, 1973.

Smith, D. E., and Matthews, B.: Aortic valvular stenosis with coarctation of the aorta. With special reference to the development of aortic stenosis upon congenital bicuspid valve. *Br. Heart J.*, **17**:198, 1955.

Taussig, H. B.: *Congenital Malformations of the Heart*. The Commonwealth Fund, New York, 1947, p. 354.

Van der Horst, R. L.; Winship, W. S.; and Gotsman, M. S.: Congenital heart malformations in the South African Indian. *Am. Heart J.*, **80**:56, 1970.

Van der Horst, R. L., and Wainwright, J.: Congenital heart disease in the Bantu: An autopsy analysis of 123 cases. *S. Adr. Med. J.*, **43**:586, 1969.

Van der Horst, R. L.; Winship, W. S.; et al.: Congenital heart disease in the South African Bantu: A report of 117 cases. *S. Afr. Med. J.*, **42**:1271, 1968.

Wada, J.: Congenital heart disease. *Jap. Circ. J.*, **27**:251, 1963.

Wallooppillai, N. J., and Jayasinghe, M. D. S.: Congenital heart disease in Ceylon. *Brit. Heart J.*, **32**:304, 1970.

Warburg, E.: Clinical statistics of congenital cardiac disease. 1,000 cases analyzed. Preliminary report. *Acta Med. Scand.*, **151**:209, 1955.

Watson, H.: The early detection of congenital malformations of the heart. *Br. Heart J.*, **34**:37, 1972.

Wauchope, G. M.: The clinical importance of variations in the number of cusps forming the aortic and pulmonary valves. *Q. J. Med.*, **21**:383, 1928.

Weiss, M. M.: Incidence of rheumatic and congenital heart disease among school children of Louisville, Ky. *Am. Heart J.*, **22**:112, 1941.

Wiland, O. K.: Extracardiac anomalies in association with congenital heart disease. *Lab. Invest.*, **5**:380, 1956.

Wood, J. B.; Serumaga, J.; and Lewis, M. G.: Congenital heart disease at necropsy in Uganda. *Br. Heart J.*, **31**:76, 1969.

Yerushalmy, J.: The California child health and development studies. Study design, and some illustrative findings on congenital heart disease. In Fraser, F. C., and McKusick, V. A. (eds.): *Congenital Malformations*. Proceedings of the third International Conference. The Hague, Netherlands, 1969. Excerpta Medica, Amsterdam, 1970, p. 299.

2

History and Physical Examination

John D. Keith

HISTORY TAKING

THE HISTORY of an infant or child with heart involvement is usually taken or elaborated after a heart defect or disease process has been suspected or identified by the finding of a heart murmur or some degree of cyanosis. Since these are usually recognized in the early weeks or months of life, the history-taking process assumes a chronologic order related to birth, pregnancy, and proceeding through the neonatal period and the first year of life on into the preschool and school years. An age-oriented or chronologic approach to history taking minimizes the chance of missing an important piece of information.

The areas of history that should be covered are as follows, although they need not necessarily be in the order set down here.

1. The mother's health and history during pregnancy, particularly during the first two or three months:

Possible rubella,
Coxsackie virus infection,
Threatened abortion,
Previous stillbirths,
Medication during pregnancy (e.g., thalidomide, etc.),
X-ray therapy,
Smallpox vaccination,
Treatment of hormonal imbalance by diethylstilbestrol.

2. The baby at birth and in the neonatal period: One should inquire regarding weight, weeks of gestation, whether full-term or premature birth, length of labor, difficulty in resuscitation of the baby at birth, cyanosis at birth (transient or persistent), breathlessness, grunting respirations, wheezing respirations, feeding difficulties, whether healthy and well, and finally the Apgar rating.

3. The baby during the first year or two of life after the neonatal period: One may inquire regarding weight gain, physical development, appetite, feeding difficulties, the developmental milestones (e.g., holding the head up, sitting up, standing, walking, first words, etc.), whether the child lacks energy compared with other infants or children, and whether he or she is easily tired.

Many mothers with normal infants think their child is cyanosed because there is a blue shading of the upper lip or the fingernails appear blue at times. A normal infant will frequently have a purple-marbling effect on the skin surface when the clothes are removed for the bath. Such changes are of course superficial and vasomotor in origin and not pathologic.

4. Preschool and school age: It is important to know whether the child is fully active or not, can run easily, whether there is tiredness, breathlessness with activity or on stair climbing, whether he can keep up with other children or wants to rest before the others and is not as active as brothers or sisters. One should also inquire regarding joint pains, possible rheumatic fever, fever of unexplained origin, sore throats, fatigue, loss of appetite, arthritis, etc. Fatigue is often difficult to evaluate because some mothers think that their child gets tired when the rest of the child population does not. Other children with heart defects are considered to be at times hyperactive by their parents in spite of the presence of a heart lesion.

5. In the presence of known congenital heart disease, especially those that have some evidence of cyanosis, one should question the parents regarding possible squatting to relieve cyanotic spells or the need to stop and rest frequently. The degree of severity of cyanotic spells should be evaluated as well as the history of dizziness or unconscious episodes.

6. When it is known that the child has congenital heart disease, the parents should be asked regarding heart defects in other members of the family. A relative may have a known congenital heart anomaly or a relative may have died early in life from a heart defect.

7. It is important to inquire regarding the presence of or history of hypertension in the family, particularly the parents, grandparents, aunts, or

uncles. It is also important to know of the presence of myocardial infarction in first-degree relatives occurring before the age of 50. If such has occurred, there may be a familial tendency to an abnormally elevated serum cholesterol. One should also inquire regarding diabetes in the family.

PHYSICAL EXAMINATION

ONE can usually tell at a glance whether the infant or child is acutely or chronically ill or essentially well. The height and the weight give one the measure of the degree of normal development. Certain abnormalities of face and figure may allow identification of common or uncommon syndromes, such as Down's syndrome, Marfan's, Turner's, Holt Oram, etc.—ones that are frequently associated with heart abnormalities. Other congenital abnormalities may be apparent, such as hare lip, cleft palate, clubbed foot, microcephaly, and hyperteleriorism, and there is a minor associated significance. One may look for evidence of the rubella syndrome, such as cataracts, deafness and heart murmurs.

The presence or absence of cyanosis is of crucial importance, and if in doubt the child should be exercised or, if an infant, made to cry (the latter preferably by the mother). The conjunctiva is frequently prominent in cyanotic children.

The tonsils may be enlarged and if large enough or obstructive enough may be the cause of intermittent hypoxia and pulmonary hypertension.

Venous or arterial pulsations in the neck should be identified. A continuous murmur may be due to an arteriovenous fistula.

The external examination of the heart involves an examination of the shape of the chest and whether or not there is any precordial bulge or deformity. Such is often the case when there is right ventricular hypertrophy. It should be remembered, however, that many normal children have asymmetry of the chest without any other underlying pathology.

The apical beat may be visible and excessively palpable. A thrill may be identified. Position and force of the apical beat may give one some indication of the heart size. Percussion of the cardiac outline was once heavily depended on. Currently, radiologic evaluation is usually available and is clearly superior.

There is a distinct tendency to start the examination of the heart with a stethoscope, but palpation and inspection as outlined above may often be rewarding.

Lungs

Examination of the lungs is important in cardiac evaluation since they are involved in various forms of heart failure. One should identify respiratory rate, ease of respiration, expiratory or inspiratory prolongation or grunt, dullness on percussion, diminished or augmented breath sounds, rhonchi, rales, atelectasis, evidence of infection, or passive congestion.

In the postoperative state, the condition of the lungs needs frequent examination to ensure adequate and rapid recovery. Adequate cough, bringing up mucus, or suction of mucus with or without the help of a physiotherapist is an important maneuver. Infection or atelectasis in the lungs must be identified and adequately treated as well as more underlying problems such as failure and congestion.

Abdomen

In a baby or child who is not crying it is usually easy to examine the abdomen very adequately. Feeding the baby or examining him in the mother's arm or on the doctor's arm may eliminate crying.

In the normal infant or child, the liver is palpable up to 3 cm below the costal margin on a line between the umbilicus and the right nipple. With congestive heart failure the margin comes down sometimes as far as 7 or 8 or 9 cm below the costal margin and may be felt to pulsate, particularly when there is right hypertrophy with tricuspid regurgitation.

When digitalis or other anticongestive medication is given, the liver frequently recedes rather promptly and thus provides a useful measure of the success of the therapy. A pen mark may be made on the abdomen at the start of the therapy at the liver margin and its recession evaluated from day to day.

The presence or absence of a palpable spleen is important as is the identification of ascites. The aorta can frequently be palpated in the normal child with a soft abdomen. A prominent or excessive pulsation may suggest an aneurysm or systemic hypertension.

Extremities

Clubbing of the fingers with cyanosis is most commonly associated with congenital heart disease, although it should be remembered that it can occur in chronic lung diseases, arteriovenous fistula of the lung, cirrhosis of the liver, bacterial endocarditis, polycythemia, or a hereditary abnormality.

In cyanotic congenital heart disease, the hands are characteristically warm and flushed and the nail bed at the site of the clubbing is shiny.

An important part of the examination is the palpation of the femoral and radial arteries. Absent femorals suggest coarctation of the aorta. A varying pulse strength may indicate premature beats or other arrhythmias. A bounding pulsation in both radial and femoral arteries occurs with aortic regurgitation, a large patent ductus, and thyrotoxicosis.

In the doctor's office if the patient is anxious, the initial examination may reveal a somewhat increased heart rate and often a bounding pulse. These usually

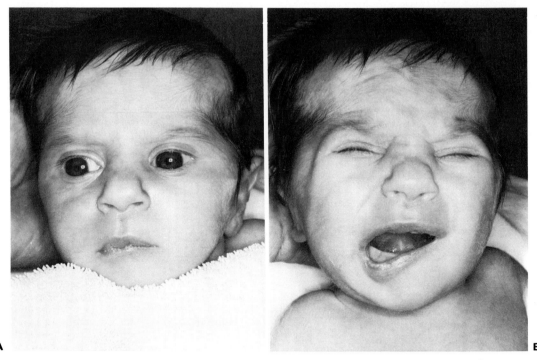

A   B

Figure 2-1. *A.* Photograph of child showing symmetric face at rest. *B.* On crying, the mouth is pulled down and to the right due to a defect on the left. (Reproduced from Pape, K. E., and Pickering, D.: Asymmetric crying facies: An index of other congenital anomalies. *J. Pediatr.*, **81**:1, 1972.)

subside during an examination, especially if the doctor is or can be reassuring to the patient.

Asymmetric Cry (Cardiofacial) Syndrome

In 1931 Parmalee described the asymmetric cry in a paper on molding due to intrauterine posture. He referred to it as partial seventh-nerve palsy. It was also noticed and reported by Hoefnagel and Penry in 1960 and Clark and McKay in 1969. However, it was Cayler in 1969 who first related the presence of congenital heart disease to the so-called cardiofacial syndrome by describing 14 infants with this sign who had heart defects as well. Chantler and McEnery (1971) added three more cases.

The largest confirmatory series was that of Pape and Pickering (1972), whose enthusiastic pursuit of the subject with findings in 44 examples of the asymmetric cry at The Toronto Hospital for Sick Children varying in age from 1 day to 16 years demonstrated a variety of other anomalies in association with this syndrome. Photographs taken from their paper are shown in Figure 2–1. The photograph labeled *A* demonstrates that at rest and composed the face is that of a normal infant. However, with crying the corner of the mouth is pulled outward and downward on the normal side but not on the abnormal side, thus producing the picture as seen in the *B* portion of Figure 2–1. To elicit this

sign the baby must be made to cry vigorously; the sign is usually not evident on smiling. They demonstrated that right-sided facial weakness occurred in 45 percent and left-sided in 55 percent of the cases.

The most significant finding was the incidence of associated defects. Fifty percent of the 44 infants had congenital cardiovascular anomalies. These were followed closely by abnormalities of the head and neck and the musculoskeletal system. A summary of these associated defects is shown in Table 2–1. It will be noted that 22 percent with the asymmetric cry had no associated abnormality.

The cause of localized facial muscle weakness is not clear. There is no good evidence that it is due to birth trauma or intrauterine posture or molding. It does not appear to be due to seventh-nerve paralysis since Nelson and Eng (1972) showed by electromyography that the nerve was intact and active but the muscle response was absent. They defined the condition as congenital hypoplasia of the depressor anguli oris muscle, thus differentiating it from congenital facial palsy.

The asymmetric cry seems to persist with the passage of time and has not disappeared in any of the cases recorded by Pape and Pickering. Furthermore, it was noted in one of their cases as late as 15 years of age. They also note that the lesion does not produce any significant cosmetic problem over the years and the individual is able to smile normally. It is only when the lips are widely contracted as in crying or an excessive grimace that the failure of the lower corner of the mouth (the anguli oris muscle) becomes apparent.

Thus, the chief value of the clinical recognition of the asymmetric cry lies in its role as an indicator of the possibility of coexistence of other congenital anomalies and especially those of congenital heart disease. Because of the overlapping involvement of the various systems listed in Table 2–1, when one identifies the asymmetric cry associated with a congenital heart defect it is well to consider also abnormalities of the head and neck, musculoskeletal system, central nervous system, and genitourinary, gastrointestinal, and respiratory tracts.

The heart defects found with this syndrome may cover a wide variety of anomalies, including tetralogy of Fallot, patent ductus, tricuspid atresia, ventricular septal defect, single ventricle, atrial septal defect, bicuspid aortic valve, double aortic arch, truncus arteriosus, and aortic stenosis. Since such a wide variety of defects have been found, it is possible that any form of congenital heart disease may be associated with the asymmetric cry.

Table 2–1. ASYMMETRIC CRYING FACIES— 44 CASES: INCIDENCE OF ASSOCIATED ANOMALIES*

Cardiovascular	22/44
Abnormalities of head, neck, ears, palate, etc.	20/44
Musculoskeletal	20/44
Genitourinary	11/44
Central nervous system	11/44
Gastrointestinal	9/44
Respiratory	5/44

* Pape, K. E., and Pickering, D.: Asymmetric crying facies: an index of other congenital anomalies. *J. Pediatr.*, **81**:21–30, 1972.

Congenital Heart Disease and Scoliosis

Scoliosis has been reported to occur with varying frequency in from 1 to 19 percent of children with congenital heart disease. Shands and Eisberg (1955), Wright and Niebauer (1956), Luke and McDonnell (1968), Wynne-Davies (1968), and Roth and associates (1973) carried out a prospective study of pediatric and adolescent children in the cardiac clinic population at the Boston Children's Hospital and found an overall incidence of 12 percent. Scoliosis was three times more common in patients with cyanotic congenital heart disease.

The apparent age of onset of scoliosis in children with congenital heart disease was reported by Beals and coworkers (1972). Eighteen percent appeared between birth and three years, 45 percent between four and nine years, and 37 percent over nine years of age on into the adolescent period. Scoliosis appears to occur earlier in children with congenital heart disease than it does when the scoliosis is an isolated phenomenon. The incidence of scoliosis in the general population has been variously reported to be between 0.03 and 6 percent.

The usual site of the curve in the spine is between the fifth and eighth vertebrae. The age of onset is frequently related to the ultimate degree of severity of the curvature; the later the onset, the milder the degree of scoliosis.

The curve site is thoracic in about half of the cases, thoracic-lumbar in 12 percent, and lumbar in 20 percent.

When scoliosis occurs as an isolated anomaly, there are rarely other congenital defects elsewhere in the body; however, when congenital heart disease occurs with scoliosis, other anomalies elsewhere in the body are not infrequent. The major ones encountered are club feet, cleft palate, tracheoesophageal fistula, mental retardation, or Down's syndrome.

The cardiac lesion most frequently encountered with scoliosis is tetralogy of Fallot, although scoliosis can occur with ventricular septal defect, atrial septal defect, patent ductus, and coarctation of the aorta.

In many cases the scoliosis is sufficiently mild that the patient can be observed for possible change over several years. Some are treated with a Milwaukee brace; others eventually need the Harrington rod or Dwyer cable instrumentation. It is interesting to note that the majority go through such surgery without difficulty even though they may have severely involved heart lesions.

Congenital scoliosis occurs as a result of an abnormality of the vertebrae. This could be a wedged-shaped body or semivertebrae or a failure in segmentation sometimes even with a bony bar joining the nearby ribs. The abnormality may be identified early in life on routine chest films. Since most children with congenital heart disease usually have an x-ray of heart and chest, it is important to look for abnormalities of the spine as well as those of the heart.

Scoliosis, whether congenital or idiopathic, may be recognized in the early years of life. The majority of these deformities remain static throughout the growth period of childhood, but some are progressive and markedly so. In order to identify those that are getting worse, it is important that the x-ray of the involved area of the spine should be taken once or twice a year. Thus, if the curvature is progressive, it can be recognized as such and treated surgically. This is usually done by a surgical fusion to prevent further deviation of the spine.

REFERENCES

Beals, R. K.; Kenney, K. H.; and Lees, M. H.: Congenital heart disease and idiopathic scoliosis. *Clini. Orthop. Related Res.*, **89**:112–16, 1972.

Cayler, G. E.: Cardiofacial syndrome. *Arch. Dis. Child.*, **44**:69, 1969.

Chantler, C., and McEnery, G.: Cardiofacial syndrome. *Proc. R. Soc. Med.*, **64**:21, 1971.

Clark, D. N.: Disease of the autonomic nervous system. In Nelson, W. E.; Vaughan, V. C., III; and McKay, R. J.: *Textbook of Pediatrics*, 9th ed. Saunders, Philadelphia, 1969, p. 1309.

Hoefnagel, D., and Penry, J. K.: Partical facial paralysis in young children. *N. Engl. J. Med.*, **262**:1126, 1960.

Luke, M. J., and McDonnell, E. J.: Congenital heart disease and scoliosis. *J. Pediatr.*, **73**:725, 1968.

McKusick, V. A. (chairman): The Fourth Conference on the Clinical Delineation of Birth Defects, June 7–11. The Johns Hopkins Medical Institutions, Baltimore, 1971.

Marden, P. M.; Smith, D. W.; and McDonald, M. J.: Congenital anomalies in the new-born infant, including minor variations. *J. Pediatr.*, **64**:357, 1964.

Nelson, K. B., and Eng, G. D.: Congenital hypoplasia of the depressor anguli oris muscle: Differentiation fron the congenital facial palsy. *J. Pediatr.*, **81**:16–20, 1972.

Pape, K. E., and Pickering, D.: Asymmetric crying facies: An index of other congenital anomalies. *J. Pediatr.*, **81**:21, 1972.

Parmelee, A. H.: Molding due to intra-uterine posture. *Am. J. Dis. Child.*, **42**:1155, 1931.

Roth, A.; Rosenthal, A.; Hall, J. E.; and Mizel, M.: Scoliosis and congenital heart disease. *Clini. Orthop. Related Res.*, **93**:95, 1973.

Shands, A. R., and Eisberg, J. B.: The incidence of scoliosis in the State of Delaware. *J. Bone Joint Surg.*, **37A**:1243, 1955.

Wright, W. D., and Niebauer, J. J.: Congenital heart disease and scoliosis. *J. Bone Joint Surg.*, **38A**:1181, 1956.

Wynne-Davies, R.: Familial (idiopathic) scoliosis. *J. Bone Joint Surg.*, **50B**:24, 1968.

3

Heart Sounds and Murmurs

John D. Keith

THE STETHOSCOPE continues to be a most valuable instrument in the diagnosis of various forms of heart disease. This is especially true in childhood, when the chest wall is thin and minor variations in heart sounds and murmurs over the precordium can be readily appreciated. Modern techniques of recording heart sounds and murmurs have provided a good deal of information regarding the events of the cardiac cycle in both normal and abnormal hearts. Early studies by Dock (1933), Orias and Braun-Menendez (1939), Rappaport and Sprague (1942), and many others, including a recent symposium (Leon and Shaver, 1975), have added much to our fundamental knowledge of this subject.

The rapid increase in our understanding of the pathology and hemodynamics of various forms of heart disease now permits a much more accurate appraisal of the clinical findings in childhood with relatively simple tools, such as the stethoscope, the electrocardiogram, and the x-ray or fluoroscope. The stethoscope never has been a more useful instrument for making a diagnosis of heart disease in infancy or childhood than at the present moment. The stethoscope was first introduced into Canada by Dr. Pierre Beautren in 1827 on his return from studying in Paris (Abbott, 1931; Segall, 1967). Although it was widely used, its full value was not appreciated for over 100 years.

The value of training in this technique was demonstrated by Butterworth and Reppert (1960) by testing two groups of physicians: one group a portion of those attending a general medical meeting, and the second from the American Heart Association meeting. Forty-nine percent of the former and 69 percent of the latter tested were able to correctly identify the pathologic heart sounds and murmurs played to them on a tape. Since medical management, diagnosis, and further specialized testing depend on the clinical examination, the importance of the stethoscope is obvious.

The detailed studies on heart sounds carried out in recent years by Feigen and summarized in 1971 indicate the characteristics of sound and the relation to recording by the human ear or by modern phonocardiographic techniques. Feigen makes the following points for the cardiographer: (1) pitch is the frequency of vibrations per second; (2) intensity is the magnitude of the sound wave; (3) harmonics and overtones modify the quality of sound; and (4) the duration of the heart sound determines whether it is recognized as a click, a snap, a tone, or a murmur, the first of these being the shortest and the last the longest.

A sophisticated sound-recording machine can better indicate changes in intensity than can the human ear. The human ear recognizes changes in pitch better than changes in intensity. However, the lower-range changes in pitch may not be recognized by the human.

Ambient noise in a quiet room may be 30 decibels, and even this may interfere with the efficiency of stethoscope reception. In a hospital ward the noise level may be up to 60 or 70 decibels. This difficulty in hearing heart sounds in the presence of noise is apparently related to the fact that the human ear is unable to detect some sounds immediately after hearing certain loud sounds. This is the masking or fatigue phenomenon.

Williams and Dodge (1926) and Butterworth (1960) have recognized that the brain of a trained observer may be able to subconsciously block out meaningless sounds such as respiration and identify faint diastolic murmurs that might not show clearly on a phonocardiograph machine as the respiratory sound is within the range of the cardiac sound as far as the machine is concerned.

Another interesting point made by Feigen (1971) relates to the well-known fact that change in hearing is common with increasing age. The higher frequencies are less well received by the older age group. This affects certain frequencies encountered in music, but rarely those encountered in auscultation of the heart. "Therefore, persons who follow an ordinary conversation with difficulty may often be well able to hear heart sounds and murmurs."

The closest splitting that can be appreciated by the ear is that of clicks at an interval of 0.02 second apart

(Johnston, 1957). The human ear is thus limited compared with the phonocardiograph, as it is in many other aspects of auscultation. However, the human brain has at its disposal many other facets that lessen the dependence on heart sounds and murmurs: the history, the general physical examination, the radiology of the heart, the electrocardiogram, angiocardiography, cardiac catheterization, ultrasound and echocardiographic technique, and many other procedures that minimize our reliance on sounds and murmurs. Thus, putting all available information together leads to a most accurate understanding of the underlying lesions. The importance of the stethoscope lies in its extraordinary usefulness in the hands of a trained observer often without the addition of many of the aids mentioned above.

HEART SOUNDS

First Heart Sound

For many years the first heart sound was considered to be composed of two components. Luisada and MacCanon, however, in 1972 demonstrated that there are several sound waves that can be recorded (see Figure 3–1). The first or zero component is inaudible and is a minor vibration that appears to be related to the muscle bundles of the left ventricle and the initial change in the shape of that chamber during systole. They have named this the zero component. The first segment of higher frequency (labeled A) occurs during the early phase of the rise of left ventricular pressure and of its first derivative (DP/DT). It appears to be caused by tension of the left ventricular structures with acceleration of the walls and deceleration of the blood within the chamber. The second component of higher frequency (labeled B) occurs at the time of opening of the aortic valve and coincides with an indentation or a second peak of the first derivatives of the left ventricular pressure curve. This sound is related to sudden acceleration of the blood and deceleration of the structures that occur immediately after the opening of the aortic valve. The C component appears at the time of the first peak of the aortic pulse when it changes from a very rapid to a less rapid rise in pressure. It coincides with the peak of the first derivative of the aortic pulse. This component is believed to be caused by vibrations of the infundibulum of the left ventricle, in the walls of the aorta, and the blood contained in these chambers. Luisada and MacCanon point out that there may be a fourth or D component, which occurs with the maximal expansion of the aortic wall and is, therefore, a vascular vibration (see Figure 3–1).

This interpretation excludes valve closure as a cause of the A component since the first sound occurs distinctly after closure has occurred. It does not exclude, but minimizes, valve tension as a cause of the first sound. It recognizes the exclusive importance of the left ventricle in causing the first sound and, therefore, minimizes or excludes the right ventricle in the normal heart. It evaluates the necessary part played by both the mitral and aortic valves in the dynamic phases of left ventricular contraction and aortic expansion, and it attributes vibrations of the first heart sound to vibrations of the left ventricular aortic system.

Thus the first significant component (A) of the heart sounds occurs at the first third of the left ventricular pressure rise. The second component (B) occurs at the opening of the aortic valve, and the third component (C) occurs at the point at which the still-rising aortic pressure curve shows a change toward the horizontal. (See Figure 3–1.)

An alternative explanation that is widely accepted suggests that both left and right heart events contribute to the production of the first heart sound. The first component is related to atrial contraction and has been called the atrial component of the first heart sound. This sound is absent whenever the QRS complex is not preceded by a P wave. It coincides with or occurs just after the Q wave. It is probably due to ventricular filling, and it can be audible in some healthy people. A second low-frequency component occurs at the time of crossover of the LV and LA pressures, and could be due to the coaptation of the mitral valve leaflets. This component is inaudible. The third component, a higher-frequency sound and the first major audible component, occurs coincident with the left atrial "c" wave and with the point of maximal posterior motion of the anterior mitral valve leaflet as seen on the echocardiogram. This is thought to be due to the tensing of the chordae tendineae and of the mitral valve. The fourth component, and the second easily audible component, occurs coincident with the right atrial "c" wave and also with the point of closure of the tricuspid valve as shown on the echocardiogram. Factors delaying tricuspid valve closure delay this component. A few inaudible "aftervibrations" may follow this last component.

The changes in magnitude of the first heart sound have been correlated with the level of left ventricular

Figure 3-1. Scheme of the cardiac cycle and of the relationship between valve openings and closures; ventricular, atrial, and arterial events; waves of the ECG; and heart sounds recorded by the phonocardiogram. *ECG*, electrocardiogram; *PCG*, phonocardiogram; *LV*, left ventricle; *RV*, right ventricle; *PA*, pulmonary artery; *LA*, left atrium; *RA*, right atrium; *AO*, aorta; *I* and *II*, first and second heart sounds; *III* and *IV*, third and fourth heart sounds; *M* and *T*, mitral and tricuspid valves; *PA* and *Ao*, pulmonary and aortic valves; *RT*, right heart; *LT*, left heart. (Reproduced from Luisada, A. A., and MacCanon, D. M.: The phases of the cardiac cycle. *Am. Heart J.*, **83**:705, 1972.)

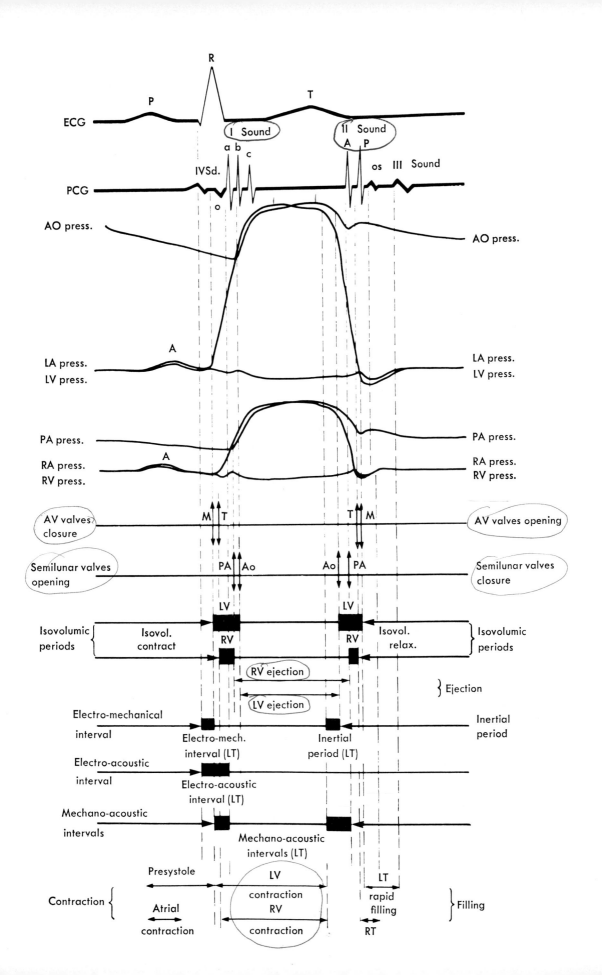

pressure and with the percentage change in amplitude of the first systolic wave of the first derivative of the left ventricular pressure. Sakamato and associates (1965) demonstrated a linear correlation between the first component of the first heart sound and the first derivative of the left ventricular pressure, suggesting a relation between the first sound and the rapidity of left ventricular contraction.

The first heart sound is increased in amplitude in hyperthyroidism or with the administration of drugs that stimulate the myocardium directly or indirectly such as epinephrine and amyl nitrite.

The first sound may be decreased in amplitude when there is weakness of the left ventricular contraction. The first heart sound varies in complete AV block, and this is related at least in part to the timing of atrial contraction in relation to ventricular contraction (Shah and Gramiak, 1970). It has also been demonstrated that the first heart sound varies with the length of the P-R interval in acute rheumatic fever in children with or without mitral insufficiency, the first sound being softened or almost absent when the conduction time in the child is between 0.18 and 0.24 second (Keith, 1937).

For some time splitting of the first heart sound has been recognized by clinical observers. In 1954 Leatham distinguished two high-frequency components of the first heart sound, which he called mitral and tricuspid, attributing them to closure or tension of the two atrioventricular valves. Luisada and Cortis (1970) demonstrated that in man tricuspid valve closure always followed mitral valve closure, but Luisada has also demonstrated by animal experimentation that the tricuspid valve plays little or no part in production of the first heart sound. In the normal phonocardiogram, splitting of the heart sound is evident in the components A and B; the separation of these two components may be very close and not identifiable by human ear.

Increased Intensity of First Heart Sound. The intensity of the first heart sound is increased when there is a rapid ventricular upstroke, increased atrioventricular flow, as in a left-to-right shunt or in high cardiac output, or shortening of the atrial ventricular filling time, as in tachycardia. There is not infrequently an increased first heart sound in the presence of a short P-R interval.

The loud first sound in mitral stenosis is usually associated with a loud opening snap.

Reduction of the intensity of the first heart sound may be due to poor conduction through the chest wall, although this is an uncommon cause in childhood. More commonly it is associated with a prolonged P-R interval or at times with myocardial disease with a slow rise of ventricular pressure pulse.

Systolic Sounds

Early systolic ejection sounds may be divided into aortic and pulmonary. The aortic ejection sounds result from aortic valve disease, aortic valvar stenosis, aortic regurgitation, or at times a bicuspid aortic valve. They also occur as a result of a dilated aorta, which may be found in marked pulmonary stenosis with a ventricular septal defect or pulmonary atresia with a ventricular septal defect, or in systemic hypertension, or in idiopathic dilatation of the aorta. The sounds also occur in syphilitic or atheromatous aortas.

The aortic ejection sounds occur approximately 0.06 second after the chief components of the first sound, and this ejection sound is well heard in the mitral area but is usually best heard in the fourth left interspace and less well at the apex. The aortic ejection sounds occur later than the pulmonary ejection sounds and do not vary much with respiration as do the pulmonary ejection sounds.

Pulmonary ejection sounds occur in pulmonary valvar stenosis and pulmonary artery dilatation. The latter may be due to pulmonary hypertension, as in Eisenmenger's syndrome, or it may be idiopathic. The pulmonary ejection sounds can usually be identified down the left sternal border, particularly in the third and fourth left interspaces, but they are very poorly transmitted to the apex. The sounds frequently diminish or disappear with inspiration, whereas the aortic ejection sounds are not affected as much by the respiratory phases.

In identifying the pulmonary ejection sound of pulmonary stenosis one may also refer to the electrocardiogram, which will usually show some evidence of right hypertrophy, a dilated pulmonary artery in the x-ray, a systolic murmur, and wide splitting of S_2.

There is usually some dilatation of the pulmonary artery in an atrial septal defect, but a pulmonary ejection sound is usually not heard in this condition until after the repair and may then be related to the dilated but somewhat slack pulmonary artery.

An aneurysm of the membranous portion of the ventricular septum may be associated with ventricular septal defect; a click may occur approximately 120 milliseconds after the Q wave of the electrocardiogram (Pieroni et al. 1971) and is highly indicative of the above pathology (it can usually be identified from pulmonary and aortic clicks).

Postejection Clicks

These sounds occur after carotid upstroke and after the rapid ejection phase is over. They are recognized by the stethoscope as occurring in mid or late systole.

Such postejection clicks have been identified occasionally in normal children, but most commonly they are noted when there is mitral valve prolapse (balloon mitral) and are usually associated with a systolic murmur, honking in type and best heard at the apex.

Prolapsed Mitral Valve

The prolapsed, or ballooning, mitral valve has received a good deal of attention in recent years and is discussed elsewhere (see page 810). This abnormality is associated with a click and a murmur. Both are best heard at the apex and inside the apex at the sternum. The murmur occurs characteristically in mid or late systole and is honking in type, but it may be blowing. The click is usually heard at the onset of the murmur.

Occasionally there may be multiple clicks or a shower of clicks, which, at times, will resemble a friction rub or the crunching-of-snow sound. If the division between the two sounds is greater than 0.05 to 0.06 second, the second component is more likely to be a click.

The importance of a correct diagnosis in relation to a prolapsed, or ballooning, mitral valve lies in the fact that in adult life some cases will be progressive and lead to increasing mitral regurgitation. This is uncommon in childhood, and a child who has minimal evidence of mitral regurgitation need not be restricted in activity. However, it is just as well to follow these children over a period of time, seeing them at two-year intervals to identify possible changes that may take place.

If the murmur is short, it may simulate the functional murmur. Correct differential diagnosis may be important in such cases to outline the underlying pathology. The character of the murmur plus the click will usually allow identification of the prolapsed mitral valve.

Second Heart Sound

The identification of aortic and pulmonary closure sounds is important since the degree of spread and the intensity of either component may be very helpful in making or confirming a variety of diagnoses. Aortic valve closure is the louder of the two components of the second heart sound in all areas, including the pulmonary area in the normal heart, and it is the sole component in the mitral area except on rare occasions in the pediatric age group. When one compares the pulmonary and aortic valve closure sounds, the pulmonary valve component is softer and confined to the pulmonary area chiefly. It is best identified on inspiration that prolongs right ventricular systole. Harris and Sutton (1968) have measured the width of splitting of the second sound in the pulmonary area in the expiratory phase and find that splitting is not audible in children in the pulmonary area on expiration in 98 percent of cases. Thus, a single second sound on expiration is a normal finding in infants and children (and in adults). In inspiration the two components of the second sound are separated by an interval varying from 0.02 to 0.06 second with an average of 0.04 second. Leatham (1970) points out that a greater separation can be achieved by slow, deep respiration in the reclining posture. He also suggests that an in-

audibility of P_2 during inspiration is rare at any age, but is usually due to low intensity rather than fusion with A_2. This is particularly true when hyperinflation of the lung is present. In infants with tachycardia, A_2 and P_2 can usually be separated with the use of the stethoscope. P_2 is almost invariably the lesser component and should be listened for in the pulmonary area since it is rarely transmitted to the mitral area. A delay in P_2 with inspiration is related to increase in stroke volume in the right ventricle during this phase of respiration. A_2 may also show slight degree of delay but not to the degree found with the pulmonary second sound.

Second Sound in Heart Abnormalities. Wide splitting of the second sound may occur in right bundle branch block, atrial septal defect, anomalous venous return, pulmonary stenosis, right ventricular failure, and myocarditis.

In right bundle branch block there is a delayed rise in the right ventricular pressure pulse resulting in a late pulmonary valve closure. Some variations with respiration can be identified.

In atrial septal defect there is increased width of splitting due to the large stroke volume and a measure of right bundle branch block. In the presence of a large defect the splitting is fixed and does not vary significantly with the phases of respiration. However, after successful surgery, although the splitting may continue it may vary with inspiration.

With anomalous venous return there is almost invariably a widely opened interatrial septal defect. With the two anomalies one then has wide fixed splitting of the two components of the second sound in the pulmonary area.

In pulmonary valve stenosis with intact ventricular septum the pulmonary component is soft and greatly delayed; however, it can usually be heard and recorded in the pulmonary area, except in the cases in which the stenosis is extreme when the pulmonary valve closure is not audible.

In pulmonary stenosis with a ventricular septal defect (tetralogy of Fallot) the pulmonary second sound is usually absent due to the markedly diminished pulmonary blood flow and pressure in the pulmonary artery. It is also related at times to the anatomy of the pulmonary valve; if there is a relatively large pulmonary blood flow and the configuration of the valve suitable, a pulmonary closure sound may at times be heard. P_2 may also be heard on occasion after a successful Blalock operation.

In ventricular septal defect with a left-to-right shunt, splitting of the second sound may be of a normal degree and the pulmonary component of normal intensity. This is because most ventricular septal defects are not large, the majority are small, and the heart is functionally normal. When the shunt is increased without increasing pulmonary vascular resistance, the splitting of the second sound may be increased in width but not fixed. This appears to be due to the fact that the ventricular septal defect, when large, may have both increased systolic and diastolic loading of both ventricles. Harris and associates (1971) have shown that the splitting of S_2 in a significant ventricular septal defect does not, as a rule, vary much more than 0.1 to 0.2 second with inspiration, and they have suggested that in such cases the diastolic shunting accounts for a substantial form of blood flow and this tends to damp the normal respiratory variation while not completely abolishing it. As the pulmonary vascular resistance rises over several years in children who are proceeding to the Eisenmenger syndrome, the degree of splitting between the A_2 and P_2 is gradually reduced until they become fused. Thus, a single-fused second sound is characteristic of a ventricular septal defect with high pulmonary vascular resistance. Splitting of the second sound in the pulmonary area may occur in pulmonary hypertension when there is a delay in the pulmonary component due to right heart failure. The pulmonary closure sound may also be delayed in systolic overloading of the right ventricle or due to right bundle branch block.

Reverse Splitting of the Second Sound. This occurs when the pulmonary valve closure is completed before the aortic valve closure. It may be found in left bundle branch block and in the Wolff-Parkinson-White syndrome when early right ventricle activation may take place. Reverse splitting is also found at times in aortic stenosis, systolic hypertension, left ventricular failure, and myocarditis.

Single Second Sound. A single second sound may occur in tetralogy of Fallot with pulmonary atresia or severe pulmonary stenosis. It may occur in the Eisenmenger syndrome with ventricular septal defect, or it may be found in a single ventricle with pulmonary atresia or with high pulmonary vascular resistance.

Uncommonly, however, a single sound may be considered to be present when the pulmonary or aortic component is inaudible.

Diastolic Sounds

There are three causes of early diastolic valve opening sounds. Perhaps the best known is that of the atrioventricular valve opening snap that occurs in mitral stenosis. The second is an atrial ventricular valve abnormality without stenosis, such as occurs in Ebstein's disease. The third is associated with increased atrial ventricular flow, which is a common phenomenon in many left-to-right shunts in children but may also occur in acute rheumatic fever and, at times, in the normal child (Margolies and Wolferth, 1932). In mitral stenosis it occurs as the result of the fused cusps, somewhat thickened, carried by rapid ventricular inflow into the left ventricle, which produces a sharp sound that can be recorded in the phonocardiogram and is referred to as the opening snap. In congenital heart disease a middiastolic murmur is much more frequently the result of a left-to-right shunt than it is due to mitral stenosis (Nadas and Alimurung, 1952).

Third Heart Sound

Rapid ventricular filling causes vibrations that are sufficiently intense to be audible as a third heart sound occurring 0.15 second after the second sound. This third sound occurs in some healthy children. Its low pitch is more readily audible with the bell rather than the diaphragm of the stethoscope. It is best heard at the apex after inspiration with the child turned on his side. The sound is heard in about 8 percent of normal children, but it is heard in approximately half of the children with rheumatic heart disease. Occasionally the third sound may appear to have some duration because of fusion of asynchronous filling sounds from each ventricle. This can mimic a middiastolic rumble.

Fourth Heart Sound

An atrial sound referred to as the fourth heart sound can be heard or recorded at times, but normally the contraction of the atrium is inaudible. A large A wave coupled with an atrial sound is a useful indication of ventricular abnormality. It is more audible in childhood when there is a summation of the atrial sound and a ventricular filling sound, as occurs in gallop rhythm.

HEART MURMURS

For many generations of physicians murmurs have assumed an increasingly important role in identifying the underlying pathology. The introduction of the cardiac catheter, coupled with techniques for identifying intracardiac and extracardiac sounds and murmurs, has paralleled our increasing understanding of the physiology of the contracting heart and movement of heart valves and has led to an augmented ability to interpret murmurs in relation to the underlying lesions.

Leatham (1958) classified heart murmurs as due to three main factors: (1) high flow through a normal or abnormal valve; (2) a forward flow through a constricted or abnormal valve into a dilated vessel or a heart chamber; and (3) regurgitant flow through an incompetent valve or a congenital heart anomaly such as patent ductus arteriosus or a ventricular septal defect.

A classification of murmurs in childhood is as follows: (1) systolic ejection murmurs, (2) systolic regurgitant murmurs, (3) diastolic murmurs, and (4) continuous murmurs.

SYSTOLIC EJECTION AND SYSTOLIC REGURGITANT MURMURS

Left ventricular outflow tract murmur
   Valvar (e.g., aortic stenosis)
   Subvalvar (e.g., discreet subvalve or aortic stenosis)
   Supravalvar (e.g., narrowing of ascending aorta)
Right ventricular outflow tract murmurs
   Valvar (e.g., pulmonary stenosis)
   Subvalvar (e.g., infundibular stenosis)
   Supravalvar (e.g., supravalvar pulmonary stenosis)
Left ventricular inflow tract systolic murmurs
   Valvar (e.g., mitral regurgitation)
Right ventricular inflow tract systolic murmurs
   Valvar (e.g., tricuspid regurgitation)

DIASTOLIC MURMURS

Regurgitation across semilunar valves
   Aortic valve regurgitation
   Pulmonary valve regurgitation
Increased flow across atrioventricular valves
Increased flow across mitral valve
   Patent ductus arteriosus
   Ventricular septal defect
   Austin Flint murmur
Increased flow across tricuspid valve
   Atrial septal defect
   Mitral regurgitation
   Tricuspid regurgitation
   Aortic regurgitation
   Ebstein's anomaly
   Hyperthyroidism
   Severe anemia
Obstruction at atrioventricular valve
   Mitral stenosis
   Parachute mitral valve
   Tricuspid stenosis
   Intracardiac tumors

CONTINUOUS MURMURS

Patent ductus arteriosus
Blalock shunt or similar surgical procedures
Arteriovenous aneurysm of the lung
Large collaterals to pulmonary artery from bronchial artery
Aortic septal defect
Coronary artery aneurysm or fistula
Total anomalous pulmonary venous return
Communication of aneurysm of aortic sinus with pulmonary artery, right atrium, or right ventricle
Traumatic arteriovenous fistula in thorax
Congenital arteriovenous fistula in chest wall
Anomalous coronary artery entering the pulmonary artery
Coarctation of pulmonary artery
Dissecting aneurysm with fistula communicating with right atrium

Systolic Murmurs

Systolic murmurs are usually divided into two categories: (1) systolic ejection murmurs and (2) systolic regurgitant murmurs. Systolic murmurs may be early or late systolic. The midsystolic starts after the first sound and ends before the second. The early systolic starts with the first sound and disappears in midsystole. Late systolic murmurs begin in midsystole and go up to and, at times, through the aortic valve closure. Regurgitant systolic murmurs are usually pansystolic, beginning with the first sound and ending at or after the aortic valve closure.

Systolic Ejection Murmurs. A midsystolic ejection murmur may occur as a result of valvular or infundibular obstruction of the right or left ventricular outflow tract, or it may be due to an increased rate of ejection through an otherwise-normal valve, or a slightly irregular valve without narrowing, or simply due to the dilatation of the pulmonary artery or aorta beyond a normal valve. A murmur from such a cause is usually described as diamond-shaped and begins after closure of the AV valve and stops before the semilunar valve closure. An ejection murmur from the right heart (e.g., pulmonic stenosis) may be diamond-shaped, with the peak or diamond occurring a little later than that of the left heart since the pressure in the right ventricle is usually less than that of the left. When there is marked ventricular obstruction, the systolic murmur is prolonged and more rounded in shape when recorded. The intensity of the aortic ejection or closure sounds is related to valve mobility and not primarily to the severity of the narrowing of the valve.

Reddy and associates (1971) point out that, regardless of the site of stenosis in the left ventricular outflow tract, significant obstruction always results in left ventricular hypertrophy with a decreased compliance. This leads to a presystolic apical expansion on palpation and an atrial diastolic gallop on auscultation. They point out that the teen-age and adult group of cases with an aortic stenosis and an atrial diastolic gallop usually have an associated left ventricular endiastolic pressure of 11 mm of mercury and a left atrial A wave peak of above 13 mm of mercury. The ventricular diastolic gallop is also heard in left ventricular outflow tract obstruction when decompensation takes place. In a differential diagnosis of left ventricular outflow obstruction one needs to consider valvular, subvalvular, and supravalvular origin as well as that due to idiopathic hypertrophic subaortic stenosis. Acquired aortic stenosis is uncommon in childhood.

The murmur significant of left ventricular outflow tract obstruction is usually best heard in the first and second right interspaces and the second and third left intercostal spaces, but not infrequently it radiates into the neck. When the murmur is well heard at the apex, a sound tracing will usually show that it has the same diamond-shaped configuration as in the aortic area, suggesting that it has the same origin as the aortic murmur and is not due to mitral regurgitation.

Right ventricular outflow tract obstruction may occur as an isolated valvar or infundibular pulmonic narrowing with an intact ventricular septum, but more commonly it occurs with a ventricular septal defect, as in tetralogy of Fallot. The details of pathologic obstruction are set down elsewhere (see page 471). In summary, however, pure valvar pulmonic stenosis causes the ejection phase to lengthen as the obstruction becomes more severe. The pulmonic closure sound is therefore progressively delayed and the splitting of S_2 widens. At the same time the pulmonic closure sound becomes fainter and finally disappears. The aortic closure sound is masked by the prolonged systolic murmur. In differentiating between valvar and infundibular stenosis the site of maximum intensity of the murmur is of questionable help. However, in the presence of infundibular obstruction the pulmonary ejection sound, or click, is never encountered and the pulmonic closure sound is not audible except in the mildest cases. When the stenosis is at the valve, a click is usually present if the gradient is less than 80 cm Hg. A sound tracing in valvar stenosis of significant severity will show a wide splitting of the second sound, wider than one would expect with infundibular stenosis.

Hultgren and associates (1969) have described the mechanism of a marked respiratory variation in the intensity of the pulmonary ejection sound or click. During expiration the sound becomes louder and later with a longer interval between it and the first heart sound. They point out that during inspiration there is a decrease in the pulmonary endiastolic pressure that parallels the change in intrathoracic pressure. In contrast there is an absolute increase in the right ventricular endiastolic pressure with equalization during the atrial filling phase. This latter is due primarily to the increased venous return during inspiration augmenting right ventricular endiastolic volume. This leads to early opening of the pulmonary valve prior to right ventricular systole, and when right ventricular systole does occur, the movement of the dome valve is minimal or absent. During expiration the pulmonary endiastolic pressure increases and exceeds right ventricular endiastolic pressure and the pulmonary valve remains in the closed position in diastole. With the onset of right ventricular systole the sudden ascent of the dome of the valve produces a loud ejection sound.

The clinical findings will usually differentiate tetralogy of Fallot from the isolated pulmonic stenosis. In the former a very clear aortic closure sound is heard but the pulmonary valve closure is inaudible.

In branch stenosis of the pulmonary artery there is a systolic ejection murmur at the upper left and right sternal borders that is widely transmitted to the right chest and back and often to the axilla. The systolic murmur may become continuous, particularly with more peripheral pulmonary artery stenosis. Sutton and associates (1968) have pointed out the presence of a loud, often palpable, pulmonic closure sound accompanied by a late ejection click in the Eisenmenger syndrome associated with a ventricular septal defect. There may be a short, rather faint systolic murmur and a pulmonary diastolic murmur as the pulmonary vascular disease progresses in severity.

The presence of increased flow across the pulmonary valve may produce a murmur as in atrial septal defects, but a flow murmur may also occur in anemia, hyperthyroidism, fever, exercise, anxiety, or excitement. Daty and Sen (1956), Rawlings (1960), and DeLeon and associates (1965) have described the straight back syndrome, in which there is a loss of normal thoracic kyphosis of the spine. Although this is not a common finding, it may occur in young people and is frequently associated with a benign systolic ejection murmur. The murmur may be associated with a wide splitting of heart sounds and a pulmonary ejection sound that varies with respiration. The diagnosis can be established by routine lateral chest film demonstrating the lack of normal thoracic kyphosis and the presence of a straight spine in the upper thoracic area.

Systolic Regurgitant Murmurs.   Such regurgitant murmurs occur in the presence of a flow of blood in retrograde fashion from one chamber or vessel of the higher pressure to a chamber of the vessel with a lower pressure during systole. A common example is that of mitral regurgitation in which the murmur usually lasts through all of systole and tends to be constant rather than diamond-shaped when recorded.

In the presence of mitral regurgitation at the onset of the left ventricular contraction, the pressure rises in the ventricle and closes the mitral valve. A murmur then begins with, or immediately after, the onset of the first heart sound. A heart sound recording will usually show the first heart sound clearly; however, with a stethoscope the murmur when loud may make it difficult to differentiate the onset of the murmur from the first heart sound. In children with rheumatic heart disease and mitral regurgitation the AV conduction time is not infrequently lengthened, and this permits the mitral and tricuspid valves to assume a closed, or a nearly closed, position before the onset of ventricular systole. This has the effect of softening, or diminishing, the first heart sound, which can be recognized by the stethoscope or demonstrated by a heart sound recording. When the regurgitation is marked, there is a large reservoir of blood in the left atrium at the beginning of each diastole and this gives rise to a rapid ventricular filling sound that is recognized as a short diastolic rumble at the beginning of diastole. This is a common finding in children with considerable mitral regurgitation, tricuspid regurgitation, atrial septal defect, and ventricular septal defects.

In tricuspid insufficiency during inspiration there is decreased intrathoracic pressure, which results in increased venous return to the right atrium. This in turn increases the flow of blood through the right side of the heart and intensifies a tricuspid murmur. The murmur of tricuspid regurgitation is best heard in the lower left sternal border area. If there is doubt about the origin, continuous deep breathing will reveal that the murmur increases with inspiration and diminishes with expiration.

In the presence of a ventricular septal defect, a characteristic pansystolic murmur is heard over the lower precordium, often with a thrill. In infants and young children, in whom the ventricular septal defect is decreasing in size, the murmur may become shorter and fainter; while it may begin with the onset of systole, it may disappear before the end of systole as the defect becomes progressively smaller before ultimately closing completely.

A midsystolic murmur may occur with mitral regurgitation due to papillary muscle dysfunction, as indicated by Burch, Depasquale, and Phillips (1963). Inadequate tension of the papillary muscle may cause a prolapse of part of the mitral valve, which produces in turn some mitral regurgitation and a midsystolic murmur. Reddy and associates (1971) point out that a fibrotic, or scarred, papillary muscle may hold down the leaflet during ventricular contraction and produce a systolic murmur. They also report that a dilated ventricle may displace the papillary muscles and prevent proper coaptation of the valve leaflets during systole and produce a murmur.

When the systolic murmur of mitral regurgitation is due to a prolapse of the anterior leaflet in the mitral valve, the flow is directed over the posterior leaflet. The murmur is then usually best heard at the apex and transmitted to the axilla. When the prolapse occurs in the posterior leaflet of the mitral valve with the flow being directed over the anterior leaflet, the murmur is more likely to be directed to the base of the heart or to the left of the sternum.

Studies by Ronan and associates (1965), Criley and colleagues (1966), and Leon and coworkers (1972) have demonstrated with left ventricular cineangiograms that the abnormal prolapse of a mitral valve leaflet usually involves the posterior cusp and the anomaly may be related to a minor papillary muscle dysfunction. The systolic murmur is often accompanied by a click or snapping sound. A variety of physical or physiologic maneuvers, exercising the patient, or administration of drugs may alter the intensity and timing of the murmurs and clicks. This type of murmur is described in greater detail on page 810.

The systolic musical honking or whooping sound appears to have a somewhat similar origin, as indicated above. Such sounds are frequently associated with clicks. Honking noises may at times be produced by transvenous pacemaker catheters situated across the tricuspid valve.

A mixture of factors may be operating in one patient, and the underlying hemodynamics must be fairly understood in order to interpret the clinical findings. A good example of this is hypertrophic obstructive cardiomyopathy, which is associated with obstruction of the outflow tract of the left ventricle and mitral regurgitation. As this condition develops in childhood, there is diminished compliance in the hypertrophied muscle of the left ventricle and this produces a prominent A wave and eventually an audible atrial gallop sound. The developing hemodynamic and pathologic problem appears to be an eccentric hypertrophy of the septum, which is progressive and at the same time is associated with an abnormal contraction of the papillary muscles that leads to an anterior displacement of the anterior leaflet in the mitral valve. Thus, during systole there is an initial period in which there is no significant obstruction of the outflow tract of the left ventricle, but with the progression of contraction of ventricle the septum deviates and bulges to the left; thus the anterior leaflet in the mitral valve is in apposition with it, producing obstruction to the outflow tract. Initially there is an ejection systolic murmur without a gradient. However, as contraction proceeds, a gradient develops in the outflow tract and a second murmur of mitral regurgitation occurs.

In summary, there is an early rapid ejection period followed by rapid upstroke of the carotid pressure tracing, and a flow murmur occurs in early systole. Thereafter a significant pressure gradient develops with the flow diminishing through the obstructive outflow tract as it narrows. This period is followed by a late systolic murmur due to mitral regurgitation. In diastole there is an atrial diastolic gallop associated with the development of decreased compliance of the left ventricle.

If there is a distention or increased volume of the left ventricle, the muscular obstruction of the outflow tract may be diminished and thus alter the murmurs. Such agents as digitalis and isoproterenol (Isuprel) increase the obstruction, and beta-adrenergic blocking agents decrease the obstruction. The straining phase of the valsalva maneuver decreases the diastolic volume and therefore increases the obstruction. Vasopressor agents may diminish the intensity of the murmur by increasing the afterload. The intensity of the murmur parallels the gradient, getting louder with more severe obstruction and fainter with diminution of the gradient.

Diastolic Murmurs

Diastolic murmurs in childhood are commonly produced by increased flow across the tricuspid or mitral valve or due to a regurgitant valve, either pulmonary or aortic. Only occasionally does one run into narrowing or obstruction of the AV valves producing a diastolic murmur as in mitral stenosis. The following list covers the majority of diastolic murmurs heard in the childhood age group: pulmonary regurgitation, aortic regurgitation, increased flow across the tricuspid valves, atrial septal defect, tricuspid regurgitation, Ebstein's disease, hyperthyroidism, anemia, increased flow across the mitral valve, patent ductus arteriosus, ventricular septal defect, mitral stenosis (congenital or acquired), tricuspid stenosis (congenital or acquired).

Aortic Valve Regurgitation. As is well recognized, the murmur of aortic regurgitation is best heard down the left sternal edge using the diaphragm end piece of the stethoscope and it is more easily found at the end of an expiration with the breath held or with the patient sitting up and leaning forward. The murmur begins after the aortic component or the second sound and usually fades away as the first sound is approached. Aortic regurgitation may also produce a diastolic murmur at the apex, referred to as the Austin Flint murmur (1862), which is regarded as due to vibrations of the mitral valve because of aortic regurgitant flow back into the left ventricle and augmented by vibrations caused by atrial systole.

Pulmonary Valve Regurgitation. Pulmonary regurgitation is commonly heard in the postoperative cases who have had total correction of tetralogy of Fallot. The valve opening has been increased by the surgeon to a degree that will allow more adequate pulmonary blood flow, and such regurgitant flow is usually minimal and rarely the cause of symptoms. Pulmonary regurgitation may also occur in Eisenmenger's syndrome, congenital anomalies of the pulmonary valve, and secondary bacterial endocarditis.

Increased Flow Across Tricuspid Valve. In the presence of an atrial septal defect or the shunt from the left atrium to the right, a flow through the tricuspid valve may be two or three times that through the mitral valve. The right ventricle is enlarged, and at the onset of diastole there is a rush of blood into the enlarged ventricle that frequently causes a diastolic murmur. A similar murmur may be heard in tricuspid regurgitation to the overloading of the right atrium. It is also heard in Ebstein's disease, hyperthyroidism, and anemia.

In the presence of a left-to-right shunt at the aortic level or the ventricular septal level there is increased flow across the mitral valve, which produces an inflow diastolic murmur and usually indicates that a considerable shunt is present.

Atrial Ventricular Valve Narrowing or Stenosis. The diastolic murmur of mitral stenosis is due to the blood propelled through the stenotic orifice of the valve. Part of the murmur may be similar to the one described above as an inflow diastolic and occurs early in diastole; the other is associated with atrial systole and is often referred to as presystolic. This latter murmur produced is the characteristic presystolic crescendo effect. In the presence of atrial fibrillation the presystolic portion of the murmur disappears and only the middiastolic murmur persists.

Continuous Murmurs

It is generally agreed that the term *continuous murmurs* refers to murmurs beginning in systole and going into diastole. The murmur need not be through the entire heart cycle in order to qualify for this definition. The majority of continuous murmurs would be included in the following list: patent ductus arteriosus, Blalock-Tausig shunt or similar surgical procedure, arteriovenous aneurysm, large collaterals to pulmonary artery from bronchial arteries, aortic septal defect, coronary artery aneurysm or fistula, total anomalous pulmonary venous return, communication of aneurysm of aortic sinus with pulmonary artery right atrium or right ventricle, traumatic arteriovenous fistula in thorax, congenital arteriovenous fistula in chest wall, anomalous coronary artery entering the pulmonary artery, coarctation of pulmonary artery, dissecting aneurysm of aorta with fistula communication into right atrium, and venous hum.

The classic type of continuous murmur is that heard with a persistent ductus arteriosus. In this condition the murmur characteristically begins just after the first sound, reaches its peak with the rise of aortic pressure, and subsides during diastole but may go right on to the next first heart sound, depending on the pressure gradient between the aorta and the pulmonary artery. If the pressure in the pulmonary artery rises, it may shorten the diastolic element of the murmur; if the pressure in the pulmonary artery equals that in the aorta, the murmur may disappear entirely or simply be heard as a short systolic murmur (see page 426).

A similar murmur is heard in the presence of a Blalock-Taussig shunt, a Potts' operation, or a Waterston operation and is due to the same cause.

In the newborn baby because of the high pulmonary artery pressure a faint murmur or no murmur at all may be present and the murmur may become continuous as the pressure in the pulmonary artery falls. The murmur disappears as the ductus closes. At times a somewhat similar murmur may be heard from large collaterals from the bronchial arteries to the pulmonary arteries. When there is an anomalous coronary artery entering the pulmonary artery, the murmur is usually absent but when present it is fainter than that heard in the patent ductus arteriosus. A coronary artery aneurysm or fistula may give a continuous murmur, but this is usually heard louder over the lower precordium than in the pulmonary area and at times it may appear to be almost inside the stethoscope. The murmur of congenital arteriovenous fistula in the chest wall may be similar.

Narrowing in coarctation of the pulmonary artery may give a continuous murmur, but such a murmur is more likely to be distributed out into the chest and is softer than the patent ductus arteriosus since the narrowing of the pulmonary artery is usually not extreme.

A venous hum may be heard over the upper precordium in many normal children due to flow of blood into large collecting veins at the entrance to the right atrium. Such murmurs are often heard above or below the right or left clavicles. They may vary with respiration and can often be obliterated or diminished by turning the head to one side or the other.

The murmur of coarctation of the aorta is rarely heard as a continuous murmur. It is recognized as a systolic murmur, usually in the pulmonary area referred through to the back, where it is identified with a stethoscope as being a systolic murmur. In spite of the stethoscope impression a sound tracing may show that it proceeds into early diastole.

Functional Heart Murmurs

The improved forms of therapy now available for children with either congenital or acquired heart disease make it increasingly important to differentiate between significant and nonsignificant heart murmurs. Furthermore, when there is a functional heart murmur, the physician must eliminate from the mind of the parent any doubt about its significance and avoid unnecessary limitation of the child's activity. An occasional child has been labeled a cardiac cripple in the presence of a perfectly normal heart.

Approximately half of normal children have a systolic murmur of some degree in some portion of the precordium (Thayer, 1925; Gibson, 1946; Friedman et al., 1949). Most functional benign murmurs in childhood can be recognized by several criteria: (1) the relatively low intensity of the murmur; (2) the fact that it is frequently limited to a small area; (3) its short duration; (4) the presence of a coarse vibratory quality in many instances; (5) the absence of other evidence of heart disease.

Short slight systolic murmurs appearing with tachycardia and disappearing when the heart rate slows to normal are obviously functional in origin. Such murmurs may appear with fever, nervousness, exercise, and infection and disappear during the resting state. These murmurs are usually recognized readily by the physician and properly categorized. Murmurs that disappear with inspiration are usually functional in origin.

There are two common types of functional murmurs that are more likely than others to cause difficulty in diagnosis in infancy and childhood. One is the so-called venous hum, best heard over the aortic area and up into the vessels of the neck; it may also, on occasion, be heard in the pulmonary area. This murmur is continuous, and, since it varies in intensity, it often simulates the murmur of a patent ductus arteriosus. However, its maximum position is usually in the aortic area. This and its softness and lack of the machinery-like quality all help to distinguish it from the patent ductus. Furthermore, it has a diastolic accentuation rather than the systolic accentuation that is characteristic of the patent doctus. It is slightly louder with inspiration (Groom et al., 1955). The venous hum appears to have its origin in the jugular vein as it joins the subclavian. It is more readily heard with the patient sitting up and with the head slightly extended or turned to the left than it is with the patient lying down and the head flexed. Pressure on the jugular vein will diminish or eliminate the murmur entirely.

The venous hum has been recognized for over 100 years. Hope identified it clearly in 1842. Graf and associates (1947), more recently, found a venous hum in 50 percent of children under the age of nine years and in 30 percent between 12 and 15 years of age.

The second type of functional murmur that may be a problem in childhood is one over the lower precordium between the apex and the sternum. It is coarse, low-pitched, and has been described as a vibratory or twanging string-type murmur. It may at times encroach on the mitral area, thus suggesting the possibility of rheumatic origin. However, it is best heard to the right of the apex and not over it. It is shorter in duration than the murmur of mitral insufficiency and has a coarser scratchy quality. It usually has a frequency of 130 cycles per second, whereas the murmur of mitral insufficiency is commonly at least double that or more. The softened first sound that is commonly heard in rheumatic heart disease in childhood may also occur with this functional type of murmur. However, the functional murmur is not transmitted to the axilla. Marienfeld and associates (1962) reported a 20-year follow-up on "innocent" murmurs and have confirmed the impression that the low-frequency vibratory murmur of childhood is indeed innocuous.

REFERENCES

Abbott, M. E. S.: History of medicine in the Province of Quebec. McGill University, 89, 38, 1931.

Argano, B., and Luisada, A. A.: The sound of the heart: innocent diastolic murmurs. *Chest*, **59**:443, 1971.

Bacon, A. P. C., and Matthews, M. B.: Congenital bicuspid aortic valves and the aetiology of isolated valvular stenosis. *Q. J. Med.*, **28**:545, 1959.

Baker, C., and Somerville, J.: Results of surgical treatment of aortic stenosis. *Br. Med. J.*, **1**:197, 1964.

Baum, D.; Khoury, G. H.; Ongley, P. A.; et al.: Congenital stenosis of the pulmonary artery branches. *Circulation*, **29**:680, 1964.

Benchimol, A.; Barreto, E. C.; and Gartlan, J. L.: Right atrial flow in patients with atrial septal defect. *Am. J. Cardiol.*, **25**:381, 1970.

Berggraf, G. W., and Craig, E.: The first heart sound in complete heart block: phono-echocardiographic correlations. *Circulation*, **50**:17, 1974.

Bigler, J. A.: Interpretation of heart murmurs. *Pediatr. Clin. North Am.*, **2**:441, 1955.

Bittar, N., and Sosa, J. A.: The billowing mitral valve leaflet: report on fourteen patients. *Circulation*, **38**:763, 1968.

Bland, E. J.; Jones, T. D.; and White, P. D.: The development of mitral stenosis in young people with a discussion of the frequent misinterpretation of a mild-diastolic murmur at the cardiac apex. *Am. Heart J.*, **10**:995, 1935.

Bonham-Carter, R. E., and Walker, C. H. M.: Continuous murmurs without patent ductus arteriosus. *Lancet*, **1**:272, 1955.

Braudo, M., and Rowe, R. D.: Auscultation of the heart—early neonatal period. *Am. J. Dis. Child.*, **101**:575, 1961.

Brigden, W., and Leatham, A.: Mitral incompetence. *Br. Heart J.*, **15**:55, 1953.

Brock, R.: Functional obstruction of the left ventricle (acquired aortic subvalvular stenosis). *Guys Hosp. Rep.*, **106**:221, 1957.

Burch, G. E.; DePasquale, N. P.; and Phillips, J. H.: Clinical manifestations of papillary muscle dysfunction. *Arch. Intern. Med.* (Chicago), **112**:112, 1963.

Butterworth, J. S., and Reppert, E. H.: Auscultatory acumen in the general medical population. *JAMA*, **174**:32, 1960.

Campbell, M.: The natural history of congenital aortic stenosis. *Br. Heart J.*, **30**:514, 1968a.

————: Calcific aortic stenosis and congenital bicuspid aortic valves. *Br. Heart J.*, **30**:606, 1968b.

Crevasse, L., and Logue, R. B.: Atypical patent ductus arteriosus. Use of a vasopressor agent as a diagnostic aid. *Circulation*, **19**:332, 1959.

Crews, T. L.; Pridie, R. B.; Benham, R.; and Leatham, A.: Auscultatory and phonocardiographic findings in Ebstein's anomaly: correlation of the first heart sound with ultrasonic records of tricuspid valve movement. *Br. Heart J.*, **34**:681, 1972.

Criley, J. M.; Lewis, K. B.; Humphries, J. O.; et al.: Prolapse of the mitral valve: clinical and cine-angiocardiographic findings. *Br. Heart J.*, **28**:488, 1966.

Currens, J. H.; Thompaon, W. B.; Rappaport, M. B.; and Sprague, H. B.: Clinical and phonocardiographic observations on the Flint murmur. *N. Engl. J. Med.*, **248**:585, 1963.

Daty, K. K., and Sen, P. K.: Incomplete aortic vascular rings. *Br. J. Surg.*, **44**:175, 1956.

Delaney, T. B., and Nadas, A. S.: Peripheral pulmonary stenosis. *Am. J. Cardiol.*, **13**:451, 1961.

DeLeon, A. C. Jr.; Perloff, J. K.; Twigg, H.; et al.: The straight-back syndrome: clinical cardiovascular manifestations. *Circulation*, **32**:193, 1965.

Dock, W.: Mode of production of the first heart sound, *Arch. Intern. Med.*, **51**:737, 1933.

Dock, W.; Grandell, F.; and Taubman, F.: The physiologic third heart sound: its mechanism and relation to protodiastolic gallop. *Am. Heart J.* **50**:449, 1955.

Dunn, F. L., and Dickerson, W. J.: Third heart sound: possible role of pericardium in its production. *Circ. Res.*, **3**:51, 1955.

Edwards, J. E.: Mitral insufficiency resulting from "overshooting" of leaflets. *Circulation*, **43**:606, 1971.

Evans, W., and Lian, C.: Use of phonocardiograph in clinical cardiology. *Br. Heart J.*, **10**:92, 1948.

Evans, J. R.; Rowe, R. D.; Downie, H. G.; and Rowsell, H. C.: Murmurs arising from ductus arteriosus in normal newborn swine. *Circ. Res.*, **12**:85, 1962.

Feigen, L. P.: Physical characteristics of sound and hearing. *Am. J. Cardiol.*, **28**:130, 1971.

Feruglio, G. A.: A new method for producing, calibrating, and recording intracardiac sounds in man. *Am. Heart J.*, **65**:377, 1963.

Feruglio, G. A., and Gunton, R. W.: Intracardiac phonocardiography in ventricular septal defect. *Circulation*, **21**:49, 1960.

Feruglio, G. A., and Screenivasan, A.: Intracardiac phonocardiogram in 30 cases of atrial septal defect. *Circulation*, **20**:1087, 1959.

Freeman, A. R., and Levine, S. A.: Clinical significance of systolic murmur: study of 1,000 consecutive "non-cardiac" cases. *Ann. Intern. Med.*, **6**:1371, 1933.

Friedman, S.; Robie, W. A.; and Harris, T. N.: Occurrence of innocent adventitious cardiac sounds in childhood. *Pediatrics*, **3**:782, 1949.

Gasul, B.; Archilla, R. A.; Fell, E.; et al.: Congenital coronary arteriovenous fistula. *Pediatrics*, **25**:936, 1961.

Gibson, G. A.: Lecture on patent ductus arteriosus. *Edinburgh Med. J.*, **8**:1, 1900.

Gibson, S.: Clinical significance of heart murmurs in children. *Med. Clin. North Am.*, **30**:35, 1946.

Goodwin, J. F.: Disorders of the outflow tract of the left ventricle. *Brit. Med. J.*, **2**:461, 1967.

Graf, W.; Möller, T.; and Mannheimer, E.: Continuous murmur; incidence and characteristics in different parts of human body. *Acta. Med. Scand.*, suppl. **196**:167, 1947.

Groom, D., and Boone, J. A.: The "dove-coo" murmur and murmurs heard at a distance from the chest wall. *Ann. Intern. Med.*, **42**:1214, 1955.

Groom, D.; Boone, J. A.; and Jenkins, M.: Venous hum in cardiac auscultation. *JAMA*, **159**:639, 1955.

Gunn, A. L., and Wood, M. C.: The amplification and recording of fetal heart sounds. *Proc. Roy. Soc. Med.*, **46**:85, 1953.

Haber, E., and Leatham, A.: Splitting of heart sounds from ventricular asynchrony in bundle branch block, ventricular ectopic beats, and artificial pacing. *Br. Heart J.*, **27**:691, 1965.

Harris, A., and Sutton, G.: Second heart sound in normal subjects. *Br. Heart J.*, **30**:739, 1968.

Harris, C.; Wise, J., Jr.; and Oakley, C. M.: 'Fixed' splitting of the second heart sound in ventricular septal defect. *Br. Heart J.*, **33**:428, 1971.

Harris, T. N., and Friedman, S.: Phonocardiographic differentiation of vibratory (functional) murmurs from those of valvular

insufficiency: further observations and application to the diagnosis of rheumatic heart disease. *Am. Heart J.*, **43**:707, 1952.

Hohn, A. R.; Van Praagh, S.; Moore, A. A. D.; Vlad, P.; and Lambert, E. C.: Aortic stenosis. *Circulation*, **32**:4, 1965.

Hope, J.: *A Treatise on the Diseases of the Heart and Great Vessels*, 3rd ed. (London). Haswell and Johnson, Philadelphia, 1842.

Hultgren, H. N.; Hubis, H.; and Shumway, N.: Cardiac function following prosthetic aortic valve replacement. *Am. Heart J.*, **77**:585, 1969.

Hunt, D., and Sloman, G.: Prolapse of the posterior leaflet of the mitral valve occurring in eleven members of a family. *Am. Heart J.*, **78**:149, 1969.

Hutchins, G. M., and Maron, B. J.: Development of endocardial valvuloids with valvular insufficiency. *Arch. Pathol.*, **93**:401, 1972.

Johnston, F. D.: Symposium on cardiovascular sound. *Circulation*, **16**:270, 1957.

Keith, J. D.: Variations in first heart sound and auriculo-ventricular conduction time in children with rheumatic fever. *Arch. Dis. Child.*, **12**:217, 1937.

Kincaid-Smith, P., and Barlow, J. B.: The atrial sound and atrial component of the first heart sound. *Br. Heart J.*, **21**:470, 1959.

Kisch, B.: Heart sounds in tachycardia. *Trans. Am. Coll. Cardiol.*, **2**:232, 1952.

Lakier, J. B.; Fritz, V. U.; Pocock, W. A.; and Barlow, J. B.: Mitral component of the first heart sound. *Br. Heart J.*, **34**:160, 1972.

Kumar, S., and Luisada, A. A.: The second heart sound in atrial septal defect. *Am. J. Cardiol.*, **28**:168, 1971.

Lakier, J. B.; Bloom, J. R.; Pocock, W. A.; and Barlow, J. B.: Tricuspid component of first heart sound. *Br. Heart J.*, **35**:1275, 1973.

Landulfo, J.: A new and original interpretation of the genesis of the "innocent" and the "functional" systolic murmurs. *Arq. bras. Cardiol.*, **25**:205, 1972.

Leatham, A.: Splitting of the first and second heart sounds. *Lancet*, **2**:607, 1954.

————: Auscultation of the heart. *Lancet*, **2**:703, 1958.

— — —: *Auscultation of the Heart and Phonocardiography*. J. & A. Churchill, London, 1970.

Leatham, A., and Segal, B.: Auscultatory and phonocardiographic signs in ventricular septal defect with left to right shunt. *Circulation*, **25**:318, 1962.

Leatham, A., and Vogelpoel, L.: The early systolic sound in dilatation of the pulmonary artery. *Br. Heart J.*, **16**:21, 1954.

Leis, T., and Grant, R. T.: Material relating to coarctation of the aorta of the adult type. *Heart*, **16**:205, 1933.

Leon, D. F., and Shaver, J. A.: *Physiologic Principles of Heart Sounds and Murmurs*. American Heart Association Monograph No. 46. The American Heart Association, Inc., New York, 1975.

Leon, D. F.; Thompson, M. E.; et al.: Hemodynamic effects of practolol at rest and during exercise. *Circulation*, **34**:46, 1972.

Lin, T. K., and Dimond, E. G.: Reliability of the grading of cardiac murmurs. *Gen. Pract.*, **8**:55, 1953.

Luisada, A.: The diastolic sounds of the heart in normal and pathological conditions. *Acta Med Scand*, **142**:685, 1952.

— — —: *The Heart Beat, Graphic Methods in the Study of the Cardiac Patient*. Paul B. Hoeber, Inc., New York, 1953.

— — —: Cardiovascular sound. *Am. J. Cardiol.*, **28**:140, 1971.

— — —: The second heart sound in normal and abnormal conditions. *Am. J. Cardiol.*, **28**:150, 1971b.

Luisada, A. A., and Aravanis, C.: Phonocardiography as a clinical method of examination. *Med. Clin. North Am.*, **41**:235, 1957.

Luisada, A. A., and Cortis, B.: The dynamic events of the normal heart in man. *Acta. Cardiol.*, **25**:203, 1970.

Luisada, A. A., and Dayem, M. D. A.: Functional diastolic murmurs. *Am. Heart J.*, **81**:265, 1972.

Luisada, A. A.; MacCanon, D. M.; et al.: New studies on the first heart sound. *Am. J. Cardiol.*, **28**:140, 1971.

Luisada, A. A., and MacCanon, D. M.: The phases of the cardiac cycle. *Am. Heart J.*, **83**:705, 1972.

Lynxwiler, C. P., and Donahoe, J. L.: Evaluation of innocent heart murmurs. *South. Med. J.*, **48**:164, 1955.

McKusick, V. A.; Murray, G. E.; Peeler, R. G.; and Webb, G. N.: Musical murmurs. *Bull. Hopkins Hosp.*, **97**:136, 1955.

McKusick, V. A.; Webb, G. N.; Humphries, J. O'N.; and Reid, J. A.: On cardiovascular sound. Further observations by means of spectral phonocardiography. *Circulation*, **11**:849, 1955.

Margolies, A., and Wolferth, C. C.: Opening snap in mitral stenosis:

its characteristics, mechanism of production and diagnostic importance. *Am. Heart J.*, 7:443, 1932.

Marienfeld, C. J.; Telles, N.; Silbera, J.; and Nordsieck, M.: A 20-year follow-up study of "innocent" murmurs. *Pediatrics*, 30:42, 1962.

Messer, A. L.; Counihan, T. B.; Rappaport, M. B.; and Sprague, H. B.: The effect of cycle length on the time of occurrence of the first heart sound and the opening snap in mitral stenosis. *Circulation*, 4:576, 1951.

Minhas, K., and Gasul, B. M.: Systolic clicks: A clinical, phonocardiographic, and hemodynamic evaluation. *Am. Heart J.*, 57:49, 1959.

Nadas, A. S., and Alimurung, M. M.: Apical diastolic murmurs in congenital heart disease. *Am. Heart J.*, 43:691, 1952.

Oakley, C. M.; Raftery, E. B.; Brockington, I. F.; et al.: Relation of hypertrophic obstructive cardiomyopathy to subvalvular mitral incompetence. *Br. Heart J.*, 29:629, 1967.

Ongley, P. A.; Sprague, H. B.; and Rappaport, E. E.: The diastolic murmur of mitral stenosis. *N. Engl. J. Med.*, 253:1049, 1955.

Orias, O., and Braun-Menendez, E.: *The Heart-Sounds in Normal and Pathological Conditions.* Oxford University Press, London, 1939.

Osler, W.: The bicuspid condition of the aortic valves. *Trans. Assoc. Am. Physicians*, 1:185, 1886.

Paget, J.: On obstruction of the branches of the pulmonary artery. *Med. Chir. Trans.*, 27:162, 1844.

Peacock, T. B.: On malformations of the aortic valves as a cause of disease. A paper from the *Monthly Journal of Medical Science* bound in the Royal Society of Medicine, London, as "Peacock on the Brain, Heart, etc." (1853).

———: On some of the causes and effects of valvular disease of the heart. Croonian Lectures, Churchill, London, 1865.

———: Very great contraction of the aortic orifice from disease of the valves. *Trans. Pathol. Soc. Lond.*, 19:163, 1868.

Perloff, J. K.: Clinical recognition of aortic stenosis. The physical signs and differential diagnosis of the various forms of obstruction to left ventricular outflow. *Prog. Cardiovasc. Dis.* 10:323, 1968.

Pieroni, D. R.; Bell, B. B.; Krovetz, L. J.; Varghese, P. J.; and Rowe, R. D.: Auscultatory recognition of aneurysm of the membranous septum associated with a small ventricular septal defect. *Circulation*, 44:733, 1971.

Pomerance, A.: Ballooning deformity (mucoid degeneration) of atrioventricular valves. *Br. Heart J.*, 31:343, 1969.

Rappaport, M. B., and Sprague, H. B.: The graphic registration of the normal heart sounds. *Am. Heart J.*, 23:591, 1942.

Ravin, A., and Bershof, E.: The intensity of the first heart sound in auricular fibrillation with mitral stenosis. *Am. Heart J.*, 41:539, 1951.

Rawlings, M. S.: The "straight-back" syndrome, a new cause of pseudoheart disease. *Am. J. Cardiol.*, 5:333, 1960.

Reddy, R. C.; Fould, L.; and Gamprecht, R. F.: Use of earophonium (tensilon) in the evaluation of cardiac arrythmias. *Am. Heart J.*, 82:742, 1971.

Reid, J. V. O.: Mid-systolic clicks. *S. Afr. Med. J.*, 35:353, 1961.

Reinhold, J. D., and Nadas, A. S.: The role of auscultation in the diagnosis and differential heart disease; a phonocardiographic study of children. *Am. Heart J.*, 47:405, 1954.

Rizzon, P.; Biasco, G.; and Maselli-Campagna, G.: The praecordial honk. *Br. Heart J.*, 33:707, 1971.

Ronan, J. A.; Perloff, J. K.; and Harvey, W. P.: Systolic clicks and the late systolic murmur; intracardiac phonocardiographic evidence of their mitral valve origin. *Am. Heart J.*, 70:319, 1965.

Rushmer, R. F. et al.: Variability in detection and interpretation of heart murmurs. *Am. J. Dis. Child.*, 83:740, 1952.

Rushmer, R. F.; Bark, R. S.; and Ellis, R. M.: Direct-writing heart-sound recorder. *Am. J. Dis. Child.*, 83:733, 1952.

Sakakibara, S.; Yokoyama, M.; et al.: Coronary arteriovenous fistula. *Am. Heart J.*, 72:307, 1966.

Sakamoto, T.; Kusukawa, R.; MacCannon, D. M.; et al.: Hemodynamic determinants of the amplitude of the first heart sound. *Circ. Res.*, 16:45, 1965.

Sears, G. A.; Movafagh, P.; and Manning, G. W.: Intracardiac phonocardiology in ventricular septal defect. *Am. J. Med. Sci.*, 243:775, 1962.

Segall, H.: Notes and events. *J. Hist. Med. Allied Sci.*, 22:414, 1967.

Shah, P. M., and Gramiak, R.: Echo-cardiographic recognition of mitral valve prolapse. *Circulation*, 41–42:III–45, 1970.

Shaver, J. A.; Nadolny, R. A.; O'Toole, J. D.; et al.: Sound pressure correlates of the second heart sound: an intracardiac sound study. *Circulation*, 49:316, 1974.

Shell, W. C.; Walton, J. A.; Clifford, M. E.; and Willis, P. W.: The familial occurrence of the syndrome of mid-late systolic clicks and late systolic murmur. *Circulation*, 39:327, 1969.

Sloan, A. W.; Campbell, F. W.; and Henderson, A. S.: Incidence of the physiological third heart sound. *Br. Med. J.*, 2:853, 1952.

Sloan, A. W., and Wishart, M.: The effect on the human third heart sound of variations in the rate of filling of the heart. *Br. Heart J.*, 15:25, 1953.

Smith, D. E., and Matthews, M. B.: Aortic valvular stenosis with coarctation of the aorta; with special reference to the development of aortic stenosis upon congenital bicuspid valves. *Br. Heart J.*, 17:198, 1955.

Spencer, M. P.; Johnston, F. R.; and Meredith, J. H.: The murmur in coarctation. *Am. Heart J.*, 56:722, 1956.

Steel, G.: The murmur of high pressure in the pulmonary artery. *Med. Chron.*, 9:182, 1888.

Sutton, G.; Harris, A.; and Leatham, A.: Second heart sound in pulmonary hypertension. *Br. Heart J.*, 30:743, 1968.

Taylor, W. C.: The incidence and significance of systolic cardiac murmurs in infants. *Arch. Dis. Child.*, 28:52, 1953.

Teare, D.: Asymmetrical hypertrophy of the heart in young adults. *Br. Heart J.*, 20:1, 1958.

Thayer, W. S.: Interpretation of systolic cardiac murmurs. *Am. J. Med. Sci.*, 169:313, 1925.

Ueda, H.; Sakamoto, T.; et al.: "Silent mitral stenosis. Patho-anatomical basis of the absence of diastolic rumble". *Jap. Heart J.*, 6:206, 1965a.

———: The Austin Flint murmur. Phonocardiographic and patho-anatomical study. *Jap. Heart J.*, 6:294, 1965b.

Vogel, J. H., and Blount, S. G.: Clinical evaluation in localizing levels of obstruction to outflow from left ventricle. *Am. J. Cardiol.*, 15:782, 1965.

Wallace, J. D.; Brown, J. R.; Lewis, D. H.; and Deitz, G. W.: Acoustic mapping within the heart. *J. Acoust. Soc. Amer.*, 1:9, 1957.

Waller, B. F., et al.: Bicuspid aortic valve. Comparison of congenital and acquired types. *Circulation*, 48:1140, 1973.

Wauchope, G. M.: The clinical importance of variations in the number of cusps forming the aortic and pulmonary valves. *Qu. J. Med.*, 21:383, 1928.

Wells, B. G.; Rappaport, M. B.; and Sprague, H. B.: The graphic registration of basal diastolic murmurs. *Am. Heart J.*, 37:586, 1949.

Weisse, A. B.; Schwartz, M. L.; et al.: Intensity of the normal second heart sound components in their traditional auscultatory areas. *Am. J. Med.*, 43:171, 1967.

Wigle, E. D., and Labrosse, C. J.: Sudden, severe aortic insufficiency. *Circulation*, 32:708, 1965.

Williams, H. B., and Dodge, A. F.: Analysis of heart sounds. *Arch. Int. Med.*, 38:685, 1926.

Wood, P.: *Diseases of the Heart and Circulation.* J. B. Lippincott Co., Philadelphia, 1956.

Yamakawa, K.; Shionoya, Y.; Kitamura, K.; Nagai, T.; Yamamoto, T.; and Ohta, S.: Intracardiac phonocardiography. *Am. Heart J.*, 47:424, 1954.

Blood Pressure and Hypertension

John D. Keith

BLOOD PRESSURE

BLOOD pressure has been studied by physicians since the time of Steven Hales in 1733. In spite of this, clinical methods of obtaining the pressure level have not yet reached the accuracy of complete reliability. In infants and children particularly, there is considerable difference of opinion as to what constitutes the best method of making these measurements. First let us refer to the mechanisms that maintain the arterial pressure.

Regulation of Blood Pressure

The arterial blood pressure in the human is regulated by a variety of mechanisms, the most important of which is the carotid sinus reflex system. This is mediated through pressure receptors located in the walls of the internal carotid arteries and the aorta. If the arterial pressure increases, the walls of these vessels are stretched and impulses flow to the medullary portion of the brain, where they inhibit the sympathetic nervous system and excite the parasympathetic. This leads to a decrease in the activity of the heart and dilatation of the peripheral arterioles. The action of the parasympathetic nerves further depresses cardiac activity, and blood pressure is reduced. Conversely, if the arterial pressure falls, the number of impulses transmitted to the medulla from the carotid and the aorta becomes reduced and this leads to stimulation of the heart and the peripheral vessels, thereby elevating the pressure. This mechanism is brought into play over a few seconds, resulting in a readjustment of the circulation. Delay in this response may lead to fainting. Neligan (1959) has studied reflex effect on blood pressure of change in position of the newborn infant and finds a modest response after four days of age. Before this there is no obvious response to change in position.

Another important circulatory reflex mechanism is the central nervous system and ischemic response. Guyton (1961) points out that this is not initiated until the blood pressure falls to approximately 20 mm of mercury. It is activated by severe shock, or marked elevation of the cerebrospinal fluid pressure, or a tumor of the brain compressing the vasomotor center. It may also be initiated in the severely cyanotic congenital heart disease cases. It contributes at times to the initial slightly elevated arterial pressure seen in the newborn in the first few minutes of life (Ashworth et al., 1959).

Another mechanism is related to the ability of smooth muscle of veins and arteries to relax or contract depending on the volume they enclose. Thus, if the blood volume increases considerably causing an increase in arterial pressure, the veins and the arteries may stretch over a few minutes until they can accommodate a new blood volume. A major response appears to lie in the veins, which can accommodate to a markedly increased blood volume in 15 to 30 minutes. This mechanism would appear to be active after the cord is tied in a newborn baby as adjustment of excess blood from the placenta takes place. It is probably also a helpful adjustment during the first six hours of life, when Sisson and associates (1959) found an increase in the circulating blood volume.

Another significant mechanism is the ability of the capillaries to shift fluid in and out of the tissues permitting more adequate adjustment to a large blood transfusion or excessive blood loss. A further mechanism that acts more slowly than those referred to above is the hemodynamic response of the kidneys to change the arterial pressure and is dependent on the renal blood flow and pressure with excretion or retention of fluids and salts. The same flow and pressure mechanisms are also affected by active reflexes in the kidney vessels. Finally, hormonal activity alters renal arterial pressure regulations through the release of glomerulotropin from the brains cells, thus affecting the secretion of aldosterone, which in turn acts on the renal tubal epithelium and causes absorption of sodium and retention of water.

Blood Pressure Apparatus

Several specialized types of apparatus have been designed to obtain more accurate blood pressure readings for investigative purposes, particularly in the newborn period. Schaffer (1955) used a plethysmograph beyond the cuff to record arterial pulsations coming through. Rice and Posener (1959) developed a differential optical pulse indicator to achieve the same purpose. Morse and associates (1960) used a microphone under the cuff, and more recently Goodman, Cumming, and Raber (1962) developed a photocell oscillometer for measuring the systolic blood pressure in newborn infants. The readings with this instrument correlated very closely with those obtained with auscultation and by direct intra-arterial blood pressures. A good review of various methods appears in *Problems of Blood Pressure in Childhood* (Moss and Adams, 1962). Recently McLaughlin and associates (1971) have shown that the Doppler gives a very close correlation with interarterial readings.

Blood pressures obtained in the newborn period are shown in Figure 4–1.

A normal, healthy newborn has an average pressure of 80 mm of mercury. This falls to a level between 60 and 65 mm of mercury and then gradually rises over a period of days and weeks until it stabilizes between 90 and 100 mm of mercury at five months. Premature levels are distinctly lower, with mean readings of 40 to 60 mm of mercury. Infants with respiratory distress as a general rule have lower systolic pressure readings during the first three weeks of life, but this is probably more related to their prematurity than to their respiratory distress

syndrome. However, when a respiratory syndrome leads to death, a lower blood pressure is characteristic and appears to be associated with a diffuse diminution in peripheral vascular resistance in both the pulmonary and systemic circulations (Rudolph et al., 1961).

The elevated arterial pressure levels in the early moments of life appear to be due to sympathetic stimulation associated with the trauma of birth. In a difficult delivery there may be the added factor of the ischemic response.

The mercury and the aneroid manometers form the chief instruments for physicians making blood pressure determinations. This part of the apparatus provides satisfactory results as long as the airways are clear and, in the case of the mercury manometer, the zero is correctly adjusted.

The chief sources of error arise in the type and size of cuff used with the manometer. The proper size for different ages is still held in some question, especially for the first year of life. The cuff sizes shown in Figure 4–2 have been used at The Hospital for Sick Children, Toronto, for the past 15 years and have proved satisfactory in giving blood pressure readings that check well with direct readings obtained at cardiac catheterization. The widths of blood pressure cuffs for the various ages are: premature, 3 cm; newborns to two years, 4.5 cm; two to four years, 7 cm; five to nine years, 10 cm; 10 to 14 years, 13 cm; and 15 cm for large children with obese arm and leg. Too small a cuff for the size of the arm gives too high a reading on the manometer.

These cuff sizes conform largely to the standard suggested by the American Heart Association Committee on Blood Pressure, with the exception

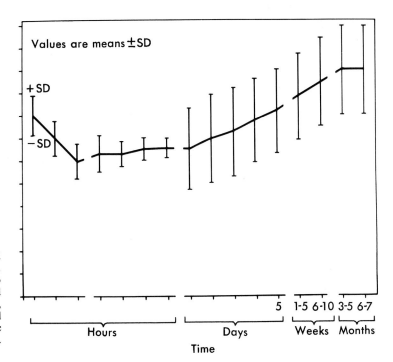

Figure 4-1. Mean systolic blood pressure in the first seven months. The mean is plotted along with two standard deviations. (Reproduced from Goodman, H. G.; Cumming, G. R.; and Raber, M. B.: Photocell oscillometer for measuring systolic pressure in newborn. *Am. J. Dis. Child.*, **103**:152, 1962.)

that we have found that larger cuffs for infants and children under the age of four give more accurate readings. This approach fits closely with that of Park and Guntheroth (1970), who recommend a cuff whose width is 25 percent greater than the diameter of the arm or leg where blood pressure is being taken. Our experience agrees with this. The cuff should fit snugly when applied since a loose fit may give a higher reading (Schaffer, 1955). The inflatable bag should come all of the way around the arm and cover completely the area overlying the artery. An infant or child is best examined in the supine or semisupine position so that he is relaxed and the arm is against a firm background. This allows auscultation of the artery to be carried out with greater ease.

A slight preliminary inflation of the cuff is often given to demonstrate to the child how simple the procedure is. Giving a feeding bottle or a sterile nipple containing cotton soaked in sugar solution is an effective method of keeping the baby quiet and permitting a satisfactory measurement.

Venous engorgement should be avoided since it may cause a failure of the sound to come through to the stethoscope at the proper level and thus yield an

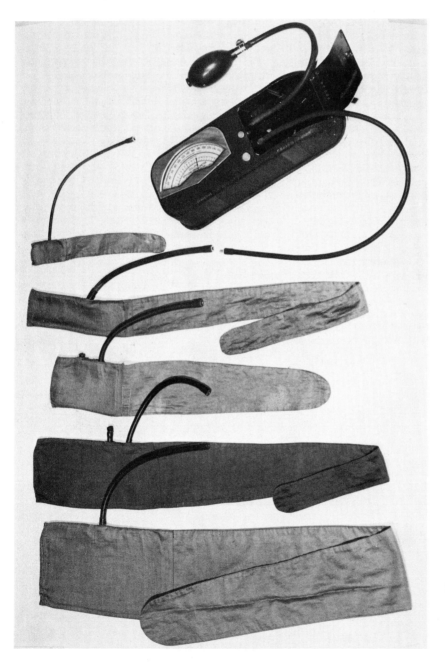

Figure 4-2. Blood pressure cuffs for various ages are shown. Premature, 3 cm; newborns to two years, 4.5 cm; two to four years, 7 cm; five to nine years, 10 cm; 10 to 14 years, 13 cm.

abnormally low reading. It can be avoided by raising the arm for 30 seconds before the cuff is inflated. It is usually better to use the small bell end of a pediatric stethoscope in determining children's blood pressure since this sits satisfactorily on the arm and excludes contact with outside air, permitting more accurate recognition of the Korotkoff sounds.

When the stethoscope is in proper position, the pressure is raised until it is approximately 20 or 30 mm of mercury above the point at which the radial pulse disappears. In a child with a normal pressure this usually means up to about 120 or 130 mm of mercury. Then the pressure is released slowly so that the needle indicates a fall of 2.3 mm per second. As the pressure falls, the Korotkoff sounds become audible over the artery below the cuff.

Blood pressure in the thigh is important in children suspected of having coarctation of the aorta or kinking of the aorta. Common usage over the years has been the application of a cuff on the leg, a size larger than the one used on the arm. The leg pressure should coincide closely with the arm pressure if the appropriate cuff is used. Park and Guntheroth (1970) recommend a cuff 25 percent wider than the diameter of the leg. This is usually easy to achieve in an infant or young child and a correct reading can be obtained. However, in the adolescent and particularly in the obese, an especially large cuff, 14 to 20 cm, may be required.

Methods

With the apparatus described, several methods for determining the blood pressure in children have been in use: (1) auscultation, (2) palpation of the artery, (3) the flush technique, (4) oscillometry, and (5) more complex electrical or mechanical devices that have been elaborated in recent years for use in both infants and older patients, such as the Doppler technique. All these methods are of value and may be used singly or together.

Auscultation. The five phases of sound are closely outlined in the Recommendations for Human Blood Pressure published by the American Heart Association.

Phase I—The period marked by the first appearance of faint, clear tapping sounds that gradually increase in intensity.
Phase II—The period during which a murmur of swishing quality is heard.
Phase III—The period during which sounds are crisper and increase in intensity.
Phase IV—The period marked by the distinct, abrupt muffling of sound so that a soft, blowing quality is heard.
Phase V—The point at which sounds disappear.

When all the sounds have disappeared, the cuff should be deflated completely.

The systolic pressure is that point at which the initial Korotkoff sounds are heard.

Muffling of the sound, or phase IV, is now regarded as the best index of diastolic pressure (Burton, 1967). Park and Guntheroth (1970) have shown that in children undergoing cardiac catheterization such muffling corresponds very closely with the diastolic pressure recorded by direct needle puncture of the brachial artery.

It is recommended by the committee of the American Heart Association that the pressure, when there is any doubt about the diastolic pressure, should be recorded as 100/80–70, the 80 referring to phase IV and the 70 to phase V when the sound disappears completely.

Palpation. With the finger on the artery just below the cuff, or at the wrist, the pressure is raised in the cuff until the pulse disappears. Then the pressure is lowered again until the pulse is felt once more. This is taken as the systolic pressure. It is not a particularly useful method in infants and children (since the pulse may be difficult to feel in either the arm or the leg in babies) and does not give a diastolic pressure. The systolic reading that is obtained is considerably lower than the true reading by direct arterial puncture (Van Bergen et al., 1954).

The Flush Technique. This method, introduced to pediatrics in 1952 by Goldring and Wohltmann, consists of placing a cuff suitable for the size and age of the child around the forearm or calf of the leg. The baby's arm is elevated and the hand grasped firmly by the examining physician so that as large an area as possible is blanched. The pressure should be sufficient for blanching but not sufficient to make the baby cry. This pressure is maintained while the cuff pressure is elevated. The cuff is slowly deflated, with the hand closely observed for signs of flushing. The point at which the flush first appears in the blanched area is taken as the blood pressure.

The chief value of this method lies in the fact that one may show the pressure differential between the arm and the leg in coarctation of the aorta. However, the method has several disadvantages: (1) It may be difficult to recognize the first sign of flushing, especially in cyanotic babies. (2) The pressure reading may vary with the rapidity with which the cuff is deflated. (3) The pressure reading obtained is more likely to be a mean pressure than a true systolic one (Moss and Adams, 1964). (4) In coarctation of the aorta, where the pressure in the arm and the leg is somewhat similar, it may be difficult to show minor differences by this technique, especially when failure is present in the young infant.

Oscillometry. With this method the pressure changes are transmitted through the arterial wall to the pressure cuff and thence to the oscillometer, where they are magnified to the observer. The oscillometer is simply a portion of the aneroid pressure indicator. The oscillations may be visualized by pressing a button at the appropriate time.

In small children using the proper size of cuff the Korotkoff sounds may be weak or inaudible. In such cases an oscillometer may help to identify when the sounds should begin to appear. It does not give as accurate an appraisal as the clear recognition of sounds with a stethoscope but with practice may be of help at times. A better way of determining blood pressure in small children is with the ultrasound Doppler technique.

Doppler Ultrasound Technique. Steinfeld and coworkers (1974) have demonstrated that for more accurate blood pressure measurements some modifications in the traditional procedure are required. They stress the need for a pneumatic bladder in the cuff that completely encircles the arm and has a minimum width-to-length ratio of 1 to 3, with an option for greater width-to-length ratio when circumstances demand it. They also recommend a greater variety in cuffs. For example, the conically shaped arm or leg, they believe, is inadequately served by the rectangular configuration of the traditional bladder and should be replaced by one that, when applied to the limb, will conform more closely to the natural contours.

Using a Doppler ultrasound transducer and sensing with a crystal microphone, the frequency analyses of the signals obtained have shown that the arterial wall oscillations cause the major components of the Korotkoff sounds. The first arterial wall oscillations begin at the moment the intrabladder pressure drops below peak intravascular pressure and terminates when the intrabladder pressure dips below the end-diastolic pressure.

They point out that the arterial wall normally gives rise to sounds detectable with a stethoscope, but at times they are not discernible because of the frequency or amplitude or both. Pediatricians frequently experience this problem in dealing with children of various ages and sizes.

Steinfeld and associates (1974) note that a suitably filtered and properly positioned Doppler ultrasound transducer is far more sensitive in directly detecting arterial wall oscillations than a stethoscope, which indirectly identifies the vibrations.

Using a pneumatic cuff bladder assembly made of heat-sealable polyolefin film, coupled with a relatively inexpensive Doppler ultrasound system, they have obtained measurements of blood pressures in infants, children, and obese adults that are more accurate than those obtained by the traditional methods.

Blood Pressure Readings at Various Ages

For general use for infants and children, a blood pressure apparatus with a mercury manometer attached is a practical instrument since it permits one to use whichever of the methods listed is most suitable for the patient concerned. The Doppler ultrasound technique is the most accurate method for infants and small children.

The determination of the blood pressure in infants and children is not as constantly useful a procedure as it is in adults; yet it has specific significance in a few conditions and is helpful in others. It therefore should always be part of the routine examination of the heart and circulation in this age group. Its chief clinical application is in coarctation of the aorta, but it is also useful in aortic insufficiency, aortic stenosis, patent ductus arteriosus, poliomyelitis, acute and chronic nephritis and essential hypertension, pheochromocytoma, head injuries, and brain tumor. Occasionally, it is helpful in vasovagal fainting attacks, shock, or myocarditis.

Woodbury and associates (1938) have obtained a few blood pressure readings on the fetus from five months to term. As would be expected, these have been lower than the pressures recorded at birth. Ashworth and coworkers (1959) found that the mean systolic pressure was elevated at birth but declined again over a period of two to three hours.

Allen-Williams (1945) and Graham and associates (1945) have presented useful data on blood pressure

Table 4-1. SYSTOLIC BLOOD PRESSURES ACCORDING TO AGE DATA BASED ON READINGS OF 795 BOYS AND 798 GIRLS*

AGE	NO. OF PTS.		MEAN		STANDARD DEVIATION		80% RANGE		90% RANGE	
	Boys	*Girls*	*Boys*	*Girls*	*Boys*	*Girls*	*Boys*	*Girls*	*Boys*	*Girls*
3	60	60	99	99	10.1	11.0	88–111	85–114	83–114	83–120
4	79	65	98	98	8.5	9.7	88–110	89–113	85–114	83–114
5	90	80	101	102	9.6	10.1	88–133	90–115	83–115	84–119
6	89	81	105	105	10.5	11.0	93–122	93–120	91–124	91–125
7	77	81	106	107	9.8	10.9	93–118	95–122	91–122	92–125
8	61	70	108	108	10.6	10.3	94–123	97–124	91–125	94–127
9	61	69	111	112	11.3	9.9	91–126	88–125	94–130	94–129
10	53	68	114	114	10.3	11.3	102–128	97–129	95–133	91–134
11	53	61	114	121	11.1	12.2	101–130	106–141	98–134	103–143
12	51	58	116	117	10.3	11.9	103–128	104–134	100–133	101–136
13	47	50	120	121	11.6	12.1	103–140	105–135	97–144	101–141
12	41	33	120	119	10.3	12.0	108–133	102–136	105–135	93–138
15	33	22	125	115	9.8	11.0	113–138	106–134	112–142	103–140
Total	795	798								

Table 4-1. DIASTOLIC BLOOD PRESSURES ACCORDING TO AGE DATA BASED ON READINGS OF 795 BOYS AND 798 GIRLS* (Cont.)

AGE	NO. OF PTS.		MEAN		STANDARD DEVIATION		80% RANGE		90% RANGE	
	Boys	Girls	Boys	Girls	Boys	Girls	Boys	Girls	Boys	Girls
3	60	60	57	58	14.2	10.9	44–75	45–74	37–80	41–77
4	79	65	57	60	9.6	10.2	42–69	45–73	40–71	41–76
5	90	80	60	60	10.2	9.2	48–74	50–73	43–75	43–75
6	89	81	60	64	10.1	92.	47–74	45–74	42–79	44–78
7	77	81	63	63	9.4	9.5	46–74	51–76	45–77	46–79
8	61	70	61	65	11.5	8.0	51–74	56–77	43–76	53–79
9	61	69	65	67	9.7	9.5	53–77	58–78	51–79	52–85
10	53	68	66	64	8.6	8.9	56–79	53–75	51–84	51–79
11	53	61	65	69	9.3	8.2	53–75	61–80	51–81	59–90
12	51	58	67	65	7.1	8.0	58–78	54–75	54–81	52–80
13	47	50	65	69	8.4	9.8	55–74	58–83	57–77	53–88
14	41	33	68	67	8.1	9.8	60–78	53–84	53–80	51–86
15	33	22	67	67	8.0	8.3	60–78	60–79	54–82	53–82
Total	795	798								

* Londe, S. M. D.: Blood pressure standards for normal children as determined under office conditions. *Clin. Pediatr.* (*Phila*) 7:401, 1968.

ranges between six months and 15 years of age.

Londe (1968) obtained blood pressure readings in 1473 boys and girls in a pediatric office practice. His data are shown in Table 4–1. The levels are similar to those of Graham and coworkers (1945), but Londe's average blood levels are a little higher as one might expect from an office visit. He also demonstrated the peak level for girls at 11 or 12 years of age, after which the level declined slightly. Moss and Adams (1962) find that boys have blood pressure slightly lower than girls at 11 or 12 years but are a little higher when they reach 16 to 18 years of age.

In the Framingham study, Kannel and colleagues (1971) found that systolic hypertension was more significant than diastolic hypertension when predicting the risk of coronary heart disease in 5127 men and women during a 14 year follow-up study. One might reasonably conclude that in childhood either systolic or diastolic hypertension should be considered sufficiently significant to justify further investigation.

SYSTEMIC HYPERTENSION

SYSTEMIC hypertension is a major problem in human disease but it is more common in adult life than in the pediatric age group. Its recognition in childhood is important since certain forms can be treated successfully when such therapy is required in the first or second decade of life. Furthermore, blood pressure readings carried out at suitable intervals may identify children who are hypertensive-prone. Such individuals may need help early in life.

Incidence

Based on a national health survey of 1962 (Wood et al., 1970), it has been estimated that nearly 20 percent of the adult population in the United States have hypertension or hypertensive heart disease. Master and associates (1950) indicated that the percentage increases in ascending age groups, being 5 percent in young adults, 20 percent in the 40-to-50 age group, and 20 to 30 percent in the 50s.

In childhood, the data are limited. Masland and associates (1956) studying 1795 outpatients, age 12 to 21 years, found that 1.4 percent had a blood pressure of 140/90 mm of mercury or more. Londe (1966) reported that 2.3 percent of 1473 children, age 4 to 15 years, seen as outpatients, had blood pressure readings over the ninety-fifth percentile for their age. It is obvious that the definition of systemic hypertension depends upon what level one regards as the upper limit of normal for the age concerned. Several reports on normal readings have appeared in the literature, and these show substantial agreement with some minor variations when one compares one group with another (Allen-Williams, 1945; Graham et al., 1945; Guntheroth and Nadas, 1955; Moss and Adams, 1962).

Blood Pressure Levels

Normal blood pressure readings for various ages are shown in Figure 4–1 and Table 4–1. If the upper limits of normal are repeatedly exceeded, hypertension is undoubtedly present. In a child who is nervous or anxious because of examination by the physician, the blood pressure may be at or above the upper limits of normal. Repeated blood pressure readings during the office visit will usually reassure both the physician and the patient. If the pressure remains elevated, readings on another day may be required; and if these appear high, it may be necessary to admit the child to the hospital for a day or two, to decide whether or not the blood pressure is continuously or abnormally elevated. Once systemic hypertension is identified, the various conditions causing raised blood pressure may be considered.

Pathologic Causes of Hypertension

The pathologic causes of hypertension in infancy and childhood may be divided into six chief groups: (1) renal, (2) cardiovascular, (3) endocrine, (4) neurologic, (5) miscellaneous, and (6) essential or primary hypertension (Rance et al., 1974).

The *renal* causes include nephritis, acute glomerular or chronic nephritis, pyelonephritis, renal tumors, lupus erythematosus, periarteritis nodosum, congenital malformation of the kidneys or its arteries, polycystic disease of the kidney and renal thrombosis, hydronephrosis, traumatic damage to the kidney, and hypoplastic kidney.

The *cardiovascular* causes include coarctation of the aorta, aortic insufficiency, aortic regurgitation, neonatal hypoxia, patent ductus arteriosus, and aortic arteritis.

Endocrine diseases may produce hypertension and are as follows: acromegaly, Cushing's disease, primary hyperaldosteronism, adrenal hyperplasia and hyperthyroidism, adrenogenital syndrome, neuroblastoma, and pheochromocytoma.

The *neurologic* conditions include intracranial tumors or abscesses, cerebral edema, encephelitis, and acrodynia.

The *miscellaneous* list would include mercury or lead poisoning, excess of licorice ingestion, radiation effects, Riley–Day syndrome, porphyria, burns, blood transfusion in patients with kidney disease, or mild preexisting hypertension.

The etiology of *essential* or *primary* hypertension is unknown.

Renal Causes. In acute glomerulonephritis of considerable severity, suppression of renal function may be accompanied by hypertensive encephalopathy and congestive heart failure. Headaches, vomiting, drowsiness, and seizures may occur, probably due to cerebral edema. When diuresis occurs, all these abnormalities rapidly disappear. Occasionally, with the marked elevation of blood pressure, the child may be dyspneic and have rales, rhonchi, and a gallop rhythm. These children usually respond satisfactorily to reserpine or hydralazine, with or without digitalis.

Renal involvement in periarteritis nodosum, scleredema, hemolytic uremic syndrome of childhood, and anaphylactic purpura with disseminated lupus erythematosus may also cause hypertensive encephalopathy. Since the underlying lesion in these instances is more serious, the prognosis is likely to be more grave than in acute poststreptococcal glomerulonephritis. Nephrosis in childhood is rarely associated with hypertension.

Pyelonephritis, causing chronic renal disease, may result in continued hypertension in childhood. This is also true for congenital anomalies of the urinary tract associated with obstructive pathology, as well as neuromuscular disorders with disturbed bladder function. A past history of urinary infection is helpful in making the diagnosis, but this may not be present and this diagnosis must be kept in mind and recognized by pyelography and occasionally renal biopsy.

RENAL ARTERY ANOMALIES. In the pediatric age group, renal ischemia may occur from congenital renal stenosis due to fibromuscular hyperplasia of one or more renal arteries and, as indicated elsewhere, it may at times be associated with coarctation of the abdominal aorta. Ljungqvist and Wallgren (1962) record renal vascular hypertension occurring in the first few weeks of life. Other causes of hypertension of renal origin include pressure of a tumor or fibrous band on renal artery, renal arteritis or aneurysm, and, on rare occasions, thrombosis of the renal artery. In 1938 Goldblatt pointed out that unilateral renal disease may give rise to systemic hypertension and may be cured by unilateral nephrectomy. Hypertension may result from Wilms' tumor in childhood, and the blood pressure can be expected to return to normal if it has been successfully removed.

Pheochromocytoma. Pheochromocytomas tend to arise in the adrenal medulla, in the chromatin tissue or in such tissue along the abdominal aorta or some other unusual site throughout the body. They are rarely seen in childhood, although Insley and Smallwood (1962) were able to collect 62 such patients under the age of 14 years. Sustained hypertension was present in the majority, although a few developed paroxysmal attacks. The majority have a single tumor that can be removed, but others have more than one, which makes surgical correction difficult. Removal of the tumor may lead to sudden drop in blood pressure, which will require infusion of norepinephrine until the body adjustments make this no longer necessary. In children, this condition is characterized by a labile blood pressure; hyperglycemia and glycosuria are occasionally present, and the urine contains increased catecholamines. Localization of tumors may be helped by intravenous pyelography, retroperitoneal aeriant sufflation, or aortography.

Neuroblastoma. Some increase of epinephrine or norepinephrine occurs in some of the cases, but the hypertension is not severe as a rule and is relieved when the tumor is removed.

Primary Aldosteronism. This condition was first described by Conn in 1955 in a patient with an adrenal corticoadenoma. This lesion leads to retention of sodium and expansion of blood volume and a depletion of potassium. Systemic hypertension is present in only a small percentage of cases. Danowsky (1962) reports a 12-year-old boy who had aldosterone-secreting tumor that was successfully removed, and hypertension, which was present, was cured. Conn and associates (1964) reported a similar case in a 3½-year-old girl with a blood pressure of 160/100. When the adenoma was removed, the blood pressure returned to normal.

Surgical treatment is required when an adenoma is identified. If no tumor is found, subtotal resection of one adrenal gland is carried out.

Cushing's Syndrome.   This is due to an adenoma or hyperplasia of the adrenal cortex or a carcinoma of the adrenal cortex. The clinical picture is characterized by a moon-facies, buffalo-hump on the back, obesity, hirsutism, muscular weakness, striae, abnormal glucose tolerance, and glycosuria. Systemic hypertension is common and may, at times, lead to heart failure or a cerebrovascular accident. In children, the growth is retarded; bilateral total or subtotal adrenalectomy with replacement therapy is indicated for hyperplasia (Hubble and Illingworth, 1957). If a tumor is present, replacement therapy is needed in the postoperative period.

Cushing's syndrome may occur with prolonged enlarged doses of corticosteroid and may be associated with hypertension. However, this complication is well recognized and is rarely allowed to proceed to a major degree of elevation of blood pressure.

Less Common Causes of Hypertension.   These include a cerebral tumor, meningitis, intracranial hemorrhage, encephalitis, Turner's syndrome (apart from coarctation of the aorta), lead poisoning, acrodynia, and familial dysautonomia.

Essential or Primary Hypertension.   This is a diagnosis that has been made infrequently in childhood in the past. The frequency increases somewhat in the teen-age group. Singh and Page (1967) reported 35 percent of hypertensive cases under 23 years of age had essential hypertension. Loggie (1969) concluded that 80 percent of children investigated at the Cincinnati Children's Hospital had hypertension secondary to some specific cause. Presumably 20 percent had essential hypertension.

The precise cause of essential or primary hypertension is unknown, but there are clues in childhood that suggest certain individuals may be hypertensive-prone. These include a history of transient blood pressure elevations on repeated observation, readings that are at or above the upper limits of normal for the age, a consistently elevated pulse rate, obesity, a family history of high blood pressure, or coronary, cerebral, or renal artery disease.

Although studies of familial incidence of hypertension in children are fairly recent, it has long been recognized that the occurrence of elevated arterial pressure is more common in certain families (Broadbent, 1898; Allbutt, 1915).

In 1934 Ayman studied 277 families and found hypertension in the children in 3.1 percent of the families when both parents were normal, in 28.3 percent when one parent was hypertensive, and in 45.5 percent when both parents were hypertensive. In 1940 Hines found that the children were hyper-reactors to the cold-pressor test in 43.4 percent when one parent was either hypertensive or a hyperreactor, and in 95 percent when both parents were affected.

Weitz (1923) found elevated blood pressure to be more frequent in siblings of hypertensive than of normotensive parents. More recently, Zinner and associates (1971) took blood pressures of 720 children, between 2 and 14 years of age, in 190 families. The result showed a clustering effect, measurable at all levels of blood pressure. Thus, a familial influence on blood pressure can be detected in children, and they considered it possible that factors responsible for hypertension are acquired in childhood. They also suggest that the tendency toward an elevated blood pressure can be detected as early as age two years.

Miall and Lovell (1967) have suggested that change of pressure with time is related to the level of pressure attained and that, once elevated, blood pressure tends to remain elevated and to rise more strikingly than blood pressure closer to the mean. Feinleib and associates (1969) also suggest that the degree of blood pressure in an individual is established fairly early in life and becomes relatively fixed by the age of 35, and in their opinion low pressures tend to remain low with time and high pressures tend to remain high. Thus, it may be that children who have a mild degree of systemic hypertension in childhood are likely to remain so throughout their life. This points to the value of Table 4–1, which indicates that the upper limit of normal may be set at two standard deviations above the mean for age and sex. Since blood pressure rises gradually from birth through adolescence, it is important to relate the blood pressure to the age and sex, rather than some single preconceived number.

The major treatment of the hypertensive-prone child or one who has essential hypertension is questionable in childhood. However, it may be proper to reduce or eliminate obesity if such is present. Occasionally it may be wise to limit excessive salt intake and, since atherosclerosis may be initiated or accelerated by hypertension, it may be suitable to control such factors as hyperlipidemia, excessive carbohydrate in the diet, and cigarette smoking. Intensive drug therapy is only indicated in those who have marked, sustained hypertension or evidence of malignant hypertension in childhood. However, mild degrees may be suitably handled by thiazides, but reserpine and hydralazine are contraindicated under such circumstances.

It has been suggested that in primary essential hypertension a reduction in pressure to normal levels, and maintenance at such levels for two or three years, may break the chain of events that leads to fixed hypertension in adult life.

In adults, Swaye and colleagues (1972) studied 717 patients with essential hypertension and 819 normotensives. No significant differences were found between the hypertensive and normotensive patients in regard to history of salt consumption. However, excessive dietary salt intake seemed to influence the severity of hypertension once it had developed.

Salt in Infant Diet and Hypertension. Dahl et al. (1968) have suggested that the salt intake of infants and children predisposes to hypertension in later life. This is based on his findings that salt feedings in early life in hypertensive-prone rats has induced hypertension more readily than when salt is provided later.

Certain societies exist for whom virtually no sodium is available (Denton, 1972). Kempner (1948) demonstrated that patients with hypertension could sustain normal activities for months on a diet containing as little as 2 mEq of sodium per day. More may be required for individuals who have had skin loss of sodium from sweating.

At the other end of the scale maximum tolerance for adults is high. Japanese and Thai farmers ingest 20 to 25 gm of salt, i.e., 400 to 500 mEq of sodium, per day (20 mEq per 100 kcal) with no sign of salt toxicity, i.e., no edema or hypernatremia.

At the present time the average consumption of salt per capita per day is 150 to 200 mEq for adults in North America. The safe tolerance for children appears to be 6 to 8 mEq of sodium per day. Because of the prevalence of essential hypertension in the adult there is a natural concern about the possible relation to salt intake. The evidence that salt intake induces hypertension is based on experimental studies in rats and epidemiologic studies in humans.

In salt-sensitive rats the blood pressure correlates with the salt intake. When such rats are fed 8 percent salt from weaning to six weeks of age, they develop hypertension by one year of age and their life-span is shortened. Extra salt increases this tendency in such rats. However, Dahl et al. (1968) found that resistant rats tolerated high-sodium intake quite well.

The conclusion reached is that salt intake is simply one of the many factors that act in varying degrees to cause hypertension in the human. Since there is little correlation between salt intake and hypertension in the human, present evidence does not provide a firm basis for advising a change in dietary salt intake for the general population. There is a reasonable possibility that a low-salt intake begun early in life may to some extent protect persons at risk from developing hypertension.

Fomon and coworkers (1970) have reviewed this evidence, and it is calculated that the maximum sodium intake for a four-month-old breast-fed infant given solid foods was 3 to 6 mEq per day. If unsalted infant foods were substituted for salted infant foods, the daily sodium intake ranged between 10 and 16 mEq per day. If infant foods with limited salt addition (0.1 percent added sodium) were used, daily sodium intake would be reduced by 17 to 34 percent depending on the source of milk. If infant foods containing added salt at 0.25 percent were substituted for infant foods, a moderate, but significant, reduction of sodium intake occurs.

The Committee on Nutrition of the American Academy of Pediatrics (1974) have found no evidence, insofar as healthy infants are concerned, that the addition of sodium chloride at current levels in infant foods is either harmful or beneficial to the infant. There is apparently no valid or scientific evidence available in support of the contention that the addition of salt to infant foods contributes to development of hypertension or other disease states in adult life, nor is there any valid evidence that the practice is harmful or that salt levels now consumed by infants in the United States overburden the excretory mechanism. Present salt intake, however, provides substantially more sodium than is required by the infant. Thus, they indicate that there is good reason to limit total intake. They point out that since salt-seasoning is primarily to satisfy the mother's taste, the addition of limited amounts of salt to processed infant foods may well be recommended even though there is no good basis for recommending any given level.

The committee therefore concludes that it seems reasonable to recommend that manufacturers add some salt to certain infant foods and that the upper level of added salt in such foods be 0.25 percent.

Diagnostic Investigations

In making a differential diagnosis of hypertension in childhood, it is not difficult to rule out coarctation of the aorta by differential blood pressures between arm and leg and feeling the femoral arteries. Diagnostic studies in the hospital should be aimed primarily at the kidney and glands of internal secretion. Such investigations, therefore, involve staying in the hospital for four or five days. Initially, one would need urinalysis, urine culture, hemoglobin, hematocrit, white blood cell count, and differential.

One would also need blood determinations for chloride, sodium, potassium, BUN creatinine, calcium, phosphorus, and carbon dioxide. A chest x-ray and electrocardiogram would be included in the routine, and in the older children, particularly, one should do a 24-hour urine collection for norepinephrine, epinephrine, metanephrines, and vanilmandelic acid (VMA).

When the above has been done, one can then turn to estimating the aldosterone secretion with a 24-hour urine specimen and the following day a 24-hour urine specimen for 17-hydroxysteroids and 17-17-keto-steroids.

An intravenous pyelogram is helpful in one-third to half of the cases that have kidney involvement, but it is usually necessary to follow this with an aortogram and a collection of blood from the renal vein for renin assay. The aortogram should be carried out in such a way as to show the renal arteries and other arteries in that segment of the aorta. The usual approach is retrograde from the femoral artery.

Renal biopsy may be required where renal surgery is contemplated in order to be certain that the kidney on the side opposite is essentially normal. Vertes and associates (1965) reported that the presence of severe generalized hypertensive vascular changes in the kidney on the opposite side of a renovascular lesion often resulted in surgical failure to relieve hypertension.

Medical Treatment

Low-Sodium Diet. A low-sodium diet of about 1 gm a day may be adequate to produce the desired effect. Severe restriction, 0.5 gm of sodium or less, is rarely necessary and may cause hyponatremia if diuretics are also used. A very low sodium diet may be contraindicated in chronic renal disease, in which there is usually inability to retain sodium. Serum electrolytes should be followed and a 24-hour urine estimated from time to time. Greater-than-normal sodium intake should not be allowed unless there is demonstrated compensatory excretion.

Antihypertensive Drugs. Antihypertensive drugs are usually used under two circumstances: (1) in hypertensive emergencies and (2) in the presence of chronic hypertension. The drugs that are readily available for parenteral administration in the treatment of hypertensive emergencies are reserpine, hydralazine, and methyldopa. Diazoxide had been used in a few medical centers in treating hypertensive emergencies occurring in children. The treatment of such emergencies is simplified if one drug is used at a time and its therapeutic potential exhausted before changing to or adding a second drug.

In chronic hypertension, if there are no symptoms resulting from the underlying condition, one may start with one agent, such as a diuretic, and gradually increase the dose and then add other drugs if necessary. If the hypertension is more severe, more potent antihypertensive agents should be used early and the dose gradually reduced as the hypertension subsides. The most commonly used drugs are the following:

ORAL DIURETICS. Oral diuretics (chlorothiazide [Diuril] and hydrochlorothiazide) cause initial contraction of extracellular and intravascular spaces and secondary reduction in cardiac output, and within several weeks the blood volumes revert to normal or near normal despite continued use. The major and prolonged antihypertensive effect is due to direct vasodilator action on the arterial wall. These drugs are very useful because the blood pressure is lowered in the supine and erect positions. Side reactions are few, antihypertensive effect is maintained even with prolonged administration, and they potentiate the action of other antihypertensive drugs. Oral diuretics are good drugs to start with if hypertension is not severe. At times they may require oral potassium supplementation. The oral dose of chlorothiazide (Diuril) is 10 to 20 mg/kg in 24 hours, given in three to four divided doses.

RAUWOLFIA ALKALOIDS. Rauwolfia (Reserpine) has a sympathetic depressant effect at the central vasomotor centers and also at the postganglionic sympathetic fibers, where it depletes catecholamine stores and thereby inhibits peripheral neural transmission. The antihypertensive effect is due primarily to its peripheral activity. In addition, it has a sedative effect. In a hypertensive crisis the dose is 0.07 mg/kg intramuscularly up to a maximum of 2.4 mg. It may be repeated every 12 to 24 hours. In chronic hypertension, a dose of 0.1 to 0.25 mg once daily by mouth is usually sufficient, and under such circumstances it is often combined with an oral diuretic or after a period of trial with hydralazine. It may cause bradycardia and nasal stuffiness, and in adults depression has been reported. Since the neonate is a nose-breather, and since deaths have been reported in newborn infants of mothers being treated with reserpine, it is not recommended in the neonate with hypertension. A few patients are very sensitive to reserpine and, therefore, where there is no emergency, it is best to start on rather small doses and work up.

HYDRALAZINE HYDROCHLORIDE (APRESOLINE). This drug acts directly on smooth muscle of the arteriolar wall. When first given, it increases stroke volume and heart rate and may at times cause palpitations of the heart. The cardiostimulatory effects can be reduced by giving reserpine as well. In hypertensive crisis, in combination with reserpine, one can give 0.1 to 0.2 mg/kg per dose intramuscularly or intravenously and repeat every four to six hours as necessary. In chronic hypertension one can use 1 mg/kg/day in divided doses, given three or four times daily, and the dose can be gradually increased to 5 mg/kg/day to a maximum of 200 mg/day. The highest doses for more than six months have caused lupus erythematosus-like syndrome with arthralgia, myalgia, and skin rash and LE cells. The syndrome is reversible when the drug is discontinued.

METHYLDOPA (ALDOMET). A decarboxylase inhibitor interferes with norepinephrine synthesis. It lowers blood pressure primarily by reducing peripheral vascular resistance without changing cardiac output or renal flow; hence it is useful in renal disease. It may cause postural hypertension. A dose of 10 mg/kg in three divided doses may be given. The adult maximum is 3 gm in 24 hours. It may cause drowsiness, hemolytic anemia, positive Coombs' test without hemolytic anemia, diarrhea, breast enlargement, and sore tongue.

GUANETHIDINE (ISMELIN). Guanethidine acts peripherally by adrenergic nerve blockade and depletion of the tissue stores of catecholamines. It causes postural hypotension and reduces renal plasma flow, glomerular filtration rate, and cerebral blood flow. Hence, it should be used with caution if accompanying cardiac or renal insufficiency is present. It is best given with an oral diuretic, which allows a lower dose of guanethidine. The dose in children is 0.2 mg/kg in 24 hours, with a range of 10 to 50 mg/day given once a day.

HYPERTENSION

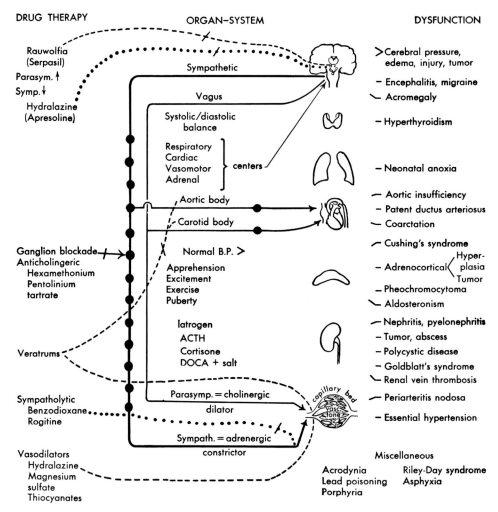

Figure 4-3. Schematic drawing of various organs and systems that may be involved in hypertension. On the right is indicated the type of dysfunction and on the left the drug therapy that might combat it. (Data in this diagram prepared by Dr. R. Slater, The Hospital for Sick Children, Toronto.)

Summary

A summary of hypertension, including a diagrammatic outline of the type of dysfunction, site of origin, and possible drug therapy, is shown in Figure 4–3.

REFERENCES

Allbutt, T. C.: *Disease of the Arterial Infundibular Angina Pectoris.* Vol 1, Macmillan, London, 1915.

Allen-Williams, G. M.: Pulse-rate and blood pressure in infancy and early childhood. *Arch. Dis. Child.,* **20**:125, 1945.

American Heart Foundation: *Recommendations for Human Blood Pressure Determinations by Sphygmomanometers.* The Association, New York, 1951.

Ashe, B. I., and Mosenthal, H. O.: Protein, salt and fluid consumption of 1,000 residents of New York. *JAMA,* **108**:1160, 1937.

Ashworth, A. M.; Neligan, G. A.; and Rogers, J. R.: Sphygmomanometer for the newborn. *Lancet,* **1**:801, 1959.

Ayman, D.: Heredity in essential hypertension: Clinical study of blood pressure of 1534 members of 277 families. *Arch. Intern. Med.,* **53**:792, 1934.

Barasanti, A. H.; Penick, R. W.; and Walsh, B. J.: "Flush" technique in the determination of blood pressure in normal infants and in infants with coarctation of the aorta. *Clin. Proc. Child. Hosp.* (Wash.), **10**:175, 1954.

Broadbent, W.: Adherent pericardium. *Trans. Med. Soc. Lond.,* **21**:109–22, 1898.

Burton, A. C.: The criterion for diastolic pressure—revolution and counterrevolution. *Circulation,* **36**:805–9, Dec. 1967.

Chapman, W. P., and Singh, M.: Evaluation of tests used in the diagnosis of pheochromocytoma. *Mod. Concepts Cardiovasc. Dis.,* **23**:221, 1954.

Clifton, W. M., and Heinz, M. O.: Survey of prenatal syphilis in Hospital for Sick Children, *JAMA,* **114**:1731, 1940.

Committee on Nutrition of the American Academy of Pediatrics: Salt intake and eating patterns of infants and children in relation to blood pressure. *Pediatrics,* **53**:115, 1974.

Conn, J. W.; Knoff, R. F.; and Nesbit, R. M.: Clinical characteristics of primary aldosteronism from an analysis of 145 cases. *Am. J. Surg.*, **107**:159, 1964.

Conn, J. W., and Louis, L. H.: Primary aldosteronism: new clinical entity. *Trans. Assoc. Am. Physicians*, **68**:215, 1955.

Dahl. L. K., and Love, R. A.: Etiological role of sodium chloride intake in essential hypertension in humans. *JAMA*, **164**:397, 1957.

Dahl, L. K.; Knudsen, K. D.; Heine, M.; and Leitl, G. J.: Effects of chronic excess salt ingestion. Modification of experimental hypertension in the rat by variations in the diet. *Circ. Res.*, **22**:11, 1968.

Danowsky, T. S.: Vascular disease in obvious and subtle endocrinopathies. *Med. Times*, **90**:175, 1962.

Denton, D.: Instinct, appetites and medicine. *Aust. N.Z. J. Med.*, **2**:203, 1972.

Downing, M. W.: Blood pressure of normal girls from age three to sixteen years of age. *Am. J. Dis. Child.*, **73**:293, 1947.

Feinleib, M., et al.: Some pitfalls in the evaluation of screening programs. *Arch. Environ. Health (Chicago)*, **19**:12–15, 1969.

Folger, G. M., Jr.; Roberts, W. C.; Mehrizi, A.; Shah, K. D.; Glancy, D. L.; Carpenter, C. C. J.; and Esterly, J. R.: Cyanotic malformations of the heart with pheochromocytoma. A report of five cases. *Circulation*, **29**:750, 1964.

Fomon, S. J.; Thomas, L. N.; and Filer, L. J., Jr.: Acceptance of unsalted strained foods by normal infants. *J. Pediatr.*, **76**:242, 1970.

Fry, D. L.; Noble, F. W.; and Mallow, A. J.: An evaluation of modern pressure recording systems. *Circ. Res.*, **5**:40, 1957a.

———: An electric device for instantaneous and continuous computation of aortic blood velocity. *Circ. Res.*, **5**:75, 1957b.

Goldblatt, H.: Studies on experimental hypertension: production of malignant phase of hypertension. *J. Exp. Med.*, **67**:809, 1938.

Goldring, D., and Wohltmann, H.: Flush method for blood pressure determinations in newborn infants. *J. Pediatr.*, **40**:285, 1952.

Goodman, H. G.; Cumming, G. R.; and Raber, M. B.: Photocell oscillometer for measuring systolic pressure in newborn. *Am. J. Dis. Child.*, **103**:152, 1962.

Gornal, A.: Personal communication, 1956.

Graham, A. W.; Hines, E. A., Jr.; and Gage, R. P.: Blood pressure in children between the ages of five and sixteen years. *Am. J. Dis. Child.*, **69**:203, 1945.

Gunteroth, W. G., and Nadas, A. S.: Blood pressure measurements in infants and children. *Pediatr. Clin. North Am.*, **2**:257, 1955.

Guyton, A. C.: Physiologic regulation of arterial pressure. *Am. J. Cardiol.*, **8**:401, 1961.

Hamilton, W. F.; Woodbury, R. A.; and Harper, H. T.: Physiologic relations between intrathoracic, intraspinal and arterial pressure. *JAMA*, **107**:853, 1936.

Hines, E. A., Jr.: Significance of hypertension as measured by cold-pressor test. *AM. Heart J.*, **19**:408, 1940.

Hinman, A. T.; Engel, B. T.; and Bickford, A. F.: Portable blood pressure recorder accuracy and preliminary use in evaluating intradaily variations in pressure. *Am. Heart J.*, **63**:663, 1962.

Hubble, D., and Illingworth, R. S.: Personal communication, 1957.

Insley, J., and Smallwood, W. C.: Pheochromocytoma in children. *Arch. Dis. Child.*, **37**:606, 1962.

Kannel, W. B., and Gordon, T.: Systolic vs. diastolic blood pressure and the risk of coronary heart disease. *Am. J. Cardiol.*, **27**:335–46, April 1971.

Kempner, W.: Treatment of hypertensive vascular disease with rice diet. *Am. J. Med.*, **4**:545–577, April 1948.

Kennedy, R. L. J.; Barker, N. W.; and Walters, W.: Malignant hypertension, cure following nephrectomy. Follow-up report of the case of a child. *Am. J. Dis. Child.*, **69**:160, 1945.

Kimmel, G. C.: Hypertension and pyelonephritis of children. *Am. J. Dis. Child.*, **63**:60, 1942.

Kumar, D.; Hall, A. E. D.; Nakashima, R.; and Gornall, A. G.: Cumulative effect of aldosterone administration in rats. *Rev. Can. Biol.* **14**:265, 1955.

Levy, P. S., and Kass, E. H.: Familial aggregation of blood pressure in childhood. *N. Engl. J. Med.*, **384**:401–404, 1971.

Ljungqvist, A., and Wallgren, G.: Unilateral renal artery hypertension in a newborn infant. *Acta Paediatr.*, **51**:575, 1962.

Loggie, J. M.: Hypertension in children and adolescents. I. Causes and diagnostic studies. *J. Pediatr.*, **74**:331–5, Mar. 1969.

———: Hypertension in children and adolescents. Diagnosis and management. *Med. Times*, **98**:163–79, April 1970.

Londe, S.: Blood pressure standards for normal children as

determined under office conditions. *Clin. Pediatr.*, **7**:401, 1968.

McLaughlin, G. W.; Kirley, R. R.; Kemmerer, W. T.; and de Lamos, R. A.: Indirect measurement of blood pressure in infants using Doppler ultrasound. *J. Pediatr.*, **79**:300–303, 1971.

Masland, R. P., et al.: Hypertensive vascular disease in adolescence. *N. Engl. J. Med.*, **255**:894, 1956.

Master, A. M.; Dublin, L. I.; and Marks, H. H.: The normal blood pressure range and its clinical implications. *JAMA*, **143**:1464, 1950.

Miall, W. E.: Follow-up study of arterial pressure in the population of a Welsh mining valley. *Br. Med. J.*, **2**:1204, 1959.

Miall, W. E.; Kensage, P.; Khosla, T.; et al.: Factors influencing the degree of resemblance in arterial pressure of close relatives. *Clin. Sci.*, **33**:271, 1967.

Miall, W. E., and Lovell, H. G.: Relation between change of blood pressure and age. *Br. Med. J.*, **2**:660, 1967.

Morse, R. L.; Brownell, G. L.; and Currnes, J. H.: The blood pressure of newborn infants: indirect determination by an automatic blood pressure recorder in 20 infants. *Pediatrics*, **25**: 50, 1960.

Moser, M.; Walters, M.; Master, A. M.; Taymor, R. C.; and Metraux, J.: Chemical blockade of the sympathetic nervous system in essential hypertension; experienced with oral therapy with 688-A (N-phenoxyisopropyl-N-benzyl-B chloroethylamine hydrochloride). *Arch. Intern. Med.*, **89**:5, 1952.

Moss, A. J., and Adams, F. H.: *Problems of Blood Pressure in Childhood.* Charles C Thomas, Springfield, Ill., 1962.

———: Flush blood pressure and intraarterial pressure. *Am. J. Dis. Child.*, **107**:489, 1964.

Neligan, G.: Systolic blood pressure in neonatal asphyxia and respiratory distress syndrome. *Am. J. Dis. Child.*, **98**:460, 1959.

Park, M. R., and Guntheroth, W. G.: Direct blood pressure measurements in brachial and femoral arteries in children. *Circulation*, **41**:231–7, Feb. 1970.

Parkinson, R. P.: A study of venous pressure in the newborn infant. *J. Pediatr.*, **50**:174, 1957.

Rance, C. P.; Arbus, G. S.; Balfe, J. E.; and Kooh, S. W.: Persistent systemic hypertension in infants and children. *Pediatr. Clin. North Am.*, **21**:801, 1974.

Reeves, T. J.; Hefner, L. L.; Jones, W. B.; Coghlan, C.; Prieto, G.; and Carroll, J.: The hemodynamic determinants of the rate of change in pressure in the left ventricle during isometric contraction. *Am. Heart J.*, **60**:745, 1960.

Rice, H. V., and Posener, L. J.: A practical method for the measurement of systolic blood pressures of infants. *Pediatrics*, **23**:854, 1959.

Roberts, L. N.; Smiley, J. R.; and Manning, G. W.: A comparison of direct and indirect blood pressure determinations. *Circulation*, **8**:232, 1953.

Robinson, M.; Hamilton, W. F.; Woodbury, R. A.; and Volpitto, P. P.: Accuracy of clinical determinations of blood pressure in children. *Am. J. Dis. Child.*, **58**:102, 1939.

Rudolph, A. M.; Drorbaugh, J. E.; Auld, P.; Rudolph, A. J.; Nadas, A. S.; Smith, C. A.; and Hubbell, J. P.: Studies on the circulation in the neonatal period. *Pediatrics*, **27**:551, 1961.

Salans, A. H., et al.: A study of the central and peripheral arterial pressure pulse in man. *Circulation*, **4**:510, 1951.

Schaffer, A. I.: Neonatal blood pressure studies. *Am. J. Dis. Child.*, **89**:204, 1955.

Semans, J. H.: Nephrectomy for hypertension in a 2½ year old child with an apparent cure for 3 years. *Bull. Hopkins Hosp.*, **75**:184, 1944.

Singh, S. P., and Page, L. B.: Hypertension in early life. *Am. J. Med. Sci.*, **253**:255–62, 1967.

Sisson, T. R. C.; Lund, C. J.; and Whalen, L. E.: The blood volume of infants. *J. Pediatr.*, **55**:163, 1959.

Snyder, C. H.; Bost, R. B.; and Platou, R. V.: Hypertension in infancy with anomalous renal artery. *Pediatrics*, **15**:88, 1955.

Steele, J. M.: Measurements of arterial pressure in man. *J. Mount Sinai Hosp. N.Y.*, **8**:1049, 1941–42.

Steinfeld, L.; Alexander, H.; and Cohen, M. L.: Updating sphygmomanometry. *Am. J. Cardiol.*, **33**:107–10, 1974.

Swaye, P. S.; Gifford, R. W., Jr.; and Berrettoni, J. N.: Dietary salt and essential hypertension. *Am. J. Cardiol.*, **29**:33, 1972.

Taussig, H. B., and Remsen, D. B.: Essential hypertension in boy of two years of age. *Bull. Hopkins Hosp.*, **57**:183, 1935.

Van Bergen, F. H., et al.: Comparison of indirect and direct methods of measuring arterial blood pressure. *Circulation*, **10**:481, 1954.

van der Tweel, L. H.: Some physical aspects of blood pressure, pulse wave, and blood pressure measurements. Original communications from the Laboratory of Medical Physics, University of Amsterdam, Amsterdam, Holland, Jan. 19, 1956.

Vertes, V.; Granel, J. A.; and Goldblatt, H.: Studies of patients with renal hypertension undergoing vascular surgery. *N. Engl. J. Med.,* **272**:186, 1965.

Weitz, W.: Zur Atiologie der genuinen oder vascularen Hypertension. 2. *Klin Med.,* **96**:151 (236, 338, 226, 286), 1923.

Wilkins, L.: Diagnosis of adrenogenital syndrome and its treatment with cortisone. *J. Pediatr.,* **41**:860, 1952.

Wood, J. E.; Barrow, S. G.; and Freis, E.: Primary prevention of hypertension. *Circulation,* **42**:39, 1970.

Woodbury, R. A.; Robinow, M.; and Hamilton, W. F.: Blood pressure studies on infants. *Am. J. Physiol.,* **122**:472, 1938.

Zinner, S. H.; Levy, P. S.; and Kass, E. H.: Familial aggregation of blood pressure in childhood. *N. Engl. J. Med.,* **284**:401, 1971.

5

Noninvasive Investigations

C. A. F. Moës, Henry M. Sondheimer, John D. Keith,
Kenneth R. Bloom, David L. Gilday, and *Richard D. Rowe*

THE CHEST ROENTGENOGRAM IN CONGENITAL HEART DISEASE

C. A. F. Moës

THE DIAGNOSIS of congenital heart disease is often difficult, especially in the neonatal period. The chest x-ray may appear relatively normal even in the presence of severe cardiac disease. One must therefore regard the x-ray with caution. To obtain the maximum amount of information from the roentgenogram, a systematic approach to film examination is essential. It may not be possible to make a definite diagnosis of congenital heart disease, although one may suggest a diagnosis by observing some fundamental principles. Of the utmost importance in evaluating the chest film are the pulmonary vascular pattern, the pulmonary artery, the heart size, the heart shape, the configuration of the aorta, the position of the heart, and the bony thorax.

Pulmonary Vascular Pattern

An evaluation of the pulmonary vascular pattern is essential in attempting to classify congenital heart disease radiologically. The vessels may be normal, increased, or decreased in size. If increased, the vascular disorder may involve either the arteries predominantly, as in left-to-right or bidirectional shunts, or the veins secondary to left-sided obstructive lesions. A shunt and obstruction may coexist. Assessment of the pulmonary vascularity is difficult at any age, although this is especially true in the first month. During the first few days of life there is frequently a persistence of the high resistance of fetal circulation and in some instances the vessels may remain small as the result of hypoxic vasoconstriction.

The size of the pulmonary arteries and veins must be assessed on both the posteroanterior and lateral chest radiographs. The *normal pulmonary arteries* (Figure 5–1*B*) are seen extending out from the hila and taper gradually toward the lung periphery. The intrapulmonary arteries within the lower lobes are normally larger in caliber than those in the upper lobes. The vessel margins are distinct. The pulmonary veins in the normal state take little part in the vascular pattern. Frequently an end-on pulmonary artery branch and companion air-containing, thin-walled bronchus are visible in the perihilar area. Normally these are of equal size (Figure 5–3*A*). On the lateral projection the normal arteries, with clear-cut margins, are readily visible in the hila and the proximal bronchi are clearly defined (Figure 5–2*B*). *Enlarged pulmonary arteries* and veins occur as a result of left-to-right shunts. The enlarged arteries are frequently seen end-on in the perihilar areas. If an end-on artery and companion bronchus are visible, the artery will be larger than the bronchus (Figure 5–3*B*). This relationship, although useful in assessing vessel size in older children, is usually not practical in infants as the bronchus cannot be readily defined. The vessels extend further into the lung periphery than in the normal (Figure 5–1*A*). In the lateral film the enlarged arteries are seen in the hila and tend to obscure the clear definition of the air-containing main stem bronchi, especially in the infant age group (Figure 5–2*A*). Enlargement of the pulmonary arteries, it must be remembered, is usually not apparent radiologically when there is a left-to-right shunt with a pulmonary-to-systemic flow ratio of less than two to one. Engorgement of the pulmonary arteries when due to left-to-right shunting at ventricular or great artery level is usually a manifestation of both increased blood flow and increased pressure in the pulmonary vascular bed. In

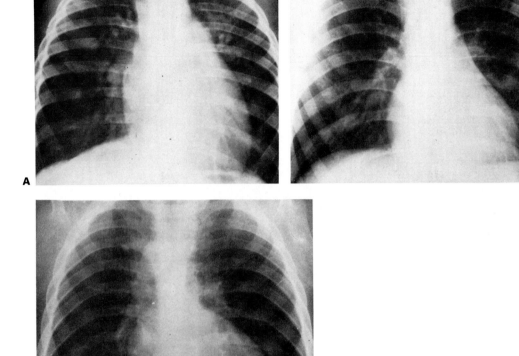

Figure 5-1. Posteroanterior views demonstrating pulmonary artery vascularity. *A*. Increased (VSD) *B*. Normal. *C*. Decreased (tetralogy of Fallot with right aortic arch).

the event of development of significant pulmonary hypertension, a decrease in the caliber of the pulmonary vascular bed is extremely difficult to recognize on the chest film in our experience in infancy and childhood.

Patients with a large left-to-right shunt may develop left-heart failure as a result of left-sided volume overloading. In its mildest form the pulmonary arteries are enlarged and the lungs are clear. At the other extreme the dilated arteries in the perihilar regions lose their distinct margins and become blurred due to leakage of fluid into the interstitial perivascular sheath. There may, in some cases, be associated clouding of the lungs due to pulmonary edema or interstitial veiling and even the development of a pleural effusion. The lungs in the infant in this situation are usually hyperinflated and the diaphragm flattened.

The presence of *pulmonary venous hypertension* may be due to left-sided obstructive lesions or primary left ventricular disorders that result in left ventricular failure. The pulmonary venous pressure is increased and these changes are reflected in the capillaries and pulmonary arteries. Radiologically these changes are initially manifest by redistribution

of blood flow such that the vascular pattern in the upper lobes is greater than that in the lower lobes (Simon et al., 1967). These changes, however, are not appreciated in infancy. As venous pressure rises, there is a leakage of fluid into the interstitial tissues and alveoli producing a reticular pattern that extends out to the lung periphery with a varying degree of interstitial veiling (Figure 5–4*A*). In the lateral film clear definition of all the vessel margins in the hila are lost and the airways are indistinct due to enlarged vessels and perivascular and peribronchial edema. Thickened interlobular septa are frequently visible as short horizontal lines abutting on the pleura in the costophrenic angles (Kerly B lines). In the neonate these are often better appreciated on the lateral film behind the sternum (Figure 5–4*B*).

Recognition of *decreased pulmonary vascularity* associated with right-to-left shunts, such as a tetralogy of Fallot, is often extremely difficult. The diameter of the pulmonary arteries is decreased and they extend into the lung periphery only to the junction of the inner and middle thirds. The main pulmonary artery is small (Figure 5–1*C*). The lateral film is frequently helpful. The pulmonary artery branches are small and the hila appear empty. The proximal bronchi and distal trachea are clearly visualized (Figure 5–2C). Pulmonary artery obstruction in its severest form, e.g., pulmonary atresia, may present a disorganized vascular pattern. Small stringy vessels representing intermingled bronchial and pulmonary arteries are visible producing a reticular appearance throughout the lungs. A normal pulmonary trunk is not present and the hila are small.

Unilateral pulmonary atresia or severe stenosis of a main pulmonary artery branch can be recognized by a decreased vascular pattern in one lung. The affected lung is usually small. The vascularity in the unaffected lung is increased. Milder degrees of main branch stenosis or peripheral branch stenosis cannot be

diagnosed without resorting to more sophisticated investigations.

Pulmonary Artery

Prominence of the main pulmonary artery may be observed as an isolated phenomenon in normal individuals, particularly in females in the pediatric age group, and is often termed idiopathic. A similar appearance is observed with pulmonary valve stenosis. Differentiation of these may be difficult radiologically. With the latter, however, dilatation of the left main branch is frequently also present

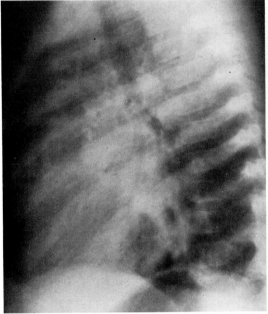

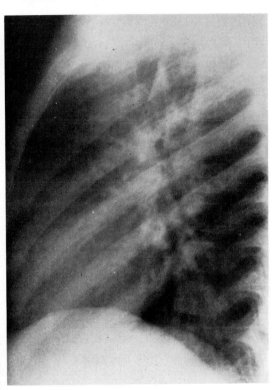

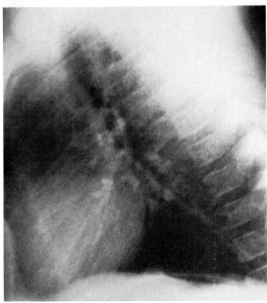

Figure 5-2. Lateral views demonstrating pulmonary artery vascularity. *A.* Increased. *B.* Normal. *C.* Decreased.

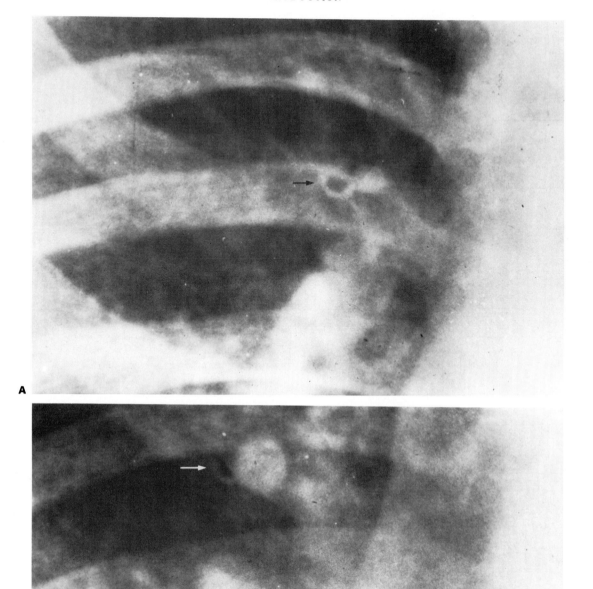

Figure 5-3. End-on pulmonary artery branch and bronchus (arrow). *A* demonstrates that the normal artery and accompanying bronchus are the same size. *B* illustrates the relationship in a left-to-right shunt. The artery is larger than the bronchus.

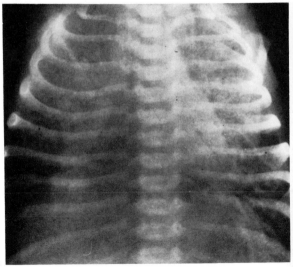
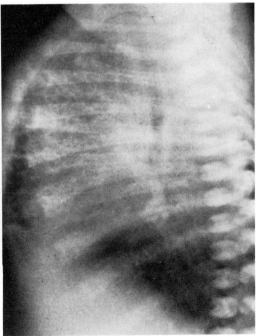

Figure 5-4. Pulmonary venous hypertension from total anomalous venous return below the diaphragm with obstruction. The anteroposterior view (*A*) shows marked pulmonary venous congestion with edema. Thickened interlobular septa are well seen on the lateral projection (*B*) behind the sternum.

and there is evidence of right ventricular enlargement.

Aneurysmal dilatation of the pulmonary arteries may occur in association with tetralogy of Fallot and absent pulmonary valve (Durnin et al., 1969; Osman et al., 1969; Lakier et al., 1974) or as an isolated lesion (Osman et al., 1969). The main pulmonary artery is grossly enlarged and there is frequently dilatation of one branch, more commonly the right. The peripheral pulmonary vessels are either normal or slightly dilated. Enlargement of a main pulmonary artery may partially obstruct a bronchus with development of emphysema.

A high course of the left pulmonary artery is described as a diagnostic feature of truncus arteriosus (Keith et al., 1967). When visible this is a clue to the diagnosis, though it has not been found to be a very helpful sign in our experience.

Heart Size and Shape

Measurements for estimation of cardiac size do exist, though even these are subject to a fairly wide range of normality (Lincoln and Spillman, 1928; Bakwin and Bakwin, 1935; Martin and Friedill, 1952; Burnard and James, 1961). In the neonate a cardiothoracic ratio of more than 58 percent on a supine film made at a 40-inch focal film distance in inspiration can probably be considered to be abnormal. During the first year the ratio gradually diminishes to approximately 50 percent on the normal 6-foot focal film distance radiograph. Despite these measurements the most reliable criterion in assessing cardiac size is experience on the part of the radiologist. Interpretation of cardiac size and shape may be complicated by the thymic silhouette in the neonate and young child (up to two years). At times oblique and lateral films will help to clear up the problem as one can appreciate that a large thymus is present anteriorly, or a subtle notch is visible separating the lower thymic margin from the heart. Should the thymus merge imperceptibly with the heart, impressions of the anterior ribs may cause scalloping of the apparent heart border. This, when present, is diagnostic of thymic tissue. If other methods fail to differentiate suspected thymic enlargement from cardiomegaly, the oral administration of steroid hormones may be used (Caffey and di Liberti, 1959). Almost complete disappearance of the thymus will occur after one week of therapy.

Estimation of individual cardiac chamber size is well described by Cooley and Schreiber (1967), Elliott and Schiebler (1968), and Swischuk (1970) and will not be discussed here. In infancy and early childhood individual chamber enlargement is often difficult to assess and, what is more, one chamber, such as the left ventricle, may enlarge and displace the right ventricle and so simulate right-sided enlargement. It is therefore better to observe the cardiac shape, which in certain instances may suggest a likely diagnosis. Table 5–1 is a list of shapes that may be associated with specific types of congenital heart disease. These are grouped according to the pulmonary vascular pattern

Table 5–1. CARDIAC SHAPES IN CONGENITAL HEART DISEASE

PULMONARY VASCULARITY	SHAPE	SUGGESTED DIAGNOSIS
Increased	"Egg shape"	Complete D-transposition of great arteries
	"Snowman," Figure of 8	Total anomalous pulmonary venous return to left vertical vein
	Triangle shape, no visible right superior vena cava	ASD (secundum)
	Discrete convex bulge left upper cardiac border	Single ventricle with ventricular inversion, absent RV sinus
		Left juxtaposition of atrial appendages
Increased or normal	Long convex left superior mediastinal contour	Congenitally corrected L-transposition of great arteries
Normal	Prominent main pulmonary artery and ? left branch	Pulmonary valve stenosis
	Scimitar syndrome	Hypoplasia right lung with anomalous pulmonary venous return
Decreased	"Coeur en sabot"	Tetralogy of Fallot

most commonly observed in each instance. A final interpretation, however, should be made in the light of such clinical finds as cyanosis, failure, etc.

Aorta

The contour of the aorta and side of the arch may play a significant role in suggesting a specific diagnosis of the type of congenital heart disease. In infancy the aorta is difficult to visualize because of the thymus. The ascending aorta in children is usually not visible on the posteroanterior film, and when seen or if there is a localized dilatation, a diagnosis of aortic valve stenosis, aortic regurgitation, or coarctation of the aorta should be suspected. The upper descending aorta is usually clearly outlined, particularly on an overpenetrated PA film. The left lateral margin is normally smooth; however, if it is notched, a coarctation of the aorta usually exists (the so-called "3 sign"). Corroborative evidence may be obtained with a barium esophagogram. The barium column in this case is indented on the left both at the level of the aortic arch and just inferior to this by the poststenotic dilated segment, the intervening protrusion of barium between the two concavities representing the coarctation site (the so-called "E sign"). The aortic arch or knob may be prominent, often due to dilatation of the root of the left subclavian artery, small in the presence of a long-segment preductal coarctation, or not clearly visible as it is obscured by a dilated left subclavian artery.

The position of the aortic arch is usually clearly visible on the frontal chest film. However, when it is not apparent its position can frequently be recognized by deviation and indentation of the trachea. Failing this, a barium esophagogram may be necessary. Although usually left-sided, a right aortic arch in the presence of levocardia is strong evidence that congenital heart disease exists. Table 5–2 shows the incidence of a right aortic arch in various types of cardiac disease encountered at The Hospital for Sick Children, Toronto.

Table 5–2. INCIDENCE OF RIGHT AORTIC ARCH CONGENITAL HEART DISEASE

TYPE OF DISEASE	INCIDENCE (PERCENT)
Tetralogy of Fallot	31
Truncus arteriosus	31
Double-outlet right ventricle	20
Tricuspid atresia	5
Isolated ventricular septal defect	2.3
Complete "D"-transposition great arteries	2.3
Congenitally corrected "L"-transposition great arteries	1

Positional Anomalies of the Heart

Cardiac malpositions may occur:

1. Secondary to anomalies of the lungs, diaphragm, or skeleton. Malpositions resulting from atelectasis or overinflation of one lung, elevation of a hemidiaphragm, or skeletal anomalies are usually easily recognized. Those due to hypoplasia of a lung as the result of absence of one pulmonary artery or anomalous pulmonary venous connection (scimitar syndrome) are often more difficult to diagnose. Congenital heart disease is not a feature of these anomalies.

2. In association with asplenia or polysplenia. In the normal individual with situs solitus of the heart and abdominal viscera the aortic arch, stomach

bubble, and spleen are situated on the left and the liver on the right. The left atrium is located on the side of the stomach and aortic arch and so is left-sided. The position of the cardiac apex is variable and, although commonly left-sided (levocardia), it may be on the right (dextrocardia). With situs inversus, the aortic arch, stomach, and spleen are on the right and the liver is left-sided. Again the left atrium follows the laterality of the aortic arch and stomach and is on the right. The cardiac apex is commonly, though not exclusively, on the right. In the presence of asplenia or polysplenia the visceral situs may be indeterminate. The liver frequently extends to both sides of the midline and the stomach bubble is central. When this visceral relationship is present, the position of the left atrium cannot be estimated and complex cardiac disease should be suspected (Rose et al., 1975).

3. Unassociated with either of the above. The incidence of cardiac abnormalities in this situation is increased (Elliott et al., 1966; Shaher et al., 1967; Elliott and Schiebler, 1968) and assessment frequently complicated. In general, one may conclude that with visceral situs inversus, a right aortic arch, and dextrocardia the incidence of severe cardiac disease is low. If there is dextrocardia with visceral situs solitus and a left aortic arch or levocardia with visceral situs inversus and a right aortic arch, the incidence of severe cardiac anomalies is high.

Bony Thorax

Specific congenital cardiac lesions may be suspected by observing the bones. Thus, with clinical and radiographic stigmata of Down's syndrome, atrioventricular canal or ventricular septal defects are suspected (Rowe and Uchida, 1961). Bone changes described are: a manubrium sterni with two separate ossification centers (Currarino and Swanson, 1964; Horns and O'Loughlin, 1965; Lees and Caldicott, 1975), absence of the twelfth ribs (Berber, 1966), and

an abnormal configuration of the lumbar vertebrae (Rabinowitz and Moseley, 1964). Similarly, in a known rubella syndrome with typical bone changes, patent ductus arteriosus and peripheral pulmonary branch stenosis are common. The proximal ends of the humeri in this instance may demonstrate irregularity and poor mineralization of the growth plate with linear and ovoid radiolucencies that alter the trabecular pattern in the metaphysis (Rabinowitz et al., 1965; Singleton et al., 1966).

Premature sternal segment fusion is well known with congenital heart disease (Fisher et al., 1973; Lees and Caldicott, 1975). Although this may occur with both cyanotic and acyanotic types, it appears to be more frequent in the former (Gabrielson and Ladyman, 1963; Fisher et al., 1973). Fisher and associates (1973) have also noted that the incidence in females is greater than in males.

Pectus carinatum may be evident in those with congenital heart disease. Corone and colleagues (1963) reported an incidence of 15 percent. Fisher and coworkers (1973) have noted that this deformity is commoner in patients with cyanotic (26 percent) than acyanotic (6.2 percent) cardiac anomalies.

Rib notching is a valuable sign in the diagnosis of coarctation of the aorta, though it is usually not seen before six or seven years of age. Most commonly the fourth to eighth ribs are involved; however, notching of the third and ninth may also be present (Boone et al., 1964). If notching is unilateral, the coarctation site may be proximal to either the left subclavian artery or an aberrant right subclavian artery. In the former the notching is confined to the right ribs; in the latter, the left.

Patients with the straight back syndrome may exhibit murmurs simulating cardiac disease (Datey et al., 1964). The spine is straight and the anteroposterior diameter of the chest is diminished. The heart may appear enlarged and the pulmonary artery prominent simulating pulmonary valve stenosis.

ELECTROCARDIOGRAPHY AND VECTORCARDIOGRAPHY
Henry M. Sondheimer and *John D. Keith*

Electrocardiography

Although the presence of an electric current in the living muscle was recognized in the eighteenth century, it was not until the time of Kölliker and Müller in 1856 that the existence of such currents was first demonstrated in the active myocardium. In 1900, Einthoven recorded this electrical activity by means of a string galvanometer, and the method was later applied clinically, evolving into the modern electrocardiograph.

The freshly isolated heart will frequently continue to beat for some time, and all heart muscle is equipped with the innate ability to contract, the atria contracting at a natural rate more rapidly than the

ventricles. It was recognized ultimately that certain portions of the myocardium, because of their greater rhythmicity, had a controlling effect on the heartbeat. The pacemaker, or sinus node, was discovered by Keith and Flack in 1907. The bundle of His had been recognized previously by His in 1893, the atrioventricular node by Tawara in 1906, and the Purkinje fibers by Purkinje in 1845. The normal beat originates in the sinus node (Lewis, 1910), passes via the intraatrial tracts to the atrioventricular node, then along the bundle of His branches to the Purkinje system of fibers, which transmit the impulse to the ventricular myocardium (Figure 5–5).

The conductivity of various portions of the heart varies as follows: atrial muscle, 1000 mm per second;

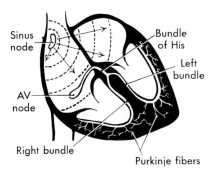

Figure 5-5. Diagrammatic outline of the conducting tissues of the heart. The impulse originates in the sinus node, then spreads over the atria. It is then conducted by the AV node, bundle of His, and the Purkinje fibers to the ventricular myocardium.

atrioventricular node, 200 mm per second; bundle of His, 200 mm per second; Purkinje network, 5000 mm per second; ventricular myocardium, 400 mm per second.

Figure 5–6 shows a drawing of electrocardiographic curve PQRST with a phonocardiogram below. The P wave indicates the spread of electrical stimulation through the atria; the QRS complex records the spread of electrical impulse through the ventricles. The T wave represents the repolarization phase of the ventricular myocardium.

The first heart sound begins after the onset of the QRS complex and reaches a maximum after the peak of the R wave. The second sound occurs at the end of the T wave.

The evaluation of intracardiac conduction has been greatly enhanced by the development of His bundle electrocardiography (Scherlag et al., 1969). Figure 5–7 shows an electrocardiographic tracing labeled PQRS and below it is an intracardiac electrogram obtained at the bundle of His and labeled A, H, and V. The A deflection represents atrial electrical activity as it approaches the AV node; the His spike (H) represents His bundle activity; and V represents ventricular activity. The P-R interval of the electrocardiographic tracing is therefore divisible into the P-A interval, representing the time taken for an impulse originating at the sinoatrial node to travel to the atrioventricular node; the A-H interval, representing the atrioventricular nodal delay; and the H-V interval, representing the conduction time from the His bundle through the bundle branches to the Purkinje system.

Electrocardiographic Leads.   The usual method of taking an electrocardiogram is to attach an electrode to each wrist and each ankle. These leads then conduct the electrical activity to the electrocardiograph machine. The potentials from right and left arms produce the tracing of standard lead I; from the right arm and left leg, standard lead II; and from left arm and left leg, standard lead III.

The unipolar limb leads are obtained by recording the difference in potential between the individual limb concerned and a central terminal that has a

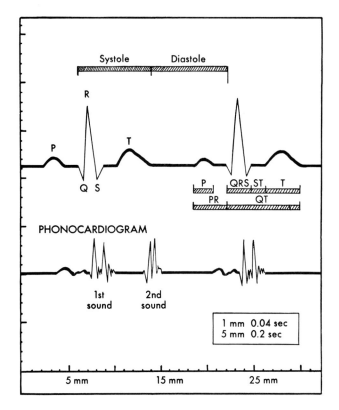

Figure 5-6. PQRST complexes of the electrocardiogram shown with the duration of various segments. Position and timing of heart sounds are also indicated.

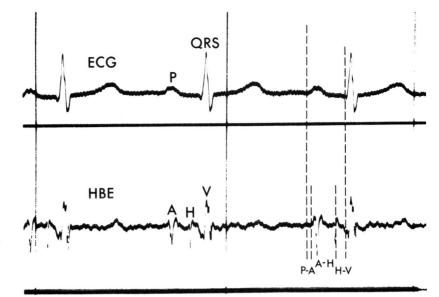

Figure 5-7. External electrocardiogram (*ECG*) and simultaneous His bundle electrogram (*HBE*) demonstrating the P–A, A–H, and H–V components of the P–R interval. (Reproduced from Roberts, N. K.: *The Cardiac Conducting System and the His Bundle Electrogram.* Appleton-Century-Crofts, New York, 1975.)

theoretical zero potential and is comprised of contacts with the other three limbs. It was demonstrated by Goldberger (1949) that one can amplify the voltage when the limb being examined is disconnected from the central terminal. Such leads are then referred to as aVR, right arm; aVL, left arm; and aVF, left leg.

The unipolar chest leads are taken in areas agreed on by a Joint Committee of the American Heart and the British Heart Associations (1938) and are referred to as V_1, V_2, V_3, V_4, V_5, and V_6. In position V_1 the exploring electrode is at the right border of the sternum in the fourth intercostal space; for V_2 the exploring electrode is at the left border of the sternum in the fourth intercostal space; for V_3 the electrode is midway along a line joining V_2 and V_4; for V_4 the electrode is at the left midclavicular line in the fifth

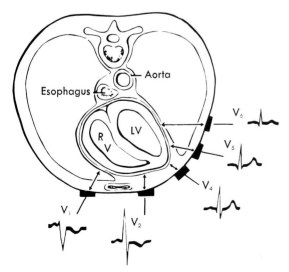

Figure 5-8. Location of the precordial leads V_1–V_6 with the normal patterns at five years of age.

intercostal space; for V_5 the exploring electrode is in the anterior axillary line at the level of V_4; for V_6 the electrode is in the midaxillary line at the same level (Figure 5–8). Similar leads over the right precordium are referred to as RV_3, RV_4, RV_5, and RV_6.

In infants and children the precordial leads are of prime importance in interpreting the electrocardiogram and its underlying pathology. The record should be obtained with care. Small pediatric electrodes should be used to avoid overlapping of electrode areas. With each application of the electrode, the paste from the previous position should be rubbed off since failure to do this may produce a distorted series of tracings (Ziegler, 1951).

In position V_1 the electrocardiograph normally registers an initially upright QRS deflection. This is due to activation of the septum, which takes place from left to right and therefore is toward the exploring electrode. This is usually followed by a major downward deflection, or S wave, during left ventricular activation. This wave is negative since the electrical activation of the left ventricle is traveling away from the electrode over the right precordium. A second R wave due to activation of the right ventricular wall frequently follows.

One of the most important electrode positions in studying the left ventricle is V_6, lying in the midaxillary line at the level of the fifth intercostal space. The activation process in this area consists initially of a downward deflection due to the activation of the septum, which is away from the electrode. As the electrical activity spreads through the left ventricle, it produces a tall upright R wave in the electrocardiogram.

Thus, over the right ventricle the R wave is chiefly due to the right ventricular activity, and the S wave is due to the left ventricular activity. Over the left ventricle the R wave is due to the left ventricular activity and the S wave chiefly to the right ventricular

Lead II

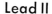

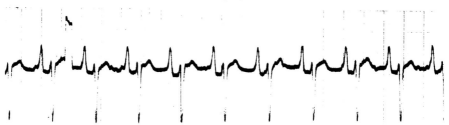

Figure 5-9. Tall peaked P waves, indicating right atrial hypertrophy.

activity. As one proceeds from the right to the left across the chest, the point where the right ventricular pattern changes to that of the left is referred to as the transitional complex.

An unusually tall R wave over the right ventricle or a deep S wave over the left ventricle is associated with right ventricular hypertrophy. An unusually deep S over the right ventricle and an abnormally tall R wave over the left ventricle are associated with left ventricular hypertrophy. In newborn babies the right ventricle is normally as large as the left and, therefore, registers a taller R than appears in older children whose left ventricular mass far outweighs the right. By comparing the tracing from V_1 to V_6, one may find a dominant right ventricular pattern, or, at times, a dominant left ventricular pattern, or a pattern that is within normal limits.

The return of the muscle cell to the resting state is inscribed by the T wave. The S-T segment of the electrocardiogram lies between the QRS and the T wave; the area enclosed by the QRS complex is equal to that enclosed by the T wave, provided the S-T segment is on the base line. When the S-T segment is elevated or depressed, the area between it and the base line is added on to the T wave area.

Electrocardiographic Deflections. The P wave records the spread of the excitation wave through the atrium from the sinus node and is usually upright in standard lead II. The P wave is normally less than 2.5 mm under one year of age and less than 3 mm from 1 to 14 years of age (Ziegler, 1951). Its duration is less than 0.07 second under one year of age and less than 0.09 second from 1 to 14 years of age. It is normally upright in leads I and II but may be inverted at times in lead III (10 percent of normal children). At times it is followed by a smaller atrial T wave (T.A.). This small T.A. wave is better seen in heart block or in atrial flutter and is best studied in lead II.

The P wave may be abnormally tall, indicating right atrial hypertrophy (Figure 5-9). This is found in a number of heart defects, such as tricuspid atresia, tetralogy of Fallot, and pulmonary stenosis with a normal aortic root. In these conditions, the P wave is characteristically narrow and pointed. It also may be somewhat elevated and broadened in mitral stenosis. Such broadening is indicative of left atrial hypertrophy (Figure 5–10).

A decrease in amplitude may occur with reflex vagal stimulation, such as pressure on the carotid sinus or in instances of sinus arrhythmia. It may also be produced by digitalis administration. The P wave in lead I is characteristically inverted in dextrocardia if the venous atrium is to the left of the midline.

The absence of a P wave may be due to its being buried in a QRS or T wave as sometimes occurs in nodal rhythm, paroxysmal tachycardia, or atrioventricular block. A P wave is not seen in atrial fibrillation.

P-R Interval. The P-R interval is usually measured in standard lead II from the beginning of the upstroke of the P wave to the beginning of the QRS complex. White et al. (1941) pointed out that this may lead to some error since lead II may not always portray the true P-R interval. Ziegler (1951), amplifying this, points out that in children the P-R segment in lead II stands a 60 percent chance of being either shorter or longer than this interval in other leads. In spite of this source of error, the measurement is of some clinical value although minor deviations should not be overstressed.

The P-R interval varies with age. At five years of age the maximum is 0.16 second (Ziegler, 1951) and

Lead II

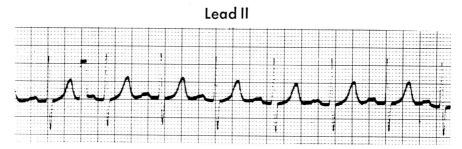

Figure 5-10. Broad biphasic P waves, indicating left atrial hypertrophy.

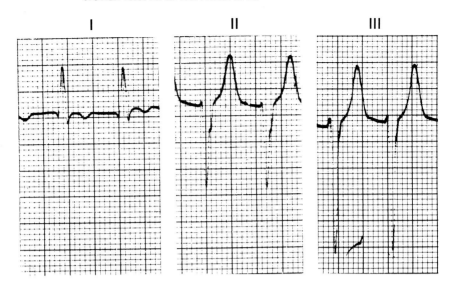

Figure 5-11. Left-axis deviation.

usually averages 0.12 second. From 5 to 16 years of age the maximum is 0.20 second and it is rarely over 0.17 second in this age group. It varies slightly with change in heart rate (Alimurung et al., 1951).

QRS Complex.   The QRS complex is due to the spread of the excitation wave through the ventricle. When an initial downward deflection is present, it is referred to as a Q wave. The first upright deflection is the R wave, whether or not there is a preceding Q wave. The downward deflection following the R wave is called the S wave. A second upright deflection in the QRS complex is called the R prime (R') wave.

A Q wave is commonly found in standard leads II and III in normal children and infants (75 percent of cases). It is less common in standard lead I (25 to 45 percent). In standard lead I the Q wave is never over 25 percent of the R wave and is rarely over 3 mm in height. It does not occur normally in the chest leads V_1 and V_2 but is present in V_6 in approximately 90 percent of normal children.

The height of the R wave should be over 5 mm in the most favorable lead. Slight notching or slowing of the R wave is common and is rarely significant.

The maximum normal duration of the QRS complex is 0.08 second from birth to three years, 0.09 second from three to eight years, and 0.10 second from 8 to 16 years. The QRS interval is prolonged in left or right bundle branch block and conditions with aberrant ventricular conduction such as the Wolff-Parkinson-White syndrome.

The frontal QRS axis is derived from the six frontal leads (I, II, III, AVR, AVL, AVF), which gives the main direction of the electrical forces. The normal frontal axis for children is between 0 and 90 degrees but lies to the right of this (60 to 150 degrees) for the first month of life. Abnormalities in electrical axis may imply right or left ventricular enlargement or even a specific anatomic diagnosis. Left-axis deviation, 270 to 360 degrees, suggests tricuspid atresia in a cyanotic infant or an endocardial cushion defect in an acyanotic one (Figure 5-11). Right-axis deviation, an axis greater than 120 degrees after one month of age, is seen with right ventricular hypertrophy in a number of conditions (Figure 5-12).

S-T Segment.   This is the short segment between the QRS complex and the T wave. It may be very brief at times—so short, in fact, that the RS wave blends immediately with the beginning of the T. The

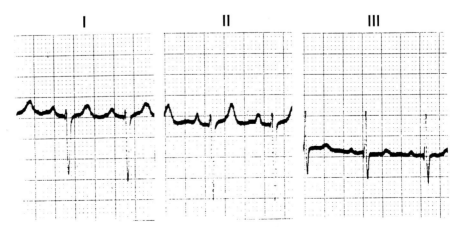

Figure 5-12. Right-axis deviation.

displacement is rarely over 1 mm and should never exceed 2 mm in the standard leads. In the precordial leads it may be displaced up to 4 mm, particularly over the right precordium.

T Wave. The T wave represents the recovery process, or repolarization, and it is normally upright in standard leads I and II but may be inverted in lead III. It should be at least 2 mm in the most favorable lead.

In the chest leads Ziegler found the T upright in V_1 in 75 percent of newborns in the first eight hours, whereas in V_6 it was upright in only 50 percent of cases during the same period. After 60 to 96 hours the T wave in V_1 is invariably inverted in normal babies, and by the end of the first week the T wave in V_6 is always upright. The T waves in V_1 are normally inverted until 12 years of age, when they may become upright. They are usually upright after 16 years of age.

Q-T Interval. The Q-T interval is measured by the interval lying between the beginning of the QRS complex and the end of the T wave. Its duration is inversely proportional to the heart rate. Kissin, Schwarzschild, and Bakst (1948) corrected the Q-T interval for heart rate and referred to it as the QT_c. The QT_c may be prolonged in hypercalcemia, rheumatic carditis, cardiac failure, and other forms of heart disease. QT_c prolongation is an essential feature of the surdocardiac syndrome.

U Wave. Following the T wave there may be a small positive deflection known as the U wave. It may be amplified by digitalis; however, its significance is not clear.

Right Bundle Branch Block. In complete right bundle branch block the septum and left ventricle are activated first. Since the septum is activated from the left side, deflections overlying the right precordium are initially positive. The following characteristics have been established as indicative of this abnormality. A widened QRS complex of 0.12 second or more is considered essential for the diagnosis in adults; in children, however, complete bundle branch block is probably present when the QRS exceeds the normal duration for the age concerned. There is a delayed activation time in the right ventricle, as one would expect, and an increased amplitude of the R' in the right precordial leads indicative of stimulus invading the right ventricle unopposed by the left, since it follows the left ventricular activation. The right precordial leads may show inverted T waves, but this is a normal finding in children in any case and is therefore not pathologic. There is a normal activation time in the left precordial leads and frequently a broad, slurred S wave (Figure 5–13).

Right bundle branch block may occur in perfectly normal children, but it is more frequently found in conjunction with congenital heart defects, especially those with right ventricular dilatation and hypertrophy, such as Ebstein's disease and double-outlet right ventricle. In addition, right bundle branch block is frequently found after surgical closure of ventricular septal defects. The anatomy of the right bundle makes it vulnerable during closure (Lev et al., 1964). Furthermore, it is now clear that right ventriculotomy alone can cause interruption of the peripheral right bundle and complete right bundle branch block on the surface electrocardiogram (Gelband et al., 1971).

INCOMPLETE RIGHT BUNDLE BRANCH BLOCK. The presence of an RSR' pattern in V_1 or RV_3 with a QRS duration that is prolonged but less than in right bundle branch block is frequently called incomplete right bundle branch block. This may be a normal finding but is usually associated with conditions that have right ventricular dilatation such as secundum atrial septal defect or atrioventricularis communis. When the increased right ventricular preload is removed, the RSR' pattern will frequently revert to normal.

V_1 V_6

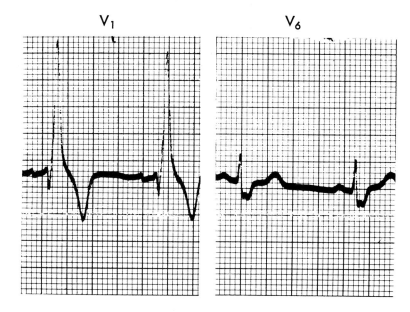

Figure 5-13. Precordial leads V_1 and V_6 in right bundle branch block.

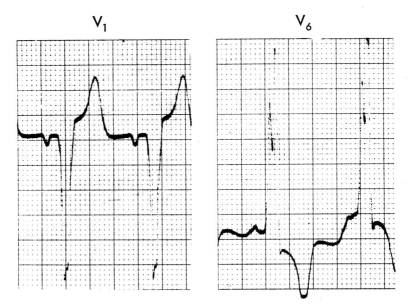

Figure 5-14. Precordial leads V_1 and V_6 in left bundle branch block.

Left Bundle Branch Block. Left bundle branch block is an uncommon finding in children. When present, it is characterized by a widened QRS interval of 0.12 second or more and a normal ventricular activation time in the right ventricle with an initially positive R followed by a deep S, which is notched. Over the left ventricle there is a delayed activation time and increased amplitude of the R'. The initial positive R over the left ventricle is due to the depolarization of the septum from right to left toward the electrode, followed by an S wave due to the spread of the stimulus from the left ventricle to the right ventricle, and a final R' due to the eventual spread of the activation to the left ventricle (Figure 5–14).

Since the bundle is blocked, stimulus in the septum is reversed, and one does not find a Q wave over the left precordium. Exceptions to this rule occur but they are rare.

Ventricular Hypertrophy or Enlargement. The normal QRS pattern derives from a balance of the potentials between the right and left ventricles. In right ventricular hypertrophy there is an increase in the mass of the right ventricle, which causes the precordial leads overlying that ventricle to show abnormally high voltage in the electrocardiographic tracing. When left ventricular hypertrophy is present, a similar abnormal pattern appears over the left ventricle.

In right ventricular hypertrophy (Figure 5–15) the following characteristics appear. (1) There is usually an increased amplitude of the R waves over the right precordium, that is, in RV_3, V_1, and V_2, due to the increase in muscle mass and size of the right ventricle.

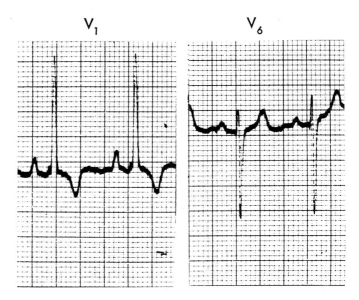

Figure 5-15. Electrocardiogram demonstrating right ventricular hypertrophy. Note the tall P in V_1 indicating that right atrial hypertrophy is also present.

$$V_1 \qquad\qquad V_6$$

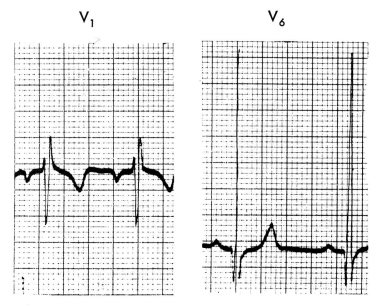

Figure 5-16. Electrocardiogram demonstrating left ventricular hypertrophy.

(2) A comparison of the height of the R and the depth of the S over the right precordial leads, the R/S ratio, will also be of value in determining the presence or absence of right ventricular hypertrophy. (3) Right-axis deviation is frequently present but is not invariably found. Also, right-axis deviation may be present in some normal individuals with a vertical electrical position of the heart. (4) Enlarged P waves may be present in right ventricular hypertrophy since the abnormality causing the increased load on the right ventricle may also increase the load on the right atrium. (5) Ziegler (1951) has demonstrated that the T wave in the right precordium is frequently upright during the first 24 hours of life; after that, in the first year, it is normally inverted in V_1. He also pointed out that the presence of an upright T after the first 24 hours of life is indicative of right ventricular hypertrophy. We have found upright T waves in V_1 in normal infants up to three days of age. Since an upright T may occur normally at 12 years of age in V_1, there is a span from the first week of life to 12 years of age where the presence of right ventricular hypertrophy may be suspected from the presence of an upright T in V_1. The upright T is significant in this age group when there is other evidence of right ventricular hypertrophy in the electrocardiographic pattern such as an R/S ratio in V_1 of 1 or greater. (6) When there is marked evidence of right ventricular hypertrophy in the electrocardiogram, the T wave is often inverted in the right precordial leads to a degree that is deeper than normal. Such is the case in children with valvular pulmonic stenosis and a normal aortic root, where the pressure in the right ventricle can be as high as 150 to 200 mm of mercury. (7) As the tall R in the right precordial leads is indicative of right ventricular hypertrophy, a deep S in the left precordial leads is of similar significance. (8) The presence of a QR pattern in the right precordial leads, R V_3 or V_1, is almost invariably associated with right

ventricular hypertrophy. A similar pattern, that of small Q, tall R, little S, big R′, is also associated with right ventricular hypertrophy.

Left Ventricular Hypertrophy. The patterns related to left ventricular hypertrophy (Figure 5–16) are as follows. (1) Left-axis deviation is frequently, but not invariably, present with left ventricular hypertrophy. (2) Over the left precordium in chest leads V_5 and V_6, one finds a tall R wave, greater than the upper limits of normal for the age of the child. Similarly, from the hypertrophied left ventricle, the S wave over the right precordium may descend to a greater depth than normal for age. (3) With minor degrees of hypertrophy of the left ventricle, the T wave may become higher over the left precordium; but, when the left ventricular hypertrophy becomes more marked, there may be flattening or inversion of the T waves in V_5 or V_6. (4) The duration of the QRS complex over the left precordium may be increased as a result of the hypertrophy of the left ventricle.

ELECTROCARDIOGRAPHIC CRITERIA FOR VENTRICULAR HYPERTROPHY. Although certain patterns, especially in the precordial leads, of the electrocardiogram are indicative or suggestive of right or left ventricular hypertrophy, it is helpful to have certain criteria that may be reasonably decisive in estimating the presence or absence of hypertrophy.

CRITERIA FOR VENTRICULAR HYPERTROPHY

RIGHT VENTRICULAR HYPERTROPHY

1. Voltage of R in V_1 greater than maximum for age (Table 5–3).
2. Voltage of S in V_6 greater than maximum for age (Table 5–3).
3. R/S ratio in V_1 greater than maximum normal for age (Table 5–3).

4. Positive T in V_1 after third day of life when R/S ratio greater than 1.0.
5. qR pattern in right precordial lead V_1.

LEFT VENTRICULAR HYPERTROPHY

1. Voltage of R in V_6 greater than maximum normal for age (Table 5–4).
2. Voltage of S in V_1 greater than maximum normal for age (Table 5–4).
3. Secondary T wave inversion in V_5 and/or V_6.
4. Deep Q wave, ≥ 4 mm, over the left precordium.

COMBINED VENTRICULAR HYPERTROPHY

1. Direct signs of right plus left ventricular hypertrophy (as above).
2. Direct signs of right ventricular hypertrophy with the following signs in left chest leads:
   a. q wave (2 mm or more)
   b. sizable R (voltage not necessarily abnormal) with tall, positive T in V_6
   c. T inversion, after a positive T in right chest leads
3. Direct signs of left ventricular hypertrophy with:
   a. sizable R or R′ in right chest leads (voltage not necessarily abnormal) or R/S ratio greater than 1.0
   b. marked clockwise rotation of QRS vector
4. Apparently normal electrocardiogram in the presence of marked true cardiac enlargement.

Examples of varying degrees of right and left ventricular hypertrophy and other characteristics of the electrocardiogram in children are shown in Figures 5–17, 5–18, 5–19, and 5–20.

Right ventricular hypertrophy is suggested if the measurements shown in Table 5–3 are exceeded.

Left ventricular hypertrophy is suggested if the measurements shown in Table 5–4 are exceeded.

LEFT VENTRICULAR HYPERTROPHY. The presence of left ventricular hypertrophy in the electrocardiogram is most useful diagnostically in infants because it narrows down the possibilities to a relatively few conditions.

If cyanosis is associated with left ventricular hypertrophy, the most common heart anomalies encountered are tricuspid atresia and pulmonary atresia with normal aortic root.

In the noncyanotic group in the first six months of life, this pattern is associated with endocardial fibroelastosis, left coronary arising from the pulmonary artery, glycogen storage disease, coronary calcinosis, aortic stenosis, and subaortic stenosis.

After one year of age, a left ventricular hypertrophy pattern is likely to be associated with coarctation of the aorta, aortic stenosis, ventricular septal defect, patent ductus arteriosus, well-established mitral insufficiency, prolonged isolated myocarditis, prolonged arterial hypertension, or aorticopulmonary septal defect.

Table 5–3.   CRITERIA FOR RIGHT VENTRICULAR HYPERTROPHY MAXIMAL MEASUREMENTS BY AGE GROUPS* (PRECORDIAL LEADS)

WAVE	AGE	MEASUREMENT, IN MILLIMETERS
R in V_1	0–24 hours	20
	1–7 days	29
	8 days–3 months	20
	3 months–16 years	19 or more
S in V_6	0–7 days	14
	8–30 days	10
	1–3 months	7
	3 months–16 years	5 or more
R/S in V_1	0–3 months	6.5
	3–6 months	4.0
	6 months–3 years	2.4
	3–5 years	1.6
	6–15 years	0.8 or more

T waves may be normally

Lead	*Inverted*	*Diphasic*
V_1	Up to 16 years	Up to 16 years
V_2	Up to 12 years	Up to 16 years
V_3	Up to 10 years	Up to 15 years
V_4	Up to 5 years	Up to 11 years
V_5	Up to 15 hours of life	Up to 14 hours of life
V_6	Up to 8 hours of life	Up to 24 hours of life

V_1 is normally upright in first 24 hours of life.
V_2 is normally upright after 12 years of age.

* Most of these measurements are adapted from standards published by Ziegler (*Electrocardiographic Studies in Infants and Children*. Charles C Thomas, Publisher, Springfield, Ill., 1951).

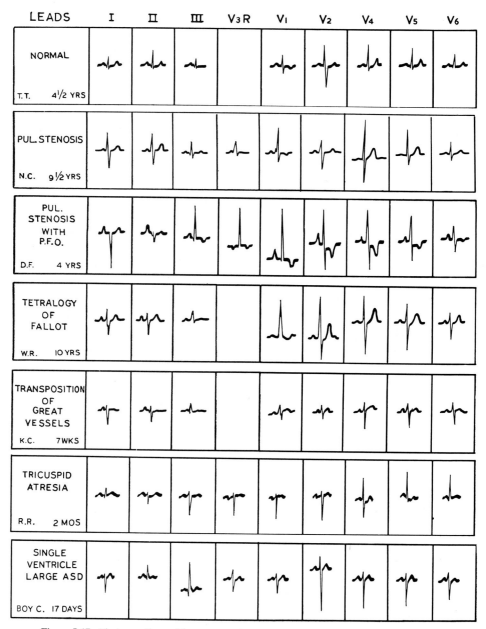

Figure 5-17. Electrocardiographic patterns of various types of heart disease in childhood.

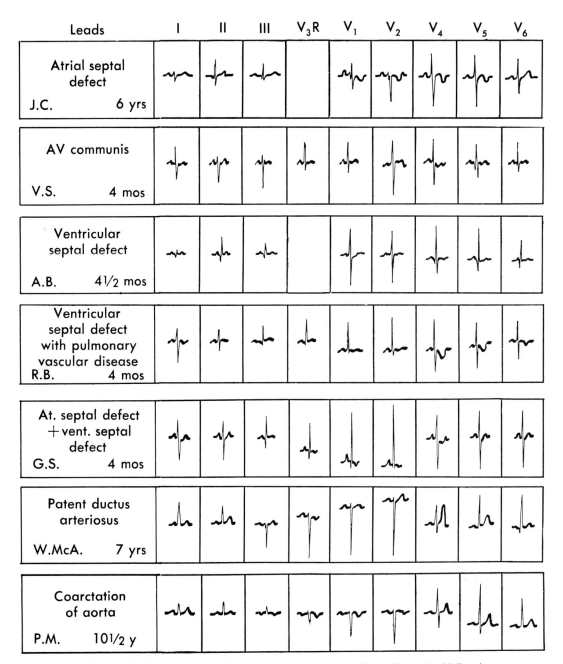

Figure 5-18. Electrocardiographic patterns of various types of heart disease in childhood.

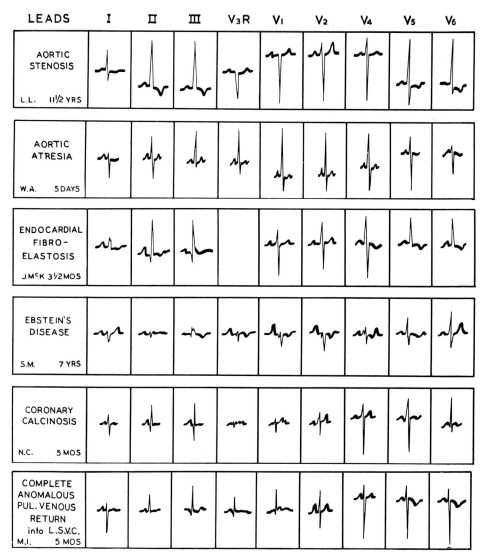

Figure 5·19. Electrocardiographic patterns of various types of heart disease in childhood.

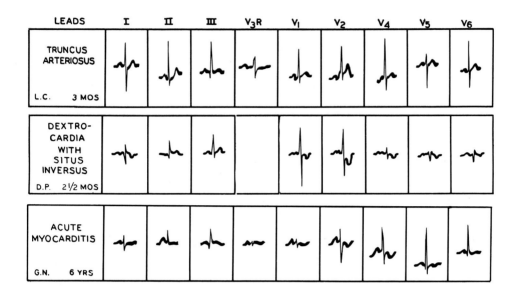

Figure 5-20. Electrocardiographic patterns of various types of heart disease in childhood.

RIGHT VENTRICULAR HYPERTROPHY. The presence of a right ventricular hypertrophy pattern is much less useful diagnostically since such a wide variety of conditions may have this finding. Right ventricular hypertrophy patterns are found commonly in the cyanotic group and include tetralogy of Fallot, transposition of the great vessels, single ventricle, aortic atresia, congenital mitral stenosis, cor pulmonale, persistent truncus arteriosus, pulmonary stenosis with patent foramen ovale, total anomalous venous drainage into the right side of the heart, Eisenmenger's complex, and primary pulmonary hypertension.

The noncyanotic group with right ventricular hypertrophy is chiefly made up of those with atrial septal defect, atrioventricularis communis, pulmonary stenosis, ventricular septal defect with pulmonary hypertension, patent ductus arteriosus with reversal of flow, coarctation of the aorta in the first six months of life, primary pulmonary hypertension, and aorticopulmonary septal defect.

COMBINED RIGHT AND LEFT VENTRICULAR HYPERTROPHY. This combination is commonly found in large ventricular septal defects, coarctation of the aorta with a large ventricular septal defect or a large patent ductus arteriosus below the coarctation, truncus arteriosus, transposition of the great vessels with associated anomalies, and single ventricle.

NO EVIDENCE OF VENTRICULAR HYPERTROPHY. There may be an absence of a ventricular hypertrophy pattern in any of the conditions listed when they are mild, such as mild aortic stenosis, small ventricular septal defect, small atrial septal defect, minimal pulmonary stenosis, minimal patency of the ductus arteriosus, and minimal coarctation of the aorta. A normal pattern may also be found in glycogen storage disease, myocarditis, and rheumatic heart disease, although characteristically these three conditions show hypertrophy.

Vectorcardiography

In addition to the electrocardiogram, we often obtain a vectorcardiogram in three planes to observe the direction and magnitude of the maximum QRS vector. This information aids in assessing ventricular hypertrophy or dilatation and can be especially useful in children with complex ventricular anatomy where the usual electrocardiographic criteria may not apply.

Various lead systems for vectorcardiography have been tested in children. The tetrahedron and cube systems have been replaced in most centers by the Frank system, which has proved to be reliable and reproducible (Pipberger and Lilienfield, 1958). Although the vectorcardiogram is classically displayed in a series of three planes; frontal, horizontal, and sagittal, each plane represents the integrated function of two of the three orthogonal leads that the system actually records. The orthogonal leads—x, right to left; y, superior to inferior; and z, anterior to posterior—can be viewed as independent entities and as such are amenable to computer analysis (Ellison and Restieaux, 1972).

If the vectorcardiographic loops are studied, their magnitude and direction can be compared with normals (Hugenholtz and Liebman, 1962). Figure

Table 5–4. CRITERIA FOR LEFT VENTRICULAR HYPERTROPHY MAXIMAL MEASUREMENTS BY AGE GROUPS* (PRECORDIAL LEADS)

WAVE	AGE	MEASUREMENT, IN MILLIMETERS
S in V_1	0–1 day	28
	1 day–1 year	19
	1 year–16 years	25 or more
R in V_5	0–3 years	30
	3–16 years	35 or more
R in V_6	0–6 months	16
	6–12 months	19
	1 year–16 years	21 or more

S–T segment depressed in V_5 or V_6
T waves inverted in left precordium may be found in severe left ventricular hypertrophy

T waves may be normally

Lead	Inverted	Diphasic
V_4	Up to 5 years	Up to 11 years
V_5	Up to 15 hours	Up to 14 hours
V_6	Up to 8 hours	Up to 24 hours

* Most of these measurements are adapted from standards published by Ziegler (*Electrocardiographic Studies in Infants and Children.* Charles C Thomas, Publisher, Springfield, Ill., 1951).

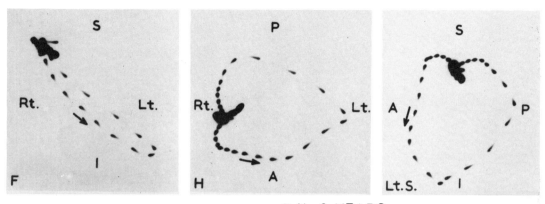

R.K. 8 YEARS

Figure 5-21. R.K., eight-year-old boy—normal heart. Axis of +50 degrees in frontal plane, counterclockwise loop in horizontal plane.

5–21 shows a normal vectorcardiogram and electrocardiogram in an eight-year-old boy.

The frontal plane is derived from the x and y leads. It is useful in determining the mean QRS axis. This does not always correlate with the scalar electrocardiogram and is usually considered to be a more accurate representation of the true direction of the electrical axis than the latter.

The horizontal loop is derived from the x and z

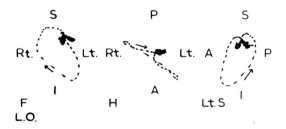

Figure 5-22. L. O., six-year-old girl—pulmonary stenosis without cyanosis with gradient between right ventricle and pulmonary artery of 110 mm of mercury. The frontal plane axis is +100 degrees. The horizontal vector shows right hypertrophy being displaced anteriorly and to the right.

leads. The loop should be counterclockwise and to the left of the E point after one year of age. An anterior loop that is clockwise or figure of eight in configuration is a clear indication of right ventricular hypertrophy (Figure 5–22).

The sagittal plane indicates whether the predominant inferior forces are being directed anteriorly or posteriorly. In left ventricular hypertrophy, a more posterior deflection will be seen (Figure 5–23) with high voltage. The y and z leads are used to derive this plane.

The magnitude of the maximum right and left vectors can be calculated in each plane from the zero or E point. However, this only represents two dimensions at a time. Ellison and Restieaux (1972) advocated the calculation of the maximal right and left vectors using the orthogonal leads and timed, simultaneous analysis. The three-dimensional maximum vector is obtained when the maximum $\sqrt{x^2 + y^2 + z^2}$ is reached with a positive x, maximum left spatial voltage; or negative x, maximum right spatial voltage.

A recent group of studies has been performed to use vectorcardiographic data to predict ventricular pressures. This has been done for the left ventricle in aortic stenosis (Fowler et al., 1972), the right ventricle

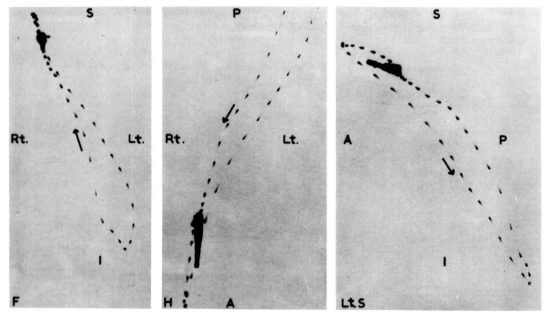

Figure 5-23. L.V.L., 14-year-old boy—ventricular septal defect plus aortic insufficiency. The vector shows marked left ventricular loading, indicated by the magnitude of the maximum spatial vectors in all planes.

in pulmonic stenosis, and the left ventricle in transposition of the great vessels (Roberts and Fowler, 1973). The usefulness of these formulae will have to be tested against other noninvasive techniques for accuracy in predicting hemodynamic data.

PHONOCARDIOGRAPHY AND SYSTOLIC TIME INTERVALS

Kenneth R. Bloom

Phonocardiography

Phonocardiography is a technique by which cardiac sounds and murmurs can be both visualized and accurately timed. This has great educational potential for the physician and student and may also aid significantly in the noninvasive assessment of the patient.

The method of performing the study is important if a record capable of adequate interpretation is to be obtained. A physician who has a thorough knowledge of the clinical problem of the patient should be responsible for the procedure. The record should be obtained in a quiet room. The phonocardiograph should be recorded simultaneously with the carotid pulse, electrocardiogram, and respiration.

The phonocardiogram can record some low-frequency sounds that are inaudible to the human ear (Kincaid-Smith and Barlow, 1959). The main clinical value, however, is in the timing of the sounds and murmurs. It may be difficult to clinically differentiate a normally split first heart sound from a fourth heart sound or an ejection or nonejection click (Fowler and Adolph, 1972). A phonocardiogram can help to differentiate these, and a patient may then either be confidently declared normal or the appropriate specific advice given.

The use of this technique to predict the severity of disease has received much attention over the years. Leatham and Weitzman (1957) showed that a good correlation existed between the expiratory splitting of the second heart sound and the right ventricular systolic pressure in valvar pulmonary stenosis. This may also be correlated with the presence of a fourth heart sound (Yahini et al., 1960), the delay of the peak, and the duration of the ejection systolic murmur in this condition (Vogelpoel and Schrire, 1960). Fixed or minimal (< 0.02 second) movement of the second heart sound on respiration has been found to occur in atrial septal defect with a moderate or large left-to-right shunt. (Aygen and Braunwald, 1962). When pulmonary hypertension complicates the atrial septal defect, the fixed wide splitting may disappear (Ibid., 1962). These findings are not invariable (Cohn et al., 1967; Myler and Sanders, 1967).

The degree of severity of valvar aortic stenosis may be assessed by the presence or absence of a left-sided fourth heart sound (Goldblatt et al., 1962) together with the measurement of the delay of the peak intensity of the systolic ejection murmur (Oakley and Hallidie-Smith, 1967).

The effects of drugs such as amyl nitrite or phenylephrine, changes in posture, and other physiologic maneuvers such as the valsalva on the murmur can be graphically assessed by use of a phonocardiogram.

Phonocardiography can be utilized successfully in children if sufficient time and care are taken over the procedure. The results, which may spare a child catheterization and may also help to plan rational therapy, are worth this effort. The preceding comments are brief references to the procedure and readers are referred to some comprehensive reviews on this subject: McKusick, 1958; Leatham, 1975; Tavel, 1972.

Systolic Time Intervals

The systolic time intervals of the left ventricle are measured as outlined in Figure 5–24.

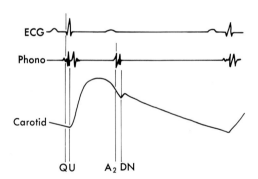

Figure 5-24. Systolic time intervals of the left ventricle.

The parameters that are usually measured are the following:

1. Total electromechanical systole: This is the time measured from the onset of the Q wave of the electrocardiogram to the aortic component of the second heart sound (Q-A$_2$).

2. The left ventricular ejection time (LVET): This is the time measured from the onset of the upstroke of the carotid pulse to the trough of the dicrotic notch (U–DN). Note that the carotid pulse is usually delayed by an average of 0.02 second compared to the intracardiac events. This does not affect the calculations.

3. The preejection period (PEP) is obtained by subtracting the LVET from the Q-A$_2$ interval.

Systolic time intervals should be recorded on strip chart recorders with paper speeds of at least 100 mm/second. The error in calculation at this rate is about 5 milliseconds. Systolic time intervals may also be measured directly from the echocardiogram (Vredevoe et al., 1974).

The systolic time intervals differ in children and they vary with both age and heart rate (Harris et al., 1964; Golde and Burstin, 1970). The ratio of the PEP/LVET is used frequently as this is not influenced by heart rate within the range of 40 to 110 beats/minute (Lewis et al., 1974). This ratio seems to correlate well with the ejection fraction as calculated at cardiac catheterization in both valvular and nonvalvular heart disease (Garrard et al., 1970).

The widest clinical use of systolic time intervals has been in aortic stenosis. In particular this method seems to have value in the assessment of the efficacy of surgery in aortic valve disease. (Benchimol and Matsuo, 1971; Parisi et al., 1971). Compensated valvar aortic stenosis results in a shortening of the PEP and lengthening of the LVET. Primary myocardial disease, however, results in a lengthening of the PEP and shortening of the LVET.

Systolic time intervals therefore provided one with a noninvasive method of evaluating and quantitating left ventricular performance in various pathologic situations. Repeated observations can be made with no distress to the patient. Valuable information can be gained concerning the initial state of the patient and his response to therapy. Comprehensive reviews on this subject have been published (Tavel, 1972; Lewis et al., 1974).

ECHOCARDIOGRAPHY
Kenneth R. Bloom

Background

Ultrasound was applied rationally to cardiac diagnosis in 1953 by Drs. Edler and Hertz. Extensive periods of research and development followed over the next years with most investigation being directed to problems involving mitral valve function, pericardial effusions, and tumors. Early use in congenital heart disease (Ultan et al., 1967) and then the use of echocardiography in the diagnosis of specific congenital heart disease

(Chesler et al., 1970; Chesler et al. 1971) showed the value of this technique in these conditions. Reliability of the findings in hypoplastic left heart syndrome has led some medical centers to regard catheterization as unnecessary when a clinical and echocardiographic diagnosis of this condition has been made (Meyer and Kaplan, 1973). The use of echocardiography in congenital heart disease has now extended to all areas and its intelligent application can add to the clinical evaluation of every patient.

Instrumentation

Safety.   Pulsed ultrasound is used for echocardiographic diagnosis. The pulse, usually about 1 microsecond in duration, is repeated one to two thousand times per second depending on the make of the ultrasonoscope. This short pulse duration with relatively long intervals between each pulse results in very low energy levels being used for the examination. These levels are at least one thousand times less than those known to produce harmful biologic effects. Extensive experimental work with ultrasound at diagnostic levels has failed to produce any reproducible damaging effects. The technique has now been used for more than 20 years with no demonstrable side effects. It would seem to be an extremely safe procedure for both the patient and the practitioner (King and Lele, 1974; Meyer, 1974).

Equipment.   A typical ultrasound machine is one capable of delivering pulses of short duration, as described, through a transducer that determines the frequency of the pulse. The returning impulse, received through the same transducer, is then electronically processed and displayed on an oscilloscope that should have a moderately long persistence phosphor. This is then recorded either by photographing the screen with a Polaroid-type camera, or by interfacing the ultrasonoscope to a strip chart recorder. The latter method is preferable in pediatric work as it enables one to record long sweeps and so to identify structural relationships. Direct photography limits one to sweeps of only a few seconds.

The ultrasound transducers vary in frequency. The higher the frequency, the less the degree of penetration, but the higher the resolution. Five-megaHertz (mHz) transducers, usually of 6-mm diameter, are used in infants; 2.5-mHz transducers with a diameter of 13 mm are commonly used in adults. The lower-frequency transducers are usually focused by an acoustic lens to minimize the divergence of the ultrasonic beam at greater tissue depths. Beam divergence is a cause of distortion of the recorded image.

It will be evident from this brief summary that the recorded echocardiogram is not a linear representation of the intracardiac anatomy. Rather, it is an electrically processed and modified image of a reflected beam of ultrasound. As such it is subject to distortion and possible misinterpretation. A full understanding of the equipment and its properties and limitations is essential to an informed use of the technique. The following are reviews on this subject: Baker, 1974; Wells, 1969; Feigenbaum, 1976.

Recent Developments.   Current work has resulted in the development of two-dimensional ultrasound imaging in real time. This includes stop action B scan (King, 1973), sector scanners (Griffith and Henry, 1974), linear phased array scan (Thurstone and von Ramm, 1974), and multicrystal arrays (Bom et al., 1973). These two-dimensional methods may well simplify echocardiographic techniques particularly

in defining the relationships of cardiac structures to each other in complex congenital heart disease (Sahn et al., 1974).

Requirements of the Normal Echocardiogram

The evaluation of the echoes obtained from a study has advanced considerably over the years that the technique has been employed. Currently, determination of ventricular volumes and function, the detection of minor abnormalities of valve motion, and also the demonstration of minor anatomic abnormalities have all required a refining of the echocardiographic technique. It is impossible to standardize the procedure completely as the echocardiographic "window" varies as does the cardiac position from person to person. An appreciation of transducer position and angulation is therefore essential if meaningful and reproducible results are to be obtained. Also, structures being compared should all be measured at the same place. An echocardiogram has become more a method of clinical evaluation than just another imaging technique.

The Technique

The child and operator must both be comfortable. The arm of the operator should be supported. The mitral valve is identified through the echocardiographic "window" usually in the fourth left interspace. The transducer should be perpendicular to the chest when defining this structure. Direction of the ultrasonic beam inferiorly and laterally should define the left ventricular free wall and left septal surface. Measurements taken at this point, just inferior to the mitral valve excursion, should give a true minor axis of the left ventricle. It may not be possible to sweep inferior to the mitral valve echo in very small children, and therefore measurements of the left ventricle in this age group may be suspect. The transducer is then rotated superiorly and medially keeping the mitral valve echo perpendicular as one sweeps up the long axis of the left ventricle. Left ventricular wall is replaced by left atrial wall, as one visualizes the left ventricular outflow tract and then into the aortic root and valve. Angulation of the transducer beam medially from this point should show the tricuspid valve. A return to the aortic valve echo with subsequent superior and lateral angulation outlines the pulmonary valve.

The continual awareness of the relation of one structure to another readily enables one to determine the normal or departures from this. It is essential to have an electrocardiogram recorded at all times to enable one to better identify structures by their movement as related to the cardiac cycle.

The Sweep (Figure 5–25).   This enables one to appreciate the relationship of the various intracardiac

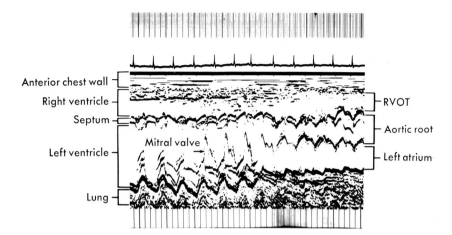

Figure 5-25. Typical findings obtained in a normal sweep. **RVOT** = Right ventricular outflow tract.

structures to each other. Mitral valve–posterior aortic root continuity, septal–anterior aortic root continuity, and the tricuspid valve at the same level as the anterior aortic root can all be assessed. Most measurements are usually made from the structures identified during a sweep as this is done in a standardized fashion.

The Ventricles. Figure 5–26 shows the features obtained from normal left and right ventricles. At birth both ventricles are approximately of equal size,

and the normal relationship is reached only after the neonatal period. The left ventricular free wall and septum are approximately of equal thickness in diastole.

Left ventricular volumes have been shown to correlate well with those obtained angiographically (Gibson, 1973). Differences in the calculations between pediatric and adult age groups must be remembered (Meyer et al., 1975). The determination of volumes is subject to error, and exquisite technique

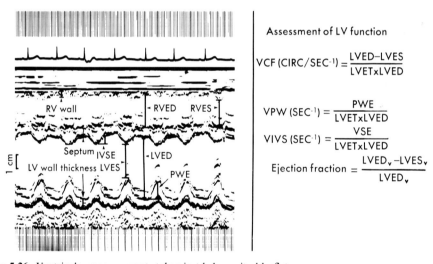

Assessment of LV function

$$VCF (CIRC/SEC^{-1}) = \frac{LVED-LVES}{LVET \times LVED}$$

$$VPW (SEC^{-1}) = \frac{PWE}{LVET \times LVED}$$

$$VIVS (SEC^{-1}) = \frac{VSE}{LVET \times LVED}$$

$$Ejection\ fraction = \frac{LVED_v - LVES_v}{LVED_v}$$

Figure 5-26. Ventricular measurements taken just below mitral leaflet.
VCF　　= Velocity of circumferential fiber shortening.
RV　　 = Right ventricle.
RVED = Right ventricular end-diastolic dimension.
RVES = Right ventricular end-systolic dimension.
LV　　 = Left ventricle.
LVED = Left ventricular end-diastolic dimension.
LVES = Left ventricular end-systolic dimension.
IVSE = Interventricular septal excursion.
VIVS = Velocity of interventricular septal excursion.
PWE = Posterior left ventricular wall excursion.
VPW = Velocity of posterior wall excursion.
LVET = Left ventricular ejection time (best calculated off the aortic valve echo).
Note: % shortening, which is the $\frac{LVED - LVES}{LVED}$, has been used with good clinical correlation. This is similar to ejection fraction but does not require conversion to volumes.

is required to provide reproducible results even in the same patient (Linhart et al., 1975).

Ventricular function has been determined by many parameters obtained from the echocardiogram. All depend on an analysis of the left ventricular posterior wall and/or left septal surface motion (Quinones et al., 1974). Some are shown in Figure 5–26.

Ventricular Septum. Septal motion is complex. The upper third of the septum moves with the aortic root, hence the left septal surface will move anteriorly in systole at this level. Normal left septal surface motion—that is, posteriorly at the onset of systole—will only be seen lower in the ventricle (Figure 5-26). Abnormal septal motion is seen when the left septal surface moves either anteriorly in systole (type A) or has little movement and appears flat (type B). These abnormalities occur in various pathologic states and may be associated with abnormal thickness of this structure (Assad-Morell et al., 1974).

Mitral and Tricuspid Valves. The idealized atrioventricular valve motion is shown in Figure 5–27. There is a wide variation in the normal, however, that has led to many difficulties in the detection of minor degrees of abnormality. The anterior mitral leaflet is not a straight structure (Pohost et al., 1975). As the ultrasonic beam is a divergent one, multiple echoes off this leaflet may be normal. The angle at which the valve is viewed will influence its systolic and diastolic slopes. Caution is therefore required in the interpretation of apparently minor variations from normal (Sahn et al., 1977).

The mitral valve is responsive to hemodynamic changes in both left and right ventricles and may appear to have abnormal movement in certain situations, although it itself is structurally normal (Kamigaki and Goldschlager, 1972; Konecke et al., 1973; Chandraratna et al., 1974).

Aortic and Pulmonary Valves. The aortic valve leaflets show a characteristic box shape (Figure 5–28). Two leaflets, probably the right and noncoronary, are usually visualized. The pulmonary valve has potentially the same pattern, but as the orientation of this valve is more directly toward the anterior chest wall, one usually sees only the posterior cusp of this valve. The visualization of the semilunar cusps enables one to determine systolic time intervals for both right and left ventricles (Stefadouros and Witham, 1975). Identification of the vessel by measurement of these intervals is of particular value in malposition (Solinger et al., 1974; Hirschfeld et al., 1975). The closure of the aortic cusps is usually near the middle of the root (Radford et al., 1976). A fine systolic fluttering of the leaflets is normal.

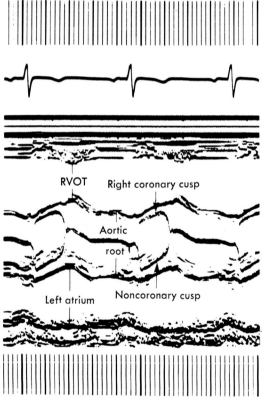

Figure 5-28. Normal aortic root.

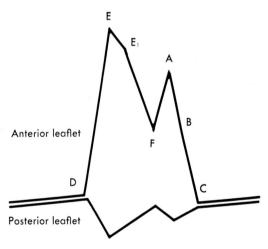

Figure 5-27. Normal AV valve motion.

C	= Onset of ventricular systole.
D	= End of ventricular systole.
E	= Maximum point of opening of anterior leaflet in early diastole.
$E–E_1$	= Early posterior movement of mitral valve ring in diastole.
$E_1–F$	= Diastolic slope of valve.
A	= Further opening of valve following atrial systole.
B slope	= Closing of valve.

Summary

Echocardiography now offers the clinician a truly noninvasive, apparently totally harmless method of visualizing intracardiac anatomy and determining cardiac function.

An enormous amount has been claimed for this technique, much of which can actually be done. Knowledge of the technical limitations of ultrasound enables a rational use that greatly contributes to pediatric cardiologic diagnosis and management. Measurements are reproducible in any one patient, and an objective dimension can be added to the clinical follow-up of the individual.

The abnormal echocardiogram will be considered under the specific abnormalities in subsequent chapters.

NUCLEAR CARDIOLOGY
David L. Gilday and *Richard D. Rowe*

THE congenital heart disease problems that can be evaluated by nuclear medicine are varied (Treves et al., 1976). For this reason several investigative methods have evolved to delineate these problems. The nuclear angiocardiogram is used to assess the route blood follows through the heart and major blood vessels. By adding computer quantification the presence and size of left-to-right shunts can be evaluated. A blood pool radiopharmaceutical for multiple gated images of the heart cavity in conjunction with a myocardial radiopharmaceutical permits assessment of overall myocardial function. The right-to-left shunt is evaluated after the injection of human serum albumin macroaggregates. The assessment of surgically created shunts uses both the previously described techniques.

Left-to-Right Shunts

The nuclear angiocardiogram is performed by injecting a small bolus (less than 1 ml) of technetium-99m albumin (12 mCi/m sq of body surface area) into the external jugular vein via a 21-gauge scalp vein needle and our extension tube stopcock and syringe is set up (Gilday, 1976). The gamma camera is set to record sequential images of the radioactive blood as it passes through the heart and lungs. The framing rate is 1 to 2 per second. The transit of this bolus is also recorded by the computer onto a disk at a rate of 4 frames per second (Medical Data Systems Modumed Trinary 32K).

The analysis of each study is divided into two parts: The first is the visual inspection and assessment of the analog images produced by the gamma camera. The second is the computer analysis of the bolus of radioactive blood as it flows through the lungs to assess any recirculation due to a left-to-right shunt.

The analog images provide a useful pictorial demonstration of the flow of the bolus through the heart and lungs (Figure 5–29). In the normal circumstance the bolus follows the expected route through the right heart to the lungs and back to the left heart and then to the aorta. This is readily seen in the images. It is often difficult to ascertain from these images whether or not a small left-to-right shunt is present. The visualization of a large left-to-right shunt or a single ventricle can usually be identified (Figure 5–30).

Computer analysis provides a much more sensitive method for detecting left-to-right shunts. The frames of data are analyzed to see whether or not the radioactive blood recirculates through the lungs due to the left-to-right shunt. An electronic cursor is placed over the right lung (Figure 5–31), and the pulmonary transit of the radioactivity is determined as a time activity histogram (Figure 5–32). The computer analyzes the transit of the radioactivity through the lungs using a least squares fit to a gamma variate function, first described by Maltz and Treves (Maltz and Treves, 1973). The method gives results that are comparable to the green dye techniques and also is more readily performed (Alderson et al., 1975). In the normal case there is a sharply rising and falling peak of activity shortly after the start of the injection. There will be no sign of a second peak due to recirculation (Figure 5–32). However, if a left-to-right shunt is present, then the second peak will become evident and the gamma variate techniques will calculate a result indicating that the pulmonary-to-systemic flow ratio is greater than the normal (range: 1 to 1.2) (Figure 5–33).

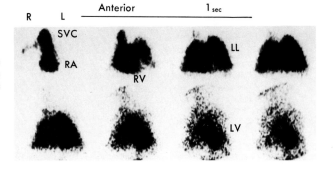

Figure 5-29. Normal heart. The normal sequence of blood flow through the heart and lungs is demonstrated in a three-day-old infant using the pinhole collimator.
SVC = Superior vena cava.
RA = Right atrium.
RV = Right ventricle.
LL = Left lung.
LV = Left ventricle.

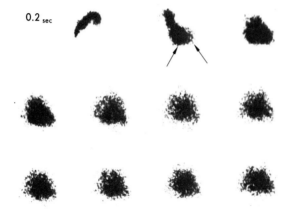

0.2 sec

Figure 5-30. Common ventricle. Blood flows into common chamber (arrow) on entering the heart in this three-day-old infant.

Right-to-Left Shunts

The quantification of right-to-left shunts is done by computing the lung perfusion compared to that of the whole body after the intravenous injection of technetium-99m-labeled macroaggregates of albumin or human serum albumin microspheres. Each part of the body is carefully imaged by the gamma camera using lead shielding to eliminate activity from the areas that are not directly in the field of view. Thus a mosaic image of the whole body can be recorded in the computer and a total count performed. Then by using the electronic cursors over each lung, a lung count can be performed. The result is a ratio of the lung to whole-body activity, which is an indication of the amount of shunted blood (Gates et al., 1973). In the abnormal case there is very high degree of

shunting, and thus one can see activity in the cerebral cortex and kidneys (Figure 5–34).

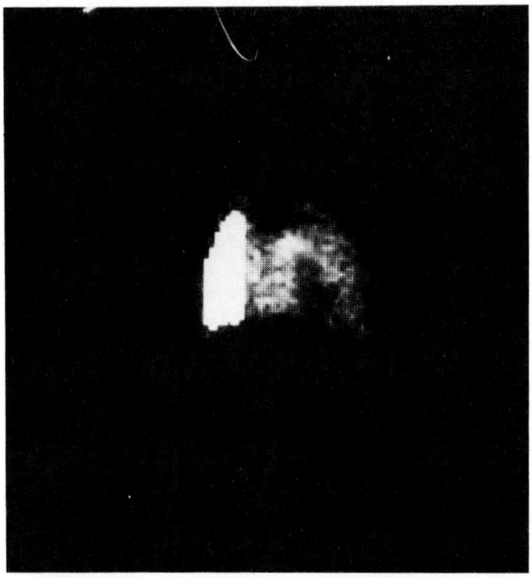

Evaluation of Surgically Created Shunts

To assess the function of surgically created shunts that are commonly used in treating congenital heart disease one makes use of both the radionuclide angiogram and the perfusion study. The choice depends upon the type of surgical shunt.

In patients with a Glenn shunt there may arise questions of its continuing patency. The situation is

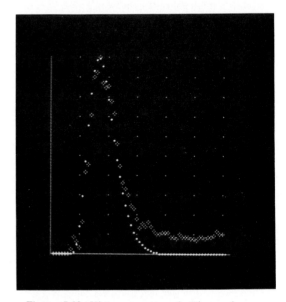

Figure 5-32. Histogram—normal. The peak represents the transit through the lung. The width of the peak must be narrow so that the clearance from the lung will be as complete as possible. The rise and fall of the activity in the superior vena cava must take less than two seconds to go from 10 percent to 10 percent for the data to be valid.

Figure 5-31. Regions of interest. The cursor has been placed over the right lung. It is set to exclude the heart and great vessels.

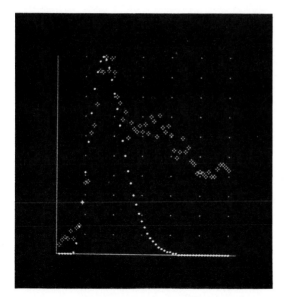

Figure 5-33. Histogram recirculation. The initial peak has a second peak starting on the downslope, indicating recirculation due to a left-to-right shunt.

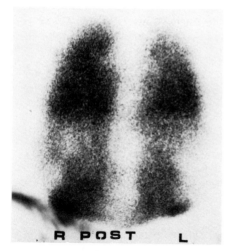

Figure 5-34. Tetralogy of Fallot. In addition to the lung radioactivity the kidneys are seen. The Tc-99m-MAA have passed through the right-to-left shunt and have temporarily occluded some of the renal arterioles.

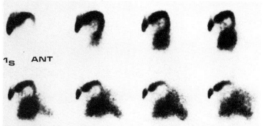

Figure 5-35. Functioning Glenn anastomosis—bolus technique. The radioactive blood passes through the superior vena cava to the right pulmonary artery to the lung, then from the pulmonary vein to the left heart and into the left lung.

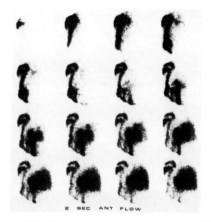

Figure 5-36. Obstructed superior vena cava and Glenn anastomosis. The radioactive blood enters the right brachiocephalic vein but does not pass into the superior vena cava. Instead the blood flows through chest wall collaterals to the inferior vena cava, then into the right heart. From there it passes into the left lung.

most readily assessed by injecting a bolus of radioactivity into the right antecubital fossa and imaging the flow of radioactive blood as it passes through the superior vena cava to the right pulmonary artery, the lungs, and then back to the left side of the heart (Figure 5–35). When venous collaterals are apparent, the implication is that there is either high backpressure from the lung or, more usually, narrowing or occlusion of the anastomosis (Figure 5–36). One can also evaluate this type of shunt by injecting technetium-99m-labeled macro-aggregates of human serum albumin, which will temporarily occlude the first capillary bed that these particles impinge upon. If injected via the superior vena cava, then these particles will lodge in the right lung, whereas if the injection is via the inferior vena cava, then they will lodge in the left lung (Figure 5–37).

In using the same technique just described one can evaluate shunts that have been created from the aorta to the pulmonary arteries. This involves the estimation of the amount of blood flow out of the left side of the heart that goes to the lungs as opposed to the whole body. This requires that the pulmonary artery at the pulmonic valve be either atretic or severely stenotic to have valid results. However, one can estimate the amount of blood flowing out of the two chambers of the heart to the pulmonary circulation by this same technique. This has proved to be valuable in Waterston and Pott's anastomoses.

Blalock shunts are the most difficult to evaluate as they cause an additional blood flow to the lung from the systemic circulation. In such circumstances the best technique requires a preoperative study and this is used as a base line for comparison to the

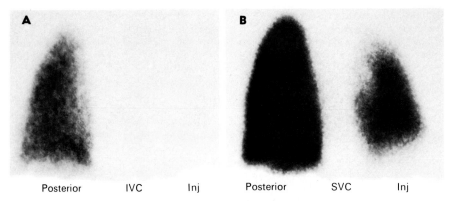

Figure 5-37. Functioning Glenn anastomosis—lung scan. When the Tc-99m-MAA is injected into the IVC the particles lodge only in the left lung (*A*). After a second injection into the SVC the particles are seen to lodge in the right lung (*B*).

postoperative surgical shunt examination (Gates et al., 1975). Thus changes in distribution of radioactivity within that lung and the comparison of the activity in the two lungs should give one an indication of the changes in blood flow through the shunt. In addition when a problem arises clinically, then the base-line examination will be valuable for comparison.

Present Status

It was an earlier expectation that the single nuclide bolus technique through a peripheral vein would provide a useful screening device to identify or exclude serious congenital heart disease in distressed newborn infants (Wesselhoeft et al., 1972; Hagan et al., 1972). It is still true today that under ideal circumstances such techniques can be useful, but three factors reduce the practicality of nuclear diagnostic studies at this age.

First, a number of noncardiac causes of right-to-left shunting cannot be resolved with the technique. Second, easy applicability of the test in nurseries has not been a widespread development: more often the infant has to be taken to the gamma camera with attendant further diagnostic delay and all the risks transportation entails at this age. Third, the development of hyperoxic blood gas testing and echocardiography now allow rapid bedside evaluation of the intracardiac defect with often quite precise anatomic information.

For all these reasons application of nuclear cardiology to this age group has not achieved widespread popularity.

On the other hand, its application to shunt evaluation, even in the very young, is quite practical and its use in evaluation of left-to-right shunts in older patients is undoubted, particularly in patients with relatively small shunts or in those who require evaluation of operative closure or creation of defects (Gates et al., 1975). There is clearly a place for combined echocardiography and nuclear methods (Rowe, 1975).

The use of nuclear angiocardiography to assess myocardial function has obvious promise for serial study of children with a variety of cardiac disorders whether operated or unoperated (Strauss et al., 1971). The techniques have not yet proved quantitatively satisfactory for infants. It seems likely that improved methods and possibly again combination with echocardiographic techniques will provide a solution.

Increasing interest is being shown in the role of myocardial ischemia in affecting the outcome of newborn patients with cardiopulmonary problems (Rowe and Hoffman, 1972) and in older infants and children with congenital heart defects before and after surgical correction (Tawes et al., 1969). Some of the newer methods of myocardial imaging at present being explored in myocardial infarction of the adult (Strauss et al., 1975) will undoubtedly soon be extended to the assessment of these areas of pediatric cardiology.

EXERCISE TESTING
Richard D. Rowe

I T has been recognized for many years that there are limitations to the assessment of cardiorespiratory health through observations made when the patient is in the resting state. Under normal circumstances any change in work from rest makes demands on energy

expenditure: exercising muscles call for a major increase in oxygen consumption and a host of adaptations affecting energy release at muscle level, and increases in heart rate, ventilation, and cardiac output occur. The great complexity of interreactions enabling adequate response to exercise means that single measures of this response are unlikely to provide a full assessment of the individual's ability to cope with the exercise demand. Nevertheless a comparison of the response of children with congenital heart disease to that of the normal offers an objective evaluation of the degree of adaptation.

Methods of Assessment

Very Young Children. The cardiovascular response of patients with congenital heart disease in infancy during crying or toddling on a carpet or running a short distance or exercising with encouragement or the use of pharmacologic agents to increase the heart rate may be crude, but they are still the only practical way in which very young patients can be examined in this sense.

Children Older Than Four Years. Given the necessary psychologic preparation and encouragement, children of this age can be exercised on bicycle ergometers and treadmills, which have been employed with increasingly sophisticated approaches to evaluate the effects of dynamic exercise in recent times. The use of the bicycle ergometer in the catheterization laboratory has provided important information available in no other way, but has obvious disadvantages for mass testing and is limited by the degree of exercise that is possible under those circumstances (Hugenholtz and Nadas, 1963; Epstein et al., 1973; Bjarke, 1974; Stone et al., 1974).

The treadmill is a feasible (Cassels and Morse, 1962; Klimt, 1971) and has been held a preferable method for study for the age group between 5 and 12 years or when it is important to obtain the maximum oxygen uptake of the patient (Åstrand, 1971).

The bicycle ergometer can achieve similar goals and has the advantage that a great amount of normal data has accumulated through its use over many years. Work output in kilopond-meters (Kpm) or kilogram-meters (Kgm) and work rate as Kpm or Kgm per minute can be calculated in bicycle testing but not on a treadmill. The measurements in the latter case must be related to the inclination of the platform (usually a 10 percent grade) and the speed (usually 1.7 to 5 mph).

The maximal oxygen uptake is obtained directly by increasing the level of work to a point above which oxygen consumption does not increase further. It is possible to obtain indirect calculation of maximal oxygen uptake by utilizing the linear relationship between heart rate and oxygen consumption (Cumming and Danziger, 1963) during a steady state response to submaximal work. Extrapolation is then possible to a predicted maximum heart rate for age. A recent recommendation from the World Health Organization is that data on oxygen uptake, workload, and electrocardiographic findings be reported for pulse rate corresponding to 75 percent of aerobic power (Lange Andersen et al., 1971). Many variables may be measured. The minimum would include the measurement of heart rate by attachment

of electrocardiographic leads. Recordings of the electrocardiogram can be made continuously through telemetry or more usually every minute, from a direct writing instrument. The ability to study changes in rate and rhythm as well as changes indicative of ischemia in children with a variety of cardiac diseases has proved most valuable (Cassels, 1966; James and Kaplan, 1974).

Although the blood pressure can be measured during exercise through programmed electrosphygmomanometers (James and Kaplan, 1974), there still remain questions of validity for such measurements when compared to direct central aortic pressure, particularly in young children with resilient vessels and marked pulse amplification.

With older children it is possible to obtain measurements of oxygen uptake and perform the procedures necessary for indirect (CO_2) method of determining cardiac output (Bar-Or and Shepard, 1971; Godfrey, 1974).

There are particular concerns in exercise testing of children that place emphasis on noninvasive methodology, in making the procedure challenging though not disturbing, and that encompass fully the ethical considerations of these studies. There are still differences of opinion as to the most satisfactory and sensitive method of exercising children. Because impairment of cardiac function may not be evident at lower levels of work, there has been a rather strong encouragement to testing of children through maximal levels of exercise (Kramer and Lurie, 1964; Goldberg et al., 1969). Techniques therefore vary (Cumming and Danziger, 1963; Kramer and Lurie, 1964; Izukawa and Drash, 1968; Goldberg et al., 1969; Bar-Or and Shepard, 1971; Thorén, 1971a; Godfrey, 1974), but the general objectives are not really dissimilar: to assess the cardiorespiratory response of a patient after warm-up through several graded levels of exercise to one specific level of exercise obtained through pretesting or by reaching an individual limit. Whether the level aimed for should be maximal (Kramer and Lurie, 1964) or submaximal (Linde, 1963; Godfrey, 1974) is still a matter for debate, there being proponents for each view. Safety of procedure is not an issue within this dialogue. What is of importance is that exercise be a true stress of measurable degree.

The Child with Congenital Heart Disease

At present it is known that the responses to exercise for many children with congenital heart disease are less than those contained in the normal population. Cyanotic patients have more striking deviations, as might be expected. There is no doubt that under submaximal exertion many children with heart malformation can perform rather well so that at this level of activity an examination of oxygen consumption or pulse rate is not particularly helpful in separating mild from severe disease (Adams and

Duffie, 1961). It is for this reason that many investigators have gone further to maximal endurance testing where it is clear that a separation point between mild and severe disease is more often obtained (Goldberg et al., 1969), or to additional data collection, particularly that which allows a determination of stroke volume at submaximal levels of exercise (Godfrey, 1974).

Though there are a large number of variables that may currently be examined in centers with appropriate facilities in a research setting (and it is important that these continue to be performed), the practical question for an individual patient may be resolved with a smaller amount of data. Until the specific and practical value of all the presently obtainable measurements is made more certain, it is unlikely that they will be sought routinely in most clinics.

For example, a normal maximal or even a submaximal exercise response alone may demonstrate convincingly to both parents and child the perhaps surprising level of exercise that can be safely permitted. Although the method may be used to avoid undue exercise limitation, it may also serve to define the limits of exercise for patients with true evidence of impaired myocardial performance (Adams and Moss, 1969). The importance of physical training in improving the response of children with chronic diseases has long been championed by Scandinavian investigators on this basis (Thorén, 1971[b]).

A simple electrocardiographic analysis during exercise may be all that is necessary for individuals with suspected effort dysrhythmias, with resting ectopic rhythms, with malformations known to be associated with a high incidence of dysrhythmia, for patients with cardiomyopathy, or for the assessment of patients with known heart disease after corrective surgery. An increasing emphasis on the electrocardiographic aspect of exercise testing in children is now apparent (Cassels, 1966; James and Kaplan, 1974).

For others—preoperatively as well as postoperatively—a more complete evaluation providing greater sensitivity in establishing the severity of cardiovascular impairment can be offered using exercise studies that include measurement of cardiac output (Epstein et al., 1973; Jonsson, 1973; Godfrey, 1974). With more input into methodology each year the ways by which blood pressure and cardiac output may be more conveniently measured is changing, and doubtless as these developments improve reliability and ease of application for children the demand for such studies will increase sharply.

The Present Situation

The present lack of agreement on the best techniques should not obscure the value that can be obtained from exercise tests for a wide variety of congenital and acquired heart disorders. More and more centers in pediatric cardiology are turning to this form of assessment in the child age range. At The Hospital for Sick Children the approach to exercise testing is made through a joint laboratory of the Respiratory and Cardiology Divisions. Both bicycle ergometry and treadmill techniques are employed and abbreviated electrocardiographic as well as more detailed evaluations are used. At present the treadmill is utilized mainly for detailed assessment of dysrhythmias or ischemic changes in the electrocardiogram or for maximum exercise performance (Ellestad et al., 1969). The bicycle ergometer is used mainly for detailed studies of the type described by Godfrey (1974). The first part of this technique is based on earlier protocols developed by a number of workers in Scandinavia and the United States (Sjostrand, 1947; Wahlund, 1948; Adams and Duffie, 1961; Godfrey et al., 1971; Jones et al., 1975) and seems best to respond to the practicalities of exercising the young child. The patients pedal a cycle at a low initial workload and increase this load by about 50–100 K pm until a maximum is reached. That point, when the exercise is stopped, is determined by the patient feeling unable to continue, but it can be stopped prior to that time in the event that cardiovascular symptoms of importance or a serious electrocardiographic change develops. The importance of encouragement to pursue the maximum effort cannot be underestimated. It usually takes between five and ten minutes to reach that maximum work rate. After completion and a rest a more detailed evaluation can then be obtained through steady state measurements made during the last two minutes of each of six minutes of exercise at one-third and two-thirds of the previously measured maximum work level. Under these conditions a detailed assessment of the ability to respond to exercise can be quite easily obtained for almost all children without great difficulty. Indirect (CO_2) Fick technique is incorporated into the study ideally so that any limitation in stroke volume can be detected.

Obviously the optimal evaluation of exercise for the patient with congenital heart disease is not yet on hand and just as clearly new methods are evolving. But the point is now firmly made: a complete evaluation of the patient with heart malformation or heart disease is no longer possible without the addition of exercise testing to the more classic ancillary studies.

REFERENCES

Chest Roentgenogram

Bakwin, H., and Bakwin, R. M.: Body build in infants. VI. Growth of the cardiac silhouette and thoracic-abdominal cavity. *Am. J. Dis Child.*, 49:861, 1935.

Berber, J. W.: A new radiographic finding in mongolism. *Radiology*, 86:332, 1966.

Boone, M. L.; Swenson, B. E.; and Felson, B.: Rib notching: its many causes. *Am. J. Roentgenol. Radium Ther. Nucl. Med.*, 91:1075, 1964.

Burnard, E. D., and James, L. S.: Radiographic heart size in apparently healthy newborn infants. Clinical and biochemical correlations. *Pediatrics*, 27:726, 1961.

Caffey, J., and di Liberti, C.: Acute atrophy of the thymus induced by adrenocorticosteroids observed roentgenographically in living human infants. *Am. J. Roentgenol. Radium Ther. Nucl. Med.*, **82**:530, 1959.

Cooley, R. N., and Schreiber, M. H.: *Heart and Great Vessels*, The Williams and Wilkins Co., Baltimore, 1967.

Corone, P.; Venntan, P.; and Emerit, I.: Deformation thoracique et communications interventriculaires. *Arch. Fr. Pediatr.*, **20**:955, 1963.

Currarino, G., and Swanson, G.: Developmental variants of ossification of manubrium sterni in mongolism. *Radiology*, **82**:916, 1964.

Datey, K. K.; Deshmukh, M. M.; Engineer, S. D.; and Dalve, C. P.: Straight back syndrome. *Br. Heart J.*, **26**:614, 1964.

Durnin, R. E.; Willner, R.; Virmani, S.; Lawrence, T.; and Fyler, D. C.: Pulmonary regurgitation with ventricular septal defect and pulmonary stenosis—tetralogy of Fallot variant. *Am. J. Roentgenol. Radium Ther. Nucl. Med.*, **106**:42, 1969.

Elliott, L. P.; Jue, K. L.; and Amplatz, K. A.: A roentgen classification of cardiac malpositions. *Invest. Radiol.*, **1**:17, 1966.

Elliott, L. P., and Schiebler, G. L.: *X-Ray Diagnosis of Congenital Cardiac Disease*. Charles C Thomas, Publisher, Springfield, Ill., 1968, pp. 45–68.

Elliott, L. P., and Schiebler, G. L.: *X-Ray Diagnosis of Congenital Cardiac Disease*. Charles C Thomas, Publisher, Springfield, Ill., 1968, p. 212.

Fisher, K. C.; White, R. I.; Jordan, C. E.; Dorst, J. P.; and Neill, C. A.: Sternal abnormalities in patients with congenital heart disease. *Am. J. Roentgenol. Radium Ther. Nucl. Med.*, **119**:530, 1973.

Gabrielson, T. O., and Ladyman, G. H.: Early closure of sternal sutures and congenital heart disease. *Am. J. Roentgenol. Radium Ther. Nucl. Med.*, **89**:975, 1963.

Horns, J. W., and O'Loughlin, B. J.: Multiple manubrial ossification centers in mongolism. *Am. J. Roentgenol. Radium Ther. Nucl. Med.*, **93**:395, 1965.

Keith, J. D.; Rowe, R. D.; and Vlad, P.: *Heart Disease in Infancy and Childhood*, 2nd ed. Macmillan Publishing Co., Inc., New York, 1967, p. 779.

Lakier, J. B.; Stanger, P.; Heymann, M. A.; Hoffman, J. I. E.; and Rudolph, A. M.: Tetralogy of Fallot with absent pulmonary valve. Natural history and hemodynamic considerations. *Circulation*, **50**:167, 1974.

Lees, R. F., and Caldicott, W. J. H.: Sternal anomalies in congenital heart disease. *Am. J. Roentgenol. Radium Ther. Nucl. Med.*, **124**:423, 1975.

Lincoln, E. M., and Spillman, R.: Studies of the hearts of normal children. II. Roentgen ray studies. *Am. J. Dis. Child.*, **35**:791, 1928.

Martin, J. F., and Friedill, H. L.: The roentgen findings in atelectasis of the newborn. *Am. J. Roentgenol. Radium Ther. Nucl. Med.*, **67**:905, 1952.

Osman, M. Z.; Meng, C. C. L.; and Girdany, B. R.: Congenital absence of the pulmonary valve. Report of eight cases with review of the literature. *Am. J. Roentgenol. Radium Ther. Nucl. Med.*, **105**:58, 1969.

Rabinowitz, J. G., and Moseley, J. E.: Lateral lumbar spine in Down's syndrome: A new roentgen feature. *Radiology*, **83**:74, 1964.

Rabinowitz, J. G.; Wolf, B. S.; Greenberg, E. I. et al.: Osseous changes in rubella embryopathy (congenital rubella syndrome). *Radiology*, **85**:494, 1965.

Rose, V.; Izukawa, T.; and Moës, C. A. F.: The syndrome of asplenia and polysplenia. A review of cardiac and non-cardiac malformations in 60 cases with special reference to diagnosis and prognosis. *Br. Heart J.*, **37**:840, 1975.

Rowe, R. D., and Uchida, I. A.: Cardiac malformations in mongolism. A prospective study of 184 mongoloid children. *Am. J. Med.*, **31**:726, 1961.

Shaher, R. M.; Moës, C. A. F.; and Khoury, G. H.: The significance of the atrial situs in the diagnosis of positional anomalies of the heart. II. An angiocardiographic study of 29 patients. *Am. Heart J.*, **73**:41, 1967.

Simon, M.; Sasahara, A. A.; and Cannilla, J. E.: The radiology of pulmonary hypertension. *Semin. Roentgenol.*, **2**:368, 1967.

Singleton, E. B.; Rudolph, A. J.; Rosenberg, H. S. et al.: The roentgenographic manifestations of the rubella syndrome in newborn infants. *Am. J. Roentgenol. Radium Ther. Nucl. Med.*, **97**:82, 1966.

Swischuk, K. E.: *Plain Film Interpretation in Congenital Heart Disease*. Lea and Febiger, Philadelphia, 1970, pp. 27–45.

Electrocardiography and Vectorcardiography

Abella, J. B.; Teixeira, O. H. P.; Misra, K. P.; and Hastreiter, A. R.: Changes of atrioventricular conduction with age in infants and children. *Am. J. Cardiol.*, **30**:876, 1972.

Abildskov, J. A., and Wilkinson, R. S., Jr.: The relation of precordial and orthogonal leads. *Circulation*, **27**:59, 1963.

Alimurung, M. M.; Joseph, L. G.; Nadas, A. S.; and Massell, B. F.: The unipolar precordial and extremity electrocardiogram in normal infants and children. *Circulation*, **4**:420, 1951.

Benjamin, J. E., and White, P. D.: Longevity with complete atrioventricular block. *JAMA*, **149**:1549, 1952.

Bristow, J. D.; Porter, G. A.; and Griswold, H. E.: Observations with the Frank system of vectorcardiography in left ventricular hypertrophy. *Am. Heart J.*, **62**:621, 1961.

Cabrera, E., and Monroy, J. R.: Systolic and diastolic loading of the heart. I. Physiologic and clinical data. II. Electrocardiographic data. *Am. Heart J.*, **43**:661, 669, 1952.

Campbell, M.: Congenital complete heart block. *Br. Heart J.*, **5**:15, 1943.

Chou, T.; Helm, R. A.; and Kaplan, S.: *Clinical Vectorcardiography*. Grune & Stratton, New York, London, 1974.

Dowling, C. V., and Hellerstein, H. K.: Factors influencing the T wave of the electrocardiogram. II. Effects of drinking iced water. *Am. Heart J.*, **41**:58, 1951.

Einthoven, W.: Ueber die Form des menschlichen Electrocardiogram. *Arch. Ges. Physiol.*, **80**:139, 1900.

Eldridge, F. L., and Hultgren, H. N.: A study of ventricular filling in complete heart block. *Stanford Med. Bull.*, **12**:257, 1954.

Elliott, L. P.; Taylor, W. J.; and Schiebler, G. L.: Combined ventricular hypertrophy in infancy. Vectorcardiographic observations with special reference to the Katz-Wachtel phenomenon. *Am. J. Cardiol.*, **11**:164, 1963.

Ellison, R. C., and Restieaux, N. J.: *Vectorcardiography in Congenital Heart Disease*. W. B. Saunders, Philadelphia, London, Toronto, 1972.

Engle, M. A.: Wolff-Parkinson-White syndrome in infants and children. *Am. J. Dis. Child.*, **84**:692, 1952.

Fowler, R. S.; Shams, A.; and Keith, J. D.: The Vectorcardiogram in Aortic Stenosis in Childhood. Proc. XI International Vectorcardiography Symposium, North-Holland Publishing Co., 1972.

Gelband, H.; Waldo, A. L.; Kaiser, G. A.; Bowman, F. O.; Malm, J. R.; and Hoffman, B. F.: Etiology of right bundle-branch block in patients undergoing total correction of tetralogy of Fallot. *Circulation*, **44**:1022, 1971.

Gillette, P. C.; Reitman, M. J.; Gitgesell, H. P.; Vargo, T. A.; Mullins, C. E.; and McNamara, D. G.: Intracardiac electrography in children and young adults. *Am. Heart J.*, **89**:36, 1975.

Goldberger, E.: *Unipolar Lead Electrocardiography*, 2nd ed. Lea & Febiger, Philadelphia, 1949.

Goldman, I. R.; Blount, S. G., Jr.; Friedlich, A. L.; and Bing, R. J.: Electrocardiographic observations during cardiac catheterization. *Bull. Hopkins Hosp.*, **86**:141, 1950.

Grant, R. P.: The relationship between the anatomic position of the heart and the electrocardiogram. A criticism of "unipolar" electrocardiography. *Circulation*, **7**:890, 1953.

Gros, G.; Gordon, A.: and Miller, R.: Electrocardiographic patterns of normal children from birth to five years of age. *Pediatrics*, **8**:349, 1951.

Hastreiter, A. R., and Abella, J. B.: The electrocardiogram in the newborn period. I. The normal infant. *J. Pediatr.*, **78**:146, 1971.
——: The electrocardiogram in the newborn period. II. The infant with disease. *J. Pediatr.*, **78**:346, 1971.

His, W.: Die Tätigkeit des embryonalen Herzens und seine Bedeutung für die Lehre der Herzbewegung beim Erwachsenen. *Arb. Med. Klin. Lpz.*, 1893, pp. 14–19.

Hugenholtz, P. G., and Liebman, J.: The orthogonal vectorcardiogram in 100 normal children (Frank system). *Circulation*, **26**:891, 1962.

Joint Recommendations of the American Heart Association and the Cardiac Society of Great Britain and Ireland: Standardization of Precordial Leads. *Am. Heart J.*, **15**:107, 1938.

Keith, A., and Flack, M.: The form and nature of the muscular connection between the primary divisions of the vertebrate heart. *J. Anat.*, **41**:172, 1907.

Khoury, G. H., and Fowler, R. S.: Normal frank vectorcardiogram in infancy and childhood. *Br. Heart J.*, **29**:563, 1967.

Kissin, M.; Schwarzschild, M. M.; and Bakst, H.: A nomogram for rate correction of the Q-T interval in the electrocardiogram. *Am. Heart J.*, **35**:990, 1948.

Kölliker, A., and Müller, H.: Nachweis der negativen Schwankung des Muskelstrome am natürlich sich contrahirenden Muskel. *Verh. Physik.-Med. Ges. Würzburg*, **6**:528, 1856.

Kreidberg, M. B., and Dushan, T. A.: Paroxysmal auricular tachycardia associated with Wolff-Parkinson-White syndrome in a newborn infant. *J. Pediatr.*, **43**:92, 1953.

Lev, M.; Fell, E. H.; Arcilla, R.; and Weinberg, M. H.: Surgical injury to the conduction system in ventricular septal defect. *Am. J. Cardiol.*, **14**:464, 1964.

Lewis, T.: Galvanometric curves yielded by cardiac beats generated in the various areas of the auricular musculature. The pacemaker of the heart. *Heart*, **2**:23, 1910.

Lown, B.; Ganong, W. F.; and Levine, S. A.: The syndrome of short P-R interval, normal QRS complex and paroxysmal rapid heart action. *Circulation*, **5**:693, 1952.

Mathewson, F. A. L., and Varnam, G. S.: Abnormal electrocardiograms in apparently healthy people. I. Long term follow-up study. *Circulation*, **21**:196, 1960.

————: Abnormal electrocardiograms in apparently healthy people. II. The electrocardiogram in the diagnosis of subclinical myocardial disease serial records of 32 people. *Circulation*, **21**:204, 1960.

Miller, R. A.: The electrocardiogram in congenital malformations of the heart. *Pediatr. Clin. North Am.*, Feb., 1954, p. 51.

Moss, A. J., and Emmanouilides, G. C.: *Practical Pediatric Electrocardiography.* J. B. Lippincott, Philadelphia and Toronto, 1973.

Myhre, J. R.: Adams-Stokes' syndrome caused by ventricular tachycardia in two cases of complete auriculoventricular block. *Acta Med. Scand.*, **147**:379, 1954.

Nagayama, T.; Hayakawa, K.; Hirayama, K.; and Kamimae, T.: Development of the circulatory organs of children, observed by electrocardiogram, vectorcardiogram and ventricular gradient. *Acta Med. Univ. Kagoshima*, **4**:271, 1962.

Pipberger, H. V.; Bialek, S. M.; Perloff, J. K.; and Schnaper, H. W.: Correlation of clinical information in the standard 12-lead ECG and in a corrected orthogonal 3-lead ECG. *Am. Heart J.*, **61**:34, 1961.

Pipberger, H. V., and Lilienfield, L. S.: Application of corrected electrocardiographic lead systems in man. *Am. J. Med.*, **25**:539, 1958.

Prinzmetal, M.: The Wolff-Parkinson-White syndrome and related phenomena. *Am. J. Med.*, **13**:121, 1952.

Purkinje, J. E.: Mikroskopisch-neurologische Beobachtungen. *Ach. Anat. Physiol.*, **12**:281, 1845.

Reynolds, R. W.: T. Wave contour in the precordial leads during childhood. *Pediatrics*, **7**:400, 1951.

Roberts, N. K., and Fowler, R. S.: Prediction of left ventricular pressure from the vectorcardiogram in transposition of the great arteries. *Am. J. Cardiol.*, **31**:736, 1973.

Roberts, N. K., and Olley, P. M.: His bundle recordings in children with normal hearts and congenital heart disease. *Circulation*, **45**:295, 1972.

————: His bundle electrogram in children. Statistical correlation of the atrioventricular conduction times in children with their age and heart rate. *Br. Heart J.*, **34**:1099, 1972.

Rosenman, R. H.; Pick, A.; and Katz, L. N.: The electrocardiographic patterns and the localization of intraventricular conduction defects. *Am. Heart. J.*, **40**:845, 1950.

Schaffer, A. I.: Unipolar electrocardiographic studies in congenital heart in infancy. *Am. J. Dis. Child.*, **80**:260, 1950.

Schaffer, A. I., and Beinfield, W. H.: The vectorcardiogram of the newborn infant. *Am. Heart J.*, **44**:89, 1952.

Schaffer, A. I.; Burstein, J.; Mascia, A. V.; Barenberg, P. L.; and Stillman, N.: The unipolar electrocardiogram of the newborn infant. *Am. Heart J.*, **39**:588, 1950.

Scherlag, B. J.; Lau, S. H.; Helfant, R. H.; Berkowitz, W. D.; Stein, E.; and Damato, A. N.: Catheter technique for recording His bundle activity in man. *Circulation*, **39**:13, 1969.

Southern, E. M.: Electrocardiography and phonocardiography of the foetal heart. *J. Obstet. Gynacol. Br. Emp.*, **71**:231, 1954.

Surawicz, B., and Lepeschkin, E.: The electrocardiographic pattern of hypopotassemia with and without hypocalcemia. *Circulation*, **8**:801, 1953.

Taran, L. M., and Szilagyi, N.: The duration of the electrical systole (Q-T) in acute rheumatic carditis in children. *Am. Heart J.*, **33**:14, 1947.

Tawara, S.: *Das Reizleitungssystem des Säugetierherzens.* Fischer, Jena. 1906.

Thomas, P., and Dejong, D.: The P wave in the electrocardiogram in the diagnosis of heart disease. *Br. Heart J.*, **16**:241, 1954.

Trethewie, E. R.: Electrocardiographic studies with varying potassium plasma levels. *Med. J. Aust.*, **2**:51, 1954.

Veasy, L. G., and Adams, F. H.: Unipolar lead electrocardiography in children. *Pediatrics*, **9**:395, 1952.

Walsh, S. Z.: Evolution of the electrocardiogram of healthy premature infants during the first year of life. *Acta Paediat.*, suppl. 145, 1963.

White, P. D.; Leach, C. E.; and Foote, S. A.: Errors in measurement of the P-R (P-Q) interval and QRS duration in the electrocardiogram. *Am. Heart J.*, **22**:321, 1941.

Widran, J., and Lev, M.: The dissection of the atrioventricular node, bundle and bundle branches in the human heart. *Circulation*, **4**:863, 1951.

Yano, K., and Pipberger, H. V.: Spatial magnitude, orientation, and velocity of the normal and abnormal QRS complex. *Circulation*, **29**:107, 1964.

Young, E.; Liebman, J.; and Nadas, A. S.: The normal vectorcardiogram of children. *Am. J. Cardiol.*, **5**:457, 1960.

Ziegler, R. F.: Characteristics of the unipolar precordial electrocardiogram in normal infants. *Circulation*, **3**:438, 1951.

————: *Electrocardiographic Studies in Normal Infants and Children.* Charles C Thomas, Publisher, Springfield, Ill., 1951.

————: Some aspects of electrocardiography in infants and children with congenital heart disease. *Dis. Chest*, **25**:490, 1954.

Phonocardiography and Systolic Time Intervals

Aygen, M. M., and Braunwald, E.: The splitting of the second heart sound in normal subjects and in patients with congenital heart disease. *Circulation*, **25**:328, 1962.

Benchimol, A., and Matsuo, S.: Ejection time before and after aortic valve replacement. *Am. J. Cardiol.*, **27**:244, 1971.

Cohn, L. H., Morrow, A. G.; and Braunwald, E.: Operative treatment of atrial septal defect: Clinical and hemodynamic assessments in 175 patients. *Br. Heart J.*, **29**:725, 1967.

Fowler, N. O., and Adolph, R. J.: Fourth sound gallop or split first sound? *Am. J. Cardiol.*, **30**:441, 1972.

Garrard, C. L., Jr.; Weissler, A. M., and Dodge, H. T.: The relationship of alterations in systolic time intervals to ejection fraction in patients with cardiac disease. *Circulation*, **42**:455, 1970.

Goldblatt, A.; Aygen, M.; and Braunwald, E.: Hemodynamic phonocardiographic correlations of the fourth heart sound in aortic stenosis. *Circulation*, **26**:92, 1962.

Golde, D., and Burstin, L.: Systolic phases of the cardiac cycle in children. *Circulation*, **42**:1029, 1907.

Harris, L. C.; Weissler, A. M.; Manske, A. O.; Danford, B. H.; White, G. D.; and Hammill, W. A.: Duration of the phases of mechanical systole in infants and children. *Am. J. Cardiol.*, **14**:448, 1964.

Kincaid-Smith, P., and Barlow, J.: The atrial sound and the atrial component of the first heart sound. *Br. Heart J.*, **21**:470, 1959.

Leatham, A., and Weitzman, D.: Auscultatory and phonocardiographic signs of pulmonary stenosis. *Br. Heart J.*, **19**:303, 1957.

Leatham, A.: *Auscultation of the Heart and Phonocardiography*, 2nd ed. Churchill Livingstone, London, 1975.

Lewis, R. P.; Leighton, R. F.; Forester, W. F.; and Weissler, A. M.: Systolic time intervals. In *Non-invasive Cardiology*, Ed. Weissler, A. M. Grune and Stratton, New York, 1974, pp. 301–68.

McKusick, V. A.: *Cardiovascular Sound in Health and Disease.* Williams & Wilkins, Baltimore, 1958.

Myler, R. K., and Sanders, C. A.: Normal splitting of the second heart sound in atrial septal defect. *Am. J. Cardiol.*, **19**:874, 1967.

Oakley, C. M., and Hallidie-Smith, K. A.: Assessment of site and severity in congenital aortic stenosis. *Br. Heart J.*, **29**:367, 1967.

Parisi, A. F.; Salzman, S. H.; and Schechter, E.: Systolic time intervals in severe aortic valve disease. *Circulation*, **44**:539, 1971.

Tavel, M. E.: *Clinical Phonocardiography and External Pulse Recording*, 2nd ed. Year Book Medical Publishers Inc., Chicago, 1972.

Vogelpoel, L., and Schrire, V.: Auscultatory and phonocardiographic assessment of pulmonary stenosis with intact ventricular septum. *Circulation*, **22**:55, 1960.

Vredevoe, L. A.; Creekmore, S. P.; and Schiller, N. B.: The measurement of systolic time intervals by echocardiography. *J. Clin. Ultrasound.*, **2**:99, 1974.

Yahini, J. H.; Dulfano, M. J.; and Toor, M.: Pulmonic stenosis: A clinical assessment of severity. *Am. J. Cardiol.*, **5**:744, 1960.

Echocardiography

Assad-Morell, J. L.; Tajik, A. J.; and Giuliani, E. R.: Echocardiographic analysis of the ventricular septum. *Prog. Cardiovasc. Dis.*, **17**:219, 1974.

Baker, D. W.: Physical and technical principles in diagnostic ultrasound. In *Diagnostic Ultrasound*, Ed. King, D. L. C. V. Mosby Co., 1974, pp. 16–51.

Bom, N.; Lancee, C. T.; Zwieten, G. V.; Kloster, F. E.; and Roelandt, J.: Multiscan echocardiography: Technical description. *Circulation*, **48**:1066, 1973.

Chandraratna, P. A. N.; Lopez, J. M.; Littman, B. B.; Gupta, J. D.; Samet, P.; and Gindlesperger, D.: Abnormal mitral valve motion during ventricular extrasystoles: An echocardiographic study. *Am. J. Cardiol.*, **34**:783, 1974.

Chesler, E.; Joffe, H. S.; Vecht, R.; Beck, W.; and Schrire, V.: Ultrasound cardiography in single ventricle and the hypoplastic left and right heart syndromes. *Circulation*, **42**:123, 1970.

Chesler, E.; Joffe, H. S.; Beck, W.; and Schrire, V.: Echocardiographic recognition of mitral-semilunar valve discontinuity. An aid to the diagnosis of the origin of both great vessels from the right ventricle. *Circulation*, **43**:725, 1971.

Feigenbaum, H.: *Echocardiography*, 2nd ed. Lea & Febiger, Philadelphia, 1976, pp. 5–53.

Gibson, D. G.: Estimation of left ventricular size by echocardiography. *Br. Heart J.*, **35**:128, 1973.

Griffith, J. A., and Henry, W. L.: A sector scanner for real time two-dimensional echocardiography. *Circulation*, **49**:1147, 1974.

Hirschfeld, S.; Meyer, R. A.; Schwartz, D. C.; Korfhagen, J.; and Kaplan, S.: Measurement of right and left systolic time intervals by echocardiography. *Circulation*, **51**:304, 1975.

Kamigaki, M., and Goldschlager, N.: Echocardiographic analysis of mitral valve motion in atrial septal defect. *Am. J. Cardiol.*, **30**:343, 1972.

King, D. L.: Cardiac ultrasonography—cross sectional ultrasonic diagnosis of the heart. *Circulation*, **47**:843, 1973.

King, D. L., and Lele, P. P.: Biologic effects of diagnostic ultrasound. In *Diagnostic Ultrasound*, Ed. King, D. L. C. V. Mosby Co., St. Louis, 1974, pp. 290–98.

Konecke, L. L.; Feigenbaum, H.; Chang, S.; Corya, B. C.; and Fischer, J. C.: Abnormal mitral valve motion in patients with elevated left ventricular diastolic pressures. *Circulation*, **47**:989, 1973.

Linhart, J. W.; Mintz, G. S.; Segal, B. L.; Kawai, N.; and Kotler, M. N.: Left ventricular volume measurements by echocardiography. Fact or Fiction. *Am. J. Cardiol.*, **36**:114, 1975.

Meyer, R. A., and Kaplan, S.: Echocardiography in the diagnosis of hypoplasia of the left or right ventricles in the neonate. *Circulation*, **46**:55, 1970.

Meyer, R. A., and Kaplan, S.: Non-invasive techniques in pediatric cardiovascular disease. *Prog. Cardiovasc. Dis.*, **15**:341, 1973.

Meyer, R. A.: Interaction of ultrasound and biologic tissues—potential hazards. *Pediatrics*, **54**:266, 1974.

Meyer, R. A.; Stockert, J.; and Kaplan, S.: Echographic determination of left ventricular volumes in pediatric patients. *Circulation*, **51**:297, 1975.

Pohost, G. M.; Dinsmore, R. E.; Rubenstein, J. J.; O'Keefe, D. D.; Grantham, R. N.; Scully, H. E.; Beierholm, E. A.; Frederiksen, J. W.; Weisfeldt, M. L.; and Daggett, W. M.: The echocardiogram of the anterior leaflet of the mitral valve. *Circulation*, **51**:88, 1975.

Quinones, M. A.; Gaasch, W. H.; and Alexander, J. K.: Echocardiographic assessment of left ventricular function. *Circulation*, **50**:42, 1974.

Radford, D. J.; Bloom, K. R.; Izukawa, T.; Moes, C. A. F.; and Rowe, R. D.: Echocardiographic assessment of bicuspid aortic valves: Angiographic and pathological correlates. *Circulation*, **53**:80, 1976.

Sahn, D. J.; Wood, J.; Allen, H. D.; Peoples, W.; and Goldberg, S. J.: Echocardiographic spectrum of mitral valve motion in children with or without mitral valve prolapse: The nature of false positive diagnosis. *Am. J. Cardiol.*, **39**:422, 1977.

Sahn, D. J.; Terry, R.; O'Rourke, R.; Leopold, G.; and Friedman, W. F.: Multiple crystal cross-sectional echocardiography in the diagnosis of cyanotic congenital heart disease. *Circulation*, **50**:230, 1974.

Solinger, R.; Elbl, F.; and Minhas, K.: Deductive echocardiographic analysis in infants with congenital heart disease. *Circulation*, **50**:1072, 1974.

Stefadouras, M. A., and Witham, A. C.: Systolic time intervals by echocardiography. *Circulation*, **51**:114, 1975.

Thurstone, F. L., and von Ramm, O. T.: A new ultrasound imaging technique employing two-dimensional electronic beam steering. In *Acoustal Holography*, Vol 5, ed. Green, Philip S. Plenum Publishing Corp., New York, 1974, p. 249.

Ultan, L. B.; Segal, B. L.; and Likoff, W.: Echocardiography in congenital heart disease—preliminary observations. *Am. J. Cardiol.*, **19**:74, 1967.

Wells, P. N. T.: *Physical Principles of Ultrasonic Diagnosis*. Academic Press, London, 1969.

Nuclear Cardiology

Alderson, P. O.; Jost, R. G.; Strauss, A. W.; Boonvisut, S.; and Markham, J.: Radionuclide angiography improved diagnosis and quantitation of left to right shunts using area ratio techniques in children. *Circulation*, **51**:1136, 1975.

Gates, G. F.; Orme, H. W.; and Dore, E. K.: Surgery of congenital heart disease assessed by radionuclide scintigraphy. *J. Thorac. Cardiovasc. Surg.*, **69**:767, 1975.

Gates, G. F.; Orme, H. W.; and Dore, E. K.: Cardiac shunt assessment in children with macroaggregated albumin technetium-99m. *Radiology*, **112**:649, 1973.

Gilday, D. L.: *Neuroradiology in Infants and Children.* (eds.): Harwood-Nash, D. C. F., and Fitz, C. R. Mosby, C. V. St. Louis 1976, p. 507.

Hagan, A. D.; Friedman, W. F.; Ashburn, W. L.; and Alazraki, N.: Further applications of scintillation scanning techniques to the diagnosis and management of infants and children with congenital heart disease. *Circulation*, **45**:858, 1972.

Maltz, D. L., and Treves, S.: Quantitative radionuclide angiocardiography determination of QP:QS in children. *Circulation*, **47**:1049, 1973.

Rowe, R. D.: The preoperative cardiac catheterization and angiocardiogram. *J. Pediatr.*, **86**:319, 1975.

Rowe, R. D., and Hoffman, T.: Transient myocardial ischemia of the newborn infant: A form of severe cardiorespiratory distress in full term infants. *J. Pediatr.*, **81**:243, 1972.

Strauss, H. W.; Harrison, K.; Langan, J. K.; Lebowitz, E.; and Pitt, B.: Thallium-201 for myocardial imaging: Relation of thallium-201 to regional myocardial perfusion. *Circulation*, **51**:641, 1975.

Strauss, H. W.; Zaret, B. L.; Hurley, P. J.; Natarajan, T. K.; and Pitt, B.: A scintiphotographic method for measuring left ventricular ejection fraction in man without cardiac catheterization. *Am. J. Cardiol.*, **28**:575, 1971.

Tawes, R. L., Jr.; Berry, C. L.; Aberdeen, E.; and Graham, G. R.: Myocardial ischemia in infants. Its role in three common congenital cardiac anomalies. *Ann. Thorac. Surg.*, **8**:383, 1969.

Treves, S., and Collins-Nakai, R. L.: Radioactive tracers in congenital heart disease. *Am. J. Cardiol.*, **38**:711, 1976.

Wesselhoeft, H.; Hurley, P. J.; Wagner, H. N., Jr.; and Rowe, R. D.: Nuclear angiocardiography in the diagnosis of congenital heart disease. *Circulation*, **45**:77, 1972.

Exercise Testing

Adams, F. H., and Duffie, E. R.: Physical working capacity of children with heart disease. *J. Lancet*, **81**:493, 1961.

Adams, F. H., and Moss, A. J.: Physical activity of children with congenital heart disease. *Am. J. Cardiol.*, **24**:605, 1969.

Åstrand, P-O.: Definitions, testing procedures, accuracy, and reproducibility. In Thorén, C. (ed.): Pediatric work physiology, *Acta Paediatr. Scand.*, Suppl **217**:9, 1971.

Bar-Or, O., and Shepard, R. J.: Cardiac output determination in exercising children—methodology and feasibility. In Thorén, C. (ed.): Pediatric work physiology. *Acta Paediatr. Scand.*, Suppl **217**:49, 1971.

Bjarke, B.: Functional studies in palliated and totally corrected adult patients with tetralogy of Fallot. *Scand. J. Thorac. Cardiovasc. Surg.*, Suppl 16, 1974.

Cassels, D. E.: Aspects of the electrocardiogram in left ventricular hypertrophy. In Cassels, D. E., and Zeigler, R. F. (eds.): *Electrocardiography in Infants and Children*. Grune & Stratton, New York, 1966, p. 235.

Cassels, D. E., and Morse, M.: *Cardiopulmonary Data for Children and Young Adults*. Charles C Thomas, Publisher, Springfield, Ill., 1962.

Cumming, G. R., and Cumming, P. M.: Bicycle ergometer studies in children. *Can. Med. Assoc. J.*, **88**:351, 1963.

Cumming, G. R., and Danzinger, R.: Bicycle ergometer studies in children. II Correlation of pulse rate with oxygen consumption. *Pediatrics*, **32**:202, 1963.

Ellestad, M. H.; Allen, W.; Wan, M. C. K.; and Kemp, G. L.: Maximal treadmill stress testing for cardiovascular evaluation. *Circulation*, **39**:517, 1969.

Epstein, S. E.; Beiser, G. D.; Goldstein, R. E.; Rosing, D. R.; Redwood, D. R.; and Morrow, A. G.: Hemodynamic abnormalities in response to mild and intense exercise following operative correction of an atrial septal defect or tetralogy of Fallot. *Circulation*, **47**:1065, 1973.

Godfrey, S. (ed.): *Exercise Testing in Children*. W. B. Saunders Co., Philadelphia, 1974.

Godfrey, S.; Davies, C. T. M.; Wozniak, E.; and Barnes, C. A.: Cardiorespiratory response to exercise in normal children. *Clin. Sci.*, **40**:419, 1971.

Goldberg, S. J.; Mendex, F.; and Hurwitz, R.: Maximal exercise capability of children as a function of specific cardiac defects. *Am. J. Cardiol.*, **23**:349, 1969.

Hugenholtz, P. G., and Nadas, A. S.: Exercise studies in patients with congenital heart disease. *Pediatrics*, **32**:Suppl 4:769, 1963.

Izukawa, T., and Drash, A.: Oxygen Consumption with Exercise. In Cheek, D. B. (ed.), *Human Growth*. Lea and Febiger, Philadelphia, 1968, p. 501.

James. F. W., and Kaplan. S.: Systolic hypertension during submaximal exercise after correction of coarctation of the aorta. *Circulation*, **50**:Suppl II–27, 1974.

Jones, N. L.; Campbell, E. J. M.; Edwards, R. H. T.; and Robertson, D. G.: *Clinical Exercise Testing*. W. B. Saunders Co., Philadelphia, 1975.

Jonsson, B.: Circulatory adaptation to exercise in congenital heart disease. *Proc. Assoc. Europ. Paediatr. Cardiol.*, 9:2, 1973.

Klimt, F.: Treadmill exertion in Children Aged Five. In Thorén, C. (ed.): Pediatric work physiology, *Acta Paediatr. Scand.*, Suppl **217**:32, 1971.

Kramer, J. D., and Lurie, P. R.: Maximal exercise tests in children. *Am. J. Dis. Child.*, **108**:283, 1964.

Lange Andersen, K.; Shephard, R. J.; Denolin, H.; Varnauskas, E.; and Masironi, R. (eds.): *Fundamentals of Exercise Testing*. World Health Organization, Geneva, 1971.

Linde, L. M.: An appraisal of exercise fitness tests. *Pediatrics*, **32**:656, 1963.

Sjostrand, T.: Changes in respiratory organs of workmen at ore smelting works. *Acta Med. Scand.*, Suppl **196**:687, 1947.

Stone, F. M.; Bessinger, F. B. Jr.; Lucas, R. V. Jr.; and Moller, J. H.: Pre- and post-operative rest and exercise haemodynamics in children with pulmonary stenosis. *Circulation*, **49**:1102, 1974.

Thorén, C. (ed.): Pediatric work physiology, *Acta Paediatr. Scand.*, Suppl 217, 1971a.

Thorén, C.: Physical training of handicapped schoolchildren. *Scand. J. Rehab. Med.*, **3**:26, 1971b.

Wahlund, H.: Determination of the physical working capacity. *Acta Med. Scand.* (Suppl.) **215**:9, 1948.

6

Cardiac Catheterization

Richard D. Rowe

THE WAY in which medicine is able to take a new idea and over time gradually reshape it from a rough if brilliant origin into a sophisticated and elaborate method of study is nowhere better demonstrated than by cardiac catheterization.

Forssman (1929) introduced the catheter into his own heart (apparently to the jeers of all but a few of his peers) in search of a method that could measure blood flow. The technique was utilized sporadically in the next decade by a number of French and Portuguese workers, but it was only after the studies of Cournand and Ranges (1941) that general interest in the method was aroused. It soon became evident that important contributions to intracardiac hemodynamics in congenital malformations of the heart were possible, and the early reports of groups under Cournand and coworkers (1949), Bing and coworkers (1947), and Dexter and coworkers (1947) provided the base line for later studies. Increasingly large numbers of infants and children were studied by the method. In particular, Ziegler (1954), Sones (1955), Downing (1959), Rowe (1960), Rudolph and Cayler (1958), and Vlad and associates (1964) reported experience using the method in infant subjects with congenital heart disease.

Over the years the injection of a variety of indicators has been added to the method, the most widely used of which has been contrast material in selective angiocardiography.

Latterly the accumulation of a quarter-century of experience has allowed publication of hemodynamic data for normal children and so permitted mathematical prediction of such values (Lucas et al., 1961; Rudolph et al., 1961; Cayler et al., 1963; Emmanouilides et al., 1964; Sproul and Simpson, 1964; Krovetz et al., 1967; Krovetz and Goldbloom, 1972a, 1972b). The last decade has also seen some outstanding technical advances in catheter and equipment design. It is now relatively simple even in infants to introduce catheters percutaneously, to float catheters through awkward angles within the normally or abnormally situated heart, to record intracardiac murmurs, to institute by special catheters surgical maneuvers such as creation of an

atrial septal defect or closure of a ductus arteriosus when needed, and to obtain rapid serial measurement of cardiac output from a single catheter. Rapid accumulation of hemodynamic data at the bedside has been accomplished by combining several of these catheter characteristics, and research into the problem of pulmonary vascular disease has been enhanced by catheters with transducers at the tip. Similarly fiberoptic catheters have facilitated intracardiac blood oxygen measurement without blood withdrawal. Computerization on a smaller or larger scale (Meester et al., 1975) has reduced the frustrations of calculations for technicians and physicians alike, and improved x-ray apparatus is showing the way to exceptionally detailed angiographic imaging of anatomic details through cine technique. The trend of development is now moving in the laudable direction of seeking information from the cardiovascular system without assault on the patient. This heady ideal we in pediatrics especially should support to the utmost (Rowe, 1975). The historic if conservative view though suggests that such a solution is incomplete as yet, and in its final form, far off. For many years we will have to rely on established, sound, invasive techniques and non- or semiinvasive methods in combination while pursuing the answers to diagnostic and research problems in children with heart disorders.

Meantime it is apparent that although the term cardiac catheterization is entrenched in usage, it is no longer a procedure involving introduction of an end hole catheter to the right side of the heart. It is now a combination of venous and arterial catheter exploration, of pressure and flow measurement, of assessment of electrical and mechanical integrity and performance, and of image and movement of chambers and vessels and of their interrelationships. Guidelines have recently been developed for institutions sponsoring cardiac catheterization laboratories that cover minimum suggested standard, and similar recommendations are available for the radiologic aspects of examination of the cardiovascular system (Reports of the Inter-Society Commission for Heart Disease Resources). The general topic of the state of cardiac catheterization has been the subject of several recent reviews (Rudolph, 1970; Forwand et al., 1971; Graham and Jarmakani, 1972; Levin, 1972; Miller, 1972; Rudolph, 1974).

INDICATIONS AND CONTRAINDICATIONS

THE Committee on Cardiac Catheterization and Angiocardiography of the American Heart Association (Cournand et al., 1953) acknowledged the difficulty of establishing indications for cardiac catheterizations. Their report merely stated that the method was being used "to complete the identification of specific congenital or acquired lesions, to establish their functional significance, to trace their physiologic course, and finally to evaluate the results of surgical procedures." We would add to this list the use of cardiac catheterization and angiocardiography in proving normality of the heart.

It is quite apparent that the diagnosis can be clinically precise for many simple common defects, but over the years it has become apparent that a proportion of even seemingly straightforward defects may have on further study a surprisingly different anatomic explanation for the clinical picture.

There has always been divergence of opinion as to whether all patients with significant congenital heart disease were to be studied fully or not. It has also been shown that detailed study of less complex cases can uncover important additional unsuspected abnormalities. More edge has been given the argument with the rapid rise of noninvasive techniques in recent years. These developments have been helpful in the sense that they permit in the elective situation a degree of screening, which adds to the classic and simpler methods of examination prior to taking the step to the more detailed catheterization procedure. Our approach that has not in essence changed in the last 15 years is to more frequent accessory studies in patients with congenital heart disease. We believe that if a patient is to be studied by cardiac catheterization and angiocardiography, that study should define the function and anatomy of the individual beyond argument.

We further no longer care to separate right heart, left heart, and angiographic studies. There is as much need to know all about the left heart in right-sided lesions as there is to determine the state of the right heart and pulmonary artery in patients presenting with left heart or aortic defects. Probably the one real restriction we hold personally about these matters is that the studies should only be performed in medical centers where full facilities exist for a really adequate study of the entire heart.

We no longer hold the view that there are any unequivocal contraindications. Patients with infective endocarditis or myocarditis one might prefer to study at a stage after the infection or congestive failure has cleared, and indeed there are other ways of obtaining information through indirect methods that are becoming perfectly acceptable and so could avoid catheterization in many cases. The same is true of the old concern about Ebstein's anomaly of tricuspid valve where the fear of arrhythmias used to act as a brake in recommending more detailed studies. We have not in recent years avoided such intervention for this disorder except in the newborn period.

This slight change of our own attitude is in keeping with the experience gained over the years by many groups working with children and simply emphasizes the comment made by Sones (1955) 20 years ago that "no patient should be denied the opportunity for precise diagnosis and possible cure or improvement because he is 'too small' or because functional severity of his lesion appears so great that death might occur during or after catheterization. For such a patient, the greatest hazard lies in continuing failure to make an exact diagnosis upon which effective treatment may be based."

MORTALITY AND COMPLICATIONS

Mortality

In any investigative procedure the factor that determines its survival as a technique is the small chance of a fatal outcome from its use. Early reports showed a very low mortality from right heart catheterization. McMichael (1951) reported 1 death in 995 catheterizations. In the report of the Committee on Cardiac Catheterization and Angiocardiography of the American Heart Association (Cournand et al., 1953) only 5 deaths were reported in 5691 cardiac catheterizations (0.1 percent). Unfortunately, neither the proportion of cases who had congenital heart disease, the condition at the time of study, nor the age distribution was given in this communication. It is known that, in our three-fourths of McMichael's studies, the catheter was placed no further centrally than the right atrium. Donzelot and D'Allaines (1954) believed a 1 percent mortality is more likely the true figure based on the experience at the Hôpital Broussais, together with that reported by Hébert, Scebat, and Lenègre (1954)—a total of 9 fatalities in 1073 cardiac catheterizations.

The mortality rate from the procedure in children, especially infants, certainly is higher than the committee's survey. Ziegler (1954) reported 4 (0.73 percent) deaths in 577 catheterizations for congenital heart disease under 15 years, the fatalities occurring in children under the age of three years. We reported 17 deaths in 3239 studies in the second edition of this book. Though the overall mortality was 0.52 percent, again in this experience the mortality was highest (1.2 percent) in the first year of life. The Cooperative Study on Cardiac Catheterization (Braunwald and Swan, 1968) found between 1963 and 1965 an overall mortality of 0.44 percent in 12,364 studies, a high mortality (6.0 percent) in the first two months of life, and an extremely low risk to life (0.14 percent) between 2 and 59 years of age. In 1859 consecutive studies in infants and children up to the age of 15 years at Johns Hopkins Hospital between 1964 and 1970 the overall mortality was 1.5 percent (Ho et al., 1972). There were no deaths in patients older than three months of age. The level of the high mortality in the first month of life varies according to the way in which mortality is defined. If only deaths in the catheterization laboratory are counted, the risk is in the order of 1 to 2 percent (Rowe, 1960), but if death within 24 hours of the study is the standard applied, then the mortality will be in the region of 10 to 19 percent (Krovetz et al., 1968; Vince, 1968; Varghese et al, 1969; Delisle et al., 1972; Ho et al., 1972; Stanger et al., 1974). For the newborn, detailed analysis shows very clearly that the most important factor involved in mortality is the severity or complexity of the malformation (Delisle et al., 1972; Ho et al., 1972). An acidotic state at catheterization was also important (Braunwald and Swan, 1968; Delisle et al., 1972). To the surprise of many there is quite convincing evidence that the injection of contrast does (not) importantly change these conclusions (Delisle et al., 1972; Ho et al., 1972). The discordance between the mortality risks during the first six weeks of life and at later ages, which seems so alarming to those unfamiliar with the true explanation, needs to be widely clarified (Table 6-1) Pediatricians especially should clearly appreciate what makes the mortality different and should be reassured that such investigations carry an extremely low mortality after the second month. It also should be apparent that some patients may die *before* they can reach the laboratory for study (Hildner et al., 1972).

Table 6–1.　MORTALITY AND CARDIAC CATHETERIZATION IN CHILDREN OF VARIOUS AGES STUDIED AT THE HOSPITAL FOR SICK CHILDREN, TORONTO

AGE GROUP	CARDIAC CATHETERIZATION N	DEATH WITHIN 24 HOURS OF STUDY* N	Percent
0–7 days	685	66	9.6
8–28 days	785	32	4.1
1–3 mo.	1073	9	0.84
3–6 mo.	942	3	0.31
6–9 mo.	572	2	0.35
9–12 mo.	355	1	0.28
>1 yr.	7843	4	0.05

* Deaths within 24 hours of study from whatever cause have been identified with specific age groups. The figures demonstrate that the highest risk of death following study occurs in the first few months after birth.

Complications

It is hardly possible to name a complication that has not been encountered in the major recent analyses (Venables and Hiller, 1963; Braunwald and Swan, 1968; Krovetz et al., 1968; Simovich et al., 1968; Tuuteri et al., 1968; Vince, 1968; Kirkpatrick et al., 1970; Ho et al., 1972; Stanger et al., 1974) or in single case reports of cardiac catheterization. It is, however, important to keep perspective in the area. One must look at both major and less serious complications and examine whether the complication is associated with the hemodynamic aspect of the investigation or whether it is related to the introduction of contrast material. It is also important, particularly in the very young, to determine whether a complication is specifically due to the catheterization-angiographic procedure or whether it is an incident in the course of the disease in a profoundly ill baby.

Major Complications. (ARRHYTHMIAS.) Transient ectopic beats of atrial or ventricular origin are extremely common (Goldman et al., 1950), and do not appear to have great importance (Zimdahl, 1951). In an earlier edition of this book we pointed out that 95 percent of 700 children catheterized at The Hospital for Sick Children showed premature systoles during the time of study, 6 percent showed transient bundle branch block, and 3 percent complete heart block. None of these disturbances seriously interfered with the studies and were almost always of brief duration. On the other hand, bouts of supraventricular tachycardia occurred in 4 percent of that series; although the outcome in all cases was a return to sinus rhythm either spontaneously or with a number of procedures invoking vagal reflexes or by administering digoxin occasionally, the complication may induce deterioration especially in the cyanotic patient or one with limited myocardial reserve. In more recent experience electrocardiographic changes lasting ten minutes or longer were recorded in less than 4 percent of 859 consecutive studies at the Johns Hopkins Hospital Pediatric Cardiac Laboratory. Although the majority of these reverted to sinus rhythm spontaneously, DC countershock was necessary for two patients, one with ventricular fibrillation and one with atrial flutter. Particular precautions are necessary when patients with left-axis deviation or right bundle branch block are being subjected to catheterization study because of the increased risk they have of developing complete heart block (Gupta and Haft, 1972). For children this is especially applicable to patients with cushion defects and those being evaluated after intracardiac surgery who not infrequently will have the legacy of conduction abnormalities. There has been disagreement about the patient risk from catheterization of the heart in Ebstein's anomaly of the tricuspid valve, but Watson's review (1974) clarifies matters. He found that 27 percent of 363 patients developed dysrrhythmias during catheterization.

Development of countershock techniques (Paul and Miller, 1962; White and Humphries, 1967) together with the capability of pacing methods in a catheterization laboratory has now largely abolished a fatal outcome from this type of complication. The importance of maintaining vigilance and attempting in every possible way to obviate the development of runs of ectopic beats or more serious arrhythmias should be the aim in every laboratory. The value of the Swan–Ganz catheter in avoiding prolonged manipulation to enter various chambers or vessels has been clearly established, and because of the cushion afforded the catheter tip by the balloon in that catheter, the potential for ectopic beats or endocardial damage is largely avoided.

PERFORATION. Perforation of the great vessel or cardiac chamber can be suspected if there is a sudden change from a positive to a negative pressure through the catheter when viewed on an oscilloscope and can be confirmed by a failure to withdraw blood or by aspiration of clear fluid from the pericardial sac. Verification is obtained by a small amount of dilute contrast material being injected. If the catheter has perforated an atrium, it should be left in place so that the surgeon may locate the perforation at thoracotomy in a bloodless field. Perforation of a ventricular chamber is not usually so serious a complication because the muscular wall tends to minimize blood loss from the right ventricle, but an outflow tract perforation can be as serious as the atrial complication. Particular care is necessary to avoid perforation of the coronary sinus (McMichael and Mounsey, 1951; Smith et al., 1951; Stern et al., 1952; Keith, 1959). Manipulation with stiff catheters is clearly the culprit in most instances (Lurie and Grajo, 1962; Pocock et al., 1963; Kazanelson et al., 1966).

AIR EMBOLISM. This is a rare but constant risk and demands that proper precautions be meticulously observed during uncoupling of catheters and the flushing apparatus. (Caverley et al., 1971).

THROMBOSES. Thromboses occurring on the venous side have been reported in recent years particularly after the use of large balloon catheters in patients with transposition of the great arteries (Kuehl et al., 1971; Ho et al., 1973). This is a serious complication not so much for the moment of occurrence, but from the viewpoint of reexamination for assessment of the cardiac repair at a later date since, in many instances, both femoral veins are thus rendered inaccessible for future study. The exact explanation is uncertain so that preventive measures cannot be certainly provided. It is our suspicion that such patients might have rather more endothelial damage to the vein on withdrawal of the balloon catheter when compared with standard catheters and that possibly the use of heparin for a longer period than only during the catheterization might help avoid the complication.

Episodes of the nature described by Johnson and associates (1947) where extensive inferior vena caval thrombosis produced serious complications are unusual. We have encountered, as previously described in this chapter, superior vena caval obstruction and a small lingular embolus in young patients in whom the precipitating factor was probably endothelial damage due to unduly long manipulation to enter the superior vena cava from the right arm and the left pulmonary artery from the main trunk.

Much more important in the overall picture of complications in cardiac catheterization is arterial thrombosis. This complication has arisen with increasing use of retrograde examination of the aorta and left heart with catheters introduced from the femoral or brachial artery. There appears little doubt that its frequency is highest in small infants where arterial cutdown techniques have been employed. In this group it is obvious that the size of the vessel and the state of the cardiac output are important factors in the development of such complications. Undoubtedly techniques of arteriotomy repair then become critical (Buckberg and Moss, 1973). The risk of thrombosis following percutaneous arterial catheterization without the use of sheaths is still high—between 15 and 20 percent for infants under 10 kg body weight (Sunderland et al., 1976). To a very large degree the actual frequency of detection of arterial thrombosis in any patient series depends upon the methods used to detect it (Johnson et al., 1975). The development of percutaneous techniques (Kirkpatrick et al., 1970; Simovich et al., 1970; Carter et al., 1975) may have decreased the risk of development of this complication in older children (Mortensen et al., 1975), and the increasing tendency for pediatric cardiologists to apply these techniques to the younger infant offers real hope that the incidence of arterial thrombosis might be further reduced within a few years. The roles of papaverine (Padmanabhan et al., 1972) or aspirin (Freed et al., 1974a) have not been entirely resolved in the preventive area. It is probable that heparin administration is helpful in this regard (Freed et al., 1974b). Although thrombosis has probably been much more common than appreciated, the fact remains that vascular insufficiency is rare despite interference with the pulse. There has been debate over whether limb shortening of significance develops in time in such patients (Bassett et al, 1968; Rosenthal et al., 1972; Bloom et al., 1974). There are real problems in interpreting minor differences in limb length that can exist normally, and as the documentation continues to mount it seems that limb shortening is not an important issue (Hawker et al., 1973b). Collateral circulation is usually very adequate in the upper extremity. The major risk to impairment of circulation comes in the lower leg following femoral arterial thromboses, and without question prompt efforts should be made to restore the arterial pathway to normal in this situation (Cahill et al., 1967; Lincoln and Deverall, 1969; Mansfield et al., 1970). It is debatable whether surgical intervention at this stage can improve matters for the small infant, but for older children there is excellent prospect of full restoration of the arterial flow to normal. We and others (Bell, 1962) have been impressed with the way in which such collateral circulation in the young can appear even sufficiently rapidly to provide normal pulses within 24 hours of the episode despite the later clear demonstration angiographically of a thrombus in the femoral artery. In the immediate newborn period the value of the use of the umbilical artery is well known and accepted, and there should be little occasion for requirement of an arterial cutdown at that age. There is no evidence to suggest later impairment of limb growth from this particular technique (Powers and Swyer, 1975; Boros et al., 1975).

OBSTRUCTION OF BLOOD FLOW. Obstruction of blood flow to the pulmonary artery, the coronary circulation, or the aorta can occur during catheterization when the catheter diameter itself critically reduces the orifice in severe pulmonic stenosis, tetralogy, or severe aortic stenosis (Paul and Rudolph, 1958; Braunwald and Swan, 1968). Such a situation may cause severe bradycardia or a hypoxic reaction, but in a modern catheterization laboratory should not produce a fatal reaction since recognition of the complication should be anticipated. Immediate withdrawal of the catheter usually improves the situation promptly. Less easily recognized at the time of catheterization but of critical importance is vasospasm of the mesenteric arteries in the ill newborn, which appears to be responsible for later perforation of the colon (Kern et al., 1971).

Less Serious Complications. Knotting of the catheter within the heart, looping in the vena cava, and embolization of shorter sheaths or catheters are complications that can be avoided but when developed can be attended to either by operation (Trusler and Mustard, 1958; Steiner et al., 1965) or more recently by the introduction of guidewires, loops, or a second catheter to assist in unknotting (Massumi and Ross, 1967; Curry, 1969; Bloomfield, 1971).

BALLOON ATRIAL SEPTOSTOMY. A number of complications have been encountered at balloon atrial septostomy, including, in addition to the thrombosis mentioned earlier, avulsion of the inferior vena cava, avulsion of the tricuspid valve, inability to deflate the balloon, and rupture of the balloon with or without embolization of balloon fragments (Ehmke et al., 1970; Ellison et al., 1970; Scott, 1970; Vogel, 1970; Williams et al., 1970; Ho et al., 1972; Hohn and Webb, 1972).

INFECTIVE ENDOCARDITIS. The development of infective endocarditis is an excessively rare complication of cardiac catheterization (Winchell, 1953; Krovetz et al., 1968). For this reason most medical centers now avoid the use of prophylactic antibiotics. For us this decision was in part the result of infections in our cases tending to be of a local nature at the incision site, and our experience continues to be that infected cutdown incisions are the most common postcatheterization infective problem.

PYROGENIC REACTIONS. Such reactions have been demonstrated to occur in somewhat over a third of infants and children after cardiac catheterization or angiocardiography; they usually last less than a day (Gilladoga et al., 1972). In this Cornell experience antibiotics did not prevent the fever developing.

EXCESSIVE RADIATION. It is obvious that excessive radiation to the patient is a concern that all connected with cardiac catheterization should avoid where possible (Hills and Stanton, 1950; Wood and Swan, 1959; Spach, 1962; Vince, 1964; Kaude and Svahn, 1974). Since all radiation is potentially harmful, every effort should be made to keep radiation to the patient at a minimum. Fluoroscopy is the principal offender in the procedure so that the cardiologist must aim to keep the amount of fluoroscopy time to a minimum and to develop techniques that permit this objective. Undoubtedly careful consideration of priorities in regard to angiocardiography and a reduction to a minimum of a number of biplane or cine filming exposures is important.

ANGIOCARDIOGRAPHY. Since cardiac catheterization is inseparable from the angiocardiographic aspects, it is important to consider the influence that the introduction of contrast might have in the morbidity and mortality. This is extremely difficult to do in the seriously ill small infant, and some observations suggest that contrast has little to do with the demise (Ho et al., 1972) of such individuals. Nevertheless it is clear that extravasation of contrast into the myocardium and cardiac rupture, though possible, are complications that can be avoided by using test injections. The neurologic complications induced by hypertonic effects of angiographic contrast material can be avoided by spacing of injections and careful avoidance of excessive amounts of contrast material. There seems to be a higher risk with pure sodium-based contrast materials than with meglumine-based media (Ho et al., 1972). Allergic responses to the material are uncommon.

Certain overall measures of a general nature in the catheterization laboratory are of great importance in maintaining the best standards of care and avoidance of complications. These include attention to the general status of the baby, particularly the metabolic status, excessive bleeding or fluid overload, or change of temperature. The body temperature, the acid-base balance, and the fluid intake should be checked frequently during cardiac catheterization and any deviation should be treated promptly (Srouji and Rashkind, 1969). All electrical outlets in the catheterization laboratory should be wired into a common ground system, so avoiding a relative potential across two apparent grounds (Burchell, 1963; Bond and Denison, 1971; Albisser et al., 1972; Arbeit et al., 1972). Appropriate availability of DC capacitance cardioconvertors (Lown et al., 1962), airways, oxygen, suction, and drugs (Table 6–2) together with appropriate training of all staff involved for cardiac resuscitation (Sasahara et al., 1959; Ryan and Cayler, 1962; Anthony et al., 1969) is really mandatory in this regard.

Table 6–2. DRUGS USEFUL IN THE CARDIAC CATHETERIZATION LABORATORY

DRUG	DOSAGE	INDICATIONS
Atropine	0.01 mg/kg IV, IM Max. dose 0.4 mg	Bradyarrhythmias

CM₃
  contains
  Largactil 6.25 mg ⎤ per
  Phenergam 6.25 mg ⎬ ml
  Demerol   25 mg ⎦ mixture
	0.1 ml/kg body weight IM
	Max. dose 2 ml
	Use 0.05 ml/kg in cyanosed children
	No CM₃ given under 1 month
		Premedication

Epinephrine (adrenaline)	Supplied as 1/1000 aqueous sol. Dilute to 1/20,000 (0.05 mg/ml) (0.5 ml of 1/1000 in 10 ml saline) 1–3 ml IV or intracardiac Repeat every 2–3 min. PRN	Anaphylactic shock Cardiac standstill

Inderal (propranolol HCl)	0.05–0.1 mg/kg IV
	Max. initial dose 1 mg
		Tachyarrhythmias
		Hypoxic spells; to assess gradient
		  lability in idiopathic hypertrophic
		  subaortic stenosis

Isoproterenol	0.2 mg/250 ml D5W Continuous infusion 1 ml (1 mcg) per min.	Inducing ⎱ LV/aortic gradient ⎰ RV/PA
Lasix (furosemide)	1 mg/kg IV Max. 40 mg	Pulmonary edema

Levophed (levarterenol bitartrate)	Dilute 2 ml of 0.2% soln. in 500 ml
	  D5W (8 mcg/ml)
	Infuse 15–60 ml/hr to maintain BP
		Maintain blood pressure in acute
		  hypotensive states

Morphine sulfate	0.1 mg/kg SCI Max. dose 5 mg	Premedication in patients with a risk of hypoxic spells
Narcan (naloxone HCl)	5 mcg/kg IV, IM (Supplied in 400 mcg/ml vials)	Narcotic respiratory depression
Priscoline (tolazoline HCl)	1 mg/kg into pulmonary artery	Evaluation of pulmonary hypertension
Sodium bicarbonate	7.5% soln. given IV 1 ml contains 0.9 mEq. Dose—Base excess × Wt. kg × 0.3 or more simply 2 ml. of 7.5% soln./kg	Metabolic acidosis
Sol-u-Cortef (hydrocortisone sodium succinate)	100 mg IV	Acute hypersensitivity reactions
Tensilon (edrophonium Cl)	0.15 mg/kg IV Max. 10 mg. Given 1/5 total dose; if no reaction in 30 sec, give rest	Supraventricular tachycardia
Valium (diazepam)	0.2 mg/kg IV, IM	Additional sedation
Xylocaine (Lidocaine HCl)	1 mg/kg IV single bolus	Ventricular tachycardia Runs of premature ventricular beats

THE METHOD

THE objective of study by cardiac catheterization in infants and children is diagnostic. Except for very young infants, in the vast majority of cases this means in effect refinement of the diagnosis. The additional input to sharpen clinical diagnosis and management that careful pressure-flow measurements, anatomic detail, and assessment of conducting or muscular function provide from this investigation is more than ever before becoming appreciated. The amount of anatomic and physiologic information necessary to achieve this end in any individual case is a matter of nice judgment.

Exploration. The tip of the venous cardiac catheter is used to explore the heart thoroughly. Attempts to enter all four chambers are made. The foramen ovale is traversed, septal defects probed,

and entry obtained into pulmonary veins and pulmonary arteries. Direct catheterization of a patent ductus arteriosus is sought. With an arterial catheter the entire thoracic aorta may be explored to the aortic valve level, and in most cases the catheter is passed through this to the left ventricle. There is advantage to individual preplanning of the exploration, and most physicians prefer certain routines of intracardiac data collection particularly in the simple malformations and in myocardial disorders. Nevertheless, it is important to maintain flexibility of approach for infants and the more complex defects or where unsuspected defects or attachment of vessels is encountered during the course of the study.

Blood Oxygen Content or Saturation. In each situation a sample of blood is taken for measurement of oxygen saturation. Nowadays this is usually accomplished photometrically through the flow cuvette oximeter (Wood et al., 1948) or separate sample instruments such as American Optical Co. and Instrumentation Laboratory oximeters. Other methods include hemoreflection (Zijlstra, 1958) or other photometric means (Gordy and Drabkin, 1957). These techniques allow for immediate information on oxygen saturation data and are superior in this respect to the older methods, but the Van Slyke technique (Van Slyke and Neill, 1925), its ultramicroequivalent (Natelson, 1951), and chromatographic methods (Lukas et al., 1961) are important, if more cumbersome, methods, one of which should be available in every laboratory for calibration of the instrumentation. The important additional checks on arterial blood oxygen saturation quite essential for infant studies can be obtained from the use of polarographic micro blood gas techniques.

Pressure Measurement. The measurement of pressure in each site explored by the cardiac catheter is achieved with strain gauges (Sutterer and Wood, 1960). The system of recording should allow an ability to rapidly alter the amplification of the pressure or the speed of recording and the obtaining of an electrical mean pressure. Visual monitoring of the pressure pulses is essential. The gold standard by which pressure measurements from conventional catheters may be judged is the catheter tip microtransducer. A conventional system that has an undamped natural frequency of about 20 cycles per second with a damping coefficient of about 0.6 is adequate for most recording. This state can be achieved for relatively large-bore catheters by use of a damping chamber (Jennings and Krovetz, 1970) but problems arise during the use of small-bore catheters such as employed in infants. The frequency response relates linearly to the internal radius of the catheter lumen so that to go from a number 6 French catheter size to a number 4 markedly reduces the response characteristics and departs from the ideal considerably. A variation of 1/10 of 1 mm in the diameter at any one point in the catheter not more than 0.5-mm diameter, such as by uneven manufacture, kinking, or fibrin formation, can obviously be quite critical. The frequency response is also inversely related to the square root of the catheter length so that going from 100- to 25-cm length will double the frequency response of the same diameter catheter. For a number 4 French 50-cm-length catheter, though one may gain from the short length, the loss of frequency response by the small diameter is an overriding consideration. Until microtransducers become cheaper and more durable, the best response possible from an imperfect system should be aimed at thorough, meticulous attention to flushing, heparinization, and periodic testing of the frequency response throughout each study (Shapiro and Krovetz, 1970).

A zero reference level is necessary. It is probably of little consequence where this is localized as long as a constant point is used, but 5 cm anterior to the skin of the back in infants and children weighing under 20 kg (10 cm for children over this weight) seems to be satisfactory reference (Blount et al., 1955).

The peak of the pressure pulse in the ventricles, pulmonary artery, and aorta is taken as the systolic level, and the level just before the systolic rise is taken as the diastolic level (Dexter et al., 1947).

Flows. Cardiac output or systemic flow may be calculated from the following formula based on the Fick principle

$$\dot{Q} = \frac{\dot{V}O_2}{C_aO_2 - C_vO_2}$$

where

$\dot{Q}$ = cardiac output (systemic flow) (L/min)
$\dot{V}O_2$ = oxygen consumption (ml/min)
C_aO_2 = content of oxygen in systemic arterial blood (ml/L)
C_vO_2 = content of oxygen in mixed venous blood (ml/L)

In the absence of shunts, the mixed venous sample is obtained from the pulmonary artery, and systemic flow (Qs) = pulmonary flow (Qp). Oxygen consumption may be measured by a number of modifications of the standard technique, but the practical difficulty of obtaining good fits of masks and mouthpieces in smaller children and infants had discouraged the routine measurement of oxygen consumption in this age group except under special circumstances (Rudolph and Cayler, 1958). Nevertheless an apparatus is available* based on the principle that the conductivity of an electrically warmed wire varies according to the composition of the surrounding gas mixture (Noyons, 1937). This approach is eminently suitable for infants because of the lack of need for tight-fitting masks or obstruction of any sort to the airways (Lees et al., 1967). Modifications of this technique employing paramagnetic oxygen analyzers rather than thermal techniques for gas measurements have been devised (Wessel et al., 1969; Kappagoda et al. 1973; Fixler et al., 1974). Predicted values for oxygen uptake have been derived using regression equations from measured values (Lucas et al., 1961; Krovetz et al. 1967; LaFarge and Miettinen, 1970), and these estimates seem reasonably satisfactory if not perfect for sedated older children (Baum et al., 1967). They are quite unsatisfactory for the infant case and the young child, and nothing short of measured values is acceptable under these conditions.

In the absence of shunts an alternative way of obtaining the cardiac output is through indicator dilution. This method is now widely used, and we have found it satisfactory even in newborn infants (Gessner et al., 1965). From the Hamilton (1932) equation:

$$\dot{Q} = \frac{60I}{ct}$$

---

* P. J. Kipp & Zonen, Delft-Holland.

where

$\dot{Q}$ = cardiac output (systemic flow) (L/min)
I = amount of injected dye (mg)
c = mean dye concentration during the primary curve (mg/L)
t = duration of primary curve (sec)

Several different calibration techniques are available (Nicholson and Woods, 1951; Emanuel et al., 1966) and details of the necessary calculations for obtaining output from the dilution curve are available (Rivera et al., 1970; Yang et al., 1972). Ways to shorten the tedium of drawing a classic semilogarithmic plot to obtain the area under the curve include the forward triangle method of Hetzel and associates (1958) and the fore-'n'-aft triangle formula (Bradley and Barr, 1969), but most simply by a nomogram (Olley et al., 1970). On-line computerization of the output (Hansen and Pace, 1962; Hara and Belville, 1963; Warner et al., 1970; Mesel and Gelfand, 1971) has gained increasing acceptance.

The technique of thermal dilution (Evonuk et al., 1961; Hosie, 1962; James et al., 1965; Branthwaite and Bradley, 1968; Ganz et al., 1971) should be of interest to the pediatrician particularly because blood withdrawal is not necessary but also because it is a method by which rapid serial measurements of flow may be made (Silove et al., 1971; Forrester et al., 1972). There is good comparability of cardiac output measured by dye and similar dilution techniques and very good correlation between the shape of curves in those patients with congenital heart disease either without shunt or having indirectional or bidirectional shunts (Paul et al., 1958; Cooper et al., 1960).

Shunts. In any discussion of the examination of systemic flow and its quantification by several methods it will be obvious that the problem for adults, where perhaps less than 5 percent of heart disease is congenital, is quite different from that in children where 90 percent of the heart disease found has a congenital basis. Furthermore, probably more than 75 percent of all congenital heart disease is complicated by a shunt of blood from one circuit to the other, the presence of which not only limits the methods available for calculation of blood flow but renders the estimation of outputs less reliable. There are several methods of estimating blood flow in shunts:

The Fick Method. Left-to-right shunts are detected by rises in oxygen saturation of blood in a chamber of the right heart or its connections. This rise commences at the site of the shunt and is sustained in chambers downstream to that site.

Then

$$\dot{Q}p \ (\text{L/min}) = \frac{VO_2}{CaO_2 - CpaO_2}$$

where $CpaO_2$ now = oxygen content of pulmonary arterial blood (ml/L) and

$$\dot{Q}s \ (\text{L/min}) = \frac{VO_2}{CaO_2 - CvO_2}$$

where CvO_2 now = oxygen content of blood from averaged caval, right atrial, or right ventricular samples, depending on the site of the left-to-right shunt. The volume of the left-to-right shunt may be expressed:

$$\dot{Q}sh \ \text{left-to-right (L/min)} = \dot{Q}p - \dot{Q}s$$

A useful approximation of the size of the shunt is commonly expressed in terms of pulmonary-to-systemic flow ratios: so if

$$\dot{Q}p = \frac{VO_2}{SaO_2 - SpaO_2}$$

where $SpaO_2$ = blood oxygen saturation in the pulmonary artery, and

$$\dot{Q}s = \frac{VO_2}{SaO_2 - SVO_2}$$

where SVO_2 = blood oxygen saturation in a site proximal to the left-to-right shunt then

$$\dot{Q}p/\dot{Q}s = \frac{SaO_2 - SVO_2}{SaO_2 - SpaO_2}$$

In addition to calculation of Qp/Qs by use of blood oxygen saturation as above, estimation of Qsh left-to-right may be expressed in terms of its contribution to pulmonary blood flow

$$Qsh \ \text{left-to-right (as percent of } Qp)$$

$$= \frac{SpaO_2 - SVO_2 \times 100}{SaO_2 - SVO_2}$$

If a right-to-left shunt exists as well, the arterial sample is not equivalent to pulmonary venous blood, as is assumed in the general formula, and the oxygen content of pulmonary venous blood is usually assumed to be 97 percent. This assumption is valid in patients with marked right-to-left shunts (Bing et al., 1947) but is not necessarily correct where left-to-right shunts exist (Kjellberg et al., 1959).

It has been customary in most laboratories when a shunt is found to calculate effective pulmonary flow (Qep). This is defined as the volume of systemic venous return that reaches the pulmonary alveoli:

$$Qep = \frac{VO_2}{CpvO_2 - CvO_2}$$

where

$CpvO_2$ = oxygen content of pulmonary venous blood (ml/L).

then

$$Qsh \ \text{left-to-right} = Qp - Qep$$

and

$$Qsh \ \text{right-to-left} = Qs - Qep$$

In simpler fashion, using blood oxygen saturation data, Qsh right-to-left may be expressed in terms of its contribution to systemic blood flow:

$$Qsh \ \text{right-to-left (as percent of } Qs) =$$

$$= \frac{SpvO_2 - SaO_2 \times 100}{SpvO_2 - SvO_2}$$

INDICATOR DILUTION. The development and refinement of indicator dilution techniques have permitted both the detection of shunts and in many instances their quantitation. Of the various methods there is little question that green dye injection with multiple sampling sites and an elaborate variety of sensing devices (less commonly now employing modified ear oximeters) (Wallgren, 1975) (Figure 6–1) is the most consistently reliable technique available. The additional information that this method supplies during the course of cardiac catheterization for congenital heart disease has

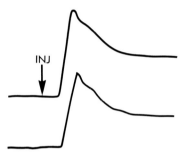

INJ

Figure 6-1. Tracings of indicator dilution patterns recorded simultaneously from the arterial system in an infant aged 11 months with a patent ductus arteriosus. Dye was injected into the main pulmonary artery. The upper curve was recorded from a Melville earpiece densitometer, while the lower curve was described as blood was withdrawn through a catheter whose tip lay in the aortic arch.

proven of great practical value. The contribution to cardiology made by those who developed these methods, particularly the Mayo group, can hardly be overemphasized.

▷ When a *left-to-right shunt* is present, injection of green dye into the central venous circulation results in early recirculation when sampling of blood is obtained from a peripheral artery. Dyed blood flows through the lung and out to the systemic circuit but a portion of it passes through the shunt and recirculates through the lung. Because the pulmonary circulation time is shorter than systemic circulation time, the shunted dye appears between the normal peak and the normal recirculation peak. In large-volume left-to-right shunts the magnitude of the deflection is reduced; i.e., the maximal concentration of dye is small and the slope of declining concentration is prolonged, no recirculation peak being identifiable. The changes are due to recirculation of dye in the heart and lungs and the resultant slow clearance of a constant proportion into the systemic circuit. Thus the disappearance time is greatly prolonged (Nicholson et al., 1969) (Figure 6–2). With smaller left-to-right shunts distortion of the dye curve is less marked, and indeed with shunts contributing less than 25 percent to the pulmonary blood flow there will usually be no obvious distortion of the disappearing slope of the curve. For these apparently normal curves calculation of the ratio of least concentration of the dye to the concentration at peak of recirculation of the dye may detect smaller shunts (Carter et al., 1960). A more precise though more laborious method of detecting shunts of between 5 and 15 percent of pulmonary blood flow by relating areas on a descending portion of the curve has been described

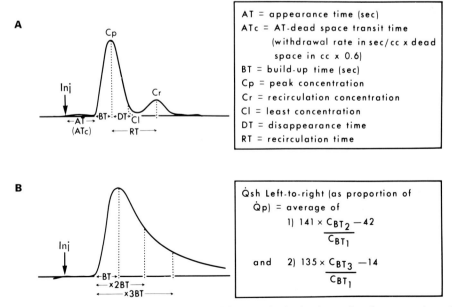

| AT = appearance time (sec) |
| ATc = AT-dead space transit time (withdrawal rate in sec/cc × dead space in cc × 0.6) |
| BT = build-up time (sec) |
| Cp = peak concentration |
| Cr = recirculation concentration |
| Cl = least concentration |
| DT = disappearance time |
| RT = recirculation time |

$\dot{Q}sh$ Left-to-right (as proportion of $\dot{Q}p$) = average of

1) $\dfrac{141 \times C_{BT_2} - 42}{C_{BT_1}}$

and 2) $\dfrac{135 \times C_{BT_3} - 14}{C_{BT_1}}$

Figure 6-2. Indicator dilution curves. *A.* Diagram of the normal. The time intervals and concentration points are those commonly employed in evaluating the curve. *B.* Diagram of a large left-to-right shunt. The rate of decline of the downslope is proportional to the magnitude of the shunt.

(Mook and Zijlstra, 1961). For quantification of left-to-right shunts the method of Carter and coworkers (1960), which is based on the rate of disappearance of dye from the circulation, is used. The method is valid for central venous injection but not for left heart injections or for infants and small children. In the latter the time of appearance of dye shunted through the pulmonary flow pathways occurs before the inscription of the concentration peak. This causes a high disappearance ratio and an erroneously high estimate of the magnitude of the shunt. An alternative formulation has been devised for infants taking this factor into consideration (Krovetz and Gessner, 1965). The detection of small left-to-right shunts requires more detailed approaches. If indicator is injected into a pulmonary vein and sampling is carried out from the pulmonary artery, the presence of a small left-to-right shunt downstream (distal to the injection site) will be confirmed by the early appearance of indicator at the pulmonary artery sampling site. It is then an easy matter to localize the site of the left-to-right shunt by further injections of green dye. There are certain problems due to mixing inadequacies and it is difficult to quantify the shunt with this technique.

Other methods that can be used to detect and localize left-to-right shunts include the hydrogen inhalation technique where a catheter with a platinum electrode at its tip is placed in the pulmonary artery and a single breath of hydrogen inhaled (Clark and Bargeron, 1959; Clark et al., 1960). This is an extremely sensitive method and has many advocates despite the fact that a negative response often requires a rather tedious technical check to ensure its validity. Furthermore, there is a potential explosive risk involved. A method that also involves inhalation of gas is that described by Amplatz and associates (1969) using a single inhalation of Freon during blood sampling from the pulmonary artery.

The quantitation of moderate to large left-to-right shunts using the N_2O method (Sanders et al., 1959) does not appear to be so widely used now while the techniques using radionuclides (Greenspan et al.,

1950; Spach et al., 1965; Flaherty et al., 1967) may perhaps be gaining in popularity (Bosnjakovic et al., 1971; Hagen et al., 1972; Weber et al., 1972; Maltz and Treves, 1973; Stocker et al., 1973). Localization of the site of the left-to-right shunt can also be obtained from certain levels of shunt with a phonocatheter (Feruglio, 1959; Lewis et al., 1959), with thermal dilution (Cooper et al., 1960), or with ascorbate (Frommer et al., 1961; Bentivoglio et al., 1967; Levy et al., 1969).

The application of roentgen video densitometry for the detection of left-to-right shunts (Armorin et al., 1971) is not a new idea but is one where improved instrumentation may eventually offer more attraction for its routine use.

In *right-to-left shunts* with indicator dilution techniques such as green dye a peripheral injection of the indicator results in a shortened appearance time and an abnormal hump in the build-up slope of the curve. The appearance time is shortened as a result of some dye being shunted into the systemic circuit through an intracardiac defect and reaching the sensing device before the dye that pass the normal longer pathway through the heart and lungs (Nicholson et al., 1951). It was soon recognized that the magnitude of the initial hump of the curve was related to the volume of shunt passing through the defect, and in many such subjects this relationship could be quantitated after a correction factor had been applied (Swan et al., 1953) (Figure 6–3). These authors showed that a right-to-left shunt time of less than 30 percent of systemic flow resulted in relatively mild arterial desaturation but that a figure of above 40 percent produced a marked fall in arterial oxygen saturation. Similar reasoning applies to the detection of early-appearing systemic evidence of other indicators following right-sided injection including selective ether (Donzelot et al., 1951; Fraser et al., 1961), ascorbate (Clark et al., 1960), or foreign gases dissolved in saline solution.

A variety of formulae based on the Fick principle are available for calculation not only of right-to-left

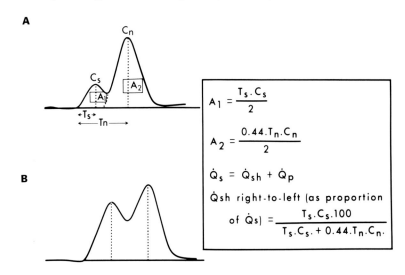

$$A_1 = \frac{T_s \cdot C_s}{2}$$

$$A_2 = \frac{0.44 \cdot T_n \cdot C_n}{2}$$

$$\dot{Q}_s = \dot{Q}_{sh} + \dot{Q}_p$$

$\dot{Q}sh$ right-to-left (as proportion of $\dot{Q}_s$) $= \dfrac{T_s \cdot C_s \cdot 100}{T_s \cdot C_s + 0.44 \cdot T_n \cdot C_n}$

Figure 6-3. Indicator dilution curves: right-to-left shunt diagrams. The ratio of the early appearing peak (shunted blood) is compared with the second peak (blood passing through the normal lung pathway). *A*. Small ($\dot{Q}_{sh} = 16$ percent of $\dot{Q}_s$). *B*. Large ($\dot{Q}_{sh} = 43$ percent of $\dot{Q}_s$).

shunts, but of mixed shunts or two shunts in one direction as well as bronchial blood flow (Bing et al., 1947; Dexter et al., 1947; Luisada and Liu, 1956; Rudolph and Cayler, 1958; Yang et al., 1972). Because phasic variation in shunt volume is not taken into account in such calculations, the concept should be regarded with some skepticism. A detailed analysis of detection and quantification of intracardiac and great vessel shunts, which emphasizes this admonition, has been made recently by Krovetz (1974).

Resistances. Calculation of vascular resistance in the systemic circulation in resistance units (mm Hg/L/min) may be obtained from the following formula:

$$Rs = \frac{SAm - RAm}{Qs}$$

where SAm = mean systemic arterial pressure and RAm = mean right atrial pressure.

For the pulmonary circulation, the vascular resistance equation reads:

$$Rp = \frac{PAm - LAm}{Qp}$$

where PAm = mean pulmonary arterial pressure and LAm = mean left atrial pressure (Figure 6–6, page 100). A healthy air of skepticism surrounds the measurement of pulmonary vascular resistance, particularly in the normal, mature pulmonary circulation (Harris and Heath, 1962; Roos, 1962) but also in patients with cardiac malformation accompanied by pulmonary hypertension (Rudolph and Nadas, 1962). It is, on the other hand, generally agreed that the calculations have practical value in most patients who have severe elevation of pulmonary vascular resistance.

Recently, because of computer developments and improved methods of hemodynamic measurement, there has been interest in reexamining the question of pressure and flow in the vascular bed. Pressure relationships, which are more applicable to pulsatile blood flow and arteries than the average flow in rigid tubes, have been assessed through the use of time-related and more accurate measurements of both variables to obtain vascular impedence (Bergel and Milnor, 1965). Although the application of these measurements to routine cardiac catheterization is some distance away, the development is exciting because of the potential for detection of abnormalities in pressure flow relationships at an earlier stage than could be revealed through simple resistance measurement.

Other formulae are available that make an approximation of orifice size and stenotic lesions of valves or the infundibulum (Gorlin and Gorlin, 1951). It is by no means certain that these derivations are valid for the child, if indeed for the adult, and they should be regarded more as steppingstones toward more accurate methods of evaluation.

There are very few laboratories where blood flows, resistances, valve orifice areas, or heart volumes are reported in absolute values. The usual practice, especially in children where the range of body size is large, is to normalize data by relating cardiac output to body surface area. The validity of this practice has been questioned, and an alternative method of comparing measured values for a particular child to a predicted value obtained through regression equations derived from normal data has been offered (Graham and Jarmakani, 1972; Krovetz and Goldbloom, 1972a).

Cardiac Volumes and Function. Increasing importance is now being attached to assessment of myocardial function in infants and children with serious heart malformation or myocardial disorders. In addition to information on pressure and flow routinely obtained is now added those relating to chamber volume and dimension. From these measurements a variety of derivatives allow assessment of myocardial performance. Although these have been in common use for the assessment of left ventricular function in adults (Dodge et al., 1960), application of the methods to children is relatively recent (Miller and Swan, 1964; Hugenholtz and Wagner, 1970). Possibly preoccupation of pediatric cardiologists with right-sided problems obscured the fact that assessment of left ventricular function has considerable importance in myocardiopathies, in a variety of left-to-right shunts, in the different forms of aortic stenosis and coarctation of the aorta, in transposition of the great arteries, and in acquired valvular lesions as well as the postoperative assessment of many malformations. Leaders in the examination of these problems have been the pediatric cardiology group from Duke University (Graham et al., 1968; Jarmakani et al., 1969; Graham et al., 1970a; Graham et al., 1971a, 1971b).

From the first cine of the catheterization left heart volumes are estimated in the levophase of pulmonary artery contrast injections. The area-length method has been utilized for left atrial and left ventricular volumes:

$$V = \frac{0.849 \, Aap \frac{1}{2} A \, lat}{LLs}$$

where

Aap = area in an anteroposterior view

$A \, lat$—area in lateral view

LLs—shortest of two longest lengths in either view

Correction factors for the overestimate of left ventricular volume resulting from such measurements have been developed for volumes of different size: small ($<15 \, cm^3$), true volume = $0.733V$; large ($>15 \, cm^3$), true volume = $0.974V - 3.1$ (Graham et al., 1971a). Formulae with corrections have also been developed for estimation of left ventricular wall mass from measuring wall thickness midway between the aortic valve and the apex in the anteroposterior view of the same angiocardiogram used to measure left ventricular volume (Graham et al., 1970a). Subtraction of left ventricular end-diastolic volume from the total end-diastolic volume gives a muscle volume, which when multiplied by 1.050 (the specific gravity of heart muscle) provides a measure of muscle mass. From normal values regression equations have been derived so that measured volumes in a given patient can be expressed as a percentage of the normal (Graham et al., 1971a). The biplane methods have been satisfactorily adapted for use with the single-plane cine-angiocardiogram (Hermann and Bartle, 1968; Sandler and Dodge, 1968).

The complex problem of assessing right ventricular volume has also been investigated more recently (Arcilla et al., 1971; Graham et al., 1973; Thilenius and Arcilla, 1974).

Inroads of noninvasive or semiinvasive techniques into the area of myocardial function through echocardiography and radionuclide cardiography are increasing, and it seems possible that further developments in these areas will permit their substitution for intracardiac methods particularly as these studies may be performed with the patient awake and can be repeated frequently (Feigenbaum et al., 1967, 1972; Mullins et al., 1969; Graham et al., 1970b; Strauss et al., 1971; Graham and Jarmakani, 1972).

The assessment of left ventricular function independent of preload or afterload through force-velocity relationships involves a number of assumptions and complex methodology. Pressure-velocity curves from the left ventricle using catheter-tip transducers to measure dp/dt and pressure have been used in children to derive an index of myocardial contractile state (Graham et al., 1971b). It is unlikely that the application of these methods will extend beyond selective investigations of children with heart disease until more certain indices of myocardial function have been established, until further miniaturization of catheter transducers has been developed, and until cost/benefit ratios have been reduced considerably.

Recent experimental work directed at assessment of regional myocardial blood flow in animals and adult humans has implications for infants and young children with severe congenital heart disease or acquired myocardial disturbances (Tawes et al., 1969; Rowe and Hoffman, 1972) where discrepancies between oxygen demands and supply for cardiac muscles are likely to be present. The proposal that a ratio of diastolic pressure time index (Buckberg et al., 1972) to tension time index (Sarnoff et al., 1958) reflects this supply/demand relationship and estimates the adequacy of subendocardial blood flow is now being examined in a variety of clinical settings. Though these approximations may eventually be supplanted by others, there is little doubt they

represent very reasonable beginnings to the search for some way to measure myocardial requirements and performance in the young as well as for older patients with heart disorders (Lewis et al., 1974; Krovetz and Kurlinski, 1976).

Intracardiac Electrocardiography. The presence of an electrode on the cardiac catheter has been recognized for years as assisting in clarification of the catheter position when certain pressure alterations occur during the course of study (Watson, 1962, 1964). The chief practical application has been in confirming the diagnosis of Ebstein's disease of the tricuspid valve. Other information that it has provided, such as knowledge of the side of pulmonary stenosis when pressure data are inconclusive, has been less useful in routine application because other methods of selective angiocardiography supplanted it.

Use of electrode catheters to record His bundle activity has a more recent application in man (Giraud et al., 1960; Watson et al., 1967; Scherlag et al., 1969).

The utilization of His electrograms together with simultaneous electrocardiograms is termed His bundle electrocardiography (Scherlag et al., 1972). There are three distinct deflections in the electrogram:

1. A (atrial) activity that occurs in the midportion of the P wave and corresponds to local atrial activity recorded in the AV node and His bundle area.

2. H (His bundle) activity that is a biphasic or triphasic potential recorded between P and QRS.

3. V (Ventricular) activity, which corresponds to ventricular activity as recorded at the AV junction. In conjunction with electrocardiographic leads it is possible to divide the P-R interval into three subintervals:

   a. The P-A interval: the time from earliest onset of P in the electrocardiogram to the onset of A in the electrogram. This interval is regarded as a measure of the conduction time from sinus to AV node.

   b. The A-H interval: the time from onset of A to the onset of H deflections. This interval is regarded as a measure of AV nodal conduction.

   c. The H-V interval: the time from the onset of H activity to the earliest onset of ventricular activity whether on an electrocardiogram or electrogram. This interval is regarded as a measure of conduction through the bundle of His and the bundle branches to the Purkinje system.

Values for these intervals have been obtained for normal children and the technique is now being used extensively in this age group (Brodsky et al., 1971; Anderson et al., 1972; Kelly et al., 1972; Roberts and Olley, 1972).

TECHNIQUE

At The Hospital for Sick Children, patients are fasted for at least four hours before study with the reservation that in small infants and particularly

cyanotic infants fluid restriction should be no more than a few hours. We do not now administer antibiotic to cover the risk of infective complications because on the balance of experience in a number of centers it would appear that the risk of bacterial endocarditis is exceptionally small and that the explanation for fever after catheterization usually has other origins (Gilladoga et al., 1972). There has been an interestingly wide range of preference for premedication of patients with congenital heart disease undergoing cardiac catheterization. In its most extreme form this has resulted in the administration of a general anesthetic (Munroe et al., 1965; Jones et al., 1972) and extended through ketamine (Faithfull and Haider, 1971) to a variety of narcotic mixtures. One of these more recently utilized is Innovar injection, which is a combination of a narcotic and analgesic (fentanyl) and a tranquilizer (droperidol) (Graham et al., 1974). Perhaps the one most widely used is the lytic cocktail (CM$_3$), in proportions developed at The Hospital for Sick Children (Smith et al., 1958) containing

Chlorpromazine	6.25 mg	
Promethazine	6.25 mg	per milliliter
Meperidine	25.00 mg	

It is given one hour before transfer to the catheterization room. The dose varies according to the age and condition of the patient. Noncyanotic infants and children receive 1 ml/10 kg of body weight up to a maximum of 1.5 ml. Deeply cyanotic infants are given only one-half, whereas slightly cyanotic infants receive two-thirds this dose. In any particular case the dose may be increased later, if necessary, by injection of a diluted solution through the cardiac catheter. Some modification of the dosage has been preferred by other centers, but for us in several different hospitals settings the above cocktail has proven to be the most consistently reliable preparation we have used over the past 15 years.

There is little question that it is preferable to use no premedication for the infant under the age of six months or 5 kg, and there are some who prefer no premedication under any circumstances. Particular care has to be exercised in patients with high pulmonary vascular resistance that alveolar hypoventilation is not induced, and again for these patients it is probably wiser to avoid any medication at all if feasible.

As usual, however, there has to be some middle ground on this matter for it is not always possible without some premedication to obtain the cooperation of the young child. There is no argument that all of the premedicants used influence the cardiovascular system through an effect on the vascular bed or myocardium (Goldberg et al., 1968; Sawyer et al., 1971) and they usually also influence oxygen consumption. For example, the administration of CM$_3$ to infants between one month and five and one-half years has been shown by Baum and associates (1967) to reduce the oxygen uptake by one-third in the period between one-half and two hours after administration of the mixture. In studies of patients with pulmonary or aortic stenosis, Hawker and

Krovetz (1974) found the depression in cardiac output from normal values to be over 15 percent after CM$_3$ premedication, whereas with Innovar it was only 5 percent. On the other hand, there is minimal effect on paO$_2$ or paCO$_2$ from the mixture (Israel et al., 1967). It should be remembered that a restless, disturbed infant or child is far from being a desirable alternative so that on balance some sedating effect is more likely to achieve meaningful information from the study. The use of premedication does not obviate the need to ensure as comfortable as possible an environment for the infant or child during the procedure by providing direct personal attention to needs at all times. A quiet atmosphere, pacifiers, music, and an understanding and reassuring nursing, technical, and medical staff are all important for this goal.

The patient is placed on the fluoroscopy table and settled in as comfortable a position as is feasible for the age. Some have used a plastic frame upon which the baby may be comfortably bundled with bandages, making sure that respiration is not interfered with. Electrocardiograph lead attachments are well-positioned and some form of respiratory monitor (Monroe et al., 1964) is desirable, and a method of maintaining body temperature for the smaller infants such as a heating pad is mandatory.

Infants usually respond to the warmth, a pacifier, and the low hum of the recording equipment or of soft music by going to sleep. Older children usually are drowsy and after the initial preparation and insertion of local anesthetic frequently doze off.

The most useful site for catheter entry is at the groin. There are some particular circumstances where that may not be the best route. Patients with a leftward and superior P axis (so-called coronary sinus rhythm) have a distinct possibility of azygos continuation of the inferior vena cava in association with polysplenia (Freedom and Ellison, 1973). In patients with congenital dislocation of the hips or with phocomelia the angulation or abbreviated limb can lead to some difficulties for insertion of the catheter, and for these situations it is probably wiser to use an arm vein or axillary vein approach (Rudolph and Cayler, 1958). In these circumstances the left arm vein is preferred unless there is reason to suspect the presence of a left superior vena cava. In newborns there are some who prefer umbilical vein entry (Linde et al., 1966; Abinader et al., 1970), although we personally have not found that to be a trouble-free route and are not entirely satisfied that there may not be some dangers from either thrombosis or other possible hepatic damage in the approach. Our preference is to enter the groin vessels whenever possible so that an adequate exploration of the atrial septum may be attained and so that a good-sized vessel is easily available for both venous and arterial sides (Figure 6–4).

At the groin the site of venous entry is usually the right femoral vein but occasionally is the left femoral vein if there has been a previous cutdown on the femoral vessels. The right saphenous vein is used for the smaller infant if a cutdown procedure is utilized

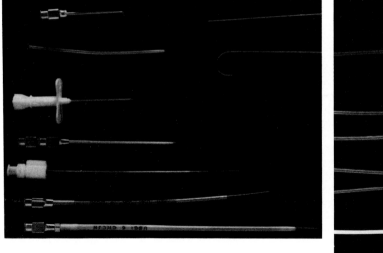
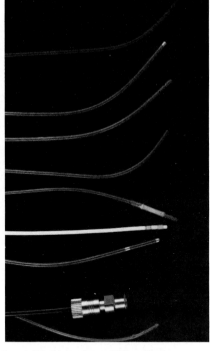

Figure 6-4. Catheter introducers and catheters. *A left* (from above down). Vlad introducer; Teflon dilator; disposable Amplatz cannula®; Longdwell cannula®; Cook cannula®; USCI arterial sheath set; USCI venous sheath set. *A right*. Straight and J-curved guide wires. *B* (from above down). Gensini catheter®; electrode catheter; NIH-type catheter®; Lehman catheter; Rashkind catheter®; Swan-Ganz catheter®; electrode catheter; umbilical arterial catheter.

and again a left saphenous vein if there has been previous entry.

Almost all arterial entry is again from the groin and the femoral artery with the obvious exception of the newborn period when the cord approach is a very happy escape from the usual cutdown alternative in the infant. The use of the umbilical artery (Sapin et al., 1963) is most successful in the first 48 hours after birth but has been used in patients up to the age of ten days. After that age there has been a variety of preferences for either the brachial artery, the axillary artery, or the femoral route for catheterization (Vlad et al., 1964).

In the past after skin preparation, draping, and local anesthetic infiltration at the right groin a cutdown was the usual method of approaching the vein and arterial routes. A few handy tips for that technique are still applicable; for infants and small veins great gentleness in handling avoids spasm, sterile glycerin is a great lubricant for a tight-catheter fit, and an introducer (Hohn and Vlad, 1959) permits separation of the lips of the vertical incision and vessels and greatly assists catheter entry. The percutaneous technique introduced by Seldinger (1953) and practiced by others (Wood and Swan, 1959; Cooley and Gianturco, 1964) was miniaturized fifteen years ago by Lurie and associates (1963). The technical difficulties inherent in working with small vessels, which this group pioneered so brilliantly, have been overcome to the degree now that the method is not only popular and widespread but is

being used for even very small infants (Boijsen and Lundstrom, 1968; Kirkpatrick et al., 1970; Simovitch et al., 1970; Takahashi et al., 1970; Viart et al., 1971; Neches et al., 1972; Carter et al., 1975; Sunderland et al., 1976).

Most commonly the femoral artery is localized by palpation of the groin and two small stab incisions of 2 mm made with a scalpel. one over each main vessel. Then a needle—for some a thinned-walled, shallow-bevel short needle or for others a Long-dwell #19 or #21 size—is passed through the vein to the bone and withdrawn slightly. For the latter we prefer a cannula of the Colonel Dickerson variety rather than the Seldinger-type bevel because its uniform spearlike tip minimizes trauma to the vessel wall and bleeding in the event of an off-center puncture. When on withdrawal blood emerges freely from the needle or plastic cannula, a guidewire of appropriate size and short length is inserted through the cannula into the vessel. For the artery we usually start by simply inserting the cannula into its full hilt and then connecting to a densitometer and strain gauge through a connecting plastic link of about 30 cm. At a later point in the study, if necessary, a dilator and sheath are used to allow entry for a cardiac catheter exactly as is done routinely on the venous side (vide infra). The technique for infants uses a #20 gauge needle and a #4-Fr catheter (White et al., 1973). For the vein the cannula is removed over the guidewire and replaced with a teflon dilator and sheath or by some similar arrangement (Desilets and Hoffman, 1965). The dilator is advanced with a rotating movement over the guide into the femoral vein and is followed by the sheath. When the sheath is free inside the vein, the guide and dilator are both removed and the cardiac catheter is inserted rapidly through the sheath. The sheath is one-half a French size larger than the catheter chosen, but the special reward for this is that its presence so minimizes trauma to the vessel from catheter manipulation that it permits the use and change of a wide variety of different types of catheter during the procedure. Various groups have minor variations in preference for catheter size and type as well as in technique but all methods are quite similar to that described above. Once catheters are in situ and connections to strain gauges and flushing systems have been made, heparin is administered in a bolus dose of 1 mg/kg and the catheterization is ready to start.

The selection of catheter size and tip configuration should depend in part on the size of the patient and the type of malformation suspected but in fact tends to become more a matter of individual preference than anything else. The important point regarding tip configuration is that three approaches to the question are possible, namely, either (1) preshaping of the catheter tip to the desired configuration, (2) use of guidewires with different distal curvatures, or (3) combinations of (1) and (2). In these ways the discordant needs for a relatively straight catheter to cross the atrial septum from the inferior approach to be followed by the necessity of turning a sharp curve downward into the left ventricle may be met. Use of guidewires or exchange of catheters is the preferred method rather than buckling the catheter tip against the wall to make a new form to the distal curve for a particular maneuver. The same general principles apply to retrograde arterial catheterization from the groin though most would prefer the use of a Gensini-type catheter for the widest possible utilization of the guidewires available for entrance into bronchial arteries, ductus arteriosus, passage across the aortic valve, and from the left ventricle into the left atrium.

On rare occasions when the retrograde approach is unsuccessful it is necessary to use the transseptal technique (Brockenbrough et al., 1962; Rovet et al., 1962; Aldridge, 1964). Left ventricle puncture to obtain a left ventricle pressure is only very rarely required (Lurie et al., 1961). The technical advances of recent years, particularly that of the balloon flotation catheter (Swan et al., 1970), have revolutionized the catheterization of the right side of the heart in complex disorders or in patients where there is particular difficulty in entering a normally connected pulmonary artery on that side. The catheter has also greatly improved the ease with which the pulmonary artery can be catheterized from the left ventricle with patients with transposition of the great arteries (Black, 1972; Kelly et al., 1972).

With the catheters in position the exploration can commence, the pressure assembly and oximeter having been previously prepared. Oscilloscopes opposite the operator indicate electrocardiographic and pressure information and the utilization of a television screen from an image amplifier is now in general usage. Probably the most useful first step in any study is to record a dilution curve from the femoral artery after injection of indicator in the inferior vena cava. We have recently preferred to inject into both venae cavae in turn. If the curve is normal, then blood oxygen sampling runs are unnecessary since if a left-to-right shunt is present it must be less than 20 percent of the pulmonary blood flow and therefore will surely not be detectable by the relatively crude blood oxygen saturation method. On the other hand, if a left-to-right shunt is visible on the curve, one can proceed to localize the shunt with blood oxygen sampling in the classic manner.

It matters little in what order the heart is explored. Sometimes it is easier to enter the left heart through a patent foramen ovale at the start and so obtain pressures and samples in pulmonary veins, left ventricle, both atria, and vena cava (Figure 6–5) before proceeding to the right ventricle and pulmonary artery. On other occasions the catheter is rapidly advanced to the pulmonary wedge position, samples and pressures then being taken in the pulmonary circuit, right ventricle (Figure 6–5) right atrium, and venae cavae before exploring the left side. Routine probing with the catheter tip should be carried out in the distal main pulmonary artery for a ductus arteriosus. Where indicated, the posteromedial position of the right ventricle requires exploration for a defect, as well as the atrial septum for a defect proper or a patent foramen ovale. Diligent gentle manipulation frequently permits success in these maneuvers.

Blood samples are taken in any desired number, preferably in at least two successive runs (Barratt-Boyes and Wood, 1957; Grayzel and Jameson, 1963). Even in the smallest infants this is safe as long as the amount of blood removed is replaced. In ordinary clinical catheterization using a cuvette oximeter we take a little over 1 ml of blood for each sample and immediately reinject after the oxygen saturation readings have been taken. Arterial samples are taken frequently, and at some stage a sample should be taken while breathing 100 percent oxygen by mask if the sample in room air is desaturated.

Over the areas for which angiocardiography or angiography will be necessary priorities should be set where more than one injection is required so that the more critically important anatomic details are clarified first. This is especially necessary for ill infants where the risk of deterioration is ever present.

Finally, additional studies where indicated such as phonocardiographic or electrophysiologic tests are performed after which the catheters and cannula are withdrawn and firm pressure applied for 15 minutes over the area if the catheterization has been percutaneous. For cut-down techniques, the vessels are reconstituted by 6-0 deknatel sutures and the skin incision closed with absorbable sutures.

Unless there have been major complications during

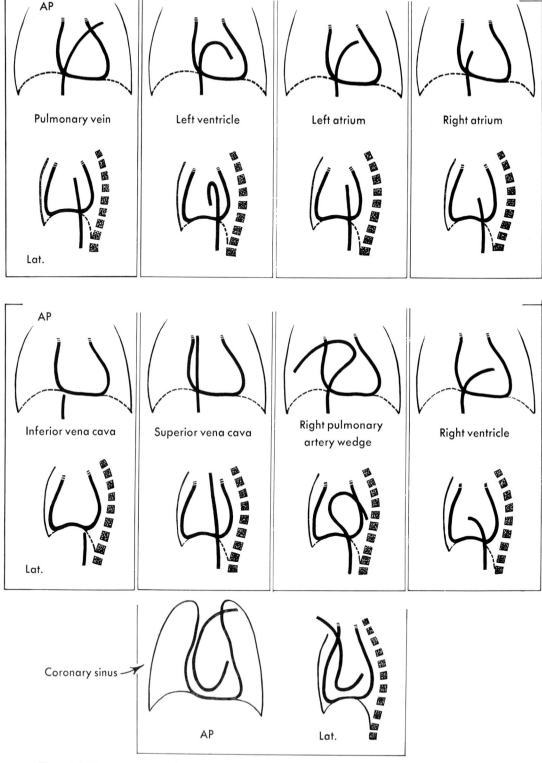

Figure 6-5. The appearance of the cardiac catheter at various positions within the normal heart of the infant.

the study, when the infant or child should be placed in an Intensive Care Unit, patients can be safely returned to a ward where vital signs may be monitored at increasing intervals for several hours and a fluid diet can be replaced by light diet as tolerated. A dorsalis pedis pulse, which is as easily palpable after study as before, means a patent artery. An absent or weak pulse by the time of return to the ward usually implies spasm or thrombosis of the vessel. An absent

pulse four hours after study is certain evidence of thrombosis at the site of catheter entry and requires surgical intervention to restore the arterial path to the leg in almost all instances except very small infants. Where further intensive medical treatment or surgical intervention is not planned immediately, the patient is usually discharged the next morning after a hematocrit has been obtained.

RESULTS

Normal

Oxygen Saturation. The normal ranges and means values of oxygen saturation in blood from the right heart and its connections have been studied in adults by Dexter and associates (1947), Holling and Zak (1950), and Barratt-Boyes and Wood (1957) and in infants and children by Kjellberg and coworkers (1959). The latter workers confirmed that in children, as in adults, there is a significantly higher oxygen saturation in blood from the inferior vena cava because of the streaming effect produced by highly oxygenated renal vein blood. They showed in their group an average difference of 6 percent ± 1.07. In a similar study on 17 infants and children, we found a mean difference of 4 percent although there were wider variations in the oxygen saturation of blood from both superior and inferior venae cavae. Eighty percent showed a higher oxygen saturation in the inferior vena cava. Kjellberg and associates (1959) have, in 31 cases, obtained two samples from the inferior vena cava—one in the usual position and one after rotational sampling. The results emphasize the effect of streaming in this area by showing a standard deviation of 5.9 percent saturation. Of interest is the observation of Fieldman and associates (1955) that, when general anesthesia is used during cardiac catheterization, these values are reversed, the oxygen saturation then becoming higher in the superior vena cava. The azygos vein may contain blood with an oxygen saturation close to that of the superior vena cava; however, in about 60 percent of patients it has a significantly higher level of oxygen saturation, presumably because of connections with the renal vein or with bronchial veins (Jain et al., 1970).

It is generally believed that normal mixing of the venous streams is not complete until the pulmonary artery or outflow tract of the right ventricle is reached, and this fact has led to considerable discussion over what constitutes an abnormal change in oxygen saturation between the venae cavae and right atrium, right atrium and right ventricle, and right ventricle and pulmonary artery. Multiple sampling theoretically could overcome some of the common difficulties, such as extracting the hepatic vein stream in the inferior vena cava and coronary sinus stream or either caval stream in the right atrium. Lasón and Alvarez (1949) take an "integrated" inferior vena caval sample by rotating the catheter tip during

withdrawal of blood for oxygen analysis. Dexter and associates (1947) prefer to ignore the highly variable inferior caval sample and rely on differences between the superior caval and right atrial oxygen content for the presence or absence of left-to-right shunt at atrial level. Others feel that a more accurate reflection of changes in oxygen saturation between the cavae and right atrium is established if the caval values are averaged (Holling and Zak, 1950; Kjellberg et al., 1959; Barratt-Boyes and Wood, 1957).

Whatever the theoretic possibilities, in practice, estimation of the difference in oxygen saturation between the inferior vena caval only and right atrial bood is unreliable in the detection of left-to-right shunts at atrial level. Either averaged caval values or the superior vena caval value by itself related to rises in oxygen saturation in the right atrium nearly always provides evidence of such shunt. It is therefore possible for inadvertent sampling of azygos vein blood at or near its vena caval junction, by giving an apparently high superior vena saturation, to falsely reduce the calculated size of an atrial left-to-right shunt (Jain et al., 1970). In our normal group the average rise in oxygen saturation between superior vena cava and right atrium was 2.1 percent, the highest value being 9.5 percent. By comparison there was an average fall in oxygen saturation between inferior vena caval and right atrial blood of 3.4 percent. Averaged caval saturations related to right atrial samples showed a fall of 0.7 percent. The saturation in right atrial samples, especially near the tricuspid valve, may be significantly affected by exit from the coronary sinus of blood of very low oxygen saturation. Samples in this region may have as little as 40 percent oxygen saturation, whereas samples from the coronary sinus itself may be as low as 25 percent (Read et al., 1955).

Lesser changes occur between right atrial and ventricular samples, over two-thirds showing an average fall of 1.3 percent and less than 30 percent having an average rise of 3 percent saturation. A further average fall of 0.3 percent occurred on sampling the pulmonary artery.

In multiple sampling Barratt-Boyes and Wood (1957) accepted as evidence for a left-to-right shunt at ventricular level a right ventricular saturation more than the right atrial saturation by approximately two standard deviations or 3 percent rise in oxygen saturation in paired samples. A different approach to such an analysis of the sampling sequence (Grayzel and Jameson, 1963) standardizes the difference in mean values between right ventricular and right atrium and determines statistical significance from the t-distribution. In this way reliability (the probability of correctly excluding the shunt) was 98.4 percent and sensitivity (the probability of diagnosing an existing shunt) was 97.1 percent at the 1 percent level of significance. Obviously any method becomes increasingly sensitive with increasing size of shunt but increasing the number of samples can improve this sensitivity for even smaller shunts. Minimum saturation changes between cardiac chambers considered indicative of left-to-right shunts in children have been published (Rudolph and Cayler, 1958) (Table 6–3). These authors have also emphasized that infants generally and some children are likely to show more variation in oxygen capacity than older subjects so that oxygen saturation changes are more reliable than alterations in blood oxygen content in the detection of shunts in this age group. They also point out the inverse relationship that mixed venous saturation level has on the least shunt detection and the siting problems in left-to-right shunts that can occur from streaming or valvular regurgitation (Rudolph and Cayler, 1958).

In 13 personally studied normal individuals and 82 from the literature for all ages, Krovetz and Goldbloom (1972a) found the mean arterial saturation at cardiac catheterization to be 96 percent with a standard deviation of 2 percent. The different blood oxygen dissociation curve for newborn infants has been examined by several groups of investigators, most recently by Oh and associates (1965). The curve may be used for estimating the percent oxygen saturation corresponding to a known oxygen tension value in neonatal blood. The mean arterial venous oxygen differences in 212 normal subjects between two months of age and 69 years was 38 ml/L with a standard deviation of 9. There was no correlation with either the age or body size (Krovetz and Goldbloom, 1972a). The one period in life when significant intracardiac and extracardiac shunts normally occur is in the first few days after birth. During the adaptation to extrauterine existence there is bidirectional duct shunting for about an hour after birth following which a left-to-right shunt of gradually diminishing size occurs through the ductus arteriosus for the rest of the first day of life. Thereafter the duct is normally closed functionally even though abnormal environmental factors may influence its reopening.

In a different fashion since the position of the free border of the foramen ovale flap varies, there may be a left-to-right shunt normally in the first 24 hours after delivery but after that time only right-to-left shunting is possible under certain physiologic (e.g., crying) as well as pathologic conditions, all of which are characterized by some transient increase in right atrial pressure. In fact, since in about 20 percent of normal persons the foramen ovale never seals, this fetal channel can become a potential site for right-to-left

Table 6–3. MINIMUM OXYGEN SATURATION CHANGES BETWEEN HEART CHAMBERS AND VESSELS REGARDED AS INDICATING THE PRESENCE OF LEFT-TO-RIGHT SHUNTS BY THAT TECHNIQUE*

SITE	NUMBERS OF SAMPLING SETS		
	1	*2*	*3*
SVC—RA	10	7	5
RA—RV	7	5	3
RV—PA	5	3	3

* Data from Rudolph and Cayler, 1958.

shunts, but, it must be emphasized, only under situations of elevated right heart pressure.

Pressures. Kjellberg and associates (1959) reported pressure measurements at cardiac catheterization in 13 normal children between 2½ and 17 years of age. The results are closely similar to those analyzed in adults by Fowler and coworkers (1953). In our series of 35 normal infants and children between 12 days and 14 years of age, the mean right atrial pressure averaged 4, right ventricular pressure 22/4, the pulmonary arterial pressure 21/10, and the pulmonary wedge pressure 7 mm of mercury. The average systolic gradient between right ventricle and pulmonary artery was 1 mm. Sixteen of thirty-two cases had identical systolic pressures in right ventricle and pulmonary artery. Of the remainder only one case (10 mm) had a gradient in excess of 5 mm of mercury, due allowance having been made for the phase of respiration. The zero level in these measurements was 5 cm above the patient's back.

For 44 normal children between two months and 15½ years Krovetz and Goldbloom (1972a) likewise found a mean right atrial pressure of 1, a right ventricular pressure of 24/3, pulmonary artery of 20/4, and a mean left atrial pressure or pulmonary arterial wedge pressure of 6 mm of mercury.

Again the situation for infants in the first few days of life is rather different. At birth the pressures in the right ventricle and pulmonary artery are at systemic level for one to four hours before decreasing. The mean pulmonary artery pressure in the first ten hours is about 40 mm of mercury (Emmanouilides et al., 1964). A decline to adult values occurs by about seven days (Krovetz and Goldbloom, 1972b) but at a rate that is quite variable. One important factor influencing atrial as well as other right heart pressure levels for some hours after birth is the amount of placental transfusion (Burnard and James, 1963; Jegier et al., 1963; Arcilla et al., 1966), and the tone of the ductus arteriosus, metabolic demands, and hypoxia also can exert important influence on individual progress to mature pressure levels.

Study of the form of the normal pressure pulses in different chambers of the heart is imperative if significance is to be attached to abnormal patterns. For this reason a fast chart speed and maximum amplification of the pulse are essential at the time of recording. Analysis of pressure pulses becomes pointless where the catheter tip is not free within the particular chamber or vessel being studied. Considerable distortion may arise in atrial tracings when the tip of the catheter rests on the atrioventricular valve or further when the tip lies against the wall of the right ventricle or main pulmonary artery. Similar distortion occurs in the systemic circuit when the arterial needle lies against the vessel wall. Most of these difficulties can be recognized and corrected. The tracing will also show damping from clotting in either catheter or cannula or at very fast heart rates.

In right atrial pressure curves of infants and children, the height of the "a" wave exceeds or equals the "v" wave in the right atrium, whereas in the left atrium it is usual for the "v" wave to be higher than "a" (Haroutunian et al., 1958). Unfortunately not all curves are sufficiently free from artefacts to allow detailed examination, and particularly in infants this is a difficulty.

The ventricular pressure pulses are normally identical in form. In each ventricle there is a short period of isovolumic contraction with almost vertical ascent of the tracing, a plateau of ejection, and then a rapid fall due to isovolumic relaxation before diastole (Figure 27–11). Recent evidence indicates average adult values for left ventricular isovolumic contraction and relaxation to be 38.1 and 81 milliseconds, respectively. Both intervals are shorter for the right ventricle and of course are influenced by the heart rate. Values for infants and children will be shorter (Luisada and McCanon, 1972).

If the catheter tip is advanced into the coronary sinus, a low pressure is encountered, but if the tip is wedged in the great cardiac vein, a pressure pulse closely similar to that of a ventricular pulse is obtained (Harris and Summerhayes, 1955). In even young infants the value may reach 75 mm of mercury in systole. Similarly, an artefactually high pressure sometimes up to 50 mm of mercury appears when the catheter tip is occluded by a contracting atrial appendage (Johansson and Ohlsson, 1961).

The pulmonary and systemic arterial pressure pulses have a distinct form.

Studies of the pulse in both systemic and pulmonary circuits of young subjects have been given impetus by the development of better instrumentation for their evaluation (catheter tip transducers; data storage and computer analysis) as well as an increasing interest in diseases of vessels in children (Rowe, 1972). On the systemic side the amplitude of the pressure wave increases as the measuring site is moved along the aorta. A prominent diastolic wave is evident in the pulse in the distal aorta and iliac arteries (O'Rourke et al., 1968). These changes during pulse transmission become progressively less evident with increasing age.

When a cardiac catheter is advanced as far as possible into the finer branches of the pulmonary artery and the tip firmly fixed (pulmonary wedge position), a reflection of the left atrial pressure is obtained (Hellems et al., 1949; Lagerlof and Werko,

1949). Connolly and associates (1953) reported that the pulmonary artery wedge pressure-pulse contour corresponds very closely to that obtained from the left atrium in regard to both magnitude and contour. Variation in results from different workers led to some questioning of the value of this measurement (Editorial, *Circulation Research*, 1953; Linden and Allison, 1963). Bell and associates (1962) found through studies employing wedge arteriography that proper alignment of the catheter in an impacted vessel was critical and that elevated left atrial pressures more often than normal were associated with satisfactory phasic wedge pressures. Unfavorable catheter tip positions were more common in patients with congenital heart disease whereas they did not occur in patients with mitral stenosis. The measurement is not only still widely employed but confidence in its value seems generally accepted. The balloon-directed catheter (Swan et al., 1970) has greatly assisted the ease with which the "wedge" is obtained. There is currently interest in estimating left ventricular end-diastolic pressure from the pulmonary arterial end-diastolic values (Bouchard et al., 1971).

Similarly, when a cardiac catheter is properly wedged in a pulmonary vein, a reflection of the pulmonary arterial pressure is obtained. Wilson and associates (1955) and Gensini and coworkers (1955) believe this relationship to be accurate at all levels of pulmonary arterial pressure, whereas Connolly and Wood (1955) found the correlation true only when the pulmonary arterial pressure was normal. We have found that, although one may occasionally obtain a good comparison between pulmonary vein wedge and pulmonary artery pressures in cases of pulmonary hypertension, there are more often gross discrepancies between the two values in such patients. Reasonably good correlation has been obtained in subjects with normal or low pulmonary artery pressures. This problem has recently been examined in children by others who reached conclusions similar to ours (Rao and Sissman, 1971; Hawker et al., 1973a). The pulmonary vein wedge is therefore an unreliable substitute for pulmonary artery pressure.

Flows. In older subjects when cardiac output is calculated from the Fick principle and related to surface area, the resulting index is relatively constant at 3.12 liters per minute per square meter (Cournand et al., 1945). In adults the actual output varies between 5.5 and 6.5 liters per minute, and is lower with the subject erect (McMichael and Sharpey-Schafer, 1944). The cardiac index in ten normal children with an average age of 12 years was 4.3 L per minute (Brotmacher and Fleming, 1957). Cardiac indices of 21 children between 6 and 16 years have been reported by Sproul and Simpson (1964). They found values of 4.1 L in the body size range of 0.7 to 1.2 M^2. In 28 children between 5 and 13 years the cardiac index by dye technique averaged 3.19 ± 0.75 L per minute and no statistically significant difference was found between the mean value for children and adults (Jegier et al., 1961). In a series of 20 normal infants, Agustsson and associates (1963) reported cardiac

Table 6–4. NORMAL LEFT HEART VOLUME VARIABLES*

	UNDER 2 YEARS	OVER 2 YEARS
LV end diastolic volume	$42 \pm 10\,cm^3/m^2$	$73 \pm 11\,cm^3/m^2$
LV ejection fraction	0.68 ± 0.05	0.63 ± 0.05
LV wall mass	All ages $88 \pm 12\,g/m^2$	
LA maximal volume	$26 \pm\ ml/m^2$	$38 \pm 8\,ml/m^2$

* Data from Graham et al., 1971a.

output ranging from 0.23 L per minute at three days to 2.3 L per minute at two years and the cardiac index from five months to 14 years averaged 4.6 L per minute per square meter. In ten normal newborn infants, indicator dilution studies with Evans blue dye have shown an average cardiac output of 548 ml per minute and an index of 2.5 liters per minute (Prec and Cassels, 1955). The validity of these measurements has recently been challenged. To avoid the influence of the ductal shunt on the upslope of dye curves, left atrial dye injections were performed in 12 newborn infants (Gessner et al., 1965). The mean left ventricular output was 4.0 L per minute per square meter. Similar values were obtained in 23 newborns by Emmanouilides and associates (1970).

Resistances.   It is obvious from the pressure-flow data in normal newborn infants that the calculated pulmonary vascular resistance is normally at a very high value in the first few days of life. It is known that during infancy and early childhood there is a steady increase in pulmonary blood flow (Lucas et al., 1961) although the pulmonary artery pressures remain constant (Rowe and James, 1957; Agustsson et al., 1963). There is a distinct hiatus in our knowledge about the detail of flow data in the first month of life. Many have questioned the validity of the extremely high values so far reported for pulmonary vascular resistance at this age. It nevertheless follows that calculated pulmonary vascular resistance must

steadily decline during infancy. Krovetz and Goldbloom (1971b) have demonstrated that the decline in calculated vascular resistance occurs in both circuits at approximately the same rate (Figure 6–6) and that both vary inversely with age, height, or weight. In their view the data cannot be interpreted as demonstrating maturation of the pulmonary vascular bed because the similar time course of calculated systemic resistance has not been demonstrated to be associated with a similar anatomic arteriolar change.

Values for normal left heart volumes in infants and children have been published (Graham et al., 1970a, 1971a; Thilenius and Arcilla, 1974). The principal variables are shown in Table 6–4. The notably decreased normalized value for left atrial and ventricular size in infants is believed due mainly to shortening of late diastolic filling. This is most likely secondary to the rapid heart rate at that age although the additional influence of reduced compliance of these chambers may also play a role (Graham and Jarmakani, 1972).

Exploration.   In most normal infants it is possible to pass the catheter tip into the left heart through a patent foramen ovale. From the left atrium the left ventricle is entered, and this is rendered more easy if the tip has a tight curve. Lesser degrees of curve usually lead to entry into the left inferior pulmonary vein. It is often possible, but rarely necessary, to enter all four pulmonary veins from the left atrium. The

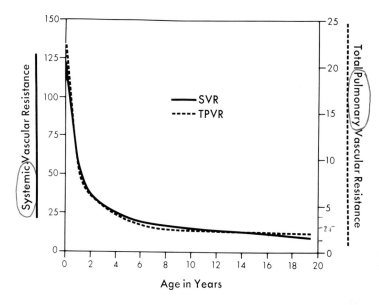

Figure 6-6. Total pulmonary and systemic vascular resistances related to age. *Both* decline in a similar time course. (Modified from Krovetz and Goldbloom, 1972.)

appearance of the catheter at fluoroscopy when the right-sided pulmonary veins have been entered almost always suggests that the vein connects with the right atrium—an illusion now widely recognized. (Folger et al., 1966).

Withdrawal of the catheter from left to right atrium usually produces a sensation of flip as the tip jerks into the right atrium through the foramen. Distinct changes in both the contour and the magnitude of the atrial pressure curve occur at this point.

Entry into vena cava opposite that through which the catheter reaches the heart may be difficult if a tight curve is being employed. Sliding the tip of the curve up the lateral wall of the atrium and then rotating it posteriorly seems the most successful maneuver to gain the entry, but replacement with a straight-tipped catheter or use of a guide wire may be necessary.

The coronary sinus is frequently entered. If a persistent left superior vena cava connects with the sinus, no harm arises. On the other hand, if a large-size catheter be advanced unrecognized into the sinus and so to the great coronary vein, serious results may develop (Read et al., 1955). Unfortunately the appearance of the catheter position in the antero-posterior view is deceptive and only by rotating the patient is fluoroscopic proof of position found (Figure 6–5). In any cardiac catheterization where, on apparently advancing through the right ventricle, the tip is held up near the "outflow" tract, a sample of blood for immediate analysis should be taken. This is always of very low oxygen saturation when taken from the sinus. The alternative is to examine fluoroscopically in the oblique position or analyze the intracardiac electrogram. No attention can be paid to the form of a high-level pressure pulse for previously stated reasons, but when an atrial level of pressure is found the decision is simple.

In normal infants the right ventricle may be entered from the inferior approach as easily as when the arm vein is used. It is only when the right atrium is very large that difficulties are encountered in reaching this chamber from below. Entry into the pulmonary artery is similarly easy. Pulmonary wedge positions from either main branch are often difficult to obtain if much curve is present on the catheter tip. If reliance is to be placed on the value of this measurement, the tip should preferably be wedged straight far out in the lung and pulmonary venous blood should be withdrawn through the catheter.

Use of the intracardiac electrogram as recorded from a unipolar electrode situated at the catheter tip has proved to be of assistance during exploration of the heart. The method is particularly helpful in detecting coronary sinus entry, for the tracing recorded from this position resembles left heart patterns (Levine and Goodale, 1950). Evidence of endocardiac injury can be detected much sooner than by the conventional electrocardiogram (Levine et al., 1949) and allows alteration of the catheter-tip position before serious complications develop. Emslie-Smith (1955) has pointed out the further advantage of assisting in later analysis of pressure

tracings recorded at cardiac catheterization. The method is not without its fallacies (Datey and Ghandi, 1961) but is generally felt to be a useful addition to catheter studies (Watson, 1962).

Abnormal

Flow. The cardiac output shows considerable variation in patients with congenital heart disease. In general, the data suggest that outputs tend to be low normal in those with severe disease when compared with subjects with either normal hearts or mild disease (Cayler et al., 1963; Rowe et al., 1966).

Oxygen Saturation. LEFT-TO-RIGHT SHUNTS. The detection of a significant rise in oxygen saturation of blood at one and subsequent levels in the right heart or its connections indicates the presence of a defect with pressure relationships permitting an arterio-venous shunt. Provided multiple samples are obtained, no difficulty usually exists in detecting gross left-to-right shunts at the various levels. In such cases problems arise only in the diagnostic interpretation of such data. For example, where the shunt is localized to the right atrial level, the anatomic possibilities are legion. Other hemodynamic and clinical data as well as further studies are necessary to reduce the possible diagnoses. Even after complete study, the precise diagnosis may remain in doubt.

In small-volume left-to-right shunts, the principal difficulty lies in deciding the significance of small rises in oxygen saturation of blood samples even after several rapid sampling runs. Under these circumstances, resort to more sensitive techniques can now be quite easily made. At all levels indicator dilution, especially using a two-catheter technique, is a very sensitive detector as is the hydrogen electrode. The nitrous oxide or krypton tests are available for older children (Sanders et al., 1959; Sanders and Morrow, 1959).

Along with others (Feruglio, 1959), we have found the phonocatheter (Lewis et al., 1959) to be of practical value in small shunts at ventricular or pulmonary arterial level, though it has not always proved as sensitive in our hands as have double-catheter dye or hydrogen techniques. It has been argued that small-volume left-to-right shunts are of no importance hemodynamically (Dexter, 1954), and this is true in the face of normal pressure relationships. However, the potential risk of subacute bacterial endocarditis is probably as high in the minor as in the more obvious defects, and for this reason it is important to establish for certain in equivocal cases whether or not a defect is present. Additionally it has become apparent that catheterization and angiocardiographic studies in such circumstances by providing detailed anatomic data may have predictive value of real benefit for future planning and management (e.g., aneurysmal transformation to small size of ventricular defect, dysplasia of the pulmonary and mitral valves, pulmonary and systemic arterial stenoses, and prolapse of aortic leaflets).

RIGHT-TO-LEFT SHUNTS. A reduced systemic arterial oxygen saturation in the presence of a congenital heart defect and absence of pulmonary disease has been generally accepted as evidence of a right-to-left shunt. Gross arterial oxygen desaturation is only rarely abolished by breathing pure oxygen, but lesser degrees may sometimes be restored to normal levels by this method. Instances of uncomplicated atrial septal defects with desaturation of arterial blood from small-volume right-to-left shunts have been revealed by indicator dilution studies (Swan et al., 1953). It is also true that certain, though not all, cases of left-to-right shunt in infancy and childhood have reduced oxygen saturation of pulmonary venous blood (Wood, 1952; Kjellberg et al., 1959). It has been suggested that this is due to an impairment of oxygen diffusion under conditions of increased pulmonary blood flow (Ordway, 1952). Breathing 100 percent oxygen usually restores the oxygen saturation to normal. Kjellberg and associates (1959) were unable in two such cases to restore the oxygen content of pulmonary venous blood to normal by 100 percent oxygen breathing and suggested as an alternative explanation that some blood might bypass the alveoli through precapillary shunts. Selective ether injection into the pulmonary circuit should reveal any small-volume right-to-left shunt of this nature, but in two cases studied in our laboratory the test was negative.

Localization of right-to-left shunts may be achieved by selective injection of ether, dye, ascorbate, or contrast material into the pulmonary artery, right ventricle, and right atrium in turn.

Pressures. ATRIAL. Recently more interest has been shown in the clinical application of detailed analysis of atrial pressure curves. Increase in the right atrial pressure with prominent x and y descents may be found in advanced congestive heart failure with large pericardial effusion or in constrictive pericarditis. In ventricular septal defect or patent ductus arteriosus, where examination of the pressure events in both atria was possible by the presence of a patent foramen ovale, the normal relationships of mean pressure and height of individual waves are preserved (Kjellberg et al., 1959). With isolated atrial septal defects, depending on the size, the right atrial mean pressure may more closely approximate that of the left but does not usually exceed it unless right ventricular failure develops. Reinhold (1955) detected a striking increase in height of the "v" wave of the jugular phlebogram of patients with this malformation. It has not appeared to be consistently so abnormal in right atrial pressure tracings of our own patients. In tricuspid stenosis, severe pulmonary stenosis, or severe pulmonary hypertension associated with high vascular resistance, the "a" wave in the right atrial tracing becomes prominent and exceeds both the "v" wave on the right side and the "a" of left atrial tracings. Severe tricuspid regurgitation produces a characteristic plateau between the "c" and "v" waves, which replaces the normal x' descent between these points. This is due to

transmission of right ventricular systolic pressure, through the incompetent valve (Bloomfield et al., 1946; Ferrer et al., 1952; McCord and Blount, 1952; Sepulveda and Lukas, 1955). In our experience the sign has been absent in some cases (confirmed at autopsy) with gross regurgitation. Minor degrees of regurgitation of this valve reveal lesser disturbances of the x' descent, and this is the more common sign in congenital heart disease complicated by tricuspid regurgitation (Shephard, 1955). In congenital or acquired mitral regurgitation, the effect of the lesion on pressure pulses in the atrium has likewise been variable. In many cases the left atrial pressure pulse shows classically a large "v" wave, but it is now clear that the important factor determining the presence or absence of pulse distortions in either atrium is the volume-elastance situation of the particular chamber (Morrow et al., 1957). Confirmation of the presence of tricuspid or mitral regurgitation may be obtained by two-catheter dye techniques, cineangiocardiography, or by the phonocatheter, but quantitation is practical only from dye or angiocardiographic methods (Sinclair et al., 1960; Gorelick et al., 1962; Miller et al., 1964).

In mitral stenosis it has been found from study of the pulmonary artery wedge pulse in adults that the "a" wave is higher than the "v" in only a third of the cases (Wood, 1954). A diastolic pressure gradient can be demonstrated in infants with mitral stenosis by catheterization of the left heart through a patent foramen ovale just as it has been in older patients (Gordon et al., 1954) with Lutembacher's syndrome (Rapaport et al., 1954) or by transseptal puncture. A diastolic pressure gradient across the mitral valve has also been observed in the absence of mitral stenosis in patients with ventricular septal defect and a high pulmonary blood flow. In small infants a further gradient may be found at the pulmonary vein–left atrial junction Noonan, 1964). A special justification for measuring pulmonary wedge pressure exists in cor triatriatum where the presence of a high value in association with a normal left atrial pressure is confirmatory (Pedersen and Therkelsen, 1954).

VENTRICULAR. *Right Ventricle.* Where right ventricular hypertension is present, both the systolic level and the form of the right ventricular pressure pulse are dependent on several factors.

1. Systolic level of the pressure pulse. Abnormalities of rhythm such as premature beats affect the height of the right ventricular systole. The principal factor governing the height of the right ventricular pressure in the presence of an intact septum and closed ductus arteriosus is the resistance to pulmonary blood flow. As this resistance is normally low, the pressure in the right ventricle is correspondingly low, and, even under conditions of increased cardiac output such as with exercise, relatively small changes in the height of this pressure take place. But increased resistance to flow resulting from obstruction at ventricular or valvular level, as in pulmonary stenosis with normal aortic root, or at the peripheral level, as in increased pulmonary vascular resistance

from a variety of causes, may alter the right ventricular pressure markedly even at rest, depending upon the degree. Under these circumstances increase in cardiac output will further elevate the right ventricular pressure within limits; e.g., in pulmonary stenosis with normal aortic root, the systolic right ventricular pressure may range from 35 to 270 mm of mercury or more depending on the tightness of the stenosis and the activity of the patient. In idiopathic pulmonary hypertension or in pulmonary hypertension secondary to lung disorders, the right ventricular pressure again varies though it usually maximally approximates and rarely exceeds systemic systolic levels in severe cases (Wood, 1952).

In cases with large ventricular septal defect, patent ductus arteriosus associated with high pulmonary vascular resistance, or in complete transposition of the great vessels, the right ventricular systolic pressure level reaches systemic level and never exceeds it.

2. Form of the pressure pulse. In patients with right ventricular hypertension and either a normal pulmonary valve or pulmonary stenosis and an overriding aorta, the right ventricular pressure pulse is, with minor differences in the slope of the ejection plateau, similar to that obtained from catheterization of the left ventricle (Figure 27–11, page 485) (Harris, 1955). On the other hand, when there is pulmonary stenosis with a normally situated aorta (i.e., an intact ventricular septum), the form of the right ventricular pressure pulse differs strikingly from the normal and from that recorded from the left ventricle in the same patient (Figure 40–6, page 773). In valvular stenosis of this type, of all except the mildest degree, there is a rounded symmetric curve, a shortened isovolumic phase, and an absence of the ejection plateau (Fineberg and Wiggers, 1936; Bouchard and Cornu, 1954; Harris, 1955; Rowe et al., 1955). Great care must be taken to exclude damping effects, which are a common cause of this form of pulse pressure. Rarely, pressure pulses mimicking this form may be seen in other conditions. The reason for these changes in cases with left heart disease remains obscure and is not necessarily related to right ventricular outflow obstruction from an extreme degree of left ventricular hypertrophy. Where infundibular stenosis is present, this contour is altered slightly by the presence of an infundibular chamber (Figure 40–6, page 773) (Harris, 1955). The pressure pulse, obtained from the outflow chamber of the right ventricle in infundibular stenosis irrespective of the aortic root position, is similar to the normal form (Figure 27–12, page 486, and Figure 40–6B and C). These concepts on the shape of right ventricular pressure pulses have been expanded by Shanahan and associates (1960). In so-called idiopathic dilatation of the pulmonary artery and in relative stenosis from an enormous pulmonary blood flow, as is seen in some cases of atrial septal defect or atrioventricularis communis, where a small pressure gradient exists between the right ventricle and pulmonary artery, the form of the pressure pulse is normal.

Left Ventricle.　Normally similar to the normal right ventricular pressure pulse, the left ventricular pressure pulse is altered in height and form by such conditions as aortic stenosis. In valvular aortic stenosis, just as in valvular pulmonary stenosis, there is a tall symmetric curve to the tracing (Wiggers, 1952).

▷*End-Diastolic Pressure.* Normal values for right ventricular end-diastolic pressure average 5 ± 1.9 mm of mercury, while for left ventricular pressure comparable figures are 7.5 ± 2.2 mm of mercury (Krovetz et al., 1967). Elevation of these levels above normal range are characteristic of ventricular failure, and this is the most usual explanation for that rise in infants and children.

PULMONARY ARTERIAL.　The pulmonary arterial pressure pulse undergoes little alteration in the presence of pulmonary hypertension beyond that of increased amplitude. A localized rise in pressure in the left pulmonary artery where the aortic stream enters the pulmonary circuit has been described in simple isolated ductus arteriosus (Levinson et al., 1951). This sign has not often been found in children with this malformation studied in our unit.

In pulmonary stenosis of moderate degree only, the form and level of the pulmonary artery pressure pulse may be entirely normal. In a proportion of these cases and in some of the so-called relative stenoses associated with large-volume left-to-right shunt, there will be a gradient on withdrawing the catheter from the pulmonary artery branches to the main trunk. Such gradient appears to be due to catheter motion artefacts as described by Wood and associates (1954). In other cases with true bilateral pulmonary arterial stenosis, an important change in the form of the main pulmonary arterial pressure pulse has been noted (Agustsson et al., 1962), as illustrated in Figure 41–8 (page 796).

In pulmonary stenosis of severe degree, the arterial form of the tracing in the pulmonary artery frequently disappears and is replaced by an irregular low pressure wave with minimal respiratory variations apparently unrelated to events in the cardiac cycle. Contrary to the opinion of Kjellberg and coworkers (1959), we believe that this type of tracing may be seen in valvular pulmonary stenosis with either normal or dextroposed aortic root. What is important is not the type of malformation present but the severity of the stenosis. In tetralogy of Fallot the form of the pulmonary arterial pulse is the only guide to the severity of stenosis because the right ventricular pressure is always at systemic level whether the stenosis be moderate or severe, quite unlike the situation in pulmonary stenosis with normal aortic root. As the catheter is withdrawn into the main pulmonary artery, in cases of severe pulmonary stenosis of valvular type, sharply negative deflections appear. These are the so-called Venturi waves and are systolic in time (Sobin et al., 1954; Bouchard and Cornu, 1955; Kjellberg et al, 1959). Venturi waves are less commonly seen in infundibular stenosis and are rare in moderate stenoses. Venturi waves are often visible in moderate to severe pulmonary arterial stenoses, are less commonly seen in infundibular stenosis, and are rare in moderate stenoses.

GRADIENTS. Withdrawal of the catheter from the pulmonary artery to the right ventricle in pulmonary stenosis produces a characteristic gradient in the pressure wave, permitting in most cases a distinction between valvular, infundibular, or combined stenosis (see Figures 27–12A, B, and C). Great care is necessary and slow withdrawal under fluoroscopic control essential if accurate conclusions are to be drawn. Recently Emslie-Smith and associates (1956) and Datey and Ghandi (1961) have shown the value of correlating changes in the intracardiac electrogram with pressure-pulse gradients in pulmonary stenosis. The use of this technique during withdrawal of the catheter from the pulmonary artery can largely obviate errors in interpretation due to motion artefact. The problem of the indefinite result is largely confined to cases of tetralogy of Fallot or to more complex types of pulmonary stenosis, which in any case are better studied in combination with selective angiocardiography. By contrast, in cases of severe pulmonary stenosis with normal aortic root, the type of stenosis can often be stated with certainty from the right ventricular pressure pulse alone, a fact of particular value in small infants in distress where it is advisable to keep manipulations to a minimum.

What gradient between the right ventricle and pulmonary artery constitutes an organic pulmonary stenosis is still a matter for debate. So long as no left-to-right shunt exists, for Soulié (1954), Kjellberg and associates (1959), and Silverman and coworkers (1956) 20 mm of mercury is the level above which organic stenosis is present. A gradient of up to 30 mm (Rudolph et al., 1954) has been present in proved cases with large left-to-right shunts and no organic stenosis. These gradients are regarded as due to dilatation of the right ventricle with relative narrowing of the pulmonary valve, bringing an increase in pressure velocity as a result. Shephard (1954) has shown that the gradient may persist even when there is a patent ductus arteriosus present in addition, a fact that argues against increased flow through the pulmonary orifice as being the significant factor in the production of the gradient.

The picture of pulmonary valve incompetence in humans is confused. There appears to be no consistent relationship between the level of diastolic pressure in the recording of pulmonary artery pressure pulse and the physical signs. Cases of proven pulmonary insufficiency may have normal or elevated diastolic levels, whereas cases with low pulmonary artery diastolic pressure have shown no murmur of pulmonary insufficiency. Ehrenhaft (1955) has described a 14-year-old boy with symptoms of at least ten years' duration and marked cardiac enlargement. At operation complete destruction of the pulmonic valve was demonstrated.

Experimentally, partial excision of a cusp of the normal pulmonic valve in dogs has produced no significant hemodynamic changes at rest but some changes after induced anoxia (Fowler et al., 1956). Complete excision of the valve in dogs has resulted in auscultatory signs of pulmonary incompetence, with some increase in heart volume in a minority after observation up to 14 months. At cardiac catheterization an average gradient between the right ventricle and the pulmonary artery of 15 mm of mercury was found, and all dogs had an abnormally low diastolic pressure in the pulmonary artery (Ellison et al., 1955). It is difficult to avoid the implication that, although mild pulmonary incompetence may never have serious effect on the heart, gross incompetence almost certainly has over a period of years.

With one of several left heart catheterization techniques available, measurement of pressure gradients between the aorta and left ventricle in aortic stenosis and between the left ventricle and left atrium in mitral stenosis now has become standard practice.

SYSTEMIC ARTERIAL. The analysis of systemic arterial pressure pulse as an accessory aid in the diagnosis of aortic stenosis and insufficiency is described in Chapter 37. Changes in height and form of the arterial pulse wave provide relatively less valuable information in other defects except where objective comparison with right heart levels or between upper and lower portions of the body is desired.

Shunt Volumes. The magnitude of shunts in cases of congenital heart disease may be calculated either from dye dilution patterns or by use of the Fick principle. With the latter method it is clear that "approximation" is the more desirable term. Dexter (1954) has emphasized that in left-to-right shunts extremely narrow arteriovenous oxygen differences and the difficulty of obtaining representative mixed venous blood samples form the major sources of error in these measurements. Kjellberg and associates (1959) have further pointed out that in large left-to-right shunts the oxygen saturation of pulmonary venous blood in children cannot be assumed to be 95 to 97 percent and, after Burchell and Wood (1950), that changes in oxygen saturation in samples from the various chambers may vary from one minute to another. Experimental (Mesel, 1970) and clinical (Schostal et al., 1972) studies in created and naturally occurring ventricular septal defects have shown an uncomfortably large error in calculations of Qp/Qs employing the Fick method particularly noticeable with the larger shunts. It is for these reasons that some prefer to define the volume of shunt more simply as small, moderate, or large on the basis of alteration in blood oxygen saturation. Despite these valid objections, shunt calculation by the Fick method gives useful approximations of the shunt size and allows comparisons in different series of cases. It is obviously important whenever possible to obtain an estimate of the shunt size by a second method in order that discrepancies may be uncovered and to give some validity to the measurement (Swan et al., 1953). The most useful, practical routine serving that purpose in our hands and in those of others has been through indicator dilution.

Resistances. As measurement of pulmonary vascular resistance hinges on measurement of pulmonary flow, the same objections apply to resistance values as to the latter measurements. A rough guide to the pulmonary resistance may be obtained by correlating pulmonary artery pressures with the size of the shunt. A very large—or a very small—volume shunt from left to right with normal or near normal pulmonary pressure implies a low vascular resistance, whereas a small-volume left-to-right shunt in association with pulmonary hypertension indicates a high vascular resistance. In the presence of marked increase in pulmonary flow from a large-volume left-to-right shunt, as in atrial septal defects, some rise in pulmonary artery pressure not necessarily related to an increase in vascular resistance follows. However, an increase in pulmonary vascular resistance is always found where the mean pressure in the pulmonary artery exceeds 50 mm of mercury (Swan et al., 1954).

The actual cause of increased pulmonary vascular resistance in cases of left-to-right shunt remains unknown, but exploration of the relation of kinetic factors involved in ejection of the shunt from high- to low-pressure areas, as in ventricular septal defect and patent ductus arteriosus (Swan et al., 1954), the persistence of fetal-type pulmonary arterioles (Civin and Edwards, 1951), and the effect of hypoxia (Burchell et al., 1953b) or drugs, needs further study. Certainly both the pulmonary and systemic vascular resistance in infants are capable of marked alteration when the subject breathes different oxygen concentrations (Eldridge and Hultgren, 1955; Janes and Rowe, 1957). In older subjects with severe pulmonary vascular disease associated with cardiac malformation the effect of enriched oxygen breathing appears to be mainly to increase systemic vascular resistance. The left-to-right shunt volume and survival are therefore highly dependent at this stage upon quite ubiquitous influences affecting the systemic circulation (Krongrad et al., 1973). The hemodynamic aspects of pulmonary vascular resistance in congenital heart disease have been well-reviewed (Rudolph and Nadas, 1962).

Exploration. A wide variety of unusual routes of passage of the catheter within the heart and great vessels has helped the physician performing cardiac catheterization to suspect specific anomalies (Taketa et al., 1975). When the heart is approached with a catheter from the left arm, the tip occasionally enters a *left superior vena cava.* This anomaly complicates further exploration of the heart. It has been found in over 40 percent of the cases with dextrocardia or isolated levocardia, but fortunately from the technical standpoint of cardiac catheterization it is less common in other cases of congenital heart disease. Campbell and Deuchar (1954) encountered the anomaly in 2 percent, whereas in our series it was present in 3 percent of 700 catheterizations. In the less complicated association the left superior vena cava communicates with the coronary sinus so that it is possible, when approaching from the left side, to enter

the right atrium and sometimes the right ventricle and pulmonary artery. The same arrangement may be met, of course, with the approach from below. Sometimes there is a communication between the two superior venae cavae, and the catheter may form a complete loop from the superior vena cava on the right, through the right atrium, coronary sinus, and left superior vena cava to the innominate vein and superior vena cava on the right. Balloon occlusion of a persistent left superior vena cava is advised to evaluate proximal connections with the right superior cava, which may have importance at the time of cardiac surgery (Freed et al., 1973). Rarely the *left superior vena cava connects with the left atrium,* a child in our series with tetralogy of Fallot having this abnormality at catheterization and autopsy.

Another rare abnormality that will be detected with the cardiac catheter is *azygos continuation of the inferior vena cava.* In this condition the catheter will be advanced from below to the level of the right atrium, but the tip cannot be directed toward the tricuspid valve and merely passes superiorly to enter the superior vena cava and then the right atrium. Manipulation beyond that point in the past has been difficult (Anderson et al., 1955; Anderson et al., 1961), but this problem has now largely been resolved by use of the Swan-Ganz catheter.

Abnormal pulmonary venous connections to the inferior vena cava, superior vena cava, or innominate vein can usually be entered with the catheter tip if approached from a favorable direction. An anomalous pulmonary vein entering the superior vena cava from the right lung is best entered by the approach from the arm. By comparison, an anomalous entry of single pulmonary vein into the inferior vena cava is likely best performed from below; and in the same way, the left superior vena cava, into which one or all four pulmonary veins drain in the total drainage anomaly, is best entered from below through the left innominate vein.

Decisions concerning connections of pulmonary veins to the right atrium are extraordinarily difficult on the basis of catheter position alone. The illusion of a pulmonary vein entering this chamber after the catheter has been advanced through an atrial defect into a pulmonary vein of the right side has been mentioned previously. Determination of the mode of pulmonary venous connection has been greatly assisted by use of indicator dilution techniques (Wood, 1962). We have been impressed by the use of selective cineangiocardiography in resolving this problem (Folger et al., 1966).

Entrance through an *atrial septal defect* is most easily made with the inferior approach. In cases of isolated atrial septal defect, it is often possible to enter the left ventricle, withdraw to the left atrium, and then probe all four pulmonary veins without leaving this chamber, in which case differentiation from pulmonary veins entering the right atrium is possible. Entrance of the catheter into the left ventricle from the right atrium has been stated to be more easily performed in cases of persistent ostium primum defects of the atrial septum (Burchell et al., 1953a; Blount et al., 1956). Inflation of balloons attached to the catheter shaft has permitted estimation of the size of smaller secundum defects (Björk et al., 1954). Insertion of a second catheter after temporary closure of the defect may then confirm abolition of the shunt (Varnauskas and Werkö, 1954) but these techniques have not come into general use. In many of the cases involving diagnostic problems at this level, the use of selective angiocardiography has been of value (Kjellberg et al., 1959; Rowe et al., 1956).

Confirmation of the presence of *ventricular septal defect* may be made directly by passage of the catheter tip through the defect itself. In such cases the catheter tip runs posteromedially in the right ventricle to a lateral position with the apex of the curve at the third or fourth thoracic vertebra before the catheter tip descends below the diaphragm. In the lateral view the catheter shaft is posteriorly placed and does not approach the anterior chest wall. A fairly stiff catheter is necessary in order to probe for a ventricular septal defect, and the tip needs to be straight when directed posteromedially in the right ventricle. During the course of probing for this defect conduction disturbances are common. In our experience only the large defects are entered with any ease. Probing for the defect is most useful, however, in the group with severe pulmonary hypertension from markedly elevated pulmonary vascular resistance where a left-to-right shunt may not be detected at cardiac catheterization.

In cases of *patent ductus arteriosus*, the catheter may be advanced from the pulmonary artery into the descending aorta. The curve described by the catheter starts laterally in the outflow tract and runs in toward the vertebral column to reach a maximal height at the fifth thoracic vertebra (see Figure 24-8, page 432). On the lateral view, the catheter curve approaches the anterior chest wall (Alvarez et al., 1949). It is best to attempt to enter a pulmonary artery branch first before probing for the ductus so that one may be sure that the catheter has in fact entered the aorta from the pulmonary artery. Otherwise occasional cases of transposition of the great vessels with e-type aorta may be confused when the catheter enters an aorta arising directly from the outflow tract of the right ventricle. It has been our experience that entry through a patent ductus arteriosus is most simply performed in the infant group, where the success rate is high under one year of age. Over that age fewer cases have been probed. The least success occurs in very small patent ductus arteriosi without pulmonary hypertension or significant shunt through the defect. Easy passage through the ductus usually indicates a large channel, but this axiom is not invariable. Perhaps the most consistent method of entry into a patent ductus is retrogradely from the aortic catheter approaching from the femoral route.

During cardiac catheterization in *aorticopulmonary window or aortic septal defect* (Adams et al., 1952; Myers et al., 1951; Downing et al., 1953; Fletcher et al., 1954; D'heer and van Nieuwenhuizen,

1956), the catheter may pass from the pulmonary artery to the aorta a short distance above the pulmonary valve. The catheter may be passed upward into the arch of the aorta and the right carotid artery as well as downward in the ascending aorta toward the aortic valves. When the catheter is placed in the latter position, it will be seen in the lateral view to lie anterior, in contrast to the posterior position seen when the catheter passes through the patent ductus arteriosus. Furthermore, the catheter traversing a patent ductus arteriosus almost always passes down into the descending aorta rather than upward toward the neck. Even if it does in rare cases pass upward after leaving the ductus arteriosus, then the left carotid artery is entered rather than the right. Samples from the brachial and femoral arteries, though theoretically a method of distinguishing from patent ductus arteriosus and aorticopulmonary septal defect, apparently are not necessarily helpful (Fletcher et al., 1954). Where the pulmonary artery systolic pressure is the same as the systemic, withdrawal from the aorta to the pulmonary artery in the window defect does not permit a differentiation from a ventricular septal defect. One technique to overcome this difficulty is to pull the catheter from the aorta to the pulmonary artery very carefully and then advance it to the pulmonary wedge position without obtaining an intervening ventricular pressure pulse (D'heer and van Nieuwenhuizen, 1956). In the occasional cases where the pulmonary artery pressure is lower than aortic, careful withdrawal may help in the decision. Localization of the shunt to the ascending aorta (and so excluding ductus arteriosus) is quite easily confirmed by sampling the dilution curve in the pulmonary artery after injections of green dye at various points distal to the aortic valve. Despite these points the problem is not simple and the use of contrast materials is probably more helpful than any other aid in making the diagnosis.

In cases of simple ventricular septal defect, entry into the pulmonary artery is usually always possible whereas entry through the ventricular defect depends upon a number of factors, more particularly the size of the defect itself. In contrast, in complicated cases of pulmonary stenosis, such as *tetralogy of Fallot*, there may be difficulty in entering one or other major vessels. Our earlier experience with catheterizations in this condition showed that the pulmonary artery was entered in almost two-thirds of the cases, but that both vessels were entered in only one-fifth of the cases. In a slightly smaller proportion neither vessel was entered.

Improved techniques in recent years have resulted in more consistent catheter entry into both great arteries from the right ventricle except when pulmonary atresia is present. Even in the latter situation the retrograde arterial approach, combined with the use of precurved catheters and guide wires, will permit selective examination of the pulmonary arteries (White, 1972).

The difficulty of entry into great vessels from a ventricular chamber in complex anomalies or where hairpin bends or other unusual courses tend to defeat catheter passage has challenged and frustrated pediatric cardiologists for many years. A number of ingenious techniques have enjoyed varying degrees of success and have usually assisted the goals of at least the originators (Celermajer et al., 1970; Pickering et al., 1971; Mullins et al., 1972; Carr et al., 1972; Berman, 1973). But clearly the most important advance toward solving this problem has been the introduction of the Swan-Ganz flow-directed, balloon-tipped catheter (Swan et al., 1970), which has literally revolutionized the approach to vessel entry for complex malformations (Kelly et al., 1971; Stanger et al., 1972), transposition of great arteries, and truncus arteriosus.

Volumes

The ratio of ejected volume to the diastolic volume of the left ventricle (ejection fraction) as derived from measurements of that chamber is perhaps one of the most reliable and useful methods available allowing a measure of ventricular function in infants and very young children. The information is derived from measurements of angiocardiographic chamber cavity area. It remains to be seen whether echocardiographic or isotopic techniques will provide as accurate results. The effect of pressure load on the left ventricle is in aortic stenosis or aortic coarctation except under conditions of frank failure does not usually either increase the left ventricular end-diastolic volume or diminish the ventricular ejection fraction. When volume loads due to ventricular or great vessel left-to-right shunts or from valvular regurgitation occur or are added to a pressure load, the left ventricular end-diastolic volume is increased (Graham and Jarmakani, 1972). Aortic and mitral valvular incompetence may be quantified reasonably well with these methods (Tyrrell et al., 1970). The largest end-diastolic volume is obtained in cardiomyopathies. In a subject in controlled failure with a pressure load plus a volume load a low ejection fraction would suggest impaired myocardial performance and the likely need for surgical intervention (Graham and Jarmakani, 1972).

Good correlation has been obtained between estimated left ventricular wall muscle mass and both the severity of obstruction in older children with aortic stenosis or coarctation of the aorta (Graham et al., 1970a) and the magnitude of left-to-right shunt in ventricular septal defect and patent ductus arteriosus (Jarmakani et al., 1969). There is more difficulty in accurately deriving left ventricular mass in infants, but a combination of left ventricular or left atrial volume measurements offers some potential for assessing relative contributions of shunts at atrial and downstream levels. One method of looking at the pulmonary flow in transposition of the great vessels comes from analysis of left ventricular systolic output (left ventricular stroke volume × heart rate) (Graham and Jarmakani, 1972).

His Bundle Electrocardiography

The His bundle electrogram has been used in adults to localize the site of conduction delay accurately, to study arrhythmias, the Wolff–Parkinson–White syndrome, and to examine the influence of intervention of these problems by pacing or through pharmacologic means (Scherlag et al., 1972). It is being used in a similar fashion to localize the site conduction delay in certain patients with congenital heart disease, to determine the prognosis for those with postoperative heart block, to demonstrate the origin of other postoperative arrhythmias and to assist in better management of tachycardias. A full appraisal of the use of His bundle electrocardiography and its limitations has not yet been determined, but clearly even now the technique is making a substantial contribution to some very difficult management areas in pediatric cardiology.

Other

It would seem desirable to study the dynamics of congenital heart under differing conditions of cardiac output. More specifically, a study of patients during exercise as well as the usual resting condition should provide better indication of the individual response to the malformation over a wide physiologic range of physical activity. This has indeed been attempted for quite a variety of disorders including congenital heart block (Ikkos and Hanson, 1960), aortic stenosis (Bache et al., 1971; Cueto and Moller, 1973), pulmonary stenosis (Johnson, 1962; Howitt, 1966; Ikkos et al., 1966; Blumenthal et al., 1971; Moller et al., 1973), coarctation of the aorta (Taylor and Donald, 1970) and postoperatively in ventricular septal defect. The hindrance to more routine use is really the logistics and inability to obtain cooperation consistently for exercise in young patients with catheters in femoral veins so that in most laboratories the procedure is reserved for older children and rather specific clinical research endeavors (Hugenholtz and Nadas, 1963). Electrical pacing or Isuprel infusion has been used in substitution but exercise cannot be mimicked exactly through these means. The development of indirect methods of assessment is more likely to expand the use of exercise tests for patients with congenital heart disease (Cumming and Danzinger, 1963; Bar-or and Shepard, 1971). (See Chapter 5.)

Although there has not been a strong trend in this direction in recent years, the importance of interaction between cardiologists and pulmonary physiologists in joint laboratories is perhaps nowhere more clearly evident than in childhood. Particular areas where real benefit has been shown and should continue to accrue is in the variety of pulmonary disorders of newborn, in patients with airways obstruction at all levels, and in patients with scoliosis and pectus excavatum.

Finally, the ingenious Mexican efforts to perform valvulotomy with a catheter (Rubio and Limon Lason, 1954), the successful introduction of the balloon catheter and catheter blade to produce atrial septostomy (Rashkind and Miller, 1966; Park et al., 1975), plastic plugs over guide wires to obliterate a patent ductus arteriosus (Porstmann et al., 1971), and the use of tissue adhesives to close collateral channels between the aorta and the lung in patients with pulmonary atresia (Zuberbuhler et al., 1974) seem likely to open the way to exploration of other major medical interventions.

REFERENCES

Abinader, E.; Zeltzer, M.; and Riss, E.: Transumbilical atrial septostomy in the newborn. *Am. J. Dis. Child.*, **119**:354, 1970.

Abrams, H. L. (Chairman), Radiologic Study Group: Optimal radiologic facilities for examination of the chest and cardiovascular system. Report and Inter-Society Commission for heart disease Resources. *Circulation*, **43**:a135, 1971.

Adams, F. H.; Diehl, A.; Jorgens, J.; and Veasy, L. G.: Right heart catheterization in patent ductus arteriosus and aortico-pulmonary septal defect. *J. Pediatr.*, **40**:49, 1952.

Agustsson, M. H.; Arcilla, R. A.; Gasual, B. M.; Bicoff, J. P.; Nassif, S. I.; and Lendrum, B. L.: The diagnosis of bilateral stenosis of the primary pulmonary artery branches based on characteristic pulmonary trunk pressure curves. A hemodynamic and angiocardiographic study. *Circulation*, **26**:421, 1962.

Agustsson, M. H.; Bicoff, J. P.; and Arcilla, R. A.: Hemodynamic studies in fifty-two normal infants and children. *Circulation*, **28**:683, 1963.

Albisser, A. M.; Jackman, W. S.; and Pask, B. A.: Management of electrical hazards in hospitals. *Can. Hosp.*, **49**:43, 1972.

Aldridge, H. E.: Transseptal left heart catheterization without needle puncture of the interatrial septum. *Am. J. Cardiol.*, **13**:239, 1964.

Alvarez, V. R.; Lason, R. L.; Borges, S.; Bouchard, F.; Canepa, A.; and Aguilar, A.: Cateterizacion del conducto arterioso. *Arch. Inst. Cardiol. México*, **19**:583, 1949.

Amorin, D. Des.; Tsakiris, A. G.; and Wood, E. H.: Use of roentgen videodensitometry for detection of left-to-right shunts in dogs with experimental atrial septal defect. In *Roentgen-, Cine- and videodensitometry. Fundamentals and applications for blood flow and heart volume determination*. Ed. Heintze, P. H., Georg Thieme, Verlag. Stuftgart, 1971, p. 99.

Amplatz, K.; Jeffery, R. F.; Gobel, F. L.; Wang, Y.; Gathman, G. E.; Moller, J. H.; and Lucas, R. V.: The Freon test. A new sensitive technic for the detection of small cardiac shunts. *Circulation*, **39**:551, 1969.

Anderson, P. A. W.; Rogers, M. C.; Canent, R. C., Jr.; Jarmakani, J. M. M.; Jewett, P. H.; and Spach, M. S.: Reversible complete heart block following cardiac surgery. Analysis of His bundle electrograms. *Circulation*, **46**:514, 1972.

Anderson, R. C.; Adams, P., Jr.; and Burke, B.: Anomalous inferior vena cava with azygos continuation (infrahepatic interruption of the inferior vena cava). Report of 15 new cases. *J. Pediatr.*, **59**:370, 1961.

Anderson, R. C.; Heilig, W.; Novick, R.; and Jarvis, C.: Anomalous inferior vena cava with azygous drainage: so-called absence of the inferior vena cava. *Am. Heart J.*, **49**:318, 1955.

Anthony, C. L., Jr.; Crawford, E. W.; and Morgan, B. C.: Management of cardiac and respiratory arrest in children. A survey of major principles of therapy. *Clin. Pediatr.*, **8**:647, 1969.

Arbeit, S. R.; Parker, B.; and Rubin, I. L.: Controlling the electrocution hazard in the hospital. *JAMA*, **220**:1581, 1972.

Arcasoy, M. M.; Guntheroth, W. G.; and Mullins, G. L.: Simplified intravascular hydrogen electrode method. *Am. J. Dis. Child.*, **104**:349, 1962.

Arcilla, R. A.; Oh, W.; Lind, J.; and Gessner, I. H.: Pulmonary arterial pressures of newborn infants born with early and late clamping of the cord. *Acta Paediatr. Scand.*, **55**:305, 1966.

Arcilla, R.; Tsai, P.; Thilenius, O.; and Ranniger, K.: Angiographic method for volume estimation of right and left ventricles. *Chest*, **60**:446, 1971.

Bache, R. J.; Wang, Y.; and Jorgensen, C. R.: Hemodynamic effects of exercise in isolated valvular aortic stenosis. *Circulation*, **44**:1003, 1971.

Bagger, Marianne; Björck, G.; Björk, V. O.; Broden, B.; Cargren, L. E.; Carlsten, A.; Edler, I.; Ejrup, B.; Eliasch, H.; Gustafson, A.; Gyllenswärd, A.; Hansson, H. E.; Holmgren. A.; Iabohrn, H.; Johnsson, S. R.; Jonsson, B.; Jönsson, G.; Karnell, J.; Kjellberg, S. R.; Krook, H.; Larsson, H.; Linden, L.; Linder, E.; Linderholm, H.; Lodin, H.; Malmström, G.; Mannheimer, E.; Möller, T.; Philipsson, J.; Radner, S.; Rudhe, U.; Ström, G.; Söderholm, B.; Ulfsparre, F.; and Werkö, L.: On methods and complications in catheterization of the heart and large vessels, with and without contrast injection. *Am. Heart J.*, **54**:766, 1957.

Bar-or, O., and Shepard, R. J.: Cardiac output determination in exercising children—methodology and feasibility. *Acta Paediatr. Scand.*, Suppl. **217**:49, 1971.

Barratt-Boyes, B. G., and Wood, E. H.: The oxygen saturation of blood in the venae cavae, right-heart chambers, and pulmonary vessels of healthy subjects. *J. Lab. Clin. Med.*, **50**:93, 1957.

Bassert, F. H., 3d; Lincoln, C. R.; King, T. D.; and Canent, R. V., Jr.: Inequality in the size of the lower extremity following cardiac catheterization. *South. Med. J.* **61**:1013, 1968.

Baum, D.; Brown, A. C.; and Church, S. C.: Effect of sedation on oxygen consumption of children undergoing cardiac catheterization. *Pediatrics*, **39**:891, 1967.

Bell, A. L. L.; Haynes, W. F., Jr.; Shimomura, S.; and Dallas, D. P.: Influence of catheter tip position on pulmonary wedge pressures. *Circ. Res.*, **10**:215, 1962.

Bell, J. W.: Treatment of postcatheterization arterial injuries. *Ann. Surg.*, **155**:591, 1962.

Bentivoglio, L. G.; Maranhao, V.; Nakhjaven, F. K.; and Goldberg, H.: Comparison of blood oximetry and the ascorbate dilution technique in the diagnosis of left-to-right shunts. *Br. Heart J.*, **29**:212, 1967.

Bergel, D. H., and Milnor, W. R.: Pulmonary vascular impedance in the dog. *Circ. Res.*, **16**:401, 1965.

Berman, M. A.: Techniques of catheterization of the pulmonary veins and pulmonary venous atrium following Mustard's operation. *Am. Heart J.*, **85**:94, 1973.

Bing, R. J.; Vandam, L. D.; and Gray, F. D.: Physiological studies in congenital heart disease. I. Procedures. *Bull. Hopkins Hosp.*, **80**:107, 1947.

Björk, V. O.; Crafoord, C.; Jönsson, B.; Kjellberg, S. R.; and Rudhe, U.: Atrial septal defects. A new surgical approach and diagnostical aspects. *Acta Chir. Scand.*, **107**:499, 1954.

Black, I. F. S.: Floating a catheter into the pulmonary artery in transposition of the great arteries. *Am. Heart J.*, **84**:761, 1972.

Blackburn, J. P.; Deucher, D. C.; Fleming, P. R.; Nuller, G. A. H.; and Morgan, D. G.: Computer storage of catheterization data—preliminary report of a cooperative study. *Br. Heart J.*, **34**:203, 1972.

Bloom, J. D.; Mozersky, D. J.; Buckley, C. J.; and Hagood, C. O. Mr.: Defective limb growth as a complication of catheterization of the femoral artery. *Surg. Gynecol. Obstet.*, **138**:524, 1974.

Bloomfield, D. A.: Techniques of nonsurgical retrieval of iatrogenic foreign bodies from the heart. *Am. J. Cardiol.*, **27**:538, 1971.

Bloomfield, R. A.; Lauson, H. D.; Cournand, A.; Breed, E. S.; and Richards, D. W., Jr.: Recording of right heart pressures in normal subjects and in patients with chronic pulmonary disease and various types of cardiocirculatory diseases. *J. Clin. Invest.*, **25**:639, 1946.

Blount, S. G., Jr.; Balchum, O. T.; and Gensini, G.: The persistent ostium primum atrial septal defect. *Circulation*, **13**:499, 1956.

Blount, S. G., Jr.; Mueller, H.; and McCord, M. C.: Ventricular septal defect. Clinical and hemodynamic patterns. *Am. J. Med.*, **18**:871, 1955.

Blumenthal, S.; Jesse, M. J.; and Hayes, C.: The natural history of pulmonary stenosis. Some observations on the hemodynamic response to exercise. In *The Natural History and Progress in treatment of Congenital heart defects*. Eds. Kidd, B. S. and Keith, J. D., Charles C Thomas, Publisher, Springfield, Ill., 1971, p. 61.

Boijsen, E., and Lundstrom, N. R.: Percutaneous catheterization and angiocardiography in infants and children. *Am. J. Cardiol.*, **22**:572, 1968.

Bond, R. D., and Denison, A. B., Jr.: Patient safety during measurement of blood flow. *Am. Heart J.*, **81**:440, 1971.

Boros, S. J.; Nystrom, J. F.; Thompson, T. R.; Reynolds, J. W.; and Williams, H. J.: Leg growth following umbilical artery catheter-associated thrombus formation: A 4-year follow-up. *J. Pediatr.*, **87**:973. 1975.

Bosnjakovic, V.; Bennett, L. R.; Vincent, W.; and Larson, J.: Dualisotope method for the determination of intracardiac shunts. *J. Nucl. Med.*, **12**:341, 1971.

Bouchard, F., and Cornu, C.: Etude des courbes de pressious ventriculaire droite et arterielle pulmonaire dans les retecissements pulmonaires. *Arch. Mal. Coeur*, **47**:417, 1954.

Bouchard, R. J.; Gault, J. H.; and Ross, J., Jr.: Evaluation of pulmonary arterial end-diastolic pressure as an estimate of left ventricular end-diastolic pressure in patients with normal and abnormal left ventricular performance. *Circulation*, **44**:1072, 1971.

Bradley, E. C., and Barr, J. W.: Fore-'n-aft triangle formula for rapid estimation of area. Dye dilution curve. *Am. Heart J.*, **78**:643, 1969.

Branthwaite, M. A., and Bradley, R. D.: Measurement of cardiac output by thermal dilution in man. *J. Appl. Physiol.*, **24**:434, 1968.

Barlee, A.; Paul, M.; Werthmann, M. W., Jr.; and Schisgall, R. M.: Femoral artery obstruction in the newborn. *Clin. Proc. Children's Hosp. D.C.*, **27**:152, 1971.

Braunwald, E., and Swan, H. J. C. (eds.): *Cooperative study on Cardiac Catheterization.* The American Heart Association, Inc. New York, Monograph No. 20, 1968.

Brockenbrough, E. C.; Braunwald, E.; Ross, J., Jr.; and Marrow, A. G.: Left heart catheterization in infants and children. *Pediatrics*, **30**:253, 1962.

Brodsky, S. J.; Mirowski, M.; Krovetz, L. J.; and Rowe, R. D.: Recordings of His bundle and other conduction tissue potentials in children. *J. Pediatr.*, **79**:61, 1971.

Brotmacher, L., and Fleming, P.: Cardiac output and vascular pressures in ten normal children and adolescents. *Guy. Hosp. Rep.*, **106**:268, 1957.

Buckberg, G., and Moss, A.: Arteriotomy in children during cardiac catheterization. *Am. J. Cardiol.*, **30**:659, 1972.

Buckberg, G. D.; Fixler, D. E.; Archie, J. P.; and Hoffman, J. I. E.: Experimental subendocardial ischemia in dogs with normal coronary arteries. *Circ. Res.*, **30**:67, 1972.

Burchell, H. B.: Electrocution hazards in the hospital or laboratory. *Circulation*, **27**:1015, 1963.

Burchell, H. B.; Helmholz, H. F., Jr.; and Wood, E. H.: Over-all experiences with cardiac catheterization. *Proc. Mayo Clin.*, **28**:1953a.

Burchell, H. B.; Swan, H. J. C.; and Wood, E. H.: Demonstration of differential effects on pulmonary and systemic arterial pressure by vanation in oxygen content of inspired air in patients with patent ductus arteriosus and pulmonary hypertension. *Circulation*, **8**:681, 1953b.

Burchell, H. B., and Wood, E. H.: Remarks on the technic and diagnostic applications of cardiac catheterization. *Proc. Mayo Clin.*, **25**:41, 1950.

Burnard, E. D., and James, L. S.: Atrial pressures and cardiac size in the newborn infant. Relationships with degree of birth asphyxia and size of placental transfusion. *J. Pediatr.*, **62**:815, 1963.

Cahill, J. L.; Talbert, J. L.; Ottesen, O. E.; Rowe, R. D.; and Haller, J. A.: Arterial complications following cardiac catheterization in infants and children. *J. Pediatr. Surg.*, **2**:134, 1967.

Calverley, R. K.; Dodds, W. A.; Trapp, W. G.; and Jenkins, L. C.: Hyperbaric treatment of cerebral air embolism: A report of a case following cardiac catheterization. *Can. Anaesth. Soc. J.*, **18**:665, 1971.

Campbell, M., and Deuchar, D. C.: The left-sided superior vena cava. *Br. Heart J.*, **16**:423, 1954.

Carr, I., and Wells, B.: Coaxial flow-guided catheterization of the pulmonary artery in transposition of the great arteries. *Lancet*, **2**:318, 1966.

Carter, G. A.; Girod, D. A.; and Hurwitz, R. A.: Percutaneous cardiac catheterization of the neonate. *Pediatrics*, **55**:662, 1975.

Carter, S. A.; Bajec, D. F.; Yannicelli, E.; and Wood, E. H.: Estimation of left-to-right shunts from arterial dilution curves. *J. Lab. Clin. Med.*, **55**:77, 1960.

Cayler, G. C.; Rudolph, A. M.; and Nadas, A. S.: Systemic blood flow in infants and children with and without heart disease. *Pediatrics*, **32**:186, 1963.

Celermajer, J. M.; Venables, A. W.; and Bowdler, J. D.: Catheterization of the pulmonary artery in transposition of the great arteries. A simple method. *Circulation*, **41**:1053, 1970.

Chun, G. M. H., and Ellestad, M. H.: Perforation of the pulmonary artery by a Swan-Ganz catheter. *N. Engl. J. Med.*, **284**:1041, 1971.

Civin, W. H., and Edwards, J. E.: The postnatal structure changes in the intrapulmonary arteries and arterioles. *Arch. Pathol.*, **51**:192, 1951.

Clark, L. C., Jr., and Bargeron, L. M., Jr.: Detection and direct recording of left-to-right shunts with the hydrogen electrode catheter. *Surgery*, **46**:797, 1959.

Clark, L. C., Jr.; Bargeron, L. M., Jr.; Lyons, C.; Bradley, M. N. and McArthur, K. J.: Detection of right-to-left shunts with an arterial potentiometic electrode. *Circulation*, **22**:949, 1960.

Conn, H. L.: Use of external counting technics in studies of the circulation. *Circ. Res.*, **10**:505, 1962.

Connolly, D. C.; Tompkins, R. G.; Lev, R.; Kirklin, J. W.; and Wood, E. H.: Pulmonary wedge pressures in mitral valve disease; relationship to left atrial pressures. *Proc. Mayo Clin.*, **28**:72, 1953.

Connolly, D. C., and Wood, E. H.: The pulmonary vein wedge pressure in man. *Circ. Res.*, **3**:7, 1955.

Cooley, J. C., and Gianturco, C.: Percutaneous introduction of closed-end cardiac catheters. *J. Thorac. Cardiovasc. Surg.*, **47**:269, 1964.

Cooper, T. E.; Braunwald, E.; Riggle, D. R.; and Morrow, A. G.: Thermal dilution curves in the study of circulatory shunts. Instrumentation and clinical applications. *Am. J. Cardiol.*, **6**:1065, 1960.

Cournand, A.; Baldwin, J. S.; and Himmelstein, A.: *Cardiac Catheterization in Congenital Heart Disease.* The Commonwealth Fund, New York, 1949.

Cournand, A.; Bing, R. J.; Dexter, L.; Dotter, C. T.; Katz, L. N.: Warren, J. V.; and Wood, E. H.: Report of Committee on Cardiac Catheterization and Angiocardiography of the American Heart Association. *Circulation*, **7**:769, 1953.

Cournand, A., and Ranges, H. A.: Catheterization of right auricle in man. *Proc. Soc. Exp. Biol. Med.*, **46**:452, 1941.

Cournand, A.; Riley, R. L.; Breed, E. S.; Baldwin, E. de F.; and Richards, D. W., Jr.: Measurement of cardiac output in man using the technique of catheterization of the right auricle or ventricle. *J. Clin. Invest.*, **24**:106, 1945.

Cueto, L., and Moller, J. H.: Haemodynamics of exercise in children with isolated aortic valvular disease. *Br. Heart J.*, **35**:93, 1973.

Cumming, G. R., and Danzinger, R.: Bicycle ergometry studies in children. *Pediatrics* (Suppl.), **32**:757, 1963.

Curry, J. L.: Recovery of detached intravascular catheter or guide wire fragments. A proposed method. *Am. J. Roentgenol.*, **105**:894, 1969.

Datey, K. K., and Ghandi, M. J.: Uses and fallacies of intracardiac electrograms at the pulmonary valve. *Br. Heart J.*, **23**:539, 1961.

Delisle, G.; Izukawa, T.; Olley, P. M.; and Kidd, B. S. L.: Risk factors in cardiac catheterization in the newborn. Canad. Cardiovasc. Soc. 25th Ann. meeting, Toronto, 1972, p. 28.

Desilets, D. T., and Hoffman, R.: A new method of percutaneous catheterization. *Radiology*, **85**:147, 1965.

Dexter, L.: Cardiac catheterization in diagnosis of congenital heart disease. *Minnesota Med.*, **37**:116, 1954.

Dexter, L.; Haynes, F. W.; Burwell, C. S.; Eppinger, E. C.; Seibel, R. E.; and Evans, J. M.: Studies on congenital heart disease: I. Technique of venous catheterization as a diagnostic procedure. *J. Clin. Invest.*, **26**:547, 1947.

D'heer, H. A. H., and van Nieuwenhuizen, C. L. C.: Diagnosis of aortic septal defects. *Circulation*, **13**:58, 1956.

Dodge, H. T.; Sandler, H.; Ballew, D. W.; and Lord, J. D.: The use of biplane angiocardiography for the measurement of left ventricular volume in man. *Am. Heart J.*, **60**:762, 1960.

Donzelot, E., and D'Allaines, F.: *Traité des Cardiopathies Congénitales.* Masson et Cie, Paris, 1954.

Donzelot, E.; Vlad, P.; Durand, M.; and Metianu, C.: Un nouveau moyen diagnostique dans les cardiopathies congénitales: l'epreuve a l'ether selective au cours du catheterisme cardiaque. *Arch. Mal. Coeur*, **44**:638, 1951.

Downing, D. F.: Cardiac catheterization in congenital heart disease. *JAMA*, **170**:770, 1959.

Downing, D. F.; Bailey, C. P.; Maniglia, R.; and Goldberg, H.: Defect of the aortic septum. *Am. Heart J.*, **45**:305, 1953.

Editorial. Pulmonary wedged catheter pressures, *Circ. Res.*, **1**:371, 1953.

Ehmke, D. E.; Durnin, R. E.; and Lauer, R. M.: Intra-abdominal hemorrhage complicating a balloon atrial septostomy for transposition of the great arteries. *Pediatrics*, **45**:289, 1970.

Ehrenhaft, J. L., in discussion of Ellison et al.: Physiologic observations in experimental pulmonary insufficiency. *J. Thorac. Surg.*, **30**:641, 1955.

Eldridge, F. L., and Hulgren, H. N.: The physiologic closure of the ductus arteriosus in the newborn infant. *J. Clin. Invest.*, **34**:987, 1955.

Ellison, R. C.; Plauth, W. H., Jr.; Gazzaniga, A. B.; and Fyler, D. C.: Inability to deflate catheter balloon: A complication of balloon atrial septostomy. *J. Pediatr.* **76**:604, 1970.

Ellison, R. G.; Brown, W. T., Jr.; Hague, E. E., Jr.; and Hamilton, W. F.: Physiologic observations in experimental pulmonary insufficiency. *J. Thorac. Surg.*. **30**:633, 1955.

Emanuel, R. W.; Hamer, J.; Chiang, B. N.; Norman, J.; and Manders, J.: A dynamic method for the calibration of dye curves in a physiological system. *Br. Heart J.*, **28**:143, 1966.

Emmanouilides, G. C.; Moss, A. J.; Duffie, E. R., Jr.; and Adams, F. H.: Pulmonary arterial changes in human newborn infants from birth to three days of age. *J. Pediatr.*, **65**:327, 1964.

Emmanouilides, G. C.; Moss, A. J.; Monset-Couchard, M.; Marcano, B. A.; and Rzeznic, B.: Cardiac output in newborn infants. *Biol. Neonate*, **15**:186, 1970.

Emslie-Smith, D.: The intracardiac electrogram as an aid in cardiac catheterization. *Br. Heart J.*, **17**:219, 1955.

Emslie-Smith, D.; Lowe, K. G.; and Hill, I. G. W.: The intracardiac electrogram as an aid in the localization of pulmonary stenosis. *Br. Heart J.*, **18**:29, 1956.

Evonuk, E.; Imig, C. J.; Greenfield, W.; and Eckstein, J. W.: Cardiac output measured by thermal dilution of room temperature injectate. *J. Appl. Physiol.*, **16**:271, 1961.

Faithfull, N. S., and Haider, R.: Ketamine for cardiac catheterization. An evaluation of its use in children. *Anaesthesia*, **26**:318, 1971.

Feigenbaum, H.; Zaky, A.; and Nasser, W. K.: Use of ultrasound to measure left ventricular stroke volume. *Circulation*, **35**:1092, 1967.

Feigenbaum, H.; Popp, R. L.; Wolfe, S. B.; Troy, B. L.; Pombo, J. F.; Haine, C. L.; and Dodge, H. T.: Ultrasound measurements of the left ventricle. A correlative study with angiocardiography. *Ann. Intern. Med.*, **129**:461, 1972.

Ferrer, M. I.; Harvey, R. M.; Cathcart, R. T.; Cournand, A.; and Richards, D. W., Jr.: Hemodynamic studies in rheumatic heart disease. *Circulation*, **6**:688, 1952.

Feruglio, G. A.: Intracardiac phonocardiography: a valuable diagnostic technique in congenital and acquired heart disease. *Am. Heart J.*, **58**:827, 1959.

Fieldman, E. J.; Lundy, J. S.; DuShane, J. W.; and Wood, E. H.: Anesthesia for children undergoing diagnostic cardiac catheterization. *Anesthesiology*, **16**:868, 1955.

Fineberg, M. H., and Wiggers, C. J.: Compensation and failure of the right ventricle. *Am. Heart J.*, **11**:255, 1936.

Fixler, D. E.; Carrell, T.; Browne, R.; Willis, K.; and Miller, W. W.: Oxygen consumption in infants and children during cardiac catheterization under different sedation regimens. *Circulation*, **50**:788, 1974.

Flaherty, J. T.; Canent, R. V.; Boineau, J. P.; Anderson, P. A. W.; Levin, A. R.; and Spach, M. S.: Use of externally recorded radioisotope dilution curves for quantitation of left to right shunts. *Am. J. Cardiol.*, **20**:341, 1967.

Fletcher, G.; DuShane, J. W.; Kirklin, J. W.; and Wood, E. H.: Aortic-pulmonary septal defect: report of a case with surgical division along with successul resuscitation from ventricular fibrillation. *Proc. Mayo Clin.*, **29**:285, 1954.

Folger, G. M., Jr.; Rowe, R. D.; and Criley, J. M.: Partial drainage of right pulmonary veins from normally connected pulmonary veins: Cineangiographic differentiation. *South. Med. J.*, **59**:389, 1966.

Forrester, J. S.; Ganz, W.; Diamond, G.; McHugh, T.; Chonette, D. W.; and Swan, H. J. C.: Thermodilution cardiac output determination with a single flow directed catheter. *Am. Heart J.*, **83**:306, 1972.

Forssmann, W.: Die Sonderrung des rechten Herizens, *Klin. Wschr.*, **8**:2085, 1929.

Forwand, S. A.; Schatzki, S. C.; and Nordberg, E. D.: Cardiac catheterization and angiocardiography. *Cardiovasc. Clin.*, **3**:No. 2: 81, 1971.

Fowler, N. O.; Mannix, E. P.; and Noble, W.: Some effects of partial pulmonary valvectomy, *Circ. Res.*, **4**:8, 1956.

Fowler, N. O.; Westcott, R. N.; and Scott, R. C.: Normal pressure in the right heart and pulmonary artery. *Am. Heart J.*, **46**:264, 1953.

Fraser, R. S.; Rossell, R. E.; Dvorkin, J.; and Valle-Cavero, C.: The identification of right-to-left shunts in the central circulation by the injection of ether. *Circulation*, **24**:1224, 1961.

Freed, M. D.; Keane, J. F.; and Rosenthal, A.: The use of heparinization to prevent arterial thrombosis after percutaneous cardiac catheterization in children. *Circulation*, **50**:565, 1974b.

Freed, M. D.; Rosenthal, A.; and Fyler, D.: Attempts to reduce arterial thrombosis after cardiac catheterization in children: Use of percutaneous technique and aspirin. *Am. Heart J.*, **87**:283, 1974a.

Freed, M. D.; Rosenthal, A.; and Bernhard, W. F.: Balloon occlusion of a persistent left superior vena cava in the preoperative evaluation of systemic venous return. *J. Thorac. Cardiovasc. Surg.*, **65**:835, 1973.

Freedom, R. M., and Ellison, R. C.: Coronary sinus rhythm in the polysplenia syndrome. *Chest*, **63**:952, 1973.

Frommer, P. L.; Pfaff, W. W.; and Braunwald, E.: The use of ascorbate dilution curves in cardiovascular diagnosis. Applications of a technic for direct intravascular detection of indicator. *Circulation*, **24**:1227, 1961.

Ganz, W.; Donoso, R.; Marcus, H. S.; Forrester, J.; and Swan, H. J. C.: A new technique for measurement of cardiac output by thermodilution in man. *Am. J. Cardiol.*, **27**:392, 1971.

Gessner, I.; Krovetz, L. J.; Benson, R. W.; Prystowsky, H.; Stenger, V.; and Eitzman, D. V.: Hemodynamic adaptations in the newborn infant. *Pediatrics*, **36**:752, 1965.

Gilladoga, A. C.; Levin, A. R.; Deely, W. J.; and Engle, M. A.: Cardiac catheterization and febrile episodes. *J. Pediatr.*, **80**:215, 1972.

Giraud, G.; Peuch, P.; Latour, H.; and Hertault, J.: Variations de potential liees a l'achvite du systeme de conduction auriculo-ventriculaire chez l'homme: Enregistremont electrocardiographique endocavitaire. *Arch. Mal. Coeur*, **53**:757, **1960.**

Goldberg, S. J.; Linde, L. M.; Gaal, P. G.; and Sachs, D.: The pulmonary and systemic hemodynamic effects produced by meperidene and hydroxyzine. *J. Pharmacol. Exp. Ther.*, **159**:306, 1968.

Goldman, I. R.; Blount, S. G., Jr.; Friedlich, A. L.; and Bing, R. J.: Electrocardiographic observations during cardiac catheterization. *Bull. Hopkins Hosp.*, **86**:141, 1950.

Gordon, A. J.; Braunwald, E.; and Ravitch, M. M.: Simultaneous pressure pulses in the human left atrium, ventricle and aorta. *Circ. Res.*, **2**:432, 1954.

Gordy, E., and Drabkin, D. L.: Spectrophotometric studies. XVI. Determination of oxygen saturation of blood by a simplified technique applicable to standard equipment. *J. Biol. Chem.*, **227**:285, 1957.

Gorelick, M. M.; Lenkei, S. C. M.; Heimbecker, R. O.; and Gunton, R. W.: Estimation of mitral regurgitation by injection of dye into the left ventricle with simultaneous left atrial sampling. A clinical study of sixty confirmed cases. *Am. J. Cardiol.*, **10**:62, 1962.

Gorlin, R., and Gorlin, S. G.: Hydraulic formula for calculation of the area of the stenotic mitral valve, other cardiac valves and central circulatory shunts. *Am. Heart J.*, **41**:1, 1951.

Graham, T. P.; Jarmakani, M. M.; Canent, R. V.; Capp, M. P.; and Spach, M. S.: Characterization of left heart volumes and mass in normal children and in infants with intrinsic myocardial disease. *Circulation*, **38**:826, 1968.

Graham, T. P.; Lewis, B. W.; Jarmakani, M. M.; Canent, R. V.; and Capp, M. P.: Left heart volume and mass quantification in children with left ventricular pressure overload. *Circulation*, **41**:203, 1970a.

Graham, T. P., Jr.; Goodrich, J. K.; Robinson, A. E.; and Harris, C. C.: Scintiangiocardiography in children. *Am. J. Cardiol.*, **25**:387, 1970b.

Graham, T. P., Jr.; Jarmakani, M. M.; Canent, R. V., Jr.; and Marrow, M. N.: Left heart volume estimation in infancy and childhood: Re-evaluation of methodology and normal values. *Circulation*, **43**:895, 1971a.

Graham, T. P., Jr.; Jarmakani, J. M.; Canent, R. V., Jr.; and Anderson, P. A. W.: Evaluation of left ventricular contractile state in childhood: normal values and observations with a pressure overload. *Circulation*, **44**:1043, 1971b.

Graham, T. P., Jr.; and Jarmakani, J. M.: Hemodynamic investigation of congenital heart disease in infancy and childhood. *Progr. Cardiovasc. Dis.*, **15**:191, 1972.

Graham, T. P., Jr.; Jarmakani, J. M.; Atwood, G. F.; and Canent, R. V., Jr.: Right ventricular volume determinations in children. Normal values and observations with volume or pressure overload. *Circulation*, **47**:144, 1973.

Graham, T. P., Jr.; Atwood, G. F.; and Werner, B.: Use of droperidol-fentanyl sedation for cardiac catheterization in children. *Am. Heart J.*, **87**:287, 1974.

Grayzel, J., and Jameson, A. G.: Optimum criteria for the diagnosis of ventricular septal defect from measurements of blood oxygen saturation. *Circulation*, **27**:64, 1963.

Greenspan, R. H.; Lester, R. G.; Marvin, J. F.; and Amplatz, K.: Isotope circulation studies in congenital heart disease. *JAMA*, **169**:667, 1950.

Gupta, P. K., and Haft, J. I.: Complete heart block complication cardiac catheterization. *Chest*, **61**:185, 1972.

Hagan, A. D.; Friedman, W. F.; Ashburn, W. L.; and Alazraki, N.: Further applications of scintillation scanning technics to the diagnosis and management of infants and children with congenital heart disease. *Circulation*, **45**:858, 1972.

Hamilton, W. F.; Moore, J. W.; Kinsman, J. M.; and Spurling, R. G.: Studies on the circulation. IV. Further analysis of the injection method, and of changes in hemodynamics under physiological and pathological conditions. *Am. J. Physiol.*, **99**:534, 1932.

Hansen, J. T.; and Pace, N.: Apparatus for automatic dye dilution measurement of cardiac output. *J. Appl. Physiol.*, **17**:163, 1962.

Hara, H. H., and Belville, J. R.: In-line computation of cardiac output from dye dilution curves. *Circ. Res.*, **12**:379, 1963.

Harris, P.: Some variations in the shape of the pressure curve in the human right ventricle. *Br. Heart J.*, **17**:173, 1955.

Harris, P., and Heath, D.: *The Human Pulmonary Circulation*. E. & S. Livingstone, Edinburgh, 1962, Chap. 7.

Harris, P., and Summerhayes, J. L. V.: Recordings of pressure obtained during catheterization of the great cardiac vein. *Br. Heart J.* **18**:453, 1955.

Harrison, D. C.; Ridges, J. D.; Sanders, W. J.; Alderman, E. L.; and Fanton, J. A.: Real-time analysis of cardiac catheterization data using a computer system. *Circulation*, **44**:709, 1971.

Haroutunian, L. M.; Neill, C. A.; and Otis, A. B.: The contour of the right atrial wave in twenty-seven cases of atrial septal defect and in other cardiac conditions. *Bull. Johns Hopkins Hosp.*, **102**:176, 1958.

Hermann, H. J., and Bartle, S. H.: Left ventricular volumes by angiography: comparison of methods and simplification of techniques. *Cardiovasc. Res*, **2**:404, 1968.

Hawker, R. E., and Celermajer, J. M.: Comparison of pulmonary artery and pulmonary venous wedge pressure in congenital heart disease. *Br. Heart J.*, **35**:386, 1973a.

Hawker, R. E.; Palmer, J.; Bury, R. G.; Bowdler, J. D.; and Celermajer, J. M.: Late results of percutanous retrograde femoral arterial catheterization in children. *Br. Heart J.*, **35**:447, 1973b.

Hawker, R. E., and Krovetz, L. J.: Depression of cardiac output by sedation in congenital semilunar valve stenosis. *Am. Heart J.*, **87**:138, 1974.

Hébert, Scebat, and Lenégre: Soc. Franç. de cardiol., 1953; quoted by Donzelot and D'Allaines (1954).

Hellems, H. K.; Haynes, F. W.; and Dexter, L.: Pulmonary capillary pressure in man. *J. Appl. Physiol.*, **2**:24, 1949.

Hetzel, P. S.; Swan, H. J. C.; Ramirez De Areliano, A. A.; and Wood, E. H.: Estimation of cardiac output from first part of arterial dye-dilution curves. *J. Appl. Physiol.*, **13**:92, 1958.

Hildner, F. J.; Javier, R. P.; Ramaswamy, K.; and Samet, P.: Near miss "pseudo-complications" of cardiac catheterization. *Am. J. Cardiol.*, **29**:270, 1972.

Hills, T. H., and Stanford, R. W.: The problem of excessive radiation during routine investigations of the heart. *Br. Heart J.*, **12**:45, 1950.

Ho, C. S.; Krovetz, L. J.; and Rowe, R. D.: Major complications of cardiac catheterization and angiocardiography in infants and children. *Johns Hopkins Med. J.*, **131**:247, 1972.

Hohn, A. R., and Vlad, P. A.: Guide for introducing catheters when cannulating small vessels. *Pediatrics*, **24**:636, 1959.

Hohn, A. R., and Webb, H. M.: Balloon deflation failure: a hazard of "medical" atrial septostomy. *Am. Heart J.*, **83**:389, 1972.

Holling, H. E., and Zak, G. A.: Cardiac catheterization in the diagnosis of congenital heart disease. *Br. Heart J.*, **12**:153, 1950.

Hosie, K. F.: Thermal-dilution techniques. *Circ. Res.*, **10**:491, 1962.

Howitt, G.: Haemodynamic effects of exercise in pulmonary stenosis. *Br. Heart J.*, **28**:152, 1966.

Hugenholtz, P. G., and Nadas, A. S.: Exercise studies in patients with congenital heart disease. *Pediatrics* (Suppl.), **32**:769, 1963.

Hugenholtz, P. G., and Wagner, R. H.: Assessment of myocardial function in congenital heart disease. In Adams, F. H.; Swan, H. J. C.; and Hall, V. E. (eds.): *Pathophysiology of congenital heart disease*. UCLA forum Med. Sc. No. 10, Univ. of California Press, Los Angeles, 1970, p. 201.

Ikkos, D., and Hanson, J. S.: Response to exercise in congenital complete atrioventricular block. *Circulation*, **22**:583, 1960.

Ikkos, D.; Jonsson, B.; and Linderholm, H.: Effect of exercise in pulmonary stenosis with intact ventricular septum. *Br. Heart J.*, **28**:316, 1966.

Israel, R.; Hohn, A. R.; Black, I. F. S.; and Lambert, E. C.: Evaluation of the sedation during cardiac catheterization of children. *Pediatrics*, **70**:407, 1967.

Jain, K. K.; Wagner, R. H.; and Lambert, E. C.: Comparison of oxygen saturation of blood in azygos vein and superior vena cava. *Circulation*, **41**:55, 1970.

James, G. W.; Paul, M. H.; and Wessel, H. U.: Thermal dilution: Instrumentation with thermistors, *J. Appl. Physiol.*, **20**:547, 1965.

James, L. S., and Rowe, R. D.: The pattern of response of pulmonary and systemic arterial pressures in newborn and older infants to short periods of hypoxia. *J. Pediatr.*, **51**:5, 1957.

Jarmakani, M. M.; Graham, T. P., Jr.; Canent, R. V., Jr.; Spach, M. S.; and Capp, M. P.: Effect of site of shunt on left heart volume characteristics in children with ventricular septal defect and patent doctus arteriosus. *Circulation*, **40**:411, 1969.

Jegier, W.; Blankenship, W.; and Lind, J.: Venous pressure in the first hour of life and its relationship to placental transfusion. *Acta Paediatr.*, **52**:485, 1963.

Jegier, W.; Sekelj, P.; Davenport, H. T.; and McGregor, M.: Cardiac output and related hemodynamic data in normal children and adults. *Can. J. Biochem. Physiol.*, **39**:1747, 1961.

Jennings, R. B., Jr., and Krovetz, L. J.: The use of a damping chamber and cine wave oscillator for optimal frequency response in pressure recording. *I.E.E.E. Trans. Indust. Electronics Control Instr.*, **17**:134, 1970.

Johansson, B. W., and Ohlsson, N.-M.: Falsely high pressure curve from the right atrial appendage. *Br. Heart J.*, **23**:281, 1961.

Johnson, A. M.: Impaired exercise response and other sidua of pulmonary stenosis after valvotomy. *Br. Heart J.*, **24**:375, 1962.

Johnson, A. L.; Wollin, D. G.; and Ross, J. B.: Heart catheterization in the investigation of congenital heart disease. *Can. Med. Assoc. J.*, **56**:249. 1947.

Johnson, R. O.; Frawley, J. E.; Wright, J. S.; and McCredie, R. M.: Ultrasound detection of femoral artery stenosis in infants and children after cardiac catheterization or surgery. *Aust. N.Z. J. Med.*, **5**:491, 1975 (Abstract).

Jones, R. S.; Meade, F.; and Owen-Thomas, J. B.: Oxygen and nitrous oxide uptake during general anaesthesia for cardiac catheterization in infants with congenital heart disease. *Br. Heart J.*, **34**:52, 1972.

Kazenelson, G.; Rowe, R. D.; Bender, H. W.; and Haller, J. A., Jr.: Non-fatal accidental atrial perforation during cardiac catheterization in the newborn. *J. Pediatr.*, **69**:127, 1966.

Kappagoda, C. T.; Greenwood, P.; Macartney, F. J.; and Linden, R. J.: Oxygen consumption in children with congenital diseases of the heart. *Clin. Sc.*, **45**:107, 1973.

Kaude, J., and Svahn, G. Absorbed, gonad and integral doses to the patient and personnel from angiographic procedures. *Acta Radio.*, **15**:454, 1974.

Keith, J. D., and Rowe, R. D.: Selective angiocardiography. In Zimmerman, H. A. (ed.): *Intravascular Catheterization*. Charles C Thomas, Publisher, Springfield, Ill., 1959, p. 710.

Kelly, D. T.; Krovetz, L. J.; and Rowe, R. D.: Double-lumen flotation catheter for use in complex congenital cardiac anomalies. *Circulation*, **44**:910, 1971.

Kelly, D. R.; Brodsky, S. J.; Mirowski, M.; Krovetz, L. J.; and Rowe, R. D.: Bundle of His recordings in congenital complete heart block. *Circulation*, **45**:277, 1972.

Kern, I. B.; Bowring, A. C.; Cohen, D. H.; Fisk, G. C.; Gupta, J. M.; and McCredie, R. M.: Spontaneous perforation of the colon following cardiac catheterization in the newborn. *Med. M. Aust.,* **2**:1022, 1971.

Kirkpatrick, S. E.; Takahashi, M.; Petry, E. L.; Stanton, R. D.; and Lurie, P. R.: Purcutaneous catheterization in infants and children. 2. Prospective study of results and complications in 127 consecutive cases. *Circulation,* **42**:1049, 1970.

Kjellberg, S. R.; Mannheimer, E.; Rudhe, U.; and Jonsson, B.: Diagnosis of congenital heart disease, 2nd ed. Year Book Publishers, Inc., Chicago, 1959.

Krongrad, E.; Helmholz, H. F., Jr.; and Ritter, D. G.: Effect of breathing oxygen in patients with severe pulmonary vascular obstructive disease. *Circulation,* **47**:94, 1973.

Krovetz, L. J.: Detection and quantification of intracardiac and great vessel shunts. In *Dye Curves. The theory and practice of indicator dilution,* (Ed.) Bloomfield, D. A. University Park Press, Baltimore, 1974, p. 119.

Krovetz, L. J., and Gessner, I. H.: A new method utilizing indicator-dilution technics for estimation of left-to-right shunts in infants. *Circulation,* **32**:772, 1965.

Krovetz, L. J., and Goldbloom, S.: Normal standards for cardiovascular data I. Examination of the validity of cardiac index. *Johns Hopkins Med. J.,* **130**:174, 1972a.

Krovetz, L. J., and Goldbloom, S.: Normal standards for cardiovascular data II. Pressure and vascular resistances. *Johns Hopkins Med. J.,* **130**:187, 1972b.

Krovetz, L. J., and Kurlinski, J. P.: Subendocardial blood flow in children with congenital aortic stenosis. *Circulation,* **54**:961, 1976.

Krovetz, L. J.; McLoughlin, T. G.; Mitchell, M. B.; and Schiebler, G. L.: Hemodynamic findings in normal children. *Pediatr. Res.,* **1**:122, 1967.

Krovetz, L. J.; Shanklin, D. R.; and Schiebler, G. L.: Serious and fatal complications of catheterization and angiocardiography in infants and children. *Am. Heart J.,* **76**:39, 1968.

Krovetz, L. J.; Grumbar, P. A.; Hardin, S.; Morgan, A. V.; and Schiebler, G. L.: Complications following use of four angiocardiographic contrast media in infants and children. *Invest. Radiol.,* **4**:13, 1969.

Kuehl, K. S.; Perry, L. W.; and Scott, L. P.: Thrombosis of the inferior vena cava in patients with cyanotic congenital heart disease. *J. Pediatr.,* **79**:430, 1971.

LaFarge, C. G., and Miettinen, O. S.: The estimation of oxygen consumption. *Cardiovasc. Res.,* **4**:23, 1970.

Lagerlöf, H., and Werkö, L.: Studies on the circulation of blood in man. VI. The pulmonary capillary venous pressure pulse in man. *Scand. J. Clin. Lab. Invest.,* **1**:147, 1949.

Lasón, R. L., and Alvarez, V. R.: Cateterismo en communication interauricular. *Arch. Inst. Cardiol. México,* **19**:545, 1949.

Lees, M. H.; Bristow, J. D.; Way, C.; and Brown, M.: Cardiac output by Fick principle in infants and young children. *Am. J. Dis. Child.,* **114**:144, 1967.

Levin, A. R.: The science of cardiac catheterization in the diagnosis of congenital heart disease. *Cardiovasc. Clin.,* **4**:No. 3:236, 1972.

Levin, A. R.; Spach, M. S.; Canent, R. V.; Boineau, J. P.; Capp, M. P.; Jain, V.; and Barr, R. C.: Intracardiac pressure-flow dynamics in isolated ventricular septal defect. *Circulation,* **35**:430, 1967.

Levin, A. R.; Spach, M. S.; Boineau, J. P.; Canent, R. V.; Capp, M. P.; and Jewett, P. H.: Atrial pressure-flow dynamics in atrial septal defects (secundum type). *Circulation,* **37**:476, 1968.

Levine, H. D., and Goodale, W. T.: Studies in intracardiac electrography in man; potential variations in coronary venous system. *Circulation,* **2**:48, 1950.

Levine, H. D.; Hellems, H. K.; Dexter, L.; and Tucker, A.: Studies in intracardiac electrography in man: II. The potential variations in the right ventricle. *Am. Heart J.,* **37**:64, 1949.

Levinson, D. C.; Cosby, R. S.; Griffith, G. C.; Meehan, J. P.; Zinn, W. J.; and Dimitroff, S. P.: A diagnostic pulmonary artery pulse pressure contour in patent ductus arteriosus found during cardiac catheterization. *Am. J. Med. Sci.,* **222**:46, 1951.

Levy, A. M.; Monrow, R.; Hugenholtz, P. G.; and Nadas, A. S.: Clinical use of ascorbic acid as an indicator of right-to-left shunts with a note on other applications. *Br. Heart J.,* **29**:22, 1969.

Lewis, A. B.; Heymann, M. A.; Stanger, P.; Hoffman, J. I. E.; and Rudolph, A. M.: Evaluation of subendocardial ischemia in valvar aortic stenosis in children. *Circulation,* **49**:978, 1974.

Lewis, D. H.; Ertugrul, A.; Deitz, G. W., Wallace, J. D.; Brown, J. R., Jr.; and Moghadam, A.-N.: Intracardiac phonocardiography in the diagnosis of congenital heart disease. *Pediatrics,* **23**:837, 1959.

Lincoln, J. C., and Deverall, P. B.: The treatment of arterial thrombosis in infants and children by balloon catheters, *J. Pediatr. Surg.,* **4**:359, 1969.

Linde, L. M.; Higashino, S. M.; Berman, G.; Sapin, S. O.; and Emmanouilides, G. C.: Umbilical vessel cardiac catheterization and angiocardiography. *Circulation,* **34**:984, 1966.

Linden, R. J.; Ledsome, J. R.; and Horman, J.: Simple methods for the determination of concentrations of carbon dioxide and oxygen in blood. *Br. J. Anaesthesia,* **37**:77, 1965.

Linden, R. J., and Allison, P. R.: The relationship between left atrial pressure and pulmonary artery "wedge" pressure in man. *Clin. Sci.,* **25**:459, 1963.

Lipp, H.; O'Donoghue, K.; and Resnekov, L.: Intracardiac knotting of a flow-directed balloon catheter. *N. Engl. J. Med.,* **284**:220, 1971.

Lown, B.; Amarasingham, R.; and Neuman, J.: New method for terminating cardiac arrythmias. Use of synchronised capacitor discharge. *JAMA,* **182**:548, 1962.

Lucas, R. V., Jr.; St. Geme, J. W., Jr.; Adams, P., Jr.; Anderson, R. C.; and Ferguson, D. J.: Maturation of the pulmonary vascular bed: a physiologic and anatomic correlation in infants and children. *Am. J. Dis. Child.,* **101**:467, 1961.

Luisada, A. A., and Liu, C. K.: *Cardiac Pressures and Pulses. A Manual of Right and Left Heart Catheterization.* Grune & Stratton, Inc., New York, 1956.

Luisada, A. A., and MacCanon, D. M.: The phases of the cardiac cycle. *Am. Heart J.,* **83**:705, 1972.

Lukas, D. S., and Ayres, S. M.: Determination of blood oxygen content by gas chromatography, *J. Appl. Physiol.,* **16**:371, 1961.

Lurie, P. R.; Armer, R. M.; and Klatte, E. C.: An apical technique for catheterization of the left side of the heart applied to infants and children. *N. Engl. J. Med.,* **264**:1182, 1961.

———: Percutaneous guide wire catheterization—diagnosis and therapy. *Am. J. Dis. Child.,* **106**:189, 1963.

Lurie, P. R., and Grajo, M. Z.: Accidental cardiac puncture during right heart catheterization. *Pediatrics,* **29**:283, 1962.

Malsky, S. J.; Roswit, B.; Reid, C. B.; and Itaff, J.: Radiation exposure to personnel during cardiac catheterization. A preliminary study. *Radiology,* **100**:671, 1971.

Maltz, D. L., and Treves, S.: Quantitative radionuclide angiocardiography. Determination of Qp:Qs in children. *Circulation,* **47**:1049, 1973.

Mansfield, P. B.; Gazzaniga, A. B.; and Litwin, S. B.: Management of arterial injuries related to cardiac catheterization in children and young adults. *Circulation,* **42**:501, 1970.

Massumi, R. A., and Ross, A. M.: A traumatic, nonsurgical technic for removal of broken catheters from cardiac cavities. *New. Eng. J. Med.* **277**:195, 1967.

McCord, M. C., and Blount, S. G., Jr.: The hemodynamic pattern in tricuspid valve disease. *Am. Heart J.,* **44**:671, 1952.

McMichael, J.: Communication in Zimdahl, W. T.: Disorders of the cardiovascular system occurring with catheterization of the right side of the heart. *Am. Heart J.,* **41**:204, 1951.

McMichael, J., and Mounsey, J. P. D.: A complication following coronary sinus and cardiac vein catheterization in man. *Br. Heart J.,* **13**:397, 1951.

McMichael, J., and Sharpey-Schafer, E.: Cardiac output in man by a direct Fick method. *Br. Heart J.,* **6**:33, 1944.

McNamara, D. G. (Chairman), Ad Hoc Committee, Council on Rheumatic Fever and Congenital Heart Disease, Amer. Heart Assoc.: Standards for a cardiac catheterization laboratory: A guide for cardiologists and for institutions sponsoring cardiac catheterization laboratories. *Circulation,* **42**:557, 1970.

Meester, G. T.; Bernard, N.; Zeelenberg, C.; Brower, R. W.; and Hugenholtz, P. G.: A computer system for real time analysis of cardiac catheterization data. *Cath. Cardiovasc. Diag.,* **1**:113, 1975.

Mesel, E.: Direct measurement of intracardiac blood flow in dogs with experimental ventricular septal defects. *Circ. Res.,* **27**:1033, 1970.

Mesel, E., and Gelfand, M.: An automated data acquisition and analysis system for a cardiac catheterization laboratory. *Comput. Biol. Med.,* **1**:199, 1971.

Miller, G. A. H., and Swan, H. J. C.: Effect of chronic pressure and volume overload on left heart volume in subjects with congenital heart disease. *Circulation*, **30**:205, 1964.

Miller, G. A. H., Brown, R.; and Swan, H. J. C.: Isolated congenital mitral insufficiency with particular reference to left heart volumes. *Circulation*, **29**:356, 1964.

Miller, G., Editorial: Cardiac catheterization. *Br. Heart J.*, **34**:117, 1972.

Mody, S. M., and Richings, M.: Ventricular fibrillation resulting from electrocution during cardiac catheterization. *Lancet*, **2**:698, 1962.

Moller, J. H.; Rao, B. N. S.; and Lucas, R. V., Jr.: Exercise hemodynamics in 64 children with pulmonary valvular stenosis. Amer. Acad. Pediat. Section on Cardiology October, 1972, New York.

Monroe, R. G.; Hauck, A. J.; and Gamble, W. J.: Simple device for the continuous recording of respiration during cardiac catheterization. *Am. J. Med. Electronics*, **3**:281, 1964.

Mook, G. A., and Zijlstra, W. G.: Quantitative evaluation of intracardiac shunts from arterial dye dilution curves. Demonstration of very small shunts. *Acta Med. Scand.*, **170**:703, 1961.

Morrow, A. G.; Braunwald, E.; Haller, J. A.; and Sharp, E. H.: Left atrial pressure pulse in mitral valve disease. A correlation of pressures obtained by transbronchial puncture with the valvular lesion. *Circulation*, **16**:399, 1957.

Mortensson, W.; Hallböök, T.; and Lundström, N-R.: Percutaneous catheterization of the femoral vessels in children. II. Thrombotic occlusion of the catheterized artery: Frequency and causes. *Pediatr. Radiol.*, **4**:1, 1975.

Mullins, C. B.; Mason, D. T.; Ashburn, W. L.; and Ross, J., Jr.: Determination of ventricular volume by radioisotope angiography. *Am. J. Cardiol.*, **24**:72, 1969.

Mullins, C. E.; Neches, W. H.; Reitman, M. J.; El-Said, G.; and Riopel, D. A.: Retrograde technique for catheterization of the pulmonary artery in transposition of the great arteries with ventricular septal defect. *Am. J. Cardiol.*, **30**:385, 1972.

Munroe, J. P.; Dodds, W. A.; and Graves, H. B.: Anaesthesia for cardiac catheterization and angiocardiography in children. *Can. Anaesth. Soc. J.*, **12**:67, 1965.

Myers, G. S.; Scannell, J. G.; Wyman, S. M.; Dimond, E. G.; and Hurst, J. W.: Atypical patent ductus arteriosus with absence of the usual aorticopulmonary pressure gradient and of the characteristic murmurs. *Am. Heart J.*, **41**:819, 1951.

Natelson, S.: Routine use of ultramicro methods in the clinical laboratory. *Am. J. Clin. Pathol.*, **21**:1153, 1951.

Neches, W. H.; Mullins, C. E.; Williams, R. L.; Vargo, T. A.; and McNamara, D. G.: Percutaneous sheath cardiac catheterization. *Am. J. Cardiol.*, **30**:378, 1972.

Nicholson, J. W., III; Burchell, H. B.; and Wood, E. H.: A method for continuous recording of Evans blue due curves in arterial blood, and its application to the diagnosis of cardiovascular abnormalities. *J. Lab. Clin. Med.*, **37**:353, 1951.

Nicholson, J. W., III, and Wood, E. H.: Estimation of cardiac output and Evans blue space in man using an oximeter. *J. Lab. Clin. Med.* **19**:588, 1951.

Nixon, P. F. G.; Hay, G. A.; Hepbron, F.; Snow, H. M.; and Addyman, R.: Amphoterle technique for recording ascorbate dilution curves and blood flow pulses. *Br. Heart J.*, **25**:173, 1963.

Noonan, J. A.: Hemodynamics of the left atrium in patients with ventricular septal defects. Soc. Ped. Res. Program & Abstracts 34th Annual meeting, Seattle, 1964, p. 63.

Noyons, A. K., M. Méthode d'enrigistrement continu de la teneur en CO_2 et en O_2 des gaz respiratoires au moyen du diaféromètre thermique, servant à l'étude du métabolisme des tissus des animaux et de l'homme. *Ann. Physiol. Physiocochim. Biol.*, **13**:909, 1937.

Oh, W.; Arcilla, R. A.; and Lind, J.: *In vivo* blood oxygen dissociation curve of newborn infants. *Biol. Neonat.*, **8**:241, 1965.

Olley, P. M.; Kidd, B. S. L.; and Zelin, S.: Cardiac output: Rapid estimation from indicator dilution curves using a new nomogram *Can. J. Physiol. Pharmacol.*, **48**:147, 1970.

Ordway, N. K.: Studies in congenital cardiovascular disease: IV. Impaired pulmonary diffusion of oxygen in persons with left-to-right shunts. *Yale J. Biol. Med.*, **24**:292, 1952.

Olley, P. M.; Kidd, B. S. L.; and Zelin, S.: Cardiac output: Rapid estimation from indicator dilution curves using a new nomogram. *Can. J. Physiol. Pharmacol.*, **48**:147, 1970.

O'Rourke, M. F.; Blazek, J. V.; Morreels, C. L., Mr.; and Krovetz, L. J.: Pressure wave transmission along the human aorta: changes with age and in arterial degenerative disease. *Circ. Res.*, **23**:567, 1968.

Padmanabhan, J.; Krovetz, L. J.; Varghese, P. J.; Izukawa, T.; Mellits, E. D.; and Rowe, R. D.: Effect of topical papaverine in preventing thrombosis following arteriotomies. A double blind study in infants and children. *J. Pediatr.*, **81**:792, 1972.

Park, S. C.; Zuberbuhler, J. R.; Neches, W. H.; Lennox, C. C.; and Zoltan, R. A.: A new atrial septostomy technique. *Cath. Cardiovasc. Diag.*, **1**:195, 1975.

Paul, M. H., and Miller, R. A.: External electrical termination of supraventricular arrythmias in congenital heart disease. *Circulation*, **25**:604, 1962.

Paul, M. H.; Rudolph, A. M.; and Rappaport, M. D.: Temperature dilution curves for the detection of cardiac shunts. *Circulation*, **18**:765, 1958 (Abstract).

Paul, M. H., and Rudolph, A. M.: Pulmonary valve obstruction during cardiac catheterization. *Circulation*, **18**:53, 1958.

Pedersen, A., and Therkelsen, F.: Cor triatriatum: a rare malformation of the heart probably amenable to surgery. *Am. Heart J.*, **47**:676, 1954.

Pickering, D.; McDonald, P.; and Kidd, B. S. L.: Catheterization of the pulmonary artery in transposition. *Pediatrics*, **47**:1068, 1971.

Pocock, W. A.; Barlow, J. B.; and Berezowski, A.: Perforation of the heart during cardioangiography. Case report of a six month old infant. *Am. J. Cardiol.* **11**:819, 1963.

Portsmann, W.; Wierny, L.; Warnke, H.; Gerstberger, G.; and Romaniuk, P. A.: Catheter closure of patent ductus arteriosus. 62 cases treated without thoracotomy. *Radiol. Clin. North. Am.*, **9**:203, 1971.

Powers, W. F., and Swyer, P. R.: Limb blood flow following umbilical artery catheterization. *Pediatrics*, **55**:248, 1975.

Prec, K. J., and Cassels, D. E.: Dye dilution curves and cardiac output in newborn infants. *Circulation*, **11**:789, 1955.

Rao, P. S., and Sissman, N. J.: The relationship of pulmonary venous wedge to pulmonary arterial pressures. *Circulation*, **44**:565, 1971.

Rapaport, E.; Rabinowitz, M.; Haynes, F. W.; Kuida, H.; and Dexter, L.: Clinical and hemodynamic observations in Lutembacher's syndrome. 2nd World Congress Cardiol., Washington, D.C., 1954.

Rashkind, W. J., and Miller, W. W.: Creation of an atrial septal defect without thoracotomy. A palliative approach to complete transposition of the great arteries. *JAMA*, **196**:991, 1966.

Read, J. L.; Bond, E. G.; and Porter, R. R.: The hazard of unrecognized catheterization of the coronary sinus. *Arch. Int. Med.*, **96**:176, 1955.

Reinhold, J.: Venous pulse in atrial septal defect: a clinical sign. *Br. Med. J.*, **1**:695, 1955.

Reports of the Inter-Society Commission for Heart Disease Resources. *Cardiovascular Diseases. Guidelines for Prevention and Care*. (Ed) Wright, I. S. and Frederickson, D. T., US Government Printing Office, Washington D.C. 1727-00035.

Resnekov, L.: Automation in cardiology. *Br. Heart J.*, **33**:Suppl: 194, 1971.

Rivera, M.; Hazelwood, P.; Gumpert, C.; and Bloomfield, D. A.: The calibration of indicator dilution curves. *Analyzer*, **1**:13, 1970.

Roberts, N. K., and Olley, P. M.: His bundle recordings in children with normal hearts and congenital heart disease. *Circulation*, **45**:295, 1972.

Roos, A.: Poseuille's law and its limitations in vascular systems. *Med. Thorac.* **19**:224, 1962.

Rosenthal, A.; Anderson, M.; Thomson, S. J.; Pappas, A. M.; and Fyler, D. C.: Superficial femoral artery catheterization. Effect on extremity length. *Am. J. Dis. Child.*, **124**:240, 1972.

Roveti, G. C.; Ross, R. S.; and Bahnson, H. T.: Transseptal left heart catheterization in the pediatric age group. *J. Pediatr.*, **61**:855, 1962.

Rowe, R. D., and Hoffman, T. Transient myocardial ischemia of the newborn infant: a form of severe cardiorespiratory distress in full-term infants. *J. Pediatr.*, **81**:243, 1972.

Rowe, R. D.: The preoperative cardiac catheterization and angiocardiogram. *J. Pediatr.*, **86**:319, 1975.

Rowe, R. D.: Cardiac catheterization in the newborn infant. *Heart Bull.*, **9**:61, 1960.

Rowe, R. D., and James, L. S.: The normal pulmonary arterial pressure during the first year of life. *J. Pediatr.* **51**:1, 1957.

Rowe, R. D.; Vlad, P.; and Keith, J. D. Atypical tetralogy of Fallot: A noncyanotic form with increased lung vascularity. Report of four cases. *Circulation*, **12**:230, 1955.

———: Experiences with 180 cases of tetralogy of Fallot in infants and children. *Can. Med. Assoc. J.*, **73**:23, 1955.

———: Selective angiocardiography in infants and children. *Radiology*, **66**:344, 1956.

Rowe, R. D.; Mehrizi, A.; Folger, G. M.; and Aleem, A.: Aspects of cardiac output in congenital heart disease. In *Human Growth*. Cheek, D. B. Lea and Febiger, Philadelphia, 1966, p. 515.

Rowe, R. D.: Stenosis of conducting arteries in infants and children. In *Birth Defects: Original article Series VIII*, No. 5; August, 1972, p. 69.

Rubio, V., and Limon Lason, R.: Treatment of pulmonary valvular stenosis and of tricuspid stenosis using a modified catheter. 2nd World Congress Cardiol., 1954, Washington. D.C. Program Abstracts II, p. 205.

Rudolph, A. M.: The changes in the circulation after birth. Their importance in congenital heart disease. *Circulation*. **51**:343, 1970.

Rudolph, A. M.: *Congenital Diseases of the Heart. Clinicophysiologic Considerations in Diagnosis and Management.* Year Book Medical Publishers, Inc., Chicago, 1974.

Rudolph, A. M., and Cayler, G. G.: Cardiac catheterization in infants and children. *Pediatr. Clin. North Am.*, **5**:907, 1958.

Rudolph, A. M.; Drorbaugh, J. E.; Auld, P. A. M.; Rudolph, A. J.; Nadas, A. S.; Smith, C. A.; and Hubbell, J. P.: Studies on the circulation in the neonatal period. The circulation in the respiratory distress syndrome. *Pediatrics*, **27**:551, 1961.

Rudolph, A. M., and Nadas, A. S.: The pulmonary circulation and congenital heart disease. Consideration of the role of the pulmonary circulation and certain systemic-pulmonary communications. *N. Engl. J. Med.*, **267**:968, 1962.

Rudolph, A. M.; Nadas, A. S.; and Goodale, W. T.: Intracardiac left-to-right shunt with pulmonic stenosis. *Am. Heart J.*, **48**:808, 1954.

Ryan, N. J., and Cayler, G. G.: Ventricular fibrillation during cardiac catheterization. Successfully treated with external defibrillation and closed chest cardiac massage. *Am. J. Cardiol.*, **10**:120, 1962.

Sanders, R. J.; Cooper, T.; and Morrow, A. G.: An evaluation of the nitrous oxide method for the quantification of left-to-right shunts. *Circulation*, **19**:898, 1959.

Sanders, R. J., and Morrow, A. G.: The identification and quantification of left to right circulatory shunts: a new diagnostic method utilizing the inhalation of a radioactive gas, Kr[85], *Am. J. Med.*, **26**:508, 1959.

Sandler, H., and Dodge, H. T.: The use of single plane angiocardiograms for the calculation of left ventricular volume in man. *Am. Heart J.*, **75**:325, 1968.

Sarnoff, S. J.; Braunwald, E.; Welch, G. H., Jr.; Case, R. B.; Stainsby, W. N.; and Macruz, R.: Hemodynamic determinants of oxygen consumption of the heart with special reference to the tension time index. *Am. J. Physiol.*, **192**:148, 1958.

Sasahara, A. A.; Rudolph, A. M.; Hoffman, J. I. E.; and Hauck, A. J.: Ventricular fibrillation during catheterization of the right side of the heart terminated successfully by external defibrillation. *N. Engl. J. Med.*, **261**:26, 1959.

Sawyer, D. C.; Lumb, W. V.; and Stone, H. L.: Cardiovascular effects of halothane, methoxyflufane, pentobarbital and thiamylar. *J. Appl. Physiol.*, **30**:36, 1971.

Scherlag, B. J.; Lau, S. H.; Helfant, R. H.; Berkowitz, W. D.; Stein, E.; and Damato, A. N.: Catheter technique for recording His bundle activity in man. *Circulation*, **39**:13, 1969.

Schostal, S. J.; Krovetz, L. J.; and Rowe, R. D.: An analysis of errors in conventional cardiac catheterization data. *Am. Heart J.*, **83**:596, 1972.

Scott, O.: A new complication of Rashkind balloon septostomy. *Arch. Dis. Child.*, **45**:716, 1970.

Seldinger, S. I.: Catheter replacement of the needle in percutaneous arteriography. *Acta Radiol.*, **39**:368, 1953.

Sepulveda, G., and Lukas, D. S.: The diagnosis of tricuspid insufficiency. *Circulation*, **11**:552, 1955.

Shanahan, R.; Myers, G. S.; Del Campo, E.; Friedlich, A. I.; and Scannel, G.: Right ventricular pressure curves in congenital and acquired heart disease. *Br. Heart J.*, **22**:457, 1960.

Shapiro, G. S., and Krovetz, L. J.: Damped and undamped frequency responses of underdamped catheter manometer systems. *Am. Heart J.*, **80**:226, 1970.

Shephard, R. J.: Pulmonary arterial pressure in acyanotic congenital heart disease. *Br. Heart J.*, **16**:361, 1954.

———: The atrial pressure tracing in congenital heart disease. *Br. Heart J.*, **17**:225, 1955.

Silove, E. D.; Cantez, T.; and Wells, B. G.: Thermodilution measurements of left and right ventricular outputs. *Cardiovasc. Res.*, **5**:174, 1971.

Silverman, B. K.; Nadas, A. S.; Wittenborg, M. H.; Goodale, W. T.; and Gross, R. E.: Pulmonary stenosis with intact ventricular septum. *Am. J. Med.*, **20**:53, 1956.

Simovitch, H.; Hohn, A. R.; Wagner, H. R.; Vlad, P.; Subramanian, S.; and Lambert, E. C.: Percutaneous right and left heart catheterization in children. Experience with 1,000 patients. *Circulation*, **41**:513, 1970.

Sinclair, J. D.; Newcombe, C. P.; Donald, D. E.; and Wood, E. H.: Experimental analysis of an atrial sampling technic for quantitating mitral regurgitation. *Proc Mayo Clin.*, **35**:700, 1960.

Sleeper, J. C.; Thompson, H. K.; McIntosh, H. D.; and Elston, R. C.: Reproducibility of results obtained with indicator-dilution technique for estimating cardiac output in man. *Circ. Res.*, **11**:712, 1962.

Smith, C.; Rowe, R. D.; and Vlad, P.: Sedation of children for cardiac catheterization with an ataractic mixture. *Can. Anaesth. Soc. J.*, **5**:35, 1958.

Smith, W. W.; Albert, R. E.; and Rader, B.: Myocardial damage following inadvertent deep cannulation of the coronary sinus during right heart catheterization. *Am. Heart J.*, **42**:661, 1951.

Sobin, S. S.; Carson, M. J.; Johnson, J. L.; and Baker, C. R.: Pulmonary valvular stenosis with intact ventricular septum: isolated valvular stenosis and valvular stenosis associated with interatrial shunt. *Am. Heart J.*, **48**:416, 1954.

Sones, F. M., Jr.: Heart catheterization in infancy. Physiological studies. *Pediatrics*, **16**:544, 1955.

Soulié, P.: In Symposium: the clinical value of instrumental methods of diagnosis in congenital heart disease. 2nd World Congress Cardiol., Washington, D.C., 1954.

Spach, M. S.: Radiation exposure in children with heart disease. *Am. Heart J.*, **64**:727, 1962.

Spach, M. S.; Canent, R. V.; Boineau, J. D.; White, A. W.; Sanders, A. P.; and Baylin, J.: Radioisotope-dilution surves as an adjunct to cardiac catheterization. I. Left to right shunts. *Am. J. Cardiol.*, **16**:165, 1965.

Spach, M. S.; Canent, R. V.; Boineau, J. D.; White, A. W.; Sanders, A. P.; and Baylin, J.: Radioisotope-dilution curves as an adjunct to cardiac catheterization. II. Right to left shunts. *Am. J. Cardiol.*, **16**:176, 1965.

Sproul, A., and Simpson, E.: Stroke volume and related hemodynamic data in normal children. *Pediatrics*, **33**:912, 1964.

Srouji, M. D., and Rashkind, W. J.: The effect of cardiac catheterization on the acid-base status of infants with congenital heart disease. *J. Pediatr.*, **75**:943, 1969.

Stanger, P.; Heymann, M. A.; Hoffman, J. I. E.; and Rudolph, A. M.: Use of the Swan-Ganz catheter in cardiac catheterization of infants and children. *Am. Heart J.*, **83**:749, 1972.

Stanger, P.; Heymann, M. A.; Tarnoff, H.; Hoffman, J. I. E.; and Rudolph, A. M. Complications of cardiac catheterization of neonates, infants and children. A three-year study. *Circulation*, **50**:595, 1974.

Starmer, C. F.; McIntosh, H. D.; and Whalen, R. E.: Electrical hazards and cardiovascular function. *N. Engl. J. Med.*, **284**:181, 1971.

Steiner, M. L.; Bartley, T. D.; Byers, F. M.; and Krovetz, L. J.: Polyethylene catheter in the heart. Report of a case with successful removal. *JAMA*, **193**:1054, 1965.

Stern, T. N.; Tacket, H. S.; and Zackary, E. G.: Penetration into pericardial cavity during cardiac catheterization. *Am. Heart. J.*, **44**:448, 1952.

Stocker, F. P.; Kinser, J.; Weber, J. W.; and Rosler, H.: Pediatric radiocardioangiography. Shunt diagnosis. *Circulation*, **47**:819, 1973.

Strangfield, D.; Gunther, K. B.; Porstmann, W.; and Buchali, K.: A new calculation method for left-to-right shunts established by radiocardiography. Comparison with dye dilution techniques. *Cardiology*, **57**:119, 1972.

Strauss, H. W.; Zaret, B. L.; Hurley, P. J.; Natarajan, T. K.; and Pitt, B.: A scintophotographic method of measuring left ventricular ejection fraction in man without cardiac catheterization. *Am. J. Cardiol.*, **28**:575, 1971.

Sunderland, C. O.; Nichols, G. M.; Henken, D. P.; Linstone, F.; Menashe, V. D.; and Lees, M. H.: Percutaneous cardiac catheterization and atrial balloon septostomy in pediatrics. *J. Pediatr.*, **89**:584, 1976.

Sutterer, W. F., and Wood, E. H.: Straingauge manometers: application to recording of intravascular and intracardiac pressures. In Glasser, O. (ed.): *Medical Physics*, vol. 3. Year Book Publishers, Inc., Chicago, 1960, p. 641.

Swan, H. J. C., and Wood, E. H.: Localization of cardiac defects by dye-dilution curves recorded after injection of T1824 at multiple sites in the heart and great vessels during cardiac catheterization. *Proc. Mayo Clin.*, **28**:95, 1953.

Swan, H. J. C.; Zapata-Diaz, J.; Burchell, H. B.; and Wood, E. H.: Pulmonary hypertension in congenital heart disease. *Am. J. Med.*, **16**:12, 1954.

Swan, H. J. C.; Zapata-Diaz, J.; and Wood, E. H.: Dye dilution curves in cyanotic congenital heart disease. *Circulation*, **8**:70, 1953.

Swan, H. J. C.; Ganz, W.; Forrester, J.; Marcus, H.; Diamond, G.; and Chonette, D.: Catheterization of the heart in man with use of a flow-directed balloon-tipped catheter. *N. Engl. J. Med.*, **283**:447, 1970.

Takahashi, M.; Petry, E. L.; Lurie, P. R.; Kirkpatrick, S. E.; and Stanton, R. E.: Percutaneous heart catheterization in infants and children. 1. Catheter placement and manipulation with guide wires. *Circulation*, **42**:1037, 1970.

Taketa, R. M.; Sahn, D. J.; Simon, A. L.; Pappelbaum, S. J.; and Friedman, W. F.: Catheter position in congenital cardiac malformations. *Circulation*, **51**:749, 1975.

Tawes, R. L., Jr.; Berry, C. L.; Aberdeen, E.; and Graham, G. R.: Myocardial ischemia in infants. Its role in three common congenital cardiac anomalies. *Ann. Thorac. Surg.*, **8**:383, 1969.

Taylor, S. H., and Donald, K. R.: Circulatory studies at rest and during exercise in coarctation of the aorta before and after operation. *Br. Heart J.*, **22**:117, 1960.

Thilenius, O. G., and Arcilla, R. A.: Angiographic right and left ventricular volume determination in normal infants and children. *Pediatr. Res.*, **8**:67, 1974.

Trusler, G. A., and Mustard, W. T.: Intravenous polyethylene catheter successfully removed from the heart. *Can. Med. Assoc. J.*, **79**:558, 1958.

Tuuteri, L.; Wallgren, E. I.; and Makinen, J.: Major complications of cardiac catheterization and angiocardiography in infants and children. *Am. Heart J.*, **76**:39, 1968.

Tyrrell, M. J.; Ellison, R. C.; Hugenholtz, P. G.; and Nadas, A. S.: Correlation of degree of left ventricular volume overload with clinical course in aortic and mitral regurgitation. *Br. Heart J.*, **32**:683, 1970.

Van Slyke, D. D., and Neill, J. M.: The determination of gases in blood and other solutions by vacuum extraction and manometric measurement. *J. Biol. Chem.*, **61**:523, 1925.

Varghese, P. J.; Celermajer, J.; Izukawa, T.; Haller, J. A.; and Rowe, R. D.: Cardiac catheterization in the newborn: Experience with 100 cases. *Pediatrics*, **44**:24, 1969.

Varnauskas, E., and Werkö, L.: Temporary occlusion of interatrial septal defect in man. *Scandinav J. Clin. Lab. Invest.*, **6**:51, 1954.

Venables, A. W., and Hiller, H. G.: Complications of cardiac investigation. *Br. Heart J.*, **25**:336, 1963.

Viart, P.; Blum, D., and Gallez, A.: La technique de microcatheterisme du coeur droit appliquee au nouveau-ne au nourrisson et a l'enfant. *Helv. Paediatr. Acta*, **26**:429, 1971.

Vince, D. J.: Medical radiation to children with congenital heart disease. *Can. Med. Assoc. J.*, **91**:1345, 1964.

Vince, D. J.: Cardiac catheterization in the first year of life. an assessment of risk. *Can. Med. Assoc. J.*, **98**:386, 1968.

Visscher, M. B., and Johnson, J. A.: The Fick principle: analysis of potential errors in its conventional application. *J. Appl. Physiol.*, **5**:635, 1953.

Vlad, P.; Hohn, A.; and Lambert, E. C.: Retrograde arterial catheterization of the left heart. Experience with 500 infants and children. *Circulation*, **29**:787, 1964.

Vogel, J. H.: Balloon embolization during atrial septostomy. *Circulation*, **42**:155, 1970.

Wallgren, C. G.: Indicator dilution studies by earpiece densitometry in infants and children with cardiovascular disease. *Acta Paediatr. Scand.*, [Suppl. 254], 1975.

Warner, H. R.; Gardner, R. M.; Pryor, T. A.; Day, W. C.; and Stauffer, W. M.: A system for on-line computer analysis of data during heart catheterization. In Adams, F. H.; Swan, H. J. C.; and Hall, V. E. (eds.): *Pathophysiology of Congenital Heart Disease*. UCLA Forum Med. Sci. No. 10, Univ. of California Press, Los Angeles, 1970, p. 409.

Watson, H.: Intracardiac electrography in the investigation of congenital heart disease in infancy and the neonatal period. *Br. Heart J.*, **24**:144, 1962.

Watson, H.: Electrode catheters and the diagnostic application of intracardiac electrography in small children. *Circulation*, **29**:284, 1964.

Watson, H.; Emslie-Smith, D.; and Lowe, K. G.: Intracardiac electrocardiogram of human atrioventricular conducting tissue. *Am. Heart J.*, **74**:66, 1967.

Waton, H.: Natural history of Ebstein's anomaly of tricuspid valve in childhood and adolescence. An international cooperative study of 505 cases. *Br. Heart J.*, **36**:417, 1974.

Weber, P. M.; dos Remedios, L. V.; and Jasko, I. A.: Quantitative radioisotopic angiocardiography. *J. Nucl. Med.*, **13**:815, 1972.

Wessel, H. U.; Rorem, D.; Muster, A. J.; Acevedo, R. E.; and Paul, M. H.: Continuous determination of oxygen uptake in sedated infants and children during cardiac catheterization. *Am. J. Cardiol.*, **24**:376, 1969.

White, R. I., Jr., and Humphries, J. O.: Direct current electroshock in the treatment of supraventricular arrhythmias. *J. Pediatr.* **70**:119, 1967.

White, R. I., Jr.: Technique and preliminary results of selective catheterization of patients with Blalock-Taussig shunts. *Radiology*, **105**:703, 1972.

White, R. I., Jr.; Giargiana, F. A.; Borushok, M.; and Harrington, D. P.: A new system for percutaneous catheterization of the pediatric patient. *Radiology*, **107**:443, 1973.

Wiggers, C. J.: Dynamics of ventricular contraction under abnormal conditions. *Circulation*, **5**:321, 1952.

Williams, G. D.; Ahrend, T. R.; and Dungan, W. T.: An unusual complication of balloon-catheter atrial septostomy. *Ann. Thorac. Surg.*, **10**:556, 1970.

Winchell, P.: Infectious endocarditis as a result of contamination during cardiac catheterization. *N. Engl. J. Med.*, **248**:245, 1953.

Wood, E. H.: Diagnostic applications of indicator-dilution technics in congenital heart disease. *Circ. Res.*, **10**:531, 1962.

Wood, E. H.; Geraci, J. E.; Pollack, A. A.; Groom, D.; Taylor, B. E.; Pender, J. W.; and Pugh, D.: General and special technics in cardiac catheterization. *Proc. Mayo Clin.*, **23**:494, 1948.

Wood, E. H.; Leusen, I. R.; Warner, H. R.; and Wright, J. L.: Measurement of pressures by cardiac catheters in man. *Minnesota Med.*, **37**:87, 1954.

Wood, E. H., and Swan, H. J. C.: Right heart catheterization. In *Cardiology* Vol. 2. McGraw-Hill Book Co., Inc., New York, 1959, Chap. 4, p. 321.

Wood, E. H.; Swan, H. J. C.; and Marshall, H. W.: Technic and diagnostic applications of dilution curves recorded simultaneously from the right side of the heart and from the arterial circulation. *Proc. Mayo Clin.*, **33**:536, 1958.

Wood, P.: Pulmonary hypertension. *Br. Med. Bull.*, **8**:348, 1952.

Yang, S. S.; Bentivoglio, L. G.; Maranhao, V.; and Goldberg, H.: *From Cardiac Catheterization Data to Hemodynamic Parameters.* F. A. Davis Company, Phila., 1972.

Ziegler, R. F.: Clinical cardiac catheterization in infants and children. *Pediatr. Clin. North Am.*, **1**:93, 1954.

Zimdahl, W. T.: Disorders of the cardiovascular system occurring with catheterization of the right side of the heart. *Am. Heart J.*, **41**:204, 1951.

Zijlstra, W. G.: *A Manual of Reflection Oximetry.* Van Gorcum & Co., Assen, 1958.

Zuberbuhler, J. R.; Dankner, E.; Zoltun, R.; Burkholder, J.; and Bahnson, H. T.: Tissue adhesive closure of aortic-pulmonary communications. *Am. Heart J.*, **88**:41, 1974.

7

Angiocardiography

C. A. F. Moës

ANGIOCARDIOGRAPHY has been available since 1937 when Castellanos, Pereiras, and Garcia first visualized the right side of the heart and Robb and Steinberg in 1938 improved the method of visualization of the left side of the heart and aorta. The modern technique of selective angiocardiography was originally developed by Chavez and associates in 1947 and further advanced by Jönsson and colleagues in 1949 and Jönsson in 1951. Since the injection is made through a cardiac catheter, a greater concentration of contrast material can be obtained at the site of the abnormal anatomy. For the most effective use of this procedure, a presumptive or at least partial diagnosis must be made beforehand, so that the catheter can be placed in the chamber most suitable to reveal the anomaly. By this procedure it has become possible to make a precise diagnosis even in the presence of complex types of congenital heart disease. The progress in cardiovascular surgery has enhanced its value, particularly since the development of intracardiac procedures that demand a more intimate knowledge of the anatomic variations present.

The development of x-ray apparatus suitable for use in angiocardiography has made great strides during recent years. Not only has the type of equipment become more versatile with sophisticated refinements being incorporated, but considerable advances have been made to decrease the radiation to the patient and personnel involved.

To study anatomic changes in angiocardiographic work, films must be taken in rapid sequence with short exposure times in order to stop cardiac motion and prevent blurring of detail. Wegelius and Lind (1953) have pointed out that a baby's heart may beat 180 times per minute, or three times per second. Systole at this rate is approximately twice the length of diastole; thus nine films per second are needed to demonstrate both systole and diastole in each cycle. To obtain this film rate, two types of apparatus are presently available; these are rapid x-ray film changers and image intensifiers with cinecamera attachments.

Numerous types of radiographic film changers

have been devised that are capable of taking 1 to 12 exposures per second. Biplane apparatus capable of taking simultaneous radiographs in two directions at right angles to each other has proved its worth. By this technique abnormalities that may be missed in one projection may become visible on films talen at right angles. Furthermore, certain anomalies are better viewed in one plane rather than the other. For example, the origin of the aorta in transposition of the great vessels is better seen in the lateral views, whereas the infundibulum of the right ventricle in tetralogy of Fallot is better studied in the anteroposterior views. Rapid film changers are basically of two types: cut film and roll film. In the cut film changers cassettes are transported into position for the x-ray exposure, then rapidly conveyed out of the way while the next cassette comes into position. The Sanchez–Perez and Picker–Amplatz are examples of changers of this type. The Schonander (A.O.T) cut film changer functions by transporting the film from a feeding magazine into the exposure area where it is compressed between the intensifying screens. After the exposure the film is ejected into a receiving magazine. Roll film is produced by the Elema, Franklin, and Amplatz see-through changers. Changers of these types can expose up to 12 frames per second in two planes simultaneously though can be programmed to work at selected slower speeds. X-ray generators of high capacity and heavy-duty x-ray tubes are recommended for use with these changers so that radiographs with high resolution can be produced. Since large film radiographs can be made, the detail presented is excellent though some image unsharpness does take place due to motion blurring from the long exposure time needed to take the films. Because valuable information may be obtained in the early films before overlapping of the chamber shadows occurs, it is important to have as many films per second during the initial period of contrast media injection, though at later stages film may be taken at a slower rate. A definite disadvantage to this type of apparatus is that once the patient is positioned over the device, no fluoroscopic check can be made with regard to centering of the patient or position of the catheter within the heart; thus any error may lead to inconclusive results and warrant repetition of the procedure. With the Amplatz or Puck see-through changers, however, it is possible to visualize the radiographic image on a television screen thus overcoming the inconvenience. The radiation dose to the patient utilizing large film apparatus is of necessity high.

In recent years the use of image intensification cinefluorography has gained considerable ground in angiocardiographic work. By this method it is possible to obtain motion pictures commonly from $7\frac{1}{2}$ to 80 frames per second, though cameras that may take pictures up to 600 frames per second have also been designed. As a result of cineradiography, hemodynamics as well as intracardiac anatomy may be studied. With present-day image intensifiers, it has become possible to obtain cine film that displays detail almost equal to that obtained on large film while keeping the radiation dose level to a minimum. The first roentgen cinephotography was performed by MacIntyre in 1896. Further studies were carried out by Reynolds (1928), Janker (1936), and others,

but advances in motion picture photography of an image produced on a fluorescent screen were slow. Cinefluorography was not practical since the light output from a conventional fluoroscopic screen is low, and to obtain motion pictures a camera with a large lens aperture is needed and the patient must of necessity be subjected to an extremely high dose of radiation. In the late 1940s and early 1950s, the work of Sturm and Morgan (1949), Moon (1950), Morgan and Sturm (1951), and others resulted in methods of intensifying the brightness of a fluoroscopic screen. With the advent of image intensification it became possible to produce a useful x-ray image that could be photographed on 35- or 16-mm film. Selective cineangiography with image intensification was first carried out by Janker (1954) in Germany and Sones (1958) in the United States. As a result of this technique it became possible to show contrast material in the various chambers of the heart following a relatively small but rapid injection. Cardiac chamber size, intracardiac and extracardiac shunts, vessel size, infundibular or valvular stenosis, and pulmonary or systemic blood flow may, therefore, be visualized.

IMAGE INTENSIFICATION SYSTEMS

SINCE selective angiocardiography is now more than ever dependent on adequate equipment, it is useful to evaluate the image intensification systems and their mode of operation. Figure 7–1 shows a patient (A) lying on an x-ray table (B). X-rays generated from the tube (C), placed under the table, pass through the patient and fall on the face of the image intensifier (D). The image produced can now be viewed by mirror optics (E), by a vidicon, plumbicon, or orthicon television camera (F), or photographed by a cine- or a still camera (G). From the television camera the signal may be relayed to a television monitor (H) or a video tape recorder (I).

Figure 7–2 shows the image-intensifying tube in more detail. This consists of a fluorescent screen (1), referred to as the input phosphor, situated at one end of an evacuated glass envelope. X-rays, after passing through the patient, strike the input phosphor and are converted into light. The light produced falls on a photoemissive layer (2), the photocathode, which is closely coupled to the input phosphor, with emission of electrons. In this way, x-rays are converted to light and light to electrons with the number of electrons emitted being proportional to intensity of the x-radiation. The electrons are accelerated through the length of the tube due to the attraction of a positively charged anode (3) at the opposite end and are electronically focused in their travel by cylindrical electrodes (4), placed about the tube. The electrons strike a small fluorescent screen (5), the output phosphor. The brightness of the image on the output phosphor is greatly enhanced over that on the input owing to acceleration of the electrons and reduction in size of the image. The increase in brightness of the

image over that seen on a conventional fluoroscopic screen is referred to as the gain of the image intensifier.

More recently a new type of image intensification tube has become available that is capable of producing an x-ray image of enhanced quality. The resolution of the image produced almost equals that of a large film-screen combination. This advance has become possible by replacing the zinc-cadmium sulfide coating of the input phosphor with sodium activated cesium-iodide crystals. With the cesium-iodide tube more of the incident x-ray photons are absorbed (50 percent) on the input phosphor, which helps to reduce the quantum mottling (noise) present in an image produced with fewer x-rays. The contrast in the output phosphor image is considerably improved over the previous intensifiers because the structure of the cesium-iodide phosphor prevents sideways scatter of light. The full benefit of the cesium-iodide phosphor can only be obtained if the electrons emitted by the photoemissive surface of the input phosphor can be accurately focused on the output phosphor. To achieve this it is necessary to perform many calculations of the electron pathways in the intensifier for different electric field configurations, and this can only be achieved by using computers. As a result of this new tube, resolution of the image is excellent and is uniform over the entire image field.

The input fields of image-intensifying tubes on the market at the present time range from 15 to 25 cm (6 to 10 in.). In more recent years intensifying tubes capable of displaying two field sizes have become available. Those presenting with a combination of 22.5 and 15 cm (9 and 6 in.), 22.5 and 12.5 cm (9 and

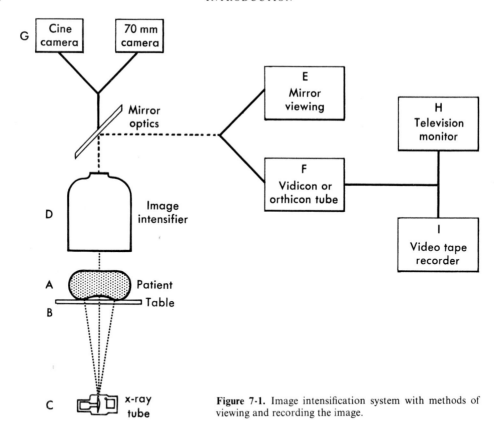

Figure 7-1. Image intensification system with methods of viewing and recording the image.

5 in.), or 25 and 17.5 cm (10 and 7 in.) are probably the most versatile. The combination type of tube is well suited to angiocardiographic examination in a children's hospital where the small field size can be used for the neonate while the larger field may be employed in older children.

In recent years the use of biplane cineangiocardio-graphy (Abrams, 1963; Pickard, 1963; Watson and Pickard, 1964) has become available in most centers. Not only is the detail extremely good, but the information obtained in one plane may be correlated with that in the other plane. This method can be most beneficial in the investigation of cardiac anomalies in the pediatric age group.

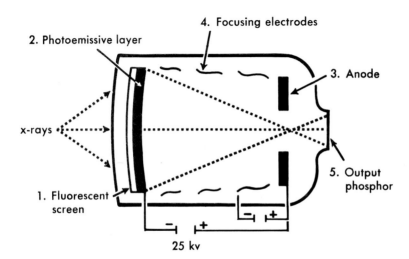

Figure 7-2. Image-intensifying tube.

VIEWING AND RECORDING OF THE IMAGE

As already mentioned, the intensified or amplified image may be viewed through a system of mirror optics or on a television monitor. Recording may be accomplished by photographing the output phosphor of the image-intensifying tube or the television monitor with cine, 70-mm, or 100-mm cameras.

A closed-circuit television system is of advantage in that it can be viewed by a large group and is therefore useful for teaching purposes. The basic components of such a system are a camera picture tube, a synchronizing generator, and a monitor. The camera picture tubes that may be used are the vidicon, orthicon or plumbicon. The vidicon tube costs less, is smaller, and is more rugged than the orthicon. It is less sensitive to light, however, and does tend to present slight stickiness or blurring of the margins of rapidly moving parts, such as the beating heart. The problem of stickiness in present-day vidicon tubes is slight, however. The image orthicon, although more sensitive to light and possessing no stickiness, is more expensive and is more complex. Because high sensitivity is no longer needed with modern image intensifiers, the image orthicon is no longer used to any extent. The plumbicon is a vidicon-type tube with a lead oxide sensitive target face, which possesses good sensitivity and hardly any stickiness. It has now become the tube of preference for image intensifier fluoroscopy.

The flexibility of television viewing can be enhanced by the technique of video tape recording of the fluoroscopic image. The image is amplified by an intensifying tube, viewed by the television camera, and the output signal recorded on video tape. The image can be simultaneously viewed on the television monitor. It is then possible to immediately replay the video tape and review the recorded image stored on the tape. This, of course, can be invaluable to one carrying out selective angiocardiography. If it is found that the patient has not been positioned properly to demonstrate an anomaly to advantage or the intracardiac catheter is improperly positioned, the examination may be repeated immediately after rectifying the mistake. The information gained is also of help in planning if further contrast injections are needed. Tape recording of the image can be performed utilizing the same low levels of radiation as are employed for television viewing alone, which is a desirable feature. However, at the present time the recording of fine detail, especially in angiocardiography, is limited; therefore, it is best to simultaneously record the examination on cine film for a definite diagnosis.

IMAGE QUALITY

METHODS of viewing and recording of the image have been described, and it would now be well to consider factors affecting the quality of the intensified image. An image of good quality is one that possesses a wide range of contrast and in which fine detail is resolved. Klatte and associates (1959), Campbell and coworkers (1960), Ter-Pogossian (1967), Rossmann (1969, 1972), and others have investigated some of the factors involved. First, consider those that affect quality of the image on the output phosphor and, second, those affecting the quality of the recording of this image.

Image Quality on the Output Phosphor. 1. KILOVOLTAGE APPLIED TO THE X-RAY TUBE. An optimum kilovoltage of approximately 80 is needed to produce radiographs of adequate contrast. This is dependent not only on the thickness of the part being examined, but on the contrast media in angiocardiography. It is therefore necessary to take into consideration the absorption curve of iodine. A kilovoltage that is too high or too low will result in an image of poor quality.

Image quality may also be reduced due to scattered radiation. Improvement may be obtained by the use of grids, though this does necessitate increasing the x-ray dose to the patient.

2. FOCAL SPOT SIZE AND MAGNIFICATION. Standard x-ray tubes use a focal spot of 1 or 2 mm in diameter and this may result in blurring of image detail due to penumbra formation. This geometric effect can be reduced by the use of tubes with a focal spot of 0.3 or 0.5 mm in diameter. Unsharpness of image detail can be further reduced by keeping the image amplifier as close to the patient as possible.

Magnification and distortion of the image vary with the distance of the x-ray tube from the patient. Both of these factors can be minimized by placing the x-ray tube as far from the subject as possible. Magnification is sometimes desirable when performing angiocardiography, especially in the pediatric patient. The central area may contain the information desired while the surrounding field contains nothing of value. By enlarging the central area, more of the individual film frame is used and thus resolution of the image is increased. In present-day image-amplifying tubes the central field can be magnified by electronic or optical means. Electronic magnification is accomplished with the combination type of image tube. Thus, in a tube such as the 6 to 9 in. only the central area of the input phosphor is utilized in the 6-in. mode with resultant improved image resolution. Optical magnification is achieved by altering the focal length of the objective lens in the cine camera so that only the central field is seen by the lens, and the image being photographed fills the whole of the cine frame. This technique is referred to as overframing. Its value is questionable, however, as it really produces only a larger picture and not one with enhanced resolution.

3. IMAGE TUBE CHARACTERISTICS. With modern image intensifiers, sensitive cine film, and television cameras, pictures may be obtained with very few x-rays. This, however, gives rise to mottling of the picture, which in turn reduces sharpness and visibility of detail. Thus, it is often necessary to use considerably more radiation than the possible minimum in order to obtain an adequate picture especially where fine detail is required.

Image Quality on Cinefilm. 1. LENS SYSTEMS. The lens system between the output phosphor of the image tube and the cine film must be properly focused or image detail will suffer.

2. IMAGE INTENSIFICATION TUBE. This must also be properly focused by adjusting the electrical focusing control or image quality will suffer.

3. FILM SIZE, TYPE, AND EXPOSURE RATE. Both 16- and 35-mm film are used in cinefluorography. Lenses presently in use with 16 mm are faster than those for 35-mm cameras. Theoretically by use of 16-mm film it should be possible to obtain cine x-rays with less radiation to the patient; however, in practice the lens must be stopped down and the radiation level increased to get rid of the x-ray mottling mentioned above. Further, although 35-mm film is less grainy than 16 mm, the x-ray mottling means that there is little practical difference between the pictures obtained on the two films.

Film for cinefluorography should possess high speed, excellent contrast, and fine grain. In practice, a film possessing all of these desirable properties at the same time is not obtainable; thus if any two factors are kept at the best possible level, the third must suffer. Speed is important in keeping the patient dosage to a minimum, contrast in providing an image with a wide range of densities, and grain in visualizing image detail.

High-speed film, however, is not always the film of choice with present-day high-brightness gain intensifying systems. With high-speed film it may be necessary to reduce the radiation output from the tube to a level where insufficient photons strike the input phosphor to produce an image of good quality. In this situation, a film of slower speed and finer grain should be considered. A high-contrast film accentuates grain and any tendency of the lens system to produce vignetting, while an increase in grain size produces an image of poor detail. Therefore, a compromise must be reached as to the type of film used for each cinefluorographic examination.

When filming a rapidly moving structure such as the heart, it is necessary to use frame rates of 30 to 80 per second, in order that intracardiac anatomy and physiology be demonstrated. A certain quality of radiation is needed to properly expose each frame; thus if exposure rate is increased, radiation to the patient is increased. When the camera shutter is synchronized with the x-ray generator, it is possible to decrease the radiation to the patient. By this method, the x-ray beam is pulsed and is shut off during the period in which the film is being transported and the shutter is closed, and is turned on while the film is stationary and the shutter is open.

4. AUTOMATIC BRIGHTNESS CONTROL. Image brightness may be kept constant by the use of a stabilizing device incorporated in the system. Once this is set, one may scan thick and thin fields without alteration in brightness levels, thus ensuring a constant fluoroscopic density. The brightness of the output phosphor is kept constant by an electronic device that senses changes in the light intensity on the phosphor and regulates the kilovoltage, milliamperage, or x-ray pulse width to compensate for these changes. The stabilizing device may also be present to maintain the brightness at a desired level for the sensitivity of the film emulsion being used, thus ensuring a constant cinefilm density.

DEVELOPING APPARATUS

THE large-size films from cut or roll film changers are best developed in automatic x-ray processors, which are available in modern x-ray departments. Cine film may also be processed in these by taping one end to a large film, which acts as a leader. Unfortunately, any alteration in the speed at which the cine film passes through the developer is difficult to alter. The ideal method is use of an automatic cine processor. To give the best results a processor of this type should have a thermostatically controlled temperature regulator, a variable speed drive so that the rate of processing of the film can be altered, and good uniform agitation of the chemicals. A replenishing system for the chemicals may be attached to the processor or the developer and fixer can be changed regularly after a certain number of feet of film have been processed. Processors of this type vary in size and as to the width of film that they can handle. It is advisable that one which is chosen should process 16- and 35-mm and probably 70-mm film.

Either photographic or x-ray developing solutions may be used in processing cine film. Although x-ray solution is commonly used, nevertheless, it increases the contrast and speed of the film emulsion though at the expense of increased film graininess.

FILM VIEWING

PROJECTORS for cinefilm viewing must have certain features not available on ordinary commercial models. These include instantaneous forward and reverse motion, variable frame speeds with flickerless motion, slow speeds, and single framing without loss of illumination or heat damage to the film. Other desirable features are large reel capacity and remote-control operation. Projection equipment for use with 16-mm film is readily available and possesses all the features listed. The choice of equipment for 35-mm film is limited and the price is considerably increased.

Some workers prefer to reduce 35-mm film to 16-mm size for viewing. In this way the original film may be kept free of scratches or damage.

PRESSURE INJECTORS, CATHETERS, AND CONTRAST MATERIAL

In selective angiocardiography the concentration and amount of the contrast material injected must be sufficient to study intracardiac anatomy and the dynamics of flow. The degree of dilution is dependent not only on the amount and rate at which the material is injected but also on the velocity of blood flow in the chamber or vessel into which it is injected. Considerable resistance to flow is encountered in forcing viscous contrast material through a thin-walled long catheter. The delivery rate can be increased by the use of pressure injections in conjunction with thin-walled catheters that are as short as is feasible and contrast media with low viscosity.

Pressure Injectors. Pressure injectors are of several basic types. Manually operated injectors, which force the contrast material through a syringe, have the disadvantage that the rate of injection tends to be too prolonged as the pressure that can be exerted is insufficient and the delivery rate is inconsistent. Compressed gas injectors such as those described by Gidlund (1956) and Amplatz (1960) must use a metal syringe because of the high pressure involved. Care must be taken with these injections so that no air enters the syringe while it is being filled with the contrast material. A mechanical injector utilizing a series of syringes has been used in the Tavaras injector produced by the Picker X-Ray Company. A stainless steel syringe is used, though this is pointed down so that any air in the system will rise to the top and also some contrast material remains in the syringe at the completion of the injection as an added safety feature to prevent air being injected. Electrically powered mechanical injectors such as the Cordis and Viamonte–Hobbs (1967) are examples of more recently developed injectors. These units can be programmed with an electrocardiogram so that injections can be made in specific phases of the cardiac cycle. The Viamonte–Hobbs unit is adequately grounded as a built-in safeguard against the hazards of ventricular fibrillation. This injector also has dials that select both the duration of the injection and the delivery rate.

To give the best results certain criteria should be fulfilled by an injector, and some of these were laid down by Gidlund (1956).

1. The injection rate should be rapid and a choice of predetermined injection speeds available. Once selected, the speed should remain constant through-out the injection to ensure uniform introduction of the contrast material.

2. The injection characteristics should be such that the chance of a catheter altering in position during the injection is minimal.

3. It is desirable that the volume of contrast material in the apparatus be sufficient to allow for several controlled injections without necessitating refilling of the syringe.

4. The contrast material within the syringe should be thermostatically heated and kept at body temperature.

5. A remote-control mechanism is preferable to protect the personnel from radiation. This may also be connected with the x-ray control and film changer or cine camera so as to commence radiography simultaneously with the dye injection or when a certain amount of dye has already been injected. To this, the more recent method of injecting the contrast media during a specific phase of the cardiac cycle through programming with the electrocardiogram should be added.

6. In pediatric work, a mechanical mechanism to prevent too large or multiple injections due to equipment malfunction should be present.

Catheters. Catheters available for present-day angiocardiography are made of Teflon, polyethylene, polyurethane, or woven dacron. The flow rate of contrast material injected is dependent not only on the inner diameter and length of the catheter, but on the viscosity of the contrast media. Of these the diameter of the catheter lumen is the most important. To obtain angiograms of the utmost quality it is recommended that a catheter with the largest possible diameter capable of insertion be used. With this, a large bolus of contrast material can be introduced in the shortest possible time. The injection pressure can be minimized resulting in less chance of catheter recoil and less risk of injury to the endothelium. In infants and children one usually uses a thin-walled catheter of size No. 5, 6, or 7. A No. 4 is too small to allow rapid discharge of contrast material. A catheter that is as short as possible will also increase the speed of injection. It is important that the catheter not be applied firmly against the wall of the ventricle as with the injection of contrast material some endocardial damage may occur. This risk can be minimized by the use of a catheter tip deflector to manipulate large-size catheters. Also, a catheter with a closed end and side holes such as the NIH will decrease the chances of this happening. Catheters of this type have the effect of diffusing the contrast material so that it does not impinge entirely on one wall with a single jet during the injection. They also minimize the whiplash effect, which tends to alter the catheter position. However, since all catheters tend to straighten to some degree during the injection, it is usually advisable to place the catheter in the chamber in such a way that it would be unlikely to slip out.

One risk is the possibility of entering the coronary sinus and making an injection into this vessel. It is, therefore, important to check the position of the catheter carefully before the injection is made by obtaining a pressure tracing. Where there is any doubt about the possibility of the catheter being within the coronary sinus, the heart should be viewed in the lateral position. It is advisable to give a small test injection of contrast material under low pressure to accurately localize the position of the catheter tip. In this way one can ascertain if the catheter end is lying free within the chamber and also the position can be optimized to demonstrate the suspected anomaly to advantage.

Contrast Material. The most common preparations in use at the present time are the diatrizoate and iothalmate compounds with a sodium or methylgluc-amine base, and metrizoates. Radiologically the compounds with a sodium base produce a more opaque appearance as they can be injected at a faster rate, being less viscid than methylglucamine compounds. They are more toxic, however (Gensine and De Giorgi, 1964; Fischer and Cornell, 1965). The amount of contrast material used in angiocardiography is calculated on the basis of body weight. In children this is usually 1 ml/kg of body weight per injection to a maximum total dose of 3 ml/kg. If more contrast media is demanded for a diagnosis, a time interval of 20 minutes should be observed before the next injection. A total maximum dose of 4 ml/kg for infants and 5 to 6 ml/kg for older children should not be exceeded.

The viscosity of the contrast material is dependent not only on temperature, but on the type of opaque medium. Therefore, not only should a contrast substance of low viscosity be used, but it should be warmed to body temperature to further lower its viscosity and increase the flow rate.

REACTIONS TO ANGIOCARDIOGRAPHY

MOST infants and children have a flushing of the skin and a feeling of heat with the injection of any of these contrast media. There is usually a transient increase in cyanosis in those who are cyanotic to begin with, or there may be a momentary pause in respiration immediately following the injection. This is usually followed by an increased depth in respiration, particularly in the babies who cry following the procedure. In the weak infants and those who are cyanotic, there may be a decreased depth in respiration for a few moments.

Certain other signs such as lacrimation, salivation, nausea, vomiting, coughing, urticaria, and headache may be seen less commonly. The more severe reactions are fortunately rare and consist of hemiplegia, convulsions, syncope, or death.

In many cases, there is a brief tachycardia with a return to normal rate in three to five minutes. Gordon and associates (1950) record a rise in venous pressure immediately following the injection of the material. There may be a slight rise in arterial pressure, but this is followed in a few seconds by a drop in systolic and diastolic pressure, which coincides with the vasodilation and flushing effect referred to previously. At the same time a rise in ventricular end diastolic pressure occurs due to the hyperosmolar effect of the contrast agent. Electrocardiographic changes are frequently noted in children during or immediately following angiocardiography but are almost invariably transient and of little consequence. They may consist of premature systoles, atrial, nodal, or ventricular in origin. Occasionally these arrhythmias may persist for as long as 25 minutes (Zinn et al., 1951). Conduction defects are not uncommon. Horger and associates (1951) studied the T wave changes that may develop in some children a few seconds after the injection is made and recorded a slight decrease in amplitude of the T wave, which may proceed to flattening or at times inversion. Such T wave changes are more likely to occur in the cyanotic child.

The toxic effects of the contrast material would appear to be due partly to the medium itself and partly to the hemodynamic alterations induced. As has been pointed out by Standen and associates (1965) and Lachlan (1970), the injection of a hyperosmolar substance into the vascular system results in an increase in the serum osmolality. This in turn causes extravascular fluid to be drawn rapidly into the vascular compartment increasing plasma volume and decreasing hematocrit values. This increase in plasma volume could be deleterious to patients in heart failure. Other aspects may also play a role in the toxicity of contrast media. Hemagglutination has been observed by Read (1959), Wiedeman (1964), and Rand and Lacombe (1965) that may result in an increase in blood viscosity. As contrast material is acid, its injection may produce acidosis. Sotos and colleagues (1962) have observed that experimentally produced prolonged hypertonicity of body fluids could disturb cellular metabolism with resulting severe metabolic acidosis. Marshall and Henderson (1968) have shown this tendency to acidosis when normal doses of contrast media are used during cerebral angiography. Large doses could therefore be expected to cause acidosis, especially if there is renal impairment, or could be harmful if the infant is already acidotic. It is thus important to correct any significant acidosis before proceeding to angiocardiography. Nogrady and Dunbar (1968) have shown that neonates have a low glomerular filtration rate and therefore might be expected to be more vulnerable to an overdose of contrast material than older children or adults.

Serious Reactions. Several studies have been reported of the serious risks involved in angiocardiography. In 1942, Pendergrass and coworkers found that in 600,000 patients who had received Diodrast intravenously, 26 deaths had occurred, a mortality rate of 0.0038 percent. These injections were made chiefly for urology and were therefore given slowly. Dotter and Jackson (1950) surveyed hospitals performing angiocardiography and collected records of 6823 such examinations with 26 deaths, or an incidence of 1 in 262 (0.38 percent). McAfee (1955) reviewed the literature and reported 37 deaths in 15,093 angiograms, or approximately 1 death in 200 angiograms. Three deaths were noted by Wennevold and coworkers (1965) among 577 patients (0.52 percent) undergoing angiocardiography. Toniolo and Buia (1966) reported a mortality rate of 1 in 4067 angiocardiograms. Recently Ansell (1970) reported on deaths in three infants occurring from an overdose of contrast material during excretory urography. About 800 to 900 angiocardiograms are performed at The Hospital for Sick Children, Toronto, each year and in the last five years two serious reactions have occurred.

Seventeen of the deaths reported by Dotter and Jackson were in children under eight years of age; 14 of them were cyanotic and were associated with multiple injections of contrast medium. In 19 of the reported fatalities sensitivity tests were done and in each case were found to be negative. Morgan (1950) reported two deaths following 1 ml of contrast medium given as a preliminary sensitivity test. Thus, sensitivity tests do not appear to be of any help in determining individual sensitivity.

TREATMENT OF SEVERE REACTIONS. One hundred percent oxygen should always be immediately available. A deep subcutaneous injection of epinephrine 1:1000 (dose 0.01 ml/kg of body weight up to a maximum of 0.5 ml) is the prime medication of choice. This may be repeated after five minutes if necessary. If not effective an intravenous injection of 100 mg of hydrocortisone is suggested. In the event of anaphylaxis with laryngeal edema and bronchial spasm, intubation of the trachea should be carried out immediately. If hypotension occurs, it should be treated with norepinephrine—4 ml of a 0.2 percent solution in 1 liter of normal saline. This is given at a rate of 30 to 60 ml per hour, though the infusion rate should be determined by the effect on the pulse rate and blood pressure. Less severe reactions may be managed with Benedryl (2 mg/kg of body weight). This is particularly beneficial for those with urticaria. It is important to have continuous electrocardiogram monitoring during the angiographic procedure to note the development of irregularities that may require special therapy. When there is cardiac arrest, cardiac massage and possible defibrillation will be needed.

Since there is some risk in selective angiocardiography, it is important to prevent serious reductions when possible by taking the following precautions:

1. Care should be taken in selection of cases to avoid those who are more likely to develop serious arrhythmias, those with primary pulmonary hypertension, or children with a history of asthma or other allergic reactions.

2. The urine should be examined for evidence of kidney disease.

3. A moderate dose of contrast medium should be used wherever possible.

4. The injection of a full dose of the contrast should not be carried out more than once on any one day.

5. Care should be taken to avoid air embolism.

6. General anesthetic appears to add to the risk of the procedure, although at times the presence of an anesthetist with an intratracheal airway readily available or in place is an advantage.

INDICATIONS FOR SELECTIVE ANGIOCARDIOGRAPHY AND SEDATION

WITH the progress in cardiac surgery that has taken place in the past 20 years not only is a knowledge of the nature of the cardiac lesion required, but an intimate understanding of the anatomy of the anomaly is essential. Therefore angiocardiography has become almost an integral part of any cardiac catheterization. These two procedures should in no way compete in arriving at an exact diagnosis, but rather should be considered as complementary.

The procedure of selective angiocardiography may be carried out without any anesthetic whatever, but usually the patient is more comfortable if given some sedative mixture. In some centers, general anesthesia is used so that the patient is unconscious. It has been our procedure in studying infants and children to use a sedative mixture (Smith et al., 1958), which consists of the following: 6.25 mg of Largactil, 6.25 mg of Phenergan, and 25 mg of Demerol per milliliter. This is administered intramuscularly at least four hours after the last feeding. Babies are usually given 0.1 ml/kg of body weight to a maximum of 2 ml in older children of this mixture one hour before the investigation is carried out. The dose is cut in half for severely cyanotic infants and to two-thirds for moderately cyanosed infants. Local anesthesia of 1 percent lidocaine (Xylocaine) is used at the site of the cutdown for insertion of the catheter. In babies and young children, this is likely to be the long saphenous or femoral vein; in older children, the medial vein at the antecubital space at the elbow is sometimes used. After the procedure no antibiotic coverage is found to be necessary.

THE NORMAL SELECTIVE ANGIOCARDIOGRAM

BEFORE one can interpret the abnormal angiocardiogram, a knowledge of the normal is essential. In an attempt to arrive at an understanding, the individual chambers, valves, and great vessels will be described as they appear on films taken in the anteroposterior and lateral projections.

A selective angiogram in a baby two years old with a normal heart is shown in the accompanying figure. The tip of the catheter is in the right ventricle (see Figure 7–3).

Normal Right Atrium. The dye-filled right atrium on the anteroposterior projection appears roughly oval in shape (see Figure 7–4*A*). Its right margin conforms to the convex right heart border. Superiorly this border may be continuous with the superior vena cava if filled either from reflux of the contrast media from the atrium or as the result of injection of dye via this route. Inferiorly the atrial border curves medially at the cardiophrenic angle to overlap the spine. Dye may regurgitate into the inferior vena cava and hepatic veins to a varying degree. The auricular appendage is not always visualized as it may be obscured by dye within the atrial body or main pulmonary artery and right branch. When demonstrated, the appendage tends to be triangular in shape with its apex directed superomedially. It lies to the left of the superior vena cava and to the right of the infundibulum of the right ventricle and proximal portion of the pulmonary artery. On occasion, it may extend to lie in front of these structures on the left. The superior border of the atrium is dome-shaped. The medial wall is formed by the interatrial septum. The septum runs superoinferiorly to join the annulus of the tricuspid valve. The annulus fibrosis overlies the left spinal margin just above the level of the diaphragm and may be recognized by a slight constriction on the superior and inferior margins and a slightly reduced dye density at this level. The septal leaflet may be seen owing to dye trapping between the leaf and the subjacent right ventricular septal surface, though the other leaflets are seldom seen.

In the lateral projection the right atrium is oval in shape (see Figure 7–4*B*). The posterior margin along with the superior portion of the inferior vena cava forms the posteroinferior cardiac border. From the superior margin, contrast substance may be continuous with the superior vena cava. Anteriorly the body is rounded and overlaps the right ventricle when this chamber is simultaneously filled. The auricular appendage is more frequently seen in this projection and appears as a trabeculated density situated anterior to the superior vena cava and overlapping the infundibulum of the right ventricle and proximal portion of the pulmonary artery.

Normal Right Ventricle. The right ventricle (see Figure 7–5*A*) is demarcated into two portions: the infundibulum or conus arteriosus superiorly, and the sinus or body, including the apical trabecular portion, inferiorly; by an incomplete ring of bulbar myocardium at the junction between these two. The posterosuperior arc of the ring is composed of the crista supraventricularis, and from this the parietal and septal bands of the crista run forward and caudally on the right and left, respectively.

The right ventricle alters in shape during the cardiac cycle. During systole on the anteroposterior view contrast media is seen streaming from the tricuspid valve in a column upward and to the left to become continuous with the pulmonary artery. During diastole, the body of the ventricle widens to extend approximately three-quarters of the way to the apparent cardiac apex. The dye-filled body is irregular in outline owing to trabeculation of its wall and the papillary muscles arising from the surfaces. The infundibulum on this projection is tubular in outline and lies to the left of the spine. Superiorly it ends in a dome at the pulmonary valve.

In the lateral projection, the ventricle occupies the

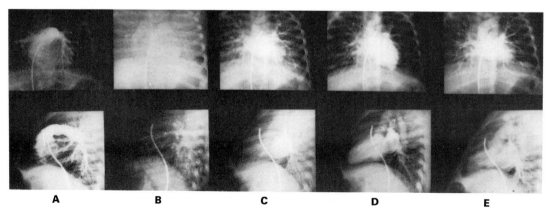

A   **B**   **C**   **D**   **E**

Figure 7-3. Normal selective angiogram. Angiogram in baby, aged two years, with normal heart. Anteroposterior view above; lateral view below. Tip of the catheter in the right ventricle. *A.* Filling of right ventricle and pulmonary artery. *B.* Diffusion of contrast medium into pulmonary capillary bed. *C.* Return of contrast to left atrium. *D* and *E.* Filling of left ventricle and aorta. Right ventricle clear.

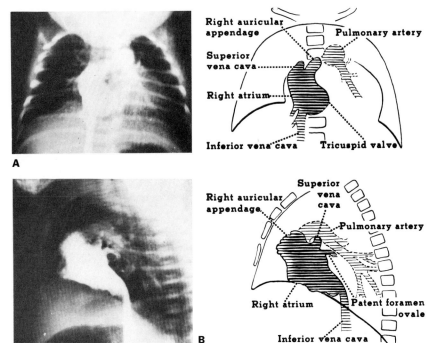

Figure 7-4. Normal angiogram of right atrium. *A.* Anteroposterior view. *B.* Lateral view. (Reproduced from Keith, J. D., and Moës, C. A. F.: Selective angiocardiography. In Zimmerman, H. A. [ed.]: *Intravascular Catheterization.* 2nd ed. Charles C Thomas, Publisher, Springfield, Ill., 1966.)

anterior and midportion of the cardiac silhouette (see Figure 7–5*B*). The anterior margin of the body extends to the anterior cardiac border and its wall is trabeculated. Inferiorly the margin conforms to the cardiac outline and rests on the diaphragm. The posterior margin is formed by the tricuspid valve. During systole, the sinus portion is seen as a narrow density situated anteriorly with contrast material streaming toward the infundibulum. In diastole, the sinus is well seen with a fairly straight posterior margin. The infundibulum is tubular and smooth in outline. It is well-delineated in this projection from middiastole to early systole and even into mid-systole if the right ventricular body is well-filled. The anterior margin is sometimes obscured by overlying right auricular appendage. The ostium of

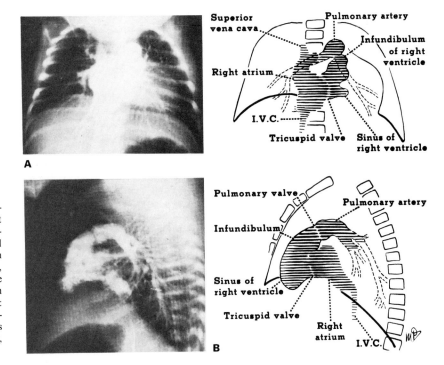

Figure 7-5. Normal angiogram of right ventricle. *A.* Anteroposterior view. *B.* Lateral view. (Reproduced from Keith, J. D., and Moës, C. A. F.: Selective angiocardiography. In Zimmerman, H. A. [ed.]: *Intravascular Catheterization,* 2nd ed. Charles C Thomas, Publisher, Springfield, Ill., 1966.)

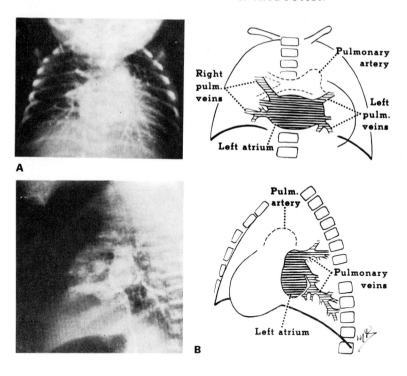

Figure 7-6. Normal angiogram of left atrium. *A*. Anteroposterior view. *B*. Lateral view. (Reproduced from Keith, J. D., and Moës, C. A. F.: Selective angiocardiography. In Zimmerman. H. A. [ed.]: *Intravascular Catheterization*, 2nd ed. Charles C Thomas, Publisher, Springfield, Ill., 1966.)

the infundibulum may be identified by a slight narrowing due to encroachment of the crista supraventricularis from behind. Distally the infundibulum ends at the pulmonary valve. The valve plane can often be identified by an area of slight waisting just proximal to the mild dilatation of the sinuses of Valsalva. Not infrequently the pulmonary valve leaflets may be seen as linear radiotranslucencies within the dye-filled pulmonary artery, the position of which correlates with the ventricular cycle.

At times, the dilatation of the sinuses of Valsalva or the valve leaflets cannot be recognized. It is then necessary to identify the valve plane by other methods. When the aorta and main pulmonary artery are simultaneously filled, the pulmonary valve lies in close relationship to the anterior margin of the proximal portion of the ascending aorta. The valve may be situated just at the anterior margin or slightly further forward. On occasion it may overlap the aorta and be obscured. When the aorta is not filled, the valve plane may be related roughly to the vena cava. If the inferior vena cava is outlined, a line projected upward and forward from the anterior margin of the superior portion of the vena cava passes through or close to the valve. On the other hand, if the superior vena cava is dye-filled, the valve lies slightly anterior to the superocardiac portion of this structure.

Normal Left Atrium. The left atrium on the anteroposterior projection is oval (see Figure 7–6*A*). The body lies below the angle formed by the main stem bronchi and is in close approximation to the left branch. The auricular appendage is often visualized. When seen it forms that portion of the left cardiac border between the main pulmonary artery superiorly and the lateral margin on the left ventricle

inferiorly. The pulmonary veins, two in number on each side, may be demonstrated entering the body of the atrium. The upper-lobe veins collect into a common trunk that runs downward and medially to enter the upper portion of the body on its posterior aspect. On the right, a horizontal vein may be seen passing from the region of the middle lobe to join the main trunk from the upper lobe, though on occasion this vein enters the atrium separately. The lower-lobe veins run upward and medially to collect in a common trunk on either side before entering the posterior surface of the atrium below the level of the upper veins. The mitral valve leaflets, although visible in this projection, are better appreciated in the lateral view.

On the lateral film, the atrium is situated posterosuperiorly (see Figure 7–6*B*). It appears as an oval density with its long axis directed superoinferiorly. The posterior margin forms the posterior cardiac silhouette above the right atrium, though the left atrium may overlap the right and extend further inferiorly, thus forming a longer segment of the posterior cardiac margin. This surface of the atrium is in intimate contact with the esophagus. Superiorly, the atrium is rounded and lies just below the left main stem bronchus. Anteriorly, the border may be obscured by contrast material in the left ventricle, though when seen it projects as far forward as the posterior aspect of the root of the aorta. The mitral valve annulus may be located by an indentation at the atrioventricular groove between the left atrium and left ventricle. The deep anterior or aortic leaflet of the valve is often visualized. Normally, it lies immediately inferior to the noncoronary leaflet of the aortic valve and runs downward and forward. The posterior leaflet is often less well defined.

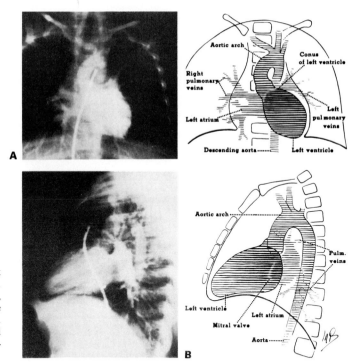

Figure 7-7. Normal angiogram of left ventricle. *A.* Anteroposterior view. *B.* Lateral view. (Reproduced from Keith, J. D., and Moës, C. A. F.: Selective angiocardiography. In Zimmerman, H. A. [ed.]: *Intravascular Catheterization*, 2nd ed. Charles C Thomas, Publisher, Springfield, Ill., 1966.)

Normal Left Ventricle. The left ventricle has only one part—the sinus or body. There is no infundibulum or conus. In the frontal plane it is somewhat elliptic in shape with the long axis running from the cardiac apex upward and to the right (see Figure 7–7*A*). The shape alters with the cardiac cycle, so that the ellipse is broad in diastole and narrows in systole. The superolateral margin is convex conforming to the lateral cardiac silhouette below the level of the pulmonary artery and left auricular appendage. This margin exhibits a smooth appearance. The inferomedial margin may display its characteristically fine trabeculation and tends to lie in a plane at approximately 45 degrees to the horizontal. This border lies to the left of the spine inferiorly, then overlaps the spine as it proceeds superiorly. Inferiorly, the medial and lateral margins converge to form a blunt point at the apparent cardiac apex. The apex is trabeculated due to numerous fine oblique trabeculae carneae joining the inferior left ventricular septal surface with the inferior free wall surface, about the base of the large anterior and posterior papillary muscles. At the base, the medial and lateral walls converge to end at the aortic valve. The aortic valve may be seen at the level of the sixth or seventh thoracic vertebra to the right of the right ventricular infundibulum.

In the lateral projection, the left ventricle has the appearance of a foot seen from the side with the toes plantar-flexed (see Figure 7–7*B*). The posterior margin is formed by the mitral valve. The superior border is convex and anteriorly curves downward toward the cardiac apex. The inferior margin is also convex, though toward the apex becomes slightly concave. The upper and lower margins converge at the apex and the characteristic fine trabeculae may be seen. The aorta is best seen in this view and projects superiorly just in front of the mitral valve site. The aortic valve plane can be recognized by an area of slight narrowing just proximal to the dilatation of the sinuses of Valsalva. The aortic valve leaflets may be identified as thin radiolucent lines within the dye-filled aorta. The tubular aortic shadow, which is smooth in outline, commences at a level approximately opposite the sixth or seventh thoracic vertebra and ascends vertically or is tilted slightly posteriorly to curve backward and form the aortic arch at the level opposite the third thoracic body.

REFERENCES

Abrams, H. L.: Present status of biplane cineangiocardiography. A roentgenographic procedure. *JAMA*, **184**:747, 1963.

Amplatz, K.: A vascular injector with program selector. *Radiology*, **75**:955, 1960.

Ansell, G.: Fatal overdose of contrast medium in infants. *Br. J. Radiol*, **43**:395, 1970.

Campbell, J. A.; Klatte, E. C.; and Shalkowski, R. A. (R. T.): Factors influencing image quality in cineroentgenography. *Am. J. Roentgenol. Radium Ther. Nucl. Med.*, **83**:345, 1960.

Castellanos, A.; Pereiras, R.; and Garcia, A.: La angiocardiographia radio opaca. *Arch. Soc. Estud. Clin. Habana*, **31**:523, 1937.

Chavez, I.; Dorbecker, N.; and Celis, A.: Direct intracardiac angiocardiography: Its diagnostic value. *Am. Heart J.* **33**:560, 1947.

Dotter, C. T., and Jackson, F. S.: Death following angiocardiography. *Radiology*, **54**:527, 1950.

Fisher, H. W., and Cornell, S. H.: The toxicity of the sodium and methylglucamine salts of diatrizoate, iothalamate and metrizoate. *Radiology*, **85**:1013, 1965.

Gensini, G. G., and DiGiorgi, S.: Myocardial toxicity of contrast agents used in angiography. *Radiology*, **82**:24, 1964.

Gidlund, A. S.: Development of apparatus and methods for roentgen studies in hemodynamics. *Acta Radiol*, Suppl., 130, 1956.

Gordon, A. J.; Brahms, S. A.; Megibow, S.; and Sussmann, M. L.: An experimental study of the cardiovascular effects of diodrast. *Am. J. Roentgenol. Radium Ther. Nucl. Med.*, **64**:819, 1950.

Horger, E. L.; Dotter, C. T.; and Steinberg, I.: Electrocardiographic changes during angiocardiography. *Am Heart J*, **41**:651, 1951.

Janker, R.: Roentgen cinematography. *Am. J. Roentgenol. Radium Ther. Nucl. Med.*, **36**:384, 1936.

———: *Roentgenotogische Funktionsdiagnostic Wupper.* Elberfeld, Garandit, 1954.

Jönsson, G.; Brodén, B.: and Karnell, J.: Selective angiocardiography. *Acta Radiol.*, **32**:486, 1949.

Jönsson, G.: Selective visualization in angiocardiography. *J. Fac. Radiol.*, **3**:125, 1951.

Klatte, E. C.; Campbell, J. A.; and Lurie, P. R.: Technical factors in selective cinecardioangiography. *Radiology*, **73**:539, 1959.

Lachlan, H.: Biochemical and other changes occurring in infants during angiocardiography. *Proc. R. Soc. Med.*, **63**:46, 1970.

McAfee, J. G.: Angiocardiography and thoracic aortography in congenital cardiovascular lesions. *Am. J. Med. Sci.*, **229**:549, 1955.

MacIntyre, J.: X-ray records for the cinematograph. *Arch. Clin. Skiagraphy*, **1**:37, 1896.

Marshall, M., and Henderson, G. A.: Tendency to acidosis following the injection of radio-opaque contrast material. *Br. J. Radiol.*, **41**:190, 1968.

Moon, R. J.: Amplifying and intensifying fluoroscopic images by means of scanning x-ray tube. *Science*, **112**:389, 1950.

Morgan, R. H.: Problems of angiocardiography. *Am. J. Roentgenol. Radium Ther. Nucl. Med.*, **64**:189, 1950.

Morgan, R. H., and Sturm, R. E.: The Johns Hopkins fluoroscopic screen intensifier. *Radiology*, **57**:556, 1951.

Nogrady, M. B., and Dunbar, J. S.: Delayed concentration and prolonged excretion of urographic contrast medium in the first month of life. *Am. J. Roentgenol. Radium Ther. Nucl. Med.*, **104**:289, 1968.

Pendergrass, E. P.; Chamberlain, G. W.; Godfrey, E. W.; and Burdick, E. O.: Survey of deaths and unfavourable sequelae following administration of contrast media. *Am. J. Roentgenol. Radium Ther. Nucl. Med.*, **48**:741, 1942.

Pickard, C.: Simultaneous bi-plane cineradiography. *Br. J. Radiol.*, **36**:939, 1963.

Rand, P. W., and Lacombe, E.: Effects of angiocardiographic injections on blood viscosity. *Radiology*, **85**:1022, 1965.

Read, R. C.: Cause of death in cardioangiography. *J. Thorac. Cardiovasc. Surg.*, **38**:685, 1959.

Reynolds, R. J.: Some experiments on production of rapid serial roentgenograms from screen image by means of cinematographic camera. *Am. J. Roentgenol. Radium Ther. Nucl. Med.*, **19**:469, 1928.

Robb, G. P., and Steinberg, I.: A practical method of visualization of the chambers of the heart, the pulmonary circulation and great blood vessels in man. *J. Clin. Invest.*, **17**:507, 1938.

Rossmann, K.: Image quality. *Radiol Clin. North Am.*, **7**:419, 1969.

———: Image quality and patient exposure. *Curr. Probl. Radiol.*, **2**:1, 1972.

Smith, C.; Rowe, R. D.; and Vlad, P.: Sedation of children for cardiac catheterization with an ataractic mixture. *Can. Anaesth. Soc. J.*, **5**:35, 1958.

Sones, J. M., Jr.: Cinecardioangiography. *Pediatr. Clin. North Am.*, **5**:945, 1958.

Sotos, J. F.; Dodge, P. R.; and Talbot, N. B.: Studies in experimental hypertonicity. II. Hypertonicity of body fluids as cause of acidosis. *Pediatrics*, **30**:180, 1962.

Standen, J. R.; Nogrady, M. B.; Dunbar, J. S.; and Goldbloom, R. B.: The osmotic effects of methylglucamine diatrizoate (Renografin 60) in intravenous urography in infants. *Am. J. Roentgenol. Radium Ther. Nucl. Med.*, **93**:473, 1965.

Sturm, R. E., and Morgan, R. H.: Screen intensification systems and their limitations. *Am. J. Roentgenol. Radium Ther. Nucl. Med.*, **62**:617, 1949.

Ter-Pogossian, M. M.: *The Physical Aspects of Diagnostic Radiology.* Harper & Row (Hoeber Medical Division), New York, 1967.

Toniolo, G., and Buia, I.: Risultati di una inchiesta nazionale sugli incidenti mortali da iniezione di mezzi di contrasto organo-iodati. *Radiol Med.*, **52**:625, 1966.

Viamonte, M., Jr., and Hobbs, J.: Automatic electric injector: development to prevent electromechanical hazards of selective angiocardiography. *Invest. Radiol.*, **2**:262, 1967.

Watson, H., and Pickard, C.: Right and left heart biplane cineangiocardiography. *Br. Heart J.*, **26**:755, 1964.

Wegelius, C., and Lind, J.: Role of exposure rate in angiocardiography. *Acta Radiol.*, **39**:177, 1953.

Wennevold, A.; Christiansen, I.; and Lindeneg, O.: Complications in 4,413 catheterizations of the right side of the heart. *Am. Heart J.*, **69**:173, 1965.

Wiedeman, M. P.: Influence of low molecular weight dextran on vascular and intravascular responses to contrast media. *Am. J. Roentgenol. Radium Ther. Nucl. Med.*, **92**:682, 1964.

Zinn, W. J.; Levinson, D. C.; Johns, V.; and Griffith, G. C.: The effect of angiocardiography on the heart as measured by electrocardiographic alterations. *Circulation*, **3**:658, 1951.

8

Embryology of Congenital Heart Disease

John W. A. Duckworth

DEVELOPMENT OF THE HEART

THE HEART develops from the progressive fusion of a pair of vessels that arise in the mesoderm covering the ventral aspect of the foregut. Directly ventral to these vessels lies the primitive pericardial cavity, which has arisen from a split in the mesoderm in this area, and directly caudal lies the septum transversum, a sheet of mesoderm lying between the primitive thoracic and abdominal cavities.

The heart tube gradually invaginates the dorsal wall of the pericardial cavity so that it comes to lie suspended in the cavity by a thin dorsal mesocardium. The rapid growth of the heart tube leads to the development of a marked flexure, which has its convex aspect facing ventrally, and also to the breakdown of the dorsal mesocardium, leaving the visceral layer of the pericardium surrounding the heart tube in continuity with the parietal pericardium, lining the fibrous pericardium, only at its arterial and venous ends.

A series of dilatations now begin to appear in the heart tube. These form from cephalic to caudal, the bulbus cordis, and the ventricle, lying on the ventrocephalic side of the loop, and the atrium, on the dorsocaudal side. The atrium and the ventricle are connected by a constricted portion of the tube, the atrioventricular canal. The bulbus cordis is connected at its cephalic end to the truncus arteriosus, from which the ventral aortae and sixth aortic arches arise. At the caudal end, the sinus venosus, which receives the whole of the venous drainage from the embryo except that from the lung buds, opens into the dorsal part of the atrium (Figure 8–1).

During the fourth week of development the bulboventricular loop twists to the right carrying the truncus arteriosus with it. The bulbus cordis now joins the right extremity of the ventricle at a sharp angle before passing up on the ventral aspect of the heart (Figure 8–4A, page 134). The turning of the ventricle to the right produces a spiral twist in the long axis of both the bulbus cordis and truncus arteriosus, which is partly responsible for the spiral course of the aorticopulmonary and bulba septa.

FORMATION OF THE SINUS VENOSUS AND ITS INCORPORATION INTO THE RIGHT ATRIUM

THE early venous drainage of the embryo consists of the following veins: the right and left anterior and posterior-cardinal veins, which drain the corresponding anterior and posterior halves of the embryo; the right and left vitelline veins, which drain the yolk sac and primitive gut; and the right and left umbilical veins, which drain the blood from the developing placenta (Figure 8–1A).

The anterior and posterior cardinal veins on each side unite to form the common cardinal veins, which enter the dorsal part of the septum transversum, and are here joined by the right and left umbilical and vitelline veins to form the right and left horns of the sinus venosus.

Subsequent growth changes, chiefly due to the growth of the liver and the development of cross anastomoses, cut down the number of veins entering the sinus. The right horn of the sinus venosus receives the right common cardinal, which becomes the terminal part of the superior vena cava, and the terminal part of the right vitelline (hepatic), which becomes the terminal part of the inferior vena cava (Figure 8–1A).

The left horn of the sinus venosus, which becomes the coronary sinus, loses all its extracardiac tributaries and persists only because the bulk of the venous drainage of the heart itself returns via this route. The left common cardinal vein (left superior

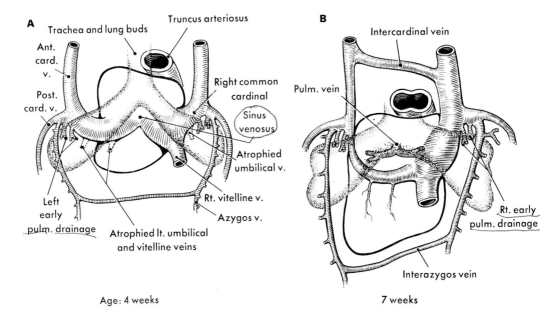

A

Trachea and lung buds

Truncus arteriosus

Ant. card. v.

Post. card. v.

Right common cardinal

Sinus venosus

Atrophied umbilical v.

Left early pulm. drainage

Atrophied lt. umbilical and vitelline veins

Rt. vitelline v.

Azygos v.

Age: 4 weeks

B

Intercardinal vein

Pulm. vein

Rt. early pulm. drainage

Interazygos vein

7 weeks

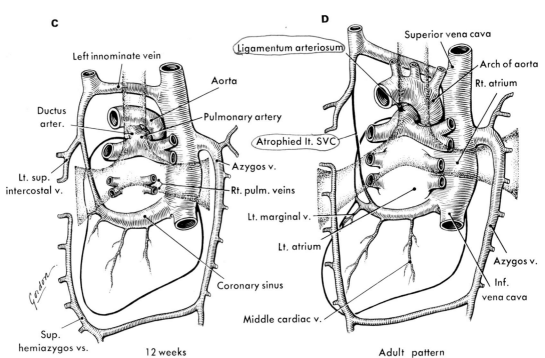

C

Left innominate vein

Ductus arter.

Aorta

Pulmonary artery

Lt. sup. intercostal v.

Azygos v.

Rt. pulm. veins

Coronary sinus

Sup. hemiazygos vs.

12 weeks

D

Ligamentum arteriosum

Superior vena cava

Arch of aorta

Rt. atrium

Atrophied lt. SVC

Lt. marginal v.

Lt. atrium

Azygos v.

Inf. vena cava

Middle cardiac v.

Adult pattern

Figure 8-1. The development of the great veins at the base of the heart.

vena cava) disappears except for a thin fibrous strand passing down from the last inch of the left superior intercostal vein, in front of the root of the left lung, to join the oblique vein of the left atrium. This strand also indicates the path taken by a persisting left superior vena cava (Figure 8–1D). The sinus venosus itself is gradually absorbed during the seventh and eighth weeks into the posterior part of the right atrium.

The cephalic part of the right valve of the sinus venosus becomes incorporated into the crista terminalis, while the caudal part forms the valve of the inferior vena cava and the valve of the coronary sinus.

The left valve of the sinus venosus becomes absorbed into the interatrial septum and disappears.

Failure of the sinus venosus to be absorbed into the right atrium results in the persistence of the sinus venosus. In this condition the right and left horns of the sinus enlarge to form a chamber that lies posterior to the right and left atria. This chamber receives the right superior and inferior venae cavae, and frequently a persisting left superior vena cava as well. It communicates with the posterior part of the right atrium through an elliptic opening guarded by the remains of the right and left valves of the sinus venosus.

During the fourth week a single pulmonary vein arises from a capillary plexus that lies on the ventral aspect of the lung buds. This vein runs ventrally to enter the venous mesocardium and penetrate the posterior aspect of the left atrium immediately to the left of the septum primum (Figure 8–1B). It is subsequently absorbed into the left atrium, together with its tributaries, the right and left pulmonary veins. These two veins are, in turn, gradually taken into the atrium. Finally absorption continues until the upper and lower tributaries of the two pulmonary veins are reached, so that it is usual to find an upper and lower vein entering the left atrium on each side (Figure 8–1C, D).

The early pulmonary venous plexus communicates freely with the posterior and common cardinal veins. The terminal part of the posterior cardinal vein becomes, on the right side, the arch of the vena azygos and, on the left side, the part of the left superior intercostal vein that lies on the left side of the arch of the aorta. Occasionally, one or more of the pulmonary veins drain by way of channels derived from their early connections with the cardinal system. In such cases they may drain directly into either the azygos vein or the right atrium on the right side or into an enlarged left superior intercostal vein, a persistent left superior vena cava, or the coronary sinus on the left side.

A greater or a lesser amount of the blood from the lungs, depending on the number of pulmonary veins that follow these abnormal routes, is thus discharged into the right atrium.

FORMATION OF THE CARDIAC SEPTA

THERE are four principal septa, which develop to bring about the formation of the four-chambered heart from the original single tube. These are: (1) the interatrial septum, (2) the septum of the atrioventricular canal, (3) the interventricular septum, and (4) the bulbar septum.

The Interatrial Septum. This is a compound septum made up of two developmentally separate septa. The first septum to form, or septum primum, develops during the fifth week of intrauterine life as a sickle-shaped fold in the dorsocephalic wall of the primitive atrium (Figure 8–2A) just to the left of the left valve of the sinus venosus. The free margin of this fold grows ventrocaudally toward the septum of the atrioventricular canal, which at this stage is formed by two mesodermal outgrowths, the anterior and posterior endocardial cushions. The passage between the growing margin of the septum primum and the endocardial cushions of the atrioventricular canal forms the foramen primum of the interatrial septum.

Finally, during the sixth week, the cephalic part of the septum primum breaks down to form the ostium secundum, and the lower margin of the septum primum fuses with the left edge of the atrial surface of the septum of the atrioventricular canal (Figure 8–2B).

The septum secundum, or second septum to form, appears during the sixth week as a thick crescentic fold on the ventrocephalic wall of the atrium between the left valve of the sinus venosus and the septum primum (Figure 8–2C, D). This septum grows in a dorsocaudal direction, gradually overlapping the ostium secundum in the septum primum and, at the same time, incorporating the left valve of the sinus venosus into the dorsal part of its right side. The septum secundum ceases to grow just after its crescentic margin has overlapped the foramen secundum. The part of the foramen primum not covered by the septum secundum forms the floor of the fossa ovalis and lies opposite the opening of the inferior vena cava, with the result that the blood entering the right atrium by this route pushes the thin septum primum to the left and passes below the thick margin of the septum secundum and through the foramen secundum into the left atrium. The aperture bounded by the lower margin of the septum secundum and the lower margin of the foramen secundum forms the foramen ovale (Figure 8–2B). The anterior part of the septum secundum fuses with the septum of the atrioventricular canal immediately to the right of the septum primum.

Defects in the normal growth pattern described above may result in any of the following abnormalities:

1. The septum primum and the septum secundum may fail to develop so that no separation of the two atria occurs.

2. The septum primum and the anterior part of the septum secundum may fail to fuse with the septum of the atrioventricular canal, giving rise to a persistent foramen primum, which may be either a single or a fenestrated aperture. The foramen secundum may be normal or absent.

3. When there is a delay in the breakdown of the septum secundum to form the foramen secundum, the septum primum may be displaced into the left atrium by the increasing blood flow and fuse across its cavity. This results in the left atrium being divided into a posterior chamber receiving the pulmonary veins and an anterior chamber communicating with the left auricular appendage, the left ventricle, and sometimes the right atrium. A small foramen primum usually connects the posterior and anterior chambers.

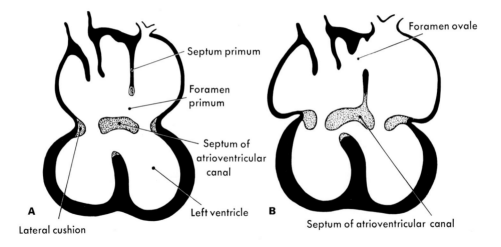

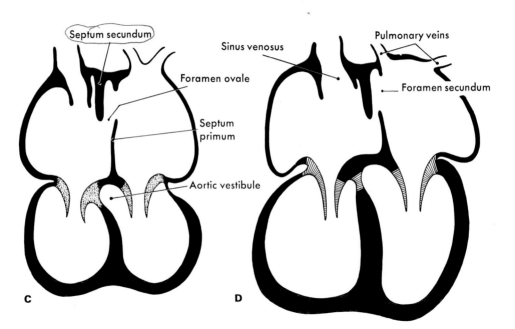

Figure 8-2. The development of the interatrial and interventricular septa.

The septum secundum may grow down to separate the atria, or it may be defective leaving a communication between either the right atrium and the posterior chamber, through a late-forming foramen secundum, or the right atrium and the anterior chamber below its crescentic lower margin, the floor of the fossa ovalis being absent due to the displaced foramen primum.

4. The septum secundum may fail to develop at all, leaving a large patent foramen secundum (Figure 8–2D).

5. The septum secundum may only partially overlap the foramen ovale, giving rise to various degrees of patent foramen ovale (Figure 8–2B).

The Septum of the Atrioventricular Canal. During the fifth week of intrauterine life two septa, which are often referred to as cushions because of their appearance, begin to grow from the dorsal and ventral aspects of the atrioventricular canal (Figure 8–4A). These broad septa are derived from the mesenchyme of the subendocardial region. As growth proceeds, fusion between the two septa occurs first on the right side and then gradually extends across toward the left, leading to the formation of a broad partition. It is with the cephalic aspect of the left side of this partition that the atrial septa fuse (Figure 8–2B).

Shortly after the appearance of the dorsal and ventral septa two lateral septa, one on each side, grow into the canal to complete the boundaries of the primitive tricuspid and mitral valves. It is from the mesenchymatous tissue of the margins of these

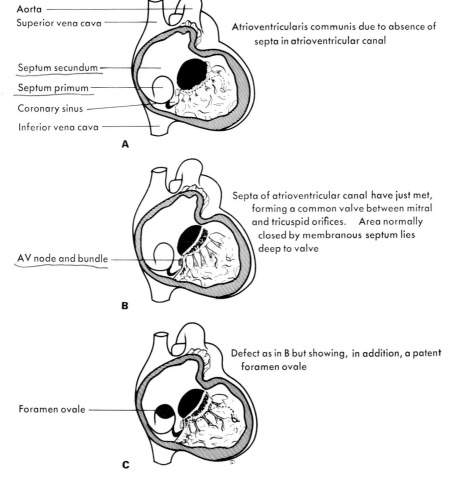

Figure 8-3. Atrioventricularis communis and associated defects.

orifices that the valve cusps develop (Figure 8–2*B*, *C*).

Defects in the normal growth pattern of the septa of the atrioventricular canal may result in any of the following abnormalities:

1. The dorsal and ventral septa may fail to fuse so that there is no division of the atrioventricular canal, although a large dorsal and ventral valve usually develops along the unfused margins of these septa (Figures 8–3 and 8–4*A*).

2. The dorsal and ventral septa may arise and fuse more to one side or the other of the atrioventricular canal, leading to a greater or lesser degree of stenosis of the mitral or tricuspid valves. This is more liable to occur on the right side because this orifice becomes closely related to the right bulbar ridge (Figure 8–4*B*, *C*) as it passes down to join the ventricular septum.

3. The dorsal and ventral septa may fuse incompletely, and, as fusion normally occurs first on the right side, this usually results in a bifid or double anterior (septal) cusp to the mitral valve (Figure 8–4*B*, *C*).

The Interventricular Septum and the Bulbar Septum. The division of the common ventricle into

right and left ventricles is intimately associated with the division of the bulbus cordis. This is to be expected since the bulbus cordis will be gradually incorporated into the right and left ventricles to form the infundibulum and aortic vestibule, respectively, and for this reason bulbar defects are often associated with interventricular septal defects.

As mentioned earlier, during the fourth week there is a sharp flexure at the junction of the bulbus cordis and the ventricle (Figure 8–4*A*). During the fifth and sixth weeks the depth of this flexure is gradually reduced, which considerably shortens the length of the posterior wall of the bulbus cordis and eventually results in its disappearance, thus bringing the aortic valve ring in contact with the ventral aspect of the fused endocardial cushions.

The disappearance of the posterior wall of the bulbus cordis as a result of the reduction of the bulboventricular sulcus also means that there will be no muscle in the posterior wall of the bulbus cordis. Whether this part of the outflow tract lies in contact with the mitral or tricuspid valve area of the endocardiol cushions or is entirely separate from

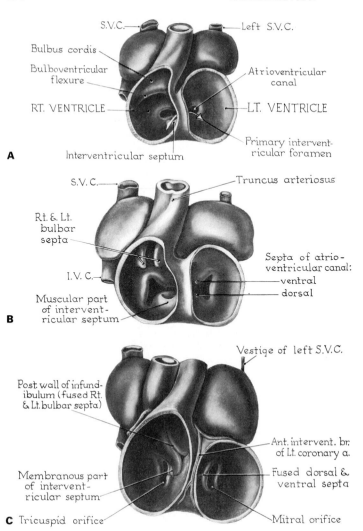

S.V.C.
Left S.V.C.
Bulbus cordis
Bulboventricular flexure
Atrioventricular canal
RT. VENTRICLE
LT. VENTRICLE
Primary interventricular foramen
A
Interventricular septum

S.V.C.
Truncus arteriosus
Rt. & Lt. bulbar septa
Septa of atrioventricular canal:
—ventral
—dorsal
I.V.C.
Muscular part of interventricular septum
B

Vestige of left S.V.C.
Post. wall of infundibulum (fused Rt. & Lt. bulbar septa)
Ant. intervent. br. of Lt. coronary a.
Membranous part of interventricular septum
Fused dorsal & ventral septa
C Tricuspid orifice
Mitral orifice

Figure 8-4. The developing heart. *A.* The fifth week of intrauterine life. *B.* The sixth week of intrauterine life. *C.* The end of the seventh week of intrauterine life.

them with muscle intervening depends upon the degree of reduction of the bulboventricular sulcus, together with the degree of right or left torsion of the bulboventricular loop.

In addition, in abnormal dextro- or levotorsion with normal reduction of the bulboventricular sulcus, whichever valve ring lies posteriorly will come to lie in contact with the endocardial cushions.

At the same time as these changes are occurring in the bulbus cordis, a low crescentic ridge appears in the common ventricle near its apex. The dorsal horn of this ridge reaches the dorsal cushion of the atrioventricular canal near its right margin, while the ventral horn extends to the ventral cushion near its left margin. The free edge of this ridge thus lies obliquely across the caudal aspect of the broad atrioventricular septum and between the two streams of blood entering the ventricle through the right and left atrioventricular orifices (Figures 8–4*A*, *B*). These streams of blood are probably one of the factors responsible for the bulging of the ventricle on either side of this ridge to form the right and left ventricles

and for the gradual increase in height of the septum. There is still a free communication between the two ventricles above the septum. This gap forms the primary interventricular foramen, which is bounded by the free margin of the ridge ventrally and the fused atrioventricular cushions dorsally (Figure 8–4*B*).

The closure of the communication between the ventricles is brought about as follows. Two ridges, a right and a left, composed of mesenchymatous tissue, grow into the cavity of the bulbus cordis, dividing it into an infundibular portion in front and an aortic vestibule behind (Figure 8–4*B, C*). As the left ridge extends caudally it passes more ventrally, and finally meets and fuses with the ventral end of the free edge of the interventricular septum along which it extends in a dorsal direction. The right ridge passes more dorsally and thus comes into relation with the ventral aspect of the tricuspid orifice, where it meets the ventral cushion of the atrioventricular canal. It does not, however, extend along the dorsal free edge of the interventricular septum, but passes directly across to

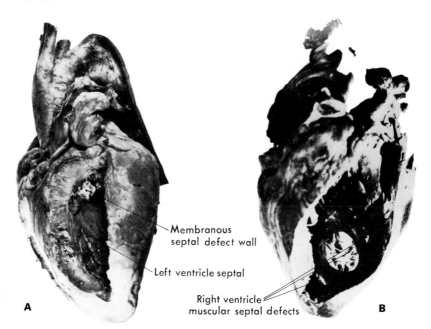

Membranous
septal defect wall

Left ventricle septal

Right ventricle
muscular septal defects

A   **B**

Figure 8-5. Abnormalities caused by defects in the normal development of the interventricular septum.

reach the free edge of the septum a short distance behind the attachment of the left bulbar ridge, with which it fuses. The greater part of the communication between the ventricles is thus cut off by the fusion of the bulbar ridges with the ventral four-fifths of the free edge of the interventricular septum (Figure 8–4C). There is still a small foramen remaining, bounded by the fused atrioventricular cushions, the dorsal margin of the right bulbar ridge, and the most posterior part of the free edge of the interventricular septum. This secondary interventricular foramen, which is the last part to close, is finally cut off by the extension of the mesenchymatous tissue from the right side of the fused atrioventricular cushions during the seventh week of intrauterine life.

The portion of the interventricular foramen closed by the extension of tissue from the fused atrioventricular cushions becomes fibrous and forms the membranous septum (Figure 8–4C).

The anterior interventricular branch of the left coronary artery develops in the subepicardial tissue in direct relation to the attached margin of the ventral end of the muscular interventricular septum, while the inferior interventricular branch of the right coronary artery is correspondingly related to the attached margin of the dorsal end. These vessels are thus in a position to supply both the muscular septum and the walls of the ventricles and throughout life accurately outline on the surface of the heart the

position of the peripheral margin of the muscular interventricular septum (Figure 8–4C).

With the final closure of the secondary interventricular foramen, which occurs during the seventh week, the aortic vestibule is bounded by the fused bulbar ridges in front, the membranous septum on the right, and the fused atrioventricular cushions behind, while on the left side it communicates with the rest of the left ventricle through the primary interventricular foramen.

Defects in the normal development of the interventricular septum may result in any of the following abnormalities:

1. The membranous septum may fail to develop. This is the commonest type of interventricular septal defect and is frequently associated with a bulbar defect due to incomplete absorption of the bulbo ventricular angle, which keeps the bulbus cordis too far to the right of the ventricular septum (Figure 8–5A).

2. The right and left bulbar ridges may fail to fuse, leading to a communication between the infundibulum and the aortic vestibule. This is usually situated close to the pulmonary valve (Figure 8–10, page 139).

3. The interventricular septum itself may be perforated in one or more places near the apex of the heart. This is due to the fact that the tissue between the early muscular trabeculae of the septum has given way (Figure 8–5B).

DEVELOPMENT OF THE INFUNDIBULUM AND AORTIC VESTIBULE

DURING the fifth week in addition to the right and left bulbar ridges, which are developing to divide the bulbus cordis into aortic vestibule and infundibulum, two further ridges of mesenchymatous tissue form,

one along the ventral wall and one along the dorsal wall, with the result that during the sixth week the bulbus cordis is largely filled with tissue derived from this source (Figure 8–6A). In the fifth week the

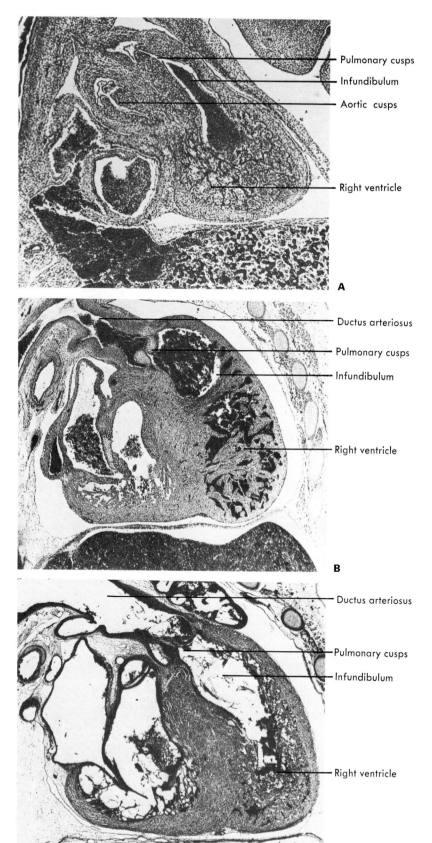

Pulmonary cusps

Infundibulum

Aortic cusps

Right ventricle

A

Ductus arteriosus

Pulmonary cusps

Infundibulum

Right ventricle

B

Ductus arteriosus

Pulmonary cusps

Infundibulum

Right ventricle

C

Figure 8-6. Sagittal sections of human hearts to show development of pulmonary valves and infundibulum. *A.* Sixth week. *B.* Seventh week. *C.* Eighth week.

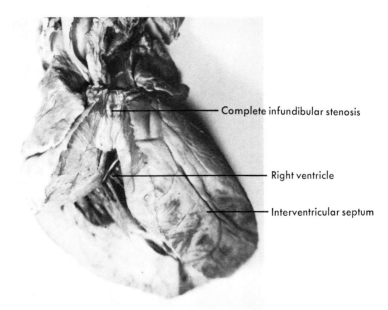

Figure 8-7. Complete infundibular stenosis.

outline of the pulmonary valve becomes demarcated at the apex of the infundibulum and of the aortic valve at the apex of the aortic vestibule as a result of the absorption of the excess mesenchymatous tissue above and below these points, with the result that the valve cusps project into the cavities as little fleshy elevations (Figure 8–6B). In the seventh week the absorption of the tissue has extended throughout the greater part of the infundibulum and aortic vestibule and the constriction between the lower end of the infundibulum and the right ventricle has begun to disappear. By the eighth week, the fleshy elevations of

the pulmonary and aortic valves have been modeled into delicate cusps and the sinuses above the valves are well-formed. The constriction between the bulbus cordis and the right ventricle has completely disappeared, and all the excess mesenchymatous tissue has been absorbed (Figure 8–6C).

Defects occurring in the development of the infundibulum and aortic vestibule may result in any of the following varieties of pulmonary stenosis:

1. The absorption of the mesenchymatous tissue in the infundibulum may fail entirely, with the result that during the later stages of intrauterine life this

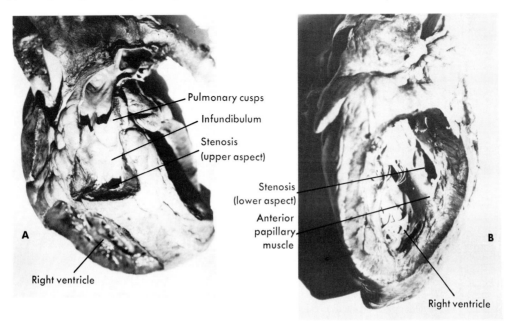

Figure 8-8. Lower infundibular stenosis.

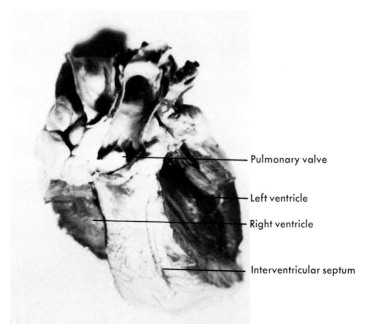

Pulmonary valve

Left ventricle

Right ventricle

Interventricular septum

Figure 8-9. Pure valvular pulmonary stenosis.

tissue becomes converted into dense fibrous tissue that runs throughout the whole length of the infundibulum, thus leading to both a valvular and infundibular stenosis (Figure 8–7).

2. The absorption may extend for a short distance below the valve cusps so that the actual valves may develop normally, but the absorption in the rest of the infundibulum is incomplete and leads to a greater or lesser degree of infundibular stenosis.

3. The absorption in the infundibulum is almost complete, but the constriction between the infundibular half of the bulbus cordis and the ventricle fails to disappear, leading to the formation of a lower bulbar stenosis in which the right ventricle and the infundibulum are separated by a thin constriction at a point just above the anterior papillary muscle (Figure 8–8).

4. The infundibulum may form normally, but the margins of the cusps of the pulmonary valve may remain adherent, giving rise to a valvular pulmonary stenosis (Figure 8–9).

5. The absorption of the mesenchymatous tissue in the aortic vestibule fails to take place, leading to a subaortic stenosis in which the aortic valve and the aortic vestibule are stenosed to a greater or lesser extent. Owing to the reduction of the depth of the bulboventricular angle and the disappearance of the greater part of the posterior wall of the bulbus cordis, the length of the stenosed portion is much shorter than that found in complete infundibular stenosis.

DISORDERS RESULTING FROM ABNORMAL DEVELOPMENT OF THE BULBOVENTRICULAR REGION OF THE HEART

THE disorders in this region are due to:

1. Incomplete reduction of the bulboventricular sulcus.

2. Reduced dextrotorsion or reduced levotorsion of the bulboventricular loop.

3. A combination of incomplete reduction of the bulboventricular sulcus and reduced dextrotorsion or reduced levotorsion of the bulboventricular loop.

If the bulboventricular angle fails to undergo reduction, the bulbus cordis will be either too far to the right (in dextrotorsion) or too far to the left (in levotorsion) of the muscular part of the interventricular septum. This will result in the outflow tracts of both great arteries arising from the morphologic right ventricle and in an interventricular septal defect, due to the inability of the bulbar part of the interventricular septum to join up with the membranous and muscular parts of the septum. If there is a reduction in the amount of dextrotorsion or levotorsion as well, the relationship of the outflow tracts of both great arteries to each other will also be altered and muscle will be found separating the posterior vessel from the endocardial cushions; e.g., when there is a reduction of 180 degrees in the amount of torsion the aorta will arise from the right ventricle anterior and to the right of the pulmonary artery, while with approximately a reduction of 125 degrees in the amount of torsion the pulmonary and aortic outflow tracts will lie side by side and there will be a right and left muscular infundibulum.

General Features:
1. The right atrium will discharge into a right-sided right ventricle.
2. The left atrium will discharge into a left-sided left ventricle.
3. The aorta and pulmonary artery will both arise from the right ventricle.
4. There will be a membranous interventricular septal defect.
5. The bulbar septum will end in the right ventricle with a free lower border that lies to the right of the interventricular septum.

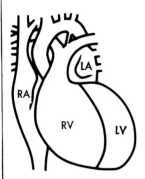 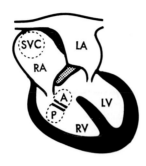

Normal Dextrotorsion.
1. Aortic vestibule lies posterior and to left of bulbar septum.
2. Pulmonary infundibulum lies anterior and to right of bulbar septum.

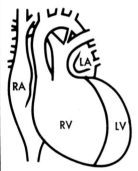 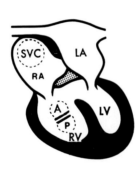

60° Reduced Dextrotorsion.
1. Aortic vestibule lies posterior and to right of bulbar septum.
2. Pulmonary infundibulum lies anterior and to left of bulbar septum.

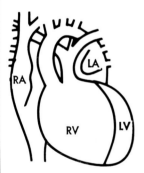 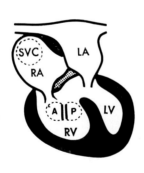

120° Reduced Dextrotorsion.
1. Bilateral infundibula. Aortic to right. Pulmonary to left.
2. Taussig-Bing anomaly.

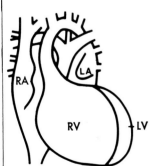 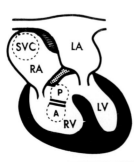

180° Reduced Dextrotorsion.
1. Aortic infundibulum lies anterior and to right of bulbar septum.
2. Pulmonary vestibule lies posterior and to left of bulbar septum.

Figure 8-10. Normal and reduced dextrotorsion of the bulboventricular loop with failure of reduction of the bulboventricular sulcus and situs solitus of the atria.

General Features:
1. A morphologic right atrium will lie on the left side and discharge into a morphologic left ventricle.
2. A morphologic left atrium will lie on the right side and discharge into a morphologic right ventricle.
3. There will be a membranous interventricular septal defect.
4. The bulbar septum will end in the morphologic right ventricle with a free lower border lying to the right of the interventricular septal defect.
5. Aorta and pulmonary artery will both arise from the right ventricle.

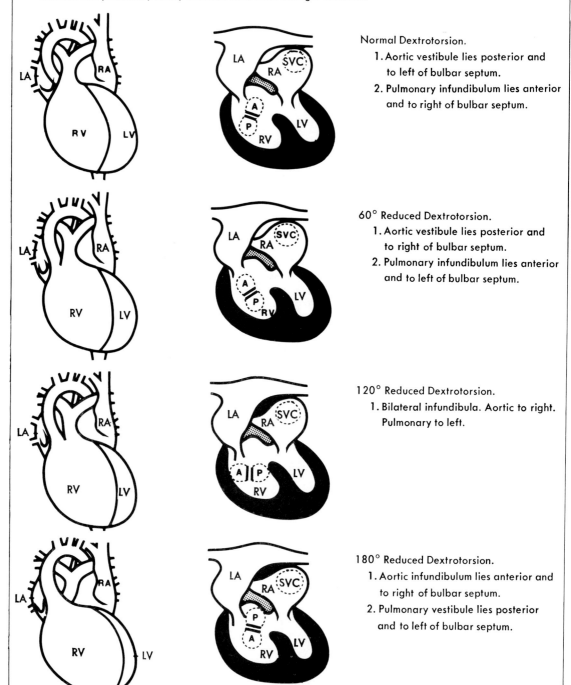

Normal Dextrotorsion.
1. Aortic vestibule lies posterior and to left of bulbar septum.
2. Pulmonary infundibulum lies anterior and to right of bulbar septum.

60° Reduced Dextrotorsion.
1. Aortic vestibule lies posterior and to right of bulbar septum.
2. Pulmonary infundibulum lies anterior and to left of bulbar septum.

120° Reduced Dextrotorsion.
1. Bilateral infundibula. Aortic to right. Pulmonary to left.

180° Reduced Dextrotorsion.
1. Aortic infundibulum lies anterior and to right of bulbar septum.
2. Pulmonary vestibule lies posterior and to left of bulbar septum.

Figure 8-11. Normal and reduced dextrotorsion of the bulboventricular loop with failure of reduction of the bulboventricular sulcus and situs inversus of the atria.

General Features:

1. On the right side a morphologic right atrium will discharge into a morphologic left ventricle.
2. On the left side a morphologic left atrium will discharge into a morphologic right ventricle.
3. There will be an interventricular septal defect.
4. The bulbar septum will end in the morphologic right ventricle with a free lower border to the left of the interventricular septal defect.
5. Aorta and pulmonary artery will both arise from a left-sided morphologic right ventricle.

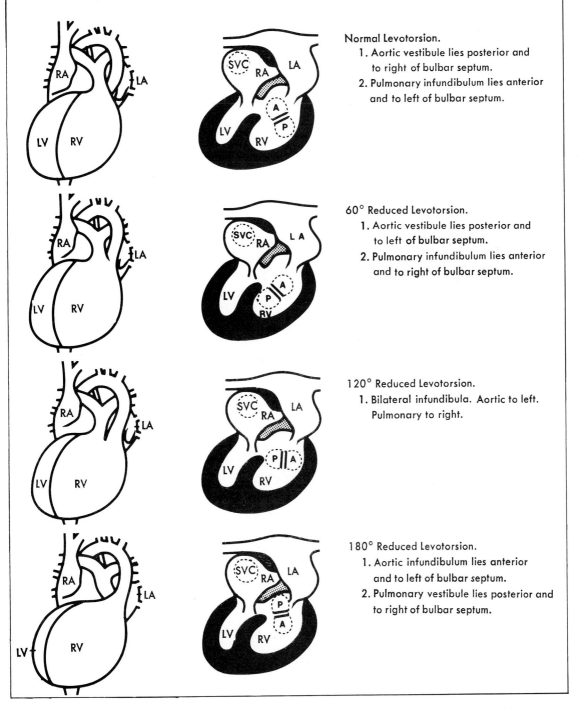

Normal Levotorsion.
1. Aortic vestibule lies posterior and to right of bulbar septum.
2. Pulmonary infundibulum lies anterior and to left of bulbar septum.

60° Reduced Levotorsion.
1. Aortic vestibule lies posterior and to left of bulbar septum.
2. Pulmonary infundibulum lies anterior and to right of bulbar septum.

120° Reduced Levotorsion.
1. Bilateral infundibula. Aortic to left. Pulmonary to right.

180° Reduced Levotorsion.
1. Aortic infundibulum lies anterior and to left of bulbar septum.
2. Pulmonary vestibule lies posterior and to right of bulbar septum.

Figure 8-12. Normal and reduced levotorsion of the bulboventricular loop, with failure of reduction of the bulboventricular sulcus and situs solitus of the atria.

General Features:
1. On the right side a morphologic left atrium will discharge into a morphologic left ventricle.
2. On the left side a morphologic right atrium will discharge into a morphologic right ventricle.
3. There will be an interventricular septal defect.
4. The bulbar septum will end in the morphologic right ventricle to the left of the interventricular septal defect.
5. Aorta and pulmonary artery will both arise from a left-sided morphologic right ventricle.

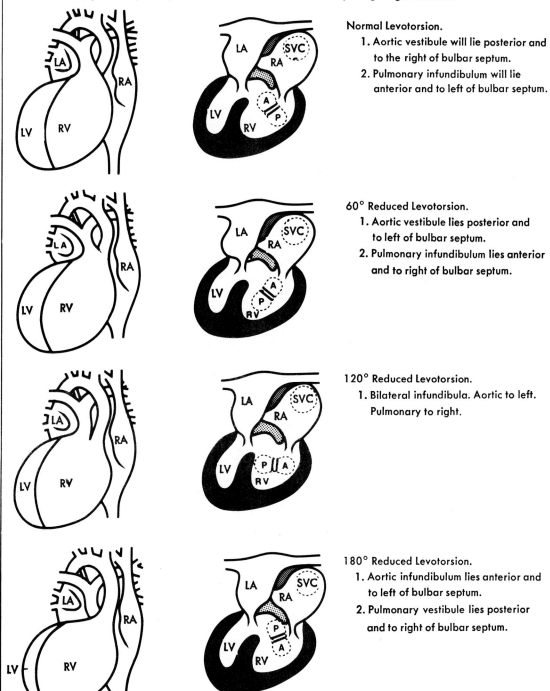

Normal Levotorsion.
1. Aortic vestibule will lie posterior and to the right of bulbar septum.
2. Pulmonary infundibulum will lie anterior and to left of bulbar septum.

60° Reduced Levotorsion.
1. Aortic vestibule lies posterior and to left of bulbar septum.
2. Pulmonary infundibulum lies anterior and to right of bulbar septum.

120° Reduced Levotorsion.
1. Bilateral infundibula. Aortic to left. Pulmonary to right.

180° Reduced Levotorsion.
1. Aortic infundibulum lies anterior and to left of bulbar septum.
2. Pulmonary vestibule lies posterior and to right of bulbar septum.

Figure 8-13. Normal and reduced levotorsion of the bulboventricular loop with failure of reduction of the bulboventricular sulcus and situs inversus of the aorta.

General Features: The atria and ventricles are orientated as in the normal heart.

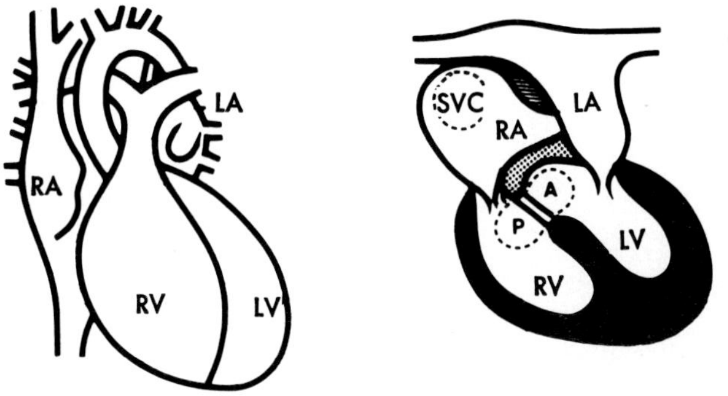

Normal Dextrotorsion.
Results in a normal heart.
1. Aorta arises from aortic vestibule of left ventricle.
2. Pulmonary artery arises from infundibulum of right ventricle.

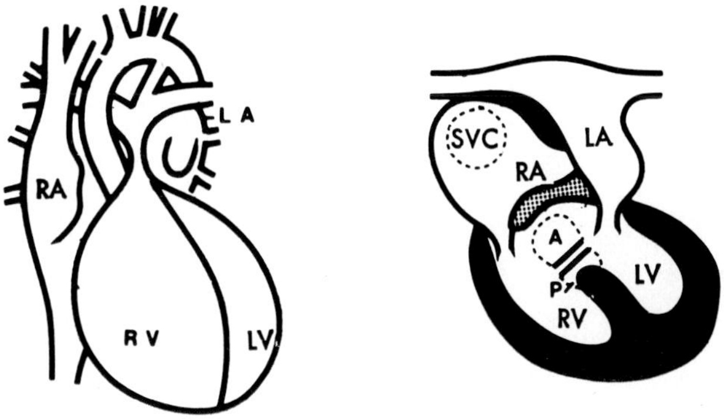

60° Reduced Dextrotorsion.
1. Aortic vestibule lies posterior and to right of bulbar septum, astride posterior edge of muscular septum.
2. Pulmonary infundibulum encroaches on anterior end of muscular septum and will be stenosed or atretic.
3. Bulbar septum lies at a right angle to muscular septum.
4. Membranous interventricular septal defect.
5. Fallot's tetralogy.

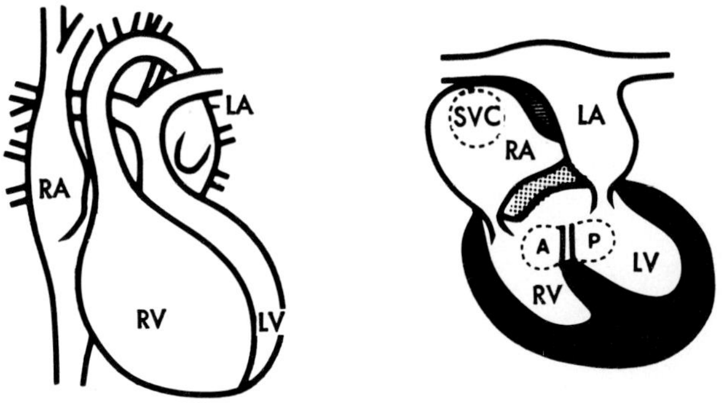

120° Reduced Dextrotorsion.
1. Bilateral infundibula. Aortic to right. Pulmonary to left of interventricular septum.
2. Membranous interventricular septal defect.
3. Partial uncorrected transposition.

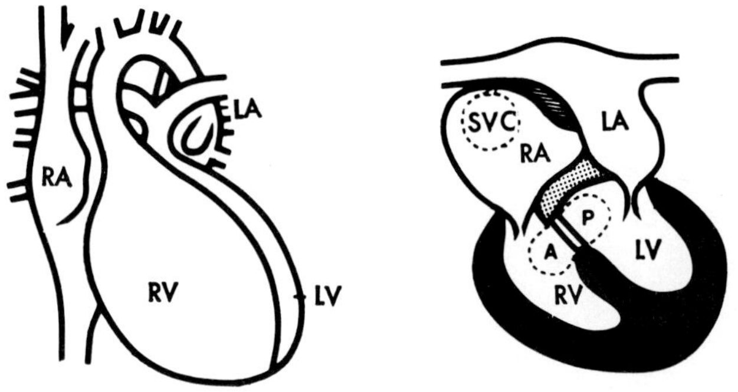

180° Reduced Dextrotorsion.
1. Aorta arises from infundibulum of right ventricle.
2. Pulmonary artery arises from pulmonary vestibule of left ventricle.
3. Complete uncorrected transposition.

Figure 8-14. Normal and reduced dextrotorsion of the bulboventricular loop with normal reduction of the bulboventricular sulcus and situs solitus of the atria.

143

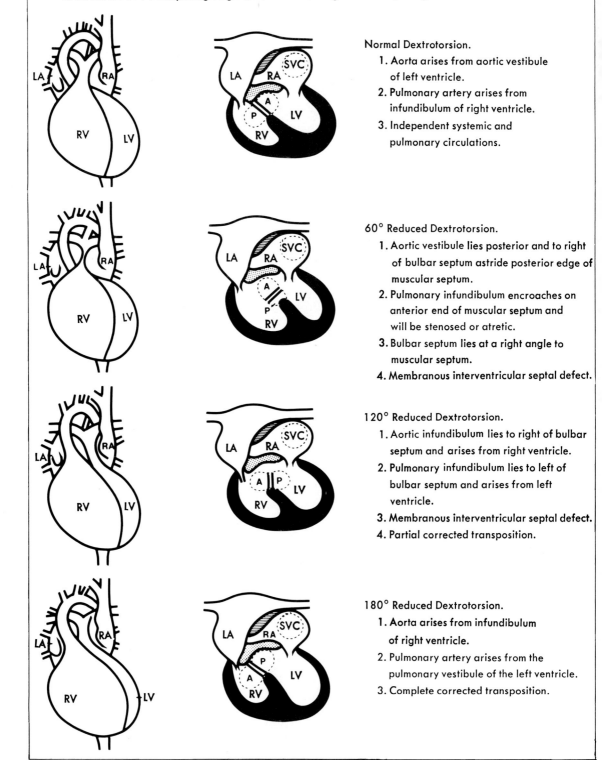

General Features:
1. On the right side a morphologic left atrium will discharge into a morphologic right ventricle.
2. On the left side a morphologic right atrium will discharge into a morphologic left ventricle.

Normal Dextrotorsion.
1. Aorta arises from aortic vestibule of left ventricle.
2. Pulmonary artery arises from infundibulum of right ventricle.
3. Independent systemic and pulmonary circulations.

60° Reduced Dextrotorsion.
1. Aortic vestibule lies posterior and to right of bulbar septum astride posterior edge of muscular septum.
2. Pulmonary infundibulum encroaches on anterior end of muscular septum and will be stenosed or atretic.
3. Bulbar septum lies at a right angle to muscular septum.
4. Membranous interventricular septal defect.

120° Reduced Dextrotorsion.
1. Aortic infundibulum lies to right of bulbar septum and arises from right ventricle.
2. Pulmonary infundibulum lies to left of bulbar septum and arises from left ventricle.
3. Membranous interventricular septal defect.
4. Partial corrected transposition.

180° Reduced Dextrotorsion.
1. Aorta arises from infundibulum of right ventricle.
2. Pulmonary artery arises from the pulmonary vestibule of the left ventricle.
3. Complete corrected transposition.

Figure 8-15. Normal and reduced dextrotorsion of the bulboventricular loop with normal reduction of the bulboventricular sulcus and situs inversus of the atria.

General Features:
1. On the right side a morphologic right atrium will discharge into a morphologic left ventricle.
2. On the left side a morphologic left atrium will discharge into a morphologic right ventricle.

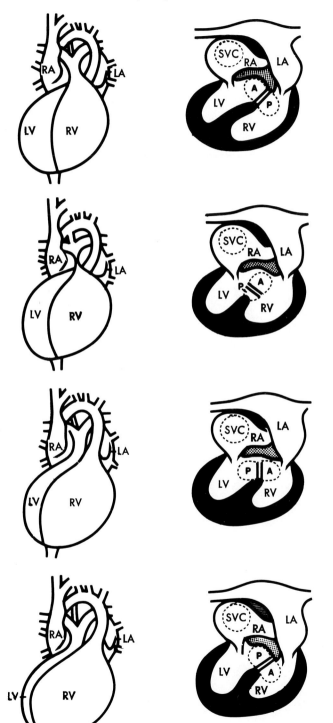

Normal Levotorsion.
1. Aorta arises from aortic vestibule of a right-sided left ventricle.
2. Pulmonary artery arises from infundibulum of a left-sided right ventricle.
3. Independent systemic and pulmonary circulations.

60° Reduced Levotorsion.
1. Aortic vestibule lies posterior and to left of bulbar septum astride posterior end of muscular septum.
2. Pulmonary infundibulum encroaches on anterior end of muscular septum and will be stenosed or atretic.
3. Bulbar septum lies at a right angle to muscular septum.
4. Membranous interventricular septal defect.

120° Reduced Levotorsion.
1. Aortic infundibulum lies to left of bulbar septum, and arises from right ventricle.
2. Pulmonary infundibulum lies to right of bulbar septum and arises from left ventricle.
3. Membranous interventricular septal defect.
4. Partial corrected transposition.

180° Reduced Levotorsion.
1. Aorta arises from infundibulum of right ventricle.
2. Pulmonary artery arises from pulmonary vestibule of left ventricle.
3. Complete corrected transposition.

Figure 8-16. Normal and reduced levotorsion of the bulboventricular loop with normal reduction of the bulboventricular sulcus and situs solitus of the atria.

General Features:
1. On the right side a morphologic left atrium will discharge into a morphologic left ventricle.
2. On the left side a morphologic left atrium will discharge into a morphologic right ventricle.

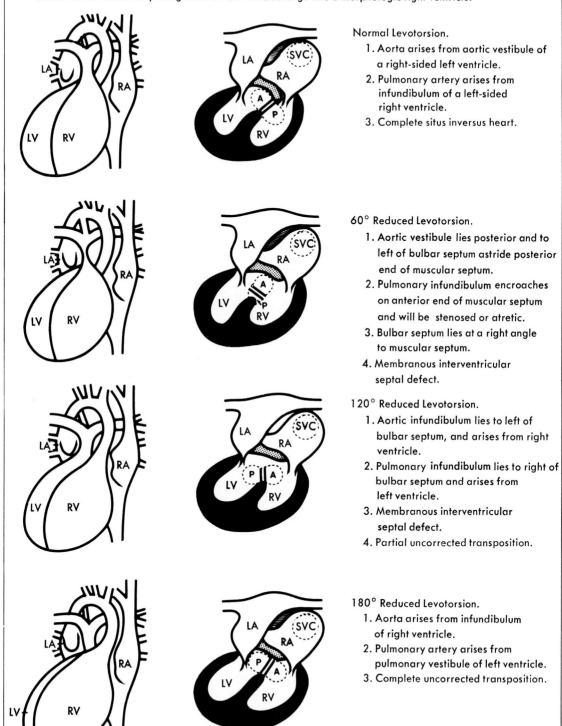

Normal Levotorsion.
1. Aorta arises from aortic vestibule of a right-sided left ventricle.
2. Pulmonary artery arises from infundibulum of a left-sided right ventricle.
3. Complete situs inversus heart.

60° Reduced Levotorsion.
1. Aortic vestibule lies posterior and to left of bulbar septum astride posterior end of muscular septum.
2. Pulmonary infundibulum encroaches on anterior end of muscular septum and will be stenosed or atretic.
3. Bulbar septum lies at a right angle to muscular septum.
4. Membranous interventricular septal defect.

120° Reduced Levotorsion.
1. Aortic infundibulum lies to left of bulbar septum, and arises from right ventricle.
2. Pulmonary infundibulum lies to right of bulbar septum and arises from left ventricle.
3. Membranous interventricular septal defect.
4. Partial uncorrected transposition.

180° Reduced Levotorsion.
1. Aorta arises from infundibulum of right ventricle.
2. Pulmonary artery arises from pulmonary vestibule of left ventricle.
3. Complete uncorrected transposition.

Figure 8-17. Normal and reduced levotorsion of the bulboventricular loop with normal reduction of the bulboventricular sulcus and situs inversus of the atria.

If the bulboventricular sulcus undergoes normal reduction but there is a reduction in the amount of dextrotorsion or levotorsion of the bulboventricular loop, various degrees of alteration in the relationships of the outflow tracts of the great arteries to each other and to the membranous and muscular parts of the interventricular septum will result. When there is a reduction of 180 degrees in the amount of torsion, the lower end of the bulbar septum will lie in the same alignment as the interventricular septum and the aorta will arise from the infundibulum of the right ventricle while the pulmonary artery will arise from the vestibule of the left ventricle. Its posterior wall will be in contact with the ventral aspect of the endocardial cushions. In this type it is unlikely that there will be an interventricular septal defect as long as the membranous septum does not fail. It is likely, however, that there will be an interventricular septal defect with lesser degrees of torsion because the alignment of the bulbar septum and the interventricular septum are not in the same plane, with the result that the various components necessary for the closure of the secondary interventricular foramen are unable to link up.

These disorders are illustrated in Figures 8–10 to 8–17.

DIVISION OF THE TRUNCUS ARTERIOSUS INTO AORTA AND PULMONARY ARTERIES

THE truncus arteriosus is the short arterial stem that connects the bulbus cordis to the caudal ends of the ventral aortae and the sixth aortic arches. The ventral aortae arise from the ventral aspect of the truncus, while the sixth aortic arches arise from the dorsal aspect.

The separation of these two sets of vessels is brought about by the growth of a right and left ridge of mesenchymatous tissue into the lumen of the truncus. As these ridges pass toward the bulbus cordis they take a spiral course, so that the right truncus ridge passes first on to the dorsal wall and then on to the left wall, while the left truncus ridge passes first on to the ventral wall and then on to the right wall. They are thus in a position to join the right and left bulbar septa at a point just above the pulmonary and aortic valves. These ridges in the truncus finally meet and fuse, leading to the formation of the aortico-pulmonary septum.

Defects in the formation of the truncus may lead to the development of any of the following abnormalities:

1. The septum may fail to develop, leading to the condition of persistent truncus arteriosus (Figure 8–18A, B). In this condition, if present as an isolated defect, the pulmonary arteries arise from the cephalic end of a common channel. It is only when the aortic and pulmonary valves are normal, with three cusps each, that we have the true common truncus arteriosus. Most of the reported cases of common truncus, in addition to the defect in the truncus, have either a defect in the aortic and pulmonary valves, which are developed from the bulbar ridges (Figure 8–18C), or are cases of aortic or pulmonary atresia.

2. The septum may only partially form, leading to the production of an aorticopulmonary fistula.

DEVELOPMENT OF THE AORTIC ARCHES

PAIRED ventral aortae arise from the ventral aspect of the apex of the truncus arteriosus and extend cephalically, ventrolateral to the primitive pharynx. From these vessels five pairs of aortic arches develop in series and pass around the pharynx in the corresponding pharyngeal arch to join paired dorsal aortae lying dorsolateral to the pharynx. A sixth pair of aortic arches develops from the dorsal aspect of the apex of the truncus arteriosus itself and passes around the pharynx to join the dorsal aortae also. Caudal to the pharyngeal part of the gut tube, the dorsal aortae fuse dorsal to the gut tube to form a single midline vessel.

The subsequent fate of these vessels is as follows (Figure 8–19):

1. The first two pairs of aortic arches degenerate as main channels once the third aortic arches have been fully established.

2. The fifth aortic arches are very rudimentary and degenerate early in development.

3. The right ventral aorta becomes the brachiocephalic artery and the right common carotid artery, while the left ventral aorta becomes the left common carotid.

4. The right and left third arches and the dorsal aortae cephalic to these arches become the right and left internal carotid arteries and extend into the cranial cavity to supply the greater part of the forebrain and its outgrowths.

5. The right and left external carotid arteries arise from the point where the third arches leave the ventral aortae, and extend cephalically ventrolateral to the pharynx to supply the whole of the inside and outside of the skull and face, except the brain.

6. The left ventral aorta forms that part of the adult arch of the aorta that lies between the origin of the innominate artery and the origin of the left common carotid artery.

7. The right fourth arch forms that part of the right subclavian artery that lies between its origin and the origin of the vertebral artery.

8. The left fourth arch forms that part of the adult arch of the aorta that lies between the origin of the left

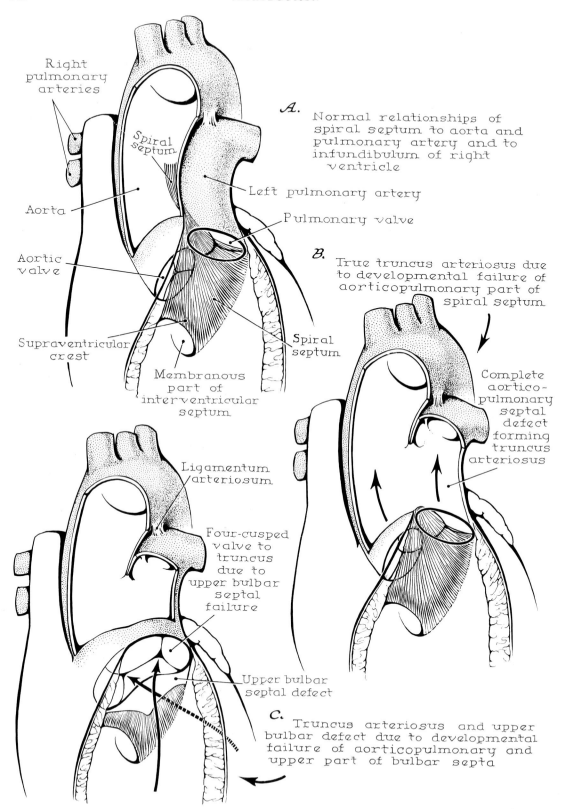

Figure 8-18. The spiral septum, developed from aorticopulmonary and bulbar septa, showing sites of developmental failure.

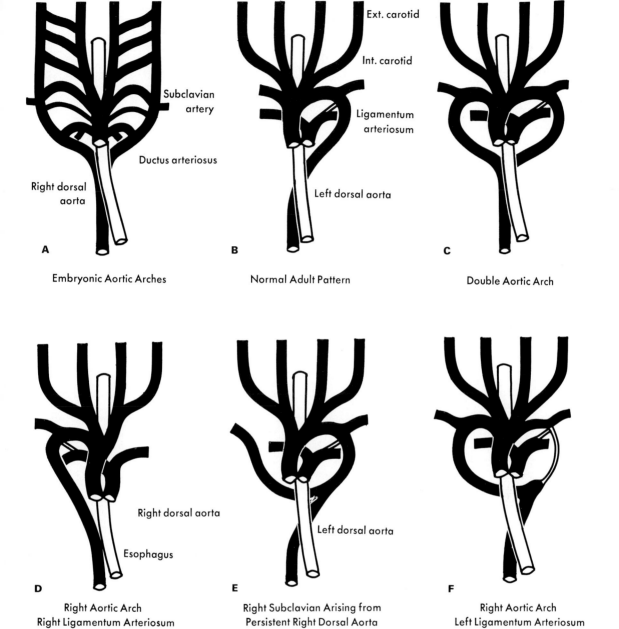

Figure 8-19. Variations in the pattern of the aortic arches, and the course of the descending aorta in relation to the esophagus.

common carotid artery and the origin of the left subclavian artery. Note that on each side the fourth arch is crossed by the vagus nerve on its lateral side.

9. The ventral part of the right sixth arch forms the commencement of the right pulmonary artery, whereas its dorsal part linking it to the right dorsal aorta disappears.

10. The ventral part of the left sixth arch forms the commencement of the left pulmonary artery, whereas its dorsal part forms the ductus arteriosus in the

embryo and fetus and the ligamentum arteriosum after birth.

11. The dorsal aortae between the third and fourth arches disappear.

12. The right dorsal aorta between the origin of the seventh intersegmental artery and its point of fusion with the left dorsal aorta disappears together with the dorsal part of the sixth arch which is linked to it.

The following abnormalities in the normal pattern may occur:

1. The right dorsal aorta caudal to the fourth arch may fail to degenerate, giving rise to a double aortic arch that completely encircles trachea and esophagus (Figure 8–19*C*).

2. The right dorsal aorta between the right fourth arch and its point of fusion with the left dorsal aorta may persist, whereas the left dorsal aorta between the origin of the left subclavian and ductus arteriosus disappears. In this type of "right aortic arch," the persistence of the left ductus arteriosus draws the right dorsal aorta behind the trachea and esophagus to the left side so that it descends on the left side of the vertebral column until it reaches the midline again at the level of the twelfth thoracic vertebra (Figure 8–19*D*). If, however, the left ductus disappears as well as the left dorsal aorta beyond the left subclavian artery and the right ductus persists, then the right dorsal aorta will descend on the right of the vertebral column to reach the midline at the level of the twelfth thoracic vertebra (Figure 8–19*F*).

3. The right fourth arch may disappear and the right dorsal aorta, from its point of fusion with the left up to the origin of the seventh intersegmental (subclavian) branch, may persist to form the first part of the right subclavian artery. The left ductus in these cases draws the persisting part of the right dorsal aorta behind the esophagus to the left side of the vertebral column so that the subclavian artery thus arises from the adult arch of the aorta just beyond the left ductus and passes behind the esophagus to reach the right side (Figure 8–19*E*).

4. Very rarely the remains of the fifth aortic arch may be present and form a small channel leaving and joining the concave aspect of the arch of the aorta, proximal to the attachment of the ligamentum arteriosum.

COARCTATION OF THE AORTA

In this condition there is a constriction of the dorsal aorta either at the aortic isthmus between the origin of the left subclavian artery and the ductus arteriosus or else in the immediate vicinity of the attachment of the ligamentum arteriosum.

In the first type the constriction, which is usually in the form of a diffuse narrowing or obliteration, probably develops early in intrauterine life due to the fact that a large volume of blood is removed from the aorta by the brachiocephalic, left common carotid, and left subclavian arteries. This leaves a much diminished flow through the portion between the origin of the left subclavian artery and the point where the caudally directed stream from the ductus arteriosus enters it. There is thus no adequate stimulus in the way of blood flow to bring about the enlargement of this portion of the dorsal aorta.

Any additional congenital defect in the heart that diminishes the aortic blood flow will further aggravate this tendency to remain narrow and may even lead to obliteration.

In those cases where the constriction is in the vicinity of the ductus arteriosus the exact etiology is less clear, but the following factors should be considered as having a bearing on the condition. In the first instance the fibrosis and contraction of the ductus arteriosus will affect the arterial wall at its point of attachment, either by involving the wall directly or by exerting traction on the wall causing a kinking at this point. In the second instance the recurrent laryngeal nerve is encircling the aorta immediately beyond the attachment of the ductus arteriosus and is exerting pressure on the wall as it is being dragged caudally.

The early disappearance of the right ductus arteriosus is probably due to the twisting of the heart as a whole to the left and the persistence of the right vitelline vein (terminal part of the inferior vena cava), which holds the right side of the heart at a lower level, including the right pulmonary artery. This means that the right recurrent laryngeal nerve will exert greater traction on the right ductus arteriosus than the left recurrent laryngeal nerve does on the left ductus arteriosus.

After disappearance of the right ductus arteriosus it will also exert considerable traction on the right fourth arch (first part of the right subclavian artery), and this fact may account for the frequent disappearance of this arch, leading to a persistence of the right dorsal aorta and thereby resulting in a retroesophageal right subclavian artery.

NERVE SUPPLY OF THE HEART

The heart, developing in the visceral mesoderm in relation to the ventral aspect of the foregut, receives its nerve supply from the parasympathetic and sympathetic divisions of the autonomic nervous system.

The parasympathetic fibers arise in the dorsal nucleus of the vagus nerve and leave the main trunk of the nerve as the superior and inferior cervical cardiac branches, and as two or more thoracic branches.

On the right side the cervical branches pass inferiorly behind the subclavian and brachiocephalic arteries to reach the deep cardiac plexus, which lies on the bifurcation of the trachea. The thoracic branches pass forward on the side of the trachea and also enter the deep plexus.

On the left side the superior cervical cardiac branch passes inferiorly behind the left common carotid artery, and joining with the thoracic branches enters the deep cardiac plexus. The inferior cervical branch passes forward across the lateral aspect of the arch of

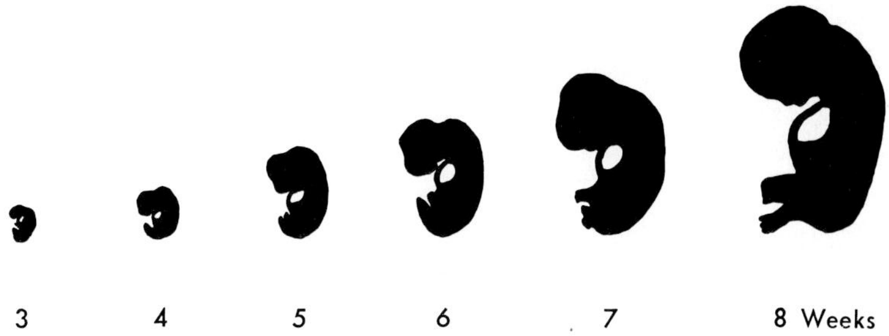

Figure 8-20. Actual size and age in weeks of the embryo, in relation to actual heart size, during the period when the cardiac septa are being formed.

3   4   5   6   7   8 Weeks

the aorta and enters the superficial cardiac plexus, which lies on the front of the ligamentum arteriosum.

After reaching the deep cardiac plexus the parasympathetic fibers pass through it and enter the heart via the venous mesocardium, and terminate on ganglion cells situated in the subepicardial tissue at the cavoauricular junction and in the posterior part of the atrioventricular groove. The postganglionic fibers are distributed to the specialized muscle of the sinoatrial and atrioventricular nodes, and to the coronary vessels.

Those reaching the superficial cardiac plexus relay in this plexus and are distributed to the smaller branches of the coronary arteries via the arterial mesocardium.

The sympathetic fibers arise as preganglionic and postganglionic neurons from the superior, middle, and inferior cervical ganglia, and the upper five thoracic ganglia of the sympathetic trunks.

On the right side they pass inferiorly in conjunction with the vagal fibers to enter the deep cardiac plexus.

On the left side the superior cervical branch passes inferiorly and crossing lateral to the arch of the aorta reaches the superficial cardiac plexus, while those from the middle, inferior, and thoracic ganglia all pass medial to the arch of the aorta and enter the deep plexus.

The sympathetic fibers enter the heart via the venous and arterial mesocardia and are distributed to the nodes and larger coronary vessels.

Afferent fibers travel in all of the cardiac branches of the vagus nerve, their cell bodies being situated in its inferior ganglion.

The sympathetic cardiac branches all carry afferent fibers, with the exception of the branches from the superior cervical ganglion, which are considered to be purely efferent. The cell bodies of the afferent fibers are situated in the seventh and eighth cervical and the upper five thoracic posterior root ganglia, which send their fibers via the inferior cervical and upper five thoracic sympathetic ganglia.

The actions of the vagus are basically a slowing of the rate of the contractions and a diminution of their force, and are probably the result of the actions of these on the specialized conducting tissue of the heart. In certain cases excessive vagal stimulation may bring about missed beats or even complete arrest of the heart. The vagal fibers to the coronary arteries normally result in vasoconstriction.

The sympathetic fibers bring about an increase in the rate and force of the contraction and dilatation of the coronary arteries. Excessive sympathetic stimulation, especially in the absence of vagal control, may bring about ventricular fibrillation.

Table 8–1. PROBABLE PERIOD DURING INTRAUTERINE LIFE WHEN THE HEART IS AFFECTED IN VARIOUS CONGENITAL CARDIAC DEFECTS

DEFECT	PERIOD
Transposition of the great vessels	3rd to 4th week
Pulmonary or aortic atresia	3rd to 5th week
Persistent sinus venosus	3rd to 6th week
Atrioventricularis communis	3rd to 6th week
Patent ductus arteriosus	3rd to 8th week
Abnormal pulmonary venous drainage	3rd to 8th week
Tricuspid or mitral atresia	3rd to 6th week
Persistent foramen primum	4th to 5th week
Triatrial heart	4th to 5th week
Complete infundibular stenosis	4th to 5th week
Muscular ventricular septal defects	4th to 6th week
Coarctation of aorta	4th week onward
Partial infundibular stenosis	5th to 6th week
Lower infundibular stenosis	6th to 7th week
Persistent truncus arteriosus	6th to 7th week
Membranous ventricular septal defects	6th to 7th week
Valvular pulmonary stenosis	6th to 8th week
Subaortic stenosis	6th to 8th week
Absent septum secundum	7th to 8th week
Persistent superior vena cava	2nd to 4th month
Persistent foramen ovale	8th week onward

REFERENCES

Bryce, T. H.: *Quain's Elements of Anatomy.* I. *Embryology.* Longmans Green & Co. Ltd., London, 1908.

Cardell, B. S.: Corrected transposition of the great vessels. *Br. Heart. J.,* **18**:186–92, 1956.

Clarkson, P. M., et al.: Isolated atrial invasion. *Am. J. Cardiol.,* **29**:887–81, 1972.

Congdon, E. D.: Transformation of the aortic arch system during development of the embryo. *Carnegie Contrib. Embryol.,* **14**:47, 1922.

Dawes, G. S.: *Foetal and Neonatal Physiology.* Year Book Medical Publishers, Inc., Chicago, 1968.

De la Cruz, M. V., and Da Rocha, J. P.: An ontogenetic theory for the explanation of congenital malformations involving the truncus and conus. *Am. Heart. J.,* **51**:782–805, 1956.

Dunkman, W. B.; Perloff, J. K.; and Roberts, W. C.: Ventricular inversion without transposition of the great arteries. *Am. J. Cardiol.,* **39**:226, 1977.

Elliott, J. P.; Neufeld, N. H.; Anderson, R. C.; et al.: Complete transposition of the great vessels. An anatomic study of sixty cases. *Circulation*, **27**:1105–17, 1963.

Frazer, J. E.: *Manual of Embryology*, 2nd ed. Balliere, Tindall & Cox, London, 1940.

Freedom, R. M.; Williams, W. G.; Dische, R.; and Rowe, R. D.: Anatomical variants in aortic atresia. *Br. Heart J.*, **38**:821, 1976.

Hamilton, W. F., and Abbott, M. E.: Coarctation of the aorta of the adult type. *Am. Heart. J.*, **3**:381, 1928.

Harris, J. S., and Farber, S.: Transposition of the great vessels with special reference to the phylogenetic theory of Spitzer's. *Arch. Pathol.*, **28**:427–502, 1939.

Keith, Sir A. K.: *Human Embryology and Morphology*, 5th ed. Edward Arnold & Co., London, 1933.

Kettler, L. H.: Persistence of truncus arteriosus communis. *Virchow Arch. Pathol., Anat.*, **304**:513, 1939.

Kramer, T. C.: The positioning of the truncus and conus and the formation of the membranous portion of the interventricular septum in the human heart. *Am. J. Anat.*, **71**:343, 1942.

McLester, J. B.; Bush, J. D.; and Du Bois, J. S.: Congenitally double left auricle. *Am. Heart J.*, **19**:492, 1940.

Melhuish, B. P. P., and Van Praag, R.: Juxtaposition of the atrial appendages. A sign of severe cyanotic congenital heart disease. *Br. Heart J.*, **30**:269–84, 1968.

Moore, K. L.: *The Developing Human*. W. B. Saunders Co., Philadelphia, 1974.

Neufeld, N. H.; Du Shane, J. W.; and Edwards, J. E.: Origin of both great vessels from the right ventricle. 2. With pulmonary stenosis. *Circulation*, **23**:603–12, 1961.

Odgers, P. N. B.: The development of the pars membranacea septi in the human heart. *J. Anat.*, **72**:247, 1938.

Patten, B. M.: *Human Embryology*, 3rd ed. Blakiston Co., New York, 1968.

Paul, M. H.; Sinha, S. N.; Muster, A. J.; et al.: Double outlet left ventricle. Report of an autopsy case with an intact ventricular septum and consideration of its developmental implications. *Circulation*, **41**:129–39, 1970.

Paul, M. H.; Van Praag, S.; and Van Praag, R.: Transposition of the great arteries. In *Paediatric Cardiology*. C. V. Mosby Co., St. Louis, 1968.

Robertson, J. I.: The Comparative Anatomy of the bulbus cordis, with special reference to abnormal positions of the great vessels in the human heart. *J. Pathol. Bact.*, **18**:191–210, 1913–14.

Shaher, R. M.: Complete and Inverted transposition of the great vessels. *Br. Heart J.*, **26**:51–66, 1964.

Symposium on coarctation of aorta. I. *Proc. Mayo Clin.*, **22**:121, 1947.

Symposium on coarctation of aorta. II. *Proc. Mayo Clin.*, **23**:321, 1948.

Tandler, J.: The development of the heart. In Keibel, F., and Mall, F. P.: *Manual of Human Embryology*, II. J. B. Lippincott Co., Philadelphia, 1912.

Tandler, J.: *Lehrbuch der Systematischen Anatomie*, 3. Band, Das Gefassystem. Leipzig, 1926.

Thilenus, D. G.; Bharati, S.; and Lev, M.: Subdivided left atrium: Our expanded concept of cor triatriatum sinistrum. *Am. J. Cardiol.*, **37**:743, 1976.

Van Mierop, L. H. S.: Transposition of great arteries. I. Classification or further confusion? *Am. J. Cardiol.*, **28**:735–38, 1971.

Van Mierop, L. H. S., and Wiglesworth, F. W.: Pathogenesis of transposition complexes 3. True transposition of the great vessels. *Am. Cardiol.*, **12**:233–39, 1963.

Van Praag, R., and Van Praag, S.: Anatomically corrected transposition of great arteries. *Br. Heart J.*, **29**:112–19, 1967.

Van Praag, R., et al.: Transposition of great arteries with posterior aorta, anterior pulmonary artery, subpulmonary conus and fibrous continuity between aortic and atrioventricular valves. *Am. J. Cardiol.*, **28**:621–40, 1971.

Van Praag, R., and Van Praag, S., Isolated ventricular inversion. A consideration of the morphogenesis definition and diagnosis of nontransposed and transposed great arteries. *Am. J. Cardiol.*, **17**:395–406, 1966.

Van Praag, R.: Transposition of great arteries. II. Transposition clarified. *Am. J. Cardiol.*, **28**:739–41, 1971.

Walmsley, T.: The heart. In Quain J.: *Elements of Anatomy*, IV, pt. 3. Longmans Green & Co. Ltd., London, 1929.

Windle, W. F.: *Physiology of the Fetus*. W. B. Saunders & Co., Philadelphia, 1940.

9

Familial Occurrence of Congenital Heart Disease

Irene A. Uchida

THE ETIOLOGY of congenital heart disease continues to intrigue both cardiologist and geneticist alike. Because of the high frequency of these defects, both sporadic and familial, prevention takes on a particularly important role. Clustering within certain families suggests that the cause of abnormal development of the heart can best be explained by a genetic predisposition made evident within the appropriate prenatal environment. On the other hand, many instances of cardiac malformations can be traced strictly to environmental insults.

Reports of the familial aspects of heart anomalies are prominent in the literature. Many of the earlier studies have been summarized by Tedesco (1933) and translated by Snelling (1937). Campbell (1949), Carleton and coworkers (1958), Chelius and associates (1962), Nora and Meyer (1966), and Zetterqvist (1972), among others, have also listed numerous familial cases. This concentration within families could be explained by the presence of the same genes, similar prenatal environment, or merely fortuitous occurrence of a very common abnormality, but the most probable explanation takes into consideration a combination of all these factors.

Clues to the importance of the many factors comprising the prenatal environment and the genetic make-up can best be revealed by careful evaluation of large series of patients with heart anomalies. Some epidemiologic studies have produced irrefutable evidence for the effect of detrimental agents during the early months of pregnancy. Others have stressed the genetic role. Between these two important contributions to our knowledge of the etiology of congenital heart disease are the controversial aspects resulting from the study of twins.

ENVIRONMENTAL FACTORS

NUMEROUS environmental factors have been scrutinized to evaluate their potential as etiologic agents. These studies stemmed mainly from the concern aroused by the all-too-frequent occurrence of heart defects as well as the puzzling discordance rate among monozygotic twins and the many attempts to delineate a suitable genetic model. It is obvious that the key to the intrinsic problem lies in maternal stress mainly during the first trimester of pregnancy. To identify the cause of this stress it is necessary to examine the data from various aspects.

Parental Age

An increase in maternal age suggests the presence of some physiologic disturbance associated with the aging process best illustrated by the striking correlation between chromosomal nondisjunction and late maternal age. Although maternal age has been found to be of etiologic significance in congenital abnormalities in general, its importance in isolated congenital heart disease is not impressive (MacMahon, 1952; Fuhrmann, 1968). Some association with late maternal age has been suggested for ventricular septal defect and tetralogy of Fallot by Campbell (1965) who found more affected children born to mothers over 35 years and 40 years of age, respectively. In a study of congenital anomalies in British Columbia, Renwick and associates (1964) reported that mothers over 39 years of age had an increased risk of producing children with congenital heart disease. Although no corrections were made for paternal age, birth order, or type of malformation, it is unlikely that they would have a significant effect upon Renwick's conclusion.

Since the age of the father has no environmental effect upon the developing fetus, a correlation between a malformation and paternal age implies a genetic event resulting from a mutation. The most frequently mentioned example is achondroplasia where an increased incidence with paternal age has been demonstrated. Campbell (1965) has suggested a similar though less striking situation for congenital heart disease but the data are not too convincing.

In general, the ages of the parents do not appear to be of significant etiologic importance.

Birth Order

Birth order is closely related to parental age, but the two roles can be separated statistically by holding one constant while examining the other. Although parity has often been examined for its etiologic significance, most reported correlations between congenital malformations and birth rank appear to be of doubtful value except for the first birth. Record and McKeown (1953) and Moss and coworkers (1964) found a higher frequency of patent ductus arteriosus among first births and suggested fetal distress as a possible cause. However, neither Anderson (1954) nor Zetterqvist (1972) found any correlation between birth rank and patent ductus arteriosus.

Teratogenic Agents

An unusual increase in frequency or seasonal variation in births of affected infants may produce clues in the identification of a teratogenic agent. Through such studies, the teratogenicity of the rubella virus was noted (Gregg, 1941). It has now been well documented that such infection during the first trimester can result in a constellation of birth defects among which is patency of the ductus arteriosus. A recent survey in Ontario (Rose et al., 1972) has added further confirmation for this association. A few cases of pulmonary stenosis following infection have also been reported (Heiner and Nadas, 1958).

Rather less conclusive have been reports suggesting cause and effect of other viral infections. A positive correlation between the mumps virus and endocardial fibroelastosis was found by St. Geme and associates (1966) but was not confirmed by Gersony and coworkers (1966). A less specific association between Coxsackie virus and a variety of cardiac malformations has been reported (Brown and Evans, 1967; Brown and Karunas, 1971).

A sudden increase in the frequency of limb malformations brought to light the teratogenic effects of the drug thalidomide (Lenz, 1965). In addition, heart lesions, mainly septal defects, were observed when this drug was ingested by the mother during a particularly sensitive period. Other drugs, such as appetite suppressants (Nora et al., 1967), anticonvulsants (German et al., 1970), and hormones (Levy et al., 1973) taken during the first trimester, have also been suspected of producing cardiac malformations.

In epidemiologic data now being gathered in Ontario (Rose, 1973), diabetes has been found to occur 11 times more frequently in mothers of children with congenital heart disease than in mothers in the general population.

Vitamin A deficiency has been shown to cause abnormalities of the heart and aortic arch in rats (Wilson and Warkany, 1950) but evidence is lacking in humans.

Hypoxia

Notable among epidemiologic studies are those conducted in Peru. Alzamora and coworkers (1960) and Penaloza and colleagues (1964) found higher frequencies of patent ductus arteriosus among populations of the Andean regions and contended that chronic exposure to lower oxygen tension at high altitudes may result in persistent patency of the ductus.

Placental Circulation

A high rate of discordance between monozygotic twins is indicative of the importance of prenatal environmental influences. This is particularly apparent in congenital heart disease where discordance appears to be the rule among monozygotic twins (see below). Since the majority of these twins develop within a single chorionic sac and share a common vascular circulation, competition between the fetuses could result in an imbalance to the disadvantage of one twin. This mechanism could also account for the excess of monozygotic twins among multiple births with one or both members affected and for differences found in the cardiac status of conjoined twins (Rossi et al., 1971). Even in single pregnancies disturbance in placental circulation at the crucial time could conceivably cause a malformation of the heart.

Of the many environmental factors examined, only rubella, thalidomide, and hypoxia have provided sufficient evidence of a detrimental influence on the development of the heart. Of these, hypoxia alone appears to have a specific effect, i.e., patent ductus arteriosus. The role of the placental circulation needs further investigation.

TWIN STUDIES

COMPARISONS of concordance and discordance rates among monozygotic (MZ) and dizygotic (DZ) twins have long been a useful method in the evaluation of hereditary and environmental influences. Since MZ twins are genetically identical, any variation between them must be environmentally determined. On the other hand, an increased frequency of concordance among MZ twins compared with DZ twins suggests the presence of genetic determinants.

In order to draw meaningful conclusions, a twin sample of sufficient size can be obtained only by pooling data from several sources. This method, however, may introduce biases arising from the reason for which interesting cases are published. Furthermore, as Miller (1969) points out, there is a risk of unwittingly using the same cases repeatedly. Only twins collected consecutively or twins found among random series of heart patients are relatively free from ascertainment biases. Table 9–1 presents these data according to the type of lesion found. Not all concordant pairs have identical malformations but they have been classified under the principal lesion. The concordance rate for MZ twins is low (17 percent), although somewhat higher than for DZ twins (3.5 percent). One notable exception is that of Nora and associates (1967), who found both members affected in 6 out of 13 MZ pairs, four pairs having identical malformations. The results of a study of 37 sets of twins by Ross (1959) have not been included because she warns that hers is not a statistically random sample and the type of lesion is not always given; 2 out of 11 MZ and 2 of 26 DZ pairs were

concordant for the presence of congenital heart disease.

The higher concordance rate among MZ twins has been interpreted as evidence for the presence of genetic factors. The explanation, however, may be more complex because of the observation of a relatively high frequency of heart defects among MZ compared with DZ twins, which is closer to a ratio of 1:1 instead of the expected 1:2. Possibly more MZ twins are being brought to the attention of investigators in spite of seemingly rigorous controls. However, since all heterosexual twins can be identified as DZ and a heart defect in one twin can cause significant physical differences between MZ twins, there may be a bias in favor of more frequent ascertainment of DZ twins in so-called random twin series. If there is a real increase in the frequency of cardiac malformations among MZ twins, the uterine environment unique to these twins, who frequently share their placental blood supply, probably plays a significant role in the etiology of congenital heart disease. The answer to this problem could lie in the investigation of twins with known placentation in order to compare MZ twins having a single chorion and a common vascular circulation with MZ twins with two chorions and independent circulations.

GENETIC FACTORS

Single Gene Inheritance

In spite of the overwhelming evidence for the importance of nongenetic influences in congenital heart disease, there is little doubt that a genetic predisposition is frequently present. This is evident in those families with a concentration of many affected relatives, particularly when the affected members have the same type of lesion. The mode of transmission appears to be autosomal-dominant in some and autosomal-recessive in others.

The most convincing evidence for single-gene inheritance is available for supravalvular aortic stenosis. Many kindreds have been reported demonstrating autosomal dominant inheritance (Zoethout et al., 1964, and Kahler et al., 1966, among others). Dominant transmission for atrial septal defect has also been suggested based on pedigrees with several affected parents and sibs (Howitt, 1961; Zetterqvist, 1972). Williamson (1969) describes a remarkable family with a mother and three of six children with atrial septal defect. Her remaining three children and four other close relatives also have congenital heart disease.

Several other cardiac conditions have been described as consistent with autosomal dominant

Table 9–1. FREQUENCIES OF CONCORDANT AND DISCORDANT CONGENITAL HEART DISEASE IN TWINS ACCORDING TO TYPE OF MALFORMATION

TYPE OF MALFORMATION	MONOZYGOTIC			DIZYGOTIC			DOUBTFUL ZYGOSITY			
	No.	Conc.	Disc.	No.	Conc.	Disc.	No.	Conc.	Disc.	
PDA	11	2	9	15	1	14	2	1	1	28
VSD	13	2	11	11	—	11	2	—	2	26
ASD	9	2	7	9	—	9	3	—	3	21
PS	8	2	6	13	1	12	—	—	—	21
Tetrad	8	1	7	9	—	9	2	—	2	19
Coarctation	2	—	2	10	—	10	1	—	1	13
Others	13	2	11	19	1	18	4	—	4	36
Total	64	11	53	86	3	83	14	1	13	164

References: Anderson, 1954; Lamy et al., 1957; Uchida and Rowe, 1957; Campbell, 1961; Nora et al., 1967; Jorgensen, 1970; Zetterqvist, 1972.

inheritance. These include familial cardiomyopathy (Treger and Blount, 1965; Sommer, 1972), familial atrial septal defect with prolonged atrioventricular conduction anomalies (Kahler et al., 1966; Bizarro et al., 1970), and hereditary prolongation of the Q-T interval (Gale et al., 1970).

An increased frequency of consanguinity among the parents of patients with dextrocardia or situs inversus has led to an interpretation of autosomal recessive inheritance by Lamy and associates (1957) and Campbell (1965). They also noted higher frequencies of parental consanguinity for other cardiac malformations, an observation that has not been supported by other investigators.

The familial nature of endocardial fibroelastosis has come to the attention of several investigators, but the most detailed study is by Chen and coworkers (1971). In a series of 119 families they found 11 affected among 62 sibs born subsequent to the proband, which gives an empiric risk figure of 18 percent. Their data did not fit either single-gene or multiple-gene inheritance.

Clustering of similar heart defects in kindreds has been demonstrated for almost all types of congenital heart disease. In many instances there is an impressive array of a variety of lesions often quite unrelated in type (Carleton et al., 1958; Zetterqvist, 1971). The same malformation may occur in isolation or as part of a syndrome. The cause may be an infection, a mutagenic agent, a gene, or a chromosome defect. Thus, the vast majority cannot be explained by simple mendelian inheritance or by specific environmental insult. Nora (1971) has suggested that subjects who are predisposed to congenital heart disease in the presence of a given environmental factor might be identified by biochemical and immunologic parameters.

Polygenic Inheritance

Many normal human traits showing a continuous gradation in variation, such as height and weight, hair and skin color and intelligence, are characterized by polygenic inheritance. This mode of transmission involves many genes sometimes with small additive effects; at other times a few genes are dominant over minor ones. Environmental influences also play a significant role.

Polygenic inheritance has been suggested for certain congenital abnormalities that do not fit a simple mode of inheritance, e.g., pyloric stenosis and cleft lip and palate. Certain epidemiologic features lead one to consider the presence of multiple genes. The trait is common and has a fairly high familial concentration. Environmental influences play an important role. The frequency of recurrence increases with each additional affected sib because of the higher concentration in some families of pertinent genetic factors and similar environmental influences. There is a lowered concordance rate among monozygotic twins because of the strong environmental component. These criteria fit well for congenital heart disease.

Clustering of similar heart defects suggests the transmission of similar genes in the presence of similar environmental factors. Even some pedigrees for which simple dominant inheritance appears obvious could be explained by the transmission of the same major genes among many minor ones. In kindreds with unrelated lesions the variation could result from the segregation of the many genes involved and/or differences in the intrauterine environment.

The concept of polygenic inheritance was succinctly stated by Wright in 1934: a continuum of both genetic and nongenetic variables is intrinsic in polygenic traits and the appearance of an abnormality depends on whether or not the combination of these variables exceeds a certain threshold. Multiple genetic and environmental influences affecting heart formation have been suspected over many years but this interpretation attained prominence and has been generally accepted because of the detailed and careful studies by Nora (1968) and Fuhrmann (1968). They give strong support to the hypothesis of multifactorial inheritance.

Any discussion of polygenic inheritance is incomplete without an attempt to assess the relative roles of heredity and environment. Basic to any conclusion is the evidence produced from twin studies. If the genetic component is strong, the majority of monozygotic twins should be concordant for the same malformation because they are genetically identical whether single or multiple genes are involved. In congenital heart disease, the pooled concordance rate is low (17 percent) and even lower if only identical malformations are considered. Thus the evidence indicates that although a susceptibility to heart defects may be genetically determined environmental influences are the stronger component.

CLINICAL SYNDROMES

Two abnormalities found frequently in association with clinically recognizable syndromes are mental retardation and congenital heart disease. Those in which chromosomes are involved are discussed in Chapter 53. Single-gene-determined syndromes are numerous. The more common abnormalities in which heart malformations are found are listed in Table 9–2. In many of these congenital heart disease occurs only occasionally, but in others cardiac defects are found with significant frequencies and may be the prime cause of death.

DERMATOGLYPHICS

I N early studies (Uchida, 1955), it was suggested that patients with congenital heart disease may have dermal configurations on the palms that deviated from the normal frequency: the axial triradius tended to be more distally displaced and simian creases appeared more frequent (see illustrations in Chapter 53). Mongoloid subjects with cardiac malformations were also found to have more distal axial triradii than those with normal hearts (Uchida and Rowe, 1961). Subsequently many reports have appeared describing the dermal patterns of the fingers and palms in congenital heart disease. The results have been contradictory (see review by Preus et al., 1970). Because multiple parameters are being measured and the differences are small even though significant, it would appear that if an association exists between dermal configurations and congenital heart disease, much more substantial data are needed for confirmation.

GENETIC COUNSELING

F O R a disease as serious and common as congenital heart disease genetic counseling is particularly important. Estimates of the frequency of cardiac defects in the general population range from eight to ten per thousand births. The parents of these children are anxious to know what are the chances that another affected child will be born. The risk of recurrence has been estimated at 1 to 4 percent after the birth of one abnormal infant, but this risk may be increased threefold after two abnormal offspring have been produced. Table 9–3 gives empiric risk figures for specific malformations as observed by Nora and associates (1970).

Empiric risk figures are also available for the

Table 9–2. GENE-DETERMINED SYNDROMES WITH CONGENITAL HEART DISEASE*

CLINICAL SYNDROME	MOST COMMON HEART DEFECT	MODE OF INHERITANCE†
	HEART DEFECT FREQUENT	
Ellis van Creveld	Atrial septal defect	Recessive
Forney	Mitral insufficiency	? Dominant
Holt-Oram	Atrial septal defect	Dominant
Hurler	Valve defect	Recessive
Hypercalcemia, idiopathic	Supravalvular aortic stenosis	? Recessive
Kartagener	Dextrocardia	Recessive
Leopard (multiple lentigines)	Pulmonary stenosis	Dominant
Noonan	Pulmonary stenosis	? Dominant
	HEART DEFECT OCCASIONAL	
Acrocephalosyndactyly (Carpenter)	Patent ductus arteriosus	Recessive
Apert	Ventricular septal defect	Dominant
	Tetralogy of Fallot	
Cerebrohepatorenal (Zellweger)	Patent ductus arteriosus	Recessive
	Ventricular septal defect	
de Lange	Ventricular septal defect	? Recessive
Fanconi pancytopenia	Patent ductus arteriosus	Recessive
Focal dermal hypoplasia (Goltz)	Atrial septal defect	? X-linked dominant
Incontinentia pigmenti (Block-Sulzberger)	Patent ductus arteriosus	X-linked dominant (lethal in males)
Klippel-Feil	Ventricular septal defect	Dominant
Laurence-Moon-Biedl	Variable defects	Recessive
Lissencephaly	Patent ductus arteriosus	Recessive
Oculoauriculovertebral dysplasia (Goldenhar)	Patent ductus arteriosus	? Recessive
	Tetralogy of Fallot	
Pierre Robin	Variable defects	? Dominant
		? X-linked recessive
Radial aplasia thrombocytopenia	Tetralogy of Fallot	Recessive
	Atrial septal defect	
Rubinstein–Taybi	Patent ductus arteriosus	? Recessive
Smith–Lemli–Opitz	Atrial septal defect	Recessive
	Tetralogy of Fallot	

* Table prepared by Drs. Celinda del Solar and Florence Char. References listed in *Birth Defects: Atlas and Compendium*, 1973.
† All autosomal unless otherwise stated.

Table 9–3. OBSERVED AND EXPECTED RECURRENCE RISKS IN SIBS OF 1405 PROBANDS WITH CONGENITAL HEART LESIONS*

| | | AFFECTED SIBS | | |
| | | *No.* | *Percent* | *Exp.* $(\sqrt{P})$ |
ANOMALY	PROBANDS			
Ventricular septal defect	212	24/543	4.4	5.0
Patent ductus arteriosus	204	17/505	3.4	3.5
Tetralogy	157	9/338	2.7	3.2
Atrial septal defect	152	11/342	3.2	3.2
Pulmonary stenosis	146	10/345	2.9	2.9
Aortic stenosis	135	7/317	2.2	2.1
Coarctation	128	5/272	1.8	2.4
Transposition	103	4/209	1.9	2.2
Tricuspid atresia	51	1/96	1.0	1.4
Ebstein's anomaly	42	1/95	1.1	0.7
Truncus	41	1/86	1.2	0.7
Pulmonic atresia	34	1/77	1.3	1.0
Total	1405	91/3225		

* Nora, J. J.; McGill, C. W.; and McNamara, D. G.: Empiric recurrence risks in common and uncommon congenital heart lesions. *Teratology*, **3**:325, 1970.

offspring of subjects with congenital heart disease. In a sample of 90 children born to affected parents studied by Campbell (1965), 4.4 percent had cardiac malformations but atrial septal defect was the only lesion identical in parent and child. More detailed studies by Nora and coworkers (1970) and Zetterqvist (1972) have yielded risk figures for specific malformations (Table 9–4). Not all lesions in parent and offspring are the same. The risks range from 2 to 4 percent and are similar to those for sibs in families in which there is one affected child.

With the development of more successful techniques for the surgical correction of heart defects, more individuals will survive to reproduce. Not only will more accurate information for genetic counseling become available, but the need for prevention will become urgent. Thus, investigations into the role of detrimental environmental factors will take on increased importance.

REFERENCES

Alzamora, V.; Rotta, A.; Battilana, G.; Abugattas, R.; Rubio, C.; Bouroncle, J.; Zapata, C.; Santa-Maria, E.; Binder, T.; Subiria, R.; Paredes, D.; Pando, B.; and Graham, G. G.: On the possible influence of great altitudes on the determination of certain cardiovascular anomalies. *Pediatrics*, **12**:259, 1953.

Anderson, R. C.: Causative factors underlying congenital heart malformations. *Pediatrics*, **14**:143, 1954.

Birth Defects: Atlas and Compendium. Daniel Bergsma (ed.) Published for The National Foundation—March of Dimes by The Williams and Wilkins Co., Baltimore, 1973.

Bizarro, R. O.; Callahan, J. A.; Feldt, R. H.; Kurland, L. T.; Gordon, H.; and Brandenburg, R. O.: Familial atrial septal defect with prolonged atrioventricular conduction. *Circulation*, **41**:677, 1970.

Brown, G. C.; and Evans, T. N.: Serologic evidence of coxsackie virus etiology and congenital heart disease. *JAMA*, **199**:183, 1967.

Brown, G. C., and Karunas, R. S.: Relationship of congenital anomalies and maternal infection with selected enteroviruses. *Am. J. Epidemiol.*, **95**:207, 1972.

Campbell, M.: Genetic and environmental factors in congenital heart disease. *Q. J. Med.*, **18**:379, 1949.

Campbell, M.: Causes of malformations of the heart. *Br. Med. J.*, **2**:895, 1965.

————: Twins and congenital heart disease. *Acta Genet. Med. Gemellol*, **10**:443, 1961(b).

Carleton, R. A.; Abelmann, W. H.; and Hancock, E. W.: Familial occurrence of congenital heart disease. *N. Engl. J. Med.*, **259**:1237, 1958.

Chelius, C. J.; Rowe, G. G.; and Crumpton, C. W.: Familial aspects of congenital heart disease. *Am. J. Cardiol*, **9**:508, 1962.

Chen, S-C.; Thompson, M. W.; and Rose, V.: Endocardial fibroelastosis: Family studies with special reference to counseling. *J. Pediatr.* 79:385, 1971.

Table 9–4. OBSERVED AND EXPECTED RISKS OF AFFECTED OFFSPRING AMONG 756 PARENTS WITH CONGENITAL HEART DISEASE*

| | PARENTS | OFFSPRING | | | |
Type of Lesion	*No. Affected*	*Total No.*	*No. Affected†*	*Percent*	*Exp.* $(\sqrt{P})$
Ventricular septal defect	57	162	6	3.7	5.0
Patent ductus arteriosus	294	607	22	3.6	3.5
Atrial septal defect	273	587	11	1.9	3.2
Pulmonary stenosis	38	102	3	2.9	2.9
Coarctation of aorta	94	191	5	2.6	2.4

* Modified from Nora et al. (1970) with additional data from Zetterqvist (1972).

† Includes 10 with lesion different from parents.

Fuhrmann, W.: Congenital heart disease in sibships ascertained by two affected siblings. *Humangenetik*, **6**:1, 1968.

Gale, G. E.; Bosman, C. K.; Tucker, R. B. K.: and Barlow, J. B.: Hereditary prolongation of QT interval: Study of two families. *Br. Heart J*, **32**:505, 1970.

German, J.; Kowal, A.; and Ehlers, K. H.: Trimethadione and human teratogenesis. *Teratology*, **3**:349, 1970.

Gersony, W. B.; Katz, S. L.; and Nadas, A. S.: Endocardial fibroelastosis and the mumps virus. *Pediatrics*, **37**:430, 1966.

Gregg, N. M.: Congenital cataract following German measles in the mother. *Trans. Ophthal. Soc. Aust.*, **3**:35, 1941.

Heiner, D. C., and Nadas, A. S.: Patent ductus arteriosus in association with pulmonic stenosis. *Circulation*, **17**:232, 1958.

Howitt, G.: Atrial septal defect in three generations. *Br. Heart J*, **23**:494, 1961.

Jorgensen, G.: Twin studies in congenital heart disease. *Acta Genet. Med. Gemellol*, **19**:251, 1970.

Kahler, R. L.; Braunwald, E.; Plauth, W. H.; and Morrow, A. G.: Familial congenital heart disease. *Am. J. Med*, **40**:384, 1966.

Lamy, M.; Grouchy, J. de; and Schweisguth, O.: Genetic and non-genetic factors in the etiology of congenital heart disease: A study of 1188 cases. *Am. J. Hum. Genet*, **9**:17, 1957.

Lenz, W.: Epidemiology of congenital malformations. *Ann. N.Y. Acad. Sci*, **123**:228, 1965.

Levy, E. P.; Cohen, A.; and Fraser, F. C.: Hormone treatment during pregnancy and congenital heart defects. *Lancet*, **1**:611, 1973.

MacMahon, B.: Association of congenital malformation of the heart with birth rank and maternal age. *Br. J. Soc. Med*. **6**:178, 1952.

Miller, R. W.: Origins of congenital heart disease: An epidemiologic perspective. *Teratology*, **2**:77, 1969.

Moss, A. J.; Emmanouilides, G. C.; Adams, F. H.; and Chuang, K.: Response of ductus arteriosus and pulmonary and systemic arterial pressure to changes in oxygen environment in newborn infants. *Pediatrics*, **33**:937, 1964.

Nora, J. J.: Multifactorial inheritance hypothesis for the etiology of congenital heart diseases: The genetic-environmental interaction. *Circulation*, **38**:604, 1968.

————: Etiologic factors in congenital heart disease. *Pediatr. Clin. North Am.*, **18**:1059, 1971.

Nora, J. J.; Gilliland, J. C.; Sommerville, R. J.; and McNamara, D. G.: Congenital heart disease in twins. *N. Engl. J. Med.*, **277**:568, 1967.

Nora, J. J.; McGill, C. W.; and McNamara, D. G.: Empiric recurrence risks in common and uncommon congenital heart lesions. *Teratology*, **3**:325, 1970.

Nora, J. J.; McNamara, D. G.; and Fraser, F. C.: Dexamphetamine sulphate and human malformations. *Lancet*, **1**:570, 1967.

Nora, J. J., and Meyer, T. C.: Familial nature of congenital heart diseases. *Pediatrics*, **37**:329, 1966.

Penaloza, D.; Arias-Stella, J.; Sime, F.; Recavarren, S.; and Marticorena, E.: The heart and pulmonary circulation in children at high altitudes. *Pediatrics*, **34**:568, 1964.

Preus, M.; Fraser, F. C.; and Levy, E. P.: Dermatoglyphics in congenital heart malformations. *Hum. Hered.*, **20**:388, 1970.

Record, R. G., and McKeown, T.: Observations relating to the aetiology of patent ductus arteriosus. *Br. Heart J.*, **15**:376, 1953.

Renwick, D. H. G.; Miller, J. R.; and Paterson, D.: Estimates of incidence and prevalence of mongolism and of congenital heart disease in British Columbia. *Can. Med. Assoc. J.*, **91**:365, 1964.

Rose, V.; Hewitt, D.; and Milner, J.: Seasonal influences on the risk of cardiac malformation: Nature of the problem and some results from a study of 10,077 cases. *Int. J. Epidemiol.*, **1**:235, 1972.

————: Personal communication.

Ross, L. J.: Congenital cardiovascular anomalies in twins. *Circulation*, **20**:327, 1959.

Rossi, P.; Bordiuk, J. M.; and Golinko, R. J.: Angiographic evaluation of conjoined twins. *Ann. Radiol.*, **14**:341, 1971.

Rowe, R. D., and Uchida, I. A.: Cardiac malformation in mongolism: A prospective study of 184 mongoloid children. *Am. J. Med.*, **31**:726, 1961.

St. Geme, J. W., Jr.; Noren, G. R.; and Adams, P., Jr.: Proposed embryopathic relationship between mumps virus and primary endocardial fibroelastosis. *N. Engl. J. Med.*, **275**:339, 1966.

Snelling, D. N.: Familial congenital heart disease. *JAMA*, **108**:1502, 1937.

Sommer, A.: Cardiovascular system: *Birth Defects*, Part XV, 1972.

Tedesco, P. A.: Su due casi di cardiopatia congenita familiare. *Cuore circ.*, **17**:76, 1933.

Treger, A., and Blount, S. G., Jr.: Familial cardiomyopathy. *Am. Heart J.*, **70**:40, 1965.

Uchida, I. A.: A comparison of the dermal patterns of congenital heart patients with those of normal controls and mongols. *Abstr. Am. Soc. Hum. Genet. Meeting*, 1955.

Uchida, I. A., and Rowe, R. D.: Discordant heart anomalies in twins. *Am. J. Hum. Genet.*, **9**:133, 1957.

Williamson, E. M.: A family study of atrial septal defect. *J. Med. Genet.*, **6**:255, 1969.

Wilson, J. G., and Warkany, J.: Cardiac and aortic arch anomalies in the offspring of vitamin A deficient rate correlated with similar human anomalies. *Pediatrics*, **5**:708, 1950.

Wright, S.: On the genetics of subnormal development of the head (otocephaly) in the guinea pig. *Genetics*, **19**:471, 1934.

Zetterqvist, P.: Accumulation of different congenital heart defects in one pedigree. *Clin. Genet.*, **2**:123, 1971.

————: *A Clinical and Genetic Study of Congenital Heart Defects*. Institute for Medical Genetics, University of Uppsala, Sweden, 1972.

Zoethout, H. E.; Carter, R. E. B.; and Carter, C. O.: A family study of aortic stenosis. *J. Med. Genet.*, **1**:2, 1964.

CARDIOVASCULAR PROBLEMS AND THEIR MANAGEMENT

10

Congestive Heart Failure

John D. Keith

HEART failure is associated with an inability of the heart to increase its output adequately to meet the normal demands of the body tissues at rest and with exercise. The heart provides the pumping energy to deliver oxygenated blood to the various organs of the body. When it fails to do so, this is evident at first only with exercise, but if the process is progressive, the signs are recognized with the individual inactive. In the first year of life, when heart failure is most frequently found in the pediatric age group, the clinical signs are usually not identified until they are evident at rest. Infection rather than activity is more likely to precipitate failure in infancy.

Fundamental Causes of Failure

There are several factors that, if sufficiently severe, will produce congestive heart failure in either infancy or childhood. These include valvular obstruction or insufficiency; mechanical obstruction of the heart as a whole, as in pericardial disease; the physical effects of large intracardiac shunts that increase the load on one or both ventricles; the presence of raised pressure in the pulmonary or systemic circulation; inflammatory reactions in the heart muscle or oxygen lack; and, finally, certain metabolic disturbances, such as hyper- or hypothyroidism. One or more of these factors may be operating in the same child, as in rheumatic fever, where myocarditis is associated with valvular insufficiency, or in congenital heart disease with pulmonary stenosis and patent foramen ovale, where the right ventricle has a high pressure to maintain and is at the same time being offered cyanotic blood from the coronaries. In reviewing the case material at The Hospital for Sick Children, Toronto, approximately 20 percent of 10,535 children with heart disease were found to have had failure at some time. Ninety percent of these were in the first year of life. A list of the various causes of heart failure in the pediatric age group is shown in Table 10–1.

Table 10–1. CAUSES OF HEART FAILURE

Aortic and ductal defects	Aortic insufficiency, congenital
	Aortic insufficiency, acquired
	Aortic valvular stenosis
	Subaortic stenosis (congenital)
	Subaortic stenosis with infundibular obstruction of right ventricular outflow (congenital)
	Supra-aortic stenosis
	Absent aortic valve
	Aortic atresia
	Patent ductus arteriosus
	Isolated aorticopulmonary septal defect
	Persistent truncus arteriosus
	Preductal coarctation of the aorta
	Postductal coarctation of the aorta
	Coarctation of the aorta:
	a. Isolated
	b. With patent ductus arteriosus
	c. With patent ductus arteriosus and ventricular septal defect
	d. With patent ductus arteriosus and atrial septal defect
	e. With patent ductus arteriosus, atrial septal defect, and ventricular septal defect
	f. With transposition of the great vessels, patent ductus arteriosus, and ventricular septal defect
	g. With transposition of the great vessels and patent ductus arteriosus

Table 10–1.   CAUSES OF HEART FAILURE (Continued)

Aortic and ductal defects	h. With ventricular septal defect
	i. With atrial septal defect
	j. With miscellaneous combinations
Arrhythmias	Complete heart block
	Complete heart block with endocardial fibroelastosis
	Paroxysmal tachycardia, supraventricular (atrial)
	Paroxysmal tachycardia, ventricular
	Persistent paroxysmal tachycardia
	Atrial flutter
	Fibrillation, atrial
	Fibrillation, ventricular
Atrial septal defects	Atrioventricularis communis
	Complete absence of atrial septum
	Persistent ostium primum
	Persistent ostium secundum
	Left ventriculo–right atrial defect
	Atrial septal defect with mitral stenosis (Lutembacher's syndrome)
Fistulae	Arteriovenous fistulae (aneurysms), systemic, congenital
	Arteriovenous fistulae (aneurysms), systemic, acquired
	Common ventricle with D-transposition (complete)
Common ventricle	Common ventricle with normal great vessels
	Common ventricle with L-transposition (corrected) of great vessels
	Common ventricle with aplasia of the right ventricle sinus (single ventricle with rudimentary outlet chamber)
	Common ventricle with hypoplasia or aplasia of the left ventricular sinus
	Common ventricle with absent or rudimentary ventricular septum
	Common ventricle with absent right and left ventricular sinuses and ventricular septum
	Common ventricle with common atrioventricular valve (with pulmonary atresia)
Mitral valve disease	Mitral atresia (aplasia)
	Mitral stenosis (congenital)
	Mitral insufficiency (congenital)
Pericarditis	Constrictive pericarditis
	Idiopathic pericarditis
	Viral pericarditis
	Rheumatic pericarditis
	Tuberculous pericarditis
	Uremic pericarditis
Pulmonary vein anomalies	Postpericardiotomy syndrome
	Anomalous pulmonary veins (total) cardiac: into coronary sinus
	Anomalous pulmonary veins (total) cardiac: into right atrium
	Anomalous pulmonary veins (total) infracardiac: into ductus venosus
	Anomalous pulmonary veins (total) infracardiac: into portal veins
	Anomalous pulmonary veins (total) mixed
	Anomalous pulmonary veins (total) supracardiac: into left superior vena cava
	Anomalous pulmonary veins (total) supracardiac: into superior vena cava
Pulmonary artery and valve anomalies	Coarctation or stenosis of the pulmonary artery branches
	Pulmonary atresia with normal aortic root
	Acute cor pulmonale (embolism)
	Chronic cor pulmonale with emphysema
	Chronic cor pulmonale with pulmonary hypertension
	Fibrocystic disease (chronic cor pulmonale)
	Primary pulmonary hypertension
	Absent pulmonary valve
Miscellaneous	Bacterial endocarditis (a precipitating factor)
	Disseminated lupus erythematosus
	Periarteritis nodosa (polyarteritis)
	Dextrocardia, levocardia, and mesocardia with various types of cardiac shunts
	Ebstein's disease
	Endocardial fibroelastosis, primary *with* valvular involvement
	Endocardial fibroelastosis, primary *without* valvular involvement
	Endocardial fibroelastosis, secondary with or without valvular involvement
	Glycogen-storage disease of the heart
	Hypertension (systemic)
	Hyperthyroidism
	Hypothyroidism
	Marfan's syndrome (arachnodactyly) *with* cardiac involvement

Table 10–1. CAUSES OF HEART FAILURE (Continued)

Miscellaneous	Muscular dystrophies, Friedreich's ataxia
	Myocarditis, viral, idiopathic, toxic
	Tumors of the heart
Rheumatic fever	Acute rheumatic fever
	Rheumatic aortic insufficiency
	Rheumatic aortic stenosis
	Rheumatic mitral insufficiency
	Rheumatic mitral stenosis
	Rheumatic mitral valvular disease
Tetralogy of Fallot	Atypical tetralogy of Fallot (acyanotic)
	Tetralogy of Fallot with tricuspid insufficiency
Transposition of the great vessels	Taussig-Bing malformation (transposition of the great vessels with overriding pulmonary artery)
	D-and L-transposition of the great vessels with cardiac shunts
Tricuspid valve anomalies	Tricuspid atresia (congenital)
	Tricuspid atresia with large ventricular septal defect
	Tricuspid atresia with dextrocardia
	Tricuspid atresia with D-transposition of the great vessels
	Tricuspid atresia with L-transposition of the great vessels
	Tricuspid stenosis (congenital)
	Tricuspid insufficiency
Ventricular septal defect	Ventricular septal defect, simple (isolated) primary condition
	Ventricular septal defect with anomalous aortic cusp
	Ventricular septal defect with tricuspid insufficiency
	Ventricular septal defect with tricuspid valvular perforation (ventriculoatrial defect, shunt LV to RA)

Certain types of heart defects develop failure in characteristic age groups. For example, during the first week of life the most common cause of heart failure is aortic atresia. From one week to one month, coarctation of the aorta leads. From one week to two months, transposition of the great vessels predominates. From two to three months, the ventricular septal defect is the chief cause of heart failure, with transposition of the great vessels second to it.

A review of the electrocardiograms and hemodynamics of the above groups suggests that 40 percent have right ventricular overload; 30 percent, right and left ventricular overload; and 30 percent, evidence of left ventricular hypertrophy. Between the two main groups of right and left hypertrophy there is a good deal of overlapping. Thus, there may be an abnormally high arterial pressure in both the systemic and pulmonary circuits, as well as the presence of an abnormal shunt, resulting in an overload of both ventricles and in the development of biventricular hypertrophy in the electrocardiogram (e.g., coarctation of the aorta with a large patent ductus arteriosus).

Heart Defect and Age of Onset of Heart Failure

Newborn. Levy and associates (1970) have listed the possible causes of congestive heart failure in the newborn infant, particularly in the first two hours of life. They include (1) volume overloading from tricuspid regurgitation and pulmonic regurgitation, (2) arterial venous fistula, (3) hypoplasia of the left heart chamber with pulmonary venous congestion

and closed foramen ovale, (4) asphyxia at birth, (5) endocardial fibroelastosis, and (6) a massive placental transfusion (the latter may occur in twins, where one twin will be plethoric and the other anemic), and (7) paroxysmal tachycardia in the first few hours of life may produce heart failure.

Birth to One Week. The most common cause of heart failure in the first week of life in our experience is aortic atresia or hypoplastic left heart syndrome (Keith, 1956; Rowe, 1959; Rowe, 1961). This is followed by transposition of the great vessels and coarctation of the aorta. Almost invariably these anomalies of the heart are grouped in a variety of combinations when failure occurs this early in life.

The left heart syndrome is accompanied by a series of handicapping anomalies. These include aortic atresia and a patent ductus, so that the only way that the blood can get to the coronary arteries is from the right heart via the ductus in a reversed direction down a small threadlike ascending aorta. The blood reaching the coronaries is not fully saturated. The patent ductus itself may constrict, thus threatening the entire circulation. The perfusion of the lung is at systemic pressure, and the blood returning from the lung enters the small left atrium, from which it may or may not be able to escape adequately through the foramen ovale. If the foramen ovale is closed, this quickly leads to pulmonary edema and early death. As has been indicated earlier, many of these cases develop hypoglycemia in the first few days of life. This sort of case illustrates the many complicating factors that may contribute to mechanical and chemical failure of the heart.

First Month. In the first month of life coarctation of the aorta is an important cause of failure and is always associated with a patent ductus arteriosus at this age. There may also be a ventricular septal defect or other anomaly increasing the possibility of a lethal defect. One must be prepared to find any one of a number of lesions in this age group, including atrioventricularis communis, paroxysmal tachycardia, total anomalous pulmonary vein drainage below the diaphragm or above it, tricuspid atresia, common ventricle, persistent truncus arteriosus, and bizarre lesions associated with dextrocardia.

Second Month. In this age group, transposition of the great vessels is a common cause of failure in one form or another. Any of the lesions mentioned above may also be found.

Second to Third Months. In this age group the ventricular septal defect comes into a place of prominence in children with large openings between the ventricles and a low pulmonary vascular resistance. When the failure is marked and there is a rapid enlargement of the heart, quite frequently other associated lesions such as an atrial septal defect and patent ductus arteriosus are associated with the ventricular septal defect. Endocardial fibroelastosis begins to make its appearance in significant proportions at this time.

Three to Six Months. The ventricular septal defect still leads as a common cause of failure in this age group, either as an isolated lesion or combined with a variety of other anomalies. Such uncommon lesions as anomalous left coronary off the pulmonary artery and truncus arteriosus with a large left-to-right shunt may begin to appear at this time.

Six to Twelve Months. By the age of six months most of the mortality curves of congenital heart disease have begun to drop significantly and the onset of congestive heart failure in any of the lesions mentioned above is much less common. A few cases of endocardial fibroelastosis have their onset in this age group, as do those with atrioventricularis communis, total anomalous pulmonary vein drainage, and certain cases of ventricular septal defect; but the problems of diagnosis are less difficult in the second half of the first year partly because the investigative techniques are more readily carried out in this age group.

Hemodynamics

There is a series of steps encountered in cardiac response leading eventually to failure. The first response to increased load on the heart is hypertrophy of the ventricle concerned, as frequently develops in coarctation without cardiac enlargement. This hypertrophy usually occurs before there is any increase in the venous pressure, but eventually such filling-pressure rise appears. This may be controlled, or kept within physiologic bounds, by increased strength of contraction of the heart muscle and also by an increased heart rate. In time, however, these mechanisms of rate and strength cease to be adequate.

When that point is reached, the one remaining compensation is by means of an increased venous filling pressure.

Venous Pressure. The first rise in venous pressure, then, may be physiologic rather than pathologic, and it does not immediately lead to signs of failure, especially if the heart muscle can respond sufficiently to the increased load. When the burden is excessive and the heart muscle becomes fatigued or weakened, the clinical signs of failure begin to appear. This state of cardiac muscle fatigue is referred to by McMichael (1952) as "hypodynamic." He also records that hypodynamic hearts are the ones most likely to respond to digitalis therapy.

Starling's law states that the contractile power of the heart muscle is a function of the initial length of the muscle fibers. In other words, the more the heart is filled in diastole, the greater is the force of the following cardiac contraction.

However, the mechanism described in Starling's law is augmented to a marked degree by humoral and neural influences that go far beyond the simple relationship between muscle fiber stretch and ventricular response originally envisaged by Starling (Sarnoff and Mitchell, 1961). In a healthy individual the ventricle can increase its output without any change, or even a reduction, in filling pressure because of these additional mechanisms (Reeves and Hefner, 1962).

Initially a slight increase in heart rate, respiration, or myocardial contractility (with or without aid from the sympathetic nerve supply to the heart) will be adequate to supply the baby's physiologic needs in heart failure. Eventually the atrial pressure will rise to a recognizable degree.

Systemic venous pressure rises in cardiac failure by several mechanisms. The primary one is due to the decreased effectiveness of the heart muscle leading to a damming back of the blood and a raised atrial pressure. Such elevation may be only a millimeter or two in the infant or child. Another factor is the reflex increase in sympathetic vasomotor tone throughout the body increasing the rate of flow through the veins to the right atrium. A third factor is the retention of fluid by the kidneys causing an augmentation of both interstitial fluid volume and blood volume.

Since we are dealing with heart muscle that is originally healthy in congenital heart disease in infants and children, the cardiac reserve is very great. As the demands on the heart increase beyond a certain point, the venous pressure rises by small increments. The augmented right atrial pressure may thus maintain the cardiac output in a satisfactory manner. The early stages of failure may increase the respiratory rate and enlarge the liver and at the same time be associated with a right atrial pressure that is close to, or a millimeter or two above, normal. In such instances digitalis will usually produce an excellent response and lead to a normal liver size and reduction in the respiratory rate.

Right Atrial Pressure. Kidd and Collins (1964) have compared the mean right atrial pressure of children with congenital heart defects, but without the signs of congestive heart failure, with the atrial pressure of children who were in failure. There was a resulting slight but distinct difference between the two groups. Those with failure averaged 9 mm of mercury and those without, 3 mm of mercury. None of those in failure had a right atrial pressure less than 6 mm of mercury. These minor degrees of rises in related pressure are of considerable significance in such patients.

Failure in infants and children is not accompanied by as much fluid retention as is characteristically seen in adults, and interstitial fluid volume and blood volume do not appear to increase to the same degree. This may be one reason the mean venous pressure is kept at a lower level. Another reason is that edema is related in some measure to the length of time that the high capillary pressure has been maintained in the body. In infants and children the process may be acute and lead more promptly to death or improvement in a large percentage of cases.

Children with more severely incapacitated hearts lead on to progressive kidney retention of fluid, which causes a deterioration of cardiac function rather than being an aid to it. It is, therefore, important to weigh infants to see if the fluid retention is occurring and to administer diuretics at appropriate times along with sodium restriction. Factors that have been listed as contributing to the disturbance of renal function in heart failure include hypoxia, myocardial metabolites, varying degrees of vasoconstriction, total circulating blood volume, and humoral and neurogenic factors.

Redistribution of Blood Flow. Another physiologic adjustment is indicated by the fact that local vasodilatation may occur in certain muscles of the body and in other areas the flow may be restricted. Reduced flow is common through the skin, liver, and kidney. In this way the aortic pressure is maintained with a selective reduction in blood flow to the less vital organs of the body. Peripheral cyanosis and cold skin constitute clinical evidence of peripheral vasoconstriction. A baby who is irritable, crying, moving arms and legs, and at the same time exhibiting dyspnea with indrawing of each inspiration must be using many muscles unnecessarily and increasing the blood flow and work of the heart to a considerable degree. It has been shown in adults with failure that a restriction in blood flow to the skin may occur. At the same time the flow to the exercising muscles may be augmented and associated with a high oxygen utilization, so much so that the venous oxygen content of the blood coming to the femoral vein in exercising leg muscles may be close to zero (Donald et al., 1957).

Downing and associates (1965) have demonstrated a positive response to norepinephrine and synthetic nerve stimulation in the newborn lamb. Blockade of beta-receptor function with agents such as propranolol eliminates these responses. Friedman and coworkers (1968) have shown diminished norepinephrine concentrations in fetal and newborn lambs by histochemical studies. This has raised the possibility of delayed innervation of the heart in the newborn and suggests that the major adrenergic support for circulatory support in the fetus and newborn is derived from the adrenal gland. Rudolph and associates (1964) have shown that left-to-right shunts are poorly tolerated in animals with beta-receptor blockade, and a norepinephrine infusion enhances the ability of the animal to tolerate the shunt. Chidsey and coworkers (1962) have shown that in congestive heart failure there is an increase in arterial catecholamines.

Woodson and coworkers (1970) have demonstrated changes in the red blood cells that allow for an internal shift in the oxyhemoglobin association so that more oxygen can be delivered to the tissues at any given level for oxygen saturation. This mechanism appears to be operative in anemia and hypoxia.

Right and Left Heart Failure in Various Defects. In the adult it is usual to divide congestive heart failure into two main groups: left heart failure and right heart failure. This is readily possible in many cases, and the clinical signs of each category are recorded below. In the pediatric age group, however, it is more difficult to make a clear differentiation. The signs of right heart failure such as liver enlargement can be identified more readily than those of the left since the latter signs may present to some degree from congestion of flow rather than definable heart failure. It has been the custom in infants and children to rely more on the signs of right heart incompetence (particularly enlargement of the liver) to make a diagnosis of failure even in the patients whose primary cause is in the left heart.

Table 10-2 may help to indicate some of the facets of the problem.

There will be little argument regarding this grouping of the cases except for ventricular septal defect and transposition of the great vessels. One may couple with them certain combined problems, such as a patent ductus arteriosus with a ventricular septal defect. One can legitimately call them causes of both right and left heart failure rather than putting them in the one column or the other. The following reasons support this conclusion.

The ventricular septal defect is primarily a burden on the left heart as long as the resistance and pressure in the pulmonary circuit are distinctly less than in the aorta. This is the case in the majority of children with ventricular septal defect. When the pressure in the pulmonary artery is the same as systemic, the work of both ventricles is similar since the cardiac output and pressure of each are then identical (excluding advanced Eisenmenger's complex, which is uncommon in childhood). Failure under such circumstances is likely to be biventricular and result in signs in the chest and enlargement of the liver at the same time.

Table 10–2. INCIDENCE OF HEART FAILURE IN VARIOUS HEART DEFECTS

PRIMARY RIGHT HEART FAILURE		PRIMARY LEFT HEART FAILURE	
Defect	*Percent with Failure*	*Defect*	*Percent with Failure*
Pulmonary stenosis	10	Aortic stenosis	8
Atrial septal defect, ostium secundum	2	Patent ductus arteriosus	5
Ostium primum, atrioventricularis communis	50	Coarctation of aorta, presenting in 1st year of life	60
Total anomalous pulmonary venous drainage	80	Endocardial fibroelastosis	90
Aortic atresia	100	Myocarditis	70
		Tricuspid atresia	15
		Paroxysmal tachycardia, 1st year of life	60
		Mitral insufficiency	
PRIMARILY BOTH RIGHT AND LEFT HEART FAILURE			
Transposition of great vessels	60	Ventricular septal defect	10

A somewhat similar argument may be set forth for transposition of the great vessels coupled with a ventricular septal defect, which occurs in over 50 percent of cases. Failure in this combination usually occurs early in life once the pulmonary vascular resistance has fallen sufficiently to greatly increase the pulmonary flow and, in doing so, with the indirect help of the arterial desaturation, creates a pressure in the left ventricle that is at systemic level. As a result, part of the left ventricular oxygenated blood is expelled into the systemic circulation. Thus a considerable systolic and diastolic load is established for both ventricles. The ventricles can bear the systolic burden alone, but when it is associated with a progressive diastolic load and a coronary supply of low oxygen tension, a fatal outcome is the rule.

In children with intracardiac or vascular shunts the pulmonary circulation may get congested without failure being present. It may be difficult at times to differentiate between the two. The use of digitalis is helpful in this regard since it would not be expected to be of help if the heart muscle has not yet begun to fail.

Volume Load; Pressure Load. Katz and associates (1955) and others have shown that myocardial efficiency is greater with an increased diastolic or blood flow load at a moderate or low pressure than in the presence of a significantly increased pressure load. It is fortunate that this is so since increased diastolic loading is so common in the congenital heart defects found in early life. The most lethal situation is a combination of systolic and diastolic loading as is found in coarctation with patent ductus when it occurs in the neonatal period. There is a very low incidence of congestive heart failure in atrial septal defect in childhood, although

the flow may be many times that of normal. When one finds a similar large shunt flow in a ventricular septal defect, failure is unlikely to occur until the pressure in the right ventricle comes up to, or near, systemic level, giving a combination of high flow and raised pressure.

The right ventricle can sustain systemic pressure readily in the pediatric age group. One rarely finds a patient with Eisenmenger's complex in failure in the childhood years. The shunt may reverse itself through an atrial septal defect, a ventricular septal defect, or a patent ductus, but the right ventricle is quite competent to withstand systemic pressure, and it is not likely to get into trouble until anoxia predominates, or the pulmonary arteries rupture with hemoptysis, or the reversed shunt adds a diastolic load to the right ventricle.

In infancy, therefore, it is a combination of the high pressure and large flow that leads to failure in the ventricular septal defects. As the small pulmonary arteries narrow and reduce the blood flow to the lungs, heart failure, if present, disappears and the heart becomes smaller.

The high-pressure defects such as aortic stenosis, pulmonary stenosis, and coarctation of the aorta do not cause failure with any frequency in childhood in the isolated form, but when these anomalies are associated with the diastolic load, the burden is frequently excessive and signs of congestive heart failure become evident. Ninety-five percent of the cases at The Hospital for Sick Children with aortic stenosis that had a fatal outcome in childhood also had other associated congenital cardiac malformations.

When there is a regurgitation of blood through the mitral or tricuspid valve, the ventricle will increase the quantity of blood being pumped to maintain an effective forward flow. Tricuspid regurgitation is probably more common than is realized in the pediatric age group and is more likely the result of insufficiency of the right ventricle than the cause of it. The anterior and posterior cusps of the tricuspid valve bear the brunt of the function of this structure in preventing reflux of blood. The septal leaflet is scanty and the other two just barely close the atrioventricular orifice in the normal subject. At cardiac catheterization a leak from the right ventricle into the right atrium is a common finding and may, in a number of cases, be induced by the catheter itself but in a fair proportion must be due to the dilated right ventricle.

Pulmonary valve regurgitation is common in severe pulmonary hypertension owing to the dilatation of the pulmonary artery. The incompetence is minimal, and if the pressure in the right ventricle is not raised, pulmonary valve insufficiency is of little consequence. If the pressure is high in the pulmonary artery and right ventricle, insufficiency in this valve is likely to precipitate failure or augment it if other causes are operating already.

Failure of the left ventricle causes a rise in left ventricular and diastolic pressure, left atrial pressure, and pulmonary venous and pulmonary capillary pressures. The lung becomes congested and less compliant, and the child breathes more heavily, which in turn causes an increase in respiratory work. Rhonchi are frequently heard in infants and children, but the rales of full-blown pulmonary edema are uncommon.

Pulmonary Vascular Bed. The pulmonary vascular bed plays a crucial role in the production of congestive heart failure, as indicated by Rudolph and coworkers (1964) in experimental animal models. A good clinical example of this is provided by comparing the severity and incidence of heart failure in Denver, Colorado, with a city at sea level. Vogel and others have shown that the slight degree of hypoxia at Denver increases the pulmonary vascular resistance and lowers the degree and prevalence of heart failure at that altitude in children with ventricular septal defects.

Ventilatory Capacity. Donald (1959) points out that in the past it has not been fully appreciated how severely ventilatory capacity may be reduced in left heart failure. Respiratory studies show a great increase in resistance to air flow. Transudate in alveolar walls, alveoli, and air passages may cause sufficient interference with oxygen transfer to reduce the arterial oxygen saturation to the point of visible cyanosis. This justifies the frequent use of oxygen under such circumstances. The arterial oxygen saturation in children with pulmonary congestion or edema may be materially helped by this procedure.

The left ventricle and right ventricle are equally powerful in many types of congenital heart disease seen in the pediatric age group, but when the left ventricle fails, the left atrium and pulmonary veins do not provide as large a reservoir as that of the systemic veins. However, the infant or young child appears to

have the ability to transmit or relieve the back pressure from the left side to the larger reservoir on the right with the result that signs of left heart failure are significantly mitigated. One may then find the pressure in the pulmonary veins or pulmonary arteries is only slightly above the normal range in children who have developed signs of right heart failure as a result of left heart incompetence.

Nocturnal dyspnea in patients who are relatively active in the daytime is infrequent in the author's experience. The infants and children are less dyspneic at night than in the daytime. This may be related to the fact that with restlessness, irritability, and crying, the activity during the waking hours may raise the blood pressure and, therefore, systemic resistance and thus tend to increase the load in the pulmonary circulation during the day. During the night when the baby is asleep, the dyspnea is frequently less obvious.

Aortic stenosis presents a special problem because the overwhelming majority of such children have relatively good exercise tolerance and show little or no elevation of the left atrial pressure at rest. The powerful left ventricle is able to expel an adequate amount of blood for average activity. The left ventricular wall is thickened and the cavity is small, especially in comparison with the hearts of children with large ventricular septal defects or patent ductus arteriosus.

Sudden exertion in the presence of a marked aortic stenosis may cause an abrupt fall in the aortic pressure so that syncope from cerebral ischemia may occur. Such spells are uncommon in childhood and sudden death is rare (1 percent).

We have found subaortic muscular stenosis likely to be accompanied by a raised left atrial and left ventricular end diastolic pressure (Wigle et al., 1962). In two instances at The Hospital for Sick Children these pressures were between 20 and 30 mm of mercury, and the only clinical sign of possible failure was dyspnea with moderate exercise. Sudden death is more likely to occur in this group than in valvular aortic stenosis.

The more classic picture of congestive heart failure when it occurs in aortic stenosis is more likely to appear in the first year of life than in the succeeding childhood years. Of 260 infants and children found to have aortic stenosis in the clinic at The Hospital for Sick Children 20 developed congestive heart failure. All but two were in the first year of life and all had additional heart malformations.

Aortic regurgitation rarely causes heart failure in the pediatric age group unless it is associated with a ventricular septal defect or some other significant lesion.

Mitral regurgitation is a regular accompaniment of the ostium primum atrial septal defect and atrioventricularis communis. It undoubtedly augments the left-to-right shunt and helps to induce failure in such infants and children. In congenital mitral insufficiency cardiac failure is common since the lesions are usually sufficiently severe to allow a large proportion of the stroke volume from the left ventricle to regurgitate into the left atrium with each systole. This can be clearly shown by angiocardiography.

Systemic Resistance in Coarctation of Aorta. Coarctation of the aorta is accompanied by vasomotor response that leads to an increased resistance in the upper part of the body of the same order as the resistance created by the coarctation and results in normal flow to all areas. On exercise or crying such patients raise their systolic pressures well over 200 mm of mercury and add to the load of the left ventricle. Donald (1959) finds an increased pulmonary wedge pressure suggesting early heart weakness or failure in the 80 adults so studied. The aortic systolic pressure in those who showed this finding was usually over 100 mm of mercury. This pressure level is less common in the infant and child group. In infants this pressure burden can usually be borne adequately, but when it is accompanied by an intracardiac shunt such as patent ductus arteriosus or ventricular septal defect, the characteristic signs of congestive heart failure are much more likely to appear, particularly in the neonatal period.

Chemical to Mechanical Energy. The process of developing, maintaining, and replenishing chemical energy and transforming it to mechanical energy is a complicated one in the heart. It involves a variety of biochemical reactions in which sodium, potassium, and calcium play a prominent part. Membrane pumps continually use energy to preserve the gradient of sodium, potassium, and calcium ions. Protein synthesis proceeds at a constant rate and maintains proper concentration of enzymes, as well as integrity of cell membranes. Substrates, in the form of carbohydrates, fats, and proteins, are taken up from the coronary bloodstream, leading to the production of adenosine triphosphate (ATP), stores of which provide the energy for cellular activity.

In the failing myocardium, there is a decrease in the maximum intrinsic velocity of shortening (V max) and a decrease in the rate of pressure rise (DP/dt). The Frank–Starling mechanism plus increased sympathetic stimulation helps to maintain the overall compensation of the circulation in the early stages of failure. However, increased stress beyond the capacity to respond adequately leads to further failure of a deepening degree. Specific biochemical limitations of cardiac function appear to be responsible. Pool (1969) points out that the uptake of substrates and oxygen is not a primary problem and energy utilization is not significantly decreased. He regards a defect in the excitation-contraction coupling as the most likely single cause of heart failure. Alterations in this mechanism may involve the release and uptake of calcium ions from the sarcoplasmic reticulum. Mason and Braunwald (1968) also conclude that the ability of digitalis to improve the contractile state of the myocardium appears to be related to the cellular action of the drug to potentiate the excitation-contraction coupling, by enhancing the concentration of calcium ions in the endoplasm enveloping the myofibrils at the moment of cardiac contraction. They suggest that the toxic manifestations of digitalis may be due to a loss of intracellular potassium.

Clinical Features

Dyspnea. Dyspnea with effort is a normal phenomenon, and it may be difficult to assess whether it is a pathologic degree or not. Children with large hearts may have dyspnea on effort without other signs of congestive heart failure.

Dyspnea at rest, on the other hand, is frequently present with heart failure in infancy. In a baby, a respiratory rate of 50 to 100 a minute is common with congestive heart failure, and it may go as high as 120 to 149 per minute on occasion. Paroxysms of tachypnea that start and stop rather suddenly are rare in childhood failure; they are much more common in the cyanotic babies without failure. A respiratory rate of over 50 per minute is usually considered abnormal in a baby.

In an infant dyspnea may be precipitated by feeding. When an effort is expended, breathing is interrupted and the process of sucking and swallowing may thus lead to exhaustion and breathlessness. Such signs make one suspect the presence of incipient failure, especially when they are associated with poor weight gain in the baby.

It should be remembered that fever, pulmonary infection, and pyelitis in infancy may produce rapid respiratory rates that simulate those of failure.

Venous Pressure. In babies in the first year or two of life, it may be possible to see the external jugular vein sufficiently clearly and under conditions that allow one to assess the problem of venous pressure. Struggling, crying, or respiratory distress on the part of the baby will increase the venous pressure. Furthermore, the amount of the vein visible may be so short that the pulsating top of the column may not be seen.

In small children, when the back of the hand is not too chubby, the venous pressure may be assessed by prominence of the veins in that area; by raising and lowering the hand above the position of the right atrium, one may notice the point at which emptying of the veins occurs. These veins should empty if the hand is held at, or just above, the sternal angle, with the child at an approximate angle of 45 degrees.

In the older children, the external jugular vein may be seen and the top of its distended pulsating column may be recognized more readily. Furthermore, in the older children the position of emptying of the veins of the back of the hand can be assessed more accurately. The top of the venous column should not exceed 3 cm above the sternal angle.

It is thus obvious that a clinical estimate of the venous pressure in babies may be especially difficult. For this reason, in the first year of life the liver size is usually of more value in assessing heart failure.

Liver Size. The liver is readily palpable in infancy and childhood; the edge can be accurately felt and measured from the costal margin. This is done preferably on a line from the right nipple to the umbilicus. If the liver is 3 to 4 cm or more from the costal margin, it is usually pathologically enlarged. It is useful to draw out the margin of the liver with a skin pencil so that one can note change in liver size from day to day. In babies there is often a marked decrease in size after 24 hours of digitalis therapy.

In infancy and early childhood liver enlargement is not commonly accompanied by pain or tenderness of that organ. Liver pulsation is usually due to impulses transmitted from the heart movement. Occasionally it is due to an atrial pressure wave during ventricular systole, especially in the presence of tricuspid insufficiency.

Pulmonary Rales. In left ventricular failure, fine pulmonary rales may be heard in the bases. This is a common finding in adults, but it is not as frequently noticed in infants and young children until a rather severe stage is reached, and a considerable degree of dyspnea is usually present before the rales appear. A complicating factor in congenital heart disease is the appearance of respiratory infections, particularly in the presence of pulmonary plethora. These may precipitate congestive heart failure, and at times it may be difficult to tell whether the rales are due to infection, to the failure, or to both.

Vital Capacity. Wilson (1940) has drawn attention over the years to the reduced vital capacity in rheumatic heart disease, even before failure appears. With the onset of failure there is a greater reduction than before due to the increased congestion in the lung fields. There have been no measurements in infants, but there is no doubt that the lung volume is considerably reduced by the congestion and edema and that the vital capacity is considerably reduced at any age (Sellers, 1962).

Radiologic Signs. Pulmonary congestion may be evident in an x-ray of the chest. This is shown in Figure 10-1 (page 175). There is a widespread increase in the density of the lung fields, especially in the hilar areas in this case, showing simple congestion. In the presence of acute pulmonary edema, a diffuse mottling appears that is evident right out to the periphery of the lung fields.

Circulation Time. The normal circulation time in an infant or young child is between 6 and 12 seconds. However, when congestive heart failure is present, the circulation time may be prolonged to 30 or 50 seconds. This delay is due in part to the engorgement of the systemic veins and the vascular bed of the lungs.

Gallop Rhythm. The presence of gallop rhythm in congenital heart disease, isolated myocarditis, and nephritic heart disease usually denotes congestive heart failure. This is not true for rheumatic heart disease where the presence of gallop is of more benign, yet significant, import.

There are a number of extra heart sounds heard in infancy and childhood that may simulate the gallop rhythm. These include the physiologic third sound, the atrial or presystolic sound (especially in the presence of a lengthened conduction time), a systolic click or systolic sounds, and, finally, the opening snap of the mitral valve in mitral stenosis.

The most commonly heard gallop in the pediatric age group is the protodiastolic sound coming 0.10 second after the second sound. It is generally thought to be due to the sudden distention of the ventricles in the rapid-filling stage of diastole. This same mechanism is believed to produce the normal third heart sound; therefore, there may be difficulty in distinguishing between a physiologic and pathologic gallop. In normal infants and in older children the physiologic third sound is usually not heard or is so faint as to be recognized as insignificant. Thus the presence of a well-heard third sound is usually considered to be pathologic and in most forms of heart disease in infancy heralds the onset of congestive heart failure.

Cyanosis. Cyanosis in infancy and childhood is usually due to one of three origins. The first is the type seen in congenital heart disease resulting from a shunt of cyanotic blood into the systemic circulation. In the presence of failure, this shunt may be augmented, bringing to the surface signs of unsaturation in the milder cases and a deepening of the cyanosis in the severe defects. Transposition of the great vessels, aortic atresia, and single ventricle are good examples of this.

The second type of cyanosis, which is referred to as central cyanosis, is that due to pulmonary congestion or disease with inadequate oxygenation in the lungs. We have studied this in babies whose failure is not accompanied by a shunt, and approximately half of these cases show a decrease in their arterial oxygen saturation, depending largely on the degree of failure present. If the failure leads to death, presumably all in this category would ultimately show cyanosis of this type in the terminal stages. Coarctation of the aorta, isolated myocarditis, and endocardial fibroelastosis may exhibit cyanosis of this category.

The third type is due to a vasomotor effect in the small vessels and capillaries, leading to a slowing of the bloodstream and desaturation of the hemoglobin. This type of cyanosis may appear in heart failure and is usually associated with cold extremities. When oximetry is carried out, the oxygen saturation of the arterial blood is found to be normal, indicating its peripheral origin. Examples of this group are seen in pulmonary stenosis without a shunt but also can be recognized at times in endocardial fibroelastosis, isolated myocarditis, and coarctation of the aorta.

It is obvious in reviewing these three common causes of cyanosis that one or more may be operating in any one child; that is, a baby with a large ventricular septal defect and pulmonary congestion may be cyanotic because of inadequate oxygenation of the blood in the lung fields, or because of a partial shunt from the right to left ventricle and aorta.

Sedimentation Rate. It has been recognized for many years that an elevated sedimentation rate in rheumatic fever not uncommonly drops to a normal reading when heart failure supervenes. We have found this effect to be related to edema and a gain in body weight in the more chronic types of failure with rheumatic heart disease. In the acute illness of rheumatic fever with an overwhelming infection and heart failure, the sedimentation rate remains high. In the chronic failures with edema, if the edema clears, the sedimentation rate returns to its previously elevated level until the infection subsides.

Blood Pressure. In the past, blood pressure in heart failure has been reported to be low or normal in the majority of cases but occasionally elevated in a few cases. We have studied this problem with some care in coarctation of the aorta in infants with heart failure; in most instances where low systolic pressure is evident on admission to the hospital, after successful treatment with digitalis, along with the relief of the failure, the blood pressure rises to the usual expected level. We have determined the blood pressure level in babies in failure from a variety of cases, and, in those that are only slightly decompensated, the pressure is usually in the normal range. When the failure has been severe and the baby's condition poor, a low systolic reading is common, somewhere between 50 and 70 mm of mercury; the normal reading for babies is between 75 and 95 mm of mercury.

Heart Rate. The heart rate is usually increased to levels over 100 to 150 in children over a year or two in age with congestive heart failure. In infants there is commonly a tachycardia of 150 to 200 beats per minute in the presence of failure. There are many causes for this response, but congestive heart failure is associated with a rise of pressure in the right atrium and great veins that sets in motion the Bainbridge reflex, by which vagal effect is diminished and the heart rate increased. This is a useful mechanism, since it produces greater cardiac output as the venous pressure and heart rates rise together.

Right Heart Failure

Right heart failure is characteristically found in aortic atresia, transposition of the great vessels, anomalous pulmonary venous drainage, atrial septal defect, and, to some degree, in ventricular septal defect, atrioventricularis communis, preductal coarctation, and others.

The signs indicative of right heart failure are increased venous pressure, dyspnea, enlarged liver, and edema. All cases will show venous distention and increased pressure, and the majority in the pediatric group with right heart failure will also show enlargement of the liver. Edema is less frequently noted; the latter may be minimal.

Left Heart Failure

Clinical Features of Left Ventricular Failure. The clinical signs of left ventricular failure are most commonly dyspnea, rales in the chest, the presence of gallop rhythm, and radiologic evidence of congested lung fields. As the left ventricle begins to fail, the venous pressure rises behind it, distending the left atrium, pulmonary veins, and lung fields. When the right ventricle fails, the venous pressure rises in the right atrium, great veins, and liver; the edema comes later. Although either ventricle may fail alone, rather commonly both are involved, one predominating over the other. Failure of the left ventricle may soon lead to a rise in pressure in the pulmonary artery, right ventricle, and pulmonary veins, thus presenting the picture of right heart failure. In babies with left heart failure, cardiac catheterization may reveal a pressure in the right ventricle and pulmonary artery varying from normal up to systemic levels. One baby with endocardial fibroelastosis had a pressure in the right ventricle of 100 mm of mercury. Another baby whose primary involvement was on the left had a pressure in the right ventricle of 32 mm of mercury when right heart failure appeared with enlargement of the liver.

Differential Diagnosis

In the first 24 hours of life there are a number of conditions that either produce congestive heart failure or simulate it.

1. In the presence of aortic or mitral atresia with a closed foramen ovale, the blood returning to the heart has little or no opportunity to escape and pulmonary edema with developing cyanosis and failure occur in a few hours, usually associated with a large heart and frequently no murmur. One may suspect the diagnosis clinically, but an angiocardiographic study will confirm it.

2. An anomalous pulmonary vein below the diaphragm produces excessive congestion of the lungs and pulmonary edema in the first few days of life. In the most severe cases, this may be in the first 24 hours. An injection of contrast medium into the pulmonary vein will show the anomalous veins.

3. The infant of a diabetic mother commonly has an enlarged heart. In most cases there is no heart failure; the liver may be slightly enlarged, thus giving the impression of congestive heart failure without the fully developed picture. However, if there is an associated ductus that is patent or severe hypoglycemia, heart failure may occur.

4. A placental transfusion at the time of birth may increase the blood volume excessively, enlarge the heart, produce a plethoric baby, and at times put an excessive load on the myocardium. This condition may be identified by finding maternal red cells in the baby's bloodstream and may require an exchange transfusion replacing some of the red cells at the same time with plasma.

5. At the time of birth, in monozygotic twins, one baby may get much more blood from the placenta than the other and be plethoric while the other is anemic. This may be associated with enlargement of the heart in the plethoric baby.

6. Idiopathic polycythemia with enlarged heart occurs with a high hematocrit over 65 percent and

may occasionally be associated with convulsions but rarely with heart failure.

7. The respiratory distress syndrome with a patent ductus may be difficult to differentiate from congestive heart failure. The latter is usually less responsive to oxygen than respiratory distress and a raised CO_2 is commonly found in respiratory distress syndrome. When in doubt, digitalis may be indicated. If heart failure is present that is not responsive to digitalis, on rare occasions a surgical closure of the ductus may be required as a lifesaving measure in the first month of life.

It is of some importance to recognize when heart failure is not present. Many babies are treated for it unnecessarily. The most common situation in which this occurs is in the child with a left-to-right shunt that might be expected at some time to produce failure but such has not yet occurred. These infants have an enlargement of the heart, tachycardia, and some elevation of the respiratory rate because of the pulmonary congestion. If the liver is not enlarged, the right atrial pressure is not elevated, and there is no edema, and the response to activity is good, failure is not considered to be present. There is a certain advantage in not giving such babies digitalis at this stage. If at a later date they do go into failure under observation, such cases respond well and give one time to plan and carry out corrective surgical procedures. If they go into failure on digitalis, they have usually reached a later stage in the downward progress of their heart reserve and surgery then is more risky. However, a good argument can be made for the prophylactic use of digitalis in patients who might go into failure, especially those who live at a distance and for whom medical supervision is not readily available.

Many infants and children with a heart defect develop a respiratory infection involving the lungs, especially those with left-to-right shunt. Such children may have an increased respiratory rate without failure. Although it is true that a number do have failure precipitated by the infection, a review of the physical signs usually makes it possible to differentiate whether or not such is present.

Finally, babies with a right-to-left shunt who are cyanotic and have a reduced blood flow to the lungs may at times have dyspnea. These infants are rarely in failure unless they have an associated tricuspid insufficiency, a rare event in this group. Their dyspnea requires morphine (1.0 mg per 5 kg [10 lb] of body weight, for infants) rather than digitalis.

Treatment

The orthopneic position is easily achieved in older children; it allows ease of breathing and diminishes the pressure in the right atrium. It is preferable to keep the patient at an angle of 45 degrees. In babies a small Gatch bed or a pillow at the back may be used. It is necessary to put a support under the thighs to keep them from sliding down in bed. At times a restriction jacket may be helpful, provided it does not interfere with breathing. The baby should be turned from side to side at regular intervals to minimize pulmonary stasis and to ascertain that a comfortable position is being maintained.

Digitalis. It used to be thought that the chief benefit of digitalis was a direct effect on the heart rate. It is now generally believed that slowing of the heart is chiefly due to restored compensation of the failing organ. Digitalis appears to have an effect on rate in certain arrhythmias, of which atrial fibrillation is the prime example. Therapeutic doses of digitalis, therefore, do not produce much slowing of a normal heart but do so in the presence of failure (Lown and Levine, 1954) as the heart improves.

The heart rate may be slowed with digitalis toxicity, but this is associated with ingestion of an unusually large amount of digitalis. Slowing of the heart with conventional doses is usually not a sign of toxicity but simply an improvement in the child's cardiac function or a moderate effect of the digitalis mediated through the vagal nerve.

While there is evidence that digitalis improves some parameters of myocardial function in patients having cardiomegaly without failure, there is no evidence that its administration improves the clinical condition. Yet, during infancy, when rapid progression of untreated heart failure is common, prophylactic digitalization of patients having enlarged hearts may prevent or minimize this complication. Such action is particularly justifiable when it is difficult to ensure close medical supervision of the infant.

In heart failure the chief effect of digitalis is on the myocardium itself. Cattell and Gold (1938) have shown that it causes an increased force of systolic contraction with more adequate emptying of the heart, resulting in improvement of the clinical condition of the patient. The exact chemical mechanism of this beneficial effect is not yet clarified but appears to be related to the cellular reaction to the drug, particularly involving potassium, sodium, and calcium ions. While there is a direct and indirect cardiac action, much depends on the hemodynamics of any particular patient (Mason and Braunwald, 1968).

One minor side effect of digitalis is its diuretic action, which is independent of its effect on the heart. Farber and associates (1951) and Lown and Levine (1954) have shown that in patients without edema or with noncardiac edema there is a slight increase in the salt and water excretion following its administration.

There are several useful digitalis agents. Lown and Levine (1954) summarized the various actions of six of these. Our chief experience has been with the digitalis leaf, digoxin, and gitaligin. Digoxin, we have found, is particularly useful in treating infants and children since it has a relatively rapid action, the duration of its effect is shorter than that of other oral preparations, and its toxic effects, if they appear, are shorter lived. Furthermore, the therapeutic effect is reached considerably before the toxic level is approached. A two-year-old brother of one of our patients swallowed 4 mg of digoxin, or approximately four times the digitalizing dose, and survived. He was desperately ill for one night and part of the next day; then he improved rapidly.

DOSE   Doherty and associates (1961) showed that digoxin absorption averaged 80 percent of the orally administered dose. Peak levels were reached in serum in 30 to 60 minutes, and a plateau curve was achieved in four to six hours. It was excreted more rapidly than digitoxin.

The common digitalizing dose of digoxin for infants and children is 0.04 to 0.08 mg/kg given in four divided doses over 24 hours. The maintenance dose is approximately one-fifth to one-fourth of the digitalizing dose. However, it is much better to give a maintenance dose on the basis of milligrams per kilogram of body weight since the weight may change as the baby grows. (See Table 10–3.)

If digitalization is a matter of urgency, the digoxin may be given intravenously, preferably by giving a fourth to a half of the digitalizing dose at the start. Subsequent portions may be given intravenously or by mouth as required. It is preferable to give only a portion of the total digitalizing dose intravenously since there is a vasoconstricting effect with a full digitalizing dose, which may occasionally precipitate pulmonary edema in a patient already in failure (McMichael, 1952).

Gitaligin is also a useful preparation since its characteristics are similar to those of digoxin. Its dose is essentially the same, as high or slightly higher amounts are well tolerated. Both these preparations have a significant difference between the therapeutic and toxic levels, thus making them safe and useful. The dosage of digitoxin is given in Table 10–3 since it has also been shown to be a useful preparation in treating infants and children.

It is probably well to pick a digitalis preparation and become thoroughly conversant with its dosage, toxicity, etc., rather than to use a variety of preparations in the treatment of heart failure.

In babies and children on the doses described, we have usually found a satisfactory digitalis effect with relief of the edema or evidence of failure. This has usually occurred without any signs of digitalis toxicity and frequently without any evidence of digitalis effect on the electrocardiogram. One cannot but conclude, therefore, that the therapeutic and toxic levels are spread fairly widely in infancy and childhood in the preparations used, and the margin of safety is considerable.

A considerable reduction in heart size may occur with digitalization and relief of heart failure (see Figure 10–1).

TOXICITY.   Anorexia, nausea, and vomiting are likely to be early signs of digitalis toxicity, and they may be followed by visual symptoms, dizziness, and headaches. There also may be ectopic beats, first-degree heart block, bundle branch block or intraventricular conduction impairment, shortening

Table 10–3. DIGITALIS DOSAGE

DRUG	DIGITALIZATION			MAINTENANCE THERAPY		
	Route	Age	Total Dose in 24 Hours	Route	Age	Total Dose in 24 Hours
Digoxin	Oral	Under 2 yr	0.05 mg/kg	Oral*	Under 2 yr	0.01 mg/kg
		Over 2 yr	0.04 mg/kg		Over 2 yr	0.008 mg/kg
	Intravenous or intramuscular	Under 2 yr	0.04 mg/kg			
		Over 2 yr	0.03 mg/kg			
Digitoxin	Oral	Under 2 yr	0.035 mg/kg	Oral	Under 2 yr	0.0035–0.007 mg/kg
		Over 2 yr	0.02 mg/kg		Over 2 yr	0.002–0.004 mg/kg
	Intravenous or intramuscular	Under 2 yr / Over 2 yr	0.02 mg/kg			
Lanatoside C		Under 2 yr	0.03 mg/kg			
		Over 2 yr	0.01–0.02 mg/kg			

The digitalizing dose should be given in divided doses over 24 hours unless an emergency arises. The lower dose is less likely to produce toxicity than the larger dose.

* Digoxin is best administered by dividing the maintenance dose into two and giving one-half in the morning and one-half in the evening.

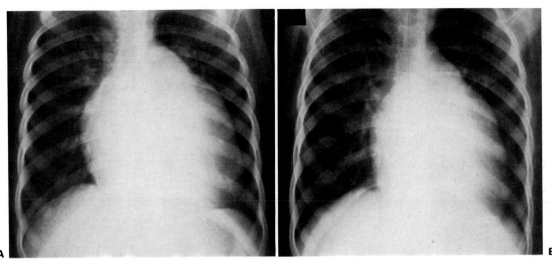

Figure 10-1. A. D., aged 12 years. Congestive heart failure. These x-rays, taken ten days apart, show heart size. *A* shows the heart before the start of therapy; *B* shows reduction in size following the use of a low-sodium diet and digitalis therapy.

of the Q-T interval, ventricular tachycardia, sinoatrial block, and intra-atrial block. These abnormalities are rare in children on digitalis. Characteristic effect on the electrocardiogram is the scooping of the S-T segment with an inversion of the first portion of the T wave. It should be remembered, however, that digitalis poisoning can occur in the absence of this electrocardiographic change.

Atrial fibrillation may be produced by an overdose of digitalis. We have seen this occur occasionally in childhood. Stopping the digitalis resulted in the return of the heart rhythm to normal. An overdose may be treated with an intravenous drip of potassium chloride (Sampson et al., 1943).

Oxygen. Most cyanotic children have their arterial oxygen level increased by the administration of oxygen. This has been tested on all varieties of congenital heart disease, and, almost invariably where there is any desaturation of the arterial blood, there is an increase with oxygen of 10 to 20 percent, depending on the type of heart defect and the severity of the cyanosis. When there is no unsaturation of the hemoglobin in congestive heart failure, it is not likely that oxygen has any beneficial effect.

The oxygen in plastic hoods and incubators should be kept at approximately 50 percent. Regular testing of oxygen content may be necessary; a flow of 4 to 5 liters a minute in incubators and 8 to 10 liters in tents may be necessary to keep the level at 50 percent.

Oxygen in high concentrations irritates respiratory mucus. Occasionally it favors the development of atelectasis by washing out the nitrogen in the pulmonary alveoli (Altschule, 1953).

In cor pulmonale, chronic hypoxia and carbon dioxide retention may be present. The respiratory center thus becomes acclimatized to the high carbon dioxide and ceases to respond, respirations being stimulated largely by hypoxia. Administration of oxygen may then depress respirations, and carbon dioxide may be retained to an excessive degree, causing drowsiness or coma. The breathing of room air rapidly reverses these effects.

Diuretics. Frank edema is not as common in children with heart failure as in adults, but fluid retention is almost invariably present. While digitalis may be all that is necessary to restore heart function and the circulation to normal, diuretics play an important part in the management regime. Most act on the tubular reabsorption mechanism in the kidney, resulting in diuresis and loss of sodium.

The mercurial diuretics have now been largely replaced by furosemide and ethacrynic acid. Both these drugs are effective in infants and children with heart failure and can be given by mouth or intramuscularly. The effects wear off in 12 to 24 hours, and one dose a day may be enough but the drug could be given twice if required. There is usually diuresis within one-half to one hour, producing a significant sodium loss and modest potassium excretion. Beneficial effects may be transient in some cases and other diuretics will then be required. Furosemide and ethacrynic acid are most effective in acute pulmonary edema and episodes of heart failure lasting days, or even on into weeks; however, if prolonged therapy is required, furosemide is better given along with other medication such as spironolactone. The doses of these various diuretic preparations are shown in Table 10–4.

Chlorothiazide (Diuril) and hydrochlorothiazide have also proved to be effective in the diuretic management of patients. Diuresis generally begins two hours after ingestion and continues for 12 hours. Quantities of sodium and potassium may be excreted, but serious potassium loss is an infrequent complication. The dosage for chlorothiazide is 20 to 40 mg/kg daily, usually given in divided doses every 12 hours.

The serum sodium and potassium levels should be monitored at intervals, since both may be depleted with the passage of time. Potassium salts should be given by mouth when the serum level falls below normal.

Table 10–4. DIURETIC AGENTS*

DRUG		DOSE
Furosemide	Intravenous	1 mg/kg/day
	Oral	2–3 mg/kg/day
Ethacrynic acid	Intravenous	1 mg/kg/day
	Oral	2–3 mg/kg/day
Chlorothiazide	Oral	20–40 mg/kg/day
Hydrochlorothiazide	Oral	2–5 mg/kg/day
Spironolactone	Oral	1–2 mg/kg/day

* See text for management details.

Treatment of Associated Pathologic Features

Electrolyte Changes in Congestive Heart Failure. When a patient with congestive heart failure is given a mercurial diuretic, the fluid eliminated contains both chloride and sodium, but more of the former than of the latter. Potassium or ammonium is excreted in place of sodium. The loss of chloride may produce alkalosis with a rise in serum bicarbonate and a fall in chloride. Such hypochloremic alkalosis rarely produces symptoms in itself in a child, but it may cause a lack of response to further mercurial diuretics. Correction of the alkalosis restores the responsiveness to mercury. The use of ammonium chloride with the administration of mercurial diuretics will usually prevent resistance from occurring.

Hyponatremia. This problem may be discussed under three headings.

DILUTIONAL HYPONATREMIA. In heart failure associated with significant edema the concentration of sodium in the blood may be lowered owing to retention of greater quantities of water. This is best treated by restricting the fluid intake to 500 to 1000 ml a day for a large child and correspondingly low amounts for small infants and children. The serum sodium will then gradually return to normal levels over a week, and the child's ability to respond to diuretics with excretion of sodium will be restored.

Acute sodium depletion may occur in the early stages of heart failure if excessive or multiple methods of diuresis are used associated with salt restriction. The symptoms include lethargy and sleepiness. By the time these are apparent the edema will have disappeared, and the serum sodium and chlorides are usually within normal limits. The symptoms will disappear when there is a freer use of the salt in the diet.

Chronic sodium depletion may occur on a strict dietary regime of low sodium plus prolonged use of diuretics. Signs include muscle weakness or cramps

and poor tissue turgor. By this time any edema that was previously present has been eliminated, and the clinical picture is associated with a lowered serum sodium and chloride. A gradual or moderate increase in use of salt in the diet will allow this electrolyte abnormality to be corrected over several days.

Acidosis. In specific cases, such as transposition of the great arteries, where failure is coupled with cyanosis, one may encounter severe degrees of acidoses, requiring prompt therapy with sodium bicarbonate. In such emergencies one may give up to 2 to 5 mEq/kg intravenously.

The amount of bicarbonate required may be arrived at by the following formula: The desired bicarbonate concentration (usually 23 mEq/L) minus existing bicarbonate concentration times 0.6 times body weight in kilograms equals milliequivalents of bicarbonate, which would be expected to totally correct the metabolic acidosis. When one is not dealing with an emergency, quarter to a half is given over a four-hour period, and if there is any doubt about the response the blood chemistry can be repeated.

In heart failure with circulatory collapse, a drip of isoproterenol (Isuprel) has occasionally proved lifesaving (0.2 μg/kg per minute). Blood pressure and heart rate should be followed closely.

Respiratory Acidosis. When there is lung pathology present with reduced pulmonary ventilation, there may be a retention of carbon dioxide, which results in high blood bicarbonate and lowered plasma chloride. The blood becomes more acid, this being revealed by a lowered pH. An electrolyte picture such as this may develop in cor pulmonale cases with congestive heart failure. The treatment is best directed against the underlying cause of the pulmonary hypertension, lung involvement, or heart failure.

Talner and associates (1965) record the presence of a respiratory acidosis in a group of 20 infants with congestive heart failure. The mean Pco_2 value was 51 mm of mercury. The mean pH was 7.3. Infants with left-to-right shunts but no failure tended to overventilate and develop a mild respiratory alkalosis.

It was of clinical significance and importance to note the finding of a Pco_2 that was reduced during failure and returned to normal or close to normal values when the failure was relieved.

Potassium Depletion. This may occur with excessive diuresis or with prolonged administration of cortisone. The importance of a lowered potassium in congestive heart failure is in association with digitalis intoxication. Friedman and Bine (1947) have shown that potassium exerts an antagonistic effect on digitalis activity. A lowered potassium allows a greater digitalis effect that may be toxic.

Potassium salts should be given by mouth in the presence of potassium depletion (1 gm daily to a child).

Edema. In adults a low-sodium diet has proved to be most helpful in clearing edema. The normal diet contains approximately 5 to 12 gm of sodium a day. A reduction to 0.5 to 1 gm daily diminishes the sodium content of the tissues to a degree that will largely prevent excessive fluid retention in the body (Schroeder, 1941; Schemm, 1942).

Most rheumatic heart disease cases in failure are placed on a fruit and fruit-juice diet when therapy is started, and since this provides a low-sodium content, it is very suitable for all children with cardiac failure and fluid depletion. If diuretics are given with a low-sodium diet, they should be given intermittently so as to avoid too great a depletion of sodium in the body. The blood chemistry should be checked under such circumstances.

For babies, a preparation of powdered milk with a low-sodium content is available (Lonalac). This is useful if the edema is obstinate and does not respond to digitalis therapy.

The fluid intake does not need to be restricted in infants and children. They are allowed the fluid quantities they wish to take, if more fluids are not forced.

PULMONARY EDEMA. Pulmonary edema may occur in many different types of congenital heart disease but is characteristic of those types that lead to marked pulmonary congestion. Four examples in this category are: (1) aortic atresia, (2) primary endocardial fibroelastosis, (3) ventricular septal defect, and (4) total anomalous pulmonary vein drainage below the diaphragm. Talner and associates (1965) suggest that wheezing respirations in an infant with congestive heart failure are characteristic of pulmonary edema.

Any of the three fundamental causes of pulmonary edema may be operating at varying degrees in each of these. First, an increased capillary permeability is suggested by the frequent finding of diapedesis of red cells and serum in histologic sections in those that have died. This is particularly common in fatalities of failure in the first few weeks of life. Second, plasma proteins may not always be of normal level, leading to a reduced blood oncotic pressure. This is more likely to occur in prematures (Domville Cook, 1960). These are much less important than the third factor, which is associated with increased capillary pressure in the pulmonary vascular bed.

Fortunately, pulmonary edema is uncommon in babies or older children. When it does occur, it is best treated with (1) orthopneic position; (2) morphine, 1 mg per year of age; (3) oxygen; or (4) oxygen bubbled through 50 percent ethyl alcohol, administered for ten minutes at a time and repeated every 20 to 30 minutes as required.

Prognosis

In a review of a large group of infants in congestive heart failure at The Hospital for Sick Children it was found that the majority died in early life. In evaluating the prognosis of any particular case, there are a number of influential factors that appear.

Cause of Failure. The underlying defect may be

successfully treated either medically or by surgical correction. When such is the case the prognosis may be good, as in coarctation of the aorta. When no medical therapy is of avail, and surgical correction is so far impossible, the prognosis is poor as in aortic atresia.

The degree of failure influences the prognosis. Those cases with rapid onset of severe failure in infancy have a poorer outlook than do those that have a milder degree coming on more slowly.

Age at Onset. The age at onset has obvious prognostic implications. The outlook is poorer if the onset is in the first week or month of life.

BIRTH TO ONE WEEK Among those that have the onset of signs and symptoms of failure in the first week of life, 85 percent will die in the next weeks or month. These cases include aortic atresia, transposition of the great vessels, and coarctation of the aorta, in that order.

ONE WEEK TO ONE MONTH When the age of onset of failure occurs between one week and one month, 66 percent will die in the near future. Coarctation of the aorta predominates in this group; transposition of the great vessels is second; endocardial fibroelastosis is third.

ONE TO TWO MONTHS When the age of onset is one to two months, 58 percent will die shortly. The leading cause of death from failure is transposition of the great vessels, with endocardial fibroelastosis second, coarctation of the aorta third, atrioventricularis communis fourth, and paroxysmal tachycardia fifth.

TWO TO SIX MONTHS When the age at onset of failure is two to three months after birth, 50 percent will die shortly. Endocardial fibroelastosis is the leading cause of death. Transposition of the great vessels is second, total anomalous pulmonary venous drainage into the right atrium or its tributaries third, and ventricular septal defect fourth.

SIX TO TWELVE MONTHS In the second half of the first year, endocardial fibroelastosis is a leading cause of death from heart failure. Ventricular septal defect is second.

ONE TO TEN YEARS After the first year of life, a variety of conditions cause heart failure but they comprise only 10 percent of the total. Of those that do develop heart failure in this age group, 40 percent die in the next few months or a year or two. This group includes ventricular septal defect, atrial septal defect, atrioventricularis communis, paroxysmal tachycardia, myocarditis, rheumatic heart disease, and anemia.

The Electrocardiogram. The electrocardiogram is of some prognostic significance. Of those with failure that showed right ventricular hypertrophy, 78 percent died shortly, whereas among those with left ventricular hypertrophy, the mortality was 44 percent. When evidence of both right and left ventricular hypertrophy was present, the mortality was 61 percent.

When right ventricular hypertrophy is present, there is a slightly higher mortality among those with a qR pattern in the right precordium than when this sign is lacking (84 per cent as compared with 60 percent).

Associated Respiratory Infection. When congestive heart failure in infancy is associated with, or precipitated by, a respiratory infection, the mortality is lower than when the failure has occurred spontaneously from the underlying defect alone. The infection can usually be treated successfully. This, coupled with therapy for the failure, causes the signs of failure to disappear completely.

Digitalis Intoxication

There are two types of digitalis intoxication: (1) therapeutic toxic levels and (2) digitalis poisoning.

Therapeutic Toxic Levels. Therapeutic but toxic levels of digitalis have been recognized from the time of Dr. William Withering over 200 years ago when he first used the drug successfully. He inferred an excessive action at times on the kidney, the stomach, the pulse, and the bowels and recommended that the drug be stopped on first appearance of any one of these effects. Over the years, the medical profession has learned to avoid most of these unpleasant side effects by the frequent observation of the patient and the use of the electrocardiogram.

In therapeutic doses, excessive effects on the kidneys, bowels, or intestine are almost unknown in childhood but occasionally electrocardiographic evidence of toxicity appears. Smith and Haber (1970) have listed the following electrocardiographic signs of digitalis intoxication. One or more may be present.

1. Supraventricular tachycardia (atrial or atrioventricular junctional) with atrioventricular block.

2. Frequent or multifocal ventricular premature beats, ventricular bigemini, or ventricular tachycardia.

3. Atrial fibrillation with high-grade atrial ventricular block (ventricular response less than 50 per minute) and ventricular premature beats.

4. Sinus rhythm with second- or third-degree atrial ventricular block.

Any one of these signs is considered to be due to digitalis effects if the rhythm disturbance disappears when the digoxin is withheld.

Signs of digitalis toxicity are reported to occur in adults by the above definition, in incidence varying from 7 to 23 percent (Rodensky and Wassermann, 1961; Sodeman, 1965; Beller et al., 1971). Digitalis toxicity is much less common in the pediatric than the adult age group, occurring in less than 2 percent of infants and children receiving a digitalis maintenance dose for chronic failure.

Fogelman and associates (1971) feel that there is sufficient degree of overlapping between toxic and nontoxic levels that this digitalis assay method is of questionable value. Recently, Smith (1971) has reviewed the subject and pointed out that 90 percent of patients without evidence of toxicity had serum levels of 2 ng/ml or below, while levels above 2 ng/ml were observed in 87 percent of patients with digitalis toxicity (which disappeared when the drug was withheld). Another series of patients studied at St. Bartholomew's Hospital and the National Heart Hospital in London by Chamberlain and associates (1970) revealed results similar to those of Smith; 21 of 22 of their patients with digitalis toxicity had serum concentrations ranging from 2 to 5.2 ng/ml. Both series had overlapping values in a modest but not negligible group of patients.

It is obvious that there are a number of factors that will affect the sensitivity of any individual to digitalis, and these include serum potassium, sodium, calcium, or magnesium, hypoxia, acid-base balance, autonomic tone, thyroid status, and associated cardioactive drugs. In children, these factors are usually brought under satisfactory control in most patients in chronic failure. The control of these elements may be more difficult in the postoperative period.

Furosemide and chlorothiazide in the treatment of chronic failure in children may promote the loss of potassium from the body. This in itself may precipitate digitalis intoxication. The potassium level should, therefore, be determined promptly and sufficient potassium administered to bring the serum levels up to normal. This caution may be of some help in treating the tachyarrhythmias induced by digitalis, but it must be remembered that it prolongs the conduction time and the refractory period of the AV node and, therefore, is contraindicated in the presence of atrioventricular block. Spironolactone in combination with usual diuretics minimizes potassium loss.

The radioimmunoassay method has given us other information, in that it has been noted after the administration of digitalis that the peak levels are usually reached in about one hour in the fasting subject and in about two hours in the nonfasting. The blood level usually becomes constant after five or six hours.

Another point of interest is that after a heart-lung pump operation, using cardiopulmonary bypass, there is a transient fall in the digitalis concentration in the serum that appears to be due to the dilution of the patient's plasma by pump-priming and transfusion, but in the postoperative period this returns to the initial levels (Coltart et al., 1971; Morrison et al., 1970).

Rogers and associates (1972) indicate that the concentrations of digitalis in the blood of pregnant mothers at term, suffering from rheumatic heart disease on maintenance digoxin, were the same as the concentrations in cord blood of the fetus at the time of delivery.

Our conclusion is that the doses recommended in Table 10–3 in infants and children will usually give blood serum levels of digitalis of less than 2 ng/ml. If any of the arrhythmias usually associated with digitalis toxicity appear, the drug should be temporarily withheld and the dose reduced to a lower level. In desperately ill babies or in infants and children in the postoperative state, it is most important to monitor the blood gases, pH, and electrolytes, as well as an occasional radioimmunoassay of serum digoxin, in order to properly manage the patient through the illness.

Bradycardia in children is rarely a sign of digitalis toxicity unless it is associated with an arrhythmia, and one need not discontinue the drug for bradycardia alone unless the rate falls below 60 per minute. In a recent report on digitalis toxicity in 179 adults (most in their 60s), Lely and Van Enter, (1970) record a great variety of signs and symptoms, but serious bradycardia occurred in only four cases, i.e., slightly over 2 percent of the total group. A slow or irregular heartbeat should indicate the need for an electrocardiogram, and if there is evidence of one of the arrhythmias listed above, the dose should be reduced or omitted temporarily. It is also important to realize that isolated prolongation of the conduction time is not considered a manifestation of digitalis toxicity in congestive heart failure. The slowing of the heart rate and elimination of the sinus tachycardia by digitalis are more related to improvement of the cardiac hemodynamics. Furthermore, the improvement initiated by digitalis is accompanied by diminution of sympathetic activity, and this may be the factor that reduces the rate, rather than the action, of digitalis on the vagus nerve or sinus pacemaker.

DRUGS IN DIGITALIS THERAPEUTIC INTOXICATION. Phenytoin and lidocaine are useful drugs in treating arrhythmias due to digitalis. Propranolol is useful in limited circumstances.

Phenytoin is particularly useful in treating tachycardia associated with digitalis toxicity, since this antiarrhythmic drug depresses the enhanced ventricular automaticity without affecting intraventricular conduction. It also tends to reverse the digitalis-induced prolongation of the P-R interval. It does not diminish the contractile effects of digitalis. Furthermore, it is useful in terminating the supraventricular arrhythmias of digitalis origin and is more effective than lidocaine in this direction. In atrial flutter or fibrillation phenytoin has little or no therapeutic effect.

Lidocaine may be effective in treating digitalis-induced ventricular tachycardia and is reported not to affect the conduction velocity of the AV node and the ventricular myocardium.

Propranolol has been used with some success in certain types of digitalis toxicity, particularly those with tachyarrhythmias. It has also proved helpful in terminating premature ventricular extrasystoles. When atrial tachycardia occurs with AV block, propranolol may restore sinus rhythm but it may depress the nodal conduction. In such cases phenytoin is preferable to propranolol. Another disadvantage of propranolol is that it depresses myocardial contractility and diminishes cardiocirculatory function since, in addition to its depressing effect on cardiac contractility and heart rate, it has a beta-blocking action that diminishes sympathetic support for the failing heart (Nayler et al., 1969).

While pediatric cardiologists may encounter a variety of degrees of sensitivity of individual children to digitalis, most children tolerate and are helped by the usual therapeutic doses. The majority of children in failure have congenital heart defects with cardiac hypertrophy. The type of heart disease encountered in the adult is more variable and the myocardium is more seriously involved, as in coronary artery disease, acute myocardial infarction, severe valvular heart disease, cor pulmonale, hypertensive heart disease, and cardiomyopathy. In many instances, the cardiac impairment has persisted for a long time.

In children, failure is usually of much shorter duration, and with energetic medical treatment the myocardium can be returned to a more healthy response in a large percentage of such patients on maintenance doses of digitalis and other supportive therapy. Arrhythmias, such as described in adults, are rare, and evidence of digitalis toxicity on a maintenance dose occurs in less than 2 percent of the pediatric age group.

The recent development of a method of determining serum digoxin levels (Smith et al., 1969) is proving helpful in establishing suitable dose levels of digitalis for children in chronic congestive heart failure. Recently, Sears, Olley, Wilson, and Mahon at The Hospital for Sick Children and the Toronto General Hospital have studied infants, children, and adults receiving therapeutic doses of digoxin. Thirteen infants in the newborn period under six weeks of age have been found to have mean serum levels of digoxin of 1.8 ng/ml. Forty-two infants and children from six weeks to two and a half years averaged 1.3 ng/ml, while 125 adults averaged 1.0 ng/ml. It is apparent from these figures that the doses of digitalis being administered to infants and children were larger on a weight basis than those given to adults. Sears and coworkers found that all cases of digitalis toxicity in the pediatric age group had serum levels of 2 ng/ml or greater. However, they also found that quite a number of infants and children were able to sustain levels of over 2 ng without evidence of toxicity.

Interest has been directed to electrical overdrive by either atrial or ventricular pacing, as a means of treating ventricular tachycardias, and it may be used for suppression of such arrhythmias induced by digitalis. The electrical stimulus is delivered at a more rapid rate than the frequency of the idiopathic ventricular focus, thus suppressing the latter. Mason and associates (1971) emphasize that ventricular pacing should not be utilized as the initial approach in the treatment of digitalis-induced ventricular tachycardia, but rather should be applied only when the standard measures fail. They point out that digitalis lowers the threshold for spontaneous repetitive ventricular extrasystoles in response to pacemaker stimuli and, therefore, may lead to further arrhythmias.

Another technique that should be kept in reserve until other measures have been tried adequately is that of countershock. Serious ventricular arrhythmias have occurred after countershock in individuals on digitalis, whether they have or have not had evidence of digitalis toxicity. Using cardioversion in such cases, it is best to keep the shock energy at lower-than-average levels, since this diminishes the possibility of shock-induced arrhythmias.

In the event of complete heart block with a progressively slower heart rate, or worsening of the heart failure, atropine and electrical pacing should be applied. (Potassium is contraindicated in complete block.)

Digitalis Poisoning. Digitalis poisoning may occur in a child receiving digitalis, either from a mistake in the dose administered or from the child's getting hold of some of the tablets. The subject has been well reviewed by Fowler and colleagues (1964) after examining the experience at The Hospital for Sick Children (Toronto) covering many years.

The majority of children who receive a poisoning dose are between one and a half and three and a half years of age, as shown in Figure 10–2. They are able to get the top off a bottle of the tablets, which may belong to the grandmother, and eat sufficient to have a serious or even lethal effect. Newer types of bottles with special tops are a great help in preventing this sort of tragedy.

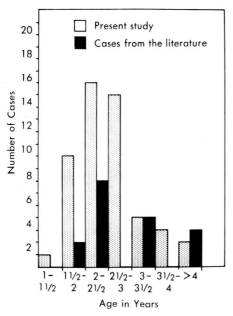

Figure 10-2. Digitalis poisoning. The age distribution of cases in this series and cases of children reported in the literature.

With the larger doses that may be taken under poisoning circumstances, the signs include the list well-known to occur with the drug. This includes nausea, vomiting, diarrhea, drowsiness, headache, confusion, convulsions, color vision, blurred vision, and other personal idiosyncrasies to the drug. The

effects on the heart have been listed previously, and these include the development of heart failure, or an arrhythmia, such as the tacharrhythmias, atrial, nodal, or ventricular, with or without varying degrees of heart block up to and including complete atrioventricular block. (See Figure 10–3.)

It is important to determine the amount and type of digitalis ingested, since a preparation such as digoxin is usually excreted rapidly from the system and the toxic effects rarely last longer than 24 or 48 hours, unless permanent damage has occurred to the brain or other organs. Digitoxin, on the other hand, or digitalis leaf may take several days longer before one is free from the deleterious effects. The following is a guide to management of a case of digitalis poisoning.

1. Determine the amount, type, and time of digitalis ingestion.

2. Empty the stomach.

3. If the child has ingested a significant amount of digitalis, place him in an intensive care unit and monitor an electrocardiogram, as well as vital signs, at frequent intervals.

4. Determine the serum electrolytes, including calcium, potassium, sodium, etc., and repeat as required.

5. Treat cardiac irregularities as described above, using phenytoin, lidocaine, or propranolol, if such is indicated.

6. Sodium ethylenediamene tetraacetic acid (EDTA) is occasionally of value in treating digitalis poisoning. It has a rapid onset of action, but its effects are rather transient and occasionally produce hypotension. However, it can be used when phenytoin and other drugs are contraindicated or ineffective.

7. Give intravenous potassium chloride if the patient is voiding and if the serum potassium is low. It is contraindicated in the presence of partial or complete heart block, or with bradycardia below 50 or 55 per minute.

8. Use an external electrical pacemaker for cardiac arrest or extreme bradycardia, i.e., below 50 per minute.

Prognosis and Mortality. The prognosis and mortality vary with the dose taken and length of time before treatment is begun, and whether or not there is underlying heart disease. The mortality in digitalis toxicity in adults has been reported to vary from 4 to 36 percent. Chung (1969) and Lown and Levine (1958) report a mortality rate of over 50 percent in patients with digitalis-induced paroxysmal atrial tachycardia with block.

However, these figures do not relate significantly to the pediatric age group. Fowler and colleagues, reporting the effects of digitalis poisoning on 48 children seen in the emergency department and wards of The Hospital for Sick Children, Toronto, with a history of accidental ingestion of digitalis or its glycocides, had only two deaths, one from cardiac arrest and the other from central nervous system toxic effects. The rest recovered with medical therapeutic assistance as outlined above.

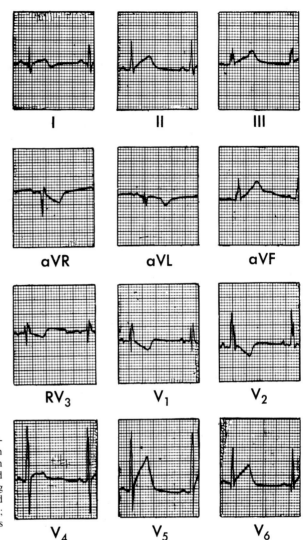

Figure 10-3. Digoxin intoxication. A full electro-cardiogram done on G. S. 48 hours after the ingestion of 10 mg of digoxin. It shows slow sinus rhythm with tall T waves and S-T segment shift. A two-year-old child died of brain damage four days after taking digitalis. The cardiac irregularities had been eliminated by suitable therapy. (Reproduced from Fowler, R. S.; Rathi, L.; and Keith, J. D.: Accidental digitalis intoxication in children. *J. Pediatr.*, **64**:188, 1964.)

Heart Failure in the Postoperative Period

Heart failure in the postoperative period may be brought on by a variety of factors. There may have been heart failure before surgery, or it may have occurred primarily following operation. When it derives from the surgical procedure itself, it may be due to the myocardial incision, pulmonary insufficiency, tricuspid insufficiency, or aortic insufficiency. It may be brought on or made worse by various types of unrelieved stenoses or shunts inadequately closed at operation. It may also be precipitated by an inadequate blood volume at the end of operation, cardiac tamponade, or acidosis.

In evaluating the state of the circulation in the recovery room one needs to consider the size of the heart, the state of the lungs, the blood pressure, the central venous pressure, the arterial oxygen saturation, the electrolytes, particularly the pH, potassium and sodium, the function of the kidneys (whether there is oliguria, azotemia, red blood cells in the urine, etc.) Electrolyte changes may occur more rapidly in the infant and are more difficult to relieve when they occur. Prevention of significant metabolic derangements is crucial in adequate management of the younger age group. The pulmonary function may be impaired by atelectasis pneumonia or hypoventilation. Infection also acts as a handicap, particularly if there is septicemia, bacterial endocarditis, or the postpericardiotomy syndrome. Other causes of difficulty are hemorrhage in any part of the body, hemorrhagic diathesis, or hemolysis.

A special problem is the low cardiac output syndrome, which is characterized by hypotension, a normal or slightly elevated central venous pressure, and vasoconstriction with peripheral cyanosis, and it usually occurs early in the postoperative period and is helped greatly by transfusion, bringing the venous pressure up as high as 12 mm of mercury.

A variety of arrhythmias must be contended with, including atrial fibrillation, flutter, heart block, nodal tachycardia, ventricular tachycardia, ventricular fibrillation, up to cardiac arrest. Digitalis toxicity must be eliminated as a cause. The arrhythmia may be corrected by a cardiovertor, by digitalis, lidocaine, or phenytoin (see Chapter 45). Atrial pacing in the first 24 hours after major cardiac surgery may be required if the heart rate is excessively slow.

In the presence of heart failure it is usually wise to have the patient digitalized before operation. The dose of digitalis is reduced if there is any evidence of renal impairment postoperatively. A low-sodium diet is given if such is necessary, depending on the history, findings, and serum sodium. The heart is helped by assisted respiration and adequate oxygen intake. Bicarbonate may be required to correct acidosis. The fluids are usually given in the form of 0.2 percent sodium chloride, 500 ml per meter squared in the first 24 hours.

REFERENCES

Ainger, L. E.: Large tonsils and adenoids in small children with cor pulmonale. *Br. Heart J.* **30**:356, 1968.

Alter, B. P.; Czapek, E. E.; and Rowe, R. D.: Sweating in congenital heart disease. *Pediatrics*, **41**:123, 1968.

Altschule, M. D.: Hazards in the treatment of cardiac decompensation. *Mod. Concepts Cardiovasc. Dis.*, **22**:190, 1953.

Batterman, R. C., and DeGraff, A. C.: Comparative study on the use of the purified digitalis glycosides, digoxin, digitoxin, and lanatoside. C., for the management of ambulatory patients with congestive heart failure. *Am. Heart J.*, **34**:663, 1947.

Batterman, R. C.; DeGraff, A. C.; and Shorr, H. M.: Further observations on the use of mercupurin administered orally. *Am. Heart J.*, **31**:431, 1946.

Batterman, R. C., and Gutner, L. B.: Increasing congestive heart failure: a manifestation of digitalis toxicity. *Circulation*, **1**:1052, 1950.

Batterman, R. C.; Rose, A.; and DeGaff, A. C.: The combined use of ouabain and digitalis in the treatmet of congestive heart failure. *Am. Heart J.*, **22**:443, 1940.

Bayliss, R. I. S.; Etheridge, M. J.; Hyman, A. L.; Kelly, H. G.; McMichael, J.; and Reid, E. A. S.: The effect of digoxin on the right ventricular pressure in hypertensive and ischaemic heart failure. *Br. Heart J.*, **12**:317, 1950.

Beller, G. A.; Smith, T. W.; Abelmann, W. H.; Haber, E.; and Hood, W. B., Jr.: Digitalis intoxication: A prospective clinical study with serum level correlations. *N. Engl. J. Med.*, **284**:989, 1971.

Belsky, H.: Use of a new oral diuretic, Diamox, in congestive heart failure. *N. Engl. J. Med.*, **249**:140, 1953.

Benzing, G., III; Schubert, W.; Hug, G.; and Kaplan, S.: Simultaneous hypoglycemia and acute congestive heart failure. *Circulation*, **40**:209, 1969.

Berliner, R. W.: Renal mechanisms for potassium excretion. *Harvey Lect.*, **55**:141, 1961.

Beyer, K. H., and Baer, J. E.: Physiological basis for the action of newer diuretic agents. *Pharmacol. Rev.*, **13**:517, 1961.

Blumenthal, S., and Andersen, D. H.: Congestive heart failure in children. *J. Chronic Dis.*, **9**:590, 1959.

Braunwald, E.; Ross, J., Jr.; and Sonnenblick, E. H.: *Mechanisms of Contraction of the Normal and Failing Heart*, 2nd ed. Little, Brown and Company, Boston, 1976.

Bristow, J. D., and Metcalfe, J.: Physical signs in congestive heart failure. *Prog. Cardiovasc. Dis.*, **10**:236, 1967.

Burch, G. E.: Disturbance of water and sodium balance in congestive heart failure. *Mod. Concepts Cardiovasc. Dis.*, **17**:(n.p.), 1948.

Castleman, B., and McNeely, B. Y.: Case records of the Massachusetts General Hospital, Case 29-1967. *N. Engl. J. Med.*, **277**:92, 1967.

Cattell, M., and Gold, H.: Influence of digitalis glucosides on force of contraction of mammalian cardiac muscle, *J. Pharmacol. Exp. Ther.*, **62**:116, 1938.

Chamberlain, D. A.; White, R. J.; Howard, M. R.; and Smith, T. W.: Plasma digoxin concentrations in patients with atrial fibrillation. *Br. Med. J.*, **3**:329, 1970.

Chidsey, C. A.; Harrison, D. C.; and Braunwald, E.: Augmentation of failure, *N. Engl. J. Med.*, **267**:650, 1962.

Chung, E. K.: *Digitalis Intoxication*. Excerpta Medica Foundation, Amsterdam, 1969, p. 174.

Clarke, N. E., and Mosher, R. E.: The water and electrolyte content of the human heart in congestive heart failure with and without digitalization. *Circulation*, **5**:907, 1952.

Coltart, D. J.; Chamberlain, D. A.; Howard, M. R.; Kettlewell, M. G.; Mercer, J. L.; and Smith, T. W.: The effect of cardiopulmonary bypass on plasma digoxin concentrations. *Br. Heart J.*, **33**:334, 1971.

Cox, M. A.; Schiebler, G. L.; Taylor, W. J.; Wheat, M. W., Jr.; and Krovetz, L. J.: Reversible pulmonary hypertension in a child with respiratory obstruction and cor pulmonale. *J. Pediatr.*, **67**:192, 1965.

Danowski, T. S.: Electrolytes and congestive failure. *Ann. Intern. Med.*, **37**:453, 1952.

Doherty, J. E.; Perkins, W. H.; and Mitchell, G. K.: Tritiated digoxin studies in human subjects. *Arch. Intern. Med.*, **108**:531, 1961.

Domville Cook, W. D.: Prognostic significance of the serum protein content in premature babies and its relation to pulmonary hyaline membrane. Preliminary communication. *M. J. Aust.*, **1**:887, 1960.

Donald, K. W.: The Bradshaw lecture, 1958, Exercise and heart disease. *Br. Med. J.*, **1**:985, 1959.

————: Hemodynamics in chronic congestive heart failure. *J. Chronic Dis.*, **9**:476, 1959.

Donald, K. W.; Wormald, P. N.; Taylor, S. H.; and Bishop, J. M.: Changes in oxygen content of femoral venous blood and leg blood flow during leg exercise in relation of cardiac output response. *Clin. Sci.*, **16**:567, 1957.

Downing, S. E.; Talner, V. S.; and Gardner, T. H.: Ventricular function in the newborn lamb. *Am. J. Physiol.*, **208**:931, 1965.

Durant, T. M., and Harvey, W. F.: The treatment of cardiac decompensation; with special reference to resistant cases. *Med. Clin. North Am.*, **37**:971, 1953.

Earley, L. E.; Kahn, M.; and Orloff, J.: Effects of infusion of chlorothiazide on urinary dilution and concentration in the dog. *J. Clin. Invest.*, **40**:857, 1961.

Edelman, I. S.: Symposium: Water and electrolytes; pathogenesis of hyponatremia: Physiologic and therapeutic implications. *Metabolism*, **5**:500, 1956.

Editorial. Diamox (Acetazoleamide). *Can. Med. Assoc.*, **72**:780, 1955.

Enselberg, C. D., and Simmons, H. G.: Clinical experience with thiomerin. Observations on its use in 205 patients. *Am. J. Med. Sci.*, **219**:139, 1950.

Farber, S. J.; Alexander, J. D.; Pellegrino, E. D.; and Earle, D. P.: Effect of intravenously administered digoxin on water and electrolyte excretion and on renal functions. *Circulation*, **4**:378, 1951.

Fishman, A. P.: Congestive heart failure. Introduction to the symposium on congestive heart failure. *J. Chronic Dis.*, **9**:417, 1959.

Fleming, W. H., and Bowen, J. C.: The use of diuretics in the treatment of early wet lung syndrome. *Ann. Surg.*, **175**:505, 1972.

Fogelman, A. M.; Finkelstein, S.; La Mont, J. T.; Rado, E.; and Pearce, M. L.: Fallibility of plasma-digoxin in differentiating toxic from non-toxic patients. *Lancet*, **2**:727, 1971.

Fowler, R. S.; Rathi, L.; and Keith, J. D.: Accidental digitalis intoxication in children. *J. Pediatr.*, **64**:188, 1964.

Friedman, M., and Bine, R., Jr.: Observations concerning the influence of potassium upon the action of digitalis glycoside (lanaotoside). *Am. J. Med. Sci.*, **214**:633, 1947.

Friedman, W. F.; Pool, P. E.; Jacobowitz, D.; Seagren, S. E.; and Braunwald, E.: Sympathetic innervation of the developing rabbit heart. Biochemical and histochemical comparisons of fetal, neonatal, and adult myocardium. *Circ. Res.*, **23**:25, 1968.

Gold, H. (ed.): Most effective application of therapeutic measures in the management of congestive failure. *Cornell Conference on Therapy*, Vol. VII. Macmillan Publishing Co., Inc., New York, 1955; also in *Am. J. Med.*, **6**:118, 1954.

Gold, H.; Cattell, M.; et al.: A comparison of the speed, the intensity, and the duration of action of four digitalis glycosides by intravenous injection in man. *Proc. Soc. Exp. Biol. Med.*, **2**:80, 1943.

Goldblatt, E.: The treatment of cardiac failure in infancy, a review of 350 cases. *Lancet*, **2**:212, 1962.

Goldring, D.; Hernandez, A.; and Hartmann, A. F.: The critically ill child: Care of the infant in cardiac failure. *Pediatrics*, **47**:1056, 1971.

Guyton, A. C.: The systemic venous system in cardiac failure. *J. Chronic Dis.*, **9**:465, 1959.

Harrison, T. R.: *Failure of the Circulation*, 2nd ed. Williams & Wilkins Co., Baltimore, 1939 (1st ed., 1935).

Hauck, A. J., and Nadas, A. S.: Cardiac failure in infants and children. *Pediatr. Clin. North Am.*, **5**:1125, 1958.

Hauck, A. J.; Ongley, P. A.; and Nadas, A. S.: The use of digoxin in infants and children. *Am. Heart J.*, **56**:443, 1958.

Herrmann, G. R.; Baxter, M. R.; Hejtmacile, M. R.; and Moran, A. R.: Diamox. New oral nonmercurial, nontoxic diuretic for the treatment of congestive heart failure. *Texas J. Med.*, **50**:209, 1954.

Hope, J. A.: *A Treatise on the Disease of the Heart and Great Vessels.* William Kidd, London, 1832.

Huffman, D. H., and Azarnoff, D. L.: Absorption of orally given digoxin preparations. *JAMA*, **222**:957, 1972.

Jaffe, H. L.; Master, A. M.; and Dorrance, W.: The salt depletion syndrome following mercurial diuresis in elderly persons. *Am. J. Med. Sci.*, **220**:60, 1950.

Katz, L. N.; Katz, A. M.; and Williams, F. L.: Metabolic adjustments to alterations of cardiac work in hypoxaemia. *Am. J. Physiol.*, **181**:539, 1955.

Keith, J. D.: Congestive heart failure. Review article. *Pediatrics*, **18**:491, 1956.

Kempner, W.: Treatment of kidney disease and hypertensive vascular disease with rice diet. *N. C. Med. J.*, **5**:125, 273, 1944; **6**:61, 117, 1945.

Kidd, B. S. L., and Collins, J.: Personal communication, The Hospital for Sick Children, Toronto, Canada, 1964.

Kirkendall, W. M., and Stein, J. H.: Clinical pharmacology of furosemide and ethacrynic acid. *Am. J. Cardiol.*, **22**:162, 1968.

Korner, P., and Shillingford, J.: The right atrial pulse in congestive heart failure. *Br. Heart J.*, **16**:447, 1954.

Kreidberg, M. B., and Chernoff, H. L.: Cardiac failure in infants. *Tufts Folia Med.*, **8**:10, 1962.

Lees, M. H.: Heart failure in the newborn infant. *J. Pediatr.*, **75**:139, 1969.

Lely, A. H., and Van Enter, C. H.: Large-scale digitoxin intoxication. *Br. Med. J.*, **3**:737, 1970.

Lesser, G. T.; Dunning, M. F.; Epstein, F. H.; and Berger, E. Y.: Mercurial diuresis in edematous individuals. *Circulation*, **5**:85, 1952.

Levy, A. M.; Hanson, J. S.; and Tabakin, B. S.: Congestive heart failure in the newborn infant in the absence of primary cardiac disease. *Am. J. Cardiol.*, **26**:409, 1970.

Lown, B., and Levine, D. H.: *Atrial Arrhythmias, Digitalis and Potassium.* Landsburger Medical Books, Inc., New York, 1958.

Lown, B., and Levine, S. A.: Medical progress; current concepts in digitalis therapy. *N. Engl. J. Med.*, **250**:771, 819, 866, 1954.

Luisada, A. A.; Goldmann, M. A.; and Weyl, R.: Alcohol vapor by inhalation in the treatment of acute pulmonary edema. *Circulation*, **5**:363, 1952.

Lyons, R. H.; Jacobson, S. D.; and Avery, N. L.: Change in plasma volume and body weight in normal subjects after low salt diet, ammonium chloride and mercupurin. *Am. J. Med. Sci.*, **211**:460, 1946.

McCue, C. M., and Young, R. B.: Cardiac failure in infancy. *J. Pediatr.*, **58**:330, 1961.

Mackenzie, J.: *Diseases of the Heart*, 3rd ed. Henry Frowde. Hodder & Stoughton, Ltd., and Oxford University Press, London, 1913 (1st ed., 1908).

McKee, P. A.; Castelli, W. P.; McNamara, P. M.; and Kannel, W. B.: The natural history of congestive heart failure: The Framingham study. *N. Engl. J. Med.*, **285**:1441, 1971.

McMichael, J.: *Pharmacology of the Falling Heart.* Charles C. Thomas, Publisher, Springfield, Ill., 1950.

———: Dynamics of heart failure. *Br. Med. J.*, **2**:525, 578, 1952.

McNamara, D. G.; Brewer, E. J., Jr.; and Ferry, G. D.: Hazards to health; accidental poisoning of children with digitalis. *N. Engl. J. Med.*, **271**:1106, 1964.

Mason, D. T., and Braunwald, E.: Digitalis; new facts about an old drug; symposium on congestive heart failure II. *Am. J. Cardiol.*, **22**:151, 1968.

Mason, D. T.; Zelis, R.; Lee, G.; Hughes, J. L.; Spann, J. F., Jr.; and Amsterdam, E. A.: Current concepts and treatment of digitalis toxicity. *Am. J. Cardiol.*, **27**:546, 1971.

Menashe, V. D.; Farrehi, C.; and Miller, M.: Hypoventilation and cor pulmonale due to chronic upper airway obstruction. *J. Pediatr.*, **67**:198, 1965.

Meriwether, W. D.; Mangi, R. J.; and Serpick, A. A.: Deafness following standard intravenous dose of ethacrynic acid. *JAMA*, **216**:795, 1971.

Morrison, J.; Killip, T.; and Stason, W. B.: Serum digoxin levels in patients undergoing cardiopulmonary bypass (abstract). *Circulation*, **42**:110, 1970.

Moss, A. J., and Duffie, E. R., Jr.: Congestive heart failure in infancy: significance of the venous pressure. *J. Pediatr.*, **60**:346, 1962.

Nadas, A. S.; Daeschner, C. W.; Roth, A.; and Blumenthal, S. L.: Paroxysmal tachycardia in infants and children. Study of 41 cases. *Pediatrics*, **9**:167, 1952.

Nadas, A. S., and Hauck, A. J.: Pediatric aspects of congestive heart failure. *Circulation*, **21**:424, 1960.

Nadas, A. S.; Rudolph, A. M.; and Reinhold, J. D. L.: The use of digitalis in infants and children. A clinical study of patients in congestive heart failure. *N. Engl. J. Med.*, **248**:98, 1953.

Nayler, W. G.; McInnes, I.; Carson, V.; et al.: The effect of lignocaine on myocardial function, high energy phosphate stores and oxygen consumption: A comparison with propranolol. *Am. Heart J.*, **78**:338, 1969.

Noonan, J. A.: Reversible cor pulmonale due to hypertrophied tonsils and adenoids. Studies in two cases. *Am. Pediatr. Soc. Inc. Abstracts* (May 6–8), p. 48, 1965.

Paul, E. A., Jr., and Hurst, J. W.: Intractable heart failure and its management, *Med. Clin. North Am.*, **54**:309, 1970.

Pool, P. E.: Congestive heart failure: Biochemical and physiologic observations. *Am. J. Med. Sci.*, **258**:328, 1969.

Redfors, A.: Plasma digoxin concentration—its relation to digoxin dosage and clinical effects in patients with atrial fibrillation. *Br. Heart J.*, **34:**:383, 1972.

Reeves, T. J., and Hefner, L. L.: The effect of vagal stimulation on ventricular contractility. *Trans. Assoc. Am. Physicians*, **74**:260, 1961.

———: Isometric contraction and contractility in the intact mammalian ventricle. *Am. Heart J.*, **64**:525, 1962.

Reeves, T. J.; Hefner, L. L.; Jones, W. B.; Coghlan, C.; Prieto, G.; and Carroll, J.: The hemodynamic determinants of the rate of change in pressure in the left ventricle during isometric contraction. *Am. Heart J.*, **60**:745, 1960.

Richardson, H.: Furosemide in heart failure of infancy. *Arch. Dis. Child.*, **46**:420, 1971.

Robinson, S. J.: Treatment of congestive failure in children. *Am. Pract.*, **2**:696, 1951.

Rodensky, P. L., and Wasserman, F.: Observations on digitalis intoxication. *Arch. Intern. Med.*, **108**:171, 1961.

Rogers, M. C.; Willerson, J. T.; Goldblatt, A.; and Smith, T. W.: Serum digoxin concentrations in the human fetus, neonate and infant. *N. Engl. J. Med.*, **287**:1010, 1972.

Rowe, R. D.: Heart disease in the first year of life—a challenge. *Manitoba Med. Rev.*, **39**:485, 1959.

———: Congenital heart disease in the neonatal period. *N.Z. Med. J.*, **60**:469, 1961.

Rudolph, A. M.; Mesel, E.; and Levy, J. M.: Epinephrine in the treatment of cardiac failure due to shunts. *Circulation*, **28**:3, 1964.

Sampson, J. J.; Alberton, E. C.; and Kondo, B.: Effect on man of potassium administration in relation to digitalis glycosides: with special reference to blood serum potassium, electrocardiogram and ectopic beats. *Am. Heart J.*, **26**:164, 1943.

Sapin, S. O.: Digitalis therapy in pediatrics. *Q. Rev. Pediatr.*, **15**:41, 1960.

Sarnoff, S. J.: Myocardial contractility as described by ventricular function curves. *Physiol. Rev.*, **35**:107, 1955.

Sarnoff, S. J., and Mitchell, J. H.: The regulation of the performance of the heart. *Am. J. Med.*, **30**:747, 1961.

Schemm, F. R.: High fluid intake in management of edema, especially cardiac edema. I. Details and basis of regime. *Ann. Intern. Med.*, **17**:952, 1942; II. Clinical observations and data. *Ibid.*, **21**:937, 1944.

———: Certain clinical aspects of the application of water balance principles to heart and kidney disease. *Ann. Intern. Med.*, **30**:92, 1949.

Schroeder, H. A.: Studies on congestive heart failure. I. The importance of restriction of salt as compared to water. *Am. Heart J.*, **22**:141, 1941.

———: Renal insufficiency caused by overhydration or depression of sodium chloride: the 'low-salt syndrome.' *J. Clin. Invest.*, **28**:809, 1949.

Schwartz, W. B., and Relman, A. S.: Electrolyte disturbances in congestive heart failure: clinical significance and management. *JAMA*, **154**:1237, 1954.

Sears, W.; Mahon, W.; Olley, P.; and Wilson, T.: Serum digoxin concentrations in infants on maintenance digoxin (Abstract). *Proc. Can. Cardiovasc. Soc.*, p. 44, 1971.

Sellers, F.: Personal communication, Department of Pediatric Cardiology, University of Saskatchewan, Saskatoon, Canada, 1962.

Sharpey-Schafer, E. P., and Wallace, J.: Circulatory overloading following rapid intravenous injections. *Br. Med. J.*, **2**:304, 1942.

Smith, T. W.: The clinical use of serum cardiac glycoside concentration measurements. *Am. Heart J.*, **82**:833, 1971.

Smith, T. W.; Butler, V. P., Jr.; and Haber, E.: Determination of therapeutic and toxic serum digoxin concentrations by radioimmunoassay. *N. Engl. J. Med.*, **281**:1212, 1969.

Smith, T. W., and Haber, E.: Digoxin intoxication: The relationship of clinical presentation to serum digoxin concentration. *J. Clin. Invest.*, **49**:2377, 1970.

Smith, T. W., and Haber, E.: Current techniques for serum or plasma digitalis assay and their potential clinical application. *Am. J. Med. Sci.*, **259**:301, 1970.

Smith, T. W., and Haber, E.: Digitalis. *N. Engl. J. Med.*, **289**:945, 1010, 1063, and 1125, 1973.

Sodeman, W. A.: Diagnosis and treatment of digitalis toxicity. *N. Engl. J. Med.*, **273**:95, 1965.

Spann, J. F., Jr.; Mason, D. T.; and Zelis, R. F.: The altered performance of the hypertrophied and failing heart. *Am. J. Med. Sci.*, **258**:291, 1969.

Starling, E. H.: *The Linacre Lecture on the Law of the Heart, Cambridge, 1915.* Longmans, Green & Co., London, 1918.

Stroud, W. D., and Wagner, J. A.: Newer preparations of mercurial diuretics in congestive heart failure. *Med. Clin. North Am.*, **38**:431, 1954.

Talner, N. S.; Sanyal, S. K.; Halloran, K. H.; Gardner, T. H.; and Ordway, N. K.: Congestive heart failure in infancy. I. Abnormalities in blood gases and acid-base equilibrium. *Pediatrics*, **35**:20, 1965.

Taylor, P. M.; Wolfson, J. H.; Bright, N. H.; Birchard, E. L.; and Egan, T. J.: Umbilical vein pressure in congestive heart failure in the newborn infant. *Acta Paediatr.*, **50**:51, 1961.

Tikoff, G., and Juida, H.: Pathophysiology of heart failure in congenital heart disease. *Mod. Concepts Cardiovasc. Dis.*, **41**:1, 1972.

Ulrich, K. J.; Kramer, K.; and Boylan, J. W.: Present knowledge of the counter-current system in the mammalian kidney. *Prog. Cardiovasc. Dis.*, **3**:395, 1961.

Urquhart, J., and Davis, J. O.: Role of the kidney and the adrenal cortex in congestive heart failure. I and II. *Mod. Concepts Cardiovasc. Dis.*, **32**:781, 1963.

Vogel, J. H. K.; McNamara, D. G.; and Blount, S. G., Jr.: Role of hypoxia in determining pulmonary vascular resistance in infants with ventricular septal defects. *Am. J. Cardiol.*, **20**:346, 1967.

Walker, W. G., and Cooke, C. R.: Diuretics and electrolyte abnormalities in congestive heart failure. I. Sodium transport and congestive failure. *Mod. Concepts Cardiovasc. Dis.*, **34**:7, 1965.

———: Diuretics and electrolyte abnormalities in congestive heart failure. III. Electrolyte disturbances in congestive heart failure. *Mod. Concepts Cardiovasc. Dis.*, **34**:17, 1965.

Walker, W. G.; Cooke, C. R.; Payne, J. W.; Baker, C. R.; and Andrew, D. J.: Mechanism of renal potassium secretion studied by a modified stop-flow technique. *Am. J. Physiol.*, **200**:1133, 1961.

Walsh, B. J., and Sprague, H. B.: Character of congestive failure in children with active rheumatic fever. *Am. J. Dis. Child.*, **61**:1003, 1941.

Weiss, A., and Steigmann, F.: Gitalin in the treatment of congestive heart failure: a clinical study. *Am. J. Med. Sci.*, **227**:188, 1954.

Wheeler, E. O.; Bridges, W. C.; and White, P. D.: Diet low in salt (sodium) in congestive heart failure. *JAMA*, **133**:16, 1947.

White, J. J.; Chamberlain, D. A.; Howard, M.; and Smith, T. W.: Plasma concentrations of digoxin after oral administration in the fasting and postprandal state. *Br. Med. J.*, **1**:380, 1971.

White, P. D.: Clinical assessment of cardiac efficiency. *Practitioner*, **169**:5, 1952.

Wigle, E. D.; Heimbecker, R. O.; and Gunton, R. W.: Idiopathic ventricular septal hypertrophy causing muscular subaortic stenosis. *Circulation*, **26**:325, 1962.

Wilson, M. G.: *Rheumatic Fever: Studies of the Epidemiology, Manifestations, Diagnosis, and Treatment of the Disease during the First Three Decades.* Commonwealth Fund, London, Oxford, 1940, p. 419.

Withering, W.: *An account of the foxglove and some of its medical uses: With practical remarks on dropsy and other disease.* M. Swinney, London, 1785.

Woodson, R. D.; Torrance, J. D.; Shappell, S. D.; and Lenfant, C.: The effect of cardiac disease on hemoglobin-oxygen finding. *J. Clin. Invest.*, **49**:1349, 1970.

CHAPTER

11

The Distressed Newborn

Richard D. Rowe and *Teruo Izukawa*

ARDIAC malformations, as well as other disturbances in patients with architecturally normal hearts, can produce cardiorespiratory distress in the newborn period. In the past two decades developments in the diagnosis and treatment of congenital heart malformation have increasingly thrust the plight of the newly born patient to the attention of nurses, physicians, and pediatric cardiologists. It has long been appreciated that there is a high mortality among patients who present in congestive heart failure or with cyanosis and with congenital heart disease at that age. In recent years, refinements in diagnostic procedures, improvement of support measures available preoperatively as well as postoperatively, and daring surgical approaches not only have clarified the best management approach for these babies but also have begun to decrease mortality significantly. It has been shown by Lambert and associates (1966) and reemphasized by others (Rowe and Vlad, 1973; Miller, 1974) that among the newborn with congenital heart disease, infants in distress in the first week of life are at greatest

risk and that even here the majority are amenable to palliative or corrective surgery.

For some malformations, particularly those in which cardiac partitioning is grossly distorted, long survival is virtually impossible and the association of major extracardiac anomalies also influences mortality (Greenwood et al., 1975). The proportion of this untreatable group of all infants with cardiorespiratory distress has never been the majority and is becoming lower (Table 11–1). For us the diagnosis after cardiac catheterization probably gives the most useful indication of the frequency with which specific cardiac disorders present in clinical practice at our Institution, for it has been our policy to study by that technique all hypoxic infants with congenital heart disease and most infants in congestive heart failure. Though new techniques such as echocardiography may reduce the necessity for this form of intervention for certain conditions, the general trends displayed in such listings will probably continue to reflect the major cardiovascular malformation problems of this age period.

Table 11–1. INCIDENCE OF CARDIAC MALFORMATIONS DELINEATED AT CARDIAC CATHETERIZATION IN THE FIRST MONTH OF LIFE IN TWO CONSECUTIVE PERIODS, 1966–1969 AND 1970–1974, THE HOSPITAL FOR SICK CHILDREN

	1966–1969		1970–1974	
MALFORMATION	*Number*	*Percent of Total*	*Number*	*Percent of Total*
Transposition of the great arteries	81	21.0	101	17.4
Tetralogy of Fallot	47	12.0	41	7.1
Ventricular septal defect	29	7.5	65	11.2
Coarctation complex	29	7.5	79	13.6
Hypoplastic left heart syndrome	25	6.5	40	6.9
Patent ductus arteriosus	23	6.0	31	5.3
Single ventricle	20	5.0	30	5.2
Transitional circulation	20	5.0	31	5.3
Hypoplastic right heart	14	3.5	44	7.6
Persistent truncus arteriosus	11	2.8	10	1.7
AV canal defect	11	2.8	17	3.0
Tricuspid valve atresia	10	2.5	12	2.1
Others	69	17.9	79	13.6
	389	100.0	580	100.0

BROAD DIAGNOSIS

Clinical Features

The distressed newborn who is deeply cyanotic or in marked congestive heart failure represents a patient in a relatively late stage of a cardiac disorder. The indications at that point of the clinical picture are self-evident to even the lay public. Part of the problem in early recognition lies in the fact that the physical signs of the cardiovascular system normally change after birth during transition of the cardiovascular system from a fetal to postnatal life. The physical signs of both the normal and the abnormal newborn infant, such as right ventricular overactivity, behavior of the second heart sound, and color of the mucous membranes, are governed largely by the level of pulmonary artery pressure, the rate of constriction of the ductus arteriosus, the metabolic status of the infant, and the amount of placental transfusion. These important variables can add to or mask physical signs in the infant with congenital heart disease.

The most severe congenital heart diseases in early infancy are not associated with loud murmurs, and many malformations that eventually are associated with loud murmurs most often do not show them immediately after birth.

Heart sounds in most patients with congenital heart disease of a serious nature are abnormal and loud; these sounds, together with a rapid rate, may constitute the first sign of serious illness. A gallop rhythm is an extremely helpful sign that indicates the presence of congestive heart failure. The presence of a single heart sound after the first 12 hours of life is almost always abnormal and should stimulate a search for other signs suggestive of cardiopulmonary disease. An ejection click is normally noted only during the first few hours of life, when it may accompany the normal hypertension that characterizes the transitional pulmonary circulation. Thereafter, the presence of a loud click may signify a large aorta, such as in pulmonary atresia, a large pulmonary artery, as in the hypoplastic left heart syndrome, or a large single vessel, as in truncus arteriosus.

In the newborn period there is a considerable propensity for peripheral cyanosis; blood arterial oxygen tensions are significantly lower shortly after birth than they will be several days later (Table 11–2, page 187). Cardiac malformations that are usually associated with severe arterial oxygen desaturation later in the neonatal period may present in the first few days of life in a relatively acyanotic form owing to the good mixing of oxygenated and unoxygenated blood that can result temporarily from continued patency of the ductus arteriosus or foramen ovale.

Reduced amplitude of arterial pulses is always an important sign in this age group and implies reduced cardiac output into the aorta; this may result from anatomic malformations, such as hypoplastic left ventricle, severe aortic stenosis, and coarctation of the aorta, or from acute left ventricular failure due to other causes, such as ischemic heart disease. Bounding pulses usually imply a large aortic run-off such as is seen with a large patent ductus arteriosus or a truncus arteriosus.

Tachypnea is a useful sign of cardiopulmonary difficulty. Respiratory rates in excess of 50 per minute usually mean that a cardiopulmonary disorder is present. Tachypnea without much respiratory effort is characteristic of congenital heart disease of the congestive type. In severe pulmonary disturbances, obvious labored respiration is a striking feature.

A large liver in addition to other signs suggesting heart disease usually indicates congestive heart failure, although enlarged livers may be encountered in a variety of other conditions in the newborn period.

The chest film has long been considered an unreliable aid in the detection of cardiac malformations. However, if good-quality films of newborn infants are obtained under optimal conditions, it may be possible to obtain very useful information about the heart (O'Hara et al., 1965). Although many patients with congenital heart disease have normal-appearing chest films, the newborn infant with serious congenital heart disease usually does not. Cardiomegaly is almost always present before the diagnosis of congestive heart failure can be made with certainty in the newborn infant. In frankly cyanotic infants, cardiomegaly or a strikingly unusual cardiac contour is often present. Because lung vascular markings are particularly difficult to evaluate in the newborn infant, roentgen interpretation may be erroneous and on occasion quite opposite to that which actually exists hemodynamically. Interpretation of such films is greatly assisted by the clinical evaluation of the baby. For example, the presence of considerable cyanosis in association with normal-appearing lung vascular markings favors the possibility of a transposition complex; the presence of severe cyanosis in association with extreme pulmonary stenosis is associated with oligemic lungs.

Moës (1975) provides a comprehensive review of the subject and readers are referred to that publication for detail. He emphasizes that although the patient with congenital heart disease does usually show abnormal cardiac configuration, important diagnostic difficulties arise because in the early newborn period the chest film may be normal and only later change (as is often the case in transposition of the great arteries) or may have an abnormal configuration in the absence of a heart malformation. Diagnostic nihilism with respect to x-ray films can be avoided by detailed consideration of cardiac contour, lung vascular pattern, abdominal and cardiac situs, and the appearance of thoracic cage, and by good communication between the clinician and the radiologist.

Electrocardiography

Severe congenital heart disease is usually associated with an abnormal electrocardiogram but in the first few days of life abnormal right ventricular hypertrophy is difficult to interpret. Reliance has then to be placed on relatively subtle changes such as an abnormal frontal plane QRS axis, the presence of q waves in V_3R and V_1, or abnormally peaked P waves. After 72 hours, an upright TV_1 is a useful sign of moderate right ventricular hypertrophy. The presence of left ventricular hypertrophy, on the other hand, is easily recognized on the newborn infant's electrocardiogram. Detailed consideration of the many variables in the abnormal tracing of newborn infants with heart disease has been given by Hastreiter and Arcilla (1971).

Blood Measurements

Particular benefit to the diagnosis and management of the distressed newborn is derived from measurement iof arterial blood gases and acid-base balance (Table 11–2). In this way arterial oxygen desaturation can be quantified and the response to high oxygen breathing evaluated and acidosis combated. There is much debate about the best site to sample because the inviting umbilical cord artery sample may be affected by a fetal direction of flow through the ductus arteriosus. Samples from the right radial or brachial artery or temporal vessels better indicate the oxygen tension of blood leaving the left heart. Hyperoxic studies can be very useful in distinguishing transitional disturbances from true major cardiac malformations of the cyanotic type when a low PaO_2 is discovered so long as the sampling is obtained in an appropriate fashion (Table 11–3). Values of PaO_2 during hyperoxia in excess of 100 mm of mercury exclude transposition of the great arteries and usually give some relief to the consideration of the need for immediate cardiac catheterization. Blood sampling for other measurements, including blood sugar, calcium, and magnesium, have likewise been useful in therapy.

Table 11–2. ARTERIAL BLOOD GASES AS MEASURED IN NORMAL NEWBORNS FROM BIRTH TO THE FIRST WEEK OF LIFE*

	BIRTH	1 HR	24 HR	7 DAYS
pH	7.26	7.30	7.39	7.4
PO_2 (mm Hg)	23	65	75	95
PCO_2 (mm Hg)	55	40	35	36
Base excess (mEq/L)	−5	−7	−4	−2

* Modified from Swyer, P. (1975).

Echocardiography

The advent of echocardiographic applications for the distressed newborn brings a new dimension to diagnosis. Indicative of its success as a tool in this area is its now almost universal application to the problem. Particularly impressive is its usefulness in hypoplastic right and left heart syndromes, tetralogy of Fallot, truncus arteriosus, and transposition of the great arteries. Serial study of left-to-right shunts, particularly patent ductus arteriosus of premature infants, is also of great help. That is not to say that the method is infallible or that in every institution the diagnostic answer will be forthcoming. A high degree of expertise and a nice judgment are required in order that there be minimum delay in proceeding to the catheterization laboratory when that route is indicated. With these reservations the importance of the method to diagnosis in this age period cannot be overestimated. Future improvements in multiscanning techniques will likely change diagnostic accuracy and the ease of its application even more.

Cardiac Catheterization and Angiocardiography

This technique is still the "gold standard" by which others may be judged. Rather than becoming less useful with the emergence of newer ancillary diagnostic procedures, cardiac catheterization has assumed a fresh importance. Other procedures are aimed at either avoiding unnecessary cardiac

Table 11–3. HYPEROXIC TEST IN THE CYANOTIC NEWBORN*

BLOOD GASES	A D-TRANSPOSITION OF THE GREAT ARTERIES		B NEONATAL SEPSIS	
	Room Air	80 percent O_2 by Hood	Room Air	80 percent O_2
PO_2 (mm Hg)	19	17	46	216
PCO_2 (mm Hg)	36	39	26	28
pH	7.22	7.27	7.38	7.44
HCO_3 (mEq/L)	22	17	15	15

* Arterial blood gases taken in room air and while breathing 80 percent oxygen by hood. *A* was 12 hours old when admitted with cyanosis. Preliminary investigations including echocardiography suggested a diagnosis of D-*transposition of the great arteries*. Despite administration of 80 percent oxygen by hood, the PO_2 remained quite low. Cardiac catheterization confirmed the diagnosis. *B* was a day-old male infant admitted lethargic, jaundiced, mildly cyanosed, and with hepatosplenomegaly. Investigations revealed infection with the *cytomegalovirus*. There was a significant rise in arterial oxygen tension with administration of oxygen.

catheterization or facilitating and shortening the procedure through narrowing the diagnostic possibilities ahead of time. The increasing ability of surgeons to palliate or repair serious congenital heart disease at this age means that more detailed anatomic information is required preoperatively. Better maintenance of infants during study, an ability to enter hitherto inaccessible areas of the central circulation, the availability of a variety of indicators for studying the circulatory pathways, the improved resolution of image intensifiers, and other technical improvements in angiocardiographic technique have all brought about great changes in the type of data that cardiac catheterization can reveal. It is now more important than ever that such sophisticated studies be performed in centers fully equipped to evaluate a baby at any hour to the fullest degree necessary. The

day of the occasional newborn cardiac catheterization in a peripheral institution is over.

It is important to appreciate that, in addition to the problems of separating severe cardiac malformation from the distressed infant with no malformation in the first week of life, there is also difficulty in deciding whether an infant with clear-cut evidence of congenital heart disease has a relatively mild or moderately severe defect or whether early absence of symptoms will soon be replaced by more important events such as congestive failure. The physical signs that assist in such cases are often subtle and sometimes may be misleading. Full utilization of blood gas studies, chest films, electrocardiography, and echocardiography, as well as serial, physical, and ancillary examinations, are important in resolving the diagnostic dilemma in such instances.

NONSTRUCTURAL HEART DISEASE

Respiratory Distress Syndrome

This respiratory disorder occurs in 14 percent (Usher, 1961b) to 33 percent (Swyer, 1974) of premature live births, but infrequently (0.2 percent) in term infants (Swyer, 1974).

A deficiency of lung surfactant, as a result of immaturity and intranatal stress, leads to alveolar atelectasis. Hypoxia resulting from perfusion of poorly ventilated areas of the lung leads to pulmonary arteriolar vasoconstriction (Dawes, 1962; Strang, 1966). Right-to-left shunting occurs at the foramen ovale, ductus arteriosus, and in the lung early in the disease because of increase in the pulmonary vascular resistance. With the collapse of alveoli, shunting becomes mainly intrapulmonary (Swyer et al., 1973). On the way to recovery, a variable left-to-right shunt may occur and persist for a time. There is some evidence, however, that left-to-right shunting may occur early in the disease in some cases (Thibeault et al., 1975).

Tachypnea will be apparent from birth or shortly after. With progression, subcostal and intercostal indrawing, edema, and sternal recession will appear. Central cyanosis occurs in a few hours. Signs of cardiac decompensation do not occur unless a large left-to-right ductal shunt occurs in the recovery phase.

In 85 percent or more cases, chest x-ray will confirm the diagnosis (Swyer, 1974). A granular pattern in inspiration or a uniform opacity in expiration along with an air bronchogram is a typical sign. The electrocardiographic changes have not been sufficiently specific to aid in the diagnosis (Keith et al., 1961; Usher, 1961a).

In treatment, oxygen, relief of acidosis, and assisted ventilation, when necessary, are most important (Swyer, 1974). To the present, drug therapy for pulmonary vasoconstriction has not altered the course (Eshaghpour et al., 1967). The need for surgery and timing in the treatment of patent ductus

arteriosus complicating respiratory distress syndrome has been controversial (Krovetz and Rowe, 1972; Lees, 1975; Neal et al., 1975; Thibeault et al., 1975), but with the advent of pharmacologic intervention may soon be an academic question (Friedman et al., 1976; Heyman et al., 1976). Maximum mortality occurs at the peak of clinical symptoms in the second day; survivors usually run a course of five days, but a more severe and prolonged course can result in lung damage particularly where oxygen and assisted ventilation have been required.

Polycythemia

In the normal newborn infant, the hemoglobin and hematocrit levels tend to be high. At birth the hemoglobin range is 13 to 20 gm percent and the hematocrit 45 to 65 percent (Nelson, 1975). Among a group of infants with polycythemia and the hyperviscosity syndrome with symptoms, the range of hematocrit was 63 to 77 percent and polycythemia was defined as a venous hematocrit of 65 percent or greater (Gross et al., 1973).

The hyperviscosity syndrome is characterized by signs and symptoms that include cyanosis and/or plethora, with the former usually peripheral. About three-quarters of one group had neurologic signs and symptoms (Gross et al., 1973; Kontros, 1972) including seizures. Fifty percent had cardiopulmonary symptoms and signs such as respiratory distress, tachycardia, and congestive heart failure. The heart is frequently enlarged (Figure 11–1 *B*, page 190). A diagnosis of cyanotic congenital heart disease was made in some patients (Gatti et al., 1966). Hyperbilirubinemia and hypoglycemia have been noted.

Laboratory investigations show increased viscosity when compared to the normal. Permanent sequelae may occur in the infants. Partial exchange transfusion will improve the viscosity.

A number of causes or associations with neonatal polycythemia are known:

1. Transfusion from the placenta (Oh et al., 1966; Moss and Monsel-Couchard, 1967; Lind, 1968), from a twin (Minkowski, 1962), or from the mother (Michael and Mauer, 1961).

2. Relative intrauterine hypoxia may increase erythropoietin production and produce polycythemia (Gatti et al., 1966).

3. Small size for gestational age (Cornblath and Schwartz, 1966).

Infants of Diabetic Mothers

Pregnancy is a hazardous period for the diabetic mother and perinatal mortality is higher in the diabetic because of the increased incidence of complications during pregnancy, cesarean sections, and premature births. The neonatal mortality has dropped from 40 percent to 10 percent (Fletcher, 1975).

The typical diabetic infant is large for gestational age (approximately one-third of the infants). Increased size of cells and their nuclei was noted in certain organs (e.g., liver, 179 percent; thymus, 137 percent; adrenal, 158 percent; lung, 127 percent; and heart, 174 percent). The heart is larger than expected for the gestational age (Naeye, 1965). Congestive heart failure due to a hypertrophic cardiomyopathy in some infants has been reported (Gutgesell et al., 1976).

Reports on the incidence of congenital anomalies vary from slightly increased (Gellis and Hsia, 1959; Pederson et al., 1964) to the 20 percent reported by Breidahl (1966). No organ system is spared, but the cardiac and spinal abnormalities appear the most frequent (Fletcher, 1975). A prospective study revealed the risk of congenital heart disease in the offspring of diabetic mothers to be 1:39 (Mitchell, 1972), whereas a retrospective study at the Joslin Clinic uncovered a 4 percent incidence of congenital heart disease, five times the incidence in the general population (Rowland et al., 1973). Ventricular septal defects and transposition of the great arteries are the common defects (Rowe and Mehrizi, 1968).

Special metabolic problems occur in the infant of a diabetic mother that influence cardiac function:

Hypoglycemia. Approximately, 50 percent of these newborn infants have glucose concentrations below 30 mg percent in the first six hours of life, (Cornblath and Schwartz, 1966). Symptoms may include jitteriness, tremors, convulsions, sweating, cyanosis, and limpness.

Hypoglycemia may accompany acute congestive heart failure (Benzing, 1969) and produce cardiac enlargement clinically and by chest x-ray (Amatayakul et al., 1970; Reid et al., 1970).

Hypocalcemia. Low calcium associated with neuromuscular irritability may occur in the infants (up to 23 percent of the group) (Warner and Cornblath, 1969).

Transient Myocardial Ischemia of the Newborn

Clinical recognition of the cardiovascular changes induced by hypoxia in the term newborn has been noted for two decades (James and Rowe, 1957; Rowe, 1959). Persisting high pulmonary vascular resistance leads to maintenance of fetal-type circulation in severe cases. Cyanosis, respiratory distress, and congestive heart failure suggested the possibility of cyanotic congenital heart disease (Robertson et al., 1967). When this condition was prolonged, fatalities occurred (Siassi et al., 1971).

A further extension of the circulatory disturbance caused by neonatal hypoxia was described in 1972 (Rowe and Hoffman, 1972). Three patients presented with signs suggestive of the hypoplastic left heart syndrome in the first day of life, with cyanosis, severe right heart failure, and low output of the left heart. Weak arterial pulses and low blood pressure with auscultatory evidence of pulmonary hypertension were present. Murmur of atrioventricular valve regurgitation was prominent. The electrocardiogram revealed variable ischemic changes with T wave inversion over the inferior or posterior or lateral leads and abnormal Q waves. Cardiomegaly and venous congestion were noted on x-ray (Figure 11–3B, page 192). There is mounting evidence that ischemic changes in the right ventricle create tricuspid regurgitation in these distressed term infants (Bucciarelli et al., 1977). Evidence supporting an ischemic basis for these findings has recently been obtained from myocardial perfusion scanning (Rowe et al., unpublished observations).

Echocardiography and isotope angiocardiography may exclude anatomic cardiac abnormalities, and cardiac catheterization most certainly does. On the cineangiocardiogram, a striking feature has been the poor contractility of the left ventricle.

Therapy with oxygen, digoxin, and a diuretic agent will support the ill neonate until the effects of hypoxia subside within days to a week. The electrocardiogram and the chest x-ray evidence of heart failure will revert to normal within three months.

HEART MALFORMATIONS

Frank Cyanosis Early in the Newborn Period (First Week)

Two of the several anatomic lesions that cause cyanosis early in the newborn period are in the first ten malformations listed in terms of frequency at cardiac catheterization in the first month of life (Table 11–1). Transposition of the great arteries ranks first in incidence and the hypoplastic right heart (ventricle) syndrome in ninth place.

Transposition of the Great Arteries. This description concerns neonates with reversal of the origin of the great arteries as the major defect. Physiologically, the systemic and the pulmonary circulations run in parallel instead of running in series. The necessary connections between the two circuits are dependent on the patency of the fetal pathways across the patent ductus arteriosus and the patent foramen ovale. Hypoxia develops when the fetal connections become inadequate or close within a few days of birth. In a few cases, the natural connections may remain adequate for one to four weeks. Additional defects such as the ventricular septal defect will allow greater obligatory mixing between the two circuits. Most patients are males of good size at birth. Associated extracardiac anomalies are rare.

Related to the inadequacy of mixing between the circuits is the degree of cyanosis, which is the major sign from birth. In those with an intact ventricular septum and without pulmonary stenosis, murmurs are absent or trivial. Congestive heart failure may appear at this time.

Classically, the chest x-ray, after the first week, shows an egg-shaped heart tilted on its side with a narrow supracardiac segment or pedicle, and increased vascularity (Figure 11–1A). In the first few days, the heart is nearly normal in size, shape, and vascular markings. The electrocardiogram in the majority without additional lesions will present with right-axis deviation and right ventricular hypertrophy. A small number may have left-axis deviation.

Arterial oxygen tension, a crucial investigation, will show values of 15 to 30 mm of mercury with little effect on breathing 80 to 100 percent oxygen.

Echocardiography, especially of the two-dimensional type, is a useful aid to diagnosis.

The normal size and apparent well-being of these infants can deceive physicians into delaying transfer, and sudden deterioration may occur due to hypoxia and acidosis. These patients constitute a major medical emergency and require prompt diagnostic confirmation and balloon atrial septostomy.

Hypoplastic Right Ventricle Syndrome. The main feature of this syndrome is a small right ventricle of varying severity usually associated with pulmonary valve stenosis. There may be accompanying hypoplasia of the tricuspid valve and ring; the smaller the right ventricle, the smaller the ring and valve.

In 20 percent, there is atresia of the main pulmonary artery without detectable pulmonary valve atresia. Although in the majority the right ventricle is small, a small group have normal or near-normal chamber sizes (Elliott et al., 1963). The enlarged right atrium has an exit route through the foramen ovale or occasionally through an atrial septal defect.

On examination, most patients are cyanotic soon after birth, but the degree of cyanosis varies with the patency and flow across the ductus arteriosus. Prominent "a" waves may be visible in the jugular veins. The liver may be enlarged as congestive heart failure develops in time. The second heart sound is

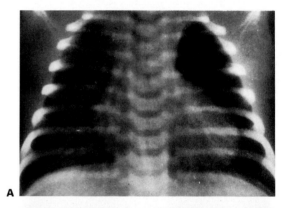

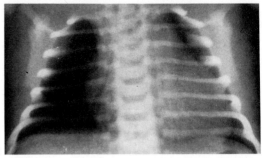

Figure 11-1. *A.* A 2-day-old infant with *D-transposition of the great arteries.* The heart is enlarged and egg-shaped and the vascular markings are increased.
B. A day-old female infant admitted with cyanosis and cardiomegaly. On the chest x-ray, there is cardiac enlargement and mild prominence of the pulmonary vessels. On the basis of a hemoglobin of 21.7 gm percent, the diagnosis of polycythemia was made along with transient myocardial ischemia, as shown by T wave inversion in the electrocardiogram leads I, aV_L, and V_1 to V_7.

single and aortic ejection clicks are common. There may be no murmur, a variable mid and late systolic murmur of tricuspid valve regurgitation, or less likely a faint continuous murmur of flow through the patent ductus arteriosus.

In the chest x-ray the majority of patients show cardiomegaly with a prominent right atrium and oligemic lung fields (Figure 11–2A). Electrocardiographic estimation of the chamber size is possible. Normal ventricular or right ventricular hypertrophy patterns indicate a reasonable-sized ventricular cavity. Left ventricular hypertrophy suggests a small right ventricle (Celermajer et al., 1968). Exceptions to these generalizations occur.

Echocardiography demonstrates the small tricuspid valve and right ventricle.

At cardiac catheterization, giant "a" waves may be present in the right atrium, and the mean right atrial pressure will exceed the mean left atrial pressure. Right ventricular pressure is elevated over the left ventricular or aortic pressure (e.g., 120 to 140 mm of mercury in the right ventricle to 60 to 70 mm of mercury systolic in the left ventricle) (Rowe and

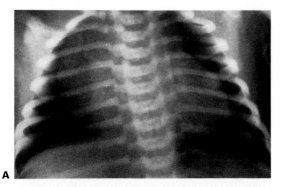

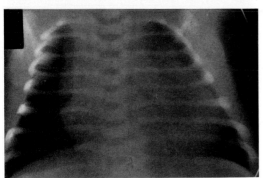

Figure 11-2. *A.* This day-old female was admitted with severe cyanosis and bradycardia. Cardiac catheterization revealed the diagnosis of *pulmonary valve atresia with intact ventricular septum* and a small right ventricle. The marked cardiomegaly is due to the large right atrium at the right border. Peripheral lung fields are clear.
B. Four-hour-old male born by elective cesarean section because of toxemia and previous cesarean sections. He was hypoxic at birth and had ascites. At a year, the heart was considered to be normal. Much of the cardiomegaly on the chest x-ray is considered due to the *thymus.* The lung fields are clear.

Mehrizi, 1968). Angiographic evidence from right and left ventricular injections is most helpful.

Others. There are several less common types of cyanotic congenital heart diseases that can present early.

Although the classic case of *Ebstein's anomaly of the tricuspid valve* may be diagnosed readily, in this period the condition may not be so apparent. Cardiomegaly, clear lung fields and right atrial hypertrophy may be of use in the diagnosis. Congestive failure is rare.

A severely ill newborn with severe cyanosis may have *total anomalous pulmonary venous return* almost always entering the systemic veins below the diaphragm. The chest x-ray is most helpful, showing pulmonary venous congestion and slight cardiomegaly (Figure 11-4*A*, page 193), and the electrocardiogram shows right ventricular dominance or hypertrophy.

Tricuspid valve atresia is a third example of a less common malformation that may present early with cyanosis. Most characteristic is the electro-cardiogram showing left-axis deviation and left ventricular hypertrophy.

Frank Cyanosis Late in the Newborn Period (One to Four Weeks)

Into this category are placed the more complex lesions with pulmonary stenosis that develop cyanosis with increasing time and obstruction.

An example is tetralogy of Fallot, where cyanosis on crying may be the first sign progressing to cyanotic spells that require urgent treatment. The heart is quiet, and the second sound is single or widely split with a soft pulmonary closure sound. An ejection systolic murmur varying with the severity of the stenosis is heard at the left sternal border. The electrocardiogram shows right ventricular hypertrophy and, in about half, a transitional zone over the right precordial leads.

When this defect is suspected, early investigation by cardiac catheterization will be helpful in future management as for example in deciding whether palliative surgery or total correction should be employed. An unfavorable anatomy will discourage early correction.

Congestive Heart Failure Early in the Newborn Period (First Week)

Two main groups of cardiac defects without significant cyanosis but which cause congestive heart failure occur in the immediate newborn group. The first includes the cases with small left ventricle and ascending aorta in the term "hypoplastic left heart syndrome." A similar broad category is incorporated in the coarctation of the aorta syndrome (Lev, 1952; Noonan and Nadas, 1958).

Hypoplastic Left Heart Syndrome. In this syndrome with small left ventricle, mitral valve and ring, and ascending aorta, the commonest group has congenital aortic valve atresia. A tiny cavity with a thick wall or only a potential cavity may constitute the left ventricle. Endocardial fibroelastosis of the endocardium is noted in half the hearts and also only in the presence of a patent mitral valve. Mitral atresia occurs in one-quarter of the patients or the mitral valve, if patent, is small. Only 10 percent of the hearts show a ventricular septal defect. In the majority (85 percent) the atrial septum is patent (15 percent with a true atrial septal defect), but in 15 percent this septum is intact (Rowe and Mehrizi, 1968).

The reported incidence of the major defect, aortic valve atresia, is 1.5 percent or 221 in 15,104 cases of congenital heart disease in Toronto. Congestive heart failure appears early and develops rapidly with the average age at death lying between four and five days (Watson and Rowe, 1962). At birth, the condition and weight of the infant appear normal. Within the first two days, varying degrees of cyanosis appear and the cyanosis becomes progressive with increasing age

(Krovetz et al., 1972). Tachypnea is invariably present from shortly after birth, but right-sided heart failure may not be apparent for two to three days. An important physical sign, along with the congestive heart failure, is the presence of poor peripheral pulses. Associated with this is an overactive precordium. On auscultation, the second sound is loud and single in the pulmonary area and a pulmonary ejection click may be present. A soft pulmonary ejection systolic flow murmur may be present at the left sternal border.

Roentgenogram of the chest demonstrates marked cardiomegaly and increased vascular markings and pulmonary congestion by the time congestive heart failure is recognized (Figure 11–3A). A barium swallow probably will show normal left atrial size and normal descending aorta despite an associated coarctation of the aorta.

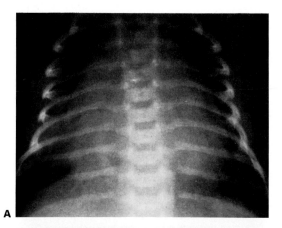

A

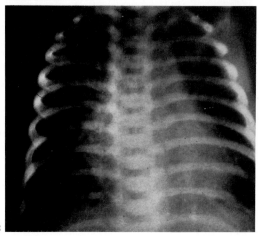

B

Figure 11-3.   *A.* Five-day-old male who developed respiratory distress and rapidly became shocked. Signs suggested the *hypoplastic left heart syndrome,* which was confirmed by echocardiography. Chest x-ray shows cardiomegaly and a hazy right border with congestion and collapse in the right lung.
B. A day-old infant with the history, signs, and clinical course of *transient myocardial ischemia.* Observe the cardiomegaly and the pulmonary venous congestion obscuring the cardiac borders.

In the majority, the electrocardiogram will show right-axis deviation, right atrial enlargement, and right ventricular hypertrophy, and a Q-R pattern in the right precordial leads. Ten percent, however, show left-axis deviation and rarely left ventricular hypertrophy, which is due to a thick left ventricular wall (Rowe and Mehrizi, 1968).

Echocardiography demonstrates the small left-sided structures nicely.

Treatment of the congestive heart failure with digitalis, diuretics, and oxygen will not improve the heart failure appreciably. In some, transient improvement may occur when the atrial connection is enlarged by creating an atrial septal defect. Physiologically, the pulmonary blood flow must be controlled and adequate systemic perfusion must be provided with banding of the pulmonary artery branches for the former and creation of a central shunt for the latter. The ascending aorta must be adequate to receive a shunt (Cayler et al., 1970; Krovetz et al., 1970). Such theoretic grounds for surgical intervention are appropriate for so very few patients that prognosis is extremely poor.

Coarctation of the Aorta Syndrome. In the newborn period, coarctation of the aorta as an isolated lesion producing heart failure is rare. However, when there are associated intracardiac defects, serious difficulties may develop early. The classification into the preductal or postductal type becomes unnecessary when it is now apparent that associated defects occur mainly with the preductal type and that in a recent theory, the anatomic setting for coarctation is produced in the fetus by the infolding of the aortic wall opposite to the entrance of the ductus arteriosus when there is abnormal flow through the ductus (Hutchins, 1971). In order of frequency, the cardiac defects associated with coarctation of the aorta are patent ductus arteriosus, ventricular septal defect, complete transposition of the great arteries, bicuspid aortic valve, mitral valve disease (Ferencz et al., 1953; Wood et al., 1975), and aortic stenosis (Smith and Matthews, 1955).

The onset of congestive heart failure in newborns with this malformation is about seven days. In the clinical diagnosis the main sign is the absence or faint pulses in the leg as compared to the arms. Small pressure difference between the leg and arm indicate that a large ventricular septal defect or patent ductus arteriosus is present. A large pressure difference with hypertension in the arm indicates an intact ventricular septum (Rowe, 1970). In the presence of a patent ductus arteriosus, the femoral pulses may change in quality from hour to hour depending on the degree of patency of the ductus arteriosus. On auscultation, a gallop rhythm may be present. There may be no murmurs, or there may be systolic murmurs of a ventricular septal defect or atrioventricular valve regurgitation.

The heart in congestive heart failure will be enlarged on the chest x-ray and there will be pulmonary congeston and increased flow in the

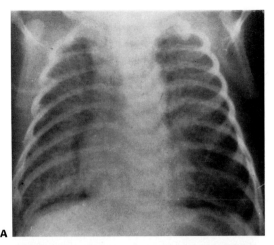

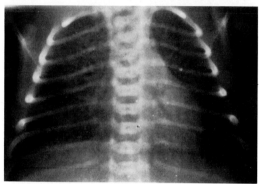

Figure 11-4. *A.* A day-old female noted to be cyanosed from birth. Postmortem examination confirmed the suspected diagnosis of *total anomalous pulmonary venous atresia*. Normal heart size with marked pulmonary venous and interstitial congestion is apparent.
B. This one-day-old premature male was admitted with tachypnea at three hours of life. A diagnosis of neonatal asphyxia and *transient tachypnea* of the newborn was made. On the chest x-ray, the normal heart size and the interstitial congestion in the upper lobes particularly are noted.

presence of a left-to-right shunt. An enlarged left atrium is common.

In cases with associated defects, the electrocardiogram almost always shows right ventricular hypertrophy. Both combined ventricular hypertrophy and left ventricular hypertrophy alone are uncommon at this age.

The echocardiogram usually shows an enlarged right ventricle and left atrial enlargement but is not specifically diagnostic.

Early investigation, after instituting antifailure measures, by cardiac catheterization is important to determine the associated malformations. In the majority with associated anomalies, early operative intervention will be required for survival. Resection of the coarctation of the aorta, ligation of the ductus, and banding of the pulmonary arteries for the control of ventricular septal defect are

necessary when the three defects are present. For patients with aortic stenosis, preliminary resection of the coarctation will be needed before dealing with the aortic stenosis.

Congestive Heart Failure Late in the Newborn Period (One to Four Weeks)

The two major malformations that produce congestive heart failure in this period, ventricular septal defect and patent ductus arteriosus, are unlikely to be diagnosed as being in heart failure before the second week of life.

Ventricular Septal Defect. Statistics from the Johns Hopkins Hospital indicate that in the first month of life in those with isolated ventricular septal defect, congestive heart failure occurred on the average at 15 days of life (Rowe, 1970). As the pulmonary vascular resistance is still elevated because of the increased pulmonary flow, the physical signs are modified. Often, the systolic murmur is not pansystolic but shortened and the pulmonary second sound is accentuated. The middiastolic murmur is not present usually. Unlike the electrocardiogram of the large shunt later in the neonatal period, when combined ventricular hypertrophy appears, only right ventricular hypertrophy may present.

In the situation where the signs of a large ventricular septal defect are atypical, cardiac catheterization is essential. If, on the angiographic measurement of a clearly delineated defect, the diameter is greater than three-fourths of the diameter of the aortic root, most cases will require surgical treatment early (Rowe, 1970).

Patent Ductus Arteriosus. Transient continuous murmurs of a patent ductus arteriosus can be detected in about 15 percent of term newborn infants up to the age of 12 hours (Braudo and Rowe, 1961). Spontaneous closure of the persistent ductus arteriosus in the term infant may occur before the third month of life; surgery will be required usually thereafter (Rowe and Neill, 1971). In one survey of 100 newborn premature infants weighing less than 2500 gm, 18 (18 percent) had murmurs of a patent ductus arteriosus apparent in the first two weeks of life usually (Clarkson and Orgill, 1974). Two of these had the idiopathic respiratory distress syndrome, only three had a significant left-to-right shunt, and only one developed heart failure. Other series of premature infants place the incidence at between 15 percent (Kitterman et al., 1972) and 19 percent (Girling and Hallidie–Smith, 1971). Of 396 newborns with respiratory distress syndrome 76 (19 percent) developed signs of a patent ductus arteriosus. Fifteen of the seventy-six (20 percent) developed congestive heart failure (Neal et al., 1975).

Onset of congestive heart failure averaged 20 days in term infants (Rowe, 1970) and 29 days in the series with respiratory distress syndrome (Neal et al., 1975). With increasing experience in surviving infants of low birth weight, it has become clear that the onset of heart failure when it occurs in such babies is now much earlier in the latter group.

Typically, the patient with patent ductus arteriosus has a continuous murmur or an abbreviated murmur of a left-to-right shunt. A minority (17 percent) had atypical murmurs that may be indications of very large or small patent ductus arteriosus (Rowe and Neill, 1970). An associated bounding pulse in all extremities is an important physical sign.

The chest x-ray will show an enlarged heart, plethoric lung fields, and left atrial and ventricular enlargement. Combined ventricular and left atrial hypertrophy will be present in the patient with heart failure. Echocardiographic assessment of the left atrial size in these patients has been a reliable guide to the size of the shunt across the patent ductus arteriosus (Baylen et al., 1974; Goldberg et al., 1975).

Medical treatment of the heart failure is indicated initially. In the term infant late spontaneous closure may occur, but after three to four months surgery is indicated when a substantial flow remains. Surgical intervention will not be required in the majority of premature infants with a patent ductus arteriosus because spontaneous closure usually occurs (Danilowicz et al., 1966; Rowe and Neill, 1970). The incidence of patent ductus arteriosus is higher again in those prematures with respiratory distress syndrome, and the method of treatment has varied. Although surgery has been resorted to and advocated early in the severe group (Kilman et al., 1974; Rittenhouse et al., 1975; Thibeault et al., 1975) the poor late results in many have been a problem (Edmunds et al., 1973; Murphy et al., 1974; Neal et al., 1975) difficult to resolve. Happily, closure of the patent ductus arteriosus with prostalandin antagonists, indomethacin, ibuprophen or acetylsalicylic acid holds promise (Friedman et al., 1976; Heymann et al., 1976; Nadas 1976).

Aortic Valve Stenosis

In The Hospital for Sick Children (Toronto) series of 11 patients with aortic valve stenosis in the first month of life, requiring surgery, the average age at valvotomy was 13 days with a range from 1 day to 28 days. Infants with less severe obstruction appear healthy at birth and the majority may not come to the attention of the cardiologist.

The typical precordial thrill of aortic valve stenosis is uncommon in the newborn, and the right ventricular thrust is the usual sign rather than the left ventricular impulse. Generally weak pulses are present in the severely obstructed patient, and the murmur, which is ejection in quality and classically best heard over the second right interspace, may in the low output state be soft or even absent and located toward the lower left sternal border. The second heart sound is usually closely split though the aortic element may be absent.

On the chest x-ray, in all patients in heart failure

there will be cardiomegaly and venous congestion with enlargement of the left atrium.

In the severely affected neonate, the electrocardiogram may show, in greater or equal proportion, right ventricular hypertrophy or left ventricular hypertrophy (Lakier et al., 1974). S-T segment and T wave abnormalities are common.

After initial treatment of cardiac failure, diagnostic cardiac catheterization and angiocardiography should be carried out. Attempts at surgical relief should be made provided contracted endocardial fibroelastosis can be ruled out. The risk is high (Lakier et al., 1974). Early surgical mortality in The Hospital for Sick Children series is 6/11 (55 percent), which is similar to other series.

Truncus Arteriosus

The average age at catheterization of ten patients investigated between 1969 and 1974 at The Hospital for Sick Children, Toronto, in the first month of life was 7.3 days. Often there may be no cyanosis. Bounding pulses, ejection click, a single second sound, and early diastolic murmur are characteristic. Very early presentation can occur with gross truncal valve regurgitation or when interrupted arch is associated. A typical feature of the chest x-ray aside from cardiomegaly and plethora is the anterior shelf seen in the lateral projection because of absence of the bulge of the main pulmonary artery. A right aortic arch is common (Taussig, 1960).

Cardiac catheterization and cineangiography carried out after beginning medical treatment for congestive heart failure will determine the anatomy and the type of pulmonary artery branching. At present, the surgical treatment of choice appears to be palliative pulmonary artery banding until the age when reconstruction of the outflow tract of the right ventricle can be carried out.

Other Heart Diseases

Arrhythmias. In the normal newborn, the autonomic nervous system control may not be fully developed. Holter (constant multihour rhythm monitoring) electrocardiographic recordings have demonstrated that rapid changes in the heart rate can occur (over a few heart beats) changing from sinus tachycardia to bradycardia (Morgan et al., 1965b). Sinus tachycardia may reach 200 beats per minute and bradycardia with nodal escape beats down to 50 beats per minute while the precipitating physiologic factors such as crying for tachycardia and defecation for bradycardia are applied. This varying heart rate with physiologic mechanisms is exaggerated and occurs in a larger percentage in the prematurely born infant (Morgan et al., 1965a).

Congenital Supraventricular Tachycardia. A concentration of first attacks of paroxysmal supraventricular tachycardia (Figure 11–5B) during the

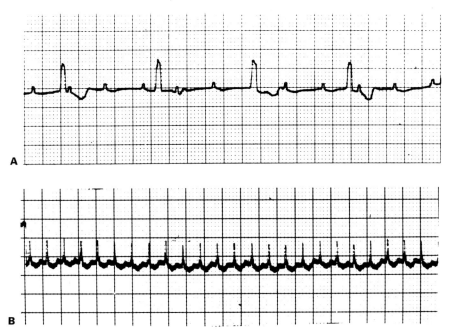

Figure 11-5. The electrocardiogram in two newborn infants with disturbances of rate.
A. A 16-day-old boy with *congenital complete heart block*. The ventricular rate is 55 per minute, the atrial rate is 150 per minute, and there is intraventricular conduction delay. The early onset of congestive failure was relieved by pacing, which has been maintained for $3\frac{1}{2}$ years.
B. A 14-day-old girl with *supraventricular tachycardia*. The ventricular rate is 300 per minute.

first few months of life has been documented (Nadas et al., 1952; Moller, Davacki, and Anderson, 1969; Jacobsen et al., 1975). Until recently the occurrence of intrauterine supraventricular tachycardia was considered unusual (Schaffer and Avery, 1971), but more recent reports suggest that congenital supraventricular tachycardia may not be rare (Lundberg, 1963; Herin and Thoren 1973; Radford et al., 1975).

Over the past 18 years, 12 cases have been diagnosed in utero or at birth, five within the past year (1975). The varied presentations such as cyanosis, cardiac failure, and marked ascites or edema may cause diagnostic difficulties unless there is awareness of the entity. Two of our patients presented as hydrops or a case of ascites. Hypoglycemia occurred in three of six cases and possibly a fourth, a disproportionately high number.

Congenital atrial tachycardia may occur in association with congenital heart disease such as atrial septal defect, Ebstein's anomaly of the tricuspid valve, transposition of the great arteries, coarctation of the aorta, and endocardial fibroelastosis (Siderides et al., 1957). Generally, no etiology may be present, but some show a Wolff-Parkinson-White pattern in the electrocardiogram.

The long-term prognosis for congenital paroxysmal atrial tachycardia in the uncomplicated case is good. Digoxin is the drug treatment of choice, but perhaps a half may not respond to it (Moller et al., 1969). In our experience, with the use of digoxin, adding early cardioversion if there is not a prompt response to digoxin, all have reverted to normal, though in one patient with the Wolff-Parkinson-White syndrome, later recurrence occurred.

Fetal electrocardiography may be helpful in diagnosing more cases in the future.

Congenital Heart Block. It is uncommon to detect complete heart block (Figure 11–5*A*) in the neonatal period, and an estimate of two cases a year in major pediatric centers has been made (Rowe and Mehrizi, 1968). Although some cases are familial (Gazes et al., 1965), most may be the result of prenatal disturbances such as infection.

Most cases have no anatomic defects, although some congenital heart malformations are associated with the slow heart rate. An example is complete or L-transposition of the great arteries. Myocardial disorders such as endocardial fibroelastosis may be accompanied by the block (Vlad et al., 1955).

Asymptomatic patients may be discovered at routine examination to have a slow heart rate. A few may be noted prenatally to have a slow rate and assumed to have fetal distress requiring emergency extraction. Congestive heart failure will occur when the heart rate remains low (30 to 50 per minute). Adams-Stokes attacks may occur. Even without a heart defect, an aortic ejection systolic murmur and apical middiastolic murmur may be heard. The only certain diagnostic sign is on a strip recording of the electrocardiogram.

For the asymptomatic neonate with congenital heart block, no treatment is indicated. For the symptomatic neonate, isoproterenol is used temporarily while an intravenous temporary pacemaker is being inserted. Permanent pacing may be necessary.

Myocarditis. Viral epidemic myocarditis in neonates was known before 1952, but in that year, Coxsackie B virus was established as a cause in Southern Rhodesia (Gear and Measroch, 1952). Ainger and associates (1966) found evidence of active myocarditis in 10 of 47 infants with the rubella syndrome who were excreting the virus after birth; of the seven in the neonatal period, four died.

Pathologically, necrosis and destruction of muscle fibers is present with round-cell infiltration. Other infectious diseases may be accompanied by minor electrocardiographic changes with or without clinical manifestations.

Clinically, the infant refuses feedings and becomes irritable. Associated fever, cyanosis, gallop rhythm, and hepatomegaly appear. Although the heart size may be normal early, with increasing severity, the heart enlarges. The classic electrocardiogram shows low QRS voltage with flattening or inversion of T waves and depression of the S-T segments. Diagnosis is made by recovery of virus from blood, stool, or throat with demonstration of rising neutralizing antibody titer against the suspected virus.

Treatment is directed toward anticongestive measures such as digitalis, diuretics, and oxygen. Prognosis is guarded.

Anemias. Congestive heart failure with volume overload in utero can occur with the severe anemia of hemolytic disease, which now is fortunately uncommon.

Tumors. Tumors of the heart are rare. At The Hospital for Sick Children, 3 of the 11 primary cardiac tumors were detected in the neonatal period. Two were rhabdomyomas and one a mesenchymal tumor at the apex (see Chapter 62).

There are obvious implications for the use of echocardiography and nuclide study in diagnosis of the above disorders (Farooki et al., 1974; Sahn et al., 1974).

MANAGEMENT

Cyanotic Heart Disease

Transposition of the Great Arteries. The neonate with this lesion presents with cyanosis and hypoxia because of inadequate communication between the two circulations. In the absence of a heart murmur, exclusion of other causes of cyanosis in this age group, particularly pulmonary and neurologic causes, is essential. The hyperoxic test is most useful (Table 11–3).

Since sudden deterioration may occur with severe hypoxia, leading to acidosis, early and urgent diagnosis by noninvasive methods as well as by cardiac catheterization is essential. Balloon septostomy is the initial and safest technique to create an adequate communication between the two circulations for this purpose (Rashkind and Miller, 1966). For technical or other physiologic reasons, some will not respond adequately to balloon septostomy, and with evidence of low arterial PO$_2$ and pH (acidosis) other surgical palliative procedures may be necessary (Fyler et al., 1969; Hawker et al., 1974). When palliative procedures fail, serious consideration to carry out placement of an atrial baffle (Mustard et al., 1964) should be given.

Pulmonary Valve Atresia and Tricuspid Valve Atresia with Pulmonary Stenosis. Among the group of neonates with pulmonary valve atresia and intact ventricular septum, the right ventricular chamber size is the critical factor in surgical management. The neonate with normal or near-normal right ventricular chamber may require a valvotomy only. In Toronto, the patients with adequate right ventricular chambers have been small in number. Until recently, medical and surgical treatment of this group of patients has been uniformly bad. Since 1967, with the use of a combination of procedures including balloon atrial septostomy, ligation of the patent ductus arteriosus, and systemic-to-pulmonary shunt (usually the Pott's anastomosis) the survival rate has been much improved (Shams et al., 1971; Trusler et al., 1975). In those patients with a closing patent ductus arteriosus, which is the main source of natural systemic-artery-to-pulmonary-artery shunt, the use of prostaglandins to promote dilatation of this channel while awaiting surgery has met with success (Olley and Coceani, 1976).

With tricuspid valve atresia and pulmonary stenosis, the initial palliative surgical treatment of choice has been the aortopulmonary artery shunt. This procedure, however, carries a variable risk in the newborn (Shams et al., 1971; Aziz et al., 1975).

Congestive Heart Failure

Digitalis. With few exceptions, the most important step in congestive heart failure in the neonate is the use of a cardiac glycoside. Even in the treatment of opposing dysrhythmias such as supraventricular tachycardia and congenital complete heart block, digitalis has a role to play, although at times secondary to use of countershock with tachycardia and electrical pacing with heart block. Of all the cardiac glycosides, digoxin has been used most effectively.

TREATMENT. The routine used at The Hospital for Sick Children, Toronto, for digoxin is:

	DIGITALIZING DOSE	MAINTENANCE DOSE
Premature infants	0.03 mg	0.003 mg b.i.d.
Newborn infants to 2 years	0.05 mg	0.005 mg b.i.d.
2 years +	0.04 mg to max 1.5 mg	0.004 mg b.i.d. to max 0.125 mg b.i.d.

The digitalizing dose is reduced by one quarter of the parenteral route of administration to be used. The total dose is divided into three equal doses. The first is given stat, the second in six hours, and the third dose eight hours after the second. The maintenance dose is started 12 hours later.

Modifications of the routine method of administration of digitalis may be considered where the heart failure is severe or the patient moribund. Engle's (1959) method is popular; the digitalizing dose is divided into two-thirds for immediate administration and one-sixth of the dose in six hours and repeated a second time, 12 hours after the initial dose.

In the past, the dosage to be used was assessed empirically on the basis of response of the heart failure. In infants, toxicity was indicated most clearly by rate and rhythm changes and therefore rhythm strips were used regularly (Rowe and Mehrizi, 1968). Since radioimmunoassay methods of measuring serum digoxin levels have been available, therapeutic and toxic levels have been defined (Sears et al., 1971; Rogers et al., 1972; Gersony, 1974). Consistent with the experience that infants tolerate a higher dosage of the digitalis glycosides, the mean serum digoxin level

in the nontoxic infant is twice that in the older children or adults (Gersony, 1974).

Diuretics. Information on the maturation of the human kidney in the early ages has been sketchy and related to work done in the animal group (Loggie et al., Part I, 1975). A similar problem arose when diuretic agents were applied to the young, but slowly the problem is being overcome. Of the various categories of diuretics available, mercurials, thiazides, saluretics, potassium-sparing diuretics, osmotic diuretics, and carbonic anhydrase inhibitors, in the neonate, the saluretics are the diuretics of choice. Furosemide is safer than ethacrynic acid in that the ototoxicity is less. The adverse effects relate to excessive diuresis and include hypovolemia, hypokalemia, and hyponatremia (Loggie et al., Parts II and III, 1975).

Potassium-sparing aldosterone antagonists such as spironolactone may be usefully used in conjunction with the saluretic diuretics.

Sodium restriction is generally not employed in this age group in the treatment of congestive heart failure, especially on a long-term basis (Rowe and Mehrizi, 1968).

The Cause. In the newborn, medical treatment alone is unlikely to solve the problem of congestive heart failure for long. Many of the congenital malformations will require surgery, whether palliative or curative (e.g., ligation of a large patent ductus arteriosus; arteriovenous fistula; resection of a coarctation of the aorta; relieving pulmonary or aortic valve stenosis; creation of an atrial septal defect in D-transposition of the great arteries with intact ventricular septum).

PROGNOSIS

THAT stage of the course of serious congenital heart malformation when it is appreciated that the baby is abnormal is obviously a very important element in the future outlook for that individual. Early detection has thus been a preeminent consideration of those concerned with reducing the infant mortality from congenital heart disease. Although the data that come from it do not guarantee a successful end result, it surely gives the best chance for such outcome by allowing a measured assessment and opportunity for precise diagnosis before the patient's condition deteriorates. There has been an unhappy experience in the past with regard to early detection in general from widely separated points of a continent having a fairly advanced medical care system (Rowe, 1972). More recently the sort of analyses possible through centralization of the care of sick infants has given encouragement that education can permit improvement in early detection. The New England Regional Cardiac Program provides a splendid demonstration of what can be accomplished by the regionalization of health care in this age group (Fyler et al., 1972). There appears to be no important discrepancy between the

State of Massachusetts death records and death from that state in the Regional Infant Cardiac Program. Case finding within the state seems to have plateaued quite early in the program indicating that communication and mutual concerns can be effective in altering the pattern of detection. Obviously, other regions could develop programs through modifications of such a plan with considerable confidence that there will be real benefit from improved survival. In the New England program the overall one-year survival rate for 1500 critically ill infants with congenital heart disease from 11 different hospitals was 65 percent. It is very probable that this figure can be even further improved (Nadas et al., 1973).

REFERENCES

Ainger, L. E.; Lawyer, N. G.; and Fitch, C. W.: Neonatal rubella myocarditis. *Br. Heart J.*, **28**:691, 1966.

Amatayakul, O.; Cumming, G. R.; and Howorth, J. C.: Association of hypoglycemia with cardiac enlargement and heart failure in newborn infants. *Arch. Dis. Child.*, **45**:717, 1970.

Aziz, K. V.; Olley, P. M.; Rowe, R. D.; Trusler, G. A.; and Mustard, W. T.: Survival after systemic to pulmonary arterial shunts in infants less than 30 days old with obstructive lesions of the right heart chambers. *Am. J. Cardiol.*, **36**:479, 1975.

Baylen, G. B.; Meyer, R. A.; Kaplan, S.; Ringenberg, W. E.; and Korfhagen, J.: The critically ill premature infant with patent ductus arteriosus and pulmonary disease—an echocardiographic assessment. *J. Pediatr.*, **86**:423, 1975.

Benzing, G. III.; Schubert, W.; Hug, G.; and Kaplan, S.: Simultaneous hypoglycemia and acute congestive heart failure. *Circulation*, **40**:209, 1969.

Braudo, M., and Rowe, R. D.: Auscultation of the heart—early neonatal period. *Am. J. Dis. Child.*, **101**:575, 1961.

Breidahl, H. D.: The growth and development of children born to mothers with diabetes. *Med. J. Aust.*, **1**:268, 1966.

Bucciarelli, R. L.; Nelson, R. M.; and Egan, E. A.: Transient tricuspid insufficiency of the newborn: a form of myocardial dysfunction in stressed newborns. *Pediatrics*, **59**:330, 1977.

Cayler, G. G.; Smeloff, E. A.; and Miller, G. E., Jr.: Surgical palliation of hypoplastic left side of the heart. *N. Eng. J. Med.*, **282**:780, 1970.

Celermajer, J. M.; Bowdler, J. D.; Gengos, D. C.; Cohen, D. H.; and Stuckey, D. S.: Pulmonary valve fusion with intact ventricular septum. *Am. Heart J.*, **76**:452, 1968.

Clarkson, P. M., and Orgill, A. A.: Continuous murmurs in infants of low birth weight. *J. Pediatr.*, **84**:208, 1974.

Cornblath, M., and Schwartz, R.: Infant of the diabetic mother. In *Disorders of Carbohydrate Metabolism in Infancy*. W. B. Saunders Co., Philadelphia, 1966.

Danilowicz, D.; Rudolph, A. M.; and Hoffman, J. I. E.: Delayed closure of the ductus arteriosus in premature infants. *Pediatrics*, **37**:74, 1966.

Dawes, G. S.: Vasodilatation in the unexpanded fetal lung. In Grover, R. F. (ed.): *Progress in Research in Emphysema and Chronic Bronchitis*. Vol. 1. *Normal and Abnormal Pulmonary Circulation*. 5th Annual Conference on Research in Emphysema. Aspen, Colorado, 1962. A. G. Basel, S. Karger, 1963, p. 152.

Edmunds, L. H. Jr.; Gregory, G. A.; Heymann, M. A.; Kitterman, J. A.; Rudolph, A. M.; and Tooley, W. H.: Surgical closure of the ductus arteriosus in premature infants. *Circulation*, **48**:856, 1973.

Elliott, L. P.; Adams, P., Jr.; and Edwards, J. G.: Pulmonary atresia with intact ventricular septum. *Br. Heart J.*, **25**:489, 1963.

Engle, M. A.: Fluid therapy in congestive circulatory failure. *Pediatr. Clin. North Am.*, **6**:241, 1959.

Eshaghpour, E.; Mattioli, L.; Williams, M. L.; and Moghadom, A. N.: Acetylcholine in the treatment of idiopathic respiratory distress syndrome. *J. Pediatr.*, **71**:243, 1967.

Farooki, Z. Q.; Henry, J. G.; Arciniegas, E.; and Green, E. W.: Ultrasonic pattern of ventricular rhabdomyoma in two infants. *Am. J. Cardiol.*, **34**:842, 1974.

Ferencz, C.; Johnson, A. L.; and Wiglesworth, F. W.: Congenital mitral stenosis. *Circulation*, **9**:161, 1954.

Fletcher, A. B.: The infant of the diabetic mother. In Averg, G. B. (ed.): *Neonatology, Pathophysiology, and Management of the Newborn*. J. B. Lippincott, Co., Philadelphia, 1975.

Friedman, W. F.; Hirschklau, M. J.; Printz, M. P.; Pittick, P. T.; and Kirkpatrick, S. E.: Pharmacologic closure of patent ductus arteriosus in the premature infant. *N. Engl. J. Med.*, **295**:526, 1976.

Fyler, D. C.; Parisi, L.; and Berman, M.: The regionalization of infant cardiac care in New England. *Cardiovasc. Clin.*, **4**:339, 1972.

Fyler, D. C.; Plauth, W. H.; Bernhard, W. F.; and Nadas, A. S.: Temporary palliation of transposition of the great arteries by balloon septostomy. *Proc. Assoc. Europ. Pediatr. Cardiol.*, **5**:47, 1969.

Gatti, R. A.; Muster, A. J.; Cole, R. B.; and Paul, M. H.: Neonatal polycythaemia with transient cyanosis and cardiorespiratory abnormalities. *J. Pediatr.*, **69**:1063, 1966.

Gazes, P. E.; Culler, R. M.; Taber, E.; and Kelly, T. E.: Congenital familial cardiac conduction defects. *Circulation*, **32**:32, 1965.

Gear, J. H. S., and Measroch, V.: *Annual Report for 1952*, South African Institute of Medical Research, p. 38.

Gellis, S. S., and Hsia, D. Y-Y.: The infant of the diabetic mother. *Am. J. Dis. Child.*, **97**:1, 1959.

Gersony, W. T.: Digitalis therapy and blood levels in pediatrics. *Pediatr. Ann.*, **3**:176, 1974.

Girling, D. J., and Hallidie–Smith, K. A.: Persistent ductus arteriosus in ill and premature babies. *Arch. Dis. Child.*, **46**:177, 1971.

Goldberg, S. J.; Allen, H. D.; Sohn, D. J.; Friedman, W. F.; and Harris, T.: A prospective 2.5 year experience with echocardiographic evaluation of prematures with patent ductus arteriosus and respiratory distress syndrome. *Am. J. Cardiol.*, **35**:139, 1975 (abstr).

Greenwood, R. D.; Rosenthal, A.; Parisi, L.; Fyler, D. C.; and Nadas, A. S.: Extracardiac abnormalities in infants with congenital heart disease. *Pediatrics*, **55**:485, 1975.

Gross, G. P.; Hathaway, W. E.; and McGaughey, H. R.: Hyperviscosity in the neonate. *J. Pediatr.*, **82**:1004, 1973.

Gutgesell, H. P.; Mullins, C. E.; Gillette, P. C.; Speer, M.; Rudolph, A. J.; and McNamara, D. G.: Transient hypertrophic subaortic stenosis in infants of diabetic mothers. *J. Pediatr.*, **89**:120, 1976.

Hastreiter, A. R., and Arcilla, J. B.: The electrocardiogram in the newborn period II. The infant with disease. *J. Pediatr.*, **78**:346, 1971.

Hawker, R. E.; Krovetz, L. J.; and Rowe, R. D.: An analysis of prognostic factors in the outcome of balloon atrial septostomy for transposition of the great arteries. *Johns Hopkins Med. J.*, **134**:95, 1974.

Herin, P., and Thoren, C.: Congenital arrhythmias with supraventricular tachycardia in the perinatal period. *Acta Obstet. Gynecol. Scand.*, **52**:381, 1973.

Heyman, M. A.; Rudolph, A. M.; and Silverman, N. H.: Closure of the ductus arteriosus in premature infants by inhibition of prostaglandin synthesis. *N. Engl. J. Med.*, **295**:526, 1976.

Hutchins, G. M.: Coarctation of the aorta explained as a branch point of the ductus arteriosus. *Am. J. Pathol.*, **63**:203, 1971.

Jacobsen, J. R.; Andersen, E. D.; Sandoe, E.; Videbaek, J.; and Wennevold, A.: Chronic supraventricular tachycardia in infancy and childhood. *Acta Pediatr. Scand.*, **64**:597, 1975.

James, L. S., and Rowe, R. D.: The pattern of response of pulmonary and systemic arterial pressures in newborn and older patients to short periods of hypoxia. *J. Pediatr.*, **51**:5, 1957.

Keith, J. D.; Rose, V.; Braudo, M.; and Rowe, R. D.: The electrocardiogram in the respiratory distress syndrome and related cardiovascular dynamics. *J. Pediatr.*, **59**:167, 1961.

Kilman, J. W.; Kakos, G. S.; Williams, T. E. Jr.; Craenen, J.; and Hosier, D. M.: Ligation of patent ductus arteriosus for persistent respiratory distress syndrome in premature infants. *J. Pediatr. Surg.*, **9**:277, 1974.

Kitterman, J. A.; Edmunds, L. H.; Gregory, G. A.; Hemann, M. A.; Tooley, W. H.; and Rudolph, A. M.: Patent ductus arteriosus in premature infants. *N. Engl. J. Med.*, **287**:473, 1972.

Kontros, S. B.: Polycythemia and hyperviscosity syndromes in infants and children. *Pediatr. Clin. North Am.*, **19**:919, 1972.

Krovetz, L. J.; Rowe, R. D.; and Scheibler, G. L.: Hemodynamics of aortic valve atresia. *Circulation*, **42**:953, 1970.

Lakier, J.; Lewis, A. B.; Heymann, M. A.; Stanger, P.; Hoffman, J. I. E.; and Rudolph, A. M.: Isolated aortic stenosis in the neonate. Natural history and hemodynamic considerations. *Circulation*, **50**:801, 1974.

Lambert, E. C.; Tingelstad, J. B.; and Hohn, A. R.: Diagnosis and management of congential heart disease in the first week of life. *Pediatr. Clin. North. Am.*, **13**:943, 1966.

Lees, M. H.: Commentary: Patent ductus arteriosus in premature infants—a diagnostic and therapeutic dilemma. *J. Pediatr.*, **86**:132, 1975.

Lev, M.: Pathologic anatomy and interrelationship of hypoplasia of the aortic tract complexes. *Lab. Invest.*, **1**:61, 1952.

Lind, J.: Placental transfusion and cardiorespiratory adaptation of the newborn infant. *Ann. Paediatr. Fenn.*, **14**:1, 1968.

Loggie, J. M. H.; Kleinman, L. I.; and Van Meanen, E. F.: Renal function and diuretic therapy in infants and children. *J. Pediatr.*, **86**:Part I, 485; Part II, 657; and Part III, 825, 1975.

Lundberg, A.: Paroxysmal tachycardia in infancy. A clinical and experimental study. *Acta Pediatr. Scand.*, **5**:143 (suppl.), 1963.

Michael, A. F., and Mauer, A. M.: Maternal-fetal transfusion as a cause of plethora in the neonatal period. *Pedatrics*, **28**:458, 1961.

Miller, G. A. H.: Congenital heart disease in the first week of life. *Br. Heart J.*, **36**:1160, 1974.

Minkowski, A.: Acute cardiac failure in connection with neonatal polycythemia (in monovular twins and single newborn infants). *Biol. Neonate*, **4**:61, 1962.

Mitchell, S. C.; Korones, S. B.; and Berendes, H. W.: Congenital heart disease in 56,109 births. *Circulation*, **43**:323, 1971.

Moës, C. A. F.: Analysis of the chest x-ray in the neonate with congenital heart disease. *Radiol. Clin. North Am.*, **13**:251, 1975.

Moller, J. H.; Davschi, F.; and Anderson, R. C.: Atrial flutter in infancy. *J. Pediatr.*, **75**:643, 1969.

Morgan, G. C., Bloom, R. S.; and Guntheroth, W. G.: Cardiac arrhythmias in premature infants. *Pediatrics*, **35**:658, 1965a.

Morgan, G. C., and Guntheroth, W. G.: Cardiac arrhythmias in normal newborn infants. *J. Pediatr.*, **61**:1199, 1965b.

Moss, A. J., and Mansel–Couchard, M.: Placental transfusion: Early versus late clamping of the umbilical cord. *Pediatrics*, **40**:109, 1967.

Murphy, D. A.; Outerbridge, E.; Stern, L.; Karn, G. M.; Jegier, W.; and Rosales, J.: Management of premature infants with patent ductus arteriosus. *J. Thorac. Cardiovasc. Surg.*, **67**:221, 1974.

Mustard, W. T.: Successful two-stage correction of transposition of the great vessels. *Surgery*, **55**:469, 1964.

Nadas, A. S.: Patent ductus revisited. *N. Engl. J. Med.*, **295**:563, 1976.

Nadas, A. S.: Doeschner, G. W.; Roth, A.; and Blumenthal, S. L.: Paroxysmal tachycardia in infants and children. Study of 41 cases. *Pediatrics*, **9**:167, 1952.

Nadas, A. S.; Fyler, D. C.; and Castaneda, A. R.: The critically ill infant with congenital heart disease. *Mod. Concepts Cardiovasc. Dis.*, **62**:53, 1973.

Naeye, R. L.: Infants of diabetic mothers: A quantitative morphologic study. *Pediatrics*, **35**:980, 1965.

Neal, W. A.; Bessinger, F. B.; Hunt, C. E.; and Lucas, R. V.: Patent ductus arteriosus complicating respiratory distress syndrome. *J. Pediatr.*, **86**:127, 1975.

Nelson, W. E.: Polycythemia. In Vaughan V. C., III, and McKay, R. J. (eds.): *Textbook of Pediatrics*. W. B. Saunders Co., Philadelphia, 1975.

Noonan, J. A., and Nadas, A. S.: The hypoplastic left heart syndrome. An analysis of 101 cases. *Pediatr. Clin. North Am.*, **5**:1029, 1958.

Oh, W.; Lind, J.; and Gessner, I. H.: The circulatory and respiratory adaptation to early and late cord clamping in newborn infants. *Acta Paediatr. Scand.* **55**:17, 1966.

O'Hara, A. E.; Wallace, J. D.; and Nerlinger, R. E.: Controlled pulmonary roentgeneographic exposure in newborn infants. *Am. J. Roentgenol.*, **95**:99, 1965.

Olley, P. M., and Coceani, F.: Prostaglandin E2 in cyanotic congenital heart disease: A new therapeutic approach. *Circulation*, **52**:(suppl. II) 11–66, 1975 (abstr.).

Olley, P. M.; Coceani, F.; and Bodach, E.: E-type prostaglandins. A new emergency therapy for certain cyanotic congenital heart malformations. *Circulation*, **53**:728, 1976.

Pedersen, L. M.; Tygstrup, I.; and Pedersen, J.: Congenital malformations in newborn infants of diabetic women. Correlation with maternal diabetic vascular complications. *Lancet*, **1**:1124, 1964.

Radford, D. J.; Izukawa, T.; and Rowe, R. D.: Congenital paroxysmal atrial tachycardia. *Arch. Dis. Child.*, **51**:613, 1976.

Rashkind, W. J., and Miller, W. W.: Creation of an atrial defect without thoracotomy. A palliative approach to complete transposition of the great arteries. *JAMA*, **196**:991, 1966.

Reid, M. Mc.; Reilly, B. J.; Murdoch, A. I.; and Swyer, P. R.: Cardiomegaly in association with neonatal hypoglycemia. *Acta Pediatr. Scand.*, **60**:295, 1970.

Rittenhouse, E. A.; Doty, D. B.; Lauer, R. M.; and Ehrenhaft, J. L.: Surgical closure of patent ductus arteriosus in premature infants. *Am. J. Cardiol.*, **35**:165, 1975 (abstr.).

Robertson, N. R. C.; Hallidie-Smith, K. A.; and Davis, J. A.: Severe respiratory distress syndrome mimicking cyanotic heart disease in term babies. *Lancet*, **2**:1108, 1967.

Rogers, M. C.; Willerson, J. T.; Goldblatt, A.; and Smith, T. W.: Serum digoxin concentrations in the human fetus, neonate and infant. *N. Engl. J. Med.*, **287**:1010, 1972.

Rowe, R. D.: Clinical observation of transitional circulations. In Oliver T. K. (ed.): Adaptation to extrauterine life. Report of the 31st Ross Conference of Pediatric Research, Columbus, Ohio, 1959, Ross Laboratories, p. 36.

Rowe, R. D.: Serious congenital heart disease in the newborn infant: Diagnosis and management. *Pediatr. Clin. North Am.*, **17**:967, 1970.

Rowe, R. D.; Finley, J. P.; Radford, D. J.; Gilday, D. L.; Howman-Giles, R. B.; Bloom, K. R.; and Chance, G. C.: Ischemic myocardial dysfunction in the newborn. Diagnostic confirmation by myocardial perfusion scintigrams. Unpublished observations.

Rowe, R. D., and Hoffman, T.: Transient myocardial ischemia of the newborn infant: A form of severe cardiopulmonary distress in full term infants. *J. Pediatr.*, **81**:243, 1972.

Rowe, R. D., and Mehrizi, A. (eds.): *The Neonate with Congenital Heart Disease.* Volume V in the Series: Major Problems in Clinical Pediatrics. W. B. Saunders Co., Philadelphia, 1968.

Rowe, R. D., and Neill, C. A.: Patent ductus arteriosus in the first year of life: Factors influencing spontaneous closure. In Kidd, L., and Keith J. D. (eds.): *Natural History and Progress in Treatment of Congenital Heart Defects*. Charles C Thomas, Springfield, Ill., 1970.

Rowe, R. D., and Vlad, P.: Diagnostic problems in the newborn. Origins of mortality in congenital cardiac malformation. In *Heart Disease in Infancy. Diagnosis and Surgical Treatment*. (Ed. B. G. Barratt-Boyes, J. M. Neutze, and E. A. Harris.) Churchill Livingstone, Edinburgh and London, 1973.

Rowland, T. W.; Hubbell, J. P.; and Nadas, A. S.: Congenital heart disease in infants of diabetic mothers. *J. Pediatr.*, **83**:515, 1973.

Sahn, D. J.; Deely, W. J.; Hagan, A. D.; and Friedman, W. F.: Echocardiographic assessment of left ventricular performance in normal newborns. *Circulation*, **49**:232, 1974.

Schaffer, A. J., and Avery, M. E.: *Disease of the Newborn*, 3rd ed. W. B. Saunders Co., Philadelphia, 1971, p. 237.

Sears, W.; Mahon, W.; Olley, P. M.; and Wilson, T. W.: Serum digoxin levels in infants and children. *Can. Cardiovasc. Soc. Progr. & Abst.*, **44**, 1971.

Shams, A.; Fowler, R. S.; and Trusler, G. A.: Pulmonary atresia with intact ventricular septum: Report of 50 cases. *Pediatrics*, **47**:370, 1971.

Siassi, B.; Goldberg, S. J.; Emmanouilides, G. C.; Higoshino, S. M.; and Lewis, E.: Persistent pulmonary vascular obstruction in newborn infants. *J. Pediatr.*, **78**:610, 1971.

Sidersides, L. E.; Antonius, N. A.; and Richlan, A.: Unusual auricular flutter in newborn infants. *J. Pediatr.*, **51**:435, 1957.

Smith, D. E., and Mathews, M. B.: Aortic valvular stenosis with coarctation of the aorta. With special reference to the development of aortic stenosis upon congenital bicuspid valves. *Br. Heart J.*, **17**:198, 1955.

Strang, L. B.: The pulmonary circulation in the respiratory distress syndrome. *Pediatr. Clin. North Am.*, **13**:693, 1966.

Swyer, P. R.: *The Intensive Care of the Newly Born. Physiologic Principles and Practice.* S. Karger, Basel, 1975.

Swyer, P. R.; Murdock, A. I.; Llewellyn, M. A.; and Bryan, M. H.: Right to left shunting in the respiratory distress syndrome of the newborn. *Bull. Physiol. Path. Resp.*, **9**:1495, 1973.

Taussig, H. B.: *Congenital Malformations of the Heart. Specific Malformation*. Vol. II. Harvard University Press, Cambridge, Mass., 1960, p. 295.

Thibeault, D. W.; Emmanouilides, G. C.; Nelson, R. J.; Lachman, R. S.; Rosengast, R. M.; and Oh, W.: Patent ductus arteriosus complicating the respiratory distress syndrome in preterm infants. *J. Pediatr.*, **86**:120, 1975.

Trusler, G. A.; Yamamoto, N.; Williams, W. G.; Izukawa, T.; Rowe, R. D.; and Mustard, W. T.: Surgical treatment of pulmonary atresia with intact ventricular septum. *Br. Heart J.*, **38**:957, 1976.

Usher, R. H.: Clinical investigation of the respiratory distress syndrome of prematurity. Interim report. *N. Y. J. Med.*, **61**:1677, 1961a.

Usher, R. H.: The respiratory distress syndrome of prematurity. *Pediatr. Clin. North Am.*, **8**:527, 1961b.

Vlad, P.; Rowe, R. D.; and Keith, J. D.: The electrocardiogram in primary endocardial fibroelastosis. *Br. Heart. J.*, **17**:189, 1955.

Warner, R. A.; and Corblath, M.: Infants of gestational diabetic mothers. *Am. J. Dis. Child.*, **117**:678, 1969.

Watson, D. G.; and Rowe, R. D.: Aortic-valve atresia. Report of 43 cases. *JAMA*, **179**:14, 1962.

Wood, W. C.; Wood, J. C.; Lower, R. R.; Bosher, L. H.; and McCue, C. M.: Associated coarctation of the aorta and mitral valve disease. *J. Pediatr.*, **87**:217, 1975.

12

Physical Growth in Infants and Children
with Congenital Heart Disease

John D. Keith

MANY pediatricians and pediatric cardiologists who have followed children over the years have noted that those with severe forms of congenital heart disease sometimes had an inadequate growth of height or weight or both. When such children were operated on successfully, they were likely to have an increase in weight and often in height as well that appeared to be greater than one would have suspected in a limited time. However, these sporadic cases do not provide statistical evidence of the overall relationship between congenital heart disease and physical growth.

One of the earliest studies on this point was that of Adams and associates (1945). Later, in 1951, Adams and Forsyth reported the effects of surgery on the growth of patients with a patent ductus arteriosus. Since then a great variety of reports have appeared in the literature. These include those of Richards (1952), Engle and associates (1958), Umansky and Hauck (1961, 1962), Krovetz (1963), and Maxwell and associates (1966).

More recently, this subject has been well reviewed and reported on by Dr. Pirkko Suoninen from Helsinki in 1971. As pointed out by Suoninen, much information is available on the follow-up of such conditions as patent ductus, coarctation of the aorta, and tetralogy of Fallot.

In the group with patent ductus arteriosus, there are many children, both boys and girls, whose height and weight are within normal limits for their age prior to surgery and who simply show normal growth rates postoperatively. However, there are others who show an accelerated gain in weight postoperatively. The greatest acceleration was seen in the case of boys and girls who had their operation early in life. In Suoninen's study, growth retardation was more marked in boys than in girls, as has been noted previously by Krovetz (1963), and a review of the literature also suggests that there is a greater lag in weight than in height. Occasionally, a child who appeared to be within the normal limits pre-

operatively showed a rapid weight gain postoperatively well above average.

The problem of nutrition in congenital heart disease becomes a somewhat more specialized one when one is dealing with infants, particularly infants who are deeply cyanosed and those with large shunts, with or without heart failure. Growth retardation of some degree is commonly noted in some of these children.

A number of hypotheses have been proposed to explain this altered growth pattern. These include chronic hypoxia, repeated respiratory infections, inadequate calories, and so forth. It has also been suggested by Lees and coworkers (1965) that such infants may be in a relatively hypermetabolic state.

Aspects of this problem have recently been studied by Huse and colleagues (1975). They also concluded that infants with congenital heart disease weighed less and gained less weight than expected for normal infants of the same age. The daily intake of calories per kilogram of body weight was either subnormal or theoretically adequate for their ages and yet the infants were underweight. These authors concluded that the growth failure seen in these infants appeared to be related to a chronically inadequate calorie intake rather than to any other factor studied.

Strangway and coworkers (1976) studied 568 infants and children at The Hospital for Sick Children in Toronto; 181 of them were less than two years old and 387 between 2 and 11 years. Dietary studies were carried out on all. The findings might be summarized as follows: Small stature was uncommon. Body weight was affected more than height or length. Retarded growth when it occurred seemed more prevalent in infants than in those surviving beyond two years. These authors found no evidence to support the contention that inadequate intake of calories or specific nutrients was an important factor in limiting growth. The patients' families appeared to be supplying an excellent standard of general care, and the investigators suspect that this included a forceful if not forced feeding. Of the various cardiac factors studied, only cyanosis appeared to affect the growth and gain in weight.

For the ordinary baby with congenital heart disease, modern formulas provide adequate water and calories and essential nutrients. However, if the infant has a large shunt or is cyanotic, the feeding management becomes somewhat more complicated. Some of the babies with large shunts appear to lose fluid through the skin excessively and need replacement of such loss. Mothers should then be instructed to keep track of the number of wet diapers and the color of the urine. Body weight should be recorded regularly, which may help in identifying the growth pattern but also indicate whether there is any overhydration taking place.

During hot summer days or during illness with fever, extra fluid or more dilute feedings may be required. Basic principles involved are that the diet should be administered with relatively high caloric density coupled with adequate fluid intake.

Kreiger (1970) found that infants with congenital heart disease had an improved weight gain if they were force-fed. The apparent increase in calorie intake was achieved by increases as little as 10 to 40 calories per kilogram per day. This may result in a total of 80 to 100 calories per kilogram in the total day's feeding. In some cases, under some circumstances, small deficits in caloric intake result in poor growth performance, particularly in the cyanosed group, and it is possible that a relatively small increase in caloric intake may produce a more adequate growth pattern. Special consideration should be given to infants who are being prepared for surgery.

In small babies, frequent small feedings may add to the total daily intake in calories and thus nourish the infant. Occasionally tube feeding may be resorted to. If the baby is anemic, Fer-in-sol in amounts of 0.3 to 0.6 ml twice a day may be needed.

Fomon (1972) recommends the use of one of the commercially obtainable liquid formulas such as Similac. An increase in caloric intake might be achieved by making up a simple formula consisting of 3 ounces of the concentrated liquid formula, 2 ounces of water, and $\frac{1}{2}$ tablespoon of Karo syrup. This gives a feeding that is approximately 9 percent protein, 60 percent carbohydrate, and 31 percent fat. The renal volume is kept low; thus the kidneys are spared while the calories are increased.

When foods other than formula are added, they should be selected with attention paid to caloric content, digestibility, and sodium content as well as renal solute load. Applesauce would fit with this regimen, but chicken with vegetables, which bears a high protein content, should perhaps be limited to one can a day.

The program outlined above pertains chiefly to infants who are in difficulty in the first few weeks or months of life from either heart failure or from excessive cyanosis. It is also helpful for those who have had palliative techniques, such as Rashkind-balloon, the Blalock-Hanlon procedure in transpo-sition of the great arteries, or a shunt operation in an infant with severe tetralogy of Fallot. In such babies, the arterial oxygen may not be adequate enough to achieve a normal weight gain with an average formula or infant diet. In cases with continued cyanosis or in the event of continued heart failure the formula and diet suggested above should be considered.

In the care of significantly cyanosed babies with congenital heart disease or those with large intracardiac shunts a number of parameters should be monitored. This applies particularly to the baby who is in hospital. The measurements should encompass daily weight and weekly length; daily urine, including output, osmolarity, and blood urea nitrogen; and skin turgor. If diuretics are being given, serum sodium potassium and chloride should be determined three times a week.

In an increasing number of instances babies are being operated on early and their weight gain improves since they become either normal or close to it following surgery. A feeding problem often evaporates after a successful correction of the cardiac lesion by the surgeons.

REFERENCES

Adams, F. H., and Forsyth, W. B.: The effect of surgery on the growth of patients with patent ductus arteriosus. *J. Pediatr.*, **39**:330, 1951.

Adams, F. H.; Lund, G. W.; and Disenhouse, R. B.: Observations on the physique and growth of children with congenital heart disease. *J. Pediatr.*, **44**:674, 1945.

Antonov, O. S.; Fufin, V. I.; Averko, N. N.; Shurgaya, A. M.; and Chernykh, N. I.: The physical development of children suffering from patent ductus arteriosus. *Pediatria*, **47**:7, 1968.

Ash, R., and Fischer, D.: Manifestations and results of treatment of patent ductus arteriosus in infancy and childhood; an analysis of 138 cases. *Pediatrics*, **16**:695, 1955.

Clatworthy, H. W., Jr., and McDonald, V. G., Jr.: Optimum age for surgical closure of patent ductus arteriosus. *JAMA*, **167**:444, 1958.

Cosh, J. A.: Patent ductus arteriosus. A follow-up study of 73 cases. *Br. Heart J.*, **19**:13, 1957.

Duffau, T. G.: Crecimiento pondo-estatural en persistencia del conducto arterioso. Estudio pre y post-operatorio de 198 casos. *Rev Chil Pediatr.*, **36**:490, 1965.

Engle, M. A.; Holswade, G. R.; Goldberg, H. P.; and Glenn, F.: Present problems pertaining to patency of ductus arteriosus. Persistence of growth retardation after successful surgery. *Pediatrics*, **21**:70, 1958.

Eppinger, E. C.; Burwell, C. S.; and Gross, R. E.; The effects of patent ductus arteriosus on the circulation. *J. Clin. Invest.*, **20**:127, 1941.

Feldt, R. H.; Strickler, G. B.; and Weidman, W. H.: Growth of children with congenital heart disease. *Am. J. Dis. Child.*, **117**:573, 1969.

Fomon, S. G.: Nutritional management of infants with congenital heart disease. *Am. Heart J.*, **83**:581, 1972.

Gasul, B. M.; Weinberg, M., Jr.; Lendrum, B. L.; and Fell, E. H.: Indication for and evaluation of surgical therapy in congenital heart disease. *Prog. Cardiovasc. Dis.*, **3**:263, 1960.

Gibson, S.: Symposium on congenital heart diseases. *Pediatrics*, **2**:325, 1948.

Gross, R. E., and Longino, L. A.: The patent ductus arteriosus. Observations from 412 surgically treated cases. *Circulation*, **3**:125, 1951.

Holman, E.; Gerbode, F.; and Purdy, A.: The patent ductus arteriosus. A review of 75 cases with surgical treatment including an aneurysm of the ductus of the pulmonary artery. *J. Thorac. Surg.*, **25**:111, 1953.

Huse, D. M.; Feldt, R. H.; Nelson, R. A.; and Novak, L. P.: Infants with congenital heart disease. Food with body weight and energy metabolism. *Am. J. Dis. Child.*, **129**:65, 1975.

Kjellberg, S. R.; Mannheimer, E.; Rudhe, U., and Jonsson, B.: *Diagnosis of Congenital Heart Disease.* Year Book Medical Publishers, Inc., Chicago, 1959.

Kreiger, I.: Growth failure and congenital heart disease. Energy and nitrogen balance in infants. *Am. J. Dis. Child.*, **120**:497, 1970.

Krovetz, L. J.: Weight gain in children with patent ductus arteriosus. *Dis. Chest*, **44**:274, 1963.

Krovetz, L. J.; Lester, R. G.; and Warden, H. E.: The diagnosis of patent ductus arteriosus in infancy. *Dis. Chest*, **42**:241, 1962.

Lynxwiler, C. P., and Wells, C. R. E.: Patent ductus arteriosus. A report of 180 operations. *South Med. J.*, **43**:61, 1950.

Lees, M. H.; Bristow, J. D.; Griswold, H. E.; et al.: Relative hypermetabolism in infants with congenital heart disease and undernutrition. *Pediatrics*, **36**:183–91, 1965.

Mahrizi, A., and Drash, A.: Growth disturbance in congenital heart disease. *J. Pediatr.*, **61**:418, 1962.

Maxwell, G. M.; Wurfel, L.; and Burnell, R. H.: A study of growth in congenital heart disease with a note on the effect of surgery. *Aust. Pediatr. J.*, **2**:188, 1966.

Potts, W. J.; Gibson, S.; Smith, S.; and Riker, W. L.: Diagnosis and surgical treatment of patent ductus arteriosus. *Arch. Surg.*, **58**:612, 1949.

Richards, M. R.: Pre- and post-operative growth patterns in congenital heart disease as shown by the Wetzel grid. *Pediatrics*, **9**:77, 1952.

Shapiro, M. J.: The preoperative diagnosis of patent ductus arteriosus. *JAMA*, **126**:934, 1944.

Sondheimer, J. M., and Hamilton, J. R.: Intestinal function in infants with severe congenital heart disease. Unpublished observations.

Strangeway, A.; Fowler, R. S.; Cunningham, R.; and Hamilton, R.: Diet and growth in congenital heart disease. *Pediatrics*, **57**:75, 1976.

Suoninen, P.: Physical growth of children with congenital heart disease. Academic dissertation, Helsinki, 1971.

Taussig, H. B.: *Congenital Malformations of the Heart.* Harvard University Press, Cambridge, Mass. 1960.

Touroff, A. S. W.: The indications for operation in patent ductus arteriosus. *N.Y. J. Med.*, **49**:1722, 1949.

Umansky, R., and Hauck, A. J.: Differential growth among children with patent ductus arteriosus. *Am. J. Dis. Child.*, **102**:563, 1961.

———: Factors in the growth of children with patent ductus arteriosus. *Pediatrics*, **30**:540, 1962.

13

Rheumatic Fever and Rheumatic Heart Disease

John D. Keith

RHEUMATIC fever is a clinical syndrome the chief manifestations of which are arthritis, heart disease, subcutaneous nodules, erythema marginatum, and chorea. The importance of this disease centers around the fact that it produces heart disease and in the past has tended to run an intermittently chronic course leading to a comparatively high mortality over the years. Recently a dramatic decrease in its incidence and severity has been witnessed in many countries, and this suggests that widespread control of its ravages is an attainable end.

Incidence

Up to the end of the first third of the twentieth century rheumatic fever was one of the chief causes of morbidity and death in childhood and early adult life. At one time 40 percent of all heart disease was considered to be of this origin. Recent statistics suggest that it is now less common than formerly. In a study of 3000 cases of heart disease in New England, White (1953) noted that rheumatic heart disease comprised 23 percent of the total, whereas a similar

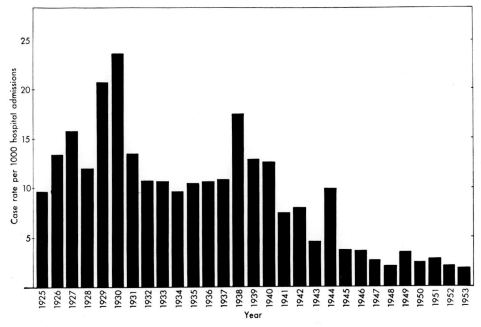

Figure 13-1. The drop in incidence of cases of rheumatic heart disease admitted to The Hospital for Sick Children, Toronto, from 1925 to 1953.

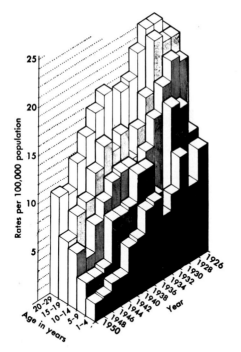

Figure 13-2. The decline in mortality that has occurred in rheumatic heart disease since 1925 in various age groups of the Canadian population.

study by White and Jones (1928) showed that rheumatic heart disease was 40 percent of the total. At The Hospital for Sick Children, Toronto, the number of cases admitted to the wards of the hospital each year has shown a gradual drop since 1925 (see Figure 13–1). At the same time, the deaths from heart disease in childhood and early adult life have shown a steady decline, dropping dramatically in all age groups up to 30 years of age (see Figure 13–2). During 1970 in the city of Toronto there was one death from rheumatic heart disease in the birth-to-15-year age group. In the same period and in the same population, there were 26 deaths from congenital heart disease. In the age group

of 10 to 15 years, rheumatic heart disease used to be second to tuberculosis among the leading fatal diseases; now it has fallen to seventh place and is a much less important cause of death in any portion of the pediatric age group. It should be pointed out, however, that although this decline has been a dramatic one, there are yet many deaths from this cause in each decade throughout the population. Furthermore, there are a large number of children with rheumatic heart disease attending our clinics who in the future may develop mitral stenosis and aortic insufficiency.

Many studies on rheumatic heart disease have been published in past years, revealing a considerable range in incidence. Several summaries of this information have appeared in the literature (Keith and Pequegnat, 1947). The prevalence then varied from 0.2 to 5 percent of the school population. More recent data, however, indicate a lower incidence. Robinson and Aggeler (1948) find 0.24 percent of their schoolchildren with rheumatic heart disease; Brownell (1955), 0.22 percent; and the Toronto Heart Registry (1970), 0.2 percent (Bland, 1960; Mayer et al., 1963).

The high incidence in certain countries is indicated by the following investigators: West Fiji (Negus and Chir, 1971); Northern India (Berry, 1972); Egypt (El-Sherif, 1971); Italy (Puddu, 1962); India (Sen et al., 1966); Israel (Borman et al., 1961); and Thailand (Chartikavanij, 1970).

Thus rheumatic heart disease is now found in only one or two schoolchildren per thousand. There are approximately an equal number who have had rheumatic fever but no residual heart involvement, which in effect doubles the number of children classed in the rheumatic category (see Figure 13–3).

Sex. In childhood approximately the same number of each sex develop rheumatic fever and rheumatic heart disease (Mayer et al., 1963). In large series, including adults, there is a slight preponderance in favor of females, in a ratio of 5:4 according to White (1951).

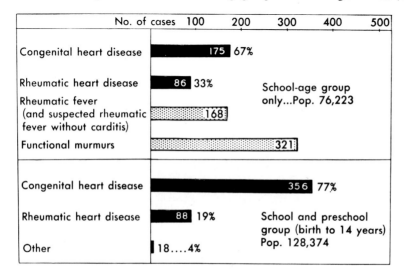

Figure 13-3. The relationship between, and prevalence of, congenital and rheumatic heart disease.

Age.   The age of onset is usually between five and ten years, but some cases do begin at two, three, or four years of age. However, it is not common to have the onset under five years of age.

Race.   All races that have been studied have been found to have some evidence of rheumatic heart disease or rheumatic fever, whether in tropical or northern climates.

Etiology

Infection.   The most important factor in the etiology of rheumatic fever is now accepted to be the group A hemolytic streptococcus. Most first attacks of rheumatic fever are preceded by streptococcal infection at an interval of a few days to five weeks. During this interval there may be an immune response to the hemolytic streptococcus, which is considered a manifestation of hypersensitivity in some cases. If penicillin is given early, within the first nine days (Rammelkamp, 1951; Houser et al., 1953), and in sufficient quantity over an adequate period of time, the patient escapes rheumatic fever. With such therapy the hemolytic streptococcus is eradicated from the throat in most instances. The administration of penicillin two weeks after the streptococcal infection does not prevent rheumatic manifestations from occurring in a susceptible individual. The administration of penicillin on the ninth day after the onset of a hemolytic streptococcal infection, although preventing the rheumatic fever, does not usually prevent the antibody rise to the organism. Thus the appearance of rheumatic fever is not dependent on the antibody rise but, more likely, is related to the persistence of the organism in the throat or other focus of infection in the body. The exact role that infection plays in producing rheumatic fever has not yet been clarified. Some special type of reaction in the collagen tissues of the body occurs, presumably in response to the streptococcal disease. A protein enzyme has been suggested as the intermediary factor (Kellner and Robertson, 1954). When the hormones were introduced, it was hoped that the etiology might be elucidated from the point of view of tissue reaction. It now appears probable that the chief effect of corticoids is in suppressing the disease temporarily. Perhaps one of the most convincing pieces of work, as far as the relation of the streptococcus to rheumatic fever is concerned, has been in prophylaxis. Kuttner and Reyersbach (1943), Coburn and Moore (1941), and others have shown that small daily doses of sulfonamides will greatly reduce the number of streptococcal infections and thus the number of rheumatic recurrences in known rheumatic patients.

Rammelkamp (1956) has found that the hemolytic streptococcus may persist much longer than previously realized in the throats of those who have suffered such an infection. Seventy-five percent of his cases have yielded positive throat cultures after 17 weeks.

If the continued activity or severity of rheumatic fever is related in any way to the persistence of group A hemolytic streptococci in the throat, it is obviously important to eradicate the organisms completely from any such focus as early as possible.

Feinstein and associates (1959), Stollerman (1961), and others have shown that in initial attacks of rheumatic fever and in recurrences some laboratory evidence of a current streptococcal infection can be found if suitable tests are carried out on the patient's serum for the various streptococcal antibodies. The chief of these is antistreptolysin O, which is found in a significant dilution in 80 percent of cases. When this antibody is not found, one should also test for antihyaluronidase, anti-DPNase, and, on rare occasions, antistreptokinase or anti-DNAse (Bernhard and Stollerman, 1959; Wannamaker and Ayoub, 1960). In rheumatic arthritis the antibody response is usually at or close to its peak. In chorea the antibody rise has fallen to a lower level—frequently within normal limits. Chorea is, therefore, an exception, and laboratory tests may be negative by the time this manifestation appears.

Individual Susceptibility.   Besides infection, an important factor in the etiology of rheumatic fever is individual susceptibility. This is clearly the case in those who have experienced one or more attacks of rheumatic fever. Then a hemolytic streptococcal infection will produce a recurrence in 50 percent of children (Swift, 1947). The susceptibility in the child population in general is certainly less than 1 percent, and in some medical centers it appears to be as low as 0.2 percent (Toronto Heart Registry, 1971).

Thus, the individual response is of paramount importance. Some cardiologists relate this to a mechanism set up by repeated streptococcal infections (Rantz, 1955); others suggest an inherited susceptibility (Wilson, 1954). If one child in a family has rheumatic fever, approximately 10 percent of the other children will develop it—an incidence that frequently is 50 to 100 times higher than in the general population in the same area. Thus, there is evidence that the susceptibility may be inherited. Studies on identical and nonidentical twins also support this conclusion (see p. 226).

The incidence of heart disease five years after the primary attack of rheumatic fever depends to a great extent on the individual susceptibility and response to the disease as revealed initially. Ninety-six percent of those who had no heart disease at the first attack have normal hearts in ten years, as do 82 percent of those who had a grade-I systolic murmur at onset, 68 percent of those who had a grade-II or -III murmur, 48 percent of those who had a diastolic murmur, and only 30 percent of those who had congestive heart failure and/or pericarditis (see Figure 13–5, page 209).

Streptococcal Antigens.   Fleischman and coworkers (1972) have demonstrated lymphocyte sensitization to streptococcal antigens in rheumatic fever or in patients who have had rheumatic heart disease. This type of hyperreactivity to streptococcal membrane antigens was noted in patients during acute rheumatic fever and in the follow-up period one to five years after the initial attack. It was also noted in those individuals with chronic valvular disease or previous history of rheumatic fever.

Fleischman and associates (1972) have further elaborated the basis of lymphocyte-mediated hyperactivity and assessed the distribution of H1-A antigens in patients with rheumatic fever and rheumatic heart disease, compared to controls. There was a definite increase in incidence of A2 in the disease group compared with controls. Detailed family studies were performed in normal families and in those with children who had rheumatic fever or rheumatic heart disease, and it was observed that the parents of children with rheumatic fever showed a significant increase in shared antigens, as compared with the parents of disease-free individuals. This may help to partially explain why rheumatic fever tends to occur in families, which may result from a predisposition to an abnormal type of reactivity to the streptococcal membrane antigens, leading to the rheumatic fever response.

Major Manifestations

The major signs and symptoms of rheumatic fever are well known but in many cases may be sufficiently

mild or vague to cast some doubt on the diagnosis. Jones (1944) helped to clarify this situation by a specific grouping of the rheumatic manifestations. His criteria have since been modified (American Heart Association, 1955) and are now the foundation of the diagnosis of acute rheumatic fever.

It is generally accepted that there are five major manifestations: arthritis, heart disease, subcutaneous nodules, erythema marginatum, and chorea. The minor manifestations are fever, elevated sedimentation rate, prolonged P-R interval in the electrocardiogram, arthralgia in the absence of typical arthritis, evidence of a preceding beta-hemolytic streptococcal infection, previous history of rheumatic fever or the presence of inactive rheumatic heart disease, presence of C-reactive protein, or a leukocytosis.

The diagnosis of acute rheumatic fever may be made when two major manifestations coexist or one major and two minor. Such a direct statement rarely misleads one, provided the manifestations are identified with clarity.

The typical picture of rheumatic fever is characterized by the onset of symptoms a few days to five weeks after a streptococcal throat infection. Heart disease, subcutaneous nodules, and erythema marginatum may accompany the arthritis or follow it

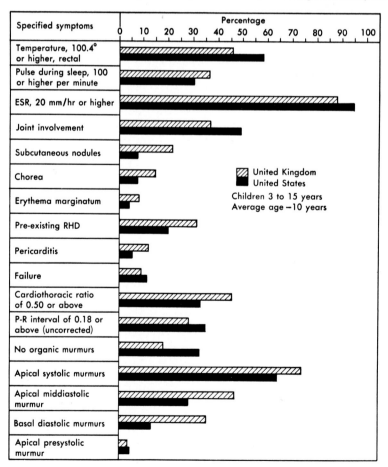

Figure 13-4. Percentage of rheumatic fever cases with specified symptoms at the start of therapy. (Data from Cooperative Rheumatic Fever Study: The treatment of acute rheumatic fever in children. A cooperative clinical trial of ACTH, cortisone and aspirin. *Circulation*, **11**: 343, 1955.)

in a matter of a few days to a few weeks. Chorea is a separate problem since it usually arises some weeks or months later. The signs and symptoms recorded in a study on 497 cases are shown in Figure 13–4 (Cooperative Rheumatic Fever Study, 1955).

Arthritis. Arthritis occurs in 75 percent of the first attacks of rheumatic fever and in between a half and two-thirds of the recurrences. The joints may appear swollen, tender, and red. Several joints are commonly involved, sometimes together and sometimes one after another—typically, the large joints such as the knees, wrists, ankles, and elbows. There is a migratory type of arthritis, moving from joint to joint during the acute illness. On occasion the involvement may be in one joint. Fever is usually present at the onset, and the sedimentation rate is elevated. As a rule, there is prompt improvement when adequate doses of salicylates are administered, but whether salicylates are given or not, it is rare for signs and symptoms to persist in any one joint longer than a week. This point is useful in differentiating rheumatoid arthritis. Rheumatoid arthritis persists longer than a week and shows less response to salicylates.

Since various forms of arthritis occur, one might expect difficulties in diagnosis. Actually, when full-blown rheumatic arthritis is present, a diagnosis is made readily in most cases. Rarely is a child with rheumatic arthritis allowed unwise activity. Errors are more commonly made in the opposite direction of keeping a child who does not have rheumatic fever in bed unnecessarily.

While arthritis in rheumatic fever frequently takes the classical form indicated above, there is a type of joint involvement that is referred to as arthralgia, which consists of aches and pains in the joints described, more as a discomfort than as direct tenderness on motion. Arthralgia is of significance in rheumatic fever because it is more likely to be associated with carditis than the more blatant joint involvement of classic arthritis (Feinstein, 1962).

A common problem in general practice is the differentiation between rheumatic and nonrheumatic leg pains in children. There is a relatively typical pattern of pain that is nonrheumatic and benign but tends to alarm the mother. This is the presence of pain in the legs after the child has gone to bed. It has usually occurred a number of times over several weeks, often months, before the mother seeks medical attention. This pain is commonly in the thighs, calves, or behind the knees, and not directly in the joints. It is gone the next morning, and the child runs about and plays normally. Heat, a little rubbing, or an aspirin tablet is all that is required in the way of therapy with this nonrheumatic type of pain. When there is any doubt, the sedimentation rate in the nonrheumatic condition would usually be found to be normal, provided there is no other source of infection. Such pain has often been referred to as "growing pain" in the past.

When an indefinite pain in the joint is accompanied by an elevated sedimentation rate, further observation is needed before a conclusion is reached. If rheumatic heart disease is present, there is usually no doubt about the diagnosis.

It is perhaps a fortunate thing that most cases of rheumatic fever that are going to develop heart disease during an attack either have previous evidence of heart disease or develop it during the first few days of the illness. Thus, joint symptoms without heart disease usually carry a good prognosis.

Heart Disease. Heart disease in rheumatic fever embodies pericarditis, myocarditis, and endocarditis. These features will be discussed under the folowing headings: pericarditis, mitral insufficiency, mitral stenosis, aortic insufficiency, and congestive heart failure.

PERICARDITIS. There may be no audible or visible signs of pericarditis, and it may appear as an incidental finding at postmortem in a case of rheumatic heart disease. Pericarditis is most commonly recognized clinically by hearing the characteristic friction rub of the fibrinous type. This is a superficial, scratchy noise that is heard over the precordium, especially near the sternum, and has a to-and-fro character in systole and diastole. It is accompanied by a fever and leukocytosis, as a rule, and sometimes an abnormal S-T segment in the electrocardiogram with flattening or inversion of the T waves in the left precordial leads. In rheumatic fever the rub lasts a few days to a week or two, whereas in the pyemic infections it is usually gone in two or three days.

Pain over the precordium is a characteristic feature of pericarditis in adults. This is rarely the case in children; they may experience a very slight degree of pain but rarely complain of it.

When the effusion forms, it produces an area of enlarged cardiac dullness and somewhat distinct heart sounds. A rapid enlargement of the cardiac shadow, clinically and by x-ray, is usually due to pericardial effusion since very rapid enlargement of the heart due to myocarditis is relatively rare. Gross enlargement due to carditis usually takes at least three to four months to occur, whereas pericardial effusion arises rapidly and commonly subsides in three to four weeks. When the cardiac shadow is markedly enlarged at the time the patient is first seen and thereafter rapidly shrinks in size, one can feel certain that he is dealing with pericardial effusion (see Chapter 15).

MITRAL INSUFFICIENCY. *Apical Systolic Murmur.* An organic apical systolic murmur is generally considered evidence of mitral insufficiency when it occurs with other rheumatic stigmata. This type of murmur occurred in 69 percent of a group of 497 children with acute, rheumatic fever (Cooperative Rheumatic Fever Study, 1955). It is prolonged, filling most of systole; is best heard at the apex; is well transmitted to the axilla; and does not change significantly with position and respirations. An organic apical systolic murmur is distinctly blowing in quality, as a rule, but it may become more high-pitched until it is described as a "seagull murmur." Mitral insufficiency is not always accompanied by its characteristic murmur since a regurgitant jet may occasionally be felt by the surgeon in cases of mitral stenosis who have no systolic murmur.

First Heart Sound. During an attack of acute rheumatic fever, there is a diminution in the first heart sound in half of the children with mitral insufficiency, due usually to the lengthened conduction time, which facilitates early closure of the mitral valve and thus diminishes the valvular component of the first sound (Dock, 1933; Keith, 1937).

Pulmonary Second Sound. The pulmonary second sound may appear slightly accentuated in acute rheumatic fever in children, but this is usually due to the relative diminution of the first sound; thus, it is not due to true accentuation of the second sound.

Third Heart Sound. A third heart sound is found in 30 percent of the cases of acute rheumatic fever with mitral insufficiency during the acute stage of the disease. The incidence falls to 8 percent by the time the active disease process has subsided (Harris et al., 1949). A few normal children also have audible third heart sounds. In adults with well-developed mitral insufficiency, Wood (1954) reports a third sound to be audible in 85 percent; however, when the insufficiency is mild, it is found in only 25 percent. The third sound has not been heard when mitral stenosis is present unless a considerable degree of insufficiency coexists. It should not be confused with the opening snap of the mitral valve, which occurs more promptly after the second sound and is indicative of mitral stenosis. Although a well-heard third sound may occasionally be noted in normal children and in inactive rheumatics, it is usually associated with active rheumatic heart disease.

Mitral Diastolic Murmur. A short diastolic murmur may be heard in children with mitral insufficiency. It usually occurs with an audible third sound, and in timing follows it immediately. It is therefore a short mid-or early diastolic murmur. It is always associated with an apical systolic murmur. It occurs in approximately one-third to one-half of the children with mitral insufficiency during the acute stage, and in approximately one-third of these cases it disappears during the ensuing year (Cooperative Rheumatic Fever Study, 1955).

A loud mitral diastolic murmur may occur in children with large hearts due to the relative stenosis of the mitral ring in the presence of a dilated left ventricular cavity.

Cardiac Impulse. The thrust of the apex due to hypertrophy of the left ventricle is described by Wood (1954) to occur in 86 percent of adults with pure mitral insufficiency. This sign is not found in children with early mitral insufficiency since the left ventricular hypertrophy is not yet developed. It does occur in the older children and in those who have had mitral insufficiency for some time. This statement is supported by our electrocardiographic findings, which showed that left ventricular hypertrophy was present in only 15 percent of the children with mitral

insufficiency. The left ventricular thrust at the apex is also found in aortic insufficiency.

Heart Size. The heart may vary in size from normal up to a grossly enlarged organ, nearly filling the chest. The largest hearts seen in childhood are usually associated with mitral insufficiency rather than with mitral stenosis. There may be thickening and scarring of the mitral valve, but the mitral ring is dilated rather than narrowed and the whole heart is enlarged.

There is usually a relationship between the degree of mitral insufficiency and the heart size. Under the fluoroscope one may see at times an enlarged left atrium with mitral insufficiency, which is similar in size and shape to that found in mitral stenosis. There may be a systolic expansion of the left atrium in the region of the esophagus, best visualized during a barium swallow. Such pulsations, when they are due to mitral insufficiency, are associated with a marked degree of insufficiency and considerable enlargement of the heart. Slight pulsations are commonly visible and are more likely transmitted from the contraction of the ventricles; these do not reflect a diagnosis of mitral insufficiency.

Electrocardiogram. In mitral regurgitation the electrocardiogram usually shows a normal tracing in the majority of children with mitral insufficiency. When we reviewed our cases of a three-year period, 15 percent of this group were found to have left ventricular hypertrophy. Left ventricular hypertrophy was more common in the older children and in those where the insufficiency had been present for some time. This is a distinguishing point from mitral stenosis, where right ventricular hypertrophy is more commonly found. Right ventricular hypertrophy in mitral stenosis appears to parallel the pulmonary resistance. In mitral insufficiency, cardiac catheterization studies frequently reveal an elevated pressure in the right ventricle and pulmonary artery as well as wedge pressure, but this is usually of a moderate degree and not sufficient to produce dominance of the right ventricle.

Differential Diagnosis. There are other murmurs that may simulate rheumatic mitral insufficiency. Perhaps the most common one in childhood is that of the functional murmur. A functional murmur may cause particular difficulty when it is heard between the apex and the sternum and has the quality referred to as the "twanging-string" type. It may simulate the rheumatic murmur sufficiently to cause difficulty in a number of children, particularly between the ages of two and seven years. It is short and coarse and not so loud as that of rheumatic heart disease. The heart is not enlarged, and the child is perfectly well. After listening to a large number of normal children, one becomes well aware of this particular murmur and can recognize it without further investigation. Other functional murmurs in the aortic or pulmonary areas or down the left border of the sternum are much less likely to be confused with those of rheumatic origin. Faint transient murmurs heard during acute illness of any origin are usually associated with tachycardia and tend to disappear when the fever subsides. The short apical systolic murmur of anemia should be ruled out.

There are a number of nonrheumatic pathologic conditions that produce an apical systolic murmur, and these should be considered in some cases. Some of these conditions have been listed by Edwards (1954): (1) an abnormal insertion of the chordae tendineae, producing insufficiency of the posterior cusp of the mitral valve; (2) congenital defect of the mitral valve with splitting and insufficiency; (3) endocardial fibroelastosis in a child who has reached the age of the rheumatic group, producing insufficiency due to either the enlarged heart or actual enlargement of the mitral valve; (4) subacute bacterial endocarditis, which may ulcerate the mitral valve near its margin and produce some degree of insufficiency; (5) congenital heart defects that produce dilatation of the ventricles and insufficiency of the mitral valve—coarctation of the aorta, ventricular septal defect, atrial septal defect, Eisenmenger's complex, to mention a few; (6) anemia; (7) isolated myocarditis; (8) cardiorespiratory murmurs; and (9) tricuspid insufficiency.

MITRAL STENOSIS. In the past 20 to 30 years the incidence of mitral stenosis has decreased in many countries of the world. Furthermore, its onset has been delayed so that it is less common in childhood. In certain countries this manifestation is still a major problem. (See Figure 13-5 and Table 13-1.)

Edwards (1954), Wood (1953), and others have pointed out that it is possible to have mitral stenosis without insufficiency. They have demonstrated at postmortem that the mitral valve may be thickened well back from the free margins, to the extent that these thickened areas meet with systole and prevent regurgitation. Such cases may have a diastolic murmur only and no systolic murmur. Another pitfall is that an apical systolic murmur may occur due to thickening and damage of the anterior cusp of the mitral valve at the outflow tract to the left ventricle, thus producing a murmur that simulates mitral insufficiency. Certain cases with this finding have been found to have stenosis only at postmortem.

The diagnosis is based on several characteristic features which are commonly, but not invariably, found. These include a presystolic murmur, an accentuated first heart sound, an accentuated pulmonary second sound, an opening snap of the mitral valve, a right ventricular heave of the precordium, some degree of enlargement of the heart, and the presence of right ventricular hypertrophy in the electrocardiogram.

Mitral Diastolic Murmur. Characteristically, there is a diastolic murmur, rather long in duration, leading up to the accentuated first heart sound. This often combines a middiastolic and presystolic murmur. As a rule, there is no interval between the murmur and the first heart sound. However, a mitral diastolic murmur, leading up to the first heart sound but with an interval between it and the first heart sound, may occur in mitral stenosis. The characteristic mitral diastolic murmur was found to be a long one in 85 percent of the cases, and in only 15 percent was it relatively short (Wood, 1953).

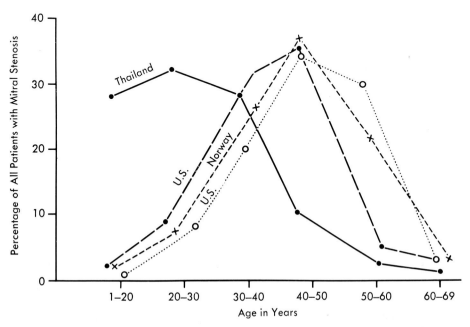

Figure 13-5. Mitral stenosis in various countries by age groups. (Reproduced from Chartikavanij, K.: Juvenile mitral stenosis. World Congress of Cardiology, London, 1970.)

Table 13–1. MITRAL STENOSIS

AUTHOR	COUNTRY	TOTAL NUMBER OF MITRAL STENOSIS	PERCENT OF JUVENILE MITRAL STENOSIS	AGE OF PATIENT IN THE SERIES (YEARS)
Logan	England (1953)	100	1	19
Goodwin	England (1955)	75	3	20
Glover	U.S.A. (1959)	1500	1	18
Ellis	U.S.A. (1959)	1000	0.6	20
Angelino	Italy (1956)	600	2	16
Reale	Italy (1966)	2000	2.4	16
Cherian	India (1965)	373	34	20
Sen	India (1966)	600	26.6	20
Borman	Israel (1961)	173	8	16
Oncharit	Thailand (1969)	143	25	20
Chartikavanij	Thailand (1970)	303	25	20

First Heart Sound. The first heart sound is almost invariably accentuated in children with mitral stenosis, although the presence of an associated mitral insufficiency may soften it to some degree. Accentuation of the first heart sound in mitral stenosis appears to be due to a sudden reversal in direction of the mitral valve with systole; previously, the valve was kept pointing into the left ventricle by high left atrial pressure. As one might expect, a loud first sound is frequently decreased as a result of valvulotomy. It has been found that the combination of the presystolic murmur leading up to a loud first heart sound is good evidence of mitral stenosis but is not indicative of the degree of stenosis.

Pulmonary Second Sound. The pulmonary second sound is frequently accentuated when the pressure is raised in the pulmonary circuit. However, the pulmonary second sound may be accentuated in the presence of a normal or only slightly elevated pulmonary resistance, with the result that the clinical value of this sign is limited.

Opening Snap. Many cases of proved mitral stenosis have an opening snap of the mitral valve. If mitral insufficiency is present, this sound is commonly not heard. The third sound is frequently heard with mitral insufficiency. Although the timing of this sound is slightly later than that of the opening snap, it may at times be difficult to tell the two apart. The third sound is rarely heard in mitral stenosis unless mitral insufficiency is also present.

Cardiac Impulse. The presence of mitral stenosis leads to elevated pressure in the left atrium, pulmonary vascular bed, the pulmonary artery, and the right ventricle. Thus, over a period of time, right ventricular hypertrophy occurs, and, when present, results in a heave over the precordial area covering the right ventricle. This heave is a useful point in making the diagnosis of mitral stenosis and can be readily distinguished from the apical thrust of mitral insufficiency.

Heart Size. Radiologically, the heart usually appears slightly to moderately enlarged, with some enlargement of the right atrium and right ventricle. In the anteroposterior view the left atrium may show on the right and left borders, and in the right anterior oblique view its dilatation may be demonstrated by a barium swallow. Wood (1953) concludes from his studies that mitral insufficiency is more likely to produce enlargement of the left atrium than is mitral stenosis. This is particularly true in children where marked insufficiency is common but advanced mitral stenosis rare.

Electrocardiogram. In mitral stenosis the electrocardiogram characteristically shows an enlarged bifid or widened P wave; this is found commonly in mitral stenosis but with considerably less frequency in mitral insufficiency. The precordial leads will usually show right ventricular hypertrophy if the pulmonary vascular resistance has been elevated sufficiently to raise the pressure in the right ventricle. Left ventricular hypertrophy is rare in pure mitral stenosis but is not uncommonly present in combined mitral stenosis and insufficiency.

Diagnosis. The diagnosis of mitral stenosis in children is usually made on the basis of a presystolic murmur leading up to a loud first sound. In the pediatric age group these signs are almost invariably associated with mitral insufficiency. A precordial impulse near the sternum points to mitral stenosis, and an apical thrust to insufficiency (mitral or aortic). An opening snap is indicative of mitral stenosis, whereas insufficiency is usually associated with a third heart sound. Stenosis has right ventricular hypertrophy in the electrocardiogram, as a rule. In established mitral insufficiency, left ventricular hypertrophy is characteristic. A short middiastolic murmur with a third heart sound is a common accompaniment of insufficiency, but this combination is not usual in pure stenosis.

AORTIC INSUFFICIENCY. The diastolic murmur of aortic insufficiency is characteristically heard down the left border of the sternum and sometimes out to the apex and above. In adult life, it is commonly associated with hypertension and a wide pulse pressure. In childhood, when first heard, it is usually not associated with hypertension, and the diastolic pressure is close to normal. However, where the insufficiency is marked, and with the passage of time, blood pressure changes occur. The high pulse pressure is vascular in origin due to a carotid sinus reflex. It occurs in the last half of systole before the regurgitation has taken place. The same phenomenon occurs in hyperthyroidism. Occasionally, in the early stages of the disease, the aortic diastolic murmur will disappear, but commonly, once it has been established for a few months, it will remain indefinitely.

Usually, the diagnosis presents no difficulty, although one should remember that nephritis, toxic myocarditis, coarctation of the aorta, and syphilis may all produce aortic insufficiency. Pulmonary insufficiency may occur in certain types of congenital heart disease, but this is commonly associated with right ventricular hypertrophy, accentuated pulmonary second sound, and, often, pulsating hilar shadows, so that the diagnosis is rarely in doubt.

CONGESTIVE HEART FAILURE. Heart failure is fortunately not common in children, occurring in 7 percent of the children in a large group with rheumatic fever (Cooperative Rheumatic Fever Study, 1955).

In general, there are two types of heart failure: the chronic type and the acute type. The former occurs in children with well-established rheumatic heart disease with marked valvular involvement and insufficiency rather than stenosis. These children commonly have distended neck veins, edema, weight gain, enlarged liver, dyspnea, rales in the chest, a sedimentation rate depressed to normal range, little or no fever, and no leukocytosis, but considerably enlarged hearts. Such children respond well to digitalis. On the other hand, acute failure is characterized by an overwhelming illness with fever, leukocytosis, a high sedimentation rate, dyspnea, tachycardia, enlarged liver, but little or no edema, moderate heart enlargement, and a poor response to digitalis.

In acute rheumatic fever with heart failure the sedimentation rate is usually high. The failure itself may lower the sedimentation rate in a patient who, prior to the failure, had an elevated level. However, this is an uncommon event, and if failure does occur and the sedimentation rate is lowered, it is usually lowered only to a minor degree. When the child is in chronic failure or when the failure is precipitated by increased physical activity, the sedimentation rate may be normal or slightly elevated. Thus, with the above-listed minor reservations, the sedimentation rate continues to be a most useful guide to the presence or absence of rheumatic activity.

There are three symptoms in congestive failure that are frequently noted in children but are uncommon in adults. These include cough, nausea, and right upper quadrant abdominal discomfort. The latter appears to be due to hepatic tenderness. Rheumatic heart disease in its most severe form in childhood is usually associated with a marked degree of mitral regurgitation and failure. In the past, this was treated with supportive therapy, digitalis, antibiotics, and so forth, and surgery was rarely attempted. Yuan and coworkers pointed out in 1964 that surgery could be most helpful. They reported a boy whose rheumatic fever started at age six and who by age 12 was a chronic invalid with congestive heart failure, atrial fibrillation, enlarged heart, and engorged lungs. A mitral anuloplasty was performed and the clinical course following this was of marked improvement. The heart was still larger than normal but was greatly reduced from its size prior to operation.

Since pericarditis may have a markedly enlarged heart shadow coupled with some dyspnea, it may be difficult to identify from heart failure. To aid in separating these three conditions, the chief differentiating points are set down in Chapter 15. A friction rub will indicate pericarditis, but one may have heart failure with pericarditis.

Subcutaneous Nodules. Subcutaneous nodules are found pushing up the skin over the elbows, knees, ankles, knuckles, back of the head, vertebrae and spinal areas, and other locations. Approximately two-thirds of the patients who have any nodules at all have them showing over the elbow. Such nodules are characteristic of rheumatic infection, and when they are present, one almost invariably finds a coexistent heart lesion. Taranta and associates (1962) report one case as an exception to this rule. For this reason, nodules do not have much diagnostic importance and may merely indicate to the observer that the infection is a severe one. They were found to occur in 21.7 percent of cases of rheumatic fever studied in England, and 7.4 percent of those of a similar group in the United States (Cooperative Rheumatic Fever Study, 1955). At the end of six weeks, two-thirds of the nodules had disappeared, and in the majority of cases the nodules disappeared completely four months after the onset of the illness.

Erythema Marginatum. Although many nondescript rashes have occurred in rheumatic fever, erythema marginatum is the only one of diagnostic significance. It is characterized by a circinate or annular rash occurring on the arms, trunk, and legs. It is usually faint with no elevation and has a dull purplish hue. If the rash is watched from hour to hour, it will be noted to change gradually. A similar rash occurs in allergic conditions, particularly in children below the usual rheumatic fever age. Here the circles of the rash may be larger, the margins raised and hivelike, and the rash redder and more palpable. The evidence at hand suggests that erythema marginatum can be classed as one of the diagnostic manifestations of the disease. In any event it is usually associated with other rheumatic stigmata.

Chorea. Chorea is a neurologic manifestation that is closely related to rheumatic fever. It is characterized by abnormal movements of the voluntary muscles, the origin of which appears to be in the basal ganglia. The onset is relatively rapid, usually a week or two in developing, and then one sees multiple purposeless movements of arms, legs, feet, facial muscles, and respiratory muscles. The original movement may be purposeful, as in reaching for an object, but the hand and arm undergo many accessory writhing movements before reaching that object. When the chorea is moderate or severe, the child is usually somewhat emotionally upset by this unusual movement over which he has no adequate control. It is not uncommon for an attack to begin in a unilateral fashion involving face, arm, and leg on one side of the body, and this is referred to as hemichorea. Eating, writing, and speech may be interfered with. The muscles tend to be hypotonic, and in severe cases the arms and legs may be thrown about in a flaillike fashion. An occasional rare case may appear almost paralyzed by the choreiform involvement of the muscle control.

In the past, about half of all cases with rheumatic fever developed chorea at some time (Bland and Jones, 1951). It seems to be decreasing in prevalence, and, in the recent study of 497 cases of rheumatic fever, only 10 percent had evidence of chorea (Cooperative Rheumatic Fever Study, 1955; Mayer et al., 1963). Approximately half of the cases of chorea develop heart disease, but it is of a milder degree, and thus the prognosis is better than in other manifestations of rheumatic fever. It must be remembered, however, that some cases may develop rheumatic valvular disease insidiously over the years. Bland (1955) found that, of those cases that showed no rheumatic stigmata other than chorea when first seen, ultimately, over a 20-year period, 25 to 30 percent developed rheumatic heart disease, particularly mitral stenosis.

A problem that arises in childhood is the differentiation between chorea and habit spasm. Many a child is considered by his parents or teacher to have chorea, when, in fact, he is simply a nervous, fidgety type or one who has a definite habit spasm. The following points are useful in differentiating between these two conditions: (1) In more than two-thirds of the cases of chorea, there is at some time a history of other rheumatic stigmata, such as heart disease, joint pains, nosebleeds, and erythema marginatum; these are lacking in habit spasm, where the most common history is one of a high-strung child who is susceptible to emotional strain. (2) The onset of chorea is relatively rapid, one to two weeks, and the parents can usually give an approximate date of the beginning; in habit spasm the onset is insidious, gradually becoming more exaggerated, and the parents cannot give an accurate time of onset. (3) In chorea the whole body usually becomes involved: face, arms, legs, and respiratory movements. It is not uncommon to have these choreiform movements limited to one side of the body, as in hemichorea; in habit spasm the movements are limited to some particular area such as the eyes, mouth, and neck, and rarely do they become generalized. (4) In chorea the movements are writhing and purposeless. A child with chorea may reach for something and that movement is purposeful, but many accessory writhing movements are made before the main movement is completed; in habit spasm the movements are spasmodic, short, and quick, and are originally purposeful, such as adjusting the collar or the hair, but become exaggerated and are made frequently without necessity. In chorea the eyebrow movement is usually upward, whereas in habit spasm the eyes may blink and the eyebrows are compressed. In chorea the writhing movements may interfere with eating, writing, and speech; these faculties are not interfered with in habit spasm, as a rule. (5) The muscles tend to be hypotonic in chorea, whereas they are either normal or hypertonic in habit spasm. (6) Chorea usually subsides in about two months; habit spasm may last for many months, although if newly acquired it may disappear rapidly.

Minor Manifestations

Fever. Approximately half the cases of children have some fever when they are first seen by the doctor. When an elevated temperature is present, it usually varies between 100° and 103° F and after a few days tends to subside to normal or slightly above normal. This fever is readily controlled by adequate administration of salicylates. Provided other causes are ruled out, an elevated temperature is accepted as evidence of rheumatic activity.

Two problems may arise in regard to fever. The first is that a child may recover completely from an attack of rheumatic fever and yet have a temperature that is between 99° and 100° F. The laboratory tests, such as the sedimentation rate and white blood count, are normal, and because of this temperature the child is kept in bed. In the management of such cases it should be remembered that some children have a normal temperature between 99° and 100° F, and if other signs of the disease have subsided, it is not an adequate reason for keeping the child in bed.

A problem in diagnosis arises when a child has a slight fever and a functional heart murmur and no other rheumatic manifestations. This may be diagnosed as rheumatic fever and lead to a prolonged stay in bed. Other causes for fever should be searched for; a careful examination of the heart and an evaluation of the history and laboratory signs should be made before a decision is reached to keep the child in bed for any significant time.

Abdominal Pain. An occasional accompaniment of rheumatic fever is abdominal pain with little or no heart involvement. The explanation of this is not entirely clear. Two recognized causes are pericarditis and enlargement of the liver, but the usual type of abdominal pain in rheumatic fever is not associated with either of these. The pain is similar to that found in acute respiratory infection and is usually vague and not too acute. As a general rule it will disappear in a day or two; however, at times it may be more severe and present a diagnostic problem when it simulates appendicitis. In such cases the presence of other rheumatic stigmata is helpful in differential diagnosis, but where one cannot be sure and the surgeons recommend operation, it rarely harms the patient to have an anesthetic and laparotomy, even though rheumatic infection with heart disease is present. The danger of withholding operation may frequently be more significant than that of performing it.

Precordial Pain. This symptom has been reported in the literature, but of late years has not been a prominent feature of the disease. It rarely occurs under the age of 15 years in children with rheumatic fever or rheumatic heart disease; even those with pericarditis do not often call attention to this symptom. In the adult patient it may occur with enlargement of the heart, pericarditis, aortic insufficiency, or aortic stenosis. It is perhaps more characteristic of aortic stenosis than of other forms of rheumatic heart disease.

Epistaxis. Nontraumatic nosebleeds are common in rheumatic fever. They appear to be less severe and less frequent than was reported 10 or 20 years ago. Nosebleeds are common in normal children; hence this finding is not of much diagnostic value.

Pulmonary Changes. Various degrees of pulmonary changes, from increased bronchial markings to complete consolidation, have been described in the literature. Children with mitral insufficiency tend to have congested lung fields and hilar areas. Increased pulmonary markings are a feature of mitral stenosis.

When an acute overwhelming infection occurs, the child may die with signs in the chest and with heart failure, and at postmortem one may find the characteristic rubbery red lung with some interstitial hyperplasia and an outpouring of epithelial cells and fluid. The x-ray may show increased bronchial markings of varying degrees and consolidation of the lung fields. This has been referred to as rheumatic pneumonia but is more a pathologic diagnosis than a clinical one. Clinically, a known rheumatic may have a primary atypical pneumonia which may be mistaken for rheumatic pneumonia, especially when it occurs in a patient who has several other rheumatic stigmata. An attack of primary atypical pneumonia is occasionally accompanied by joint symptoms in the early stages of the disease.

Elevated Sedimentation Rate. The sedimentation rate and white blood count remain abnormally elevated for longer than the other signs mentioned above and therefore are most useful in deciding how long a patient should be kept in bed. The sedimentation rate in the early acute stages of the disease is usually over 30 mm in one hour, and thus a relatively high reading may be of some diagnostic value although the test itself is nonspecific.

Comparing the sedimentation rate and the white blood count, Massell and Jones (1938) found that the average time for an abnormal reading is about the same in both tests; however, the sedimentation rate has certain advantages over the white blood count. The chief one is that its degree of alteration from normal is greater than the white blood count; the blood count is often just a little bit above the upper limits of normal, and, since a 10 to 15 percent error may occur, the method is not so useful as the sedimentation rate.

When the blood sedimentation rate returns to normal, it is taken as evidence that the rheumatic process has subsided. By experience, it has been found that this is generally true and that the patient then may be allowed up safely for increasing periods of time,

depending on the severity of his previous infection.

It should be remembered that this is a nonspecific test and may be elevated by any infection or by a tonsillectomy. The notable exception in its use in rheumatic fever is the fact that in heart failure the sedimentation rate may be normal in spite of the fact that active rheumatic disease is present.

Finally, it should be remembered that rheumatic heart disease may be histologically active with no symptoms, no leukocytosis, no fever, and no raised sedimentation rate. Sections of the left atrium of such cases at operation for mitral valvular disease have shown pathologic changes, including various stages of Aschoff bodies.

Electrocardiogram. A sinus tachycardia is commonly found in the acute stage of the illness, especially with fever. With the administration of aspirin, the temperature and the pulse rate fall, and by the end of the second or third week less than 10 percent show a tachycardia as demonstrated by the sleeping pulse (tachycardia being defined as a sleeping pulse of 100 or over).

A bradycardia of less than 60 (sleeping pulse) occurs in a number of cases between the second and fourth weeks. This is more likely to occur in those with no heart disease, or a relatively mild degree, than in those with severe heart involvement. It is interesting that such bradycardia is apparent considerably before the white blood count, sedimentation rate, and other signs of activity subside completely (24.7 percent showing bradycardia in the second week, of those on cortisone; and 10 percent in the second and third weeks, of those on aspirin) (Cooperative Rheumatic Fever Study, 1955; Keith, 1938).

P-R INTERVAL. It has been recognized for many years that the conduction time, or P-R interval, is frequently increased in children with acute rheumatic fever. In general usage, the upper limit of normal in a child has been taken as 0.2 second. This, however, does not indicate minor degrees of lengthening of the conduction time. For example, if the child's conduction time is normally 0.12 second and increases to 0.16, this is a significant increase. Clarke and Keith (1972) have devised a P-R index that is a simplified method for demonstrating these changes. They were able to show that in 84 percent of 508 patients with acute rheumatic fever, abnormalities of conduction occurred. (See Figures 13–6 and 13–7.) Simple streptococcal infection or acute glomerulonephritis per se were not associated with similar abnormalities of conduction.

Slight or moderate lengthening of the conduction time may occur in certain forms of congenital heart disease; for example, it is present in 57 per cent of L-transposition of the great arteries, 50 percent of Ebstein's anomaly, 43 percent of children with atrial septal defects, 12 percent of cases of coarctation of the aorta, 8 percent with total anomalous pulmonary vein drainage, 6 percent in cases of ventricular septal defect, 3.4 percent in patent ductus, 3 percent in pulmonary stenosis, and 3 percent in tetralogy of

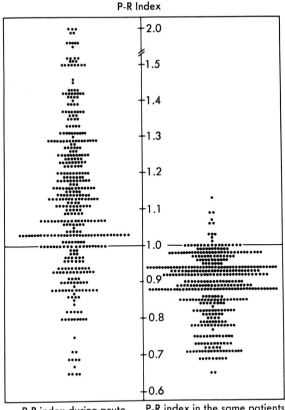

P-R Index

P-R index during acute
rheumatic fever
(445 patients)

P-R index in the same patients
when rheumatic fever inactive

Figure 13-6. P-R index in 445 patients with acute rheumatic fever in sinus rhythm, compared with the same patients when convalescent. (Reproduced from Clarke, M., and Keith, J. D.: Atrioventricular conduction in acute rheumatic fever. *Br. Heart J.*, **34**:472, 1972.)

Fallot. It rarely occurs in otherwise-normal children.

It appears, therefore, that lengthening of the P-R interval, when the above congenital heart anomalies are ruled out, is relatively specific for rheumatic fever, either with or without carditis, particularly when the conduction lengthening is reversible. It is suggested, therefore, that a significantly reversible P-R interval prolongation could well be used as a major criterion among the Jones criteria in the diagnosis of rheumatic fever.

In chronic rheumatic heart disease the conduction time is characteristically longer than the average for the child's age, usually between 0.18 and 0.21 second, and does not change much during the acute stages, as a rule, although occasionally a child with a grossly enlarged heart, in the third or fourth attack, will show marked prolongation of the P-R interval. This lengthening of conduction time is rare in diseases other than rheumatic fever and therefore has some diagnostic significance when the other findings are in doubt.

Varying degrees of lengthening conduction time, up to complete heart block, are apparent. Complete heart block is relatively uncommon, but a number of cases have been reported in the literature. It has been

encountered several times at The Hospital for Sick Children.

Abnormal T waves, either flattened or inverted, over the left precordium have been described and are a characteristic finding of acute rheumatic pericarditis. Such findings usually return to normal when the pericarditis subsides.

Several studies have been reported on the Q-T interval measurement of electrical systole. When this is corrected for rate (QTC), it has been suggested that a lengthened value is evidence of active rheumatic heart disease. Unfortunately, the measurement of the QTC involves several possible errors. Normal standards differ with different workers, and there may be lengthening of the Q-T interval from drugs, electrolytic changes, congestive heart failure, ventricular hypertrophy, and dilatation. Abnormal values may occur in cases with inactive rheumatic heart disease, and normal values may occur in the presence of gross carditis. Thus, this measurement is of very doubtful value.

Premature beats may occur with acute rheumatic heart disease and have been noted particularly in aortic valvular disease, pericarditis, and mitral valvular disease. They are not particularly common in rheumatic fever, and, since they may occur in

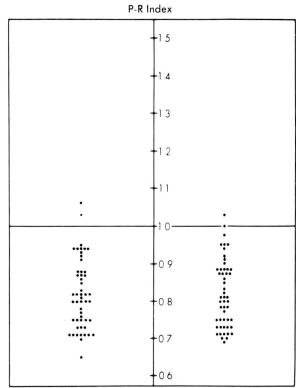

Figure 13-7. P-R index in 51 patients with streptococcal infection: acute stage compared with 2 to 6 weeks later. (Reproduced from Clarke, M., and Keith, J. D.: Atrioventricular conduction in acute rheumatic fever. *Br. Heart J.*, **34**:472, 1972.)

perfectly normal people, one must be guarded in interpreting them as evidence of myocarditis.

Atrial fibrillation is likely to occur when mitral stenosis is present, but since mitral stenosis is uncommon in childhood, atrial fibrillation is a relatively rare finding in this age group. In mitral stenosis the electrocardiogram commonly shows some evidence of right ventricular hypertrophy, with high R waves over the right precordium and in unipolar limb lead aVR. When mitral insufficiency is present, one is likely to find either no evidence of hypertrophy or left ventricular hypertrophy, with tall R waves over the left precordium. In the absence of aortic insufficiency, this becomes a useful aid to the diagnosis.

Left-axis deviation and left ventricular hypertrophy may be found in mitral insufficiency, especially in those children who have a moderately severe involvement of the valve. The presence of right axis in itself is of little help in the diagnosis of mitral stenosis.

Other Manifestations. Obtaining a good growth of group A hemolytic streptococci from the throat of a patient with rheumatic fever is highly suggestive of a streptococcal infection. More precise evidence is immunologic change indicative of such antecedent infection. It is apparent that more emphasis should be placed on this form of investigation since it is now

clear that all original attacks and apparently the recurrences as well are initiated by the beta-hemolytic streptococcus. Thus one can find an increased titer to one of several streptococcal antibodies—antistreptolysis O, antihyaluronidase, antistreptokinase, anti-DPNase (Bernhard and Stollerman, 1959; Wannamaker and Ayoub, 1960). Eighty percent of children with acute rheumatic fever will show increased levels of antistreptolysis O; in the other 20 percent tests for the other antibodies will be required. After a hemolytic streptococcal infection, these antibodies show a sharp and steady rise, usually for the first four weeks, and then a gradual drop extending over several months. Thus, when rheumatic fever follows the streptococcal infection, the antistreptolysis O titer does not usually reach its peak until about two to four weeks after the onset of rheumatic symptoms. Several estimations of this antibody, showing a progressive rise or fall, may be of diagnostic value.

Another test is the detection of C-reactive protein in the serum of patients with rheumatic fever. The presence of even small amounts of this protein in the blood is indicative of a pathologic state and suggestive of rheumatic activity. One of the advantages of this test is that C-reactive protein is completely absent from normal blood. However, a positive reaction may be obtained in certain diseases other than rheumatic fever. These include malignant tumors, acute nephritis, and rheumatoid arthritis.

Evidence of Active Rheumatic Fever

Active rheumatic fever is considered to be present when two major manifestations are present. Major manifestations are arthritis, carditis,* subcutaneous nodules, erythema marginatum, and chorea. Active rheumatic fever is also indicated by the presence of one major and two minor manifestations. Minor manifestations are fever, arthralgia (in the absence of arthritis), prolonged P-R interval, elevated sedimentation rate, presence of C-reactive protein in the blood serum, evidence of preceding beta-hemolytic streptococcal infection, previous history of typical acute rheumatic fever, or presence of inactive rheumatic heart disease.

Treatment

Since the heart valves on the left side of the heart have the most work to do, it is not unexpected that they should show the most damage when rheumatic fever is present. It would also seem reasonable, therefore, to rest both valves and heart muscle during the active stage of the disease and keep the amount of work done by these structures to a minimum.

The first requisite for treatment, therefore, is rest in bed. This is usually best achieved in the beginning in a children's hospital where experienced nurses can supervise the child in bed and establish a routine that he can follow for many weeks. There he can best be treated during the active stages of fever, arthritis, and tachycardia with frequent administration of drugs. Medical and nursing care are constantly at hand.

The one drawback to a children's hospital is that respiratory infections are not uncommon, and some of these may be streptococcal in origin. Certain basic considerations should therefore be established in a children's hospital to guard the health of the child in the early stages of acute rheumatic fever. Preferably, he should be nursed in a room with only one or two other patients so as to avoid contact with infection. It is useful to have one other child for company in the room since the bed stay is usually a fairly long one. The other occupant should, of course, be one who is free from respiratory infection. Visitors should be supervised so that they are kept to a minimum, and no one should be allowed to visit who has had a

respiratory infection in the last week or two. To prevent streptococcal infections in rheumatic fever patients in the hospital as well as to clear their throats of such organisms, the following regime is adequate: 1,200,000 units of benzathine penicillin intramuscularly on admission, then once a week for three weeks. After that the same dose is given once a month in the hospital and after the child has gone home. This allows for the maximum benefit over the period of the first year since it has been demonstrated that this form of prophylaxis is the most effective in preventing recurrences. For the children who resent and cannot put up with such monthly intramuscular injections, oral prophylaxis is recommended—200,000 units of penicillin twice a day, or 0.5 gm of sulfisoxazole or sulfadiazine daily for those under 25 kg and 1 gm daily for those over 25 kg.

When a suitable routine has been well established and the more acute stages have begun to subside satisfactorily, the child may be sent home. This will depend largely on the progress he has made in the early stages of the disease as well as on the facilities at home and the ability of the mother to look after him during a relatively prolonged stay in bed.

A general practice is to keep the patient in bed until the sedimentation rate is normal. If the heart damage has been considerable, it may be wise to keep the child in bed for two to four weeks after the sedimentation rate returns to normal. If there is no heart damage at all, one may begin to let the child up as soon as the sedimentation rate returns to normal. When heart damage has been present, one can increase the activity by ten minutes each day, by allowing the child up ten minutes the first day, 20 minutes the second, 30 minutes the third, and so on, adjusting the time as the child responds to slight increase in activity, permitting him to walk around the room and to amuse himself quietly around the house. When no heart disease is present, the time up may be increased 15 or 20 minutes a day. When the child has been allowed up all day, he may go outside on fine days and play quietly. His activity can then be gradually increased over the next two to three months, depending on the severity of the heart damage. Most children who have had rheumatic heart disease and make a good recovery can undertake a great deal in the way of activity; hence one cannot base one's recommendations on actual performance but on what would seem wise for the heart to withstand. Five categories are therefore suggested:

1. No restrictions whatever.
2. Slight restriction, which would involve abstaining from races, basketball, football, and hockey, but being allowed to play baseball, swim, and participate in the ordinary corner-lot games with the other children.
3. Moderate restriction, wherein the child would not be allowed baseball or running but might ride a bicycle on level ground, swim a little, and lead a quiet, average life.

---

* Carditis, as evidenced by any one of the following: (1) the new appearance of a significant apical systolic murmur, apical middiastolic murmur, or aortic diastolic murmur in an individual without a history of rheumatic fever or preexisting rheumatic heart disease, or a change in the character of any of these murmurs under observation in an individual with previous history of rheumatic fever or rheumatic heart disease; (2) obvious increasing cardiac enlargement by x-ray; (3) pericarditis manifested by a definite friction rub or pericardial effusion; or (4) congestive heart failure, in a child or in a young adult under 25, in the absence of other causes.

4. Fairly marked restriction of activity in that the child would be allowed no games or bicycle riding but could take part in short walks only.

5. Semi-invalidism, where a good part of the day would be spent on a couch with a minimum of physical activity.

Occupational Therapy. While keeping up the morale of a rheumatic patient is chiefly dependent on companionship, occupational therapy runs this a close second. Occupational therapy in a children's hospital is a great asset since there are so many things available these days to interest and entertain children in the way of games, sewing, leatherwork, etc. An excellent list is provided by the American Heart Association booklet, *Have Fun—Get Well.*

Schooling. In many cities a visiting teacher is available to provide schooling for children who are convalescent but well enough to accept some teaching. This helps the child to keep abreast of the work going on in the class at school and is also a means of occupying some of his hours during the day.

Drug Therapy. SALICYLATES. Since 1876, when Maclagan and Strickler first administered salicylates in the treatment of rheumatic fever, this has been a widely used form of therapy. Many papers have been published supporting their value in this disease, but few have assessed their results critically. In spite of the fact that most of a century has passed since the first treatment, the possible beneficial results have not been clarified adequately. This was indicated in an excellent review by Illingworth and coworkers (1954) in Sheffield.

The efficacy of salicylates has been judged by the effects on the following manifestations of the disease during the past few decades: (1) fever, (2) arthritis, (3) sedimentation rate, (4) murmurs, (5) heart size, (6) erythema marginatum, (7) chorea, (8) nodules, (9) heart failure, and (10) conduction time in the electrocardiogram. Only in the first three—fever, arthritis, and sedimentation rate—has there been reasonably good evidence of a beneficial effect with the use of salicylates, when compared with no therapy. There is no significant evidence that the other manifestations are altered by this form of treatment. Most important of all, there is no clear-cut evidence that heart disease is prevented or diminished by salicylate therapy, although some investigators feel that there is some slight evidence to indicate such an effect (Illingworth et al., 1954). However, since salicylates do control fever and arthritis and appear to return the sedimentation rate to normal sooner than would otherwise be expected, one cannot but conclude that this is a useful drug in the treatment of acute rheumatic fever.

The question of dosage is a pertinent one, and many authors have urged the use of very large doses. Of these, Coburn (1943), Wilkinson (1937), Illingworth and coworkers (1954), and others have advocated a dosage schedule that not uncommonly produces toxic symptoms. It has yet to be shown that levels that continuously approach toxicity are better than those that are somewhat lower and avoid unpleasant side

effects. It is possible that the daily administration of $\frac{1}{2}$ gr per pound (0.065 gm per kilogram) of body weight, without the use of sodium bicarbonate, is adequate to achieve all that is possible with this drug. Such doses produce blood levels that are rarely toxic and yet control the symptoms. However, since each individual shows a different blood level to the same dose, occasionally it may be necessary to determine blood levels at intervals and to raise or lower the dose accordingly. A blood level of 20–25 mg per 100 ml is safe and yet effective (Markowitz and Gordis, 1972).

Although more investigation is needed to clarify the problem in the light of currently recommended large doses, a backward glance over the past 80 years does not suggest that this is a dramatically beneficial form of therapy. In any disease where it is so difficult, with a particular form of therapy, to demonstrate clinical improvement as a result of such therapy, one cannot but conclude that the margin of benefit is a narrow one.

Acetylsalicylic acid, or aspirin, is a useful form of salicylate since it contains no sodium and can be readily used in failure. The following starting dose schedule is recommended: 0.5 gm per pound (0.065 gm per kilogram) of body weight for the first 48 hours, given in divided doses every four hours times five; this dose is to be kept up until the sedimentation rate has been normal for two weeks in those cases without heart disease and for four to eight hours in those that have evidence of heart disease.

On such doses one rarely encounters toxic symptoms. One need not stop or reduce such therapy for deafness or tinnitus in children. If nausea or vomiting occurs, the use of milk as a chaser for each dose of salicylates will usually help, as will a diet for 24 to 48 hours of milk and fruit juices.

If toxic signs such as acidosis or tachypnea develop, one should stop the salicylates until one can determine whether there is an individual idiosyncrasy to the drug or simply a slightly lowered threshold of toxicity. If the latter is the case, one can restart therapy at a lower dosage; if the former, one should use gentisic acid, sodium gentisate, or ethanolamide of gentisic acid, giving 1 gm every three hours six times daily. This rarely produces any toxic effects.

HORMONES. Since Hench and associates in May, 1949, first used cortisone in the treatment of rheumatic fever, numerous publications on the subject have appeared in the literature. Some investigators interpreted the evidence as indicative of a marked beneficial effect on the heart; others were more skeptical. It is difficult to carry out a well-controlled clinical experiment on rheumatic fever patients. Several reports are available, but perhaps the best prototype is that of the Cooperative Rheumatic Fever Study of 1955 and 1960 when cortisone, ACTH, and salicylate therapy were compared.

The temperature was equally well controlled by ACTH and aspirin. Sedimentation rate decreased much more rapidly in the hormone groups than in those treated with aspirin. There was a rise in sedimentation rate, sharp, though temporary, in the hormone groups after treatment was stopped. At the same point, there was a similar but less significant change in the aspirin group. Finally, all three groups reached the same level at 13 weeks and at one year. There was not much difference in heart rate between the three groups while they were on treatment; however, when treatment was stopped, those on the hormones showed a higher level for the observation period. Furthermore, there was a greater proportion with bradycardia during treatment in the aspirin group than in those who were treated with hormones. Arthritis responded in the same way in all groups.

Nodules took longer to disappear in the cases treated with aspirin. There was no evident difference in the response to treatment in the cases with chorea. Neither the appearance nor the disappearance of erythema marginatum was related to therapy.

During the first three to four weeks of treatment, a larger proportion of those treated with hormones showed an increase in heart size than did those treated with aspirin. However, at the end of one year, there was no significant difference in heart size. There seems little difference in the response to the three treatment groups when failure is present. In those cases with pericarditis, the response to therapy was similar in all groups.

Of the children who had no heart disease on admission to the hospital, only 15 percent subsequently developed a heart murmur during the course of the illness and the one-year follow-up, regardless of the type of therapy. In the children with a grade-2 apical systolic murmur, a larger proportion had this murmur disappear during the course of treatment in the hormone group than in the salicylate group. However, this difference disappeared at the end of one year. The loud apical systolic murmurs rarely change during therapy or follow-up. The P-R interval in the electrocardiogram decreased more rapidly in the hormone group during the early stages of therapy, but by the end of nine weeks there was no difference between the treatment groups.

Only six deaths occurred in 497 cases under 16 years of age during the illness and one-year follow-up. There were deaths in each treatment group, and thus no difference in response to such therapy.

In summary, all three forms of therapy appeared to have some beneficial effect on the rheumatic process. In most instances there was little to choose between the three treatment groups. Subsequent studies by several investigators have revealed similar findings or slight evidence favoring either hormones or salicylates.

Massell (1955), Dorfman and associates (1961), and Gilbert and associates (1960) have presented findings that suggest hormones are slightly superior to salicylates. Kuttner finds no difference between her two modes of therapy, and if anything, the data favor salicylates. Illingworth and associates' investigations (1957) point to a slight superiority of salicylates combined with hormone over either used separately. One cannot but conclude that the margin of superiority of one of these forms of therapy over the other is small. However, each may have its own place in the treatment regime. The steroids are useful in the early stages in making the patient feel better, improving appetite, and speeding up the disappearance of murmurs. The salicylate, on the other hand, is useful is suppressing rheumatic activity in all stages but particularly when the steroid therapy is stopped and one wishes to prevent or minimize the rebound phenomenon. Salicylates also permit one to use the sedimentation rate as a guide to activity in the later stages of the disease. This is not possible when the patient is receiving steroids.

In regard to the early starting of treatment, there was no difference in the Cooperative Rheumatic Fever Study (1955) between the hormone-treated group and those on salicylates in groups treated early or late. However, it would appear reasonable that any form of therapy in rheumatic fever should be started as early as possible.

Disadvantages of the Hormones. From a practical point of view, the hormones are more expensive than salicylates; they may produce unwanted side effects such as excessive hirsutism, weight gain, hypertension, ruptured duodenal ulcer, unfavorable response to infection or trauma or surgery, and, with the cessation of therapy, a rebound that may be a miniature recurrence of rheumatic fever.

In considering the problem as a whole, in view of the fact that rheumatic fever cases without heart disease on admission rarely develop heart disease during that attack, it might appear reasonable to use salicylate therapy rather than hormone therapy in such children. Since the murmurs disappear more effectively and more rapidly in the hormone-treated group, one could withhold the use of cortisone in such children until a significant apical systolic murmur does appear.

Summary of Antirheumatic Therapy. Once the diagnosis has been clarified, it is recommended to start with salicylates when there is no evidence of cardiac involvement using the dosage schedule given above. In the more seriously ill patient with significant heart disease, hormones may be given as well as the salicylates in the following dosage schedule shown in Table 13–2.

The continued administration of salicylates will minimize any rebound when the hormone is stopped. The salicylate therapy does not suppress the sedimentation rate in the manner of the hormones, and this laboratory test may then be helpful in estimating rheumatic disease activity in the later stages of the illness.

If heart failure is present, salt restriction and diuretics should be used to avoid sodium retention.

Recurrences

In earlier decades it was thought that much of the rheumatic heart disease process developed insidiously without the presence of an active recurrence.

Table 13–2 ANTIRHEUMATIC DRUG THERAPY

1. 1,200,000 units benzathine penicillin, intramuscularly, on admission and on the seventh and the fourteenth days, and once a month for one year thereafter.
2. Aspirin, $\frac{1}{2}$ gr per pound (0.065 gm per kilogram) daily for three months.
3. Prednisone dosage:

DAY	PREDNISONE
1–7	60 mg (15 mg six-hourly)
8	50 mg (12.5 mg six-hourly)
9	40 mg (10 mg six-hourly)
10	30 mg (7.5 mg six-hourly)
11	20 mg (5 mg six-hourly)
12	15 mg (5 mg eight-hourly)
13	10 mg (5 mg twice daily)
15	5 mg (2.5 mg twice daily)

(Prednisone may be omitted if no heart disease present.)
4. After one year start oral prophylaxis of 200,000 units of penicillin G twice daily or 0.5 to 1.0 gm of sulfisoxazole or sulfadine once daily. This may be substituted before the first year is up if benzathine penicillin intramuscularly cannot be continued because of discomfort to the child.

More recent studies, such as those of Thomas (1961), Feinstein and Arevalo (1964), and Tompkins and associates (1972), indicate that the more carefully patients are followed, the more evidence there is that recurrences do occur if there is any progression of the cardiac involvement. Tompkins and coworkers (1972) conclude, "Thus it appears that rheumatic heart disease frequently disappears clinically, usually regresses and seldom worsens in the first ten to twenty years if recurrences of acute rheumatic fever or episodes of bacterial endocarditis are prevented."

For many years it has been recognized that the tendency for rheumatic recurrence to take place lessens as the child grows older and as the time from the original attack lengthens.

Although rheumatic fever is intimately related to streptococcal infections, the exact relationship has never been clearly delineated; however, it does appear that there is a constitutional, possibly genetic, susceptibility that may antedate the first attack, or it may be that the susceptibility to the streptococcus with a rheumatic type of reaction is acquired, or it may be a combination of these two things.

Spagnuolo and associates (1971) have demonstrated that rheumatic recurrences are more frequently found after severe streptococcal infections than after mild ones. Their evidence suggests that recurrence is indeed due to the severity of the infection rather than the magnitude of the ASO titer rise, which has been implicated at times in the past. Their data suggest that rheumatic fever is the result of two components—one decaying rapidly after a rheumatic attack leading to fewer and fewer recurrences, and the other decaying slowly or not at all, maintaining some degree of individual susceptibility. The greater concordance of rheumatic fever in monozygous than in dizygous twins in consistent with the concept of a genetic predisposition.

Prevention of Rheumatic Fever

In the control of rheumatic fever, there are two main problems to consider. The first is the prevention of the initial attack of rheumatic disease, which usually occurs between five and ten years of age, and the second is the prevention of recurrences once a child has had his first attack. The first measure of success in prevention of recurrences was achieved after the sulfonamides were discovered over 30 years ago; small daily doses reduced the incidence of subsequent rheumatic activation (Coburn and Moore, 1939). The prevention of initial attacks had to wait until penicillin was discovered.

Initial Attacks. In attempting to prevent the initial attack of rheumatic fever following a streptococcal infection, sulfonamides were soon discovered to be ineffective. Since the end of World War II, however, several studies using penicillin to achieve this have been successful. Massell, Rammelkamp, Houser, and others have demonstrated the effectiveness of adequate penicillin, given at the time of the hemolytic streptococcal infection, in reducing the number of patients who develop rheumatic fever.

In the school population of Chicago, Siegel and coworkers (1961) carried out a controlled study comparing penicillin-treated children suffering from streptococcal nasopharyngitis with symptomatically treated children with the same type of infection. There were no rheumatic fever attacks in those treated with penicillin and only two in those treated symptomatically. These two occurred in the 14 percent of the group that were considered severe and comparable to epidemics in service personnel.

It appears, therefore, that the attack rate of rheumatic fever in children is modified by a decrease in the virulence and contagion of the strains of streptococcus in the throats of schoolchildren. The widespread and early use of penicillin by pediatricians and general practitioners in treating many respiratory infections in the pediatric age group may well have contributed to this control of virulence. For adequate treatment of a hemolytic streptococcal infection, however, one should give as a minimum 600,000 units of benzathine penicillin intramuscularly (Breese, 1960). When oral penicillin is employed, 800,000 units a day must be given for ten days to achieve comparable results.

If all hemolytic streptococcal infections could be so treated, there is good evidence that the incidence of rheumatic fever could be reduced. However, the problem is difficult since one-third of the children presenting with rheumatic fever have no history of preceding illness. Of the two-thirds who do have a preceding upper respiratory infection, many have no clinical evidence suggesting a streptococcal origin. The hemolytic streptococcal infections are commonly associated with fever, headaches, sore throat, exudation of the throat, and enlarged cervical glands. When these are present, one should certainly administer enough penicillin to ensure control of the infection and complete eradication of the organism. This appears to be good pediatric practice for any child between 3 and 15 years of age who has a throat infection suggesting that caused by the hemolytic streptococcus. However, such clinical signs are not commonly present in children with upper respiratory infections; hence the diagnosis may be in doubt. Since penicillin is administered mainly to combat a streptococcal infection, it would seem reasonable to give it in a dosage or by a method that is sufficient to eliminate the organism from the respiratory tract. This preferably requires an injection of the long-acting preparation, 600,000 units of benzathine penicillin.* This type of penicillin permits the doctor to treat average cases with one house call. Since it is rarely necessary or possible for the doctor to make two or more calls on a patient with respiratory infection, such type of therapy would appear to be the optimum in controlling streptococcal infections in rheumatic fever attacks.

Prevention of Recurrences. The second problem is that of the child who is a known rheumatic patient. Many studies have indicated that approximately 50 percent of these children will develop a rheumatic recurrence if they have a hemolytic streptococcal infection. Once susceptibility is recognized by the original rheumatic attack, such children should be put on prophylaxis. Coburn and Young (1949), Kuttner (1951), Thomas (1952), and others have demonstrated the value of sulfonamides in preventing streptococcal infections and thus rheumatic recurrences. A summary of these studies shows that 2 percent of the rheumatic recurrences have occurred among known rheumatic children receiving sulfonamide prophylaxis, whereas among children without such prophylaxis there have been recurrences in 44 percent.

Bland and Jones (1951) found in a follow-up of a large rheumatic group that 70 percent developed recurrences over a ten-year period when not receiving prophylaxis. It is clear, therefore, that such prophylaxis should be kept up for ten years at least. Wilson and Lubschez' (1944) data suggest that the recurrence rate is more common in the younger children. In their group between 4 and 13 years, there was a 25 percent recurrence rate, but between 14 and 16 years, the rate had fallen to 8.6 percent, and at 17 years to 5.3 percent. Thus, in childhood every child who has had clear-cut rheumatic fever should be given a daily dose of prophylactic antibiotic.

The problem of prevention in adolescence and adult life has been dealt with by several investigators (Stollerman, 1962). Some have suggested that prophylaxis be kept up for life. Recently Johnson, Stollerman, and Grossman (1960) have followed a group of patients who have been free of active rheumatic fever for five years at least and for whom prophylaxis has consisted of penicillin in therapeutic doses when symptomatic streptococcal disease occurred. Immunologic titers obtained bimonthly

revealed that three-quarters of the streptococcal infections were asymptomatic and therefore not treated with penicillin during the active disease process. In the adolescent group with a mean age of 19 years, 27 percent each year contracted a streptococcal infection. Considering the asymptomatic infections that were therefore not treated, 5 percent were followed by rheumatic recurrences. The recurrence rate per patient year of follow-up totaled only 1.3 percent, however.

The annual incidence of streptococcal infections in the adults whose mean age was 39 years was approximately 15 percent. Among these infections that were either untreated or treated too late to prevent a strong immune response, the recurrence rate was approximately 5 percent, but this only involved two recurrences following 40 streptococcal infections. The rheumatic recurrence rate per patient year of follow-up in this group was 0.7 percent.

Thus there is a decline in streptococcal disease in advancing years, but if a sore throat of hemolytic streptococcal origin does occur, it would appear just about as likely to cause a recurrence in adult life as in the earlier years, especially if there is an epidemic or evidence of severe streptococcal infection being passed around.

The fundamental factor, however, remains that of individual susceptibility. This may be measured by a patient's response to previous attacks, as has been indicated previously, but the subject has been evaluated from another aspect recently by the group at Irvington House. This involved an investigation of the magnitude of the immune response following a streptococcal infection and relating it to the presence or absence of cardiac involvement in known rheumatic patients. In the young rheumatic subjects without heart disease and a feeble antibody response a 4 percent recurrence rate occurred compared with 28 percent when an immunologic response of the same magnitude occurred in those with demonstrable rheumatic heart disease. A strong immune response resulted in a 36 percent recurrence rate in the former group and a 65 percent rate in the latter.

There are, therefore, many factors to be taken into consideration in planning prophylactic measures for any one individual. These include the age of the person concerned, the prevalence of streptococcal epidemics, the climate, the presence of previous rheumatic heart disease, the likelihood of contact with groups of people harboring hemolytic streptococci, the length of time since the last previous attack.

One can conclude, therefore, that prophylaxis should be given daily to children and adolescents covering the susceptible age groups. In adult life the program of control of streptococcal infections will depend on an evaluation of the individual and his environment. But if daily prophylaxis is not administered, each infection suggestive of a hemolytic streptococcal origin should be treated with therapeutic doses of penicillin.

Oral penicillin has proved to be effective prophylactically; the suitable dose will probably vary

---

* An alternative would be to give aqueous procaine penicillin and the long-acting variety combined (all-purpose Bicillin, Wyeth).

from one individual to another depending on how well it is absorbed. There is good evidence (Tidwell, 1954), however, that 200,000 units of oral penicillin of the type buffered with sodium citrate, administered twice daily, will usually keep the throat clear of hemolytic streptococci and thus prevent an infection.

Stollerman (1954) has investigated the use of benzathine penicillin, giving 1,250,000 units once a month by injection. In a group of children in a convalescent home, this maintained a significant blood level for most of the month, and the throats were persistently negative for hemolytic streptococci for 95 percent of the cases. Penicillin reactions were rare, occurring in approximately 1 percent, and did not require stopping such prophylaxis.

In the doses recommended previously, sulfisoxazole prophylaxis rarely produces toxic symptoms. Less than 1 percent of children develop a rash. Occasionally, where the mother complains that the child has a poor appetite or seems slightly unwell while receiving sulfonamide prophylaxis, it is better to discontinue the drug. In the United States Navy during World War II, toxic reactions occurred in approximately 0.5 percent of the young adults so treated.

Oral penicillin rarely causes toxic reaction; occasionally urticaria may develop, but even in the long-acting type of penicillin it usually clears up and does not recur. If the urticaria is severe or associated with an angioneurotic edema, penicillin should not be continued. There is a significant local reaction to the long-acting penicillin, causing some degree of discomfort. This is a minor disadvantage, which is usually more than balanced by the beneficial effects.

The control of rheumatic fever, then, is obviously the control of streptococcal infections, and to achieve this in childhood one of three prophylactic regimes is usually adopted in childhood: (1) monthly injection of 1,200,000 units of benzathine penicillin, (2) 200,000 units of oral penicillin given twice daily, or (3) 0.5 to 1 gm of sulfadiazine once a day (0.5 gm to child under 25 kg). The first regimen has proved to be the most effective. The oral method is less reliable because the patient may forget to take a dose. However, young children resent the intramuscular injection of the benzathine penicillin and frequently become sufficiently disturbed to cause the physician to change to the oral preparation. The older patients also prefer

the oral regimen. The physician must therefore select the routine that is most suitable and effective for his patient. The important thing is that the drug should be administered regularly, and at each visit this should be impressed on the parents and child.

It is always a problem for the doctor to know how regularly children with rheumatic fever actually take prophylactic penicillin or sulfadiazine as prescribed by their physician. Gordis and coworkers (1969) report that two-thirds of their patients appeared to be taking oral penicillin regularly and one-third were taking the penicillin only one-fourth of the time, as demonstrated by a urine examination. Morrow and Rabin (1965) found similar degree of compliance or lack of compliance in a study of self-medication with isoniazid.

Tonsillectomy. Although many authors have published investigations and opinions on the question of tonsillectomy in children with rheumatic fever, it still remains a moot question. Nearly 50 years ago, Kaiser (1930) published data and doubted the validity or necessity of removing tonsils, except under exceptional circumstances. More recently, Feinstein and Levitt (1970) carried out a study on tonsil size in 532 children, all of whom had previous attacks of rheumatic fever. These children were examined frequently and the size of the tonsils related to the streptococcal infections and rheumatic recurrences. In rheumatic patients who faithfully maintained effective prophylaxis, the size of the tonsils did not seem to influence the development of streptococcal infections in rheumatic recurrences. However, if such prophylaxis was not maintained, large tonsils appeared to increase the patient's susceptibility to these hazards. These results tended to support the argument in favor of performing tonsillectomy for young rheumatic patients who had major cardiac damage and persistently large tonsils and who could not be trusted to maintain continuous anti-streptococcal prophylaxis. (For grading tonsil size, see Figure 13–8.)

Prognosis

There has been a clinical impression in recent years that rheumatic fever is becoming milder. An increasing amount of evidence supports this view and

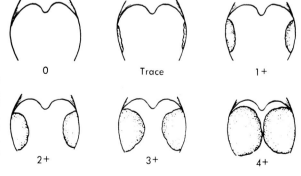

Figure 13-8. The size of tonsils did not affect the incidence of infection or rheumatic recurrences when good prophylaxis was maintained. In the individuals who did not keep up the prophylaxis there was an increase in staphylococcal infection and rheumatic recurrences. (Reproduced from Feinstein, A. R., and Levitt, M.: Tonsil size. *N. Engl. J. Med.*, **282**:285, 1970.)

0   Trace   1+

2+   3+   4+

suggests that both the prevalence of the disease and the mortality are diminishing steadily. In the Cooperative Rheumatic Fever Study (1955) there were only six recorded deaths in the group of 497 children with rheumatic fever and rheumatic heart disease, during the acute illness and a follow-up of one year. At The Hospital for Sick Children, in the past 20 to 30 years a gradual decrease has been shown in the deaths related to the admissions. Perhaps even more striking has been the fall in Canadian mortality figures in the age group from 1 to 30 years during the past 25 years. In Figure 13–2 (page 204) one sees a drop in each age group, but it is most marked between the ages of 5 and 15, the childhood years that concern us particularly. Hedley (1939) was one of the first to point out this decrease in mortality.

Findlay and Fowler (1966) compared two groups of patients treated 20 years apart. The outstanding difference was found in the mortality from acute carditis in the initial episode of rheumatic fever. The rate for the group seen in the 1930s was 15 percent compared with 2 percent for those seen in the 1950s.

The figures on the prevalence of rheumatic fever are as indicative as those on mortality. Most children's hospitals in North America have noticed a decrease in the number of patients suffering from rheumatic fever in their wards. This is reflected in the figures shown; when related to the number of daily admissions, it will be seen that there has been a significant decrease at The Hospital for Sick Children over the past 15 years (Figure 13–1, page 203).

Considering the mortality in rheumatic fever in greater detail, we must turn to figures of published articles on the natural history of rheumatic fever during the past 10 to 30 years. These figures may not apply accurately today, but several excellent investigations have been reported that serve as a useful guide in assessing the prognosis.

Table 13–3. OVERALL MORTALITY OF 1000 RHEUMATIC FEVER CASES, BOSTON, 1930–1950

	NO RHEU- MATIC HEART DISEASE	RHEU- MATIC HEART DISEASE	DEATHS
Original status (average age: 8 years)	347	653	—
Ten years later (average age: 18 years)	323	475	202
Twenty years later (average age: 28 years)	319	380	301

In 1921–1922 at the Good Samaritan Hospital in Boston the mortality over the first five years from the first attack of rheumatic fever was 24 percent. In succeeding decades it fell dramatically, until by 1950–1951 the figure was down to 3 percent (Bland, 1960).

There are certain signs and symptoms by which one judges the severity of the illness, and Bland and Jones (1952) pointed out that these are intimately related to the prognosis.

Findlay and Fowler (1966) showed marked decrease in mortality in recent years (Table 13–4).

Table 13–4. MORTALITY IN RHEUMATIC HEART DISEASE*

	CASES WITH CARDITIS	EARLY DEATH
1937–1940	82	15%
1957–1960	96	2%

* Data from Findlay and Fowler, 1966.

Morton and Lichty (1970), reporting the morbidity and mortality from rheumatic fever and rheumatic heart disease in Colorado in a lower economic group, found that the morbidity did not alter when the period 1949–1951 was compared with the period 1959–1961. However, the mortality dropped to one-third during the same interval. Pilapil and Watson (1971) reported on a series of 104 cases in Mississippi, which showed a mortality of 34 percent during the period 1956–1965.

Prognosis by Decades. PROGNOSIS 1920–1950. Bland and Jones (1951) reported a follow-up study of 1000 cases of rheumatic fever, followed an average period of 20 years, many of them for 30 years or more. This is one of the best and most representative studies of the time. A summary of their overall mortality figures is shown in Table 13–3. These figures reveal a 20 percent mortality in ten years, probably reflecting the situation in the 1920s, but followed by a 30 percent mortality in 20 years, which would include the 1930s and beyond. Most of these cases died with congestive heart failure (80 percent), and it is important to note that one-tenth of them died as a result of subacute bacterial endocarditis or acute bacterial endocarditis. It is now known whether the majority of these bacterial infections may be either prevented or cured, and deaths are uncommon from this cause in the 1970s.

As mentioned above, Bland (1960) points out that in 1921 and 1922 at the Good Samaritan Hospital in Boston, the mortality from the first attack of rheumatic fever was 24 percent. In succeeding decades it fell dramatically, until by 1950–1951 the figure was down to 3 percent in the same institution.

PROGNOSIS 1950–1960. In the cooperative study carried on in 13 medical centers in Canada, Great Britain, and the United States, which included in-hospital treatment and careful follow-up with prophylaxis over ten years, the results are shown in Figure 13–9. The mortality was down to 3.9 percent. The ultimate prognosis was markedly influenced by the severity of the cardiac involvement when the child first entered the study. When no heart disease was found at the beginning, 94 percent had no heart disease at the end of ten years. If a grade-1 mitral

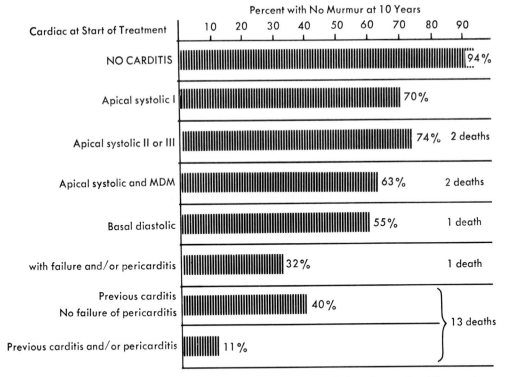

Figure 13-9. Ten-year follow-up study of 497 children with acute rheumatic fever. International Cooperative Study, 1950–1960, conducted in 13 medical centers in Canada, Great Britain, and the United States. (Reproduced from *Circulation*, **32**:457, 1965.)

systolic murmur was heard at the beginning, 70 percent had no heart disease at the end of ten years. With a grade-2 or grade-3 apical systolic murmur, 74 percent had no murmur in ten years. When a basal diastolic murmur was present with a systolic one, 55 percent had no murmur after ten years. The most severe group comprised those who had previous heart disease with failure and/or pericarditis. At the end of ten years in this latter group only 11 percent were free of heart disease. (See Figure 13–9.)

In this cooperative study involving three countries the improved prognosis is clearly evident, when compared with the earlier findings of Bland and Jones. The latter, in presenting the results of a follow-up study on 653 patients with well-defined rheumatic heart disease, showed that after ten years all signs had disappeared in only 11 percent; at the end of 20 years, signs had disappeared in 16 percent. Most of these had an apical systolic murmur but some were described as having a diastolic rumble as well.

PROGNOSIS 1960–1970. Tompkins and associates (1972) record the prognosis on 115 rheumatic fever patients receiving regular intramuscular penicillin prophylaxis once a month with an average follow-up of 9.3 years. There were no known deaths in this group during this period. None developed mitral stenosis and none developed bacterial endocarditis. Those with no carditis at the beginning of the study

had no carditis at the end. Of those who started out with mitral regurgitation, 74 percent had no murmur at the end of nine years. Among those with aortic regurgitation, 27 percent had no such murmur at the end of nine years. This study probably represents a favorable cross-section of rheumatic fever patients, since they were selected because they had kept on their prophylactic program and received benzathine penicillin once a month by injection rather than oral prophylaxis. It is thus a more favorable group than that seen in the general cardiac clinic. It does reveal, however, that an excellent prognosis is available to those willing and able to be seen regularly by the physician and maintained on a good prophylactic program. The results are similar to those shown in Figure 13–9.

Pericarditis. Pericarditis has always been considered a serious form of heart involvement in rheumatic fever. The mortality has varied greatly. At The Toronto Hospital for Sick Children the mortality in rheumatic pericarditis has fallen from 70 percent to 40 percent during the past 30 years. However, the prognosis appears to be considerably better in older persons, as shown by Massie and Levine (1939), who found that only 16 percent of their patients succumbed to acute rheumatic pericarditis. Schlesinger (1930) collected reports of seven children who recovered completely from pericarditis. On the other hand, Massie and Levine (1939) reported that 25 percent of 135 adult patients who recovered have no signs or symptoms of the disease. Bland (1960) notes a decrease in the percentage of rheumatic fever patients with pericarditis in recent years.

Arthritis. Mackie (1926), Findlay (1931), and Coombs (1924) reported an incidence of heart disease between 60 and 75 percent in the first attack of arthritis. For two or more attacks, this incidence rose to 70 to 80 percent. Of 410 patients with arthritis occurring at some time, 22 percent died in the first ten years and 27 percent over a period of 20 years (Bland and Jones, 1951). Thus arthritis is not the most severe manifestation of the disease.

This has been supported by Feinstein and Spagnuolo (1961), who pointed out that the incidence of carditis increased with decreasing severity of the joint symptoms. Carditis was found in 26 percent of rheumatic fever patients with red, hot, or swollen joints but occurred in 40 percent of those with only tender joints. Furthermore, the severity of the carditis could be related inversely to the severity of the arthritis, the most severe forms of heart disease usually occurring in the patients who had no evidence of arthritis.

Heart Size. Bland and Jones's (1951) figures show a high mortality among those cases that have greatly enlarged hearts. Campbell (1939), of the New York Life Insurance Company, noted that where there was just slight enlargement the mortality was 37 percent and with moderate enlargement it was 73 percent (where 100 percent is taken as the normal or expected death rate).

Valvular Lesions. White (1953) recorded the frequency with which heart valves were involved in rheumatic heart disease. Sixty-two percent of his cases had mitral disease alone, 5 percent had aortic valvular disease alone, and 33 percent had both. In children, the aortic valve involvement is less frequently demonstrated, with mitral disease predominating, usually mitral regurgitation. In the City of Toronto Heart Registry (1971) among the children with rheumatic heart disease, 81 percent had mitral regurgitation and 10 percent aortic regurgitation with mitral regurgitation. Six percent had aortic regurgitation alone, 1 percent mitral regurgitation and early stenosis, and 1 percent pericarditis.

Bland and Jones (1951) reported that only one-third of their rheumatic fever patients who developed mitral stenosis had clear evidence of recurrent activity. Walsh and associates (1940) found, however, that 85 percent of their cases with mitral stenosis had definite recurrences but they appeared to be associated with a milder form of rheumatic fever initially and with apparently mild recurrences. At The Hospital for Sick Children (Toronto) we have had similar findings. The cases that developed mitral stenosis appear to have followed a relatively mild course for the disease but were slowly progressive over the years. The long-term follow-up at the Toronto General Hospital shows mitral stenosis

appearing between 20 and 50 years of age many years after the initial attack that occurred in early childhood.

The age at which mitral stenosis may develop varies from one country to another. In Western countries it is usually between 20 and 50, but it will be seen that in Thailand many develop this lesion in their teens (see Figure 13–5).

Mitral stenosis cases tend to develop atrial fibrillation and congestive heart failure, whereas the aortic regurgitation group more frequently provide a site for bacterial endocarditis. Now that bacterial endocarditis can either be prevented or be treated more adequately, the prognosis in this latter group has markedly improved.

The prognosis for mitral stenosis has also improved considerably, and many lives have been lengthened as a result of the valvotomy techniques and prophylactic measures. Aortic regurgitation may be treated surgically by a variety of procedures, and it is obvious, therefore, that if the myocardium itself remains competent, the problems created by valvular disease can frequently be managed with success.

Chronic Rheumatic Carditis. This is a term reserved for those patients who, following an attack of rheumatic fever, continue to show evidence of active infection and active carditis for more than six months and at times extending over years. Taranta and associates (1962) point out that this term does not include cases whose only sign of activity is an elevated sedimentation rate since this group does well, nor does it include the prolonged cases of chorea. It does refer to those children or adults who have progressive signs of carditis as well as a raised sedimentation rate. Usually they have had three or four previous attacks, but the continued activity is not accompanied by immunologic evidence of fresh streptococcal infection. The mortality is high in this group, and they need constant antirheumatic treatment—preferably salicylates because of the long administration required. Taranta and associates note that Aschoff's bodies were not seen in the majority of such patients who died and who had a histologic examination made of their hearts. Fresh valvular disease was identified frequently, however.

Functional Ability. Ninety-five percent of children who have recovered from their attack of rheumatic fever are able to lead an essentially normal life. Approximately 5 percent lead a somewhat restricted life, but the majority are able to go to school and take part in the ordinary activities. Those with significant mitral or aortic valve disease are kept out of strenuous and competitive sports.

The improvement in prognosis in the past two decades has been caused by a number of factors, including a reduced severity of hemolytic streptococcal infections in the community. This is due to frequent and regular treatment of throat infections with penicillin in the population, improved social and economic conditions, and prophylaxis in known rheumatics with sulfonamides and penicillin.

Familial Incidence

Irene A. Uchida

Although the appearance of more than one case of rheumatic fever in the same family is noted from time to time, the role of genetics as an etiologic factor remains to be clarified. There is no doubt about the intimate association between group A hemolytic streptococcus and rheumatic fever, and the spread of the latter can often be traced to its origin in crowded conditions that favored the spread of streptococcal infections. However, only a relatively small proportion of the subjects thus exposed developed rheumatic fever. Attempts to assess the role of inheritance should, therefore, take into consideration the interplay of an inherent susceptibility and an infective agent.

Familial Occurrence. Apparently the earliest statement supporting heredity was made by Cheadle in 1889: "The tendency to rheumatism is transmitted as strongly as the tendency to gout." Since then this statement has been given a great deal of support. Of 200 rheumatic patients studied by Faulkner and White (1924), 35.5 percent had a positive family history. Gauld and associates (1939, 1940) found 73.3 percent of 96 rheumatics with a positive family history, whereas only 21.9 percent of 33 tuberculosis patients had relatives with rheumatic fever. Sampson and coworkers (1945), however, found no significant difference in the frequency of positive family histories between rheumatics and nonrheumatics in school populations: 5.8 percent of 88 rheumatics and 3.6 percent of 3614 controls.

The basis for the familial tendency has aroused much discussion. Irvine-Jones (1933) stated: ". . . the undoubted familial occurrence of rheumatism would seem to be due to a specific and contagious agent than to certain familial characteristics . . . ." In a series of three studies, Read, Gauld, and others (1938, 1939, 1940) concluded that, although exposure to rheumatic infection is shown to be of importance, they prefer a genetic interpretation of their observations. Paul (1943) is of the same opinion.

Possible Modes of Inherited Susceptibility. Some authors have suggested a definite mode of inheritance. Draper and Seegal (1923) and Irvine-Jones (1933) believed that the inherited susceptibility was influenced by sex, but this has not been confirmed in more recent studies. A single autosomal dominant gene with complete penetrance is the method of inheritance suggested by Beers (1948), who was able to trace rheumatic individuals through four generations. Another impressive pedigree of five generations, indicating the same type of inheritance, was published by Pickles (1943), and a similar family was examined by Bradley (1950).

That a single autosomal recessive gene determines the susceptibility to rheumatic fever is the theory proposed by Wilson, Schweitzer, and coworkers

(1937, 1940, 1943) and corroborated by Mallen and Castillo (1952). The former authors examined 112 families and found close agreement between the observed and expected values except for the offspring of parents who both had rheumatic fever where, under a recessive hypothesis, all should be affected. On the basis of reduced penetrance in this latter group the frequencies for affected offspring in the other types of matings were too high. The same discrepancies were found in 40 families studied by Gray and associates (1952), which led them to conclude that, if heredity is an etiologic factor, it does not follow a specific genetic pattern. Similar conclusions were reached by Stevenson and Cheeseman (1953) after examining 462 families. They felt that heredity was a major factor, but a definite mendelian mechanism could not be established. In all these studies the frequencies of rheumatic offspring were higher in families where one parent was affected.

Subsequently Wilson and Schweitzer (1954) reported the results of a further study on the inheritance of rheumatic fever, giving support to their previous conclusion of a recessive inheritance. This study is particularly interesting since it began with selected parents rather than selected children. The observations are, therefore, more readily interpreted.

Family Studies at The Hospital for Sick Children. In a study of 58 rheumatic patients and their families no simple genetic mechanism could be determined (Uchida, 1953). In an attempt to produce more substantial evidence, this sample was extended to include 104 families with a total of 420 offspring (Table 13–5). All patients, sibs, and parents were examined by the Cardiac Service of The Hospital for Sick Children in Toronto. The sample was restricted to "white" families of the lower-income group and children under the age of two years were excluded.

The percentage frequencies of affected children for the different types of matings are given in Table 13–6. There are no significant differences among these frequencies.

Table 13–5. NUMBER OF AFFECTED AND UNAFFECTED INDIVIDUALS IN 104 FAMILIES EXAMINED AT THE HOSPITAL FOR SICK CHILDREN, TORONTO

	SEX	AFFECTED	UNAFFECTED	TOTAL
Offspring	♂	64	153	217
	♀	54	149	203
	Total	118	302	420
Parents	♂	5	99	104
	♀	13	91	104
	Total	18	190	208

Since this sample is biased by the presence of at least one affected child in every family studied, the corrected incidence of rheumatic fever among the offspring was estimated by a method developed by

Table 13–6. DISTRIBUTION OF RHEUMATIC OFFSPRING OF AFFECTED AND UNAFFECTED PARENTS

TYPE OF MATING	NUMBER OF MATINGS	TOTAL NUMBER OF OFFSPRING	AFFECTED OFFSPRING	
			Number	*Percent*
Both parents unaffected	87	350	98	28.0
One parent affected	16	65	19	29.3
Both parents affected	1	5	1	20.0

Haldane (1932, 1938) and simplified by Finney (1949). The resulting values were 8 percent for families with neither parent affected and 11 percent for families with one parent affected. These two frequencies obviously differ from the 25 percent and 50 percent expected on a recessive hypothesis. However, the higher frequency of rheumatics among the offspring of affected parents is consistent with the other studies reported above and supports the conclusion that a genetic factor may be present. On the other hand, from these studies a simple hereditary mechanism cannot be demonstrated.

It soon became evident that merely analyzing and comparing frequencies of affected subjects in rheumatic and nonrheumatic families would not produce definitive results. A new approach was suggested by the progress being made in studies of the infective agent. Serologic analyses showed significant rises in antistreptolysin-O or antihyaluronidase levels in rheumatic patients (Wannamaker and Ayoub, 1960). This lead was followed by Quinn and Fekerspiel (1967) in a five-year study of rheumatic and nonrheumatic families. They looked for differences in sensitivity to streptococcal infections, but although additional rheumatic patients were found in rheumatic families only, the frequency and severity of infections were similar. They concluded that a susceptibility to rheumatic fever was inherent in the host but were unable to explain the mechanism involved.

Matanoski and colleagues (1968) also tried to appraise the immune response that placed children from rheumatic families at higher risk and arrived at similar conclusions. The overall rate of streptococcal infections did not differ between rheumatic and nonrheumatic families but the mean level of antistreptolysin-O was found to be higher in the former. They drew no conclusion regarding transmission of host susceptibility.

Twin Studies.   The largest series of twins with rheumatic fever have been recorded in German literature. Kaufmann and Scheerer (1938), Brandt and Weihe (1939), and Claussen (1955) studied a total of 226 twin pairs of which 99 were monozygotic and 127 dizygotic. Of the monozygotic pairs, 30 percent were concordant for rheumatic fever whereas in only 9 percent of the dizygotic twins was rheumatic fever present in both.

In a series of 56 twin pairs, 16 monozygotic and 40 dizygotic, reported by Taranta and coworkers (1959), three monozygotic pairs were concordant for both the presence of rheumatic fever and the type of manifestation. Among the dizygotic twins, 1 out of 23 same-sexed pairs and 1 out of 17 heterosexual pairs were concordant. The latter pair, however, had different clinical manifestations.

The low concordance rate in monozygotic twins indicates that environmental factors are important in the etiology of rheumatic fever. These data, therefore, are consistent with the hypothesis that an inherent susceptibility is present in the host, but it is less important than the environmental agent.

Association with Blood Groups.   Because of the precision with which blood group antigens can be identified, they are particularly useful in testing for a possible association with the development of disease. The ABO blood group has been shown to be associated with duodenal ulcers, gastric carcinoma, and pernicious anemia. A similar association with blood groups has been proposed for rheumatic fever.

Glynn and colleagues (1956) suggested an association between streptococcal infections and the composition of throat secretions. After examining the saliva of rheumatic fever patients, they postulated that these patients carried the nonsecretor gene. (The secretor gene allows ABO antigens to be secreted in the saliva but this gene is not linked with the ABO genes.) Other studies associated a susceptibility to rheumatic fever with the ABO blood group (Clarke et al., 1960) and Rh and MN groups (Buckwalter et al., 1962). Further investigations, however, did not confirm these results (Addis, 1959; Lim et al., 1965). Whether or not an association exists between blood groups and rheumatic fever thus remains open to question.

Conclusion.   The evidence presented indicates that environmental factors, specifically group A hemolytic streptococcal infection and the conditions that favor its spread, combine with an inherited susceptibility to produce rheumatic fever. Better control over environmental agents has resulted in a marked decrease in incidence. The exact method of genetic transmission, however, remains unknown, but as the nongenetic factors are brought increasingly under control, the emphasis should shift to investigations of inherited susceptibility.

Definite risk figures for rheumatic susceptibility are difficult to assess accurately. In general, however, the chance of having a second rheumatic child, after one has been so diagnosed in the family, must be based upon the figure derived from the above analysis, which is approximately 10 percent.

Stevenson and Cheeseman (1953), by using only children born subsequently to the index case, found a risk of approximately 5 percent for families with neither parent affected and 9 percent for families with one parent affected.

In occasional cases where dominant inheritance is demonstrated, the risk of having an affected child may be close to 50 percent, penetrance being almost complete.

REFERENCES*

Adebonojo, F. O.: Monoarticular arthritis: an unusual manifestation of infectious mononucleosis. *Clin. Pediatr.*, **11**: 549, 1972.

Alexander, W. D., and Smith, G.: Disadvantageous circulatory effects of salicylate in rheumatic fever. *Lancet*, **1**: 768, 1962.

American Heart Association: Jones's criteria (modified) for guidance in the diagnosis of rheumatic fever. *Mod. Concepts Cardiovasc. Dis.*, **24**: 291, 1955.

Angelino, P. F.; Levi, V.; Brusca, A.; and Actis-Dato, A.: Mitral commissurotomy in younger age group. *Am. Heart J.*, **51**: 916, 1956.

Ash, R.: Prognosis of rheumatic infection in childhood. *Am. J. Dis. Child.*, **52**: 280, 1936.

————: Rheumatic infection in childhood: fifteen to twenty year follow-up: caution against early ambulant therapy. *Am. J. Dis. Child.*, **76**: 46, 1948.

Ayoub, E. M., and Dudding, B. A.: Streptococcal group A carbohydrate antibody in rheumatic and non-rheumatic bacterial endocarditis. *J. Lab. Clin. Med.*, **76**: 322, 1970.

Bernhard, G. C., and Stollerman, G. H.: Serum inhibiton of streptococcal diphosphopyridine nucleotidase in uncomplicated streptococcal pharyngitis and in rheumatic fever. *J. Clin. Invest.*, **38**: 1942, 1959.

Berry, J. N.: Prevalence survey for chronic rheumatic heart disease and rheumatic fever in Northern India. *Br. Heart J.*, **34**: 143, 1972.

Besterman, E.: The changing face of acute rheumatic fever. *Br. Heart J.*, **32**: 579, 1970.

Bi-Regional Workshop on the Prevention of Rheumatic Fever: Sponsored by the Council on Rheumatic Fever and Congenital Heart Disease, the Committee on Community Program, the New England and Upper Atlantic Regions, and the Connecticut Heart Association, Hartford, Connecticut: The Community Control of Streptococcal Infections, 1971.

Bland, E. F.: Personal communication, 1955.

————: Declining severity of rheumatic fever. *N. Engl. J. Med.*, **262**: 597, 1960.

Bland, E. F., and Jones, T. D.: Rheumatic fever and rheumatic heart disease. A twenty year report on 1000 patients followed since childhood. *Circulation*, **4**: 836, 1951.

————: Natural history of rheumatic fever; twenty year perspective. *Am. Intern. Med.*, **37**: 1006, 1952.

Borman, J. B.; Stern, S.; Shapita, T.; Milwidsky, H.; and Braun, K.: Mitral valvotomy in children. *Am. Heart J.*, **61**: 763, 1961.

Boyd, A. R. J.: City of Toronto, Department of Public Health, 1969 Annual Statement.

Breese, B. B.: Beta hemolytic streptococcal infections in children. *Pediatr. Clin. North Am.*, **7**: 843, 1960.

Breese, B. B.; Disney, F. A.; Talpey, W. B.; et al.: β-Hemolytic streptococcal infection: comparison of penicillin and lincomycin in the treatment of recurrent infections of the carrier state. *Am. J. Dis. Child.*, **117**: 147, 1969.

Brownell, K. D.: Personal communication, 1955.

Bunim, J. J.: Current evaluation of the diagnosis, treatment and prevention of rheumatic fever. *Bull. Rheum. Dis.*, **13**: 293, 1962.

Campbell, E. J.: New York Life Insurance Company Report, 1939.

Chamovitz, R.; Catanzaro, F. J.; Stetson, C. A.; and Rammelkamp, C. H.: Prevention of rheumatic fever by treatment of previous streptococcal infections. *N. Engl. J. Med.*, **251**: 466, 1954.

Chartikavanij, K.: Juvenile mitral stenosis. World Congress of Cardiology, London, 1970, page 27.

Cherian, G.; Vytilingan, K. I. Sukumar, I. P.; and Gopinath, N.: Mitral valvotomy in young patients. *Br. Heart J.*, **26**: 157, 1964.

Clarke, G. M., and Robinson, J. S.: Group A beta-haemolytic streptococcal septicaemia, complications and management. *Med. J. Aust.* **1**: 324, 1971.

Clarke, M., and Keith, J. D.: Atrioventricular conduction in acute rheumatic fever. *Br. Heart J.*, **34**: 472, 1972.

Clarke, N. E., and Mosher, R. E.: Phenolic compounds in the treatment of rheumatic fever. II. The metabolism of gentisic acid and the ethanolamide of gentisic acid. *Circulation*, **7**: 337, 1953.

Coburn, A. F.: Salicylate therapy in rheumatic fever. A rational technique. *Bull. Hopkins Hosp.*, **73**: 435, 1943.

Coburn, A. F., and Moore, L. V.: The prophylactic use of sulfanilamide in streptococcal respiratory infections, with special reference to rheumatic fever, *J. Clin. Invest.*, **18**: 135, 1939.

————: A follow-up report on rheumatic subjects treated with sulphanilamide. *JAMA*, **107**: 176, 1941.

Coburn, A. F., and Pauli, R. H.: Studies on immune response of rheumatic process. VI. Significance of rise of antistreptolysin level in development of rheumatic activity. *J. Clin. Invest.*, **14**: 769, 1935.

Coburn, A. F., and Young, D. C.: *The Epidemiology of Hemolytic Streptococcus.* Williams & Wilkins Co., Baltimore, 1949.

Collis, W. R. F., and MacDonald, A. J.: The beta streptococcal theory of rheumatic fever in the modern treatment of the condition. *Acta Paediatr.*, **100**(suppl): 54, 1954.

Combined Rheumatic Fever Study Group: A comparison of the effect of prednisone and acetylsalicylic acid on the incidence of residual rheumatic heart disease. *N. Engl. J. Med.*, **262**: 895, 1960.

Coombs, C. F.: *Rheumatic Heart Disease.* William Wood & Co., New York, 1924.

Cooperative Rheumatic Fever Study: The treatment of acute rheumatic fever in children. A cooperative clinical trial of ACTH, cortisone, and aspirin. *Circulation*, **11**: 343, 1955.

————: The treatment of acute rheumatic fever in children. A cooperative clinical trial of ACTH, cortisone, and aspirin. *Circulation*, **22**: 503, 1960.

Crea, M. A., and Mortimer, E. A., Jr.: The nature of scarlatinal arthritis. *Pediatrics*, **23**: 879, 1959.

DeGraff, A. C., and Lingg, C.: The course of rheumatic heart disease in adults. I. Factors pertaining to age at initial infection, the development of cardiac insufficiency, duration of life and cause of death. *Am. Heart J.*, **10**: 459, 1935a.

————: The course of rheumatic heart disease in adults. II. The influence of the type of valvular lesion on the course of rheumatic heart disease. *Am. Heart J.*, **10**: 478, 1935b.

Diehl, A. M.; Hamilton, T. R.; and Keeling, I. C.: Long-acting repository penicillin in prophylaxis of recurrent rheumatic fever. *JAMA*, **155**: 1466, 1954.

Dock, W.: Mode of production of first heart sound. *Arch. Intern. Med.*, **51**: 737, 1933.

Dorfman, A.; Gross, J. I.; and Lorinez, A. E.: The treatment of acute rheumatic fever. *Pediatrics*, **21**: 692, 1961.

Edwards, J. E.: Differential diagnosis of mitral stenosis: a clinicopathologic review of simulating conditions. *Lab. Invest.*, **3**: 89, 1954.

Ellis, F. H. Jr.; Brandenburg, R. O.; Callahan, J. A.; and Marshall, H. W.: Open heart surgery for acquired mitral insufficiency. *Arch. Surg.*, **79**: 222, 1959.

Ellis, F. H., Jr., and Bulbulian, A. H.: Prosthetic replacement of the mitral valve. I. Preliminary experimental observations. *Proc. Mayo Clin.*, **33**: 532, 1959.

Ellis, L. B., and Ramirez, A.: The clinical course of patients with severe rheumatic mitral insufficiency. *Am. Heart J.*, **78**: 406, 1969.

El-Sherif, N.: Rheumatic tricuspid stenosis a haemodynamic correlation. *Br. Heart J.*, **33**: 16, 1971.

Evans, R. P. C.: Rheumatic involvement of all four heart valves. *Guy Hosp. Rep.*, **102**: 146, 1953.

Favara, B. E.; Hoyum, B.; and Franciosis, R. A.: The antistreptolysin O latex test. *Am. J. Dis. Child.*, **123**: 462, 1972.

Feinstein, A. R.: The stethoscope: a source of diagnostic aid and conceptual errors in rheumatic heart disease. *J. Chronic Dis.*, **11**: 91, 1960.

Feinstein, A. R., and Arevalo, A. C.: Manifestations and treatment of congestive heart failure in young patients with rheumatic heart disease. *Pediatrics*, **33**: 661, 1964.

Feinstein, A. R., and Levitt, M.: Tonsil size. *N. Engl. J. Med.*, **282**: 285, 1970.

* References for the section on Familial Incidence appear on pages 230–31.

Feinstein, A. R., and Spagnuolo, M.: Mimetic features of rheumatic fever recurrences. *N. Engl. J. Med.*, **262**:533, 1960.

——: The clinical patterns of acute rheumatic fever. *Medicine*, **41**:279, 1962.

Feinstein, A. R.; Taranta, A.; and Di Massa, R.: Errors in the diagnosis of acute rheumatic fever. *N. Y. J. Med.*, **60**:2835, 1960.

Feinstein, A. R.; Wood, H. F.; Epstein, J. A.; Taranta, A.; Simpson, R.; and Tursky, E.: A controlled study of three methods of prophylaxis against streptococcal infection in a population of rheumatic children. II. Results of the first three years of the study, including methods for evaluating the maintenance of oral prophylaxis. *N. Engl. J. Med.*, **260**:697, 1959.

Findlay, I. I., and Fowler, R. S.: The changing pattern of rheumatic fever in childhood. *Can. Med. Assoc. J.*, **94**:1027, 1966.

Findlay, L.: *The Rheumatic Infection in Childhood*. Longmans, Green & Co., Inc., New York, 1931.

Fischel, E. E.; Frank, C. W.; and Ragan, C.: Observations on treatment of rheumatic fever with salicylate, ACTH and cortisone. I. Appraisal of signs of systemic and local inflammatory reaction during treatment, the rebound period and chronic activity. *Medicine*, **31**:331, 1952.

Fischel, E. E., and Pauli, R. H.: Serologic studies in rheumatic fever: I. 'Phase' reaction and detection of autoantibodies in the rheumatic state. *J. Exp. Med.*, **89**:669, 1949.

Fleischman, J.; Falk, J. A.; Zabriskie, J.; and Falk, R. E.: A study of HL-A antigen phenotype in rheumatic fever and rheumatic heart disease patients. Canadian Cardiovascular Society, 1972.

Foltz, E. L.; Roberts, E.; Steers, E.; Milliken, M. A.; and Norris, R. F.: The effect of penicillin prophylaxis on the colonization of the nasopharynges of rheumatic fever patients by staphylococci. *Am. J. Med. Sci.*, **77**:683, 1963.

Friedman, S.; Hallidie-Smith, K. A.; and Harris, T. N.: Congenital deformity of the atrioventricular valve leaflets simulating rheumatic mitral insufficiency. *Am. J. Med. Sci.*, **238**:79/557, 1959.

Gil, J. R.; Rodriguez, H.; and Ibarra, J. J.: Incidence of asymptomatic, active rheumatic cardiac lesions in patients submitted to mitral commissurotomy and the effect of cortisone on these lesions; clinical and histopathologic study of sixty cases. *Am. Heart J.*, **50**:912, 1955.

Gilbert, G.; Aerichide, N.; Lamontagne, R.; Allard, C.; and David, P.: Diagnosis, treatment and prophylaxis of rheumatic fever evaluated over a twelve-year period. Institute of Cardiology, Montreal, Canada.

Gilbert, G.; David, P.; Aerichide, N.; and Lefebvre, M.: Treatment and prevention of rheumatic carditis. *Can. Med. Assoc. J.*, **83**:179, 1960.

Glaser, R. J., and Smith, D. E. (eds.): Aortic insufficiency with cardiac failure and recurrent abdominal pain. Clinic-pathologic conference, Barnes Hospital. *Am. J. Med.*, **11**:507, 1951.

Glover, R. P.: Mitral surgery in a young girl. *Am. J. Cardiol.*, **4**:132, 1959.

Glover, R. P., and Gadboys, H. L.: The role of the left ventricle in the surgical management of aortic stenosis. *Angiology*, **10**:1, 1959.

Goodwin, J. F.; Hunter, J. D.; Cleland, W. P.; Davies, L. G.; and Steiner, R. E.: Mitral valve disease and mitral valvotomy. *Br. Med. J.*, **2**:573, 1955.

Gordis, L.; Markowitz, M.; and Lilienfeld, A. M.: Studies in the epidemiology and preventability of rheumatic fever. IV. A quantitative determination of compliance in children on oral penicillin prophylaxis. *Pediatrics*, **43**:173, 1969.

Gross, M., and Greenberg, L. A.: *The Salicylates*, Hillhouse Press, New Haven, Conn., 1948.

Harris, T. N.; Friedman, S.; and Haub, C. F.: Phonocardiographic differentiation of the murmur of mitral insufficiency from some commonly heard adventitious sounds in childhood. *Pediatrics*, **3**:845, 1949.

Hedley, O. F.: Trends, geographical and racial distribution of mortality from heart disease among persons five to twenty-four years of age in the United States during recent years (1922–36). *Public Health Rep.*, **54**:2271, 1939.

Hench, P. S., et al: Effects of adrenal cortical hormone (17-hydroxy-11-dehydro-corticosterone (compound E) on acute phase of rheumatic fever: preliminary report. *Proc. Mayo Clin.*, **24**:227, 1949.

Hench, P. S.; Kendall, E. C.; Slocumb, C. H.; and Polley, H. F.: Effects of cortisone acetate and pituitary ACTH on rheumatoid arthritis, rheumatic fever, and certain other conditions: study in clinical physiology. *Arch. Intern. Med.*, **85**:545, 1950.

Hench, P. S.; Slocumb, C. H.; Polley, H. F.; and Kendall, C.: Effects of cortisone and pituitary adrenocorticotropic hormone (ACTH) on rheumatic disease. *JAMA*, **144**:1327, 1950.

Henderson, L. L.: Sodium salicylate in rheumatic fever; effect of adjuvant medication. *Am. J. Med. Sci.*, **225**:480, 1953.

Houser, H. B.: Treatment and prophylaxis of streptococcal infections for prevention of rheumatic fever. *J. Michigan Med. Soc.*, **52**:1289, 1953.

Houser, H. B.; Clark, E. J.; and Stolzer, B. L.: Comparative effects of aspirin, ACTH and cortisone on the acute course of rheumatic fever in young adult males. *Am. J. Med.*, **16**:168, 1954.

Houser, H. B.; Eckhardt, G. C.; Hahn, E. O.; Denny, F. W.; Wannamaker, L. W.; and Rammelkamp, C. H.: Effect of aureomycin treatment of streptococcal sore throat on the streptococcal carrier state, the immunologic response of the host, and the incidence of acute rheumatic fever. *Pediatrics*, **12**:593, 1953.

Howie, V. M., and Ploussard, J. H.: Treatment of group A streptococcal pharyngitis in children. *JAMA*, **121**:477, 1961.

Illingworth, R. S.; Burke, J.; Doxiadis, S. A.; Lorber, J.; Philpott, M. G.; and Stone, D. G. H.: Salicylates in rheumatic fever: an attempt to assess their value. *Q. J. Med.*, **23**:177, 1954.

Illingworth, R. S.; Lorber, J.; Holt, K. S.; Rendle-Short, J.; Jowett, G. H.; and Gibson, W. M.: Acute rheumatic fever in children. A comparison of six forms of treatment in 200 cases. *Lancet*, **2**:653, 1957.

Jacobs, A. L.; Leitner, Z. A.; Moore, T.; and Sharman, I. M.: Vitamin I in rheumatic fever. *J. Clin. Nutr.*, **2**:155, 1954.

Jarcho, S.: Rheumatic carditis: Bouillaud and some unknown Irish precursors. *Am. J. Cardiol.*, **1**:514, 1958.

Johnson, A. L., and Ferencz, C.: The effect of cortisone therapy on the incidence of rheumatic heart disease. *N. Engl. J. Med.*, **248**:845, 1953.

Johnson, E. E.; Stollerman, G. H.; and Grossman, B. J.: Streptococcal infections in adolescents and adults after prolonged freedom from rheumatic fever. *N. Engl. J. Med.*, **263**:105, 1960.

A Joint Report by the Rheumatic Fever Working Party of the Medical Research Council of Great Britain and the Sub-Committee of Principal Investigators of the American Council on Rheumatic Fever and Congenital Heart Disease, American Heart Association: The natural history of rheumatic fever and rheumatic heart disease. *Can. Med. Assoc. J.*, **93**:519, 1954.

Jones, T. D.: The diagnosis of rheumatic fever, *JAMA*, **126**:481, 1944.

Jones, T. D., and Bland, E. F.: Clinical significance of chorea as a manifestation of rheumatic fever: a study in prognosis. *JAMA*, **105**:571, 1935.

——: Rheumatic fever and heart disease: completed ten-year observations on 1,000 patients. *Trans. Assoc. Am. Physicians*, **57**:267, 1942.

Jones, T. D.; White, P. D.; Roche, C. F.; Perdue, J. J.; and Ryan, H. A.: The transportation of rheumatic fever patients to a subtropical climate. *JAMA*, **108**:1308, 1937.

Kaiser, A. D.: Results of tonsillectomy. A comparative study of twenty-two hundred tonsillectomized children with an equal number of controls three and ten years after operation. *JAMA*, **95**:837, 1930.

Keith, J. D.: Variations in the first heart sound and the auriculoventricular conduction time in children with rheumatic fever. *Arch. Dis. Child.*, **12**:217, 1937.

——: Over-stimulation of vagus nerve in rheumatic fever. *Q. J. Med.*, **7**:29, 1938.

——: Rheumatic heart disease—a public health problem. *Can. J. Public Health*, **32**:95, 1941.

——: Modern trends in acute rheumatic fever. *Can. Med. Assoc. J.*, **83**:789, 1960.

Keith, J. D., and Brick, M.: Changes in the size of the heart in children with rheumatic fever. *Am. Heart J.*, **24**:289, 1942.

Keith, J. D., and Pequegnat, L. A.: Some observations on the prevalence of rheumatic heart disease in Canada. *Can. J. Public Health*, **38**:111, 1947.

Keith, J. D., and Ross, A.: Observations on salicylate therapy in rheumatic fever. *Can. Med. Assoc. J.*, **52**:554, 1945.

Kelley, V. C.; Ely, R. S.; Done, A. K.; and Ainger, L. E.: Studies of 17-hydroxycorticosteroids. *Am. J. Med.*, **18**:20, 1955.

Kellgren, J. H.: Diagnostic criteria for population studies. *Bull. Rheum. Dis.*, **13**:291, 1962.

Kellner, A. A., and Robertson, T.: Cardiac lesions induced by a proteolytic enzyme isolated from filtrates of group A streptococci. Paper presented at the 2nd International Congress of Cardiology, 1954.

Kloth, H. H.; Reed, G. E.; and Spagnuolo, M.: Open heart surgery in active rheumatic carditis: report of a case. *Pediatrics*, **43**:613, 1969.

Kuschner, M., and Levieff, L.: Correlation between active rheumatic lesions in the left auricular appendage and elsewhere in the heart. *Am. J. Med. Sci.*, **226**:290, 1953.

Kuttner, A. G.: Prevention of rheumatic fever and rheumatic heart disease. *Postgrad. Med.*, **14**:429, 1951.

————: Personal communication, 1955.

————: Paper presented at 28th Annual Meeting of the American Academy of Pediatrics, Chicago, October 3–8, 1959.

Kuttner, A. G., and Reyersbach, G.: The prevention of streptococcal upper respiratory infections and rheumatic recurrences in rheumatic children by the prophylactic use of sulfonamide. *J. Clin. Invest.*, **22**:77, 1943.

Lanier, J. C., and Gyland, S. P.: Preventive value of diagnosing and treating streptococcal throat infections. *Clin. Pediatr.*, **10**:566, 1971.

Logan, A., and Turner, R.: Mitral stenosis, diagnosis and treatment. *Lancet*, **1**:1007–1018 and 1957–1064, 1953.

McCarty, M.: Nature of rheumatic fever. *Circulation*, **14**:1138, 1956.

McEwen, C.: The treatment of rheumatic fever. *Am. J. Med.*, **17**:794, 1954.

McIntosh, R., and Wood, C. L.: Rheumatic infections occurring in the first three years of life. *Am. J. Dis. Child.*, **49**:835, 1935.

Mackie, T. T.: An analytical study of three hundred and ninety-three cases of rheumatic fever and eighty-nine cases of chorea. *Am. J. Med. Sci.*, **172**:199, 1926.

Maclagan, T. J.: The treatment of acute rheumatism by salicin. *Lancet*, **1**:342, 383, 1876.

Maresch, G. J.; Dodge, H. J.; and Lichty, J. A.: Incidence of heart disease among Colorado school children. *JAMA*, **149**:802, 1952.

Margileth, A. M.; Mella, G. W.; and Zilvetti, E. E.: Streptococci in children's respiratory infections: diagnosis and treatment. *Clin. Pediatr.*, **10**:69, 1971.

Margileth, A. M., and Puig, J. R.: Streptococcal surveillance during 1970. *Clin. Proc. Child. Hosp. D.C.*, **26**:194, 1970.

Markowitz, M., and Gordis, L.: *Rheumatic Fever*. 2nd ed. W. B. Saunders Company, Philadelphia, 1972.

Markowitz, M., and Kuttner, A. G.: Effect of intensive and prolonged therapy with cortisone and hydrocortisone in first attacks of rheumatic carditis. *Pediatrics*, **16**:325, 1955.

————: Treatment of acute rheumatic fever. *Am. J. Dis. Child.*, **104**:313, 1962.

Massell, B. F.: Salicylates, hormones, and penicillin in the treatment of rheumatic fever. *Med. Clin. North Am.*, **34**:1419, 1950.

————: The medicinal treatment of acute rheumatic fever. *Med. Clin. North Am.*, **37**:1215, 1953.

————: ACTH and cortisone therapy of rheumatic fever and rheumatic carditis. *N. Engl. J. Med.*, **251**:183, 221, 263, 1954.

————: Hormone treatment of rheumatic carditis. *Bull. Rheum. Dis.*, **6**:99, 1955.

Massell, B. F., et al.: Prevention of rheumatic fever by prompt penicillin therapy of hemolytic streptococcal respiratory infections: progress report, *JAMA*, **146**:1469, 1951.

Massell, B. F.; Jharveri, S.; Czoniczer, G.; and Barnet, R.: Treatment of rheumatic fever and rheumatic carditis. *Med. Clin. North Am.*, **45**:1349, 1961.

Massell, B. F., and Jones, T. D.: The effect of sulfanilamide on rheumatic fever and chorea. *N. Engl. J. Med.*, **218**:876, 1938.

Massell, B. F.; Mote, J. R.; and Jones, T. D.: The artificial induction of subcutaneous nodules in patients with rheumatic fever. *J. Clin. Invest.*, **16**:125, 1937.

Massell, B. F., and Warren, J. E.: Effect of pituitary adrenocorticotropic hormone (ACTH) on rheumatic fever and rheumatic carditis. *JAMA*, **144**:1335, 1950.

Massie, E., and Levine, S. A.: The prognosis and subsequent developments in acute rheumatic pericarditis. *JAMA*, **112**:1219, 1939.

Mayer, F. E.; Doyle, E. F.; Herrera, L.; and Brownell, K. D.: Declining severity of first attack of rheumatic fever. *Am. J. Dis. Child.*, **105**:146, 1963.

Morrow, R., and Rabin, D. L.: Reliability in self-medication with isoniazed (abst.). *Clin. Res.*, **13**:362, 1965.

Mortimer, E. A., Jr.; Vaisman, S.; Givnau, I.; Guasch, J. L.; Schuster, C.; Rakita, L.; Krause, R. M.; Roberts, R.; and Rammelkamp, C. H., Jr.: The effect of penicillin on acute rheumatic fever and valvular heart disease. *N. Engl. J. Med.*, **260**:101, 1959.

Morton, W. E., and Lichty, J. A.: Rheumatic heart disease epidemiology. *Am. J. Epidemiol.*, **92**:113, 1970.

Morton, W. E.; Warner, A. L.; Weil, J. V.; Schmock, C. L., Jr.; Snyder, J.; and Lichty, J. A.: Rheumatic heart disease epidemiology. *Am. J. Epidemiol.*, **41**:773, 1970.

Morton, W. E., et al.: Rheumatic heart disease epidemiology. III. The San Luis Valley prevalence study. *Circulation*, **41**:773, 1970.

Murphy, G. E.: The characteristic rheumatic lesions of striated and of nonstriated or smooth muscle cells of the heart. *Medicine*, **42**:73, 1963.

Mustard, W. T.: Personal communication, 1954.

Negus, R. M., and Chir, B.: Rheumatic fever in Western Fiji: the female preponderance. *Med. J. Aust.*, **2**:251, 1971.

Oncharit, Thailand: World Congress of Cardiology, London, 1970.

Palmieri, M. R.; Costas, M.; and Rivera, R. S.: Rheumatic fever in the tropics. *Am. Heart J.*, **63**:18, 1962.

Paul, J. R.: Pleural and pulmonary lesions in rheumatic fever. *Medicine*, **7**:383, 1928.

Perlman, L. V.; Ostrander, L. D.; Keller, B. J.; and Chiang, B. N.: An epidemiologic study of first degree atrioventricular block in Tecumseh, Michigan. *U. Mich. School Public Health*, **59**:40, 1971.

Perry, L. W.; Poitras, J. M.; and Findlan, C.: Rheumatic fever and rheumatic heart disease among U.S. college freshmen, 1956–65. *Public Health Rep.*, **83**:919, 1968.

Pilapil, V. R., and Watson, D. G.: Rheumatic fever in Mississippi. *JAMA*, **215**:1626, 1971.

Prevention of Rheumatic Heart Disease. Report of the Inter-Society Commission for Heart Disease Resources. *Circulation*, **41**:A-1, 1970.

Puddu, V.: Cardiovascular diseases in Italy. *Am. J. Cardiol.*, **10**:341, 1962.

Rammelkamp, C. H., Jr.: Hemolytic streptococcal infections. In Harrison, T. R. (ed.): *Principles of Internal Medicine*. Blakiston Co., Philadelphia, 1951, pp. 799–825.

————: Present status of streptococcal infections in relation to rheumatic fever and glomerulo-nephritis. *Am. J. Clin. Pathol.*, **26**:555, 1956.

Rammelkamp, C. H., Jr.; Houser, H. B.; Hahn, E. O.; Wannamaker, L. W.; Denny, F. W.; and Eckhardt, G. C.: The prevention of rheumatic fever. In Thomas, L. (ed.): *Rheumatic Fever*. University of Minnesota Press, Minneapolis, 1952.

Rammelkamp, C. H., Jr., and Stolzer, B. L.: The treatment and prevention of rheumatic fever. *Pediatr. Clin. North Am.*, **1**:265, 1954.

Rammelkamp, C. H., Jr.; Wannamaker, L. W.; and Denny, F. W.: Epidemiology and prevention of rheumatic fever. *Bull. N.Y. Acad. Med.*, **28**:321, 1952.

Randolph, M. F., and DeHaan, R. M.: A comparison of lincomycin and penicillin in the treatment of group A streptococcal infections: speculation on the 'L' form as a mechanism of recurrence. *Delaware Med. J.*, **41**:51, 1969.

Randolph, M. F.; Redys, J. J.; and Hibbard, E. W.: Streptococcal pharyngitis. *Delaware Med. J.*, **42**:29, 62, 87, 1969.

Rantz, L. A.: The streptococcal etiology of rheumatic fever. *Med. Clin. North Am.*, **39**:339, 1955.

Rapkin, R. H.: The diagnosis of epiglottitis: simplicity and reliability of radiographs of the neck in the differential diagnosis of the croup syndrome. *J. Pediatr.*, **80**:96, 1972.

Rapkin, R. H., and Eppley, M. L.: The recognition of streptococcal pharyngitis. *Clin. Pediatr.*, **10**:706, 1971.

Reale, A.: The stenosi aortiche congenite. *Atti Soc. Ital. Cardiol.*, **1**:103, 1966.

Robinson, S. J.; Aggeler, D. M.; and Daniloff, G. T.: Heart disease in San Francisco school children. *J. Pediatr.*, **33**:49, 1948.

Rowe, R. D.; McKelvey, A. D.; and Keith, J. D.: The use of ACTH, cortisone and salicylates in the treatment of acute rheumatic fever. *Can. Med. Assoc. J.*, **68**:15, 1953.

Rutstein, D. D.: Need for a public health program in rheumatic fever and rheumatic heart disease. *Am. J. Public Health*, **36**: 461, 1946.

Sarrouy, C.; Sendra, L.; and Duboucher, G.: Considerations on the evolution of heart diseases in Algeria. *Am. Heart J.*, **61**: 145, 1961.

Saslaw, M. S.; Ross, B. D.; and Dobbin, M.: The incidence of rheumatic heart disease in native school children of Dade County, Florida. *Am. Heart J.*, **40**: 760, 1950.

Schaefer, L. E.; Rashkoff, I. A.; and Megibow, R. S.: Sodium gentisate in the treatment of acute rheumatic fever. *Circulation*, **2**: 265, 1950.

Schlesinger, B.: The relationship of throat infection to acute rheumatism in childhood. *Arch. Dis. Child.*, **5**: 411, 1930.

Sen, P. K.; Panday, S. R.; Parulkar, G. B.; and Biswas, P. K.: Mitral stenosis in the young. *Dis. Chest*, **49**: 384, 1966.

Shackman, N. H.; Heffer, E. T.; and Kroop, I. G.: The C-reactive protein determination as a measure of rheumatic activity. *Am. Heart J.*, **48**: 599, 1954.

Shoung Lin, J.: Appendectomy in children with acute rheumatic fever. *Pediatrics*, **43**: 573, 1969.

Siegel, A. C.; Johnson, E. E.; and Stollerman, G. H.: Controlled studies of streptococcal pharyngitis in a pediatric population. I. Factors related to the attack rate of rheumatic fever. *N. Engl. J. Med.*, **265**: 559, 1961.

Spagnuolo, M., and Feinstein, A. R.: Congestive heart failure and rheumatic activity in young patients with rheumatic heart disease. *Pediatrics*, **33**: 653, 1964.

Spagnuolo, M.; Gavrin, J.; and Ryan, J.: A day hospital for children with rheumatic fever. *Pediatrics*, **45**: 276, 1970.

Spagnuolo, M.; Pasternack, B.; and Taranta, A.: Risk of rheumatic fever recurrences after streptococcal infections. *N. Engl. J. Med.*, **285**: 641, 1971.

Stillerman, M.; Isenberg, H. D.; and Moody, M.: Streptococcal pharyngitis therapy. *Am. J. Dis. Child.*, **123**: 457, 1972.

Stollerman, G. H.: Rheumatogenic and nephritogenic streptococci. *Circulation*, **43**: 915, 1971.

Stollerman, G. H.: Repository benzathine penicillin for the control of rheumatic fever. *Bull. Rheum. Dis.*, **5**: 79, 1954.

―――: The use of antibiotics for the prevention of rheumatic fever. *Am. J. Med.*, **17**: 757, 1954.

―――: Factors determining the attack rate of rheumatic fever. *JAMA*, **177**: 823, 1961.

―――: Current evaluation of the diagnosis, treatment and prevention of rheumatic fever. *Bull. Rheum. Dis.*, **13**: 293, 1962.

Stollerman, G. H.; Glick, S.; Patel, D. J.; Hirschfeld, I.; and Rusoff, J. H.: Determination of C-reactive protein in serum as a guide to the treatment and management of rheumatic fever. *Am. J. Med.*, **15**: 645, 1953.

Stollerman, G. H.; Siegel, A. C.; and Johnsson, E. E.: Variable epidemiology of streptococcal disease and the changing pattern of rheumatic fever. *Mod. Concepts Cardiovasc. Dis.*, **34**: 45, 1965.

Stricker, J. S.: Ueber die resultate der behandlung der polyarthritis rheumatica mit salicylsaure. *Berl. Klin. Wchr.*, **13**: 1, 15, 99, 1876; abst. in *Dublin J. Med. Sci.*, **52**: 395, 1876. Cited by Gross and Greenberg (1948).

Svane, S.: Peracute spontaneous streptococcal myositis. *Univ. Inst. Pathol.*, **137**: 155, 1971.

Swift, H. F.: The relationship of streptococcal infections to rheumatic fever. *Am. J. Med.*, **2**: 168, 1947.

Taranta, A.; Fiedler, J. P.; Gilson, B. S.; Gordis, L.; Hufnagel, C. A.; Kloth, H. H.; Markowitz, M.; and Wannamaker, L. W.: Community resources for the diagnosis and acute care of patients with rheumatic fever. *Regional Med. Programs Service*, **4**: 197, 1971.

Taranta, A., et al.: Community resources for the diagnosis and acute care of patients with rheumatic fever. *Circulation*, **44**: A197, 1971.

Taranta, A.; Spagnuolo, M.; and Feinstein, A. R.: "Chronic" rheumatic fever. *Ann. Intern. Med.*, **56**: 367, 1962.

―――: The occurrence of rheumatic-like subcutaneous nodules without evidence of joint or heart disease: report of a case. *N. Engl. J. Med.*, **266**: 13, 1962.

Thomas, C. B., and France, R.: A preliminary report of the prophylactic use of sulfanilamide in patients susceptible to rheumatic fever. *Bull. Hopkins Hosp.*, **64**: 67, 1939.

Thomas, C. B.; France, R.; and Reichsman, F.: The prophylactic use of sulfanilamide in patients susceptible to rheumatic fever. *JAMA*, **116**: 551, 1941.

Thomas, G.: Heart failure in children with active rheumatic carditis. *Br. Med. J.*, **2**: 205, 1954.

Thomas, G. T.: Five-year follow up on patients with rheumatic fever treated by bedrest, steroids, or salicylate. *Br. Med. J.*, No. 5240: 1635, 1961.

Thomas, L.: Recent advances in research on rheumatic fever. *Minnesota Med.*, **35**: 1105, 1952.

Tidwell, R. A.: Rheumatic fever prophylaxis. *Northwest Med.*, **53**: 470, 1954.

Todd, E. W.: Antigenic streptococcal hemolysin. *J. Exp. Med.*, **55**: 267, 1932.

Tompkins, D. G.; Boxerbaum, B.; and Liebman, J.: Long-term prognosis of rheumatic fever patients receiving regular intramuscular benzathine penicillin. *Rainbow Rheumatic Fever Clin.*, **45**: 543, 1972.

United Kingdom and United States Joint Report: Treatment of acute rheumatic fever in children: cooperative clinical trial of ACTH, cortisone and aspirin. *Circulation*, **22**: 503, 1960.

Wallace, H. M., and Rich, H.: Changing status of rheumatic fever and rheumatic heart disease in children and youth. *Am. J. Dis. Child.*, **89**: 7, 1955.

Wallgren, A. J.: The prognosis of rheumatic fever in childhood. Paper given at III Congresso Internazionale di Medicina Dell'assicurazione Vita, 1949.

Wallis, A. D.: Dietary eggs and rheumatic fever. *Am. J. Med. Sci.*, **227**: 167, 1954.

Wallis, A. D., and Viergiver, E.: Serum phospholipid and rheumatic fever. *Am. J. Med. Sci.*, **227**: 171, 1954.

Walsh, B. J.; Bland, E. F.; and Jones, T. D.: Pure mitral stenosis in young persons. *Arch. Intern. Med.*, **65**: 321, 1940.

Wannamaker, L. W.: and Ayoub, E. M.: Antibody titres in acute rheumatic fever. *Circulation*, **21**: 598, 1960.

Wannamaker, L. W.; Denny, F. W.; Perry, W. D.; Rammelkamp, C. H., Jr.; Eckhardt, G. C.; Houser, H. B.; and Hahn, E. O.: The effect of penicillin prophylaxis on streptococcal disease rates and carrier state. *N. Engl. J. Med.*, **249**: 1, 1953.

Wedum, B. G.; Darley, W.; and Rhodes, P. H.: Prevalence of rheumatic heart disease at high altitudes. *Am. J. Dis. Child.*, **79**: 205, 1950.

Wegria, R., and Smull, K.: Salicylate therapy in acute rheumatic fever. *J. Pediatr.*, **26**: 211, 1945.

Westerman, G.: A comparison of penicillin and Dalacin C in streptococcal pharyngitis and tonsillitis therapy. *JAMA*, **198**: 173, 1970.

Wheatley, G. M.: Rheumatic fever. A summary of present concepts. *Pediatrics*. **3**: 680, 1949.

White, P. D.: Acute heart block occurring as the first sign of rheumatic fever. *Am. J. Med. Sci.*, **152**: 589, 1916.

―――: *Heart Disease*, 4th ed. The Macmillan Co., New York, 1951.

―――: Changes in relative prevalence of various types of heart disease in New England, *JAMA*, **152**: 303, 1953.

White, P. D., and Jones, T. D.: Heart disease and disorders in New England. *Am. Heart J.*, **3**: 302, 1928.

Wilkinson, K. D.: Personal communication, 1937. Birmingham Children's Hospital.

Wilson, M. G.: Pattern of hereditary susceptibility in rheumatic fever. *Circulation*, **10**: 699, 1954.

Wilson, M. G.; Helper, H. N.; Lubschez, R.; Hain, K.; and Epstein, N.: Effect of short-term administration of corticotropin in active rheumatic carditis. *Am. J. Dis. Child.*, **86**: 131, 1953.

Wilson, M. G., and Lubschez, R.: Recurrence rates in rheumatic fever. The evaluation of etiologic concepts and consequent preventive therapy. *JAMA*, **126**: 447, 1944.

Wood, P.: Appreciation of mitral stenosis: investigations and results. *Br. Med. J.*, **1**: 1113, 1954.

World Health Organization Technical Report Series, No. 126: Prevention of rheumatic fever, second report of the Expert Committee on Rheumatic Diseases, 1957.

Yuan, S. H.; Doyle, E. F.; Pisacano, J. C.; and Reed, G. E.: Severe rheumatic mitral insufficiency in childhood amenable to surgery. *Pediatrics*, **33**: 571, 1964.

Familial Incidence

Addis, G. J.: Blood groups in acute rheumatism. *Scott. Med. J.*, **4**: 547, 1959.

Beers, C. V.: Four generations of rheumatic heart disease (proceedings of the Eighth International Congress of Genetics). *Hereditas*, **35** (suppl.): 534, 1948.

Bradley, W. H.: The mechanism and prevention of the rheumatic state. *Proc. Roy. Soc. Med.*, **43**: 979, 1950.

Brandt, G., and Weihe, F. A.: Polyarthritis rheumatica bei Zwillingen. *Z. Menschl. Vererb. Konstitutionsl.*, **23**: 169, 1939.

Buckwalter, J. A.; Naifeh, G-S.; and Auer, J. E.: Rh fever and the blood groups. *Br. Med. J.*, **2**: 1023, 1962.

Cheadle, W. B.: *The Various Manifestations of the Rheumatic State as Exemplified in Childhood and Early Life.* Smith, Elder & Co., London, 1889.

Clarke, C. A.; McConnell, R. B.; and Sheppard, P. M.: ABO blood groups and secretor character in rheumatic carditis. *Br. Med. J.*, **1**: 21, 1960b.

Claussen, F.: Beitrage der Zwillings-Forschung zum Rheuma-Problem. *Z. Rheumaforsch.*, **14**: 145, 1955.

Draper, G., and Seegal, D.: The importance to the clinician of the study of genetics. *Eugenic News*, **8**: 63, 1923.

Faulkner, J. N., and White, P. D.: The incidence of rheumatic fever, chorea and rheumatic heart disease. *JAMA*, **83**: 425, 1924.

Finney, D. J.: The truncated binomial distribution. *Ann. Eugenics*, **14**: 319, 1949.

Gauld, R. L.; Ciocco, A.; and Read, F. E. M.: II. Further observations on the occurrence of rheumatic manifestations in the families of rheumatic patients. *J. Clin. Invest.*, **18**: 213, 1939.

Gauld, R. L.; and Read, F. E. M.: Studies of rheumatic disease. III. Familial association and aggregation in rheumatic disease. *J. Clin. Invest.*, **19**: 393, 1940.

Glynn, A. A.; Glynn, L. E.; and Holborow, E. J.: The secretor status of rheumatic fever patients. *Lancet*, **II**: 759, 1956.

Gray, F. G.; Quinn, R. W.; and Quinn, J. P.: A long-term survey of rheumatic and nonrheumatic families. *Am. J. Med.*, **13**: 400, 1952.

Haldane, J. B. S.: A method for investigating recessive characters in man. *J. Genetics*, **25**: 251, 1932.

————: The estimation of the frequencies of recessive conditions in man. *Ann. Eugenics*, **8**: 255, 1938.

Irvine-Jones, E.: Acute rheumatism as a familial disease. *Am. J. Dis. Child.*, **45**: 1184, 1933.

Kaufmann, O., and Scheerer, E.: Uber die Erblichkeit des akuten Gelenkrheumatismus. *Z. Menschl. Vererb. Konstitutionsl.*, **21**: 687, 1938.

Lim, W. N.; Kelkner, A.; Schweitzer, M. D.; Smith, D.; and Wilson, M. G.: Association of secretor status and rheumatic fever in 106 families. *Am. J. Epidemiol.*, **82**: 103, 1965.

Mallen, M. S., and Castillo, F.: Genetica del reuma cardio-articular. *Arch. Inst. Cardiol. Mexico*, **22**: 136, 1952.

Matanoski, G. M.; Price, W. H.; and Ferencz, D.: Epidemiology of streptococcal infections in rheumatic and nonrheumatic families. *Am. J. Epidemiol.*, **87**: 179, 1968.

Paul, J. R.: *The Epidemiology of Rheumatic Fever and Some of its Public Health Aspects.* Metropolitan Life Insurance Co., New York, 1943.

Pickles, W. N.: A rheumatic family. *Lancet*, **245**: 241, 1943.

Quinn, R. W., and Fekerspiel, C. F.: Rheumatic fever and rheumatic heart disease. A five-year study of rheumatism and nonrheumatic families. *Am. J. Epidemiol.*, **85**: 120, 1967.

Read, F. E. M.; Ciocco, A.; and Taussig, H. B.: The frequency of rheumatic manifestations among the siblings, parents, uncles, aunts and grandparents of rheumatic and control patients. *Am. J. Hyg.*, **27**: 719, 1938.

Sampson, J. J.; Hahman, P. T.; Halverson, W. L.; and Shearer, M. C.: Incidence of heart disease and rheumatic fever in school children in three climatically different California communities. *Am. Heart J.*, **29**: 178, 1945.

Stevenson, A. C., and Cheeseman, E. A.: Heredity and rheumatic fever. *Ann. Eugenics*, **17**: 177, 1953.

Taranta, A.; Torosdag, S.; Metrakos, J. D.; and Uchida, I.: Rheumatic fever in monozygotic and dizygotic twins. *Circulation*, **20**: 778, 1959.

Uchida, I. A.: Possible genetic factors in the etiology of rheumatic fever. *Am. J. Hum. Genet.*, **5**: 61, 1953.

Wannamaker, L. W., and Ayoub, E. M.: Antibody titres in acute rheumatic fever. *Circulation*, **21**: 598, 1960.

Wilson, M. G.: *Rheumatic Fever.* The Commonwealth Fund, New York, 1940.

Wilson, M. G., and Schweitzer, M. D.: Rheumatic fever as a familial disease. *J. Clin. Invest.*, **16**: 555, 1937.

————: Pattern of hereditary susceptibility in rheumatic fever. *Circulation*, **10**: 699, 1954.

Wilson, M. G.; Schweitzer, M. D.; and Lubschez, R.: The familial epidemiology of rheumatic fever: Genetic and epidemiologic studies. *J. Pediatr.*, **22**: 468, 1943.

14

Bacterial Endocarditis
(Infective Endocarditis)

John D. Keith

ONE OF the most satisfying medical achievements in the past 30 years has been the dramatic drop in mortality in bacterial or infective endocarditis. Since the advent of the antibiotics, the mortality has fallen from approximately 100 percent to 20 to 30 percent. Furthermore, the deaths are now usually due to complications of the disease, such as heart failure or embolus, rather than the infection itself. Many excellent reviews of the condition in adults are available: Bloomfield (1950), Cates and Christie (1951), Finland (1954, 1972), Keefer (1953), Macaulay (1954), Lerner and Weinstein (1966), Weinstein and Rubin (1973), and Weinstein and Schlesinger (1973).

Kelson and White (1945) have pointed out that the division of bacterial endocarditis into acute and subacute forms is not exact, and they suggest that the designation of the causative organism is a preferable method. This applies most pointedly to those cases over two years of age where the causative organism is usually cultured. In bacterial endocarditis in infants under two years of age, the condition is often not suspected until it is found at postmortem, and frequently the etiologic agent is not cultured. The clinical pattern is not as clear-cut as in the children over two years of age. For these reasons we have divided bacterial endocarditis in infancy and childhood into two age groups.

Rheumatic endocarditis has for a long time been recognized as a common site for the seeding of a bacterial infection, and in the past the majority of cases have had such underlying lesions. Recently, however, particularly in children and young adults, congenital heart malformations presented themselves more obviously in this connection, although as long ago as 1844 Paget drew attention to the fact that congenital malformations of the heart may be predisposed to accept bacterial infections.

The terms *acute* and *subacute bacterial endocarditis* remain very useful in the pediatric age group, but in the adult such a classification has become indistinct since a great variety of organisms of widely different virulence and some nonbacterial in origin have been identified, many with a paradoxic clinical response. The name *infective endocarditis* has thus come into fashion. Although the majority of cases in childhood fit into the old classification, occasionally this is not so and bizarre infective organisms of varying potency can occur. At such times prolonged observation of cultures and appropriate use of special media and serologic methods are required.

BACTERIAL ENDOCARDITIS IN INFANTS UNDER TWO YEARS OF AGE

IN the first two years of life there is a group of cases, with acute infection superimposed on one or more heart valves, that is distinct from other forms of bacterial endocarditis. This type has been well described by White (1926), Macaulay (1954), and Ward (1971). The latter author not only summarized the literature from 1852 to 1953 but also collected data on 106 cases. In his own material he found that this type of bacterial endocarditis in infants occurred in 0.8 percent of 1501 autopsies on babies under the age of two years. All of the cases reported had acute endocarditis, involving the mitral valve in 64 instances, tricuspid valve in 35, aortic valve in 18, and pulmonary valve in seven. Organisms were cultured in only 30 cases, and these were as follows: streptococcus, 13; staphylococcus, five; pneumococcus, four; gonococcus, two; tubercle bacillus, two; and others, four. The bacterial endocarditis in many instances may have been the cause of death, but in a large number of infants it was of secondary importance to infection elsewhere in the body and was, therefore, not of major clinical significance. This was especially true of the cases with miliary tuberculosis, severe enteritis, and pneumonia.

The significant difference from the older children with bacterial endocarditis was noted in the incidence of the underlying lesions. In only 8 percent was there evidence of congenital heart disease, and since all cases were under the age of two years there was no rheumatic valvular disease present. The largest proportion of these babies were in the first weeks or months of life.

The clinical picture is that of an acute infection with fever and a progressively severe illness. In a large proportion there was evidence of infection or sepsis elsewhere in the body, such as skin lesions, pneumonia, enteritis, empyema, osteomyelitis, and tuberculosis. The spleen was palpable in a few cases, and embolic phenomena were relatively rare, occurring in only 18 percent. There was a marked tachycardia in some, usually out of proportion to the fever. In a few there was a precordial murmur, which appeared as the disease progressed. The diagnosis was usually not made until after death, when the heart was opened (Ward, 1971; Blieden et al., 1972).

This type of lesion has always been rare, and it will undoubtedly be rarer in the future since the antibiotics are now given freely with any signs of infection in infancy, and usually with curative effect.

BACTERIAL ENDOCARDITIS IN CHILDREN OVER TWO YEARS OF AGE

THE age incidence of 408 cases of bacterial endocarditis was reported by Cates and Christie (1951) and Lerner and Weinstein (1966). The rarity of this infection in early childhood will be readily appreciated, since only 4 percent were under the age of 15 years in the Cates and Christie series. Small groups of cases, usually due to a variety of organisms, have been reported in the pediatric literature (Aubert and Lerche, 1950; Cutler et al., 1958), but no large series in childhood has been presented. For this reason our own findings will also be given.

Weinstein and Rubin (1973) have summarized the age distribution of cases of infective endocarditis in the literature for 1927 to 1967. The average age has crept up from 31 years to 47 years. They also recorded that the mortality statistics for the United Kingdom have indicated that while the mean age of those dying of the disease in 1945 was 39.2 (18.4 percent over 60), it was 55.5 years in 1963 (46.8 percent over 60 years).

At The Hospital for Sick Children, Toronto, we have seen and are following each year in the cardiac clinic 8000 children with rheumatic or congenital heart involvement. The follow-up system makes it unlikely that development of subacute bacterial endocarditis in any child in this population would go unrecorded. In spite of a large increase in population in the past 25 years the incidence of infective endocarditis has not increased. (See Table 14–1.)

During the past 25 years at The Hospital for Sick Children there have been 82 children over the age of two years with bacterial endocarditis. During this period there have been 450,000 admissions to this hospital. The organisms found are listed in Table 14–1.

Thayer (1926) found that *Str. viridans* or a nonhemolytic streptococcus was the causative agent

Table 14–1.   **ORGANISMS FOUND IN INFECTIVE ENDOCARDITIS**

	IN CHILDREN			IN ADULTS AND OLDER CHILDREN	
	Keith et al. (HSC),		*Cutler et al.,*	*Geraci,*	*Vogler et al.,*
	1950–1964	*1965–1971*	*1958*	*1958*	*1962*
Streptococcus viridans	13	11	13	91	41
Nonhemolytic streptococcus, including enterococcus	7	0	1	28	24
Staphylococcus pyogenes	14	8	2	24	45
Staphylococcus albus	9	0	0	4	0
Hemolytic streptococcus	2	1	1	1	5
Streptococcus (Diplococcus) pneumoniae	1	0	1	0	0
Escherichia coli	1	0	0	3	0
Pseudomonas	1	1	1	5	1
Haemophilus influenzae	0	0	1	0	0
Klebsiella pneumoniae	1	0	0	0	1
Others	1	0	0	2	7
Unknown	10	1	4	14	19
	60	+22 = 82	24	172	143

in two-thirds of the adult cases and that the staphylococcus was the etiologic factor in only 9 percent. Phipps (1932) reported that, in the less acute form of the disease, *Str. viridans* was the cause in 90 percent of the cases; in the more acute form the beta-hemolytic streptococcus accounted for approximately one-half and the staphylococcus for one-fourth of the cases in adults.

Until 1958 at The Hospital for Sick Children and at the Boston Children's Hospital *Str. viridans* was found most commonly (Nadas, 1963). This was also true for Geraci (1958), whose patients were chiefly adults. However, Vogler and associates, who summarized their data for the period 1948 to 1960, found that staphylococcus most frequently was the etiologic factor although the incidence over the years was relatively constant. In recent years, since extensive heart surgery has become a routine procedure, the staphylococcus has appeared more prominently as a cause of bacterial endocarditis in many medical centers. It should be pointed out, however, that Robinson and Ruedy (1962) isolated the enterococcus more commonly than any other organisms in their patients between 1950 and 1960. This has not been the pediatric experience, since this particular microorganism is rarely an etiologic factor in children. Any of the common or uncommon organisms may be encountered, but 80 percent are either *Str. viridans* or nonhemolytic streptococcus (pyogenic or nonpyogenic).

As in the other forms of bacterial endocarditis, these children may have a history of preceding congenital or rheumatic heart disease. Before 1958 half of our cases had rheumatic valve disease as the underlying lesion. Since then we have only had one child with a rheumatic basis for endocarditis. Ninety-eight percent had a congenital heart defect prior to the bacterial infection. In adults, White (1951) reported that 80 percent of the cases of infective endocarditis occurred after rheumatic valvular disease, 10 percent with congenital heart disease, and 10 percent with otherwise-normal valves. Since then rheumatic heart disease as a factor has declined in adults. Involvement of the mitral valve is seen less frequently and the aortic valve more frequently in the adult age group.

Infections of the teeth, tonsils, and glands have long been considered to be predisposing factors in the production of this disease. In only four of our cases was there any history of a dental extraction preceding the onset of the subacute bacterial endocarditis. Kelson and White (1945) have estimated that the risk of the susceptible cardiac patient's having an attack of bacterial endocarditis after a tooth extraction is 1 in 533 chances.

The problems of this disease spectrum have altered, as a result of the introduction of cardiac surgery and hemodialysis and, more recently, the use of intravenous narcotics. For a number of reasons the incidence for childhood appears to have dropped while the age distribution has shifted toward the latter half of life.

Clinical Features

The diagnostic problems in all forms of bacterial endocarditis are similar, and the complete diagnosis is dependent on culturing the organism. However, certain clinical signs may sometimes suggest the more acute staphylococcal type of the disease. One of these signs is the presence of a high septic type of fever rising to 103° to 104° F in the early stages of the illness. A high leukocyte count of 15,000 to 25,000 is also suggestive. It should be pointed out, however, that the white blood cell count may be within normal limits even in the presence of a staphylococcal septicemia. This was true in one of our cases; it has also been pointed out by Fisher and coworkers (1955). Four of our staphylococcal cases occurred before suitable antibiotics were available, and they ran the usual short course from onset to death. The duration of the illness varied from three days to three weeks. Since the problems of diagnosis and management of acute and subacute bacterial endocarditis in childhood are essentially the same, the two will be discussed together.

The ages of our cases varied from nine months to 18 years. There seemed to be no particular age more susceptible than any other, except that the disease was much less common in infants and in very early childhood.

Signs of illness were less severe, as a rule, in those cases due to *Str. viridans* than in those due to the staphylococcus. Fever was always present in some degree but did not reach as high a peak as it did with the septic organisms. Insidious onset, with loss of appetite and some degree of pallor, was common in the beginning. Usually the preexisting heart disease had been recognized before, and with the onset of fever and malaise the parents sought medical advice.

Anemia was present to a slight extent in our cases but was not usually marked. None of our children had any clubbing of the fingers attributed to the bacterial infection, but splenomegaly occurred in two-thirds of the cases. Petechiae of the skin, which are commonly found in normal children, were difficult to appraise, especially since many children have small spots that resemble petechiae; large numbers on the skin usually suggest a severe bacteremia. Obvious embolism was uncommon.

Osler's nodes were usually not seen in our children. These nodes consist of tiny, raised red nodules, 0.625 cm ($\frac{1}{4}$ in.) in diameter on the skin of the fingers and toes.

The erythrocyte count was usually around 4,000,000, and the hemoglobin was 70 percent. The leukocyte count was rarely over 10,000 in children with infections due to *Str. viridans*. In staphylococcal infections the white blood cell count varied from 15,000 to 25,000, except in one case where it was 800.

Hematuria should be looked for as a possible embolic phenomenon. The mouth should be examined for evidence of infected gums or alveolar abscesses. Sinus x-ray films may be indicated. The echocardiograph may also be used to identify vegetations (Martinez et al., 1974).

Diagnosis

Vogler and associates (1962) have pointed out that recognition of the bacterial endocarditis is the single most important factor influencing survival. The diagnosis is usually made on the basis of the presence of an underlying heart lesion, whether rheumatic or congenital, accompanied by a fever lasting for a few days to a few weeks, with evidence of embolic phenomena such as petechiae, a palpable spleen, and a positive blood culture. Certain predisposing events also may lead one to suspect the possibility of subacute bacterial endocarditis. These include not only a recent tooth extraction, after which one may have a superimposed endocarditis due to *Str. viridans*, but also the presence of paronychiae or impetigo, which suggests either a streptococcal or a staphylococcal infection. Exposure to rats may lead to a *Spirillum* or *Streptobacillus moniliformis* infection and a cat bite to a *Pasteurella* infection. An operation involving the intestinal tract may cause a *Str. faecalis* (enterococcus) or *Escherichia coli* infection, but this source is uncommon in childhood. What is more common is the association with a recent heart operation. When the diagnosis of bacterial endocarditis is suspected, a series of blood cultures is taken with the minimum of delay. They should be started on the day of the patient's admission to the hospital. Although organisms may be cultured from the blood in many cases at any time in the day, the best time to take blood is one to two hours before the temperature begins to rise. This point is often difficult to estimate accurately, but a look at the temperature chart may give the time the temperature might be expected to rise, or one may wait until the temperature begins to rise and then take a series of blood cultures 10 to 15 minutes apart. Six are usually an adequate number in children. This process can be repeated in 24 hours if previous cultures are negative. It is preferable to take a relatively large number of cultures during the first 24 to 28 hours rather than to have sporadic cultures scattered over several days. This is especially important in cases of rheumatic heart disease with bacterial involvement of the aortic or mitral valves since embolism or heart failure is more likely to take place. In those severely ill, suitable treatment should be started as promptly as possible, preferably within 48 hours after admission. When the underlying cause is congenital heart disease with a lesion on the right side of the heart, pulmonary embolism is less important since it is of relatively little significance in childhood. It is usually safe to wait 48 hours to determine the presence or absence of organisms in blood cultures and to determine their sensitivity before proceeding with antibiotic therapy. Finland (1954) recommends the following methods of culturing the blood in suspected cases of subacute bacterial endocarditis: (1) Routine broth media are ordinarily used. Also employed are (2) sugar agar pour plates and (3) special media that permit the growth of fastidious organisms, including anaerobes and fungi, with incubation and observation of these cultures for as long as three weeks before they are discarded as negative. When other approaches fail, attempts may be made to obtain cultures from bone marrow, arterial blood, and urine. Two or three positive cultures from such sources are required to establish a causal relationship. In children there is no evidence that culturing arterial blood will yield organisms that cannot be isolated from the venous portion of circulation. Urine culture under aseptic precaution may on rare occasions reveal causative organisms. Most investigators have not found it necessary to culture by catheterization when right-sided bacterial endocarditis is involved. Ninety-seven percent of the positive blood cultures show up as such within the two days of culturing (Levinson et al., 1950).

Dillon and colleagues (1973) and Martinez and coworkers (1974) have carried out echocardiograms on patients with bacterial endocarditis. They demonstrated shaggy or fuzzy echoes resulting from vegetations that had a distinctive appearance, and both groups of authors conclude such findings should arouse suspicion in making an early diagnosis of bacterial endocarditis.

Treatment

Bacteria. A summary of the therapy is shown in Table 14–2 (page 238). Such therapy must kill the organism seeded in the heart valves; consequently, it is generally recommended that bactericidal drugs rather than bacteriostatic ones should be used. When penicillin first became available, early successes were reported in the treatment of bacterial endocarditis due to *Str. viridans* (Loewe et al., 1944; Hobbey and Dawson, 1944). It was soon discovered that penicillin could penetrate fibrin, was bactericidal in its action, and sterilized the lesions in 95 percent of cases. The majority of the early cases due to *Str. viridans* responded to such therapy in relatively small doses. Later it was noted that a few of the organisms were capable of long survival, and these survivors were usually eliminated by the addition of streptomycin (Spicer and Blitz, 1948). This led to the combined therapy in the cases that did not respond to penicillin alone.

The success of therapy often depends on the identification of the organism and its sensitivity to penicillin primarily but may depend on sensitivity to streptomycin, methicillin, oxacillin, etc. Since most cultures of *Str. viridans* are sensitive to penicillin, bacteriologic cure is usually achieved. Staphylococci are more likely to be resistant to penicillin, and early and intensive therapy is important with the most suitable antibiotic.

In treating *Str. viridans* infection, short-term courses of two weeks in larger doses are frequently curative, but failures can occur, which makes the longer term preferable. Oral therapy may also be successful, but not all children absorb penicillin as completely as others, thus leading to failures from time to time (Santos-Buch et al., 1957). This approach is not recommended in children unless excessive difficulties are encountered in giving frequent injections intramuscularly or because of multiple thromboses due to intravenous therapy, but even then, if the drug is given by mouth, it is important to obtain the same levels as with the intravenous or intramuscular approach.

In dealing with organisms, such as *Str. viridans*, that are very sensitive to penicillin (inhibited by 0.1 unit of penicillin per milliliter), a total of not less than 2,400,000 units of penicillin intravenously may be administered daily to children. This is best given in four divided doses. Such treatment should be continued for one month. When the organisms are resistant to 0.2 to 0.4 unit or more of penicillin per milliliter, 8,000,000 to 24,000,000 units of penicillin in four to eight divided doses should be administered (see Table 14–2, page 238). If the clinical response is not adequate, probenecid (Benemid) should then be added to heighten the blood level of penicillin (20 mg per pound per day, given in four divided doses).

The authors have referred to the synergistic action of streptomycin and penicillin in combating *Str. viridans*. This combination is particularly useful in treating enterococcal infections. Furthermore, such a combination may prevent or delay the development of resistance of organisms to either penicillin or streptomycin or both. If eighth-nerve involvement appears, the dose of streptomycin should be halved and penicillin increased. It may become necessary to stop the streptomycin entirely.

Sensitive staphylococci can be treated successfully with penicillin, provided the organism is fully sensitive. Since resistant colonies may appear during the course of therapy, it is considered wise to give a fairly large dose of penicillin intravenously in six divided doses during the 24 hours; a total daily dose of 6,000,000 units should be adequate in fully sensitive organisms. It is important to give the penicillin dose into the intravenous tubing so that a high peak is reached when the penicillin therapy should be maintained for four weeks at least.

The most useful antibiotic available at the present time to treat staphylococcal bacterial endocarditis resistant to penicillin is methicillin or cephalothin. The former may be given to a child in doses of 400 mg/kg, the total daily dose being given in six divided doses intravenously into the tubing and kept up for four weeks after the infection is controlled. If this fails to control the infection, the alternative is cephalothin in doses as indicated in Table 14–2 (page 238).

Fisher and associates (1955) have shown that there is no close relationship between the sensitivity of the staphylococci to penicillin and the dose required for successful therapy. Dosage, therefore, should be based primarily on response to therapy, and with the new antibiotics available, it is unlikely that one needs to turn to a number used in the past, such as erythromycin and ristocetin, which occasionally have been successful in difficult staphylococcal infections. Johnson and Hurst (1954) used erythromycin successfully in treating a three-year-old boy with a penicillin resistance to staphylococcal infection superimposed on congenital heart disease.

The hemolytic streptococcus and *Str. (D.) pneumoniae* are usually quite sensitive to penicillin, and 2,400,000 units daily of the combined repository type (penicillin G and procaine penicillin) for four weeks should be adequate.

The disadvantage of chlortetracycline, ocytetra-cycline, and chloramphenicol is that these antibiotics are essentially bacteriostatic rather than bactericidal. They have been tried with various types of bacterial endocarditis but are much less effective than the antibiotics listed above; furthermore, they do not appear to be synergistic when applied in combination with penicillin. They therefore have little place in the treatment of bacterial endocarditis. One might resort to their use in cases that do not respond to those regimens that are usually effective. Their use has been suggested in allergic individuals. Penicillin-allergic patients are better treated with penicillin plus an antihistamine, such as chlorpheniramine (Chlor-trimeton) (Beck, 1953), or by desensitizing doses or with the help of corticosteroids.

Green and associates (1967) record a history of penicillin allergy in 18 percent of 400 cases of infective endocarditis. Three-quarters required penicillin therapy, and of these 39 percent had an allergic reaction. In contrast, only 6 percent of those with no history of penicillin allergy had any reaction to penicillin therapy. A total of 40 cases had an allergic response. In all but eight of these, the prescribed dose of penicillin therapy was completed with the aid of antihistamines and corticosteroid therapy.

Alternative drugs can be given for *Str. viridans*. Cephalothin, along with streptomycin, is effective in this situation, or erythromycin and streptomycin. For staphylococci, clindamycin can be given effectively parenterally.

Bacteroides comprise the majority of organisms in the intestine, and they may enter the bloodstream following manipulation of the bowel of any sort but more frequently in diabetes or neoplastic disease. The drugs of choice for combating this infection are clindamycin, erythromycin, and chloramphenicol. Weinstein and Schlesinger (1973) recommend therapy for four to six weeks but point out that these drugs are bacteriostatic rather than bacteriocidal for the above-listed organisms.

Diphtheroids may be difficult to identify because they may need anaerobic cultures. Successful therapy has been reported with chloramphenicol and tetracycline (Davis et al., 1961; Merzbach et al., 1965.

Pseudomonas aeruginosa responds to a combination of gentamicin and arteriocillin (Lerner, 1971).

Escherichia coli, Proteus, and enterobacteria may be sensitive to ampicillin, cephalothin, and gentamicin. However, many strains of enterobacteria may not be susceptible to these drugs. Sensitivity of the organism to various antibiotics is therefore most important in this group.

Yeasts and Fungi. Infections of this type are uncommon in childhood but may be found in young people who have become heroin addicts or in patients with indwelling catheters. In spite of the use of broad-spectrum antibiotics in childhood such patients rarely get endocarditis due to yeasts or fungi. Although it has some limitations, amphotericin B appears to be the drug of choice in this group (see Table 14–2, page 238).

Blood Cultures. In judging the effectiveness of mixed antibiotic therapy, it is usually best to test the organism against the patient's serum a day or two after such therapy has been begun.

NEGATIVE BLOOD CULTURES. The patient whose blood cultures are repeatedly sterile presents a special problem. There may be all the classic signs of bacterial endocarditis (including later postmortem confirmation), yet no organism can be obtained from the bloodstream or from the vegetations. Such a case appears to have the worst prognosis. Reasons for negative blood cultures have been summarized by Lerner and Weinstein (1966) and include: (1) the use of antibiotics in undefined febrile illnesses; (2) right-sided endocarditis; (3) prolonged duration of bacterial endocarditis, producing a "bacteria-free" state; (4) presence of renal disease; and (5) difficulties in obtaining and culturing blood.

In the study reported by Feinberg (1950) of 140 patients with signs of subacute bacterial endocarditis treated with penicillin, 114 had positive blood cultures and 26 had persistently negative blood cultures. Of the former, 72 percent recovered, but of the latter only 38 percent survived. From the findings of Cates and Christie (1951) in a cooperative study in England, it was determined that 52 percent of 408 patients with positive blood cultures recovered, whereas only 18 percent of 34 patients with negative blood cultures survived. Both groups were treated with penicillin.

In most children with infective endocarditis it is quite safe to wait 48 hours for the results of blood culture before starting therapy. After that time, in the face of a negative culture, it may be necessary to start antibiotic therapy if the clinical signs warrant it.

A suitable combination under such circumstances would be ampicillin and gentamicin (ampicillin, 400 mg/kg/day, in six divided doses, intravenously; gentamicin, 3 mg/kg/day, intramuscularly).

If such treatment controls the temperature and blood cultures remain negative, ampicillin may be reduced to 200 mg/kg/day and the gentamicin to 1 mg/kg/day. This therapy should be effective for a variety of organisms, excluding some penicillin-resistant staphylococci. It should also affect all streptococci and most enterobacteriaceae.

POSITIVE BLOOD CULTURES. The value of a positive blood culture is obvious. First, it allows one to decide with accuracy what antibiotic should be used and what dose is suitable, and the sensitivity of the organisms helps in deciding the length of therapy. The prognosis is poorer if the disease has been present for several weeks before therapy has been instituted. This is mainly because heart failure and other complications, such as embolism, are more likely to occur. Although heart failure may occasionally appear in the rheumatic group, embolism is the most frequent serious complication in childhood and has occurred in approximately one-third of our patients with lesions on the left side of the heart. It is exceedingly important to see these patients as early as possible and treat them adequately. Thus, regardless of whether the blood culture is negative or positive, therapy should not be postponed more than 48 hours.

It is important that the patient be admitted to the hospital during this initial period until treatment is well established. In the majority of cases it is wise to keep the patient hospitalized until the treatment has been completed and a suitable observation period experienced. However, when the organism is a highly sensitive one and arrangements can be made for therapy at home, the patient may occasionally be treated there. There is more justification for home therapy in the presence of congenital heart disease with a lesion on the right side of the heart, since less supervision of activity is needed. When the mitral or aortic valve is involved, however, strict bed rest and nursing supervision are important. These cases should probably be hospitalized until cured.

Finally, when the period of therapy has been completed, the patient should be observed for a period of three to four weeks for signs of returning fever or other manifestations suggestive of relapse. Fortunately, relapses are uncommon in children when an adequate dose of the proper antibiotic has been used. It is important to keep the child in bed for a month after the completion of the antibiotic treatment as it seems possible that activity may increase the chance of cerebral embolism during the healing stage.

Results of Therapy. ACUTE BACTERIAL ENDOCARDITIS. Before the advent of the antibiotics, children with staphylococcal bacterial endocarditis survived only three days to three weeks from the time of onset of symptoms. Now many lives are saved, even when relatively resistant organisms are present. Fisher and associates (1955) report successful therapy in 54 percent of 13 cases of staphylococcal endocarditis. At The Hospital for Sick Children there have been 19 in this category treated with antibiotics. Eight survived (42 percent). All but two of these had a staphylococcal organism sensitive to penicillin. Among the 11 that died only three had organisms sensitive to penicillin. This covered a period before some of the new, more efficacious antibiotics were available.

SUBACUTE BACTERIAL ENDOCARDITIS. In the "adult" literature, approximately 70 percent of the cases recovered from the bacterial infection and

Table 14-2. BACTERIAL ENDOCARDITIS

CAUSATIVE ORGANISMS	ANTIBIOTIC	TOTAL DAILY DOSE	BLOOD LEVEL OF PENICILLIN REQUIRED	DURATION OF THERAPY
1. Sensitive *Str. viridans.* Hemolytic streptococcus or *Str. (D.) pneumoniae* are sensitive to 0.1 unit/ml of penicillin or less	Combined procaine and aqueous penicillin or aqueous penicillin	2,400,000 units intramuscularly divided into 3 doses. If child objects to repeated intramuscular injections, give 2,400,000 units aqueous penicillin in 4 divided doses into intravenous tubing	Doses recommended will give adequate blood levels	4 weeks
2. Comparatively resistant streptococcus, enterococcus, or nonhemolytic streptococcus or *Str. viridans* requiring more than 0.1 unit/ml of penicillin to inhibit growth but sensitive to concentrations of penicillin attainable in blood and tissues	Aqueous penicillin by intravenous drip and streptomycin intramuscularly	8,000,000 to 64,000,000 units in 4–8 divided doses depending on the sensitivity of the organism and the weight of the patient intravenously. 2.0 gm streptomycin intramuscularly (40 mg/kg) if child less than 50 kg. This dose may be maintained for 1–2 weeks. It should then be reduced by half or earlier if signs of 8th-nerve involvement occur.	Serum should inhibit organism when diluted 5–10 times	4 weeks Full doses 1–2 weeks ½ doses to complete course of 4 weeks
3. Staphylococcus, fully sensitive organisms (not producing penicillinase)	Aqueous penicillin intravenously	6,000,000 to 15,000,000 units intravenously in 6 divided doses into tubing	5–10 times sensitivity of organism	4 weeks
4. Staphylococcus not fully sensitive to penicillin; resistant	Methicillin* (Celbenin) (Staphcillin)	(400 mg/kg). Total daily dose given in 6 divided doses intravenously into tubing	5–10 times sensitivity of organism	4 weeks after infection is controlled
	Cloxacillin* (Orbenin) or	(100–400 mg/kg) intramuscularly or intravenously daily		4 weeks
	Cephalothin	200 mg/kg intravenously daily		4 weeks

5. Unknown organisms   In most children with infective endocarditis it is quite safe to wait 48 hours for the results of blood culture before starting therapy. After that time, in the face of a negative culture, It may be necessary to start antibiotic therapy if the clinical signs warrant it.   *[4 weeks from time infection is controlled]*

   A suitable combination under such circumstances would be ampicillin and gentamicin (ampicillin, 400 mg/kg/day, in six divided doses, intravenously; gentamicin, 3 mg/kg/day intramuscularly).

   If such treatment controls the temperature and blood cultures remain negative, ampicillin may be reduced to 200 mg/kg/day and the gentamicin to 1 mg/kg/day. This therapy should be effective against a variety of organisms, excluding some penicillin-resistant staphylococci. Most infections due to streptococci and enterobacteriaceae should respond.

6. Uncommon organisms   In children the most common organisms cultured are *Str. viridans* and the staphylococcus. Uncommon organisms are more rarely encountered than in adult life. They include *Escherichia coli*, the *Enterobacter-Klebsiella* group, *Pseudomonas*, and *Candida albicans*.

   Candida albicans   This type of infection may occur from time to time as a result of intensive antibiotic therapy and the increased use of intravenous methods. The agent preferred to combat this organism is amphotericin B. It may prove inadequate for the job in bacterial endocarditis in spite of the fact that it is effective against the acute systemic infections. Surgical removal of the lesion may be required (Kay et al., 1961). The dose of amphotericin B starts with 0.25 mg/kg the first day, increasing by 0.25 mg/kg daily until a maximum of 1 mg/kg daily is reached. It is a somewhat toxic agent that may produce chills, fever, vomiting, phlebitis, anemia, leukopenia, and renal damage. Because of this the dose described above should be given by gradual increments.

   Pseudomonas   For this type of infection carbenicillin is given with gentamicin (carbenicillin, 500 to 1000 mg/kg/day; gentamicin, 3 to 5 mg/kg/day). The upper dose is preferred provided the renal function is normal.

   Escherichia coli   For this organism a combination of a penicillin or cephalosporin and an aminoglycoside to which the organism is sensitive is the treatment of choice, e.g., ampicillin and gentamicin.

   Such therapy also applies to other related enterobacteria, e.g., the *Enterobacter-Klebsiella* group, *Proteus* species, and *Serratia*.

carried on with whatever degree of cardiac involvement existed before the infection. Approximately 30 percent died from the infection itself or from heart failure, cerebral hemorrhage, or embolism. It is now generally realized that although the bacterial infection may be eradicated, the underlying heart condition or embolism may prove fatal.

At The Hospital for Sick Children, out of a total of 82 cases, 63 percent recovered and 37 percent died. The mortality was higher between 1958 and 1962 than between 1952 and 1957. This was chiefly due to the increase in staphylococcal endocarditis, often occurring in the postoperative period when the heart muscle is functioning at a disadvantage and any infection is more difficult to control (Zakrzewski and Keith, 1965). In the past seven years the mortality has fallen slightly to 30 percent. The prognosis in the presence of a *Str. viridans* infection, as one would expect, is better than with *Staph. aureus*. Similarly, about one third of 149 episodes of bacterial endocarditis between 1933 and 1972 encountered at the Children's Hospital Medical Center in Boston ended fatally (Johnson et al., 1975).

A few patients recover from subacute bacterial endocarditis and develop a recurrence later. This is estimated to occur in roughly 2 percent of adults. We have observed this only once in childhood cases.

One of the youngest successful treated cases of subacute bacterial endocarditis was reported by Aubert and Lerche (1950) in a ten-month-old baby whose infection was due to *Haemophilus hemolyticus*. The infant was treated with streptomycin and sulfathiazole over a period of nine days.

In estimating the prognosis in any one case, it is of prime importance to know where the lesion is and what bacterial organism is involved. If it is within the tricuspid or pulmonary valves or on the ventricular septum, the prognosis is usually good since emboli of the brain are most unlikely to occur and pulmonary embolism will usually do no harm. If the lesion is in the mitral or aortic valve, there is always the serious risk of cerebral embolism, whether the antibiotic therapy has been successful or not. The heart size is of importance since one can evaluate the possibility of heart failure occurring. The presence of signs of activity of rheumatic disease is also significant since the rheumatic infection may proceed during the course of subacute bacterial endocarditis.

However, in the past few years there has been an attempt to combine very large doses of antibiotics with a shorter treatment period. Hamburger and Stein in 1952 cured 10 out of 12 patients with bacterial endocarditis in slightly under two weeks by the daily administration of 16,000,000 units of crystalline penicillin. All of these cases harbored organisms highly sensitive to penicillin. In 1953, Geraci and Martin cured 18 out of 23 patients with bacterial endocarditis due to penicillin-sensitive streptococci by using daily, in divided doses, 1,200,000 to 2,400,000 units of penicillin and 1.2 to 2.4 gm of dihydrostreptomycin. They reported (1953) treating all cases of streptococcal endocarditis with sensitivity to 0.1 unit of penicillin per milliliter or less with 1,200,000 units of aqueous penicillin and 0.5 gm each of streptomycin and dihydrostreptomycin, intramuscularly, every 12 hours for two weeks.

Although these forms of therapy have undoubtedly shortened the length of treatment, there have been some failures with each regimen, and this discourages one from using short-term therapy since any failure necessitates the repetition of therapy. This method is most suitable in the presence of a penicillin-sensitive strain of *Str. viridans*. Further studies on dosage and the development of new antibiotics may make the shorter forms of therapy more feasible in the future.

Prophylaxis

It has been confirmed by numerous studies that a significant number of cases of bacterial endocarditis follow a tooth extraction in an individual who has congenital or rheumatic heart disease. Other forms of surgery or manipulation also appear to bear a causative relationship at times. The removal of the tonsils and adenoids, conditions of the antepartum and postpartum periods, prostatectomies, genitourinary operations, and certain diagnostic procedures such as cardiac catheterization have been implicated.

In children we are chiefly concerned with dental extractions and removal of tonsils and adenoids. Several investigators have studied the incidence of positive blood cultures immediately following the removal of one or more teeth and have found that it varies between 16 and 75 percent. As indicated previously, Kelson and White (1945) have calculated that the risk of bacterial endocarditis following a tooth extraction in a patient with congenital or rheumatic heart disease is approximately 1 in 533.

At The Toronto Hospital for Sick Children in the past 25 years there have been 82 cases of bacterial endocarditis, and four have followed a tooth extraction. From this experience and from the interpretation of the literature, one has the impression that bacterial endocarditis following a tooth extraction is much less common in children than in adults.

It is now generally agreed that some form of prophylaxis should be given at the time of dental extractions or the other manipulative procedures or operations listed above to children who have congenital or rheumatic heart disease. The hospital dental clinic does nearly 3000 extractions a year and this is only a fraction of the number done in the area served by the hospital. It is well to remember, however, that at least four failures of prophylaxis, using penicillin before and after the specific procedure, have been reported. Because of the diversity of opinion as to how prophylaxis should best be done, a Committee on Prevention of Rheumatic Fever and Bacterial Endocarditis of the American Heart Association was appointed. Their recommendation is listed below.

Prophylaxis for Dental Procedures and Also for Tonsillectomy, Adenoidectomy, and Bronchoscopy:
See revised recommendations (Kaplan et al., 1977).
1. For most patients: *penicillin*
   a. Intramuscular: 600,000 units of procaine penicillin G mixed with 200,000 units of crystalline penicillin G one hour prior to procedure and once daily for two days following the procedure.
   b. Oral: (1) 500 mg of penicillin V or phenethicillin one hour prior to the procedure and then 250 mg every six hours for the remainder of that day and for the two days following the procedure, or (2) 1,200,000 units of penicillin G one hour prior to procedure and then 600,000 units every six hours for the remainder of that day and for the two days following the procedure.
2. For patients suspected to be allergic to penicillin or for those on continual oral penicillin for rheumatic fever prophylaxis, who may harbor penicillin-resistant *Str. viridans*: *erythromycin*—oral:
   For adults: 500 mg one and one-half to two hours prior to the procedure and then 250 mg every six hours for the remainder of that day and for the two days following the procedure.
   For children: The dose for small children is 20 mg/kg orally one and one-half to two hours prior to the procedure and then 10 mg/kg every six hours for the remainder of that day and for the two days following the procedure.
   Note: Erythromycin preparations for parenteral use are also available.

Prophylaxis for Gastrointestinal and Genitourinary Tract Surgery and Instrumentation and Also for Any Surgery of Infected Tissues:
1. For most patients: *penicillin*
   600,000 units of procaine penicillin G mixed with 200,000 units of crystalline penicillin G intramuscularly one hour prior to the procedure and once daily for the two days following the procedure.
   Plus *streptomycin*
   1 to 2 gm intramuscularly, one hour prior to the procedure and once daily for the two days following the procedure.
   For children: 40 mg/kg intramuscularly one hour prior to the procedure and once daily for the two days following the procedure (not to exceed 1 gm each 24 hours).
   Or *ampicillin*
   25 to 50 mg/kg given orally or intravenously one hour prior to the procedure and then 25 mg/kg every six hours for the remainder of that day and for the two days following the procedure.
   Plus *streptomycin* (as above)
2. For patients suspected to be allergic to the penicillins,
   erythromycin can be given (instead of penicillin or ampicillin)
   Plus *streptomycin* (as above)
   Vancomycin can be given as an alternative to

erythromycin, 0.5 gm to 1.0 gm intravenously every six hours for the remainder of that day and for the two days following the procedure.
Plus *streptomycin*
For children: 20 mg/kg one hour prior to the procedure and then 10 mg/kg every six hours for the remainder of that day and for the two days following the procedure.

CONTRAINDICATIONS TO ABOVE REGIMEN. The main contraindication is sensitivity to penicillin. All patients should be carefully questioned for previous history suggesting penicillin sensitivity. If such a history is obtained, even if equivocal, penicillin should not be given. Under such circumstances, lincomycin should be used in a dose of 250 mg by mouth four times daily for older children. For small children, a dosage of 40 mg/kg/day divided into three or four evenly spaced doses may be used. The total dosage should not exceed 1 gm per day. It may be given the day of the procedure and the day following.

Prophylaxis in Relation to Catheterization of the Heart and to Heart Surgery. There are numerous factors that predispose to infective endocarditis. These include an underlying heart lesion, cardiac surgery (whether open or closed), cardiac catheterization, the use of polyethylene intravenous catheters, drug administration or addition, debilitating diseases, prolonged steroid administration, and bone marrow depression. Finland (1972) indicates that infective endocarditis is now more common in older patients than in the past, and in the pediatric field it is a little less common than it used to be.

Prophylaxis During Cardiac Catheterization. Prophylaxis during cardiac catheterization has involved a good deal of study and discussion in recent years. Kreidberg and Chernoff (1965) reported fever in approximately 30 percent of children having cardiac catheterization, with the same incidence whether or not they were receiving penicillin prophylaxis. Transient bacteremia was noticed in both groups, occurring in about 4 to 5 percent; none developed infective endocarditis. In the cooperative prospective study involving 12,367 cardiac catheter-angiocardiograph procedures, Swan (1968) reported bacteremia in only three cases, two due to a *Staph. aureus* and the third due to *Strep. viridans*. There were no cases of infective endocarditis. Most major catheter laboratories now do not use prophylactic chemotherapy but reserve the antibiotic for use on any infection appearing in the postcatheter period, which fortunately is an infrequent occurrence.

Endocarditis and Cardiac Surgery. Much has been written in current journals regarding endocarditis following cardiac surgery. Amoury and coworkers (1966) found an incidence of 3.3 percent. Fraser and associates (1967) in Canada reported 2.7 percent among 520 patients who survived cardiopulmonary bypass. Of their 14 patients with this complication *Staph. albus* occurred in ten, *Staph. aureus* in three. They record that only two patients survived the endocarditis, death being associated with infection on the prosthesis as a rule. Carey and

Hughes (1970) reported only two incidents of infective endocarditis among 863 cardiac operations, and both of these occurred in heroin addicts. These authors have made a habit of soaking the prosthesis in a solution containing a high concentration of penicillin and methicillin and consider this important in reducing postoperative infection on the valves.

In the adult imposition of endocarditis is usually related to the use of prosthetic valves or patches. Most instances of postcardiotomy endocarditis in 1950–1963 followed repair of heart defects or valvotomies. The risk appears higher when the operation involves the aortic valve, especially when foreign material is implanted, but it is relatively low when congenital defects are corrected. The frequency of endocarditis following incision of the aortic valve has been recorded as 3.8 percent by Koiwai and Nanas (1956). Yeh and coworkers (1967) recorded an incidence of 3.5 percent of endocarditis following an insertion of ball valve. It was 9.5 percent in those in whom a Starr-Edwards valve was inserted. The risk of infective endocarditis in 12,367 cardiac catheterizations was 0.02 percent (352) (Braunwald and Swan, 1968).

The organisms for deposit on prosthetic valves vary with the time interval following surgery. Shortly after operation *Staph. aureus* or *albus* or *Str. viridans* may be involved, as may *Candida*, *Aspergillus*, or diphtheroids. However, after a prolonged interval any of the usual or unusual viruses may be encountered. Replacement of the prosthesis may then be required. The risk of endocarditis in such cases is no different from that associated with any other type of valvar disorder. Hemodialysis may lead to infection not only at the arteriovenous shunt but also on the cardiac valves. In heroin addicts *Staph. aureus* endocarditis and *Staph. epidermidis* endocarditis have been reported.

In the past decade several investigators have questioned the value of chemoprophylaxis at the time of, and following, heart surgery, whether open or closed (Kittle et al., 1961; Goodman et al., 1968; Conte et al., 1972). The latter carried out a double-blind study with no significant difference between the two groups. At the same time other reports have supported the use of antibiotics prophylactically (Nelson et al., 1965; Stein et al., 1966; Gooch et al., 1967).

One result of the above observations has been that physicians and surgeons are more conscious of the various sources or routes of infection, as well as the possibility of resistant organisms. Greater efforts are now made to ensure sterile extracorporeal circulation fluids, reduction of air contaminants in operating rooms, more concerted efforts to identify offending organisms when infection occurs, and the use of specific therapy when possible to control and eliminate the infection process.

Fortunately, however, very few prosthetic valves are inserted in children, and this problem is not a major one in the pediatric age group. In the adult field, however, this complication has led to the evaluation and practicality of surgery during active infective endocarditis. When a surgical procedure is available, it may be important to reoperate if medical treatment fails to sterilize the bloodstream, as is occasionally the case with a patent ductus. It may be important to do this when yeast or fungal infections are present to remove as much of the central infective lesion as possible. When bacterial endocarditis occurs in the postoperative period and medical treatment cannot eliminate the offending organism, reoperation must be considered in spite of the high risk involved at this vulnerable stage. The adequacy of medical therapy, the response of the patient, and severity of the illness must be balanced against the risks of a second operation under difficult circumstances.

INDICATIONS FOR REOPERATION IN INFECTIVE ENDOCARDITIS FOLLOWING CARDIAC SURGERY. The most common is cardiac failure that does not respond to medical therapy. This is most frequently due to aortic regurgitation but may be caused by mitral valve incompetence. There is considerable urgency in the presence of acute aortic insufficiency associated especially with low cardiac output, a diastole that is shorter than systole, soft murmurs, a lack of appreciable enlargement of left ventricle, or diminished intensity of the first heart sound secondary to high left ventricular diastolic pressure.

Fowler and coworkers (1967) and Griffin and associates (1972) have emphasized the need for emergency aortic valve replacement. Eight patients died in whom the procedure was not carried out, whereas of seven patients with a similar lesion who were repaired surgically only three died.

REFERENCES

Aceves, S., and Cesarman, T.: Estudio clinico de algunos aspectos de la endocarditis bacteriana (en especial de la curva termica). *Arch. Inst. Cardiol. México,* **23**:235, 1953.

American Heart Association: Bacterial endocarditis—revisited. *Mod. Concepts Cardiovasc. Dis.,* **33**:831, 1964.

————: Prevention of bacterial endocarditis. A statement for physicians and dentists prepared by the Rheumatic Fever Committee and the Committee on Congenital Cardiac Defects of the Council on Rheumatic Fever and Congenital Heart Disease of the American Heart Association, 1972.

Amoury, R. A.; Bowman, F. O., Jr.; and Malm, J. R.: Endocarditis associated with intracardiac prostheses: diagnosis, management and prophylaxis. *J. Thorac. Cardiovasc. Surg.,* **51**:36, 1966.

Andriole, V. T., and Kravetz, H. M.: The use of amphotericin B in man. *JAMA,* **180**:269, 1962.

Andriole, V. T.; Kravetz, H. M.; Roberts, W. C.; and Utz, J. P.: *Candida* endocarditis: clinical and pathologic studies. *Am. J. Med.,* **32**:251, 1962.

Antel, J. J.; Rome, H. P.; Geraci, J. E.; and Sayre, G. P.: Toxic-organic psychosis as a presenting feature in bacterial endocarditis. *Proc. Mayo Clin.,* **30**:45, 1955.

Aubert, A., and Lerche, C.: Subacute bacterial endocarditis in a child, ten months old, successfully treated with streptomycin. *Am. Heart J.,* **39**:141, 1950.

Bacterial endocarditis: a changing pattern. *Lancet,* **11**:146, 1967.

Bain, R. C.; Edwards, J. E.; Scheifley, C. H.; and Geraci, J. E.: Right-sided bacterial endocarditis and endarteritis. *Am. J. Med.,* **24**:98, 1958.

Barratt-Boyes, B. G.: Surgical correction of mitral incompetence resulting from bacterial endocarditis. *Br. Heart J.,* **25**:415, 1963.

Barratt-Boyes, B. G., and Roche, A. H. G.: A review of aortic valve homografts over a six and one-half year period. *Ann. Surg.*, **170**:483, 1969.

Bastin, R.; Frottier, J.; Vilde, J. L.; et al.: Bacterial endocarditis. Data from a study of 276 cases. *Lyon Med.*, **225**:61, 1971.

Beck, C. A.: Subacute bacterial endocarditis in penicillin-sensitive patient. *JAMA*, **153**:1170, 1953.

Blakemore, W. S.; McGarrity, G. J.; Thurer, R. J.; Wallace, H. W.; MacVaugh, H., III; and Coriell, L. L.: Infection by air-borne bacteria with cardiopulmonary bypass. *Surgery*, **70**:830, 1971.

Blieden, L. C.; Morehead, R. R.; Burke, B.; and Kaplan, E. L.: Bacterial endocarditis in the neonate. *Am. J. Dis. Child.*, **124**:747, 1972.

Block, P. C.; De Sanctis, R. W.; Weinberg, A. N.; and Austen, W. G.: Prosthetic valve endocarditis. *J. Thorac. Cardiovasc. Surg.*, **60**:540, 1970.

Bloomfield, A. L.: The present status of treatment of subacute bacterial endocarditis. *Circulation*, **2**:801, 1950.

———: Diagnosis and prevention of bacterial endocarditis. *Circulation*, **8**:290, 1953.

Braunwald, E., and Swan, H. J. C.: Co-operative study on cardiac catheterization. *Circulation* (suppl.), **3**:27, 1968.

Brunsdon, D. F. V.; Enticknap, J. B.; and Milstein, B. B.: A case of subacute bacterial endocarditis due to Pseudomonas pyocyanea complicating valvotomy for advanced mitral stenosis. *Guy Hosp. Rep.*, **102**:303, 1953.

Brunson, J. G.: Coronary embolism in bacterial endocarditis. *Am. J. Pathol.*, **19**:689, 1953.

Buckley, M. J.; Mundth, E. D.; Daggett, W. M.; and Austen, W. G.: Surgical management of the complications of sepsis involving the aortic valve, aortic root, and ascending aorta. *Ann. Thorac. Surg.*, **12**:391, 1971.

Bunn, P. A., and Cook, E. T.: Treatment of subacute bacterial endocarditis. *Ann. Intern. Med.*, **41**:487, 1954.

Caldwell, R. L.; Hurwitz, R. A.; and Girod, D. A.: Subacute bacterial endocarditis in children. *Am. J. Dis. Child.*, **122**:312, 1971.

Carey, J. S., and Hughes, R. K.: Control of infection after thoracic and cardiovascular surgery. *Ann. Surg.*, **172**:916, 1970.

Cates, J. E., and Christie, R. V.: Subacute bacterial endocarditis. A review of 442 patients treated in 14 centers appointed by the Penicillin Trials Committee of the Medical Research Council. *Q. J. Med.*, **20**:93, 1951.

Cherubin, C. E., and Neu, H. C.: Infective endocarditis at the Presbyterian Hospital in New York City from 1938–1967. *Am. J. Med.*, **51**:83, 1971.

Chiles, N. H.; Smith, H. L.; Christensen, N. A.; and Geraci, J. E.: Spontaneous healing of subacute bacterial endarteritis with closure of patent ductus arteriosus. *Proc. Mayo Clin.*, **28**:520, 1953.

Committee on Prevention of Rheumatic Fever and Bacterial Endocarditis of the American Heart Association: Prevention of rheumatic fever and bacterial endocarditis through control of streptococcal infections. *Circulation*, **21**:151, 1960.

Conte, J. E., Jr.; Cohen, S. N.; Roe, B. B.; and Elashoff, R. M.: Antibiotic prophylaxis and cardiac surgery: a prospective double-blind comparison of single-dose versus multiple-dose regimens. *Ann. Intern. Med.*, **76**:943, 1972.

Cutler, J. G.; Ongley, P. A.; Schwachman, H.; Massell, B. F.; and Nadas, A. S.: Bacterial endocarditis in children with heart disease. *Pediatrics*, **22**:706, 1958.

Danilowicz, D. A.; Reed, G. E.; and Silver, W.: Ruptured mitral chordae after subacute bacterial endocarditis in a child with a secundum atrial septal defect. *Johns-Hopkins Med. J.*, **128**:45, 1971.

Davis, A.; Binder, M. J.; Burroughs, J. T.; Miller, A. B.; and Finegold, S. M.: Diphtheroid endocarditis after cardiopulmonary bypass surgery for repair of cardiac valvular defects. *Antimicrob. Agents Chemother.*, **3**:643, 1961.

Davis, J. M.; Moss, A. J.; and Schenk, E. A.: Tricuspin *Candida* endocarditis complicating a permanently implanted transvenous pacemaker. *Am. Heart J.*, **77**:818, 1969.

Dillon, J. C.; Feigenbaum, H.; Konecke, L. L.; Davis, R. H.; and Chang, S.: Echocardiographic manifestations of valvular vegetations. *Am. Heart J.*, **86**:698, 1973.

Feigenbaum, H.: *Echocardiography*. Lea & Febiger, Philadelphia, 1972, p. 74.

Feinberg, S. M.: Antihistaminic drugs—5 years of experience. *Illinois Med. J.*, **97**:54, 1950.

Finland, M.: Treatment of bacterial endocarditis. *Circulation*, **9**:292, 1954.

———: Treatment of bacterial endocarditis. *N. Engl. J. Med.*, **250**:372, 1954.

———: Current problems in infective endocarditis. *Mod. Concepts Cardiovasc. Dis.*, **41**:53, 1972.

Finland, M., and Barnes, M. W.: Changing etiology of bacterial endocarditis in the antibacterial era. *Ann. Intern. Med.*, **72**:341, 1970.

Fisher, A. M.: A method for the determination of antibacterial potency of serum during therapy of acute infections: preliminary report. *Bull. Hopkins Hosp.*, **90**:313, 1952.

Fisher, A. M.; Wagner, H. N., Jr.; and Ross, R. S.: Staphylococcal endocarditis: some clinical and therapeutic observations on thirty-eight cases. *Arch. Intern. Med.*, **95**:427, 1955.

Fowler, N. O.; Hamburger, M. H.; and Bove, K. E.: Aortic valve perforation. *Am. J. Med.*, **42**:539, 1967.

Fraser, R. S.; Rossall, R. E.; and Dvorkin, J.: Bacterial endocarditis occurring after open heart surgery. *Can. Med. Assoc. J.*, **96**:1551, 1967.

Friedberg, C. K.: The diagnosis and treatment of subacute bacterial endocarditis. *Am. Pract.*, **4**:444, 1953.

———: The use of drugs in the treatment of bacterial endocarditis. *Med. Clin. North Am.*, **38**:385, 1954.

Garrido Lecca, G.; and Tola, A.: Subacute bacterial endocarditis treated with chloramphenicol and oxytetracycline. *JAMA*, **152**:913, 1953.

Geraci, J. E.: The antibiotic therapy of bacterial endocarditis. *Med. Clin. North Am.*, **42**:1101, 1958.

Geraci, J. E.; Heilman, F. R.; Nichold, D. R.; and Wellman, W. E.: Antibiotic therapy of bacterial endocarditis. VII. Vancomycin for acute micrococcal endocarditis: preliminary report. *Proc. Mayo Clin.*, **33**:172, 1958.

Geraci, J. E., and Martin, W. J.: Antibiotic therapy of bacterial endocarditis. IV. Successful short-term (two weeks) combined penicillin-dihydrostreptomycin therapy in subacute bacterial endocarditis caused by penicillin-sensitive streptococci. *Circulation*, **8**:494, 1953.

———: Antibiotic therapy of bacterial endocarditis. V. Therapeutic considerations of erythromycin. *Proc. Mayo Clin.*, **29**:109, 1954.

———: Antibiotic therapy of bacterial endocarditis. VI. Subacute enterococcal endocarditis: clinical, pathologic and therapeutic consideration of 33 cases. *Circulation*, **10**:173, 1954.

Gooch, A. S.; Maranhao, V.; Alblaza, S.; and Goldberg, H.: Medical complications following open-heart surgery. *Arch. Intern. Med.*, **120**:672, 1967.

Goodman, J. S.; Schaffner, W.; Collins, H. A.; Battersby, E. J.; and Keonig, M. G.: Infection after cardiovascular surgery: clinical study including examination of antimicrobial prophylaxis. *N. Engl. J. Med.*, **378**:117, 1968.

Green, G. R.; Peters, G. A.; and Geraci, J. E.: Treatment of bacterial endocarditis in patients with penicillin hypersensitivity. *Ann. Intern. Med.*, **67**:235, 1967.

Grehl, T. M.; Cohn, L. H.; and Angell, W. W.: Management of *Candida* endocarditis. *J. Thorac. Cardiovasc. Surg.*, **63**:118, 1972.

Griffin, F. M. Jr.; Jones, G.; and Cobbs, C. G.: Aortic insufficiency in bacterial endocarditis. *Ann. Intern. Med.*, **76**:23, 1972.

Griffiths, S. P.: Bacterial endocarditis associated with atrial septal defect of the ostium secundum type. *Am. Heart J.*, **61**:543, 1961.

Hamburger, M., and Stein, L.: Streptococcus viridans subacute bacterial endocarditis: 2 week treatment schedule with penicillin. *JAMA*, **149**:542, 1952.

Hatcher, C. R., Jr.; Symbas, P. N.; Logan, W. D.; and Abbott, O. A.: Surgical aspects of endocarditis of the aortic root. *Am. J. Cardiol.*, **23**:192, 1969.

Hawe, A. J., and Hughes, M. H.: Bacterial endocarditis due to Chromobacterium prodigiosum: report of a case. *Br. Med. J.*, **1**:968, 1954.

Henderson, J., and Nickerson, J. F.: Bacterial endocarditis with candida albicans superinfection. *Can. Med. Assoc. J.*, **90**:452, 1964.

Hobby, G. L., and Dawson, M. H.: Effect of rate of growth of bacteria on action of penicillin. *Proc. Soc. Exp. Biol. Med.*, **56**:181, 1944.

Hunter, T. H.: Bacterial endocarditis. *Am. Heart J.*, **42**:472, 1951.

Johnson, D. H.; Rosenthal, A.; and Nadas, A. S.: A forty-year review of bacterial endocarditis in infancy and childhood. *Circulation*, **51**:381, 1975.

Johnson, T. D., and Hurst, J. H.: Bacterial endocarditis due to a penicillin-resistant staphylococcus. *N. Engl. J. Med.*, **251**:219, 1954.

Kaplan, E. L.; Anthony, B. F.; Bisno, A.; Durack, D.; Houser, H.; Millard, H. D.; Sanford, J.; Shulman, S. T.; Stillerman, M.; Taranta, A.; and Wenger, N.: Prevention of bacterial endocarditis. AHA Committee report. *Circulation*, **56**:135A, 1977.

Kaplan, E. L., and Taranta, A. V.: Infective endocarditis—An American Heart Association Symposium. American Heart Association Monograph Series No. 52, American Heart Association, Dallas, Texas, 1977.

Kay, J. H.; Bernstein, S.; Feinstein, D.; and Biddle, M.: Surgical cure of *Candida albicans* endocarditis with open-heart surgery. *N. Engl. J. Med.*, **264**:907, 1961.

Keefer, C. S.: Present day treatment of subacute bacterial endocarditis. *JAMA*, **152**:1397, 1953.

Keith, J. D.: Bacterial endocarditis. In Gaisford, W., and Lightwood, R. (eds.): *Pediatrics for the Practitioner*. Butterworth and Co., Ltd., London, 1953, Vol. I, pp. 485–88.

Kelson, S. R., and White, P. D.: Notes on 250 cases of subacute bacterial (streptococcal) endocarditis studied and treated between 1927 and 1939. *Ann. Intern. Med.*, **22**:40, 1945.

King, L. H.; Bradley, K. P.; Shires, D. L.; Donohue, J. P.; and Glover, J. L.: Bacterial endocarditis in chronic hemodialysis patients: a complication more common than previously suspected. *Surgery*, **69**:554, 1971.

Kittle, C. F., and Reed, W. A.: Antibiotics and extracorporeal circulation. *J. Thorac. Cardiovasc. Surg.*, **41**:34, 1961.

Kleid, J. J.; Kim, E. S.; Brand, B.; Eckles, S.; and Gordon, G. M.: Heart block complicating acute bacterial endocarditis. *Chest*, **61**:301, 1972.

Koiwai, E. K., and Nahas, H. C.: Subacute bacterial endocarditis following cardiac surgery. *Arch. Surg.*, **73**:272, 1956.

Kreidberg, M. B., and Chernoff, H. L.: Ineffectiveness of penicillin prophylaxis in cardiac catheterization. *J. Pediatr.*, **66**:286, 1965.

Kretschmer, K. P., and Lawrence, G. H.: Valve replacement in patients with bacterial endocarditis. *Am. J. Surg.*, **118**:273, 1969.

Lerner, A. M.: In Discussion IV. Second International Symposium on Gentamicin. *J. Infect. Dis.*, **124S**:210, 1971.

Lerner, P. I., and Weinstein, L.: Infective endocarditis in the antibiotic era. *N. Engl. J. Med.*, **274**:199, 1966.

Levin, J.: Diphtheroid bacterial endocarditis after insertion of a Starr valve. *Ann. Intern. Med.*, **64**:396, 1966.

Levinson, D. C.; Griffith, G. C.; and Pearson, H. E.: Increasing bacterial resistance to antibiotics; study of 46 cases of streptococcus endocarditis and 18 cases of staphylococcus endocarditis. *Circulation*, **2**:668, 1950.

Lewis, I. C.: Bacterial endocarditis complicating septicaemia in an infant. *Arch. Dis. Child.*, **29**:144, 1954.

Libman, E.: A study of the endocardial lesions of subacute bacterial endocarditis: with particular reference to healing or healed lesions; with clinical notes. *Am. J. Med. Sci.*, **144**:313, 1912.

Lillehei, C. W.; Wargo, J. D.; and Hammerstrom, R. N.: Experimental bacterial endocarditis and proliferative glomerulon-ephritis: description of method of production utilizing bilateral lower extremity or single aorta-vena cava arteriovenous fistulas. *Dis. Chest*, **24**:421, 1953.

Loewe, L.; Rosenblatt, P.; Greene, H. J.; and Russell, M.: Combined penicillin and heparin therapy of subacute bacterial endocarditis. *JAMA*, **124**:144, 1944.

Louria, D. B.: The treatment of endocarditis. *Am. Heart. J.*, **66**:429, 1963.

Macaulay, D.: Acute endocarditis in infancy and early childhood. *Am. J. Dis. Child.*, **88**:715, 1954.

McGeown, M. G.: Bacterial endocarditis: the process of healing. *Ulster Med. J.*, **23**:39, 1954.

MacKay, D. N., and Kaye, D.: Serum concentrations of colistin in patients with normal and impaired renal function. *N. Engl. J. Med.*, **270**:394, 1964.

Maramba, L. C.; Hildner, F. J.; Samet, P.; and Greenberg, J. J.: Tricuspid valve subacute bacterial endocarditis complicating tetralogy of Fallot. *Chest*, **59**:227, 1971.

Martin, W. J.; Nichols, D. R.; Svien, H. J.; and Ulrich, J. A.: Cryptococcosis: Further observations with amphotericin B. *Arch. Intern. Med.*, **104**:4, 1959.

Martinez, E. C.; Burch, G. E.; and Giles, T. D.: Echocardiographic diagnosis of vegetative aortic bacterial endocarditis. *Am. J. Cardiol.*, **34**:845, 1974.

Meleney, F. L.; Johnson, B. A.; and Teng, P.: Further experiences with local and systemic bacitracin in treatment of various surgical and neuro-surgical infections and certain related medical infections. *Surg. Gynecol. Obstet.*, **94**:401, 1952.

Merzbach, D.; Freundlich, E.; Metzker, A.; and Falk, W.: Bacterial endocarditis due to corynebacterium. *J. Pediatr.*, **67**:792, 1965.

Miller, G.; Hansen, J. E.; and Pollock, B. E.: Staphylococcus endocarditis. *Am. Heart J.*, **47**:453, 1954.

Murdoch, J. M.; Allan, R.; Ishiyama, S.; and Weinstein, L.: Panel discussion of severe gram-positive infections. *Postgrad. Med. J.*, **47**(suppl. 94):102, 1971.

Nadas, A. S., and Fyler, D. C.: *Pediatric Cardiology*, 3rd ed. W. B. Saunders Co., Philadelphia, 1972.

Nelson, R. M.; Jenson, C. B.; Peterson, C. A.; and Sanders, B. C.: Effective use of prophylactic antibiotics in open heart surgery. *Arch. Surg.*, **90**:731, 1965.

Newman, W.; Torres, J. M.; and Guck, J. K.: Bacterial endocarditis: an analysis of fifty-two cases. *Am. J. Med.*, **16**:535, 1954.

O'Hare, M. M., and Stevenson, J. S.: Specific bacteriolysin in subacute bacterial endocarditis caused by a haemolytic Staphylococcus albus. *Br. Med. J.*, **2**:1086, 1953.

Okies, J. E.; Viroslav, J.; and Willieams, T. W., Jr.: Endocarditis after cardiac valvular replacement. *Chest*, **59**:198, 1971.

Okies, J. E.; Williams, T. W., Jr.; Howell, J. F.; Crawford, E. S.; Morris, G. C.; and DeBakey, M. E.: Valvular replacement in bacterial endocarditis. *Cardiovasc. Res. Cent. Bull.*, **8**:126, 1970.

Paterson, P. Y.: Status of prevention of subacute bacterial endocarditis. American Heart Association Prevention Committee, Atlanta, Ga., 1968.

Phipps, C.: Acute bacterial endocarditis. *N. Engl. J. Med.*, **207**:768, 1932.

Quinn, R., W., and Brown, J. W.: Bacterial endocarditis: unusual case with blood cultures positive for brucella abortus and viridans streptococcus. *Arch. Intern. Med.*, **94**:679, 1954.

Rabens, R. A.; Geraci, J. E.; Grindlay, J. H.; and Karlson, A. G.: Experimental bacterial endocarditis due to Streptococcus mitis. *Circulation*, **11**:199, 1955.

Rabens, R. A.; Karlson, A. G.; Geraci, J. E.; and Edwards, J. E.: Experimental bacterial endocarditis due to Streptococcus mitis. II. Pathology of valvular and secondary lesions. *Circulation*. **11**:206, 1955.

Rantz, L. A.: Combined antibiotic therapy in subacute bacterial endocarditis. *Stanford Med. Bull.*, **12**:26, 1954.

Rantz, L. A.; Carnes, W. H.; and Bernhard, R. W.: Bacterial endocarditis with repeatedly negative blood cultures. *Stanford Med. Bull.*, **12**:266, 1954.

Roantree, R. J., and Rantz, L. A.: Fatal staphylococcal endocarditis treated with erythromycin. *Arch. Intern. Med.*, **95**:320, 1955.

Robbins, W. C., and Tompsett, R.: Treatment of enterococcal endocarditis and bacteremia: results of combined therapy with penicillin and streptomycin. *Am. J. Med.*, **10**:278, 1951.

Roberts, N.: Mimics of bacterial endocarditis. *Am. J. Cardiol.*, **26**:529, 1970.

Robinson, M. J., and Ruedy, J.: Sequelae of bacterial endocarditis. *Am. J. Med.*, **32**:922, 1962.

Roth, O., et al.: Chlortetracycline (Aureomycin) in prevention of bacteremia following oral surgery: attempt to prevent subacute bacterial endocarditis in patients with heart disease. *Arch. Intern. Med.*, **92**:485, 1953.

Saldanha, L. F.; Goldman, R.; Adashek, K.; and Mulder, D. G.: Treatment of bacterial endocarditis: complicating haemodialysis. *Br. Med. J.*, **3**:92, 1972.

Sallam, I.; Sammon, A.; McGeachie, J.; and Bain, W. H.: Prophylactic antibiotics in closed heart surgery. *Chest*, **60**:252, 1971.

Sande, M. A.; Johnson, W. D., Jr.; Hook, E. W.; and Kaye, D.: Sustained bacteremia in patients with prosthetic cardiac valves. *N. Engl. J. Med.*, **286**:1067, 1972.

Sanger, M. D., and Stein, I.: The treatment of subacute bacterial endocarditis in a patient sensitive to aqueous procaine penicillin. *N.Y. J. Med.*, **53**:1237, 1953.

Santos-Buch, C. A.; Koenig, M. G.; and Rogers, D. E.: Oral treatment of subacute bacterial endocarditis with phenoxymethyl penicillin (penicillin V) *N. Engl. J. Med.*, **257**:249, 1957.

Saslaw, S.: Cephalosporins. *Med. Clin. North Am.*, **54**:1217, 1970.

Shah, P.; Sinch, W. S. A.; Rose, V.; and Keith, J. D.: Incidence of bacterial endocarditis in ventricular septal defects. *Circulation*, **34**:127, 1966.

Sharkey, B., and McGovern, V. J.: Advanced chronic endocarditis with mitral stenosis and aortic stenosis in a child of three years. *Med. J. Aust.*, **1**:668, 1953.

Shinebourne, E. A.; Cripps, C. M.; Hayward, G. W.; and Shooter, R. A.: Bacterial endocarditis, 1956–1965: analysis of clinical features and treatment in relation to prognosis and mortality. *Br. Heart J.*, **31**:536, 1969.

Shnider, B. L., and Cotsonas, N. J., Jr.: Embolic mycotic aneurysms, a complication of bacterial endocarditis. *Am. J. Med.*, **10**:246, 1954.

Smith, I. M.: Cephalosporin therapy of staphylococcal infections in adults. *Postgrad. Med. J.*, **47**(suppl. 78):87, 1971.

Spicer, S., and Blitz, D. A.: A study of the response of bacterial populations to the response of penicillin: a quantitative determination of its effect on the organisms. *J. Lab. Clin. Med.*, **33**:417, 1948.

Stason, W. B.; DeSanctis, R. W.; Weinberg, A. N.; and Austen, W. G.: Cardiac surgery in bacterial endocarditis. *Circulation*, **38**:514, 1968.

Stein, P. D.; Harken, D. E.; and Dexter, L.: The nature and prevention of prosthetic valve endocarditis. *Am. Heart. J.*, **71**:393, 1966.

Sussman, I., and Price, P.: Right-sided endocarditis on a patent foramen ovale associated with periarteritis nodosa. *Ann. Intern. Med.*, **37**:614, 1952.

Swan, H. J. C.: Infectious, inflammatory, and allergic complications. In Braunwald, E. and Swan, H. J. C. (eds.): Cooperative Study on Cardiac Catheterization. *Circulation*, **37**: Suppl. 111, 111–49, 1968.

Thayer, W. S.: Studies on bacterial (infective) endocarditis. *Hopkins Hosp. Rep.*, **22**:1, 1926.

Touroff, A. S. W., and Vesell, H.: Subacute streptococcus viridans endarteritis complicating patent ductus arteriosus. *JAMA*, **115**:1270, 1940.

Turk, D. C., and Wilson, C. T. M.: A case of enterococcal endocarditis. *Guy Hosp. Rep.*, **103**:260, 1954.

Vogler, W. R.; Dorney, E. R.; and Bridges, H. A.: Bacterial endocarditis; a review of 148 cases. *Am. J. Med.*, **32**:910, 1962.

Wallach, J. B.; Glass, M.; Lukash, L.; and Angrist, A. A.: Bacterial endocarditis and mural thrombi in the heart. *Circulation*, **10**:524, 1954.

Ward, A. M.: Endocarditis in the neonatal period. *Arch. Dis. Child.*, **46**:249, 1971.

Weinstein, L., and Rubin, R. H.: Infective endocarditis—1973. *Prog. Cardiovasc. Dis.*, **16**:239, 1973.

Weinstein, L., and Schlesinger, J.: Treatment of infective endocarditis. *Prog. Cardiovasc. Dis.*, **16**: 275, 1973.

Wessler, S., and Avioli, L. V.: Enterococcal endocarditis. *JAMA*, **204**:916, 1968.

Whipple, R. L.: The cure of a patient with a very resistant Streptococcus viridans endocarditis with massive penicillin therapy. *Am. Heart J.*, **42**:414, 1951.

Whipple, R. L., and Bloom, W. L.: The occurrence of false positive tests for albumin and glucose in the urine during the course of massive penicillin therapy. *J. Lab. Clin. Med.*, **36**:635, 1950.

White, P. D.: The incidence of endocarditis in earliest childhood. *Am. J. Dis. Child.*, **32**:536, 1926.

———: *Heart Disease*, 4th ed. The Macmillan Co., New York, 1951.

Williams, T. W.; Viroslav, J.; and Knight, V.: Management of bacterial endocarditis. *Am. J. Cardiol.*, **26**:186, 1970.

Wilson, D.: Personal communication, 1964.

Winchell, P.: Infectious endocarditis as a result of contamination during cardiac catheterization. *N. Engl. J. Med.*, **248**:245, 1953.

Wise, J. R., Jr.; Cleland, W. P.; Halldie-Smith, K. A.; et al.: Urgent aortic valve replacement for acute aortic regurgitation due to infective endocarditis. *Lancet*, **2**:115, 1971.

Wood, W. S., and Hall, B.: Rupture of spleen in subacute bacterial endocarditis: mycotic aneurysm of splenic artery and spontaneous rupture of spleen in subacute bacterial endocarditis. *Arch. Intern. Med.*, **93**:633, 1954.

Wray, T. M.: The variable echocardiographic features in aortic valve endocarditis. *Circulation*, **52**:658, 1975.

Yeh, T. J.; Anabtawi, I. N.; Cornett, V. E.; Stern, H.; and Ellison, R. G.: Bacterial endocarditis following open heart surgery. *Ann. Thorac. Surg.*, **3**: 29, 1967.

Zakrzewski, T., and Keith, J. D.: Bacterial endocarditis in infants and children. *J. Pediatr.*, **67**:1179, 1965.

15

Pericarditis

John D. Keith

W HITE (1951) points out that pericarditis was first described in the Middle Ages before other forms of heart disease were known. At the present time it is found with some frequency among adults but is a less common finding among children.

Incidence

In 1932, Smith and Willius found pericarditis in 4.2 percent of 8912 postmortems of all ages at the Mayo Clinic. Griffith and Wallace in 1949 reported the finding of pericarditis in 5.4 percent of 13,353 autopsies. The most common type was nonspecific idiopathic pericarditis.

During the 29-year period from 1924 to 1952 there were 294,129 admissions to The Hospital for Sick Children, Toronto. During the same period there were 235 cases of pericarditis recorded, an incidence of 1 in every 1250 admissions. Table 15–1 classifies these cases according to etiology. It will be noted that rheumatic pericarditis is first, accounting for 55

percent of all cases. Next in frequency is purulent or septic pericarditis with 28 percent. All the other causes together account for only 17 percent.

Clinical Features

Precordial pain in childhood is not as frequently a feature of pericarditis as it is in adults. It occurred in 70 of our 129 cases of rheumatic pericarditis but was rarely referred to in the group of septic origin. When it did occur in the latter group, it was not a marked feature of the illness and usually lasted only a day or two.

It has been shown by Capps (1943) that the visceral and inner surfaces of the parietal pericardium are insensitive to pain. The pain is caused chiefly by involvement of the pleura, either mediastinal, diaphragmatic, or costal.

Most children with pericarditis develop a moderate effusion which in itself does not usually produce symptoms. If the effusion is marked, there may be interference with the diastolic filling of the

Table 15–1. PERICARDITIS IN CHILDREN

| PERICARDITIS TYPE | TORONTO HOSPITAL FOR SICK CHILDREN | | BOSTON CHILDREN'S HOSPITAL |
	1924–1952, O'Hanley	*1955–1964,* Khoury	*1949–1959,* Nadas and Levy
Rheumatic	129	5	6
Purulent	67	2	6
Idiopathic (acute, benign)	13	18	4
Coxsackie	—	3	—
Rheumatoid	8	5	5
Constrictive	1	3	—
Tuberculous	7	—	2
Traumatic	—	1	—
Miscellaneous*	10	8	9
Total	235	45	32

* Miscellaneous includes: uremia, periarteritis nodosa, disseminated lupus, postoperative pericardial tamponade, thrombocytopenic purpura, congenital hypoplastic anemia, Cooley's anemia, glycogen-storage disease, Friedreich's ataxia, ulcerative colitis, chronic nonspecific, rupture aorta in pericardium, meningococcal infection, Gaucher's disease.

heart as well as a resulting congestion of the great veins with distention of the neck vessels and enlargement of the liver. Thus it may be difficult to differentiate the clinical picture from heart failure. The characteristic feature of pericarditis is the friction rub, which was present in 84 percent of the 129 cases of rheumatic pericarditis, 15 percent of the 67 cases of septic pericarditis, 87 percent of the seven cases of tuberculous pericarditis, and 85 percent of the 13 cases of benign idiopathic pericarditis. Thus a friction rub was present in nearly nine-tenths of our cases with a rheumatic, tuberculous, or idiopathic basis, but in comparison only 15 percent of those with septic pericarditis exhibited this sign.

The friction rub was usually heard best along the left sternal border, but in many cases it was audible over the entire precordium. The thin chest wall in a child allows one to hear, with greater ease than in adults, the rough, superficial sound of the rubbing together of the two pericardial surfaces. The sound is well imitated by placing the diaphragm of the stethoscope into the palm of the hand and rubbing the back of the hand in a to-and-fro motion. In children it is usually loud and well heard, but it may occasionally be faint or intermittent, especially as the effusion increases. The sound may persist after a large collection of fluid has accumulated in the pericardial sac, possibly because of adhesions or because the heart is held anteriorly against the pericardium. Eventually the developing effusion separates the adhering surfaces and causes the rub to disappear. Complete adherence of the pericardial layers or normal healing may also be responsible for

its disappearance. The friction rub must be distinguished from a pleuropericardial rub and also from mediastinal emphysema such as occasionally occur in pneumonia in children. At times the bulging pulmonary artery of cor pulmonale may produce a rubbing sound against the pericardium that simulates pericarditis.

The heart sounds are usually difficult to hear in the presence of the friction rub, whether or not effusion is present. As the effusion develops and the rub disappears, the sounds will be distant and faint.

With developing pericardial effusion, the lung is pushed back posteriorly and laterally, and in many instances bronchial breathing becomes audible at the left base posteriorly (Ewart's sign). When this is a marked feature, there may also be some dullness of percussion in the same area.

With marked effusion the pulse becomes weaker, especially during inspiration, producing the so-called paradoxic pulse.

Tachycardia is common, the majority of children with rheumatic fever having a rate between 120 and 150. In babies with pericarditis the rate varies between 120 and 190 during the more acute stages of the illness.

Radiologic Examination

As the effusion increases, the cardiac borders fill out and produce a somewhat pear-shaped shadow, and the cardiophrenic angles become less acute. Thus the usual contours of the heart chambers and

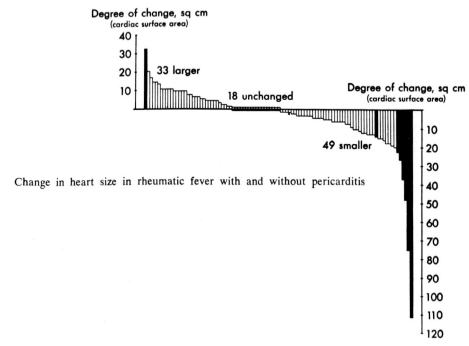

Change in heart size in rheumatic fever with and without pericarditis

Figure 15-1. The individual change in heart size in 100 cases of acute rheumatic fever. The vast majority had only a modest decrease in size during the illness. Those who did show a marked change all had pericarditis with effusion. (Pericarditis shown in black.)

great vessels tend to disappear into a smooth outline. When an x-ray is taken with the patient lying down, the shadow of the heart and pericardium has a globular shape forming somewhat acute angles with the diaphragm. With the patient sitting up, the shadow becomes more triangular. The heart shadow itself can rarely be distinguished within the outline of the pericardial effusion. However, an angiocardiogram may reveal the size and position of the chambers of the heart and demonstrate the distended pericardial sac. The same information can be obtained by cardiac catheterization. Under the fluoroscope the shape and size of the cardiac shadow, coupled with the absence of the usual pulsations of the borders, will permit one to suspect the presence of pericarditis when the friction rub is absent.

In rheumatic fever, when no friction rub is heard and the cardiac outline is suggestive, diagnosis can be made with considerable assurance when marked change of the shadow size takes place in a month or less. Although this does not occur in all cases of rheumatic pericarditis, when present it is a reliable sign of effusion (see Figure 15-1). Change in heart size due to myocarditis is a more gradual process and usually takes several months to accomplish.

Electrocardiography

In the early acute stage of the illness the S-T interval may be elevated, usually in the leads over the left precordium. This change may be of a minor degree at times and is best recognized by serial electrocardiograms. The S-T interval may be concave rather than convex as seen in myocardial infarction. The T waves are normal at first and then become flattened and frequently inverted. In children all of the left precordial leads and commonly two, if not three, of the standard leads may show T wave changes. These changes last from two to three weeks in most cases but may persist for several months or occasionally years in tuberculous pericarditis.

The amplitudes of the QRS and T waves are frequently diminished when effusion is present.

The alterations in the electrocardiogram are considered to be due to: (1) involvement of the myocardium immediately under the pericardium, causing S-T and T wave changes; and (2) the pericardial effusion, causing a diminution in voltage.

Diagnosis

The most reliable signs of pericarditis are: (1) a friction rub; (2) rapid and significant change in heart size, occurring over a period of one to four weeks; (3) the detection of fluid by pericardial tap or echocardiography; (4) electrocardiographic changes.

The diagnosis of pericarditis is based primarily on finding the typical friction rub over the peri-

cardium. If this is lacking, one turns to the size and shape of the cardiac shadow and the relatively rapid change in heart size over a few weeks. The presence of faint heart sounds and bronchial breathing at the left base are additional suggestive signs. One cannot rely greatly on the size and shape of the heart alone. A number of years ago, out of 22 cases considered, by the use of these criteria alone, to have pericardial effusion during life, the diagnosis was confirmed at postmortem in only nine; in the other 13 the increase in the cardiac shadow was due to enlargement of the heart itself and not to effusion. Ultrasound or echocardiography has now proved to be valuable in recognizing pericardial effusion (Feigenbaum, 1970).

Echocardiography is an accurate method of detecting pericardial fluid (Feigenbaum et al., 1967). Normally both visceral and parietal layers of pericardium are slightly separated (1 to 2 mm) at the peak of anterior motion of the posterior ventricular wall. As fluid accumulates, the parietal pericardium flattens and separates from the visceral pericardium. These changes are usually best seen at the level of the posterior wall of the left ventricle. Anterior fluid may be seen as an echo-free space just posterior to the anterior chest wall. The sweep up the left ventricle will usually show a progressive decrease in the amount of fluid with apposition of the layers of the pericardium as one approaches the left atrium. Careful attention to the identification of these details is required to avoid false-positive diagnoses. In particular, one must differentiate the normally occurring echo-free space just posterior to the pericardium from an effusion.

It is usually not difficult to differentiate a pleural friction rub occurring in the general area of the pericardium. Such a rub may be altered at times by the force of the heartbeat and thus resemble pericarditis. However, it is usually simple to eliminate this possibility by having the patient hold his breath.

The electrocardiogram may show a raised S-T segment, inverted T waves over the left precordium, and diminished QRS and T voltage. Their diagnostic significance is limited by the fact that similar patterns are seen in myocarditis.

One of the most difficult problems in pericarditis, when it occurs in rheumatic fever, is the differentiation of acute pericarditis from acute heart failure or chronic heart failure. The following points are of use in distinguishing these three conditions:

1. *Edema and weight gain* are usual in chronic heart failure, but they are rare in acute heart failure and do not occur in pericarditis.
2. The presence of *dyspnea* is of no value since it is frequently present in all three conditions.
3. A *friction rub*, of course, is characteristic of pericarditis and not of heart failure.
4. Although the *heart shadow* may appear enlarged in all three conditions, there is a rapid increase or decrease in the heart size when effusion is present; such is not the case with chronic or acute heart failure.
5. *Hilar shadows* may be congested in all three but

are more likely to be so with heart failure.

6. With chronic heart failure there is a long history of *previous rheumatic fever activity*; such is usually not the case with pericarditis.

7. In chronic heart failure there is usually evidence of *marked valvular involvement*; this may or may not be present in acute heart failure, but it is often not present with pericarditis.

8. Patients with acute failure are usually *acutely and seriously ill*, whereas those with pericarditis are often less seriously ill.

9. The *sedimentation rate* may be elevated or normal in chronic failure; it is usually high in acute failure and pericarditis.

10. The *neck veins* are distended with acute or chronic failure; they may be distended with pericarditis but not uncommonly are normal.

11. *Rales in the chest* are common when failure is present but are usually absent in pericarditis.

12. The *response to digitalis* is good when chronic failure is present; there may be a slight response with acute failure and no response with pericarditis.

13. Finally, it is well to remember that *pericarditis and failure may occur together*: such was the case in 71 of our 129 cases of rheumatic fever with pericarditis.

Differential Diagnosis. In childhood when pericarditis is found to be present, one has to differentiate between rheumatic pericarditis, septic pericarditis, rheumatoid pericarditis, tuberculous pericarditis, uremic pericarditis, periateritis nodosa, disseminated lupus erythematosus, chronic constrictive pericarditis, idiopathic benign pericarditis, and hemopericardium. Another type should now be added, and that is the pericarditis occurring after a surgical operation when the pericardium has been opened, as in the performance of a Brock valvulotomy.

As in all pediatric problems, the age is of considerable significance in diagnosis. This is illustrated by Table 15–2. If there are signs of pericarditis in a baby under two years, it is not rheumatic in origin but is most probably septic. If the child is three to five years of age, it is much more likely to be a rheumatoid basis. If over five years, rheumatic fever is the foremost probability.

Pyogenic pericarditis is frequently missed because it occurs as a secondary complication of pneumonia, osteomyelitis, or other purulent infections; although this type is seen most commonly in the first two years of life, it may occur at any age in childhood. A friction rub may be present, but more commonly the diagnosis is suspected by the appearance of the cardiac shadow.

Pericarditis in rheumatoid arthritis occurs almost invariably in the first five years of life, usually between the ages of two and five. There is usually high fever uncontrolled by salicylates, pericardial friction rub, and transient arthritis eventually followed by typical joint swellings.

There is rarely difficulty in the diagnosis of uremic pericarditis because of the underlying nephritis. Cases of periarteritis nodosa have usually run a prolonged course of illness before the pericardial friction rub appears.

The diagnosis of acute idiopathic benign pericarditis is made by exclusion. A friction rub is noted in a child who is usually over five years of age, is not desperately ill, and has no evidence of rheumatic fever or pyogenic infection. One may suspect rheumatic fever, but no other rheumatic stigmata develop. One may at times suspect rheumatoid arthritis, but no other signs of rheumatoid arthritis appear. The course is variable but usually benign, and it is difficult to be certain about the diagnosis until the course is run.

Chronic constrictive pericarditis presents a separate problem in diagnosis. Since there is no friction rub, the heart usually is not enlarged to a significant degree. The diagnosis as a rule is not difficult unless, as happens occasionally, the condition has come on rapidly following a recent acute pericarditis. Traumatic pericardial effusion and tamponade may occur from a swallowed safety pin (Norman and Cass, 1971).

Treatment

The underlying disease must be treated primarily, whether it be rheumatic fever, pyogenic infection, tuberculosis, etc. Rheumatic fever therapy has been outlined elsewhere (see Chapter 13). Pyogenic pericarditis is best treated when the organism has been cultured either directly from the pericardial fluid by aspiration or, if this is not obtainable, from a sputum or blood sample. Sensitivity to various antibiotics can be tested and the proper drug given in suitable doses. Since these patients are almost invariably severely ill with a primary infection in the lung, the bone, or some other focus throughout the body, therapy should be prompt and adequate. Among the pyogenic organisms, *Staphylococcus aureus* is most commonly the causative agent (see Table 15–5, p. 250). *Streptococcus (Diplococcus)*

Table 15–2. RELATIVE INCIDENCE BY AGE GROUPS

TYPE	UNDER 2 YEARS	2–5 YEARS	5–10 YEARS	OVER 10 YEARS
Rheumatic (129 cases)	0	6	56	67
Rheumatoid (8 cases)	2	6	0	0
Septic (67 cases)	30	11	17	9
Tuberculous (7 cases)	1	3	3	0
Nonspecific (13 cases)	0	7	5	1

pneumoniae and the hemolytic streptococcus are the second and third most commonly found. Thus, if purulent pericarditis is suspected and the etiology has not been or cannot be determined, therapy should be aimed primarily to cover these three organisms. Such therapy should be maintained until the illness has resolved and convalescence is well established. Methicillin (Celbenin, Staphcillin) will frequently be the treatment of choice. It may be given, 100 mg per kilogram of body weight total daily dose, in six divided doses intravenously in tubing of continuous intravenous.

. At the time that antibiotic therapy is initiated, a pericardial paracentesis may need to be performed if there is a large effusion that is producing a high degree of tamponade. This may be estimated by the presence of marked tachycardia, enlargement of the liver, and engorgement of the vessels. Surgical intervention and the introduction of a drainage tube into the pericardium may be necessary if the patient does not respond to the therapy outlined.

Aspiration is best performed in a child in the fourth or fifth left interspace approximately 1 cm inside the border of the pericardial margin. This can be estimated from x-ray or fluoroscopic examination. It is sometimes advantageous to do the paracentesis on the fluoroscopic table.

Pericardial paracentesis is rarely needed in rheumatic pericarditis since the prime difficulty is in the myocardium rather than the pericardium, and the pericardial effusion is rarely sufficient to interfere seriously with cardiac function. Pericardial paracentesis is of more value in pyogenic pericarditis for both diagnosis and the relief of cardiac tamponade when such is present.

Cardiac tamponade was seen in one of our cases who ruptured the base of the aorta into the pericardial sac. Death occurred a few hours later in spite of surgical attempts to control the source of hemorrhage.

The prognosis in rheumatic fever with pericarditis is best illustrated in Table 15–3 (page 249), which shows the mortality over a 29-year period at The Hospital for Sick Children. It will be noted that the mortality dropped from 70 percent in 1924 to 1928 to 40 percent in 1949 to 1952.

A similar table has been prepared for septic pericarditis (Table 15–4, page 250), and it will be noticed that the mortality was 100 percent in the 1924-to-1928 period and there have been relatively few survivors over the years since. Fifty-eight of sixty-seven cases died, or approximately 13 percent have survived, and the recoveries have been evenly distributed over the years.

Tuberculous pericarditis has had a mortality of approximately 75 percent in the past (Table 15–7, page 254). It may be reduced in the future with the newer drugs.

There have been no deaths in this series from benign idiopathic pericarditis, and such patients have had no apparent residual defects, although it is possible that some of them may eventually develop constrictive pericarditis. Constrictive pericarditis has a poor prognosis without operation; with surgery the majority of cases do well, but there is an 18 percent mortality.

RHEUMATIC PERICARDITIS

RHEUMATIC pericarditis has become steadily less frequent. From 1924 to 1928 there were 27 cases of rheumatic fever with pericarditis; from 1955 to 1963 the figure had fallen to five, although admissions to The Hospital for Sick Children had trebled during this interval (Table 15–3).

Table 15–3. INCIDENCE AND MORTALITY OF RHEUMATIC FEVER WITH PERICARDITIS*

TIME INTERVAL	INCIDENCE	DEATHS	PERCENT MORTALITY
1924–1928	27	19	70
1929–1933	31	16	50
1934–1938	20	12	60
1939–1943	24	14	60
1944–1948	14	5	35
1949–1952	13	5	40
1955–1963	5	0	0
Total	134	71	55

* O'Hanley, J.: Hospital for Sick Children, Toronto, 1953.

Although the incidence of rheumatic pericarditis has been diminishing, the mortality has also been decreasing—from 70 percent to 40 percent from 1924 to 1952. Findlay in 1931 had a mortality rate of 47 percent, and Ash in 1936 had a rate of 58 percent.

Rheumatic pericarditis is associated with an irregular accumulation of fibrin over the pericardium that becomes adherent primarily to one surface but not uncommonly develops on both surfaces, and this often leads to complete obliteration of the pericardial sac. At postmortem the pericardium presents a shaggy, rough appearance. Normally there is a small amount of fluid in a child's pericardium—10 to 15 ml—but with pericarditis and effusion there may be several hundred milliliters.

The rheumatic patients with pericarditis usually appear acutely ill at the onset and as a rule present other signs of rheumatic fever. Furthermore, 84 percent of our cases with pericarditis had an audible friction rub. Many also exhibited a rapid change in heart size; usually there was considerable increase in the cardiac outline when the diagnosis was made so that the change was associated with a decrease in size over a one-to four-week period (see Figure 15–1).

The electrocardiographic changes are similar to those described, but the pattern may be altered by the underlying myocarditis of rheumatic infection. Elevation of the S-T segment, followed later by low or inverted T waves, is a common finding.

Pericarditis does not in itself affect the long-term prognosis since the latter is more dependent on the degree of myocarditis and endocarditis. However, those children who have pericarditis are likely to have more underlying disease and, therefore, a poorer prognosis. It is interesting to note that the outlook is improving in this regard.

There is no evidence that rheumatic pericarditis leads to constrictive pericarditis in later years in this group. Steroids are rarely needed in this situation.

SEPTIC PERICARDITIS (PURULENT)

SEPTIC pericarditis has also fallen in frequency over the years. From 1924 to 1928 there were 20 cases admitted to The Hospital for Sick Children; from 1949 to 1952 there were only three (Table 15–4). The deaths have declined with the incidence, while the mortality percentage has remained approximately the same.

Table 15–4. INCIDENCE AND MORTALITY OF SEPTIC PERICARDITIS*

TIME INTERVAL	INCIDENCE	DEATHS
1924–1928	20	20
1929–1933	12	10
1934–1938	17	13
1939–1943	7	7
1944–1948	8	5
1949–1952	3	3
1955–1964	2	2
Total	69	60

* O'Hanley, J.: Hospital for Sick Children, Toronto, 1953.

Septic pericarditis leads to the formation of a purulent exudate of varying degrees of consistency, thick or thin. Coagulated masses of fibrin, adhering to the visceral and parietal surfaces and covered with a purulent coating, are seen at postmortem. A variety of organisms have been recovered from our cases of septic pericarditis and are listed in Table 15–5. *Staphylococcus aureus*, *Str. (D.) pneumoniae*, and the hemolytic streptococcus were the chief offending organisms. With the control of *Str. (D.) pneumoniae* and the hemolytic streptococcus by modern antibiotics, these bacteria will probably be less of a problem in the future. The staphylococcus may continue to be a cause of this complication, especially in young children. Where staphylococcal pericarditis is suspected, antibiotics that deal with the less sensitive strains should be used.

Most of our cases of septic pericarditis are associated with pneumonia, empyema, or osteomyelitis. In the face of such infection one's attention may be drawn to the heart by a friction rub, but only 15 percent exhibited this sign. There may be a large or enlarging cardiac shadow shown by x-ray. Where there is any suspicion of pericarditis, an electro-cardiogram may help in the diagnosis: It may show S-T or T wave changes, which can appear early before the purulent exudate has accumulated sufficiently to alter the cardiac outline or produce tamponade.

The prognosis with this form of pericarditis is usually grave. A pericardial aspiration is important for the determination of the organism and the initiation of appropriate antibiotic therapy. Open drainage may be required at times if the response to therapy is not satisfactory (Benzing and Kaplan, 1963).

Table 15–5. SEPTIC PERICARDITIS, CAUSATIVE ORGANISMS*

ORGANISMS	NUMBER OF CASES
Staphylococcus aureus	25
Streptococcus (Diplococcus) pneumoniae	15
Hemolytic streptococcus	12
Staphylococcus aureus and hemolytic streptococcus	5
Staphylococcus aureus and *Streptococcus (Diplococcus) pneumoniae*	1
Haemophilus influenzae	2
Escherichia coli	1
Pseudomonas aeruginosa	1
Streptococcus anaerobius	1
Organism undetermined	4

* O'Hanley, J.: Hospital for Sick Children, Toronto, 1953.

Table 15–6. PERICARDITIS AS A MANIFESTATION OF VARIOUS SYSTEMIC DISEASES*

DISEASE	TOTAL NUMBER OF CASES	CASES WITH PERICARDITIS	ASSOCIATED PERICARDIAL EFFUSION
Uremia	72	7	5
Rheumatoid arthritis	130	8	1
Periarteritis nodosa	9	1	0
Tuberculosis	136	7	0

* Hospital for Sick Children.

MENINGOCOCCAL PERICARDITIS

PERICARDITIS complicating meningococcal meningitis is rarely encountered in children. Scott and coworkers (1971) have summarized the limited literature in this regard, which comprises seven cases in children, 43 cases when adults are included. Morse and associates (1971) have added six cases in army personnel.

Infants and children receiving treatment for meningococcal infections must therefore be observed closely for signs of pericarditis, and in patients known to have meningococcal infection one should look for evidence of friction rub, chest pain, electrocardiographic changes, or occasionally progressive pericardial compression, which at times may necessitate pericardial tap. In the latter situation, removal of pericardial effusion will show an immediate improvement in the patient. Recovery in these cases may be slow but is usually complete over several weeks or months. The heart function and size return to normal and the ultimate prognosis is good. Large doses of aqueous penicillin will usually control the infection adequately. Constrictive pericarditis may occur occasionally, as reported by Weis and Silber (1961).

Digitalis may occasionally be required, since Hardman and Earle (1969) report a significant incidence of interstitial myocarditis in 200 patients with fatal meningococcal infections.

PERIARTERITIS NODOSA

OUT OF nine cases of periarteritis nodosa diagnosed at The Hospital for Sick Children, we have had one with signs of pericarditis. This was a baby boy of five months who was ill for four weeks and developed a pericardial friction rub during the fourth week of illness. He died the day after the rub was heard, and a sterile pericarditis was confirmed at postmortem. The microscopic examination of organs throughout the body showed lesions typical of periarteritis nodosa.

UREMIC PERICARDITIS

IN 72 cases of uremia at The Hospital for Sick Children, there have been seven with pericarditis; a similar proportion of uremic cases in adult life have pericarditis. All of our cases were in the terminal stage of chronic nephritis, and death took place within three weeks after the appearance of the pericardial friction rub. The lesion was always recognized by the rub; there was no pain. A small amount of pericardial effusion was usually present at the time of death.

The electrocardiogram usually does not show the typical changes seen in the other forms of pericarditis, but minor elevation of S-T or lowering of T waves may occur. The cause of uremic pericarditis is unknown.

RHEUMATOID ARTHRITIS

THERE have been 130 cases of rheumatoid arthritis admitted to The Hospital for Sick Children during a 29-year period, and eight of these had pericarditis. All but one were diagnosed by hearing the characteristic friction rub. In the eighth case the diagnosis was made at postmortem.

The ages of these children were 15 months, 20 months, three years (three cases), $3\frac{1}{2}$ years, four years, and 13 years. All of these cases had their pericarditis at the age of four years or under. In the 13-year-old boy, rheumatoid arthritis appeared at four years of age with signs suggestive of pericarditis; an adherent pericardium was found at postmortem at 13 years. Lietman and Bywaters (1963) found pericarditis more common in the 10-to-15-year age group. They also report an incidence of pericardial involvement similar to ours (7 to 8 percent).

The illness almost invariably began with a high, spiking fever of no obvious origin, which persisted. This was soon accompanied by occasional joint pains or a stiff neck of a degree that was not sufficient to make a diagnosis of rheumatoid arthritis. The pericardial friction rub was usually heard at this stage, approximately a month after the onset of fever and illness. Typical periarticular swellings of rheumatoid arthritis appeared later, as a rule, usually six to eight weeks after the beginning of the illness and approximately a month after the friction rub was first heard.

In the early stages it may be difficult to determine the cause of the fever or pericarditis, but once the pericarditis has occurred, there are certain diagnostic points of value.

1. A maculopapular rash suggestive of rheumatoid arthritis may appear.
2. Joint pains suggestive of rheumatic infection may occur. Those with a fever that does not respond to salicylates suggest rheumatoid arthritis. Furthermore, the age (three to five years) is a little young

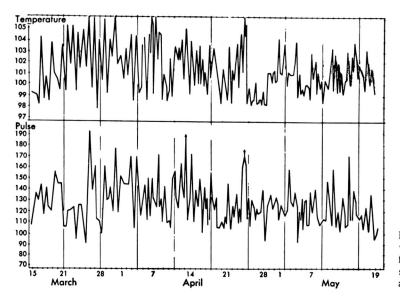

Figure 15-2. K. P., 3½-year-old with pericarditis who had high fever for ten weeks. She subsequently developed rheumatoid arthritis six years later.

for rheumatic fever. The leukocyte count is generally quite high, 30,000 to 40,000, but may be 10,000 to 15,000 on occasion. The fever shows a favorable response to cortisone in suitable doses. When doubt exists about the presence of pericarditis, an x-ray of the heart may show effusion, and the electrocardiogram may show typical changes.

It would appear barely possible that some cases of rheumatoid arthritis may have fever and pericarditis and not develop arthritis. They might then be listed among the acute benign type of pericarditis. One of our cases did not develop typical signs of rheumatoid arthritis for six years. The temperature during her original illness is shown in Figure 15–2.

Most children with pericarditis and rheumatoid arthritis recover from the attack, as far as the pericarditis is concerned, and have no residual cardiac signs. Postmortem findings suggest that many of those who survive develop an adherent pericardium. A number of these children are seriously ill when they have pericarditis and offer a clear-cut situation for the use of hormones as a lifesaving measure.

IDIOPATHIC PERICARDITIS

THE number of cases grouped under the title of idiopathic pericarditis is diminishing as the virology techniques improve. The association with pericarditis has been noted in Coxsackie infection as well as influenza, mumps, herpes zoster, varicella, and Asian influenza. A thorough investigation should be made in each case of pericarditis to identify the etiology if possible.

There were 31 cases in our series in which the etiology was unknown; all survived and have no residual evidence of heart disease. On reviewing the histories one wonders whether a few cases may have been rheumatic in origin, in spite of the fact that no arthritis or endocarditis occurred and the recovery from pericarditis was complete. One case (not included) was ten months old, and it is possible that this one was due to a pyogenic infection, although no evidence of this was available.

Smith and coworkers (1955) have described acute benign pericarditis in 20 percent of 24 children with Cooley anemia who had had splenectomy. No cases occurred in the 14 cases who retained their spleens.

Clinical Features

The majority of our cases appeared to fit the classification of Barnes and Burchell (1942). These varied in age from 3 to 11, usually being a little older than the patients with rheumatoid arthritis. Chest pain was not uncommon but was not the marked feature it is in adults. It was marked in 3 of the 13 cases; in one it was referred to the neck and shoulder, and in the other two to the abdomen to a sufficient degree to require surgical consultations. The onset of pain was usually insidious, but in one case it occurred suddenly at night. Some increase in respiratory rate was common.

Fever was usual in the early stages, frequently between 101° and 102° F; it subsided after a week in the majority of cases, but in some it continued to be the most prominent feature of the illness with a sawtooth type of swing up to 104° F and down to normal again daily for several weeks. One case had no fever or tachycardia at any time, and the pericardial effusion gradually subsided over six months.

All but two had the characteristic pericardial friction rub; the friction rub in these cases lasted for one to ten days. One of the cases with no friction rub had a pericardial effusion that was verified by paracentesis. The other had a tremendous cardiac shadow that ultimately returned to normal size.

The electrocardiographic changes were the same as for the other forms of pericarditis and usually persisted for one to three months but occasionally lasted for longer periods of time. X-ray findings were also similar to those in the other forms of pericarditis.

Laboratory Findings

On paracentesis the fluid is serosanguineous as a rule. The leukocyte count varies between 7000 and 25,000, but in our cases it was usually over 12,000. The sedimentation rate was elevated; in the milder forms it returned promptly to normal within one to three weeks, and in the more severe cases or prolonged illnesses the elevation lasted throughout the illness.

Clinical Course and Prognosis

The course in children is extremely variable; some of our cases were better in two weeks, others were very ill with high fever for nearly three months. In spite of this, all survived, and are now active and well with normal hearts.

In the literature there has been one reported death; this patient was being treated with anticoagulants because of suspected myocardial infarction. Hemorrhage into the pericardial sac occurred with tamponade.

Recurrences did not appear in our group; however, they have been reported to occur in 15 percent of adults.

Diagnosis

The diagnosis is made by exclusion of other forms of pericarditis. In this group it is difficult to exclude rheumatic fever entirely even when there are no other signs of the disease (arthritis, endocarditis, nodules, chorea, or erythema marginata), because it is a well-known fact that rheumatic fever may show no signs other than heart disease and it is possible that signs of heart disease may be limited to the pericardium. Thus, in years in which there are a large number of rheumatic patients appearing, it is possible that some cases of rheumatic fever may have been grouped in this category.

Septic pericarditis must be ruled out. This usually occurs in a younger age group among children who are more desperately ill. The response to antibiotics is more likely to be satisfactory and, on paracentesis, a purulent exudate is obtained; on occasion the organism is cultured.

Tuberculous pericarditis is usually painless, and a friction rub may last for a long time—several weeks to several months. There should be evidence of tuberculosis elsewhere in the body, most commonly in the lungs.

Treatment

Symptomatic treatment with rest in bed until the illness has subsided is the usual therapy. Penicillin is without effect in this infection, but Friedman and associates (1952) have reported a shortening of the course by the administration of ACTH and cortisone to four children. We have also noted significant improvement with this therapy.

TUBERCULOUS PERICARDITIS

TUBERCULOUS pericarditis may occur at any age but is more common after ten years of age than before. At The Hospital for Sick Children there have been seven cases. Five of these were examined at the postmortem table; the other two are still alive and well. Out of 136 postmortem studies on children dying from tuberculosis there have been five with pericarditis (Boyd, 1953).

Pathology

Primary invasion of the pericardium by the tubercle bacillus is considered to be an uncommon event in children, if it occurs at all. Almost invariably the lesion is due to a direct extension from the lung. It may spread from infected hilar glands or directly from caseous lung tissue. In adults it may appear as the only manifestation of the disease, but in all probability it will spread in the same way from the lung or hilar glands. Tubercles may be scattered over the visceral or parietal pericardium, but usually there is a diffuse pericardial reaction with considerable fibrosis. The fibrosis may predominate on either the visceral or parietal side initially, but eventually there is obliteration of the pericardial sac as such. Early, the tubercles are small and scattered, but ultimately they coalesce into a fibrotic reaction. The early acute stage usually proceeds into one characterized by effusion, but if the patient survives, the fluid is absorbed and the fibrotic reaction remains.

The pericardial fluid is watery (specific gravity, 1.018); the white blood cells in the pericardial fluid vary between 500 and 1000 per milliliter, and there is a lymphocytosis. Red blood cells can be present, and in a few cases tubercle bacilli may be demonstrated in the fluid itself. In the past the mortality has been reported to be between 65 and 90 per cent.

Clinical Features

The ages of our seven cases varied from 22 months to ten years. They all had evidence of pulmonary tuberculosis; besides this, two had miliary tuberculosis infection and two had tuberculous meningitis. The duration of signs and symptoms preceding the onset of pericarditis varied from two weeks to seven months in the five cases that died. The duration of the illness preceding pericarditis in the two cases that survived was two years in one and four years in the other. The onset was rather slow and insidious.

The temperature in some cases increased to between 99° and 103° F. The pulse rate was usually elevated and varied between 90 and 160; it was more closely related to the degree of fever than to the state of the pericarditis.

No pericardial friction rub was heard in the cases that died and came to postmortem. The two cases that survived had pericardial friction rubs that lasted for six weeks in each case. The heart sounds were sometimes slightly muffled, and occasionally a third sound suggesting a gallop was present. A mitral systolic murmur was present in one case. Pericardial effusion indicated by x-ray was present in one of the seven cases.

Heart failure is a common finding among the cases reported in the literature; it was present in only one of our cases and was associated with venous congestion, enlargement of the liver, and edema.

The leukocyte count varied between 15,000 and 21,000 in all but one case; in the latter the count was 6000 to 8000 while the child was on isoniazid. The sedimentation rate was usually elevated but was normal occasionally.

Diagnosis

These children have evidence of tuberculosis elsewhere in the body, usually in the lung. Associated with such infection one may find evidence of pericarditis. The most diagnostic sign is the pericardial rub, which may last for weeks; in other forms of pericarditis it rarely lasts longer than ten days to two weeks. When rheumatic fever is present, other rheumatic stigmata aid in making the diagnosis. In benign idiopathic pericarditis one may suspect a tuberculous origin. The absence of tuberculous infection in other parts of the anatomy will usually eliminate this diagnosis.

The appearance of pericardial effusion suggested by x-ray size and shape of the heart is indicative of tuberculous pericarditis when it occurs in a patient already suffering from active tuberculosis. The presence of a significant tachycardia occurring in a tuberculous patient without other explanation will make one suspect pericarditis. The appearance of heart failure in tuberculous infection is suggestive of pericarditis since heart failure is reported in half the adult cases with tuberculous pericarditis. It appears to be much less common in children.

The appearance of the electrocardiographic changes of pericarditis are suggestively diagnostic. There may be elevation of the S-T portion in the very early stages, but this is quickly followed by inverted T waves in leads I, II, or III in the standard leads and over the left precordium in the precordial leads. Thus, some of the signs indicated above are indefinite; the presence of typical electrocardiographic alterations in a child with evidence of tuberculosis will allow one to make the diagnosis with reasonable assurance.

Finally, in certain cases the diagnosis may be made only at postmortem since no signs suggesting this lesion may appear during life.

Treatment

Boyd (1953) has reported the treatment with isoniazid of two children with tuberculous pericarditis. The response was favorable in both instances and the patients have recovered and are doing well. In this investigator's experience in treating tuberculosis, this was a more effective therapy than streptomycin, chloramphenicol, or paraaminosalicylic acid. The dose of isoniazid was 10 mg per kilogram of body weight, and such therapy was maintained in these two cases for six to nine months. The treatment was maintained until all signs of active tuberculous infection had subsided, long after the pericardial friction rub had disappeared entirely.

Prognosis

In the past the mortality in tuberculous pericarditis has been high. Table 15–7 indicates the mortality in six reports in the literature.

The mortality recorded in the past has varied from 65 to 92 percent, which indicates that the appearance of a friction rub is an ominous sign. The fact that two

Table 15–7. MORTALITY IN TUBERCULOUS PERICARDITIS

REFERENCE	PERCENT MORTALITY	NUMBER OF CASES	YEAR
Clarke	70	13	1929
Harvey and Whitehill	80	37	1937
Keefer	90	20	1937
Stepman and Owyan	92	37	1934
Andrews, Pickering, and Sellors	69	16	1948
Wood	65	41	1951

cases have survived on being treated with isoniazid is very encouraging and suggests that early and effective treatment may, in the future, save a good many lives.

One crucial point in prognosis remains to be discussed: that of the possible development of chronic constrictive pericarditis in these cases as a sequel to successful therapy or in cases where the pericarditis has not been recognized at the time of its occurrence. In 41 cases of tuberculous pericarditis reported by Wood (1951), studied during their acute episode, six progressed steadily into the chronic constrictive stage with no symptomatic period between the resorption of effusion and the development of constrictive

pericarditis. In all there was a gradual onset of symptoms varying from a few weeks to two years, and all died eventually. The sixth patient died after pericardiectomy and had been observed eight years after the acute episode before developing constrictive pericarditis. None of Wood's surviving patients has developed clinically obvious constrictive pericarditis.

In our seven cases one died in heart failure and at postmortem showed evidence of marked fibrosis of the parietal pericardium. Part of the cardiac embarrassment may well have been due to some degree of constriction from the pericardial involvement.

CHRONIC CONSTRICTIVE PERICARDITIS

WHITE (1951) points out that Lowen in 1669 was the first to describe a constrictive pericardium at postmortem. He also quotes the excellent clinical description of chronic pericarditis published by Chevers in 1842. Pick did not present his description of the disease until 1896.

Several excellent reviews of the subject among adults are available. Chronic constrictive pericarditis is an uncommon disease at any age but is very rare in childhood. Among 213 cases in the literature, 48 were found to be under 20 years of age. The youngest reported was two and one-half years of age (Vining, 1955). Approximately 2 percent of the routine postmortems among adults reveal hearts with adherent pericardia, and between 1 and 10 percent of cases with adherent pericardia have some evidence of constriction. Less than 40 cases have been reported in the literature in children under the age of 15 years (Shea et al., 1957; Caddell et al., 1960). At The Hospital for Sick Children in the 40-year period from 1924 to 1964, there have been 280 cases of pericarditis. Two of these were clear-cut cases of chronic constrictive pericarditis; a third was of tuberculous origin and had some evidence of constrictive effect. Two others have occurred more recently and have developed more rapidly than is usually the case. Simcha and Taylor (1971) describe five cases and present an excellent review of the problem in childhood.

Etiology

Most cases have an insidious onset without any clear-cut relationship to specific etiologic factors. Some develop following acute respiratory infection; others develop after tuberculous infection; still others follow a nonspecific pericarditis or a suppurative lesion. Thus, although the etiologies are various, tuberculosis appears to be the most common cause.

A summary of the literature reveals the following figures:

ETIOLOGIC FACTORS IN CHRONIC CONSTRICTIVE PERICARDITIS

Idiopathic	60 percent
Tuberculous	30 percent
Other: pyogenic infection, tularemia, meningococcus, trauma, tumor, Coxsackie virus	10 percent

Constrictive pericarditis has been known to occur following acute nonspecific pericarditis, tularemia, trauma, tumor, and pyogenic infection. As is shown above, it follows tuberculous infection most commonly; approximately 30 percent of all cases of chronic constrictive pericarditis have clinical or histologic evidence of tuberculous infection. This leaves a large group of cases under the heading of idiopathic, and it is difficult to say to which category they belong. A number of cases have been allocated to this group, but on postmortem at a later date they have been found to be tuberculous. Therefore, some observers feel that the majority of cases classified as idiopathic chronic constrictive pericarditis are actually tuberculous. Where a child has no clinical evidence of tuberculosis and the tuberculin test is negative, it is difficult to believe that tuberculosis is the cause. Further study of this problem is needed.

Pathology

There is a fibrous thickening of the visceral pericardium and parietal pericardium with varying degrees of involvement of each. The pericardial sac itself is usually obliterated, but this is not a necessary accompaniment of the disease. Constriction may occur from visceral pericarditis alone. The fibrosed pericardium is usually 1 to 5 mm thick, covers the whole of the pericardium, and may involve the great veins as well. In adults calcification of the pericardium is present in nearly one-half of the cases, but this has not been reported in childhood.

The heart muscle is usually not affected; however, as Harvey and coworkers (1953) point out, myocardial involvement may at times contribute to the clinical picture to some degree. When the heart has been compressed by the constricting pericardium for a considerable period, the myocardium is reduced in power. When the heart is freed and normal diastolic filling can take place, it may be some time before the myocardium regains its former strength.

When tuberculosis is the etiologic factor, there may be evidence of direct extension from the hilar glands or from a caseous pulmonary infection close to the pericardium.

Clinical Features

Dyspnea with effort, ascites, edema, and orthopnea are frequently found and have usually developed insidiously over a period of time without any acute onset. Heart murmurs are usually absent, being present in only 5 percent of cases, according to Chambliss and associates (1951). In such instances there may be a moderate systolic murmur heard at the apex. Schrire and coworkers (1968) have noted that absence of murmurs is the rule, and the only patients with murmurs among their first 220 cases of constrictive pericarditis had unrelated valve disease. However, they point out that diastolic murmurs may occasionally be produced by calcium penetrating into the heart, producing valve narrowing, or by constricting bands around the edges of the ventricular grooves. A third sound is commonly present due to rapid inflow filling at the beginning of diastole because of the high venous pressure. Venous pressure is always elevated and varies between 150 and 400 mm of water; thus, one will usually have evidence of distended neck veins, and under the fluoroscope the superior vena cava may appear enlarged.

The blood pressure is normally low and decreases with inspiration, producing the so-called paradoxic pulse. The patient may appear well. One-third of the cases are cyanosed in the adult group, but this is not a feature in childhood. The pulse rate is usually over 100 per minute in childhood.

There is no precordial thrust of the heart, such as one expects to find in many cases with heart failure, and the heart sounds are frequently distant although at time they may be normal. Ascites is more common than pitting edema, the former occurring in two-thirds and the latter in one-fourth of all patients

Laboratory Findings

Serum proteins are frequently reduced, and the A/G ratio may be reversed. The vital capacity is reduced, and the venous pressure varies from 150 to 400 mm of water. Measurement of the cardiac output shows the stroke volume to be reduced slightly in most cases.

Electrocardiography

The most characteristic findings are a P wave that is broad and notched, T waves that are inverted over the left precordium, and diminished voltage of the QRS. Thus, the electrocardiogram is of considerable value in diagnosis since T wave changes occur in practically all reported cases. Although the T waves are usually inverted over the left precordium, occasionally the alteration may be limited to a low or depressed T segment. Abnormalities of rhythm, such as atrial fibrillation, extrasystoles, and flutter, are commonly reported in adults; paroxysmal tachycardia is rare. If the patient is not treated, these electrocardiographic changes persist. They may disappear or improve following pericardiectomy, but in many cases they remain unaltered.

Radiologic Examination

The heart may be triangular, globular, or boot-shaped, but the most striking feature of this condition under the fluoroscope is the absence or diminution of cardiac pulsations. This is illustrated most vividly by comparing fluoroscopic shadows before and after operation when the increase in degree of pulsations will be evident.

The cardiac shadow remains fixed during inspiration and expiration. The size is within normal limits in half the cases; the rest may be slightly or moderately enlarged. After operation there may be an increase or a decrease in the size of the cardiac shadow or it may remain unchanged.

The superior vena cava may appear widened due to the great-vein engorgement, and the normal outlines of the aorta and pulmonary artery are frequently obscured. Vascular markings of the lungs may be increased due to passive congestion.

Calcification is an unusual finding in the radiographic examination in childhood but was reported in two of the eight cases in the pediatric age group presented by Shea and coworkers (1957).

Diagnosis

Problems in differential diagnosis include heart failure from other causes, cirrhosis of the liver, and idiopathic benign pericarditis.

In childhood, heart failure is usually due to congenital heart disease, which can be readily differentiated from chronic constrictive pericarditis. The presence of ascites, a heart that is of normal size or only slightly enlarged, lack of cardiac activity under the fluoroscope, the characteristic electrocardiogram, the congested veins, and the raised venous pressure all suggest the correct diagnosis. In doubtful cases cardiac catheterization is of aid since this will reveal not only a high right atrial pressure but also a precipitous fall in pressure in the right ventricle at the end of systole, proceeding to a sharp dip in diastole and then rising to an elevated diastolic pressure, which corresponds to the pressure in the right atrium.

The major diagnostic problem in recent years has been the identification of acutely developing constrictive pericarditis. This may occur in as brief an interval as 21 days (Weis and Silber, 1961) or a month (Caddell et al., 1960). The most likely lesions producing signs and symptoms so quickly are those of purulent origin, especially the meningococcal infections. We have also noted the condition following Coxsackie virus infection. The signs are those of tamponade without significant pericardial effusion. Early treatment is imperative.

An occasional case begins with a chronic subacute effusion and ends up as a constrictive pericarditis. Hancock (1971) has summarized the literature on this subgroup and presented observations on 13 patients. The results of surgery usually proved satisfactory.

Treatment

Medical treatment depends upon the severity of constriction of the pericardium. Bed rest may be necessary for some, whereas moderate restriction of activity will suffice for others. The use of diuretics and a low-sodium diet is indicated when there are considerable ascites and edema, although it should be pointed out that prolonged use of a low-sodium diet may occasionally lead to a salt deficit and may be deleterious at the time of operation. Paracentesis should be resorted to when the ascites does not respond to therapy. Digitalis may be of help if the myocardium is weak, but it is probably more likely to be useful in the immediate postoperative period when the myocardium is subjected to increased diastolic length after a prolonged period of inability to expand.

The most satisfactory treatment is that of pericardiectomy, and many series, totaling 400 to 500 cases altogether, have been reported since the first

operation was performed by Delorme (1898). At the operation the pericardium is removed by blunt dissection, freeing as much of the cardiac surface as possible, including the point of entrance of the great veins when they appear to be constricted. Roshe and Shumacher in 1959 reported their experience in children with chronic cardiac tamponade.

The surgical maneuvers required for this operation involve some risk of hemorrhage or cardiac irregularity. Ventricular fibrillation and cardiac arrest have occurred. The preoperative use of digitalis may decrease cardiac irregularity and reduce the possibility of failure. Hemorrhage may occur from incising the right or left atria during pericardiectomy or from postoperative bleeding. Postoperative complications such as hemorrhage, wound infection, and cardiac failure are not common. The mortality at operation is approximately 18 percent but has varied from 4 to 45 percent (Portal et al., 1966; Dayem et al., 1967; Jones et al., 1970; Simcha et al., 1971; Wychylis et al., 1971).

The more acute cases developing over a few weeks or months should be identified and operated on promptly. It seems likely that some of those can be prevented in the purulent group by adequate antibiotic therapy, which also may include a pericardostomy, as recommended by Benzing and Kaplan (1963).

Vining (1955) has reported the successful pericardiectomy on a child of four years who had had signs and symptoms of constrictive pericarditis for two years. The child returned to normal health after the procedure.

Among those who survive, the results of therapy are usually good. Most patients have an increased exercise tolerance, and the responses are satisfactory or excellent in three-fourths of the cases. The pulse rate and venous pressure fall; the stroke volume and pulse pressure increase; the ascites and edema disappear. Occasionally paracentesis is required during the few days following operation. Mortality is higher and the response is less favorable among those patients who are cyanotic before operation or have definite evidence of tuberculosis.

COXSACKIE VIRUS PERICARDITIS

FOR many years it was suspected that idiopathic pericarditis may at times have a virus origin. Epidemics of Bornholm disease, now considered to be essentially Coxsackie in origin, were frequently associated with incidences of pericarditis. It may well have been this condition that Bing was describing in 1933 when he reported six cases with a pericardial friction rub that also had pleurodynia. Weinstein (1957) reported a case of benign pericarditis with a high antibody titer to Coxsackie virus group B5. Kagan and Bernkopf (1957) published data on a ten-month-old baby in which type B3 was isolated from the stool and pericardial fluid. Since then several

series have been recorded clearly identifying the Coxsackie virus with acute pericarditis (McLean, Walker and Bain, 1958; Bell and Meis, 1959; Gillett, 1959; Null and Castle, 1959; Howard and Maier, 1968). McLean points out that one needs to demonstrate a significant antibody titer to the infection or a positive culture before the diagnosis can be made with certainty. Coxsackie types B5 and B3 are the ones most frequently reported. Clinical signs or symptoms should be those usually associated with Coxsackie infection. Least important but helpful, Coxsackie virus should be recovered for the patient.

There are a multiplicity of signs and symptoms relating to Coxsackie infection. These include fever, malaise, headache, tachycardia, pleurodynia, lymphadenopathy, splenomegaly, meningeal signs, cardiac enlargement, congestive heart failure, and pericardial friction rub.

Myocarditis is an uncommon complication of Coxsackie infection apart from the first few weeks of life. In this age group it commonly precipitates heart failure with fatal results. However, it is recorded from time to time among the older children and adults and may be present with or without pericardial signs and symptoms (Null and Castle, 1959).

Myocarditis with failure superimposed on the pericarditis is indicated by gallop rhythm, cardiac enlargement (apart from pericardial effusion), congestive heart failure with enlarged liver, and visible jugular venous pulse.

The friction rub may persist for a few hours or for several days. In children it is rarely accompanied by precordial pain.

Occasionally the Coxsackie infection leads to chronic constrictive pericarditis. Those recovering from this infection should therefore be reviewed after the recovery from the initial illness.

Treatment

Strict bed rest seems to be the most important factor in treating these cases, and early activity appears to prolong the period of convalescence. Steroids have not been found to alter the course of this disease significantly. Gillett (1959) found the salicylates were helpful in relieving symptoms and reducing fever in the acute stages of the disease.

The prognosis appears to be good in the vast majority of cases, with complete recovery being the rule. Even when myocarditis is present, recovery is usually complete. The outcome is likely to be in doubt when there is meningoencephalitis or when myocarditis occurs in the first two or three weeks of life (see Chapter 51). Surgery is occasionally needed if chronic constrictive pericarditis appears as a sequela to this infection.

POSTPERICARDIOTOMY SYNDROME

THIS syndrome occurs as a sequela of cardiac surgery and appears to be a delayed response to the opening of the pericardium. It is characterized by fever, chest pain, and signs of pleural or pericardial reaction with or without a friction rub. The chest pain is likely to be minimal or absent in children (Johnson, 1959; Engle and Ito, 1961; McGuiness and Taussig, 1962).

The onset of the signs or symptoms of this syndrome usually occurs two or three weeks following the episode of cardiac surgery but may occur a few days or up to several months later. When the clinical signs listed above appear, an x-ray of the chest will almost invariably reveal abnormalities of the heart or lungs. The cardiac shadow may show enlargement or lack definition in outline. Pleural involvement may be evident with effusion, thickening of pleural layer, and tenting of the diaphragm. Both pericardium and pleura appear to be involved together more often on the left side of the chest than the right (McGuiness and Taussig, 1962).

The electrocardiogram may show T or S-T changes, but the presence of conduction defects, right bundle branch block, and digitalis effect frequently makes it difficult to defend this approach to diagnosis.

McGuiness and Taussig (1962) have suggested that early ambulation is responsible for either causing or prolonging the syndrome and present evidence that the patients who were left in bed until all signs and symptoms of a convalescence had subsided were less likely to develop any of the complicating manifestations referred to above.

It is recommended that patients with a friction rub or with x-ray signs of pleural or pericardial disease be kept in bed until these signs have disappeared. In some cases this convalescence may be completed at home if the patient has otherwise had a good result from his cardiac surgery.

Steroids have been used with some evidence of success, but occasionally the patient appears to become dependent on them and the course of the disease is prolonged. Then it may be difficult to stop such therapy (Connolly and Burchell, 1961). If they are used, a short course with moderate doses for a few days would appear to be all that is indicated.

CONGENITAL ABSENCE OF THE PERICARDIUM

IT is believed that Columbus (1559) was the first to describe congenital absence of the pericardium. An occasional case was reported in the succeeding centuries (Baille, 1793). Ladd (1936a, 1936b) was the first to recognize a case in life during the surgical repair of a diaphragmatic hernia. In 1959, Ellis and associates reported the first case recognized radiologically. Since then, the condition has been recognized sporadically and diagnostic items have steadily increased.

Most cases have no symptoms. This is particularly true when there are no other anomalies present. When symptoms do occur, the most common one is a vague chest pain. Occasionally, dizziness has been recorded.

Systolic ejection murmurs have been noted in most patients, usually along the left sternal border. The apical impulse is shifted to the left and apical precordial activity may be somewhat obvious.

In complete absence of the left pericardium the heart is usually shifted to the left with the trachea in the midline. There is prominence of the pulmonary artery segment, and the right heart border may not be visible or may appear rather indistinct and is usually hidden by the spine. Lung tissue may be seen between the left hemidiaphragm and the inferior border of the heart. Radiologists have recognized a tongue of lung projecting between the aorta and the main pulmonary artery in the left anterior oblique view.

In partial pericardial defects, the heart is usually in the normal position and the abnormality consists of prominence of the pulmonary artery or left atrial appendage, with the latter herniating through the left upper heart border. An angiogram will clearly show its relationship to the rest of the heart. Pernot and coworkers (1972) have recently reviewed the problem of the partial pericardial defects.

The electrocardiographic changes usually consist of right-axis deviation, incomplete right bundle branch block, and leftward displacement of the transitional zone in the precordial leads. Some children have sinus bradycardia. One patient had complete heart block (Varriale et al., 1967).

Prognosis

The absence of the left pericardium does not interfere with a normal life unless other cardiac anomalies are present. This may not be true of the smaller defects or partial defects of the pericardium, which permit a herniation of the left atrium with consequent strangulation of the portion of the heart. Three reports have been published as sudden death with herniation (Boxall, 1887; Sunderland and Wright-Smith, 1944; Bruning, 1962).

Treatment

No treatment is needed for a complete absence of the pericardium, but in the presence of symptoms or the possibility of sudden death in partial defects, the surgical procedures include a left atrial appendectomy, division of adhesions, a pericardioplasty, or extension of the defect to prevent herniation. The very small defects that are unlikely to produce herniation do not require surgical intervention.

REFERENCES

Alexander, J.; Macleod, A. G.; and Barker, P. S.: Sensibility of the exposed human heart and pericardium. *Arch. Surg.*, **19**:1470, 1953.
Andrews, G. W.; Pickering, G. W.; and Sellors, T. H.: The etiology of constrictive pericarditis, with special reference to tuberculous pericarditis together with a note on polyserositis. *Q. J. Med.*, **41**:291, 1948.
Ash, R.: Prognosis of rheumatic infection in childhood; statistical study. *Am. J. Dis. Child.*, **52**:28, 1936.

Bain, H. W.; McLean, D. M.; and Walker, S. J.: Epidemic pleurodynia (Bornholm disease) due to coxsackie B-5 virus: interrelationship of pleurodynia, benign pericarditis and aseptic meningitis. *Pediatrics*, **27**:889, 1961.
Barnes, A. R., and Burchell, H. B.: Acute pericarditis simulating acute coronary occlusion. *Am. Heart J.*, **23**:247, 1942.
Bell, J. F., and Meis, A.: Pericarditis in infection due to coxsackie virus group B, type 3. *N. Engl. J. Med.*, **261**:126, 1959.
Bellet, S., and McMillan, T. M.: Electrocardiographic patterns in acute pericarditis. *Arch. Intern. Med.*, **61**:381, 1938.
Benzing, G., III, and Kaplan, S.: Purulent pericarditis. *Am. J. Dis. Child.*, **106**:89, 1963.
Beresford, O. D.: Fugitive pericarditis. *Arch. Dis. Child.*, **24**:135, 1949.
Bing, C.: Epidemic pericarditis. *Acta Med. Scand.*, **80**:29, 1933.
Bower, B. D.: Acute benign pericarditis: a report of 4 cases in childhood. *Br. Med. J.*, **1**:244, 1953.
Boxall, R.: Incomplete pericardial sac escape of heart into left pleural cavity. *Trans. Obstet. Soc. Lond.*, **28**:209, 1887.
Boyd, G. L.: Tuberculous pericarditis in children. *Am. J. Dis. Child.*, **86**:293, 1953.
Brown, M. G.: Acute benign pericarditis. *N. Engl. J. Med.*, **244**:666, 1951.
Bruning, E. G.: Congenital defect of the pericardium. *J. Clin. Pathol.*, **15**:133, 1962.
Burchell, H. B.: Acute nonspecific pericarditis. *Mod. Concepts Cardiovasc. Dis.*, **16**:(n.p.), 1947.
———: Problems in the recognition and treatment of pericarditis. *J. Lancet*, **74**:465, 1954.
Burchell, H. B.: Barnes, A. R.; and Mann, F. C.: The electrocardiographic picture of experimental localized pericarditis. *Am. Heart J.*, **18**:133, 1939.
Caddell, J. L.; Friedman, S.; and Johnson, J.: Constrictive pericarditis. *Am. J. Dis. Child.*, **100**:850, 1960.
Capps, J. A.: Pain from pleura and pericardium. *Res. Nerv. Ment. Dis. Proc.* (1942), 23:263, 1943.
Carmichael, D. B.; Sprague, H. B.; Wyman, S. M.; and Bland, E. F.: Acute nonspecific pericarditis. Clinical, laboratory, and follow-up considerations. *Circulation*, **3**:321, 1951.
Chambliss, J. R.; Jaruszewski, E. J.; Brofman, B. L.; Martin, J. F.; and Feil, H.: Chronic cardiac compression (chronic constrictive pericarditis): a critical study of sixty-one operated cases with follow-up. *Circulation*, **4**:816, 1951.
Clarke, J. A.: Clinically primary tuberculous pericarditis. *Am. J. Med. Sci.*, **177**:115, 1929.
Connolly, D. C., and Burchell, H. B.: Pericarditis: a ten year survey. *Am. J. Cardiol.*, **7**:7, 1961.
Crandell, W. B.; Yeomans, A.; Hoffman, D. L.; and Stueck, G. H.: Electrolyte studies in pericardial resection. *J. Thorac. Surg.*, **26**:486, 1953.
Dayem, M. K.; Wasfi, F. M.; Bentall, H. H.; Goodwin, J. F.; and Cleland, W. P.: Investigation and treatment of constrictive pericarditis. *Thorax*, **22**:242, 1967.
Delorme, E.: Sur un traitement chirurgical de la symphyse cardiopéricardique. *Bull. Mém. Soc. Chir. Paris*, **24**:918, 1898; *Gaz. Hôp.*, **72**:1150, 1898.
Deterling, R. A., and Humphreys, G. H.: Factors in the etiology of constrictive pericarditis. *Circulation*, **12**:30, 1955.
Ellis, K.; Leeds, N. E.; and Himmelstein, A.: Congenital deficiencies in pericardium. *Am. J. Roentgenol.*, **82**:125, 1959.
Engle, M. A., and Ito, T.: The postpericardiotomy syndrome. *Am. J. Cardiol.*, **7**:73, 1961.
Evans, J. M.; Walter, C. W.; and Hellems, H. K.: Alterations in the circulation during cardiac tamponade due to pericardial effusion. *Am. Heart J.*, **39**:181, 1950.
Feigenbaum, H.: Echocardiographic diagnosis of pericardial effusion. *Am. J. Cardiol.*, **26**:475, 1970.
Feigenbaum, H.; Zaky, A.; and Waldhausen, J. A.: Use of reflected ultrasound in detecting pericardial effusion. *Am. J. Cardiol.*, **19**:84, 1967.
Findlay, L.: *Rheumatic Infections in Childhood*, Edward Arnold & Co., New York, 1931.
Fowler, N. O., and Manitsas, G. T.: Infectious pericarditis. *Prog. Cardiovasc. Dis.*, **16**:323, 1973.
Freeman, M. E., and Parker, G. F.: Treatment of staphylococcic pericarditis with bacitracin. *J. Pediatr.*, **43**:720, 1953.
Friedberg, C. K., and Gress, L.: Pericardial lesions in rheumatic fever. *Am. J. Pathol.*, **12**:183, 1936.

Friedman, S.; Ash, R.; Harris, T. N.; and Lee, H. F.: Acute benign pericarditis in childhood; comparisons with rheumatic pericarditis, and therapeutic effects of ACTH and cortisone. *Pediatrics*, 9:551, 1952.

Fuller, C. C., and Quinlan, J. W.: Acute pneumonitis and pericarditis. *N. Engl. J. Med.*, 229:399, 1943.

Gibbons, J. E.; Goldbloom, R. B.; and Dobell, A. R. C.: Rapidly developing pericardial constriction in childhood following acute nonspecific pericarditis. *Am. J. Cardiol.* 15:863, 1965.

Gibson, S., and Demenholz, E. J.: Rheumatic heart disease in childhood. *J. Pediatr.*, 9:505, 1936.

Gillett, R. L.: Acute benign pericarditis and the coxsackie virus. *N. Engl. J. Med.*, 261:838, 1959.

Goldman, M. J., and Lau, F. Y. K.: Acute pericarditis associated with serum sickness. *N. Engl. J. Med.*, 250:278, 1954.

Goyette, E. M.: Acute idiopathic pericarditis. *Ann. Intern. Med.*, 39:1032, 1953.

Griffith, G. C., and Wallace, L.: The etiology of pericarditis. Abstract, Third Inter-American Cardiological Congress. *Am. Heart J.*, 37:636, 1949.

Hancock, E. W.: Subacute effusive-constrictive pericarditis. *Circulation*, 43:183, 1971.

Hansen, A. T.; Eskildsen, P.; and Gotzsche, H.; Pressure curves from the right auricle and the right ventricle in chronic constrictive pericarditis. *Circulation*, 3:881, 1951.

Hardman, J. M., and Earle, K. M.: Myocarditis in 200 fatal meningococcal infections. *Arch. Pathol.*, 87:318, 1969.

Harvey, R. M.; Ferrer, M. I.; Cathcart, R. T.; Richards, D. W.; and Cournand, A.: Mechanical and myocardial factors in chronic constrictive pericarditis. *Circulation*, 8:695, 1953.

Harvey, R. M. and Whitehill, M. R.: Tuberculous pericarditis. *Medicine*, 16:45, 1937.

Herrmann, G. R.; Marchand, E. J.; Greer, G. H.; and Hejtmancik, M. R.: Pericarditis. *Am. Heart J.*, 43:641, 1952.

Hodges, R. M.: IV. Idiopathic pericarditis (case record of the Massachusetts General Hospital, from the service of Dr. M. S. Perry). *Boston, Med. Surg. J.*, 51:140, 1854.

Howard, E. J., and Maier, H. C.: Constrictive pericarditis following acute Coxsachie viral pericarditis. *Am. Heart J.*, 75:247, 1968.

Jaiyesimi, F.; Monaghan, J.; Moes, C. A. F.; and Rowe, R. D.: Constrictive pericarditis in childhood: Analysis of the discriminating features and the causes of delay in diagnosis. Unpublished observations.

Johnson, J. L.: Postpericardiotomy syndrome in congenital heart deformities. *Am. Heart J.*, 57:643, 1959.

Jones, J. E.; Bernhard, W. F.; LaFarge, C. G.; and Gross, R. E.: Results of surgery of constrictive pericarditis in pediatric patients. *Am. J. Surg.*, 119:465, 1970.

Kagan, H., and Bernkopf, H.: Pericarditis caused by coxsackie virus B. *Ann. Paediatr.*, 189:44, 1957.

Katz, L. N., and Gauchat, H. W.: Observations on pulsus paradoxus. *Arch. Intern. Med.*, 33:350, 1924.

Keefer, C. S.: Tuberculosis of the pericardium. *Ann. Intern. Med.*, 10:1085, 1937.

Keith, N. M.; Pruitt, R. D.; and Baggenstoss, A. H.: Electrocardiographic changes in pericarditis associated with uremia. *Am. Heart J.*, 31:527, 1946.

Kotte, J. H., and McGuire, J.: Pericardial paracentesis. *Mod. Concepts Cardiovasc. Dis.*, 20:102, 1951.

Ladd, W. E.: Congenital absence of pericardium with report of case. *N. Engl. J. Med.*, 214:183, 1936a.

————: Surgical diseases of alimentary tract in infants. *N. Engl. J. Med.*, 215:705, 1936b.

Lawrence, W.; Adams, W. E.; and Cassels, D. E.: Constrictive pericarditis with obstruction of pulmonary veins. *J. Thorac. Surg.*, 17:832, 1948.

Lietman, P. S., and Bywaters, E. G.: Pericarditis in juvenile rheumatoid arthritis. *Pediatrics*, 32:855, 1963.

Lin, S. F.: Acute idiopathic pericarditis. *Con. Serv. Med. J.*, 10:159, 1954.

Logue, R. B., and Wendkos, M. H.: Acute pericarditis of benign type. *Am. Heart J.*, 36:587, 1948.

Lundstrom, R.: Purulent pericarditis and empyema caused by hemophilus influenzae, type B. *Am. Heart J.*, 49:108, 1955.

McCord, M. C., and Taguchi, J. T.: Nonspecific pericarditis. A fatal case. *Arch. Intern. Med.*, 87:727, 1951.

McGuiness, J. B., and Taussig, H. B.: The postpericardiotomy syndrome, its relationship to ambulation in the presence of "benign" pericardial and pleural reaction. *Circulation*, 26:500, 1962.

McGuire, J.; Kotte, J. H.; and Helm, R. A.: Acute pericarditis. *Circulation*, 9:425, 1954.

McLean, D. M.; Walker, S. J.; and Bain, H. W.: Coxsackie B5 virus in association with pericarditis and pleurodynia. *Can. Med. Assoc. J.*, 79:789, 1958.

Marks, P. A., and Roof, B. S.: Pericardial effusion associated with myxedema. *Ann. Intern. Med.*, 39:230, 1953.

Massell, B. F., and Warren, J. E.: Effect of pituitary adrenocorticotropic hormone (ACTH) on rheumatic fever and rheumatic carditis. *JAMA*, 144:1335, 1950.

Massie, E., and Levine, S. A.: The prognosis and subsequent developments in acute rheumatic pericarditis. *JAMA*, 112:1219, 1939.

Metcalfe, J.; Woodbury, J. W.; Richards, V.; and Burwell, C. S.: Studies in experimental pericardial tamponade. *Circulation*, 5:518, 1952.

Miller, H.; Uricchio, J. F.; and Phillips, R. W.: Acute pericarditis associated with infectious mononucleosis. *N. Engl. J. Med.*, 249:136, 1953.

Morgan, J. R.; Rogers, A. K.; and Forker, A. D.: Congenital absence of the left pericardium. *Ann. Intern. Med.*, 74:370, 1971.

Morse, J. R.; Oretsky, M. I.; and Hudson, J. A.: Pericarditis as a complication of meningococcal meningitis. *Ann. Intern. Med.*, 74:212, 1971.

Nadas, S. A., and Levy, J. M.: Pericarditis in children. *Am. J. Cardiol.*, 7:109, 1961.

Nay, R. M., and Boyer, N. H.: Acute pericarditis in young adults. *Am. Heart J.*, 32:222, 1946.

Norg, R. M.: The electrocardiogram in acute pericarditis. *J. Indiana Med. Assoc.*, 42:222, 1949.

Norman, M. G., and Cass, E.: Cardiac tamponade resulting from a swallowed safety pin. *Pediaetrics*, 48:832, 1971.

Null, F. C., and Castle, C. H.: Adult pericarditis and myocarditis due to coxsackie virus group B, type 5. *N. Engl. J. Med.*, 261:937, 1959.

Pernot, C.; Hoeffel, J-C.; Henry, M.; Frisch, R.; and Brauer, B.: Partial left pericardial defect with herniation of the left atrial appendage. *Thorax*, 27:246, 1972.

Portal, R. W.; Besterman, E. M. M.; Chambers, R. J.; Holmes Sellors, T.; and Somerville, W.: Prognosis after operation for constrictive pericarditis. *Br. Med. J.*, 1:563, 1966.

Powers, P. R.; Read, J. L.; and Porter, R. R.: Acute idiopathic pericarditis simulating acute abdominal disease. *JAMA*, 157:224, 1955.

Preble, R. B.: Etiology of pericarditis. *JAMA*, 37:1510, 1901.

Rabiner, S. F.; Specter, L. S.; Ripstein, C. B.; and Schlecker, A. A.: Chronic constrictive pericarditis as a sequel to acute benign pericarditis. *N. Engl. J. Med.*, 251:425, 1954.

Reeves, R. L.: The cause of acute pericarditis. *Am. J. Med. Sci.*, 225:34, 1953.

Roberts, W. C., and Fredrickson, D. S.: Gaucher's disease of the lung causing severe pulmonary hypertension with associated acute recurrent pericarditis, *Circulation*, 35:783, 1967.

Robertson, R.: Chronic constrictive pericarditis. *Am. J. Surg.*, 88:76, 1954.

Roshe, J., and Shumacher, H. B., Jr.: Pericardiectomy for chronic cardiac tamponade in children. *Surgery*, 46:1152, 1959.

Rubenstein, J. J.; Goldblatt, A.; and Daggett, W. M.: Acute constriction complicating purulent pericarditis in infancy. *Am. J. Dis. Child.*, 124:591, 1972.

Schrire, V.; Gotsman, M. S.; and Beck, W.: Unusual diastolic murmurs in constrictive pericarditis and constrictive endocarditis. *Am. Heart J.*, 76:4, 1968.

Scott, L. P.; Knox, D.; Perry, L. W.; and Pineros-Torres, F. J.: Meningococcal pericarditis. *Am. J. Cardiol.* 29:104, 1971.

Shabetai, R.; Fowler, N. O.; and Guntheroth, W. G.: The hemodynamics of cardiac tamponade and constrictive pericarditis. *Am. J. Cardiol.*, 26:480, 1970.

Shapiro, J. B., and Weiss, M.: Tuberculous pericarditis with effusion: the impact of antimicrobial therapy. *Am. J. Med. Sci.*, 225:229, 1953.

Shea, D. W.; Kirklin, J. W.; and DuShane, J. W.; Chronic constrictive pericarditis in children. *Am. J. Dis. Child.*, 93:430, 1957.

Simcha, A., and Taylor, J. F. N.: Constrictive pericarditis in childhood. *Arch. Dis. Child.*, **46**:515, 1971.

Smalley, R. E., and Ruddock, J. C.: Acute pericarditis: a study of 18 cases among service personnel. *Ann. Intern. Med.*, **25**:799, 1946.

Smith, H. L., and Willius, F. A.: Pericarditis. I. Chronic adherent pericarditis. II. Calcification of pericardium. III. Pericarditis with effusion. IV. Fibrinous pericarditis and "soldier's patches." V. Terminal pericarditis. *Arch. Intern. Med.*, **50**:171, 184, 192, 410, and 415, 1932.

Stepman, T. R., and Owyan, E.: Clinically primary tuberculous effusion. *Med. Clin. North Am.*, **18**:201, 1934.

Sunderland, S., and Wright-Smith, R. J.: Congenital pericardial defects. *Br. Heart J.*, **6**:167, 1944.

Sutton, L. P.: Paracentesis of the pericardium as a therapeutic measure. *Am. J. Dis. Child.*, **48**:44, 1934.

Thomas, G. T.; Besterman, E. M. M.; and Hollman, A.: Rheumatic pericarditis. *Br. Heart J.*, **15**:29, 1953.

Vander Veer, J. B., and Norris, R. F.: Electrocardiographic changes in acute pericarditis. *Am. Heart J.*, **14**:31, 1937.

Varriale, P.; Rossi, P.; and Grace, W. J.: Congenital absence of the left pericardium and complete heart block. *Chest*, **52**:405, 1967.

Venner, A.: Constrictive pericarditis associated with rheumatic valve disease. *Guy Hosp. Rep.*, **103**:59, 1954.

Vining, C. W.: Constrictive pericarditis in early childhood. *Proc. Roy. Soc. Med.*, **48**:1103, 1955.

Volpe, R., and Charles, W. B.: A case of tuberculous pericarditis treated with streptomycin and para-amino salicylic acid, *Bull. Acad. Med. Toronto*, **7**:71, 1954.

Wacker, W., and Merrill, J. P.: Uremic pericarditis in acute and chronic renal failure. *JAMA*, **156**:764, 1954.

Weinstein, S. B.: Acute benign pericarditis associated with coxsackie virus group B, type 5. *N. Engl. J. Med.*, **257**:265, 1957.

Weis, E. I., and Silber, E. N.: Acute constrictive pericarditis. *J. Pediatr.*, **58**:548, 1961.

White, P. D.: Chronic constrictive pericarditis. *Circulation*, **4**:288, 1951.

Williams, C., and Soutter, L.; Pericardial tamponade. *Arch. Intern. Med.*, **94**:571, 1954.

Williams, R. G., and Steinberg, I.: The value of angiocardiography in establishing the diagnosis of pericarditis with effusion. *Am. J. Roentgenol.*, **61**:41, 1949.

Wilson, R. H.; Hoseth, W.; Sadoff, C.; and Dempsey, M. E.: Pathologic physiology and diagnostic significance of the pressure pulse tracings in the heart in patients with constrictive pericarditis and pericardial effusion. *Am. Heart J.*, **48**:671, 1945.

Wolff, L.: Acute pericarditis, with special reference to changes in heart size. *N. Engl. J. Med.*, **229**:423, 1943.

Wood, F. C.: Observations on pericardial disease. *Med. Clin. North Am.*, **37**:1639, 1953.

Wood, J. A.: Tuberculous pericarditis: a study of forty-one cases, with special reference to prognosis. *Am. Heart J.*, **43**:737, 1951.

Wood, P.: Chronic constrictive pericarditis. *Am. J. Cardiol.*, **7**:48, 1961.

Wychulis, A. R.; Connolly, D. C.; and McGoon, D. C.: Surgical treatment of pericarditis. *J. Thorac. Cardiovasc. Surg.*, **62**:608, 1971.

Yu, P. N. G.; Lovejoy, F. W.; Joos, H. A.; Nye, R. E., Jr.; and Simpson, J. H.: An unusual case of massive pericardial effusion with hemodynamic studies. *Ann. Intern. Med.*, **39**:928, 1953.

CHAPTER

16

Cor Pulmonale

Richard D. Rowe and *Michael J. Godman*

COR PULMONALE has been defined by the World Health Organization (1963) as right ventricular hypertrophy developing from diseases affecting the functional structure of the lung, except when these alterations are the consequence of disease of the left side of the heart or of congenital diseases. As the mechanisms involved in producing cor pulmonale have become clearer in recent times, it has become evident that right ventricular hypertrophy, a pathologic definition, is not clinically apparent at an early stage of the disease. Similarly, congestive heart failure is a late manifestation and right ventricular hypertrophy may be present for a long time prior to its onset. Finally, reversibility of pulmonary hypertension in the commonest form of cor pulmonale (chronic obstructive pulmonary disease) emphasizes that the clinical course of cor pulmonale can be related to the changes in pulmonary artery pressure. In the very mildest cases pulmonary hypertension is present only during exercise. As the disease progresses it becomes evident at rest and finally will be associated with right ventricular failure. These considerations have led many authorities in the field to prefer the term *chronic pulmonary heart disease* (Thomas, 1972; Ferrer, 1975).

The term describes a variety of clinical entities since pulmonary hypertension, an essential feature of each, may arise from (1) diseases of the lung parenchyma and airways, (2) inadequate ventilatory drive, (3) disorders of the chest wall and neuromuscular apparatus, and (4) pulmonary vascular disease.

In the first three of these disorders alveolar hypoventilation is the major stimulus to produce pulmonary vasoconstriction and set in train a sequence of events that may ultimately result in right ventricular hypertrophy. Exactly how hypoxia initiates pulmonary arterial constriction is not totally clear (Fishman, 1961) but local constriction rather than reflex constriction is now regarded as the important mechanism. Barer (1963) and Bergofsky and Holtzman (1967) have shown that alveolar hypoxia produces the major vasoconstrictive response in the lung, but a reduction in arterial oxygen tension in the blood of the pulmonary artery can also produce a lesser degree of vasoconstriction. Conversely the alveolar response can be smaller if the pulmonary arterial blood is well oxygenated. Acidemia alone may result in a significant rise in the pulmonary vascular resistance (Fishman et al., 1960), and it is probable that acidosis acts synergistically with hypoxia to produce this change in man.

It is not surprising that most clinical investigation of pulmonary heart disease has been performed in adult patients since chronic obstructive pulmonary disease is so common in that age group. It has become apparent that the pulmonary hypertension that develops is not a consequence of anatomic obliteration of vessels by parenchymal disease but simply a functional response to alveolar hypoventilation and respiratory acidosis. The importance of this changing viewpoint is that in this form of pulmonary heart disease, right ventricular failure can be repeatedly reversed and probably to some extent avoided through appropriate therapy.

While there has been little argument about the role of pulmonary hypertension and right ventricular function in the advanced forms of the disorder, the position of left ventricular function has been the subject of much more debate (Rao et al., 1968; Foraker et al., 1970; Fishman, 1971; Kharja and Parker, 1971; Ishikawa et al., 1972; Ferrer, 1975). Current views tend to minimize the importance of that possibility in the adult group. Several comprehensive reviews of cor pulmonale as it applies to the young have been published (Morgan, 1967; Noonan, 1971; Monset-Couchard et al., 1975).

DISEASES OF THE LUNG PARENCHYMA AND AIRWAYS

Cystic Fibrosis

Although there are a number of conditions in the young that can produce alveolar hypoventilation, the only disease that commonly causes pulmonary heart disease is cystic fibrosis (Andersen, 1938; Royce, 1951; Bodian, 1952; Nadas et al., 1952). The frequency with which pulmonary heart disease complicates this disease at autopsy has varied between 20 and 70 percent in early reports (Royce, 1951; Bodian, 1952). The longer life produced by improved therapy of the disease over the past decade might have been expected to result in a relatively high incidence of cor pulmonale at eventual autopsy. Such would appear to be the case from the data of Ryland and Reid (1975) who found 30 of 36 patients dying of cystic fibrosis to have right ventricular hypertrophy. On the other hand, their data showed that the cardiac changes could not be related directly to age since there was no significant difference for the age at death between those with mild or severe right ventricular hypertrophy and those with none. The muscle of the small pulmonary arteries was increased in all the cases but was more marked in those who showed right ventricular hypertrophy. Whether the more recent major improvement in mortality, brought about by early diagnosis and highly individualized treatment under close evaluation through pulmonary function and blood gas studies, will eventually provide a different pathologic picture with less involvement of the heart reflecting a significantly lower degree of pulmonary hypertension during life remains to be seen (Crozier, 1974).

Clinical Features. The principal manifestations of chronic pulmonary heart disease relate to the lung. The pathophysiology in these patients is that of airway obstruction, air trapping, loss of lung elasticity, uneven ventilation, and ventilation-perfusion inequalities (Featherby et al., 1969). The influence of these defects on lung function is revealed in blood gas assessment as well as in ventilatory studies. Arterial hypoxemia is extremely common and undoubtedly is a primary cause of pulmonary arterial hypertension. Because of the gross pulmonary disease that may be present in many cases it is extremely difficult to identify features that in patients without frank pulmonary disease would permit the diagnosis of an elevated pulmonary arterial pressure. In other words, the pulmonary signs overshadow the cardiac signs. The heart sounds are faint and the pulmonary component of the second heart sound is often unimpressive. The chest is barrel-shaped, and the patient has rales and often clubbing of the fingers and toes.

Dyspnea, obvious distention of neck veins, a palpable liver, and edema do not necessarily indicate the presence of congestive heart failure under these circumstances.

Development of cor pulmonale may be extremely early as it was with one infant who developed a cough at three days, congestive heart failure at 11 days, and died at 47 days (Royce, 1951). Usually, however, the late stages of pulmonary heart disease are not manifest in infancy.

Radiologic Examination. A decreasing cardiothoracic ratio with progression of the lung disease has been noted (Caffey, 1951), and it is usually impossible to make any judgments about the state of the major pulmonary artery vessels because of the advanced parenchymal changes in the lungs. Some cases do show cardiomegaly, especially in the late phases with heart failure. Serial changes may be useful in this regard.

Electrocardiography. Contrary to the situation where the electrocardiogram is reasonably helpful in the diagnosis of pulmonary heart disease in the adult with chronic obstructive pulmonary disease (Kilcoyne et al., 1970; Padmavati and Raizada, 1972), the electrocardiogram in children with cystic fibrosis has proved disappointing as an aid to the diagnosis of the development of chronic pulmonary heart disease. As an isolated investigation seeking information on the state of the pulmonary circulation, the electrocardiogram has, in fact, been singularly unhelpful (Siassi et al., 1971) and even the application of vectorcardiography to the problem has not proved useful when attention has focused on right ventricular forces (Liebman et al., 1967; Siassi et al., 1971). By contrast, Fowler and coworkers (1974) found that as the respiratory function studies deteriorated or the PaO_2 fell, the voltage over the left ventricle in the Frank vectorcardiogram became less. They recommended that simple hand measurements of left voltage be used to follow patients with cystic fibrosis in order to detect the development of cor pulmonale. It is interesting that Siassi and colleagues (1971) noted in their studies that the ratio of R/S in V_1 became lower with more severe cor pulmonale in cystic fibrosis. One can conclude from these electrical studies that it is not feasible to identify mild cor pulmonale in its earliest forms by the electrocardiogram.

Other Noninvasive Tests. Increased right ventricular dimension determined echocardiographically was shown by Rosenthal and associates (1976) in 80 percent of 61 patients with varying stages of severity of cystic fibrosis. The more severe the cervical manifestations of the disease, the greater was the likelihood of right ventricular enlargement. Marked elevation of the ratio of the right ventricular preejection period to the right ventricular ejection time obtained echocardiographically is usually a reliable indication of the presence of pulmonary hypertension (Hirschfeld et al., 1975), but abnormal chest configuration renders its application less satisfactory for patients with chronic obstructive lung disease. On the other hand myocardial perfusion scanning with thallium-201 appears to be a very useful technique to assess the effects of chronic pulmonary hypertension on the right ventricular myocardium. In patients with pulmonary hypertension the normally poor visualization of the right ventricular free wall is clearly shown by the scan, and there is noticeable thickening (Cohen et al., 1976).

Cardiac Catheterization. A limited number of studies have been performed in patients with cystic fibrosis (Goldring et al., 1964; Kelminson et al., 1967; Siassi et al., 1971; Whitman et al., 1975). As with other forms of chronic obstructive pulmonary disease, it has been found that the pulmonary artery pressure relates to the degree of arterial hypoxemia. A condition such as sleep, which reduces alveolar ventilation, will increase the pulmonary artery pressure. The studies of Kelminson and associates (1967) indicate that vasodilating drugs reduce the mean pulmonary artery pressure as well. The obvious inference is that improvement in the airways obstruction can relieve the pulmonary hypertension. The studies of Siassi and others (1971), which contain the largest reported number of patients undergoing investigation, had 17 subjects with normal pulmonary artery pressure, 12 with pulmonary artery mean pressures between 21 and 28 mm Hg and five with pulmonary artery pressures in excess of 38 mm Hg. Those with the more severe degree of change were over the age of ten years, and those with the greater severity of pulmonary heart disease had the greatest severity of cystic fibrosis as a whole when assessed by clinical score (Shwachman and Kulczycki, 1958). In the few patients studied serially there was no major change in the pulmonary artery pressure, but in follow-up over a period of seven years the mortality was clearly greatest in the group with severe pulmonary hypertension.

Prognosis and Treatment. A vigorous approach to the management of the pulmonary disturbance and the general status of the patient recognized by many investigators as having importance is now well clarified for children with cystic fibrosis (Crozier, 1974). It is apparent from the studies of Whitman and associates (1975) that acute induction of diuresis for patients with cor pulmonale reduces right atrial pressure appreciably and is probably related to contraction of central blood volume. The treatment of established pulmonary heart disease with diuretics, digoxin, and other measures is not usually successful for long. The greater challenge lies in attempts to prevent the development of cor pulmonale. The relationship between those who respond to alveolar hypoxia by vasoconstriction and "nonresponding" and survival, demonstrated for adults by Lindsay and Read (1972), has not been expanded to date for children.

Other Lung Disorders

Most of the other conditions that occasionally may be implicated in the production of cor pulmonale in children are excessively rare. Interstitial lung disease of the *Hamman-Rich* variety has been reported (Donohue et al., 1959), and even in infancy these patients at autopsy may show right ventricular hypertrophy (O'Shea and Yardley, 1970).

Chronic pulmonary heart disease has been implicated as a late consequence of *bronchopulmonary dysplasia* where severe fibrotic changes occur in the lungs of some infants who have been mechanically ventilated for treatment of idiopathic respiratory distress syndrome (Northway et al., 1967). The disorder is under suspicion of being primarily the consequence of mechanical stresses caused by high positive airway pressure during the acute phase of the disorder. A related problem is the *Wilson-Mikity syndrome* in premature infants who develop late progressive respiratory difficulty and may die from progressive impairment. Their problem appears to be related to uneven airways obstruction from a variety of possible causes (Burnard et al., 1963).

Idiopathic pulmonary hemosiderosis, an uncommon disorder of unknown etiology, is characterized by recurrent intra-alveolar hemorrhage with deposition of hemosiderin in the lung. A small number of affected cases may develop cor pulmonale as a consequence of chronic pulmonary fibrosis, though more often the development of congestive heart failure in this condition is a consequence of myocarditis, which is found in about 10 percent of the patients at autopsy (Williams and Phelan, 1975).

Pulmonary lymphangiectasis is a rare developmental abnormality of the newborn in which dilated lymphatics markedly impair ventilation. Severe hypoxemia and CO_2 retention lead to cor pulmonale and usually early death (Avery and Fletcher, 1974).

Frank Airways Obstruction

Upper Airways Obstruction. Chronic obstruction of the airways with cor pulmonale may result from a lesion anywhere in the respiratory tract between the posterior nares and the late divisions of the bronchial tree. Those at a high level are usually correctable conditions though perhaps the most urgent of these is the patient with choanal atresia at birth, for whom the provision of an oral airway is critical and can usually relieve the immediate symptoms. One of the most dramatic forms of reversible upper airways obstruction that can be associated with pulmonary hypertension and congestive heart failure is *hypertrophied tonsils and adenoids*. It is rather remarkable that this condition was not recognized by pediatricians until the early 1960s (Menashe et al., 1965; Noonan, 1965; Luke et al., 1966; Levy et al., 1967; Ainger, 1968; Cayler et al., 1969; Levin et al., 1975).

Characteristically, these are young children who have been noted to snore from early infancy and who go through periodic exacerbations of airway obstruction with somnolence, which often culminate in edema and frank heart failure, including pulmonary edema. Although the exact pathogenesis is not certain, there are two principal features contributing to the symptoms. First, alveolar hypoventilation produces pulmonary vaso-constriction and, second, major intrathoracic pressure swings occur. There have been more males than females affected in the reports to date and more black than white children. There has been a suggestion that the syndrome is associated with mental retardation, but we believe, as do others (Levin et al., 1975), that the occurrence of this finding is an overestimate. In our view, the reason for apparent retardation is that most cases come from disadvantaged social groups. The majority of children are between two and four years of age but infants as young as three months have been affected.

The eyelid edema and proteinuria that are common accompaniments of the severely symptomatic patient may be so striking as to raise the question of renal disease on the initial examination. The electro-cardiogram characteristically shows P pulmonale with or without right ventricular hypertrophy. The P wave is not only the first sign to appear but it is the first to disappear after relief of the airways obstruction.

Cardiac catheterization has demonstrated pul-monary hypertension, sometimes, but not com-monly, to systemic levels. Left atrial and left ventricular end-diastolic pressures may be elevated. The striking feature about the pressure is a remarkable respiratory swing so that on inspiration pressures become negative with respect to atmos-pheric zero. In one child we studied, a transient right atrial pressure of minus 100 mm Hg developed at one point. Myocardial contraction as judged by ejection fractions has been normal. The wide excursion of the pressure tracings can be immediately reversed by the introduction of an airway. Needless to say, sedation is an absolute contraindication in such patients.

Blood gases at the height of a particular episode may reveal, in addition to reduction in PaO_2, hypercapnea, but on a number of occasions the blood gases in our patients have been normal at a time when there has been frank heart failure.

It is important to recognize the condition because it responds dramatically to the institution of an adequate airway and to adenoidectomy and/or tonsillectomy. It is of considerable interest that most reviews of the continuing controversy for that operation only very recently have mentioned this disorder—probably the most crucial indication for the operation! If the true diagnosis is not recognized patients can die.

A number of other conditions may produce similar symptoms. In patients with the *Pierre Robin syndrome* with a cleft palate and hypoplastic mandible, the tongue tends to obstruct the pharynx and special measures are necessary to assist these infants during the first few weeks after birth. Instances of frank pulmonary edema and heart failure have been reported (Cogswell et al., 1974). We have seen milder forms of the disorder in children with *cleft palate alone, Down's syndrome,* and *mucopolysaccharidosis.*

The syndrome can develop in patients with *laryngomalacia* (Cox et al., 1965) and in broncho-malacia, and a very severe form of respiratory insufficiency in pulmonary heart disease can develop, usually ending in death in late infancy (Williams and Campbell, 1960). We studied one infant with that complication where the diagnosis remained uncertain until autopsy and have been privileged to see another severely affected older patient studied by Dr. David Watson of Jackson, Mississippi.

Bronchial Asthma. Some years ago the possibility of there being an important cardiac component to bronchial asthma was raised (Griffin et al., 1959; Blitz et al., 1961; Dees 1961). In 1965 Richards and Patrick analyzed 24 asthmatic deaths at the Children's Hospital in Los Angeles and found evidence of right ventricular hypertrophy in 2 of the 24 autopsies. Both those children died rather unexpectedly. In five other children with long-standing asthma there was no evidence of a pathologic lung change and the authors felt it was unreasonable to label asthmatics as potential candidates for cor pulmonale. In a study of the electrocardiogram and vectorcardiogram in children with severe bronchial asthma Quivers and coworkers (1964) assessed 30 children in a home for asthmatic patients and noted that their electrocardio-grams showed right ventricular hypertrophy in only two patients. These were the most severely affected of the 30. The vectorcardiogram showed right atrial hypertrophy in 30 percent and, in addition, revealed a posterior orientation of the QRS loop in the horizontal plane, which could not be related to the severity of the asthma. Right atrial hypertrophy was present in five of nine adult asthmatic patients studied by Gunstone (1971), but low or normal right heart pressures were found in all nine at cardiac catheterization.

Thus, though most investigators conclude that cor pulmonale in association with bronchial asthma is a rare event, there are obviously stresses on the circulation induced by asthmatic attacks that have many similarities to those seen in upper airways obstruction. We are indebted to Dr. James Robotham for the following comment in that regard:

Conventional considerations of hemodynamic events in asthma have not been rewarding but if one considers transmural (relative to intrathoracic pressure) rather than the traditional measurements relative to atmosphere, an entirely different con-ceptual approach can be developed (Schrijen et al., 1975). The greater relevance of transmural pressures is readily appreciated when considering the right atrial pressure during an inspiratory effort, during which the right atrial volume increases. An elastic chamber whose volume is increased with an incompressible fluid has increased its transmural pressure. Traditional measurement of right atrial pressure shows a fall with inspiration. Clearly, the events are reflected by the transmural rather than the traditional pressures relative to atmosphere. Carry-ing this concept to examine the pressures on both sides of the heart, the markedly negative inspiratory and the overall mean negative intrathoracic pressures lead to the conclusion that both right and left ventricles are increasingly afterloaded as the asthmatic attack progresses. This hypothesis is supported by the finding of pulmonary venous congestion on the chest x-ray of acute asthmatic patients. During a Mueller maneuver (closed glottis inspiratory effort) a chest film of a normal subject shows cardiomegaly and marked pulmonary venous congestion. Echocardiographic evaluation during a Mueller maneuver reveals a marked increase in left atrial size with

decreased left ventricular stroke volume and ejection fraction. Both left and right heart transmural pressures are elevated during inspiration with canine models of asthma. The right ventricle is additionally afterloaded when forced to pump blood "uphill" from the negative pressure intrathoracic cavity through the pulmonary capillary bed, which is compressed by the much higher alveolar pressure.

In summary, utilizing transmural pressures, the hemodynamic events of asthma suggest that significant afterloading of both ventricles is a major factor impairing cardiac performance.

INADEQUATE VENTILATORY DRIVE

MARKED obesity with hypoventilation may give rise to cor pulmonale and right ventricular failure. The term *pickwickian syndrome* has been used to describe these patients (Burwell et al., 1956; Auchincloss and Gilbert, 1963). Mechanical interference with ventilation seems unlikely to be the sole explanation for hypoventilation in these patients, and a decreased sensitivity of the central nervous system to CO_2 inhalation, returning to normal after weight reduction, has been demonstrated (Bates et al., 1964). The therapy for the syndrome is weight loss. It is important to emphasize that it is a rare problem, even

in very obese children (Jenab et al., 1959; Cayler et al., 1961).

Alveolar hypoventilation may occur secondary to central nervous system disorders, particularly those involving the hypothalamus and brain stem (Fishman et al., 1957). The evocative term *Ondine's curse* has been applied to the syndrome of failure of automatic control of ventilation (Severinghaus and Mitchell, 1962; Mellins et al., 1970). Treatment of such cases may be difficult, and mechanical ventilation is usually required. Phrenic nerve stimulation may prove a promising approach in the long term.

ABNORMALITIES OF THE CHEST WALL AND NEUROMUSCULAR APPARATUS

A NUMBER of musculoskeletal and neuromuscular disorders can give rise to generalized hypoventilation. Neuromuscular disorders such as the *Werdnig-Hoffman syndrome, Guillain-Barré syndrome, myasthenia gravis,* and *poliomyelitis* may be associated with general alveolar hypoventilation. In these diseased states hypoventilation usually has to be of long standing, and of moderate to marked severity, before leading to pulmonary hypertension and right ventricular hypertrophy and failure. In such cases, serial blood gas tension determinations may be helpful in deciding when the patient requires mechanical ventilatory support.

Kyphoscoliosis may be severe enough to result in chest wall restriction and alveolar hypoventilation. The pulmonary complication is more often a problem in adults than in children (Berkofsky et al., 1959), but the work of Davis and Reid (1971) showed that the restriction of both lung and blood vessel growth and the late development of right ventricular hypertrophy would argue that the spinal curve should be straightened as early as possible.

Pectus excavatum is a genetically determined abnormality of the sternum and related portions of the diaphragm and occurs in the general population in a proportion of 0.13 percent to 0.4 percent. In patients

in whom it is a solitary abnormality, it seems more common in boys, it is often associated with a pulmonary ejection systolic murmur, and it is associated with small RS complexes in V_1 more frequently than in age-matched controls (Guller and Hable, 1974). The heart tends to be flattened and some observers believe there is impairment of cardiac function that can be relieved by surgical repair of the deformity (Beiser et al., 1972). Detailed studies contrasting operated and untreated children followed for more than ten years support the more traditional conservative approach (Gyllenswärd, 1975). Others maintain that safe, effective relief of severe pectus deformity when performed before the age of three years argues in favor of a preventive approach (Ravitch, 1977).

In infants, a rare deformity of the thoracic cage that results in respiratory failure is that known as *asphyxiating thoracic dystrophy.* In this condition death usually results in infancy or early childhood. Treatment by tracheostomy and assisted ventilation may result in some improvement, but the problem does not usually resolve and the thoracic disorder is part of a generalized chondrodystrophy (Jeune et al., 1954).

PULMONARY VASCULAR DISEASE

INCLUDED in this heading are a limited number of disorders, most of them quite rare, in which there is primary abnormality within the wall of the small arteries of the lung. They include transient pulmonary vasoconstriction of the newborn, primary pulmonary hypertension, miscellaneous pulmonary vascular disorders, and thromboembolic pulmonary vascular disease.

Transient Pulmonary Vasoconstriction in the Newborn

A large number of different labels have been applied to this disease entity—persistent fetal circulation, persistent pulmonary vascular obstruction of the newborn, persistent transitional circulation, progressive pulmonary hypertension, early respiratory distress syndrome, and transient myocardial ischemia (Rowe, 1959; Keith et al., 1961; Prod'hom et al., 1965; Roberton et al., 1967; Gersony et al., 1969; Siassi et al., 1971; Sundell et al., 1971; Burnell et al., 1972; Rowe and Hoffman, 1972; Brown and Pickering, 1974; Levin et al., 1975). Profusion of nosology indicates, first, that the pathogenesis of the disorder is still uncertain and, second, that the full clinical spectrum of the disease is not yet widely appreciated.

The most common form of the disorder is reflected in disturbed right heart hemodynamics. Many of the early descriptions (Rowe, 1959; Keith et al., 1961; Prod'hom et al., 1965; Roberton et al., 1967) referred to an occasional striking disturbance of pulmonary circulation that could occur in *term* infants and drew attention to the distressed breathing, hypoxia, and fetal direction of ductal flow, which was later followed by trends toward normal transitional hemodynamics in the pulmonary circulation, i.e., lowering of the pulmonary arterial pressure to mature levels, left-to-right shunt through the ductus, and eventual closure of both duct and foramen ovale. The much more marked pressure change that results from hypoxia in the newborn when contrasted with the response of older infants provided evidence of the mechanism (James and Rowe, 1957; Moss et al., 1964). Data from cardiac catheterization in the later reports rounded out this picture, confirmed the role of high pulmonary vascular tone in the disorder, and strongly suggested hypoxia was the trigger mechanism. The presence of murmurs suggesting atrioventricular valve regurgitation was later reported by Rowe and Hoffman (1972) though right heart failure has been a known association for many years.

Investigators in their clinical descriptions drew attention to the essentially right-sided effect of high pulmonary vascular resistance until it was recognized that left heart disease could form an additional part of the disease. In a series of patients reported by Rowe

and Hoffman (1972) the evidence of a syndrome of left ventricular failure in addition to the right heart stress was produced. There was reasonable electrocardiographic evidence of myocardial ischemia or infarction during the recovery phase in these patients. It was postulated that intense pulmonary vasoconstriction imposed a very major load on right ventricular work with resultant ischemia of the right ventricle as well as that of the posterior wall of the left ventricle, an area frequently supplied by the branches of the right coronary artery. To draw attention to the role of subendocardial ischemia in the clinical picture, this form of the disorder was labeled transient myocardial ischemia but it is probably simply one form of the syndrome described under the various terms mentioned above.

It is conceivable that a third category of the disease exists in which relatively selective and less extensive subendocardial ischemia of the posterior wall of the left ventricle occurs without striking right-sided manifestations. One of our patients with mild cardiomegaly, signs of minimal mitral regurgitation compatible with a prolapsed mitral valve leaflet, and electrocardiographic changes indicating posterior myocardial damage at the age of five days fitted this concept. The murmur disappeared by the end of the first month of life and the cardiac examination at six months was entirely normal.

Clinical Features.　In its usual form the affected infant is born at term but commonly there will be a history of perinatal stress. Tachypnea and cyanosis are present within 24 hours of delivery. The development of respiratory distress and the appearances of the chest x-ray are not characteristic of the idiopathic respiratory system of the syndrome of the premature infant. The breathing is more akin to that encountered in severe cardiac disease than the distressed and labored respirations characteristic of the idiopathic respiratory distress syndrome. There is frequently a right ventricular lift parasternally, and though there may be no murmurs, the second heart sound is always accentuated and usually is split. In the more severe forms of the disorder there will be gallop rhythm and a tricuspid regurgitant murmur at the lower left sternal border. The liver is often enlarged and frank failure present. The chest x-ray is often unremarkable, although with increasing severity of the disease and the development of congestive failure, there is often cardiomegaly. Overdistended lungs may be seen but the granular appearance of the premature with respiratory distress syndrome is not present (Sundell et al., 1971). The hemoglobin and hematocrit values are normal, and though hypocalcemia and hypoglycemia may be present, these are not invariable. Arterial blood gas analysis will show hypoxemia and varying levels of PCO_2 though high values of that measurement are usually not obtained. The hypertoxic test often will show an increase in

PaO_2 values obtained from the right arm or temporal artery, but in very severe cases the response to high ambient oxygen may be surprisingly limited.

The electrocardiogram shows right ventricular dominance or right ventricular hypertrophy and is only occasionally helpful in demonstrating abnormal T wave changes suggesting myocardial damage. QRS voltage in the tracings is usually normal but may exceed normal values.

The main clinical problem is to distinguish those disorders that may produce hypoxia but are extracardiac, such as birth asphyxia, tracheo-esophageal fistula, aspiration pneumonia, diaphragmatic hernia, from cyanotic congenital heart disease. Echocardiography is especially useful in demonstrating normal cardiac anatomy, but in cases of doubt cardiac catheterization and angiocardiography must be employed. The catheterization data show systemic, or close to systemic, levels of pressure in the right ventricle and pulmonary artery, right-to-left shunting at both duct and foramen levels, and usually normal left atrial pressures. The angiocardiograms following right ventricular injection frequently show tricuspid regurgitation, a wide-open duct with pulmonary artery-to-aorta contrast shunting, and normal pulmonary venous return to the left atrium.

In the less common but most severe form of the disorder where, in addition to gross congestive heart failure, there is left ventricular failure, the presenting symptoms are similar to the usual case for the first 12 to 24 hours. As left ventricular failure develops, pulses weaken and, though the change is probably not an abrupt one, the clinical picture is more one of an abrupt development of vascular collapse from a previously reasonable status. Patients therefore present at this stage of the illness in a manner similar to those who have hypoplastic left heart syndrome with aortic outflow obstruction or interruption of the aortic arch and are usually initially diagnosed as such on admission (Rowe and Hoffman, 1972). Blood gas measurements are very often similar to the usual form but the chest x-ray almost always shows cardiomegaly and may show pulmonary venous congestion. The electrocardiogram often shows severe right ventricular hypertrophy with evidence of subendocardial ischemia more often present in records obtained during recovery than at the height of the illness. Echocardiography demonstrates reduced left ventricular wall movement and other indices of myocardial function. Serial studies most often indicate improvement of ventricular performance. Cardiac catheterization and angiocardiography reveal findings similar to the more usual form of the disease with the addition that raised left ventricular function is further emphasized by sluggish contraction of the left ventricle in left-sided angiocardiograms.

Treatment. In the usual form of the disease oxygen is probably the most important therapy. Attention should be paid to normalizing glucose and calcium levels and acid-base balance. In patients with congestive heart failure, digitalis and diuretics are usually employed. It has been our experience that caution should be utilized in those cases because of a tendency of the patients to develop toxic effects from the drug with the usual doses of digoxin employed for congestive failure at this age.

For probably the vast majority of patients with the disease, these relatively simple measures are sufficient. For the more severe cases and perhaps in order to attempt more rapid resolution of the disorder, a number of workers have attempted to lower pulmonary vascular resistance by the administration of vasodilating drugs. Theoretically such medication would best be administered directly into a major pulmonary artery division since the right-to-left shunting at pulmonary artery level might otherwise produce undesirable hypotensive changes on the systemic side. In practice, careful monitoring of the patient and cautious administration of the drug intravenously have appeared to be quite effective in a relatively limited experience (Korones and Eyal, 1975; Goetzman et al., 1976), but the exact role of these preparations in treatment is currently still uncertain.

Clearly, if the pulmonary vascular resistance is totally unresponsive to any of the above forms of therapy, the patient's condition may continue to deteriorate. Gross hypoxia ultimately causes acidosis and death. Possibly for these patients a more radical form of support should be employed such as those that have been instituted for deteriorating premature infants with respiratory distress syndrome (White et al., 1971). It should be emphasized, however, that the majority of patients can be managed adequately on relatively conservative therapy.

The course of the average case is one of progressive improvement with these measures over a period of several days with fairly prompt response of the congestive aspects within 48 hours. In the case of the patients with the unusually severe form involving left heart failure the response is often dramatic and almost unbelievable to those who witness the change. The development of a loud mitral regurgitant murmur and continuing left ventricular failure are ominous (Richart and Benirschke, 1959). Confirmation of an ischemic basis for the clinical picture has recently been obtained through myocardial imaging techniques (Rowe et al., unpublished observations).

Follow-up information on this group of patients is scanty, although in most group experience the babies appear quite well at a later date. This indeed may be the case, but patients with this very severe form of the disease certainly deserve a detailed later assessment for more subtle signs of ventricular dysfunction, particularly of the left side.

Primary Pulmonary Hypertension

In adults this condition accounts for 3 percent of chronic pulmonary heart disease (Hood, 1968). The incidence in infancy and childhood is more difficult to assess. At The Hospital for Sick Children, Toronto, among 22,000 cases of heart disease we have records on 29 patients (<0.2 percent) with this disorder. At the Children's Hospital Medical Center in Boston, pulmonary hypertension or pulmonary vascular obstruction of unknown etiology occurred in 165 patients forming 1.6 percent of the total experience. There have been a number of reports in this age group (Herdenstam, 1949; Maxwell and Wilson, 1954; Berthrong and Cochrane, 1955; Husson and Wyatt, 1956; Rosenberg and McNamara, 1957; Kjellberg et al., 1959; Farrar et al., 1961; Thilenius et al., 1965). The term should probably be used fairly specifically for the distinctive syndrome that is associated with intrinsic, idiopathic obstructive disease in the small terminal arterioles and arteries of the pulmonary vascular bed.

Etiology. In the vast majority of cases, a satisfactory explanation has not been found, and it is probably not etiologically a homogeneous disorder. In older patients, it is mainly a disease of young women, but there is no sex preponderance in infancy or early childhood. It has been suggested that the disease may represent persistence of the fetal type of pulmonary vasculature, with secondary intimal proliferative changes. In the immediate postnatal period, the elastic fibers in the pulmonary artery are arranged in a parallel manner, similar to those in the aorta. After birth, with a fall in pulmonary artery pressure, this arrangement of the elastic fibers normally becomes distorted, but if pulmonary hypertension persists postnatally, then the fetal type of histologic pattern in the pulmonary trunk is retained. Farrar and associates (1961) and Roberts (1963) found that the histologic pattern in the pulmonary trunk was varied, some cases having the adult type and others fetal pattern. An autoimmune basis has also been suggested, and familial occurrences have been reported (Husson and Wyatt, 1956; Coleman et al., 1959; Farrar et al., 1961; Melman and Braunwald, 1963; Rogge et al., 1966).

Wagenvoort and Wagenvoort (1970), from a detailed pathologic study of the lung vessels in 156 clinically diagnosed cases of primary pulmonary hypertension, emphasized that the changes are identical to those seen in congenital heart disease complicated by pulmonary hypertension as in large ventricular septal defects. On the basis of these findings, they speculated that the alterations in primary pulmonary hypertension are initiated by vasoconstriction, produced by a variety of stimuli.

Pathology. At autopsy, the right atrium and right ventricle are considerably dilated and hypertrophied. The foramen ovale may be open or closed. The chief findings occur in the small vessels of the lungs and have been extensively reviewed by Wagenvoort and Wagenvoort (1970). There is usually medial hypertrophy, laminar intimal fibrosis, and often fibrinoid necrosis, arteritis, and plexiform lesions. In some cases, thrombosis or thromboembolism complicates

the picture. Occasionally, a necrotizing arteritis is present.

Clinical Features. The principal features are dyspnea, fatigue, and syncope, and these may be particularly related to exertion. Syncope may mimic a convulsive disorder (Noonan, 1971). In infancy dyspnea may interfere with feeding and weight gain may be poor. Chest pain may occur in infants as well as in older children (Maxwell and Wilson, 1954). Most fatal cases in childhood develop symptoms before the age of five years.

Cyanosis when present is due to associated intracardiac shunting, usually via a patent foramen ovale, or from intrapulmonary shunting. Clubbing rarely occurs unless there is a significant right-to-left shunt. A prominent "a" wave is visible in the neck. All patients have a right ventricular lift and a markedly increased pulmonary component of the second heart sound. There is usually a loud pulmonary ejection click. Murmurs are commonly absent. Some patients have a soft midsystolic murmur at the left sternal edge. With progress in the severity of pulmonary hypertension, a pulmonary early diastolic murmur may develop, and as right ventricular decompensation occurs, murmurs of tricuspid regurgitation appear. Congestive heart failure is a terminal feature, and arrhythmias usually herald the decline of the patient.

Electrocardiography. The QRS axis is deviated rightward, usually in excess of $+100°$. Right ventricular hypertrophy, commonly of a marked or extreme degree, is present in the precordial leads, with a tall R wave in V_1, or a qR complex in V_1 and deep T wave inversion in the right precordial leads. Early in the disease, the tracing may be normal. The P waves usually are tall and peaked but can be normal, and the P-R interval is usually normal. Serial tracings may be valuable in following the progression of the disease. The appearance of T inversion in II, III, and aVf is a late sign.

Radiologic Examination. Prominence of the main pulmonary arteries and some degree of cardiac enlargement with normal peripheral pulmonary vascularity are the classic x-ray appearance in the child with this disease. The vascular markings at the hilum occasionally are normal. The right atrial enlargement is usually slight, but may increase when heart failure and tricuspid incompetence occur. Barium swallow is normal and the lung parenchyma is always normal.

Pulmonary Function Tests. A decrease in PaO_2 is found if there is right-to-left shunting at intracardiac or pulmonary level. Since there is not usually a primary disturbance of pulmonary ventilation, or alveolar capillary gas exchange, $PaCO_2$, PaO_2, and pH are commonly normal or are altered only by dyspnea and hyperventilation of heart failure.

Echocardiography. In the patient with apparent primary pulmonary hypertension the echocardiogram can be very useful. In the first instance it can assess the chamber dimensions and particularly assist in the exclusion of left atrial and mitral obstructive lesions. Patients with high pulmonary vascular resistance and congenital heart defects, such as in the Eisenmenger complex, should be clarified by the sweep from the ventricular septum to the aorta to search for overriding of that vessel.

The recent contributions of Hirschfeld and associates (1975) employ the ratio of the right ventricular preejection periods/right ventricular ejection time as obtained from the right heart and pulmonary valve echocardiogram to determine the presence of pulmonary hypertension. Whenever the pulmonary artery diastolic pressure or the pulmonary vascular resistance is increased, this ratio rises above the normal value of about 0.25.

Cardiac Catheterization. This always demonstrates elevated right ventricular and pulmonary artery pressures. Calculated levels of pulmonary vascular resistance are extremely high. The pulmonary artery wedge pressure is always normal, but may be difficult to obtain. The cardiac output is usually low in contrast to a low normal or even slightly increased output when pulmonary hypertension is due to disorders of pulmonary function or parenchymal lung disease. If right ventricular failure is present, the right ventricular end-diastolic and right atrial pressures are elevated. Angiocardiography shows dilated pulmonary vessels with a "pruned" appearance and slow passage of the contrast through the lungs. There is a risk of sudden death associated with right-sided injections of contrast in these circumstances, so that the decision to proceed with that step of the study requires nice judgment (Berthrong and Cochrane, 1955; Watson, 1964; Sasahara and Mark, 1976).

We have had the opportunity of following one male patient with the disorder over a period of four years, following the onset of symptoms at the age of three. Initially quite modest hypertension was present, but serial studies revealed a progressive increase in pulmonary arterial pressure to the point where the values eventually exceeded systemic level. Dramatic decreases in the level of pulmonary artery pressure were demonstrated after the administration of acetylcholine and oxygen during the initial studies, but the acute responses to drugs over the period of observation diminished. At the last study performed, the only way in which the pulmonary artery pressure could be altered was by the administration of 100 percent oxygen.

Diagnosis. The differential diagnosis of primary pulmonary hypertension may be difficult, for there is a wide variety of diseases associated with an elevated pulmonary vascular resistance. The clinical picture in many of these may be identical. Recognition of the secondary forms of pulmonary hypertension is important, since many may be remediable, and it is a sound principle always to consider the possibility of a remediable lesion underlying what appears to be primary pulmonary hypertension.

Patients with severe pulmonary hypertension and the Eisenmenger syndrome with intracardiac or intervascular communications are usually cyanosed.

Occasionally, however, the clinical picture may be indistinguishable from that seen in primary pulmonary hypertension, and cardiac catheterization may be required to establish whether an intracardiac or intervascular shunt is present. Lesions associated with pulmonary venous hypertension, such as pulmonary venous stenosis, and malformations affecting the left side of the heart may give rise to an elevated pulmonary vascular resistance. The radiologic findings of interstitial or alveolar edema may be helpful. A slightly enlarged left atrium may indicate congenital mitral stenosis. An elevated pulmonary arterial wedge pressure at cardiac catheterization may help in confirming the presence of pulmonary vein stenosis or a left heart obstructive lesion. Echocardiography would seem to be the appropriate preliminary step prior to catheterization or angiocardiography to clarify the anatomic type of obstruction, whether it is cor triatriatum, supravalvular stenosing ring, mitral valve stenosis, mitral atresia, disease of the left ventricular myocardium, or aortic outflow tract obstruction. Evaluation of the clinical picture, and of the x-ray, helps to rule out diseases of the pulmonary parenchyma, and pulmonary function tests are not usually required. The pulmonary artery elevation seen in pulmonary parenchymal disease is not as marked as that in primary pulmonary hypertension. Evidence of thromboembolic disease, or of an associated systemic disease process, should also be sought for carefully.

Prognosis and Treatment. The condition is progressive, and the average duration of life after onset of symptoms in childhood is usually less than one year. Occasional exceptions to this rule occur (Thilenius et al., 1965). Survival longer than seven years is not reported. Infants have been known to die at less than six months of age. In older children, frequent and severe syncopal episodes usually precede sudden death. Death may also follow progressive right ventricular failure. Trial of a variety of therapies including long-term oxygen, anticoagulants, and steroids leads to the conclusion that no effective treatment is available. Digitalis and diuretics may be of some help, but are unlikely to influence the natural history of the disease when there are fixed pulmonary vascular changes.

Miscellaneous Pulmonary Vascular Disorders

Sickle cell anemia may be associated with occlusive pulmonary vascular disease, with pulmonary infarction, and with vascular changes occurring secondary to aggregation of the abnormal red blood cells (Moser and Shea, 1957). Arteritis of the small pulmonary arteries is a feature of some *connective tissues disorders*, especially lupus erythematosus. The major clinical manifestations in such cases are usually related to involvement of other organs. Primary thrombosis of the pulmonary artery has been reported in some patients with a *nephrotic syndrome* on steroid therapy and seems particularly related to the diuretic phase of their disease (Gootman et al., 1964). Pulmonary hypertension has been reported in adults following ingestion of an *anorexigenic drug*, aminorex (Gurtner et al., 1971). Progressive pulmonary hypertension can occur in association with *portal hypertension*, with death resulting from right heart failure. The cause of this complication in such patients is unknown but it has been considered likely that some substance, possibly released from

platelets, can enter the pulmonary circuit under these circumstances and produce pulmonary vasoconstriction (Levine et al., 1973).

Pulmonary arterial pressures in apparently normal children residing at high altitude can be significantly elevated secondary to hypoxia (Penaloza, 1964; Vogel et al., 1964). These children are usually asymptomatic. The pulmonary artery pressure may fall on descent to sea level.

THROMBOEMBOLIC PULMONARY VASCULAR DISORDERS

THROMBOEMBOLIC pulmonary vascular disease can present acutely or occur insidiously as progressive pulmonary hypertension. Both forms are an uncommon problem in childhood.

Acute Thromboembolism.   In adults, occlusion of the pulmonary artery by a massive clot is the principal cause of acute cor pulmonale. Such an event in childhood is rare and usually follows immobilization or some diagnostic or therapeutic intervention (Johnson et al., 1947; Wilson and Rowe, 1952; Haber and Bennington, 1962; Gootman et al., 1964). Multiple pulmonary emboli are also uncommon. Emery (1962) found only three patients among two thousand autopsies in children with gross evidence of pulmonary embolism. In the same series, however, there were 21 patients in whom emboli were only found on microscopy. About a third of the cases had died dramatically, the others having had an abrupt onset of severe respiratory symptoms, and many were undiagnosed, or believed clinically to have pneumonia. Primary causes for these emboli were sepsis of the lower abdomen, cachexia, and Spitz Holter valves inserted for the management of hydrocephalus. Wise and associates (1973) reported 28 cases of venous thrombosis in childhood, which were unrelated to previous cardiac catheterization, and in whom local infection or trauma was the main precipitating factor. Three of these cases had emboli to the lung.

Pulmonary emboli are associated with a number of hemodynamic changes. There may be a decreased cardiac output, systemic hypotension, and an increased pulmonary artery pressure, and pulmonary arteriolar resistance. Probably both mechanical and vasoconstrictive factors are responsible for the pulmonary hypertension (Sasahara, 1974).

In massive pulmonary embolism the clinical picture is dramatic. There is usually sudden collapse with hypotension, cyanosis, tachypnea, distended neck veins, a prominent third or fourth heart sound, gallop, and accentuation of the pulmonary component of the second heart sound. The patient may die immediately due to ventricular fibrillation. In some cases, marked slowing of the heart rate together with a low stroke volume produces poor tissue perfusion, with acidosis and cardiac arrest. The patient, however, may survive massive or recurrent emboli

and demonstrate an ability to lyse and reabsorb these.

The electrocardiogram, almost invariably, shows sinus tachycardia. Right bundle branch block may occur, but is often only a transient finding. In adults an $S_1Q_3T_3$ pattern is a commonly reported association, but the most frequently observed abnormalities are nonspecific T wave changes (Oram, 1966; Stein et al., 1975). It is important to emphasize that the electrocardiogram may be normal. The chest x-ray may show vascular blanching and prominence of the main pulmonary artery, but lobar atelectasis, consolidation, and elevation of the diaphragm are more frequent findings. Pulmonary angiograms provide more reliable evidence of embolism than do pulmonary perfusion scans (Bell and Simon, 1976).

Management is usually conservative. External cardiac massage may be necessary if cardiac arrest or circulatory collapse occurs. Noradrenalin and Isoprenaline both have powerful inotropic effects, and the vasoconstrictive effects of the former may also be beneficial. Removal of a massive embolus under cardiopulmonary bypass can be carried out, but should be deferred until after pulmonary angiography, if there is any doubt about the diagnosis. Lung scanning is now used increasingly in the diagnosis of pulmonary embolism in adults, with a high degree of sensitivity, but not the specificity of pulmonary angiography. In infants and children, phlebothrombosis virtually never occurs, unless there is severe paralysis, immobilization, or trauma to the lower limbs (Wise et al., 1973). Heparinization should probably be started in these exceptional cases in the acute stage following an embolus. Thereafter the patient should be continued on a coumadin derivative for three to six weeks. Urokinase and streptokinase are thrombolytic agents that have recently been tested widely, but their current role in the management of pulmonary embolism is not yet certain. The results of recent clinical trials have suggested, however, that massive pulmonary emboli will lyse more rapidly in patients treated with these agents, followed by heparin, as compared to those treated with heparin alone (Fratantoni et al., 1975).

Chronic Thromboembolism.   Recurrent embolism with progressive pulmonary hypertension can complicate endocarditis, rheumatic fever, and schistosomiasis (Garcia-Palmidri, 1964). Pulmonary hypertension has also been well-documented as a complication of ventriculovenous shunts for the treatment of hydrocephalus (Talner et al., 1961; Noonan and Ehmke, 1963; Sperling et al., 1964; Hougen et al., 1975). In such cases, pulmonary hypertension may be advanced before being recognized. Infective emboli, from the superior vena cava and right atrium, spontaneous thrombosis, and an autoimmune reaction of the pulmonary vessels to cerebrospinal fluid have all been postulated. The valve should be removed and replaced, probably by a ventriculoperitoneal shunt (Favara and Paul, 1967).

The symptoms and signs of chronic thromboembolic pulmonary vascular disease may be identical to those seen in primary pulmonary hypertension.

With chronic embolic disease the therapeutic principle should be to prevent further embolism, and to allow regression of the vascular changes, secondary to the previous emboli.

Fat Embolism. This disorder is extremely rare in childhood. Drummond and associates (1969), reviewing the experience of The Hospital for Sick Children, Toronto, found only nine cases of clinical fat embolism between 1951 and 1968. Three occurred in patients with advanced systemic connective tissue diseases. In such cases, even minimal trauma may initiate a rapid, fulminating clinical course characterized by sudden onset of dyspnea, tachypnea, tachycardia, and cyanosis. In some cases, the clinical picture may not occur until 24 to 48 hours after the trauma, and systemic rather than pulmonary manifestations may predominate. There is no specific treatment for fat embolism, and the important principle is to maintain pulmonary function. Arterial hypoxemia is almost invariably present, and assisted ventilation may be necessary. Massive doses of corticosteroids have been shown to be useful and lifesaving (Fischer et al., 1971).

Air Embolism. A rare cause of acute cor pulmonale in childhood, air embolism may complicate a variety of medical and surgical procedures, including simple maneuvers such as changing intravenous bottles. The lethal dose varies with the age, condition, and position of the patient, and rapidity with which air enters the circulation. It may be as little as 5 cc per kilogram. Death usually results either from an air lock within the right ventricle or from embolism to the lungs, with secondary reflex pulmonary vasoconstriction (Berglund et al., 1970). The infant or child usually becomes suddenly cyanosed and stops breathing. A loud, continuous murmur or noise may be heard over the precordium from the air and blood trapped in the right ventricle. Treatment consists of turning the patient onto the left side (Durant et al., 1947) with the head in the dependent position, and the administration of 100 percent oxygen. Aspiration of air through a needle or catheter inserted into the right ventricle may be helpful.

REFERENCES

Ainger, L. E.: Large tonsils and adenoids in small children with cor pulmonale. *Br. Heart J.*, **30**:356, 1968.

Andersen, D. H.: Cystic fibrosis of the pancreas and its relation to celiac disease: clinical and pathological study. *Am. J. Dis. Child.*, **56**:344, 1938.

Auchincloss, J. H., and Gilbert, R.: The cardiorespiratory syndrome related to obesity: clinical manifestations and pathologic physiology. *Prog. Cardiovasc. Dis.*, **1**:413, 1959.

Avery, M. E., and Fletcher, D. B.: *The Lung and Its Disorders in the Newborn Infant*, 3rd ed. W. B. Saunders Co., Philadelphia, 1974.

Barer, G. R.: The circulation through collapsed adult lungs. *J. Physiol.*, **168**:10P, 1963.

Bates, D. V., and Christie, R. V.: Respiratory function in disease. In *Primary Alveolar Hypoventilation Syndrome*. W. B. Saunders Co., Philadelphia, 1964.

Beiser, G. D.; Epstein, S. E.; Stampfer, M.; Goldstein, R. E.; Noland, S. P.; and Levitsky, S.: Impairment of cardiac function in patients with pectus excavatum with improvement after operative correction. *N. Engl. J. Med.*, **287**:267, 1972.

Bell, W. R., and Simon, T. L.: A comparative analysis of pulmonary perfusion scans with pulmonary angiograms. *Am. Heart J.*, **92**:700, 1976.

Berglund, E., and Josephson, S.: Pulmonary air embolization in the dog. *Scand. J. Clin. Invest.*, **26**:97, 1970.

Bergofsky, E. J.; Turino, G. M.; and Fishman, A. P.: Cardiorespiratory failure in kyphoscoliosis. *Medicine*, **38**:263, 1959.

Bergofsky, E. H., and Holtzman, S.: A study of the mechanisms involved in the pulmonary pressor response to hypoxia. *Circ. Res.*, **20**:50b, 1967.

Berthrong, M., and Cochrane, T. H.: Pathological findings in nine children with primary pulmonary hypertension. *Bull. Hopkins Hosp.*, **97**:69, 1955.

Blitz, D.; Balboni, F. A.; and Stanchi, E. A.: Acute bronchial asthma in children. A cardiopulmonary problem? *N.Y. State J. Med.*, **61**:4259, 1961.

Bodian, M.: *Fibrocystic Disease of the Pancreas*. William Heinemann, Ltd., London, 1952.

Brown, R., and Pickering, D.: Persistent transitional circulation. *Arch. Dis. Child.*, **49**:883, 1974.

Burnard, E. D.; Grattan-Smith, P.; Picton-Warlow, C. G.; and Cranang, A.: Pulmonary insufficiency in prematurity. *Aust. Pediatr. J.*, **1**:12, 1963.

Burnell, R. H.; Joseph, M. C.; and Lees, M. H.: Progressive pulmonary hypertension in newborn infants. *Am. J. Dis. Child.*, **123**:167, 1972.

Burwell, C. S.; Robin, E. D.; Whaley, R. D.; and Bickelmann, A. G.: Extreme obesity associated with alveolar hypoventilation: A Pickwickian syndrome. *Am. J. Med.*, **21**:811, 1956.

Caffey, J.: Cited by Royce (1951).

Cayler, G. G.; Johnson, E. J.; Lewis, B. E.; Kortzeborn, J. D.; Jordan, J.; and Fricker, G. A.: Heart failure due to enlarged tonsils and adenoids. *Am. J. Dis. Child.*, **118**:708, 1969.

Cayler, G. G.; Mays, J.; and Riley, H. D.: Cardiorespiratory syndrome of obesity (Pickwickian syndrome) in children. *Pediatrics*, **27**:237, 1961.

Cogswell, J. J., and Easton, D. M.: Cor pulmonale in Pierre Robin syndrome. *Arch. Dis. Child.*, **49**:905, 1974.

Cohen, H. A.; Baird, M. G.; Rouleau, J. R.; Fuhrmann, C. F.; Bailey, I. K.; Summer, W. R.; Strauss, H. W.; and Pitt, B.: Thallium 201 myocardial imaging in patients with pulmonary hypertension. *Circulation*, **54**:790, 1976.

Coleman, P. N.; Edmunds, A. W. B.; and Tregillus, P.: Primary pulmonary hypertension in three sibs. *Br. Heart J.*, **21**:81, 1959.

Cox, M. A.; Schiebler, G. L.; Taylor, W. J.; Wheat, M. W., Jr.; and Krovetz, L. L.: Reversible pulmonary hypertension in a child with respiratory obstruction and cor pulmonale. *J. Pediatr.*, **67**:192, 1965.

Crozier, D. N.: Cystic fibrosis. A not-so-fatal disease. *Pediatr. Clin. North Am.*, **21**:935, 1974.

Davies, G. M., and Reid, L.: Effect of scoliosis on growth of alveoli and pulmonary arteries and on right ventricle. *Ach. Dis. Child.*, **46**:623, 1971.

Dees, S. C.: Asthma in infants and young children. *JAMA*, **175**:365, 1961.

Donohue, W. L.; Laski, B.; Uchida, I.; and Munn, J. D.: Familial fibrocystic dysplasia and its relation to the Hamman-Rich syndrome. *Pediatrics*, **24**:786, 1959.

Drummond, D. S.; Salter, R. B.; and Boone, J.: Fat embolism in children. *Can. Med. Assoc. J.*, **101**:200, 1969.

Durant, T. M.; Long, J.; and Oppenheimer, M. J.: Pulmonary (venous) air embolism. *Am. Heart J.*, **33**:269, 1947.

Emery, J. L.: Pulmonary embolism in children. *Arch. Dis. Child.*, **37**:591, 1962.

Farrar, J. F.; Reye, R. D. K.; and Stuckey, D.: Primary pulmonary hypertension in childhood. *Br. Heart J.*, **23**:605, 1961.

Favara, B. E., and Paul, R. N.: Thromboembolism and cor pulmonale complicating ventriculo-venous shunt. *JAMA*, **199**:162, 1967.

Featherby, E. A.; Weng, T-R.; Crozier, D. N.; Duic, A.; Reilly, B. J.; and Levison, H.: Dynamic and static lung volumes, blood-gas tensions and diffusing capacity in patients with cystic fibrosis. Proc 5th International Cystic Fibrosis conference, Cambridge. Cystic Fibrosis Research Trust, London, 1969, p. 232.

Ferrer, M. I.: Cor pulmonale (pulmonary heart disease): Present-day status. *Am. Heart J.*, **89**:657, 1975.

Fischer, J. E.; Turner, B. H.; Herndon, J. J.; and Riseborough, E. J.: Massive steroid therapy in severe fat embolism. *Surg. Gynecol. Obstet.*, **132**:667, 1971.

Fishman, A. P.: Respiratory gases in the regulation of the pulmonary circulation. *Physiol. Rev.*, **41**:214, 1961.

————: The left ventricle and "chronic bronchitis and emphysema." *N. Engl. J. Med.*, **285**:402, 1971.

Fishman, A. P.; Fitts, H. W.; and Cournand, A.: Effects of breathing carbon dioxide upon the pulmonary circulation. *Circulation*, **22**:220, 1960.

Fishman, A. P.; Turino, G. M.; and Bergofsky, E. H.: Syndrome of alveolar hypoventilation. *Am. J. Med.*, **23**:333, 1957.

Foraker, A. G.; Bedrossian, C. W. M.; and Anderson, A. E., Jr.: Myocardial dimensions and proportions in pulmonary emphysema. *Arch. Pathol.*, **90**:344, 1970.

Fowler, R. S.; Rappaport, H.; Cunningham, K.; Crozier, D. N.; and Levison, H.: Reduced left voltage in the vectorcardiogram as an indicator of cor pulmonale in cystic fibrosis. *Pediatr. Res.*, **8**:349, 1974.

Fratantoni, J. E.; Ness, P.; and Simon, T. L.: Thrombolytic therapy: current status. *N. Engl. J. Med.*, **293**:21, 1975.

Garcia-Palmieri, M. R.: Cor pulmonale due to schistosoma mansoni. *Am. Heart J.*, **68**:714, 1964.

Gersony, W. M.; Duc, G. V.; and Sinclair, J. C.: "P.R.C." syndrome (persistence of the fetal circulation). *Circulation*, **40**(suppl. 3):84, 1969.

Goetzman, B. W.; Sunshine, P.; Johnson, J. D.; Wennberg, R. P.; Hackel, A.; Merten, D. F.; Bartaletti, A-L.; and Silverman, N. H.: Neonatal hypoxia and pulmonary vasospasm: response to tolazoline. *J. Pediatr.*, **89**:617, 1976.

Goldring, R. M.; Fishman, A. P.; Turino, J. M.; Cohen, H. I.; Denning, C. R.; and Andersen, D. H.: Pulmonary hypertension and cor pulmonale in cystic fibrosis of the pancreas. *J. Pediatr.*, **65**:501, 1964.

Gootman, N.; Gross, J.; and Mensch, A.: Pulmonary artery thrombosis. A complication occurring with prednisone and chlorothiazide therapy in two nephrotic patients. *Pediatrics*, **34**:861, 1964.

Griffin, J. T.; Kass, I.; and Hoffman, M. S.: Cor pulmonale associated with symptoms and signs of asthma in children. *Pediatrics*, **24**:54, 1959.

Guller, B., and Hable, K.: Cardiac findings in pectus excavatum in children: review and differential diagnosis. *Chest*, **66**:165, 1974.

Gunstone, R. F.: Right heart pressures in bronchial asthma. *Thorax*, **26**:39, 1971.

Gurtner, H. P.; Gertsch, M.; Salzmann, C.; Scherrer, M.; and Stucki Pand Wyss, F.: Haufen sich die primar vascularen Formen des chronischen Cor Pulmonale? *Schweiz. Med. Wochenschr.*, **98**:1579, 1968.

Gyllensward, Å.; Irnell, L.; Michaëlsson, M.; Qvist, O.; and Sahlstedt, B.: Pectus excavatum. A clinical study with long term postoperative followup. *Acta Paediatr. Scand.*, Suppl. 255, 1975.

Haber, S. L., and Bennington, J. L.: Pulmonary embolism in an infant. *J. Pediatr.*, **61**:759, 1962.

Herdenstam, C. G.: Primary pulmonary vascular sclerosis in infancy. *Acta Pediatr.*, **38**:284, 1949.

Hirschfeld, S.; Meyer, R.; Schwartz, D. C.; Korfhagen, J.; and Kaplan, S.: The echocardiographic assessment of pulmonary artery pressure and pulmonary vascular resistance. *Circulation*, **52**:642, 1975.

Hood, W. B., Jr.; Spencer, H.; Lass, R. W.; and Daley, R.: Primary pulmonary hypertension: familial occurrence. *Br. Heart J.*, **30**:336, 1968.

Hougen, T. J.; Emmanouilides, G. C.; and Moss, A. J.: Pulmonary valvular dysfunction in children with ventriculovenous shunts for hydrocephalus: a previously unreported complication. *Pediatrics*, **55**:836, 1975.

Husson, G. S., and Wyatt, T. C.: Primary pulmonary hypertension in siblings. *Am. J. Dis. Child.*, **92**:506, 1956.

Ishikawa, S.; Fattal, G. A.; Popiewicz, J.; and Wyatt, J. P.: Functional morphometry of myocardial fibers in cor pulmonale. *Am. Rev. Resp. Dis.*, **195**:358, 1972.

James, L. S., and Rowe, R. D.: The pattern of response of pulmonary and systemic arterial pressures in newborn and older infants to short period of hypoxia. *J. Pediatr.*, **51**:5, 1957.

Jeune, M.; Carron, R.; Berand, C.; and Loaec, Y.: Polychondrodystrophie avec blocage thoracique d'evolution fate. *Pediatrie*, **9**:39, 1954.

Johnson, A. L.; Wollin, D. G.; and Ross, J. B.: Heart catheterization in the investigation of congenital heart disease. *Can. Med. Assoc. J.*, **56**:249, 1947.

Keith, J. D.; Rose, V.; Braudo, M.; and Rowe, R. D.: The electrocardiogram in the respiratory distress syndrome and related cardiovascular dynamics. *J. Pediatr.*, **59**:167, 1961.

Kelminson, L. L.; Cotton, E. K.; and Vogel, J. H. K.: The reversibility of pulmonary hypertension in patients with cystic fibrosis. Observations on the effects of tolazoline hydrochloride. *Pediatrics*, **39**:24, 1967.

Kharja, F., and Parker, J. O.: Right and left ventricular performance in chronic obstructive lung disease. *Am. Heart J.*, **82**:319, 1971.

Kilcoyne, M. M.; Davis, A. L.; and Ferrer, M. I.: A dynamic electrocardiographic concept useful in the diagnosis of cor pulmonale. Result of a survey of 200 patients with chronic obstructive pulmonary disease. *Circulation*, **42**:903, 1970.

Kjellberg, S. R.; Mannheimer, E.; Rudhe, U.; and Jönsson, B.: *Diagnosis of Congenital Heart Disease*. Year Book Publishers, Inc., Chicago, 1959.

Korones, S. B., and Eyal, F. G.: Successful treatment of "persistent fetal circulation": with tolazoline. *Pediatr. Res.*, **9**:367, 1975.

Levin, D. L.; Muster, A. J.; Pachman, L. M.; Wessel, H. U.; Paul, M. H.; and Koshaba, T.: Cardiac catheterization, immunologic and psychosomatic evaluation in nine patients. *Chest*, **68**:166, 1975.

Levine, O. R.; Harris, R. C.; Blanc, W. A.; and Mellins, R. B.: Progressive pulmonary hypertension in children with portal hypertension. *J. Pediatr.*, **83**:964, 1963.

Levy, A. M.; Tabakin, B. S.; Hanson, J. S.; and Narkewicz, R. M.: Hypertrophied adenoids causing pulmonary hypertension and severe congestive heart failure. *N. Engl. J. Med.*, **277**:506, 1967.

Leibman, J.; Doershuk, C. F.; Rapp, C.; and Matthews, L.: The vectorcardiogram in cystic fibrosis—diagnostic significance and correlation with pulmonary function tests. *Circulation*, **35**:552, 1967.

Lindsay, D. A., and Read, J.: Pulmonary vascular responsiveness in the prognosis of chronic obstructive lung disease. *Am. Rev. Resp. Dis.*, **105**:242, 1972.

Luke, M. J.; Mehrizi, A.; Folger, G. M., Jr.; and Rowe, R. D.: Chronic naopharyngeal obstruction as a cause of cardiomegaly, cor pulmonale and pulmonary edema. *Pediatrics*, **37**:762, 1966.

Maxwell, I., and Wilson, R.: Cor pulmonale in infancy stimulating congenital heart disease. *Pediatrics*, **41**:587, 1954.

Mellins, R. W.; Balfour, H. H.; Torino, G. M.; and Winters, R. W.: Failure of automatic control of ventilation (Ondine's curse): report of an infant born with this syndrome and a review of the literature. *Medicine*, **49**:487, 1970.

Melman, K. L., and Braunwald, E.: Familial pulmonary hypertension. *N. Engl. J. Med.*, **269**:770, 1963.

Menashe, V. D.; Farretii, C.; and Miller, M.: Hypoventilation and cor pulmonale due to chronic upper airway obstruction. *J. Pediatr.*, **67**:199, 1965.

Monset-Couchard, M.; Mason, C. V.; and Moss, A. J.: Cor pulmonale in children. *Current Problems Pediatr.*, **5**:1, 1975.

Morgan, A. D.: Cor pulmonale in children: review and etiological classification. *Am. Heart J.*, **73**:550, 1967.

Moser, K. M., and Shea, J. G.: The relationship between pulmonary infarction, cor pulmonale, and the sickle cell states. *Am. J. Med.*, **22**:561, 1957.

Moss, A. J.; Emmanouilides, G. C.; Adams, F. H.; and Chuang, K.: Response of ductus arteriosus and pulmonary and systemic arterial pressure to changes in oxygen environment in newborn infants. *Pediatrics*, **33**:937, 1964.

Nadas, A. S.; Cogan, G.; Landing, B. H.; and Schwachman, H.: Studies in pancreatic fibrosis; cor pulmonale: Clinical and pathological observations. *Pediatrics*, **10**: 319, 1952.

Noonan, J. A.: Reversible cor pulmonale due to hypertrophied tonsils and adenoids. Studies in two cases. *Circulation*, **32**: 11–164, 1965.

———: Pulmonary heart disease. *Pediatr. Clin. North Am.*, **18**: 1255, 1971.

Noonan, J. A., and Ehmke, D. A.: Complications of ventriculovenous shunts for control of hydrocephalus. Report of three cases with thromboemboli to the lungs. *N. Engl. J. Med.*, **269**: 70, 1963.

Northway, W. J., Jr.; Rosan, R. C.; and Port, D. Y.: Pulmonary disease following respirator therapy of hyaline membrane disease. Bronchopulmonary dysplasia. *N. Engl. J. Med.*, **276**: 357, 1967.

Oram, S., and Davies, P.: The electrocardiogram in cor pulmonale. *Prog. Cardiovasc. Dis.*, **9**:341, 1967.

O'Shea, P. A., and Yardley, J. H.: The Hamman-Rich syndrome in infancy: report of a case with virus-like particles by electron microscopy. *Johns Hopkins Med. J.*, **126**:320, 1970.

Padmavati, S., and Raizada, V.: Electrocardiogram in chronic cor pulmonale. *Br. Heart J.*, **34**:658, 1972.

Penaloza, D.; Arias-Stella, J.; Sime, F.; Recavarren, S.; and Marticoven, E.: Heart and pulmonary circulation in children at high altitudes. Physiological, anatomical and clinical observations. *Pediatrics*, **34**:568, 1964.

Prod'hom, L. S.; Levison, H.; Cherry, R. B.; and Smith, C. A.: Adjustment of ventilation, intrapulmonary gas exchange, and acid-base balance during the first day of life. Infants with early respiratory distress. *Pediatrics*, **35**:662, 1969.

Quivers, W. W.; Linde, L. M.; Sapin, S. O.; and Heimlich, E. M.: The electrocardiogram and vectorcardiogram in children with severe bronchial asthma. *Am. J. Cardiol.*, **14**:616, 1964.

Rao, B. S.; Cohn, K. E.; Eldridge, F. L.; and Hancock, E. W.: Left ventricular failure secondary to chronic pulmonary disease. *Am. J. Med.*, **45**:229, 1968.

Ravitch, M. M.: Editorial. Repair of pectus excavatum in children under 3 years of age: a twelve-year experience. *Ann. Thorac. Surg.*, **23**:301, 1977.

Richards, W., and Patrick, J. R.: Death from asthma in children. *Am. J. Dis. Child.*, **110**:4, 1965.

Richart, R., and Benirschke, K.: Myocardial infarction in the perinatal period. *J. Pediatr.*, **55**:706, 1959.

Roberton, N. R. C.; Hallidie-Smith, K. A.; and Davis, J. A.: Severe respiratory distress syndrome mimicking cyanotic heart-disease in term babies. *Lancet*, **2**:1108, 1967.

Roberts, W. C.: The histologic structure of the pulmonary trunk in patients with primary pulmonary hypertension. *Am. Heart J.*, **65**:230, 1963.

Rogge, J. D.; Mishkin, M. E.; and Genovese, P. D.: Familial occurrence of primary pulmonary hypertension. *Ann. Intern. Med.*, **65**:672, 1966.

Rosenberg, H. S., and McNamara, D. G.: Primary pulmonary hypertension. *Pediatrics*, **20**:408, 1957.

Rosenthal, A.; Tucker, C. R.; Williams, R. G.; Khaw, K. T.; Striedor, D.; and Schwachman, H.: Echocardiographic assessment of cor pulmonale in cystic fibrosis. *Pediatr. Clin. North Am.*, **23**: 327, 1976.

Rowe, R. D.: Clinical observations of transitional circulations, in Oliver, T. K. Jr. Ed. Adaptation to extrauterine life, Report of the thirty-first Ross Conference on Pediatric Research, Columbus, Ohio, 1959, Ross Laboratories, p. 36.

Rowe, R. D.; Finley, J. P.; Radford, D. J.; Gilday, D. L.; Howman-Giles, R. B.; Bloom, K. R.; and Chance, G. W.: Ischaemic myocardial dysfunction in the newborn. Diagnostic confirmation by myocardial perfusion scintigram. Unpublished observations.

Rowe, R. D., and Hoffman, T.: Transient myocardial ischemia of the newborn infant: a form of severe cardiorespiratory distress in full-term infants. *J. Pediatr.*, **81**: 243, 1972.

Royce, S. W.: Cor pulmonale in infancy and early childhood. Report on 34 patients with special reference to the occurrence of pulmonary heart disease in cystic fibrosis of the pancreas. *Pediatrics*, **8**:255, 1951.

Ryland, D., and Reid, L.: The pulmonary circulation in cystic fibrosis. *Thorax*, **30**:285, 1975.

Sasahara, A. A.: Current problems in pulmonary embolism. *Prog. Cardiovasc. Dis.*, **17**:161, 1974.

Sasahara, A. A., and Mark, E. J.: Case records of the Massachusetts General Hospital. Rapidly progressive pulmonary hypertension in a 15-year-old girl. *N. Engl. J. Med.*, **294**:433, 1976.

Schrijen, F.; Ehrlich, W.; and Permutt, S.: Cardiovascular changes in conscious dogs during spontaneous deep breaths. *Pfluegers Arch.*, **355**:205, 1975.

Severinghaus, J. W., and Mitchell, R. A.: Ondine's curse—failure of respiratory centre automaticity while awake. *Clin. Res.*, **10**:122, 1962.

Shwachman, H., and Kulczycki, L. L.: Longterm study of one hundred and five patients with cystic fibrosis. *Am. J. Dis. Child.*, **96**:6, 1958.

Siassi, B.; Moss, A. J.; and Dooley, R. R.: Clinical recognition of cor pulmonale in cystic fibrosis. *J. Pediatr.*, **78**:794, 1971.

Sperling, D. R.; Patrick, J. R.; Anderson, F. M.; and Fyler, D. C.: Cor pulmonale secondary to ventriculoauriculostomy. *Am. J. Dis. Child.*, **107**:308, 1964.

Stein, P. D.; Dalen, J. E.; McIntyre, K. M.; Sasahara, A. S.; Wenger, N. K.; and Willis, P. W.: The electrocardiogram in acute pulmonary embolism. *Prog. Cardiovasc. Dis.*, **17**:247, 1975.

Sundell, H.; Garrott, J.; Blankenship, W. J.; Shepard, F. M.; and Stahlman, M. T.: Studies on infants with type II respiratory distress syndrome. *J. Pediatr.*, **78**:754, 1971.

Talner, N. S.; Lin, H-Y.; Oberman, H. A.; and Schmidt, R. W.: Thromboembolism complicating Holter valve shunt. A clinicopathologic study of four patients treated with this procedure for hydrocephalus. *Am. J. Dis. Child.*, **101**:602, 1961.

Thilenius, A. G.; Nadas, A. S.; and Jockin, H.: Primary pulmonary vascular obstruction in children. *Pediatrics*, **36**:75, 1965.

Thomas, A. J.: Chronic pulmonary heart disease. *Br. Heart J.*, **34**:653, 1972.

Vogel, J. H. K.; Pryor, R.; and Blount, S. G.: The cardiovascular system in children from high altitude. *J. Pediatr.*, **64**:315, 1964.

Wagenvoort, C. A., and Wagenvoort, N.: Primary pulmonary hypertension. A pathologic study of the lung vessels in 156 clinically diagnosed cases. *Circulation*, **42**:1163, 1970.

Watson, H.: Severe pulmonary hypertensive episodes following angiocardiography with sodium metrizoate. *Lancet*, **2**:732, 1964.

White, J. J.; Andrews, H. G.; Risemberg, H.; Mazur, D.; and Haller, J. A.: Prolonged respiratory support in newborn infants with a membrane oxygenator. *Surgery*, **70**:288, 1971.

Whitman, V.; Stern, R. C.; Bellet, P.; Doershuk, C. F.; Liebman, J.; Boat, T. F.; Borkat, G.; and Matthews, L. W.: Studies on cor pulmonale in cystic fibrosis. I. Effects of diuresis. *Pediatrics*, **55**:83, 1975.

WHO Report: Cor pulmonale. *Circulation*, **27**:594, 1963.

Williams, H., and Campbell, P.: Generalized bronchiectasis associated with deficiency of cartilage in the bronchial tree. *Arch. Dis. Child.*, **35**:182, 1960.

Williams, H. E., and Phelan, P. D.: Respiratory illness in children. Blackwell Science Publications, Oxford, 1975, p. 340.

Wilson, R., and Rowe, R.: Some special problems in the use of ACTH and cortisone therapy in children. *J. Pediatr.*, **40**:164, 1950.

Wise, R., and Todd, J. C.: Spontaneous lower extremity venous thrombosis in children. *Am. J. Dis. Child.*, **126**:766, 1973.

17

Cardiac Arrhythmias

Peter M. Olley

INTRODUCTION

ALTHOUGH cardiac arrhythmias are not uncommon in infancy and childhood, their current prevalence is unknown. Previous estimates of their incidence have been based on electrocardiographic studies not primarily designed to detect arrhythmias. Increasing use of electronic monitoring devices suggests that their incidence is much higher than previously thought (Church et al., 1967). Many childhood arrhythmias are either too benign to cause symptoms or too transient to permit accurate electrocardiographic identification. Others such as atrial fibrillation and flutter are undoubtedly less common in childhood than in adult life.

Various forms of cardiac surgery have increased the incidence of all types of arrhythmias.

A knowledge of expected heart rates under resting conditions in different age groups is helpful in detecting departures from the normal (Table 17–1).

Table 17–1. NORMAL HEART RATES IN INFANTS AND CHILDREN*

AGE	HEART RATE		
	Average	*Minimum*	*Maximum*
0–24 hours	125	88	166
1 day–1 week	138	100	188
1 week–1 month	162	125	188
1–3 months	161	115	215
3–6 months	147	125	215
6 months–1 year	147	115	188
1–3 years	130	100	188
3–5 years	105	68	150
5–8 years	102	75	150
8–12 years	88	51	125
12–16 years	83	38	125

* Ziegler, R. F.: *Electrocardiographic Studies in Normal Infants and Children.* Charles C Thomas, Publisher, Springfield, Ill., 1951.

Normal rhythmic cardiac contraction is initiated by spontaneous depolarization of the sinoatrial node. This depolarization generates an impulse that spreads sequentially through the atrial wall and specialized internodal tracts to the atrioventricular node, and then to the His bundle and its branches to reach the Purkinje network and to excite the ventricular muscle.

The sinoatrial node first described by Keith and Flack (1907) lies within the right atrial wall adjacent to the superior vena cava. Measuring approximately 5 by 20 mm, it consists of muscle cells surrounding a central artery; close to its center, distinctive rather primitive "P" cells are identifiable, while more peripherally both Purkinje-like fibers and undifferentiated cells are found (James and Sherf, 1968). These "P" or pale cells are probably the pacemaking cells of the sinus node and similar cells can be found in the AV node. The central artery is derived from the right coronary artery in 60 percent of hearts and from the left coronary in the remainder. The sinoatrial node is generously innervated with both sympathetic and parasympathetic fibers.

First described early in the present century, the atrial internodal tracts have only recently been accepted as an integral part of the conducting system and their precise importance remains ill-defined. Three internodal pathways connect the sinoatrial and atrioventricular nodes (James, 1966) and a further tract connects the sinoatrial node to the left atrium. First described some 50 years ago (Wenckebach, 1907; 1908; Thorel, 1909; Bachmann, 1916), their possible role in atrial conduction was minimized when Lewis's theory of uniform atrial impulse transmission gained wide acceptance. Recent electrophysiologic and biochemical studies (de Carvalho et al., 1959; Wagnar et al., 1966) have confirmed that these tracts do in fact conduct impulses more rapidly than the surrounding atrial myocardium thus favoring their role as specialized conducting pathways.

Fibers of all three internodal tracts intermingle near the atrioventricular node, but James (1961) and Sherf and James (1969) have suggested that the "input" area of the atrioventricular node be considered in two main divisions. Most fibers enter the crest of the node delivering impulses that must traverse the entire node; in contrast some fibers enter much more distally bypassing most of the central nodal fibers and connecting almost directly with the His bundle. Impulses carried in this latter pathway may avoid the normal delay inherent in conduction through the atrioventricular node. In theory at least these are potential pathways for abnormal conduction and possible reentry mechanisms. The physiologic significance of this divided input is unclear.

The atrioventricular node lies subendocardially just inferior to the coronary sinus ostium and the medial leaflet of the tricuspid valve, connected above with the internodal tracts and below with the His bundle, which penetrates the fibrous skeleton of the heart. Hoffman and Cranefield (1964) have shown that true atrioventricular nodal fibers do not show spontaneous depolarization and are therefore nonautomatic and cannot normally assume pacemaker function. Automaticity can develop in the coronary sinus portion of the node and in the adjacent junctional tissue between the node and the bundle. His bundle and Purkinje cells can also assume pacing function. The nodal and junctional region is supplied by a specific artery derived from the right coronary artery in 92 percent of hearts and from the left circumflex in the remainder. The AV node is less well innervated than the sinoatrial node and its supply is largely parasympathetic from the left vagus. The His bundle and its branches are also plentifully supplied with vagal fibers.

The His bundle penetrates the cardiac skeleton to reach the crest of the muscular portion of the interventricular septum. From the point where it emerges it gives off fasciculi of the left bundle, which divides into two major and discrete branches.

The anterior branch runs anterosuperior to ramify over the anterior half of the left septal surface and endocardium of the anterior left ventricle. The posterior branch is directed posteroinferior over the posterior half of the septum and the posterior inferior surface of the left ventricle (Lev, 1968).

These two branches run to their respective papillary muscles merging peripherally with the Purkinje network, which facilitates the rapid spread of excitation. From the Purkinje subendocardial plexus an extensive intramyocardial network carries the impulse through the septum and free ventricular wall.

The right bundle branch forms a distinct tract along the lower margin of the crista supraventricularis to the moderator band. Close to the anterolateral papillary muscle it divides into three terminal rami continuous with the Purkinje networks of the inferior, anterior, and lower septal surfaces of the right ventricle.

The right bundle branch and the anterior division of the left bundle derive their blood supply from the left anterior descending coronary artery while the posterior division of the left bundle is usually supplied by the posterior descending coronary artery.

James (1970) has shown that the atrioventricular node and the His bundle arise as separate structures in the embryo and normally fuse in the first gestational month. In patients with congenital complete heart block, there appears to be a failure of fusion although both structures may be present (Huntingford, 1960). Lev and others (1971) have described absence of communication between the atrial musculature and the AV node or His bundle (in the absence of the AV node) in seven patients with congenital atrioventricular block. They suggest that this may be due to a malformation of the central fibrous body during absorption of the bulbus.

The conducting system in congenital heart malformations may have an abnormal course, its continuity may be interrupted, or there may be accessory communications in addition to or in place of the usual pathways (Lev, 1968). Complete or partial atrioventricular block, right bundle branch block, left hemiblock, and Wolff-Parkinson-White syndrome may relate to these abnormalities.

Both persistent atrioventricularis communis and tricuspid atresia are usually associated with characteristic early excitation of the posterior parts of the left ventricle. Feldt and coworkers (1970) have studied the conduction system in atrioventricularis communis and observed that the posterior left bundle branch fascicles have a relatively early origin from the common bundle and that the anterior fascicles appear deficient; furthermore, the right bundle branch appears to have an abnormally prolonged course. Guller and associates (1969) found similar abnormalities in two patients with tricuspid atresia. Anderson and others (1974) studied 11 cases of congenitally corrected transposition. In all, the connecting AV node was situated anteriorly in the right atrium at the lateral junction of pulmonary and mitral valves. An anteriorly situated bundle descended into the morphologic left ventricle (right-sided) and encircled the anterolateral quadrant of the pulmonary outflow tract before descending on the anterior septum and bifurcating. The bundle branches were inverted. In cases with a ventricular septal defect the bundle was related to the anterior quadrants of the defects.

Surgical attempts to correct single ventricle have stimulated studies of the conducting system in this malformation. In single ventricles (both atrioventricular valve orifices opening into a single ventricular sinus, which is associated with two coni leading to the two great arteries) the normal posterior AV node is rudimentary while an accessory anterior AV node is found in the roof of the right atrium. This latter node gives rise to an AV bundle descending in the outflow tract of the posterior vessel to lay in the right margin of the foramen between the main and outlet chambers. The bundle bifurcates astride the septum between the chambers to give a typical left bundle to the main ventricular chamber and right bundle tissue to the outlet chamber (Anderson et al., 1974; Bharati and Lev, 1975). In contrast in true common ventricles in which the AV orifices enter separate sinuses slightly subdivided by a remnant of posterior ventricular septum, the conducting tissue usually lies on a posterior muscular ridge (Lev, 1968).

PHYSIOLOGY

THE microelectrode technique for recording intracellular potentials in cardiac cells has greatly increased our understanding of normal cardiac physiology and the pathophysiology of many cardiac arrhythmias. Several excellent reviews of the subject have been published (Hoffmann and Cranefield, 1964; Pick, 1973). In general, arrhythmias may result from abnormalities of impulse formation or impulse conduction, or both.

Under normal physiologic conditions most cardiac fibers are nonautomatic and a steady potential difference of approximately 90 mv can be recorded across the cell membrane, the interior being negative with respect to the exterior. This resting membrane potential (RMP) is abolished by excitation, becoming momentarily reversed; RMP is then restored in three distinct phases of repolarization. This whole sequence of electrical events is termed the action potential. An external electrical stimulus provokes an action potential only if the stimulus is sufficient to lower the RMP to a critical threshold potential, approximately 65 mv in normal cardiac fibers.

Automatic cardiac fibers are self-excitatory, and their action potentials are characterized by slow spontaneous depolarization during the resting phase probably due to a time-dependent decrease in potassium efflux (Vassalle, 1966). This diastolic depolarization is unique to pacemaker fibers. When the threshold potential is reached, an action potential is generated and a wave of excitation spreads to adjacent nonautomatic fibers. Such automatic cells are found in the sinoatrial node, in the interatrial tract, in the coronary sinus portion of the atrioventricular node, in the junctional region, and in the His-Purkinje system. Under appropriate conditions many of these automatic cells may assume pacemaker capacity, but this function normally resides in the sinoatrial node and all other latent pacemaker cells are suppressed by the wave of excitation originating from the sinoatrial region.

Vassalle (1971) has reviewed the control of automaticity and pointed out that it is more complex than the traditional view that sinoatrial activity is enhanced by sympathetic discharge and suppressed by vagal discharge. Experiments in dogs suggest that right stellate ganglion stimulation accelerates sinus nodal discharge at all frequencies but that low-frequency stimulation of the left stellate ganglion produces slowing of the sinus rate even after bilateral vagotomy. In both cases cardiac contractility is enhanced. These findings suggest a mechanism for increasing cardiac contractility with simultaneous cardiac acceleration.

Both right and left sympathetic nerves apparently enhance ventricular pacemakers to an equal degree.

Increased vagal activity slows spontaneous diastolic depolarization and increases the resting membrane potential of the sinus node. Excessive vagal stimulation may arrest both sinoatrial and atrial activity. Direct vagal control of Purkinje and ventricular pacemakers is probably of little importance. West (1961) and Lange (1965) have performed experiments that suggest that latent pacemakers are subject to a frequency dependent suppression. Pacemaker tissue stimulated at a frequency in excess of its intrinsic rate exhibits a temporary inhibition of its pacemaker ability when stimulation ceases. This overdrive suppression accounts for temporary ventricular standstill occurring during excessive vagal stimulation or following the sudden onset of complete heart block.

Many arrhythmias result from changes in automaticity that may be influenced by alterations in the rate of diastolic depolarization, maximum diastolic potential, and the threshold potential. Catecholamines increase the rate of spontaneous depolarization in the His-Purkinje system, therefore enhancing their pacemaker potential. A rise in temperature, hypoxia, elevated PCO_2, and stretching of the myocardium all tend to augment automaticity and increase the risk of latent pacemakers usurping the sinus node.

Other dysrhythmias especially premature beats and some ectopic tachycardias may result from reentry pathways secondary to areas of abnormal refractoriness coupled with entry and exit block.

Finally, defects of conduction may result in temporary or permanent forms of heart block of varying degree.

SPECIFIC ARRHYTHMIAS

THE following discussion is not intended to be an exhaustive review of all cardiac arrhythmias but rather to highlight some of the special arrhythmias problems seen in children.

Disorders of Impulse Formation

Sinus Tachycardia. The heart rate in normal infants varies considerably from 80 up to 200 beats/minute. It rarely exceeds 200 even with crying or infection and certainly not for prolonged periods. Sinus tachycardia is a persistently elevated heart rate above the expected for age; it often shows slight variations in rate over a period of hours and usually slows slightly during carotid sinus massage returning to the original rate when the pressure is released. Sinus tachycardia is often a compensatory response and has numerous causes including exercise, emotion, anemia, fever, infections, heart failure, hemorrhage, shock, and thyrotoxicosis. Adrenaline, atropine, and other drugs may accelerate the heart.

Lyon and Rauh (1939) reported ten cases of sinus tachycardia (110 to 115 beats/minute) in children persisting for months or years with no evidence of heart disease and no apparent interference with normal activities. One patient at The Hospital for Sick Children, Toronto, was a 13-year-old boy who had a heart rate that was persistently between 130 and 140 even when he was asleep; his tachycardia continued as long as he was followed (between three and four years), but he was able to lead a normal life although he tired more rapidly than many of his friends and was not quite so active. No evidence of heart disease developed.

The ECG shows normal P waves each followed by a normal QRS complex; the P wave duration, P-R and Q-T intervals are usually shortened; S-T depression and flattening or inversion of the T wave may develop if the tachycardia is prolonged and may persist for 12 to 24 hours after the tachycardia ceases.

Treatment of sinus tachycardia is directed toward the underlying cause rather than to the heart rate itself. Attempts to slow the heart with digoxin in the absence of heart failure are nearly always misguided.

Sinus Bradycardia. A persistent heart rate below 90 in infants and below 60 in children may be due to sinus bradycardia (Figure 17–1). This may occur in healthy individuals, especially trained athletes. Bradycardia is less common in children than tachycardia but may occur in some infectious fevers, such as scarlet fever during convalescence. Sinus bradycardia may also arise reflexly in acute nephritis with hypertension and in raised intracranial pressure and jaundice. It also occurs in 20 percent of patients with acute rheumatic fever (Keith, 1938).

The ECG is normal apart from the slow rate, each normal P wave being followed by a normal QRS complex.

Sinus bradycardia requires no treatment per se but the presence of heart block should always be excluded by an ECG.

Sinus Arrhythmia. Irregular impulse formation by the sinus node is called sinus arrhythmia and is present in some degree in most children and young adults but may be difficult to detect in infants. A normal phenomenon, it is occasionally so marked as to suggest a more serious arrhythmia. Its presence does not exclude significant heart disease.

Two varieties can be distinguished. In one the heart rate increases toward end inspiration and slows again during expiration. This variation is related to diminished vagal tone during inspiration. In the other, less common type the arrhythmia bears no relationship to respiration and most often occurs during the administration of digoxin or morphine.

Sinus arrhythmia requires no treatment.

Premature Beats. Premature beats (extrasystoles, ectopic beats) may be atrial, junctional, or ventricular in origin. Although no single mechanism can explain all such beats most are due to reentry pathways. A small area of myocardium remains refractory and consequently unresponsive to the next normal impulse, which bypasses the area; later retrograde conduction returns to the area, which is now responsive, forming the focus for a premature systole. Less commonly a true ectopic focus due to heightened automaticity or the existence of a parasystolic focus may account for premature beats.

The true incidence in childhood is difficult to determine. Robinson (1959) found an incidence of 1 to 2 percent in normal children and between 4 and 6 percent in those with heart disease. Lyon and Rauh (1939) in a large study and literature review found an incidence of 0.06 percent in newborns, 2.2 percent in normal schoolchildren, and 4.3 percent in children with heart disease. All types of premature beats were observed and most were transient.

Although premature beats may be seen in patients with acute rheumatic fever and other forms of myocarditis, they are much less often a feature of digitalis intoxication than in adults.

Most children with premature beats are asymptomatic but some may be conscious of the heart "missing a beat" or may be referred because of the cardiac irregularity.

The ECG is diagnostic; atrial premature beats are typified by a distorted or inverted P wave and normal QRS complexes except when they are very premature and fail to be conducted. Premature junctional beats are recognized by inversion of the P wave, which just precedes, coincides with, or just follows the QRS. Ventricular premature beats may originate anywhere in the ventricles and cause sequential activation of the ventricles resulting in slurred, wide QRS complexes and T waves of the opposite polarity. No preceding P wave is observed. Ventricular premature beats are usually followed by a full compensatory pause.

RESPIRATORY SINUS ARRHYTHMIA L.D., Aged 11 years
Rate   75/min   53/min

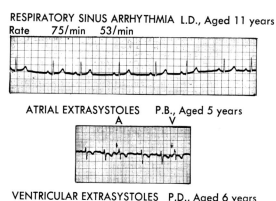

ATRIAL EXTRASYSTOLES   P.B., Aged 5 years
A   V

VENTRICULAR EXTRASYSTOLES P.D., Aged 6 years
A   V

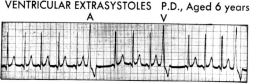

Figure 17-1. Electrocardiograms showing respiratory sinus arrhythmia, atrial premature beats, and ventricular premature beats.

Exercise tends to abolish premature systoles in patients with normal hearts while in heart disease they tend to become more frequent.

No treatment except reassurance of the patient and parents is required when there is no underlying heart disease. Frequent or symptomatic premature beats often respond to oral propranolol, and mild sedation may help to relieve anxiety.

Paroxysmal Supraventricular Tachycardia. Sudden rapid regular rhythm originating in the atria or atrioventricular junctional region with a ventricular rate of between 140 to 240 beats/minute is usually done to supraventricular tachycardia, which may be paroxysmal, repetitive, or occasionally sustained. Paroxysmal supraventricular tachycardia can be regarded as a series of rapidly repeated premature beats. The paroxysms usually start suddenly, last seconds, hours, or days, and end abruptly.

A Greek physician, Claudius Galenas, A.D. 130, practicing in Rome seems to have recognized the existence of paroxysmal tachycardia (Lindqvist, 1956). According to Willius and Dry (1956), the first case described in the literature was by Charles J. B. Williams in 1835.

Stokes in 1854 and Bristowe in 1887 were also among the first to describe recurrent palpitation of extreme rapidity in persons otherwise healthy. Gradually over the years an increasing number of cases have been reported in the medical literature, so that now there is information on several hundred cases in childhood. Taran and Jennings (1937) from 1912 to 1927 reported 52 cases in children under 15 years. Nadas and associates in 1952 reported on 41 cases. Our present series adds another 74 cases and Lundberg's (1963) 39 more. In evaluating the frequency of various heart anomalies in childhood by comparison with certain congenital heart defects, we have estimated that paroxysmal tachycardia occurs once in every 25,000 children.

Etiology

Paroxysmal supraventricular tachycardia may occur in association with many conditions. During most cardiac catheterizations transient arrhythmias are common, especially during manipulations close to the tricuspid valve and in the right ventricular outflow tract. Such arrhythmias are seldom prolonged and rarely serious and usually stop spontaneously when the catheter is withdrawn from the heart. The occasional bout of tachycardia that fails to terminate spontaneously can often be stopped by provoking a ventricular ectopic beat with the catheter tip in the right ventricular outflow tract.

Cardiac surgery may be similarly complicated by rhythm changes both during the operation and in the postoperative period when hypoxia, electrolyte disturbances, and changes in pH may contribute. Digitalis toxicity may produce paroxysmal supraventricular tachycardia with atrioventricular block, although this arrhythmia is uncommon in children.

Seventy percent of patients with Wolff-Parkinson-White syndrome experience one or more episodes of paroxysmal tachycardia. Other factors that have been implicated are emotional stress, hyperthyroidism, hemochromatosis, cardiac tumors, childhood infections, congenital heart disease (especially Ebstein's anomaly), skull fracture, blow on the chest, and rheumatic heart disease.

In our patients omitting those due to cardiac catheterization, anesthesia, and surgery, the etiology of paroxysmal tachycardia was as follows: unknown, 51; Wolff-Parkinson-White syndrome, 14; congenital heart disease, 6; sinus tumors, 2: A similar etiologic incidence was reported by Nadas and coworkers (1952).

Lundberg (1963) found a slightly higher incidence of neuroses, syncope, or peptic ulcer in one or other parent than is found in the general population. He also records the association of attacks with infection in one-sixth of his cases but points out that it is frequently difficult to differentiate between some of the signs of infection and those of heart failure.

Mechanism

Two main theories have been proposed to explain paroxysmal supraventricular tachycardia (PST). The circus movement or gross reentry theory and the unifocal or run of atrial ectopics theory. The available evidence strongly favors the former explanation for most cases.

First proposed by Mines (1913), the circus movement theory has considerably supportive evidence (Durrer et al., 1967; Massumi et al., 1967; Goldreyer et al., 1969; Goldreyer and Bigger, 1970). His bundle recordings taken during onset of PST (paroxysmal supraventricular tachycardia) have helped to document its initiation following atrial premature beats. PST due to reentry has the following features: (1) it is initiated or terminated by an atrial premature beat, (2) during its establishment there is a regular sequence of cycle lengths, and (3) once established the paroxysm has a fixed cycle length (Bellet, 1971).

Lewis (1925), Scherf (1947), and Printzmetal (1952) have been the major proponents of the unifocal theory of origin of PST regarding it as consisting of a run of supraventricular ectopic beats from a single ectopic focus of enhanced automaticity. Acceptance of the circus theory does not exclude the possibility that a unifocal explanation may underlie some cases of clinical PST (Bellet, 1971; Gilette, 1976; Gilette and Garson, 1977).

Clinical Features

Clinical signs and symptoms vary a good deal but depend largely on the presence or absence of cardiac disease, the state of the heart muscle, the duration of the attack, and the patient's emotional state. There are some children who can have an attack of paroxysmal tachycardia without being aware of its occurrence and without showing any symptoms. The examining physician may notice a fast, regular rate, or he may demonstrate it on the electrocardiographic tracing. Such cases usually have a rate less than 200.

The majority of children over the age of five or six are aware of the sudden onset of the tachycardia and usually stop whatever activity they have undertaken and sit or lie down. They may appear slightly pale. Occasionally the tachycardia may proceed for many days or even weeks without showing more signs or symptoms. The children are usually aware of a need for keeping quiet; at least they do not wish to move about and are likely to show some anxiety.

The cases arising in infancy show the most dramatic signs and symptoms. By the time they are brought to the hospital they are frequently quite ill. Most have an ashen complexion; slight cyanosis of the lips is common; the skin may be cold and clammy, the temperature subnormal; irritable movements of the head and arms are common, as is enlargement of the liver. Some may have a few rales in the chest and evidence of edema. Fever may occur as the illness progresses, especially if it is associated with the infection. In atrial tachycardia the heart sounds are extremely constant in intensity. A short, faint systolic murmur is heard in a number of cases, but this disappears when the rate decreases. Pain is frequently reported among adults during an attack but is not commonly present in childhood. The leukocyte count may be markedly elevated (up to 25,000 in our series). Infants in the first two weeks of life have been shown to have a lower ventricular rate than those above this age (Lundberg, 1963).

Nadas and associates (1952) have shown that failure is usually related to the duration of the attack in infancy. If the duration is less than 24 hours, failure rarely occurs; a fifth of the cases show failure in 36 hours, and half of them in 48 hours. The heart rate also influences the onset of failure in that it rarely occurs with rates less than 200. A rate over 200 is not always a decisive factor in the appearance of failure.

Congestive heart failure occurred in 36 percent of our cases in the first year of life but only rarely in those over that age. We had one child of 13 years whose heart rate continued at 210 beats per minute for three weeks. She developed heart failure during the second week. This cleared rapidly when her heart rate returned to normal (Keith and Brown, 1940). Another problem was a boy of 14 years whose tachycardia persisted at 165 for six months and finally ended in death in spite of a variety of forms of therapy. His electrocardiogram showed occasional bursts of normal rhythm occurring under quinidine therapy. The lack of response may have been due to an associated Coxsackie virus infection.

Prolonged PST may produce a fall in stroke output and systemic blood pressure; in the presence of significant heart disease profound cardiovascular collapse may ensue. In those children with normal hearts, failure is most likely to occur in infants with extremely fast rates and prolonged duration of the paroxysm.

The chest x-ray may show significant cardiomegaly with or without pulmonary edema and it may take several days for the heart size to return to normal.

Electrocardiography

The ECG reveals a ventricular rate ranging from 140 to 240 beats/minute; the ventricular complexes are usually normal in contour although occasionally aberrant conduction may widen the QRS complex and make the differentiation from ventricular tachycardia difficult. If P waves are discernible, their configuration differs from that in normal sinus beats; frequently the P wave is buried in with the preceding T wave and is impossible to distinguish. Secondary S-T depression and T wave inversion may occur and may persist for hours or days after termination of the paroxysm. Once normal sinus rhythm is restored, the ECG may show atrial premature beats coupled to the preceding normal beat; the syndrome of Lown-Ganong-Levine, i.e., short P-R interval with normal width QRS; or the Wolff-Parkinson-White syndrome.

Diagnosis

Paroxysmal supraventricular tachycardia must be differentiated from sinus tachycardia, from atrial flutter, and, when aberrant QRS complexes are present, from ventricular tachycardia. Carotid sinus massage may assist the differential diagnosis. In cases where P waves are difficult to detect, an ECG recorded with an esophageal or intra-atrial electrode will often reveal the atrial mechanism and permit distinction between atrial tachycardia with aberrancy and ventricular tachycardia.

Treatment

Many attacks terminate spontaneously. It is usually worth attempting conversion by reflex stimulation of the vagus nerve. This can be achieved by unilateral carotid sinus massage; simultaneous bilateral pressure should not be performed since fatalities have occurred (Nadas et al., 1952). The exact technique is important and should be performed only when monitoring and resuscitative equipment is available. The patient should be recumbent with the head tilted backward and to one side; the artery is compressed against the vertebral column as high up in the neck as possible while the heartbeat is monitored with a stethoscope on the precordium. As soon as the arrhythmia stops, pressure should be released. If massage on one side is unsuccessful the opposite side should be tried.

Steady eyeball pressure applied just below the supraorbital ridge also produces vagal stimulation and may terminate the tachycardia; however, detachment of the retina has occurred as a complication (Figure 17–2). Induction of vomiting or the Valsalva maneuver is occasionally effective in terminating an attack. Failure of any of these procedures in a given attack does not rule out their possible effectiveness in subsequent episodes.

In infants and young children digoxin is undoubtedly the treatment of choice. In our experience and in those cases reported in the literature, 80 percent of attacks in this age group were terminated by this drug usually within one or two days and commonly after the first dose. We use digoxin, 0.06 mg/kg of body weight, giving half this dose immediately (IM), a fourth in four to six hours, and another fourth in 8 to 12 hours. One-tenth of the total digitalizing dose is then given every 12 hours as a maintenance dose. A few patients in the first year of life fail to respond to digoxin, especially those associated with the Wolff-Parkinson-White syndrome or congenital heart anomalies. In these patients propranolol, 0.1 mg/kg given as slow IV injection, is often effective and is the second drug of choice unless failure is severe.

In the desperately ill patient or the resistant patient who failed to respond to digoxin or propranolol, electrical DC countershock should be tried. Paul and Miller (1962) and Pryor and Blount (1964) first reported its successful use for paroxysmal tachycardia in the pediatric age group. In our hands this has proved safe and usually effective and we now regard it as the primary form of treatment in the urgent or resistant case. An initial shock of 10 watt/sec is usually effective in infancy.

Parasympathomimetic drugs such as neostigmine and edrophonium (Tensilon) may be effective either alone or combined with carotid sinus massage; other drugs in this group such as acetyl-β-methylcholine and acetylcholine cause profound hypotension and should be avoided. Edrophonium can only be given IV and is a specific inhibitor of cholinesterase. In infancy 0.5 mg is given over a 30-second period while the patient's cardiac rhythm is monitored. In older children 2 mg is given initially, and if this is ineffective, a further 5 mg can be tried after a ten-minute interval.

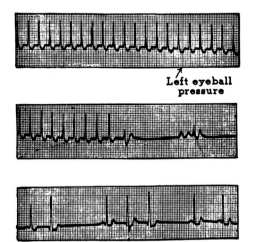

Figure 17-2. D. W., aged nine years, who had occasional attacks of tachycardia. The electrocardiogram (continuous lead II) shows pressure on left eyeball, bringing attack under control.

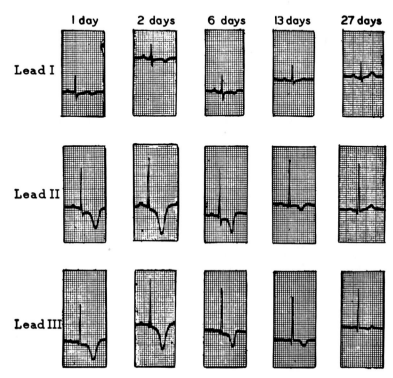

Figure 17-3. T. B., aged 13 years. This tracing shows the inverted T waves that sometimes persist in the electrocardiogram after the paroxysmal tachycardia has returned to normal rhythm. Tracings are shown from the first to the twenty-seventh day after cessation of tachycardia. On the twenty-seventh day the T waves appear normal for the first time.

Toxic effects include excessive vagal stimulation, nausea, diarrhea, excessive salivation, and muscle twitching. Hypotension and both atrial and ventricular asystole may be observed. The duration of action and toxic effects following edrophonium administration are of short duration. Should AV block be produced it may be reversed by 0.5 to 1.0 mg of atropine IV. In our experience recurrences after edrophonium are common and it is unlikely to replace digoxin as the drug of choice.

Quinidine and procainamide have also been used successfully in the past but both have a significant incidence of serious side effects and should probably be reserved for the most resistant cases.

The physician should remember that in older children many attacks terminate spontaneously and may not require overenthusiastic treatment. Many patients can be taught little tricks, such as blowing up a balloon or sticking a finger down their throat, that will often end an attack.

Prevention of Recurrences

Although most infants have only one attack, we usually continue maintenance of digoxin for six months; if there is no recurrence in that period it can be discontinued. If paroxysms are occurring only once or twice a year, no preventive therapy is necessary. In children who experience repeated attacks of paroxysmal tachycardia precipitating causes can seldom be identified but when present should be eliminated as far as possible. Maintenance digoxin may prevent recurrences, but if it is ineffective propranolol, 5 to 10 mg, tid PO alone or in combination with digoxin, may help. In more resistant patients quinidine, 60 to 200 mg daily, or procainamide, 30 to 50 mg/kg/24 hours in divided doses, should be tried.

Conversion of supraventricular tachycardia to sinus rhythm by an appropriately timed atrial or ventricular premature beat induced by an implanted pacemaker has been described in adults as has the control of frequent PST in the Wolff-Parkinson-White syndrome by a permanently implanted pacemaker with electrodes attached to the left atrium. The pacemaker was set to pace at 108/minute and was turned on during a paroxysm by holding a magnet over the implanted unit and converted each paroxysm back to sinus rhythm (Preston and Kirsh, 1970). Dreifus and others successfully treated a five-month-old infant with a similar problem with a permanently implanted radiofrequency pacemaker.

Prognosis

In paroxysmal supraventricular tachycardia the prognosis is good in the vast majority of cases. The mortality is low, probably less than 5 percent (Nadas et al., 1952); our figure is 2 percent. Lundberg (1963) records a mortality of 9 percent in infants in the first year of life, but four of his five deaths were associated with infection or congenital heart disease. The presence of underlying congenital heart disease increases the risk if it is the cyanotic variety. As a group, Nadas and associates (1952) did not find these cases more liable to heart failure during the attacks.

Among those who were successfully treated, 74 percent had one or more recurrences and 26 percent had no recurrence in their follow-up of 1 to 20 years (Nadas et al., 1962). In the group with recurrences, slightly over half had many recurrences, whereas the rest had only one to three return episodes.

The most striking prognostic feature revealed in Nadas and associates' study (1952) was the relation to the age of onset. If the onset occurred in the first four months of life, the recurrence rate was only 22 percent; if it was after the fourth month, the recurrence rate was 83 percent. Lundberg (1963), investigating cases with onset in the first year of life, reported subsequent attacks common in the first year but appearing in only 7 to 12 percent after that. Of over 44 cases with onset in the first year of life, 34 percent had recurrences during the first year. Later they were uncommon. In over 26 cases with onset after the first year of life, the recurrence rate was 58 percent.

PAROXYSMAL VENTRICULAR TACHYCARDIA

This arrhythmia is fortunately rare in childhood and when it does occur, apart from cardiac catheterization, is likely to be associated with serious heart disease. Many examples previously described as ventricular tachycardia in otherwise-normal hearts are undoubtedly examples of supraventricular tachycardia with aberrant ventricular conduction (Radford et al., 1977).

Bellet (1971) has summarized the electrocardiographic features that make the diagnosis of paroxysmal ventricular tachycardia likely:

1. The beats of the paroxysms must be ectopic in origin and conform to those observed as isolated ventricular premature beats before onset of the paroxysms (Figure 17-4).

2. The QRS complexes should be widened (0.12 second or more) and notched.

3. The first step of the paroxysm should bear the same relationship to the preceding normal beat as a ventricular premature beat bears to the previous beat.

4. Ventricles beat regularly or only slightly irregularly at 130 to 180/minute while the atria beat more slowly, regularly, and independently.

5. Occasional ventricular captures are observed (conducted beats from atria with narrow QRS).

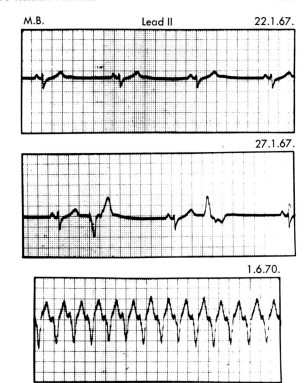

Figure 17-4. Electrocardiograms showing sinus bradycardia (22.1.67), sinus bradycardia with ventricular premature beats (27.1.67), and paroxysmal ventricular tachycardia (1.6.70) in the same patient. Note that the QRS morphology during the tachycardia resembles that of the first premature beat in the second strip.

6. Ventricular fusion beats (from combined ectopic and sinus beats). If all the above are present the diagnosis of a ventricular origin is highly likely; in difficult cases a His bundle electrogram showing His potentials related only to atrial activity will be diagnostic.

This arrhythmia is seldom tolerated for long without developing signs of an inadequate cardiac output; substernal pain, dyspnea, shock, syncope, and congestive cardiac failure may all occur especially if there is serious underlying heart disease.

Treatment depends on the underlying cause and the patient's general condition.

Lidocaine is especially effective in ventricular arrhythmias and is the preferred treatment. Given as an intravenous bolus (1 to 2 mg/kg) it is commonly effective within one or two minutes and suppresses ventricular irritability for up to 20 minutes. If the arrhythmia recurs, a continuous intravenous infusion at a rate of 15 mcg/kg is usually effective in suppressing ventricular ectopic activity and may be continued for many hours if required.

Intravenous quinidine or procainamide may also revert ventricular tachycardia to sinus rhythm but both are associated with a significantly higher incidence of side effects than is lidocaine.

With the exception of ventricular arrhythmias due to digoxin toxicity, which are uncommon in children, phenytoin and propranolol are usually ineffective in the treatment of paroxysmal ventricular tachycardia.

Electric countershock with the DC converter is the treatment of choice for drug-resistant episodes of paroxysmal ventricular tachycardia not due to digoxin.

REPETITIVE PAROXYSMAL TACHYCARDIA

A GROUP of 40 cases with this type of tachycardia was collected by Parkinson and Papp in 1947. These cases all had continuously recurrent runs of paroxysmal tachycardia with intermittent return to normal sinus rhythm for a few beats. Although their ages varied from 4 to 75 years, seven of them were in the pediatric age group. The atrial form was the most common, but a few instances of atrial flutter, atrial fibrillation, and ventricular tachycardia were described.

This form of paroxysmal tachycardia may persist for many months or years. Over half of the cases have an eventual return of normal rhythm, and Parkinson (1947) points out that this is one group in which you can tell the mother that there is a good chance that the child will "grow out of it."

The average rate, including the bursts of tachycardia and normal sinus rhythm, is usually between 120 and 180 per minute. Most children withstand this rate very well, do not go into failure, and are able to lead a normal existence.

We have had one such case, first seen at six years of

age. In his electrocardiogram bursts of sinus rhythm occurred interrupting runs of tachycardia. His average heart rate was between 140 and 150. He attended school, played all sports with the other children, and on occasion walked 3 to 4 miles.

Treatment

Digitalis is indicated where there is an excessive rate and the heart is enlarged or if failure appears, but usually treatment is not required and digitalis is rarely needed. Such therapy does not seem to alter the rate to a significant degree, and its use has been described as disappointing by Parkinson and Papp (1947). Cardioversion or electrical countershock should also be tried in this group.

Prognosis

The prognosis appears to be good in children with this condition, and most cases eventually return to normal sinus rhythm. In any event, the tachycardia does not usually interfere with a normal life.

PERSISTENT PAROXYSMAL ATRIAL TACHYCARDIA

SHACKNOW and coworkers (1954) have published details of 14 cases of persistent paroxysmal atrial tachycardia: 13 cases collected from the literature and one of their own. Three-fourths of these cases were in the pediatric age group at the onset of their tachycardia.

Persistent paroxysmal atrial tachycardia constitutes one of the most difficult problems among the arrhythmias. Fortunately, most cases of tachycardia subside in a few hours to a few days, some with and some without treatment. Persistent cases, however, are refractory to all forms of therapy. In most instances a great variety of drugs have been tried without apparent effect.

In our series we have had one such case: a three-year-old girl who suddenly developed paroxysmal atrial tachycardia and in whom the tachycardia persisted despite treatment with a variety of drugs. During the early stages of her investigation, her heart was considerably enlarged and there was evidence of failure with hepatomegaly and jugular venous distention. Although digitalis did not return the rate to normal, it reduced the rate to around 150/minute partly by slowing the heart and partly by producing occasional intervals of sinus rhythm for one to two beats. However, to do this a large daily dose, approximately 0.5 mg, was required; a larger dose produced extrasystoles and dropped beats. While she was on this form of therapy, her heart was reduced in size to near-normal. She eventually developed nephrosis and died four years after the onset.

In the 14 cases reviewed by Shacknow and associates (1954), palpitation and awareness of the heartbeat were the most common symptoms, usually accompanied by slight shortness of breath on exertion. However, five of these patients were asymptomatic and the arrhythmia was discovered during examination for other reasons. Obviously the rate must have been slow enough so that no enlargement of the heart or heart failure had occurred. There was no evidence in these cases to indicate that the arrhythmia had been present from birth. This is what one would expect since most arrhythmias occurring in the first few months of life cease and do not recur. One patient was said to have tachycardia at six months of age; another patient was 34 years of age when his tachycardia was first noticed. Cardiac enlargement was noted in only 3 out of the 14. No associated disease, such as myocarditis or hyperthyroidism, was found in this group. Congestive heart failure occurred in four but was readily controlled. In Shacknow's own case, the atrial rate remained between 200 and 300 per minute and the ventricular rate varied between 120 and 180 with differing degrees of atrioventricular block.

It is most important to try electrical countershock (cardioversion) in children with this arrhythmia.

Prognosis

The ultimate prognosis in this group is difficult to assess, but some of the cases are asymptomatic and probably have a good outlook; others either have a mild disability or their rate can be controlled with digitalis; a number eventually return to normal after a period of many months or many years. The tachycardia may at times be a contributory cause of death.

ATRIAL FLUTTER

ATRIAL flutter is rare in children. Moller and colleagues (1969) have presented details of six personally observed infants with this arrhythmia and have reviewed published data on 30 other infants. Hoyer and Lyon (1946) were able to collect ten cases from the literature four of whom ranged in age from two to ten years.

Atrial flutter may develop any time from fetal life up through childhood. The majority, however, appear in infancy and a number of reports have dealt with the newborn. Moller and colleagues suggest that two types of atrial flutter may occur. Type I (congenital atrial flutter) is recognized prenatally or within the first week of life; it is more common, has a nearly equal sex distribution, and responds to digitalis in about half the cases. Type II (paroxysmal atrial flutter) is first recognized after age three weeks; it occurs predominantly in males and infrequently responds to digitalization. Of the 36 patients reviewed only three had associated cardiac malformations. There were nine deaths in all. The prognosis for both types was poor either if periods of atrial fibrillation occurred or if a coexistent cardiac defect was present.

The clinical manifestations of atrial flutter are variable and may be quite mild when 2:1 or 3:1 AV block is present. The atrial rate varies between 200 and 450, the ventricular rate being half or one-third or a fourth depending on the degree of block. Consequently the ventricles frequently beat at a rate that does not produce heart failure.

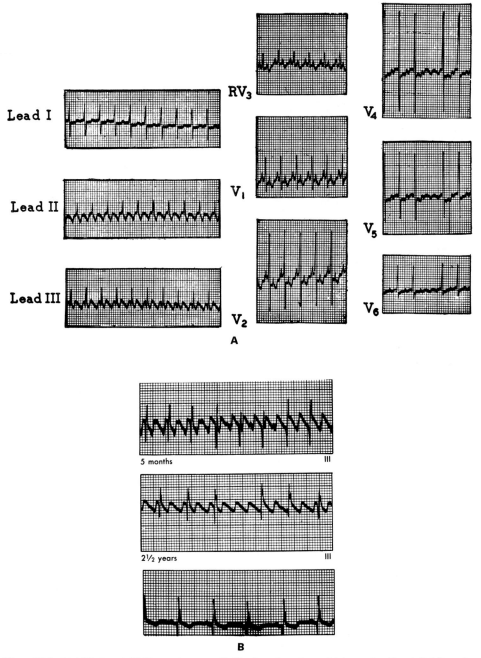

Figure 17-5. Atrial flutter. *A*. W. K., aged one month. Tracings show the ventricles contracting at slightly under 200 per minute and the atria at approximately twice this rate. *B*. Tracings taken at five months and two and one-half years.

Diagnosis

The diagnosis is established by finding typical "F" waves in the electrocardiogram giving a regular, sawtoothed appearance to the tracing. The ventricular rate may be regular with a fixed degree of block or may vary if the degree of block changes (Figure 17–5).

Treatment

Electrical DC countershock is the preferred treatment and has been reported as being particularly successful in this group (Lown et al., 1962; Brown et al., 1964).

Prognosis

In those patients with normal hearts, with onset before birth or within the first week of life, and who respond to digoxin, the prognosis appears to be good. When the onset is later, there is a poor response to therapy, and when associated cardiac disease is present or periods of atrial fibrillation occur, the prognosis should be guarded. In the 36 patients reviewed by Moller and associates there were nine deaths.

ATRIAL FIBRILLATION

ATRIAL fibrillation is uncommon in childhood. It occurs occasionally in older children with advanced rheumatic heart disease and may occur on rare occasions as the result of digitalis intoxication, especially if the serum potassium is lowered. Tumors of the heart involving the atria, such as hamartomas, may also precipitate this arrhythmia. Its appearance as a spontaneous functional disorder occurring suddenly in paroxysms during childhood is very rare. In adults, approximately a fifth of all cases of atrial fibrillation of this latter type are paroxysmal in origin. The two most common etiologic factors in adults are rheumatic heart disease and coronary heart disease. It may also be precipitated by the presence of an atrial septal defect in an adult. Such a cause is uncommon in childhood (Radford and Izukawa, 1977).

Diagnosis

Atrial fibrillation may be suspected in a child when the heartbeat is rapid and continuously irregular, with varying intensity of heart sounds and a marked variability of the cardiac impulse. Heart failure may or may not accompany it. The pulse may be so weak that only a few beats are felt. The heart rate should be measured by stethoscope or electrocardiogram.

The diagnosis is best made by the use of the electrocardiogram (Figure 17–6), which clearly defines the irregularity of the ventricular beats and usually reveals small "F" waves occurring at 300 to 500 per minute, representing the abnormal atrial contractions. The ventricles cannot respond to this rate of stimulation and usually beat at approximately 150 per minute. Both the rapid ventricular rate and the loss of atrial contribution to the ventricular filling impair cardiac output especially during exercise.

Treatment

This arrhythmia usually responds well to digitalis in full doses. Digoxin (0.06 mg/kg) given in divided doses over several hours, as rapidly as required, slows the ventricular rate in the majority of cases. If the ventricular rate is very rapid and an emergency exists, one-fourth of the digitalizing dose may be given intravenously and repeated in 15 to 30 minutes, until digitalization is completed; then the digitalization may be carried on with one-fifth of the digitalizing dose as long as it is necessary to control the rate. Some cases will revert to normal rhythm; others will need such therapy continuously.

Electrical countershock may be effective in converting atrial fibrillation to sinus rhythm although recurrences are common in adults (Brown et al., 1964).

WOLFF – PARKINSON – WHITE SYNDROME AND ITS VARIANTS (PREEXCITATION; WPW SYNDROME)

IN 1930 Wolff, Parkinson, and White first described an entity characterized by paroxysmal tachycardia and between attacks electrocardiographic abnormalities including a short P-R interval, widening of the QRS interval, and a delta wave, the latter being a slurring of the initial portion of the QRS complex and representing premature ventricular excitation. In adults the criteria for diagnosis include a P-R interval that is 0.12 second or less and a QRS of 0.11 second or more. Mannheimer (1946) pointed out that 0.09 second is probably the upper limit of normal for the QRS duration in children and consequently a QRS of 0.10 second is a criterion of this condition for this age group. Its importance lies in the susceptibility of such patients to paroxysmal tachyarrhythmias and because the electrocardiogram may simulate that of serious heart disease. The WPW syndrome has recently been reviewed by Narula (1973).

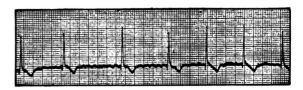

Figure 17-6. Atrial fibrillation. D. B., aged 11 years.

WPW syndrome results from premature excitation (preexcitation) of one or other ventricles occurring when the sinus impulse partially or completely bypasses the normal atrioventricular junctional pathways. Several potential anomalous pathways have been described. Kent (1914) first described anomalous atrioventricular pathways, and their existence has more recently been confirmed anatomically by Lev (1966) and electrophysiologically by mapping during cardiac surgery (Durrer and Roos, 1967). James (1966) has described bypass fibers around the AV node. Maheim and Clerc (1932) have reported fibers connecting the conducting bundles to the ventricular septum. The existence of these pathways, which may be involved alone or in combination, allows rational explanations to be made of the ECG features of classic WPW and its variants.

These variants include a normal P-R with a prolonged QRS and prominent delta wave or a short P-R with a delta wave but normal QRS duration. Lown and coworkers (1952) described the association of a short P-R interval and a normal QRS duration and configuration. All these variants may be associated with paroxysmal tachycardia. Unlike classic WPW the Lown–Ganong–Levine syndrome is more common in females.

The true incidence of the preexcitation syndromes in the general nonhospital population is unknown. Most authors suggest an incidence of about 0.1 percent of unselected children (Landtman, 1947; Joseph et al., 1958). Tamm (1956) discovered 17 cases in 5500 children, while Swiderski and associates (1962) reported an incidence of 0.5 percent in children with suspected heart disease. Approximately 40 percent of children with WPW have associated congenital heart disease, most commonly Ebstein's anomaly, L-transposition of the great arteries, and familial or primary myocardial disease. About 70 percent of the patients are males.

Because WPW is often transient or intermittent it has been difficult to determine the role of heredity in its etiology. Although there have been several reports of its familial occurrence, Warner and McKusick (1958) concluded that heredity was not a significant factor on the basis of their detailed study of 14 families including 80 members. Certainly no pattern of inheritance has yet been established.

Classic WPW syndrome has been divided into types A and B (Rosenbaum et al., 1945). Type A is

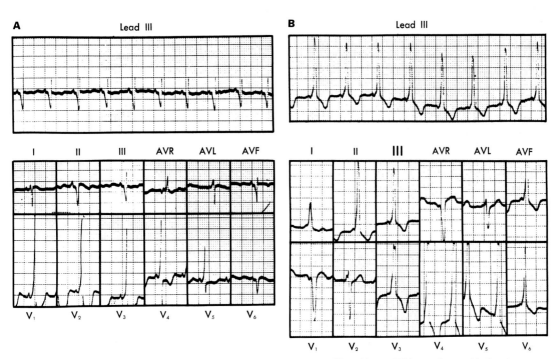

Figure 17-7. Electrocardiograms showing type A and type B Wolff-Parkinson-White syndrome. Notice the short P-R interval and wide QRS complexes with a slurred upstroke (delta wave).

characterized by large R waves in the right precordial leads while type B shows large negative deflections in the same leads (Figure 17–7). These findings suggest that the anomalous pathway in type A involves the left bundle and left ventricle and the right bundle and ventricle in type B. Although the combination of WPW with true bundle branch block is uncommon, it may occur and in such cases the vectorcardiogram may be helpful. In both conditions there is relative delay in activation of one ventricle, which is manifested in the VCG by increased proximity of the dots in the vector loop. In WPW this delay always involves the initial portion of the loop, while in left or right bundle branch block the delay is seen in the midsection of the loop.

Premature beats and tachyarrhythmias occur in about 70 percent of patients with the Wolff-Parkinson-White syndrome. Paroxysmal atrial tachycardia is most common but atrial fibrillation and flutter also occur. Occasionally ventricular fibrillation may cause sudden death (Wood et al., 1943). Durrer and Roos (1967) suggested that retrograde conduction via the anomalous pathway with reactivation of the atria was the basic mechanism underlying the arrhythmia. Epicardial mapping at surgery has confirmed retrograde conduction through these pathways.

Prognosis

The prognosis depends on the frequency and severity of attacks of paroxysmal tachycardia and on the presence or absence of associated cardiac disease. Infants with otherwise normal hearts who first develop PAT under six months have the best prognosis; although the WPW pattern may persist, the bouts of tachycardia usually cease. Patients presenting for the first time at an older age are more likely to suffer recurrences. When an associated heart defect is present, the prognosis becomes that of the basic lesion. Giardina and associates (1972) reviewed 62 infants and children with WPW. In 29 patients and six children treated for paroxysmal supraventricular tachycardia, digoxin relieved the episodes in all but one and prevented recurrences in all but four. Only 4 of 46 patients followed as children and adolescents had tachyarrhythmias. These authors concluded that

the prognosis into adult life for infants and children with WPW with or without episodes of tachycardia is good.

Treatment of Paroxysmal Supraventricular Tachycardia in WPW Syndrome

As indicated previously, digoxin is the preferred drug in children with paroxysmal supraventricular tachycardia. Propranolol may also effectively terminate the tachycardia and prevent recurrences. Quinidine and procainamide have been used successfully to terminate attacks but are not recommended in children.

Atropine, by enhancing normal conduction, and quinidine or procainamide, by increasing refractoriness of the accessory pathway, may all tend to normalize the ECG between attacks. Propranolol is probably the most valuable agent for preventing recurrences.

Amiodarone, initially introduced as an antianginal drug, has shown some promise in controlling recurrent tachyarrhythmias in adults with WPW syndrome (Rosenbaum et al., 1974).

In drug-resistant episodes cardioversion is frequently successful in terminating attacks but is naturally of no value in prevention.

An intracardiac electrode catheter used to provoke premature atrial depolarization or retrograde atrial depolarization by ventricular stimulation may terminate the supraventricular tachycardia by interrupting the reentry pathway (Durrer and Roos, 1967; Massumi et al., 1967). Dreifus and others (1971) reported successful treatment of a five-week-old infant with recurrent WPW tachycardia using a radio frequency pacemaker (permanently implanted). During attacks the pacemaker was switched on by a magnet held near the generator. The fixed-rate competitive pacing terminated the episodes.

The techniques of epicardial mapping has resulted in successful surgical interruption of anomalous conduction pathways (Cobb et al., 1968). Gallager and coworkers (1975) have recently reviewed the evaluation and surgical prevention of recurrent tachycardia in patients with the WPW syndrome.

ATRIOVENTRICULAR JUNCTIONAL RHYTHMS

AV junctional rhythms are uncommon and usually transient in children. If the sinus node fails to pace the heart or if its intrinsic rate falls below that of the AV junctional region, the AV junction may assume pacemaker function usually with a rate between 40 and 60. Occasionally AV junctional automaticity may be enhanced so that its rate exceeds that of the sinus node resulting in junctional tachycardia. Finally, should the AV node fail to conduct atrial

impulses, the AV junction may again assume pacemaking. Automatic fibers also lie close to the coronary sinus ostium and are capable of assuming pacemaker function producing coronary sinus rhythm.

Junctional rhythms are most often a transient feature in rheumatic and other myocarditis, during cardiac catheterization and surgery, or during therapy with digoxin or parasympathomimetic drugs. Junctional rhythms are not uncommon following the Mustard operation for transposition when they may be permanent.

Bacos and associates (1960) described the familial occurrence of junctional rhythm. In children with congenital heart disease the presence of coronary sinus rhythm suggests partial anomalous venous return to the right atrium or a persistent left superior vena cava associated with an atrial septal defect (Hancock, 1964).

The electrocardiogram is usually diagnostic; the P wave may precede, coincide with, or follow the QRS and is inverted or abnormal in shape. Occasionally P waves are absent. The QRS is usually of normal width and configuration but occasionally shows aberrant conduction. In coronary sinus rhythm the P-R is normal or slightly short (0.10 to 0.17 second); the P wave is negative in leads II and III and often peaked. Its axis is deviated to the left.

Junctional and coronary sinus rhythms are usually transient and treatment is directed toward the underlying cause. AV junctional tachycardia is sometimes paroxysmal when the causative factors, clinical picture, and management are similar to paroxysmal atrial tachycardia.

DEFECTS OF CONDUCTION: ATRIOVENTRICULAR HEART BLOCK

ATRIOVENTRICULAR heart block may be partial or complete. Partial block is further divided into first and second degree. All types may be temporary, intermittent, or permanent.

The P-R interval represents total conduction time of the cardiac impulse from the sinoatrial node, through the atria, atrioventricular node, bundle of His, and its branches to the onset of ventricular activation. Since Scherlag and colleagues (1969) demonstrated the feasibility of direct recordings of His bundle electrical activity in patients it has become possible to separate conduction into four components: intra-atrial; AV nodal; bundle of His; and the bundle of branches and Purkinje network. All degrees of block may develop at any of these sites.

First-Degree Heart Block

First-degree heart block most commonly involves abnormal delay in the AV nodal region and manifests as a prolongation of the P-R interval in the standard ECG. The P-R interval varies with both age and heart rate (Ziegler, 1951; Sodi Pallares et al., 1958), and there exist several studies of P-R intervals in normal children. The values published by Ziegler (1951) do not allow for heart rate changes. Ashman and Hull's (1937) figures were considered inadequate by Alimurung and Massell (1956) but their own figures are unreliable because of the small numbers of patients in many of the groups. Clarke and Keith (1972) have published maximum P-R intervals according to heart rate and age based on their study of 672 normal children whose ages ranged from 5 to 15 years. They confirmed the linear relationship between P-R interval and heart rate first observed by Alimurung and Massell. First-degree heart block may be defined as P-R prolongation greater than the maximum P-R interval for heart rate and age.

The P-R interval may be abnormally prolonged during rheumatic fever (Parkinson et al., 1920; Keith, 1938; Mirowski et al., 1964). In a study of 445 patients with acute rheumatic fever using their new criteria for maximum P-R interval Clarke and Keith (1972) found that 75 percent of the patients had P-R prolongation. There was no difference between those with carditis and those without cardiac involvement.

Viral infections, diphtheria, vagal stimulation, digoxin, and propranolol may all be associated with first-degree heart block, which may also follow cardiac surgery or occur during catheterization. Certain congenital cardiac anomalies listed in Table 17–2 tend to have abnormally long P-R intervals.

Table 17–2. P-R INTERVAL IN CONGENITAL HEART DISEASE IN CHILDHOOD

DIAGNOSIS	P-R INTERVAL WITH 0.18 SECOND OR MORE
	Percent
L- or corrected transposition of great arteries	57
Ebstein's disease	50
Atrial septal defect	43
Coarctation of the aorta	12
Complete anomalous pulmonary vein drainage	8
Ventricular septal defect	6
Patent ductus arteriosus	3.4
Pulmonary stenosis	3
Tetralogy of Fallot	2
Transposition of great vessels	0
Tricuspid atresia	0

While usually an electrocardiographic diagnosis, first-degree heart block may be suspected clinically by softening of the first heart sound. Although it may have diagnostic implications, it does not cause symptoms nor does it require treatment per se.

Second-Degree Heart Block

Second-degree heart block may result from progressive lengthening of the P-R interval in succeeding cycles until the impulse fails to be conducted to the ventricles and a ventricular beat is "dropped." The cycle then repeats. Usually the P-R interval increments get smaller until the beat is dropped. This phenomenon first described by Wenckebach (1914) retains his name but is alternatively referred to as Mobitz type-I block. The Wenckebach phenomenon occurs in association with the same conditions that cause first-degree heart block.

In a less common form of second-degree block ventricular beats are dropped without previous P-R prolongation and the P-R interval is usually constant for conducted beats. The dropped beats may occur periodically or constantly when ventricular complexes occur only after every second, third, or fourth atrial beat resulting in 2:1, 3:1, or 4:1 AV block, 2:1 is most common. This form of second-degree block is usually due to bilateral bundle branch problems. This is often called Mobitz type-II heart block and indicates a more serious prognosis often progressing to complete heart block. The pathophysiology of second-degree atrioventricular block has been reviewed by El Sherif and coworkers (1975).

Unless the heart rate is slow, second-degree heart block seldom causes symptoms. On auscultation the first heart sound may progressively diminish in intensity. Exercise or atropine may abruptly double the ventricular rate in 2:1 heart block. If they do not do so, and the ventricular rate is below 60, complete atrioventricular block should be suspected.

Complete Atrioventricular Heart Block

Complete atrioventricular heart block results from absolute failure of the atrial impulse to be transmitted to the ventricles. The atria and ventricles beat independently, the former usually in response to the sinus node and the latter at a slower rate responding to a pacemaker situated in the lower AV junctional region, the bundle of His, or more distally. In general, the lower the pacemaker lies in the conducting system, the slower the idioventricular rate. Complete AV block may result from lesions proximal to, within, or distal to the His bundle and may involve a single lesion within the bundle or multiple lesions in each of the three fascicles.

Complete heart block in childhood may be congenital or acquired and be temporary or permanent. Our overall experience at The Hospital for Sick Children is summarized in Table 17–3.

Table 17–3. COMPLETE ATRIOVENTRICULAR HEART BLOCK

Congenital	Isolated	67
	Associated congenital heart disease	23
Acquired	Postoperative	40
	Acute rheumatic fever	2
	Acute streptococcal infection	1

Pathogenesis

Strictly speaking, congenital atrioventricular heart block is that which is known to be present at birth; however, heart block discovered in early childhood in the absence of any known cause and in which no previous examination has revealed sinus rhythm is usually regarded as congenital. Morquio (1901), in describing a family in which several siblings had bradycardia, syncope, and died in childhood, first suggested that complete heart block may be congenital. Several cases have been recognized in utero. Lev (1972) has reviewed with examples the origins of congenital AV block, which may be due to (1) discontinuity between the atrial musculature and the more peripheral conducting system, (2) interruption of the His bundle, and (3) pathologic changes in an aberrant conduction system.

While congenital block is more commonly seen in an otherwise normal heart, it may occur in association with other cardiac defects especially L-transposition of the great arteries but also with atrioventricularis communis, endocardial fibroelastosis, and ventricular septal defect. Temporary complete heart block has been attributed to mumps (Rosenberg, 1945). Diphtheria and rheumatic fever may cause complete heart block while certain drugs such as digoxin and quinidine may produce it temporarily.

Clinical Features

Although congenital complete heart block may be detected in utero suggesting fetal distress, it is more often not discovered until the child is a few years old. Of 67 children with isolated complete heart block seen at The Hospital for Sick Children the mean age of referral and recognition was 4.9 years and the mean heart rate, 60. All were recognized by eight years. Congenital heart block seldom causes symptoms and is usually compatible with normal growth and development (Miller and Rodriguey-Cororel, 1968). Most patients lead active lives (Campbell and Emanuel, 1967), and Ikkos and Hanson (1960) have shown that these patients have a normal physical working capacity. Sixty-four percent of our patients were completely asymptomatic while 30 percent tired easily on exertion. Kenmore and Cameron (1967) described normal pregnancy and delivery in a patient with congenital complete heart block. Symptomatology and prognosis depend on (1) the site and stability of the idioventricular pacemaker and (2) the presence or absence of associated congenital heart disease. In the isolated form problems such as congestive heart failure or syncope are most likely to occur in infancy. However, two patients of ours developed syncope for the first time at ages 10 and 12 years, respectively.

There is a clear association between syncopal attacks and heart rate. If the rate falls below 40 to

45/minute such attacks are likely, and untreated the prognosis is grave (Taussig, 1960).

Systolic ejection murmurs are common probably as a result of the increased stroke volume. The first heart sound varies in intensity, as noted by Dock (1933). Faint atrial sounds may be heard during the longer diastolic pauses and a rapid inflow type of mitral diastolic murmur was present in 17 percent. Venous pressure is elevated and venous cannon waves can be seen whenever the right atrium contracts against a closed tricuspid valve.

The slow ventricular rate results in an increased stroke volume and end-diastolic heart volume. Consequently, the cardiothoracic ratio on chest x-ray was greater than 55 percent in over half our patients. The ECG shows complete heart block and in 50 percent of the patients left ventricular hypertrophy was present (Figure 17–8).

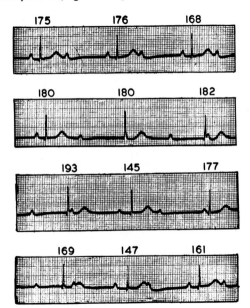

Figure 17-8. M. M., aged seven years, who had complete heart block. The electrocardiogram (continuous lead II) shows the ventricular rate varying from 35 to 45 per minute, and the atrial rate varying from 60 to 68 per minute (figures equal milliseconds since preceding QRS).

Prognosis

Fortunately, the ventricular pacemaker in congenital heart block is usually a single stable focus in the AV junctional or His bundle tissue. The QRS complexes in the ECG are narrow and of normal contour. The resting rate is usually from 45 to 60/minute and many patients can increase their rate by 10 to 20 beats/minute on exertion. Such patients do well.

Four of our patients with isolated complete heart block died, one from drowning possibly due to an Adams-Stokes attack. Three had definite Adams-Stokes episodes as the terminal event. The four deaths occurred at two days, two months and two at 30 months. Molthan and associates (1962) report three cases of congenital heart block in children with repeated Adams-Stokes attacks ultimately causing death. They stressed the importance of wide QRS complexes with a left bundle branch block pattern in suggesting a poor prognosis. Ventricular rates at birth under 30 beats/minute with multifocal QRS complexes carry an especially unfavorable significance and suggest prenatal toxic or inflammatory etiology rather than the more usual developmental causes.

Acquired complete heart block in childhood is almost always a surgical problem and may especially follow closure of a ventricular septal defect or intracardiac repair of Fallot's tetralogy. It may also complicate atrial septal defect closure, Mustard's operation, and procedures on the aortic and mitral valve. Although usually an immediate and permanent complication, it may occur temporarily in the immediate postoperative period. Although such patients usually recover normal sinus rhythm within a few days, it has recently been recognized that some of these patients may develop complete heart block months or even years after their surgical procedure. The pattern of left anterior hemiblock associated with right bundle branch block and a prolonged P-R interval may provide a clue to those patients at risk of developing late complete heart block (Moss et al., 1972).

Acquired heart block is usually associated with a slower idioventricular rate, wider QRS complexes often of abnormal contour, less response to exercise, congestive heart failure, and syncope. The prognosis is grave and treatment is nearly always required.

Treatment

Congenital heart block requires no treatment unless syncope or unremitting heart failure develops. Temporary acquired heart block due to drugs, acute rheumatic fever, or renal failure can be managed with a temporary transvenous pacing catheter lodged in the right ventricle. The power unit may be either a fixed rate or demand unit according to the clinical situation. Permanent congenital heart block or acquired heart block causing symptoms should be managed by insertion of a permanent pacing unit. In older children the most satisfactory combination is a demand unit buried in the axilla and attached to a transvenous pacing catheter in the right ventricular apex. In small children the unit is better attached to epicardial electrodes because of possible displacement by growth. The chief advantage of the demand unit is that it avoids competition with the patient's own rhythm; whenever the patient's heart accelerates above the preset pacemaker rate, an inhibitory circuit is activated that prevents further stimulus discharge until the ventricular rate once more falls below the critical level.

While pacemakers are becoming increasingly reliable and efficient, there are considerable problems involved in the mangement of children with permanent pacemakers. The need for frequent hospital visits, the problems of growth, and the psychologic stresses on both child and parents can be almost overwhelming. The indications for such therapy should be strictly observed.

Although isoproterenol given intravenously or sublingually may increase the heart rate in complete heart block there is little place for its use therapeutically. Its effect is too unpredictable, the risk of ventricular tachyarrhythmias too great, to permit its use except under emergency circumstances where temporary pacing is not possible.

Artificial Pacemakers

Attempts to control the heartbeat by direct electrical stimulation were described in the early 1800s. In 1952 Zoll restored effective cardiac action in patients with Adams-Stokes attacks by transthoracic pacing. This successful demonstration stimulated further research culminating in Chardack's (1960) completely implantable system powered by a mercury cell battery. The basic principles of this technique have been widely accepted and pacemaker units have become increasingly sophisticated. While the earlier models relied on epicardial electrodes attached to the myocardium at thoractomy, Furman and Schwedel showed that a permanently implanted transvenous catheter could be used to stimulate the right ventricle, and this method has been adapted to a completely implanted transvenous pacing system. Semiflow-directed pacing catheters have made this a relatively simple procedure. Direct transvenous endocardial pacing has become the preferred method in most adult centers and may be used temporarily or permanently. In children growth may displace the transvenous pacing catheter from the apex of the right

ventricle, and at present epicardial electrodes placed during thoracotomy are preferred in this age group.

Pacemaker units are of two major types. One is fixed-rate units in which pacing is independent of the electrical activity of the heart. Although these pacemakers are relatively simple and less prone to premature failure, they carry the risk of competition with the patient's intrinsic rhythm especially if sinus rhythm is restored. If the pacemaker stimulus falls during the vulnerable period of ventricular de-polarization, ventricular fibrillation may be induced. Noncompetitive pacemakers have been designed to avoid this problem and are of several subtypes. Ventricular-inhibited demand pacemakers stimulate only when the patient's ventricular rate falls below the preset pacemaker rate; otherwise the patient's own QRS complex is fed back to the unit and the generator suppressed. Ventricular-triggered standby pace-makers sense normally occurring QRS complexes and immediately discharge into the absolute refractory period of these beats; if there is no spontaneous beat, the pacer will discharge at its preset escape interval.

Atrial synchronous pacing requires two electrodes. An atrial electrode senses the P wave and the heart is paced after a suitable delay by a ventricular electrode. A long refractory period prevents rapid ventricular pacing in the event of atrial tachycardia, flutter, or fibrillation.

Early models of demand (ventricular-inhibited) pacemakers could be inhibited by external electrical equipment such as electric shavers, radar sources, cautery, and microwave grills; however, improved generator screening has reduced the risk in later models. The present functional life for all types of generator is about 24 to 36 months, but there are strong hopes of extending this period with newer designs such as the lithium-based cell and the nuclear power source, which hopefully may last eight to ten years.

CARDIOAUDITORY SYNDROME

JERVELL and Lange-Nielsen (1957) first described the curious association of congenital deafness with Q-T prolongation in the ECG, episodes of syncope, and risk of sudden death. Subsequent reports (Ward, 1964) have described Q-T prolongation and the other features in the absence of deafness. Both syndromes may occur on a familial basis although the exact model of inheritance is not clear. James has reviewed the various forms of Q-T prolongation and its relationship to arrhythmias.

The incidence of Q-T prolongation in congenitally deaf children seems to vary between 0.1 to 1.0 percent (Frazer et al., 1964). Syncopal attacks begin early but generally after the first year of life and are due to paroxysmal ventricular fibrillation or short periods of asystole (Olley and Fowler, 1970). Attacks are often

precipitated by fear or other emotional stimuli and may be fatal.

The pathogenesis is unknown. Most probably this syndrome represents an abnormal response to adrenergic stimulation. A certain amount of experimental evidence supports this view. Alternative hypotheses have included abnormalities in the vascularization of the sinus node or in myocardial metabolism.

The possible relationship of this condition to abnormal sympathetic activity suggests possible therapy. Schwartz and colleagues (1975) reviewed the world experience with this condition. They were able to obtain data on 220 patients. They concluded that untreated patients have a poor prognosis (mortality rate 73 percent) and that in patients treated with drugs

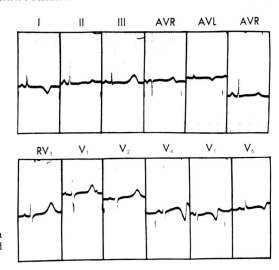

Figure 17-9. Cardioauditory or Surdo-cardiac syndrome in a 6-year-old boy. Note the long Q-T interval (0.56 second) and the abnormal T-wave inversion.

other than beta blockers the prognosis is equally bad; beta blockers clearly reduce the mortality (to 6 percent) and are effective in the majority of patients. In the few patients in whom medical treatment was only partially suppressive left sympathectomy was completely effective and also shortened the Q-T interval (3/3 patients).

This condition should be suspected in any deaf child who suffers from "convulsions." The ECG is diagnostic (Figure 17–9).

POSTOPERATIVE ARRHYTHMIAS

CHANGES in cardiac rhythm are common and extremely varied in the immediate postoperative period. Fortunately most are temporary and secondary to surgical trauma, anesthetic agents, disturbances in acid-base status, electrolyte imbalance, or digoxin. They may, however, seriously interfere with cardiac function and usually require prompt treatment. Of more long-term significance is the appreciation that certain operations are associated with a significant incidence of late rhythm problems (Figure 17–10).

Surgically Induced Right Bundle Branch Block with Left Anterior Hemiblock

Right ventriculotomy as employed in the surgical correction of tetralogy of Fallot and frequently in closing simple ventricular septal defects is commonly followed by the electrocardiographic pattern of complete right bundle branch block (RBBB). This may be due to either proximal or distal damage to the right bundle branch (Gelband et al., 1971; Krongrad et al., 1974). Postventriculotomy right bundle branch block may increase the risk of complete heart block in these patients later in life when acquired left bundle disease becomes not uncommon. In some patients RBBB is associated with left anterior hemiblock (LAH), and the incidence of this bifascicular block pattern has been variously reported as being from 8 to 22 percent of patients undergoing tetralogy or

ventricular septal defect correction. RBBB with left anterior hemiblock may be considered to be present when RBBB is associated with a QRS axis of 240 to 360° in the frontal plane. The true significance of this electrocardiographic finding remains uncertain. In coronary artery disease and cardiomyopathies this pattern is a known percursor of complete heart block. Wolff and coworkers (1972) reported a high incidence of late-onset complete heart block in postsurgical patients with bifascicular block. Sudden death occurred in 12 percent of these patients compared with 2 percent in a control group with RBBB alone. The overall late mortality was 25 percent compared with 2 percent for the control group. Subsequent reports have been less pessimistic about the significance of this finding.

Experience at The Hospital for Sick Children, Toronto, suggests that the prognosis for patients with this electrocardiographic lesion may be much better than first reported. Of 382 patients undergoing correction of tetralogy of Fallot, 24 percent developed right bundle branch block with left anterior hemiblock postoperatively. However, the long-term morbidity and mortality for these patients was no worse than for those with right bundle branch alone. The single most predictive factor in determining a high risk of late complete block was the occurrence of temporary complete heart block in the immediate postoperative period. Twelve of forty-seven patients with immediate postoperative complete heart block suffered late dysrhythmic problems; there were three deaths, eight in complete block were

D.G.   Lead II   5.12.63.

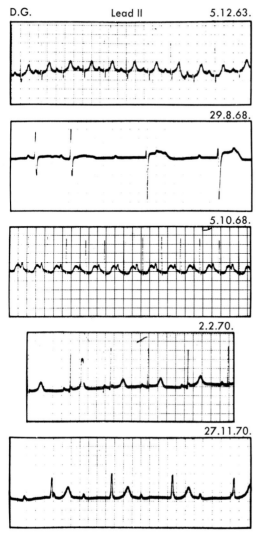

29.8.68.

5.10.68.

2.2.70.

27.11.70.

Figure 17-10. Electrocardiograms from a girl who underwent surgical closure of a ventricular septal defect on August 28, 1968. The top tracing shows sinus rhythm present to the time of surgery. The immediate postoperative tracing, August 29, 1968, shows periods of complete block with an idioventricular rhythm. Four weeks later sinus rhythm returned and persisted for two years. In November, 1970, complete heart block recurred and has persisted. The patient has a permanent pacemaker.

treated with permanent pacemakers, and one with RBBB-LAH was given a demand pacemaker because of syncope. Only 2 of the 354 patients without temporary postoperative complete heart block have died because of late onset arrhythmia (Sondheimer et al., 1976). Denes and others (1975) performed electrophysiologic studies in 119 adults with chronic bifascicular block (RBBB and LAH). Although they found a higher two-year cumulative mortality in those patients with prolonged His bundle to ventricular conduction than those with normal conduction, the difference was not statistically

significant. The follow-up period was, however, relatively short. At the present time, it seems inappropriate to recommend long-term pacemakers in patients with either the ECG pattern of RBBB and LAH or those with a history of temporary complete block in the immediate postoperative period.

Postsurgical complete heart block requires insertion of a permanent artificial pacemaker, as discussed previously.

Disease of the sinoatrial node or injury secondary to suturing or cannulation of the superior vena cava during cardiac bypass may result in the sick sinus syndrome. The general features of this syndrome has been reviewed by Moss and Davis (1974) and by Ferrer (1974). Failure of impulse formation in the sinus node or failure of transmission of the sinus impulse to depolarize the atrial myocardium causes bradycardia, but symptoms are unlikely unless there is also failure or delay in the onset of escape rhythms originating in the junctional region. Symptomatic sinus node disease therefore usually implies additional conducting-tissue disease beyond the sinus node. Periods of sinus arrest, sinus bradycardia, slow or rapid junctional rhythms, supraventricular ectopic beats, and supraventricular tachycardia including atrial flutter or fibrillation may all occur in the same patient although ventricular ectopic activity is uncommon. The occurrence of both bradycardia and tachycardia in the same patient gives rise to the alternative name of the brady-tachyarrhythmic syndrome.

Sick sinus syndrome is essentially an electrocardiographic diagnosis and has been subclassified by Easley and Goldstein (1971) into type I, in which sinus bradycardia or sinus arrest predominates, and type II in which paroxysmal tachycardia predominates. Radford and Izukawa (1975) reviewed 20 patients with symptomatic sick sinus syndrome requiring treatment. Fifteen of these patients had had preceding cardiac surgery, most commonly a Mustard correction of transposition; however, the syndrome was also seen after patch closure of an atrial septal defect (three patients) repair of total anomalous pulmonary venous return (one), and correction of tetralogy of Fallot (two). In the five patients who had symptomatic sick sinus syndrome without preceding surgery the most common etiology appeared to be viral myocarditis. Symptoms included syncope, palpitations, dyspnea, pallid spells, and nonanginal chest pain.

Treatment of this condition is frequently difficult and is indicated only for patients with significant symptoms or if the arrhythmia is producing congestive heart failure. Drug therapy with digoxin or propranolol may suppress paroxysmal tachycardia but may cause more profound bradycardia between such episodes. Cardioversion carries an increased risk in these patients (Lown, 1967) but it is often necessary to terminate persistent tachycardia. Patients with syncope or intractable heart failure due to the bradycardia require the insertion of a permanent cardiac pacemaker.

HIS BUNDLE ELECTROGRAMS

PIONEERED by Scherlag and colleagues (1969), His bundle electrograms (HBE) have been the subject of numerous recent reports (Scherlag et al., 1972; Haft, 1973) that have reviewed the use and limitations of this technique and suggested standardization of both methodology and nomenclature. More recently techniques for recording atrioventricular nodal, right bundle branch, and left bundle branch potentials have been described.

Coupled with simultaneous recordings of the surface ECG, the HBE can provide more precise localization of the site of block or delay in patients with conduction defects. HBEs have proved useful in analyzing certain arrhythmias and in studying the WPW syndrome (Castellanos et al., 1971). Roberts and Olley (1972) and Abella and coworkers (1972) have established normal conduction times for children of different ages.

Several ECG patterns may be associated with a risk of developing subsequent complete heart block, e.g., right bundle branch block with left-axis deviation, left bundle branch block with right-axis deviation, and left bundle branch block. HBEs recorded from these patients may eventually prove predictive in indicating which patients are at highest risk by unmasking conduction problems inapparent in the surface ECG.

In addition to the above uses, the HBE has been used by several groups to study the effect of various drugs on the conducting system. Largely an investigative technique at present, the clinical indications for His bundle electrocardiography will become more clearly defined in the future.

DRUGS IN ARRHYTHMIAS

Digoxin

In addition to its positive inotropic action, digoxin has several effects on heart muscle important in understanding its action in management of certain arrhythmias.

High doses of digoxin produce slowing of conduction velocity especially through the AV node and His bundle, this action being partly direct and partly vagal. P-R prolongation seen in the ECG reflects this action, which also explains the frequent occurrence of AV dissociation and complete heart block in digoxin toxicity.

Digoxin in therapeutic doses shortens the refractory period of atrial and ventricular muscle while prolonging the functional refractory period of the AV node; these combined effects underlie the slowing of the heart rate in atrial fibrillation. The shortened ventricular refractory period is reflected in the reduced Q-T interval seen in patients receiving digoxin.

Automaticity is induced in Purkinje fibers by digoxin and in toxic doses is increased in all areas of the heart except the sinoatrial node. Occasional ventricular premature beats may occur with moderate doses; with increasing doses ventricular bigeminy is seen eventually leading to ventricular tachycardia and ventricular fibrillation.

Digoxin is indicated for supraventricular ectopic rhythms associated with rapid ventricular rates, which often convert to sinus rhythm after digitalization. Atrial fibrillation responds to digoxin with slowing of the ventricular rate and some patients may revert to normal sinus rhythm; similarly the degree of block in atrial flutter is usually increased by digoxin thereby reducing the ventricular rate. Digoxin is frequently effective in preventing recurrence of paroxysmal supraventricular tachycardia especially in infants.

Almost every known arrhythmia has been caused by digoxin toxicity in both children and adults; however, in children ventricular premature beats are less common than conduction disturbances such as sinoatrial block, atrioventricular dissociation, or AV junctional ectopic rhythms. When digoxin toxicity is suspected, the drug should be discontinued and the electrolyte and acid/base of the patient determined. Hypokalemia and any metabolic acidosis should be corrected. In patients with advanced degree of AV block due to digoxin, potassium salts are contraindicated because of their action of prolonging the AV node refractory period. Both lidocaine and phenytoin are effective in suppressing ventricular tachycardia due to cardiac glycosides, phenytoin being particularly useful in that it reverses the glycoside-induced prolongation of AV conduction. Phenytoin is also the most effective drug for suppressing supraventricular tachyarrhythmias due to digoxin. Junctional or His bundle conduction disturbances due to digoxin may respond to atropine.

Lidocaine

Lidocaine is of value in the treatment of ventricular arrhythmias especially those complicating cardiac surgery, myocardial infarction, and digitalis intoxication. The need for parenteral administration and its short duration of action limit its use to acute situations. Lidocaine has little effect on atrial arrhythmias.

It acts by reducing ectopic rhythm formation in the ventricles.

Paroxysmal ventricular tachycardia, paroxysmal ventricular fibrillation, and frequent ventricular premature beats occurring postoperatively or during cardiac catheterization usually respond to lidocaine. Quickly metabolized in the liver, its action, when given intravenously, is rapid in onset and of short duration (except in patients with depressed hepatic function). Following intramuscular administration therapeutic levels are reached in 10 to 15 minutes and its action is over within two hours. The margin between effective therapeutic doses and those causing toxicity is wide. Like many antiarrhythmic drugs myocardial depression may occur with large doses. Drowsiness, muscle twitching, hallucinations, and seizures may occur. Hypotension and rhythm disturbances such as sinus tachycardia, sinus bradycardia, and arrest are rare.

The recommended doses are:

IV (bolus)	1–2 mg/kg given over 30–60 seconds
IV (continuous infusion)	15–25 mcg/kg/min

Quinidine

Long established as an effective treatment for several arrhythmias quinidine is a naturally occurring alkaloid in cinchona bark where it is found with quinine. Although both substances depress skeletal and cardiac muscle, quinidine is most effective on cardiac muscle. Quinidine depresses myocardial contractility, reduces its excitability, and slows conduction velocity.

Most experience with quinidine in the management of arrhythmias has been in adults; its use in children has been less and is poorly documented in the literature. Quinidine has been used to convert atrial fibrillation to sinus rhythm and to prevent its recurrence and to suppress paroxysmal tachyarrhythmias of both supraventricular and ventricular origin. Although premature systoles do not normally require treatment, quinidine will often effectively suppress them.

Side effects and toxic reactions are relatively common and individual patient response often unpredictable. Nausea, vomiting, and diarrhea are most common; tinnitus, vertigo, and other features of cinchonism can develop. Serious thrombocytopenia has been reported. Sudden death due to ventricular fibrillation may occur even with the usual therapeutic doses. Paroxysmal ventricular tachycardia or fibrillation may occur in 3 to 4 percent of patients on the recommended doses (Selzer and Wray, 1964). Serious hypotension often complicates the intravenous use of quinidine. Great caution should be exercised in giving quinidine to patients already receiving digoxin as the effects on the cardiac rhythm may be quite unpredictable.

The ECG in patients receiving quinidine may show widening of the QRS with Q-T prolongation and sinus bradycardia with P-R prolongation.

At The Hospital for Sick Children, Toronto, we feel that quinidine has very little place in the treatment of arrhythmias in children except for a trial in patients with paroxysmal tachyarrhythmias refractory to other drugs.

The recommended oral dose is 6 mg/kg q3h (maximum 0.2 G q3h).

Procainamide

The cardiac actions and indications for use of procainamide resemble those of quinidine. Like quinidine it produces significant depression of myocardial contractility with a fall in cardiac output and blood pressure.

It may be given orally, intramuscularly, or intravenously but probably only orally in childhood. Both cardiac and other side effects may occur. Somnolence, hallucinations, and convulsions may be produced while prolonged administration may cause a lupus-like syndrome that subsides spontaneously on withdrawing the drug. Thrombocytopenia, severe anemia, and agranulocytosis have been reported. Intravenous administration is hazardous and should be slow. Hypotension, ventricular fibrillation, or asystole can develop.

In children, procainamide should be limited to oral administration in the prevention of recurrent tachyarrhythmias resistant to other therapy. For the urgent treatment of ventricular arrhythmias lidocaine and electrical countershock are safer than IV procainamide.

The recommended oral dose is 30 to 50 mg/kg/24 hours divided into four to six doses.

Edrophonium Chloride (Tensilon)

Tensilon is a rapidly acting cholinesterase inhibitor with an extremely short duration of action. It has been used successfully to convert paroxysmal supraventricular tachycardia to sinus rhythm. Reported side effects have been few and subside quickly; transient bradycardia and hypotension may be seen. There has, as yet, been no systematic evaluation of its role in pediatric arrhythmias. We have used edrophonium for the conversion of paroxysmal supraventricular arrhythmias but successful conversion is frequently transient and other measures often necessary.

Recommended initial dose for infants is 0.5 mg given IV over 30 seconds. Adult dose is 10 mg IV.

Propranolol

Propranolol is the most widely available beta-adrenergic blocking drug whose electrophysiologic effects are due not only to beta-adrenergic blockade but also to a direct myocardial action. This direct action is independent of both circulating catecholamines and sympathetic nervous activity and resembles the action of quinidine and procainamide.

It is mainly responsible for the antiarrhythmic action of these drugs.

With the exception of recurrent supraventricular tachycardia associated with the WPW syndrome, where propranolol may be extremely effective, it is not usually the drug of first choice. Propranolol should be tried in patients with supraventricular tachycardia who are refractory to digoxin and it is often effective in preventing recurrences. Used in combination with digoxin it may help to slow the ventricular rate in patients who do not respond to digoxin alone. Propranolol is also quite useful in treating arrhythmias due to digoxin toxicity except those associated with AV conduction disturbances in which it may increase the degree of block.

Propranolol may cause undue bradycardia and hypotension but its major disadvantage lies in its myocardial depressant action, which may precipitate congestive heart failure. Finally, it should not be used in asthmatics as it causes bronchial constriction.

Recommended dosage:

IV   0.1 mg/kg given slowly
PO   1.0 mg/kg per day divided q6h

Phenytoin (Diphenylhydantoin)

Originally introduced as an anticonvulsant phenytoin (diphenylhydantoin) is of value in the management of certain arrhythmias. Phenytoin decreases sinoatrial node automaticity and increases AV conduction velocity. It reverses the prolongation of AV conduction produced by digoxin. Automaticity in the His-Purkinje system is depressed by phenytoin. This drug is effective in suppressing ventricular arrhythmias following anesthesia, catheterization, and cardiac surgery especially when digoxin is implicated in their cause. The bulk of the evidence suggests that it has little effect against supraventricular arrhythmias.

Phenytoin can be given IV or orally. The IV route should be used only in emergencies and under ECG control; oral administration is preferable. Maximum plasma levels are reached in about 12 hours after oral administration. Metabolized in the liver, the drug should be given in reduced dosage to patients with liver disease.

Sleepiness, nystagmus, ataxia, confusion, and disorientation may complicate therapy with phenytoin. Hypotension, bradycardia, and occasionally cardiac arrest have been reported but ventricular arrhythmias are rare. Like several other anti-arrhythmics phenytoin is a myocardial depressant.

Recommended dose:

PO   1–3 mg/kg/q8h
IV   1–3 mg/kg under ECG control

ELECTRICAL METHODS OF TREATMENT

Defibrillation

In 1956 Zoll and associates demonstrated that closed-chest defibrillation using an AC defibrillator was clinically practical. This demonstration assumed great importance when closed-chest cardiopulmonary resuscitation became established. In 1962 Lown and coworkers introduced the DC defibrillator, which is more effective in defibrillating the hypoxic heart. This equipment is now standard in all hospitals.

Ventricular fibrillation is uncommon in children and most often occurs after cardiac surgery especially in association with hypoxia, acidosis, and electrolyte disturbances. Ventricular fibrillation occasionally complicates cardiac catheterization. In the intensive care unit or the catheter laboratory a defibrillator is readily available, but when fibrillation occurs on the open ward life can be maintained by external cardiac massage and assisted ventilation until a defibrillator is obtained. Attempted defibrillation is most likely to be successful if applied immediately and if a high-energy, unsynchronized discharge between 50 and 400 watts/second is combined with correction of both acidosis and hypoxia. For children over five years external electrodes measuring 10 cm in diameter wrapped in saline-soaked gauze and applied one to the apical region and the other to the right infraclavicular region are most effective. Smaller electrodes (5.5 cm diameter) are available for young children and infants. Following successful defibrillation possible precipitating causes should be corrected; the child's ECG should be monitored continuously; and if multiple ventricular premature beats suggest recurrence is likely, a continuous infusion of lidocaine, 1 to 3 mg per minute, may prevent further fibrillation.

Electrical Countershock

Both Lown and coworkers (1961) and Zoll (1962) reported their successful use of an AC discharge to terminate ventricular tachycardia. Lown (1962) extended the application of DC countershock from conversion of ventricular fibrillation to convert various refractory arrhythmias to normal sinus rhythm. Cardioversion or synchronized electrical countershock has now been used successfully in atrial fibrillation, atrial flutter, paroxysmal supraventricular, and ventricular tachyarrhythmias. Paul and Miller (1962) and Pryor and Blount (1964) first reported the successful conversion of paroxysmal atrial tachycardia in children.

The DC converter delivers a synchronized shock to the heart usually coinciding with the peak of the R wave thereby avoiding the vulnerable period of the ventricle (occurring at the peak of the T wave) in which ventricular fibrillation may be induced. The shock simultaneously discharges all fibers excitable at that instance, abolishes all reentry pathways, and, provided the sinus node is healthy, restores normal sinus rhythm. While depolarizing the heart, counter-shock also stimulates both parasympathetic and sympathetic cardiac nerves and causes catecholamine release. This autonomic stimulation may be responsible for postconversion tachy- or brady-arrhythmias, which can be minimized by keeping the stimulus strength low and can be blocked with atropine or propranolol. Attempted cardioversion of arrhythmias due to digitalis toxicity is often followed by serious postconversion arrhythmias especially ventricular tachycardia or fibrillation, and DC countershock is therefore contraindicated in arrhythmias secondary to excessive digoxin, which are better treated by potassium salts and diphenyl-hydantoin and the withdrawal of digoxin.

DC countershock in children is indicated for paroxysmal supraventricular tachycardia resistant to carotid sinus massage, digoxin, and edrophonium, for atrial fibrillation and flutter, and for paroxysmal ventricular tachycardia.

Relative contraindications include recent onset of the arrhythmia, repetitive arrhythmia, and recent systemic or pulmonary embolus. Arrhythmia secondary to digoxin toxicity is an absolute contraindication.

Except when extremely urgent, cardioversion in children is best performed under light general anesthesia; digoxin is withheld for 24 hours preceding conversion and there is no need for anticoagulation. The patient is connected to the cardioverter, which should be provided with an oscilloscope so the ECG can be viewed continuously. General anesthesia can be induced with methohexital IV (2 mg/kg) combined with atropine (0.015 mg/kg). Alternatively, thiopentone, up to 5 mg/kg, can be used. It is not usually necessary to intubate the patient. The electrodes are amply smeared with electrode jelly and positioned as for ventricular defibrillation. The patient is well-oxygenated by the anesthetist. An initial low-energy discharge of 10 watt/sec is applied, which if ineffective is followed by a 50 watt/second shock. Lown has stressed the advantages of minimal energy shocks in preventing postconversion arrhythmias.

Defibrillation and IV lidocaine should be available in case ventricular tachycardia or fibrillation supervenes. Other complications such as pulmonary edema, elevated serum enzymes, and transient S-T elevation, all seen in adults, appear to be rare in children. DC countershock with its rapid reliable conversion and relative safety has rightly become established as a major therapy in many arrhythmias.

Following conversion the patient should be nursed in the anesthetic recovery room and the ECG monitored for four hours—if there are no complications, the patient may then be discharged or returned to the general wards.

THE DIAGNOSTIC APPROACH TO AN ARRHYTHMIA IN CHILDHOOD

THE detection of an arrhythmia in a child usually engenders considerable parental anxiety and always requires careful evaluation. Fortunately most arrhythmias can be diagnosed by accurate observation using a single-channel ECG strip and simple interventions such as carotid sinus massage.

Arrhythmias may be benign, symptomatic but non-life-threatening, or life-threatening. Asymptomatic arrhythmias are usually detected because of an irregular pulse or by an electrocardiogram taken for

other indications. Any doubts as to the significance of such a finding will usually be resolved by the nature of the rhythm change and an exercise ECG. Benign arrhythmias usually disappear during exercise and regular sinus tachycardia is seen.

Carotid sinus massage (CSM) can be used to differentiate tachyarrhythmias (Table 17–4). Both the diagnostic and therapeutic effectiveness of such massage can be enhanced by pretreatment with edrophonium (Tensilon) 45 seconds prior to applying

Table 17–4.   EXPECTED EFFECTS OF CAROTID SINUS MASSAGE IN THE COMMON TACHYARRHYTHMIAS

TACHYARRHYTHMIA	CAROTID SINUS MASSAGE
Sinus tachycardia	Slight slowing, rapid rate returns on release
Paroxysmal supraventricular tachycardia	Abrupt termination or no effect
Paroxysmal supraventricular tachycardia with AV block	Slows, increase in AV block, rapid rate returns on release
Atrial flutter	Vent. rate may halve due to increase in AV block. Occ. converts to atrial fibrillation
Ventricular tachycardia	Atrial slowing, ventricular rate unchanged. May help to detect P waves

massage. Gentle but firm compression is applied to the carotid sinus with the patient supine and the neck hyperextended while a continuous ECG strip is recorded.

Patients with symptoms suggestive of an arrhythmia but in whom the resting cardiogram is normal pose a difficult diagnostic problem. Sometimes the arrhythmia may be provoked by a graded exercise test while recording a single ECG lead continuously. Younger children find a treadmill easier to handle than a bicycle ergometer, and the exercise program can be adjusted to the child's age and physical state. If significant arrhythmias are provoked by exercise, it is often helpful to use repeat tests to assess the effectiveness of therapy. The introduction of portable systems allowing continuous recording of a single-lead ECG for periods of up to 24 hours has facilitated the investigation of elusive intermittent arrhythmias. The recorder is suitable for children down to five years old while ambulant and for all ages when confined to bed. It takes approximately 30 minutes to scan the tape and suspect segments can be recorded on paper for more detailed study.

Invasive electrophysiologic studies only seldom provide information that significantly alters the management of patients with rhythm problems. His bundle electrograms certainly permit more precise localization of conduction defects, and atrial pacing may unmask an unsuspected impairment of atrioventricular conduction. Measurement of sinus node recovery times can confirm the presence of impaired sinus node function suspected from surface recordings. However, in most patients this type of investigation is unnecessary for precise diagnosis and good management.

Once an arrhythmia has been identified its significance must be determined. Benign asymptomatic arrhythmias require no treatment except adequate explanation and reassurance. Whether symptomatic arrhythmias require treatment will depend on the frequency and severity of the symptoms and on the type of arrhythmia. Life-threatening problems will require the appropriate treatment outlined in the sections on specific arrhythmias. Finally, in instituting therapy the clinician must be perfectly clear as to the objectives of such treatment and possible adverse effects.

REFERENCES

Abella, J. B.; Teixeira, O. H. P.; Misra, K. P.; and Hastreiter, A. R.: Changes of atrioventricular conduction with age in infants and children. *Am. J. Cardiol.*, **30**:876, 1972.

Alexander, S.; Kleiger, R.; and Lown, B.: Use of external electric countershock in the treatment of ventricular tachycardia. *JAMA*, **177**:916, 1961.

Alimurung, M. M., and Massell, B. F.: The normal PR interval in infants and children. *Circulation*, **13**:257, 1956.

Anderson, R. H.; Arnold, R.; Thapar, M. K.; Jones, R. S.; and Hamilton, D. I.: Cardiac specialised tissue in hearts with an apparently single ventricular chamber (double inlet left ventricle). *Am. J. Cardiol.*, **33**:95, 1974.

Anderson, R. H.; Becker, A. E.; Arnold, R.; and Wilkinson, J. L.: The conducting tissues in congenitally corrected transposition. *Circulation*, **50**:911, 1974.

Ashman, R., and Hull, E.: *Essentials of Electrocardiography*. The Macmillan Co., New York, 1937.

Bachmann, G.: Inter-auricular time interval. *Am. J. Physiol.*, **41**:309, 1916.

Bacos, J. M.; Eagan, J. T.; and Orgain, E. S.: Congenital familiar nodal rhythm. *Circulation*, **22**:887, 1960.

Bellet, S.: *Clinical Disorders of the Heart Beat*, 3rd ed. Lea & Febiger, Philadelphia, 1971.

Bharati, S., and Lev, M.: The course of the conduction system in single ventricle with inverted (L) loop and inverted (L) transposition. *Circulation*, **51**:723, 1975.

Bigger, J. T., Jr., and Goldreyer, B. N.: The mechanism of supraventricular tachycardia. *Circulation*, **42**:673, 1970.

Bristowe, J. S.: On recurrent palpitation of extreme rapidity in persons otherwise apparently healthy. *Brain*, **10**:164, 1887–88.

Brown, K. W. G.; Whitehead, E. H.; and Morrow, J. D.: Treatment of cardiac arrhythmias with synchronised electrical countershock. *Can. Med. Assoc. J.*, **90**:103, 1964.

Campbell, M., and Emanuel, R.: Six cases of congenital complete heart block followed for 34–40 years. *Br. Heart J.*, **29**:577, 1967.

Castellanos, A.; Castillo, C. A.; and Agha, A. S.: Contribution of His bundle recordings to the understanding of clinical arrhythmias. *Am. J. Cardiol.*, **28**:499, 1971.

Chardack, W. M.; Gage, A. A.; and Greatbatch, W.: A transistorized self-contained implantable pacemaker for the long-term correction of complete heart block. *Surgery*, **48**:643, 1960.

Church, S. C.; Morgan, B. C.; Oliver, T. K., Jr.; and Guntheroth, W. G.: Cardiac arrhythmias in premature infants. An indication of autonomic immaturity? *J. Pediatr.*, **71**:542, 1967.

Clarke, M., and Keith, J. D.: Atrioventricular conduction in acute rheumatic fever. *Br. Heart J.*, **34**:472, 1972.

Cobb, F. R.; Blumenschein, S. D.; Sealy, W. C.; Boineau, J. P.; Wagnar, G. S.; and Wallace, A. G.: Successful surgical interruption of the bundle of Kent in a patient with Wolff-Parkinson-White syndrome. *Circulation*, **38**:1018, 1968.

de Carvalho, A. P.; Demello, W. C.; and Hoffman, B. F.: Electrophysiological evidence for specialised fiber types in rabbit atrium. *Am. J. Physiol.*, **196**:483, 1959.

Denes, P.; Dhingra, R. C.; Wu, D.; Chuquima, R.; Amat-Y-Leon, F.; Wyndham, C.; and Rosen, K. M.: H-V interval in patients with bifascicular block (right bundle branch block and left anterior hemiblock): clinical, electrocardiographic and electrophysiologic correlations. *Am. J. Cardiol.*, **35**:23, 1975.

Dock, W.: Mode of production of first heart sound. *Arch. Intern. Med.*, **51**:737, 1933.

Dreifus, L. S.; Arriaga, J.; Watanabe, Y.; Downing, D.; Haiat, R.; and Morse, D.: Recurrent Wolff-Parkinson-White syndrome (type B). *Circulation*, **28**:586, 1971.

Durrer, D., and Roos, J. P.: Epicardial excitation of the ventricles in a patient with Wolff-Parkinson-White syndrome (type B). *Circulation*, **35**:15, 1967.

Durrer, D.; Schoo, L.; Schuilenburg, R. M.; and Wellens, H. J. J.: Role of premature beats in the initiation and termination of supraventricular tachycardia in the Wolff-Parkinson-White syndrome. *Circulation*, **36**:644, 1967.

Easley, R. M., and Goldstein, S.: Sino-atrial syncope. *Am. J. Med.*, **50**:166, 1971.

El Sherif, N.; Scherlag, B. J.; and Lazzara, R.: Pathophysiology of second degree atrioventricular block: a unified hypothesis. *Am. J. Cardiol.*, **35**:421, 1975.

Fay, J. E.; Olley, P. M.; Partington, M. W.; Kavety, V. B.; and Ahmad, G.: Surdocardiac syndrome: incidence among children in schools for the deaf. *Canad. Med. Assoc. J.*, **105**:718, 1971.

Feldt, R. H.; Dushane, J. W.; and Titus, J. L.: The atrioventricular conduction system in persistent common atrioventricular canal defect: correlations with electrocardiogram. *Circulation*, **42**:437, 1970.

Ferrer, M. I.: The sick sinus syndrome. *Circulation*, **47**:635, 1973.

Frazer, G. R.; Froggatt, P.; and James, T. N.: Congenital deafness associated with electrocardiographic abnormalities, fainting attacks and sudden death. A recessive syndrome. *Q.J.Med.*, **33**:131, 1964.

Furman, S., and Schwedel, J. B.: An intracardiac pacemaker for Stokes-Adams seizures. *N. Engl. J. Med.*, **261**:943, 1959.

Gallagher, J. J.; Gilbert, M.; Svenson, R. H.; Sealy, W. C.; Kasell, J.; and Wallace, A. G.: Wolff-Parkinson-White syndrome. The problem, evaluation, and surgical correction. *Circulation*, **51**: 767, 1975.

Gelband, H., and Rosen, M. R.: Pharmacologic basis for the treatment of cardiac arrhythmias. *Pediatrics*, **55**: 59, 1975.

Gelband, H.; Waldo, A. L.; Kaiser, G. A.; Bowman, F. O.; Malm, J. R.; and Hoffman, B. F.: Etiology of right bundle branch block in patients undergoing total correction of tetralogy of Fallot. *Circulation*, **44**: 1022, 1971.

Giardina, A. C. V.; Ehlers, K. H.; and Engle, M. A.: Wolff-Parkinson-White syndrome in infants and children. A long-term follow-up study. *Br. heart. J.*, **34**: 839, 1972.

Gilette, P. C.: The mechanisms of supraventricular tachycardia in children. *Circulation*, **54**: 133, 1976.

Gilette, P. C., and Garson, A.: Electrophysiologic and pharmacologic characteristics of automatic etopic atrial tachycardia. *Circulation*, **56**: 571, 1977.

Goldreyer, B. N.; Bigger, J. T., Jr.; and Heissenbuttel, R.: Reentrant supraventricular tachycardia. *Clin. Res.*, **17**: 243, 1969.

Guller, B.; Dushane, J. W.; and Titus, J. L.: The atrioventricular conduction system in two cases of tricuspid atresia. *Circulation*, **40**: 217, 1969.

Haft, J. I.: The His bundle electrogram. *Circulation*, **47**: 897, 1973.

Hancock, E. W.: Coronary sinus rhythms in sinus venosus defect and persistent left superior vena cava. *Am. J. Cardiol.*, **14**: 608, 1964.

Hoffman, B. F.; and Cranefield, P. F.: The physiological basis for cardiac arrhythmias. *Am. J. Med.*, **37**: 670, 1964.

Hoyer, B., and Lyon, R. A.: Auricular flutter with block in children. *Am. J. Dis. Child.*, **72**: 734, 1946.

Huntingford, P. J.: The aetiology and significance of congenital heart block. *J. Obstet. Gynaecol. Br. Common W.*, **67**: 259, 1960.

Ikkos, D., and Hanson, J. S.: Response to exercise in congenital atrioventricular block. *Circulation*, **22**: 583, 1960.

James, T. N.: Morphology of the human atrioventricular node, with remarks pertinent to its electrophysiology. *Am. Heart J.*, **62**: 756, 1961.

―――: *The Specialised Conducting Tissue of the Atria in Mechanisms and Therapy of Cardiac Arrhythmias*. Grune & Stratton, Publishers, New York, p. 97, 1966.

―――: Cardiac conduction system: foetal and postnatal development. *Am. J. Cardiol.*, **25**: 123, 1970.

James, T. N., and Sherf, L.: Ultrastructure of myocardial cells. *Am. J. Cardiol.*, **22**: 389, 1968.

Jervell, A., and Lange-Nielson, F.: Congenital deaf-mutism, functional heart disease with prolongation of the Q-T interval, and sudden death. *Am. Heart J.*, **54**: 59, 1957.

Joseph, R.; Ribierre, M.; and Najean, Y.: Le syndrome de Wolff-Parkinson-White dans la premiere enfance; ses repports avec la tachycardie paroxysims du nourisson. *Sem. Hop. (Paris)*, **34**: 552, 1958.

Keith, A., and Flack, M. W.: The form and nature of the muscular connections between the primary divisions of the vertebrate heart. *J. Anat. Physiol.*, **41**: 172, 1907.

Keith, J. D.: Overstimulation of vagus nerve in rheumatic fever. *Q. J. Med.*, **1**: 29, 1938.

Keith, J. D., and Brown, A.: Paroxysmal tachycardia report of two cases. *Am. J. Dis. Child.*, **59**: 362, 1940.

Kent, A. F. S.: The right lateral auriculo-ventricular junction of the heart. *J. Physiol.*, **48**: 22, 1914.

Krongrad, E.; Hefler, S. E.; Bowman, F. O.; Malm, J. R.; and Hoffman, B. F.: Further observations on the etiology of right bundle branch block pattern following right ventriculotomy. *Circulation*, **50**: 1105, 1974.

Landtman, B.: Heart arrhythmias in children, *Acta Paediatr. (Suppl. 1)*, **34**: 1, 1947.

Lange, G.: Action of driving stimuli from intrinsic and extrinsic sources on in situ cardiac pacemaker tissues. *Circ. Res.*, **17**: 449, 1965.

Lev, M.: The pre-excitation syndrome: anatomic considerations of anomalous AV pathways. In *Mechanisms and Therapy of Cardiac Arrhythmias*, edited by Dreifus, L. S., Likoff, W. S. Grune & Stratton, New York, 1966, p. 665.

―――: Conduction system in congenital heart disease. *Am. J. Cardiol.*, **21**: 619, 1968a.

―――: The conduction system, In Gould, S. E. (ed.): *Pathology of the Heart and Blood Vessels*, 3rd ed. Charles C Thomas, Publisher, Springfield, Ill., 1968b, p. 180.

―――: Pathogenesis of congenital atrioventricular block. *Prog. Cardiovasc. Dis.*, **15**: 145, 1972.

Lev, M.; Cuadros, H.; and Paul, M. H.: Interruption of the atrioventricular bundle with congenital atrioventricular block. *Circulation*, **43**: 703, 1971.

Lewis, T.: *The Mechanism and Graphic Registration of the Heart Beat*, 3rd ed. Shaw and Son, London, 1925.

Lindqvist, T.: Paroxysmal tachycardia. *Svensk. Lakartidn.*, **53**: 2917, 1956.

Lown, B.: Electrical reversion of cardiac arrhythmias. *Br. Heart J.*, **29**: 469, 1967.

Lown, B.; Amarasingham, R.; and Neuman, J.: A new method for terminating cardiac arrhythmias; use of synchronized capacitor discharge. *JAMA*, **182**: 548, 1962.

Lown, B.; Ganong, W. F.; and Levine, S. A.: Syndrome of short PR interval, normal QRS complex and paroxysmal rapid heart action. *Circulation*, **43**: 693, 1952.

Lown, B.; Neuman, J.; Amarasingham, R.; and Berkovits, B. V.: Comparison of alternating current with direct current electroshock across the closed chest. *Am. J. Cardiol.*, **10**: 223, 1962.

Lundberg, A. K. E.: Paroxysmal tachycardia in infancy. A clinical and experimental study. *Acta Paediatr. (Suppl.)*, **143**: 1, 1963.

Lyon, R. A., and Rauh, L. W.: Extrasystoles in children. *Am. J. Dis. Child.*, **57**: 278, 1939a.

―――: Simple tachycardia in children. *JAMA*, **113**: 1121, 1939b.

Mahaim, I., and Clerc, A.: Nonvelle forme anatomique de bloc du Coeur a substituer au bloc dit d'aborisations (bloc bilateral manque), *C.R. Soc. Biol. (Paris)*, **109**: 183, 1932.

Mannheimer, E.: Paroxysmal tachycardia in infants. *Acta Paediatr.*, **33**: 383, 1946.

Massumi, R. A.; Kistin, A. D.; and Tawakkol, A. A.: Termination of reciprocating tachycardia by atrial stimulation. *Circulation*, **36**: 637, 1967.

Miller, R. A., and Rodriguez-Coronel, A.: Congenital atrioventricular block. In *Heart Disease in Infants, Children and Adolescents*, edited by Moss, A. J., and Adams, F. H. Williams & Wilkins Co., Baltimore, 1968.

Mines, G. R.: On dynamic equilibrium in the heart. *J. Physiol.*, **46**: 349, 1913.

Mirowski, M.; Rosenstein, B. J.; and Markowitz, M.: A Comparison of atrioventricular conduction in normal children and in patients with rheumatic fever, glomerulonephritis and acute febrile illness. *Pediatrics*, **33**: 334, 1964.

Moller, J. H.; Davachi, F.; and Anderson, R. C.: Atrial flutter in infancy. *J. Pediatr.*, **75**: 643, 1969.

Molthan, M. E.; Miller, R. A.; Hastreiter, A. R.; and Paul, M. H.: Congenital heart block with fatal Adams-Stokes attacks in childhood. *Paediatrics*, **30**: 32, 1962.

Morquio, L.: Sur une maladie infantile et familiale caracterisee par des modifications permanentes du pouls, des modifications syncopales et epiléptiformes. *Arch. Méd. Euf.*, **4**: 467, 1901.

Moss, A. J., and Davis, R. J.: Brady-Tachy syndrome. *Prog. Cardiovasc. Dis.*, **16**: 439, 1974.

Moss, A. J.; Klyman, G.; and Emmanouilides, G. C.: Late onset complete heart block: newly recognized sequela of cardiac surgery. *Am. J. Cardiol.*, **30**: 884, 1972.

Nadas, A. S.; Daeschener, C. W.; Roth, A.; and Blumenthal, S. L.: Paroxysmal tachycardia in infants; study of 41 cases. *Pediatrics*, **9**: 167, 1952.

Narula, O. S.: Wolff-Parkinson-White syndrome. *Circulation*, **47**: 872, 1973.

Olley, P. M., and Fowler, R. S.: The Surdo-cardiac syndrome and therapeutic observations. *Br. Heart J.*, **32**: 467, 1970.

Parkinson, J.; Grosse, A. H.; and Gunson, E. B.: The heart and its rhythm in acute rheumatism. *Q. J. Med.*, **13**: 363, 1920.

Parkinson, J., and Papp, C.: Repetitive paroxysmal tachycardia. *Br. Heart J.*, **9**: 241, 1947.

Paul, M. H., and Miller, A. R.: External electrical termination of supraventricular arrhythmias in congenital heart disease. *Circulation*, **25**: 604, 1962.

Pick, A.: Mechanisms of cardiac arrhythmias: from hypothesis to physiologic fact. *Am. Heart J.*, **86**: 249, 1973.

Preston, T. A., and Kirsh, M. M.: Permanent pacing of the left atrium for treatment of WPW tachycardia. *Circulation*, **42**: 1073, 1970.

Prinzmetal, M., et al.: *The Auricular Arrhythmias.* Charles C Thomas, Publisher, Springfield, Ill., 1952.

Pryor, R., and Blount, S. G., Jr.: Refractory supraventricular tachycardia in infancy. *Am. J. Dis. Child.,* **107**:428, 1964.

Radford, D. J., and Izukawa, T.: The sick sinus syndrome: symptomatic cases in children. *Arch. Dis. Child.,* **50**:879, 1975.

Radford, D. J., and Izukawa, T.: Atrial fibrillation in children. *Pediatrics,* **59**:250, 1977.

Radford, D. J.; Izukawa, T.; and Rowe, R. D.: Congenital paroxysmal atrial tachycardia. *Arch. Dis. Child.,* **51**:613, 1976.

Radford, D. J.; Izukawa, T.; and Rowe, R. D.: Evaluation of children with ventricular arrhythmias. *Arch. Dis. Child.,* **52**:345, 1977.

Roberts, N. K., and Gelband, H.: *Cardiac Arrhythmias in the Neonate, Infant, and Child.* Appleton-Century-Crofts, New York, 1977.

Roberts, N. K., and Olley, P. M.: His bundle electrogram in children. Statistical correlation of the atrioventricular conduction times in children with their age and heart rate. *Br. Heart J.,* **34**:1099, 1972.

Robinson, S. J.: Arrhythmias in children. *Med. Times,* **87**:870, 1959.

Rosenbaum, F. F.; Hecht, H. H.; Wilson, F. N.; and Johnston, F. D.: The potential variation of the thorax and the esophagus in anomalous atrioventricular excitation (W-P-W syndrome). *Am. Heart J.,* **29**:281, 1945.

Rosenbaum, M. B.; Chiale, P. A.; Ryba, D.; and Elizari, M.: Control of tachyarrhythmia associated with Wolff-Parkinson-White syndrome by Amiodarone Hydrochloride. *Am. J. Cardiol.,* **34**:215, 1974.

Rosenberg, D. H.: Acute myocarditis in mumps (epidemic parotitis). *Arch. Intern. Med.,* **76**:257, 1945.

Scherf, D.: Studies on auricular tachycardia caused by aconitine administration. *Proc. Soc. Exp. Biol.,* **64**:233, 1947.

Scherlag, B. J.; Lau, S. H.; Helfant, R. H.; Berkowitz, W. D.; Stein, E.: and Damato, A. N.: Catheter technique for recording His bundle activity in man. *Circulation,* **39**:13, 1969.

Scherlag, B. J.; Samet, P.; and Helfant, R. H.: His bundle electrogram. A critical appraisal of its uses and limitations. *Circulation,* **46**:601, 1972.

Schwartz, P. J.; Periti, M.; and Malliani, A.: The long Q-T syndrome. *Am. Heart J.,* **89**:379, 1975.

Selzer, A., and Wray, H. W.: Quinidine syncope. Paroxysmal ventricular fibrillation occurring during treatment of chronic atrial arrhythmias. *Circulation,* **30**:17, 1964.

Shacknow, N.; Spellman, S.; and Rubin, I.: Persistent supraventricular tachycardia. Case report with review of the literature. *Circulation,* **10**:232, 1954.

Sherf, L., and James, T. N.: A new electrocardiographic concept: synchronized sino-ventricular conduction. *Dis. Chest,* **55**:127, 1969.

Sodi-Pallares, D.; Portillo, B.; Cisneros, F.; de la Cruz, M. V.; and Acosta, A. R.: Electrocardiography in infants and children. *Pediatr. Clin. North Am.,* **5**:871, 1958.

Sondheimer, H. M.; Izukawa, T.; Olley, P. M.; Trusler, G. A.; and Mustard, W. T.: Conduction disturbances after total correction of tetralogy of Fallot. *Am. Heart. J.,* **92**:278, 1976.

Stokes, Sir W.: Observations on some cases of permanently slow pulse. In *Diseases of the Heart and the Aorta.* Hodges & Smith, Dublin, 1954, p. 333.

Swiderski, J.; Lees, M. H.; and Nadas, A. S.: The Wolff-Parkinson-White syndrome in infancy and childhood. *Br. Heart J.,* **24**:561, 1962.

Tamm, R. H.: Das Wolff-Parkinson-White syndrom eine haufige Erkvaukimg im Kindesalter. *Helv. Pediatr. Acta,* **11**:78, 1956.

Taran, M. L., and Jennings, K. G.: Paroxysmal atrio-ventricular nodal tachycardia in a newborn infant. *Am. J. Dis. Child.,* **54**:557, 1937.

Taussig, H. B.: *Congenital Malformations of the Heart.* Harvard University Press, Cambridge, Mass., 1960, p. 275.

Thorel, C.: Vorlaufige Mitteilung uber eine besondere Muskel Verbindung zwischem der Cava superior und dem Hisschem Bundel. *Munchen. Med. Wschr.,* **56**:2159, 1909.

Vassalle, M.: Analysis of cardiac pacemaker potential using a "voltage clamp" technique. *Am. J. Physiol.,* **210**:1335, 1966.

———: Automaticity and automatic rhythms. *Am. J. Cardiol.,* **28**:245, 1971.

Wagnar, M. L.; Lazzara, R.; Weiss, R. M.; and Hoffman, B. F.: Specialized conducting fibers in the interatrial band. *Circ. Res.,* **18**:502, 1966.

Ward, O. C.: New familial cardiac syndrome in children. *J. Irish Med. Assoc.,* **54**:103, 1964.

Warner, A. O., and McKusick, V. A.: Wolff-Parkinson-White syndrome: a genetic study. *Clin. Res.,* **6**:18, 1958.

Wenckebach, K. F.: Beitrage zur Kenntris der menschlichen Herztatigkeit. *Arch. Anat. Physiol.,* **102**:1, 1907.

———: Beitrage zur Kenntris der menschlichen Herztatigkeit. *Arch. Physiol. 3 (Suppl.):* 53, 1908.

———: Die Therapie des Vorhoffimmerns. Die unregelmassige Herztatigkeit und ihre Klinische Bedeutung. W. Engelmann, Leipzig and Berlin, 1914, p. 125.

West, T. C.: Effects of chronotropic influences on sub-threshold oscillations in the sino-atrial node. In *The Specialized Tissues of the Heart* (Paes do Carvalho, A., De Mello, W. C., Hoffman, B. F., eds.). Amsterdam, Elsevier, 1961, p. 81.

Willius, F. A., and Dry, T. J.: *A History of the Heart and the Circulation.* W. B. Saunders, Co., Philadelphia, 1956.

Wolff, L.; Parkinson, J.; and White, P. D.: Bundle branch block with short PR interval in healthy young people prone to paroxysmal tachycardia. *Am. Heart J.,* **5**:685, 1930.

Wolff, G. S.; Rowland, T. W.; and Ellison, R. C.: Surgically induced right bundle branch block with left anterior hemiblock. An ominous sign in postoperative tetralogy of Fallot. *Circulation,* **46**:587, 1972.

Wood, F. C.; Wolferth, C. C.; and Geckeler, G. D.: Histologic demonstration of accessory muscular connections between auricle and ventricle in a case of short PR interval and prolonged QRS complex. *Am. Heart J.,* **25**:454, 1941.

Ziegler, R. F.: *Electrocardiographic Studies in Normal Infants and Children.* Charles C Thomas, publisher, Springfield, Ill., 1951.

Zoll, P. M.: Resuscitation of the heart in ventricular standstill by external electrical stimulation. *N. Engl. J. Med.,* **247**:768, 1952.

Zoll, P. M., and Linenthal, A. J.: Termination of refractory tachycardia by external countershock. *Circulation,* **25**:596, 1962.

Zoll, P. M.; Linenthal, A. J.; Gibson, W.; Paul, M. H.; and Norman, L. R.: Termination of ventricular fibrillation in man by externally applied countershock. *N. Engl. J. Med.,* **254**:727, 1956.

18

Sudden Death: Treatment of Cardiac Arrest

John D. Keith and *Rodney S. Fowler*

SUDDEN DEATH

SUDDEN or unexpected death during infancy and childhood is well known to the laity and to the medical profession since it is commonly publicized in the daily press. A number of studies have been carried out on this subject in the pediatric age group, and different patterns have been emphasized by different authors. Etiologic factors have undoubtedly changed with passing generations. Many publications have appeared on the subject in recent years: Adelson and Kinney (1956), Vital Statistics of the U.S. (1960), Wedgewood and Benditt (1966), O'Reilly and Whiley (1967), Steele and coworkers (1967), Harris and Chan (1969), Lambert and associates (1974), and Thornback and Fowler (1975).

Incidence

The incidence of sudden infant death syndrome is shown in Table 18–1 as varying from 1.4 to 3 for 1000 live births. It occurs more commonly in large cities, less frequently in the country.

General Causes

In the newborn period, the weak immature babies may die suddenly from their prematurity alone or death may result from the aspiration of vomitus. Bizarre congenital defects of the diaphragm, lungs, gastrointestinal tract, heart, and central nervous system have also been implicated. Hyperadrenalism or hypoadrenalism is a rare cause of sudden death.

In the past, direct suffocation has been a common cause of death (Davison, 1945), due chiefly to infants sleeping in the same bed as older persons. Deaths of this origin have now become rare.

The syndrome of sudden death in infancy remains an enigma in spite of the intensive studies of the last five or ten years. No clear-cut etiologic factors have been discovered. However, the findings do indicate a characteristic age distribution, with a peak at two to three months of age, as well as a preponderance in males, low-birth-weight babies, and lower socioeconomic group of families. Nearly all the infants died during sleep in a silent fashion, usually in the early morning. Both the epidemiologic findings and some virus studies suggest that such an infection may play a contributory role, but it seems likely that several factors may be involved. Caddell (1972) suggests the hypothesis of magnesium deprivation in this syndrome. She points out that magnesium deprivation may occur in a rapidly growing infant, particularly in a mother who has also had a diet poor in magnesium. Morgan (1969), who had a long experience in pediatric practice, points to the fact that

Table 18–1. INCIDENCE OF SUDDEN INFANT DEATH SYNDROME

			NUMBER PER 1000 LIVE BIRTHS
Ministry of Health of Great Britain	1965	England and Wales (overall)	1.4
Carpenter	1965	England and Wales (overall)	2.2
Peterson	1966	Seattle	2.87
Steele et al.	1967	Canada	3.00
Froggatt et al.	1968	Northern Ireland	2.3
Valdes-Dapena et al.	1968	Philadelphia	2.55
Fitzgibbons et al.	1969	Olmstead Co., Minn. (Mayo Clinic)	1.2

almost invariably one finds these babies lying face down and suggests that an infant on raising the head may have had a vasovagal effect that could produce sudden death, particularly one who is recovering from a respiratory infection.

Sudden Death of Cardiac Origin

Sudden death may occur in acute myocarditis, endocardial fibroelastosis, congenital pulmonary stenosis, congenital aortic stenosis, paroxysmal tachycardia, congenital heart block with Adams–Stokes attack, and bacterial endocarditis with cerebral embolism. Ventricular fibrillation, pulmonary embolism, and certain drugs are also implicated in unexpected fatalities in childhood.

Sudden death from acute myocarditis has been emphasized by several authors (Goldbloom and Wiglesworth, 1938; Bowden, 1951; Werne and Garrow, 1953). Sudden death from endocardial fibroelastosis has been referred to by Adams and Katz (1952) and Adelson and Kinney (1956).

Congenital pulmonary stenosis may lead to sudden death. In these babies relatively minor events, such as breath holding, vomiting, and minor infections, may produce sudden death. This is more likely to occur in the first year of life than after that period. A similar danger occurs with aortic stenosis. The margin of safety is possibly a little greater with aortic stenosis, and one is more likely to have evidence indicative of a severely narrowed opening, as revealed in the electrocardiogram, and thus can issue a warning against violent exercise. Sudden deaths from aortic stenosis may occur during a game of football or while walking up a hill.

Sudden death from Adams–Stokes attack in congenital heart block is very uncommon but has been reported (see Chapter 17). In addition, sudden death from arrhythmia associated with prolapse of the mitral valve may occur in childhood (see Chapter 43). Any particular patient who is under treatment for bacterial endocarditis, especially when the aortic or mitral valve is involved, is under risk of sudden death from cerebral embolism.

Certain drugs are at times dangerous to the heart. The heart becomes more irritable with hypoxia and therefore more sensitive to digitalis, and fibrillation may result. The heart is also more sensitive to digitalis when there is diminished potassium content. The administration of potassium may cause heart block if given too rapidly or in too large quantities. When intravenous potassium penicillin is being given to patients in whom renal function may be impaired, this should be borne in mind.

Recently Thornback and Fowler (1975) at The Hospital for Sick Children, Toronto, have reviewed the hospital experience. They point out that sudden unexpected death is uncommon in the child with cardiac disease. Sudden death among adults with cardiac disease is commonplace. Kuller and co-workers (1966) observed a population of 550,000 in the Baltimore area over a ten-month period, and 336 died suddenly in the age group of 25 to 65, most of whom had arteriosclerotic heart disease.

Sudden death for our purposes was defined as death occurring instantaneously or within an estimated 24 hours of the onset of acute signs or symptoms in a child who was ambulatory with congenital heart disease.

Among 18,000 patients with heart disease seen at The Hospital for Sick Children in the past 25 years, 3055 died before the age of 21. However, only 33 of these fitted the definition of sudden death. Four main groups accounted for the majority of these deaths:

Left ventricular outflow tract obstruction	14
Pulmonary vascular disease	7
Heart block	7
Transposition of great arteries	3
Disease or anomalies of the coronary arteries	1
Other	1

Left Ventricular Outflow Tract Obstruction. In left ventricular outflow tract obstruction, such as aortic valvar stenosis or discrete subvalvar stenosis, there were 14 sudden deaths out of a total of 916 cases; thus approximately 1 percent of this group died suddenly or unexpectedly. However, in the majority of cases of those that died suddenly, the electrocardiogram showed left ventricular hypertrophy with strain, or they were symptomatic or had a decreased exercise tolerance and occasional dyspnea or syncope. Only one child was asymptomatic and died suddenly after climbing a hill on a tree-planting expedition.

These cases contrasted with the 30 children who had diffuse muscular obstruction. There were eight deaths, five of them sudden. Thus, 17 percent of cases with idiopathic hypertrophic muscular obstruction die suddenly in childhood.

Pulmonary Vascular Disease. Of 93 patients with significantly increased pulmonary vascular resistance, 33 had primary pulmonary hypertension and 60 developed the disease in association with a ventricular septal defect. Thirty-one percent of these patients died before the age of 21. Seven of the deaths were sudden. The overall incidence of sudden death from this cause was, therefore, 7.5 percent.

Heart Block. During the surgical repair of a ventricular septal defect, the procedure may damage the left anterior fascicle of the left bundle branch, giving left anterior hemiblock that has a characteristic pattern following surgery with right bundle branch block and a swing of the axis from a positive one to a negative one, usually minus 60 degrees. Sudden death occurred in five children with this type of electrocardiographic pattern postoperatively in our series and has been a continuing problem (Sondheimer et al., 1976).

Another cause of sudden death in the cardiac group is failure of a pacemaker. We had two deaths from this complication.

Table 18–2. MEDICAL DEATHS (NO PREVIOUS SURGERY)*

DIAGNOSIS	PATIENTS No.	Percent of Total
Aortic stenosis	33	18
Eisenmenger's syndrome	28	15
Cyanotic heart disease with pulmonary stenosis	20	10
Obstructive cardiomyopathy	17	9
Nonobstructive cardiomyopathy	12	7
Endocardial fibroelastosis	12	7
Ebstein's disease	11	6
Myocarditis	10	5
Congenital atrioventricular block	8	4
Primary pulmonary hypertension	4	2
Miscellaneous	31	17
Total	186	100

* Lambert, E. C.; Menon, V.; Wagner, H. R.; and Vlad, P.: Sudden unexpected death from cardiovascular disease in children—a co-operative international study. *Am. J. Cardiol.*, **34**:89, 1974.

Transposition of Great Arteries. In children with transposition of the great vessels, the Mustard procedure has been carried out in 105, and three of these children have died postoperatively, suddenly and unexpectedly—one after four years and the other two after one year. None had documented evidence of arrhythmia or heart failure, although all had needed digitalis in the immediate postoperative period.

Anomalous Coronary Artery. We have had one child die suddenly while playing football, and he was found at autopsy to have an anomalous left coronary artery arising from the right sinus of Valsalva in conjunction with the right coronary. From this unusual origin it passed anteriorly between the aorta and the main pulmonary artery before dividing into its two branches. The vessel was somewhat narrowed at the point where it passed between the two great arteries.

Twenty-two children have had an anomalous coronary arising from the pulmonary artery, and of the 13 deaths with this cause only one has been sudden.

Lambert and associates (1974) conducted an international study that included 254 cases that fitted the diagnosis of sudden death between the ages of 1 and 21. Their figures were similar to those of Thornback and Fowler (1975). See Tables 18–2 and 18–3.

Possible Prevention. In the case of aortic stenosis it is important to know the severity of the narrowing, and once this is determined it can be easily recognized which patients are the ones at risk. They should be restricted in activity until surgery has been carried out, if such is indicated.

In relation to the Eisenmenger syndrome it is obviously important to identify the cases that may lead to pulmonary vascular disease early in life and see that they are corrected surgically before the damage has been done to the pulmonary branches. Cyanotic congenital heart disease with pulmonary stenosis

Table 18–3*. LATE POSTOPERATIVE SUDDEN DEATH UNRELATED TO AND IN SPITE OF SURGERY

DIAGNOSIS	PATIENTS (NO.)	CARDIAC SURGICAL PROCEDURES (NO.) Closed Heart	Open Heart
Cyanotic heart disease with pulmonary stenosis	13	15	2
Eisenmenger's syndrome	9	7	3
Aortic stenosis	3	1	3
Aortic stenosis and coarctation	2	2	
Coarctation of aorta	3	3	
Transposition of great arteries	4	4	
Congenital atrioventricular block	1	1	
Miscellaneous	5	2	3
Total	40	35	11

* Lambert, E. C.; Menon, V.; Wagner, H. R.; and Vlad, P.: Sudden unexpected death from cardiovascular disease in children—a co-operative international study. *Am. J. Cardiol.*, **34**:89, 1974.

obviously needs surgical treatment in the majority of cases, and one is continually balancing the risk of surgery versus the risks of continuing with medical therapy.

Pacemakers will usually prevent Adams–Stokes attacks, thus prolonging life in children with complete heart block.

Many other conditions are becoming amenable to operation, including Ebstein's malformation, the aortic valve deformity seen in Marfan's syndrome, and the accessory conduction tissue of the Wolff-Parkinson-White and related syndromes. Advances in these areas will reduce the liability to sudden death under such conditions. The efficacy of mitral valve replacement in relief of refractory ventricular arrhythmias associated with mitral valve prolapse, remains to be established.

Physical Activity. There is a continuous responsibility on the part of the doctor to advise the parents regarding physical activity of the child in relation to the heart defect present. Thus, the doctor may review a long list of activities with the parents, including hockey, football, soccer, baseball, races, bicycling, skating, swimming, basketball, running, and stair climbing. The threat of sudden death is one of the reasons for restricting children to some degree from the more strenuous sports and activities. However, the majority of sudden deaths referred to above occurred when the children were sleeping or at rest. Only 10 per cent of the series reported by Lambert and associates (1974) had been taking part in sports of some kind at the time of their demise. Half of these had severe aortic stenosis or obstructive cardiomyopathy of a degree that would suggest that they were serious risks at the time. Thus, one can determine at a glance from Tables 18–2 and 18–3 what patients are likely to be at risk, and these obviously should be restricted in their physical activity. Others that are not at risk should be guided into a more normal form of life.

TREATMENT OF CARDIAC ARREST IN INFANTS AND CHILDREN BY CARDIAC MASSAGE

IN the newborn and young infant the heart is less prone to develop ventricular fibrillation with hypoxemia than in the adult, so that the problem of defibrillation does not arise as frequently. Thus, cardiac arrest in this age group is not as likely to be associated with this arrhythmia, and this enhances the possibility of successful cardiac massage when cardiac arrest does occur.

The myocardium of an arrested heart is usually severely hypoxic, especially in the asphyxiated infant, and it is important that the myocardium be well oxygenated and regain its tone in order to maintain an adequate cardiac beat. A clear airway and ventilation of the lungs constitute an integral part of successful resuscitation. Kouwenhoven and associates (1960) clearly demonstrated the effectiveness of closed-chest cardiac massage in maintaining the blood pressure and resuscitating patients with cardiac arrest. Since then there have been numerous reports of successful closed-chest resuscitation, both in hospital and outside. Enthusiasm for this technique has been tempered by the fact that trauma to the ribs, liver, heart, lungs, and other organs has occurred during this procedure (Thaler and Krause, 1962) and has led to a study of techniques that eliminate trauma to the heart or neighboring structures. Thaler and Stobie (1963) have developed an improved technique of external cardiac massage in infants and young children. This is carried out as is shown in the accompanying Figure 18–1. The body is held with the head toward the operator, tilting slightly downward. The thumbs are superimposed over the middle of the sternum, a point determined by quick palpation of the sternal notch and xiphisternal junction. (It is the correct selection of this pressure point that avoids damage to the liver. If pressure is applied to the xiphisternum, the latter may occur.) For additional support the fingers are linked behind the back of the infant. Pressure is applied to the sternum by the ball of the lower thumb, assisted if necessary by pressure from the upper thumb. The ribs are left free to expand during artificial ventilation. Pressure should be applied slowly and released rapidly, at the rate of 1 compression per second, or slightly faster, producing 60 to 90 pulsations per minute. Circulatory pressures may be followed on a sphygmomanometer attached to the infant's arm or can be checked by feeling the femoral pulses. The size of the pupils gives an estimate of effective cerebral flow. After each five compressions the thumbs are lifted off the chest, and the lungs ventilated by artificial means. If only one operator is available, mouth-to-mouth ventilation may be administered without difficulty or confusion. As soon as possible an electrocardiographic tracing should be obtained. If ventricular fibrillation is present, defibrillation by means of an external defibrillator should be carried out immediately. When electrocardiographic patterns return to normal, external compression should be continued until effective circulatory pressures can be maintained by the unassisted heart.

Closed-chest massage and defibrillation may be required as a cardiac emergency in the cardiac catheterization laboratory. Such procedures are likely to be highly successful since the arrest or the fibrillation can be identified as soon as it occurs and proper measures instituted as indicated above. Thus, the heart, brain, or other organs are given little time to develop hypoxemic changes and resuscitation is most likely to be successful. An oxygen-enriched atmosphere of course is useful. If the above measures prove ineffective, 1 to 2 ml of calcium chloride, 10 percent

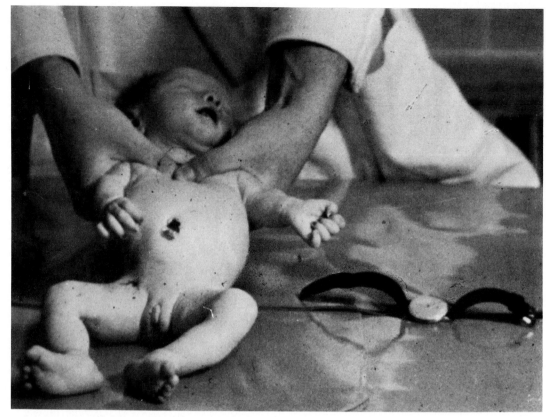

Figure 18-1. Superimposed thumbs compressing the midsternum. Note the bulging of the abdomen as the liver descends. (Reproduced from Thaler, M. M., and Krause, V. W.: Serious trauma in children after external cardiac massage. *New Engl. J. Med.*, 267: 500, 1962.)

solution, or epinephrine, 1 in 10,000, may be injected directly into one of the cardiac chambers and massage continued.

REFERENCES

Sudden Death

Adams, F. H., and Katz, B. L.: Endocardial fibroelastosis. Case reports with special emphasis on the clinical findings. *J. Pediatr.*, **41**: 141, 1952.

Adelson, L., and Kinney, E. R.: Sudden and unexpected death in infancy and childhood, *Pediatrics*, **17**: 663, 1956.

Bergman, A. B.; Ray, C. G.; Pomeroy, M. A.; Wahl, P. W.; and Beckwith, J. B.: Studies of the sudden infant death syndrome in King County, Washington. *Pediatrics*, **49**: 860, 1972.

Bowden, K. M.: Unexpected death in infants and young children. *Med. J. Aust.*, **1**: 925, 1951.

Caddell, J. L.: Magnesium deprivation in sudden unexpected infant death. *Lancet*, **11**: 258, 1972.

Davison, W. H.: Accidental infant suffocation. *Br. Med. J.*, **2**: 251, 1945.

Donohue, W. I.: Personal communication, 1956.

Eisinger, G.: The mystery of sudden infant death. *Clin. Pediatr.*, **10**: 189, 1971.

Fitzgibbons, J. P., Jr.; Nobrega, F. T.; Ludwig, J.; Kurland, L. T.; and Harris, L. E.: Sudden, unexpected, and unexplained death in infants. *Pediatrics*, **43**: 980, 1969.

Friedberg, C. K.: Syncope: pathological physiology, differential diagnosis and treatment. *Mod. Concepts Cardiovasc. Dis.*, **40**: 55, 1971a.

———: Syncope: pathological physiology, differential diagnosis and treatment (II). *Mod. Concepts Cardiovasc. Dis.*, **40**: 61, 1971b.

Froggatt, P.; Lynas, M. A.; and Marshall, T. K.: Sudden death in babies: Epidemiology. *Am. J. Cardiol.*, **22**: 457, 1968.

Garrow, I., and Werne, J.: Sudden apparently unexplained death during infancy. III. Pathologic findings in infants dying immediately after violence, contrasted with those after sudden apparently unexplained death. *Am. J. Pathol.*, **19**: 833, 1953.

Gee, D. J.: A glycoprotein in cardiac conducting tissue. *Br. Heart J.*, **31**: 588, 1969.

Goldbloom, A., and Wiglesworth, F. W.: Sudden death in infancy. *Can. Med. Assoc. J.*, **38**: 119, 1938.

Green, J. R.: A pathological basis for sudden death in eight generations. Abstract of paper, 1964.

Harris, L. E., and Chan, J. C. M.: Infant feeding practices. *Am. J. Dis. Child.*, **117**: 483, 1969.

James, T. N.: Sudden death in babies: new observations in the heart. *Am. J. Cardiol.*, **22**: 479, 1968.

———: QT prolongation and sudden death. *Mod. Concepts Cardiovasc. Dis.*, **38**: 35, 1969.

Kuller, L.: Sudden and unexpected non-traumatic deaths in adults: a review of epidemiological and clinical studies. *J. Chronic Dis.*, **19**: 1165, 1966.

Lambert, E. C.; Menon, V.; Wagner, H. R.; Vlad, P.: Sudden unexpected death from cardiovascular disease in children—a cooperative international study. *Am. J. Cardiol.*, **34**: 89, 1974.

Minuck, M., and Perkins, R.: Long-term study of patients successfully resuscitated following cardiac arrest. *Can. Med. Assoc. J.*, **100**: 1126, 1969.

Morgan, E. A.: Crib deaths. *Can. Med. Assoc. J.*, **100**: 968, 1969.

O'Reilly, M. J., and Whiley, M. K.: Cot deaths in Brisbane, 1962 to 1966. *Med. J. Aust.*, **2**: 1084, 1967.

Ray, C. G.; Beckwith, J. B.; Hebestreit, N. M.; and Bergham, A. B.: Studies of the sudden infant death syndrome in King County, Washington, *JAMA*, **211**: 619, 1970.

Salk, L.: Sudden infant death: impact on family and physician. *Clin. Pediatr.*, **10**:248, 1971.

Schwartz, C. J., and Walsh, W. J.: The pathologic basis of sudden death. *Progr. Cardiovasc. Dis.*, **13**:465, 1971.

Second International Conference on Causes of Sudden Infant Death, Seattle, 1969.

Sondheimer, H. M.; Izukawa, T.; Olley, P. M.; Trusler, G. A.; and Mustard, W. T.: Conduction disturbances after total correction of tetralogy of Fallot. *Am. Heart J.*, **92**:278, 1976.

Steele, R.; Kraus, A. S.; and Langworth, J. T.: Sudden unexpected death in infancy in Ontario. Part I. Methodology and findings related to the host. *Can. J. Public Health*, **58**:359, 1967.

Thornback, P., and Fowler, R. S.: Sudden unexpected death in children with congenital heart disease. *Can. Med. Assoc. J.*, **113**:745, 1975.

U.S. Department of Health, Education and Welfare: Vital Statistics of the United States, 1960, Vol. 1-Natality. Washington, D.C.: Public Health Service, National Vital Statistics Division, 219.

Wedgewood, R. J., and Benditt, E. P.: *Sudden Death in Infants*. PHS Publication No. 1412, Washington, D.C.: U.S. Department of Health, Education, and Welfare, Public Health Service III, 1966.

Werne, J., and Garrow, I.: Sudden apparently unexplained death during infancy. I. Pathologic findings in infants found dead. *Am. J. Pathol.*, **29**:633, 1953.

———: Sudden apparently unexplained death during infancy. II. Pathologic findings in infants observed to die suddenly. *Am. J. Pathol.*, **29**:817, 1953.

Cardiac Arrest

Adelson, L.: A clinicopathologic study of the anatomic changes in the heart resulting from cardiac massage. *Surgery*, **104**:513, 1957.

Adrouny, Z. A.; Stephenson, M. J.; Straube, K. R.; Dotter, C. T.; and Griswold, H. E.: Serum glutamic oxaloacetic and pyruvic transaminases in a case of cardiac arrest resuscitated by external cardiac massage. *Circulation*, **27**:571, 1963.

Altemeier, W. A., and Todd, J.: Studies on the incidence of infection following open chest cardiac massage for cardiac arrest. *Ann. Surg.*, **158**:596, 1963.

Baringer, J. R.; Salzman, E. W.; Jones, W. A.; and Friedlich, A. L.: External cardiac massage. *N. Eng. J. Med.*, **265**:60, 1961.

Bellegie, N. J.; Seldon, T. H.; and Judd, E. S., Jr.: Cardiac massage for cardiac arrest during surgery. *Proc. Mayo Clin.*, **27**:305, 1952.

Bellville, J. W.; Artusio, J. F., Jr.; and Glenn, F.: The electroencephalogram during cardiac manipulation. *Surgery*, **38**:259, 1955.

Bynum, W. A.; Connell, R. M.; and Hawk, W. A.: Causes of death after external cardiac massage: analysis of observations on fifty consecutive autopsies. *Cleveland Clin. Quart.*, **30**:147, 1963.

Clark, D. T.: Complications following closed-chest cardiac massage. *JAMA*, **181**:127, 1962.

Cohen, A. I.; Sumner, R. G.; Whalen, R. E.; Brown, I.; and McIntosh, H. D.: Closed-chest cardiac massage. Survival after fifty-five minutes of ventricular fibrillation without apparent sequelae. *Arch. Intern. Med.*, **110**:57, 1962.

Cole, F.: Cardiac massage in the treatment of arrest of the heart. A study of three hundred fifty cases, with two original case reports. *Arch. Surg.*, **64**:175, 1952.

Dawson, B.; Moffitt, E. A.; Glover, W. J.; and Swan, H. J. C.: Closed-chest resuscitation in a cardiac catheterization laboratory. *Circulation*, **25**:976, 1962.

Haight, C., and Sloan, H.: Successful cardiac resuscitation despite perforation of the heart during massage. *Ann. Surg.*, **141**:240, 1955.

Hurwitt, E. S., and Seidenberg, B.: Rupture of the heart during cardiac massage. *Ann. Surg.*, **137**:115, 1953.

Kouwenhoven, W. B.; Jude, J. R.; and Knickerbocker, G. G.: Closed-chest cardiac massage, *JAMA*, **173**:1064, 1960.

Moya, F.; James, L. S.; Burnard, E. D.; and Hanks, E. C.: Cardiac massage in the newborn infant through the intact chest. *Am. J. Obstet. Gynecol.*, **84**:789, 1962.

Neri, L., and Stevenson, D. L.: Cardiac massage. A new approach. *Lancet*, **2**:1207, 1954.

Nikishin, I. F.: Cardiac rupture during heart massage. Ventricular standstill following administration of procaine amide. *J. Int. Coll. Surg.*, **22**:535, 1954.

Nixon, P. G. F.: The arterial pulse in successful closed-chest cardiac massage. *Lancet*, **2**:844, 1961.

Peddie, G. H.; Creech, O., Jr.; and Halpert, B.; Structural changes in the heart resulting from cardiac massage. *Surgery*, **40**:481, 1956.

Portal, R. W.; Davies, J. G.; Robinson, B. F.; and Leatham, A. G.: Notes on cardiac resuscitation, including external cardiac massage. *Br. Med. J.*, **1**:636, 1963.

Rahter, P. D., and Herron, J. R.: Cardiac resuscitation of the newborn infant. *Am. J. Obstet. Gynecol.*, **79**:249, 1960.

Schweizer, O.; Howland, W. S.; Miller, T.; and Bellville, J. W.: Rupture of the auricle during cardiac resuscitation with complete recovery. *N.Y. J. Med.*, **58**:104, 1958.

Thaler, M. M., and Krause, V. W.: Serious trauma in children after external cardiac massage. *N. Engl. J. Med.*, **267**:500, 1962.

Thaler, M. M., and Stobie, G. H. C.: An improved technic of external cardiac compression in infants and young children. *N. Engl. J. Med.*, **269**:606, 1963.

Vetten, K. B.; Wilson, V. H.; Crawshaw, G. R.; and Nicholson, J. C.: Experimental studies in cardiac massage with special reference to aortic occlusion. *Br. J. Anaesth.*, **27**:1, 1955.

Weale, F. E., and Rothwell-Jackson, R. L.: The efficiency of cardiac massage. *Lancet*, **1**:990, 1962.

Yanoff, M.: Incidence of bone-marrow embolism due to closed-chest cardiac massage. *N. Engl. J. Med.*, **269**:839, 1963.

19

Cerebral Complications in Congenital Heart Disease

Douglas A. McGreal

MANY pathologic changes may be found in the brains of children dying from congenital heart disease. These include venous congestion, petechial hemorrhages, inflammatory reactions, focal necrosis and encephalomalacia, patchy demyelination, vascular occlusions, and cerebral abscess (Cohen, 1960).

From a clinical point of view, cerebral complications have become less frequent but are still seen and may be classified as:

1. Hypoxic episodes with or without loss of consciousness or convulsions.
2. Cardiovascular accidents.
3. Cerebral abscess.

Hypoxic Episodes

Brief "blue spells" or apneic episodes with or without evident loss of consciousness or convulsions may be seen in the child with congenital cyanotic heart disease, related to low arterial oxygen content and precipitated by febrile illness or by other more obscure factors. Most such spells occur in the under-two age group, but they are not unknown in older age groups. Tyler and Clark (1958) reviewed the subject and correlated the arterial oxygen levels with degrees of disturbance of consciousness and convulsions. It is possible that severe or repeated hypoxic insults to the brain will cause damage, which in turn may give rise to convulsions and hence the need for anticonvulsant medication. However, this is uncommon in the young child.

Hypoxic attacks are treated with oxygen, the correction of anemia, and, where possible, cardiac surgery.

Cerebrovascular Accidents

Cerebrovascular accidents (CVA) in congenital heart disease have been recognized for many years (Garrod et al., 1913; Abbott, 1936; Taussig, 1947).

The latter emphasized the relationship to hypoxia and to the higher red blood cell count. Tyler and Clark (1957) reviewed the subject and found that 3.8 percent of their children with congenital heart disease (14.5 percent cyanotic) had this complication. Phornphutkul and associates (1973) found the overall incidence of CVA in children with cyanotic congenital heart disease to be 1.6 percent, the majority of the children being under two years of age, and 70 percent of episodes occurring under the age of four years. They noted that the accidents in those under four years of age were associated with anemia and hypoxemia but that in the older children the association was with polycythemia and hypoxemia. Tetralogy of Fallot and transposition of the great vessels accounted for 90 percent of the patients.

Pathologically there are areas of infarction related to arterial or venous occlusion.

The prognosis is better with the older children, but sequelae are common and include hemiplegia, seizures, and mental retardation.

The diagnosis lies in exclusion of bacterial endocarditis and cerebral abscess, and the age range (younger patients) is helpful in this respect. Investigations such as computer-assisted tomography (CAT), the radionuclide brain scan, the electroencephalogram (EEG), blood culture, and the progression of the clinical picture are useful diagnostically. Treatment is symptomatic. Preventive measures include early correction of relative anemia and early corrective surgery where possible.

Cerebral Abscess

Brain abscess as a complication of congenital heart disease has been recognized for many years. Farre, in 1814, was the first to describe the association, and the reports in the early literature were summarized by Newton (1956). The reported incidence of brain abscess with congenital heart disease varies with the population studied, but at The Hospital for Sick Children, Toronto, over a 15-year period the percentage has been 0.8. With cyanotic congenital heart disease a 2 percent incidence of brain abscess is reported by Fischbein and coworkers (1974). When brain abscess is considered from all causes, about 10 percent have an associated congenital heart lesion, but in the childhood years "cyanotic congenital heart disease remains the single common correlate with brain abscess formation" (Calkins and Bell, 1967).

Brain abscess with congenital heart disease is rare under the age of two (Hoffman et al., 1970); about half the cases occur between the ages of three and ten, with a third between the ages of 10 and 20. It is of interest that brain abscess is rarely associated with bacterial endocarditis (Fontana and Edwards, 1962).

Clinical Features. The clinical features have been reviewed by Matson and Solam (1961), Raimondi and associates (1965), and Samson and Clark (1973). Development of the abscess may be preceded by recognized infection, such as otitis, pharyngitis, generalized upper respiratory infection, or rarely dental infection, but more commonly the onset is insidious. Headache, which may become severe, vomiting, and focal neurologic signs including convulsions are most likely to be present, while the signs of infection such as fever, raised white count, and raised sedimentation rate may be minimal or absent. The signs of increased intracranial pressure—papilledema, split sutures on the skull x-ray, slowing of the pulse, and so forth—are late features and indicate an abscess of considerable size and duration. It should be emphasized that in the presence of cyanotic congenital heart disease in a child over two years of age, any cerebral symptoms or signs should be considered to indicate the presence of an abscess until proven otherwise.

Investigations should initially be noninvasive since these are most helpful; the CAT scan, the radionuclide scan, and the EEG all provide useful and likely diagnostic information that may be supplemented by cerebral angiography when necessary. In suspected cases, lumbar puncture should not be performed. The very rare posterior fossa or brain stem abscess may be difficult to diagnose clinically.

Pathology. With rare exceptions, cerebral abscess is found in the cyanotic congenital heart group, with a right-to-left shunt, Fallot's tetralogy, and transposition of the great vessels providing most of the patients. Fischbein and associates (1974) record the frequency of brain abscess as 2.8 percent of Fallot's tetralogy and double-outlet right ventricle, 1.9 percent of complete AV canal, 1.3 percent of tricuspid atresia, and 1 percent of dextrotransposition. The abscess, or abscesses, may occur in any part of the brain but rarely in the posterior fossa or brain stem. Clearly, since most of the patients are over three years of age, the rates of incidence will reflect both the total numbers and the numbers of those who survive long enough possibly to develop cerebral complications. Culture of the organisms involved in abscess formation shows a great variety of bacteria, both aerobic and anaerobic, and it is not uncommon for no organism to be identified. It has been suggested (Matson and Solam, 1961) that two conditions are prerequisite for abscess formation: (1) intermittent bacteremia and (2) focal encephalomalacia. It is logical to assume that because of the presence of a right-to-left shunt, there is an absence of the normal phagocytic-filtering action of the pulmonary vascular bed so that transient bacteremia may result in infection reaching the brain. Focal encephalomalacia is increased by hypoxia and decreased cerebral blood flow. Infection may also reach the brain by direct extension from ears and sinuses. Fischbein and coworkers (1974) correlate morbidity and mortality in brain abscess as inversely related to oxygen saturation levels. High blood viscosity may also play a part by decreasing blood flow and predisposing to arterial or venous occlusion (Berthrong and Sabiston, 1951).

Treatment. As already stated, it should be considered axiomatic that any child with congenital heart disease and cerebral symptoms has a brain abscess until proven otherwise, especially if the child is over two years of age. Once the diagnosis is made, treatment is neurosurgical and generally repeated aspirations will be satisfactory. The use of antibiotics is routine, but the value of these is uncertain once abscess formation has begun. The prognosis is better with early diagnosis, depending on the cardiac condition, but about 50 percent of survivors will have some neurologic sequelae.

Prevention. In view of the etiologic factors involved—age, right-to-left shunt, hypoxia, and decreased cerebral blood flow—it might be expected that corrective (as opposed to palliative) surgery in the first two years of life would reduce the incidence of brain abscess at a later date.

REFERENCES

Abbott, M. E.: *Atlas of Congenital Cardiac Disease.* American Heart Association, New York, 1936.

Beller, H.: The syndrome of brain abscess with congenital cardiac disease. Report of a case with complete recovery. *J. Neurosurg.,* **8**:239, 1951.

Berthrong, M., and Sabiston, D. C., Jr.: Cerebral lesions in congenital heart disease. A review of autopsies on one hundred and sixty two cases. *Bull. Hopkins Hosp.,* **89**:384, 1951.

Calkins, R. A., and Bell, W. E.: Cerebral abscess and cyanotic congenital heart disease. *Lancet,* **87**:403, 1967.

Cohen, I.; Bergman, P.; and Malis, L.: Paradoxic brain abscess in congenital heart disease. *J. Neurosurg.,* **8**:225, 1951.

Cohen, M. M.: The central nervous system in congenital heart disease. *Neurology,* **10**:452, 1960.

Ehni, G., and Crain, E. L.: "Paradoxical" brain abscess; report of a unique case in association with Lutembacher's syndrome. *JAMA,* **150**:1298, 1952.

Faris, A. A.; Guth, C.; Youmans, R. A.; and Poser, C. M.: Internal carotid artery occlusion in children. *Am. J. Dis. Child.,* **107**:188, 1964.

Farre, J. R.: *On Malformations of Human Heart.* Longman, Hurst, Rees, Orme and Brown, Ltd., London, 1814.

Fischbein, C. A.; Rosenthal, A.; Fischer, E. G.; Nadas, A. S.; and Welch, K.: Risk factors for brain abscess in patients with congenital heart disease. *Am. J. Cardiol.,* **34**:97, 1974.

Fontana, R. S., and Edwards, J. E.: *Congenital Cardiac Disease. A Review of 357 Cases Studied Pathologically.* W. B. Saunders Co., Philadelphia, 1962.

Garrod, A. E.; Batten, F. E.; and Thursfield, H.: *Diseases of Children.* E. Arnold and Co., London, 1913.

Gluck, R.; Hall, J. W.; and Stevenson, L. D.: Brain abscess associated with congenital heart disease. *Pediatrics*, **9**:192, 1952.

Hanna, R.: Cerebral abscess and paradoxic embolism associated with congenital heart disease. Report of 7 cases with review of the literature. *Am. J. Dis. Child.*, **62**:555, 1941.

Hoffman, H. J.; Hendrick, E. B.; and Hiscox, J. L.: Cerebral abscess in early infancy. *J. Neurosurg.*, **33**:172, 1970.

McGreal, D. A.: Brain abscess in children. *Can. Med. Assoc. J.*, **86**:261, 1962.

Maronde, R. F.: Brain abscess and congenital heart disease. *Ann. Intern. Med.*, **33**:602, 1950.

Martelle, R. R., and Linde, L. M.: Cerebrovascular accidents with tetralogy of Fallot. *Am. J. Dis. Child.*, **101**:206, 1961.

Matson, D. O., and Salam, M.: Brain abscess in congenital heart disease. *Pediatrics*, **27**:772, 1961.

Moncrieff, A., and Evans, P.: *Diseases of Children*, 5th ed. E. Arnold Co., London, 1953.

Newton, E. J.: Brain abscess in congenital heart disease. *Q. J. Med.*, **25**:201, 1956.

Phornphutkul, C.; Rosenthal, A.; Nadas, A. S.; and Berenberg, W.: Cerebrovascular accidents in infants and children with cyanotic congenital heart disease. *Am. J. Cardiol.*, **32**:329, 1973.

Raimondi, A. J.; Matsumoto, S.; and Miller, R. A.: Brain abscess in children with congenital heart disease. *J. Neurosurg.*, **23**:588, 1965.

Robbins, S. L.: Brain abscess associated with congenital heart disease. *Arch. Intern. Med.*, **75**:279, 1945.

Samson, D. S., and Clark, K. A.: A current review of brain abscess. *Am. J. Med.*, **54**:201, 1973.

Smolik, E. A.; Blattner, R. J.; and Heys, F. M.: Brain abscess associated with congenital heart disease. Report of case with complete recovery. *JAMA*, **130**:145, 1946.

Sweeney, D. B., and Patton, W. B.: Surgical management of cerebral abscess associated with congenital heart disease. *South. Med. J.*, **43**:799, 1950.

Taussig, H. B.: *Congenital Malformations of the Heart*. The Commonwealth Fund, New York, 1947.

Tyler, H. R., and Clark, D. B.: Cerebrovascular accidents in patients with congenital heart disease. *Arch. Neurol.*, **77**:483, 1957.

————: Loss of consciousness and convulsions with congenital heart disease. *Arch. Neurol.*, **79**:506, 1958.

CHAPTER

20

The Heart in Anemia

Peter D. McClure, M. Renate Dische, and *John D. Keith*

I T H A S long been recognized that the heart may be affected in anemia. In infants and children, iron deficiency, hemorrhage, blood dyscrasias, and infection are the most common causes of a lowered hemoglobin. In spite of the fact that approximately 60 cases with the principal diagnosis of anemia are admitted each year to The Hospital for Sick Children, Toronto, only 1 or 2 percent have clinical evidence of cardiac involvement.

When the hemoglobin drops below 7 gm percent, an increase in cardiac output occurs (Blumgart and Altschule, 1948). When it drops below 3.5 gm percent, cardiac enlargement is usually found, with or without congestive heart failure (Tung et al., 1937). The increased cardiac output is associated with a reduction of total peripheral resistance. The blood volume is reduced (Sharpey-Schafer, 1944), and the venous pressure is increased.

At postmortem following severe and prolonged anemia, cardiac enlargement is the rule. The heart is increased in size and weight, particularly the left ventricle. Fatty degeneration and microscopic foci of myocardial necrosis have been described (Friedberg and Horn, 1939). Dilatation of the heart and hypertrophy are both found. The former is more common in the acute anemias, and the latter appears in the more chronic types. There are several factors that contribute to the enlargement of the heart: the degree of the anemia, the rapidity with which the anemia develops, the ability of the patient's cardiovascular system to adjust physiologically to the anemia, and the presence of underlying disease.

When the hemoglobin falls below 7 gm percent, the cardiac output increases and gives more work to the myocardium. At the same time, the blood supplying the heart has a diminished oxygen-carrying capacity, producing some degree of hypoxemia in the tissues. Thus, these two factors lead to cardiac hypertrophy. Although the severer cases have the largest hearts, there is no exact parallel between the degree of anemia and the heart size.

Clinical Features

Pallor is, of course, a cardinal feature of children with cardiac involvement due to anemia. It is frequently accompanied by lassitude, hyporexia, and sometimes dizziness. There may be a history of dyspnea with effort, due to the anemia alone or at times associated with congestive heart failure.

Part of the clinical picture of heart disease in anemia may be the underlying cause, such as hemorrhage, leukemia, chronic hemolytic anemia, or severe iron deficiency. In the presence of such etiologic factors, careful examination of the heart should be made.

The heart rate is usually increased 10 to 30 beats per minute over the usual rate for the age concerned. The hands are usually warm and moist. Blood pressure is slightly lower than normal, with a widened pulse pressure that may be associated with capillary pulsations. The apical beat is more forceful than usual; the pulse is fuller and more readily palpable. The first heart sound may be normal or booming and distinctly increased, at times simulating that of mitral stenosis. The second heart sound is clear-cut and finely split, and frequently there is a third heart sound present.

Heart murmurs are the rule but may occasionally be absent. The apical systolic murmur, transmitted to the axilla, is a common finding, but just as frequently one may hear a systolic murmur down the left sternal border. At times a rapid-inflow type of diastolic murmur follows the third sound just inside the apex. On relatively rare occasions an aortic diastolic murmur may be recognized down the left sternal border and is considered to be due to dilatation of the aortic valve ring. This disappears when the anemia is completely corrected.

The murmur is not closely related to heart size. Hunter (1946) reports that well-heard murmurs may be present when the heart is normal in size, and occasionally may be absent when enlargement is present. The murmur appears to be due to the accelerated blood flow and reduced viscosity. It usually persists after the cardiac enlargement has disappeared and is more intimately related to the hemoglobin level of the blood. The murmur usually disappears when the hemoglobin level has returned to normal.

A third of the patients reported by Hunter (1946) with anemia showed cardiac enlargement. Return to normal size occurred in all but three with treatment. The rapidity with which normal size is reached varies markedly, depending on the cause of the anemia and the patient's response to therapy. In children the return to normal size may occur within one week after the beginning of therapy.

Heart failure may occur in the severe cases. This has been found more frequently in adults since other factors causing cardiac damage are frequently associated. In children, heart failure due to anemia is rare. Anemia is one of the few causes of high-output heart failure. The others are beriberi, hyperthyroidism, and arteriovenous aneurysm. Heart failure is usually associated with dyspnea, enlargement of the liver, a mild degree of edema, enlargement of the heart, a systolic murmur, or a well-heard third heart sound followed by an inflow diastolic murmur proceeding at times to a distinct gallop rhythm.

Electrocardiographic Changes

A variety of electrocardiographic changes have been reported, nonspecific and usually minor in degree. Flattening or inversion of the T wave may occur; low amplitude of the T, prolongation of the P-R interval, depression of the S-T segment, and increased voltage over the left precordium indicative of left ventricular hypertrophy also may appear. Some of these changes may disappear with therapy; others will persist for some weeks or months. The

evidence of hypertrophy is likely to persist for many months before disappearing.

A three-year-old boy who had a hemoglobin of 3.3 gm percent and a markedly enlarged heart with a systolic murmur at the apex had an electrocardiogram showing a left ventricular hypertrophy pattern in the precordial leads. Two transfusions caused the murmur to disappear and the heart to reduce in size slowly.

The electrocardiogram is shown (Figure 20–1) of a boy 13 years of age with a hemoglobin of 1.7 gm percent, who was found to have leukemia as well as anemia. It was of interest that, in spite of the underlying disease and the severe anemia, the heart was only slightly enlarged and measured 11.5/21.5 cm. With two transfusions and one week's observation, the heart had returned to within normal limits in size and measured 10.5/21.5 cm. Gallop rhythm, which was present on admission, disappeared three days after repeated transfusions. The electrocardiogram showed left ventricular hypertrophy with depression of the S-T segment. On admission 12 days later, when the hemoglobin was 5 gm percent, the S-T segment had returned to normal, and the signs of left ventricular hypertrophy had diminished.

Treatment

For infants or children with heart involvement in anemia, transfusion is the treatment of choice, but the blood must be given cautiously to avoid overloading the circulation and precipitating acute congestive failure or death.

Small transfusions of 5 ml per pound of body weight, given slowly and repeated as often as required to bring the hemoglobin up close to normal, are usually a safe method of proceeding. Packed cells rather than whole blood should be used if many transfusions are indicated. Iron medication or specific

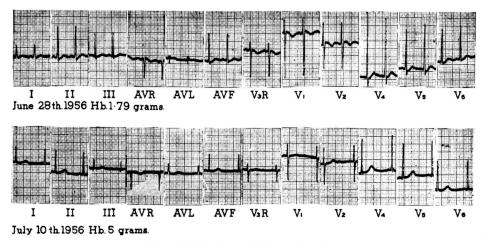

I   II   III   AVR   AVL   AVF   V₃R   V₁   V₂   V₄   V₅   V₆
June 28th.1956 Hb.1·79 grams.

I   II   III   AVR   AVL   AVF   V₃R   V₁   V₂   V₄   V₅   V₆
July 10th.1956 Hb.5 grams.

Figure 20-1. L. H., aged 13 years. Anemia.

therapy for any underlying disease may be needed at the same time.

Prognosis

Once the anemia is corrected, provided there is no other cause, the cardiac involvement will rapidly or gradually disappear and the heart will return to normal. Gallop rhythm usually disappears in two or three days, the heart size decreases as the dilatation is relieved, and later, the hypertrophy diminishes over a period of several months.

The murmur will disappear rapidly as the hemoglobin returns to normal level.

SPECIFIC DISEASE

Sickle Cell Anemia

Sickle cell anemia, or homozygous S disease, is a chronic form of severe anemia with onset early in life. It predominantly afflicts the black population; approximately 8 percent of American Negroes are heterozygous for the sickle gene. About 1 in 150 marriages will unite two heterozygotes, with the possibility that 24 percent of their offspring will be homozygous for hemoglobin S and will therefore present the clinical picture of sickle cell anemia.

Sickle cell anemia was the first molecular disease elucidated in man (Pauling et al., 1949). It depends on the substitution of a nonpolar amino acid, valine, for a polar amino acid, glutamic acid, in the six position of the beta chain of the hemoglobin molecule. Alterations in the folding and aggregation of hemoglobin S molecules during reducing oxygen tension produce the sickling phenomenon.

The sickling of red cells was first described in 1910 by Dr. Herrick, a Chicago cardiologist, in a severely anemic West Indian student with cardiac enlargement and a murmur (Herrick, 1910). Since then it has been recognized that cardiac disease is a frequent and early complication of sickle cell anemia.

Symptoms of sickle cell anemia can occur as early as the first few months of life, or as soon as cessation of hemoglobin F synthesis causes a rise in the level of hemoglobin S. There is, characteristically, severe arterial hypoxemia to which the heart adjusts by increased minute output (Lindsay et al, 1974). This increase in cardiac output usually occurs at levels of hemoglobin below 7 gm per 100 ml of blood.

The heart is therefore under considerable long-term stress, and congestive heart failure may occur early in life. The work of the heart is further increased by repeated focal occlusions of small pulmonary vessels. These are favored by local tissue hypoxia in the frequent pulmonary infections, particularly pneumococcal pneumonia, to which patients with sickle cell anemia are prone.

Clinical Features. Children with sickle cell anemia frequently have evidence of cardiovascular involvement. The clinical findings resemble those in chronic anemia of other causes, but are more prominent and earlier in onset, reflecting the severity of the disease and the difficulties met in its control. The heart generally shows signs of great activity dependent on its increased stroke volume. There is a prominent, often enlarged sustained apical impulse, and a left parasternal lift may be felt. The first heart sound is modestly accentuated; the second heart sound is prominent and frequently split. A systolic, typically ejection-type murmur is transmitted over the precordium of virtually all patients. In a young child, rheumatic heart disease may be difficult to distinguish, because of the coincident findings of swollen painful hands, the precordial murmur, and mitral regurgitation.

Chest x-ray discloses diffuse cardiac enlargement of variable degree with some enlargement of the pulmonary artery and increase in pulmonary vascular markings in most children.

Electrocardiographic findings of cardiac hypertrophy are usually present. Prolongation of the P-R and Q-T interval, nonspecific changes in the S-T segment and the T waves may be present, but none of these are specific for the disease.

Life expectancy is considerably shortened in sickle cell anemia. In the United States a median survival of 20 years was calculated on the basis of data from the Bureau of Vital Statistics. Cause of death in children is usually a fulminant infection.

Pathology. A variety of pathologic findings have been reported, but none are pathognomonic for the disease. A consistent finding is cardiac enlargement. The ratio of cardiac weight to body weight was increased from 20 percent to over 100 percent with an average of 60 percent. In a large series of autopsies on children, varying in age from a few months to 14 years, cardiac hypertrophy predominantly of the left ventricle was present in every case (Webber and Kaufman, 1975). Right ventricular hypertrophy, secondary to advanced pulmonary vasculo-occlusive disease, can occur in older patients. Focal myocardial fibrosis, an inconstant finding in sickle cell anemia, has been related to ischemic sequelae of intravascular sickling in intramyocardial coronary arterial branches. Arteritis and nonocclusive intimal thickening with an increase of mucoid interstitial material have been noted. Not surprisingly 25 percent of young children dying with fulminant sepsis had a variable degree of myocarditis.

Thalassemia Major

Thalassemia major, one of the more common hereditary hemolytic anemias, was first recognized as a distinct entity by Dr. Thomas Cooley in 1925

(Cooley and Lee, 1925). Although best known for its incidence among the Eastern Mediterranean population, it also afflicts Southeast Asians and has been reported in Chinese, blacks, and others. It is worldwide in distribution.

Thalassemia is inherited as a single autosomal, incompletely dominant gene: in the homozygous state two incompletely dominant abnormal alleles are present. When two heterozygotes with thalassemia minor mate, there is a 25 percent chance for a homozygous offspring with thalassemia major.

The basic biochemical defect in the thalassemia syndromes is an imbalance in globin synthesis (prevalent in peoples of Italian and Greek origin): there is a decrease in beta-chain synthesis with normal alpha-chain production (Kacian et al., 1973). Several intracellular defects have been found. The most important one is decreased production of normal messenger RNA responsible for beta-chain synthesis and resulting in a substitution of the beta chain by chains typical of hemoglobin F and hemoglobin A_2.

The effects of this disordered globin synthesis are manyfold. In general, decreased levels of hemoglobin are present in the maturing red blood cells. Intracellular accumulation of excessive free alpha chains has been linked to cellular deformation in the spleen and bone marrow with the ensuing rapid destruction of red blood cells characteristic of thalassemia. This is poorly compensated by excessive but ineffectual hematopoiesis.

Clinical Features.   In contrast to the heterozygous individual with thalassemia minor whose symptoms are absent or mild, the majority of individuals homozygous for thalassemia suffer from severe disease. The typical patient with thalassemia major presents in the first two years of life with profound anemia and failure to thrive. In older children severe bone pain and disfiguring facial changes secondary to exuberant erythropoiesis are troublesome symptoms. There is usually marked splenic enlargement due to extramedullary hematopoiesis and massive trapping of erythrocytes in the splenic sinusoids. The disease is palliated by splenectomy and blood transfusions at frequent intervals. Both procedures entail their own brand of iatrogenic misfortune. Splenectomy is followed by reduced resistance to infection, particularly pneumococcal sepsis and meningitis. Prolonged blood transfusions eventually lead to severe iron overload of all organs with marked parenchymal damage in some and gradual appearance of functional abnormalities in most. Clinically these become overt as cirrhosis of the liver, diabetes mellitus, endocrine abnormalities, and heart disease.

Improved management of infectious episodes, adjustment of the transfusion schedule to symptomatic requirements, and removal of excessive iron stores by chelating agents have gradually led to survival of patients with thalassemia major well into their third decade. The majority succumb to heart disease.

Cardiac involvement increases in incidence and severity with advancing age of the patient. Only about one-fourth of the children between six and ten years of age have signs of cardiac abnormalities, while virtually all suffer some form of cardiac disease by the end of their second decade. Recurrent pericarditis, cardiac arrhythmias, and congestive heart failure are the major presenting forms of cardiac involvement.

Pericarditis, more often without pericardial effusion, is a benign and self-limiting complication of thalassemia major and tends to recur (Master et al., 1961). The average patient experiences his first attack when about 11 years old. Precordial pain accompanied by transient fever may usher in the illness. The etiology of the recurring pericarditis remains unexplained. No causative agent has been identified although the frequent history of antecedent upper respiratory or gastrointestinal disturbance suggests a viral background.

Cardiac arrhythmias are a more serious complication and afflict practically every patient somewhat later in the course of his disease. They may precede congestive heart failure by months or even years. The average age of onset in a series of 38 cases was 13 to 14 years (Canale et al., 1975). The most frequently encountered arrhythmias are atrial and ventricular premature contractions, incomplete bundle branch block, and first-degree heart block. Shifting pacemaker and sinus arrhythmia are likely to occur in the younger patient. Prolonged conduction, atrial flutter and fibrillation, paroxysmal atrial tachycardia, and occasionally ventricular tachycardia and AV dissociation are more typical of advanced disease and may accompany heart failure. Early recognition of cardiac arrhythmia and prompt treatment have a favorable influence on the course of the disease.

Congestive heart failure is usually preceded by evidence of cardiac enlargement, which increases with the onset of failure. The initial episode of cardiac failure occurred at about 14 to 15 years of age in a large number of cases under study (Canale et al., 1975). Until recently it was thought to be an ominous sign of impending death. However, improved cardiac management has permitted survival from 1 to 12 years after the first episode of congestive heart failure. Nevertheless, congestive heart failure with or without severe arrhythmia is the leading cause of death in thalassemia major.

Pathology.   At autopsy the heart is much enlarged with both right and left ventricular hypertrophy. The myocardium is deep brown and often flabby. Diffuse iron incrustation of myocardial fibers accompanied by variable degree of focal atrophy and fibrosis is present in both ventricles and the interventricular septum. Subepicardial fibrosis not clearly related to epicardial scarring is a frequent finding. The subendocardial areas are relatively normal. However, there is focal iron and calcium incrustation of the endocardial elastic fibrils, most conspicuous in the left atrium. The papillary muscles, particularly the posterior one, may be extensively replaced by fibrous tissue. The affected myocardial fibers frequently display bizarre nuclear and cytoplasmic distortion.

Muscle giant cells and binucleate muscle fibers are not infrequent. Myocardial damage was most severe in a patient receiving the greatest amount of iron (179 gm in 22 years), but the relation between tissue injury and the amount of iron administered is not clear-cut in most cases (Canale et al., 1975). The coronary arteries, particularly the small muscular intramyocardial branches, often display iron pigment in their thickened muscular walls and intima. However, no occlusive changes have been observed and there was little relation to the degree of myocardial fibrosis. The conduction system is also affected by the general iron incrustation, but generally to a lesser degree than the surrounding myocardium. The sinoatrial node is generally spared.

HEMATOLOGIC COMPLICATIONS

POLYCYTHEMIA is invariably present in those patients who are cyanosed due to a right-to-left shunt. In fact, a normal hemoglobin in a cyanosed patient should make one suspect concomitant iron deficiency (Rudolph et al., 1953). Hemoglobins of more than 20 gm per 100 ml (hematocrits greater than 60 per cent) are not uncommon. The rise in hematocrit is due to an increased red cell mass with plasma volume remaining in a normal range. Blood viscosity rises exponentially once the hematocrit exceeds 50 per cent. This leads to sluggish circulation, excessive deoxygenation, aggravation of peripheral cyanosis, and tissue hypoxia. In extreme cases the patient may experience headache, dizziness, and general malaise. Fortunately, thrombosis is rare, but it is a distinct danger in patients with hematocrits over 70 percent who become dehydrated or are subjected to excessive temperatures. The tendency to thrombosis may also be aggravated by the presence of iron deficiency (Martelle and Linde, 1961).

The advantage in oxygen-carrying capacity gained by a high hemoglobin may be outweighed by the disadvantages resulting from high blood viscosity and secondary decreased oxygen transport to tissues. For this reason, some have suggested phlebotomies in patients who are symptomatic or are going to surgery. However, acute phlebotomies have been reported to cause vascular collapse, seizures, and cerebral vascular accidents and should therefore be discouraged. A safer procedure is the selective removal of red cells with their replacement by plasma or albumin. This has been shown to decrease viscosity, increase peripheral blood flow, improve oxygen availability to tissues, and reduce bleeding at surgery (Rosenthal et al., 1970).

A wide variety of *hemostatic defects* in coagulation factors has been described, including deficiencies of vitamin K–dependent factors (prothrombin; factors VII, IX, and X) and consumable factors (fibrinogen; factors V and VIII) (Wedemeyer et al., 1972). In many cases, coagulation factors have been normal (Johnson et al., 1968; Wedemeyer et al., 1972), while at the opposite extreme cases with frank disseminated intravascular coagulation have been described (Dennis et al., 1967). Deficiencies of vitamin K–dependent factors might be explained on the basis of liver deficiency secondary to vascular sludging and hypoxia. However, the mechanism leading to minor deficiencies of one or more factors such as factor V or fibrinogen seems less poorly defined. Coagulation defects are much more likely to be found in cyanotic patients than acyanotic. Since no set pattern exists, patients need to be assessed individually. Postoperatively, the defects are often more severe and a fall in factor VIII and fibrinogen can be expected.

Thrombocytopenia is a common finding in cyanotic patients, and its severity is related to the degree of hypoxia and polycythemia. Turnover studies have shown that platelet survival is diminished while production is normal or increased. These changes are associated with increased platelet stickiness and aggregation to adenosine diphosphate (ADP). There appear to be at least two mechanisms whereby hypoxia brings about these changes. Tissue hypoxia results in lactic acidemia, which causes increased platelet adhesiveness (Goldschmidt and Kun, 1973). Second, platelet adhesiveness increases in direct proportion to the red cell volume, as shown in both in vivo and in vitro studies by Hellen (1960). The increased red cell breakdown causes increased release of ADP into the circulation with resultant increased platelet aggregation and reduced survival.

Thrombocytopenia is further aggravated by destruction and loss of platelets during extracorporeal circulation. This state may persist for one to two days postoperatively. When platelet counts drop below 50,000 per cubic millimeter, a platelet transfusion should be considered. In the severely thrombocytopenic patient, preoperative reduction of red cell mass may improve the situation.

Increased *fibrinolysis* has been reported in some patients both before and during surgery. Although there is controversy as to whether this leads to increased bleeding during surgery, some studies have shown that epsilon-aminocaproic acid (an inhibitor of fibrinolysis) reduced bleeding in cyanotic patients on prolonged extracorporeal circulation (McClure and Izsak, 1974).

Blood Changes Secondary to Cardiac Surgery. Hemolytic anemia due to traumatic damage to red cells is not infrequent following surgery in which prosthetic valves or Teflon patches are inserted (Marsh and Lewis, 1970). Damage is due to the high shear forces and abnormal hemodynamics created by such operations. The degree of hemolysis can vary from barely detectable shortened red cell survival to severe incapacitating disease requiring multiple transfusions. Damaged red cells are readily apparent in the peripheral blood as fragmented cells (schistocytes) and spherocytes. An elevated reticulocyte count, polychromasia, elevated indirect bilirubinemia, and reduced serum haptoglobin are other evidences of increased hemolysis. Hemoglobin released into the plasma results in hemoglobinemia, hemosiderinuria, and hemoglobinuria. Large quantities of iron may be lost in the urine resulting in iron deficiency. Some improvement may occur with time as the abnormal surfaces become covered with endothelium. In many cases, however, it may be necessary to give long-term iron therapy to compensate for urine losses, and in severe cases it may be necessary to reoperate.

Platelet survival is also reduced in patients with prosthetic heart valves. This does not appear to be part of a general consumptive coagulopathy since fibrinogen turnover is normal (Harker and Slichter, 1970). Platelet consumption is not active enough to prevent thrombopoiesis from maintaining a normal platelet count. However, it may well be related to the high incidence of thromboembolic complications. The administration of dipyridamole and aspirin has returned platelet survival to normal (Harker and Slichter, 1970) and may be a useful drug regimen to prevent embolization.

REFERENCES

Abramson, D. I.; Fierst, S. M.; and Flachs, K.: Resting peripheral blood flow in the anemic state. *Am. Heart J.*, **25**:609, 1943.

Blumgart, H. L., and Altschule, M. D.: Clinical significance of cardiac and respiratory adjustment in chronic anemia. *Blood*, **3**:329, 1948.

Bradley, S. E., and Bradley, G. P.: Renal function during chronic anemia in man. *Blood*, **2**:192, 1947.

Canale, V.; Engle, M. A.; and Dische, M. R.: Personal communication, 1975.

Case, R. B.; Berglund, E.; and Sarnoff, S. J.: Ventricular function. VII. Changes in coronary resistance and ventricular function resulting from acutely induced anemia and the effect thereon of coronary stenosis. *Am. J. Med.*, **18**:397, 1955.

Cooley, T. B., and Lee, P.: A series of cases of splenomegaly in children with anemia and peculiar bone changes. *Trans. Am. Pediatr. Soc.*, **37**:29, 1925.

Dennis, L. H.; Stewart, J. L.; and Conrad, M. E.: A consumption coagulation defect in congenital cyanotic heart disease and its treatment with heparin. *J. Pediatr.*, **71**:407–10, 1967.

Ellis, L. B., and Faulkner, J. M.: The heart in anemia. *N. Engl. J. Med.*, **220**:943, 1939.

Friedberg, C. K., and Horn, H.: Acute myocardial infarction not due to coronary occlusion. *JAMA*, **112**:1675, 1939.

Goldschmidt, B., and Kun, E.: Platelet adhesiveness in cyanotic congenital heart disease. *Acta Paed. Acad. Scient. Hung.*, **14**:99–103, 1973.

Harker, L., and Slichter, S. J.: Studies of platelet and fibrinogen kinetics in patients with prosthetic heart valves. *N. Engl. J. Med.*, **283**:1302–1305, 1970.

Hatcher, J. D.; Halperin, M. H.; Hudson, W. E.; and Stanton, J. R.: Cardiovascular adjustments in anemia. *Proc. N. Engl. Cardiovasc. Soc.*, **10**:31, 1951–52.

———: The physiological responses of the circulation to anaemia. *Mod. Concepts Cardiovasc. Dis.*, **23**:235, 1954.

Hatcher, J. D.; Sunahara, F. A.; Edholm, O. G.; and Woolner, J. M.: The circulatory adjustments to post-haemorrhagic anaemia in dogs. *Circ. Res.*, **2**:499, 1954.

Hellen, A. J.: The adhesiveness of human blood platelets in vitro. *Scand. J. Clin. Lab. Invest. Suppl.* 51, 1960.

Herrick, J. B.: Peculiar elongated and sickle-shaped red blood corpuscles in a case of severe anemia. *Arch. Int. Med.*, **6**:517, 1910.

Heyman, A.; Patterson, J. L., Jr.; and Duke, T. W.: Cerebral circulation and metabolism in sickle cell and other chronic anemias, with observations on the effects of oxygen inhalation. *J. Clin. Invest.*, **31**:824, 1952.

Hunter, A.: The heart in anemia. *Q. J. Med.*, **15**:107, 1946.

Johnson, C. A.; Abildguard, C. F.; and Schulman, L.: Absence of coagulation abnormalities in children with cyanotic congenital heart disease. *Lancet*, **2**:660–62, 1968.

Kacian, D. L.; Gambino, R.; Dow, L. W.; Groschard, E.; Motta, C.; Ramirez, F.; Speigelman, S.; Marks, P. A.; and Bank, A.: Decreased globin messenger RNA in thalassemia detected by molecular hybridization. *Proc. Nat. Acad. Sci.*, **70**:1886, 1973.

Komrower, G. M., and Watson, G. H.: Prognosis in idiopathic thrombocytopenic purpura of childhood. *Arch. Dis. Child.* **29**:502, 1954.

Lindsay, J., Jr.; Meshel, J. C.; and Patterson, R. H.: The cardiovascular manifestations of sickle cell disease. *Arch. Intern. Med.*, **133**:643, 1974.

McClure, P. D., and Izsak, J.: The use of epsilon-aminocaproic acid to reduce bleeding during cardiac bypass in children with congenital heart disease. *Anesthesiology*, **40**:604–608, 1974.

Marsh, G. W., and Lewis, S. M.: Cardiac hemolytic platelet and fibrinogen kinetics in patients with prosthetic heart valves. *N. Engl. J. Med.*, **283**:1302–1305, 1970.

Martelle, R. R., and Linde, L. M.: Cerebral vascular accidents with tetralogy of Fallot. *Am. J. Dis. Child.*, **101**:206–209, 1961.

Master, J.; Engel, M. A.; Stern, G.; and Smith, C. H.: Cardiac complications of chronic, severe, refractory anemia with hemochronatosis. I. Acute pericarditis of unknown etiology. *J. Pediat.*, **58**:455, 1961.

Melrose, D. G., and Shackman, R.: Fluid mechanics and dynamics of transfusion. Rapid replacement of severe blood-loss. *Lancet*, **1**:1144, 1951.

Pauling, L.; Itano, H. A.; Singer, S. J.; and Wells, I. C.: Sickle cell anemia and molecular disease. *Science*, **110**:543, 1949.

Rosenthal, A.; Nathan, D. G.; Marty, A. T.; Button, L. N.; Miettinen, O. S.; and Nadas, A. S.: Acute hemodynamic effects of red cell volume reduction in polycythemia of cyanotic congenital heart disease. *Circulation*, **42**:297–307, 1970.

Rudolph, A. M.; Nadas, A. S.; and Borges, W. H.: Hematologic adjustment to cyanotic congenital heart disease. *Pediatrics*, **11**:454–64, 1953.

Schulman, I.; Smith, C. H.; and Stern, G. S.: Studies on the anemia of prematurity. *Am. J. Dis. Child.*, **88**:567, 1954.

Sharpey-Schafer, E. P.: Cardiac output in severe anemia. *Clin. Sci.*, **5**:125, 1944.

———: *Shock and Circulatory Homeostasis*. Josiah Macy Jr. Foundation, New York, 1952.

Stead, E. A., Jr., and Warren, J. V.: Cardiac output in man. An analysis of the mechanisms varying the cardiac output based on recent clinical studies. *Arch. Intern. Med.*, **80**:237, 1947.

Terry, R.: Erythrocyte sedimentation in anemia. *Br. Med. J.*, **2**:1296, 1950.

Tung, C. L.; Bien, W. M.; and Chu, Y-C.: The heart in severe anemia. *Chinese Med. J.*, **52**:479, 1937.

Videbaek, A.: Low plasma-potassium levels in acute leukemia. *Lancet*, **2**:912, 1951.

Webber, C. M., and Kaufman, S.: Personal communication, 1975.

Wedemeyer, A. L.; Edson, J. R.; and Krivit, W.: Coagulation in cyanotic congenital heart disease. *Am. J. Dis. Child.*, **124**:656–60, 1972.

Winsor, T., and Burch, G. E.: The electrocardiogram and cardiac state in active sickle cell anemia. *Am. Heart J.*, **29**:685, 1945.

Wintrobe, M. M.: The cardiovascular system in anemia. With a note on the particular abnormalities in sickle cell anemia. *Blood*, **1**:121, 1946.

21

Ventricular Septal Defect

John D. Keith

IN 1879, Roger first described the clinical signs of ventricular septal defect and indicated the underlying pathology. Although this was done with scant pathologic evidence at the time, subsequent studies have borne out the validity of his report and have identified the anomaly with a harsh systolic murmur over the fourth interspace to the left of the sternum. Some medical centers use the term *maladie de Roger* in referring to the mildest form of the anomaly.

Maude Abbott (1932) gives credit to Dalrymple as the first to describe Eisenmenger's complex in 1847 by reporting a postmortem study on a 45-year-old woman who had cyanosis for several years before her death. Eisenmenger recorded the findings of a similar case in 1897. Later Maude Abbott gathered a number of case records together from the literature and established the use of the term *Eisenmenger's complex.* Eisenmenger's complex is now considered simply a ventricular septal defect with pulmonary hypertension and a pulmonary vascular resistance sufficient to force blood from the right side of the heart to enter the aorta (Blount et al., 1955; Wood et al., 1954).

This chapter includes a classification of the ventricular septal defect, a discussion of its anatomy and possible embryologic origins, and a reference to its incidence with or without other cardiac anomalies. It also covers the clinical and hemodynamic data that aid in making a diagnosis of the presence of the defect and the complications that may arise in consequence. It concludes with an outline of the prognosis and a discussion of the indications for surgical correction.

Prevalence

It is difficult to arrive at an accurate estimate of the frequency of ventricular septal defect for a number of reasons. Postmortem studies reported in the literature have been from various age groups, and many of the ventricular septal defects have been complicated by other anomalies. If the isolated ventricular septal defect is compared in frequency with other congenital heart anomalies based on autopsy figures, a distorted picture is obtained because the ventricular septal defect is more benign than many other severe heart lesions found in infancy and early childhood. Thus postmortem figures give a low percentage of ventricular septal defects. However, if a patient with the classic signs is seen repeatedly over several years, many of the conditions that might simulate the ventricular septal defect will be ruled out. Pulmonary stenosis, aortic stenosis, and patent ductus arteriosus are examples of this.

As an isolated lesion it has been reported in certain recent clinical studies in relation to live births. Four such references are summarized as follows:

INCIDENCE PER LIVE BIRTHS

AUTHOR		RATE PER 1000 LIVE BIRTHS
Hoffman and Rudolph	1965	1.35
Rose and Keith	1970	1.37
Mitchell et al.	1971	2.26
Yerushalmy	1970	2.47

It will be seen that it occurs in between 1.3 and 2.4/1000 live births.

It is not found as commonly in autopsy series. Gelfman and Levine (1942) found it occurred in 1/1000 of autopsies and Kaplan and associates (1961) in approximately 0.5/1000, a distinctly lower figure than those above relating to live births.

INCIDENCE PER AUTOPSIES

AUTHOR		RATE PER 1000 AUTOPSIES
Gelfman and Levine	1942	1.09
Selzer	1949	(a) 0.4
Selzer and Laqueur	1951	(b) 0.65
Kaplan et al.	1961	0.57
Bloomfield	1964	0.25

The ventricular septal defect occurs with many congenital heart anomalies. These are listed in Table

21–1 and include: tetralogy of Fallot, common ventricle, persistent truncus, mitral atresia, atrioventricularis communis, transposition of the great vessels and many others. The frequency is shown in the table, and it can be seen that in association with other anomalies the ventricular septal defect makes up another group that is approximately 26 percent of all congenital heart disease. Thus, as an isolated or combined lesion the ventricular septal defect is present in approximately 50 percent of all congenital anomalies of the heart.

To clarify the problem of incidence more adequately, one may divide ventricular septal defect into three groups: (1) those where it exists as an isolated lesion; (2) those where it occurs as the prime lesion with or without another defect, such as patent ductus or mitral insufficiency; and (3) those cases in which the other lesion appears to be primary but the ventricular septal defect makes up part of the picture. A good example of the third category is tetralogy of Fallot. Table 21–1 indicates that the ventricular septal defect occurs in approximately 23 percent as an isolated lesion. If one estimates the prevalence as in category 2 the figure would be that shown in Table 1–3 (page 4)—28.3 percent.

Since many cases close during infancy and childhood and even on into adult life, a true incidence can only be obtained by following every case from birth for many decades. This is obviously impossible to do but the figures shown above present an approximation of the true prevalence.

Classification

The ventricular septum develops between the fifth and seventh weeks of fetal life and is formed by a complex union of the muscular partition, which is evolved between the ventricles and the bulbar ridges that divide the great vessels. In the center of the heart the endocardial cushions contribute to the union of these structures (see Chapter 22).

Grant (1961) presented evidence based on dissection studies indicating that ventricular septal defects in the outflow tract in the right ventricle were frequently due to a failure of certain muscular components to develop in fetal life. The anomalous opening is then related to the particular muscle segment affected and the size of the defect to the degree of involvement. Furthermore, he pointed out that muscular hypertrophy occurred in specific portions of muscle bundles of the outflow tract, with abnormal hyperplasia being the predominant feature in certain cases, particularly tetralogy of Fallot. He concluded that either the anomalous septal opening or the abnormal muscular hyperplasia may be the result of primordial injury, and this is dependent upon the timing and severity of the damage to specific muscle bundles in fetal life. In addition, he suggested that a variety of combined defects are due to somewhat similar episodes in other portions of the heart. Endocardial cushion defects cause the lesion of the atrioventricularis communis and ostium primum, both the defects and the left-axis deviation associated with these lesions being explained on the basis of faulty fusion of the bulboventricular septa producing a disturbance in development of the left conducting bundle branch, particularly the anterior branch. Another syndrome that he suggested is due, at least in part, to an abnormality of junction tissue in the bulbomusculature is Ebstein's anomaly, which leads to displacement of the tricuspid valve toward the apex. This coincides with Goerttler's suggestion in

Table 21–1. INCIDENCE OF VENTRICULAR SEPTAL DEFECT ISOLATED OR ASSOCIATED WITH OTHER CARDIAC ANOMALIES

ASSOCIATED CARDIAC ANOMALY	PERCENTAGE WITH VENTRICULAR SEPTAL DEFECT	PERCENTAGE OF ALL FORMS OF CONGENITAL HEART DISEASE
Isolated ventricular septal defect	100	23
Tetralogy of Fallot	100	11
Common ventricle	100	2
Persistent truncus	100	1
Mitral atresia	100	0.1
Atrioventricularis communis	100	2
Aortic insufficiency	100	0.1
Left ventricle into right atrium	100	—
Double-outlet right ventricle	100	—
Pulmonary stenosis and VSD	100	—
Tricuspid atresia	90	2.7
Absent isthmus	80	—
L-transposition of great vessels	65	0.1
D-transposition of great vessels	56	4.5
Coarctation of aorta and VSD	16	1.0
Atrial septal defect (ostium secundum) and VSD	10	0.7
Patent ductus arteriosus and VSD	5	0.8
Mitral stenosis and VSD	Rare	—
Mitral insufficiency and VSD	Rare	—
Aortic stenosis and VSD	Rare	—

1958 that this syndrome is due to a defect in growth during the stage of invagination of the ventricular loop associated with a deformed septum.

The defect in the ventricular septum may appear in a variety of areas (see Figure 21–1). From the clinicians' point of view, the position of the defect, its size, and its relation to the conduction mechanism of the heart, to the heart valves, and to other lesions are the important points to be elucidated in any classification. Figure 21–1 shows the four areas most frequently involved in the isolated form of ventricular septal defect.

Bécu and coworkers have devised a classification of ventricular septal defect based on a division of the right ventricle into outflow and inflow tracts. In an arbitrary manner they define the outflow tract as the portion of the ventricular septum that lies between the pulmonary valve above and the nearest part of the tricuspid valve below (or papillary muscle of the conus). The inflow tract is referred to as the portion of the septum that lies below the anterior and medial leaflets of the tricuspid valve. The crista supraventricularis, or ridge of septal tissue that originates from the septum that lies below the anterior and medial divide the outflow tract into superior and inferior portions. Lesions lying above the crista are relatively uncommon. The greatest number of ventricular septal defects lie between the crista and the medial leaflet of the tricuspid valve. In this position they are in close proximity to the aortic valve, and many are directly continuous with it. A number have a small band of tissue separating them from the aortic valve. While such openings are in the area of the membranous portion of the septum. Bécu has demonstrated that the defect is more often in the muscular tissue adjoining the membranous portion of the septum rather than in the latter structure itself (see Figure 21–1).

Defects may appear in area C (Figure 21–1) under the posterior leaflet of the tricuspid valve. This occurs in about 15 percent of cases, and its chief significance clinically is that it can be readily approached by a surgeon from the right atrium through the tricuspid valve and closed without ventriculotomy. Defects may also occur in that portion of the right heart as indicated by position D (Figure 21–1) and pierce the muscular portion of the septum in various positions down to and including the apex.

Bécu and associates' terminology (1956) of inflow and outflow tracts of the right ventricle is open to question since their outflow tract includes defects of the retrocristal junction, which is in reality inflow and outflow since it occurs at the junction of both. Others who have considered the anatomy of the area and details of the defect in recent years include Goor and associates (1970) and Rosenquist and Sweeney (1974).

In any classification of ventricular septal defect one must take into account the great variety of anomalies that are associated with it. Many such anomalies of the heart develop as a result of a variety of underlying deficiencies or malalignments, which also alter the position and character of the ventricular opening. In an effort to classify the numerous types that may occur the following grouping is set down (Van Praagh, 1965).

From the embryologic and anatomic standpoints, the ventricular septum in reality is a union for four septa: (1) the bulbar septum; (2) the ventricular sinus septum; (3) the retrocristal septum; and (4) the atrioventricular septum.

Defects involve all four septa. Hence, there are four general types of ventricular septal defects:

1. Bulbar septal defects *(supracristal)*
2. Ventricular sinus septal defects *(muscular)*
3. Retrocristal defects *(membranous)*
4. AV septal defects

Just as the vectorcardiogram permits understanding of the scalar electrocardiogram, an appreciation

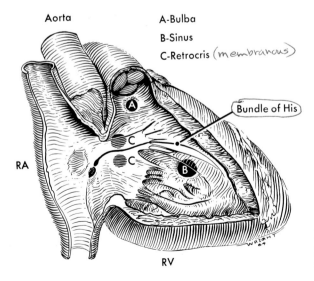

Aorta

A-Bulba
B-Sinus
C-Retrocris *(membranous)*

Bundle of His

RA

RV

Figure 21-1. The position and types of the ventricular septal defect are shown. *A.* Bulbar septal defects. *B.* Sinus septal defects. *C.* Membranous region defects. AV canal defects are discussed in Chapter 22.

of the relevant embryology facilitates an understanding of the various anatomic types of ventricular septal defect.

Bulbar Septal Defects. The bulbar septum is the intracardiac portion of the bulbotruncal septum. There is no definite embryologic distinction between the bulbar and the truncal portions of this septum; hence the bulbotruncal septum is regarded as one structure.

The bulbotruncal septum is absent in truncus arteriosus. Therefore, a high, large anterior defect is present, limited superiorly by the semilunar valves of the truncus and inferiorly by the crest of the ventricular sinus septum anteriorly.

Defects, due probably to muscle deficiency, may involve the bulbar septum and may be associated with absence of the moderator band.

In the Taussig-Bing malformation, the defect is high, large, and anterior, with the same boundaries superiorly and inferiorly as the defect in true truncus arteriosus (semilunar valves superiorly, crest of sinus septum anteroinferiorly). But the bulbar septum is not absent. On the contrary, it may be well-formed, but it is markedly malaligned relative to the ventricular sinus septum. The bulbar septum is displaced to the right and lies in an approximately anteroposterior plane, whereas the sinus septum is further to the left and makes an angle of approximately 40 degrees to the left, relative to the anteroposterior plane.

Defects in the Ventricular Sinus Septum. The ventricular sinus septum is the common party wall that remains between the excavations or evaginations of the right and left ventricular sinuses. The ventricular sinus septum does not grow upward, as has been believed. Indeed, the crest of the sinus septum is the oldest portion; the ventricular septum "grows" downward, with the progressive outpouching of the ventricular sinuses.

Muscular defects occur in any portion of the sinus septum. They may be small or large, single or multiple. The ventricular septum may be absent or rudimentary, resulting in an infrequent type of single or common ventricle.

When neither ventricular sinus develops, the common party wall between the sinuses, that is, the ventricular septum, also is absent, this also being an infrequent type of single or common ventricle.

The "Swiss cheese" ventricular septum, with multiple muscular defects, appears to be related to a deficient septal musculature, a deficiency of stratum compactum, the ventricular septum being composed of a mesh of trabeculae carneae of stratum spongiosum; hence the numerous defects.

In cases of tricuspid atresia without transposition, a muscular sinus septal defect, characteristically small, but occasionally large, is the only communication between the left ventricle and the hypoplastic right ventricle and pulmonary artery.

Junctional Defects in the "Membranous" Region (Retrocristal). The region of the membranous septum lies posterior to the crista supraventricularis. This is a "tripartite" septum, formed by its three neighbors:

1. The bulbar ridges (right and left), which also form the bulbar septum.
2. The right tubercles (dorsal and ventral) of the AV endocardial cushions, which also form the tricuspid valve.
3. Endocardial cushion tissue on the crest of the muscular ventricular septum.

Hence, the retrocristal region is a functional area among the bulbar septum, the ventricular sinus septum, and the atrioventricular canal (right side of). This junction appears vulnerable to abnormalities involving any of its three sources. Hence, it is to be anticipated that retrocristal junctional defects are by far the most frequent type.

Defects involving the retrocristal "membranous" junction occur in the following malformations:

1. As isolated, retrocristal defects;
2. In the tetralogy of Fallot;
3. In origin of both great arteries from the right ventricle (excluding the Taussig-Bing malformation);
4. In the transpositions (D- and L-) of the great arteries;
5. In the left ventricular–right atrial defects; and in
6. Single (left) ventricle with rudimentary (bulbar) outlet chamber.

Junctional Atrioventricular Septal Defects. The atrioventricular junction is posterior (inferior), relative to the immediately retrocristal region. This junction normally is formed by the most inferior portion of the atrial septum, which is the septum of the atrioventricular canal, and by the crest of the ventricular sinus septum posteriorly (inferiorly).

Defects at the atrioventricular septal junction are as follows:

1. With patent AV canal, complete or partial (absence of AV canal septum);
2. With displacement of the ventricular sinus septum (to the right, left, anteriorly, or posteriorly), in association with hypoplasia or absence of either ventricular sinus;
3. With both 1 and 2; and
4. With neither 1 nor 2. In the latter situation, there is a high, long, posterior defect of the "AV canal type," but without patency of the AV canal and without displacement of the posterior portion of the ventricular sinus septum. This defect appears to represent a failure of union of the posterior sinus septal crest with the AV canal septum, without other abnormalities (Neufeld et al., 1961).

324

The incidence of the various types of ventricular septal defect listed above was obtained by autopsy study of Bécu and associates (1956) (see Table 21–2). More recently, Cooley, Garrett, and Howard (1962), reporting 300 surgically treated cases, found that 79 percent occurred in the membranous portion of the septum. This is slightly higher than the 70 percent recorded by Bécu in 1958.

Pathology

The ventricular septal defect in infancy or childhood has a considerable range in size, varying from 1 mm in diameter up to 25 mm. It may be circular, elliptic, or eccentric. The rim may be smooth and rounded, or firm and fibrotic, or ridgelike. Figure 21–2 indicates the marked variation in size, shape, and position that can occur. The very small defects suggest that spontaneous closure could take place, especially when it is remembered that experimental surgeons have found it difficult to keep open defects 5 mm or less produced artificially in dogs (Kay et al., 1953). Twenty-eight percent of the hearts with this anomaly examined at The Hospital for Sick Children had defects of 4.5 mm or less. Figure 21–3 indicates in graph form the size ranges found in the pediatric age group. As one might expect, the defects are smaller in infancy than in later childhood, but such size change with body growth is relatively minimal compared with the body weight or surface area or lung capacity change occurring during the same period. When the size of the defect-body surface area ratio is related to age, the relative size decreases markedly with advancing years. Rarely the defect may increase in size 25 to 50 percent or slightly more as the child grows from birth to ten years. The pulmonary blood flow normally increases nearly 1000 percent during the same period. The capacity of the lung to accept an increased blood flow grows much more rapidly in the normal individual than any increase in ventricular septal defect size. This is a favorable hemodynamic adjustment on the part of the patient as long as the defect remains smaller than the aorta. There is frequently a relative decrease in size of the defect when its diameter is related to body surface area (see Figure 21–4), lung volume, or heart size. Approximately 50 percent of isolated ventricular septal defects in childhood have diameters 75 percent of aortic diameter or less (Sherman, 1963). The overriding of dextraposed aorta has been the cause of much discussion in the past but is no longer considered of much consequence now in relation to the hemodynamics or degree of cyanosis. Its importance probably lies in the fact that when the aorta is dextraposed, the ventricular defect is usually a large one and hence is associated with an augmented pulmonary blood flow and increased pressure with the consequent pathology if left uncorrected over the years. Dextraposition of the aorta is characteristic of tetralogy of Fallot, and Selzer and Laquer (1951) compared the size of the ventricular septal defect in three groups: (1) tetralogy, (2) ventricular septal defect with dextraposition of the aorta, and (3) simple ventricular septal defect. The first two had the largest defects.

The most characteristic response to the increased pulmonary flow and pressure as a result of the ventricular defect is in the pulmonary arteries. The prognosis both immediate and remote is intimately

Table 21–2. ANATOMIC AND EMBRYOLOGIC CLASSIFICATION OF VENTRICULAR SEPTAL DEFECTS

TYPES	MALFORMATIONS	POSSIBLE EMBRYOLOGIC PATHOGENESIS
Bulbar septal defects, 8 percent	1. Isolated ventricular septal defect 2. Taussig-Bing malformation 3. Truncus arteriosus	1. Deficient bulbar myocardium 2. Malalignment of bulbar septum relative to ventricular sinus septum, ± bulbar septal deficiency 3. Absent bulbar septum
Sinus septal defects, 12 percent	1. Isolated muscular VSD, single, multiple, small, large 2. Tricuspid atresia	Deficiency myocardium of sinus septum
Membranous region VSD 70 percent	1. Isolated ventricular septal defect 2. Tetralogy of Fallot 3. Transpositions of great arteries (D and L) 4. LV → RA defect	Deficient closure of this junctional zone by bulbar ridges (right and left), by right tubercles (dorsal and ventral) of AV endocardial cushions, and by endocardial cushion tissue on crest of sinus septum
AV canal region VSD 8 percent	1. Isolated 2. With patent AV canal, complete, partial	Defective junction between atrial and ventricular sinus septa, ± malalignment of ventricular septum relative to atrial septum, ± patent AV canal (absent AV canal septum)
Combinations of the above, 2 percent		

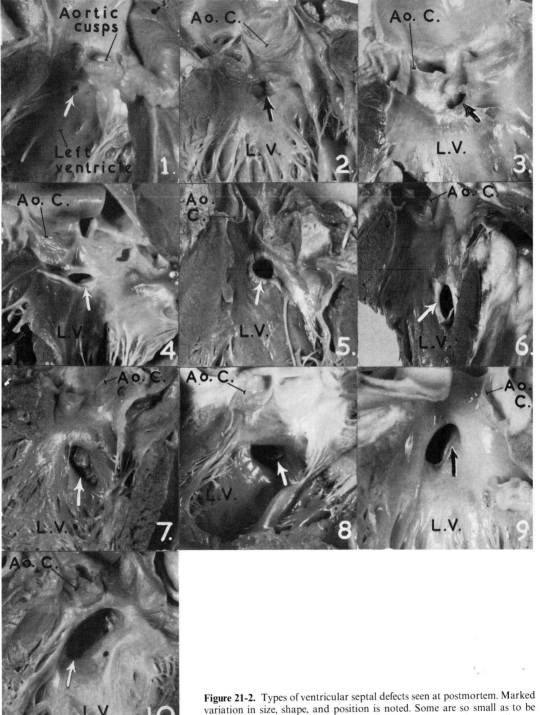

Figure 21-2. Types of ventricular septal defects seen at postmortem. Marked variation in size, shape, and position is noted. Some are so small as to be unimportant; others are so large that marked pulmonary hypertension or congestive heart failure is inevitable.

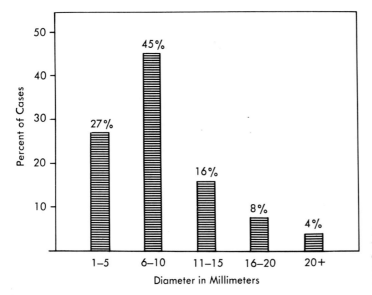

Figure 21-3. The variation in size of the ventricular septal defect in 94 children examined at autopsy (Toronto Hospital for Sick Children). (Fowler and Keith, 1964.)

related to reaction of these vessels. It is therefore important to study the pulmonary vascular response in some detail in both the normal and abnormal individual. The pulmonary arteries have three main divisions: (1) the elastic arteries, (2) the muscular arteries, and (3) the arterioles. The elastic arteries are 1000 μm or greater in diameter. The media of these vessels consist predominantly of elastic fibrils with some smooth-muscle fibers, collagen, and ground substance. The elastic tissue in the pulmonary trunk changes from that of fetal life and infancy as the child matures. The adult pattern is established by the end of the second year and consists of a thinning out of the

media and a breaking up of the elastic tissue so that it becomes more irregular and sparse than in the aorta with short fibrils branching in all directions. This is different from the appearance in infancy when there are long, parallel fibrils with a more symmetric distribution as is found in the aorta. If pulmonary hypertension persists from birth, this elastic tissue retains its infantile appearance.

The normal muscular arteries are between 100 and 1000 μm in diameter. They are hypertrophied in the newborn with a lumen-to-wall ratio of 1:1 or 1:2 but thin out rapidly during the first year of life and then more gradually during childhood until they become

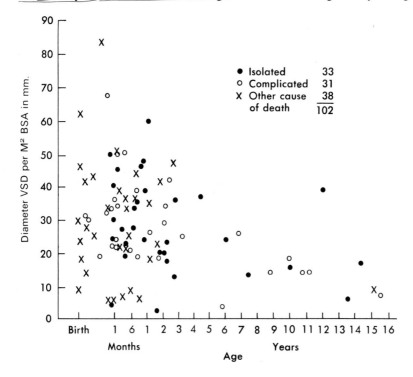

Figure 21-4. The diameter of the ventricular septal defect is related to body surface area and age of the child. There is a relative decrease in size of the defect as the child grows older. (Autopsy data.) (Fowler and Keith, 1964.)

the thin-walled structure that is characteristic of the adult.

Pulmonary arterioles normally have a distinct muscular media only at the point of origin from the parent muscular artery. The remaining course of the arteriole is structured with a single elastic lamina. In the presence of pulmonary hypertension there is a muscular media present and hypertrophied in many small arteries down to 30 mm in diameter.

It is worth pointing out that there may be some relative increase in thickness of the media of the pulmonary muscular arteries in the region of the lingula. This is important when taking biopsies since this area of the lung should be avoided in order to get a true sample of the pulmonary anatomy.

In the presence of a small ventricular septal defect, maturation of the pulmonary arteries proceeds in normal fashion with a normal thinning of the wall. If a big defect is present with a large blood flow and increased pressure in the pulmonary artery, a number of changes may occur. First, the normal hypertrophy of the small muscular arteries may persist on into infancy and childhood instead of regressing in a normal fashion. During the first month of life it is impossible to tell normal pulmonary vascular structure from that associated with a large ventricular septal defect. After the first month or two of life, however, the difference between the normal and pathologic begins to be apparent.

There are four grades of response of the pulmonary artery to the increased flow and pressure, and these are as follows (Edwards, 1957):

Grade 1: Hypertrophy of the medial wall of the small muscular arteries (media may be 25 percent of diameter of external elastic lamina [normal = 2.8 to 3.1 percent]). (See Figure 21–5.)

Grade 2: Hyperplasia of the intima. (See Figure 21–6.)

Grade 3: Hyperplasia and fibrosis of the intima to the point of obstruction in many small pulmonary arteries. At this stage the pulmonary arteries tend to become tortuous. (See Figure 21–7.)

Grade 4: Dilatation lesions. A thinning of the wall beyond the site of obstruction in the small arteries. This may reach such proportion of saccular formation when such dilated vessels lie near the air spaces that they may herniate into them and rupture causing hemoptysis. Plexiform lesions may form at the site of obstruction, resulting in small, thin-walled blood vessels that appear to proceed in and out of the obstruction area.

Since some of the occluded vessels reach a diameter of 0.2 to 0.3 mm, it can be readily seen that as soon as these lesions are widespread a marked decrease in the pulmonary blood flow results. In the presence of a ventricular septal defect this may cause a reversal of flow through the anomalous opening of the aorta and clinically produce cyanosis on exercise or at rest.

Dammann and associates (1961) report that all patients over the age of two years examined by lung biopsy who had pulmonary artery pressures 75 percent of the aortic pressure or greater had obvious hypertrophy of the pulmonary artery wall coupled with intimal change, some in grade 2, others in grade 3 (see Figure 21–8).

The original dynamic responses obviously put a load on the left ventricle when the pulmonary flow is large and the resistance low. The load shifts gradually

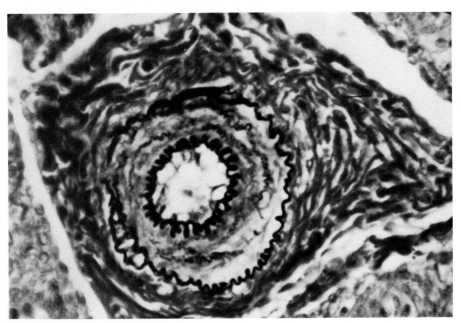

Figure 21-5. Hypertrophy of the medial wall of a small muscular artery.

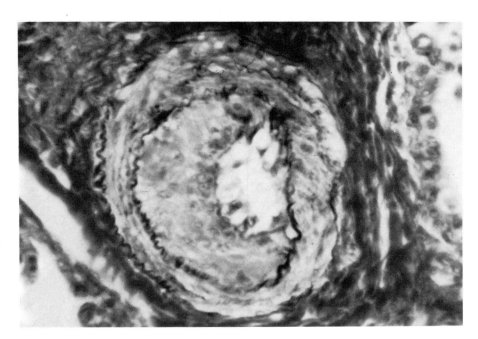

Figure 21-6. Hyperplasia of intima of small muscular artery.

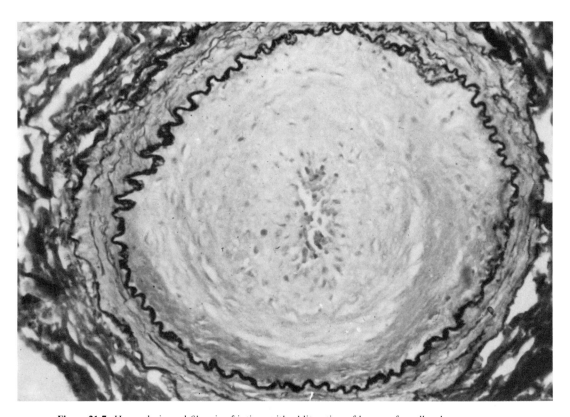

Figure 21-7. Hyperplasia and fibrosis of intima with obliteration of lumen of small pulmonary artery.

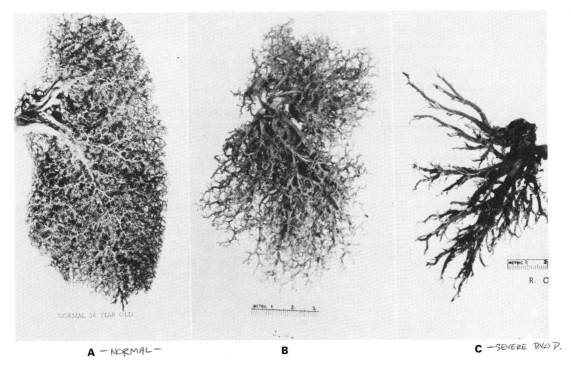

Figure 21-8. Plastic cast of arterial pulmonary circulation showing three grades of pulmonary vasculature. *A.* Normal 16-year-old girl. *B.* J. J., two years after banding operation in child with ventricular septal defect; moderate pulmonary vascular obstruction shown. *C.* R. C., ten years, patient with marked pulmonary vascular disease secondary to large ventricular septal defect. (Reproduced from Dammann, J. F., Jr.; McEachen, J. A.; Thompson, W. M., Jr.; Smith, R.; and Muller, W. H.: The regression of pulmonary vascular disease after the creation of pulmonary stenosis. *J. Thorac. Cardiovasc. Surg.*, **42:**722, 1961.)

to the right as the resistance rises and the blood flow to the lungs decreases. The changing dynamics are reflected in the size and thickness of the ventricular walls as well as in the pulmonary arteries.

The infants and children who have died with ventrical septal defects fall into four groups that help to clarify the problem of cause of death to some degree. These groups are: (1) those with isolated ventricular septal defects; (2) those with other cardiac defects; (3) those with noncardiac congenital defects (e.g., mongolism); (4) those whose death was associated with other causes such as pneumonia.

An analysis of the cases seen at The Hospital for Sick Children indicates that there are frequently several factors operating contributing to a fatal outcome (see Figure 21–9). These include prematurity, mongolism, tracheoesophageal fistulae and syndrome, respiratory infections, atelectasis, and

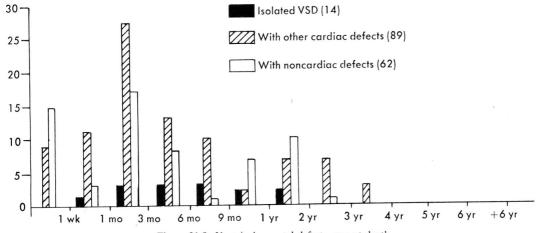

Figure 21-9. Ventricular septal defect—age at death.

finally congestive heart failure. Each of these may play a primary or secondary role.

On reviewing our cases of isolated ventricular septal defect in an effort to determine the chief cause of death, it appeared likely that only 20 percent died of congestive heart failure per se. There were others who died of prematurity, mongolism, or pneumonia, where failure was undoubtedly a contributing factor. But it was abundantly clear that the overwhelming majority of these children do not die of the ventricular septal defects. The highest mortality was in the first year of life. After the first year death due to a ventricular septal defect is uncommon. Out of our 2427 cases of isolated ventricular septal defect 5.5 percent died in infancy or childhood. Under the age of one year there were usually important contributory factors. Some will ultimately die of Eisenmenger's complex with slowly progressive pulmonary vascular obstruction. Death from this latter cause is rare in the pediatric age group. A low incidence has been noted by Lyndfield and associates (1961).

Bundle of His.   It is of considerable importance for the surgeon to know the path followed by the bundle of His so that he may avoid damaging the conducting tissue during correction of the ventricular septal defect. This has been studied by Titus, Daugherty, and Edwards (1963). They demonstrated that the bundle followed a path along the posterior rim of the ventricular septum and was intimately related to the margin of a septal defect in 13 of 14 cases in which the anomaly was in the area of the membranous portion. In its course along the posterior or inferior aspect of the ventricular septal defect the bundle gave off the left bundle branches. The latter fanned out over the left ventricular surface so that most of these fibers were not intimately related to the defect itself.

The right bundle continued on its anterior-inferior course. In some instances it was associated with the margin or rim of the septal defect, while in others it was definitely inferior to the margin.

In the area where the bundle pathway presents a problem to the surgeon the position of the bundle was in the central portion of the rim of the hearts studied, closer to the left side in six, and closer to the right in one. If the defect was a very small one, the conducting tissue did not appear to be intimately related to the margin of the defect. Lev (1959) has shown that in tetralogy of Fallot the bundle was situated to the left side of the septum and below the defect in the cases studied.

The surgeons have learned to avoid this crucial margin of the anomalous opening by placing their sutures with care and, when a patch is used, suturing the posterior-inferior part of the patch on to the right ventricular side of the septal defect (Kirklin et al., 1957).

Hemodynamics

Newborn Period.   The most characteristic pathologic change in a child with a ventricular septal defect is centered on the pulmonary arteries. These vessels are frequently affected to some degree by the resultant hemodynamics and follow an evolutionary process, which may be rapid or slow depending on the size of the defect and the response to it. The normal infant also follows an evolutionary course in both systemic and pulmonary circulations, which must be understood to evaluate the pathologic changes that occur when an intracardiac shunt is present.

In the normal fetus at term the blood flow through the lungs is thought to be 5 to 10 percent depending on the stage of fetal development. This flow, accompanied by a systemic pressure in the pulmonary artery, indicates a pulmonary vascular resistance of $40,000$ dynes/sec/cm^{-5}. Within a few hours of birth in some cases or, at most, two or three days, the mean pressure in the pulmonary artery has fallen to less than 50 percent of systemic mean pressure. The flow in the pulmonary artery rises to 8 ml per second (Rowe, 1959; Rudolph et al., 1958, 1961), which yields a pulmonary vascular resistance of 4800 dynes/sec/cm^{-5}, one-tenth of that during fetal life. During the next week or two there is a further drop in the pulmonary resistance to 2500 dynes/sec/cm^{-5}. Thereafter there is a decline extending in a curve over infancy and early childhood that brings the mean pulmonary vascular resistance to 300 dynes at four to six years and 200 at six to eight years of age (Lucas et al., 1961). After that the level continues to drop slowly as long as the child is growing and the pulmonary artery pressure is unchanged (see Figure 21–10).

There must always be a marked drop in pulmonary vascular resistance at birth when the lungs expand and the postnatal cardiovascular adjustments begin. There are several excellent reasons for this, the chief ones being the following: (1) the straightening out of the coiled distal pulmonary arteries with lung expansion; (2) the increased blood flow through the capillaries, which distends them and thus tends to reduce the resistance; (3) the rise in oxygen content of arterial blood, which in a reflex fashion helps to lower pulmonary vascular resistance (Rowe and James, 1957); (4) the elasticity of the pulmonary arteries, which are naturally more distensible than the systemic arteries; and (5) vasomotor reflex response that may vary from hour to hour (Cassin et al., 1964).

The opposing factors creating pulmonary vascular resistance include the thickened muscular arteries with diminished lumens, the contractile response of the pulmonary vasculature to increased flow and pressure, and the reflex effect of diminished arterial oxygen content, which may occur under a variety of circumstances. Any classification of the reaction of the pulmonary arterial system to a ventricular septal defect must take into account the above factors.

The systemic circulation also goes through a maturation process but appears to be more adapted to physiologic adjustments than to anatomic change since the systemic arteries have a wider range of response to the sympathetic nervous system.

At the time of birth the systemic resistance based on a flow of 8 ml per second and a mean pressure of

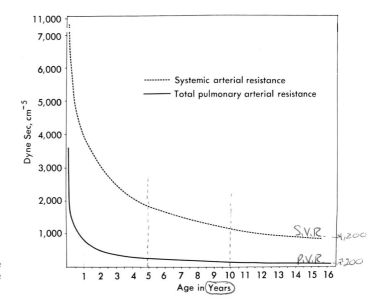

Figure 21-10. A comparison between the systemic and pulmonary vascular resistance from birth to adolescence.

62 mm of mercury is 10,000 dynes. As the tissues' need for blood increases, the resistance gradually falls, but the rate of fall does not appear to be as precipitous as in the pulmonary circulation (using data from Rowe et al., 1957, 1959, 1964; Lucas et al., 1961). The curve of systemic resistance was shown by Lucas and associates in 1961. It will be seen that it drops to 4000 to 5000 dynes at six months and 3000 to 4000 dynes in the second year of life, reaching 1500 to 2500 dynes at five years of life, but it continues to decline until adolescence is reached (see Figure 21–10).

Thus, during the first day or two of life the systemic-to-pulmonary vascular resistance ratio is approximately 2.5 to 1, at two to three weeks it is 2.8 to 1, at one month it is 3 to 1, at six months 4 to 1, and at one year 5 to 1. After this it varies between 5 to 1 and 10 to 1 or greater.

The anatomic changes in the pulmonary arteries coincide with, but do not exactly parallel, the physiologic adjustments. In the neonatal period there is a decrease in the thickness of the media of the small pulmonary arteries followed by a further recession over a period of two to six months. Edwards (1957), Wagenvoort et al. (1961), and Ferguson and associates (1960) have produced histologic evidence that the maturation of the pulmonary vascular tree is not complete until four years of age. Thus, while the anatomic and physiologic data point to the same general conclusion, the initial drop in pressure in the first week of life is greater than the change in the pulmonary artery anatomy.

When the lumen of the arteriole of normal lungs is related to the body surface area, or the age of the infant or child, an evolutionary maturation curve similar to that comparing age and pulmonary vascular resistance is obtained (Lucas et al., 1961). Another parameter of interest is the elastic resistance of the pulmonary arteries, which provides an indication of the vascular distensibility of the

pulmonary circulation (Deuchar and Knebel, 1952). Lucas finds this to be 20,000 dynes/sec/cm^{-5} in the neonatal period and 700 dynes/sec/cm^{-5} at 12 to 16 years. Thus, a modest increase in pulmonary blood flow in an infant is accompanied by a much greater rise in pulmonary artery pressure than one will find at a later age. In this way the clinical and anatomic observations of the limited pulmonary vascular capacity to accommodate a large blood flow or volume are again supported by physiologic data.

Pathophysiology. The pathologic results of the ventricular septal defect are mediated through two main avenues. Both stem from the effect of the shunt on the pulmonary arteries. The first is associated with diminished pulmonary vascular resistance and congestive heart failure, and the second with increased pulmonary vascular tone hypertrophy of wall coupled with subsequent muscular and endothelial change that may lead to reversal of flow and inoperability. During the first two to four weeks of life there do not appear to be significant differences between the appearance of the pulmonary arteries of the infant with ventricular septal defect and the normal. After the first month, however, the baby with a large ventricular septal defect will almost invariably show a medial layer in the pulmonary artery that is thicker than the normal (Wagenvoort et al., 1961). Intimal proliferation in the pulmonary arteries occurs. Fry (1968) indicates that a pulmonary blood flow three times normal may produce shearing forces that yield pathologic changes in the intima.

The thinning out of medial thickness, or maturation process, that occurs normally in the first weeks of life has been described by Dammann and Ferencz to occur more slowly or not at all in the infants with large ventricular septal defects. Contrary to such data, a few cases have been reported with very thin pulmonary arteries and flooded lung fields leading to early death. The more common response, however, as was indicated above, has been one of hypertrophy of the medial layer associated with varying degrees of increase in pulmonary vascular resistance.

After birth the pulmonary vascular resistance does not fall as rapidly in an infant with a ventricular septal defect as in the normal newborn. Furthermore, when it does fall, it may not recede to normal levels. This type of a response explains the delayed onset of heart failure in ventricular septal defect in the interval following birth. Failure does not usually appear in the healthy newborn for 4 to 12 weeks but may appear earlier in the premature, since there is a more rapid decline in the pulmonary vascular resistance.

Vogel and associates (1967) showed that hypoxia of altitude diminishes the incidence of heart failure in infants with such defects born in Denver, at an altitude of 5280 feet above sea level. A larger percentage go into failure if born at sea level.

Studies of Rudolph and coworkers (1961) are also of interest, since they demonstrate that with an increased pulmonary blood flow, as in ventricular septal defect, the normal regression of medial muscle layer in the pulmonary arterioles is often prevented. When they perform a left pneumonectomy in puppies, the flow through the remaining lung was associated with the development of pulmonary hypertension. The latter did not occur when unilateral pneumonectomy was carried out in adult animals. Vogel (1967) ligated the left pulmonary artery of calves at Denver and another group at sea level. In the latter, there was no effect on the pulmonary artery pressure, but in the former (born in Denver) there was a marked progressive pulmonary hypertension.

In evaluating the hemodynamic relationships interest focuses on pressure, flow, and resistance in both the pulmonary and systemic circulation. By hydraulic studies in an artificial circulation, Brostoff and Rodbard (1956) have investigated the pressure curves of a variety of types of ventricular septal defect with or without associated shunts, stenosis, or insufficiencies.

There are two major factors responsible for the flow through a small septal opening—the size of the defect and the *pressure gradient between the two sides*. In addition to these obvious conclusions, Brostoff showed that in a small defect the shunt is minimal and ceases before the end of the systole. In a moderate defect the flow is predominantly systolic and is associated with an early but slight diastolic shunt. When the defect is a large one, the pressure is usually the same in both ventricles and the shunt depends on the differences in resistance between the two circuits. When the flow is large, an appreciable diastolic flow is present in addition to that occurring during systole.

The level of systemic arterial pressure can produce a significant effect on the magnitude of the shunt. Rarely does one find a marked systemic hypertension with a ventricular septal defect, but when the pressure does rise in the systemic circuit with this anomaly, it is associated with an increased pulmonary artery flow and pressure. In such cases the systemic pressure level may have developed in order to compensate for the pulmonary vascular resistance and force more blood through the lung fields. Whatever the cause, there is a further burden on the arterial tree of the lung likely to lead to the development of sclerosis in the pulmonary vessels.

Flow through the defect may be affected by additional factors: (1) The margins of the ventricular septal defect may contract during systole, thus reducing the shunt; (2) Rodbard and associates (1954) showed that contraction of the pulmonary infundibulum may produce some degree of narrowing of the outflow tract of the right ventricle during strong systolic contractions. We have demonstrated this by angiocardiogram and showed that occasionally the narrowed outflow tract may act as a resistance to further flow from the right ventricle to the pulmonary artery. Gasul et al. (1957) suggested that this process may proceed to anatomic infundibular stenosis over several years and thus alter the dynamics of a simple ventricular septal defect to those of tetralogy of Fallot.

As has been indicated, the newborn infant makes certain adaptations and adjustments to the presence of ventricular septal defect. These may be described as acute or chronic. While there is an acute element in the newborn during the first few days of life, there is a further adjustment over several weeks or months that may be described as chronic. From experimental work these factors have been well summarized by Lillehei, Bobb, and Visscher (1950) and by Siegel (1961). Chronic adjustments included a gradual increase of blood volume, plasma volume, total body water, and pulmonary blood volume even in the absence of cardiac failure. In the acute stage of an experimentally produced ventricular septal defect there is an increased heart rate and cardiac output and an increased peripheral venous and arterial constriction with the result that there is a shift of the circulating blood volume toward the cardiopulmonary area. There is also an increased pulmonary vascular resistance, which, coupled with the increased blood volume, tends to diminish the shunt through the defect. Siegel also demonstrated an adjustment of ventricular myocardial function to a more efficient curve. The latter enables the heart to handle more efficiently the increased work demands placed on it by the shunt through the ventricular septal defect. It is suggested by Siegel that these mechanisms of compensation of acute intraventricular shunt are in most part brought into play by the indirect action of the shunt on the baroreceptors of the aortic arch and carotid sinus. Evidence of most of these compensating adjustments appears in the neonatal period and the early months of life when a ventricular septal defect is present.

Lucas and associates (1961) have correlated the diameter of ventricular septal defect with body surface area. Those patients with openings of less than 1 cm per meter square body surface area had only minor alteration in the cardiac dynamics or none at all. Over a period of observation of several years little or no change took place. On the other hand, when the openings were greater than 1 cm per meter square body surface area, two changes were noted in part of the group. Some patients had a decrease in the size of the opening and thereby a reduction in blood flow to the lungs. Others, who had large defects, showed a higher mortality with surgery.

Dammann and Ferencz (1956) and many others have pointed out that during the first year excessive pulmonary blood flow may manifest itself by dyspnea, frequent respiratory infections, or frank heart failure. At the end of the first year or in the second year the baby begins to improve, with a diminution in pulmonary congestion, increased physical activity, and less dyspnea. Their anatomic studies suggest that this physiologic improvement is associated with hypertrophy of the media of the muscular arteries of the lung with diminution in the size of their lumen by hypertrophy as well as constriction and endothelial change. This improved state may last for years, but it is believed that in many cases it will eventually lead to persistent pulmonary hypertension, high pulmonary vascular resistance, reversal of flow through the defect with clinical cyanosis, and ultimately death from heart failure, pulmonary hemorrhage, or infarction. This final phase has been described as Eisenmenger's syndrome and is referred to below.

Postoperative Response in Distal Pulmonary Arteries. Once pulmonary hypertension with an increased pulmonary vascular resistance has been established for several years, surgery for correction of the primary cause has rarely produced any significant change in pulmonary vascular resistance in the short-term studies reported so far on ventricular septal defect. A number of such investigations have been presented in detail in the literature.

Lucas and associates (1961) found a postoperative drop in pressure in nine cases of ventricular septal defect but saw little change in resistance. Braunwald (1964) similarly recorded a fall in pulmonary artery pressure after successful surgery in eight patients with ventricular septal defect whose average age was 19 years. As in the other studies, there was minimal change in the pulmonary-to-systemic vascular resistance ratio in the interval of 1 to 12 months that elapsed from the time of operation to the time of postoperative catheterization. The findings were similar in a group of nine cases of atrial septal defect. It was noteworthy, however, that the children who had a patent ductus arteriosus or aortic window closed did have a significant drop in both pulmonary artery pressure and resistance in most cases.

In the group operated on for correction of the ventricular septal defect that has had pre- and postoperative catheter studies, the age at operation has usually been four years or over. Earlier operation would probably favor a postoperative decline in pulmonary vascular resistance. Individual case reports suggest that this does occur (Lillehei, 1963; Blount and Woodward, 1960; Braunwald, 1964). It will also be of interest to note whether the pulmonary vascular resistance will decline two, three, or four or more years postoperatively. No one has yet established at what time in the life of an infant or child pulmonary vascular resistance will return to normal once it becomes increased as a result of a ventricular septal defect.

The postoperative physiology in atrial septal defect is also of significance when assessing the pathologic dynamics of ventricular septal defect. Burchell (1959) recorded no change in pulmonary vascular resistance in four patients with atrial septal defect who had pre- and postoperative catheterization examinations. The fifth had a slight increase in resistance two weeks postoperatively. Beck and associates (1960), from the same institution, followed Burchell's report with seven additional cases of atrial septal defect. Three of these had some drop in resistance. There was the usual fall in pressure in all cases, but even the pulmonary vascular resistance fell, as it did in these three instances, the pulmonary-to-systemic resistance ratio did not decline significantly.

It is quite clear that the newborn has an immediate reduction in resistance, and it appears likely that over the next few weeks all cases of ventricular septal defect have a further decline in this function of the pulmonary arteries. In some instances the fall in resistance may be so marked as to cause failure, and in others it may be minimal and thus prevent excessive flooding of the lungs.

It is important, however, to recognize at an early age which patients are likely to establish an irreversible high resistance in their pulmonary arteries so that they may be singled out and corrected surgically before it is too late to do so successfully. Such patients have been referred to as hyperreactors.

Hyperreactors and Hyporeactors (Including Pulmonary Vascular Obstruction, Eisenmenger's Complex). Eisenmenger described the end stage of the hyperreactor first in 1897 and, based on postmortem findings, pointed out the association of a ventricular septal defect with atherosclerosis of the pulmonary artery. A better understanding of the hemodynamics had to wait until the catheterization era (Bing et al., 1947), which coincided with the intensive pathologic studies of Edwards, Heath, Dammann, Ferencz, and others. Wood's classic monograph on the subject brought all the available data together in 1958 and emphasized the diversity of underlying lesions that could lead to pulmonary vascular obstruction. These included all the causes of increased pulmonary flow and pressure, ventricular septal defect, patent ductus arteriosus, aorticopulmonary septal defect, persistent truncus arteriosus, transposition of the great vessels with ventricular septal defect, L-transposition of the great vessels with ventricular septal defect, common ventricle, atrioventricularis communis, single atrium, atrial septal defect, anomalous pulmonary vein drainage (either partial or total), and a number of other less common lesions.

A number of definitions could be given, but Wood defined the Eisenmenger syndrome as pulmonary hypertension at systemic level due to a high pulmonary vascular resistance (over 800 dynes/sec/cm^{-5}), with reversed or bidirectional shunt through a large ventricular septal defect.

Edwards (1953), Brewer and Heath (1959), and others have indicated that the primary changes are those found in association with long-standing pulmonary artery hypertension and consist of hypertrophy of the media of the small muscular pulmonary arteries with fibroelastosis of the intima causing thickening or occlusion. In the pulmonary arterioles these findings point to the presence of a distinct media between the two elastic laminae and intimal fibrosis. With these findings there are associated certain secondary changes that help to maintain an adequate blood flow through the alveolar capillaries by the formation of branches of the muscular pulmonary arteries that lead into thin-walled structures resembling veins. These branches may arise at, or proximal to, the site of the obstruction in the parent artery and may end as capillaries in the alveolar walls (Harris and Heath, 1962). Such collateral channels may be the basis of pulmonary hemorrhage.

The fully developed pathologic picture described above is uncommon in childhood and does not usually make its appearance until the late teens or the twenties, leading to an average length of life between 20 and 35 years (Wood, 1958; Bloomfield, 1964), but it may occur as early as three or four years. However, there is a steady progression of histologic change that has been labeled as having five grades: grade 1, hypertrophy of the media of the small muscular arteries; grade 2, medial hypertrophy and intimal fibroelastosis; grade 3, fibrosis and, ultimately, obstruction of the vessel; grade 4, evolution of the plexiform collateral channels referred to above; and grade 5, an uncommon response, characterized by a necrotizing arteritis.

When the diagnostic criteria referred to by Wood (1958) in his definition of Eisenmenger's syndrome are present in adult life, the pathologic criteria of grades 3 or 4 are also satisfied. This, however, is not the case in childhood and particularly the first year of life when hypertrophy of the media of the small muscular arteries is a normal finding. Furthermore, from the hemodynamic point of view an infant with a ventricular septal defect may have a pulmonary vascular resistance of 2000 dynes/sec/cm^{-5} and yet, subsequently, have a drop in resistance to the normal level by the age of one, two, three, or four years. For these reasons, fully developed Eisenmenger's syndrome is rare in early childhood. In the normal infant and in the infant with a ventricular septal defect there is always a drop in pulmonary vascular resistance at birth and in the first few weeks of life. This is borne out by a series of 191 cardiac catheterizations at The Hospital for Sick Children (Kidd et al., 1965) performed on ventricular septal defects in the first year of life, as well as those recorded in the literature in similar age groupings. The onset of cardiac failure corresponds with this drop in resistance, and it is therefore commonly found when it does occur in ventricular septal defect between the ages of one and six months. It is rarely seen in the first week or two of life unless some complicating lesion is present. Cassin and associates (1964) have shown that the fetal lamb, before birth, can lower its pulmonary vascular resistance on occasion to levels similar to those found some weeks after birth when the postnatal adjustments of the pulmonary circulation have been completed. Such a drop in resistance appears to be transitory in the fetal lamb.

Frequency of Hyperreactors. If Eisenmenger's syndrome is defined in ventricular septal defect as having pulmonary hypertension at systemic level, a pulmonary vascular resistance of 800 dynes/sec/cm^{-5} or more, and bidirectional flow through the defect, then 10 percent of our cases over two years of age studied by cardiac catheterization in childhood fell into this category (see Figure 21–11). It is of interest to reiterate that all of these patients were over two years of age.

Wood (1958) suggested that Eisenmenger's complex dates from birth, with a marked reactive pulmonary hypertension from that time onward. The evidence at hand (Kidd, 1965) indicates that all infants have a drop in pulmonary vascular resistance in early life in the presence of a ventricular septal defect. Some with a relatively high resistance after birth have it decline slowly, others rapidly. After the age of two years the patterns declare themselves more precisely. Normal pulmonary artery pressures and resistances are likely to remain unchanged (Lyndfield et al., 1961; Arcilla et al., 1963; Griffiths et al., 1964). These are almost invariably associated with small defects. High pressures and raised resistances usually lead to a slow increase in pulmonary vascular resistance and obstruction. In only a few patients is this rise in resistance rapidly progressive. The Eisenmenger syndrome occurs with only a few exceptions among the patients with large defects usually over 2 cm in diameter. Those that fall into this category are likely to come from the cases that have a relatively large flow in childhood and a moderately high pulmonary vascular resistance (Kidd et al., 1965). Those with low flow and high resistance initially will usually have a satisfactory decline in resistance by one year of age. The pattern is similar in both ventricular septal defect and atrial septal defect, but the speed with which Eisenmenger's syndrome may develop may be grossly different in these two lesions. High pulmonary vascular resistance of a permanent nature appears early in the hyperreactors with a large ventricular septal defect and late in those with atrial septal defects. The fundamental factor appears to be the reaction of the pulmonary arteries to the flow-pressure stimulus. Hyperreactivity has now been shown to be present in certain individuals and certain species.

Grover and associates (1963), using a variety of data, evaluate the response in the human, the cow,

Figure 21-11. This figure portrays the hemodynamic groups in 400 infants and children who have had cardiac catheter studies at The Hospital for Sick Children, Toronto. Those under two years have been separated from those over two years. Group I all had a low flow and low resistance, a pulmonary/systemic flow ratio of less than 2:1, and a systemic-to-pulmonary resistance ratio of over 7:1. Group II had a pulmonary/systemic flow ratio of more than 2:1 and a systemic/pulmonary resistance ratio of greater than 7:1. Group III had a pulmonary/systemic flow ratio of more than 2:1 with a slightly altered systemic-to-pulmonary resistance ratio of 5–7:1. Group IV had a pulmonary/systemic flow ratio greater than 2:1 and a systemic/pulmonary resistance ratio of less than 5:1.

Groups V and VI have low pulmonary blood flow and high resistance, pulmonary/systemic flow ratios of less than 2:1, and systemic-to-pulmonary resistance ratios of less than 5:1. Group VI cases have reversal of flow through the defect.

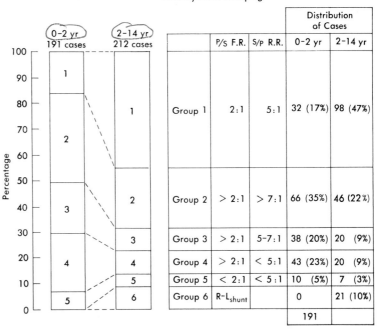

Ventricular Septal Defect
Hemodynamic Grouping

	P/S F.R.	S/P R.R.	Distribution of Cases	
			0-2 yr	2-14 yr
Group 1	2:1	5:1	32 (17%)	98 (47%)
Group 2	> 2:1	> 7:1	66 (35%)	46 (22%)
Group 3	> 2:1	5-7:1	38 (20%)	20 (9%)
Group 4	> 2:1	< 5:1	43 (23%)	20 (9%)
Group 5	< 2:1	< 5:1	10 (5%)	7 (3%)
Group 6	R-L$_{shunt}$		0	21 (10%)
			191	

and the sheep. The cow appears to be the most reactive and the sheep the least. Man is between these two with both hyper- and hyporeactors.

Anyone studying infants and children with cardiac catheterization techniques in the presence of left-to-right shunts will realize the wide range of difference in pulmonary vascular response. Wood (1958) noted that mitral stenosis led to severe pulmonary hypertension in 25 to 30 percent of cases, whereas another 30 percent with equal left atrial and pulmonary venous pressures had little or no pulmonary vascular reaction. In humans with congenital absence of one pulmonary artery there is double the blood flow to one lung and 19 percent of such cases develop severe pulmonary hypertension (Pool et al., 1962). Five percent of our infants with large ventricular septal defects will have so little pulmonary vascular resistance that they will die of congestive heart failure in the first year of life. Others with similar-sized defects will constrict their pulmonary arteries and survive.

When cattle are taken to 10,000-ft altitude for the summer months, one-third develop severe pulmonary hypertension, but at 12,400 ft all become hypertensive (Grover et al., 1963). Lambs at the same altitude retain normal pulmonary artery pressures (Reeves et al., 1963). Ligation of one pulmonary artery in newborn calves produces severe pulmonary hypertension, but this never occurs in lambs (Pool et al., 1963).

The reason for the difference in response of the individual humans has not become apparent. Bedford finds a much higher incidence of pulmonary hypertension in females than males with atrial septal defect, much greater than the normal sex difference in this congenital anomaly. He also finds infection more common in the severe hypertensive group. Hypoxia has long been identified as a factor in pulmonary hypertension, and the administration of oxygen is a standard method of reducing the pressure at catheterization in responsive cases. Vogel and associates (1962) found 20 percent of high school students at 10,000-ft altitude developed severe pulmonary hypertension with exercise, whereas the remaining portion of the group had virtually no rise in pulmonary artery pressure when given 13 percent of oxygen at rest and had very little rise with exercise.

Discussing the hyperreactive type, Lillehei (1963) records 40 cases of pulmonary hypertension with high pulmonary vascular resistance averaging 1358 dynes with an average age of 4.5 years. Postoperatively, after the ventricular defect had been closed at an average age of 7.2 years, the pulmonary vascular resistance was 944 dynes. This is a decline in resistance, but it also coincides with a growth in height and weight, which may have increased the volume flow to the lungs but not significantly altered the original pulmonary vascular pathology. To determine whether the resistance will continue to fall will require a follow-up of several years, and it seems highly probable that a number of these children will ultimately develop chronic pulmonary vascular disease of the Eisenmenger type. His figures were averages, and those patients with a significant postoperative drop in resistance may have been between two and four years of age, who would be expected to have such a response in the normal course of events.

One of our children had a ventricular septal defect with increased flow and pressure at three and one-half months of age (see Table 21–5, page 355). The right ventricle systolic pressure was 55 and the aortic systolic 75 mm of mercury. She was recatheterized at two years of age, and the pressure in the right ventricle and aorta were identical. The ventricular septal defect was closed surgically at this time, and the pressure in the right ventricle dropped 20 percent when measured on the operating table. Postoperatively this child ran a course of progressive pulmonary vascular obstruction, and at seven years the systolic pressure in the right ventricle was 130 mm of mercury, while that in the aorta was 94 mm of mercury. At death in her eighth year she had overwhelming diffuse pulmonary vascular obstruction with multiple grade 3 and 4 lesions in the pulmonary arteries (see Figure 21–7).

There have been cases reported in the literature that have had significant pulmonary hypertension and heart failure in the first year or two of life but subsequently had the ventricular septal defect close spontaneously. Initially these children were catheterized, and on repeat catheterization, besides showing closure of the defect, the study revealed normal right ventricular pulmonary artery pressures in all (Keith et al., 1971). Thus pulmonary hypertension aggravated by the stimulus of flow and failure was readily reversible in this group.

Arcilla and associates (1963), investigating 75 infants and children with ventricular septal defect, found normal or slight pulmonary hypertension in two-thirds of their cases on repeat catheterization. When no hypertension existed initially, a similar normotensive finding was almost invariably present subsequently. Three-quarters of cases with mild hypertension and two-thirds of those with moderate or severe hypertension showed a significant drop in both pressure and flow after a significant intervening period. This was interpreted as a relative reduction of the size of the ventricular septal defect during early childhood. Only 8 percent had evidence of persistent pulmonary vascular disease with high resistance.

Kidd and associates (1965) present the data on 405 catheter studies on infants and children with isolated ventricular septal defects (Figure 21–11). They found no cases of Eisenmenger's complex (high pulmonary vascular resistance with reversal of flow) under two years. Twenty percent had high or moderately high pulmonary vascular resistance, and the rest, or 80 percent, had low or slightly elevated pulmonary vascular resistance. A summary of the data is shown in the accompanying figure (see Figure 21–11).

Under two years, 17 percent had small defects with low flow and normal pulmonary vascular resistance. Another 25 percent moved to this group after the age of two years, bringing the percentage up to 43 percent.

Obviously the septal defect must have decreased in relative size so that flow and pressure were diminished (six of the cases closed completely). In the period covered, which extended over several years, 17 percent were found to develop a high pulmonary vascular resistance–low flow. None of the infants in the first year had such a hemodynamic pattern.

From the accumulated evidence in the human it is fair to conclude that closure of the ventricular septal defect any time in the first year of life will result in the return of pulmonary pressure and resistance to normal in all but a rare exception. This may be true for the second year of life also, but the evidence is less adequate as yet. There are a number with high or moderate flow with high resistance that, given time, may eventually proceed to the fully developed Eisenmenger picture. Following a fully representative group over the years is essential before the natural history and prognosis are apparent. In the meantime, studies at various ages will provide useful information. In this regard the data of Evans and associates (1964) are of interest. In a group of 78 adults with ventricular septal defect and an average age of 23 years, 20 percent had a pulmonary vascular resistance greater than 800 dynes/sec/cm^{-5}. Keith and associates (1971) found that in 295 adults 9.5 percent had developed the Eisenmenger syndrome.

Our data would suggest that Wood (1958) was incorrect in stating that Eisenmenger's disease dates from birth since none of our cases that had cardiac catheterization in the first year of life fell into this category. Furthermore, in most instances it appears unlikely that the hyperreactive cases can be clearly identified before two years of age in this regard. Those with hyporeactive pulmonary arteries are unlikely to become a problem. In between these two groups are the children who eventually yield cases of pulmonary vascular disease over a period of many years, as do some of the patients with atrial septal defect in later life (Bedford, 1960).

A review of these data leads one to the conclusions that it is important to catheterize each case of ventricular septal defect with increased flow and increased resistance once a year in the first two or three years of life. It is also important to catheterize the large-flow cases of low resistance at similar intervals. In infancy it is this latter group that is more likely to have heart failure but such children may develop pulmonary vascular disease of the Eisenmenger type eventually if the flow is large enough.

It would appear important to operate on the hyperreactors as early as they can become clearly identified early in life and before they have developed diffuse pulmonary artery disease that is irreversible. A raised pulmonary vascular resistance in an infant or child in the first year or two of life is more likely to recede with a normal maturation of the pulmonary arteries if the defect is closed during this physiological labile period.

Cardiac Catheterization

As has been indicated above, cardiac catheterization has provided a most useful tool in assessing the hemodynamics of a ventricular septal defect (Bing et al., 1947; Wood et al., 1954; Kay et al.; 1953; Fowler, 1954; Blount et al., 1955; Adams et al., 1955). See Figure 21–12.

A rise in oxygen content of 1 volume percent on going from the right atrium to the right ventricle is usually considered as reliable evidence of an interventricular shunt. Lesser shunts may occur with smaller rises, as indicated in one of our cases that had a rise of only 0.5 volume percent in the right ventricle, and yet was found to have a small ventricular septal defect postmortem. A source of error is in the position of the right ventricle from which the samples of blood are taken. Those taken from the infundibulum are more significant and more closely resemble those of the pulmonary artery than samples that are taken from the body of the right ventricle. Wood and coworkers (1954) have shown that in one-third of their cases the oxygen content of the blood taken from the body of the right ventricle more closely resembled the right atrial samples in spite of the fact that a significant ventricular septal defect was found.

Clinical Features

In the vast majority of children with this anomaly the lesion is discovered in the first year of life since periodic examinations in infancy are now the rule.

Since the ventricular septal defect is the most common heart anomaly identified in childhood, its diagnosis should be made with relative ease. In the classic case the defect is not a large one. The characteristic murmur over the lower precordium permits its identification with considerable regularity. This has been checked with cardiac catheterization studies in approximately half our cases with the result that several additional useful diagnostic points emerge. Besides the loud, harsh pansystolic over the lower precordium maximum in the third and fourth left interspaces, many are accompanied by a thrill. The cardiothoracic ratio may be normal or increased. The electrocardiogram is frequently normal. The hilar shadows may be normal or a little prominent. In making a clinical diagnosis, one is correct in a high percentage of such cases by depending on the typical murmur. Further evidence is provided if the patient is seen on several visits to the office or hospital since repeated inspections over a period of time tend to rule out such overlapping diagnoses as aortic stenosis, pulmonary stenosis, atypical or acyanotic tetralogy of Fallot, persistent truncus arteriosus, transposition of the great vessels with a ventricular septal defect, right ventricular infundibular stenosis, coarctation of the aorta with a ventricular septal defect, and other combined lesions. However, the most convincing evidence is a rise in percentage oxygen saturation on going from right atrium into right ventricle during a cardiac catheterization or a positive angiogram into the left ventricle.

Exercise Tolerance. The exercise tolerance is usually good, and limitation of activity is slight. Dyspnea occurs only with vigorous effort. Even in

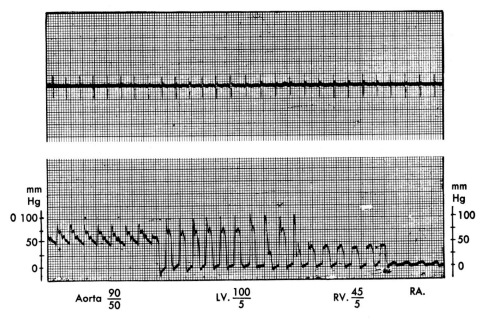

Figure 21-12. T. R., aged four years. Ventricular septal defect with a 15 percent rise of oxygen saturation in the right ventricle. The tip of the catheter entered the left ventricle and the aorta from the right ventricle. The withdrawal pressure curve is shown above.

children with enlarged hearts and enlarged pulmonary blood flow, it is surprising how well and how active they are. The same may be said of those with pulmonary hypertension and high pulmonary resistance. Their exercise tolerance is usually good unless they show a lowering of the oxygen saturation with effort. A special group are the babies with a very large pulmonary blood flow, many of whom are dyspneic at rest. If they survive the first year of life, they usually begin to show marked improvement in their respiratory rate and in response to exercise. This is presumably associated with a rise in pulmonary resistance (Adams et al., 1955).

Clinical Appearance. These children have a normal color as a rule. It is only in children with advanced pulmonary vascular resistance or congestive heart failure that there is any evidence of clinical cyanosis. In severe cases the face, chest, and body are thin, and there may be prominence of the precordium. This is especially true of those who have marked pulmonary hypertension with enlargement of the right ventricle. The babies with large defects appear undernourished and are dyspneic at rest. Their respirations vary from 35 to 100 per minute.

Cardiac Impulse. In mild cases with small defects the heart is quiet and there is no abnormal thrust at the apex or over the right ventricle. In those with rather large ventricular septal defects and low pulmonary resistance, there is commonly an increase in force of the apex beat due to hypertrophy of the left ventricle. When pulmonary hypertension is present, there is frequently a heave of the right ventricle that can be palpated over the precordium on the left sternal border. When both ventricles are hypertrophied, one may feel both an apical thrust and precordial heave.

Thrill. A thrill over the lower precordium is an important clinical sign of ventricular septal defect since its presence is confirmatory evidence of the underlying anomaly. A thrill was present in many of our cases catheterized where the pressure in the right ventricle was less than systemic. It was present in only 25 percent of those in which the pressure was the same in right and left ventricles.

Heart Murmurs. Roger's main contribution in 1879 was to link a particular murmur with a ventricular septal defect. His original description has been sustained by the passage of time. The murmur is loud and harsh and extends all through systole, appearing to include both the first and second sounds in its scope. The point of maximum intensity is between the third and fifth interspaces near the left sternal border. This was so in 90 percent of our cases

confirmed by catheterization. In 10 percent it was best heard in the second and third left interspaces.

A systolic murmur may be accompanied by a middiastolic murmur due to the rapid inflow at the beginning of diastole. The presence of this diastolic murmur is related to the volume of left-to-right shunt, and it is therefore more common with large blood flows and large hearts. Wood and coworkers (1954) find it present in 90 percent of their severe cases with large blood flow, in 60 percent of the moderate ones, and in 10 percent of the mild cases.

Heart Sounds. The pulmonary second sound is accentuated when pulmonary hypertension is present. In the severe and moderately severe cases the third heart sound in the mitral area is a frequent occurrence. As in mitral insufficiency it is considered to be due to rapid inflow of blood in early diastole from left atrium to left ventricle.

Because of the length of the systolic murmur, it is sometimes difficult to distinguish the second heart sound clearly, but it may be heard, as a rule, in the pulmonary area and part way down the left sternal border. When it is clearly heard, one may recognize a normally split second sound. In those children with pulmonary hypertension the pulmonary component of the second sound may be so loud as to overshadow the aortic component. The splitting may then only be recognized by phonocardiography. A systolic click may be heard up the left sternal border in some cases of pulmonary hypertension.

Radiologic Examination

The x-ray has proved the most useful method of estimating the size and severity of the ventricular septal defect and the reaction of the pulmonary vasculature to the shunt through it. Coupled with the physical findings and the electrocardiogram, it is a most helpful guide over the years to prognosis and therapy. Frequently cardiac catheterization cannot be repeated with ease, but the x-rays may be taken at intervals and are thus helpful in the management of the infants and children with various degrees of ventricular septal defect (Figures 21–13 to 21–18).

Heart enlargement may be due to excessive pulmonary blood flow, increased pressure in the pulmonary artery and right ventricle, congestive heart failure, pulmonary insufficiency, or tricuspid insufficiency.

In a study of 1000 cases of isolated ventricular septal defect the cardiothoracic ratios were as shown in Table 21–3.

Table 21–3. CARDIOTHORACIC RATIO IN VENTRICULAR SEPTAL DEFECT—1000 CASES

	50% OR LESS	51–55%	56–60%	61–65%	66%+
Birth–2 yr	6%	26%	37%	23%	8%
2–5 yr	21%	35%	29%	10%	5%
6–9 yr	41%	35%	16%	6%	2%
10 yr +	52%	28%	10%	8%	2%

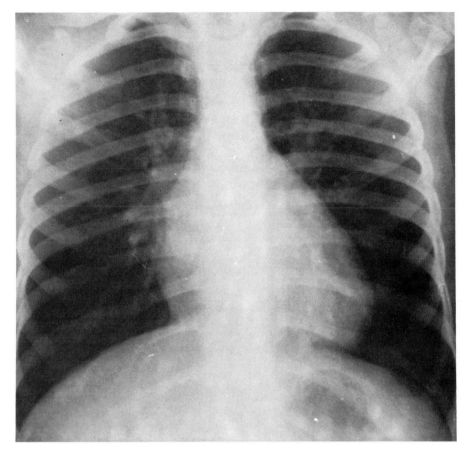

Figure 21-13. D. S., aged six years. Small ventricular septal defect demonstrated at cardiac catheterization. Heart shape shows minor variations only. Essentially normal size.

It will be noted that approximately 70 percent had a cardiothoracic ratio over 55 percent in the first two years of life, but by the time ten years was reached this figure had fallen 20 percent. This reduction in relative heart size appears to be due to four chief factors: (1) As any child grows there may be a slight reduction in the cardiothoracic ratio as the lung volume and chest size increase in proportion to the cardiac outlines. (2) There may be an absolute decrease in the size of the ventricular septal defect. (3) There may be a relative reduction in size of the ventricular septal defect when it is compared with the increased lung volume and heart size that occurs as the child develops in the years between two and ten, thus improving the ability to cope with left-to-right shunt. (4) In some cases there is a gradual development of progressive pulmonary vascular obstruction leading to reduced pulmonary blood flow, a reduced diastolic load on the left ventricle, and consequently a diminution in heart size. The latter response is present to a significant degree and occurs in approximately a tenth of the children in the pediatric age group with this anomaly. A relative or absolute decrease in size of the ventricular septal defect appears to occur in at least 65 per cent.

The typical radiologic features are generalized enlargement of the heart coupled with prominence of the main pulmonary artery and its major branches. Under the fluoroscope the chamber size and the hilar shadows can be studied very readily. This method is particularly useful in identifying intrinsic hilar vessel pulsation and in estimating the size of the left atrium. The left ventricle shows enlargement in those cases that have large blood flows, whereas in those that have marked pulmonary hypertension the right ventricle is predominant and there is little or no enlargement of the left. The largest hearts are found when the two factors of maximum flow and pressure occur together.

The left atrium is enlarged slightly or moderately in those cases that have large shunts, partly owing to the excessive blood flow and partly owing to the generalized enlargement of the heart.

When the defect is small or moderate in size, the right atrium appears normal. The right atrium is more likely to be enlarged when there is pulmonary hypertension or congestive heart failure. Even more marked enlargement appears when there is insufficiency of the tricuspid valve.

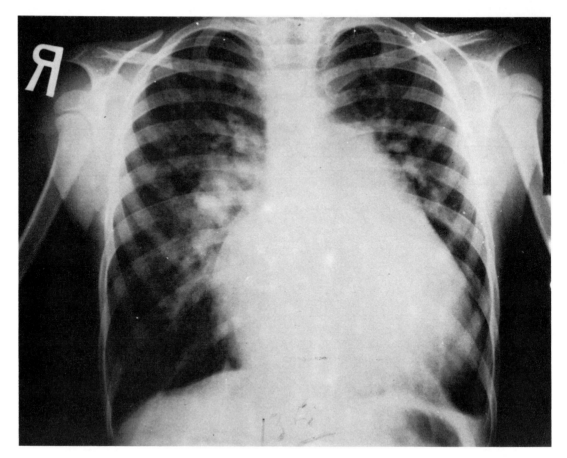

Figure 21-14. J. H., aged eight years. Large ventricular septal defect with large left-to-right shunt, dilated main pulmonary artery, and frank pulmonary plethora. Enlarged left-to-right ventricles.

The hilar shadows usually give useful information regarding the degree of blood flow and pressures in the pulmonary artery. They are normal and show no pulsations with small shunts. When the blood flow is moderate and the pressure in the pulmonary artery definitely less than systemic, the hilar shadows usually show a modest degree of pulsation. When the pressure and blood flow are high, the hilar shadows usually show marked pulsation. When the pressure is high and the flow reduced, the pulsations diminish again. This lack of hilar response is seen more frequently in adults with prolonged hypertension (Blount et al., 1955) and is relatively rare in children. The pulmonary artery is prominent but not bulging in those with a moderate pressure in this vessel, but with more marked pulmonary hypertension, bulging of the artery is the rule.

In the younger age group, under one year of age, a diversity of shape and size of the cardiac outline is seen. The heart varies from being normal in size to extending to the left chest wall. The apex appears raised in some and in others is depressed downward and out to the left. No characteristic outline is found.

Angiocardiography

In small defects after right ventricular contrast injection the right ventricle, pulmonary artery, and left heart chambers are slightly enlarged, if at all, and reopacification of the pulmonary artery may be minimal or absent. Injection from the right ventricle in large defects may show transient passage of contrast to the left ventricle and major reopacification of the pulmonary artery on the levophase. Generally, the best appearance to visualization of the defect is from selective left ventricular injection. The position and diameter of the defect can often be satisfactorily demonstrated in standard LAO or lateral projection (see Figure 21–19), but special projections recently described explore the whole length of the septum and give excellent anatomic detail (Soto et al., 1976). To complete the study an aortogram is essential, not only to exclude associated ductus arteriosus patency or coarctation of the aorta but to clarify whether aortic valve prolapse exists. Right ventricular injections should always be performed when there is systemic pressure in the right ventricle or in the presence of

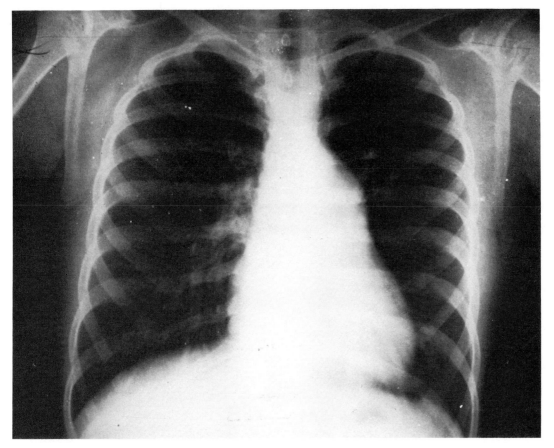

Figure 21-15. W. A., aged 12 years. Ventricular septal defect with high pulmonary vascular resistance, obstructive lesions in small pulmonary arteries, reduced pulmonary blood flow, and reversal of flow through ventricular septal defect. Cyanotic at rest and with slight exercise (Eisenmenger's complex).

pressure gradients across the right ventricular outflow or pulmonary artery bifurcation in order that associated anomalies such as double outlet right ventricle, pulmonary, valvular, or infundibular stenosis, or pulmonary artery stenosis can be clearly defined.

Electrocardiography

As our knowledge of the physiology, pathology, and prognosis of ventricular septal defect increases over the years, we find that the electrocardiogram is becoming more useful as a tool in estimating the size of the ventricular septal defect and the type of pulmonary vascular response to it. It is also helpful in estimating the prognosis over the years as well as estimating the optimum time for surgery in any particular case. Many studies have been reported previously (Sodi-Pallares et al., 1958; Adams, 1959; Char et al., 1959; DuShane et al., 1960; Scott, 1961; and Vince and Keith, 1961).

It is well recognized that the electrocardiogram should not be used as an isolated method of evaluation but should be considered with the information available from a variety of sources, clinical, radiologic, as well as hemodynamic.

There are four basic hypertrophy or loading patterns, which may be labeled (1) normal, (2) left ventricular loading, (3) right ventricular loading, and (4) combined loading. The criteria for identifying these patterns are given in Chapter 5. The hypertrophy patterns in a thousand cases of ventricular septal defect studied at The Hospital for Sick Children are as follows:

	NORMAL	LEFT VENTRICULAR HYPERTROPHY	COMBINED HYPERTROPHY	RIGHT HYPERTROPHY
Under 2 years	16%	18%	52%	14%
Over 2 years	32%	34%	21%	13%

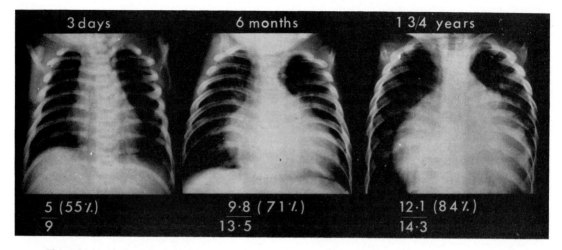

Figure 21-16. H. G. This child had an x-ray of the chest and heart at three days of age. The presence of a ventricular septal defect coupled with an atrial septal defect caused rapid and progressive enlargement of the heart with ultimate failure and death. The tremendous cardiomegaly is shown at one and three-quarter years.

In the infant the predominant pattern is combined right ventricular loading due to increased flow from the defect associated with either normal or abnormal increase in pulmonary vascular resistance. Thus, in this age period both ventricles have extra work to do. As the child grows older and the pulmonary vascular resistance diminishes, the lung capacity increases, and, in many cases, the defect becomes smaller either relatively or absolutely, the patterns change so that the predominant patterns over two years of age are either normal or left ventricular hypertrophy in type. When a normal electrocardiographic pattern is present, the pulmonary artery pressure is usually close to or within normal range and the pulmonary-to-systemic flow ratio is most frequently less than two to one. In the presence of a left ventricular hypertrophic pattern the pressure in the pulmonary artery is either normal or slightly or moderately elevated, has a low pulmonary vascular resistance, and the flow ratio is commonly less than two to one or between two to one and three to one.

When the flow ratio is above two to one and the resistance in the pulmonary circuit has increased significantly, combined hypertrophy is the usual pattern. When the flow is less than two to one and the pulmonary vascular resistance has become quite high, a right ventricular hypertrophy pattern predominates with little or no evidence of left. When a full-blown Eisenmenger complex is clinically evident, marked right ventricular hypertrophy is clearly present.

Kidd and coworkers (1965) have set forth six hemodynamic groups in ventricular septal defect, which have been described (Figure 21–11). When the hypertrophy patterns are linked to each of the hemodynamic groups, a revealing relationship is indicated that is helpful in clinical assessment. In hemodynamic group I with low flow and low resistance a normal electrocardiographic pattern predominates (54 percent), left hypertrophy occurs in

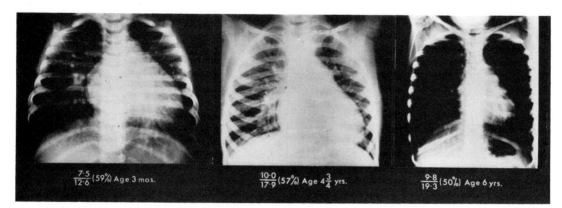

Figure 21-17. S. M. This child had a large shunt through ventricular septal defect at three months with low pulmonary vascular resistance. Pulmonary/systemic flow ratio was 8:1. At six years repeat catheterization showed the resistance had risen, pulmonary artery flow ratio was high, and flow was reduced. Pulmonary/systemic flow ratio was then 1.4:1.

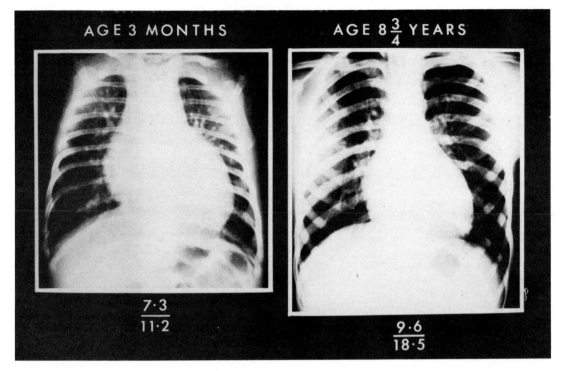

Figure 21-18. D. S., aged three months and eight years. Moderately large defect shown by catheter study at three months. Very small defect shown by repeat study at eight years. Child now leading a normal life. The reduction in heart size parallels the reduction in defect size.

some (24 percent), and combined or pure right patterns occur in the remainder, are relatively uncommon, and are usually found in infancy in this category.

At the other end of the scale is hemodynamic group VI (Eisenmenger complex) with high pulmonary vascular resistance and reversal of flow through the defect. A pure right ventricular hypertrophy pattern is found in an overwhelming proportion of cases. A few show combined loading. An exceptional case presents with minimal evidence of right ventricular hypertrophy that might be considered within normal limits.

Hemodynamic groups II to V lie between these two extremes.

QRS Axis. When the mean QRS frontal axis is related to the hemodynamic groups, the findings are as follows:

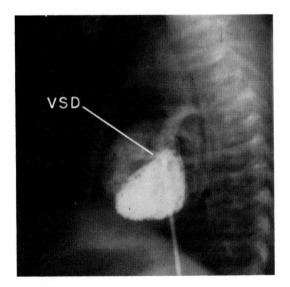

Figure 21-19. J. M., aged three weeks. Selective angiocardiogram performed in the left ventricle shows ventricular septal defect.

HEMODYNAMIC GROUP	MEAN FRONTAL QRS AXIS
I (low flow, low resistance)	31 degrees
II (increased flow, low resistance)	53 degrees
III (increased flow, slightly increased resistance)	70 degrees
IV (good flow, greater resistance)	84 degrees
V (low flow, high resistance)	114 degrees
VI (high resistance, reversal of flow)	146 degrees

It is quite apparent, when one identifies the mean frontal QRS axis with the various hemodynamic groups, that the low-flow and low-resistance cases have an axis that is within the normal limits and to the left. As the flow and resistance increase, the mean QRS axis shifts around to a point where it is deviated markedly to the right.

While the range of mean QRS axis in each of the hemodynamic groups varies considerably, it is almost invariably less than 90 degrees after the age of two years in groups I and II. In group III it is also usually less than 90 degrees, but a few cases may range between 90 and +120. In hemodynamic group IV the majority are 90 degrees or less, but a number of cases may be found between +90 and +180. In hemodynamic group V the majority fall between +90 and +180, but a few cases may still be seen with an axis between +30 and +90. However, in group VI, all the cases have an axis above the horizontal and have an axis of −150 or −120. Thus, the direction of the mean QRS axis in conjunction with the other clinical data may give one a good clue as to the state of the pulmonary vasculature and the height of the pulmonary vascular resistance.

However, perhaps more valuable than a single electrocardiograph reading is the repeated study of the direction of the QRS axis of the electrocardiogram over the first year of life and at intervals thereafter. The normal QRS axis in the newborn is frequently between +90 and +150, and if over the next few months this axis is changing steadily to a more leftward position, approaching +75 or +60 or +30, one may be certain that the resistance is falling and the hemodynamic group into which the patient will fall is likely to be a favorable one. Whenever we had repeated electrocardiograms in any child in hemodynamic group I, II, or III, with the passage of time, the mean QRS axis either shifted to the left or

remained the same within the limits of normal (see Figure 21–20). In hemodynamic groups V and VI the QRS axis showed evidence of shifting to the right. This was most noticeable in group VI. In group IV, on the other hand, in some instances the electrocardiogram shifted toward the left and in other cases shifted to the right. Obviously group IV is an intermediary group, and these patients may be developing either diminished or increased pulmonary vascular resistance in the early stages of life. These findings are portrayed in Figure 21–20. An example of an individual case followed from shortly after birth to 13 years of age is demonstrated in Figure 21–21. This child had developed the clinical and hemodynamic picture of Eisenmenger's complex by 12 years of life.

P WAVE. In reviewing our catheter-proved cases of ventricular septal defect, we find that the P-R interval is within normal limits in 95 percent of cases. The P wave duration was found to be slightly prolonged in 30 percent of the cases; the height of the P wave was within normal limits, and significant notching of P in leads I or II was noted in approximately 30 percent. Notching and broadening were shown only in groups with either left loading or combined loading, and within these groups this sign was usually accompanied by a tall R or a deep Q. It appeared, therefore, simply to offer additional evidence of diastolic loading of the left atrium and left ventricle.

An electrocardiographic pitfall occurs when a child with a ventricular septal and high pulmonary vascular

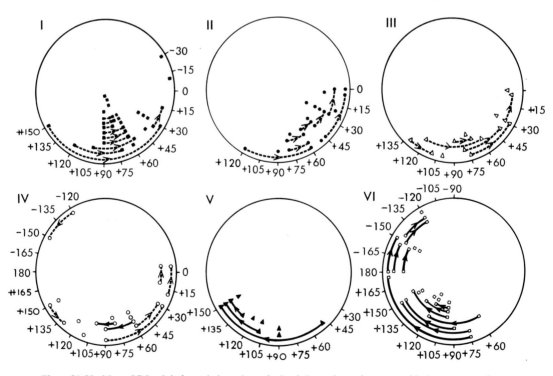

Figure 21-20. Mean QRS axis in frontal plane shown in the six hemodynamic groups with changes occurring as the infant grows into childhood and approaches adolescence. Hemodynamic groups I, II, and III all shift to the left with a more favorable axis. Groups V and VI shift to the right with an unfavorable axis.

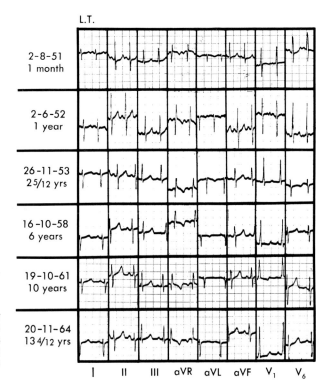

Figure 21-21. L. T. This child with a ventricular septal defect gradually developed the high pulmonary vascular resistance of Eisenmenger's complex. Note the progressive change of the QRS frontal axis from early life to 13 years of age. Axis shifts steadily to the right.

resistance also has an associated mitral valve anomaly with insufficiency. Such cases may show a broad-notch P wave in the electrocardiogram and evidence of left ventricular loading with increased height of the R wave in V_6 or a significant Q wave and yet have pulmonary vascular changes that are irreversible and unlikely to permit survival at the time of operation.

COUNTERCLOCKWISE VECTOR. As would be expected, the direction of the frontal vector followed the direction of the axis as a rule. A third of our cases had a counterclockwise vector and 82 percent of these had an axis of less than 90 degrees. There were, however, a few cases that had a counterclockwise vector with an axis of 90 degrees or more. When we reviewed these separately, it was obvious that they had other evidence of relatively good pulmonary blood flows and would, therefore, fall into the moderate or low pulmonary vascular resistance group.

TALL PEAKED T WAVES. Tall, broad R waves in V_6 are often followed by tall T waves in the same lead and are usually a sign of diastolic ventricular loading. Tall, broad QRS complexes over the right precordium with tall T waves following them are indicative of marked right ventricular loading, and in such cases the prognosis is poor and almost invariably associated with increased pulmonary vascular resistance.

Q WAVE. Twenty-five percent of our cases with ventricular septal defect showed a Q wave in V_6 of 4 mm or more. Sixty percent had a Q wave of 2 mm or more. A Q wave of 4 mm or more was usually associated with other evidence of left ventricular

diastolic loading such as a tall R in V_6, a deep S in V_1, or notching of the P wave. There was left-axis deviation or a pulmonary-to-systemic blood flow ratio of two to one.

Vectorcardiography

The vectorcardiogram may at times prove superior to the routine scalar lead. This is because the horizontal vector gives a more complete picture of electrical impulse from the heart since the ordinary precordial leads do not go all the way around the chest as a rule and may not as accurately reflect maximal positions of electrical activity.

The mean QRS axis in the frontal plane may be determined with greater accuracy from vectorcardiogram and from the scalar leads. A comparison of vectorcardiograms over a period of several months or years may more accurately reflect the changes occurring in the relationship of one ventricle to the other and therefore further reflect the changes in pulmonary vasculature.

The horizontal plane vector in the normal heart or in the presence of a small ventricular septal defect reveals a counterclockwise loop and a voltage pattern that is within normal limits for the age. The axis of this vector is usually between 0 and +60 degrees.

In the right ventricular hypertrophy or loading pattern the horizontal vector is usually clockwise and its dominant portion is anterior and to the right. The axis, therefore, is between +70 and +150 degrees and the direction of the vector is clockwise.

In left ventricular loading or hypertrophy the vector is counterclockwise in direction and to the left, somewhat similar to the normal pattern but with increased voltage, and the axis of the vector may be within the normal range or veer round beyond 0 degrees to a negative axis.

The combined loading or hypertrophy pattern in the horizontal vector shows a wide variety of loops since many combinations of both right and left loading may be apparent; thus there may be a clockwise or a counterclockwise loop, or it may be a figure of eight usually with the terminal portion clockwise. Examples of these patterns are shown in the accompanying illustrations (Figures 21–22 to 21–25).

It is of interest that the initial forces (0.01, 0.02 vector) correlated well the pulmonary/systemic flow ratio. This was also true of the maximum QRS forces. The latter were increased in hemodynamic groups II, III, and IV, where the shunt was large, and

reduced again in groups I and VI, where the shunt was small.

As would be expected, the maximum spatial vector increases with rising pulmonary vascular resistance. These changes are clearly displayed in the vectorcardiogram and reflect the underlying pathology with greater accuracy than does the axis in the frontal plane, although the latter is a most useful measurement and easier to obtain.

Echocardiography

Left-to-right shunting at ventricular level produces a volume overload of the left atrium and ventricle. This is shown echocardiographically as increased left atrial and left ventricular dimensions. The degree of left atrial enlargement is related to the measured left-to-right shunt (Lewis and Takahashi, 1976; Bloom et al., 1977). This enables one to separate large (>2:1)

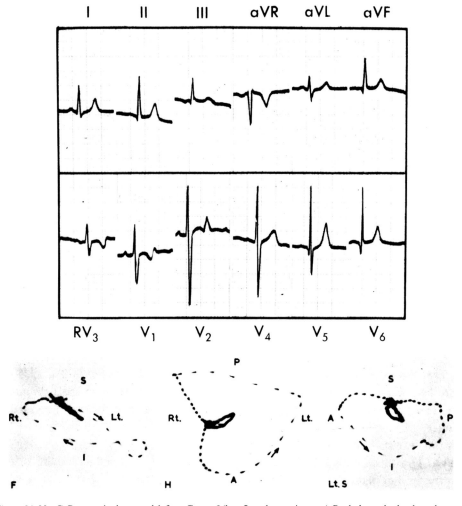

Figure 21-22. G. B., ventricular septal defect. Group I (low flow, low resistance). Both the scalar leads and vector loops are within normal limits. (The horizontal vector appears slightly enlarged because it was increased photographically.)

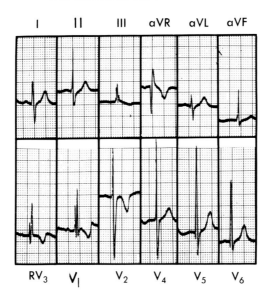

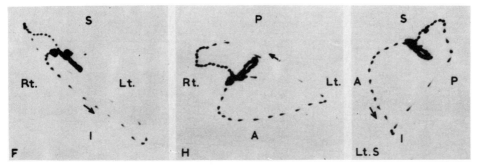

Figure 21-23. M. K., 5½ years—ventricular septal defect. Group II (increased flow, low resistance). Scalar leads show left ventricular hypertrophy and right bundle branch block and slight right hypertrophy. The vector horizontal loop corroborates this.

from small (<2:1) shunts (Bloom et al., 1977). These findings are similar to those seen in patent ductus arteriosus.

Aneurysmal transformation of ventricular septal defect may be recognized by abnormal echoes appearing on the right septal surface (Assad-Morell et al., 1974; Sapire and Black, 1975).

Loss of septal echoes may occur in any patient due to the varying plane of the septum and has not been a reliable diagnostic feature in most investigators' experience using either single crystal or cross-sectional techniques (Goldberg et al., 1975).

The association of pulmonary hypertension may be recognized by an enlarged, thick-walled right ventricle and abnormal systolic time intervals as determined by pulmonary valve leaflet motion (Hirschfeld et al., 1975).

The echocardiogram thus provides the clinician with noninvasive evidence of the degree of left-to-right shunting and pulmonary vascular resistance. As such, it is of value in the initial assessment and long-term clinical follow-up of the patient with ventricular septal defect.

Diagnosis

There is abundant pathologic and cardiac catheterization evidence that a ventricular septal defect is usually present when there is a loud, harsh systolic murmur maximum in the third and fourth left interspaces with or without a thrill, in a child who has no obvious cyanosis. The presence of increased hilar shadowing is of some value in confirming the diagnosis. The electrocardiogram may show left ventricular hypertrophy, right ventricular hypertrophy, biventricular hypertrophy, or a normal tracing. The heart is enlarged to some degree in many cases. The cardiac catheterization will usually show a rise in oxygen content on entering the right ventricle; however, in certain instances there may be an insignificant rise even in the presence of a definite ventricular septal defect. A hydrogen electrode in the right ventricle or a left ventricular angiogram will usually locate such minimal shunts.

Even with these techniques a shunt may not be recognized and it may be necessary to augment them with norepinephrine or angiotensin, as described by

348 SHUNTS

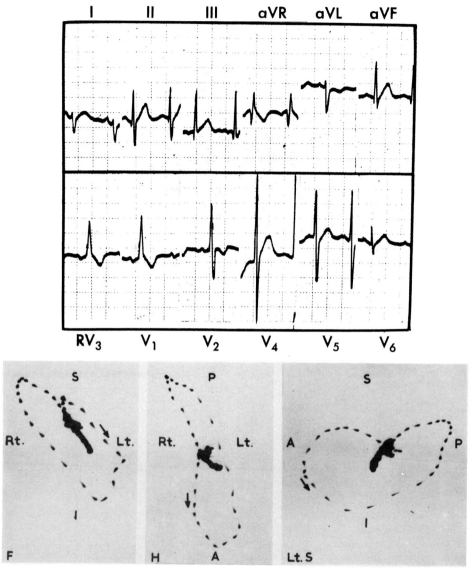

Figure 21-24. D. B., one-year-old boy—ventricular septal defect. Group IVB (increased flow, moderately increased resistance). Pulmonary artery pressure is two-thirds systemic with a pulmonary-to-systemic flow ratio of 2.5:1. Systemic/pulmonary resistance ratio is 3.7:1; axis is +60 in frontal plane. The horizontal vector indicates confined hypertrophy, which is not evident in scalar leads. Thus vector loop is more indicative of hemodynamics than scalar leads.

Cumming (1965). These drugs raise the left ventricular pressure and force a sufficient shunt through a small defect to permit its identification with certainty.

Since all these refined techniques cannot be carried out on all patients suspected of having a ventricular septal defect, some criteria are required for making a diagnosis. Among the patients referred to in the various charts and figures on the accompanying pages we have included those selected on the following bases:

1. Those with cardiac catheter or angiocardiographic evidence of a ventricular septal defect.

2. Those with a well-heard systolic murmur maximum in the fourth left interspace and in whom with the passage of time the various defects listed below are ruled out.

These criteria will not include all cases having such defects especially the very small ones as shown by Cumming (1965), but they do cover the vast majority. It would appear likely that many of the children with well-heard systolic murmurs maximum in the fourth left interspace near the sternum do in fact have small ventricular septal defects even though the heart is not enlarged, there is no thrill, and the electrocardiogram is normal.

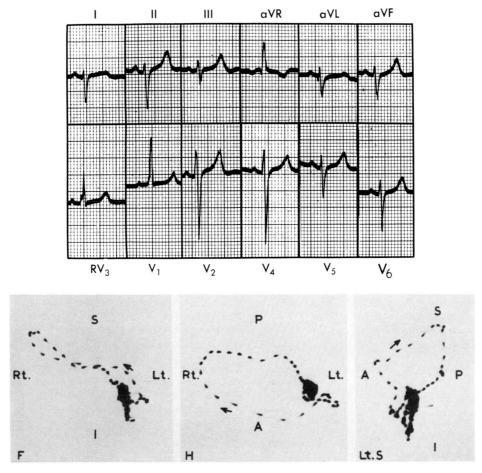

Figure 21-25. J. G., 18-year-old girl—ventricular septal defect. Group VI (low flow, very high resistance). This is an example of advanced pulmonary vascular disease (Eisenmenger's complex). Axis is −150 degrees. The vector is almost entirely to the right in the precordial leads (horizontal) and is clockwise. R in V_1 is of moderate height. T in V_1 is upright. There are a small R and a deep S in V_6.

In making a diagnosis it is necessary to rule out certain conditions that may simulate a ventricular septal defect at certain ages. These are listed below. This is usually possible with repeated observations and selected cardiac catheter studies.

Differential Diagnosis. The following conditions have presented some difficulties in differential diagnosis of ventricular septal defect. This is chiefly a list that includes some of the mistakes the authors have made in the past and hope to avoid in the future. It includes:

1. Pulmonary stenosis.
2. Aortic stenosis.
3. Infundibular stenosis.
4. Ventricular septal defects associated with certain noncyanotic anomalies.
5. Tetralogy of Fallot.
6. Endocardial fibroelastosis.
7. Transposition of the great vessels.
8. Common ventricle.
9. Mitral regurgitation.

PULMONARY STENOSIS. Occasionally it may be difficult to differentiate between a ventricular septal defect and pulmonary stenosis. This is sometimes the case in the first six months of life when the point of maximum intensity of the murmur is difficult to define and may be misleading. If cyanosis is present and the murmur is maximum in the pulmonary area, or if there is poststenotic dilatation in the pulmonary artery and right ventricular hypertrophy in the electrocardiogram, there is usually a little difficulty in making the diagnosis of pulmonary stenosis and differentiating between the two. Without cyanosis and minimal right ventricular hypertrophy, observation over many months or a year or two will usually settle the problem. In doubtful cases cardiac catheterization is required.

AORTIC STENOSIS. It is well recognized that aortic stenosis can produce a systolic murmur that is best heard over the precordium or at the apex and thus simulate a ventricular septal defect. In babies in the first year of life it is not uncommon to hear a murmur over the left precordium rather than the aortic area in this condition. As time goes on, however, a high percentage of such cases will have the murmur shift to its more characteristic location in the aortic area. The aortic murmur may be shorter and more stenotic in type; the ventricular septal defect not uncommonly in childhood produces a similar effect. Systolic click or split first sound is more characteristic of aortic stenosis, and the electrocardiogram in the latter condition is more likely to show a deep S in V_1 when left ventricular hypertrophy is present. However, in doubtful cases a left heart catheterization is required.

INFUNDIBULAR STENOSIS. Localized stenosis of the outflow tract of the right ventricle occurs occasionally and produces a murmur low in the precordium and is often accompanied by a thrill. Right ventricular hypertrophy in the electrocardiogram is a characteristic finding as well as lack of pulsations in the hilar shadows. Second sound is likely to be fainter in the pulmonary area than with a ventricular septal defect, and the persistence of this and other signs indicated above with repeated observations suggests the need for cardiac catheterization, which will permit one to make the differential diagnosis with accuracy.

VENTRICULAR SEPTAL DEFECT ASSOCIATED WITH AN ATRIAL SEPTAL DEFECT. When an atrial septal defect accompanies the ventricular septal defect, the combination may be difficult to recognize, but the following points may arouse one's suspicions: (1) an unusually large heart with a bulging pulmonary artery and large pulsating hilar shadows associated with a murmur that is characteristic of ventricular septal defect but with signs being more severe than in the majority of cases when the defect is isolated; (2) electrocardiographic evidence of a very marked right ventricular hypertrophy pattern with strain, deeply inverted T waves over the right precordium, and depressed S-T segment in the same leads, with right-axis deviation in the standard leads; (3) a large right atrium; (4) the presence of congestive heart failure associated with a very large heart. In the presence of any of these findings, one should do a cardiac catheterization.

PATENT DUCTUS ARTERIOSUS WITH VENTRICULAR SEPTAL DEFECT. This association may be suspected if there is a continuous murmur in the pulmonary area coupled with characteristic murmur over the lower precordium. However, a number of cases of patent ductus arteriosus may have a murmur that is systolic in time and best heard over the lower precordium. This is true in some infants in the early months of life, and when the heart is enlarged or there is any evidence of failure, cardiac catheterization should be performed and surgical closure of the ductus carried out if necessary.

COARCTATION OF THE AORTA WITH VENTRICULAR SEPTAL DEFECT. This is not an uncommon finding. During routine examination of a child with characteristic septal murmur, one should check the femoral arteries and blood pressures for signs of coarctation. The raised pressure in the left ventricle usually produces a very intense murmur.

TETRALOGY OF FALLOT. Approximately 15 percent of our cases of tetralogy of Fallot have no history of cyanosis during the first year of life while at rest. However, most of these, when studied carefully, show some slight degree of cyanosis with crying or breath holding. A few, however, have arterial oxygen saturations over 90 at rest and show little or no drop with exercise. Such cases have a loud, harsh systolic murmur in the third and fourth left interspaces, and superficial examination strongly suggests a ventricular septal defect. These children usually have a fairly marked right ventricular hypertrophy on electrocardiogram that suggests the true diagnosis. When there is any doubt, a cardiac catheterization should be performed. The presence of a right aortic arch is helpful in making the diagnosis.

ENDOCARDIAL FIBROELASTOSIS. A few of these cases have murmurs over the lower precordium simulating ventricular septal defects. Such murmurs are usually due to either aortic or mitral valve disease, and the presence of a marked left ventricular hypertrophy pattern with strain would make one highly suspicious of endocardial fibroelastosis. Cardiac catheterization will help to clarify the diagnosis.

TRANSPOSITION OF THE GREAT VESSELS. When this anomaly is present with tricuspid atresia, there may be only slight cyanosis at times with large pulsating hilar shadows. Left ventricular hypertrophy is seen in this defect and commonly failure. The signs are usually sufficiently severe to warrant an angiocardiogram or cardiac catheterization, and this will clarify the diagnosis.

COMMON VENTRICLE. Common ventricle will frequently be associated with the murmurs similar to ventricular septal defect since there is a narrowing at the entrance of the outflow tract to the aorta. However, the majority of these cases will show cyanosis at rest, which increases with activity. Eighty percent of them have evidence of transposition of the great vessels. Many of them have radiologic evidence of L-transposition, which may be characteristic. Angiocardiographic studies may be required to clarify the diagnosis.

Ventricular Septal Defect with Congestive Heart Failure

Of 1000 cases of ventricular septal defect, 93 had clinical evidence of congestive heart failure with dyspnea, enlarged liver, and pulmonary congestion. Breathlessness per se was not considered as frank failure since, in many cases, this was due to increased pulmonary flow alone rather than myocardial insufficiency.

Incidence of Congestive Heart Failure. The incidence figures vary with the group studied. Of 1000 cases, 9.3 per cent had congestive heart failure.

However, if these are divided by age and by cardiac catheter study, the figures are as follows:

CATHETERIZED	CONGESTIVE HEART FAILURE (Percent)
Under 1 year	25
Over 1 year	12
NOT CATHETERIZED	
Under 1 year	10
Over 1 year	3.4

It is obvious that the heart is most likely to fail in the first year of life. This has previously been demonstrated by Morgan, Griffiths, and Blumenthal (1960), Engle (1954), and Sherman (1963), but the mortality from this cause has declined in the past decade, as indicated by comparing the data of Mehrizi, Hirsch, and Taussig (1964), Ober and Moore (1955), and Rowe and Cleary (1960). The first two groups—one in Baltimore and the other in Boston—found a high incidence of deaths from ventricular septal defect in their records studied from 1930 to 1950, while Rowe and Cleary found a lower mortality from ventricular septal defect in the recent decade.

It is not fully realized how difficult it is to decide the cause of death in infants with a ventricular septal defect. Among the 54 cases that died with isolated ventricular septal defect among 1000 cases the following classification of cause of death was made in 1964.

Operative deaths	24
Operative deaths with recent heart failure	2
Failure and pneumonia	7
Failure per se	11
Pneumonia per se	3
Others	7

The others include cases that died of aspiration, tracheal abnormality, anemia, mongolism, or multiple noncardiac defects. Since 1964 operative deaths have declined as have those with failure and pneumonia.

Prematurity. It is of interest that 17 percent of our infants and children with ventricular septal defects and congestive heart failure were premature at birth. Prematurity apparently leads to either a weaker myocardium or lower pulmonary vascular resistance, or it may simply be that prematures are more likely to have a ventricular septal defect.

Treatment of Congestive Heart Failure. Therapy consists of digitalization, oxygen administration, Fowler's position with use of a supporting seat, diuretics, antibiotics as required, and oxygen when necessary.

The administration of oxygen is of value in the early, acute stages and appears to be of help when the lung is congested, especially when there is any evidence of arterial desaturation. In such instances, ear oximetry shows that oxygen therapy will raise the arterial oxygen saturation slightly. The oxygen is usually not required for more than a few days at a time. This is especially true when the response to the other drugs mentioned above is satisfactory. In the presence of pulmonary edema, diuretics are most helpful in controlling heart failure and in relieving the edema. Furosemide is particularly useful in this regard, 0.1 mg/kg. Serum potassium should be checked and, at suitable intervals, the other electrolytes, especially sodium and chlorides.

One of the major problems in the management of an infant or child with a ventricular septal defect and congestive heart failure concerns the problem of whether to resort to surgery. Most children who show evidence of myocardial inadequacy will eventually need surgical closure, but many facets need to be examined in any individual case before proceeding with operative therapy. The following points may offer guidance in this regard:

1. Many of these infants with failure can be managed medically through such illness and maintained successfully on digitalis until the optimum time for surgery arrives.

2. Failure precipitated by respiratory infection can frequently be managed with the aid of antibiotics and decongestive therapy until the acute illness is over, and then marked improvement is often apparent. Operative mortality is significant in the early weeks of life. Operation in the face of inadequately controlled failure is associated with a higher mortality. The presence of associated cardiac anomalies commonly precipitates congestive heart failure in the first year or two of life, and when such anomalies are present, surgical intervention may be more urgent but it is important to identify the additional anomalies.

3. Finally, knowledge of the actual defect diameter is useful in prognosis: moderate-sized defects commonly become much smaller during infancy whereas larger ones do not (Rowe, 1973).

Spontaneous Closure of Ventricular Septal Defect

That spontaneous closure of the ventricular septal defect was occurring has been suspected for many years. In 1918 French described the clinical findings in a young boy whose murmur and thrill disappeared at five years of age. Montanini (1932) presented the first anatomic evidence that closure could occur naturally by an adherent medial leaflet of the tricuspid valve. A similar case was also reported by Majka and associates (1960), and more recently three additional cases by Coles et al. (1962). This mode of closure was obviously rare, and it was not until recent years that the suggestion was made that closure of the defect may be occurring in larger numbers than had previously been realized (Keith et al., 1958; Evans et al., 1960). Good reviews of several aspects of the subject have appeared recently (Evans et al., 1960; Soulie et al., 1960; Nadas et al., 1961; Agustsson et al., 1963; Bloomfield, 1964; Moore et al., 1965).

Evans, Rowe, and Keith (1960) presented evidence of closure of the anomalous opening in a patient who initially had cardiac failure and obviously had a large defect. Their chief emphasis, however, was placed on the disappearance of the murmur and obliteration of the defect when the shunt was small initially. Thus 37 children were described who had a systolic murmur in early life that gradually diminished and eventually disappeared.

Kavanagh-Gray (1962) presented cardiac catheter as well as angiographic evidence of a defect closing between the ages of three weeks and three months. Hoffman and Rudolph (1965) recorded a relatively high incidence (8 out of 26 cases) of defect closure in the first year of life using serial catheter studies. If special catheter techniques are used early in life, a higher incidence of very small defects will undoubtedly be disclosed. This was emphatically demonstrated by Cumming (1965) who found that there may be no hemodynamic evidence of the defect until either norepinephrine or angiotensin is administered.

Since spontaneous closure of the ventricular septal defect begins in the early weeks of life, incidence figures must be based on early diagnosis and a long follow-up. At The Hospital for Sick Children, we have recorded 630 infants with ventricular septal defect, seen first in the first year of life and followed for an average of seven years. A summary of the spontaneous closure in this group is shown in Table 21–4. As one might expect, the smallest defects (e.g., the clinical group) had the highest incidence of closure (26 percent).

Table 21–4. SPONTANEOUS CLOSURE OF VENTRICULAR SEPTAL DEFECT

	630 CASES FOLLOWED FROM INFANCY	
	Number of Cases	Number of Spontaneous Closures
A. Catheter and surgery	104	0
B. Catheter study only	208	22 (11%)
C. Clinical	318	82 (26%)

295 CASES FOLLOWED IN ADULT CLINIC (ALL BORN BEFORE 1955)	
NUMBER OF CASES	NUMBER OF SPONTANEOUS CLOSURES AFTER THE AGE OF 13 YEARS
295	12 (4%)

Besides the infant and childhood group, there are those that have been followed into the teens and twenties. Four percent of these have closed spontaneously after leaving the Cardiac Clinic at The

Hospital for Sick Children, the oldest being 31 years. Thus, one may add these cases to those closing in the pediatric ages.

The age when closure takes place is recorded in Figure 21–26. It will be seen that the majority close in the first seven years of life, with the numbers falling off in the teens. However, the process continues on into adult life. The latest age we have encountered of disappearance of the murmur has been 31 years. Reviewing the evidence, one can conclude that if a baby is born with a small ventricular septal defect, the chance of it closing completely by adult life is probably 60 to 70 percent.

Alpert and coworkers (1973) followed 55 infants who had small ventricular septal defects for a five-year period. Fifty-eight percent closed spontaneously in that period. The incidence of closure varied with the type and position of the defect. Sixty-five percent with a muscular defect were obliterated and 25 percent of the membranous ones. Where the anatomic position could not be determined, the incidence was 58 percent.

Shaher and colleagues (1965) reported a case of spontaneous closure of the ventricular septal defect in a case of transposition of the great vessels. The authors have a similar experience later proven at autopsy.

Several mechanisms may be postulated for spontaneous closure. These include: (1) fibrosis of margins of defect with ultimate closure; (2) an adherent tricuspid valve cusp that seals off the defect; (3) fistulous tracks surrounded by reactive fibrosis (Bloomfield, 1964); and (4) low defects in the muscular portion of the septum that close as the muscle bundles hypertrophy. Apart from the adherent tricuspid valve evidence of the precise mechanism, closure is not well-documented. This problem will undoubtedly receive more attention in the near future. Bloomfield (1964) suggested that a careful examination of hearts at autopsy in later life may show evidence of prior closure. (See Simmons and associates [1966].)

The question of spontaneous closure after childhood deserves special attention.

Aneurysm of the Membranous Septum

Aneurysm of the membranous septum was first described by Laennec (1826). Since then many authors have identified this pathologic finding, either as an isolated phenomenon or associated with other cardiac anomalies, particularly the ventricular septal defect. It has also been described with a variety of arrhythmias and conduction defects. Many theories concerning the origin of this malformation have been proposed. Mall (1912) suggested that it was associated with a congenitally weakened state arising from a mildly dextraposed aorta. This theory was supported by Lev and Saphir (1938). However, other authors have been unable to document an abnormal

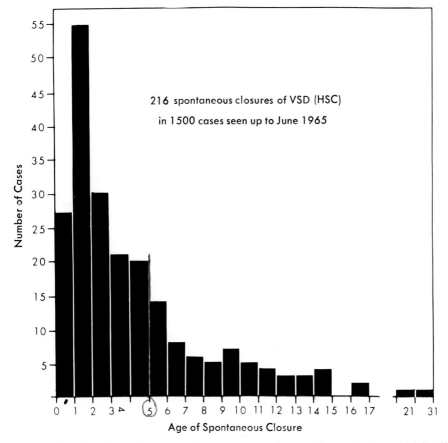

Figure 21-26. The above figure, demonstrates that spontaneous closure of the ventricular septal defect, if it is going to occur, is most likely to occur in the first five years of life. However, it may occur in subsequent years. The latest age we have demonstrated closure is 30 years.

position of the membranous septum or the aorta root in such children (Baron et al., 1964). Although there may be different etiologies, the more likely explanation is that which involves adherence of some portion of the tricupsid valve to the area of the ventricular defect (Tandon and Edwards, 1973).

Such aneurysms were first demonstrated during life by Steinberg (1957) who reported an angiocardiograph of an aneurysm in a 60-year-old housewife. The majority of such aneurysms, when associated with a ventricular septal defect, usually have a small left-to-right shunt. Several authors have suggested that the presence of an aneurysm may facilitate spontaneous closure of the ventricular septal defect (Varghese, 1969). Recent information makes the case for the development of aneurysm of the muscular septum to be an extremely common situation in the natural history of ventricular septal defect (Freedom et al., 1974).

Pieroni and associates (1971) presented evidence of auscultatory recognition of aneurysm of the membranous septum associated with ventricular septal defects. An early systolic sound preceding the pansystolic murmur with a clicky quality is localized between the lower left edge of the sternum and the apex and is best heard in expiration in patients with angiographic evidence of aneurysm. Phonocardiograms show this sound to be 100 to 130 milliseconds after the Q wave of the electrocardiogram. This clinical finding has proven a very reliable method for clinical diagnosis. Pickering and Keith (1971) later presented confirmatory data. Additionally the systolic murmur has late systolic accentuation (Linhart and Razi, 1971; Pieroni et al., 1971).

Recently Freedom and colleagues (1974) studied 56 unselected children with isolated ventricular septal defects to determine the occurrence and natural history of the syndrome. Each child had two cardiac catheterizations, four years apart. Twenty children, who had an aneurysm of the membranous ventricular septum at first catheterization, at second catheter had little change in their findings. Twelve children were noted on the second study to have developed an aneurysm when the pulmonary blood flow was relatively small; the incidence of membranous septal aneurysm was overall 70 percent.

Spontaneous closure of the usual ventricular septal defect has been estimated by various authors to be somewhere between 25 and 40 percent, if patients are followed from birth for five or ten years. Although

[handwritten margin note: 25% to 40% V.S.D's close spontaneously]

closure may occur in the presence of an aneurysm of the membranous septum, such event appears to be uncommon (Varghese and Rowe, 1969). No satisfactory figure has been arrived at yet, but appears to be less than 5 percent. No instance of spontaneous closure was observed in the study of Freedom and associates (1974). It seems likely that the majority of older children now being followed for many years with little or no change in heart size, murmur, or electrocardiogram frequently have an aneurysm in the membranous portion of the septum associated with their murmurs. Whether prolonged follow-up of 16 and 20 years will increase the incidence of closure in this particular group is something that remains to be determined. (See Figure 21–27.)

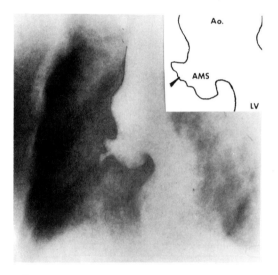

Figure 21-27. Aneurysm of the membranous septum. Left ventricular angiocardiogram showing the aneurysm (*AMS*) and a small junction through it.

Decrease in Size of the Defect Without Complete Closure

One may carry this discussion a step further since during childhood years a considerable number of children show clinical and laboratory evidence of a decrease in the size of the ventricular septal defect without complete closure. The evidence for this is as follows:

1. When the pulmonary artery pressure and the shunt through the defect both decrease, one must conclude that the defect has become smaller. Arcilla and coworkers (1963) have presented data indicating that, when both pressure and flow were increased initially, both pressure and flow were diminished in 70 percent of their patients of one to seven years on whom repeat cardiac catheter studies were made. The studies were made chiefly during the first five or six years of life, and from the data one can conclude, therefore, that there was a decrease in size of the defect in 70 percent of their children. Our own data (Kidd

and coworkers, 1965) lead to a similar conclusion, although the incidence is not as high. Sandoe (1963) reports a decrease in defect size in 50 percent of cases followed an average of six years.

2. Laboratory data coincide closely with the clinical evidence using heart size and the electrocardiogram as parameters. Sixty-eight percent of the children under two years of age in our 1000 cases studied had cardiothoracic ratios over 55 percent. Only 26 percent over the age of five years had cardiothoracic ratios of 55 percent or less. At the same time, electrocardiographic data showed a change in a similar direction. Under two years of age only 34 percent had normal or left ventricular hypertrophy patterns, which are usually associated with normal or close-to-normal pulmonary artery pressures. Over the age of two the incidence of these benign patterns had risen to 68 percent. A decrease in heart size associated with an improvement in electrocardiographic pattern strongly suggests a decrease in both pressure and flow, which in turn indicates a reduction in the size of the defect.

It has been indicated previously that the murmurs disappeared and the defect apparently closed in approximately 25 percent of cases. It now appears likely that in approximately one-half of the remainder a reduction in the size of the defect occurred in early childhood. This may have been an absolute reduction in some cases; in others it may have been due to increase in the muscular development of the septum, and during ventricular systole the defect itself may contract significantly. Decrease in size is more likely to occur in the defects that are not large to begin with. In other words, it is more likely to occur in those defects that are less than 5 mm in the infants and less than 10 mm in diameter in the rest of childhood.

Development of Infundibular Pulmonary Stenosis

Since Gasul and associates (1957) first described the development of infundibular stenosis in a child who had previously had an isolated ventricular septal defect, a number of investigators have attempted to determine the true incidence of this developing complication. As we have demonstrated (Keith et al. 1971), it appears to vary with the hemodynamic group concerned. It did not occur in hemodynamic groups I, V, or VI. It did occur in five to 10 percent of the cases in groups II, III, and IV that had been seen first in infancy, catheterized, and followed for five or six years. All of these had a flow ratio greater than 2:1 initially. Tyrrell and coworkers (1973) had presented the data on 22 cases from The Hospital for Sick Children, Toronto, which initially had a gradient across the pulmonary outflow tract of less than 20 mm of mercury. All increased significantly with follow-up and at the second catheter several years later ten had evidence of tetralogy of Fallot, three had anomalous right ventricular muscle bundle, one had a prolapsed aortic valve with infundibular stenosis, and the other eight had developed simple infundibular narrowing with the ventricular septal defect.

Specific angiographic measurements appear useful in detecting early on those cases who had certain anatomic features of tetralogy of Fallot but without the coronal gradient across the outflow tract of the right ventricle. In these cases, as a result of the underdevelopment of the distal pulmonary infundibulum, a deviation of the crysta supraventricularis in the outflow tract and the pulmonary valve give rise to an increased right ventricular outflow tract angle. This angle has proved to be useful in recognizing those patients who will ultimately develop a typical tetralogy of Fallot picture over a period of time. An example of a normal angle of the outflow tract of the right ventricle is shown in Figure 21–28 and is usually in the neighborhood of 40 degrees.

In tetralogy of Fallot, on the other hand, the outflow tract is more horizontal in relation to the ventricle and makes an angle of approximately 65 degrees (see Figure 21–29).

A right aortic arch is associated with ventricular septal defect and is also helpful in identifying those that are likely to have progressive infundibular stenosis (Varghese et al., 1970). Ten out of fourteen patients with this combination developed progressive infundibular stenosis.

Deaths

In 630 infants followed from the first five years of life for an average of 7.5 years, the deaths amounted to 6.7 percent during that period (Table 21–5).

Table 21–5. DEATHS FROM VENTRICULAR SEPTAL DEFECT

GROUP	NO. OF CASES	DEATHS
Clinical evaluation	318	(0)
Catheter study only	208	15 (7%)
Catheter and surgery	104	27 (26%)
Total	630	42 (6.7%)

There were no deaths in the very small ventricular septal defects diagnosed by clinical evaluation. There was a 7 percent mortality in those that had a catheter study only and did not require surgery; however, among those that did require surgery the mortality was 26 percent. The majority of the latter were in

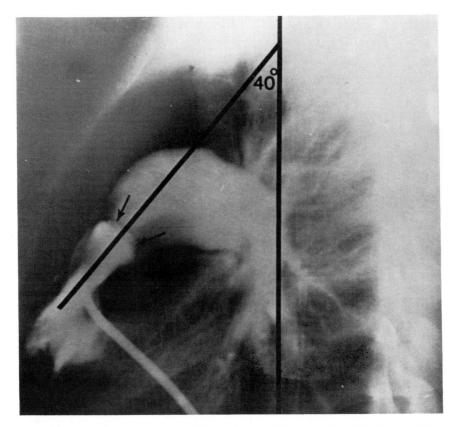

Figure 21-28. Right ventricular outflow angle. The usual normal right ventricular outflow is shown. The normal range is usually between 20° and 46° (mean 33°).

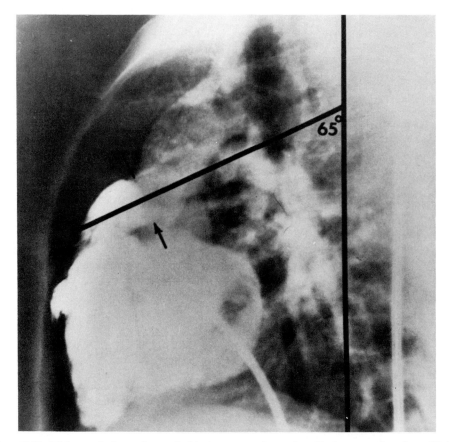

Figure 21-29. Right ventricular outflow angle. Much greater angles are found in the group of tetralogy of Fallot ranging from 52° to 80° (mean 66°). Children who are likely to acquire increasing outflow tract gradients are likely to have outflow angles similar to those found in the tetralogy of Fallot.

intractable failure and required either banding operation or an attempt at direct closure. In either case the risk was high in the first six months of life. The mortality in this latter category has been falling steadily and it is hoped that it will be largely eliminated in the future.

In the 295 cases, all of whom were born before 1955 and followed until the present time, ten or 3.4 percent have died in the late teens and 20s. Most of these deaths have been due to progressive pulmonary vascular disease, but two of them were associated with attempts at surgery.

The Clinical Syndrome of Eisenmenger's Reaction

The monograph of Wood (1958), which has been referred to previously, defines the Eisenmenger syndrome as pulmonary vascular disease with reversal of flow through the defect and a pulmonary vascular resistance of 800 dynes/sec/cm^{-5}. It is a phase of the ventricular septal defect spectrum that is more characteristic of the second and third decades of life than the first since the vascular changes tend to occur at a slow pace.

Incidence. This diagnosis does not fit the newborn period or the first year of life because, with a few exceptions, the pulmonary vasculature shows nothing more than hypertrophy with minimal narrowing of the lumen at this stage. If a defect such as a patent ductus arteriosus is closed during this period, the pulmonary vascular resistance falls and there is no progressive disease. After the first birthday, however, signs of raised resistance may become increasingly significant over the next few years if the defect is not treated and the pulmonary arteries are reactive.

A review of hemodynamic groups of patients with ventricular septal defect in the literature, 1958–1964, indicated the incidence of pulmonary vascular disease with high pulmonary vascular resistance, Eisenmenger complex, varying from 10 to 20 percent. In children it was approximately 10 percent and in adults 16 to 20 percent Wood, 1958; Lyndfield, 1960; Lucas, 1961; Arcilla, 1963; Leachman, 1963; Evans, 1964; Kidd, 1964.

In the past the incidence of this complication was considerably higher in adults than in childhood. Wood (1958) found it in 16 percent. Evans (1964) in 19 percent. Both these study groups had an average age of 22 years. Recently, however, a review of our data on teen-age and adult cases shows an incidence of 9.4 percent (Table 21–7, page 361).

Clinical Features. The fully developed clinical picture of the Eisenmenger syndrome is slow in appearing in childhood, and most of the children who ultimately develop it lead a relatively active life for many years. As they grow older, the clinical signs and symptoms begin to appear with diminished exercise tolerance, cyanosis, first only with exercise and later at rest, failure to thrive, retarded growth, clubbing of the fingers, and polycythemia.

Obvious clinical cyanosis during childhood is uncommon before the age of ten years, but ear oximetry may more frequently show a drop in arterial oxygen saturation with exercise. Griffiths and associates (1964) suggest that those who develop cyanosis early are more likely to run a stable course and, therefore, have a slightly improved prognosis.

Clubbing of the fingers develops gradually and, when present, is usually minimal in childhood. Polycythemia is also minimal. Squatting is not seen in this group in our experience unless it is associated with some degree of infundibular narrowing.

A pulmonary diastolic murmur of valve insufficiency begins to develop, particularly in those with dilated pulmonary arteries and slowly progressive pulmonary vascular disease. Wood (1958) found such a murmur present in 50 percent of the adult age group. Only on rare occasions have we encountered a right aortic arch in this category, although Wood records it in 16 percent of his cases. This may have been due to the inclusion of some cases with acyanotic tetralogy of Fallot who more characteristically have a right aortic arch.

Radiologic Examination. The radiologic findings are particularly useful, and since, in recent years, most cases with murmurs are being followed from birth, changes then become evident. Observation over several years, plus suitable investigations, catheter studies, and angiocardiography, will rule out such defects as patent ductus with reversal of flow through it, persistent truncus arteriosus, common ventricle, and transposition of the great vessels, D or L type. The radiologic findings are likely to show a decrease in the cardiothoracic ratio from that noted in the first year or two of life. At the same time the pulmonary artery will bulge more prominently, the central hilar shadows will pulsate, but the lung fields beyond the hilar areas will clear in the majority of cases. In the advanced stages heart failure, pulmonary valve insufficiency, and tricuspid valve insufficiency may cause some enlargement of the heart. (Progressive enlargement of the heart is characteristic of the relatively small group of cases that continue to have pulmonary vascular disease after the ventricular septal defect has been closed surgically.)

Complications. As the pathologic process continues, a variety of related complications may appear. These include congestive heart failure, pulmonary thrombosis, hemoptysis, bacterial endocarditis, brain abscess, paroxysmal tachycardia, and other arrhythmias.

Course and Prognosis. Since pulmonary vascular disease usually develops in those cases with large ventricular septal defects, the initial signs and symptoms are related to engorgement of the pulmonary vascular circulation, dyspnea, and, frequently, congestive heart failure. During the first year or two of life these symptoms are controlled by the progressive thickening, narrowing, and endothelial change in the pulmonary arteries until a balance of circulation is achieved, but with an adequate pulmonary blood flow to permit such children a relatively good exercise tolerance and no cyanosis. In this way they may lead an active life for many years, but gradually, as the pulmonary vasculature changes narrow the lumen of the small arteries diffusely throughout the lung field, cyanosis first appears with exercise and then at rest. During adolescence and early life, or later, heart failure associated with pulmonary valvular insufficiency may occur, or hemoptysis may precipitate a downward trend in the course of the patient or sudden death.

The prognosis of patients with advanced pulmonary vascular disease is indicated by Clarkson and colleagues from the Mayo Clinic (1968), who presented a follow-up of 58 cases, five years after the initial diagnostic catheter study. All of these patients fitted the category of the Eisenmenger's syndrome. Eighty percent were still alive but the probability of survival varied with each group as follows:

AGE GROUP	SURVIVAL AFTER FIVE YEARS, %
10–19 years	95
20 years and over	56

Management. Management or treatment to be effective in children whose pulmonary arteries are hyperreactive should be preventive. An infant with evidence of a ventricular septal defect, significant cardiac enlargement, and electrocardiographic changes with or without dyspnea or heart failure should have a cardiac catheterization carried out in the first few months of life. The electrocardiogram and clinical findings may then be used to decide what hemodynamic studies should be repeated. The continued presence of heart failure, the persistence of a large shunt over many months, and a progression of a shift of the QRS axis to the right in the electrocardiogram with right hypertrophy indicate the need for recatheterization and possible surgery. If the resistance is rising significantly, surgery will probably be called for. With the newer techniques, profound hypothermia, and approach to closure of the defect through the right atrium, surgery may be carried out in the first 6 or 12 months of life with a significantly low mortality in cases where such procedure is justified. If this is done successfully, one rarely encounters progressive pulmonary vascular disease at a later date.

To underline the need for surgery in the first year of life, it may be pointed out that if the operation is delayed until after the child is two years old, there are few children who will have progression of their pulmonary vascular disease, even though the ventricular septal defect has been completely closed (Friedli et al., 1973).

In these hyperreactors, this may lead on to progressive pulmonary vascular change and a clinical picture that is similar to progressive idiopathic pulmonary hypertension. We have had one such case (see Table 21–5). Similar cases have been reported in the literature (Lillehei et al., 1964). Progressive dyspnea and enlargement of the heart, congestive heart failure, cyanosis, hemoptysis, and sudden death may characterize the downhill course. Our case described in Table 21–5 was operated on at approximately two years of age. If surgery had been done in the first six months of life, it seems likely that the pulmonary vascular changes would have been avoided.

Even though careful assessment of clinical and physiologic data correlates well with evidence of increased pulmonary blood flow and with a reduction of pulmonary artery systolic pressure following operation, it may be difficult to predict the long-term outlook with regard to progressive pulmonary vascular obstructive disease (DuShane, 1971). Of 46 patients with ventricular septal defect with pulmonary hypertension, all but one had a significant drop of the pulmonary artery pressure immediately after surgery. Fifteen of these patients, all over two years of age, had evidence of increased pulmonary vascular resistance (RP greater than 9 units/meter^2)

at the time of postoperative cardiac catheterization one-half to seven years later. Nine of the fifteen had significant symptoms. However, in those who were under two years of age at the time of surgery, none showed any evidence of progressive or increased pulmonary vascular resistance when recatheterized some time after corrective surgery.

In his detailed monograph on the subject, Wood concludes that the average length of life of these cases is approximately 35 years. The maximum age reached for an individual with a ventricular septal defect he records as 65 years. Bacterial endocarditis as a cause of death in the Eisenmenger group occurred in only 5 percent (Wood, 1958). Fourteen percent died abruptly, a figure substantiated by Young and Mark (1971). Syncopal attacks are an ominous sign.

Surgical closure of the ventricular septal defect in the classic Eisenmenger syndrome carries a surgical mortality that is prohibitive. Furthermore, even if the patient does survive, there may be no benefit and the vascular disease is not impeded. It may at times be speeded up (see Figure 21–30).

Pregnancy and Pulmonary Vascular Disease

Neilson et al. (1971) conclude that the Eisenmenger syndrome is a strong contraindication to pregnancy. This is supported by the data of Jones and Howitt (1965) and Naeye (1967). Among 45 cases there were 15 maternal deaths and a mortality of 33 percent. This compared unfavorably with a maternal death among cases of tetralogy of Fallot (4.2 percent) and

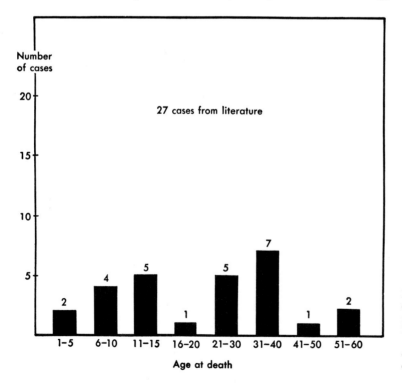

Figure 21-30. Age at death in 27 cases of ventricular septal defects reported in the literature as Eisenmenger's complex (Selzer, 1949). Many of these must have developed their pulmonary vascular changes later in life.

coarctation of the aorta (4.3 percent). All contraceptives are also contraindicated in Eisenmenger syndrome. Sterilization is usually recommended.

Bacterial Endocarditis

Bacterial endocarditis has always been an infrequent but significant complication of congenital heart disease. Since the ventricular septal defect is the most common anomaly in this category, it is important to assess the magnitude of the problem in this particular defect (see Table 21–6). This is especially so now that surgical closure is being recommended by some authorities solely on the basis of the risk of bacterial endocarditis developing during the course of a lifetime.

It is necessary to have a knowledge of the incidence of bacterial endocarditis in ventricular septal defect as well as to know the natural history of the anomaly before one can form an adequate opinion of the problem. We have therefore attempted to evaluate the risks both in childhood and in adult life (Shah et al., 1966).

Autopsy studies were reported by Gelfman and Levine (1964) who reviewed 34,023 such examinations in the Boston area and observed 31 cases over the age of two years who had uncomplicated ventricular septal defect. Thirteen, or 42 percent, had bacterial endocarditis, the highest incidence being in the second and third decades of life. Only two of these were over the age of 40. Selzer (1949) gathered autopsy data on 73 cases of ventricular septal defect and added 12 cases from his own autopsy record. He reported that 18 out of the total 85 cases (21 percent) died of bacterial endocarditis. More recently Bloomfield (1964) assembled autopsy findings of 17 cases of ventricular septal defect and observed bacterial endocarditis in five (28 percent). If these three studies are added together, one finds an incidence of approximately 25 percent as having developed bacterial endocarditis. It is obvious that this is not a proper estimate of the situation since the autopsy figures lean heavily toward the critically ill patients and give us no true indication in relation to those that have survived.

Table 21–6. BACTERIAL ENDOCARDITIS IN VENTRICULAR SEPTAL DEFECT

AUTHORS	PATIENT YEARS	SUBACUTE BACTERIAL ENDOCARDITIS
Wood (Bloomfield, 1964)	638	0
Griffiths et al. (1964)	837	4
Bloomfield (1964)	222	1
Walker et al. (1965)	1407	6
Total	3104	11

These groups taken together indicate one case of bacterial endocarditis in 282 patient years.

At The Hospital for Sick Children in Toronto we have seen 1041 cases of uncomplicated ventricular septal defect during a 15-year period, 1950 to 1964, in the ages between 2 and 17 years. During the same period only seven cases with bacterial endocarditis were observed from among this group. In terms of the follow-up period it can be stated that the seven cases of bacterial endocarditis occurred in 8223 patient years, or approximately 1 in 1000 patient years.

We have approached this problem from yet another point of view. It is obviously important to obtain figures on the incidence of the ventricular septal defect in various groups of the population. Rose and Keith have done this for the pediatric age group in the city of Toronto proper and found that during the early years of life the incidence of the ventricular septal defect is approximately 0.8 in 1000 in a population of birth to five years of age. This figure corresponds well with that reported recently by Rudolph (1965) who estimated an incidence of 1 in 1000 among children in the first year of life. In the school-age group in Toronto it was found the incidence fell to 1 in 2000.

We have reviewed the case notes of all patients with ventricular septal defect seen over a ten-year period from 1955 to 1964 in all major Toronto hospitals. In the city of Toronto proper there was a school population of 96,397 children between the ages of 5 and 14 years, and there were 47 that had good evidence of ventricular septal defect. In this age group only one patient developed bacterial endocarditis in a ten-year period, that is 1 in 470 patient years. This would place the risk of the infection at 2.1 per thousand patient years. An extension of this approach would indicate that a child of five years had a 13.6 percent risk of developing bacterial endocarditis by the age of 70 years, and the calculated risk for a 15-year-old to a similar age would be 11.5 percent. These figures only pertain if the incidence of bacterial endocarditis in ventricular septal defect is unchanged over the years. The risk appears to diminish with advancing age, since this particular anomaly is an uncommon finding after the middle years of adult life.

In the city of Toronto proper with a population of 562,134 among the individuals between the ages of 5 and 69 years, there were four cases of ventricular septal defect with bacterial endocarditis in a ten-year period. These figures may be compared with those of metropolitan Toronto with a population of 1,360,048 in which there were eight cases. Such data indicate an incidence of bacterial endocarditis in the ventricular septal defect population of 1.3 to 1.4 per 1000 patient years, provided the incidence of ventricular septal defect remains the same in adult life as at 14 years of age. An important observation was recorded that not a single case of ventricular septal defect with bacterial endocarditis was found above the age of 35 years in either the city of Toronto or the wider metropolitan Toronto area. The possibility that many of these may close spontaneously in adult life must be reasonably considered, but whatever the explanation is, it must be emphasized that bacterial endocarditis superimposed on a ventricular septal defect is not a significant cause of death in the latter half of life.

Risk of Death. It is also important to estimate the actual risk of death from such infection. All the seven cases seen at The Hospital for Sick Children were cured of the infection with no apparent deterioration of cardiac function. In the metropolitan Toronto population studies, all the eight cases but one recovered from the infection, and this individual had preexisting mitral and aortic valve disease and might well have recovered if such valve involvement had not been coexistent with the ventricular septal defect. From these figures it would appear that the risk to a five-year-old child with uncomplicated ventricular septal defect of dying as a result of bacterial endocarditis over a period of 65 years would be approximately 2.7 percent, and a similar risk to a 15-year-old over the next 55 years would be 2.3 percent. This is certainly no higher than the operative mortality for ventricular septal defect in most centers.

It must also be pointed out that surgery itself may initiate the occurrence of bacterial endocarditis. Lind et al. (1964) reported five cases developing bacterial endocarditis in the early postoperative period out of 205 cases of heart pump surgery for congenital heart disease. Three of these had isolated ventricular septal defects. Our experience at The Hospital for Sick Children is somewhat similar. Surgical closure of the ventricular septal defect has been undertaken in 200 patients. Three of these developed bacterial endocarditis in the early postoperative period.

Another factor that must be considered is the influence of the antibiotics on the incidence of bacterial endocarditis initially. The incidence of bacteremia is certainly less with the prompt use of antibiotics during infections and at dental care. Most of the autopsy figures referred to above were derived from material before 1940. These data would not appear to be applicable to this day and age since the means of prevention and early treatment in bacteremia are available.

It is possible to conclude, therefore, that modern therapy for bacterial endocarditis in the presence of a ventricular septal defect is highly effective. One may also reasonably conclude on the basis of available data that the incidence of bacterial endocarditis with death is approximately the same or less than the mortality from the operative procedure of closure of the ventricular septal defect, and there is insufficient evidence to designate the risk of future bacterial endocarditis as an adequate reason for surgical closure of the anomaly.

Summary of Prognosis in Ventricular Septal Defect

There are a number of factors that shape the clinical course of the child with the ventricular septal defect. Primarily, and of crucial significance, is the size of the defect itself. Next in importance is the response of the pulmonary vascular system to increased flow and pressure. This includes postnatal changes as well as those of childhood and later years. The prognosis is also related to the presence or absence of associated defects whether they be cardiac or noncardiac and the patient's response to pneumonia, congestive heart failure, and bacterial endocarditis.

From the studies of Lucas and associates (1961), Arcilla and associates (1963), and Kidd and associates (1965), it is obvious that the natural history of the ventricular septal defect is frequently a dynamic process that is improving at various rates in infancy and childhood. The most important building blocks of information in this field have appeared in the past 15 years in the work of Wood (1958), Nadas and associates (1960), Kirklin and DuShane (1961), Lucas and associates (1961), Lynfield and associates (1961), Stanton and Fyler (1961), Howitt and Wade (1962), Arcilla and associates (1963), Auld and associates (1963), Weidman and associates (1963), Kidd and associates (1964), Sigmann and associates (1967), Horiuchi and associates (1967), Barratt-Boyes and associates (1971), Dillard and associates (1971), DuShane (1971), Fontan and associates (1971), Keith and associates (1971), Corone and associates (1977), and Weidman and associates (1977).

Although there are more details or ramifications of the natural history that remain to be elaborated on, the main features of the outcome at various stages are becoming increasingly apparent. One may summarize the available information as follows:

The prognosis in the isolated ventricular septal defect in childhood appears to be good on the whole. The favorable responses far outweigh those that are unfavorable. The possible courses that may be followed by a child with a ventricular septal defect in infancy and childhood are as follows:

1. The defect may get smaller.
2. The defect may close entirely.
3. The defect may remain the same size as the individual grows. In effect, number 3 is a reduction in size of the anomaly provided it is less than the diameter of the aorta, or less than 1 cm per meter body surface area.
4. The defect may get larger as the child grows.
5. Progressive pulmonary vascular obstruction may occur rapidly over a period of two to four years in the severe cases, or more slowly over a period of 10 to 60 years. The response is likely to be more rapid if the defect is a particularly large one.
6. The patient may develop congestive heart failure and have either a favorable or unfavorable response to digitalis therapy—the former is more likely. The patient may be particularly susceptible to pneumonia or highly resistant to it.
7. The course may be unfavorable if there are associated noncardiac anomalies of a serious nature, particularly in the neonatal period.
8. Bacterial endocarditis may occur (one in a thousand patient years).
9. Infundibular narrowing of a minor degree may

be present at birth, which will progressively narrow the outflow tract of the right ventricle and thus protect the pulmonary vasculature.

10. The child with an isolated ventricular septal defect may be operated on successfully. The mortality with such procedures is reaching an acceptably low level in the age group over two years. Further advance is needed in the treatment of the infant.

11. It should be remembered that a few patients with moderately elevated pulmonary vascular resistance or high resistance may go on to develop progressive pulmonary vascular disease with a fatal termination after they have been operated on successfully and the septal defect closed.

Infants with Long-Term Follow-up. Any study of the ventricular septal defect must begin in the early part of the first year of life and follow a large group through many years. We have attempted to do this at The Hospital for Sick Children with 630 infants seen originally early in the first year and being reviewed at intervals since. To identify the prognosis in various categories, we have used the physiologic classification suggested by Kidd (1965). This hemodynamic classification indicates various degrees of severity of involvement of the heart and the pulmonary vasculature in ventricular septal defect.

In the review of Keith and coworkers (1971) the 630 cases seen originally in the first year of life were followed for an average of 7.5 years. At the same time these authors reviewed a group of teen-agers and adults (295 cases) followed for an average of 15 years. A summary of these three groups is shown in Table 21–7.

Hemodynamic group 5 is a unique group in the first year of life with a high resistance and low flow, and all of those identified at this early stage in this category have subsequently revealed a decline in the pulmonary vascular resistance to normal levels. Presumably these infants are characterized by a persistence in the fetal pulmonary vascular response

after birth, which lasts for several months, but declines in the latter half of the first year of life. Those in this category appear to have small defects to begin with, or become so fairly rapidly, and therefore have a favorable response in spite of the initial high resistance in the lung fields.

Cases that evolve into group 5 after the first year of life do so because of progressive increase in pulmonary vascular resistance and are totally different from the benign group referred to above in early infancy. After the first year, group 5 cases have a poor prognosis, eventually joining the children in group 6. Fortunately, the numbers in these two categories are steadily decreasing with the modern approach and techniques for surgical correction.

Once a child with a ventricular septal defect has reached the teen-age or adult group, the prognosis is usually good and at least 80 percent have small defects and are leading normal lives, fully active with no functional disability. Furthermore, it is worth reemphasizing that 4 percent close spontaneously after they have reached adolescence or adult life, and only 1 percent have developed endocarditis. In the future, with proper investigation, management, or surgical correction, almost all cases with ventricular septal defect should reach adult life with a good prognosis and leading normal lives.

Surgery for Ventricular Septal Defect

The modern technique for closure of the ventricular septal defect involves cardiopulmonary bypass with the aid of a pump oxygenator, but successful results have been reported by hypothermia (Horiuchi et al., 1963). The combination of the two methods has also been employed at times (Cooley et al., 1962; Barratt-Boyes, 1971; Barratt-Boyes et al., 1976; Subramanian, 1976; Rein et al., 1977). A median sternotomy incision is the one preferred since

Table 21–7. VENTRICULAR SEPTAL DEFECT GROUPS COMBINED

HEMODYNAMIC GROUP	FIRST SEEN IN 1ST YEAR: 630 CASES (%)	FOLLOW-UP AT 7.5 YEARS: 630 CASES (%)	TEEN-ADULT GROUP: 295 CASES (%)
1. Pulmonary-to-systemic flow ratio of less than 2:1 and a normal pulmonary vascular resistance	50.0	71.0	80.0
2. Pulmonary-to-systemic flow ratio of greater than 2:1 with a normal pulmonary vascular resistance	26.5	14.0	5.0
3. Pulmonary-to-systemic flow ratio greater than 2:1 with slight increased resistance	16.0	12.0	1.7
4. Pulmonary-to-systemic flow ratio greater than 2:1 with a moderate increase in resistance	6.0	4.0	3.7
5. Pulmonary-to-systemic flow ratio of less than 2:1 with high pulmonary vascular resistance but no reversal of flow	1.5	0.6	0.2
6. Pulmonary-to-systemic flow ratio of less than 2:1 with high pulmonary vascular resistance and reversal of flow through the defect	0.0	0.3	9.4

it provides an easier, quicker approach and is better for pulmonary function postoperatively. The defect is usually repaired by a Teflon or Dacron patch.

If heart block occurs during the suturing process, the suture is removed and replaced further away from the bundle area. Since the first attempts were made to correct the ventricular septal defect 15 or more years ago, the surgical techniques have improved steadily with the mortality dropping each year to new lower levels. In the over-two-years-of-age group the mortality in 1959 to 1961 was approximately 10 percent. Since then it has fallen to less than 3 percent, or lower, if there is a proper selection of cases. The operative deaths are related to shock, low cardiac output syndrome, hemorrhage, heart block, incomplete repair, excessive pulmonary vascular disease, or postoperative pulmonary problems.

Heart block used to be a major cause of death until recent years but with increasing knowledge of the position of the bundle of His and its branches, this complication has declined to less than one-half of 1 percent among children operated on. The other factors include myocardial anoxia and low cardiac output. Transient block may occur during, or immediately following, surgery without harm to the patient. If the block persists, however, it may lead to death subsequently and thus continued heart block usually requires the implantation of a pacemaker. The prognosis of pacemakers in children is improving as the techniques and pacemakers are refined.

Trifascicular block may occur in a child following surgical closure of the ventricular septal defect. This is associated with evidence of complete right bundle branch block, left anterior hemiblock, and a negative axis in the electrocardiogram. Such cases are leading normal lives from long-time postoperative follow-up. A few fatal cases have been reported but have occurred in the immediate postoperative period and with evidence of complete heart block.

If the preoperative physiologic studies indicate that the patient has a pulmonary-to-systemic flow ratio greater than two to one and a low pulmonary vascular resistance, the mortality should be approximately 1 per cent (Kirklin and DuShane, 1963); with a moderately raised pulmonary vascular resistance, it should be in the order of 3 percent; with a high pulmonary vascular resistance but not quite at systemic levels, 25 percent; and with pulmonary vascular resistance at systemic levels, 50 to 70 percent (Cooley et al., 1962; Kirklin and DuShane, 1963). These figures refer to children over the age of one year and not in congestive heart failure.

Incomplete repair as reported by Lillehei (1964) occurred in 14 percent of his cases. This occurs as a rule only in the children with pulmonary hypertension with large defects. The incidence of such cases may be as high as 25 percent (Theye and Kirklin, 1963). Kirklin and DuShane (1963) point out that only 10 percent of these defects are likely to be hemodynamically significant and suggest that improved techniques will reduce this figure to less than 5 percent.

In hemodynamic groups II to IV (without increased pulmonary vascular resistance) in the first three years of life, the postoperative exercise tolerance is excellent and such patients are then able to lead normal, active lives. There does not appear to be any progression of the pulmonary vascular disease process in these groups in the follow-up data available. However, when the pulmonary vascular resistance is high and the pulmonary blood flow low, as in groups V and VI, the resistance remains high postoperatively with rare exceptions. Such children have a poor exercise tolerance as a rule after they have recovered from their surgery, and they experience little or no improvement in their cardiovascular status in the years following operation. Late sudden deaths occur at times in this group. The most extreme case in this latter category at The Hospital for Sick Children was a child of two and one-half years operated on successfully, but without any decline in the pulmonary vascular resistance. Continued observation indicated that the pulmonary vascular disease process was progressive until the time of death at six years of age. Only rarely does one find such an unfavorable response.

Friedli and associates (1974) have presented data on 57 children with septal defects who have been operated on and have various degrees of pulmonary vascular disease. The results of a follow-up study averaging five years are shown in Figure 21–31.

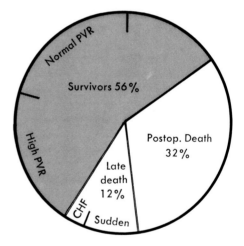

Figure 21-31. Fate of 57 patients after surgical closure of ventricular septal defect in the presence of increased pulmonary vascular resistance (PVR). Eighteen (32 percent) died at, or shortly after, surgery. Seven (12 percent) died one to seven years after surgery from Eisenmenger syndrome; sudden death occurred in five, while two died in congestive heart failure (CHF). Of the 32 long-term survivors, 11 have high PVR (more than 400 dynes sec cm^{-5}/M^2) proven by catheterization; 12 have normal PVR; the others were not recatheterized. Return to normal PVR was only found in patients with mild elevation of resistance preoperatively. (Reproduced from Friedli, B.; Kidd, B. S. L.; Mustard, W. T.; and Keith, J. D.: Surgical closure of ventricular septal defect with elevated pulmonary vascular resistance: Late results. Am. J. Cardiol., **33**:403, 1974 [Abstract].)

At the very opposite pole is the child whose excessively high pulmonary vascular resistance is due to an unusual degree of vascular spasm producing systemic resistance in the pulmonary artery. Such cases may respond to oxygen or Priscoline at the time of cardiac catheter study. They also respond to successful cardiac surgery with a drop in pulmonary vascular resistance. A case illustrating this was reported by Blount and Woodward (1960). Unfortunately, it is a rare event to encounter such a favorable reaction in children with high pulmonary vascular resistance, but it is more likely to occur in the age group under two years (Friedli et al., 1974).

Pulmonary Artery Banding.   For many years it has been recognized in tetralogy of Fallot that a modest degree of pulmonary stenosis has a protective effect on the pulmonary vasculature and yet may permit a relatively good exercise tolerance with a minimum of cyanosis. The shunt through the ventricular septal defect is controlled by the pulmonary stenosis. The principle involved in this situation was put into clinical practice by Muller and Dammann (1952) when they placed a constricting band around the pulmonary artery in an infant with a ventricular septal defect who was in congestive heart failure. This approach has been widely used since. A summary of a few of the reports in the literature indicate that the mortality varies from 5 to 35 percent depending on the selection of cases and techniques used (Dammann and Muller, 1961; Willman et al. 1962; Albert et al., 1961; Morrow and Braunwald, 1961; Gammelbaard et al., 1961; European Pediatric Cardiology Conference, 1964; Goldblatt et al., 1965; and DuShane, 1971). Recently pulmonary artery banding has been downgraded in favor of direct and complete repair at an early age, (Kirklin, 1975; Subramanian, 1976).

Surgery for Ventricular Septal Defect in the First Year of Life.   The modern technique for closure of ventricular septal defects in infancy involves cardiopulmonary bypass usually with the aid of a pump oxygenator, but successful results have been reported by profound hypothermia (Barratt-Boyes, 1971; Horiuchi et al., 1963; Subramanian, 1973). A combination of the two methods is also employed at times using a moderate degree of hypothermia (Cooley et al., 1962).

Recent reports (Horiuchi et al., 1967; Dillard et al., 1971) have indicated some disadvantages to the heart-lung pump machine that are related to a nonpulsatile perfusion and can be avoided by the technique of surface-induced deep hypothermia and circulatory arrest. At the end of the operation the left ventricle is vented as is the aorta to prevent air embolism, and then rewarming can be quickly carried out using the cardiopulmonary bypass technique. If evidence of any disassociation is present, pacemaker wires are inserted.

Subramanian (1973) prefers to use the transatrial approach in which the tricuspid valve is pulled aside and does not need to be incised or detached. Under hypothermia the heart is relaxed and the defect can then be closed with a Dacron velour patch with a continuous suture. Using this approach both Barratt-Boyes (1971) and Subramanian (1973) have reported successful results with a low mortality. The latter has closed 15 recently with no deaths; 11 have been available for follow-up of greater than six months and all have shown progressive increase in weight percentiles. All of these 15 were under one year of age at the time of surgery.

If a child with ventricular septal defect is going to require surgery, it is usually evident in the first year of life, either because of heart failure or enlargement of the heart with some progressive increased pulmonary vascular resistance. Those early in life with persistent heart failure and pulmonary artery hypertension will eventually develop increased resistance in their pulmonary vasculature and will have a better outlook and a lower mortality, if operated on rather than left to hazards of intercurrent respiratory infections. The risks of chronic failure, repeated chest infections, or progressive increase in pulmonary vascular resistance, with ultimate development of the Eisenmenger syndrome, are well documented.

Thus, it appears likely that approximately 5 percent of babies in the first year of life with isolated ventricular septal defect should have the operation in the first year unless there is some evidence of pulmonary valve stenosis or infundibular stenosis that protects the lung fields and diminishes or eliminates the possibility of failure.

Banding operation for a child in chronic congestive heart failure usually involves a mortality of at least 10 percent. The second operation to remove the band and close the ventricular septal defect is not without risk and appears to be approximately 10 percent, but may go as high as 25 percent, thus closure of the defect directly in the first year of life in a single operation is probably safer than the two procedures combined.

There may be certain circumstances in which banding operation is required. These would include multiple, large, Swiss cheese holes in the ventricular septum, or when there is a complicated defect present such as coarctation of the aorta with a ventricular septal defect and a double operation to completely correct both anomalies would require excessive time and excessive risk.

The management of a child with a large ventricular septal defect requires first of all observation and catheterization to outline the pathology and anatomy present; the child should be adequately treated medically, and if the response is good, the operation can be postponed or delayed until the latter half of the first year, when the risk of surgery would be minimal. If the defect shows evidence of marked diminution in size, surgery may become unnecessary. If, on the other hand, medical treatment is inadequate to contain the failure, the complete correction operation is indicated within a few days, or few weeks, depending on the infant's progress.

It is important to recatheterize the child during the second half of the first year of life in those who have, or had, heart failure whether the heart remains large or becomes smaller, in order to be certain about the pulmonary vascular resistance. If the latter is increasing, surgery is required even though the baby looks improved and failure is absent.

A few reports emphasized the reduction of pulmonary vascular resistance that may occur following direct closure of the ventricular septal defect (or banding of the pulmonary artery) (Wada and Iwa, 1969; Samaan, 1970; Burkes, 1971; Castaneda et al., 1971; Mikolov, 1971). As has been indicated previously, most postserial cardiac catheterization studies have shown no change in the pulmonary vascular resistance or, if they occur, it has been to a minimal degree. However, further studies are needed to clarify this point, particularly in older children. In the younger age groups, especially infants, a drop in resistance is likely to occur in our experience (Keith et al., 1971) and can be shown by serial catheter studies, particularly when the first catheter study was carried out in the first year of life. Among 93 infants with increased pulmonary vascular resistance initially, 7 percent had a decrease in resistance when they were recatheterized one to five years later. However, if increased pulmonary vascular resistance is encountered after the first year of life, and the degree is greater than 800 dynes/sec/cm^{-5}, it is unlikely to drop significantly with surgery. There may be a few exceptions to this in the second year of life, especially when the pulmonary blood flow is greater than 2:1, but they may be due to inadequacy—the catheterization technique rather than true changes. However, after two years of age, successful closure of the ventricular septal defect may cause a drop in pulmonary artery pressure, but rarely in resistance. The data are thus overwhelmingly in favor of early surgery when the complicating effects of flow and pressure can be controlled or prevented, or reversed. Modern techniques indicate a lowering mortality for surgical correction in the first year of life.

One may summarize the selection of ventricular septal defect cases for surgery as follows:

1. The optimum age for closure of the uncomplicated ventricular septal defect is from one to three years, but many will require surgical correction in the first year of life. All cases with a pulmonary-to-systemic flow ratio of 2.5 to one or greater at two years of age may be considered suitable for closure at the optimum time. Direct closure of the defect is indicated in early life when the infant is in congestive heart failure that will not respond to medical management, especially in the first six months of life. Direct closure is preferable to banding when a balancing of the risks warrants it (Rowe and Trusler, 1977).

2. Children with pulmonary-to-systemic flow ratios of under 2.5 to one with normal pulmonary artery pressure should wait until new low levels in operative mortality are reached.

3. Children with congestive heart failure in the first year of life may require surgery; many will respond to medical therapy. Approximately 20 percent are intractable and need surgical correction.

4. Each infant with a ventricular septal defect with cardiac enlargement or electrocardiographic abnormalities should be catheterized in the first year of life, and if there is evidence that the pulmonary vascular resistance is rising, catheterization should be repeated yearly, until the course is clarified. (A significant increase in resistance over the normal level for the age should be indication for corrective surgery at that time. If the resistance falls or remains at a level that is not excessive for the age, operation may be postponed to a more optimum time.)

5. Children who have a high pulmonary vascular resistance and a low pulmonary blood flow, with obstructive pulmonary vascular disease over the age of two years are a poor risk for surgical correction and have an excessively high mortality rate at operation (70 to 80 percent). If they do survive surgery, they usually show minimal change in either pulmonary artery pressure or resistance postoperatively and are likely to have progressive increase in the pulmonary vascular disease.

6. Children with high pulmonary vascular resistance whose vasoconstriction is relaxed by the use of oxygen or relaxant drugs are suitable patients for surgical correction. Such cases are more likely to occur in the younger age group.

COARCTATION OF THE AORTA AND VENTRICULAR SEPTAL DEFECT WITH OR WITHOUT A PATENT DUCTUS ARTERIOSUS

COARCTATION with a ventricular septal defect has been mentioned infrequently in the medical literature. In a series of 200 cases of coarctation of the aorta reported by Dr. Maud Abbott (1936) only one was found to have a ventricular septal defect. Calodney and Carson (1950) reported 21 postmortem cases of coarctation of the aorta; nine of them had an associated ventricular septal defect and all of them had the preductal type of coarctation. Individual cases were reported with this combination (Campbell and Cardell, 1953; Rossall and Thompson, 1958; Seaman and Goldring, 1955).

At The Hospital for Sick Children we have had 24 cases in which the coarctation of the aorta was associated with ventricular septal defect. The ductus was proved to be patent in eight of these. Eleven of the total group died between the ages of five days and five months, and the rest are still alive, suggesting that if an infant survives the first six months of life with this combination, it is likely to live on for several years at least.

In the neonatal period the attention of the examining physician is drawn to the heart by the presence of a loud systolic murmur heard over the precordium, and such a murmur was present in 22 of the 24 cases at The Hospital for Sick Children. It was considered to be grade II or greater in all but two cases. A third of the murmurs were described as ejection type and two-thirds were described as pansystolic murmurs. A thrill was coexistent in 65 percent.

When examined in the Cardiology Department these infants were not usually considered to be cyanotic, but in a few instances cyanosis was noted when the baby cried. The majority were dyspneic, and this is understandable, since at least 60 percent have all the clinical signs of congestive heart failure with enlarged hearts, enlarged livers, and dyspnea. The cardiothoracic ratios varied from 50 to 82 percent with an average of 61 percent. The hilar shadows were increased in the x-rays of all of the infants.

The blood pressure readings were those usually found in infants with coarctation of the aorta, with the aortic systolic pressure ranging from 70 to 140 mm of mercury. The femoral arteries were rarely palpable, but when they were, the pulse was feeble and showed little systolic variation. The electrocardiogram appeared to be within normal limits for the age in one case only, a left loading pattern was present in five, a right loading pattern in ten, and combined right and left ventricular loading in eight.

Twelve of the twenty-four cases had cardiac catheterization performed, and in three-quarters of these the oxygen rise in the right ventricle was between 10 and 20 percent above that of the right atrium. There were two cases in which the level was between 5 and 10 percent higher in the right atrium and two in which it was 1 to 5 percent higher. One of the infants with little or no oxygen rise in the right ventricle had the tricuspid valve plastered over the septal defect so that the flow through the defect was practically nil. The pressure in the right ventricle was less than 50 percent of the systemic level in three, 50 to 60 percent in two, and 90 percent in seven. Among the 11 patients who died and were examined at postmortem, eight

had a widely patent ductus arteriosus and in three the ductus was closed. When the ductus was opened, it ranged between 3 and 8 mm in diameter with a mean of 5 mm. The size of the ventricular septal defect varied from 2 by 2 mm up to 5 by 18 mm, the average size being approximately 5 by 6 mm. The coarcted segment almost invariably had an internal diameter of 1 to 2 mm when examined at the autopsy table.

Of a group of 108 infants in the first year of life having coarctation of the aorta at The Hospital for Sick Children reported by Glass and associates (1960), 25 percent had ventricular septal defects. When one divides this group of 108 cases into preductal and postductal, it is found that 46 percent of the preductal coarctation infants had ventricular septal defects and only 10 percent had defects of the postductal type.

It is obvious that this combination of lesions is a particularly lethal one since the mortality in the first six months of life is over 50 percent; the downhill course is associated with progressive enlargement of the heart and liver, dyspnea, and rapid respirations characteristic of congestive heart failure. The problem is a difficult one for the physician since at least half of these patients will not respond adequately to digitalis, and yet the extensive surgery required for a baby with two or three major defects is accompanied by a high mortality, especially in the first six months of life. However, as techniques are simplified and made safer, it may be that a larger proportion of these babies who do not respond medically can be corrected partly or totally in the crucial periods of the first year of life. The diagnosis of multiple defects can be suspected by the clinical signs and the murmur with a thrill, and the blood pressure differential between the arms and the legs may be confirmed by cardiac catheterization or selective angiogram with the tip of the catheter in the left ventricle.

ABSENCE OF THE AORTIC ISTHMUS

THIS extreme form of aortic arch anomaly is not common and is usually fatal after a few weeks of life but as a rule runs a course that is similar to that of coarctation of the aorta with a patent ductus below the coarctation.

Seidel (1818) left a record of a case in the museum index at Kiel. Sporadic reports have occurred in the medical literature since then including cases mentioned by Maud Abbott (1936), Peacock (1866), Gaspar (1929), and Evans (1933). A useful review of the problem was published in 1959 by Everts-Suárez and Curzon. They make the observation that absent aortic isthmus is associated with a ventricular septal defect and a patent ductus in 80 percent, thus producing triad of anomalies. All of these patients have of necessity a patent ductus arteriosus to carry the blood to the lower part of the body. From the management and surgical point of view it should also be remembered that 80 percent have a ventricular septal defect.

Although some observers have expected otherwise, the clinical findings are similar to those of coarctation, ventricular septal defect, and patent ductus arteriosus with a preductal type of coarctation. Cyanosis is rarely seen in these infants except on crying or in the terminal stages of congestive heart failure. There does not appear to be any differential in skin color between the upper and lower parts of the body, a finding that was expected because of the patent ductus communicating with the descending aorta. On the contrary, however, there appears to be a collateral circulation from the upper part of the body to the thoracic aorta below the entrance to the ductus, which contributes to the maintenance of a fairly adequate blood pressure in the lower part of the body and probably in the flow from the descending aorta toward the pulmonary artery in a fair proportion of these cases. Others may have a balanced flow so that the resistances may be similar in systemic and pulmonary circulations and the collateral flow will, therefore, be as the descending aorta to the lower limbs and the pulmonary flow to the pulmonary artery branches. In the infants and children who have survived more than a few days or a few weeks a good collateral flow between the two segments of the thoracic aorta has been established. This was present in the case reported by Merrill et al. (1957). The case of Kjellberg and associates had only a slight increase in oxygen content in the descending aorta. Dorney Fowler, and Mannix (1955) reported a five-year-old girl who exhibited unilateral clubbing of the fingers presumably due to nonoxygenated blood coming from the left superior venae cavae from the lower segment of the aorta. Her condition was confirmed by thoracotomy but no attempt was made to correct it. However, Merrill, Webster, and Samson (1957)

reported a three-and-one-half-year-old girl who was successfully treated by surgery. Marston and associates (1957) quote Chamberlain as having performed a successful operation on one of these children by using a graft. Shumacker (1957) also surgically treated a child with this defect by using an autograft from the subclavian artery to the descending aorta.

Until quite recently most successful operative repairs were accomplished in older children. Although surgery for newborns with this condition still carries a high mortality there have been some spectacular successes even at this age (Barratt-Boyes et al., 1972; Murphy et al., 1973; Trusler and Izukawa, 1975).

VENTRICULAR SEPTAL DEFECT AND AORTIC INSUFFICIENCY

ONE of the most challenging combinations of lesions is the ventricular septal defect associated with aortic insufficiency, since it presents special anatomic, hemodynamic, and surgical problems that have not yet been adequately mastered.

The first recorded description of this lesion is that of Breccia (1906) in the Italian literature and Laubry and Pezzi (1921) in the French literature. Since then numerous cases have either been reported or been referred to in the literature; the present authors have encountered 50 cases proved by autopsy, operation, or cardiac catheterization. This constitutes 2 percent of our total group with ventricular septal defect, a somewhat lower incidence than that of 5 percent previously reported (Nadas, 1964). The importance of this syndrome is that it almost invariably leads to a decreased exercise tolerance and later heart failure, after a period of relative freedom from symptoms. This latent period may vary from 2 to 50 years, but after the onset of significant symptoms associated with progressive dyspnea, a fatal outcome is likely to occur. Several factors influence the course of this lesion (Keane et al., 1977).

Anatomy

Anatomically the syndrome is characterized by a high ventricular septal defect with little or no tissue separating the defect from the aortic valve. The right aortic cusp is the one most frequently defective. It has a dilated pouch appearance and sags into the left ventricular outflow tract over the area occupied by the ventricular septal defect. Its margin is usually thickened. The contents of the aorta may spill into the left ventricle or through the ventricular septal defect into the right ventricle during each diastolic pause. Occasionally the deformed aortic cusp is prolapsed into the ventricular septal defect in such a manner that it protrudes into the right ventricle sufficiently to partly obstruct the ventricular shunt. A probe can be

readily passed from the right ventricle into the aorta. The posterior cusp may be involved either alone or associated with a deformed right coronary cusp (Ash and Murphy, 1957). Occasionally the anomalous cusp is pulled down by a fibrous band attached to it from below (Laubry, 1933).

With these valvular deformities there are an enlarged, hypertrophied left ventricle and an enlarged and somewhat hypertrophied right ventricle. Between one-quarter and one-half of the cases have a modest degree of hypertrophic obstruction of the outflow tract of the right ventricle (Nadas et al., 1962; Keck et al., 1963). The pulmonary valve is rarely stenosed, but obstruction is likely to occur in the infundibulum. It was of a slight or modest degree in 8 of the 18 cases reported by Keck but was severe in one. This defect is a suitable site for development of bacterial endocarditis. Three of the twenty-two postmortem cases reported by Scott had such secondary infection.

While the usual cause of aortic insufficiency is an elongation and inversion of the margin of one cusp, at times there may be other defects such as fenestrations of the aortic valve or a diffuse involvement of all three valvular cusps. Occasionally the syndrome is accompanied by calcification of the aortic valve. The size of the ventricular septal opening has been reported by a number of authors and ranges from 3 or 4 mm up to 30 mm in size. It may be smaller than the isolated ventricular septal defect, and the prolapsed aortic valve may partly obliterate it.

There have been very few reports on the pulmonary arteries of the cases that have come to autopsy. Among those that have been recorded some have had a moderate degree of medial hypertrophy in the small muscular arteries of the lung and in others the change has been minimal (Scott et al., 1958). Full-blown pulmonary artery obstruction as is seen in Eisenmenger's complex has not been a feature of this syndrome.

Classification

In 1968 Van Praagh and McNamara proposed a classification for ventricular septal defect with aortic regurgitation based on autopsy findings. They suggested that there were two principal anatomic categories: (1) the subcrystal type associated with a protruding right, or noncoronary, cusp of the aortic valve; and (2) a supracrystal type occurring below the pulmonary valve but through which the prolapsed right coronary cusp of the aortic valve appeared. The subcrystal type I was further divided into two subgroups: (a) without pulmonary infundibular stenosis and (b) with infundibular stenosis. Tatsuno and associates (1973) suggested further divisions. In the subpulmonary types he indicated there were two subdivisions, one adjacent to the pulmonary valve and the other a few millimeters away from it. The infracrystal type he divided into three categories: (1) adjacent to the right coronary cusp, (2) adjacent to the noncoronary cusp, and (3) midway between the two. He pointed out that infundibular stenosis could occur with a subpulmonary as well as the infracrystal type of ventricular septal defect.

Clinical Features

The murmur may be noted early in infancy on routine examination but is considered to be due to a simple ventricular septal defect, since the baby is free of symptoms at this age and congestive heart failure is unlikely to occur until the second decade. Failure has been reported as early as at four years.

On examination there is a loud, harsh systolic murmur, often accompanied by a thrill maximum in the second and fourth left interspaces. It is accompanied by a blowing diastolic murmur down the left sternal edge. Several experienced observers have reported a continuous murmur heard over the left precordium. This is the exception, however, and in most instances one can readily recognize the typical systolic diastolic character of the two components. The heart is enlarged to the left with a forceful apical beat, and an inflow diastolic murmur may be noted inside the apex.

The early diastolic murmur of aortic insufficiency down the left sternal border is rarely heard before two or three years of age. It is almost invariably present, if it is going to occur at all, by the age of 14. In other words, the insufficiency develops as the child gets a little older and appears to be related to the inadequacy of a cusp of the aortic valve, which gradually becomes everted. A systolic murmur well heard in the first and second left interspaces and accompanied by a thrill is indicative of the additional lesion of infundibular stenosis.

Frequently the peripheral signs of aortic insufficiency are present with a Corrigan pulse, increased systemic systolic pressure, and decreased diastolic pressure—the latter often being down to zero. The systemic systolic pressure readings in 23 postmortem proven cases varied from 100 up to 175 mm Hg. These may be compared with the systolic pressure in the pulmonary artery. In each case the pulmonary artery systolic pressure was lower than the system systolic. On the average the pulmonary systolic was approximately half that of the systemic, although it varied up and down from this level.

There were no cases reported with clubbing, and only those that had severe congestive heart failure showed slight cyanosis—the rest were entirely free from cyanosis and had normal coloring. This is to be expected since the pressure in the left ventricle always exceeds that of the right ventricle and pulmonary artery.

The exercise tolerance is good in the majority, and congestive heart failure appears only in a modest percentage in the pediatric age group. We have had three children under 15 develop failure, one at ten, one at 11 and the other at 14 years. Nadas' experience was similar with failure occurring most frequently in the teens. Two cases are recorded by Bahnson that are exceptions to the rule: one child had failure at four and the other at six years of age.

Electrocardiography

The characteristic electrocardiographic tracing shows a left ventricular hypertrophy loading pattern with deep S waves in V_1 or tall R waves in V_6, and this is frequently associated with an increased depth of the Q in V_6. Occasionally the T wave in V_6 is depressed. On the whole, the latter is lower than the average normal for the age. Left ventricular hypertrophy loading pattern is present in 95 percent of cases (100 percent of Keck's cases) combined with right ventricular hypertrophy in 35 percent and a normal tracing in less than 5 percent. Isolated right ventricular hypertrophy has not been demonstrated in recent reports in the literature and is most unlikely to occur even when pulmonary infundibular stenosis is present. However, this electrocardiographic pattern occurred in one of our cases having associated pulmonary stenosis. In two others with catheter evidence of moderate pulmonary stenosis, the electrocardiogram presents a combined hypertrophy tracing. The right loading pattern appears related to the right ventricular pressure, which in turn may be affected by obstruction at the outflow tract of the right ventricle, but of the 18 cases reported by Keck, only one had a right ventricular overloading pattern and only one had an axis greater than 90 degrees. The axis varied, in our experience, from 0 to +150 degrees. Eighty percent had an axis of less than 90 degrees. Of our three cases with an axis of 90 degrees or over, two had pulmonary infundibular stenosis and the other had congestive heart failure.

When the combined ventricular loading pattern occurs, the left ventricular element almost invariably predominates over the right.

The majority of cases in Keck's series were over the pediatric age group, whereas our average age was over nine years.

Radiologic Examination

Radiologically there is an apparent generalized enlargement of the heart with the left ventricle being chiefly involved. The right ventricle is slightly to moderately enlarged. The pulmonary artery is usually somewhat prominent on the left border. The peripheral pulmonary vessels are increased in all children, and in a few patients the major vessels are seen to pulsate. The ascending aorta is prominent and pulsates more vigorously than usual owing to the high systolic and low diastolic systemic pressure.

Cardiac Catheterization

Cardiac catheterization should be carried out in any case with clinical findings that suggest a diagnosis of ventricular septal defect with aortic insufficiency. A left heart catheter should also be inserted. One will find an oxygen rise on entering the right ventricle, usually in the order of 15 or 20 percent, and this may vary between 5 and 30 percent. Careful sampling in the outflow tract of the right ventricle and the pulmonary artery is necessary to avoid the misleading results of streaming. These figures indicate a flow ratio between the pulmonary and systemic circulations of approximately 2.5:1 to 1.2:1. Very large shunts appear uncommon either because the defect is not large enough or because there is interference with the flow through it by the anomalous aortic cusp.

There may be a moderately elevated systolic pressure in the right ventricle and pulmonary artery at times, but as a rule pulmonary systolic pressure will not exceed 35 mm of mercury. The accompanying figures show the relationship between the systemic pressure and the pulmonary artery pressure, and, as was mentioned above, it will be seen that none of the cases had systemic pressure in the right ventricle or pulmonary artery. There is always a wide difference. The low diastolic pressure in the systemic circuit permits a more ready discharge of blood from the left ventricle into the aorta at the beginning of systole, thus avoiding some of the systolic shunt that is usually seen in the conventional isolated ventricular septal defect. Furthermore, the systolic peak of the left ventricular pressure curve is of short duration and may not be adequately transmitted through to the pulmonary artery, which may have a sparing effect on the medial and intimal coats of the small muscular branches. The resistance in the pulmonary circuit is frequently within normal range and is less than one-fifth systemic resistance in 85 percent of cases. This figure is based on our own data and that of Keck (1963). A gradient between RV and PA of more than 15 mm of mercury suggests infundibular stenosis, especially when the L-R shunt is not large.

Treatment

Slight aortic regurgitation is sometimes seen at the time of open correction of an isolated ventricular septal defect, usually occurring through the center of the valve at the confluence of the commissures (Spencer et al., 1962). We have noted this and have reviewed our clinical findings before operation as well as making careful examination after. No murmur is heard in such cases, and no evidence of progressive aortic valve lesion has appeared in follow-up. It seems certain, therefore, that the cases we are considering now have arisen as a result of an anomaly of the aortic valve or its supporting structures as well as a ventricular septal defect. In this combination of lesions it is apparent from the cases reviewed from the literature, as well as our own, that death may occur at

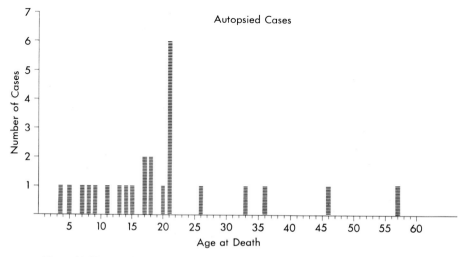

Figure 21-32. Ventricular septal defect with aortic insufficiency showing age at death.

any time up to 57 years of age (see Figure 21–32). It is also apparent that many of these cases have a mild degree of involvement of valve opening, and the prognosis, therefore, is not uniformly poor. Some cases, of course, are rapidly progressive in early childhood with a fatal outcome, but this is the exception rather than the rule (see Figure 21–32). The largest number of deaths appear to occur in the late teens and early twenties.

Each case must be evaluated on its own merits in estimating prognosis and in reaching a decision regarding surgical intervention. As surgical techniques improve for this particular combination of defects, and as the risks diminish, more children will be operated on at a relatively early age. Since most cases do not present with evidence of a double lesion before the age of four years, the question of surgery for the two anomalies rarely arises in infancy. This is important since the mortality risk is higher in the first year or two of life.

The children with fairly large hearts and evidence of congestive heart failure should be operated on promptly, since prolonged medical management of such cases will probably not be satisfactory. Among those who are in no difficulty, the age for elective surgery will depend on the development of more ideal techniques dealing with each of the two lesions when they are found combined.

Surgical correction was first successfully performed in 1960 by Garamella and colleagues. Subsequently Spencer (1962), Ellis (1963), Plauth (1965), Gonzalez-Lavin and Barratt-Boyes (1969), and Treasure and associates (1971) have all reported successful surgical corrective procedures, plus many others listed below.

The surgical techniques suggested in the past have varied from simple closure of the ventricular septal defect with no intervention in relation to the aortic valve up to closure of the ventricular septal defect plus complete replacement of the aortic valve with a prosthetic or homograft valve. Hartmann and Weldon (1972) recommend reconstruction of the aortic valve by shortening the free edge of the cusp so that all distances from the corpra arantii to the commissural attachments are equal. Somerville and coworkers (1970) presented medical-surgical data on 20 cases with direct closure of the ventricular septal defect through the aorta and repair and/or replacement of the aortic valve. Homograft replacement of the aortic valve was preferred to repair and was associated with less aortic regurgitation postoperatively. In six of their twenty cases, or 30 percent, all of the aortic cusps were abnormal suggesting that the prolapse of one cusp is not necessarily the prime cause of aortic regurgitation although it is possible that once a leak has occurred because of malposition of one cusp, the others may become old and thickened because of the trauma of the regurgitant jet.

Thus, there is still a diversity of opinion in regard to the optimum form of anatomic correction. Treasure

and associates (1971) recommend that children with ventricular septal defect and mild aortic regurgitation should be treated by closure of the ventricular septal defect alone as soon as they reach sufficient size for elective open heart operation. They recommend early surgery since with the passage of time aortic regurgitation gradually becomes more severe and, therefore, more difficult to treat adequately from the surgical point of view. For those that have severe aortic regurgitation they recommend a ventricular septal defect closure with an aortic valvuloplasty as an acceptable compromise rather than total replacement of the aortic valve.

Trusler (1973) at The Hospital for Sick Children, Toronto, has used valvuloplasty as the method of choice. He measures each cusp accurately, with particular attention being paid to the prolapse leaflet, in regard to depth, length, and quality of the free margins. In the presence of severe valvular cusp prolapse he plicates both commissures. When the prolapse is less severe, the plication is done at one commissure only. The sutures are usually reinforced with Teflon felt pledgets. After closure of the aorta a right ventricular incision is made and this allows inspection of the reconstructed aortic valve from below and assessment of valve competence. The ventricular septal defect can then be closed with a Dacron patch.

Trusler (1973) reports that of ten children with subcrystal ventricular septal defects, six had an excellent result with disappearance of the aortic regurgitant murmur, three continued to have a grade one diastolic murmur. The pulse pressure was reduced in all ten, but one had a well-heard diastolic murmur after a second operation. The children with supracrystal septal defects have shown a reduction in heart size and blood pressure and pulse pressure. Two continued to have grade one aortic diastolic murmurs following corrective procedures. A repeat angiogram on seven children show that four now have completely competent aortic valves and three have slight evidence of insufficiency.

Van Praagh and McNamara (1968) pointed out that a number of the subcrystal defects were associated with commissural malformations or bicuspid valves. In such cases the operative therapy is made more difficult and the ultimate result less satisfactory. It is in this sort of case that Somerville and coworkers (1970) have recommended replacement of the aortic valve. This may be indicated in certain selected children by the use of either a homograft or a prosthetic valve, but undoubtedly it should be reserved for very severe aortic regurgitation and a markedly deformed cusp that is incapable of adequate correction by other means.

Valvuloplasty has been favored also by Spencer and colleagues (1973). They emphasize that aortic valve replacement was not necessary in any of their 20 patients. Their observation period of 1 to 12 years suggests no progression of the aortic regurgitation beyond the first few months after operation.

VENTRICULAR SEPTAL DEFECT WITH
VENTRICULOATRIAL COMMUNICATION

THIS usually consists of a ventricular septal defect coupled with an anomalous opening in the tricuspid valve, which permits a communication between the left ventricle and the right atrium. It is frequently oval in shape and is most commonly associated with a fusion of the tricuspid valve to the margins of the ventricular septal defect so that neither the left ventricle nor the right atrium communicates with the right ventricle through the anomaly. With each ventricular systole, blood is forced in a jetlike stream into the right atrium. Several authors have reported excellent examples of this problem (Perry et al., 1949; Stallman et al., 1955; Lynch et al., 1958; Braunwald et al., 1960; Levy et al., 1962).

Perry and associates (1949) suggested a classification for this subgroup of anomalies as follows:

A. Defect between outflow tract of left ventricle and right atrium above the annulus of the tricuspid valve.

B. Defect as in A and a defect in the ventricular septum below the anomalous valve.

C. Defect just below the annulus of the tricuspid valve so that the left ventricle communicates with the right atrium through a segment of the septal leaflet of the tricuspid valve fused to the margins of the septal defect.

D. Defects in both the tricuspid valve and ventricular septum but not fused together (see Figure 21–33).

Of the 21 cases that have been reported in the literature the majority have presented for examination and special studies between the ages of four and ten years, although they range in age from six weeks to 31 years. More than half the cases reported have not been in failure and have not been severely incapacitated. On the contrary, many have had a relatively good exercise tolerance and only a few had pulmonary congestion or were severely restricted in physical ability. The youngest case in congestive heart failure was six weeks old (Levy et al., 1962).

On physical examination the heart beat may be normal or slightly increased in force at the apex, and an exceptional case will have a right ventricular heave if pulmonary hypertension is present. Characteristically, there is a harsh systolic murmur best heard in the third and fourth left interspaces and accompanied by a thrill. All the cases reported in the literature as well as our own have had a systolic murmur. The thrill was absent in only one instance. In one of our children at The Hospital for Sick Children it was faintly palpable. In the others it could be readily felt.

The heart size is usually moderately increased, and only a few cases have had marked enlargement of the heart with massive hilar shadow markings. The left atrium may be slightly enlarged, but a more characteristic finding is a dilatation of the right atrium, which is noted in more than half the children. This creates a cardiac silhouette that is "ball-like" (Levy et al., 1962).

Cardiac Catheterization

There is a rise in oxygen content on passing from the venae cavae into the right atrium, usually between 5 and 40 percent (1 to 3 volumes percent). There may be a further rise on proceeding into the right ventricle, as one finds in some instances of simple atrial septal defect because of inadequate mixing in the right atrium, or because there is a shunt both into the right atrium and into the right ventricle at the same time.

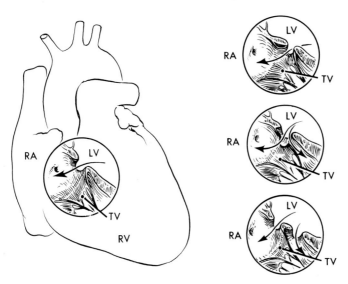

Figure 21-33. Ventricular septal defect with ventriculoatrial communication.

The right atrial pressure is normal or slightly elevated and rarely exceeds 10 mm of mercury. The right ventricular pressure is normal or slightly elevated in about half the cases; in the rest it will vary up to levels that are close to systemic. However, no case has been reported in which the pressure in the right ventricle was at systemic level. A typical case may have a pulmonary-to-systemic blood flow ratio of 2 to 1 but occasionally this may range as high as 4 to 1. After a cardiac catheterization in which an oxygen rise has been identified in the right atrium, the majority of these children are diagnosed as having an atrial septal defect.

Electrocardiography

There is considerable variation in the electrocardiogram—some patients have tracings within normal limits, and others show left ventricular loading with right bundle branch block or combined hypertrophy. Enlarged P waves of right atrial hypertrophy are noted in two-thirds of cases. No characteristic pattern has been identified.

Angiography and Dye Dilution Curves

The radiologic picture has been reported by Nordenstrom and Ovenfors (1960) and Braunwald and coworkers (1960).

An angiocardiogram performed with the tip of the catheter in the left ventricle reveals a characteristic shadow with immediate filling of the right atrium from the left ventricle before the right ventricle shows opacification. It may also reveal enlarged heart chambers, especially the right atrium, as well as dilatation of the central and peripheral branches of the pulmonary artery.

The underlying pathology may be suspected by a dye dilution curve if an injection is made into the left ventricle after an oxygen rise has been noted in the right atrium. A tracing characteristic of a left-to-right shunt will be demonstrated. A suitable injection into the left ventricle with a hydrogen-sensitive catheter in the right atrium will show an immediate response in a typical curve.

Differential Diagnosis

As has been noted in the chapter on atrial septal defect, several diagnostic possibilities present themselves when arterialization of the right atrial blood is found during cardiac catheterization, such as an atrial septal defect, and intraventricular septal defect with tricuspid insufficiency, a left ventricular right atrial defect with or without tricuspid valve involvement, and aneurysm of the sinus of Valsalva with an opening into the right atrium.

A long, harsh systolic murmur with a thrill is rarely found in ostium secundum but may occur in atrial ventricularis communis. However, the latter is likely to have a characteristic electrocardiographic pattern, and one can usually pass the catheter from the right atrium into the left atrium without difficulty as well as demonstrate evidence of mitral insufficiency. Aneurysm of the sinus of Valsalva is frequently accompanied by a rapid onset of failure when a sudden opening occurs between this sinus and the right atrium. Furthermore, a diastolic murmur of aortic insufficiency is usually heard. A more difficult differential diagnosis is that between the lesion under discussion and a ventricular septal defect with tricuspid insufficiency. Tricuspid insufficiency with a ventricular septal defect is more likely to occur if failure is present, and this is an uncommon event in left-ventricle-to-right-atrium anomalies. One of the most illuminating forms of investigation is the angiocardiogram with injection of the left ventricle. This will clearly show filling of the right atrium before the right ventricle is opacified and thus clarifies the diagnosis. However, when type B or D is present and the defect communicates with both chambers, the findings may be indistinguishable; then the final diagnosis may not be possible until operation or postmortem.

A somewhat similar anomaly has been reported by Dr. Charlotte Ferencz (1957). This case had a left ventricular right atrial communication with a malformed mitral valve. The tricuspid valve was normal and there was no ventricular septal defect. Postmortem examination indicated this was a variant of the atrioventricular canal defect group and there was left-axis deviation in the electrocardiogram suggestive of such a lesion. This selective angiocardiogram into the left ventricle in such a case will show the communication into the right atrium but will also reveal insufficiency in the mitral valve. This, coupled with left-axis deviation, may suggest the correct diagnosis in such cases.

Treatment and Prognosis

Surgical correction has been attempted in several centers (Stallman et al., 1955; Lynch et al., 1958). The first successful report was that of Kirby and associates (1957). Since then a number of successful closures of these defects have been recorded (Gerbode et al., 1958; Nordenstrom and Ovenfors, 1960; Braunwald and Morrow, 1960; Levy et al., 1962).

The problem arises as to what the precise prognosis is in these cases and whether or not they should be presented for surgical correction. Because of the position of the defect when type A or C is present, modern techniques should permit closure without difficulty and with success. Indications for operation should be similar to those in the simple ostium secundum. If type B or D is present, indications are similar to those with combined ventricular and atrial septal defects. In these more severe cases the history, the presence of heart failure, enlargement of the heart, increase with pressure and increased flow—all suggest that operative closure of both the ventricular septal defect and the anomalous opening of the tricuspid valve should be carried out.

It appears now that all of these patients should be operated on in early childhood. Accurate diagnosis has not usually been achieved in the past, but such recognition should be possible in the majority of cases in the future. The optimum age for surgery would be after the age of two unless failure or marked cardiomegaly is present, and then operation should be carried out after the maximum benefit is achieved by medical management.

These children may have the cardiotomy performed under hypothermia or by artificial heart-lung pump. The former approach is adequate if the defect is a small one, but if it is large or accompanied by a separate defect in the ventricular septum, the latter procedure is required.

At operation the atrial defect can be repaired with satisfactory results. The opening is closed and further shunt prevented. A tricuspid leak is repaired. If a thrill is present over the right ventricle after an atrial defect has been closed, it is necessary to explore the right ventricle for a second defect.

There have been approximately 14 patients reported in the literature corrected surgically. The overall mortality is approximately 10 percent, but this includes some infants and children with large defects. When the defect is small, the risk would appear to be insignificant. Postoperatively the patients do well with rare exceptions (Levy et al., 1962).

REFERENCES

Abbott, M. E.: Congenital heart disease. In *Nelson's Loose-Leaf Medicine*, 4:207, 1932. Thomas Nelson & Sons, New York.

Abbott, M. E.: *Atlas of Congenital Cardiac Disease*. Plate XV, p. 36. The American Heart Association, 1936.

Abbott, M. E.; Lewis, D. E.; and Beattie, W. W.: Differential study of case of pulmonary stenosis of inflammatory origin (ventricular septum closed) and 2 cases of (a) pulmonary stenosis and (b) pulmonary atresia of developmental origin with associated ventricular septal defect and death from paradoxical cerebral embolism in 3 cases, aged respectively 14, 10 and 11 years. *Am. J. Med. Sci.*, 165:636, 1923.

Adams, F. H.: Pulmonary hypertension in children due to congenital heart disease. *J. Pediatr.*, 40:42, 1952.

————: Comments on the early diagnosis and treatment of patients with congenital heart disease. *Dis. Chest*, 36:426, 1959.

Adams, P., Jr.; Kiely, B.; Cohen, M.; and Lillehei, C. W.: Ventricular septal defect in infants and children; results of direct closure in 25 patients. *Abstract, Combined Meeting of the American, British and Canadian Pediatric Societies and the Society for Pediatric Research*. Quebec, 1955, p. 30.

Adams, P., Jr.; Lucas, R. V.; Ferguson, D. J.; and Lillehei, C. W.: Significance of pulmonary vascular pathology in ventricular septal defect as determined by lung biopsy. Abstract. Society for Pediatric Research Transactions, *Am. J. Dis. Child.*, 94:476, 1957.

Agustsson, M. H.; Arcilla, R. A.; Bicoff, J. P.; Moncada, R.; and Gasul, B. M.: Spontaneous closure of ventricular septal defects in 14 children demonstrated by serial cardiac catheterizations and angiocardiography. *Pediatrics*, 31:958, 1963.

Albert, H. M.; Fowler, R. L.; Craighead, C. C.; Glass, B. A.; Atik, M.: Pulmonary artery banding. A treatment for infants with intractable cardiac failure due to interventricular septal defects. *Circulation*, 23:16, 1961.

Alpert, B. S.; Mellits, E. D.; and Rowe, R. D.: Spontaneous closure of small ventricular septal defects. *Am. J. Dis. Child.*, 125:194, 1973.

Arcilla, R. A.; Agustsson, M. M.; Bicoff, J. P.; Lynfield, J.; Weinberg, M., Jr.; Fell, H. G.; and Gasul, B. M.: Further observations on the natural history of isolated ventricular septal defect in infancy and childhood. *Circulation*, 28:560, 1963.

Ash, R., and Murphy, L.: High ventricular septal defect and slight dextroposition of the aorta (Eisenmenger type) associated with deformed aortic valve simulating patent ductus arteriosus. *Am. Heart J.*, 54:788, 1957.

Ash, R.; Wolman, I. J.; and Bromer, R. S.: Diagnosis of congenital cardiac defects in infancy: a study of thirty-two cases with necropsies. *Am. J. Dis. Child.*, 58:8, 1939.

Assad-Morell, J. L.; Tajik, A. J.; and Giuliani E. R.: Aneurysm of interventricular septum. Echocardiographic features. *Mayo Clin. Proc.*, 49:164, 1974.

Auld, P. A. M.; Johnson, A. L.; and Gibbons, J. E.: Changes in pulmonary vascular resistance in infants and children with left-to-right intracardiac shunts. *Circulation*, 27:257, 1963.

Auld, P. A. M.; Johnson, A. L.; Gibbons, J. E.; and McGregor, M.: Changes in pulmonary vascular resistance in infants and children with left-to-right intracardiac shunts. *Circulation*, 15:857, 1957.

Azevedo, A. de C.; Toledo, A. N.; Carvalho, A. A. de; Zaniolo, W.; Dohmann, H.; and Roubach, R.: Ventricular septal defect; an example of its relative diminution. *Acta Cardiol. (Brux.)*, 13:513, 1958.

Bahnson, H. T.: Discussion of Kirklin, J. W.; McGoon, D. C.; and DuShane, J. W.: Surgical treatment of ventricular septal defect. *J. Thorac. Cardiovasc. Surg.*, 40:805, 1960.

Bailey, C. P.; Lacy, M. H.; Neptune, W. B.; Weller, R.; Arvanitis, C. S.; and Karasic, J.: Experimental and clinical attempts at correction of inter-ventricular septal defects. *Ann. Surg.*, 136:919, 1952.

Barger, J. D.; Cressman, R. W.; and Edwards, J. E.: Bilateral ductus arteriosus associated with interruption of the aortic arch. *Am. J. Clin. Pathol.*, 24:441, 1954.

Barratt-Boyes, B. G.; Neutze, J. M.; Clarkson, P. M.; Shardey, G. C.; and Brandt, P. W. T.: Repair of ventricular septal defect in the first two years of life using profound hypothermia-circulatory arrest techniques. *Ann. Surg.*, 184:376, 1976.

Barratt-Boyes, B. G.; Nicholls, T. T.; Brandt, P. W. T.; and Neutze, J. M.: Aortic arch interruption associated with patent ductus arteriosus, ventricular septal defect and total anomalous pulmonary venous connection. *J. Thorac. Cardiovasc. Surg.*, 63:367, 1972.

Barratt-Boyes, B. G.; Simpson, M.; and Neutze, J. M.: Intra-cardiac surgery in neonates and infants using a deep hypothermia with surface cooling and limited cardiopulmonary bypass. *Circulation*, 43:1, 1971.

Beck, W.; Swan, H. J. C.; Burchell, H. B.; and Kirklin, J. W.: Pulmonary vascular resistance after repair of atrial septal defects in patients with pulmonary hypertension. *Circulation*, 22:938, 1960.

Bécu, L.; Fontana, R. S.; DuShane, J. W.; Kirklin, J. W.; Burchell, H. B.; and Edwards, J. E.: Anatomics and pathologic studies in ventricular septal defect. *Circulation*, 14:349, 1956.

Bedford, D. E.: The anatomical types of atrial septal defects, their incidence and clinical diagnosis. *Am. J. Cardiol.*, 6:568, 1960.

————: Personal communication, 1963.

Benchimol, A., and Dimond, G. E.: Phonocardiography in ventricular septal defect. *Am. J. Med.*, 28:347, 1960.

Benvenuto, R., and Lewis, F. J.: Gradual closure of interventricular septal defects. *J. Thorac. Cardiovasc. Surg.*, 37:673, 1959.

Bernhard, W. F.; Litwin, S. B.; Williams, W. W.; Jones, J. E.; and Gross, R. E.: Recent results of cardiovascular surgery in infants in the first year of life. *Am. J. Surg.*, 123:451, 1972.

Bing, R. J.; Vandam, L. D.; and Gray, F. D., Jr.: Physiological studies in congenital heart disease; results of preoperative studies in patients with tetralogy of Fallot. *Bull. Hopkins Hosp.*, 80:121, 1947.

Bircks, W., and Reidemeister, C.: Results of surgical treatment of ventricular septal defect. *Br. Heart J.*, 33:88, 1971.

Bleifer, S.; Dorioso, E.; and Grishman, A.: The auscultatory and phonocardiographic signs of ventricular septal defects. *Am. J. Cardiol.*, 5:191, 1960.

Bloom, K. R.; Rodrigues, L.; and Swan, E. M.: Echocardiographic evaluation of left-to-right shunt in ventricular septal defect and persistent ductus arteriosus. *Br. Heart J.*, **39**:260, 1977.

Bloomfield, D. K.: The natural history of the ventricular septal defect in patients surviving infancy. *Circulation*, **29**:914, 1964.

Blount, S. G.; Mueller, H.; and McCord, M. C.: Ventricular septal defect. *Am. J. Med.*, **18**:871, 1955.

Blount, S. G., Jr., and Woodward, G. M.: Considerations involved in the selection for surgery of patients with ventricular septal defect. *Am. J. Cardiol.*, **5**:223, 1960.

Bonnet, L. M.: Sur la lésion dite stenose congénitale de l'aorta, dans la région de l'isthme. *Rev. Méd.*, *Paris*, **23**:481, 1903.

Borst, M. G.; McGregor, M.; Wittenberger, J. L.; and Berglund, E.: Influence of pulmonary arterial and left arterial and left atrial pressures on pulmonary vascular resistance. *Circ. Res.*, **4**:393, 1956.

Braunwald, E. Personal communication, 1964.

Braunwald, E.; Brockenbrough, E. C.; Frahm, C. J.; and Ross, J. Jr.: Left atrial and left ventricular pressures in subjects without cardiovascular disease: observations in eighteen patients studied by transeptal left heart catheterization. *Circulation*, **24**:267, 1961.

Braunwald, E., and Morrow, A. C.: Ventricular-right atrial communication diagnosed by clinical hemodynamic and angiocardiographic methods. *Am. J. Med.*, **28**:913, 1960.

Braunwald, N. S.; Braunwald, E.; and Morrow, A. G.: The effects of surgical abolition of left shunts on the pulmonary vascular dynamics of patients with pulmonary hypertension. *Circulation*, **26**:1270, 1960.

Breccia, G.: Sopra un caso di morbo del Roger complicato con insufficienza aortica, decorso senza sintomi. *Gazz. Osp. Milano*, **27**:625, 1906.

Brewer, D. B., and Heath, D.: Pulmonary vascular changes in Eisenmenger's complex. *J. Pathol. Bact.*, **77**:141, 1959.

Brostoff, P., and Rodbard, S.: Hydrodynamics in ventricular septal defects. *Am. Heart J.*, **51**:325, 1956.

Brown, J. W.: *Congenital Heart Disease*, 2nd ed. Staples Press, Ltd., London, 1950.

Burchell, H. B.: Regression of pulmonary vascular hypertension after cure of intracardiac defects. In Adams, W. R., and Veith, I.: *Pulmonary International Symposium.* Grune & Stratton, Inc., New York, 1959, p. 245

Burchell, H. B.; DuShane, J. W.; and Brandenburg, R. O.: The electrocardiogram in patients with atrioventricular cushion defects (defects of the atrioventricular canal). *Am. J. Cardiol.*, **6**:575, 1960.

Burchell, H. B.; Edwards, J. E.; and Morgan, E. H.: Aortic sinus aneurysm with communications into the right ventricle and associated ventricular septal defect. *Proc. Mayo Clin.*, **26**:336, 1951.

Calodney, M. M., and Carson, M. J.: Coarctation of the aorta in early infancy. *J. Pediatr.*, **37**:46, 1950.

Campbell, M., and Cardell, B. S.: A case of Eisenmenger's complex with coarctation of the aorta. *Guy Hosp. Rep.*, **102**:4, 1953.

Cassin, S.; Dawes, G. S.; and Ross, B. B.: Pulmonary blood flow and vascular resistance in immature foetal lungs. *J. Physiol.* (Lond.), **171**:80, 1964.

Castaneda, A. R.; Zamora, R.; Nicoloff, D. M.; Moller, J. H.; Hunt, C. E.; and Lucas, R. V.: High pressure, high-resistance ventricular septal defect. *Ann. Thorac. Surg.*, **12**:29, 1971.

Char, F.; Adams, P.; and Anderson, R. C.: Electrocardiographic findings in one hundred verified cases of ventricular septal defect. *AMA J. Dis. Child.*, **97**:48, 1959.

Clark, J., and White, P. D.: Congenital aneurysmal defect of the membranous portion of the ventricular septum (associated with heart block, ventricular flutter. Adams-Stokes syndrome and death). *Circulation*, **5**:725, 1952.

Clarkson, P. M.; Frye, R. L.; DuShane, J. W.; Burchell, H. B.; Wood, E. H.; and Weidman, W. H.: Prognosis for patients with ventricular septal defect and severe pulmonary vascular obstructive disease. *Circulation*, **38**:129, 1968.

Clawson, B. J.: Types of congenital heart disease in 15,597 autopsies. *Lancet*, **64**:134, 1944.

Claypool, G.; Ruth, W.; and Lin, T. K.: Ventricular septal defect with aortic incompetence. Simulating patent ductus arteriosus. *Am. Heart J.*, **54**:788, 1957.

Clelland, W. P.; Bentall, H. H.; and Bromley, L. L.: Ventricular septal defects. *Proc. Roy. Soc. Med.*, **54**:785, 1961.

Coleman, E. N.; Reid, J. M.; Barclay, R. S.; and Stevenson, J. G.: Ventricular septal defect repair after pulmonary artery banding. *Br. Heart J.*, **34**:134, 1972.

Coles, J. C.; Carroll, S. E.; and Gergeley, N.: The diagnosis and treatment of congenital heart disease. II. Treatment of congenital heart disease in the infant and neonate. *Can. Med. Assoc. J.*, **87**:318, 1962.

Collins, G.; Calder, L.; Rose, V.; Kidd, L.; and Keith, J.: Ventricular septal defect: Clinical and hemodynamics changes in the first five years of life. *Am. Heart J.*, **84**:695, 1972.

Cooley, D. A.: Inter American Cardiology Conference, Montreal (1964). (1961 reports included.)

Cooley, D. A.; Garrett, H. E.; and Howard, M. S.: The surgical treatment of ventricular septal defect. An analysis of 300 consecutive surgical cases. *Prog. Cardiovasc. Dis.*, **4**:312, 1962.

Cooley, D. A., and Hallman, G. L.: Cardiovascular surgery during the first year of life. Experience with 450 consecutive operations. *Am. J. Surg.*, **107**:474, 1964.

Cooley, D. A.; Hallman, G. L.; and Hammam, A. S.: Congenital cardiovascular anomalies in adults. *Am. J. Cardiol.*, **17**:303, 1966.

Coppoletta, J. M., and Wolbach, S. B.: Body weights and organ length in infants and children; study of body length and normal weights of more important vital organs of body between birth and 12 years of age. *Am. J. Pathol.*, **9**:55, 1933.

Corone, P.; Doyon, F.; Gaudeau, S.; Guerin, F.; Vernant, P.; Ducam, H.; Rumeau- Rouquette, C.; and Gaudeul, P.: Natural history of ventricular septal defect: A study involving 790 cases. *Circulation*, **55**:908, 1977.

Cournand, A.; Baldwin, J. S.; and Himmelstein, A.: *Cardiac Catheterization in Congenital Heart Disease: A Clinical and Physiological Study in Infants and Children.* The Commonwealth Fund, New York, 1949, p. 59.

Cournand, A.; Riley, R. L.; Himmelstein, A.; and Austrian, R.: Pulmonary circulation and alveolar ventilation perfusion relationships after pneumonectomy, *J. Thorac. Surg.*, **19**:80, 1950.

Cross, R. E.: The patent ductus arteriosus. Observations on diagnosis and therapy in 225 surgically treated cases. *Am. J. Med.*, **12**:472, 1952.

Cumming, G. R.: Confirmation of closure of ventricular septal defects. Value of pressor agents. *Am. J. Cardiol.*, **15**:259, 1965.

Daicoff, G. R., and Miller, R. H.: Congestive heart failure in infancy treated by early repair of ventricular septal defect. *Circulation*, **41**:110, 1970.

Dammann, J. F., Jr., and Ferencz, C.: The significance of the pulmonary vascular bed in congenital heart disease. III. Defects between the ventricles of great vessels in which both increased pressure and blood flow may act upon the lungs and in which there is a common ejectile force. *Am. Heart J.*, **52**:210, 1956.

Dammann, J. F., Jr., and Muller, W. H.: The regression of pulmonary vascular disease after the correction of pulmonary stenosis. *J. Thorac. Cardiovasc. Surg.*, **42**:722, 1961.

Dammann, J. F., Jr.; McEachen, J. A.; Thompson, W. M., Jr.; Smith, R.; and Muller, W. H.: The regression of pulmonary vascular disease after the creation of pulmonary stenosis. *J. Thorac. Cardiovasc. Surg.*, **42**:722, 1961.

Dawes, G. S., and Mott, J. C.: The vascular tone of the fetal lung. *J. Physiol.*, **164**:469, 1962.

De la Cruz, M. V., and da Rocha, J. P.: An ontogenetic theory for the explanation of congenital malformations involving the truncus and conus. *Am. Heart J.*, **51**:782, 1956.

Dentin, G., and Pappas, E. G.: Ventricular septal defect and aortic insufficiency. Report of three cases. *Am. J. Cardiol.*, **2**:544, 1958.

Deuchar, D. C., and Knebel, R.: The pulmonary and systemic circulations in congenital heart disease. *Br. Heart J.*, **14**:225, 1952.

Diehl, A. M.; Kittle, C. F.; and Crockett, J. E.: Spontaneous complete closure of a high-flow, high pressure, ventricular septal defect. *Lancet*, **81**:572, 1961.

Dillard, D. H.; Mohri, H.; and Merendino, K. A.: Correction of heart disease in infancy utilizing deep hypothermia and total circulatory arrest. *J. Thorac. Cardiovasc. Surg.*, **61**:64, 1971.

Dooley, K. J.; Parisi-Buckley, L.; Fyler, D. C.; and Nadas, A. S.: Results of pulmonary arterial banding in infancy:—Survey of five years' experience in the New England Regional Infant Cardiac Program. *Am. J. Cardiol.*, **36**:484, 1975.

Dorney, E. R.; Fowler, N. O.; and Mannix, F. P.: Unilateral clubbing of the fingers due to absence of the aortic arch. *Am. J. Med.*, **18**:150, 1955.

Doyle, J. T.; Wilson, J. S.; and Warren, J. V.: The pulmonary vascular responses to short-term hypoxia in human subjects. *Circulation*, **5**:263, 1952.

Drorbaugh, J. E.; Auld, P. A. M.; Rudolph, A. J.; Nadas, A. S.; Smith, C. A.; and Hubbell, J. P.: Studies on the circulation in the neonatal period; the circulation in the respiratory distress syndrome. *Pediatrics*, **27**:551, 1961.

DuShane, J. W.: Total anomalous pulmonary venous connection. *Proc. Mayo Clin.*, **31**:167, 1956.

DuShane, J. W.; Krongrad, E.; Ritter, D. G.; and McGoon, D. C.: The fate of raised pulmonary vascular resistance after surgery in ventricular septal defect. In Kidd, B. S. L., and Rowe, R. D. (eds.): *The Child with Congenital Heart Disease after Surgery*. Futura Publishing Co. Inc., Mount Kisco, New York, 1976, p. 299.

DuShane, J. W.; Krongrad, E.; Ritter, D. G.; and McGoon, D. C.: The fate of raised pulmonary vascular resistance after surgery in ventricular septal defect. Read at the International Symposium on the Child with Congenital Heart Disease After Surgery, Toronto, 1975.

DuShane, J. W.; Weidman, W. H.; Brandenburg, R. O.; and Kirklin, J. W.: The electrocardiogram in children with ventricular septal defect and severe pulmonary hypertension. Correlation with response of pulmonary arterial pressure to surgical repair. *Circulation*, **22**:49, 1960.

Ebert, P. A.; Canent, R. V. Jr.; Spach, M. S.; and Sabiston, D. C., Jr.; Late cardiodynamics following correction of ventricular septal defects with previous pulmonary artery banding. *J. Thorac. Cardiovasc. Surg.*, **60**:516, 1970.

Edwards, J. E.: Congenital malformations of the heart and great vessels. In Gould, S. E. (ed.): *Pathology of the Heart*. Charles C Thomas, Publisher, Springfield, Ill., 1953, p. 288.

———: Symposium on cardiovascular diseases: functional pathology of congenital cardiac disease. *Pediatr. Clin. North Am.*, **1**:13, 1954.

———: Functional pathology of the pulmonary vascular tree in congenital cardiac disease. *Circulation*, **15**:164, 1957.

Edwards, J. E; Douglas, J. M.; Burchell, H. E.; and Christensen, N. A.: Pathology of intrapulmonary arteries and arterioles in coarctation of aorta associated with patent ductus arteriosus. *Am. Heart J.*, **38**:205, 1949.

Eisenmenger, V.: Die angeborenen Defecte de Kammerscheidewand des Herzens. *Ztschr. f. klin. Med.*, **32**, Suppl. 1, 1897.

———: Ursprung der Aorta aus Seichen Ventrikeln beim defecte des Septum Ventriculorum. *Wien. Klin. Wschr.*, **11**:25, 1898.

Ellis, F. H., Jr.; Ongley, P. A.; and Kirklin, J. W.: Ventricular septal defect with aortic valvular incompetence. *Circulation*, **27**:789, 1963.

Engle, M. A.: Ventricular septal defect in infancy, *Pediatrics*, **14**:16, 1954.

European Pediatric Cardiology Conference, Holland, 1964. Meeting Abstracts.

Evans, J. R.; Rowe, R. D.; and Keith, J. D.: Spontaneous closure of ventricular septal defects. *Circulation*, **22**:1044, 1960.

Evans, J. R., and associates: Personal communication, 1964.

Evans, W.: Congenital stenosis (coarctation) atresia and interruption of the aortic arch (a study of twenty-eight cases). *Q. J. Med.*, **2**:1, 1933.

———: Heart murmurs. *Br. Heart J.*, **9**:225, 1947.

Everts-Suárez, E. A., and Carson, C. P.: The triad of congenital absence of aortic arch (isthmus aortae), patent ductus arteriosus and interventricular septal defect—a trilogy. *Ann. Surg.*, **150**:1, 1959.

Ferencz, C.: Transposition of the great vessels: Pathophysiologic considerations based upon a study of the lungs. *Circulation (Suppl. 11)*, **33**:232, 1966.

———: Atrio-ventricular defect of membraneous system: left ventricular–right atrial communication with malformed mitral valve stimulating aortic stenosis; report of a case. *Bull. Hopkins Hosp.*, **100(S)**:209, 1957.

Fergulio, G. A.: Intracardiac phonocardiography. A valuable diagnostic technique in congenital and acquired heart disease. *Am. Heart J.*, **58**:827, 1959.

———: A simple method for intracardiac acoustic auscultation and phonocardiography. *Circulation*, **27**:578, 1963.

Fergulio, G. A., and Gunton, R. W.: Intracardiac phonocardiography in ventricular septal defect. *Circulation*, **21**:49, 1960.

Ferguson, D. J.; Adams, P.; and Watson, D.: Pulmonary arteriosclerosis in transposition of the great vessels, *Am. J. Dis. Child.*, **99**:653, 1960.

Fontan, F.; Bricaud, H.; Simmoneau, J.; et al.: Closure under extra-corporeal circulation of poorly tolerated ventricular septal defects in infants. *Arch. Mal. Coeur*, **64**:48, 1971.

Fowler, N.; Westcott, R. N.; and Scott, R. C.: Normal pressures in the right heart and pulmonary artery. *Am. Heart J.*, **46**:264, 1953.

Fowler, N. O.: Some variations in the clinical picture of congenital defect of the interventricular septum. *Am. J. Med.*, **17**:322, 1954.

Fowler, R. S., and Keith, J. D.: Personal communication, 1964.

Freedom, R. M.; White, R. D.; Pieroni, D. R., Varghese, P. J.; Krovetz, L. J.; and Rowe, R. D.: The natural history of the so-called aneurysm of the membranous ventricular septum in childhood. *Circulation*, **49**:375, 1974.

French, H.: The possibility of a loud congenital heart murmur disappearing when a child grows up. *Guy Hosp. Gaz.*, **32**:87, 1918.

Friedli, B.; Kidd, B. S. L.; Mustard, W. T.; and Keith, J. D.: Surgical closure of ventricular septal defect with elevated pulmonary vascular resistance: late results of surgical closure. (Abst.) *Am. J. Cardiol.*, **33**:403, 1974.

Fritts, H. W., and Cournand, A.: Physiological factors regulating pressure, flow and distribution of blood in the pulmonary circulation. In Adams, W. R., and Veith, I.: *Pulmonary Circulation: An International Symposium*, Grune & Stratton, Inc., New York, 1959, p. 62.

Fry, J.: Acute Myocardial infarction. The pre-hospital phase. *Schweiz. Med. Wochenschr.*, **98**:1210, 1968.

Gammelgaard, A.; Therkelsen, A.; and Boesen, I.: Surgical treatment of coarctation of the aortal and hypoplasia of the aortic arch in infants. *Acta Chir. Scand.*, **117**:137–45, 1959.

Gammelgaard, A.; Therkelsen, F.; Boesen, I.; and Terslev, E.: Ventricular septal defects in infancy treated with surgical narrowing of the pulmonary artery. A follow-up examination. *Acta Chir. Scand.* (Suppl.), **283**:84, 1961.

Garamella, J. J.; Cruz, A. B.; Heupel, W. H.; Dahl, J. C.; Jensen, N. K.; and Berman, R.: Ventricular septal defect with aortic insufficiency. Successful surgical correction of both defects by the transaortic approach. *Am. J. Cardiol.*, **5**:266, 1960.

Gardiner, J. H., and Keith, J. D.: Prevalence of heart disease in Toronto children; 1948–1949 Cardiac Registry. *Pediatrics*, **7**:713, 1951.

Gaspar, I.: Two of the rarer congenital anomalies of the heart. *Am. J. Pathol.*, **5**:285, 1929.

Gasul, B. M.; Dillon, R. F.; and Vrla, V.: Further observations of the natural course of ventricular septal defects: new clinical and physiologic data. (Abstract.) *Circulation*, **16**:885, 1957.

Gasul, B. M.; Fell, E. H.; and Casas, R.: The diagnosis of aortic septal defect by retrograde aortography. Report of a case. *Circulation*, **4**:251, 1951.

Gelfman, R., and Levine, S. A.: Incidence of acute and subacute bacterial endocarditis in congenital heart disease. *Am. J. Med. Sci.*, **204**:324, 1942.

Gerbode, F.; Hultgren, H.; Melrose, D.; and Osborn, J.: Syndrome of left ventricular–right atrial shunt: successful surgical repair of defect in 5 cases with observation of bradycardia on closure. *Ann. Surg.*, **148**:433, 1958.

Gibson, S., and Clifton, W. M.: Congenital heart disease: a clinical and postmortem study of one hundred and five cases. *Am. J. Dis. Child.*, **55**:761, 1938.

Glass, I. H.; Mustard, W. T.; and Keith, J. D.: Coarctation of the aorta in infants. A review of twelve years experience. *Pediatrics*, **26**:109, 1960.

Glenn, W.; Tole, A.; Lougo, E.; Hume, M.; and Gentsch, T.: Induced fibrillatory arrest in open heart surgery. *N. Engl. J. Med.*, **262**:852, 1960.

Glover, R. P.; Henderson, A. R.; Margutti, R.; and Gregory, J.: The fate of intracardiac pericardial grafts as applied to the closure of septal defects and to the relief of mitral insufficiency. In *Surgical Forum of the American College of Surgeons*. W. B. Saunders Co., Philadelphia, 1952.

Goerttler, K.: *Normale und pathologische entwicklung des menschlichen herzens.* Georg Thieme, Stuttgart, 1958, p. 71.

Goldberg, J. J.; Allen, H. D.; and Sahn, D. J.: *Pediatric and Adolescent Echocardiography. A Handbook.* Year Book Medical Publishers, Inc., Chicago, 1975, p. 293.

Goldblatt, A.; Bernhard, W. S.; Nadas, A. S.; and Gross, R. E.: Pulmonary artery banding. Indication and results in infants and children. *Circulation,* 32:172, 1965.

Gonzalez-Lavin, L., and Barratt-Boyes, B. G.: Surgical considerations in the treatment of ventricular septal defect associated with aortic valvular incompetence. *J. Thorac. Cardiovasc. Surg.,* 57:422, 1969.

Goor, D. A.; Lillehei, C. W.; Rees, R.; and Edwards, J. E.: Isolated ventricular septal defect. Developmental basis for various types and presentation of classification. *Chest,* 58:468, 1970.

Gorlin, R., and Gorlin, S. G.: Hydraulic formula for calculation of area of stenotic mitral valve, other cardiac valves, and central circulatory shunts. *Am. Heart J.,* 41:1, 1951.

Graham, T. P.; Cordell, G. D.; and Bender, H. W.: Ventricular function following surgery. In Kidd, B. S. L., and Rowe, R. D. (eds.): *The Child with Congenital Heart Disease after Surgery.* Futura Publishing Co. Inc., Mount Kisco, N.Y., 1976, p. 277.

Grant, R. P.: The architecture of the right ventricular outflow tract in the normal human heart and in the presence of ventricular septal defects. *Circulation,* 24:223, 1961.

Grieg, D.: Case of malformation of the heart and blood vessels of the foetus. *Monthly J. Med. Soc. Bd.,* 15:28, 1852.

Griffiths, S. P.; Blumenthal, S.; Jameson, A. E.; Ellis, K.; Morgan, B. C.; and Malm, J. R.: Ventricular septal defect: Survival in adult life. *Am. J. Med.,* 37:23, 1964.

Grosse-Brockhoc, F.; Loogen, F.; and Schaede, A.: Angeborene Herz-und Gefässmissbildungen: Ventrikelseptumdefekt mit Aortenklappeninsuffizienz (ohne und mit Pulmonalstenose). In *Handbuch der Inneren Medizin.* Springer-Verlag, Berlin, 1960, vol. 9, part 3, p. 244.

Grover, R. F.; Reeves, J. T.; Will, D. H.; and Blount, S. G., Jr.: Pulmonary vasoconstriction in steers at high altitudes. *J. Appl. Physiol.,* 18 (May), 1963.

Hallidie-Smith, K. A.; Olsen, E. G. J.; Oakley, C. M.; Goodwin, J. F.; and Cleland, W. P.: Ventricular septal defect and aortic regurgitation. *Thorax,* 24:257, 1969.

Hallman, G. L., and Cooley, D. A.: Surgery of the heart and great vessels in the newborn period. *Postgrad. Med.,* 34:48, 1963.

Hamburger, L. P., Jr.: Congenital cardiac malformation presenting complete interruption of the isthmus aortae with transposition of the great arteries. *Bull. Hopkins Hosp.,* 61:421, 1937.

Hamilton, W. F., and Abbott, M. E.: Complete obliteration of the descending arch at insertion of the ductus in a boy of fourteen; bicuspid aortic valve; impending rupture of the aorta; cerebral death, *Am. Heart J.,* 3:381, 1928.

Harned, H. S., and Peters, R. M.: Spontaneous closing of ventricular septal defects: two case reports. *Circulation,* 22:760, 1960.

Harris, P., and Heath, D.: In *The Human Pulmonary Circulation. Its Form and Function in Health and Disease.* E. & S. Livingstone, Edinburgh, 1962.

Hartmann, A. F., Jr., and Weldon, C. S.: Surgical management of aortic insufficiency associated with interventricular septal defect. *Circulation* (Suppl. 3), 41 & 42:1972.

Heath, D., and Best, P. V.: The tunica media of the arteries of the lung in pulmonary hypertension, *J. Pathol. Bact.,* 76:165, 1958.

Hirschfeld, S.; Meyer, R.; Schwartz, D. C.; Korfhagen, J.; and Kaplan, S.: The echocardiographic assessment of pulmonary artery pressure and pulmonary vascular resistance. *Circulation,* 52:642, 1975.

Hoffman, J. I. E., and Rudolph, A. M.: Natural history of ventricular septal defect in infancy. *Circulation,* 28:737, 1963.
——: The natural history of ventricular septal defects in infancy. *Am. J. Cardiol.,* 16:634, 1965.

Honda, T.; Horiuchi, T.; Abe, T.; Koyamada, K.; Ishitoya, T.; and Ishizawa, Y.: Histometrical study of the pulmonary arteries in normal postnatal development and in patients with ventricular septal defect. *Tohoku. J. Exp. Med.,* 102:403, 1970.

Horiuchi, T.; Koyamada, K.; Matano, I.; Mohri, H.; Komatsu, T.; Honda, T.; Abe, T.; Ishitoya, T.; Sagawa, Y.; Matsuzawa, A.; Matsumura, M.; Tsuda, T.; Ishizawa, E.; Ishikawa, S.; Suzuki, H.; and Saito, Y.: Radical operation for ventricular septal defect in infancy. *J. Thorac. Cardiovasc. Surg.,* 46:180, 1963.

Horiuchi, T.; Koyamada, K.; Ishitoya, T.; Honda, T.; Abe, T.; and Sagawa, Y.: Radical operation under hypothermia for ventricular septal defect in infancy. A report of 64 consecutive cases. *J. Cardiovasc. Surg.,* 8:85, 1967.

Howitt, G., and Wade, E. G.: Repeat catheterization in ventricular septal defect and pulmonary hypertension. *Br. Heart J.,* 24:649, 1962.

Hultgren, H.; Selzer, A.; Purdy, A.; Holman, E.; and Gerbode, F.: The syndrome of patent ductus arteriosus with pulmonary hypertension. *Circulation,* 8:15, 1953.

Hurst, W. W., and Schemm, F. R.: High ventricular septal defect with slight dextroposition of the aorta (Eisenmenger type) which presented the clinical features of patent ductus arteriosus. *Am. Heart J.,* 36:144, 1948.

Ingham, D. W.: Congenital heart disease: incidence at the Mayo Clinic. *J. Tech. Methods,* 18:131, 1938.

Jacobius, H. L., and Moore, R. A.: Incidence of congenital cardiac anomalies in autopsies at New York Hospital. *J. Tech. Methods,* 18:133, 1938.

James, L. S.: Physiology of respiration in newborn infants and in the respiratory distress syndrome. *Pediatrics,* 24:1069, 1959.

James, L. S., and Rowe, R. D.: The pattern of response of pulmonary and systemic arterial pressures in newborn and older infants to short periods of hypoxia. *J. Pediatr.,* 51:5, 1957.

Jew, E. W., Jr., and Cross, P.: Aortic origin of the right pulmonary artery and absence of the transverse aortic arch. *Arch. Pathol.,* 53:191, 1952.

Jones, L. O., and Wheeler, R. M.: Isolated interventricular septal defect simulating mitral stenosis. *Southern Med. J.,* 47:1070, 1954.

Jones, A. M., and Howitt, G.: Eisenmenger syndrome in pregnancy. *Br. Med. J.,* 1:1627, 1965.

Kaplan, S.; Daoud, G. I.; Benzing, G., III; Devine, F. J.; Glass, I. H.; and McGuire, J.: Natural history of ventricular septal defect. *Am. J. Dis. Child.,* 105:581, 1963.

Kaplan, S.; Daoud, G. I.; Glass, I. H.; Shemtob, A.; and McGuire, J.: Natural course of ventricular septal defect. *Circulation,* 24:968, 1961.

Kavanagh-Gray, D.: Spontaneous closure of a ventricular septal defect. *Can. Med. Assoc. J.,* 87:868, 1962.

Kay, E. B., and Zimmerman, H. A.: Surgical repair of interventricular septal defects. *JAMA,* 154:986, 1954.

Kay, J. H.; Thomas, V.; and Blalock, A.: The experimental production of high interventricular septal defects. A physiological and pathological study. *Surg. Gynecol. Obstet.,* 96:529, 1953.

Keane, J. F.; Plauth, W. H., Jr.; and Nadas, A. S.: Ventricular septal defect with aortic regurgitation. *Circulation,* 56:(Suppl. 1), 1–72, 1977.

Keck, E. W.; Ongley, P. A.; and Kincaid, O. W.: Ventricular septal defect with aortic insufficiency. A clinical and hemodynamic study of 18 proved cases. *Circulation,* 27:203, 1963.

Keith, J. D.; Rowe, R. D., and Vlad, P.: *Heart Disease in Infancy and Childhood.* Macmillan Publishing Co., Inc., New York, 1958.

Keith, J. D.; Rose, V.; Collins, G.; and Kidd, B. S. L.: Ventricular septal defect, incidence, morbidity, and mortality in various age groups. *Br. Heart J.,* 33:81, 1971.

Kidd, L.; Rose, V.; Collins, G.; and Keith, J.: Ventricular septal defect in infancy—a hemodynamic study. *Am. Heart J.,* 69:4, 1965.
——: The hemodynamics in ventricular septal defect in childhood. *Am. Heart J.,* 70:732, 1965.

King, H.; Shumacker, H. B.; and Deniz, N.: Experimental surgical repair of ventricular septal defects. *Surgery,* 3:1100. 1953.

Kirby, C. K.; Johnson, J.; and Ziusser, H. F.: Successful closure of a left ventricular–right atrial shunt. *Ann. Surg.,* 145:392, 1957.

Kirklin, J. W.: Personal communication, 1956.

Kirklin, J. W.; Applebaum, A.; and Bargeron, L. M.: Primary repair vs. banding for ventricular septal defects in infants. In Kidd, B. S. L., and Rowe, R. D. (eds.): *The Child with Congenital Heart Disease after Surgery.* Futura Publishing Co. Inc., Mount Kisco, New York, 1976, p. 3.

Kirklin, J. W., and DuShane, J. W.: Repair of ventricular septal defect in infancy. *Pediatrics,* 27:961, 1961.

Kirklin, J. W., and DuShane, J. W.: Indications for repair of ventricular septal defects. *Am. J. Cardiol.,* 12:75, 1963.

Kirklin, J. W.; Harshbarger, H. G.; Donald, D. E.; and Edwards, J.

E.: Surgical correction of ventricular septal defect; anatomic and technical considerations. *J. Thorac. Surg.*, 33:45, 1957.

Kirklin, J. W.; McGoon, D. C.; and DuShane, J. W.: Surgical treatment of ventricular septal defect. *J. Thorac. Cardiovasc. Surg.*, 40:763, 1960.

Kjellberg, S. R.; Manheimer, E.; Rudhe, U.; and Jonsson, B.: *Diagnosis of Congenital Heart Disease*, Year Book Publishers, Inc., Chicago. 1955, p. 307.

Kramer, T. C.: The partitioning of the truncus and conus and the formation of the membranous portion of the interventricular septum in the human heart. *Am. J. Anat.*, 71:343, 1942.

Laennec, R. T. H.: *Traite de L'auscultation Mediate et des Maladies des Poumons et du Coeur*, 2nd ed. J. S. Chaude, Paris, 1926.

Laubry, C., and Pezzi, C.: *Traité des Maladies Congénitales du Coeur*. Baillière, Paris, 1921.

Laubry, C.; Routier, D.; and Soulie, P.: Les souffles de la maladie de Roger. *Rev. Med.*, 50:439, 1933.

Leachman, R. D.: Observations on the pulmonary vascular resistance following surgical closure of high resistance ventricular septal defect. *Cardiovasc. Res. Cent. Bull.*, 2:23, 1963.

Leckert, J. T., and Sternberg, S. S.: Congenital aneurysm of the membranous interventricular septum with unique anomaly of the pulmonary vessels. *Am. Heart J.*, 39:768, 1950.

Leech, C. B.: Congenital heart disease: clinical analysis of seventy-five cases from the Johns Hopkins Hospital. *J. Pediatr.*, 7:802, 1935.

Lessof, M.: Heart sounds and murmurs in ventricular septal defect. *Guy Hosp. Rep.*, 108:361, 1959.

Letterer, E.: Kongenitaler defekt des aortenbogens. *Centrabl. Allg. Path. Anat.*, 33:155, 1923.

Lev, M.: The pathologic anatomy of ventricular septal defects. *Dis. Chest*, 35:1, 1959.

———: The architecture of the conduction system in congenital heart disease—III Ventricular septal defect. *Arch. Pathol.*, 70:529, 1960.

Lev, M.; Joseph, R. H.; Rimoldi, H. J. A.; Paiva, R.; and Arcilla, R. A.: The quantitative anatomy of isolated ventricular septal defect. *Am. Heart J.*, 81:315, 1971.

Lev, M., and Saphir, O.: Congenital aneurysm of the membranous septum. *Arch. Pathol.*, 25:819, 1938.

Levine, S. A.: *Clinical Heart Disease*, 4th ed. W. B. Saunders Co., Philadelphia, 1951.

Levy, M. J.; Amplatz, K.; and Lillehei, C. W.: Transthoracic left heart catheterization and angiocardiography for combined assessment of mitral and aortic valves. *Radiology*, 78:638, 1962.

Levy, M. J.; DeWall, R.; Elliott, L. P.; and Cuello, L.: Origin of both great arteries from the right ventricle and pulmonary stenosis. A propos case successfully corrected. *Dis. Chest*, 42:372, 1962.

Levy, M. J.; De Wall, R.; and Lillehei, C. W.: Left ventricular-right atrial canal and subaortic stenosis. Report of a case diagnosed preoperatively. *Am. Heart J.*, 64:392, 1962.

Lewis, A. B., and Takahashi, M.: Echocardiographic assessment of left-to-right shunt volume in children with ventricular septal defect. *Circulation*, 54:78, 1976.

Li, M. D.; Collins, G.; Disenhouse, R.; and Keith, J. D.: Spontaneous closure of ventricular septal defect. *Can. Med. Assoc. J.*, 100:737, 1969.

Lillehei, C. W.; Levy, M. J.; and Adams, P.: High pressure ventricular septal defects. *JAMA*, 188:949, 1964.

Lillehei, C. W.; Bobb, J. R. R.; and Visscher, M. B.: Effect of arteriovenous fistulas upon pulmonary arterial pressure, cardiac index, blood volume, and the extracellular fluid space. *Surg. Forum*, 1:275, 1950.

Lillehei, C. W.; Cohen, M.; Warden, H. F.; and Varco, R. L.: The direct vision intercardiac correction of congenital anomalies by controlled cross circulation; results in 32 patients with ventricular septal defects, tetralogy of Fallot, and atrioventricularis communis defects. *Surgery*, 38:11, 1955.

Lillehei, C. W.; Cohen, M.; Warden, H. E.; Ziegler, N. R.; and Varco, R. L.: The results of direct vision closure of ventricular septal defects in eight patients by means of controlled cross circulation. *Surg. Gynecol. Obstet.*, 101:447, 1955.

Linde, L. M.; Goldberg, S. J.; and Seigel, S.: The natural history of arrhythmias following septal defect repair. *J. Thorac. Cardiovasc.*

Surg., 48:303, 1964.

Linhart, J. W., and Razi, B.: Late systolic murmur: A clue to the diagnosis of aneurysm of the membranous ventricular septum. *Chest*, 60:283, 1971.

Lucas, R. V., Jr.; Adams, P., Jr.; Anderson, R. C.; Meyne, N. G.; Lillehei, C. W.; and Varco, R. L.: The natural history of isolated ventricular septal defect. A serial physiologic study. *Circulation*, 24:1372, 1961.

Luisada, A. A., and Liu, C. K.: Simple methods for recording intracardiac electrocardiograms and phonocardiograms during left or right heart catheterization. *Am. Heart J.*, 54:531, 1957.

Lynch, D. L.; Alexander, J. K.; Hersherger, K. L.; Mise, J.; Dennis, F. W.; and Cooley, D. A.: Congenital ventriculoatrial communication with anomalous tricuspid valve. *Am. J. Cardiol.*, 1:404, 1958.

Lyndfield, J.; Gasul, B. M.; Arcilla, R.; and Luam, L. L.: The natural history of ventricular septal defect in infancy and childhood. *Am. J. Med.*, 30:357, 1961.

McGinn, S., and White, P. D.: Progress in the recognition of congenital heart disease. *N. Engl. J. Med.*, 214:763, 1936.

Majka, M.; Ryan, J.; and Bondy, D. C.: Spontaneous closure of a ventricular septal defect. *Can. Med. Assoc. J.*, 82:317, 1960.

Mall, F. P.: Aneurysm of the membranous septum projecting into the right atrium. *Anat. Rec.*, 6:291, 1912.

Malm, J. R.; Blumenthal, S.; Jameson, A. G.; and Humphreys G. H.; II: Observations on coarctation of the aorta in infants, *Surgery*, 86:1, 1963.

Marquis, R. M.: Ventricular septal defect in early childhood. *Br. Heart J.*, 12:265, 1950.

Marshall, H. W.; Swan, H. J. C.; Burchell, H. B.; and Wood, F. H.: Effect of breathing oxygen on pulmonary artery pressure and pulmonary vascular resistance in patients with ventricular septal defect. *Circulation*, 23:241, 1961.

Marston, F. L.; Bradshaw, H. H.; and Meredith, J. H.; A genesis of the aortic isthmus. *Surgery*, 42:352, 1957.

Mason, D., and Hunter, W.: Localized congenital defects of the cardiac interventricular septum. *Am. J. Pathol.*, 13:835, 1937.

Mehrizi, A.; Hirsch, M. S.; and Taussig, H. B.: Congenital heart disease in the neonatal period. *J. Pediatr.*, 65:721, 1964.

Merrill, D. L.; Webster, C. A.; and Samson, P. C.: Congenital absence of the aortic isthmus. *J. Thorac. Surg.*, 33:311, 1957.

Mitchell, S. C.; Korones, S. B.; and Berendes, H. W.: Congenital heart disease in 56,109 births, incidence and natural history. *Circulation*, 43:323, 1971.

Montanini, N.: Di un raro meccanismo di completa riparazione in caso di difetto del setto interventricolare. *Med. Ital.*, 13:449, 1932.

Moore, D.; Vlad, P.; and Lambert, E. C.: Spontaneous closure of ventricular septal defect following cardiac failure in infancy. *J. Pediatr.*, 66:712, 1965.

Morgan, B. C.; Griffiths, S. P.; and Blumenthal, S.: Ventricular septal defect. I: Congestive heart failure in infancy. *Pediatrics*, 25:54, 1960.

Morgan, F. H., and Burchell, H. B.: Ventricular septal defect simulating patent ductus arteriosus. *Proc. Mayo Clin.*, 25:69, 1950.

Morrow, A. G., and Braunwald, N. S.: The surgical treatment of ventricular septal defect in infancy. The technique and results of pulmonary artery constriction. *Circulation*, 26:34, 1963.

———: The surgical treatment of ventricular septal defect in infancy. *Circulation*, 24:34, 1961.

Muir, D. C., and Brown, J. W.: Patent interventricular septum. *Arch. Dis. Child.*, 9:27, 1934.

Muller, W. H., Jr., and Dammann, J. F., Jr.: The treatment of certain congenital malformations of the heart by the creation of pulmonic stenosis to reduce pulmonary hypertension and excessive blood flow. *Surg. Gynecol. Obstet.*. 95:213, 1952.

Murphy, D. A.; Lemire, G. G.; Tessler, I.; and Dunn, G. L.: Correction of type B aortic arch interruption with ventricular and atrial defects in a three-day-old infant. *J. Thorac. Cardiovasc. Surg.*, 65:882, 1973.

Murray, G.: Closure of defects in the cardiac septa. *Am. Surg.*, 128:843, 1948.

Mustard, W. T., and Thomson, J. A.: Clinical experience with the artificial heart lung preparation. *Can. Med. Assoc. J.*, 76:4, 1957.

Nadas, A. S.: *Pediatric Cardiology*, W. B. Saunders Company, Philadelphia, 1957, p. 319.

————: The natural history of certain congenital cardiovascular manifestations. *Pediatrics,* 33:993, 1964.

Nadas, A. S.; Rudolph, A. M.; and Gross, R. E.: Editorial, Pulmonary arterial hypertension in congenital heart disease. *Circulation,* 33:1041, 1960.

Nadas, A. S.; Scott, L. P.; Hauck, A. J.; and Rudolph, A. M.: Spontaneous functional closing of ventricular septal defects. *N. Engl. J. Med.,* 264:309, 1961.

Nadas, A. S.; Van Der Hauwaer, L.; Huck, A. J.: and Gross, R. E.: Combined aortic and pulmonic stenosis. *Circulation,* 25:346, 1962.

Nadas, A. S.; Thilenius, O. G.; LaFarge, C. G.; and Hauck, A. J.: Ventricular septal defect with aortic regurgitation. *Circulation,* 24:862, 1964.

Naeye, R. L.: Arterial changes during the perinatal period. *Arch. Pathol.,* 71:12, 1961.

Naeye, R. L.: The pulmonary arterial bed in ventricular septal defect: Anatomic features in childhood. *Circulation,* 34:962, 1966.

Neilson, G.; Galea, E. G.; and Blunt, A.: Eisenmenger's syndrome and pregnancy. *Med. J. Aust.,* 1:431, 1971.

Neufeld, H. N.; Titus, J. L.; DuShane, I. W.; Burchell, H. B.; and Edwards, J. E.: Isolated ventricular septal defect of the persistent common atrioventricular canal type. *Circulation,* 23:685, 1961.

Nicholson, M. M.: Relative incidence of cardiac anomalies found in autopsies performed in Washington hospitals. Abstract 28th Annual Meeting of the Int. A. M. Museums. *J Tech Methods,* 15:100, 1936.

Nicoloff, D. M.; Zamora, R.; et al.: Transatrial closure of high-pressure, high-resistance ventricular septal defects. *J. Pediatr. Surg.,* 6:650, 1971.

Nogueira, C. Zimmerman, H. A.; and Kay, E. B.: Results of surgery for ventricular septal defects. *Am. J. Cardiol.,* 5:239, 1960.

Nordenstrom, B., and Ovenfors, C.: Septal defect between the left ventricle and the right atrium diagnosed by cardioangiography. *Acta. Radiol.,* 56:393, 1960.

Ober, W. B., and Moore, T. E., Jr.: Congenital cardiac malformation in the neonatal period. An autopsy study. *N. Engl. J. Med.,* 253:271, 1955.

Okada, R.; Glagov, S.; and Lev. M.: Relation of shunt flow and right ventricular pressure to heart valve structure in atrial septal defect. *Am. Heart J.,* 78:781, 1969.

Olsen, E. G. J., and Valentine, J. S.: Case report-anomalous bands in the heart. *Br. Heart J.,* 34:210, 1972.

Pagtakhan, R. D.; Hartmann, A. F.; Goldring, D.; and Kissane, J.: The valve-incompetent foramen ovale. *J. Pediatr.,* 71:848, 1967.

Patterson, M. W. H.: A radiopaque pulmonary artery band. *J. Thorac. Cardiovasc. Surg.,* 61:975, 1971.

Peacock, T. B.: *On Malformation of the Human Heart.* J. Churchill & Sons, London, 1866, p. 153.

Perry, C. B.: Congenital anomalies of the heart in elementary school children. *Arch. Dis. Child.,* 6:265, 1931.

————: Congenital heart disease as seen in elementary school children. *Bristol Med.-Chir. J.,* 48:41, 1931.

Perry, C. B., et al.: Discussion on course and management of congenital heart disease. *Proc. Roy. Soc. Med.,* 30:693, 1937.

Perry, E. L.; Burchell, H. B.; and Edwards, J. F.: Congenital communication between the left ventricle and the right atrium: co-existing ventricular septal defect and double tricuspid orifice. *Proc. Mayo Clin.,* 24:198, 1949.

Philpott, N. W.: Relative incidence of congenital cardiac abnormalities in Montreal hospitals. *J. Tech. Methods,* 15:96, 1931.

Pickering, D., and Keith, J. D.: Systolic clicks with ventricular septal defects: A sign of aneurysm of ventricular septum? *Br. Heart J.,* 33:538, 1971.

Pieroni, P.; Bell, B. B.; Krovetz, L. J.; Varghese, P. J.; and Rowe, R. D.: Ausculatory recognition of aneurysm of the membranous ventricular septum associated with small ventricular septal defect. *Circulation,* 44:733, 1971.

Plauth, W. H.; Braunwald, E.; Rockoff, S. D.; Mason, D. T.; and Morrow, A. G.: Ventricular septal defect and aortic regurgitation. *Am. J. Med.,* 39:552, 1965.

Pool, P. E.; Averill, K. H.; and Vogel, J. H. K.: Effect of ligation of left pulmonary artery at birth on maturation of pulmonary vascular bed. *Med. Thorac.,* 19:362, 1963.

Rannels, H. W., and Propst, J. H.: Incidence of congenital cardiac

anomalies found at autopsies performed in Hospital of University of Pennsylvania. *J. Tech. Methods,* 17:113, 1937.

Reeves, J. T.; Grover, E. B.; and Grover, R. F.: Pulmonary circulation and oxygen transport in lambs at high altitude. *J. Appl. Physiol.,* 18 (May), 1963.

Rehder, K.; Kirklin, J. W.; and Theye, R. A.; Physiologic studies following surgical correction of atrial septal defect and similar lesions. *Circulation,* 26:1302, 1962.

Rein, J. G.; Freed, M. D.; Norwood, W. I.; and Castaneda, A. R.: Early and late results of closure of ventricular septal defect in infancy. *Ann. Thorac. Surg.,* 24:19, 1977.

Richards, D. W., and Cohn, I.: Interventricular septal defect, pulmonary artery aneurysm with thrombosis, "cyanose tardive," and paradoxical systemic arterial embolizations. *Am. Heart J.,* 47:313, 1954.

Riley, R. L.; Himmelstein, A.; Motley, H. L.; Weiner, H. M.; and Cournand, A.: Studies of the pulmonary circulation at rest and during exercise in normal individuals and in patients with chronic pulmonary disease, *Am. J. Physiol.,* 152:372, 1948.

Ritter, D. G.; Feldt, R. H.; Weidman, W. H.; and DuShane, S. W.: Ventricular septal defect. *Circulation* (Suppl. 111), 32:42, 1965.

Roberts, J. T.: Incidence of congenital heart disease in Charity Hospital of New Orleans. *J. Tech. Methods,* 17:108, 1937.

Roberts, W. C.; Morrow, A. C.; Masson, D. T.; and Braunwald, E.: Spontaneous closure of ventricular septal defect. Anatomic proof in an adult with tricuspid atresia. *Circulation,* 27:90, 1963.

Rodbard, S.; Shaffer, A.; and Brostoff, P.: Contraction of the pulmonary infundibular ring as a mode of stenosis in man. *J. Lab. Clin. Med.,* 44:917, 1954.

Roe, B. B.: A simplified technique for closure of interventricular septal defects. *J. Thorac. Cardiovasc. Surg.,* 40:232, 1960.

Roger, H.: Recherches cliniques sur la communication congénitale des deux coeurs, par inocclusion du septum interventriculaire. *Bull. Acad. Méd., Paris,* 8:1074, 1189, 1879.

Rogers, H. M.; Evans, I. C.; and Domeier, L. H: Congenital aneurysm of the membranous portion of the ventricular septum: report of two cases. *Am. Heart J.,* 43:781, 1952.

Rogers, H. M., and Rudolph, C. C.: Congenital ventricular septal defects with acquired complete heart block. *Am. Heart J.,* 41:770, 1951.

Rose, V.: Personal communication, 1964.

Rose, V.; Boyd, A. R.; and Ashton, T.: Incidence of heart disease in children in the city of Toronto. *Can. Med. Assoc. J.,* 9:95, 1964.

Rosenberg, S. Z., and Braun, K.: Ventricular septal defect with aortic insufficiency, acute rheumatic carditis and Asian influenza, *Am. J. Cardiol.,* 7:273, 1961.

Rosenquist, G. C., and Sweeney, L. J.: The membranous ventricular septum in the normal heart. *Johns Hopkins Med. J.,* 135:9, 1974.

Rossall, R. E.; Shiel, F. O'M.; and Shoesmith, J.: Coarctation of the aorta with patent ductus arteriosus and multiple intracardiac defects. *Am. J. Cardiol.,* 2:502, 1958.

Rossall, R. E.; and Thompson, H.: Formation of new vascular channels in the lungs of a patient with secondary pulmonary hypertension. *J. Pathol. Bact.,* 76:593, 1958.

Rowe, R. D.: Neonatal pulmonary hypertension. In Oliver, T. K. (ed.): *Adaptation to Extrauterine Life.* Report of the 31st Ross Conference on Pediatric Research, Columbus, Ohio, Ross Laboratories, 1959, p. 30.

Rowe, R. D., and Cleary, T. E.: Congenital cardiac malformation in the newborn period. Frequency in a children's hospital. *Can. Med. Assoc. J.,* 83:299, 1960.

Rowe, R. D., and James, L. S.: The normal pulmonary arterial pressure in the first year of life. *J. Pediatr.,* 51:1, 1957.

Rowe, R. D.: Angiocardiography in the prognosis for young infants in congestive failure with ventricular septal defect: the value of the defect/ascending aorta diameter ratio. In Barratt-Boyes, B. G.; Neutze, J. M.; and Harris, E. A. (eds.): *Heart Disease in Infancy: Diagnosis and Surgical Treatment.* Churchill Livingstone, Edinburgh, 1973, p. 119.

Rowe, R. D., and Lowe, J. B.: Auscultation in the diagnosis of persistent ductus arteriosus in infancy: a study of 50 patients. *New Zeal. Med. J.,* 63:195, 1964.

Rowe, R. D., and Trusler, G. A.: Considerations pronostiques chez les enfants opérés ou non-opérés durant la première année de la vie. *Coeur,* 8 (No. 3, Numéro spécial). Journées internationales de cardiologie pédiatrique. October 1976, Bendor.

Rowe, R. D.; Vlad, P.; and Keith, J. D.: A typical tetralogy of Fallot. *Circulation*, **12**:230, 1955.

Rudolph, A. M.: The infant with heart disease. *Pediatrics*, **33**:990, 1964.

Rudolph, A. M.; Drorbaugh, J. E.; Auld, P. A. M.; Rudolph, A. J.; Nadas, A. S.; Smith, C. A.; and Hubbell, J. P.: Studies on the circulation in the neonatal period. The circulation in the respiratory distress syndrome. *Pediatrics*, **27**:551, 1961.

Rudolph, A. M.; Mayer, F. E.; Nadas, A. S.; and Gross, R. E.: Patent ductus arteriosus. A clinical and hemodynamic study of 23 patients in the first year of life. *Pediatrics*, **22**:892, 1958.

Samaan, H. A.: Surgery of ventricular septal defect and pulmonary vascular resistance. *Thorax*, **25**:665, 1970.

Sandoe, E.: Congenital isolated ventricular septal defect: Haemodynamics, clinical features and prognosis after the age of 2 years. (*Thesis*) Munksgaard, Copenhagen, p. 136, 1963.

Sapire, D. W., and Black, I. F. S.: Echocardiographic detection of aneurysms of the interventricular septum associated with ventricular septal defect. A method of non-invasive diagnosis and follow-up. *Am. J. Cardiol.*, **36**:797, 1975.

Sarnoff, S. J.: Myocardial contractility as described by ventricular function curves: observations on Starling's law of the heart. *Physiol. Rev.*, **35**:106, 1955.

Scott, R. C.: The electrocardiographic diagnosis of right ventricular hypertrophy: correlation with the anatomic findings. *Am. Heart J.*, **60**:659, 1960.

———: The electrocardiogram in atrial septal defects and atrioventricular cushion defects. (Annot.) *Am. Heart J.*, **62**:712, 1961.

Scott, R. C.; McGuire, J.; Kaplan, S.; Fowler, N. O.; Green, R. S.; Gordon, Z.; Shabetai, R.; and Davolos, D. D.: The syndrome of ventricular septal defect with aortic insufficiency. *Am. J. Cardiol.*, **2**:530, 1958.

Seaman, W. B., and Goldring, D.: Coarctation of the aorta with patent ductus arteriosus. *J. Pediatr.*, **47**:588, 1955.

Seidel, J. F.: Index musei anatomici kiliensis kiel. C. F. Mohr, Kiliae, p. 61, 1818.

Selzer, A.: Defect of the ventricular septum: Summary of the twelve cases and review of the literature. *Arch. Intern. Med.*, **84**:798, 1949.

Selzer, A., and Laqueur, G. L.: The Eisenmenger complex and its relation to the uncomplicated defect of the ventricular septum: review of 35 autopsied cases of Eisenmenger's complex, including two new cases. *Arch. Intern. Med.*, **87**:218, 1951.

Senning, A.: Ventricular fibrillation during extracorporeal circulation used as a method to prevent air embolus and to facilitate intracardiac operation. *Acta Chir. Scand. (Supp.)*, **17**:1, 1952.

Shah, P.; Singh, W. S. A.; Rose, V.; and Keith, J. D.: Incidence of bacterial endocarditis in ventricular septal defects. *Circulation*, **34**:127, 1966.

Shaher, R. M.; Fowler, R. S.; Kidd, B. S. L.; Moes, C. A. F.; and Keith, J. D.: Spontaneous closure of a ventricular septal defect in a case of complete transposition of the great vessels. *Can. Med. Assoc. J.*, **93**:1037, 1065.

Shepard, J. T.; Semler, H. J.; Helmholz, H. F., Jr.; and Wood, E. H.: Effects of infusion of acetylcholine on pulmonary vascular resistance in patients with pulmonary hypertension and congenital heart disease, *Circulation*, **20**:381, 1959.

Sherman, F. E.: *An Atlas of Congenital Heart Disease*. Lea & Febiger, Philadelphia, 1963.

Shumacker, H. B., Jr.; Kajikuri, H.; Grice, P.; Rodriguez, R.; Rikeri, A.; Moore, T. C.; and Siderys, H.: Comparative experimental study of aortic grafts. *Surgery*, **41**:943, 1957.

Siegel, J. H.: A study of the mechanisms of cardiovascular adaptation to an acute ventricular septal defect. *J. Thorac. Cardiovasc. Surg.*, **41**:524, 1961.

Sigmann, J. M.; Stern, A. M.; and Sloan, H. E.: Surgical closure of ventricular septal defect in infants. *Am. J. Cardiol.*, **13**:13, 1964.

Sigmann, J. M.; Stern, A. M.; and Sloan, H. B.: Early surgical correction of large ventricular septal defects. *Pediatrics*, **39**:4, 1967.

Simmons, R. L.; Moller, J. H.; and Edwards, J. E.: Anatomic evidence for spontaneous closure of ventricular septal defect. *Circulation*, **34**:38, 1966.

Skirpan, P. J.; McCormack, L. J.; and Sones Mason, F., Jr.: Coarctation of the aorta associated with a defect of the muscular portion of the interventricular septum in an infant, *Cleveland Clin. Quart.*, **23**:36, 1956.

Sodi-Pallares, D.; Pileggi, F.; Cisneros, F.; Ginefra, P.; Portello, B.; Medrano, G. A.; and Bisteni, A.: The mean manifest electrical axis of the ventricular activation process (AQRS) in congenital heart disease; a new approach in electrocardiographic diagnosis. *Am. Heart J.*, **55**:681, 1958.

Somerville, J.; Brandao, A.; and Ross, D. N.: Aortic regurgitation with ventricular septal defect. *Circulation*, **31**:317, 1970.

Soto, B.; Bargeron, L. M., Jr.; and Barnes, G. T.: Special projections for angiographic study of various congenital heart malformations. Scientific Exhibit. Program for American Heart Association, 49th Scientific Sessions, 1976, p. 169.

Soulie, R.; Corone, R.; Bouchard, F.; and Cornue, C.: Fermeture spontanee d'une communication interventriculaire. *Arch. Mal. Coeur Vaiss.*, **53**:802, 1960.

Spencer, F. C.; Bahnson, H. T.; and Neill, C. A.: The treatment of aortic regurgitation associated with a ventricular septal defect. *J. Thorac. Cardiovasc. Surg.*, **43**:222, 1962.

Spencer, F. C.; Doyle, E. F.; Danilowicz, D. A.; Bahnson, H. T.; and Weldon, C. S.: Long-term evaluation of aortic valvuloplasty for aortic insufficiency and ventricular septal defect. *J. Thorac. Cardiovasc. Surg.*, **65**:1, January, 1973.

Spitzer, A.: Ueber den Bauplan des normelen und missbildeten Herzens: Versuch einer phylogenetischen theorie. *Virchow Arch. Pathol. Anat.*, **243**:81, 1923.

Stallman, M.; Kaplan, S.; Helmsworth, J. A.; Clark, L. C.: and Scott, H. W.: Syndrome of left ventricular–right atrial shunt resulting from high interventricular septal defect associated with defective septal leaflet of the tricuspid valve. *Circulation*, **12**:813, 1955.

Stanton, R. E., and Fyler, D. C.: The natural history of pulmonary hypertension in children with ventricular septal defects assessed by serial right-heart catheterization. *Pediatrics*, **27**:621, 1961.

Starr, A.; Menashe, V.; and Dotter, C.: Surgical correction of aortic insufficiency associated with ventricular septal defect. *Surg. Gynecol. Obstet.*, **3**:71, 1960.

Steinberg, I.: Diagnosis of congenital aneurysm of the ventricular septum during life. *Br. Heart J.*, **19**:8, 1957.

Stewart, M.: Congenital interruption of the aortic arch, *Arch. Dis. Child.*, **23**:63, 1948.

Streetar, G. L.: Developmental horizons in human embryos. Descriptions of age groups XV, XVI, XVII and XVIII. *Carnegie Inst. Contrib. Embryol.*, **32**:133, 1948.

Subramanian, S.; Wagner, H.; Vlad, P.; and Lambert, E.: Surface-induced deep hypothermia in cardiac surgery. *J. Pediatr. Surg.*, **6**:612, 1971.

Subramanian, S.: Primary definitive intracardiac operations in infants: ventricular septal defects. In Kirkland, J. W. (ed.): *Advances in Cardiovascular Surgery*. Grune & Stratton, New York, 1973, p. 141.

Subramanian, S.: Ventricular septal defect: Problems of repair in infancy. In Kidd, B. S. L., and Rowe, R. D. (eds.): *The Child with Congenital Heart Disease After Surgery*. Futura Publishing Co., Inc., Mount Kisco, N.Y., 1976, p. 11.

Swann, W. C.: Interventricular septal defect complicated by pregnancy. *Am. Heart J.*, **43**:900, 1952.

Szypulski, J. T.: Study of congenital heart disease at Philadelphia General Hospital. *J. Tech. Methods*, **17**:119, 1937.

Tandon, R., and Edwards, J. E.: Aneurysm-like formations in relation to membranous ventricular septum. *Circulation*, **47**:1089, 1973.

Tatsuno, K.; Konno, S.; and Sakakibara, S.: Ventricular septal defect with aortic insufficiency. *Am. Heart J.*, **85**:13, 1973.

Taufic, M., and Lewis, F. J.: A device for the experimental creation of ventricular septal defects. *J. Thorac. Surg.*, **25**:413, 1953.

Taussig, H. B.: *Congenital Malformations of the Heart*. The Commonwealth Fund, New York, 1947.

Taussig, H. B., and Semans, J. H.: Severe aortic insufficiency in association with a congenital malformation of the heart of the Eisenmenger type. *Bull. Hopkins Hosp.*, **66**:156, 1940.

Terplan, K., and Sanes, S.: The incidence of congenital heart lesions in infancy. *J. Tech. Methods*, **15**:86, 1936.

Theye, R. A., and Kirklin, J. W.: Physiologic studies following surgical correction of ventricular septal defect. *Circulation*, **27**:530, 1963.

Titus, J. L.: Daugherty, G. W.; and Edwards, J. E.: Anatomy of the atrioventricular conduction system in ventricular septal defect. *Circulation*, **28**:72, 1963.

Treasure, R. L.; Hopeman, A. R.; Jahnke, E. J.; Green, D. C.; and Czarnecki, S. W.: Ventricular septal defect with aortic insufficiency. *Ann. Thorac. Surg.*, **12**:411, 1971.

Trusler, G. A.: Repair of ventricular septal defect with aortic insufficiency. *J. Thorac. Cardiovasc. Surg.*, **66**:394, 1973.

Trusler, G. A., and Izukawa, T.: Interrupted aortic arch and ventricular septal defect. Direct repair through a median sternotomy incision in a 13-day-old infant. *J. Thorac. Cardiovasc. Surg.*, **69**:126, 1975.

Trusler, G. A.; Moes, C. A. F.; and Kidd, B. S. L.: Repair of ventricular septal defect with aortic insufficiency. *J. Thorac. Cardiovasc. Surg.*, **66**:3, 1973.

Trusler, G. A., and Mustard, W. T.: A method of banding the pulmonary artery for large isolated ventricular septal defect with and without transposition of the great arteries. *Ann. Thorac. Surg.*, **13**:351, 1972.

Tyrrell, M. J.; Kidd, B. S. L.; and Keith, J. D.: Diagnosis of tetralogy of Fallot in the acyanotic phase. *Circulation*, **42**:(Suppl. III), 113, 1970.

Van Der Hauwaert, L., and Nadas, A. S.: Auscultatory findings in patients with a small ventricular septal defect. *Circulation*, **23**:886, 1961.

Van Praagh, R.: Personal communication, 1965.

Van Praagh, R., and McNamara, J. J.: Anatomic types of ventricular septal defect with aortic insufficiency. *Am. Heart J.*, **75**:604, 1968.

Varghese, P. J.; Allen, J. R.; Rosenquist, G. C.; and Rowe, R. D.: Natural history of ventricular septal defect with right-sided aortic arch. *Br. Heart J.*, **32**:537, 1970.

Varghese, P. J.; Izukawa, T.; Celermajer, J.; Simon, A.; and Rowe, R. D.: Aneurysm of the membranous ventricular septum: A method of spontaneous closure of small ventricular septal defects. *Am. J. Cardiol.*, **24**:531, 1969.

Vogel, J. H. K.; Grover, R. F.; and Blount, S. G.: Pathophysiologic correlations in patients with ventricular septal defect and increased pulmonary vascular resistance (abstract). *Am. J. Cardiol.*, **19**:154, 1967.

Vogel, J. H. K.; McNamara, D. G.; and Blount, S. G.: Role of hypoxia in determining pulmonary vascular resistance in infants with ventricular septal defects. *Am. J. Cardiol.*, **20**:346, 1967.

Wada, J., and Iwa, T.: Two-stage treatment of ventricular septal defect with pulmonary hypertension. *Ann. Thorac. Surg.*, **8**:415, 1969.

Wade, G., and Wright, J. P.: Spontaneous closure of ventricular septal defects. *Lancet*, **1**:737, 1963.

Wagenvoort, C. A.; Neufeld, H. N.; DuShane, J. W.; and Edwards, J. E.; The pulmonary arterial tree in ventricular septal defect.

Circulation, **23**:740, 1961.

Walker, W. J.: Spontaneous closure of traumatic ventricular septal defect. *Am. J. Cardiol.*, **15**:263, 1965.

Walker, W. J.; Garcia-Gonzalez, E.; Hall, R. J.; Czarnecki, S. W.; Franklin, R. B.; Das, S. K.; and Cheitlin, M. D.: Interventricular septal defect: Analysis of 415 catheterized cases, ninety with serial hemodynamic studies. *Circulation*, **31**:54, 1965.

Weber, F. P.: Congenital heart disease. *Br. J. Child. Dis.*, **15**:113, 1918.

Weidman, W. H.; Blount, S. G.; DuShane, J. W.; Gersony, W. M.; Hayes, C. J.; and Nadas, A. S.: Clinical course in ventricular septal defect. *Circulation*, **56**:(Suppl. 1), 1–56, 1977.

Weidman, W. H.; DuShane, J. W.; and Kincaid, O. W.: Observations concerning progressive pulmonary vascular obstruction in children with ventricular septal defects. *Am. Heart J.*, **65**:148, 1963.

Weisman, D., and Kesten, H. D.: Absence of transverse aortic arch with defects of cardiac septum. *Am. J. Dis. Child.*, **76**:326, 1948.

Weiss, E.: Congenital ventricular septal defect in man, aged 79. *Arch. Intern. Med.*, **39**:705, 1927.

White, P. D.: *Heart Disease*, 4th ed. The Macmillan Co., New York, 1951.

Willius, F. A., and Keys, T. E.: *Cardiac Classics*. C. V. Mosby Co., St. Louis, 1941.

Willman, V. L.; Cooper, T.; Mudd, J. G.; and Hanlon, C. R.: Treatment of ventricular septal defect by constriction of pulmonary artery. *Arch. Surg. (Chicago)*, **85**:745, 1962.

Wood, P.: *Diseases of the Heart and Circulation*, 2nd ed. Eyre and Spottiswoode, London, 1956.

———: Aortic stenosis. *Am. J. Cardiol.*, **1**:553, 1958.

———: The Eisenmenger syndrome. II. *Br. Med. J.*, **2**:755, 1958.

———: As quoted by Bloomfield, D. K.: Natural history of ventricular septal defect in patients surviving infancy. *Circulation*, **29**:914, 1964.

Wood, P.; Magidson, O.; and Wilson, P. A. O.: Ventricular septal defect, with note on acyanotic Fallot's tetralogy. *Br. Heart J.*, **16**:387, 1954.

Wood, P. H.: Congenital heart disease: review of its clinical aspects in light of experience gained by means of modern techniques. *Br. Med. J.*, **2**:639, 1950.

———: Pulmonary hypertension. *Br. Med. Bull.*, **8**:348, 1952.

Yerushalmy, J.: The California Child Health and Development Studies. Study design and some illustrative findings on congenital heart disease. Congenital Malformation. In Fraser, F. C., and McKusick, V. A. (eds.): *Congenital-Malformations*. Proceedings of the Third International Conference. The Hague, Netherland, 1969. Excerpta Medica, Amsterdam, 1970.

Young, D., and Mark, H.: Fate of the patient with the Eisenmenger syndrome. *Am. J. Cardiol.*, **28**:658, 1971.

22

Atrial Septal Defect: Ostium Secundum, Ostium Primum, and Atrioventricularis Communis (Common AV Canal)

John D. Keith

HE ATRIAL septal defect has assumed a position of prominence and great interest in the congenital heart field because of its prevalence and because it can now be operated on so successfully. There have been several excellent reviews on this anomaly in the past by McGinn and White (1933), Roesler (1934), Bedford and associates (1941), Taussig (1947), Dexter (1956), DuShane and associates (1960), Besterman (1961), Hastreiter and associates (1962), and others, covering several decades. Thus, in the past, the postmortem data and clinical findings have been studied in detail, but more recently the hemodynamics have been thoroughly investigated (Van Meirop and associates, 1962; Hoffman et al., 1965; Burchell, 1971; Parisi and Nadas, 1971; Feldt, 1976).

This chapter will deal with atrial septal defect, ostium secundum, ostium primum, and atrioventricularis communis (common AV canal). (See Figure 22–1.)

Ostium Secundum. This defect may be divided into six subgroups (see Figure 22–2). The central defect is most common, comprising two-thirds of the ostium secundum group. The inferior vena caval type is next in frequency—approximately a quarter of the group. The superior vena caval or sinus venosus type is less frequent, but when it occurs it is usually associated with anomalous veins from the upper and middle lung fields.

The endocardial cushion defects are in a special group and will be dealt with separately under ostium primum and atrioventricularis communis.

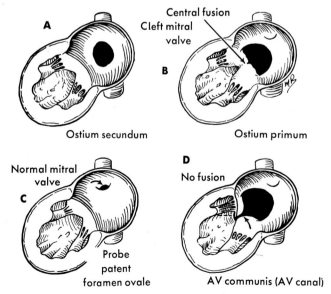

Figure 22-1. Chief types of atrial septal openings. Each group has many variations. See text for details.

A Cleft mitral valve Central fusion

Ostium secundum

B Ostium primum

Normal mitral valve

C Probe patent foramen ovale

D No fusion

AV communis (AV canal)

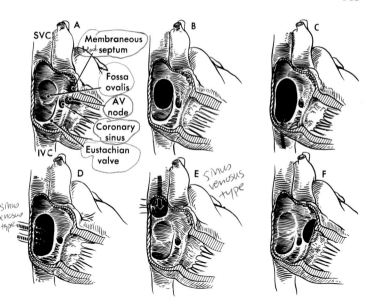

Figure 22-2. Anatomic types of atrial septal defect. *A.* Normal atrial septum, patent foramen ovale. *B.* Central fossa ovalis defect. *C.* Inferior caval defect (large eustachian valve). *D.* Large inferior vena cava defect (no posterior margin). *E.* Superior caval defect. Anomalous right upper and middle pulmonary veins. *F.* Atrioventricular defect. (Modified from Bedford, D. E.; Sellors, T. H.; Sommerville, W.; Belcher, J. R.; and Besterman, E. M. M.: Atrial septal defect and its surgical treatment. *Lancet,* **1**:1255, 1957.)

Mitral   Tricuspid

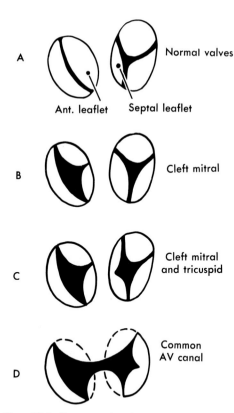

Figure 22-3. Shown are the mitral and tricuspid valves. *A.* Normal valves. *B.* Cleft mitral but normal tricuspid. *C.* Cleft mitral and cleft tricuspid. *D.* Complete common atrioventricular canal with completely cleft mitral and tricuspid valves. (Modified from Bedford, D. E.; Sellors, T. H.; Sommerville, W.; Belcher, J. R.; and Besterman, E. M. M.: Atrial septal defect and its surgical treatment. *Lancet,* **1**:1255, 1957.)

Ostium Primum (Figure 22–1*B*). There is an opening in the lower portion of the septum that may be either large or small; the lower margin of this opening is valve tissue at the point of meeting of the mitral and tricuspid valves. There is usually a cleft in the mitral valve. Developmentally this category is described as a partial endocardial cushion defect.

Atrioventricularis Communis (Common AV Canal) (Figure 22–1*D*). This consists of an opening in the lower portion of the atrial septum, as in the ostium primum, but is associated with a failure of fusion of the valve tissue at the center of the atrioventricular canal resulting in a variety of atrial and ventricular septal defects and mitral and tricuspid valve defects.

The general arrangements of the mitral and tricuspid valves in the normal, in ostium primum, and in atrioventricularis communis are shown in Figure 22–3. Other types of combinations of atrial septal defects may be found. There may be multiple openings in the septum, complete absence of the interatrial septum, or combinations and degrees of ostium secundum and ostium primum.

There may be a great variety of congenital heart anomalies associated with atrial septal defects or with a pathologic degree of patency of the foramen ovale. These may be divided into two groups: (1) those that are usually noncyanotic, which would include ventricular septal defect, patent ductus arteriosus, coarctation of the aorta, and defects of the mitral valve, and (2) the usually cyanotic conditions, such as pulmonary stenosis, pulmonary valve atresia, tricuspid atresia, transposition of the great vessels, tetralogy of Fallot, anomalous pulmonary veins (partial or complete), and Ebstein's disease (see MacKrell and Ibanez, 1958). (See Table 22–1.)

A patent foramen ovale is not an uncommon finding at any postmortem. This valvelike structure closes functionally shortly after birth but may maintain a slotlike opening for life (Figure 22–1*C*). In

Table 22–1. ATRIAL SEPTAL DEFECTS, INCIDENCE OF SUBGROUPS, THE HOSPITAL FOR SICK CHILDREN, TORONTO

DEFECT		NUMBER OF CASES	PERCENT OF TOTAL
Ostium secundum		561	53
Ostium primum		171	16
Ostium primum with assoc. defects		21	2
Atrioventricularis communis		267	27
Atrioventricularis communis with assoc. defects		20	2
	Total	1075	100
Ostium secundum			
Isolated form			68.4
With pulmonary stenosis			10.0
With partial anomalous pulmonary vein drainage			7.0
With mitral stenosis			1.0
With rheumatic mitral insufficiency			0.3
With ventricular septal defect			5.0
With patent ductus arteriosus			3.0
With coarctation of the aorta			0.3
Other			5.0
	Total		100.0

one postmortem series it was found to occur in 17 percent of individuals with otherwise normal hearts. It is, therefore, not considered a pathologic occurrence. It may, however, be forced open by other defects, such as pulmonary stenosis, tricuspid atresia, and Ebstein's disease, and then it contributes to the functional pathology of the anomaly concerned (Tandon and Edwards, 1974) (Table 22–2).

Table 22–2. POSTMORTEM INCIDENCE OF ATRIAL SEPTAL DEFECT IN HEART ANOMALIES USUALLY CYANOTIC

ANOMALY	PERCENT
Tricuspid atresia	33
Common ventricle	33
Tetralogy of Fallot	17
Transposition of great vessels	12
Pulmonary atresia	0
Pulmonary stenosis with normal aortic root	8
Truncus arteriosus	0

It is the purpose of this chapter to deal chiefly with ostium secundum, ostium primum, and atrioventricularis communis and briefly to consider the association with patent ductus arteriosus, coarctation of the aorta, ventricular septal defect, and mitral valve defects as well as pulmonary hypertension, pulmonary stenosis, and partial anomalous pulmonary vein drainage. Where atrial openings occur with cyanotic groups, they will be dealt with separately in other chapters.

Prevalence

Among adults Bedford and associates (1941) and Brown (1950) reported that the atrial septal defect is the most common congenital anomaly of the heart. This view was also supported by Wood and coworkers (1954), who found it was first in frequency and comprised 17 percent of their total cases of congenital heart disease. It should be pointed out that its incidence is not as common in any age group as the bicuspid aortic valve, which occurs once in every 100 routine autopsies. (See Chapters 1 and 38.)

At the Toronto Hospital for Sick Children, Rose (1976) reports that out of 15,004 children with congenital heart disease those in the atrial septal defect category accounted for 11 percent of the total and occurred once in every 1548 live births.

There are also a number of cases that do not present with sufficient signs or symptoms to lead to medical consultation in the first decade of life and are later recognized for the first time in their teens or twenties.

In the total atrial septal defect group, ostium secundum occurs in 53 percent of cases, ostium primum in 18 percent, and atrioventricularis communis in 29 percent. These figures are in the same range as those of other reports in the literature (Cooley, 1960; Parisi and Nadas, 1971).

Familial Occurrence

Ostium Secundum and Prolonged Atrioventricular Conduction Time. Bizarro and coworkers at the Mayo Clinic (1969) report the familial occurrence of atrial septal defects with prolonged atrioventricular conduction times in the electrocardiogram. Sixteen members of a family had atrial septal defects, 11 of whom had evidence of prolonged atrioventricular conduction time in the electrocardiograms. Five other members of this family had prolonged AV conduction without atrial septal defects. Their pedigree suggests that the syndrome of atrial septal defects with prolonged P-R interval is a manifestation of a single mutant autosomal gene with a high degree of penetrance. The usual type of atrial septal defect is sporadic with little likelihood of recurrence in subsequent sibs or children. However, when the defect is accompanied by a long P-R interval, the genetic prognosis is dramatically changed and the risk is almost 50 percent that the condition will recur in subsequent sibs or children of affected persons.

Familial Atrial Septal Defects of the AV Canal Variety. Yao and associates, in 1968, presented data of four cases in one sibship. Also, in 1968, Emanuel and coworkers carried out a study of 92 cases of atrioventricular septal defect. Nineteen percent of the 92 propositi had one or more relatives with congenital heart disease. Only three of these, however, had relatives with concordant lesions. (See also Table 9–1.)

Holt-Oram Syndrome. Anomalies of the osseous system occurring in conjunction with an atrial septal defect were first reported by Oppenheimer and colleagues in 1949. In 1960, Holt and Oram elaborated on the association and reported four members of the same family with such a combination of lesions. The disorder is transmitted as an autosomal dominant (Nora and Fraser, 1974). These children can have their atrial septal defects corrected in the usual manner. However, a number of authors have reported a high incidence of rhythm abnormalities in these patients.

Pathology

Ostium Secundum. At postmortem the heart appears generally enlarged. The right atrium is distended. The right ventricle shows an enlarged cavity, considerably larger than the left ventricle. The right ventricular wall is hypertrophied to a moderate degree. The left ventricular wall may be of normal thickness, but in some cases, particularly those that have any mitral insufficiency, the left ventricular wall may be thicker than normal and thicker than the right ventricular wall. The pulmonary artery is almost invariably larger than the aorta, though occasionally they are equal, and rarely the aorta is larger than the pulmonary artery in adults. In adults, the atrial septal defect varies from 1 to 4 cm in diameter, the average defect usually being about 2 cm (Edwards, 1953). It is commonly slightly elliptic. In infants and children we have found the defect varies from 2 to 4 mm up to 15 by 17 mm in size, being somewhat smaller than the opening in atrioventricularis communis or ostium primum. When the opening is 2 by 2 cm or more, the two atria are considered to be functioning as a common atrium (Dexter, 1956).

The defect may be simply a failure of the valve of the foramen ovale with broadening of the opening. It may take the form of fenestrations of the septum. Occasionally, the opening may be high up near the entrance of the superior vena cava. Where this is the case, it is almost invariably associated with partial anomalous pulmonary vein drainage with one or both of the pulmonary veins entering the right atrium or

superior vena cava (see Chapter 32). In such cases it seems probable that the anomalous veins maintained an abnormal atrial opening in the upper portion of the septum during embryologic development and resulted in its continued patency in postnatal life.

Table 22–3.　TYPE OF ATRIAL SEPTAL DEFECT*

Foramen ovale defect	6%
Central fossa ovalis	62%
Superior vena cava	6%
Inferior vena cava	24%
Total (superior and inferior) (common atrium)	2%

* Data from Bedford and Besterman (1963).

There may be combinations of defects in the atrial septum as in Table 22–3. Ostium secundum may occur with a great variety of other malformations of the heart. Probably the most important of these is prolapse of the mitral valve. Polysplenia may occasionally coexist. Cooksey (1970) reported calcification of the tricuspid valve in a case of atrial septal defect in a man 44 years old.

Endocardial Cushion Defects: Ostium Primum and Atrioventricularis Communis. In 1955 Watkins and Gross suggested the term *endocardial cushion defects* to include all anomalies resulting from abnormal development of the endocardial cushions. Van Mierop and colleagues (1962) have indicated the natural course of development of the endocardial cushions and the periods in fetal life when abnormalities may occur. A useful classification has been obtained by Feldt (1976).

The partial form is referred to as ostium primum and consists of an opening in the lower portion of the atrial septum that may be either large or small. The lower margin of this opening is the valve tissue at the point of meeting of the mitral and tricuspid valves. A cleft in the anterior leaf of the mitral valve is commonly present, but the tricuspid and ventricular septa are usually intact.

The more severe form of endocardial cushion defect is a persistent atrioventricularis communis (common AV canal), which is characterized by a defect in the lower part of the atrial septum and an associated defect in the proximal part of the ventricular septum with abnormalities of the atrioventricular valves. There are various subgroups described by Van Mierop (1962). The most common arrangement is to have both atrial and ventricular septal defects with a cleft tricuspid and cleft mitral valve. The next in frequency is an intact tricuspid valve associated with the atrial and ventricular septal defects and a cleft mitral valve. Next in order is a ventricular defect but no atrial defect, a cleft mitral but intact tricuspid valve. There may be an atrial septal defect but no ventricular septal defect, a mitral cleft but an intact tricuspid valve. A rare case is a left-ventricle-to-right-atrial defect with a cleft tricuspid but normal mitral valve. (See Figures 22–4 and 22–5.)

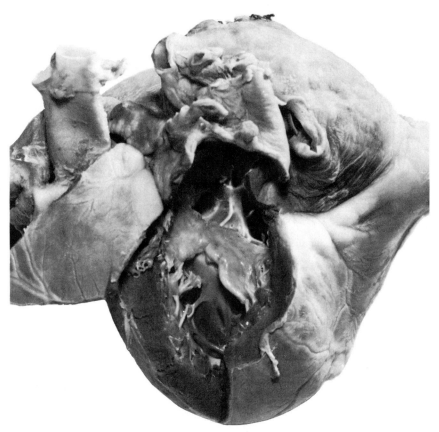

Figure 22-4. A. P., aged five years. Ostium primum. The left ventricle is shown with a cleft, incompetent mitral valve.

Atrio-ventricularis Communis

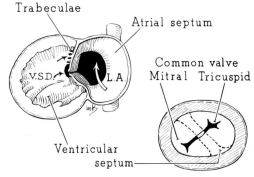

Figure 22-5. Diagrammatic illustration of atrioventricularis communis showing a large atrial septal defect, a moderate-sized ventricular septal defect partially obstructed by trabeculae, and a common atrioventricular valve.

At The Hospital for Sick Children, Toronto, there have been 287 cases of atrioventricularis communis recognized clinically, surgically, or at autopsy. The pulmonary artery is nearly always larger than the aorta, and the right ventricular capacity is greatly increased. The wall is usually as thick as or thicker than that of the left ventricle just below the pulmonary valve in two-thirds of the hearts. The others have a thick wall in this area, so that all cases show an external fullness in the region of the infundibulum that can usually be recognized radiologically in the plain x-ray of the heart or by angiocardiogram. This feature may be of value diagnostically. The right atrium is large, and the pulmonary artery branches are dilated.

Thus, anatomically, at postmortem there is evidence of a shunt from left atrium to right atrium with gross overloading of the right side of the heart and pulmonary circulation. The hemodynamics may be altered by various valve anomalies.

The atrial septal defect in most instances is a large one in the lower portion of the septum with no tissue between the defect and the common mitral and tricuspid valve structure. There is usually a crescentic piece of tissue constituting the remnant of the atrial septum, which protrudes down into the heart from the upper portion of the atrium.

When the mitral and tricuspid valves are prodded into a closed position in a specimen with this anomaly, it will be seen that there is usually a communication between the left and right ventricles over the upper and anterior portions of the ventricular septum. This opening is sometimes obstructed to some degree by a meshwork of fine trabeculae proceeding from the valve to the septal margin. In some cases these trabeculae may be so short and so bound down to the septum that the defect is minimal and a minimal passage of blood with systole can occur. In the majority of cases there is a smooth opening of considerable proportions that permits a large blood flow from left ventricle to right with each systole.

Rogers and Edwards (1948) have summarized the findings of 55 cases of atrioventricularis communis from the literature and have included five cases of their own. Altogether, there were six cases with major associated anomalies plus 19 with a relatively minor associated defect. Down's syndrome was present in 30 percent. These findings are substantiated in our group by the presence of Down's syndrome in 37 percent of our postmortem group.

Without surgery the majority of these babies die in the first year of life, as is indicated in Figure 22–6. That the prognosis has improved markedly with modern surgical techniques is quite evident. However, because of the multiple defects many of the AV canal cases do poorly. Parisi and Nadas (1971) report a 45 percent survival after ten years from the time of the catheterization procedure, which was usually done in the first year of life.

Hemodynamics

The shunt from left atrium to right atrium is identified chiefly by the rise in oxygen saturation in the right atrium over that of the superior vena cava, but is also recognized by angiocardiography, indicator dilution curves, or radionuclide angiography.

In the presence of a small atrial septal defect, there is a pressure difference between the atria that is usually not more than 3 mm of mercury (Dexter, 1956). With a large defect when the opening is greater than 2 sq cm in cross-sectional area, the two atria function as one and there is then no pressure difference discernible. Under this circumstance, the characteristic shunt from left atrium to right atrium

does not appear to be due to a difference in pressure, and since there is then a common filling pressure for both ventricles, the relative receptiveness of the ventricles must be the decisive factor.

In the series at The Hospital for Sick Children the systolic pressure in the pulmonary artery exceeded 50 mm of mercury in 5 percent. Liddle and associates (1960) reported an incidence of 8 percent. Bedford and Besterman (1963), studying a group of adults, found that pulmonary hypertension was present in 35 percent by age 40. Blount and associates (1954) recognized pulmonary hypertension in 50 percent of their patients with ostium secundum (chiefly adults). It is well-established that one may have normal pressures in the pulmonary circuit in elderly individuals or one may have pulmonary hypertension in the young, yet the analysis of any large group indicates there is an obvious tendency for the percentage of patients with raised pulmonary vascular resistance to increase with advancing years, even in the presence of relatively benign anomaly (Bedford, 1960).

The administration of oxygen is helpful in differentiating between various categories of response of the pulmonary vasculature in atrial septal defect. Inhalation of oxygen will reduce the pulmonary vascular resistance and thus the pulmonary pressure in the majority of children who have hypertension from this cause. Heath and associates (1958) demonstrated the same effect on adults and related the response to the degree of anatomic pulmonary artery obstruction present. The small shunts with low resistance showed minimal response to oxygen, and a similar finding was noted in the most advanced stages of vascular change. An intermediate group between these two extremes most commonly exhibited a significant drop in pressure and resistance when oxygen was inhaled. Thus there are two main categories of pulmonary vascular resistance: (1) a functional one, which responds to oxygen, and (2) an obstructive organic one, which shows little or no response to oxygen.

McGoon and associates (1959), in discussing the atrial defect, have demonstrated that even those with

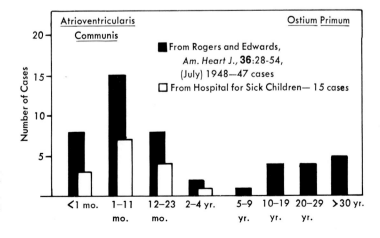

Figure 22-6. Atrioventricularis communis (cases without other major defects). Age of patients at time of death. Compare with age at death in ostium primum.

apparently normal pulmonary artery pressure may have a significant drop in pressure when receiving oxygen. This was not found in normal individuals.

P.V.R.
< 5 wood u

By measurement the pulmonary vascular resistance in atrial septal defect is usually in the normal range below 400 dynes/sec/cm^{-5}. A few cases fall between 400 and 800, but a figure exceeding 800 is exceptional and is associated with organic obstruction (Heath et al., 1958; Bedford, 1960).

As long as the right ventricular output is maintained, cyanosis is unlikely to occur because the systemic venous blood returning to the heart is carried out continuously through the pulmonary circulation. If the right ventricular output falls, as it may in heart failure, mixing of the blood from the two atria may occur, and some of the desaturated blood may get into the systemic circulation. Pulmonary venous engorgement may occasionally be the cause of unsaturated blood returning to the left atrium, but this is not a prominent factor in atrial septal defect in children and is probably not a prominent factor at any age.

Dexter (1956) has presented evidence that when the right ventricle fails in atrial septal defect, there is no relationship between the venous filling pressure and the right ventricular output. On the other hand, when the left ventricle fails, the left ventricular output remains relatively constant by means of the help of a rising venous pressure. Clinically, right ventricular failure is indicated by a lowered right ventricular output and the appearance of cyanosis or by a distinct but less obvious fall in the oxygen content of the arterial blood. It may be brought on by excessive blood flow through the right side of the heart, marked increase in pulmonary vascular resistance, or tricuspid insufficiency.

Left ventricular failure is indicated by further congestion of the pulmonary vascular bed and systemic venous system and is most likely to occur when mitral insufficiency or mitral stenosis complicates an atrial septal defect. Digitalis increases the cardiac output of right ventricular failure without altering the venous pressure, but with left ventricular failure, digitalis appears to reduce the venous pressure while maintaining the output.

Heath and Edwards (1958) divided the histologic changes in the pulmonary arteries into six grades of severity and related them to the hemodynamics of the intracardiac shunt. In the atrial septal defect the pulmonary blood flow was larger in grades 1 to 3 (4 to 12 L per minute per square meter). In grades 5 and 6 the pulmonary blood flow was reduced to less than 4 L per minute per square meter, and this is coincidental with organic obstruction within the pulmonary arteries.

The ratio of pulmonary to systemic blood flow is two to one or greater in 90 percent of patients with atrial septal defect in adults (Bedford, 1963). The ratio is two to one or greater in 95 percent of children, thus indicating what is already well-known, that the pulmonary pressure and resistance are characteristically low in this particular anomaly.

In both childhood and adult life the development of pulmonary vascular obstruction is a reasonably slow process even in those individuals whose arteries appear more susceptible than those of the rest of the population.

The response of the pulmonary arteries in children with atrial septal defect is apparently different in children with large ventricular septal defect since in the latter there is rarely any drop in pulmonary vascular resistance within a year or two after successful closure of the defect. In the atrial defect, Beck and associates (1960) report 3 out of 12 cases showed some decline postoperatively. (See also Burchell, 1971.)

When the atrial defect is combined with another anomaly such as ventricular septal defect or patent ductus arteriosus, or both, arterial changes are more likely to occur in childhood, and the Eisenmenger syndrome with reversal of flow and cyanosis may then occur. This syndrome is rarely found in children with the simple ostium secundum.

Clinical Features—Ostium Secundum

Most congenital anomalies of the heart are recognized early in life. But this is not the case with a simple atrial septal defect (ostium secundum). In the past few were recognized as abnormal hearts under three years of age (Nakamura and associates, 1964). In many instances the family doctor heard a heart murmur and suspected a heart defect, but because the murmur was not loud he considered it functional for some time until it increased in intensity or the heart became enlarged and its precordial thrust more obvious. Now, however, most murmurs are identified early and a diagnosis arrived at.

Among the group at The Hospital for Sick Children 60 percent were females and 40 percent males. Some of the patients are noticeably thin, but the others have an average physique without obesity. The average height is within normal limits. These findings are in keeping with the observations frequently expressed in the literature that such patient may at times have a thin, emaciated appearance (Bedford et al., 1941; White, 1951). The point of interest, however, is that this is not always the case. Parisi and Nadas (1971) found a failure to thrive in 30 percent of patients with secundum defects. It was much more common in the endocardial cushion defects (60 to 90 percent).

Exercise Tolerance. The exercise tolerance is good in the majority of the children. It was considered good in 57 percent of our cases, moderate in 24 percent, and poor in 19 percent. Many of these children have been able to lead a relatively normal life as far as their physical activities are concerned, but they are a little more quiet and less strenuous in their play, dyspnea with effort being common. Parisi and Nadas (1971) found fatigue or dyspnea in 60 percent. Their endurance is limited, as judged by improvement following corrective surgery.

Cyanosis. Rarely do children with simple atrial septal defect show any signs of cyanosis except as a terminal event, when heart failure supervenes, or when a left superior vena cava is attached to the left atrium. One girl of ten years had intermittent episodes of failure, and with each episode slight cyanosis appeared that cleared when the failure was relieved. The arterial oxygen saturations by oximetry in our cases showed normal or close-to-normal readings. All had a resting level of over 90 percent, a few had a slight drop during exercise, and all showed a rise with oxygen up to approximately 100 percent.

More recently Rasmussen and associates (1973) reported that 50 percent have a slight decrease in arterial oxygen saturation. Nadas and Fyber (1972) found 98 percent have an arterial oxygen saturation of 90 percent or greater (chiefly children in their study). Blount and associates (1954) reported a 30-year-old patient who had been cyanotic for several years and at postmortem was found to have a simple atrial septal defect as an isolated anomaly. It was associated with a widespread pulmonary artery hypertrophy and narrowing. Selzer and Lewis (1949) collected data on 11 such cyanotic cases reported in the literature. They accounted for 7 percent of 180 autopsy-proved cases of atrial septal defect. All were adults. Wood (1958) recorded the incidence of Eisenmenger's complex in this anomaly as 6 percent.

Cardiac Impulse. Ninety percent of our children over three years of age had some increase in force of the heartbeat. This was best elicited by having them sit up and lean forward slightly; then, with the palm of the hand over the precordium in the left parasternal area, one can readily appreciate the increased force of the right ventricle through the relatively thin chest wall.

A thrill was present in the pulmonary area in only 2 percent of our cases of simple atrial septal defect (ostium secundum) without pulmonary stenosis. Bedford and coworkers (1941) found it in 25 percent of their clinical cases. Disenhouse and associates (1954) found it in 30 percent of a group of infants and children. Braudo and associates (1954) reported 32 cases of atrial septal defect in children and noted a thrill in the pulmonary area only in those with a mild associated pulmonary stenosis. Five percent of our cases had pulmonary stenosis, and all but one of them had a thrill.

The thrill noted in some of the atrioventricularis communis and ostium primum group is usually in the third to fourth left interspaces and not in the pulmonary area. One can conclude that a thrill in the first to second interspaces is uncommon in a simple atrial septal defect (ostium secundum) in childhood and, when present, should lead one to suspect a pulmonary stenosis.

Heart Murmurs. Braudo and associates (1954) reported that only 18 percent of their children gave a history of murmur from birth. They all developed murmurs eventually, but in 20 percent the murmurs were not recognized until after infancy.

In our group 98 percent had murmurs up the left

border of the sternum, being maximum in the first to second left interspaces in two-thirds and second to third interspaces in one-third. The murmur was usually grade 2, of moderate intensity, and not widely distributed. The murmur was present in three-quarters of the cases. In the other quarter the intensity might be described as grade 3, slightly harsher, and more widely distributed. It is in this group with the harsher murmurs that one may expect to find cases with associated pulmonary stenosis. Occasionally the murmur had a faint, low-pitched quality suggesting functional origin rather than a congenital anomaly. Rarely was the murmur absent.

A middiastolic murmur was frequently heard between the apex and the sternum and was most commonly noted in those who had large defects rather than in those with the smaller ones. It is believed to be due to the rapid inflow from the right atrium to the right ventricle during diastole. This type of murmur is present in 85 percent of children with this anomaly (Braudo et al., 1954). Five percent of our cases also had the murmur of pulmonary insufficiency.

Splitting of the second sound can be recognized in these patients, and the pulmonary component is always of normal or slightly increased intensity. The width of splitting is characteristically fixed and does not vary with respiration; occasionally it does in children with smaller defects with only a slight increase in pulmonary blood flow.

Electrocardiography (Ostium Secundum). The characteristic electrocardiographic findings combine evidence of right ventricular hypertrophy with incomplete right bundle branch block. This pattern was present in 85 percent of our cases. Those that did not show right bundle branch block were those that had right ventricular hypertrophy over the right precordial leads, usually with a qR pattern; they may well have had an isoelectric R that was not apparent (see accompanying chart, Figure 22–7, showing a segment from the right precordium in each of 30 cases). The P wave was elevated slightly in 25 percent. The P-R interval was lengthened to 0.19 second or more in 36 percent; it was between 0.16 and 0.18 second in 48 percent; it was under 0.16 second in 16 percent. Since most normal children have P-R intervals of less than 0.16 second, this measurement is of some diagnostic importance. The electrocardiogram of a typical case is shown in Figure 22–8.

Left-axis deviation in the standard leads may occur on rare occasions with simple ostium secundum. Tan and associates (1975) record that 2 percent of their ostium secundum cases had an electrical axis between 270° and 330°. The characteristic axis is shown in Figure 22–9 and is most commonly between 90 and 150 degrees.

The characteristic tracing, therefore, in simple atrial septal defect, has right-axis deviation in the standard leads and evidence of right ventricular hypertrophy in the precordial leads, a lengthened P-R interval, and incomplete right bundle branch block.

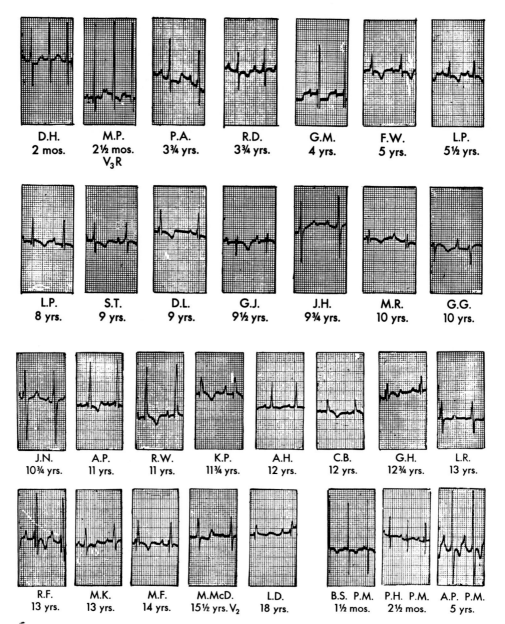

Figure 22-7. Precordial lead V_1 in atrial septal defects (proved by cardiac catheterization), showing considerable variation from one case to the next. Some show marked right ventricular hypertrophy patterns (e.g., M. P., aged $2\frac{1}{2}$ months; R. W., aged 11 years); others show minor degrees of right ventricular hypertrophy (e.g., M. K., aged 13 years). Bundle branch block of some degree is present in most cases.

Radiologic Examination. In infants and young children with atrial septal defect there may be equivocal cardiomegaly and relatively normal vascularity in the chest film. However, most patients with a large shunt at any age show heart enlargement, a full pulmonary artery segment, and increased arterial markings in the lungs. The aorta is of normal size and left sided, and the left atrium is not enlarged, an important differentiating point from posttricuspid shunts with intact atrial septum. A vertical shadow on the left side of the mediastinum suggests the association of a left superior vena cava. Occasionally an azygos continuation of the superior vena cava or anomalously connected right pulmonary veins can be suspected by a prominence above the superior cava–right atrial junction.

Echocardiography. Almost all patients with a detectable left-to-right shunt have an enlarged right ventricular end-diastolic dimension (Diamond et al., 1971; Tajik et al., 1972). An enlarged right ventricular end-diastolic dimension may be the only echocardiographic feature of an atrial septal defect. This, in

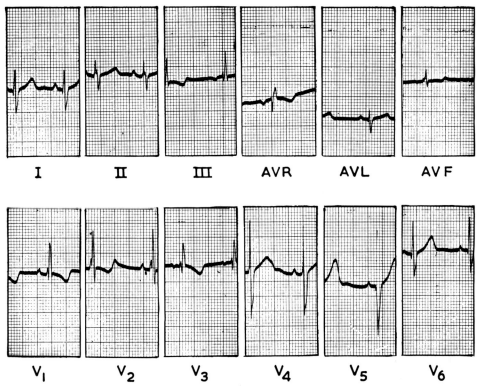

Figure 22-8. D. L., aged nine years. Right-axis deviation with moderate evidence of right ventricular hypertrophy and incomplete right bundle branch block.

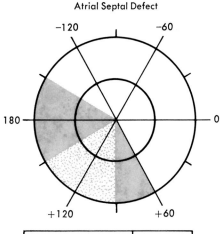

Mean Axis	Percent
+60° to +90°	9
+90° to +150°	75
+150° to +180°	9
Indeterminate	7

Figure 22-9. Mean frontal axis of the QRS complex in 96 patients with ostium secundum defects of the atrial septum showing range of +60 to −150 degrees with peak incidence between +90 and +150. In seven patients the mean axis was indeterminate.

itself, is not diagnostic of the condition and should be assessed together with the relevant clinical information.

Septal motion may be normal, intermediate (type B), or reversed (type A) (Meyer et al., 1972). The septal motion tends to be related to the size of the shunt. It is usually reversed in those patients with the largest shunts and largest right ventricular dimensions (Kerber et al., 1973; Laurenceau and Dumsenil, 1976); Radtke et al., 1976).

The echocardiogram may also be used to detect associated anomalies such as mitral valve prolapse.

Angiocardiography (Ostium Secondum). In general, the purpose of angiocardiography, after preliminary hemodynamic study, is to confirm that a left-to-right shunt is occurring at atrial level and to obtain an indication of the extremes of defect size, i.e., trivial versus absent atrial septum. Other applications include further assessment of any pressure gradients detected across the pulmonary valve or bifurcation of the main pulmonary artery and examination of mitral valve and left ventricular anatomy and function. Where applicable, anatomy of right or left pulmonary veins or of a left superior vena cava and their connections can be clarified. These objectives are best realized through selective angiography. Selective left atrial injection in LAO projection will allow identification and localization of the defect. In the case of sinus venosus defect, contrast will spill over into the superior vena cava. Caval injections may outline unsuspected drainage into the left atrium. There is seldom a practical need to provide precise dimensions of the atrial defect, but when occasionally that is desirable a balloon catheter filled with increasing amounts of contrast can be slowly and repeatedly drawn across the communication. When a point of balloon resistance and mild deformity is reached during the traverse, one can assume the defect to be roughly the diameter of the balloon when inflated to that degree.

Contrast injection into the main pulmonary artery with the patient supine gives on levophase the most consistent visualization of an atrial left-to-right shunt and allows indirect assessment of defect size. Tilted projections can demonstrate the entire length of the main pulmonary artery in the same anteroposterior plane and more sharply reveal branch stenosis. Right ventricular injections of contrast in lateral projections will show an abnormal pulmonary valve, while left ventricular injections in anteroposterior and right anterior oblique projections clarify the mitral anatomy, particularly prolapse of the mitral leaflets (see Chapter 43).

Pulmonary Hypertension (Ostium Secundum). Pulmonary hypertension with a pulmonary artery systolic pressure greater than 50 mm of mercury is present in 5 percent of the children with isolated secundum atrial septal defect. The clinical features of this particular group are different from the rest. All of them have significant cardiac symptoms, and an occasional case will have cyanosis with effort. On examination the intensity of the pulmonary valve closure sound is noticeably increased and frequently palpable. A few have a pulmonary diastolic murmur down the left sternal border, and when this is associated with a hyperkinetic pulmonary hypertension, it may disappear postoperatively. A dominant "a" wave will sometimes be observed in the jugular venous pulse; the heart tends to be larger than in the rest of the group; and in all of our patients the cardiothoracic ratio exceeded 65 percent. In the electrocardiogram the height of the R wave in V_1 exceeded 16 mm in every case.

As might be expected, the incidence of pulmonary hypertension is higher when the atrial septal defect is complicated by a second lesion such as a ventricular septal defect, or partial anomalous vein drainage, or patent ductus arteriosus. Those with pulmonary hypertension appear to have a higher incidence of respiratory infections, and the latter may have contributed to the pulmonary vascular state.

Bedford (1960) has analyzed 300 cases of atrial septal defect in adults and finds pulmonary hypertension in 4.3 percent below 20 years of age, 18.2 percent in those aged 20 to 40 years, and 40.5 percent in those over 40 years. In 75 percent the hypertension was obstructive and in the remainder it was hyperkinetic. In the obstruction group the pulmonary vascular resistance average 1024 dynes/sec/cm^{-5} with a pulmonary-to-systemic blood flow ratio of 1.35:1. In the hyperkinetic group the pulmonary

vascular averaged 243 dynes/sec/cm^{-5} with a pulmonary-to-systemic blood flow ratio of 4:1.

When the obstructive type of pulmonary hypertension develops, the heart may be enlarged, normal, or small in size (Bedford, 1960). All the children investigated have had a significantly large shunt and enlarged hearts except those who have a very small opening between the atria (the latter do not develop the Eisenmenger complex). The heart becomes smaller as the pulmonary blood flow decreases and before the right atrial pressure rises and failure develops.

Clinical Features—Combined or Complicated Ostium Secundum Defects

Pulmonary Stenosis with Atrial Septal Defect with Left-to-Right Shunt. The association of pulmonary stenosis with atrial septal defect and a persistent left-to-right shunt occurred in 10 percent of the cases at The Hospital for Sick Children (see Table 22–1). This association is usually with the secundum type of atrial defect but may occasionally occur with ostium primum or atrioventricularis communis.

Cyanosis on exertion confirmed by oximetry was present in 40 percent of these patients. A systolic thrill was felt in the pulmonary area in all but one. Closure of the pulmonary valve was usually delayed and soft, but in two instances it was delayed and snappy in character. A middiastolic murmur was heard in only one patient, being a rare finding in this group. A dominant A wave was observed in the jugular venous pulse and in half of the children.

The heart size tended to be small except for one patient in whom a deformed tricuspid valve resulted in tricuspid regurgitation and dilation of the right atrium. The cardiothoracic ratio was 55 percent or less in the vast majority. In a few the left pulmonary artery was dilated and its origin was usually high, as was seen in pulmonary stenosis with intact septum. The pulmonary vascular markings may be increased occasionally and pulsatile in a few, but as a rule they appear normal.

The electrocardiogram in these patients is very similar to that in the isolated atrial septal defect as far as the P-R interval or the P wave or the QRS axis is concerned. The R wave in V_1, however, was 16 mm or more in 80 percent of this group.

The systolic gradient across the pulmonary valve ranges from 20 to 70 mm of mercury at cardiac catheterization. The right ventricular pressure curve is usually symmetric with a pointed peak in keeping with valvular stenosis. In every case the small or moderate left-to-right shunt is present at the atrial level but no right-to-left shunt can be detected under resting conditions.

We have recommended surgical treatment of the pulmonary stenosis in our children who have a pressure gradient exceeding 50 mm of mercury. In the others with a smaller gradient the atrial defect was closed without attempting to deal with the pulmonary stenosis. This has resulted in a significant reduction in the gradient but does not always eliminate it.

Atrial Septal Defect with Partial Anomalous Vein Drainage. Partial anomalous pulmonary drainage to the right atrium with a superior vena cava was present in 7 percent. In each case the right pulmonary veins were at fault. The atrial septal defect was unusually small and located at the entrance of the superior vena cava (sinus venosus defect) in half the cases, and in the other half, it was in the center of the septum. (See Chapter 32.)

There were no distinctive features which permit recognition of this anomaly prior to cardiac catheterization, although the incidence of cyanosis with exertion and pulmonary hypertension was likely to be more common than in the isolated septal defect. X-rays of the chest did not usually reveal the anomalous veins entering the superior vena cava of the right atrium, as was frequently the case with adults (Bedford, 1960).

At cardiac catheterization the pulmonary drainage into the superior vena cava can be probed in almost every case. When the veins enter the right atrium directly, it is more difficult to be certain that the connection is anomalous. Indirect evidence can be obtained by differential dilution studies (Braunwald et al., 1959), or, more simply, by a small injection of contrast medium. A gradient across the atrial septum in the presence of a large left-to-right shunt suggests a small atrial septal defect and partial anomalous pulmonary vein drainage.

Atrial Septal Defect and Mitral Valve Prolapse. This combination of defects is being recognized with increasing frequency. Indeed, mitral valve prolapse may be the most common anomaly associated with secundum atrial septal defect (see Chapter 43). The degree of prolapse is usually minor, having little hemodynamic influence. The physical findings of the mitral valve deformity are often obscured until after repair of the atrial defect is accomplished. However, at times significant mitral regurgitation may be present, producing a pansystolic murmur at the apex.

Under such circumstances, the differential diagnosis of ostium primum defect with cleft mitral valve and atrial septal defect with rheumatic mitral incompetence must be entertained. The electrocardiogram usually shows a superior QRS axis when the ostium primum defect is present. In addition, the echocardiogram should be very helpful in separating the ostium primum defect from the atrial septal defect–mitral valve prolapse combination. Fortunately, rheumatic mitral incompetence is now a rare association with atrial septal defect.

Significant mitral regurgitation may have an important bearing on the hemodynamics of the atrial septal defect. Closure of the atrial septal defect without appropriate treatment of the mitral valve may result in the perplexing situation of congestive failure postoperatively. Clear definition of the mitral valve anatomy before surgery is important. First,

parents can be warned in advance of the existence of the anomaly so that a clear understanding of the need for continued follow-up is gained. Second, control of mitral regurgitation secondary to mitral valve prolapse can often be obtained by valvuloplasty, whereas the rheumatic form may require mitral valve replacement. These have different management problems and prognostic implications.

Atrial Septal Defect and Mitral Stenosis (Lutembacher's Syndrome). This syndrome was thoroughly reported by Roesler (1934) and Bedford and coworkers (1941). At that time the association of mitral valvular disease was shown to occur in one-third to two-thirds of the cases that came to postmortem. In the past 30 years this situation has changed dramatically, and Cosby and Griffith (1949) reported finding only 2 out of 19 cases with the associated lesions of atrial septal defect and mitral stenosis. Nadas and Alimurung (1952) reviewed and summarized the findings of 25,000 consecutive autopsies in five Boston hospitals and found only five instances of atrial septal defect with mitral stenosis. This association has occurred in four of the patients at The Hospital for Sick Children. In the era in which we live now the mitral valve involvement is rarely rheumatic in origin and is, therefore, almost invariably congenital in origin in the pediatric age group. Fatigue and dyspnea on exertion appear to be the rule, but congestive heart failure and atrial fibrillation are uncommon in the pediatric age group. On physical examination the outstanding feature is the extreme accentuation of the first heart sound, which is readily palpable at the apex. Even in the pulmonary area the first sound is louder than in the uncomplicated atrial septal defect. The opening snap was not heard in our cases or recorded phonographically. The jugular venous pulse of one patient showed a giant "a" wave, and a QR pattern was recorded in lead V_1 of the electrocardiograms of two of our patients. This was encountered only twice in 134 other patients with ostium secundum atrial septal defects. The R in V_1 exceeded 16 mm in one patient. A left atrial hypertrophy was not detected. On fluoroscopy the cardiothoracic ratio exceeded 65 percent and the pulmonary conus was unusually prominent. The left atrium was slightly enlarged in one patient and normal in another.

The findings at cardiac catheterization varied with the size of the atrial septal defect and the severity of the mitral stenosis. The left atrial pressure pulse may show a large "a" wave, while the right atrial tracing may be within normal limits if the atrial defect is small.

SURGICAL TREATMENT. Muller and coworkers (1966) point out that fewer than 50 operations for this complex lesion have been reported. Most cases of Lutembacher's syndrome are more than 30 years of age by the time they become symptomatic. This is particularly true when the mitral stenosis is acquired. However, when the mitral stenosis is congenital in origin, symptoms may appear very early in life.

Atrial and Ventricular Septal Defects Combined. This combination of anomalies has been reviewed by several authors (Evans, Rowe, and Keith, 1961). All are agreed that it results in a pathologic entity that is more severe than either defect alone.

Separate defects of the atrial and ventricular septum were encountered together in 16 of our patients and confirmed at the operation or autopsy. The heart disease was recognized in the first year of life in every case since the disability was almost always severe. In half the cases congestive heart failure developed, and 40 percent had cyanosis with crying.

The physical findings were those of a ventricular septal defect or pulmonary hypertension. A systolic thrill was felt in two-thirds. Radiologically the heart was always large, and in the majority it exceeded 65 percent in the cardiothoracic ratio. The left atrium was slightly enlarged in a few and moderately enlarged in an occasional case but was commonly within normal limits. In the electrocardiogram a tall R in V_1 and left ventricular hypertrophy combined with right ventricular hypertrophy were characteristic of the majority. The mean axis in the QRS complex resembled secundum atrial septal defect in most instances, being in the range of $+60$ to $+150$ degrees in two-thirds, but in one-third left axis with counterclockwise frontal vector was found.

Cardiac catheterization revealed an atrial septal defect readily by probing and by a large left-to-right shunt at the atrial level. A ventricular septal defect, however, was rarely probed, and in most instances there was no significant further rise in oxygen saturation on entering the right ventricle. The systolic pressure in the right ventricle or pulmonary artery was at or near systemic level in every case. For these reasons the diagnosis of this combination is frequently difficult to make, and an angiocardiogram into the left ventricle may be helpful in delineating the anomalies present. It must always be remembered that a ventricular septal defect with tricuspid insufficiency may give somewhat similar cardiac catheter findings.

Clinical Features—Ostium Primum and Atrioventricularis Communis (Common AV Canal)

The clinical features vary with the degree of the underlying pathology. When there is a primum atrial septal defect with a cleft mitral valve, the physiologic effects are less severe than when the tricuspid valve is cleft as well. For this reason the clinical findings can be divided into four groups: (1) those pertaining to a primum atrial septal defect with cleft mitral valve, (2) those related to a primum atrial septal defect with cleft mitral and tricuspid valves, (3) those with common atrium and cleft mitral valve, and (4) those with common atrial ventricular canal (atrioventricularis communis).

Isolated Ostium Primum Atrial Septal Defect. Three of our patients had an atrial septal defect of the ostium primum type with no recognizable cleft in the mitral or tricuspid valves at surgery. Cooley (1960) reports seven such cases. There were no physical signs of mitral incompetence on examination, and radiologically the left atrium appeared slightly enlarged in one patient and normal in the other. Electrocardiogram showed no evidence of left atrial or left ventricular hypertrophy. In one patient the mean axis of the QRS was -70 degrees with a counterclockwise frontal vector, and in another the axis was indeterminate where the flat vector loop was across the horizontal plane. At catheterization the low position of the defect was noted in one patient. Dye dilution curves in the left ventricle were normal. A third patient with a small primum atrial septal defect and no deformity of the atrioventricular valves had in addition a moderately large secundum defect and pulmonary stenosis. Electrocardiographic axis was -130 degrees with a counterclockwise frontal vector. No clinical, electrocardiographic, or radiologic evidence of mitral valve disease was detected in the valve, and it appeared normal at operation.

Occasionally an atrial septal defect of the secundum variety may occur with a cleft mitral valve. This has been reported by Billig and associates (1968) and Pifarre and coworkers (1968). At The Hospital for Sick Children in Toronto we have had three such cases.

Ostium Primum Atrial Septal Defect with Cleft Mitral Valve. This group comprised approximately 10 percent of the total atrial septal defect group. Symptomatically cardiac disability was more common than in the isolated secundum. Dyspnea or easy fatigability was present in 50 percent; the other half had few or no symptoms. Congestive heart failure occurred in approximately 7 percent. Cyanosis with exertion was observed in a similar percentage. Stethoscope examination revealed evidence of mitral incompetence in three-quarters of the patients, and in many a distinct left ventricular impulse was noted. In 25 percent of the children in this group a separate pansystolic murmur at the apex could not be distinguished.

The cardiothoracic ratio exceeded 65 percent in half the cases—the size of the left atrium was assessed in the majority and found to be normal, slightly enlarged, or moderately enlarged in equal proportions.

The electrocardiogram showed a counterclockwise inscription on the frontal vector with a mean QRS axis between -50 and -130 degrees in all but one patient who had a figure-of-eight loop with a mean axis of -20 degrees (see Figures 22–10 and 22–11). Evidence of left ventricular hypertrophy combined with right ventricular hypertrophy was found in the majority. Right ventricular hypertrophy alone was present in a few of the remaining, and one patient had a normal ventricular balance. Left atrial hypertrophy was seen in a third.

At cardiac catheterization pulmonary arterial pressures are usually in the normal range, and pulmonary hypertension is quite uncommon. Left

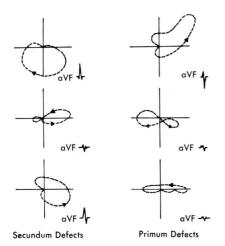

Secundum Defects   Primum Defects

Figure 22-10. Frontal vector of the QRS complex computed from the electrocardiograms of six patients showing clockwise loop usually seen with secundum defects and counterclockwise loop above the horizontal plane typical of ostium primum defects. Vectors with a figure-of-eight pattern or flat loop closely applied to the horizontal axis may be seen with either secundum or primum defects. The configuration of the QRS complex in lead aVF is shown alongside the vector loop. (Reproduced from Evans, J. R.; Rowe, R. D.; and Keith, J. D.: The clinical diagnosis of atrial septal defect in children. *Am. J. Med.*, **30**:345, 1961.)

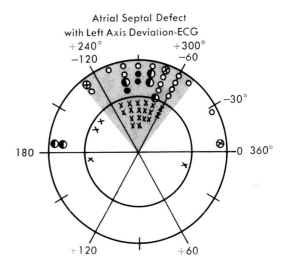

⊗   ASD
○   ASD + cleft mitral valve
◖   ASD + cleft mitral and tricuspid valves
●   Common atrium
✕   Common atrioventricular canal

Figure 22-11. Mean axis of the QRS complex in 50 patients with ostium primum syndrome showing tendency to left-axis deviation. Patients with atrial defect with or without cleft mitral and tricuspid valves are shown in outer circle and those with common atrioventricular canal in the inner circle. (Reproduced from Evans, J. R.; Rowe, R. D.; and Keith, J. D.: The clinical diagnosis of atrial septal defect in children. *Am. J. Med.*, **30**:345, 1961.)

atrial pressure tracings rarely provided convincing evidence of mitral regurgitation. Dye dilution curves with left ventricular injection proved to be a better method of detecting regurgitation (see Figure 22–12).

A primum atrial septal defect may occur with clefts in both mitral and tricuspid valves without the ventricular septal defect that is found in atrioventricularis communis. This combination is less common than the primum atrial septal defect with cleft mitral valve alone. Congestive heart failure may develop in this group, and such children are a little more likely to have a mild cyanosis with exertion, although at times no symptoms may arise.

An apical systolic murmur suggestive of a mitral or tricuspid incompetence is unlikely to be present, although the reason for this is not clear. The second heart sound is usually narrowly split with marked accentuation of the pulmonary component due to pulmonary hypertension.

Significant cardiac enlargement and dense hilar shadows are the rule. Electrocardiographic evidence of right ventricular hypertrophy is usually found in this group, and at times it is associated with left ventricular hypertrophy. As in the other categories, the mean QRS axis is negative and usually in the range between −70 and −110 degrees, although on occasion it may follow a figure-of-eight pattern around the horizontal.

On echocardiography, the features of right ventricular volume overload, as described for secundum defects, are also seen. In addition, the abnormal anterior displacement of the mitral valve

results in prolonged diastolic apposition of the anterior mitral valve leaflet to the septum (Williams and Rudd, 1974; Pieroni et al., 1975). The left ventricular outflow tract appears narrowed. Marked reduplication of the systolic image of the mitral valve is usually seen (Pieroni et al., 1975).

At cardiac catheterization a large left-to-right shunt is always present, and moderate pulmonary hypertension is a characteristic finding. Atrial pressure tracings do not appear to facilitate recognition of mitral or tricuspid incompetence.

Common Atrium and Cleft Mitral Valve. Total absence of the atrial septum producing a common atrium associated with a cleft mitral valve was present in three of four patients. This condition has previously been reported by McGoon and associates (1959). Contrary to expectation, the murmur of mitral incompetence is usually not present. Commonly, but not always, there are left-axis deviation and a counterclockwise vector. Right ventricular dominance is usually present, but combined ventricular loading may also occur.

Cyanosis at rest is unusual in these children but may be apparent with exercise. In our experience the mean axis of the P wave is direct at −60 degrees in the frontal plane, whereas in all but 1 of the other 47

Atrial Septal Defect

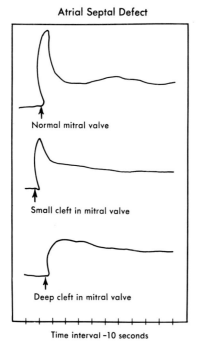

Normal mitral valve

Small cleft in mitral valve

Deep cleft in mitral valve

Time interval ~10 seconds

Figure 22-12. Dye dilution curves recorded by ear oximetry following left ventricular injection of Cardio-Green in three patients with ostium primum defects of the atrial septum. No evidence of mitral regurgitation was noted in first patient in whom no abnormality of the mitral valve was found at surgery. In the two patients with a cleft mitral valve the dye curves suggest mild and gross regurgitation, respectively. (*Arrow* marks time of injection.) (Reproduced from Evans, J. R.; Rowe, R. D.; and Keith, J. D.: The clinical diagnosis of atrial septal defect in children. *Am. J. Med.*, **30**: 345, 1961.)

patients with variants of the ostium primum syndrome, the mean axis fell between − 10 and + 80 degrees. This may at times lead one to suspect common atrium, but it should be noted that the finding was not present in the electrocardiogram of two patients reported by Ellis and associates (1960). **Atrioventricularis Communis (Common AV Canal).** In this group one is usually dealing with babies in the first year or two of life, and failure to thrive is invariable. Cyanosis with crying is noted in the majority, and congestive heart failure is a common event but may not have appeared in those who die early from other causes. Although mitral incompetence must be surprising as it may seem only one part of a constant dynamic event in these children, only one of four patients had physical signs that would lead one to suspect its presence. The second sound is usually closely split with an accentuated pulmonary component.

Radiologically the heart is greatly enlarged with a cardiothoracic ratio of over 65 percent in over half the cases. The outflow tract to the right ventricle is particularly prominent; the left atrium is slightly enlarged or moderately enlarged in the majority. The electrocardiogram characteristically shows com-

bined right and left ventricular hypertrophy although right ventricular hypertrophy with an isolated pattern is almost as common. Left atrial hypertrophy is seen in only 10 percent. The mean QRS axis is usually between − 60 and − 140 degrees, but occasionally it is close to the horizontal plane and in one case was + 20 degrees and in another + 170 degrees. However, in each case the frontal vector was counterclockwise with the bulk of the loop above the horizontal axis.

In the echocardiogram the anterior leaflets of the mitral and tricuspid valves are contiguous in the plane of the ventricular septum in diastole when the septal echoes appear deficient (Williams and Rudd, 1974). A single leaflet appearing predominantly mitral may pass through the septum and merge with the tricuspid valve. Multiple systolic echoes are seen in the mitral valve (Pieroni et al., 1975). The prolonged apposition of the anterior mitral valve leaflet to the septum, as described for primum atrial septal defect, is usually not seen in complete canal defects. Marked narrowing of the left ventricular outflow tract is usually seen.

Chamber size depends to a large extent on the degree of valvar regurgitation and shunting. Hagler (1976) found an enlarged right ventricle in 85 percent, a large left ventricle in 29 percent, a small left ventricle in 33 percent, and a large left atrial/aortic root ratio in most.

Cardiac catheterization reveals pulmonary hypertension at or near the systemic level in the majority. Similar findings were reported by Lambert and associates (1955). Both the ventricular and atrial openings are important, but the hypertension and the mortality appeared to be associated with the size of the ventricular septal defect since those with an insignificant ventricular communication survive longer and run a milder course.

The arterial oxygen saturation of the systemic blood at rest varies from 60 to 90 percent; most of the readings have been in the normal or close-to-normal range when the baby is quiet. There is frequently a decrease with crying on exercise revealing a latent reversal of flow between the atria. This is supported by the fact that none of these babies showed cyanosis at birth but nearly all of them became cyanotic later. Baron and associates (1964) have pointed out that left-sided angiocardiograms will usually display certain features that are characteristic of atrioventricularis communis or endocardial cushion defects.

The frontal angiocardiogram reveals the anomalies that occur to advantage. The outflow tract of the left ventricle in these cases is bounded on the right by the abnormal leaflet of the mitral valve, which is usually cleft. Because of the multiple abnormal chordae that are incorporated in this leaflet, the right border appears serrated or scalloped rather than smooth as in a normal heart. The line of attachment of the superior segment of the cleft anterior leaflet extends anteriorly on to the ventricular septum beneath the non-coronary aortic cusp, where the membranous septum is present in the normal.

There may be a horizontal cleft or filling defect seen in systole where the free margins of the superior and inferior segments of the abnormal anterior mitral leaflet meet. The apparent filling defect is due to the thickened margins of the valve segments. (See Figure 22–4.) When these segments do not coapt adequately, contrast material refluxes into the left atrium demonstrating mitral insufficiency, which is characteristic of atrioventricularis communis.

In diastole the superior segment of the cleft mitral valve bulges into the left ventricular outflow tract, giving it an elongated, narrowed appearance. This impingement on the right border of the outflow tract gives it a more horizontal position than is normally present, so that it has a somewhat gooseneck appearance.

Differential Diagnosis

In the differential diagnosis of atrial septal defect there are a number of cardiac anomalies that cause an increase in oxygen saturation in the right atrium and as such need to be considered in assessing the diagnostic problem after a cardiac catheterization. These anomalies include ostium secundum, ostium primum, atrioventricularis communis, and the possible association of these lesions with pulmonary stenosis, pulmonary hypertension, mitral stenosis, mitral insufficiency, ventricular septal defect, or patent ductus arteriosus. Other anomalies with similar catheterization findings are total anomalous pulmonary vein drainage into the right atrium or its tributaries, aneurysm of aortic sinus entering into the right atrium, left ventricular right atrial defect, coronary artery fistula into the right atrium, coronary sinus, and mitral or aortic atresia with left-to-right flow through an open foramen ovale.

The accurate diagnosis of an atrial septal defect is important for surgical management, especially in centers where they find it more expeditious to carry out the ostium secundum closure by means of hypothermia, reserving the extracorporeal circulation for the more major defects.

The electrocardiogram provides a most reliable method in differentiating ostium secundum from ostium primum defects. When the mean axis and QRS complex lie between +60 and −150 degrees and the frontal vector rotates in a clockwise manner, the defect is almost certainly of the secundum type. Left-axis deviation and counterclockwise vector are characteristic of primum defects. Very rarely a secundum defect may present these findings. When the mean axis is indeterminate and the frontal vector forms a flat loop or figure-of-eight pattern closely applied to the horizontal axis, it is not possible to designate the site of the defect from the electrocardiogram. In such cases evidence of mitral or tricuspid incompetence strongly favors a primum defect. The mean axis in common atrial ventricular canal may fall beyond the range of primum defect in a few instances, but counterclockwise rotation of the

frontal vector with the major portion of the loop above the horizontal axis is a consistent finding in our experience.

As is indicated above, the clinical features of the secundum defect in children follow a relatively uniform pattern. Severe disability and congestive heart failure are uncommon and cyanosis on exertion is rare. The dominant "a" wave exceeding the V wave by 3 cm, or more, is not seen in the jugular venous pulse or in the right atrial pressure tracing at cardiac catheterization. Cardiothoracic ratio is almost invariably below 65 percent, and electrocardiographic evidence of left atrial or left ventricular hypertrophy is only seen occasionally. In V_1 the R wave seldom exceeds 16 mm, and a qR pattern in this lead is uncommon.

Pulmonary hypertension occurs in 5 percent of children with isolated ostium secundum atrial septal defect. One can usually recognize this combination by the presence of a loud pulmonary component of the second sound and a tall R in V_1 of the electrocardiogram. A very modest murmur is heard over the pulmonary artery area. Some of these children have cyanosis with exertion, a dominant "a" wave in the jugular venous pulse, and unusually prominent pulmonary arteries. When pulmonary hypertension is found with an ostium secundum defect, one should search carefully for associated lesions since the incidence of pulmonary hypertension is greater in the presence of combined anomalies.

When pulmonary stenosis is associated with an atrial septal defect and a persistent left-to-right shunt, its presence may be suspected by a systolic thrill and the altered pulmonary component of the second heart sound. Closure of the pulmonary valve is delayed and usually soft, although on rare occasions, it may have a snapping quality (Wood, 1958). Cyanosis with exertion or a dominant "a" wave in the jugular venous pulse may also be seen. The heart is smaller than expected with an isolated atrial septal defect, and the hilar shadows may be normal or slightly increased. The R wave in lead V_1 in the electrocardiogram exceeds 16 mm in the majority of cases. If the systolic pressure gradient across the pulmonary valve is greater than 40 or 50 mm of mercury, surgical relief of the stenosis may be warranted at the time of closure of the atrial septal defect.

Partial anomalous pulmonary vein drainage is difficult to recognize by clinical means in patients with atrial septal defect and is best identified at cardiac catheterization by careful exploration of the superior vena cava and right atrium with the tip of the catheter and with dye dilution curves injecting into the right and left pulmonary arteries or right and left atria and pulmonary veins (Braunwald et al., 1960).

When mitral stenosis occurs with atrial septal defect, it may be congenital or rheumatic in origin; the latter cause is uncommon in childhood, since rheumatic mitral valve obstruction takes considerable time to develop. The physical signs draw attention to the mitral stenosis, particularly when sinus rhythm is present. The middiastolic and presystolic murmurs are louder, and the first heart sound is of remarkable intensity at the apex and in the axilla. A giant "a" wave may be seen in the jugular venous pulse. Radiologically, the heart is significantly enlarged and the pulmonary conus unusually prominent. In the electrocardiogram a qR pattern or a dominant R wave is seen in lead V_1. The size of the atrial septal defect may explain the variation in physical and radiologic signs in patients with Lutembacher's syndrome. When the atrial septal defect is large, the physical signs of mitral stenosis are less impressive. A giant "a" wave occurs in the jugular venous pulse in the left atrium and is not appreciably enlarged at fluoroscopy. On the other hand, when the defect is small, the signs of mitral stenosis are striking, the jugular venous pulse is normal, and the left atrium is detectably enlarged.

The clinical picture presented by patients with both secundum atrial septal defect and a ventricular septal defect is rarely confused with that of the isolated septal defect. Severe disability, congestive heart failure, and cyanosis on exertion are all common and usually occur in the first year of life. A systolic murmur and thrill at the lower sternal border are physical signs of pulmonary hypertension that may be found on detailed examination. The heart is almost always markedly enlarged, the QRS axis and frontal vector resemble secundum atrial septal defect in the majority of patients, but the R wave in V_1 usually exceeds 16 mm, the evidence of left atrial and left ventricular hypertrophy may be present. The ostium primum group of atrial septal defects is distinguished by left-axis deviation and counterclockwise rotation of the vector loop in the frontal plane. These electrocardiographic characteristics are not related to the degree of mitral incompetence since they may occur in patients with typical primum defects who have no clinical, hemodynamic, or anatomic evidence of mitral incompetence. Furthermore, when rheumatic mitral regurgitation occurs in association with secundum atrial septal defect, a right-axis deviation, clockwise inscription, and a frontal vector are found. It would appear, therefore, that this distinctive pattern of an electrical excitation is due to an embryologic defect in the development of the conduction system.

Common atrium resulting from complete absence of the atrial septum should be considered when cyanosis is noticed at rest in patients with ostium primum syndrome. Marked left-axis deviation of the P wave (−60 degrees) in the frontal plane with a relatively short P-R interval has been a characteristic finding in our experience but was not present in the electrocardiograms of two patients reported elsewhere (Ellis et al., 1959). Such changes in the P wave should arouse suspicion of common atrium since they are seldom encountered in other types of primum defect.

The clinical presentation of patients with common atrial ventricular canal rarely simulates atrial septal defect. Severe disability, congestive failure, and cyanosis are common, and only a few patients survive early childhood. The grave prognosis of this malformation may be exaggerated by the coexistence of mongolism, but in spite of this association most of the children with this severe common atrial ventricular canal defect have died by the age of five or six (see Figure 22–6). Clinical signs are variable but more commonly suggest ventricular septal defect than uncomplicated atrial septal defect or mitral incompetence. The heart is markedly enlarged, and in half the patients the electrocardiogram shows evidence of combined ventricular hypertrophy. The feature that links common atrial ventricular canal to the various forms of ostium primum septal defects is the consistent finding of counterclockwise rotation of the frontal vector above the horizontal axis.

Atrial septal defect and patent ductus arteriosus may present a problem in diagnosis because, although the continuous murmur of patent ductus arteriosus may be heard, one may not suspect atrial septal defect. Thus, catheterization is in order in cases of patent ductus arteriosus when there is evidence of right ventricular hypertrophy.

Coarctation of the aorta may occur with atrial septal defect. This possibility stresses the necessity to regularly feel the femoral arteries and to obtain blood pressure in the arms and legs of all patients with anomalies of the heart.

Total anomalous pulmonary vein drainage into the right atrium or its tributaries can be differentiated by the right-to-left shunt at atrial level with diminished oxygen content of arterial blood and inability to enter any pulmonary veins from the left atrium. An angiogram into the pulmonary artery will usually reveal the anomalous common collecting vein leading into either a left superior vena cava, coronary sinus, right atrium, or infradiaphragmatic channel.

The sudden onset and the diastolic murmur will usually suggest the presence of aortic sinus–right atrial fistula. In doubtful cases an angiogram in the aortic root will clarify the diagnosis.

A communication between the left ventricular outflow tract and the right atrium produces cardiac catheter findings similar to those of an atrial septal defect. However, the former is almost invariably accompanied by a thrill over the lower precordium. A left ventricular angiocardiogram will show immediate filling of the right atrium.

A difficult problem may present itself when a ventricular septal defect occurs with tricuspid insufficiency. The right atrial pressure tracing may suggest tricuspid insufficiency with a large "v" wave, but such hemodynamic contours may be within normal limits and one may need to resort to the double-catheter technique, injecting a dye into the right ventricle and withdrawing from the right atrium to clarify the diagnosis.

Prognosis

In infancy and childhood death from ostium secundum is distinctly uncommon. An occasional death occurs in the first year of life and is usually associated with a respiratory infection. In a comparison of this problem with those in other children's centers in North America, a similar low mortality in childhood was recorded (Nakamura et al., 1964). The deaths reported in six medical centers in the infant and child group are shown in Figure 22–13. Kavanagh-Gray (1963) has reviewed this problem as it relates to infancy, and she records patients with atrial septal defect who developed signs or symptoms in the first year of life. Only one patient was in failure. There were two patients who died—both suddenly. One patient had other congenital anomalies. Others have reported similar incidents as uncommon events (Brinton and Campbell, 1953; Disenhouse et al., 1954; Ober and Moore, 1955).

The prognosis in infancy and early childhood is good, but it should be remembered that an atrial septal defect may occur in conjunction with another heart anomaly and the latter may be masked by the former. The prognosis in major combined lesions is often poor.

The data available on adults suggest that the prognosis is better than 40 years ago. Roesler summarized available literature up until 1934, and the average length of life was 36 years. Bedford and associates (1941) found a similar life-span. Since then, Cosby and Griffith (1949) reported an average length of life of 49 years, 13 years longer than the average reported by Roesler. The difference in mortality between the group of Cosby, on the one hand, and those of Roesler and Bedford, on the other, may well be explained by the presence of mitral valvular disease. Both Bedford and Roesler found mitral stenosis in 40 to 50 percent of their cases (1934 and 1941), whereas Cosby found it in only 10 to 15 percent in 1949. A further reduction has undoubtedly taken place in recent years with the progressive decline in rheumatic fever and rheumatic heart disease.

In uncomplicated ostium secundum, death rarely occurs in infancy and childhood, the heart is not particularly handicapped as a rule, the pressure in the right ventricle and pulmonary artery is only slightly elevated, and in the absence of mitral valvular disease

the life expectancy may, on the average, be around 50 years although an occasional case may live to be 80. In the final stages of life with this defect, there is a slight impairment of exercise tolerance over a period of 10 to 20 years. This leads to a slowly progressive heart failure, the majority dying of this complication (Bedford, 1963). The rest die of embolism, thrombosis, subacute bacterial endocarditis, or from natural causes (Mark and Young, 1965).

natural history of untreated A.S.D.

After the childhood years are past, various potential causes of death begin to appear leading to congestive heart failure, hyperkinetic pulmonary hypertension, mitral stenosis or incompetence, and atrial fibrillation. A few may die of obstructive pulmonary vascular disease (Eisenmenger's complex). Infection may add its effects to any of these. Several authorities have indicated the incidence of the complications listed above is greatly increased after 35 or 40 years of age, occurring in two-thirds of older patients, whereas they are present in only 10 to 15 percent of children or young adults (Coulshed and Littler, 1957; Kelly and Lyons, 1958; Colmers, 1958; Kavanagh-Gray and Mather, 1959; Ellis et al., 1960; Chiong, 1960; Bedford and Besterman, 1963; Rahimtoola et al., 1968). (See Figure 22–14.)

In ostium secundum there appears to be no urgency for surgery, but as with patent ductus arteriosus, since the operation has become remarkably safe, the overwhelming majority should be corrected surgically. The prognosis is not as good if there is another heart anomaly with the atrial septal defect. Of those that die in early life two-thirds have other associated anomalies, such as patent ductus arteriosus, ventricular septal defect, coarctation of the aorta, or mitral stenosis.

The ages at death in each of the two groups of patients with ostium primum and atrioventricularis communis are shown in Figure 22–6. Since these data are based on postmortem studies, they do not include the few cases in each category that may have survived longer. However, there is little doubt we are correct in assuming that children with atrioventricularis communis usually die before the sixth year of life and that a large percentage of patients with ostium primum succumb before the age of 30. Constant

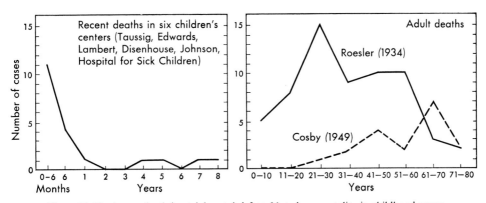

Figure 22-13. Age at death in atrial septal defect. Note low mortality in childhood group.

Atrial Septal Defect

Ost. secundum — 381 cases
Ost. primum — 59 cases

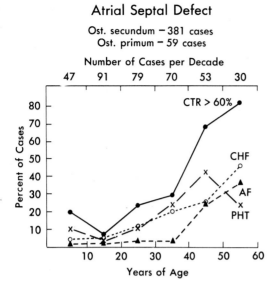

Figure 22-14. Complications in 440 patients with atrial septal defects, chiefly ostium secundum. *CTR*, cardiothoracic ratio; *CHF*, congestive heart failure; *AF*, atrial fibrillation; *PHT*, pulmonary hypertension. After the age of 40 years these complications increase significantly (Bedford and Besterman, 1963).

supervision, careful medical management, and early surgery are required to salvage children with atrioventricularis communis. Since the prognosis is much better in ostium primum, correction of that defect may be carried out as an elective procedure, preferably under five years of age.

Treatment

In 1947, Cohn described an ingenious method of closing the interatrial septum in dogs, by inverting the wall of the right atrium. In 1948, Murray reported his work in attempting to close atrial septal defects in humans by passing a silk suture through the plane of the atrial septum, thus buckling the septal region in an effort to obliterate the opening completely. Swan and associates (1950) devised a method of placing a plastic button across the septal defect but found that it was not satisfactory in humans. Bailey and his group (1953) used a modification of the Cohn technique and sewed the wall of the right atrium to the rim of the defect, thus obliterating its lumen. Gross and associates (1952) developed a rubber well that could be sewed into the side of the right atrium so as to permit the sewing together of the rim of the septal opening, working down through a pool of blood in the artificial well. Kirklin (1956) reported good results with a low mortality using this method. Following Bigelow's studies (1950), Lewis and Taufic (1953) reported the use of hypothermia with successful closure of the atrial septal defect. This has been supported by the work of Swan and coworkers (1955). In this technique the patient was cooled either by

means of a blanket or with a tub of ice water under anesthesia, until the temperature approximated 30° C. Both the venous return and the great arterial vessels were clamped for a period of five to eight minutes while the right atrium was opened and the defect closed by direct suturing.

These methods are now superseded in most medical centers by the cardiopulmonary bypass technique using a pump oxygenator. The surgical closure of an atrial septal defect has now become a very safe and effective procedure. This applies particularly to ostium secundum, in which the surgical mortality in childhood is less than 1 percent. There is a little more risk with the ostium primum anomaly, but surgical correction for it is also a very safe procedure. Risks are at their lowest level in the first decade of life with only a minimal increase in the second decade, but as one proceeds on into middle age and the elderly, the risks and complications of surgery steadily mount. They are related to pulmonary hypertension, pulmonary vascular disease, heart failure, arrhythmias, and presence or absence of other associated illness with the advance of years.

In the first and second decades of life the surgical correction is complete and satisfactory. The child may then lead an active, energetic life. Arrhythmias are rare before or after surgery.

Postoperatively children have a good exercise tolerance and proceed to lead normal lives. In adults a diminished exercise tolerance may persist if the pulmonary vascular resistance is elevated prior to surgery. Catheterization may show a moderate decrease but not to normal. Embolic episodes are a possibility, and these may include fatal cerebrovascular accidents (Hawe et al., 1968). Ten to fifteen percent of adults have some form of atrial arrhythmia postoperatively. These may include atrial flutter, atrial fibrillation, nodal rhythm, or heart block.

Lueker and associates (1969) reported that 9 out of 26 cases of postoperative atrial septal defect repairs have some persistence of the opening between the atria. Vlad (1975) has recatheterized 18 cases postoperatively and rarely found evidence of an opening persisting one to ten years later.

It seems likely that in the future the vast majority of cases will be operated on in the first 10 or 20 years of life, which will result in the lowest mortality and minimize the possibility of postoperative complications.

Selection of Cases for Surgery. In a baby who is one to two years of age with an atrial septal defect and in whom one thinks there is a possibility that spontaneous closure may occur, it is obvious that surgery need not be resorted to at that time. Since spontaneous closure almost invariably takes place in the first five years it would seem reasonable to postpone operation until four or five years when correction can be carried out with great safety.

Moss (1971) summarized the current opinion among pediatric cardiologists regarding surgical closure of the atrial septal defect, secundum type, in the asymptomatic child. All agreed that the defect should be closed at a suitable age when the pulmonary-to-systemic flow ratio was 2.5:1 or greater. There was almost complete unanimity when the flow ratio was greater than 2:1. Approximately 30 percent had some reservation when the flow ratio was between 1.5 and 2:1. However, with the current very safe surgical closure techniques it is obvious that the latter group can also be recommended for surgery at a suitable age.

In the adult over the age of 20 or 30 new factors come into play. Burchell (1971) has indicated that the first high-risk marker is a high ratio of pressure to flow in the pulmonary circulation and the second high-risk marker is congestive heart failure. Over the years considerable attention has been paid to age as a factor in selection of cases for operation, but in the absence of severe hypertension or heart failure the mortality has not exceeded that of the younger patients and the results are satisfactory. Rahimtoola and colleagues (1968) report that out of 83 adult patients operated on in the 1954–1960 period 77 survived operation, and of these 46 were known to have good health five years or more after the operation.

Ostium Primum and Atrioventricularis Communis (Common AV Canal). Since the lesions associated with the ostium primum and atrioventricularis communis are usually multiple, surgical techniques are directed toward repairing each anomalous segment as adequately as possible. Extracorporeal circulation is required with complete body perfusion and interruption of the patient's heart function long enough to deal with these defects. With atrioventricularis communis this may be quite prolonged.

The floating leaflets of the atrioventricular valves are united in the midportion and sewn firmly together. They may then be stitched to the upper margin of the ventricular septum. The clefts in the mitral or tricuspid valves are repaired with silk sutures. The interatrial communication is closed with an adequate patch. Usually the surgeon finds it necessary to open the right ventricle in order to patch or repair the ventricular septal defect but at times it may be achieved through the atrium.

Edwards has pointed out that frequently in endocardial cushion defects abnormal chords attach to the mitral valve near the site of the cleft. After the cleft has been repaired, these chords must be cut to release the valve and permit normal function. The septal leaflet of the tricuspid valve is frequently deficient in structure as well as having a broad cleft. The lack of tissue may be compensated for, if and when the anterior and posterior leaflets of the tricuspid valve are ballooned out and of sufficient area to prevent reflux. If not, a chronic state of tricuspid incompetence persists.

The operative mortality in ostium primum is relatively low and only a little higher than that in ostium secundum. This is a safe operation, and the results are usually satisfactory, although frequently a systolic murmur persists at the apex indicating some degree of mitral incompetence. If such patients are recatheterized, the hemodynamics will usually show

minimal regurgitation. Functionally, the heart appears to be in the normal range in the vast majority of those that have survived operation in this particular category.

In the atrioventricular communis cases the operative mortality is higher than in the ostium primum. It is well to remember that the natural mortality of these cases without surgery is overwhelming, with the majority failing to survive the first five or six years of life; those who do survive may develop either heart failure or the Eisenmenger complex with chronic pulmonary hypertension and a reversal of flow and eventual death in the second decade unless they have a minor form of this complex defect.

As one might expect, the surgical mortality is higher in the infant if the atrioventricular valves are diffusively defective and the heart functions largely like a common ventricle, if intractable failure has preceded operation, or if pulmonary vascular disease is present in a significant degree.

Since one of the above-listed factors is present in a large percentage of cases, the difficulty in the selection of patients for operation becomes obvious—those who develop major symptoms in the first few months of life are difficult to salvage.

Since the mortality is so high in babies with this anomaly, those who present signs and symptoms in the first year of life should be seriously considered for surgery. One of our first cases was operated on in 1954. This was a baby of one year of age who had an enlarged heart shadow, dyspnea with crying or slight effort, an electrocardiogram that showed the classic pattern, and diagnosis confirmed in the catheterization laboratory. This baby has done exceedingly well and is now leading a normal life. X-rays of the heart before and after operation are shown in Figure 22–15.

Not all cases need surgery in the first year of life. If they have no symptoms, the heart is not excessively enlarged, and the flow and pressure are minimal, operation should be postponed as in the group with simple atrial septal defect and the patient should be kept under close observation.

In the medical management of babies with atrioventricularis communis one finds that they are more susceptible to respiratory infection than the average baby and require antibiotics more frequently. If failure develops, they will need digitalis and other forms of supportive therapy.

Arrhythmias. Sealey and coworkers (1969) point out that there are three main internodal tracts in the right atrium. The anterior tract is the shortest; the middle is next in length and courses along the limbus of the fossa ovale to the AV node. The longest is posterior and follows the crista terminalis through the valve of the inferior vena cava to the AV node. At surgery these tracts can be damaged either by the incision in the auricle or septum, or by replacement of sutures. Sealey and colleagues refer to an interesting observation of Bowman and Malm (1965), who approached the interior of the heart through a transverse right atriotomy followed by a mid or low

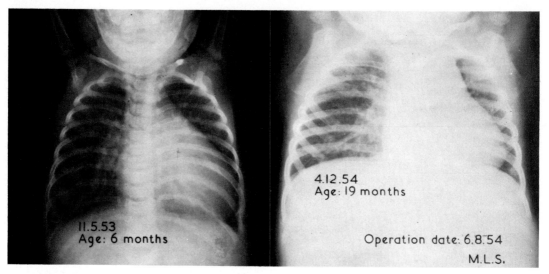

Figure 22-15. M. L. S., with atrioventricularis communis, operated on at 15 months with closure of the atrial and ventricular defects. X-ray at six months shows grossly enlarged heart. X-ray at 19 months shows much less enlargement.

transverse atrial septal incision. In this group of 16 patients, 14 developed nodal rhythm after surgery and two required temporary pacing in order to maintain cardiac output. Thus, it is suggested that to preserve at least one of the tracts the atriotomy incision should be made parallel to the crista terminalis. If a transverse incision through the atrial septum is needed for an approach to the left atrium or mitral valve, it should be placed as high as possible so as to preserve the pacemaking tissue superior to and in the region of the coronary sinus.

Chen and coworkers (1968) record an incidence of dysrhythmia or conduction defect of 52 percent with no significant difference in the incidence between the cases of ostium secundum and primum defects. Thirty percent of these defects were associated with some increase in the right bundle branch block. One developed complete AV block, which had persisted over a year at the time of reporting. Petersson (1967), in recording electrocardiograms in 107 patients before and after operation, half of whom were children, found that postoperatively arrhythmias occurred in 55 percent.

Sealey (1969) studied arrhythmias in atrial secundum defects before and after surgery. Preoperative dysrhythmias were encountered in 32 patients, or 29 percent of the group. The incidence in those under 20 years was 17 percent, over 20 years 43 percent, and over 30 years 57 percent. They demonstrated a relationship between age and the degree of shunting through the atrial septal defect but no relation to the pulmonary artery pressure.

Postoperatively, 35 percent had arrhythmias, including atrial fibrillation, atrial flutter, auricular tachycardia, fibrillation, and flutter and nodal rhythm, atrial fibrillation being the most common. Sixteen of the patients who had normal sinus rhythm

before operation developed atrial fibrillation or flutter afterward. In over a third of the 36 patients who had dysrhythmia after surgery, such irregularities persisted, chiefly atrial fibrillation or flutter.

Evans and Bedford (1961) found dysrhythmias in the 15 percent of patients having noncardiac operations of the thorax over the age of 59. Cohen and Pastor (1957) found an incidence of 23 percent in men over the age of 50 having noncardiac thoracic operations. It is obvious that several factors contribute to the development of cardiac irregularities, especially in the older patient.

Postoperative arrhythmias can usually be controlled by digoxin, which may be required for several weeks or more, depending on the type and persistence of the irregularity. Where the arrhythmia is endangering the life or successful recovery of the patient, cardioversion countershock is indicated. The latter may be followed by a modest dose of quinidine for a few weeks as a prophylactic measure.

Spontaneous Closure. Although spontaneous closure of the ventricular septal defect and patent ductus arteriosus are well-documented, only recently has spontaneous closure of the atrial septal defect been described (Cayler, 1967; Cumming, 1968; Mascarinas, 1969; El-Said et al., 1971; Mody, 1973). All these investigators have shown that such an event does occur in this particular cardiac anomaly, with a modest degree of frequency.

At The Hospital for Sick Children, Toronto, among 445 patients with a catheter diagnosis of an atrial septal defect secundum, 15, or 3 percent, had 3% spontaneous closure. At the time of the original diagnosis, four patients had some evidence of congestive heart failure. Cardiomegaly was seen in the x-ray of the heart in eight, or approximately 50 percent. All of the children showed evidence of right ventricular hypertrophy in the electrocardiogram originally. All have returned to normal appearance with a follow-up of several years. The evidence from our studies and those elsewhere suggest that in spontaneous closure of the atrial septal defect the closure tends to occur early in life, usually in the first five years. Although one cannot elaborate on the mechanism of closure, it seems likely that the foramen ovale was stretched open and subsequently the hemodynamics of the atria allowed less stretch and normal growth permitted functional closure.

REFERENCES

Abbott, M., and Kaufmann, J.: Report of an unusual case of congenital cardiac disease. Defect of the upper part of the interauricular septum (persistent ostium secundum) for comparison with a report of a case of persistent ostium primum. *J. Pathol. Bact.*, **14**:525, 1910.

Abbott, M. F.: *Atlas of Congenital Cardiac Disease.* American Heart Association, New York, 1936, pp. 13, 50.

Adams, C. W.: A reappraisal of life expectancy with atrial shunts of the secundum type. *Dis. Chest*, **48**:66, 1965.

Ainger, L. E., and Pate, J. W.: Ostium secundum atrial septal defects and congestive heart failure in infancy. *Am. J. Cardiol.*, **15**:380, 1965.

Albers, W. H.; Hugenholtz, P. G.; and Nadas, A. S.: Constrictive pericarditis and atrial septal defect, secundum type. *Am. J. Cardiol.*, **23**:860, 1969.

Aldridge, H. E., and Yao, J.: Secundum atrial septal defect in the adult. *Can. Med. Assoc. J.*, **97**:269, 1967.

Anderson, P. A. W.; Jones, R. H.; and Sabiston, D. C.: Quantitation of left-to-right cardiac shunts with nuclide angiography. *Circulation*, **49**:512, 1974.

Ashby, D. W.; Chada, J. S.; and Henderson, C. B.: Associated skeletal and cardiac abnormalities: the Holt-Oram syndrome. *Q. J. Med.*, **38**:267, 1969.

Auld, P. A. M.; Jegier, W.; Morales, F.; Gibbone, J. E.; and McGregor, M.: Increased pulmonary vascular tone in acyanotic congenital heart disease with "normal" vascular resistance. Paper presented at the Canadian Cardiovascular Society Fifteenth Annual Meeting, Quebec City, Canada, Nov. 30, 1962.

Bailey, C. P.; Bolton, H. E.; Jameson, O. L.; and Neptune, W. B.: Atrio-septo-prxy. for interatrial septal defects. *J. Thorac. Surg.*, **26**:300, 1953.

Barger, J. D.; Edwards, J. E.; Parker, R. L.; and Dry, T. J.: Atrial septal defect: presentation of a case with obstructive pulmonary vascular lesions caused by metastatic carcinoma. *Proc. Mayo Clin.*, **23**:182, 1948.

Barnard, C. N., and Schrire, V.: Surgical correction of endocardial cushion defects. *Surgery*, **49**:500, 1961.

Baron, M. G.; Wolf, B. S.; Steinfeld, L.; and Van Mierop, L. H. S.: Endocardial cushion defects. Specific diagnosis by angiocardiography. *Am. J. Cardiol.*, **13**:162, 1964.

Beck, W.; Swan, H. J. C.; Burchell, H. B.; and Kirklin, J. W.: Pulmonary vascular resistance after repair of atrial septal defects in patients with pulmonary hypertension. *Circulation*, **22**:938, 1960.

Bedford, D. E.: The anatomical types of atrial septal defect, their incidence and clinical diagnosis. *Am. J. Cardiol.*, **6**:568, 1960.

——: Personal communication, 1963.

Bedford, D. E., and Bestermann, E. M. M.; Personal communication, 1963.

Bedford, D. E.; Papp, C.; and Parkinson, J.: Atrial septal defect. *Br. Heart J.*, **3**:37, 1941.

Bedford, D. E., and Sellors, T. H.: Atrial septal defect. In *Modern Trends in Cardiology.* Butterworth, London, 1969, p. 138.

Bedford, D. E.: Atrial septal defect. *Proc. Roy. Soc. Med.*, **54**:779, 1961.

Besterman, E.: Atrial septal defect with pulmonary hypertension. *Br. Heart J.*, **23**:587, 1961.

Bigelow, W. G.; Callaghan, J. C.; and Hopps, J. A.: General hypothermia for experimental intracardiac surgery. *Ann. Surg.*, **132**:531, 1950.

Bigelow, W. G.; Lindsay, W. K.; and Greenwood, W. F.: Hypothermia: its possible role in cardiac surgery. *Ann. Surg.*, **132**:849, 1950.

Bigelow, W. G.; Lindsay, W. K.; Harrison, R. C.; Gordon, R. A.; and Greenwood, W. F.: Oxygen transport and utilization in dogs at low body temperatures. *Am. J. Physiol.*, **160**:125, 1950.

Billig, D. M.; Hollman, G. L.; Bloodwell, R. D.; and Cooley, D.: Surgical treatment of atrial septal defects in patients with angina pectoris. *Ann. Thorac. Surg.*, **5**:566, 1968.

Bizarro, R. O.; Callahan, J. A.; Feldt, R. H.; Kurland, L. T.; Gordon, H.; and Brandenburg, R. O.: Familial atrial septal defect with prolonged atrioventricular conduction. *Circulation*, **41**:677, 1970.

Bjork, V. O.; Craafoord, C.; and Varnauskas, E.: Closure of an atrial septal defect and pulmonary valvulotomy in a 49-year-old man. *Ann. Surg.*, **140**:212, 1954.

Blount, S. G.; Balchum, O. J.; and Gensini, G.: The persistent ostium primum atrial septal defect. *Circulation*, **13**:499, 1956.

Blount, S. G.; McCord, M. C.; and Swan, H.: Surgical closure of atrial septal defect: the response in a patient with severe pulmonary hypertension. *Am. Surg.*, **20**:305, 1954.

Blount, S. G.; Swan, H.; Gensini, G.; and McCord, M. C.: Atrial septal defect. Clinical and physiologic response to complete closure in five patients. *Circulation*, **9**:801, 1954.

Bowman, F. O., and Malm, J. R.: The transseptal approach to mitral valve repair. *Arch. Surg.*, **90**:329, 1965.

Braudo, J. L.; Nadas, A. S.; Rudolph, A. M.; and Neuhauser, E. B. D.: Atrial septal defects in children. A clinical study with special emphasis on indications for operative repair. *Pediatrics*, **14**:618, 1954.

Braunwald, E.; Lombardo, C. R.; and Morrow, A. G.: Drainage pathways of pulmonary veins in atrial septal defect. *Br. Heart J.*, **22**:385, 1960.

Braunwald, E., and Morrow, A. C.: Ventriculo–right atrial communication diagnosed by clinical hemodynamic and angiographic methods. *Am. J. Med.*, **28**:913, 1960.

Braunwald, E.; Morrow, A. G.; and Cooper, T.: Left ventricular angiocardiography in the diagnosis of persistent atrioventricular canal and related anomalies. *Am. J. Cardiol.*, **4**:862, 1959.

Bredt, H.: Die Missbildungen des menschlichen Herzens. *Ergebn. Allg. Pathol.*, **30**:77, 1936.

Brinton, W. D., and Campbell, M.: Necropsies in some congenital diseases of the heart, mainly Fallot's tetralogy. *Br. Heart J.*, **15**:335, 1953.

Brown, J. W.: *Congenital Heart Disease*, 2nd ed. Staples Press, Ltd., London, 1950.

Buchman, J.; Kah, A., Jr.; and Hara, M.: Lutembacher syndrome successfully treated by mitral commissurotomy. *Ann. Surg.*, **139**:497, 1954.

Burchell, H. B.: Atrial septal defect—prognosis in adult life-risks and benefits of surgery. In Kidd, B. S. L., and Keith, J. D. (eds.): *The Natural History and Progress in Treatment of Congenital Heart Defects.* Charles C Thomas, Springfield, Ill., 1971.

Calazel, P.; Gerrard, R.; Daly, R.; Draper, A.; Foster, J.; and Bing, R.: Physiological studies in congenital heart disease. XI. A comparison of the right and left auricular capillary and pulmonary artery pressures in nine patients with auricular septal defects. *Bull. Hopkins Hosp.*, **88**:20, 1951.

Campbell, M., and Polani, P. E.: Factors in the etiology of atrial septal defect. *Br. Heart J.*, **23**:477, 1961.

Cascos, A. S.: Genetics of atrial septal defect. *Arch. Dis. Child.*, **47**:254, 1972.

Cayler, G. G.: Spontaneous functional closure of symptomatic atrial septal defects. *N. Engl. J. Med.*, **65**:276, 1967.

Chen, S. C.; Arcilla, R. A.; Moulder, P. V.; and Cassels, D. E.: Postoperative conduction disturbances in atrial septal defect. *Am. J. Cardiol.*, **33**:636, 1968.

Chen, S. C.; Arcilla, R. A.; Cassels, D. E.; Thilenius, O. G.; and Ranniger, K.: Abnormal initial QRS vectors in atrial septal defect. *Am. J. Cardiol.*, **24**:346, 1969.

Chiong, M. A.: Interatrial septal defect longevity. *Can. Med. Assoc. J.*, **83**:1012, 1960.

Coelho, F.; Paiva de E.; and Nunes, A.: Selective angiocardiography in the diagnosis of atrial septal defect (ostium secundum type). *Am. J. Cardiol.*, **7**:167, 1961.

Cohen, M. G., and Pastor, B. H.: Delayed cardiac arrhythmias following non-cardiac thoracic surgery. *Dis. Chest*, **32**:435, 1957.

Cohn, R.: An experimental method for the closure of interauricular septal defects in dogs. *Am. Heart J.*, **33**:453, 1947.

Coles, J.; Sears, G.; and MacDonald, C.: Atrial septal defect complicated by pulmonary hypertension—A long term follow up. Annual Mtg., American Surgical Assoc., 1967.

Colmers, R. A.: Atrial septal defects in elderly patients—report of three patients aged 68, 72 and 78. *Am. J. Cardiol.*, **1**:768, 1958.

Cooksey, J. D.; Parker, B. M.; and Weldon, C. S.: Atrial septal defect and calcification of the tricuspid valve. *Br. Heart J.*, **32**:409, 1970.

Cooley, D. A.: Results of surgical treatment of atrial septal defects. Particular consideration of low defects including ostium primum and atrioventricular canal. *Am. J. Cardiol.*, **6**:605, 1960.

Cosby, R. S., and Griffith, G. C.: Interatrial septal defect. *Am. Heart J.*, **38**:80, 1949.

Coulshed, N., and Littler, T. R.: Atrial septal defect in the aged. *Br. Med. J.*, **1**:76, 1957.

Cournand, A.: Motley, H. L.; Himmelstein, A.; Dresdale, D.; and Baldwin, J.: Recording blood pressure from the left auricle and the pulmonary veins in human subjects with interauricular septal defects. *Am. J. Physiol.*, **150**:267, 1947.

Craig, R. J., and Selzer, A.: Natural history and prognosis of atrial septal defect. *Circulation*, **37**:805, 1968.

Cumming, G. R.: Functional closure of atrial septal defects. *Am. J. Cardiol.*, **22**:888, 1968.

Curtin, J. Q.: Congenital cardiac anomaly: persistent common atrioventricular ostium. *Am. Heart J.*, **44**:884, 1952.

Daicoff, G. R.; Brandenburg, R. O.; and Kirklin, J. W.: Results of operation for atrial septal defect in patients forty-five years of age and older. *Circulation*, **35** Suppl. 1:42, 1967.

Dexter, L.: Atrial septal defects. *Br. Heart J.*, **18**:209, 1956.

Diamond, M. A.; Dillon, J. C.; Haine, C. L.; Chang, S.; and Feigenbaum, H.: Echocardiographic features of atrial septal defect. *Circulation*, **43**:129, 1971.

Disenhouse, R. B.; Anderson, R. C.; Adams, P.; Novick, R.; Jorgen, J.; and Levin, B.: Atrial septal defect in infants and children. *J. Pediatr.*, **44**:269, 1954.

Donald, D. E.; Kirklin, J. W.: and Grindlay, J. H.: The use of polyvinyl sponge plugs in the closure of large atrial septal defects created experimentally. *Proc. Mayo Clin.*, **28**:288, 1953.

DuShane, J. W.; Weidman, W. H.; Brandenburg, R. O.; and Kirklin, J. W.: Differentiation of interatrial communications by clinical methods. Ostium secundum, ostium primum, common atrium, and total anomalous pulmonary venous connection. *Circulation*, **21**:1960.

Edwards, J. E.: Congenital malformations of the heart and great vessels. A. Malformations of the atrial septal complex. In Gould, S. E. (ed.): *Pathology of the Heart*. Charles C Thomas. Publisher. Springfield, Ill., 1953, p. 266.

——: The problem of mitral insufficiency caused by accessory chordae tendinae in persistent common atrioventricular canal. *Proc. Mayo Clin.*, **35**:299, 1960.

Ellis, F. H., Jr.; Brandenburg, R. O.; and Swan, H. J. C.: Defect of the atrial septum in the elderly. Report of successful surgical correction in five patients sixty years of age or older. *N. Engl. J. Med.*, **262**:219, 1960.

Ellis, F. H., Jr.; Kirklin, J. W.; Swan, H. J. C.; DuShane, J. W.; and Edwards, J. E.: Diagnosis and surgical treatment of common atrium (cor triloculare-biventriculare). *Surgery*, **45**:160, 1959.

Ellis, F. H., Jr.; McGoon, D. C.; and Kirklin, J. W.: Surgical management of persistent common atrioventricular canal. *Am. J. Cardiol.*, **6**:598, 1960.

El-Said, G.; Galioto, F. M., Jr.; Williams, R. L.; and McNamara, D. G.: Spontaneous functional closure of isolated atrial septal defect. *Am. J. Dis. Child.*, **122**:353, 1971.

Emanuel, R.; Nichols, J.; Anders, J. M.; Moores, E. C.; and Somerville, J.: Atrioventricular defects—A study of 92 families. *Br. Heart J.*, **30**:645, 1968.

Engle, M. A.: Ventricular septal defect in infancy. *Pediatrics*, **14**:16, 1954.

Esplugas, E.; Kidd, B. S. L.; Olley, P. M.; and Trusler, G.: Hemodynamic results following complete atrioventricular canal defect repair. (Abst.) *Am. J. Cardiol.*, **35**:135, 1975.

Evans, J. R.; Rowe, R. D.; and Keith, J. D.: The clinical diagnosis of atrial septal defect in children. *Am. J. Med.*, **30**:345, 1961.

Feldt, R. H.: *Atrioventricular Canal Defects*. W. B. Saunders Co., Philadelphia, 1976.

Filho, J. B.; Benchimol, A. B.; and Anache, M.: O fonocardiograma nos defeitos do septo auricular. Correlacão dos dados de escuta com a hemodinãmica. *Arq. Brasil Cardiol.*, **13**:273, 1960.

Gault, J. H.; Morrow, A. G.; Gay, W. A.; and Ross, J., Jr.: Atrial septal defect in patients over the age of forty years. *Circulation*, **37**:261, 1968.

Gibbon, J. H., Jr.; Hopkinson, M.; and Churchill, F. D.: Changes in circulation produced by gradual occlusion of pulmonary artery. *J. Clin. Invest.*, **11**:543, 1932.

Gibson, S., and Clifton, M. M.: Congenital heart disease: a clinical and postmortem study of one hundred and five cases. *Am. J. Dis. Child.*, **55**:761, 1938.

Griffiths, S. P.; Ellis, K.; Burris, J. O.; Bumenthal, S.; Bowman, F. O.; and Malm, J. R.: Postoperative evaluation of mitral valve function in ostium primum defect with cleft mitral valve (partial form of atrioventricular canal). *Circulation*, **40**:21, 1969.

Gross, R. E.; Pomeranz, A. A.; Watkins, E.; and Goldsmith, E. I.: Surgical closure of defects of the interauricular septum by use of an atrial well. *N. Engl. J. Med.*, **247**:455, 1962.

Gunn, F. D., and Dieckmann, J. M.: Malformations of the heart including two cases with common atrioventricular canal and septum defects and one with defect of the atrial septum (cor triloculare biventriculosum). *Am. J. Pathol.*, **3**:595, 1927.

Hagler, D. J.: Echocardiographic findings in atrioventricular canal defect. In Feldt, R. H. (ed.): *Atrioventricular Canal Defects*. W. B. Saunders Co., Philadelphia, 1976, p. 100.

Hancock, E. W.; Oliver, G. C.; Swanson, M. J.; and Hultgren, H. N.: Valsalva's maneuver in atrial septal defect. *Am. Heart J.*, **65**:50, 1963.

Hastreiter, A. R.; Wennemark, J. R.; Miller, R. A.; and Paul, M. H.: Secundum atrial septal defects with congestive heart failure during infancy and early childhood. *Am. Heart J.*, **64**:467, 1962.

Hawe, A.; Rastelli, G. C.; Brandenburg, R. O.; and McGoon, D. C.: Late embolic complications after repair of atrial septal defects. *Circulation*, **38**:1–97, 1968.

Hawker, R. E.; Freedom, R. M.; and Krovetz, J.: Preferential shunting of venous return from normally connected left pulmonary veins in secundum atrial septal defect. *Am. J. Cardiol.*, **34**:339, 1974.

Heath, D., and Edwards, J. E.: The pathology of hypertensive pulmonary vascular disease: a description of six grades of structural changes in the pulmonary arteries with special reference to congenital cardiac septal defects. *Circulation*, **18**:533, 1958.

Heath, D.; Helmholz, H. F., Jr.; Burchell, H. B.; Du Shane, J. W.; and Edwards, J. E.: Graded pulmonary vascular changes and hemodynamic findings in cases of atrial and ventricular septal defects and patent ductus arteriosus. *Circulation*, **18**:1958.

Hoffman, J. I. E.; Danilowicz, D.; and Rudolph, A. M.: Hemodynamics, clinical features, and course of atrial shunts in infancy. *Circulation*, **32**:1965.

Holt, M., and Oram, S.: Familial heart disease with skeletal malformations. *Br. Heart J.*, **22**:236, 1960.

Hufnagel, C. A., and Gillespie, J. F.: Closure of interauricular septal defects. *Bull. Georgetown Univ. Med. Cent.*, **4**:137, 1951.

Hull, F.: The cause and effects of flow through defects of the atrial septum. *Am. Heart J.*, **38**:350, 1949.

Kavanagh-Gray, D.: Atrial septal defect in infancy. *Can. Med. Assoc. J.*, **89**:491, 1963.

Kavanagh-Gray, D., and Mathur, B. B.: Atrial septal defect as it appears in patients over the age of forty. *Can. Med. Assoc. J.*, **80**:350, 1959.

Keith, A.: Malformations of the heart. *Lancet*, **2**:433, 1909.

Keith, J. D., and Forsyth, C. C.: Auricular septal defect in children. *J. Pediatr.*, **38**:172, 1951.

Kelly, J. J., Jr., and Lyons, H. A.: Atrial septal defect in the aged. *Ann. Intern. Med.*, **48**:267, 1958.

Kerber, R. E.; Dippel, W. F.; and Abboud, F. M.: Abnormal motion of the interventricular septum in right ventricular volume overload. Experimental and clinical echocardiographic studies. *Circulation*, **48**:86, 1973.

Kirklin, J. W.: Personal communication, 1956.

Kjellberg, S. R.; Mannheimer, E.; Rudhe, U.; and Jönsson, B.: *Diagnosis of Congenital Heart Disease*. Year Book Publishers, Inc., Chicago, 1955.

Krabbenhoft, K. L., and Evans, W. A., Jr.: Some pulmonary changes associated with intracardiac septal defects in infancy. *Radiology*, **63**:498, 1954.

Kramer, T. C.: The partitioning of the truncus and conus and the formation of the membranous portion of the interventricular septum in the human heart. *Am. J. Anat.*, **71**:343, 1942.

Lambert, E. C.; MacManus, J. E.; and Paine, J. R.: Indications for the results of cardiac surgery in infants. *N.Y. J. Med.*, **55**:2471, 1955.

Laurenceau, J. L., and Dumesnil, J. G.: Right and left ventricular dimensions as determinants of ventricular septal motion. *Chest*, **69**:388, 1976.

Leech, C. B.: Congenital heart disease, clinical analysis of 75 cases from the Johns Hopkins Hospital. *J. Pediatr.*, **7**:802, 1935.

Levin, A. R.; Spach, M. S.; Boineau, J. P.; Canent, R. V., Jr.; Capp, M. P.; and Jewett, P. H.: Atrial pressure-flow dynamics in atrial septal defects (secundum type). *Circulation*, **37**:476, 1968.

Levy, M. J.; DeWall, R.; and Lillehei, C. W.: Left ventricular–right atrial canal and subaortic stenosis. Report of a case diagnosed preoperatively. *Am. Heart J.*, **64**:392, 1962.

Lewis, F. J., and Taufic, M.: Closure of atrial septal defects with aid of hypothermia; experimental accomplishment and report of one successful case. *Surgery*, **33**:52, 1953.

Lewis, F. J.; Varco, R. L.; and Taufic, M.: Repair of atrial septal defects in man under direct vision with the aid of hypothermia. *Surgery*, **36**:538, 1954.

Liddle, H. V.; Meyer, B. W.; and Jones, J. C.: The results of surgical correction of atrial septal defect complicated by pulmonary hypertension. *J. Thorac. Cardiovasc. Surg.*, **39**:35, 1960.

Lillehei, C. W.; Cohen, M.; Warden, H. E.; and Varco, R. L.: The direct vision intracardiac correction of congenital anomalies by controlled cross circulation: results in 32 patients with ventricular septal defects, tetralogy of Fallot, and atrioventricularis communis defects. *Surgery*, **38**:11, 1955.

Lillehei, C. W.; Anderson, R. C.; Ferlic, R. M.; and Bonnabeau, R. C., Jr.: Persistent common atrioventricular canal. *J. Thorac. Cardiovasc. Surg.*, **57**:83, 1969.

Lind, J., and Wegelius, C.: Atrial septal defects in children. *Circulation*, **7**:819, 1953.

Lueker, R. D.; Vogel, J. H. K.; and Blount, S. G.: Cardiovascular abnormalities following surgery for left-to-right shunts: observations in atrial septal defects, ventricular septal defects, and patent ductus ateriosus. *Circulation*, **40**:85, 1969.

Lutembacher, R.: De la stenose mitrale avec communication interauriculare. *Arch. Mal. Coeur*, **9**:237, 1916.

McDonald, L.; Emanuel, R.; and Towers, M.: Aspects of pulmonary blood flow in atrial septal defect. *Br. Heart J.*, **21**:279, 1959.

McGinn, S., and White, P. D.: Interauricular septal defects associated with mitral stenosis. *Am. Heart J.*, **9**:1, 1933.

McGoon, D. C.; DuShane, J. W.; and Kirklin, J. W.: The surgical treatment of endocardial cushion defects. *Surgery*, **46**:185, 1959.

McGoon, D. C.; DuShane, J. W.; and Kirklin, J. W.: Surgical treatment of atrial septal defect in children. *Pediatrics*, **24**:992, 1959.

McGoon, D. C.; Swan, H. J. C.; Brandenburg, R. O.; Connolly, D. C.; and Kirklin, J. W.: Atrial septal defect: factors affecting the surgical mortality rate. *Circulation*, **14**:1959.

McMullan, M. H.; Wallace, R. B.; Weidman, W. H.; and McGoon, D. C.: Surgical treatment of complete atrioventricular canal. *Surgery*, **72**:905, 1972.

MacKrell, J. S., and Ibanez, R.: Atrial septal defects, a clinicopathologic appraisal. *Am. J. Cardiol.*, **2**:665, 1958.

Manning, J.: Personal communication, 1956.

Mark, H., and Young, D.: Congenital heart disease in the adult. *Am. J. Cardiol.*, **15**:293, 1965.

Mascarinas, T. C.; Shankar, K. R.; Lauer, R. M.; and Diehl, A. M.: Atrial septal defect—spontaneous obliteration of a significant left to right atrial shunt: documentation by serial catheterization and angiocardiography studies. *J. Kans. Med. Soc.*, **70**:7, 1969.

Meeker, L.: Congenital defect of the heart in a mongolian idiot: persistent ostium atrioventriculare commune without other grave anomalies. *J. Tech. Methods*, **14**:72, 1935.

Meyer, R. H.; Schwartz, D. C.; Benzing, G.; and Kaplan, S.: Ventricular septum in right ventricular volume overload. *Am. J. Cardiol.*, **30**:349, 1972.

Mody, M. R.: Serial hemodynamic observations in secundum atrial septal defect with special reference to spontaneous closure. *Am. J. Cardiol.*, **32**:978, 1973.

Morrow, A. G.; Gilbert, J. W.; Baker, R. R.; and Collins, N. P.: The

closure of atrial septal defects utilizing general hypothermia. *J. Thorac. Cardiovasc. Surg.*, **40**:776, 1960.

Mortensen, J. D.; Veasey, L. G.; and Toronto, A. F.: Clinical and physiological changes following surgical closure of atrial septal defect. *Dis. Chest*, **40**:1961.

Moss, A. J., and Siassi, B.: The small atrial septal defect—operate or procrastinate? *J. Pediatr.*, **79**:854, 1971.

Muller, W. H. Jr.; Littlefield, J. B.; and Beckwith, J. R.: Surgical treatment of Lutembacher's syndrome. *J. Thorac. Cardiovasc. Surg.*, **51**:66, 1966.

Murray, G.: Closure of defects in cardiac septa. *Ann. Surg.*, **128**:843, 1948.

Mustard, W. T.; Baird, R. J.; and Trusler, G. A.: The use of hypothermia in the closure of atrial septal defects in children. *Surgery*, **50**:301, 1961.

Mustard, W. T., and Keith, J. D.: Unpublished data, 1963.

Mustard, W. T., and Keith, J. D.: Unpublshed data, 1964.

Nadas, A. S., and Alimurung, M. M.: Apical diastolic murmurs in congenital heart disease. *Am. Heart J.*, **43**:691, 1952.

Nadas, A. S., and Ellison, R. C.: Phonocardiographic analysis of diastolic flow murmurs in secundum atrial septal defect and ventricular septal defect. *Br. Heart J.*, **29**:684, 1967.

Nakamura, F. F.; Hauck, A. J.; and Nadas, A. S.: Atrial septal defects in infants. *Pediatrics*, **34**:101, 1964.

Neal, W. A.; Moller, J. H.; Varco, R. L.; and Anderson, R. C.: Operative repair of atrial septal defect without cardiac catheterization. *J. Pediatr.*, **86**:2, 1975.

Neptune, W. B.; Bailey, C. P.; and Goldberg, H.: The surgical correction of atrial septal defects associated with transposition of the pulmonary veins. *J. Thorac. Surg.*, **25**:623, 1953.

Nora, J. J., and Fraser, F. C.: *Medical Genetics: Principles and Practice.* Lea & Febiger, Philadelphia, 1974.

Ober, W. B., and Moore, T. E., Jr.: Congenital cardiac malformation in the neonatal period. An autopsy study. *N. Engl. J. Med.*, **253**:271, 1955.

Opdyke, D. F.; Duomarco, J.; Dillon, W. H.; Schrieber, H.; Little, R. C.; and Seely, R. D.: Study of simultaneous right and left atrial pressure pulses under normal and experimentally altered conditions. *Am. J. Physiol.*, **154**:258, 1948.

Parisi, L. F., and Nadas, A. S.: In Kidd, B. S. L., and Keith, J. D. (eds.): *Natural History of Atrial Septal Defects. The Natural History and Progress in Treatment of Congenital Heart Difects.* Charles C Thomas, Springfield, Ill., 1971.

Patten, B. M.: Developmental defects at the foramen ovale. *Am. J. Pathol.*, **14**:135, 1938.

Petersson, P. O.: Atrial septal defect of secundum type. *Acta Paediatr. Scand.*, **5**:174, 1967.

Philpott, N. W.: Relative incidence of congenital cardiac anomalies in Montreal hospitals. *J. Tech. Methods.* **15**:96, 1936.

Pieroni, D. R.; Homey, E.; and Freedom, R. M.: Echocardiography in atrioventricular canal defect: A clinical spectrum. *Am. J. Cardiol.*, **35**:54, 1975.

Pifarre, R.; Dieter, R. A.; Hoffman, F. G.; and Neville, W. E.: Atrial secundum septal defect and cleft mitral valve. *Ann. Thorac. Surg.*, **6**:373, 1968.

Radtke, W. E.; Tajik, A. J.; Gan, G. T.; Schattenberg, T. T.; Giuliani, E. R.; and Tancredi, R. G.: Atrial septal defect: Echocardiographic observations. Studies in 120 patients. *Ann. Intern. Med.*, **84**:246, 1976.

Rahimtoola, S. H.; Kirklin, J. W.; and Burchell, H. B.: Atrial septal defect. *Circulation*, **37, 38**:2, 1968.

Rainer, W. G.; Sadler, T. R.; Dirks, D. W.; and Swan, H.: Holt-Oram syndrome. *J. Thorac. Cardiovasc. Surg.*, **63**:478, 1972.

Rasmussen, K.: Prediction of hemodynamic data in atrial septal defects of secundum type from simple and combined vectorcardiographic data. *Am. Heart J.*, **87**:4, 1974.

Rasmussen, K.; Simonsen, S.; Storstein, O.: Quantitative aspects of right-to-left shunting in uncomplicated atrial septal defects. *Br. Heart J.*, **35**:894, 1973.

Rehder, K.; Kirklin, J. W.; and Theye, R. A.: Physiologic studies following surgical correction of atrial septal defect and similar lesions. *Circulation*, **26**:1962.

Reid, J. M., and Stevenson, J. C.: Cardiac arrhythmias following successful surgical closure of atrial septal defect. *Br. Heart J.*, **29**:742, 1967.

Reinhold, J. D.: The child with congenital heart disease. *Med. World*, **83**:118, 1955.

Robinson, D. W.: Persistent common atrioventricular ostium in a child with mongolism. *Arch. Pathol.*, **32**:117, 1941.

Robson, G. W.: Congenital heart disease, a persistent ostium atrioventriculare commune with septal defects in a mongolian idiot. *Am. J. Pathol.*, **7**:229, 1931.

Roesler, H.: Interatrial septal defect. *Arch. Intern. Med.*, **54**:339, 1934.

Rogers, H. M., and Edwards, J. E.: Incomplete division of the atrioventricular canal with patent interatrial foramen primum (persistent common atrioventricular ostium). Report of five cases and review of the literature. *Am. Heart J.*, **36**:28, 1948.

Rogers, H. M.; Evans, I. C.; and Domeier, L. H.: Congenital aneurysm of the membranous portion of the ventricular septum: report of two cases. *Am. Heart J.*, **43**:781, 1952.

Rogers, H. M., and Rudolph, C. C.: Persistent common atrioventricular canal. *Am. Heart J.*, **45**:623, 1953.

Rowe, G. G.; Castillo, G. A.; Maxwell, G. M.; Clifford, J. E.; and Crumpton, G. W.: Atrial septal defect and the mechanism of shunt. *Am. Heart J.*, **61**:369, 1961.

Sanchez, J.; Rodriguez-Torres, R.; Lin, J. S.; Goldstein, S.; and Kavety, V.: Diagnostic value of the first heart sound in children with atrial septal defect. *Am. Heart J.*, **78**:467, 1969.

Scott, L. P.; Hauck, A. J.; Nadas, A. S.; and Gross, R. E.: Endocardial cushion defect: preoperative and postoperative survey. *Circulation*, **26**:1962.

Sealey, W. C.; Farmer, J. C.; Young, W. G.; and Brown, I. W.: Atrial dysrhythmia and atrial secundum defects. *J. Thorac. Cardiovasc. Surg.*, **57**:245, 1969.

Seldon, W. A.; Rubinstein, C.; and Fraser, A. A.: The incidence of atrial septal defect in adults. *Br. Heart J.*, **24**:557, 1962.

Selzer, A., and Lewis, A. M.: The occurrence of chronic cyanosis in cases of atrial septal defect. *Am. J. Med. Sci.*, **218**:516, 1949.

Shah, C. V.; Patel, M. K.; and Hastreiter, A. R.: Hemodynamics of complete atrioventricular canal and its evolution with age. *Am. J. Cardiol.*, **14**:326, 1969.

Shumacker, H. B., and King, H.: Septum primum atrial septal defects. *J. Thorac. Cardiovasc. Surg.*, **43**:366, 1962.

Siltanen, P.: Atrial septal defect of secundum type in adults. Clinical and hemodynamic studies of 129 cases before and after surgical correction under cardiopulmonary bypass. *Acta Med. Scand. (Suppl.)*, **497**:1, 1968.

Somerville, J.; Stark, A. J.; Waterston, D. J.; Aberdeen, E.; Carter, R. E. B.; and Waich, S.: Banding of the pulmonary artery for common atrioventricular canal. *Br. Heart J.*, **29**:816, 1967.

Sondergaard, T.: Closure of atrial septal defects. *Acta Chir. Scand.*, **107**:492, 1954.

Swan, H.; Moresh, G.; Johnson, M. E.; and Warner, C.: The experimental creation and closure of auricular septal defects. In some surgical aspects of cardiovascular research. A symposium. Federal Security Agency, Washington, D.C., 1950.

Swan, H.; Virtue, R. W.; Blount, S. G.; and Kircher, L. I.: Hypothermia in surgery. Analysis of 100 clinical cases. *Ann. Surg.*, **142**:382, 1955.

Tajik, A. J.; Gan, G. T.; Ritter, D. G.; and Schattenberg, T. T.: Echocardiographic pattern of right ventricular diastolic volume overload in children. *Circulation*, **46**:36, 1972.

Tan, King-Twok; Takao, A.; Hashimoto, A.; and Sato, T.: Electrocardiogram of secundum type atrial septal defect simulating endocardial cushion defect. *Br. Heart J.*, **37**:209, 1975.

Tandon, R., and Edwards, J. E.: Atrial septal defect in infancy. Common association with other defects. *Circulation*, **49**:1005, 1974.

Taussig, H. B.: *Congenital Malformations of the Heart*. The Commonwealth Fund, New York, 1947.

Terplan, J., and Sanes, S.: The incidence of congenital heart lesions in infancy. *J. Tech. Methods*, **15**:86, 1936.

Tikoff, G.; Keith, T. B.; Nelson, R. M.; and Kuida, H.: Clinical and hemodynamic observations after surgical closure of large atrial septal defect complicated by heart failure. *Am. J. Cardiol.*, **23**:810, 1969.

Uhley, M. H.: Lutembacher's syndrome and a new concept of the dynamics of interatrial septal defect. *Am. Heart I.*, **24**:315, 1942.

Van Mierop, L. H. S.; Alley, R. D.; Kausel, H. W.; and Stranahan, A.: The Anatomy and Embryology of Endocardial Cushion Defects. *J. Thorac. Cardiovasc. Surg.*, **43**:1, 1962.

Watkins, E., Jr., and Gross, R. E.: Experiences with surgical repair of atrial septal defects. *J. Thorac. Surg.*, **30**:469, 1955.

Wheat, M. W., and Burford, T. H.: Digitalis in surgery: extension of classical indications. *J. Thorac. Cardiovasc. Surg.*, **41**:162, 1961.

White, P. D.: *Heart Disease*, 4th ed. The Macmillan Company, New York, 1951.

Williams, R. G., and Rudd, M.: Echocardiographic features of endocardial cushion defects. *Circulation*, **49**:418, 1974.

Wolf, P. S.; Vogel, J. H. K.; Pryor, R.; and Blount, S. G., Jr.: Atrial septal defect in patients over 45 years of age. *Br. Heart J.*, **30**:115, 1968.

Wood, P.: The vasoconstrictive factor in pulmonary hypertension. *Br. Heart J.*, **20**:557, 1958.

Wood, P.; Magidson, O.; and Wilson, P. A. O.: Ventricular septal defect, with note on acyanotic Fallot's tetralogy. *Br. Heart J.*, **16**:387, 1954.

Yao, J.; Thompson, M. W.; Trusler, G. A.; and Trimble, A. S.: Familial atrial septal defect of the primum type. *Can. Med. Assoc. J.*, **98**:217, 1968.

Zakrzewski, T. K.; Slodki, S. J.; and Luisada, A. A.: The first heart sound in atrial septal defect. *Am. Heart J.*, **78**:476, 1969.

Zetterqvist, P.: The syndrome of familial septal defects, heart arrhythmias, and hand malformations (Holt-Oram) in mother and son. *Acta Paediatr. Scand.*, **52**:115, 1963.

23

Single Ventricle

B. S. Langford Kidd

[handwritten] TYPES A, B, C, D

SINGLE ventricle is a condition that has been well defined pathologically for many years (Farre, 1814; Holmes, 1824; Favorite, 1934; Abbott 1936; Taussig, 1939), but only recently has its clinical recognition been achieved with any ease and accuracy (Van Praagh et al., 1965). It has also been bedeviled with a confusing and variable nomenclature.

Here the term "single ventricle" is used to describe that condition where one ventricular chamber receives both the mitral and tricuspid valves, or a common atrioventricular valve. This definition excludes mitral and tricuspid atresia. In its commonest form the single ventricle is a single left ventricle with a small outflow chamber. Both D- and L-transposition are common.

Other terms used to describe this condition have included cor triloculare biatriatum (Favorite, 1934; Rogers and Edwards, 1951), which means "three-chambered heart with two atria," and hence a single ventricle; and cor biloculare (Wood and Williams, 1928; Conn et al., 1950), a term that indicates that the atrial septum is also missing. "Common ventricle" was used interchangeably with "single ventricle" by Abbott (1936), Taussig (1939), and Edwards (1960); Lev (1953) and Lev and coworkers (1962) used the term "single ventricle" when there was an outlet chamber, and "common ventricle" when this was absent. Another term is "single ventricle with rudimentary or diminutive outlet chamber" (Lambert, 1951; Megevand et al., 1953). Abbott (1936) used the term "Holmes heart" (Holmes, 1824) to describe single ventricle with normally related great vessels and pulmonary stenosis (Kraus et al., 1969; Marin-Garcia et al., 1974b). More recently, Elliott and Morgan (1968) prefer "common," while both Engle (1968) and Nadas and Fyler (1972) express a preference for "single." Lev and associates (1969) use "single (primitive) ventricle" to describe only the commonest variety of this condition. The present author has chosen "single" because it seems slightly more preponderant and because "common" seems to have no significant superior virtues.

Anatomy and Embryology

Although the entity of single ventricle had been recognized for many years, controversy existed as to what single ventricle really was, with some support for the theory that the basic problem was really a large ventricular septal defect (Taussig, 1960). Since Van Praagh and colleagues in 1964 applied the principles of Lev (1954) to the recognition of what chambers (defined morphologically) were represented in a series of 60 unselected postmortem cases of single ventricle, the situation has become somewhat clearer. They defined four types, one of which was nearly four times more common than the other three combined.

The most frequent variety of single ventricle is a single left ventricle. This variety, termed type A by Van Praagh and associates, was present in 78 percent of their series (Table 23–1) and was as frequent in the experience of Engle (1968) and Lev (1969). In this type, the right ventricular sinus or inflow tract is generally believed to be absent. There is, however, a small rudimentary outflow chamber, which represents the right ventricular infundibulum communicating with the single left ventricle through the bulboventricular foramen. This chamber lies anteriorly and either to the right (if there is a D-loop) or to the left (if there is an L-loop) and so ventricular inversion (Figure 23–1). This diminutive outflow chamber usually gives rise to the aorta since transposition is nearly six times more common than the normal relationship of the great arteries in single ventricle. In these cases the pulmonary artery arises from the large left ventricle. *[handwritten margin: high incidence of transposition = single ventricle]*

Van Praagh's other three types were much less frequent. Single right ventricle with complete absence of the left ventricular sinus was present in 5 percent of cases (type B). In 7 percent of cases approximately equal amounts of right and left ventricular sinus myocardium were present, but were not divided by a ventricular septum; this group (classified type C) is nearest to the "huge ventricular septal defect" concept. In a final group of 10 percent (type D) there was development of neither ventricular sinus. Engle

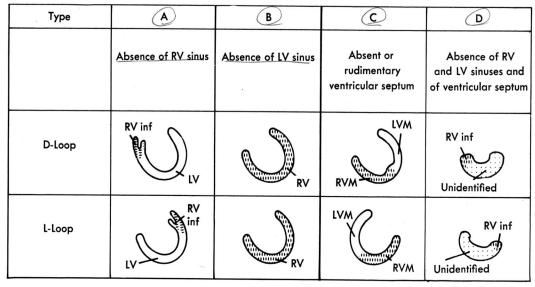

Type	A	B	C	D
	Absence of RV sinus	Absence of LV sinus	Absent or rudimentary ventricular septum	Absence of RV and LV sinuses and of ventricular septum
D-Loop	RV inf — LV		LVM — RVM	RV inf — Unidentified
L-Loop	RV inf — LV		LVM — RVM	RV inf — Unidentified

Figure 23-1. Diagram of Van Praagh's classification of single ventricle.

(1968) in a series of 41 cases (12 of whom, however, had tricuspid or mitral atresia) found 61 percent to be type A, 17 percent type B, 3 percent type C, and 17 percent uncertain.

Table 23–1   TYPES OF SINGLE VENTRICLE IN A POSTMORTEM SERIES*

Type A, single LV	78%
Type B, single RV	5%
Type C, undivided Vs	7%
Type D, infund. only	10%

* Van Praagh, R.; Ongley, P. A.; and Swan, H. J. C.: Anatomic types of single or common ventricle in man. Morphologic and geometric aspects of 60 necropsied cases. *Am. J. Cardiol.*, **31**: 367, 1964.

It is important in describing the characteristics of a condition with a complex embryologic basis to deal in turn with each of the major cardiac segments, atria, ventricles, and great arteries (Van Praagh, 1972). In Van Praagh's series, 83 percent were in visceroatrial situs solitus (Table 23–2) (that is, in the usual position), with the right atrium on the right along with the liver, and the left atrium on the left along with the stomach. Only 3 percent had visceroatrial situs inversus. In 13 percent of cases the visceroatrial situs was indeterminate ("heterotaxy"); all these cases had asplenia. The direction of ventricular looping determines the relative position of the right and left ventricles. A D-loop is seen in the situs solitus normal and in D-transposition, with the right ventricle on the right; and the L-loop is seen in the situs inversus individual and in L-transposition, with the right ventricle on the left. In Van Praagh's series, 57 percent had a D- or dextro loop and 43 percent an L- or levo loop.

Table 23–2.   SEGMENTAL RELATIONSHIP IN SINGLE VENTRICLE*

VISCEROATRIA VS. SITUS		VENTRICULAR LOOP		GREAT ARTERY POSITION	
Solitus	83%	D-	57%	Solitus normal	15%
Inversus	3%	L-	43%	D-TGA	42%
Indeterminate	13%			L-TGA	43%

* Van Praagh, R.; Ongley, P. A.; and Swan, H. J. C.: Anatomic types of single or common ventricle in man. Morphologic and geometric aspects of 60 necropsied cases. *Am. J. Cardiol.*, **31**: 367, 1964.

The great artery position was also determined in this series. This was solitus normal in 15 percent of cases, 42 percent in the D-transposition position, and 43 percent in the L-transposition. It is justified to call these cases D- and L-transposition since the great vessels are, in fact, "transposed" and the aorta arises above the right ventricular outflow tract. In cases without an outflow chamber this same relationship between the great arteries is more accurately described as "malposition." Because most cases have an outflow chamber, albeit not always clearly demonstrable, all cases are referred to as "transposed" (Lev et al., 1968). Lev and coworkers (1969) in his series of 46 cases—all with single left ventricle with an infundibular chamber—found 17 with D-transposition and 23 with L-transposition. Three cases were uncertain, and only three had a normal position.

There were 11 cases of dextrocardia in Van Praagh's series; six of them had visceroatrial situs solitus, and only one had situs inversus. In four with asplenia the situs was uncertain. In Lev's series 83 percent had levocardia and 15 percent dextrocardia, with one mesocardia.

These large clinical and pathologic experiences of Van Praagh, Engle, and Lev demonstrate that most cases are in levocardia with visceroatrial situs solitus, although heterotaxy with asplenia and situs inversus do occur. Atrioventricular discordance is present in nearly half of the cases and normally related great vessels are rare. D-Transposition and L-transposition are of equal frequency.

The concept of single ventricle as faulty development of ventricular septation has been challenged by de la Cruz and Miller (1965 and 1968), who introduced the concept of "double-inlet left ventricle." They proposed that the terms "single" and "common" ventricle (and also cor biatriatum triloculare) be confined to the entity in which the ventricular septum is absent or represented only by a small muscular ridge, and in which both atria empty into, and both great vessels arise from, the same chamber. The definition fits the "common ventricle" of Lev (1969) and Van Praagh's type C single ventricle (absence or rudimentary development of the sinus portion of the ventricular septum) (1965). These cases are rare. On embryologic ground, de la Cruz and Miller feel that the most frequent form of this sort of anomaly (type A single ventricle of Van Praagh and the single [primitive] ventricle of Lev) is a double-inlet left ventricle. They described two cases. In one the tricuspid valve straddled the ventricular septum (as it did in some of Van Praagh's type A single ventricles), and the right ventricle, although small, contained landmarks of both sinus and infundibular portions. In the other, both atrioventricular valves opened entirely into the left ventricle, and the right ventricle was represented solely by the infundibulum as in the classic most frequent variety of single ventricle. Mehrizi and associates (1966) described 11 further cases in all of which the right ventricle was represented by both the sinus region and the infundibular outflow tract. In at least three of these cases, the tricuspid valve straddled the ventricular septum. Liberthson and coworkers (1971) described a further 14 cases in which the atrioventricular orifices straddled or were displaced in relation to the ventricular septum. In all 14 cases the left ventricle was large, but the small right ventricle contained both sinus and conus portions; and this was almost certainly so in the three cases described briefly by Keith and colleagues (1958).

Recently, Quero (1970, 1972) has reopened the question of whether there can be "single" ventricle with atresia of one atrioventricular valve. This viewpoint has some merit, and also the agreement of Cabrera and associates (1974), and the morphologic support of Rosenquist and coworkers (1970) and Anderson and Becker (1974). There is no unanimity of opinion as to what constitutes a single or primitive ventricle. Is the single ventricle, type A, of Van Praagh a morphologically left ventricle, or is it a morphologically primitive ventricle? This is the question that Anderson and his colleagues have posed (1976, 1977). Their conclusion is that the distinctive feature of the primitive ventricle is absence of the posterior ventricular septum, i.e., that portion which interposes between the atrioventricular valves. Thus, in their terminology, the type A single ventricle of Van Praagh is not a morphologically left ventricle, but rather is a primitive ventricle with an outlet chamber. At the present time, this difference of opinion has not been resolved.

It is likely, then, that the embryologic basis of this group of anomalies is the faulty alignment of the atrioventricular canal in relationship to the two developing ventricles. On completion of the formation of the bulboventricular loop, both atria relate only to the primitive ventricular part of the tube, that is, the part that is going to form the left ventricle. In order for the atrioventricular canal to relate to the right ventricle, which is going to form from the bulbus cordis part of the tube, the atria must expand to the right and the ventricular part of the loop move to the left. As the right atrium makes more complete functional contact with the right ventricle, this ventricle develops more normally. However, if this movement is incomplete, the tricuspid valve may straddle the ventricular septum and the right ventricle will be hypoplastic. If it does not take place at all, both atrioventricular valves relate solely to the left ventricle and the right ventricle will be represented solely by the infundibulum (de la Cruz and Miller, 1968; Asami, 1969; Lev, 1969).

Quero and coworkers (1973) have recently described seven patients and postulated that the other end of this spectrum does exist: that double-inlet right ventricle (Classification of Heart Disease in Childhood), single right ventricle (Van Praagh et al., 1964), and straddling mitral valve are examples of *excessive* displacement of the atrioventricular canal toward the bulbus cordis. In two of their cases both valves opened into a large right ventricle, as in Van Praagh's type B single ventricle. However, in these cases a hypoplastic left ventricle was seen. This was not found in the cases of Van Praagh and colleagues.

The nomenclature and the anatomic or embryologic groups of these diverse series of cases are far from clearly defined at the present time. It would seem reasonable to call the most frequent type, with large left ventricle and small right ventricular outflow tract, "single ventricle," and to confine the term double-inlet left ventricle to the cases in which both sinus and infundibulum of the right ventricle are clearly present. The even rarer cases with straddling and displaced atrioventricular valves and single or double-inlet right ventricle should probably be defined in descriptive rather than in nominative terms.

Associated Anomalies

The common and uniting feature in this condition is that both venous returns pass into a common chamber from which the mixed blood is ejected into the great arteries. Whether or not these great arteries are transposed is of little functional significance. However, obstruction to this ventricular outflow is frequent and will affect the clinical picture.

outflow obstruction

Table 23–3.   PERCENTAGE INCIDENCE OF VENTRICULAR OUTFLOW OBSTRUCTION IN SINGLE VENTRICLE*

| SERIES | PULMONARY OUTFLOW OBSTRUCTION | | | SYSTEMIC OUTFLOW OBSTRUCTION | | | |
	PS	PA	Total	AS	AA	Total	Coarct. Ao.
Van Praagh (1964)	27	20	47	35	—	35	23
Engle (1968)	17	17	34	17	17	34	10
Lev (1968)	30	11	41	48	—	48	23
Average (n–147)			41 %			39 %	19 %

* PS, PA, AS, AA = pulmonary and aortic stenosis and atresia.

As can be seen from Table 23–3, the incidence of obstruction to both pulmonary and systemic outflow is approximately equal. It had previously been suggested (Brown, 1950; Taussig, 1960) that the artery arising from the outflow chamber was usually stenosed while that from the single ventricle was not. The clinical and postmortem series of Van Praagh and associates (1965) did not support this, in that the outflow chamber great artery was stenosed in only 48 percent while the single ventricle great artery was not stenosed in only 65 percent. So while there is a tendency in this direction, it is not the rule. However, it was noted in this series that all the cases of D-transposition had some degree of subaortic stenosis at the site of the bulboventricular foramen, together with preductal coarctation or atresia of the aortic isthmus. None had pulmonary obstruction. On the other hand, with L-transposition subaortic obstruction occurred only in 73 percent, while 50 percent had obstruction of the pulmonary outflow tract.

Other lesions found in association with single ventricle are: atrial septal defect (both primum and secundum), single atrium, and anomalous pulmonary venous drainage, these last two occurring in association with asplenia.

Prevalence

This is an uncommon congenital defect occurring 222 times in 15,104 clinical cases of congenital heart disease seen at The Hospital for Sick Children, Toronto, between 1950 and 1973, representing 1.5 percent of the total cases. Fifty-six percent of the cases were boys, a male/female ratio of 1.25:1. Using an incidence figure of 0.8 percent for congenital heart disease among live births, these figures would suggest an incidence for single ventricle of 1 in 6500 live births.

Clinical Features

Because of the major circulatory derangement in these children, they commonly present early in childhood. The ages at referral to The Hospital for Sick Children of 182 children who had single ventricle are shown in Figure 23–2, 42.3 percent presenting in the first week of life and 56 percent by the end of the

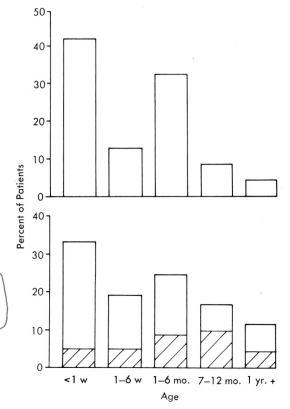

Figure 23-2. Age at presentation (above) and age at death (below) of cases of single ventricle series of The Hospital for Sick Children, Toronto. Hatched areas in deaths associated with surgery.

first month; 88.4 percent had been seen at this center before the age of six months.

The clinical course in any infant is determined by the hemodynamics. Although some streaming does occur, there is more or less complete mixing of the systemic and pulmonary venous returns in the common ventricular chamber (Rahimtoola et al., 1966; Marin-Garcia et al., 1974b; Macartney et al., 1976), and since the blood is ejected into the great arteries by a common ejectile force, the hemodynamic state of the patient will be determined by the resistance to outflow into the two circulations. In the case of the systemic circulation, as well as the systemic vascular resistance, there may be additional obstruction at the aortic valve, at a coarctation, or at the bulboventricular foramen if there is transposition. In the case of the pulmonary circulation, as well as the pulmonary vascular resistance, there may be valvular or subvalvular pulmonary stenosis.

Since it is the changes in the pulmonary circulation that will have the greater impact, the clinical picture is determined by whether the net intracardiac shunt is left-to-right or right-to-left, or, to put it another way, by the dimension of the pulmonary blood flow, since systemic blood flow is less variable.

In the first major clinical group, pulmonary blood flow is small in the fetus because of the collapsed lungs and high pulmonary vascular resistance; after birth, when there is no pulmonary stenosis, pulmonary blood flow will start to increase markedly as pulmonary vascular resistance falls. This circulatory overload will give rise to rapid breathing, fatigue, poor feeding, failure to gain weight, respiratory distress, and congestive heart failure. Cyanosis is not especially prominent in these children: indeed in 53 of the 182 children seen at this hospital (29.1 percent), cyanosis was not noted at the time of initial referral, although systemic desaturation was always present when it was measured. In addition 17.6 percent of The Hospital for Sick Children series were in frank congestive failure, with tachycardia and liver enlargement. The chest usually showed a hyperactive precordium with a diffuse cardiac impulse, the first heart sound was usually described as loud, and the second either as single or as narrowly split. There was usually a murmur described as either pansystolic or long-ejection in type, and in addition a middiastolic flow murmur of rapid ventricular filling—or a third heart sound—was noted.

In the second group, those with limited pulmonary blood flow, cyanosis will be the prominent presenting feature and heart failure rare. Children in this group will resemble those with tetralogy of Fallot and will either have been cyanosed from birth or have become more cyanosed with time. The depth of the cyanosis will vary, being most severe when pulmonary blood flow is least, and less marked if the pulmonary blood flow is increased. The cyanosis always increases with crying or exertion and was noted at first referral in 70 percent of the 182 children seen in our clinic. In children with small pulmonary blood flow, the precordium will be quiet, with a localized cardiac impulse. There will sometimes be a systolic thrill. The first sound will be normal, and the second sound single. There will usually be a harsh grade III–IV ejection systolic murmur best heard at the base of the heart, and frequently as well in the second right as in the second left interspace due to the often more medial position of the pulmonary artery.

Radiologic Examination

Single ventricle has no typical radiographic characteristics that make it easily recognizable

(Hallerman et al., 1966). In those cases where there is increased pulmonary blood flow, the chest x-ray always shows an enlarged heart with pulmonary plethora. Although there is no characteristic cardiac shape associated with single ventricle, abnormalities of the great arteries may sometimes be suspected from the basal shadows. A narrow pedicle may suggest D-transposition, while L-transposition may be suggested by a prominence on the upper left border with a sloping shoulder formed by the ascending aorta.

As indicated above, the presence or absence of pulmonary stenosis is of great hemodynamic, prognostic, and therapeutic importance. This may be suspected from the plain chest x-ray. With unobstructed pulmonary blood flow, there are cardiomegaly and prominence of the pulmonary vasculature and a large left atrium; in the majority of cases with pulmonary stenosis, the pulmonary vascularity appears normal and the heart is only mildly enlarged or may be normal (Van Praagh et al., 1966). Only where the obstruction to pulmonary outflow is very severe, or where there is pulmonary atresia, is there pulmonary oligemia.

In the later stages in single ventricle with unobstructed pulmonary blood flow, obliterative changes take place in the peripheral pulmonary vasculature. With the increase in pulmonary vascular resistance, pulmonary blood flow falls. Here the heart will decrease in size, and the peripheral lung fields will clear. However, the proximal hilar pulmonary arteries will appear prominent with tortuous branching.

Echocardiography

Ultrasound can be of great value in the study of single ventricle. The most striking feature is that (as might be expected) there is no ventricular septum in the usual location. In some cases, however, a small septum may be located high and anterior in the outflow area, and probably represents the bulbar septum demarcating the outlet chamber. The great arteries can be seen, and may be recognized as transposed or not. The question of whether there is one or two atrioventricular valves is more difficult to answer: two valves may be visualized at two different sites or levels in the main chamber, but this is not always so. The demonstration of two distinct atrioventricular valves simultaneously without an intervening ventricular septum is diagnostic, however (Figure 23–3).

Electrocardiography

Study of the electrocardiogram and vectorcardiogram in cases of single ventricle has not proven to be very useful prospectively, either in indicating the diagnosis of single ventricle or in delineating the type of single ventricle present, the position of the outlet chamber and great arteries, or the presence or absence

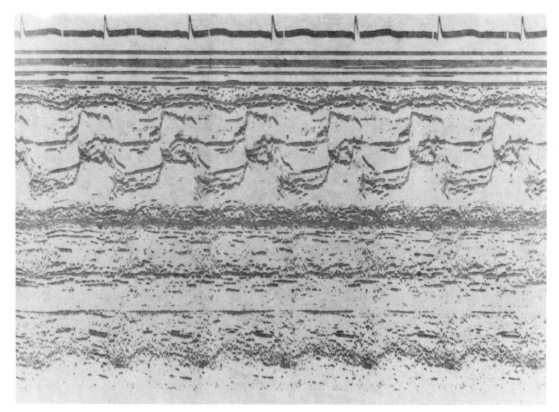

Figure 23-3. Echocardiogram from a patient with single ventricle. Mitral and tricuspid valves are seen without any intervening septum.

of pulmonary stenosis. When the heart specimen is in one's hand, the electrocardiogram can often be interpreted logically, but, unfortunately, the reverse is not true (Van Praagh et al., 1965; Engle, 1968). However, minor discrepancies in the electrocardiogram from what is expected from the more commonly occurring lesions may alert one's suspicions to this diagnosis.

As has been pointed out by Sodi-Pallares and coworkers (1959), the initial forces in the QRS axis are generated by septal depolarization. Therefore, in cases where this does not occur in its customary left-to-right manner—producing initial electrical forces anteriorly and to the right and Q waves confined to the left chest—one can assume either that the ventricular septum is not in its usual place or that the conducting system is not normally situated. Thus, a pattern with Q waves in the right chest (as may be seen in L-transposition) is suspicious; additionally, however, Q waves may either be absent completely or present in all leads (Elliott et al., 1964).

The mean QRS vector in the frontal plane may vary widely (Davachi and Moller, 1969) although Marin-Garcia and associates (1974) described left axis deviation in 9 of 13 patients with single ventricles and normally related great arteries.

Ventricular hypertrophy patterns again may not be helpful: on anatomic grounds one might suspect that an undifferentiated pattern across the chest might be common, and indeed large RS waves from V_1 through V_6 is one of the more usual patterns (Figure 23–4). However, both right and left ventricular hypertrophy pattern can be seen separately. In other cases the electrical forces are directed posteriorly and QS waves are seen (Keith et al., 1958; Morgan et al., 1965; Van Praagh et al., 1965). High-voltage midprecordial RS complexes (the Katz–Wachtel sign) have been reported by Shaher (1963) and by Elliott and coworkers (1963), but are not specific.

Abnormal atrioventricular conduction may also occur with first and second degree heart block (Marin-Garcia et al., 1974a). This is yet another feature in common with both single ventricle and corrected transposition, in both of which the conducting pathways are abnormally located.

Hemodynamics

As indicated above, the diagnosis of single ventricle is made by cardiac catheterization and angiocardiography. Commonly the catheter, passing up the inferior vena cava to the right atrium, enters a large ventricular cavity through the tricuspid valve. There is a step-up in oxygen saturation, which may vary from location to location in the ventricular chamber

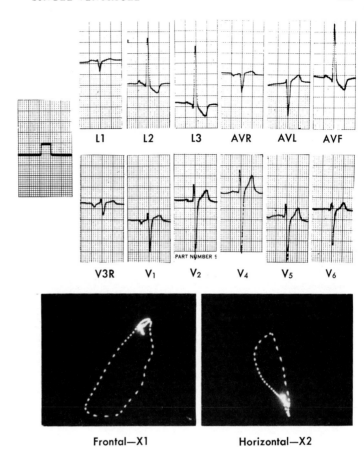

Figure 23–4. Electrocardiogram and vector loops from a child with single ventricle. Note absence of Q waves and the similarity of the ventricular complexes in the precordial leads.

Frontal—X1   Horizontal—X2

and which is at systemic pressure. Entry into the great arteries may be easy or may necessitate the use of a Swan-Ganz balloon catheter. If the atrial septum is crossed, the catheter enters the same ventricular chamber through the left atrioventricular valve. A catheter passed retrogradely into the heart via the aorta will either lie in the anterior outflow chamber or, passing through the bulboventricular foramen, enter the common ventricular chamber.

The aortic oxygen saturation will be reduced, mostly depending on the level of pulmonary blood flow. Rahimtoola et al., (1966) reported that complete mixing in the common chamber was rare and that "favorable" streaming—that is, streaming of the pulmonary venous blood to the aorta and of the systemic venous blood to the lungs—was more likely to occur when there was L-transposition; more complete mixing was noted when there was pulmonary stenosis. These findings were supported by Marin-Garcia and associates (1974a). More recently, however, Macartney and coworkers (1976) were unable to confirm this: using stepwise regression analysis they were unable to improve on the prediction of systemic arterial oxygen saturation from the measurement of pulmonary and systemic blood flows by including additional anatomic information such as the position of the great arteries.

It is of major importance to assess the pulmonary outflow tract, to measure the pressure there (if necessary using a Swan-Ganz balloon catheter), and to determine whether there is pulmonary stenosis or whether a low pulmonary blood flow is due to progressive pulmonary vascular disease. When the hemodynamic measurements have been made and flows, resistances, and outflow gradients calculated, good angiocardiography will be vital.

Angiocardiography

As indicated above, angiocardiography is the basic element in the successful and detailed diagnostic assessment in single ventricle. This has become even more important with the advent of successful repair of this condition (Edie et al., 1973; Ionescu et al., 1973).

There are seven important questions to which the cardiologist and cardiovascular surgeon need answers:

1. Can You Identify What Type of Single Ventricle Is Present? It is generally agreed that two types of single ventricle can and should be identified angiocardiographically: single ventricle with and without an outflow chamber (Marin-Garcia et al., 1974; Macartney et al., 1976). This distinction is best made by an injection into the major chamber, with the

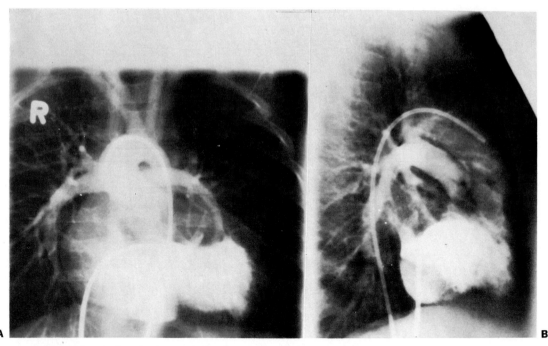

A

B

Figure 23-5. Injection with the ventricular chamber in a case of single ventricle, type C. The great arteries are in D-malposition.

catheter traversing either the left or right atrioventricular valves. The injection should be made at a high flow rate through the largest possible catheter to ensure good visualization; and, especially in those cases where there is increased pulmonary blood flow, the volume injected should be at least 1.5 ml/kg. Serial radiography should be performed in the biplane mode either with a large film changer or with a ciné camera.

In the most common type, the ventricular chamber into which the atrioventricular valves open is demonstrated as large and fairly smooth-walled, and there is filling of the outlet chamber through the bulboventricular foramen (Figure 23–5). In the no-outflow chamber group, both great arteries arise from this major chamber. Cineangiography in the left anterior oblique projection may resolve uncertainty about the presence or absence of the ventricular septum.

2. Where Is the Outflow Chamber? This chamber is usually situated anteriorly, and may be medial and anterior—as is commonly the case when there is D-transposition (Figure 23–6)—or lateral and anterior where there is L-transposition (Figure 23–7). The chamber (which may be small and restrictive, or large and contain elements of the sinus of the right ventricle) is often fairly well seen following injection in the large chamber. However, a retrograde approach via the femoral artery, with injection just below the aortic valve, may be necessary to define it completely.

3. What Is the Relationship of the Great Arteries? These are usually well-defined from the

injection in the major ventricle with filming in the biplane mode. They may be transposed. With D-transposition, the aorta arising anteriorly from the outlet chamber will be on the right, and the pulmonary artery posteriorly on the left. With L-transposition, the aorta will be anterior and on the left, the ascending aorta will form the upper left cardiac border, and the pulmonary artery arise posteriorly and to the right. When the relationship of the great arteries is normal, this is usually clearly seen.

4. Is There Obstruction to Pulmonary Outflow? The presence or absence of pulmonary stenosis is of major importance, and angiography may be very useful if it has not proved possible to catheterize the pulmonary artery either with a regular or a Swan-Ganz balloon catheter. Pulmonary stenosis may be either valvular or subvalvular (Macartney et al., 1976) and is best seen in the biplane injections below the pulmonary valve. Where there is no transposition, the obstruction may be at the bulboventricular foramen.

5. Is There Obstruction to Systemic Outflow? Again this is best demonstrated from the biplane study performed in the major chamber. Commonly the obstruction is at the bulboventricular foramen or in the restrictive outflow chamber. Although these obstructions may be well seen in the anteroposterior and lateral projections, oblique projections may be necessary to see the bulboventricular septum in profile.

6. What Is the State of the Atrioventricular Valves? This question is also of major importance from

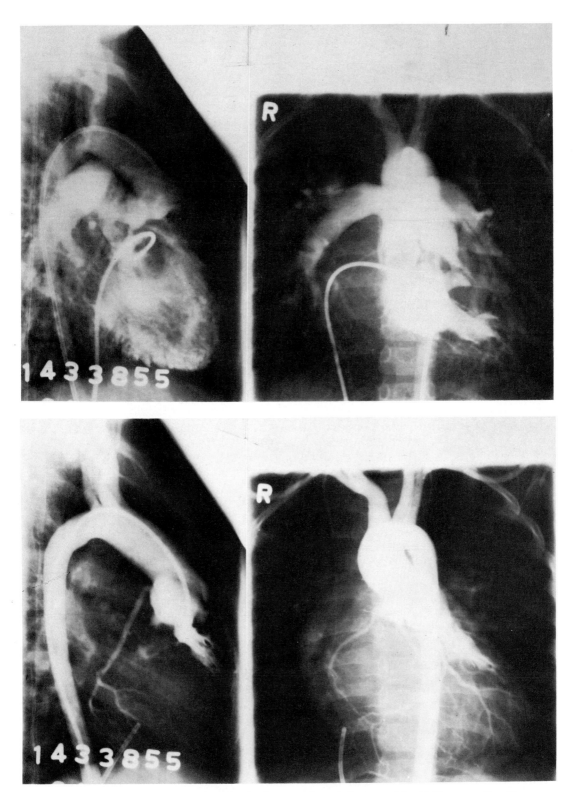

Figure 23-6. Injection into the outflow chamber in a case of type A single ventricle with D-transposition. The common ventricle and pulmonary arteries fill with contrast refluxing through the bulboventricular foramen.

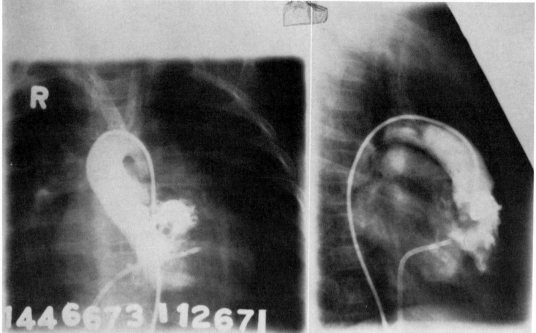

A   B

Figure 23-7. Injection into the common ventricular chamber (*A*) and into the outflow chamber (*B*) in a case of single ventricle with L-transposition. Note the small outflow chamber.

the point of view of reconstructive surgery. The atrioventricular valves may be normal, inverted as in L-transposition, or common as in the atrioventricular canal type of defect. Furthermore, one or other may be absent (Quero, 1972; Macartney et al., 1976), for although these cases of mitral and tricuspid atresia are not included in the definition of single ventricles used in this chapter, the presence or absence of both valves must be established in any case of apparent single ventricle under study. Finally, the valve may straddle the bulboventricular septum (Liberthson et al., 1971). The techniques used to distinguish these possibilities are: (1) during diastole following the ventricular injection either (a) the limbus of two separate valves may be seen, or (b) nonradiopaque blood may be seen entering the chamber already opacified with dye through two different locations, or in an area remote from the valve the catheter has passed through; (2) small injections into both atria may demonstrate two valve mechanisms; (3) injections into the pulmonary circulation may demonstrate that the pulmonary venous return enters the ventricle from a different position; (4) passing the catheter into the ventricle through an atrioventricular valve in two apparently different positions is less helpful. This differentiation is the most difficult part of the diagnostic procedure. In some cases resolution may not be possible short of surgery. However, with the demonstration of Danielson and associates (1974) that a common atrioventricular valve can be successfully replaced by two prosthetic valves, it is possible that this may be less important in the future.

7. Are There Associated Lesions?   Other anomalies, such as coarctation of the aorta or a persistent ductus arteriosus, should be sought and excluded.

Diagnosis

The diagnosis of single ventricle is most commonly made in a newborn or in a young infant who is probably mildly cyanosed and in respiratory distress, if not in frank congestive heart failure. However, as indicated above, this picture will vary. In the group with large pulmonary blood flow, the differential diagnoses are from complete transposition of the great arteries with a ventricular septal defect, from double-outlet right ventricle, from persistent truncus arteriosus, or from a large left-to-right shunt such as a ventricular septal defect and a persistent ductus arteriosus with pulmonary hypertension. The chest x-ray and electrocardiogram may suggest corrected transposition. In the second group, with pulmonary stenosis and diminished pulmonary blood flow, the most common differential diagnoses are with tetralogy of Fallot or transposition with pulmonary stenosis, or double-outlet right ventricle with pulmonary stenosis.

As mentioned above, the slightly discrepant electrocardiographic findings and the difficulty in delineating the ventricular septum on echocardiogram will suggest the diagnosis. The basis of accurate diagnosis is good selective angiocardiography.

Prognosis

This is a serious malformation. Of The Hospital for Sick Children series of 182 patients seen between 1950 and 1973 with single ventricle, 117 (64.3 percent) are dead, 50 percent within the first month of life and 74 percent within the first six months. Fourteen of the twenty-seven deaths among older children were associated with surgery, either palliative or attempted correction. In recent years, however, the prognosis has improved, with demonstration in a number of centers that surgical "correction" is feasible (Sakakibara et al., 1972; Edie et al., 1973; Ionescu et al., 1973a; Danielson et al., 1974; McGoon et al., 1976).

The initial problem, however, is in the newborn period. Here the prognosis is worse if there is pulmonary atresia, as pulmonary blood flow (and so life) is dependent on the continued persistence of the ductus arteriosus. Early and successful systemic-pulmonary anastamosis, possibly preceded by prostaglandins infusion (Olley et al., 1976), will be lifesaving.

Severe obstruction to left-sided outflow, whether at the subaortic, bulboventricular foramen level, or at the valve or aortic isthmus, is of more serious prognosis.

If the infant, either by palliation or by the natural balance of lesions, can survive past the first few years, surgical repair may be possible (Edie and Malm, 1976).

Treatment

Treatment initially is of the distressed, cyanosed newborn. Digitalis and diuretics should be administered if heart failure is present, and any concurrent chest infections treated with appropriate antibiotics. In those cases where the cyanosis is marked, and after digitalization in other cases, cardiac catheterization should be carried out and diagnosis established by biplane selective angiocardiography. At this point the diagnosis should be as complete as possible, especially identifying additional lesions such as coarctation.

If, following accurate diagnosis, heart failure persists, pulmonary artery banding should be carried out to limit pulmonary blood flow, relieve heart failure, and protect the pulmonary vasculature from the development of progressive pulmonary vascular disease. Freedom et al. (1977) have documented progressive narrowing of the bulboventricular foramen in 4 of 31 patients with single ventricle, outlet chamber, and transposition of the great arteries who underwent palliative pulmonary arterial banding. This narrowing results in functional subaortic stenosis as the aorta originates above the outlet chamber and was documented to occur following the banding procedure. It was suggested that concentric muscular hypertrophy in response to the pulmonary artery band may initially narrow the bulboventricular

foramen, especially in those defects that initially appear relatively small, or those associated with obstructive anomalies of the aortic arch with progressive narrowing of the bulboventricular foramen. Fibrous tissue might proliferate about the margins of the now restrictive defect, further compromising aortic blood flow. Clinical recognition of this development may be predicated on presence of symptoms such as angina, lack of continued clinical improvement in a patient whose pulmonary arterial band has significantly reduced pulmonary blood flow, and on the development of ventricular strain. Severe restriction at the bulboventricular foramen has been documented three months following banding. If there is a persistent ductus or a coarctation, these can be dealt with at the same time. Pulmonary stenosis, on the other hand, may need a systemic-pulmonary anastamosis to improve pulmonary blood flow. This may be postponed for a period if the cyanosis is not marked; if, on the other hand, it is severe (as in pulmonary atresia), shunting should be carried out as an emergency.

Until recently a "corrective" procedure for single ventricle was not available. There was lack of information about whether an artificially partitioned ventricular cavity could function as two separate ventricles. In addition, there was a lack of accurate preoperative diagnosis and a high incidence of complicated associated lesions such as D- and L-transposition. A further factor was the unknown and variable position of the conducting tissue in these primitive ventricles. Two steps made progress possible. First, Seki and associates (1972) demonstrated that a partitioned heart would function. Second, Anderson and coworkers (1974) reported that the conducting pathway between the atria and ventricles in single ventricle (double-inlet left ventricle) was from an anterior node, and that the atrioventricular bundle came down in the front of the outflow of the posterior great artery and on the right margin of the bulboventricular foramen; there it split, the right bundle coursing into the outflow chamber and the left bundle into the main chamber. This is different from the course in "huge ventricular septal defect" type C single ventricle where the bundle runs posteriorly.

The development of a technique of mapping the conduction tissue intraoperatively (Kaiser et al., 1970) has made it possible for surgeons to avoid it and consequent complete heart block. These steps made septation of the ventricular cavity feasible and this has now been carried out successfully at a number of centers (Edie et al., 1973; Ionescu et al., 1973; McGoon et al., 1976), both in the common variety with an outlet chamber and where there is no outlet chamber. Edie and Malm (1976) believe that the main features of successful repair are mapping of the conducting system, stable fixation of the prosthetic septum, and relief of pulmonary outflow obstruction—whether natural as in pulmonary stenosis or iatrogenic as in pulmonary artery banding. Complete transposition can be dealt with by the Mustard procedure. Recently Danielson and colleagues (1974) reported successful repair of single ventricle in association with complete atrioventricular canal; so this former contraindication to separation of the ventricles seems not so important.

Long-term follow-up on these cases is not yet available, but evidence suggests that the artificially partitioned ventricular chamber functions as two separate chambers at different pressures. Normal cardiac outputs can be maintained and other postoperative complications are rare, provided the conducting tissue has not been damaged.

In conclusion, there is now the possibility that the child who has survived infancy (either by fortunate anatomy or by successful palliation) may be a candidate for successful repair of single ventricle. Much longer follow-up will be necessary to assess this management fully, although at present it looks hopeful.

REFERENCES

Abbott, M. E.: *Atlas of Congenital Cardiac Disease*. American Heart Association, New York, 1936, p. 60.

Anderson, R. H.; Arnold, R.; Thapar, M. K.; Jones, R. S.; and Hamilton, D. I.: Cardiac specialized tissue in hearts with an apparently single ventricular chamber (double inlet left ventricle). *Am. J. Cardiol.*, 33:95, 1974.

Anderson, R. H., and Becker, A. E.: Morphological observation in specimens of tricuspid atresia with reference to bulboventricular morphogenesis. *Br. Heart J.*, 37:552, 1975.

Anderson, R. H.; Becker, A. E.; Wilkinson, J. L.; and Gerlis, L. M.: Morphogenesis of univentricular hearts. *Br. Heart J.*, 38:558, 1976.

Anderson, R. H.; Wilkinson, J. L.; Gerlis, L. M.; Smith, A.; and Becker, A. E.: Atresia of the right atrioventricular orifice. *Br. Heart J.*, 49:414, 1977.

Asami, I.: Beitrag zur Entwicklung des Dammerseptums in menschlichen Herzed mit besonderer Berucksichtigung der sogenannten Bulbusdrehung. *Z. Anat. Entwicklungsgesch.*, 128:1, 1969.

Brown, J. W.: *Congenital Heart Disease*, 2nd ed. Staples Press, London, 1950.

Cabrera, A.; Azunca, J. I.; and Bilbao, F.: Single primitive ventricle with D-transposition of the great vessels and atresia of the left A-V valve. *Am Heart J.*, 88:225, 1974.

Classification of Heart Disease in Childhood. International Society of Cardiology, V.R.B. Offsetdrukkerij-Kleine de A4, Groningen, 1970.

Conn, J. J.; Clark, T. E.; and Kissane, R. S.: Cortriloculare. *Am. J. Med.*, 8:187, 1950.

Danielson, G. K.; Giuliani, E. R.; and Ritter, D. G.: Successful repair of common ventricle associated with complete atrioventricular canal. *J. Thorac. Cardiovasc. Surg.*, 67:152, 1974.

Davachi, F., and Moller, J. H.: The electrocardiogram and vectorcardiogram in single ventricle. Anatomic correlations. *Am. J. Cardiol.*, 23:19, 1969.

de la Cruz, M. V., and Miller, B. L.: Double inlet left ventricle. Report of two cases with embryological consideration. *Circulation*, 32:75, 1965 (Abstr.).

de la Cruz, M. V., and Miller, B. L.: Double inlet left ventricle: two pathological specimens with comments on the embryology and on its relation to single ventricle. *Circulation*, 37:249, 1968.

Edie, R. N.; Ellis, K.; Gersony, W. M.; Krongrad, E.; Bowman, F. O.; and Malm, J. R.: Surgical repair of single ventricle. *J. Thorac. Cardiovasc. Surg.*, 66:350, 1973.

Edie, R. N., and Malm, J. R.: Surgical repair of single ventricle. In: *The Child with Congenital Heart Disease After Surgery*. Ed. by B. S. L. Kidd and R. D. Rowe. Futura Press, New York, 1976.

Edwards, J. E.: Congenital malformations of the heart and great vessels. In: *Pathology of the Heart*, 2nd ed. Ed. by S. E. Gould, Charles C. Thomas, Publisher, Springfield, Ill., 1960, p. 335.

Elliott, L. P.; Amplatz, K.; Anderson, R. L.; and Edwards, J. E.: Cor triloculare biatriatum with pulmonary stenosis in normally related great vessels. *Am. J. Cardiol.*, 11:469, 1963.

Elliott, L. P., and Morgan, A. D.: Common ventricles. In: *Heart Disease in Infants, Children and Adolescents*. Ed. by A. J. Moss and F. H. Adams. The Williams & Wilkins Co., Baltimore, 1968, p. 589.

Elliott, L. P.; Ruttenberg, H. D.; Eliot, R. S.; and Anderson, R. C.: Vectorial analysis of the electrocardiogram in common ventricle. *Br. Heart J.*, 26:302, 1964.

Engle, M. A.: Single ventricle. In: *Paediatric Cardiology*. Ed. by H. Watson. Lloyd Luke Ltd., London, 1968, Chap. 43, p. 633.

Farre, J. R.: Pathological research. In: *Malformations of the Heart*. Longman, Hurst, Orme and Brown, London, 1814, Essay 1, p. 28.

Favorite, G. O.: Cor biatriatum triloculare with rudimentary right ventricle, hypoplasia of transposed aorta, and patent ductus arteriosus terminating by rupture of dilated pulmonary artery. *Am. J. Med. Sci.*, 187:663, 1934.

Freedom, R. M.; Sondheimer, H.; Dische, R.; and Rowe, R. D.: Development of "subaortic stenosis" after pulmonary arterial banding for common ventricle. *Am. J. Cardiol.*, 39:79, 1977.

Hallerman, F. J.; Davis, G. D.; Ritter, D. G.; and Kincaid, O. W.: Roentgenographic features of common ventricle. *Radiology*, 87:409, 1966.

Holmes, A. F.: Case of malformation of the heart. *Trans. Med. Chir. Soc. Edinburgh*, 1:252, 1824.

Ionescu, M. I.; Macartney, F. J.; and Wooler, G. H.: Intracardiac repair of single ventricle with pulmonary stenosis. *J. Thorac. Cardiovasc. Surg.*, 65:602, 1973.

Kaiser, G. A.; Waldo, A. L.; Beach, P. M.; Bowman, F. O.; Hoffman, B. F.; and Malm, J. R.: Specialized cardiac conduction system: Improved electrophysiologic identification techniques at surgery. *Arch. Surg.*, 101:673, 1970.

Keith, J. D.; Rowe, R. D.; and Vlad, P.: *Heart Disease in Infancy and Childhood*. Macmillan Publishing Co., Inc., New York, 1958, p. 477.

Kraus, A. P.; Smith, R. M.; Schneider, A. B.; and Parker, B. M.: Single ventricle with normal relationship of the great vessels and pulmonic stenosis. *Am. Heart J.*, 78:530, 1969.

Lambert, E. C.: Single ventricle with a rudimentary outlet chamber. Case report. *Bull. Johns Hopkins Hosp.*, 88:231, 1951.

Lev, M.: *Autopsy Diagnosis of Congenitally Malformed Hearts*. Charles C Thomas, Publisher, Springfield, Ill., 1953, p. 154.

Lev, M.: Pathologic diagnosis of positional variations in cardiac chambers in congenital heart disease. *Lab. Invest.*, 3:71, 1954.

Lev, M.; Liberthson, R. R.; Kirkpatrick, J. R.; Eckner, F. A. P.; and Arcilla, R. A.: Single (primitive) ventricle. *Circulation*, 39:577, 1969.

Lev, M.; Paul, M. H.; and Miller, R. A.: A classification of congenital heart disease based on the pathological complex. *Am. J. Cardiol.*, 10:733, 1962.

Liberthson, R. F.; Paul, M. H.; Muster, A. J.; Arcilla, R. A.; Eckner, F. A. O.; and Lev, M.: Straddling and displaced atrioventricular orifices and valves with primitive ventricles. *Circulation*, 43:213, 1971.

Macartney, F. J.; Partridge, J. B.; Scott, O.; and Deverall, P.: Common or single ventricle. An angiocardiographic and hemodynamic study of 42 patients. *Circulation*, 53:543, 1976.

Marin-Garcia, J.; Tandon, R.; Moller, J. H.; and Edwards, J. E.: Common (single) ventricle with normally related great vessels. *Circulation*, 49:565, 1974a.

Marin-Garcia, J.; Tandon, R.; Moller, J. H.; and Edwards, J. E.: Single ventricle with transposition. *Circulation*, 49:994, 1974b.

McGoon, D. C.; Marcelletti, C.; Denielson, G. K.; Wallace, R. B.; Ritter, D. C.; and Maloney, J. D.: The problems of correcting single or common ventricle. (Abstr.) *Circulation*, (Suppl. II), 54:11–101, 1976.

Megevand, R. M.; Paul, R. M.; and Parker, J.: Single ventricle with diminutive outlet chamber associated with coarctation of the aorta and other cardiac anomalies. *J. Pediatr.*, 43:687, 1953.

Mehrizi, A.; McMurphy, D.; Ottesen, O. E.; and Rowe, R. D.: Syndrome of double inlet left ventricle: Angiocardiographic differentiation from single ventricle with rudimentary outlet chamber. *Bull. Johns Hopkins Hosp.*, 119:255, 1966.

Morgan, A. D.; Krovetz, L. J.; and Schiebler, G.: Electrovector-cardiographic analysis of nine cases of single ventricle with the great vessel arrangement of corrected transposition. In: Hoffman, B. F. (ed.): *Vectorcardiography.* North-Holland, Amsterdam, 1966.

Nadas, A. S., and Fyler, D. C.: Communications between systemic and pulmonary circuits with predominantly left to right shunts. In: *Pediatric Cardiology.* Ed. by A. S. Nadas and D. C. Fyler. W. B. Saunders Co., Philadelphia, 1972, p. 396.

Olley, P. M.; Coceani, F.; and Bodach, E.: E-type prostaglandins. A new emergency treatment for certain cyanotic congenital heart malformations. *Circulation,* **53**:728, 1976.

Quero, M.: Atresia of the left atrioventricular orifice associated with a Holmes heart. *Circulation,* **42**:739, 1970.

Quero, M.: Coexistence of single ventricle with atresia of one atrioventricular orifice. *Circulation,* **46**:213, 1971.

Quero, M.; Martinez, V. M. P.; Azcarate, M. J. M.; Batres, G. M.; and Granados, F. M.: Exaggerated displacement of the atrioventricular canal towards the bulbus cordis (rightward displacement of the mitral valve). *Br. Heart J.,* **35**:65, 1973.

Rahimtoola, S. H.; Ongley, P. A.; and Swan, H. J. C.: The hemodynamics of common (or single) ventricle. *Circulation,* **34**:14, 1966.

Rogers, H. M., and Edwards, J. E.: Cor triloculare biatriatum: An analysis of the clinical and pathologic features of nine cases. *Am. Heart J.,* **41**:299, 1951.

Rosenquist, G. C.; Levy, R. J.; and Rowe, R. D.: Right atrial-left ventricular relationship in tricuspid atresia. Position of the pressure D site of the atretic valve as determined by transillumination. *Am. Heart J.,* **80**:495, 1970.

Sakakibara, S.; Tominaga, S.; Imai, Y.; Whara, K.; and Matsumero, M.: Successful total correction of common ventricle. *Chest,* **61**:192, 1972.

Seki, S.; Tsakiris, A. G.; Mair, D. D.; and McGoon, D. C.: Radical correction of single ventricle in an experimental model. *Am. Surg.,* **176**:748, 1972.

Shaher, R. M.: The electrocardiogram in single ventricle. *Br. Heart J.,* **25**:465, 1963.

Sodi-Pallares, D.; Bostami, A.; Fishlader, B. L.; and Medramo, G. A.: Importance of the unipolar morphologies in the interpretation of the electrocardiogram. *Am. Heart J.,* **57**:590, 1959.

Taussig, H. B.: A single ventricle with a diminutive outlet chamber. *J. Tech. Methods,* **19**:120, 1939.

Taussig, H. B.: *Congenital Malformation of the heart: Specific Malformations.* Harvard University Press, Cambridge, Mass., 1960; Vol. II.

Van Praagh, R.; Ongley, P. A.; and Swan, H. J. C.: Anatomic types of single or common ventricle in man. Morphologic and geometric aspects of 60 necropsied cases. *Am. J. Cardiol.,* **31**:367, 1964.

Van Praagh, R.; Van Praagh, S.; Vlad, P., and Keith, J. D.: Diagnosis of the anatomic types of single or common ventricle. *Am. J. Cardiol.,* **15**:345, 1965.

Van Praagh, R.: The segmental approach to diagnosis in congenital heart disease in Birth Defects. Original Article Series, The Cardiovascular System 8, 4. The Williams & Wilkins Co., Baltimore, 1972.

Wood, R. H., and Williams, G. A.: Primitive human hearts: Cor "biloculare" and triloculare; report of cases. *Am. J. Med. Sci.,* **175**:242, 1928.

CHAPTER

24

Patent Ductus Arteriosus

Richard D. Rowe

ANATOMIC description of the ductus arteriosus and acknowledgment of its postnatal closure were made by Galen in the second century (Siegel, 1962), though most observations of the structure and function of this vessel have been accumulated in the last 30 years (Cassels, 1973).

At an early stage of fetal development in human and other mammals the sixth aortic arch, then paired, is formed by connection between the pulmonary arteries growing from the truncus arteriosus and paired sprouting vessels from the dorsal aortae. On the right side the pulmonary arch so formed eventually loses connection with the right dorsal aorta, but on the left side the corresponding distal segment of the pulmonary arch remains to constitute the ductus arteriosus. The ductus of the mature human fetus is closely similar on gross examination to the appearance found in many mammals. It is a large vessel connecting the distal portion of the main pulmonary artery to the ventrolateral aspect of the aorta just distal to the left subclavian artery or to the brachiocephalic branches of the aortic arch. Though a large structure in fetal life, the ductus arteriosus normally is obliterated after birth and eventually becomes a fibrous ligament.

Anatomy

Ductus Arteriosus. The angle of entrance of the ductus into the aorta is acute, about 32 degrees, the degree not changing significantly at the time of constriction in the neonatal period (Mancini, 1951). The prominent aortic lip or "valve" of the ductus arteriosus of animals is not generally believed to have functional significance in man (Fay and Travill, 1967). A large structure during fetal life, it then has an internal diameter equal to that of the aorta and pulmonary artery (Lind and Wegelius, 1954). The mean inner diameter increases with fetal age (Hornblad, 1969). Autopsy examination of stillborn or newborn infant specimens shows a large ductus (Figure 24–1*A*). By contrast, at the end of the

newborn period the ductus is usually thick, its lumen being much narrower (Figure 24–1*B*). Lumen contraction has been variously stated to be maximal at the pulmonary end (Hoffman, 1964; Keith et al., 1967), the aortic end (Everett and Johnson, 1951; Quiroga, 1961), and at both ends of the ductus arteriosus (Barnard, 1939), but most evidence favors the first of these three as the normal sequence. Later, fibrosis converts the ductus into the ligamentum arteriosum, a small intimal dimple marking the pulmonary connections in about one-fourth of adult autopsies. Calcification of the ligamentum is relatively common in children (Currarino and Jackson, 1970). Usually there is no evidence of a previous communication on the aortic wall of adult cadavers (Greig et al., 1954).

The size and shape of the persistent ductus arteriosus vary remarkably. It may be long and narrow or very short and wide. The wall is usually thin (Figure 24–1*C*). Since normal closure begins at the pulmonary artery end of the duct, there frequently is a conical formation to the persistently patent channel, the aortic end forming the mouth, findings frequently encountered in aortograms of young infants with transposition of the great vessels or at operation for small isolated patent ductus arteriosus. The reverse also occurs. In partial persistence of the ductus arteriosus, demonstrated angiographically (Quiroga, 1961), the portion remaining open is at the pulmonary artery end of the duct. This variant seems to be associated with some degree of pulmonary stenosis, e.g., tetralogy of Fallot, simple pulmonary stenosis, stenosis of pulmonary arteries. Aneurysmal changes have been found in the ductus most often at autopsy in infants under the age of two months (Falcone et al., 1972), but occasionally in a clinically recognizable form in older children (Tutassaura et al., 1969). Right-sided ductus arteriosus occurs but is rare. We have one specimen in our collection with bilateral ductus arteriosi to add to others reported (Kelsey et al., 1953).

The broad histologic view of the ductus arteriosus in liveborns is that of a conducting artery differing substantially from either the pulmonary artery or aorta by having a relatively thick intima, a media with a single elastic lamina, variable "mucoid" material, and an intricate helicoid spiral muscular arrangement. A specific feature that has attracted the attention of all workers in the field has been the intimal mounds so characteristic of the ductus arteriosus after birth. These structures first appear in the sixth month of fetal life (Barnard, 1939; Jager and Wollenman, 1942; Danesino et al., 1955; Collela et al., 1963) and are clearly composed of smooth muscle fibers together with mucoid substance projecting through deficiencies in the elastic lamina. These developments have long been considered a likely prerequisite for ductal closure. Recently, Bakker (1962) has observed that the single elastic lamina in the human ductus arteriosus shows points of rupture, reduplication, and fragmentation as early as the fourth month of fetal life. These changes precede the formation of intimal mounds and, together with signs of hyperplasia of smooth muscle cells in the media at the base of the mound, constitute evidence for the view that mounding is a secondary reparative process for damage created in the elastic layer during fetal existence.

All observers are agreed that a strong contraction of muscle is the main factor responsible for postnatal closure of the duct. Von Hayek (1935) noted that the arrangement of the muscle spirals in the ductus was uniquely suitable for obliteration of the lumen with very little shortening of the channel. There is general consensus that in the contracted state the intimal mounds form longitudinal ridges, that the wall becomes thicker, and that the muscle bundles in the media and intima are separated by a structureless material resembling mucoid degeneration. According to Bakker (1962), the contraction of smooth muscle in the intimal mounds after birth causes not only the longitudinal ridges within the lumen but also traction on the underlying media resulting in medial muscle disorganization. It is this latter change that is believed to produce the characteristic mucoid lakes.

Subsequently a slower change involving cytolysis of the dead cells and replacement of much of the media with fibrous tissue occurs and eventually this itself shrinks to obliterate the lumen. A considerable time range for full achievement of this process is evident from available histologic studies. Furthermore, there appears to be a species difference in respect to the beginnings of closure antenatally (Hörnblad, 1967). The most striking prenatal closure tendency is seen in the guinea pig (Sciacca and Condorelli, 1960), as might be predicted from the extremely early postnatal occlusion of the ductus in this species. There is no reason to consider that clot formation in the duct lumen contributes to normal closure (Barnard, 1939), and in fact fibrinolytic activity is higher in the duct wall than in either aorta or pulmonary artery (Gennser and Åstedt, 1971). The role of vasa vasorum in the process is uncertain. There seems little doubt that a marked increase in vascularization of the duct media from expansion of adventitial vasa occurs during the first month after birth (Clarke, 1965). These changes would appear more likely secondary than primary in nature, but the question remains open at present (Allan, 1961; Hoffman, 1964). Although a considerable search by

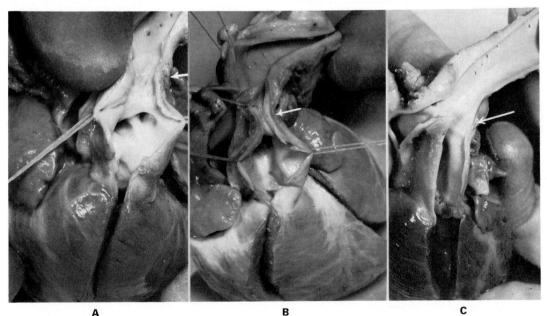

A　　　　　　　　　　**B**　　　　　　　　　　**C**

Figure 24-1. Normal and abnormal patency of the ductus arteriosus. *A.* The specimen from an infant who died with adrenogenital syndrome at four days. Notice the widely patent ductus but roughened ductal endothelium. *B.* The specimen from an infant who died at 28 days from thrush and bronchopneumonia. The ductus is thick-walled and only probe patent. *C.* The persistently patent ductus arteriosus. Note the thin wall and uniformly wide diameter.

light microscopy for nervous elements in the ductus failed to reveal fibers in the media (Barnard, 1939; Danesino et al., 1955; Holmes, 1958), more recent evidence is that neural elements do penetrate into the media and are distributed in relation to muscle cells in a manner indicating that the morphologic framework for a neuroeffector is present (Silva and Ikeda, 1971).

The most striking feature on gross inspection at autopsies of individuals dying with solitary persistent patency of the ductus arteriosus when contrasted with the normal neonatal ductus at say three weeks of age is the thinness of the vessel wall. Despite this, it is usually possible to see some evidence of intimal ridging from mound formation. Microscopic sections show striking reduction in muscle fibers and elastin (Edwards, 1960; Harris and Heath, 1962; Keith et al., 1967). Occasionally elastic fibers in the media are thicker and more abundant than normal (Desligneres and Larroche, 1970). Such appearances may be seen in *large* duct patencies not only in older individuals but in infants as young as three weeks. But they can hardly be said to be characteristic of the usual anatomic situation and undoubtedly represent one extreme of the spectrum of pathologic patency. The findings from cardiac catheterization, aortography, and at surgical correction would argue that most individuals with persistent patency have relatively small ducts, which therefore must be partially constricted channels. Biopsy data from this group have not been systematically examined, but in sporadic examples similar changes though of lesser degree than the more blatant unconstricted patent ductus have been encountered.

The Heart. The left atrium, left ventricle, aorta, and pulmonary artery are frequently enlarged as a result of the abnormal left-to-right shunt. In the rare type of the malformation, where reversal of the shunt is a predominant feature, right ventricular hypertrophy and right atrial hypertrophy are seen alone.

Closure of the Ductus Arteriosus

Animals. Sequences in closure of the ductus arteriosus and observations on the environment producing it were studied by Barclay and associates (1942) in lamb fetuses, Kennedy and Clark (1942) in the guinea pig, and Everett and Johnson (1951) in puppies. Subsequently the group headed by Dawes (Dawes and associates, 1953, 1955) and Hatcher (1960) expanded this information. It became clear that following the onset of respiration there was a major fall in pulmonary vascular resistance and that the ductus tended to constrict to approximately half its previous diameter in short order, a left-to-right shunt developing through the ductus for at least 12 hours and sometimes up to two days. It was obvious to these early workers that a continuous murmur would be the result of this hemodynamic change, and such was detected in the left chest in many species, including the lamb (Dawes et al., 1955), the calf and foal (Amoroso et al., 1958), the puppy (Handler,

1956), and newborn swine (Evans et al., 1963). Relatively little information is available about the anatomic state of the duct in animals at this stage after delivery, and few attempts have been made to study the natural history of duct closure in large series of newborn animals. In the guinea pig, anatomic closure is complete within 24 hours, and studies by Italian workers indicate that reduction in duct lumen in this species is well advanced in late pregnancy (Sciacca and Conderelli, 1960). In the dog and swine major contraction seems to occur at about eight hours, but anatomic closure is not complete for two or three weeks (House and Ederstrom, 1968; Rowe and Neill, 1971).

Humans. In a classic study involving 558 consecutive autopsies of infants under one year of age with normal hearts, Christie (1930) found anatomic closure of the ductus arteriosus in 35 percent at age two weeks, in 56 percent at four weeks, and in 88 percent at eight weeks. Subsequent examination of the question has placed more emphasis on the degree of constriction of the ductus arteriosus at autopsy during the first month of life. Mitchell (1957) found, for example, that by the end of the first week of life the "normally closing ductus" would admit no more than a snugly fitting 2-mm probe although the proportion of anatomically closed ducts at age two to four weeks in her series (57 percent) agrees closely with the data of Christie (1930). Wilson (1958) went even further in examining the ductus arteriosus of stillbirths and early neonatal deaths. He showed that in 70 percent of stillborn infants there was no evidence of contraction of the ductus arteriosus from its fetal diameter and that less than 10 percent of the 37 stillborns examined had constricted ductus arteriosi. By comparison only 17 percent of 63 infants dying during the early neonatal period had uncontracted ducts. One concludes from his communication that the major time for ductal constriction in his material was in the first 48 hours of life and that premature infants were likely to have more advanced closure than mature infants by that time. Unfortunately, data of this nature in humans, while useful for the latter part of the neonatal period, will always be inconclusive in respect to the first week or two of life for the very nature of disturbances causing death at this age is such as to favor delayed closure of the ductus arteriosus.

Early serial angiographic studies in newborn infants (Keith and Forsyth, 1950; Lind and Wegelius, 1954) suggested that very rapid closure of the ductus arteriosus occurred in the human. The small number of babies examined in these studies, the use of serial angiography rather than cine techniques, the knowledge that none of the subjects were truly normal, and the unstated environmental conditions all tend to decrease the value of the observations.

Early studies using an ear oximeter to register dilution patterns following intravenous injection of Evans blue dye showed that about two-thirds of 29 infants examined in this way on the first day of life had a left-to-right shunt, one-quarter had a bidirectional shunt, and one-third had no shunt at all (Prec and

Cassels, 1955). The uncertainties of ear oximetry in the neonate and the fact that the rapid circulation time at this age erroneously exaggerates left-to-right shunts following venous injections of dye (Krovetz and Gessner, 1965) leave data of this sort in question. The first direct evidence of left-to-right shunt through the ductus arteriosus in humans was obtained in cardiac catheterization studies of mongoloid infants with normal hearts by Rowe and James (1957) and in normal infants or mongoloid infants by Adams and Lind (1957). These authors found evidence through blood oxygen sampling methods of a left-to-right shunt through the ductus in four out of six infants under 12 days of age and in three of four under four days of age, respectively. The shunt was not large, pulmonary/systemic flow ratios averaging 1.5/1 and 1.8/1 in the two series. Some years later Rudolph and associates (1961) studied eight apparently normal infants under the age of 30 hours (including some infants of diabetic mothers and some mongoloid infants) and found even smaller left-to-right shunts. Using blood oxygen sampling techniques and the method of retrograde umbilical artery catheterization initiated by Saling (1960), Moss and associates (1963) examined 30 healthy newborn infants and showed that a bidirectional shunt existed for the first six hours of life and a significant left-to-right shunt through the ductus for the first 15 hours after delivery. Beyond that time the shunt became insignificant or was not detectable with their methods.

In the light of subsequent evidence it becomes apparent that the earlier studies simply established that the ductus in the human does not close functionally immediately after birth. Subject selection (with a propensity to hypoxic influences) probably affected the duration of the shunting mechanism in these reports. The latest data, still subject to criticism on the grounds of overestimating shunt volume because mixed pulmonary arterial samples were obviously not obtained, nevertheless show that in healthy term babies significant left-to-right shunting through the ductus arteriosus probably stops by the latter part of the first day of life. Whether under usual conditions with a variety of thermal environments or for other reasons the initially closed ductus may later reopen temporarily, as is suggested by the data of Jegier and colleagues (1964), is still uncertain.

There is particular interest in the behavior of the ductus arteriosus in the low-birth-weight infant born prematurely. Evidence from hemodynamic measurements and clinically shows that the ductus arteriosus in these babies can be entirely normal and quite similar to larger babies born at term (Moss et al., 1965; Wallgren et al., 1967; Jones and Pickering, 1977). However, in the late phase of the respiratory distress or after apneic episodes develop, as commonly occurs in this group, the normal circulatory transition, including closure of the ductus arteriosus, is often significantly delayed. A left-to-right shunt of variable size is a frequent complication. When pharmacologic or surgical intervention is not required for treatment of left-to-right shunts in such patients, there is a distinct tendency for closure to occur at an age equivalent to term gestation.

Etiology

Delay in closure or failure to close of the ductus arteriosus after birth has been examined from a functional standpoint in a number of different aspects in man and animals.

Prenatal Factors. Important breeding experiments in dogs with hereditary ductus arteriosus have produced animals without ductus, with partial persistence (aortic diverticulum), or with true ductus. This graded phenotypic expression of the defect suggests a threshold trait with a high degree of penetrability (Patterson et al., 1972). A number of reports indicating familial aggregation of patent ductus arteriosus in man suggest a genetic influence (Walker and Ellis, 1940–41; Ekstrom, 1952; Joyce and O'Toole, 1954; Burman, 1961). Recurrence of cardiac defects in later-born sibs of patients with patent ductus arteriosus has been calculated to be 2 percent (Record and McKeown, 1953; Anderson, 1954; Polani and Campbell, 1960). Nora and associates (1967) documented from the literature and their own experience four concordant members of eight monozygotic twin pairs; only one was concordant for this malformation. These data argue for a significant genetic role in etiology of ductus even though the lack of 100 percent concordance indicates a contribution to the final expression by environmental factors. The incidence of persistent ductus arteriosus in children of affected parents in Stockholm supports multifactorial causation (Zetterqvist, 1970).

Maternal rubella during the first trimester has been known to lead to patent ductus arteriosus in a number of offspring of such mothers (Gregg, 1941), but why some are spared despite other vascular disorders due to rubella is at present uncertain. There is evidence to support the view that where patent ductus arteriosus results in such circumstances the actual amount of smooth muscle in the duct wall may be reduced (Varghese et al., 1968).

In premature infants delayed but eventual closure of the ductus arteriosus may occur. It was appreciated earlier that this was so for large as well as relatively trivial left-to-right shunts (Burnard, 1959; Usher, 1962; Auld, 1966; Danilowicz et al., 1966; Rowe and Neill, 1971). Improved early survival of low-birth-weight babies has been associated recently with a much higher incidence of patent ductus arteriosus in the premature, many with large left-to-right shunts. The explanation for this new picture is at present uncertain but hypoxia, fluid overload (Stevenson, 1977), enzyme deficiency (Molnar et al., 1962), and reduced smooth muscle bulk have at various times been suggested as the cause. That most premature ducts do close, that closure tends to occur spontaneously at a point in time corresponding to what would have been term for that particular pregnancy (Powell, 1963; Jones and Pickering, 1977), and that treatment with prostaglandin synthetase inhibitors usually closes the ductus promptly in the newborn period whatever the gestational age of the baby (Friedman et al., 1976; Heymann et al., 1976; Friedman et al., 1977) argue that muscle mass is not deficient and that hypoxia is not the continuing factor of importance in keeping such ducts open. Rather the evidence now much more strongly favors some maturational cause, probably related to pro-staglandin function or to the final chain of initiation of smooth muscle contraction (Heymann and Rudolph, 1975; Coceani and Olley, 1977). The relationship of other types of congenital heart malformation and patent ductus arteriosus has not been analyzed in great detail despite the fact that Taussig (1960) long ago suggested that the ductus arteriosus closure can be delayed in severe congenital heart disease such as tetralogy of Fallot. Mitchell (1957) noted little difference in the time of closure of the ductus in neonates between those with and those without congenital heart malformation. A re-trospective study by Bass and Rowe (1967) of patients with severe congenital heart malformation who underwent detailed diagnostic investigation showed that patent ductus arteriosus is an associated finding in almost 40 percent of such patients in the first 15 months of life after which time there is an abrupt decrease in its frequency.

Postnatal Period. HYPOXIA. In some early angiographic studies Barclay, Franklin, and Prichard (1944) found in lambs that the ductus arteriosus sometimes reopened after an initial functional closure. They made the important observation that this sequence when present appeared to be related to general deterioration of the fetal preparation. The influence of acute asphyxia in the immediate postnatal situation in lambs was extensively examined by the Oxford group of investigators (Born et al., 1956). In their important paper it was shown that either in the naturally born partially asphyxiated state or in underventilated and anesthetized lambs with low arterial oxygen saturation (about 30 percent) the ductus constricted possibly due to the effect of the catecholamine release. If oxygenation of such animals was improved by ventilation, the duct was observed to dilate as arterial oxygen saturation levels reached the order of 65 to 70 percent and then finally constricted when arterial saturation reached 85 percent. These elegant studies indicating the importance of oxygen in accomplishing closure show that in addition to the oxygen, catecholamines may play a role in duct constriction. The work of Burnard (1959) in showing the early appearance of a ductal murmur in asphyxiated humans at birth is corroborative though the data from studies in newborn piglets suggest that catecholamines may have an opposite effect under certain circumstances and so suggest a more complex interaction than previously indicated (Rowe and Neill, 1971). Certainly exclusion of catechol action by experimental design in fetal lamb preparations favors

the important action on the ductus being high blood oxygenation (Reis and Anderson, 1964). More recent experiments in lamb fetuses using an artificial placenta where flow, pO_2, and pCO_2 are controlled have shown that within 20 minutes of raising fetal pO_2 from 13 to 20 mm of mercury to 40 to 60 mm of mercury the ductus constricts markedly, a response that is unaffected by metabolic or respiratory acidosis (Zapol et al., 1971). Earlier physiologic studies in newborn infants demonstrated that acute hypoxia produced marked pulmonary hypertension, some lowering of systemic blood pressure, and conditions favorable to the development of a right-to-left shunt through the ductus arteriosus (James and Rowe, 1957; Rowe, 1957, 1959). The ability to reduce ductal shunting by 100 percent oxygen breathing was first demonstrated in a patient with hemolytic disease of the newborn at the age of four weeks by Kjellberg and associates (1959) who concluded that asphyxia retarded ductal closure. Saling (1960) detected increase of right-to-left shunts with hypoxia in infants under two hours of age. Later more detailed examinations on 13 term infants by Moss and associates (1964) clearly demonstrated that the hypoxic state always caused a rise in pulmonary artery pressure in humans and that, at least in the early postnatal hours, there was a return of left-to-right shunts, which had been previously abolished by 100 percent oxygen breathing. Despite unequivocal demonstration of oxygen effect, the relationship of postnatal age to this effect or paradoxic responses to appropriate oxygen environments have received relatively scant attention (Born et al., 1956; Moss et al., 1964; Keith et al., 1967).

The influence on the ductus function after short exposures to hypoxia might prolong the dilating response of the more acute reaction. Support for this view came from studies on the epidemiology of persistent patent ductus arteriosus. Alzamora and associates (1953) and Penaloza and associates (1964) demonstrated that though the incidence of patent ductus arteriosus in schoolchildren born at sea level in Peru (0.05 percent) was similar to that in North American children, there was a progressive rise (to 0.72 percent) in the incidence among children born at altitudes of between 3.5 and 5 km in Peru. Such relationships between the reduced oxygen pressure of altitude and the incidence of patent ductus arteriosus have not been apparent in caucasian populations in Denver or Leadville, Colorado, raising questions of genetic or at least multifactorial influence to explain the South American observations. Experimental aspects of chronic hypoxia have considered the hemodynamic consequences of pulmonary vascular and right heart muscle mass alterations more often than answering the problem of ductal response. Isolated muscle strips from the ductus arteriosus or whole ductus specimens from lambs and other species have been shown to contract and relax by increasing and decreasing respectively oxygen concentration of a surrounding Tyrode's or Ringer's solution (Kovalcic, 1963; Gillman and Burton, 1966). The initial level of pO_2 at which this constriction occurs and the maximal degree of constriction increase with advancing gestational age in the lamb (McMurphy et al., 1972). Studies of the guinea pig ductus suggest that oxygen triggers duct constriction by increasing the rate of oxidative phosphorylation within smooth muscle cells (Fay, 1971). Noradrenaline, adrenaline, and acetylcholine also cause the isolated ductus to contract, responses that can be abolished by appropriate drug antagonists without affecting the response of the ductus to oxygen. A number of metabolic blocking agents including sodium cyanide have no effect on the oxygen response of the ductus, but the fact that amytal and phenothiazines do so suggested that these drugs may produce their effect by inhibition of a flavoprotein oxidase (Kovalcic, 1963). The experiments of Assali's group in intact fetal lambs indicate that catechol effect on ductal flow appears to be secondary to changes produced by these drugs on the systemic and pulmonary vascular beds whereas acetylcholine appears to exert its effect on blood flow through the ductus by direct constrictive action on the vessel wall. These results emphasize the importance of modifying factors on in vivo action of drugs and indicate the need for considerably more exploration of pharmacologic action in experimental situations. Pertinent to this matter is the possible role of bradykynin, a vasoactive peptide, in neonatal circulatory adjustments. Dawes (1966) first indicated the potential role of this substance by injecting it into fetal lambs. There was an immediate increase in pulmonary vascular conductance. Subsequently, Heymann and associates (1967) have revealed that bradykynin is increased in plasma from left atrial samples of fetal lambs following ventilation with 100 percent oxygen. Both bradykynin and acetylcholine augment oxygen-induced ductal constriction (McMurphy et al., 1972). By contrast, E-type prostaglandins appear to maintain patency of the ductus arteriosus (Coceani and Olley, 1973; Elliott and Starling, 1972).

With the exception of prostaglandin $F_{2\alpha}$ all the prostaglandins relax the smooth muscle of the fetal ductus arteriosus under low oxygen tension. Ductus sensitivity is most marked to prostaglandin (PG) E_2, is probably maximal at the beginning of the last trimester of gestation, and declines thereafter, while the contractile response to oxygen increases as term is approached. It is thought that the fetal ductal arteriosus is maintained open by a continuous endogenous production of PGE_2 acting on the highly responsive ductal smooth muscle. When arterial pO_2 rises at birth, ductal sensitivity to PGE_2 is markedly reduced and the ductus constricts. In cyanotic infants paO_2 never rises high enough to cause complete loss of sensitivity to E_2, the duct remains partially open and can be further dilated by infusion of exogenous PGE_2 or E_1. In the premature infant prostaglandin responsiveness remains relatively dominant, and although paO_2 rises at birth, the duct is still responsive to PGE_2 in many infants and remains patent. Prostaglandin synthetase inhibitors (e.g.,

indomethacin) cause ductus constriction under these conditions by blocking the production of endogenous PG. This ability to close the patent ductus with a PG synthetase inhibitor is strong evidence again $PGE_{2\alpha}$, a weak contractor of ductus smooth muscle, being the mediator of physiologic closure of the ductus arteriosus (Olley, P. M., personal communication, 1977).

Recent perfusion studies in dogs with hereditary persistent ductus arteriosus have shown a lack of constrictive effect from oxygen or norepinephrine in the face of histologic evidence of a marked reduction in muscle cells in the duct wall (Patterson et al., 1972). Current research on ductal closure places increasing emphasis upon the pathway of the oxygen effect or noneffect so that the enigma that has surrounded the reaction of this unique vessel over the centuries appears likely to be resolved.

Incidence

Anderson (1954) estimated the incidence of patent ductus arteriosus in the general population to be between 1 in 2500 and 1 in 5000. In the Toronto Heart Registry (Gardiner and Keith, 1951) the incidence was 1 in 3850. From the latter source isolated patent ductus arteriosus accounted for 12 percent of all congenital heart disease. This compares with 14.5 percent found by Wood (1950) and 9.2 percent in Maude Abbott's series (1936).

Several practical difficulties enter into the determination of the true incidence of patent ductus arteriosus when one includes newborn material. It is difficult to conclude from autopsies whether the patency of a given ductus was likely to have persisted had the infant survived or whether with survival the duct might have shut. No study is really free of this problem. There are three recent studies on incidence that suggest that patent ductus arteriosus is more common than previously reported in the pediatric population. One is an analysis of patent ductus arteriosus in 58,314 liveborn infants from Gothenberg, Sweden, by Calgren (1969). His figure from a closely knit population was 1 in 1881 live births. In 13,653 live births from the National Womens Hospital in New Zealand, an incidence of 1 in 1365 was found for ductus arteriosus. In the perinatal cooperative study of the United States National Institutes of Health, Mitchell and associates (1969) in 54,033 births found an incidence of ductus arteriosus of 1 in 1543. The exact frequency of persistent ductus arteriosus in prematurely born babies is uncertain. There can be little question that the overall incidence of persistently patent ductus arteriosus in the first few months of life when compared with term babies is higher and has recently increased from causes which are currently being debated. It seems likely that most of this increase is in premature infants who develop the respiratory distress syndrome. In that circumstance the incidence is approximately 15 percent (Kitterman et al., 1972; Neal et al., 1975). Many of the ducts in this group also close spontaneously, or can be closed by medical means, so that the proportion that need surgical closure later in infancy or childhood is quite difficult to estimate.

It is well known that the malformation is more common in females than in males. Ekstrom (1952), analyzing the sex distribution in reports up to 1950, found that of 557 cases 69 percent were female. This female preponderance has been confirmed in subsequent series (Gross, 1952; Ash and Fischer, 1955; Polani and Campbell, 1960; Krovetz and Warden, 1962). The last-mentioned authors have pointed out that the sex ratio is equal in most series of rubella-related patent ductus arteriosus. Such has been the recent experience in 50 infants with patent ductus arteriosus from Green Lane Hospital: 9/17 were female in those with rubella history, whereas 20/33 were female in those where pregnancy was apparently normal. In a Birmingham analysis it was found that the male incidence is fairly constant throughout the year but that there is an increase in numbers of female patients born in the summer months. The slight seasonal increase in numbers found in our 812 cases occurred in the same period as this latter group (Rose et al., 1972). Not much more than 2 percent of ductus arteriosus is believed to be explained by rubella infection in utero (Campbell, 1961), but the exact influence of this virus on the number of cases is really uncertain (Rutstein et al., 1952) and operative series in children usually show a higher percentage (Hospital for Sick Children, 1968; Panagopoulos et al., 1971).

Hemodynamics

Before birth, blood is directed from the pulmonary artery through the ductus into the aorta because of the high pulmonary vascular resistance. After birth there is an alteration in pressure relationships between the pulmonary and systemic circuits, resulting in a left-to-right shunt through the patent ductus. The chief factors that influence the flow of blood through a persistent ductus arteriosus are the diameter of the ductus arteriosus and the pressure relationships on either side although in the newborn period the vasomotor tone of the duct itself can contribute much more to pressure flow variations (Bromberger-Barnea et al., 1965). In the majority of patients with classic relatively asymptomatic patent ductus arteriosus it seems likely, though it has not been proven, that the chief resistance to excessive left-to-right shunt occurs at the ductus itself and that the factor of tone no longer enters into the picture. In those with a larger duct diameter the pulmonary vascular resistance becomes a more important factor. In the small number with pronounced pulmonary hypertension and large ducts it is probable that there is not a normal fall in pulmonary vascular resistance after birth but that some alteration will occur allowing a left-to-right shunt of relatively small volume. Evidence suggests that the retention of a very high

pulmonary vascular resistance in younger infants may be related to a history of recurrent hypoxia, usually from pulmonary disturbances (Prec et al., 1962).

Clinical Features

History. Certain information from the history in infants with patent ductus arteriosus has value. It is well-recognized that a background of congenital rubella is frequently associated with ductus arteriosus. The birth months of rubella babies in North America lie between October and March so that the delivery month has some importance in drawing attention to that etiologic possibility. Furthermore, premature infants seem to have a higher risk of developing persistent ductus arteriosus, especially if prematurity is associated with birth asphyxia or the respiratory distress syndrome. These details about the pregnancy and delivery are important pointers toward diagnosis and management just as the presence of a difficult delivery, cesarean section, or upper gastrointestinal anomalies may be helpful in the baby at term with clinical signs of persistent ductus arteriosus.

Symptoms. Only very occasionally is there a history of significant disability in children with persistent ductus arteriosus. This is probably because the great majority of these youngsters have small rather than large degrees of patency. Those who have symptoms such as fatigue or cyanosis usually will not be found to have any sinister explanation, for in most cases they are probably iatrogenic in origin.

By contrast, infants presenting with ductus arteriosus are much more likely to have serious disability again undoubtedly related to the size of the pulmonary blood flow. Forty-one percent of 208 infants operated on under the age of two years at The Hospital for Sick Children (Trusler et al., 1968) had congestive failure or cardiothoracic ratios in excess of 0.60. A similar proportion with congestive failure was found in 41 infants from the Johns Hopkins Hospital (Rowe and Neill, 1971). In all these babies, failure to thrive was common and pulmonary infections were not infrequent.

Physical Signs. Substandard physical development in childhood occurred in one-third of our cases and in 38 percent of those reported by Ash and Fischer (1955). Muir and Brown (1932), Gilchrist (1945), Adams and Forsyth (1951), and Gross (1952) found similar changes. Krovetz (1963) found that 90 of 342 patients with a surgically corrected patent ductus arteriosus exhibited severe preoperative growth failure manifested by weights below the third percentile for age and sex. Ekstrom (1952) reported that the heights and weights of 111 patients with patent ductus arteriosus lay within normal limits in all cases. The reason for this seems to be the fact that only one of these patients was under one year of age. Often, in young patients with large shunts, there is major improvement in growth following surgical treatment, but it has been a disconcerting fact that many patients with more moderate or small shunts do not progress so favorably in terms of growth postoperatively. Engle and colleagues (1958) found growth retardation continued in one-half to one-third of their patients operated upon between 3 and 14 years. This suggested that surgery was advisable before the age of three in order to avoid stunting during a period of rapid growth that would not subsequently be corrected. Of nine infants followed 11 months or more after surgery below the age of two years, Bauersfeld and coworkers (1957) found that only two showed any improvement, and in one of the two the improvement was trivial. The remainder continued in their preoperative percentile category. The view of Umansky and Hauck (1962), based on the response to surgery in 422 children under eight years, was that the major determinant of poor growth in patients with patent ductus arteriosus more likely lay in prenatal factors. Mehrizi and Drash (1962) did not find that surgery before three years resulted in spectacular resumption of normal growth. They were undecided whether this was because of a short follow-up or because of other, presumably prenatal, factors. The continued failure of a proportion of patients to grow adequately postoperatively was examined by Krovetz (1963), who found statistically significant relationships between those who did catch up and those who did not in the preoperative presence of congestive failure and the presence of additional noncardiac anomalies. Feldt and associates (1969) in examining the birth of children with congenital heart disease as a whole included a small number of patients with ductus arteriosus in their analysis. Their conclusions were that preoperative congestive heart failure was frequently associated with severe growth failure, that most children had growth acceleration after surgery, and that those who did not either had abnormal growth preoperatively, were beyond the age where growth could be accelerated, or had significant residual cardiac or extracardiac defects.

Cardiovascular. The presence of permanent cyanosis rules out patent ductus arteriosus as a simple lesion. Apart from a few cases in failure in infancy, or with bidirectional flow through the ductus arteriosus from pulmonary hypertension, even transient cyanosis is absent. In our experience employing oximetry, the simple case in childhood never has alteration of arterial oxygen saturation, either with exercise or with respiratory infections, and it is likely that the cases reported as exhibiting cyanosis at such times fall into the group with pulmonary hypertension due to high pulmonary vascular resistance.

A precordial thrill, usually systolic in time, less often continuous or rarely systolodiastolic, is palpable in the pulmonary areas in about three-fourths of the patients in childhood. Thrills are less frequently detected in the infant group. Femoral and radial arterial pulses are usually equally brisk. The femoral pulse may, in occasional cases, be slightly weaker than normal but not to a degree seen in true coarctation of the aorta. (Laubry and Routier, 1930).

Pulsation in the suprasternal notch is frequently seen, and the thrill often extends to this area.

The accuracy of resting blood pressures recorded with a sphygmomanometer by different examiners is open to question. Nevertheless, it is of practical importance that 75 percent of our older patients and 95 percent of the infant patients have had pulse pressures exceeding 45 mm of mercury when measured by this method. Recent literature has rightly condemned the exercise test (Bohn, 1938) as frankly misleading. Taylor and associates (1950) and Lewes (1952) have shown that exercise is more likely to lower the diastolic blood pressure-level of healthy subjects and raise the same level in cases with a patent ductus arteriosus. But a wide pulse pressure at rest is obviously very common and therefore a valuable sign (Krovetz et al., 1962). It must, though, be used in conjunction with other features of the malformation, for a similar change occurs in cases of mitral insufficiency (Wood, 1954) and in ventricular septal defect (Goldbloom et al., 1953).

The most important aid to diagnosis from physical examination in this malformation is obtained by auscultation. Three main types of murmur have been described:

CONTINUOUS MURMUR (Figure 24–2). In the vast majority of patients there is a continuous or machinery murmur in the pulmonary area. As described by Gibson, "it begins after the commencement of the first sound . . . it persists through the second sound and dies away gradually during the long pause. The murmur is rough and thrilling. It begins softly and increases in intensity so as to reach its acme just about, or immediately after, the incidence of the second sound, and from that point gradually wanes until its termination. The second sound can be heard to be loud and clanging."[*] Phonocardiography confirms this excellent description (Routier, 1937; Levine and Harvey, 1949; Haring et al., 1954; Reinhold and Nadas, 1954). The latter workers emphasize that the crescendo systolic element in the pulmonary area is late in onset and that this feature of timing is not present in other congenital defects that may have murmurs maximal in this area.

Occasionally the continuous murmur in a young patient will alter strikingly from one examination to another or even during the one examination. Two such cases were reported by Taussig (1960), another by Keith and Sagarminaga (1961), and one by Hyrske and associates (1965), where a valvelike structure within the ductus was believed to have been responsible for the intermittent obliteration of the shunt. In a four-year-old patient at Green Lane Hospital great variation in auscultatory findings, ranging from a loud continuous murmur to no murmur at all, could be produced by a variety of postural changes. At operation an unusually long, thin patent ductus arteriosus was found, suggesting that kinking of the channel in different body postures

---

[*] *Edinburgh Med. J.*, **8** : 1, 1900.

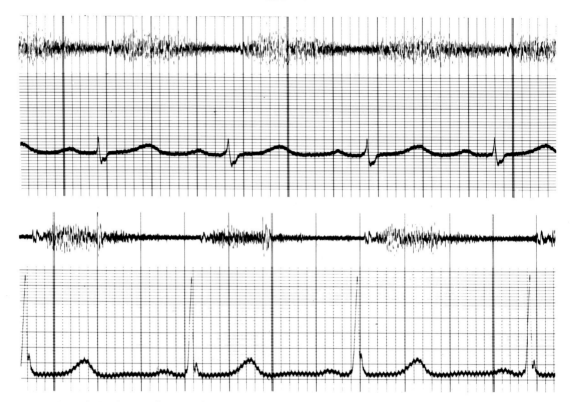

Figure 24-2. Phonocardiograms from patients with persistent ductus arteriosus to demonstrate two presentations of sound recognizable as having origin in the duct. *Upper*, the classic continuous murmur shown "wrapped" around the second heart sound (here obliterating the latter). *Lower*, the abbreviated duct murmur; the prominent noise is in systole. The diastolic component is short and of low intensity.

might have been responsible for the changing signs.

Spontaneous disappearance of the established, continuous murmur is rare. It may occur with closure of the ductus arteriosus. This is rather commonly noted in newborn infants, especially prematures, but has less commonly been observed in older children and adults (Gilchrist, 1945; Bishop, 1952; Taussig, 1954; White, 1954). Two infants were seen at each of Green Lane Hospital and the Johns Hopkins Hospital with a definite rubella background in whom an established patent ductus arteriosus closed spontaneously in the latter half of the first year of life. In the two from the Johns Hopkins Hospital, pulmonary-to-systemic flow ratios at the end of the first month of life were 1.7 and 1.8/1, respectively. It was considered at that time that the anatomic size of the ductus by angiography in each patient was small. By contrast, disappearance of a continuous murmur may be the result of the development of severe pulmonary hypertension, secondary to pulmonary vascular obstruction (Keys and Shapiro, 1943; Benn, 1947; Campbell and Hudson, 1952; Evans and Heath, 1961). The latter authors describe a patient who, after having a typical continuous murmur at 30 years, was found at age 38 to have no murmur and signs of severe pulmonary hypertension. Autopsy revealed a widely patent ductus arteriosus, and histologic examination of the main pulmonary artery

provided evidence of acquired pulmonary hypertension. At Green Lane Hospital are records of one premature infant born after a rubella pregnancy who developed congestive heart failure on the third day of life, which responded to medical management. A typical continuous murmur was evident and still present one month later. By one year this girl had an unimpressive systolic murmur, pulmonary ejection click, and pulmonary early diastolic murmur. Combined ventricular hypertrophy was present in the electrocardiogram. At operation a moderate-sized ductus was ligated. Pressures in pulmonary artery and aorta were 100/58 and 110/62 (mm of mercury) before ligation and 87/48 and 103/62 after. Postoperatively the infant developed tachycardia, peripheral cyanosis, tricuspid regurgitation, and distended neck veins and died within 24 hours. At autopsy the right ventricle was dilated and hypertrophied and the lung vascular bed revealed grade-3 hypertensive changes (Figure 24–3).

ABBREVIATED MURMUR (Figure 24–2). This is a murmur that is identical with the classic continuous murmur until the second sound after which it fades away quite abruptly. The intensity of this murmur is not appreciably different from the classic murmur, and eddy sounds, which are common in the high-velocity situation of the small- to moderate-sized ductus, are particularly helpful in

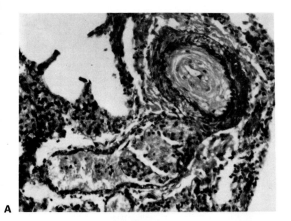

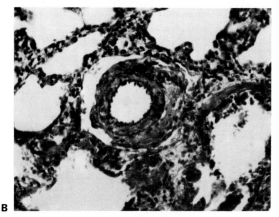

Figure 24-3. Changes in the lung vascular bed of patients with persistent ductus arteriosus. *A.* D. B., a female infant, who died in the immediate postoperative period of acute right heart failure at age 13 months. Grade 4 changes at autopsy. *B.* R. H., a female Maori infant, with a large shunt surgically obliterated at age three weeks (see Figure 24-13). Lung biopsy shows reasonably advanced maturation of the vascular bed for this age.

diagnosis in this type (Hubbard and Neis, 1960; Rowe and Lowe, 1964).

NONSPECIFIC MURMUR. Under this heading would be included all murmurs that have no clear evidence of a ductal origin in patients who have proven isolated ductus arteriosus. The majority of these murmurs are low-intensity, midsystolic ejection murmurs maximal in the pulmonary area. Occasionally, one finds a systolic murmur suggesting tricuspid or mitral regurgitation, or an early diastolic murmur of pulmonary incompetence. Rarely, there is no murmur. In our experience the soft ejection murmur proved to be the most frequently encountered. These features are confined to patients who have an extremely large duct or who have a trivial communication, and clearly the diagnosis can only be confirmed by further investigation. In fact, the diagnosis is seldom achieved prior to such studies.

Special Points. There is an overall relationship between the presence of pulmonary hypertension and

absence or shortening of the diastolic murmur in patent ductus arteriosus (Adams et al., 1952; Ziegler, 1952; Krovetz and Warden, 1962). Exceptions to this rule have been noted. The author's experience with the murmur in newborn animals particularly, but also in normal newborn infants, suggests that at the time when an external murmur may be only early systolic or may even be absent, a trivial flow through a greatly constricted ductus may be occurring (Evans et al., 1963; Rowe and Lowe, 1964).

When the murmur is soft or intermittent, it may be more certainly recognized by the administration of vasopressor drugs such as mephentermine or phenylephrine (Crevasse and Logue, 1959; Beck et al., 1961). It has been shown by the technique of intracardiac phonocardiography that, in patients in whom a quite innocent sounding ejection murmur in the pulmonary area may be present in association with normal electrocardiogram and x-ray, a continuous murmur may be recorded in the main pulmonary artery where the shunt is really quite trivial in nature (Wennevold, 1968). Likewise, at the other extreme, it is possible to utilize intracardiac phonocardiography to clarify the diagnosis in patients with extremely large ducts and rise in oxygen saturation in the right ventricle, which may lead to difficulties in diagnosis between ductus and ventricular septal defect or both (Moghadam et al., 1965; Bouchard et al., 1967).

In patients with large volume left-to-right shunts an apical middiastolic murmur has been noted in from one-fourth to one-half (Ravin and Darley, 1950; Storstein et al., 1952). Middiastolic murmurs were encountered in 8 of 22 patients with large flow, reported by Neill and Mounsey (1958). Five of these eight had an opening snap, a sign also observed by Gray (1956). The authors have been impressed by the high proportion with middiastolic murmurs in their patients, finding it unusual not to detect an apical flow murmur in all except patients with small shunts.

The Second Sound. In the average young child the second heart sound, though often having slightly accentuated pulmonary valve closure, has a normal degree of splitting and responds normally during the respiratory cycle. Eddy sounds mentioned previously are commonly noted in the pulmonary area in patients with large shunts (Neill and Mounsey, 1958). With high pulmonary vascular resistance the second heart sound becomes accentuated but not single (Leatham, 1969) and pulmonary ejection sounds may become audible in the advanced case.

Paradoxic splitting (Gray, 1956) is confined to patients with large shunts and is usually clinically obvious only in older children and adults.

Features of Very Young Infants. There is rather special diagnostic difficulty in the case of the newborn infant symptomatic from the presence of a large ductus arteriosus. The main reason for the assessment problem is that practically all newborn infants dying within the first few days of life will be found to have a widely patent duct (Mitchell, 1957). In many of these there are clearly other factors responsible for death.

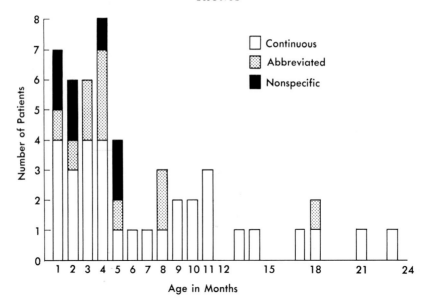

Figure 24-4. Histogram showing the relationship between age and the type of murmur encountered in 50 infants with patent ductus arteriosus.

We have had the experience of occasional patients dying in congestive failure in the first week of life without massive left-to-right shunt where investigations had demonstrated an anatomically widely patent duct alone. At autopsy, no other cause for death could be found. Prec and coworkers (1962) reported a rather similar experience in an older infant in whom surgical closure of the ductus resulted in cure.

Rarely newborns may present in pulmonary edema in the first few days of life. Histologic evidence of unusually rapid maturity of the pulmonary vascular bed was observed in such cases by Heath and coworkers (1958), but this has not always been the finding. More of the newborn patients who present with difficulty and congestive failure have signs that support the clinical diagnosis of ductus arteriosus. One-half of 41 infants recently seen at the Johns Hopkins Hospital with patent ductus arteriosus were examined during the first month of life. The population consisted of premature infants, on the one hand, who had a high incidence of birth asphyxia or respiratory distress syndrome and so-called term infants or infants with low birth weight for gestational age where birth difficulties were not notable. Premature babies had either the continuous murmur or the abbreviated murmur; of the term babies, nonspecific murmurs were present in 17 percent (Rowe and Neill, 1970). There may be more difficulty in distinguishing these murmurs when premature infants are being mechanically ventilated.

In a study of 50 infants under two years with persistent ductus arteriosus seen at Green Lane Hospital, a true continuous murmur was found in 32, abbreviated murmurs in 12 (Figure 24–4), and a nonspecific murmur in six. Scott and Gearty (1960) found a similarly high proportion (78 percent) where

a ductal murmur could be recognized in the first year.

The crackling crescendo nature of the murmur in systole and short spillover into diastole should go far to making the diagnosis of patent ductus arteriosus in the infant without a frank continuous murmur. While accepting that the occasional patient will have either a short noncrescendo systolic murmur or no murmur from a large ductus, the authors believe that detailed auscultation proves that presentation with these atypical signs is exceptional. Our figures suggest that murmurs unrecognizable as ductal occur in only 15 percent, and that this incidence is not appreciably higher than obtains for older patients.

There is regrettably still a commonly held belief that a nonspecific systolic murmur, making bedside diagnosis difficult or impossible (Dammann and Sell, 1952; Gross, 1952; Krovetz and Warden, 1962), is the frequent presentation during infancy (Figure 24–4). Accessory confirmatory studies may still be desired for many patients of this group, but careful auscultation can very frequently provide initial help in diagnosis. Further investigation is mandatory for symptomatic infants masquerading with signs suggestive of ventricular defect, atrioventricular canal, or mitral regurgitation since some will be proved to have a large isolated ductus (Cruze et al., 1963).

Radiologic Examination

Heart Size. In 133 operated cases at The Hospital for Sick Children between the ages of 3 and 15 years, 20 percent had a cardiothoracic ratio exceeding 0.55, and 12 percent had a cardiothoracic ratio exceeding 0.60. In our cases there was a very clear-cut relation between large ductus, cardiac enlargement, and the electrocardiogram (Figure 24–5). In these cases left ventricular hypertrophy was invariable. At the Hopital Broussais, Donzelot and associates (1954) reported in 60 operated cases: gross enlargement in 10 percent, slight to moderate enlargement in 65 percent, and normal heart size in 25 percent. Ash and Fischer (1955) reported a normal heart size in only one-third of 124 cases in childhood. Of 20 babies operated on at The Hospital for Sick Children before the age of three years, the average cardiothoracic ratio was 0.63.

Contour. The cardiac contour is often normal in simple patent ductus arteriosus. In the infant or older patient with substantially large shunt or with pulmonary hypertension, there is almost always a pulmonary artery bulge in the left midborder of the heart and often combined ventricular hypertrophy. The aorta is usually prominent, and in over half the cases, the angle between the aortic knuckle and the main pulmonary artery is filled in. Barium swallow usually confirms the size of the left aortic arch and also can determine the degree of enlargement of the left atrium. The incidence of left atrial enlargement ranges from 50 percent (Gross and Longino, 1951) to 10 percent (Donzelot and Heim de Balsac, 1948). Left atrial enlargement is very common in children, is almost invariable in the symptomatic infant group, and permits exclusion of atrial septal defect.

Attention has been drawn to a transient mass visible in the chest roentgenograms of term infants in the first day of life that has been referred to as the ductus bump (Berdon et al., 1965). This mass usually disappears by the third day of life and is quite benign. The presence of calcification in the region of the ductus in children with congenital heart disease is

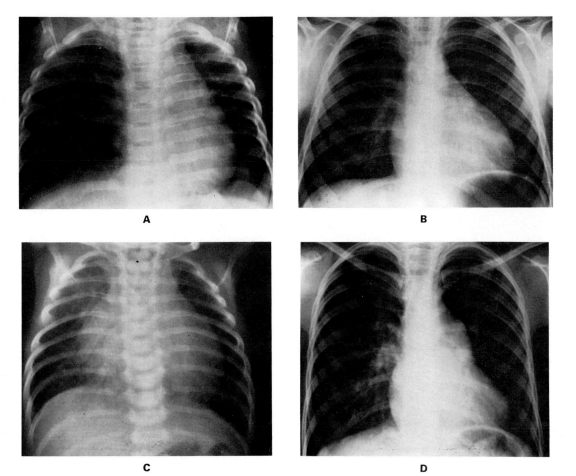

A

B

C

D

Figure 24-5. The cardiac contour at x-ray in patent ductus arteriosus.

A. S.M., an 8-month-old girl with a small patent ductus arteriosus. At cardiac catheterization the pulmonary arterial pressure was normal and the pulmonary/systemic flow ratio was 1.3:1.

B. L. D., a 5-year-old boy with patent ductus arteriosus. At cardiac catheterization the pulmonary arterial pressure was 35/15 mm Hg and the pulmonary/systemic flow ratio was 2:1.

C. F. M., a 4-week-old male infant with patent ductus arteriosus. At cardiac catheterization the systolic pulmonary arterial pressure was at systemic level and the pulmonary/systemic flow ratio was large.

D. P. R., a 6-year-old girl with a large ductus complicated by severe pulmonary hypertension, small volume aorticopulmonary shunt, predominant right ventricular hypertrophy, and slight cardiac enlargement.

against patency of the ductus arteriosus (Currarino and Jackson, 1970).

Lung Vascularity. Some increase in lung vascular markings is usual. The majority of our cases had a grade-2 increase (1 to 4), and in most this has been evenly distributed throughout the lungs. In the preterm infant with left-to-right ductal shunt pulmonary plethora in sequential radiographs is as reliable as echocardiography in establishing severity (Rausch et al., 1976). The development of pulmonary vascular disease has been shown to produce a disproportionately large main pulmonary artery, and in the majority of cases there is only slight enlargement of the lobar and segmental arteries and reduction of peripheral vascularity (Rees, 1968). Calcification in the pulmonary arteries may be seen when there is long-standing shunt reversal (Timpanelli and Steinberg, 1961), but actual calcification of the duct is more likely to be associated with closure or aneurysm (Figure 24–6).

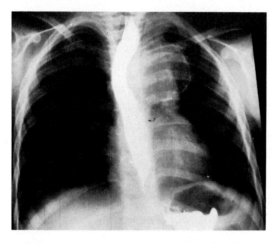

Figure 24-6. The chest film of a four-and-a-half-year-old girl with an ejection systolic murmur in the pulmonary area showing a circumscribed mass with a calcified margin in the left superior mediastinum. The ductal aneurysm was open at its aortic end and was removed successfully under cardiopulmonary bypass.

Electrocardiography

Many publications have maintained that in an uncomplicated patent ductus arteriosus, the electrocardiogram is normal (Ash, 1946; Benn, 1947; Gilchrist, 1948; Lynxwiler and Wells, 1950; Gross, 1952). More recently Donzelot and associates (1954) have felt that a normal electrocardiogram is present in only one-third of the patients. A normal tracing was present in 20 percent of Hospital for Sick Children cases.

ÂQRS. Left-axis deviation has been reported as rare until adolescence but was present in 15 percent of our cases. A normal axis was present in 83 percent. Ash and Fischer (1955) reported a normal axis in 91 percent.

Atrial Hypertrophy. About 5 percent of our cases had left atrial hypertrophy as the sole abnormality in their electrocardiogram, and about the same percentage showed left atrial hypertrophy in association with left ventricular hypertrophy.

Ventricular Hypertrophy. Slight left ventricular hypertrophy in the older cases has been reported by Soulié (1952) in 68 percent and by Donzelot and coworkers (1954) in 55 percent. Of 13 infants operated before three years at The Hospital for Sick Children all electrocardiograms were abnormal, seven showing left ventricular hypertrophy and six combined ventricular hypertrophy (Figure 24–7). In a total of 95 electrocardiograms in cases confirmed at operation, left ventricular hypertrophy was evident in over 60 percent, and there were only two instances of right ventricular hypertrophy. This contrasts with a recently reported group of 246 operated cases over one year in which 63 percent had no evidence of ventricular hypertrophy (Krovetz and Warden, 1962.)

Other. The presence of an upward concavity in S-T segments of leads II, III, AV_F, V_5, and V_6, originally described by Sodi-Pallares and colleagues (1958), was confirmed in the tracings of 63 percent of patients over one year of age by Krovetz and Warden (1962). This would appear to be a useful diagnostic point since it is uncommon in other forms of congenital heart disease. Incomplete bundle branch block has been reported as an uncommon finding in between 2 and 4 percent of the cases.

Correlation. Correlation of the electrocardiogram with the other features of the malformation is interesting. Only one of our cases with a "normal" electrocardiogram had an abnormal cardiothoracic ratio, but large ducti were found in a few of the cases showing no electrical disturbances. The cases with left atrial hypertrophy as the sole abnormality had small hearts and relatively small ducti. The cases with right ventricular hypertrophy showed severe pulmonary hypertension. In the infant group, by definition severe cases, the ducti were all large and the heart was grossly enlarged.

In electrocardiographic studies on young infants with patent ductus arteriosus mostly aged under six months, Marcano and Goldberg (1969) failed to obtain good correlation between either the degree of right ventricular hypertrophy and level of mean pulmonary arterial pressure or the degree of left ventricular hypertrophy and shunt size.

Electrocardiographic reversion after operation was much more delayed in infants than in older children. In older children prompt postoperative reduction in voltage of Q and R in V_6 has been noted by Watson and Keith (1962). The evolution of the electrocardiogram in infants and children has not been studied in detail. We have a few tracings that were taken from infancy in children operated on at a later age. For example, one case, which showed a normal tracing at 11 months and at two years, developed left ventricular hypertrophy by three years. A moderate-sized ductus was ligated at four years of

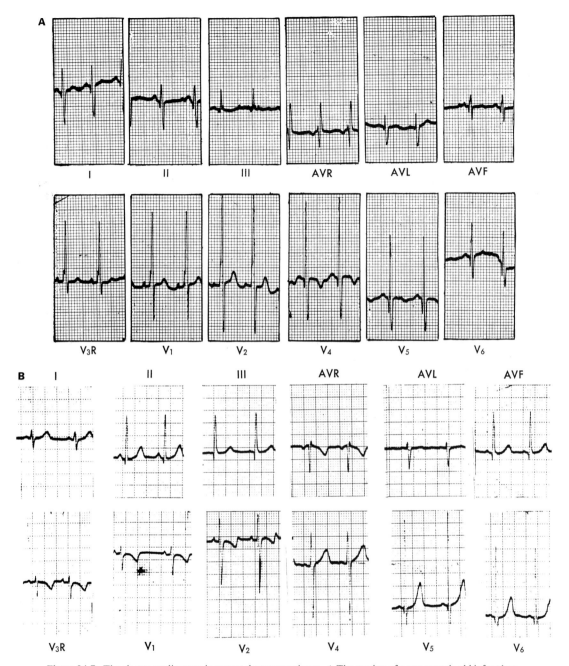

Figure 24-7. The electrocardiogram in patent ductus arteriosus. *A.* The tracing of a one-month-old infant boy with autopsy-confirmed simple patent ductus arteriosus. Combined ventricular hypertrophy is present. In other neonates in gross failure the degree of right overloading may mask all signs of left ventricular overload. *B.* The tracing of a four-year-old girl with a small left-to-right shunt. There is modest left ventricular overload.

age. Another case at 14 months of age had complete right bundle branch block only, but by two years had left ventricular hypertrophy as well. One month postoperatively, incomplete right bundle branch block was the remaining abnormality in the electrocardiogram.

Echocardiography

Though not diagnostic, the echocardiogram can give an indication of the degree of hemodynamic disturbance. Varying degrees of left atrial and left ventricular enlargement will be found. In our experience there is good correlation between left atrial diameter and left-to-right shunt size (Bloom et al., 1977). There has been considerable interest recently in using the technique for this purpose in the respiratory distress syndrome of premature infants (Silverman et al., 1974; Bayley et al., 1975).

Cardiac Catheterization

The hemodynamics of the ordinary case of patent ductus arteriosus have been previously described (Cournand et al., 1949). Confirmation of the clinical diagnosis may be obtained in the ordinary case either by demonstration of a rise of oxygen content of blood in the pulmonary artery over that obtained from the right ventricle by aortic injection of indicators, by direct probing of the duct (Figure 24–8) (Alvarez et al., 1949), or by phonocatheter techniques. It has been

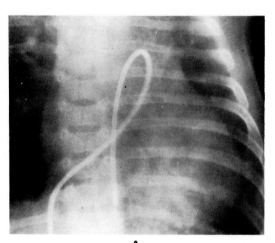

A

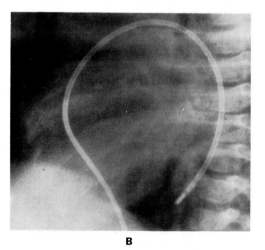

B

Figure 24-8. The course of the venous catheter in patent ductus arteriosus. *A.* Anteroposterior radiograph. *B.* Lateral radiograph.

shown by various workers that the flow through the ductus averages 40 percent of the left ventricular output but varies considerably (Eppinger et al., 1941; Keys and Shapiro, 1943; Taylor et al., 1950; Adams et al., 1952; Bing, 1952). Except in cases with elevated left atrial pressure at rest when exercise decreases pulmonary blood flow, in the ordinary patient there does not seem to be an important change in pulmonary blood flow with effort. Because of the difficulty of obtaining representative sampling from pulmonary artery branches, quantitation of the shunt may be more accurately obtained from simultaneous left atrial and systemic arterial sampling after aortic root or left ventricular injection of indicator. The pressure in the pulmonary artery is not usually raised in the ordinary case to any significant degree. Swan and associates (1954), in a group of 24 cases, found a mean pressure in the pulmonary artery of more than 40 mm of mercury in ten instances. It is possible that the high incidence of pulmonary hypertension in this group and other reported cases is from the selection of cases, as it is not usual to perform the investigation as a routine measure in this malformation. Although there is little doubt that the vast majority of cases of patent ductus arteriosus do not require cardiac catheterization preoperatively, the method has considerable value in the infant group with symptoms or in cases exhibiting the effects of pulmonary hypertension. Important contributions in the infant group have been made with regard to cardiac catheterization by Adams and coworkers (1952), Dammann and Sell (1952), Ziegler (1952), Lyon and Kaplan (1954), Rudolph and coworkers (1958), and Krovetz and coworkers (1962). The infants with symptoms, cardiac enlargement, and electrocardiographic evidence of left or combined ventricular hypertrophy show a large aorticopulmonary shunt and frequently high pressures in the pulmonary artery (Figure 24–9). In half of the cases in which the aorta was entered through the patent ductus arteriosus by Ziegler, the mean pulmonary arterial pressure was 75 percent of that in the aorta. This presence of pulmonary hypertension, so common in the infant cases, seldom has the same serious import as hypertension in the older cases.

There are a number of problems that arise in the interpretation of the catheterization findings. These are chiefly in relation to oxygen saturation data: a significant rise in blood oxygen saturation data may occur at atrial or ventricular level in patients with large ductal shunts, especially infants, owing to dilatation of a patent foramen ovale, pulmonary or tricuspid regurgitation, or all three (Rudolph et al., 1958; James et al., 1961). The problem then is whether the findings are due to these relatively innocent complications or whether the patient has true septal defects in addition to the ductus.

Measurement of the interatrial pressure gradient and use of the phonocatheter are two simple maneuvers that usually clarify matters in regard to the atrial and ventricular septa, respectively, although resort to more complex double-catheter techniques

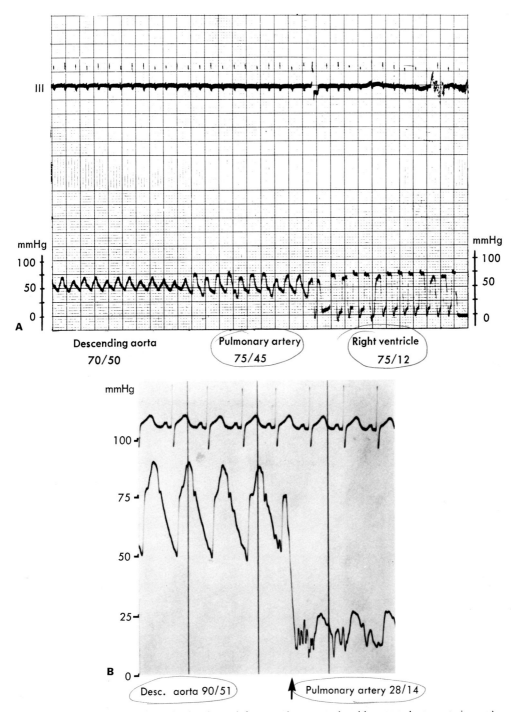

Figure 24-9. *A*. Cardiac catheterization in an infant, aged one month, with patent ductus arteriosus. A continuous withdrawal pressure record taken after direct probing of the ductus with the catheter. Note the difference in pressure pulse between aorta and pulmonary artery and the marked pulmonary and right ventricular hypertension.

B. Pressures recorded during withdrawal of a catheter from the descending aorta to the right ventricle in an 8-month-old infant girl with isolated patent ductus arteriosus. The Qp/Qs was 3.5/1 and the mean wedge pulmonary artery pressure 12 mm Hg. The *arrow* marks the point at which the catheter has flipped through the ductus into the pulmonary artery.

with indicators or selective angiography may be necessary for complete diagnosis.

When the shunt is clearly confined to the pulmonary artery, the remaining question is usually whether there is an aortic septal defect or patent ductus arteriosus present. This is more often solved simply by direct catheterization of the ductus and descending aorta in the classic manner. Rarely the position of entry may appear unusual because of cardiac rotation or because the catheter passes upward to a carotid vessel. The authors have found the routine retrograde passage of a catheter from the femoral artery to the main pulmonary artery to obviate any such confusion by the site of entry. This technique permits confirmation of a single aortico-pulmonary defect by cineangiography or by making possible examination of arterial dilution patterns after indicator injection at increasingly distal sites from the aortic root (Braunwald et al., 1957).

The arterial oxygen saturation in the average case is normal, and it is only in cases with pulmonary hypertension and bidirectional flow or in the infant cases with marked pulmonary hypertension that there is any alteration in this respect. In these cases there is a lower saturation of blood from the femoral artery than that obtained from the brachial artery analysis, a difference that can be augmented when the patient breathes a mixture containing 10 percent oxygen.

To show this situation even more clearly, right ventricular injection of indicator with arterial sampling in both right brachial and a femoral artery or the descending aorta will result in the description of dissimilar dilution curves, early-appearing dye being visible in the trace from descending aorta or femoral artery. Cineangiocardiography provides similar information.

Studies from The Hospital for Sick Children and elsewhere (Swan et al., 1954; Kidd et al., 1968; Leachman et al., 1971) have shown in older children that patent ductus arteriosus occupies a position intermediate between ventricular and atrial septal defects in regard to the development of pulmonary vascular disease. Values of more than 5 resistance units per M^2 were found in 25 percent of 680 patients with ventricular septal defect, 11 percent of 183 patients with patent ductus arteriosus, and 2 percent of 327 patients from The Hospital for Sick Children with atrial septal defect. Since the majority of our patients under the age of two years demonstrated normal evolution of pulmonary vascular resistance with age, it can be assumed that measurable alterations of the pulmonary vascular bed are not usually established until after infancy.

Angiocardiography

Aortography also can clarify the diagnosis (Keith and Forsyth, 1950). Its particular advantage is that in the young patient, in the presence of shunts of comparable magnitude, it can define the different duct

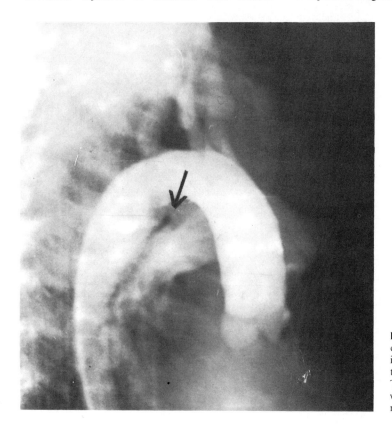

Figure 24-10. The lateral aortogram of C. B., a 12-month-old female Maori infant, with a large left-to-right shunt through a patent ductus arteriosus. The *arrow* points to the ductus, which was confirmed as large at surgery one month later.

diameters quite conclusively. Nowadays the technique involves injection of contrast from a catheter (Jonsson et al., 1948) placed retrogradely near the aortic isthmus from either the umbilical or femoral arterial route (Figure 24–10). Occasions still arise where the original brachial arterial method is preferred (Figure 24–11). The venous angiocardiogram of earlier years (Lind and Wegelius, 1954) has been largely replaced by more selective techniques to show shunts in either direction through the ductus.

Complications

Congestive Heart Failure. At The Hospital for Sick Children, 86 of 208 infants operated under the age of two years had either congestive failure or very large hearts. At the Green Lane Hospital, 13 infants of 43 with patent ductus arteriosus seen under the age of 12 months had congestive failure, while at the Johns Hopkins Hospital, comparable figures were 17 out of 41. Krovetz and coworkers (1962) found a similarly high proportion with congestive heart failure in a series of 39 infants operated on for patent ductus arteriosus during the first year of life. The clinical features are then similar to that of the symptomatic

infant group in general with the addition of definite signs of right heart failure—dyspnea, gallop rhythm, and enlarged liver. There is usually some response to medical treatment, but surgery is strongly advised after the initial benefit unless the infant falls into certain categories—particularly into the premature birth group—to be discussed later. There is real danger in deferring surgical therapy especially after the first few months of life, and the authors have observed unexpected death in a number of such infants prior to adopting the more aggressive approach. Similar recommendations have been reached by others and the value of this approach is now widely recognized (Ash and Fischer, 1955; Bauersfeld et al., 1957; Clatworthy and McDonald, 1958; Rowe et al., 1961; Krovetz et al., 1962; Ochsner et al., 1962).

Congestive heart failure, while not the most important complication of the patient with extreme pulmonary vascular disease, in ductus arteriosus may occur as a terminal feature.

Subacute Bacterial Endocarditis. Reports of groups comprising mainly adults have suggested a high incidence of subacute bacterial endocarditis. Less than 2 percent of 515 surgically treated patients with patent ductus arteriosus developed this

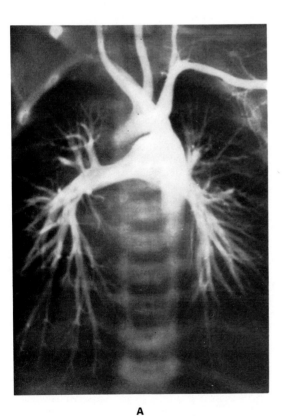
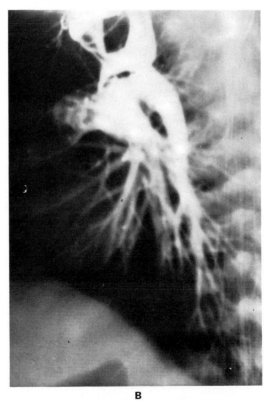

| A | B |

Figure 24-11. The retrograde aortogram (*A*, anteroposterior view; *B*, lateral view) of K. H., a female infant aged 77 hours, with cardiomegaly and gross congestive failure due to patent ductus arteriosus. Death occurred at 80 hours. The autopsy showed solitary large (uncontracted) ductus arteriosus and normal histologic appearance of lung parenchyma, vascular bed, and myocardium.

complication in a recent survey covering 20 years (Krovetz and Warden, 1962), and the disorder seems to be much less common in young children and infants. This is also the experience at the Johns Hopkins Hospital where between 1956 and 1965, among 51 episodes of bacterial endocarditis in 46 patients with congenital heart disease, there was not a single instance of isolated ductus arteriosus. Campbell (1968) suggests an incidence of 0.5 to 1.0 percent per annum after the first decade of life in patients with ductus arteriosus. At The Hospital for Sick Children, two children who developed subacute bacterial endocarditis at 4 and 12 years, respectively, were successfully treated with penicillin and had their ducti ligated several months later. One other girl of nine years died in the prepenicillin era from an infected ductus. The vegetations tend to proliferate at the pulmonary end of the ductus and in the pulmonary artery. Embolization of the lungs is a consequence. Thus it may mimic pneumonia or miliary tuberculosis (Gilchrist, 1945). It follows that patients with this malformation and a persistent fever should have blood cultured with the possibility of this infection in mind.

Current opinion favors treating bacterial endo-carditis with penicillin in the usual manner in these cases, delaying surgery until the infection has been overcome. There may be rare exceptions to this regime in a few cases where the infection is far-advanced, but the mortality rate is much higher when closure of the ductus is undertaken during the time of sepsis (Shapiro, 1947; Gross and Longino, 1951).

Disturbing reports of staphylococcal septicemia, presumably resulting from preoperative infection of the ductus area, have appeared (Fleming and Seal, 1955; Ross et al., 1961). In one such case at The Hospital for Sick Children, a four-year-old girl underwent an uneventful suture ligation for simple patent ductus arteriosus. One month postoperatively, at home, she developed malaise and high fever. Penicillin-resistant *Staphylococcus aureus* was isolated on blood culture. Clinically, there was a return of the continuous murmur and evidence of an aneurysm of the ductus arteriosus, and she eventually died from massive hemorrhage following rupture of this aneurysm into the left main bronchus.

Aneurysm of the Ductus. Aneurysm of the ductus is held to be relatively common. Sellors (1945) noted 29 instances, of which 24 were children. Cruickshank and Marquis (1958) and Falcone and associates (1972) refer to 60 cases in the literature, mostly in infants. Several reports of rupture of an aneurysm in infants have emerged. The postmortem material at The Hospital for Sick Children includes 12 neonates with definite aneurysm of the ductus but no rupture. Many of the aneurysms reported are associated with subacute bacterial endocarditis and are, therefore, mycotic in nature. Many are based on operative reports only. It is thus doubtful if true aneurysm of the ductus is common; consequently a realistic figure may be in the vicinity of 1 to 2 percent. Similarly, dilation of the pulmonary arterial system is very frequent, but true aneurysm of the pulmonary artery is much less common.

Pressure effects from such aneurysms may occur. Recurrent laryngeal nerve palsy has been reported from stretching of this structure by aneurysm of the ductus or aneurysm of the left main branch of the pulmonary artery. Apart from these it is unwise to imply that pressure effects are the result of an enlarged pulmonary artery even though its size may be enormous. One infant under our care with patent ductus arteriosus and persistent left lower lobe collapse had aneurysmal dilatation of the pulmonary artery, normal pulmonary arterial pressure, and a localized aortic aneurysm below the ductal insertion, which was compressing the bronchus in question. It is probable that the pressure in the pulmonary artery is a more important factor than the actual size of the vessel in producing compression effects.

Aortic Embolism. In the absence of dehydration, polycythemia, or sepsis, a fatal aortic thrombosis originating in the otherwise normal ductus arteriosus of a ten-day-old infant has been reported (Stout and Koehl, 1970). A literature review by these authors found ten similar patients all under two weeks of age. The pathogenesis of the complication is unclear.

Ductus Arteriosus with Other Congenital Heart Disease

Patency of the ductus arteriosus is a common finding in a wide variety of congenital malformations of the heart. In some of these—notably in the pulmonary stenosis or atresia accompanying tetralogy of Fallot; less strikingly in tricuspid atresia, pulmonary atresia with intact ventricular septum, or single ventricle—the presence of the aortico-pulmonary communication is of some benefit to the patient. Indeed, the aim of shunt operations for these conditions is to mimic this natural circumstance, and closure of the ductus is then contraindicated. But in some situations the association of a patent ductus arteriosus with existing lesions only adds further cardiac strain frequently to an already overburdened heart.

There is no evidence either that persistence of the ductus arteriosus is more common in the types of cardiac malformation that would benefit from its presence or less common in malformations to which it clearly imposes additional hemodynamic strain (Bass and Rowe, 1967).

A wide variety of heart defects of the acyanotic group have been found in association with patent ductus arteriosus. The extent of this problem in practical terms is shown when 15 percent of 515 patients undergoing surgery for patent ductus arteriosus at the University of Minnesota Hospitals had additional cardiac defects (Krovetz and Warden, 1962).

A similar group of patients had been encountered at The Hospital for Sick Children, and there have been a number of other publications describing the various combinations. The incidence of the complicating anomaly tends to vary, but the chief lesions appear to be ventricular septal defect, coarctation of the aorta, aortic stenosis, pulmonary stenosis and pulmonary artery stenosis, and mitral regurgitation.

Ventricular Septal Defect. A relatively small number of this group have the classic continuous murmur in the pulmonary area and a pansystolic murmur with thrill in the third to fourth left intercostal space. In such cases the ventricular septal defect is of small size, pulmonary vascular resistance is normal, and the pulmonary artery pressure is normal or only slightly elevated. There is usually no difficulty in distinguishing the pansystolic murmur of the ventricular septal defect from transmission to the lower left sternal border of the crescendo systolic component of the murmur from the isolated ductus. The rare type-I ventricular septal defect where pansystolic murmur is maximal over the pulmonary area may be completely obscured by the duct murmur.

Difficulty in diagnosis of the combination arises more often when there is substantial pulmonary hypertension, murmurs due to one or both defects having become atypical. Fortunately this is the type of case where accessory studies are almost always performed. Both defects in these cases are usually large, but this is not always so and one defect may have a substantially greater diameter than the other. Reliance on the presence of an important rise in oxygen saturation of pulmonary artery blood over that obtained in the right ventricle cannot be made in these circumstances. Probing of the duct with the catheter and the demonstration or exclusion by aortic dye or contrast injection have been useful in the authors' hands, while others prefer aortography (Elliott et al., 1962). It is evident from the experience with the combination that where a ventricular septal defect and patent ductus arteriosus exist with pulmonary hypertension, the ventricular septal defect is the dominant lesion. There is no sure clinical method of separating isolated ventricular septal defect from the combination, yet the presence of a ductus has important surgical implications and failure to detect it preoperatively can lead to disaster during perfusion. Sasahara and coworkers (1960) showed in their cases not only a lack of improvement but an increase in pulmonary vascular resistance following division of the duct, and consequently they prefer to tackle both conditions at the one operation. Elliott and coworkers (1962), although observing similar resistance changes, did not find that preliminary duct surgery influenced later closure of the ventricular septal defect adversely, believing rather that the overall risk of operation is lowered by using a two-stage repair.

Coarctation of the Aorta. In many young infants in congestive heart failure with obvious coarctation of the aorta, signs of patent ductus arteriosus may be lacking and yet substantial aorticopulmonary shunts are evident on catheterization or at operation. In other patients the duct murmur is clearly audible.

Sometimes there is a widespread continuous murmur in the pulmonary area, axilla, and back simulating patent ductus arteriosus but created from passage of blood through the coarctation itself. In older patients a similar murmur may be produced by collateral vessels.

Aortic Stenosis. Seven of an earlier group of personal cases of complicated patent ductus arteriosus had aortic stenosis, and the authors found the combination a particularly difficult one to diagnose with certainty. Recognition of the association from the presence of an ejection systolic murmur in the aortic area with a separate thrill in this region and in the neck was reported by Mark and coworkers (1958) in nine patients with aortic stenosis among 90 operations for patent ductus arteriosus. They suggested that since all had small ducts the disproportionate enlargement of the left ventricle and aorta should arouse suspicion. No doubt careful auscultation may permit clinical diagnosis in many, but the authors have encountered several patients with large-flow patent ductus arteriosus who had a loud ejection systolic murmur in the aortic area and a coarse thrill in carotid vessels where all signs disappeared after division of the duct. The signs were presumably due to a high left ventricle stroke volume. We have also noted the silent ductus in some infants with severe aortic stenosis where marked pulmonary hypertension was present.

Pulmonary Stenosis and Pulmonary Artery Stenoses. The combination of simple pulmonary stenosis with patent ductus arteriosus was reported in six patients by Heiner and Nadas (1958). In three there was a history of maternal rubella and in one the right ventricle–pulmonary artery gradient was masked before division of the ductus. The association can sometimes be suspected by the presence of prominent jugular "a" waves and right ventricular hypertrophy in the electrocardiogram, even though the ejection systolic murmur characteristic of pulmonary stenosis is masked by the louder continuous murmur of the ductus. Rowe (1963) later reported the association of stenosis of the pulmonary artery with rubella syndrome. In these cases the continuous murmur of a duct may mask the complicating anomaly, but clues will be present from the wide transmission of the stenotic murmur to the anterolateral aspects of the thorax, as well as some degree of right ventricular overload in the electrocardiogram. This association is extremely common in patients with rubella background, but the authors have encountered male sibs with the combination of coarctation of the aorta, patent ductus arteriosus, and peripheral pulmonary artery stenosis.

Mitral Regurgitation. The first report of patent ductus arteriosus with mitral regurgitation described three children all with pulmonary hypertension and mitral systolic murmur (Linde and Adams, 1959). After large ducts were interrupted surgically, the apical murmur remained. An experience of this malformation at Green Lane Hospital concerns 16 patients. All have had very large ducts at operation and usually, but not always, pulmonary hypertension. In one patient the mitral regurgitation disappeared immediately after surgery. In another patient who died at operation a large dilated mitral ring but normal valve and left ventricular endocardium were found at autopsy. The other 14 have distinct residual mitral regurgitation, although the murmur has become less intense after duct division. No lengthy follow-up has yet been reported, and it is not known whether the pathologic basis is the same in all cases. None of the patients had associated corrected transposition of the great vessels, and not included was one patient who had a definite rheumatic episode or AV canal defects to account for the mitral leak. One of the earlier patients from The Hospital for Sick Children series had a small ductus in association with gross endocardial fibroelastosis with mitral regurgitation, but the clinical picture was unlike the above-mentioned cases.

The Problem of Ductus Arteriosus with Pulmonary Hypertension

Although in patent ductus arteriosus there is ordinarily an increase in pulmonary blood flow because of continuous left-to-right shunt through the aorticopulmonary communication, it is uncommon to find as a result much alteration in pulmonary artery pressure. Experimental studies (Levy and Blalock, 1938; Eppinger et al., 1941; Leeds, 1942) and clinical measurements (Eppinger et al., 1941; Cournand, 1947; Dexter et al., 1947; Storstein et al., 1952) have confirmed that the pulmonary circulation can accommodate very considerable increases in blood volume without change in pressure. Nevertheless, numerous reports of pulmonary hypertension associated with patent ductus arteriosus have emerged. Recent interest has centered around these patients showing *marked* pulmonary hypertension because of their different clinical features, the practical problem they pose in regard to surgery, and the academic questions raised in relation to etiology (Chapman and Robbins, 1944; DuShane and Montgomery, 1948; Griswold et al., 1949; Johnson et al., 1950; Pritchard et al., 1950; Campbell and Hudson, 1951; Myers et al., 1951; Adams et al., 1952; Bothwell et al., 1952; Dammann and Sell, 1952; Taussig et al., 1952; Burchell et al., 1953; Cosh, 1953; Dammann et al., 1953; Holman et al., 1953; Hultgren et al., 1953; Shephard, 1954; Yu et al., 1954; Anderson and Coles, 1955; Marquis and Gilchrist, 1955; Shepherd et al., 1955; Ellis et al., 1956; Heath et al., 1958a; Jose et al., 1961; Leachman et al., 1971).

The actual incidence of pulmonary hypertension in isolated patent ductus arteriosus is not known. The published data probably indicate too high a frequency because of the selective nature of the case material. The catheterization experience at The Hospital for Sick Children is likewise affected by this factor. An approximation may be made on grounds other than catheterization data if only severe cases of

pulmonary hypertension are to be estimated. It is reasonable to postulate that such severe cases will have atypical murmurs, that there will be *some* right ventricular hypertrophy in the electrocardiogram, and that some will have come to autopsy. On this basis of calculation in an experience with 168 cases of isolated ductus arteriosus seen at The Hospital for Sick Children, severe pulmonary hypertension was encountered in 11 percent of the cases from one month to 15 years.

Theoretically there are three possible mechanisms in which the pulmonary artery pressure may become elevated in patent ductus arteriosus:

1. From markedly increased pulmonary blood flow. There is some experimental (Ekström et al., 1951) and clinical (Dexter et al., 1950) evidence that shows that beyond a certain volume of flow in the pulmonary circuit the pulmonary artery pressure becomes elevated.

2. From increased pulmonary venous pressure. It is known (Hickam, 1949; Dexter et al., 1950) that left ventricular failure from whatever cause (or any similar obstruction of blood flow in the left heart such as mitral stenosis, endocardial fibroelastosis, or triatrial heart) by increasing the pressure in the pulmonary veins will result in elevation of pulmonary arterial pressures, sometimes to an extreme degree. In such cases the pulmonary "wedge" or "capillary" pressure will be abnormally high.

3. From increased pulmonary vascular resistance. While the cause of such constriction is uncertain at the present time, a number of theories have been suggested and some important contributions made to this problem (Edwards et al., 1949; Burchell et al., 1953; Swan et al., 1954; Heath et al., 1958a; Jose et al., 1961).

Structural changes, principally thickening of the walls of arterioles and small muscular pulmonary arteries with associated intimal changes, are fairly constantly encountered in the reported cases. This led Civin and Edwards (1951) to suggest that a persistence of the fetal structure in pulmonary small vessels might be the cause of pulmonary hypertension in some instances of patency of the ductus arteriosus. Swan and associates (1954) believe that kinetic effects of the pulmonary artery pressure pulse may promote degenerative changes in the pulmonary small vessels in other cases. That a functional element exists as well is provided by the work of Burchell and coworkers (1953), who demonstrated that the magnitude and occasionally even the direction of a right-to-left shunt through the ductus may be altered in cases of marked pulmonary hypertension. The effect is produced by varying the vascular resistance with differing oxygen tensions in inspired air.

Hyperkinetic Pulmonary Hypertension. Not all infants with symptoms due to ductus arteriosus in infancy will be found to have pulmonary hypertension at cardiac catheterization, and it is surprising how many can accommodate very large pulmonary blood flows without elevating their pulmonary artery pressure. Furthermore, the element of selection enters into the available information on the subject. In a group of 26 babies catheterized under one year of age with ductus arteriosus, which excluded all infants in the premature group but included all other cases with ductus arteriosus and cardiomegaly or symptoms at the Johns Hopkins Hospital in a recent period, patients were equally distributed between those with normal pressure, mild, moderate, or severe pulmonary hypertension. The higher the pressure in the pulmonary artery, the less classic the murmur and the more serious the symptoms. Most with moderate to severe pulmonary hypertension had congestive failure. In six patients with the abbreviated murmur studied at the Green Lane Hospital, there was a large shunt in four cases and a moderate shunt in two. The average systolic, diastolic, and mean pulmonary artery aortic pressure ratios were 0.64, 0.80, and 0.71, respectively. This compares with five patients from that study where classic continuous murmur was present and where the shunt was large in two, moderate in two, and smaller in one. The average systolic, diastolic, and mean pulmonary artery aortic pressure ratios were 0.43, 0.45, and 0.44, respectively. Frequently, the pulmonary wedge or left atrial pressure is elevated moderately in the cases with large shunts. Most of these findings can be readily transferred to the older child with large-volume left-to-right shunt. Abolition of the shunt surgically leads in these instances to a drop in the pulmonary artery pressure to normal range, and no instances have been reported under these circumstances where a late development of pulmonary vascular disease has become evident.

Pulmonary Vascular Disease. PATIENTS WITH CLEAR EVIDENCE OF ACQUIRED PULMONARY VASCULAR DISEASE. A few reported adult cases in earlier life have had the classic physical signs of isolated patent ductus arteriosus, in particular the loud continuous murmur, but have shown with increasing age disappearance of the diastolic element of the murmur. Autopsy has revealed pronounced right ventricular hypertrophy and small vessel occlusive changes in the lungs. Examples of this group have been reported by Campbell and Hudson (1952), Evans and Heath (1961), and Jose and coworkers (1961). It must be concluded from these descriptions that pulmonary hypertension was either absent or only moderate in childhood and that a true increase in pulmonary vascular resistance has resulted as a secondary effect of prolonged aorticopulmonary shunting. These cases then initially have left-to-right shunt, then bidirectional, and, possibly, finally predominantly right-to-left shunting through the ductus.

Electrocardiographically this group will undergo changes corresponding to the direction of ductus flow: at first, normal tracings or left ventricular hypertrophy, changing at a later age to combined hypertrophy, and then right hypertrophy alone. Examination of the elastic tissue architecture of the main pulmonary artery in these cases may give variable results, depending on whether or not there was hyperkinetic pulmonary hypertension in early life.

The theory of progressive damage to pulmonary small vessels by kinetic factors in the pulmonary artery pressure pulse, as postulated by Swan and associates (1954), seems to be particularly applicable to this group.

PATIENTS WITHOUT CLEAR EVIDENCE OF ACQUISITION OF PULMONARY VASCULAR DISEASE. This group embraces all ages. They are categorized in this fashion because most of the reported incidents have involved patients in or beyond the second decade of life. Marquis (1968) has reported three children of this picture between the ages of seven and nine years. It is almost certain that these patients have had pulmonary hypertension from a very early stage, and while it is obvious that the fully developed picture of pulmonary vascular disease was not present at that time, it is highly likely that pulmonary vascular resistance was markedly elevated even then, for in none of the reported cases has there ever been a typical continuous murmur or electrocardiographic evidence of left ventricular hypertrophy. The reason why some patients behave in this fashion with relatively high vascular tone even in infancy is not clear. The relationship between these patients and symptomatic infants with pulmonary vascular disease is uncertain (Siassi et al., 1971; Burnell et al., 1972). Holman (1937) has suggested that such a picture could result if a predominant proportion of blood entering the right atrium flowed through the right ventricle and pulmonary artery during fetal life.

Exertional dyspnea is the commonest symptom in these cases. Cyanosis may be early but more often does not become obvious or generalized for many years. As it is confined to the legs alone or left arm and legs, a superficial examination may fail to disclose its presence. Clubbing is correspondingly a localized phenomenon when present.

Murmurs are "atypical." There is never a continuous murmur as in the ordinary case without or with only slight pulmonary hypertension. Systolic frequently, diastolic alone, or both systolic and diastolic murmurs may be present. Rarely there is no murmur. The second pulmonic sound is virtually always greatly accentuated, often palpable and split. An obvious pulmonary ejection click is invariably present. Heart failure is a terminal complication, but sudden death, bacterial endocarditis, and hemoptysis are all part of the general symptomatology in the late stages.

Radiologically the heart is most often of normal size or only slightly increased until failure appears. The pulmonary artery segment bulges greatly while the hilar vascularity is not really remarkable. The electrocardiogram shows right-axis deviation and right ventricular hypertrophy of moderate or marked degree, but many records have shown relatively mild right ventricular hypertrophy or combined ventricular hypertrophy and suggested left ventricular hypertrophy even in the face of very advanced pulmonary vascular obstruction in a manner not usually seen in septal defects with high pulmonary vascular resistance (Lowe, 1963).

Accessory studies are essential for accurate diagnosis. Indeed, frequently the condition is first revealed during such investigations in a puzzling case.

Cardiac catheterization permits demonstration of the malformation by direct probing of the ductus arteriosus. There is pronounced pulmonary hypertension, the systolic levels equaling or exceeding the systemic level. Any left-to-right shunt present through the ductus is of small volume, the shunt being wholly or predominantly right-to-left. Occasionally the left-to-right shunt may be of larger volume in younger patients. Samples of blood from the right radial artery are much more highly saturated with oxygen than femoral arterial samples. The calculated pulmonary vascular resistance is markedly elevated.

Indicator dilution techniques will reveal more strikingly the functional hemodynamics, and pulmonary arteriography shows clearly opacification of the descending aorta in these circumstances (Campbell and Hudson, 1951; Lukas et al., 1954; Yu et al., 1954).

At autopsy there is marked right ventricular hypertrophy with pulmonary artery dilatation and atheroma. Microscopically, changes in the pulmonary arteries are invariable, and the architecture of the elastic lamellae in the main pulmonary artery is identical with the arrangement found in the aorta (Heath et al., 1958).

Diagnosis

The Uncomplicated Case. There is not usually any great difficulty with diagnosis in the ordinary case of isolated patent ductus arteriosus. A well child, free of any symptoms and cyanosis, is found on routine auscultation to have a continuous machinery murmur in the second left interspace. Roentgen examination may show normal size or slight cardiac enlargement, and the lung vascularity is usually slightly increased. An electrocardiogram will show no axis deviation and, in most, some degree of left ventricular hypertrophy.

Of these features the continuous murmur is the most important single sign, but the minimum investigation should include electrocardiogram and x-ray as well. In 94 percent of Ekström's (1952) series of 290 cases of patent ductus arteriosus, in 95 percent of 160 operated cases at The Hospital for Sick Children, in 94 percent of 126 cases seen by Ash and Fischer (1955), and in 86 percent of 515 patients in a Minnesota series (Krovetz and Warden, 1962), the diagnosis was based essentially on this auscultatory sign.

The continuous murmur is most frequently heard at the first consultation, even in infants. Ash and Fischer (1955) had 24 infants under one year with a

continuous murmur in their series. There is a fairly general tendency to regard a nonspecific systolic murmur as being more usual in infancy. The exact percentage in which this occurs is not known; the belief that it is common is always open to the suspicion that under perhaps more satisfactory circumstances some spillover into diastole might not have been recognized.

Why it often takes a period of months or even a year for the continuous murmur to become "classic" in some infants is unknown. It is unlikely that this is due either to the general decline in pulmonary vascular resistance during this period or to major change in duct diameter. Possibly the gradual rise of systemic pressure has a bearing on this matter.

A number of conditions that simulate patent ductus arteriosus by their murmur require differentiation.

VENOUS HUM. A venous hum, very commonly found in young children, may in some cases be loud enough to confuse. It may be heard over the base of the heart and be maximal to the right or left of the sternum. Characteristically, movement of the neck to one side or digital compression of the jugular vein abolishes the hum, whereas extension of the neck increases its intensity. In those patients with a faint continuous murmur and true ductus arteriosus these maneuvers do not change the murmur, and the second pulmonic sound by its accentuation frequently assists in excluding a venous hum.

PULMONARY ARTERIOVENOUS FISTULA. Pulmonary arteriovenous fistulae produce a distant continuous murmur, but the position of the murmur in the chest is frequently alone sufficient to exclude ductus arteriosus as its cause. In very young children such a fistula in the left upper lobe may result in confusion. Other features that make a possible error unlikely are the cyanosis and clubbing in association with normal heart size and normal electrocardiogram present in all except a very few with pulmonary arteriovenous fistula. In two cases seen at The Hospital for Sick Children, patency of the ductus arteriosus was not considered in the diagnosis in either.

AORTICOPULMONARY WINDOW. Aorticopulmonary window may give rise to a typical, continuous machinery murmur in the second left interspace in association with left ventricular hypertrophy. This has inevitably resulted in a number of cases undergoing thoracotomy for ligation of a suspected ductus arteriosus. Practically all large operative series of ductus arteriosi will have one or two such examples. Other cases of aortic window reported in the literature have not mimicked the picture of ductus arteriosus so closely. In these cyanosis has been present, the murmur has not been continuous, and right ventricular hypertrophy has been present in the electrocardiogram. Cardiac catheterization has not always been helpful although several reports (Dexter, 1949; Adams et al., 1952; D'heer and van Nieuwenhuizen, 1956) have shown the value of the technique in demonstrating the window directly.

Aortography would seem the best method at present available for visualizing the defect. With this technique and using cine methods, separation from the ductus arteriosus will usually be possible in infants. A study of arterial dilution patterns after central, followed by more distal, injections of indicator has real value in dealing with this problem. A ductus arteriosus is not infrequently associated (Deverall et al., 1969).

RUPTURED SINUS OF VALSALVA. This is a rare condition in young children, being much more frequently seen in adults where the dramatic clinical picture following the time of rupture lends to relatively easy diagnosis. Nevertheless, cases have been recorded in the younger age group where the continuous murmur may lead to errors of interpretation. The case of Fowler and Bevil (1951) had a sudden onset of symptoms at four years, a machinery murmur in the sixth left interspace and left ventricular hypertrophy in the electrocardiogram. Cardiac catheterization revealed a left-to-right intracardiac shunt commencing at ventricular level. The authors have encountered a six-year-old boy who ruptured a sinus of Valsalva aneurysm into his left ventricle during the course of subacute bacterial endocarditis. His physical signs suggested aortic stenosis and regurgitation, and at operation there was a 40-mm systolic gradient between the left ventricle and the sinus and an 80-mm systolic gradient between the left ventricle and ascending aorta. The aortic valve, though bicuspid, was not stenotic and the sinus aneurysm appeared to be distorting the aortic valve. In most patients there is a progressive downward course following rupture of the sinus into the right ventricle. Aortography seems the most certain method of confirming the diagnosis.

OTHERS. Continuous murmurs over the precordium have also been noted in coronary arterial fistulae, traumatic or congenital thoracic wall fistulae, surgically created or congenital aorticopulmonary arterial anastomosis, mitral atresia, aortic regurgitation, coarctation of the aorta, the supracardiac form of total anomalous pulmonary venous return, and pulmonary artery stenosis (Zuberbuhler et al., 1975).

The Complicated Case. ASSOCIATED DEFECTS. Cyanotic Cases. The presence of a continuous murmur in association with cyanotic congenital heart disease is an indication either of patent ductus arteriosus or of the presence of collateral circulation to the lung through bronchial arteries. Some of these patients will be only slightly cyanosed if the collateral flow is large, but, with the exception of tricuspid atresia, they show evidence of right ventricular hypertrophy in the electrocardiogram. This important hint toward the true role of a ductus arteriosus in cases of complicated pulmonary stenosis or atresia should make it possible to avoid errors of interpretation. Rarely, tetralogy of Fallot

may be associated with such a large flow through the ductus that not only is the arterial oxygen saturation normal on exercise but the heart is enlarged, pulmonary vascularity is increased, and combined ventricular hypertrophy is present in the electrocardiogram (Figure 24–12).

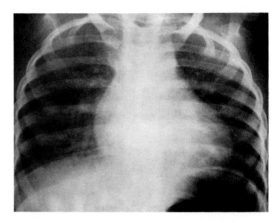

Figure 24-12. Tetralogy of Fallot with patent ductus arteriosus. The x-ray of a two-year-old noncyanotic child with normal arterial oxygen saturation on effort. A loud, continuous murmur with thrill was present. The electrocardiogram showed combined ventricular hypertrophy; the x-ray, moderate cardiac enlargement (cardiothoracic ratio, 0.57) with increased lung vascularity. Cardiac catheterization revealed tetralogy of Fallot with valvular stenosis to be the important malformation.

Noncyanotic Cases. Mention has already been made of cases of patent ductus arteriosus in association with aortic stenosis, coarctation of the aorta, and ventricular or atrial septal defects. In previous years clarification by recognition of each malformation and its individual contribution to the total picture was difficult, but with present investigative techniques there should be no difficulty about this task once the decision for further study has been made. *Ventricular septal defect with aortic insufficiency* occasionally causes confusion (Laubry and Pezzi, 1921; Soulie et al., 1949; Wood, 1950; Wood et al., 1954), but the to-and-fro murmur accompanying this anomaly in the presence of left ventricular hypertrophy in the electrocardiogram and the angiographic findings should allow its separation from ductus arteriosus. Roughly one-third of symptomatic infants with patent ductus arteriosus and considerable cardiac enlargement will have atypical murmurs. In these, clinical examination may be only suggestive of patent ductus arteriosus. Cardiac catheterization and angiography are then of value. The great problem in these patients is to separate the isolated malformation from *combined defects. Truncus arteriosus* with pulmonary arteries arising from the common trunk may prove a difficult problem in differential diagnosis in infants. Usually the patients are clinically noncyanotic, there is a harsh, systolic murmur over the precordium, and heart failure unresponsive to digitalis develops early in infancy. The second sound is usually loud and single but not always so, and an early diastolic murmur of incompetence of the truncus valve is common (Deely et al., 1962). The pulse is often bounding. The electrocardiogram not uncommonly shows left ventricular hypertrophy or biventricular hypertrophy. An aortogram will demonstrate filling of the pulmonary arteries with contrast material. At one time or another practically all types of malformation producing large hearts in noncyanotic infants have been labeled possible ductus arteriosus. Certainly, because of the high mortality in untreated cases, no infant in this group should be denied the investigation when there is any doubt at all about the diagnosis.

A firm clinical diagnosis of patent ductus arteriosus is impossible without accessory investigation in cases of patent ductus arteriosus with severe pulmonary hypertension associated with high pulmonary vascular resistance. Very occasionally a history of intermittent cyanosis of left arm and both legs is obtained or differential clubbing of these areas is seen. Cyanosis may be entirely absent clinically and the murmur, even if present, unhelpful. The only unequivocal feature on auscultation usually is the loudness of the pulmonic second sound indicative of marked pulmonary hypertension. Yet even in this regard, two of the eight cases reported by Bouchard and associates (1950) had normal second basal sounds. The electrocardiogram varies considerably, but where *predominant* reversal of ductal flow is present, right ventricular hypertrophy is the rule. Such cases are clinically considered as ventricular septal defect, aorticopulmonary window, patent ductus arteriosus with reversal of flow, primary pulmonary hypertension, and transposition of the great vessels "complexes." Calcification of the pulmonary artery in the roentgenogram, so characteristic of this situation in adults (Timpanelli and Steinberg, 1961), has not been a feature of the young patient.

Spontaneous Closure of the Ductus Arteriosus

In a channel that normally is patent both functionally and anatomically for a period after birth it becomes a matter of semantics as to what really represents spontaneous closure. For practical purposes it is here assumed that the great majority of healthy babies will have no shunt through the ductus after 24 hours. It has long been clear, however, that delay in accomplishing the relatively mature pulmonary circulation in the first month is associated with a delay in the normal closure of the ductus arteriosus. What is probably most important is to take for analysis those patients who have clinical features compatible with the picture of an abnormally

patent ductus arteriosus and so include in the question of spontaneous closure only those ducts where there is important hemodynamic upset. In examining this type of population it has been found that spontaneous closure is particularly likely to occur in premature infants with clinical evidence of patent ductus arteriosus after the first few days of life. More than 75 percent of ducts in premature infants in this category will undergo spontaneous closure within four months of birth. The possibility for spontaneous closure in term infants is less striking but is again maximal in the first two to three months. In them earlier hypoxic episodes can often be held responsible for the delay. A certain number, however, close later as instanced by some infants with a rubella background and others even with genetic history of ductus arteriosus. The possibility of spontaneous closure for term infants after the third month has been calculated as less than 10 percent.

More debate, of course, surrounds the possibility of spontaneous closure of the ductus arteriosus after infancy. This matter has been discussed rather fully by Campbell (1968), who has used a rather small number of series for his extrapolations. He concludes that the ductus closes spontaneously in 0.6 percent per annum, at least for the first four decades, which would suggest that about 20 percent will have closed by the age of 60. This finding was not offered as a reason for deferring the curative operation except in a few subjects where the flow was extremely small, and even that recommendation could be debated.

Prognosis

There has been considerable argument in the literature relating to prognosis in the untreated case of patent ductus arteriosus. Pathologic evidence has been criticized as weighting the picture toward too short a life expectancy. Abbott (1936) recorded 20 of 92 such autopsies as occurring before five years, the mean age of her group being 24 years. Keys and Shapiro (1943) in 60 autopsies found that after 17 years the life expectancy of patients was only half that of the general population. Certainly the very small number of cases reported as surviving 65 years is evidence of reduction in life-span produced by the malformation. Campbell (1955) concluded that serious symptoms result in later life in practically all nontreated cases. He calculated that by the age of 30, about one-fifth of the patients with persistent ductus would have died; by age 60, over 60 percent will have succumbed (Campbell, 1968). An assessment of unselected material over a very long period of time would be necessary before accurate figures for prognosis could be obtained. Unfortunately that possibility can no longer be realized. Nonetheless, the present evidence is strongly suggestive that patent ductus arteriosus leads to premature death. The prognosis for the premature infant with patent ductus arteriosus is a more complex matter and is currently under study.

Treatment

Medical Management. PROPHYLAXIS. The suggestion of routine therapeutic abortion for mothers affected by rubella during the first trimester of pregnancy remains controversial, although the 1964 epidemic in the United States with its tragic consequences has again brought the whole question under critical review. Much more intensive examination of affected offspring produced a considerable body of evidence for widespread damage to fetal tissues from the infection and changed the views of many physicians who formerly opposed termination of pregnancy after maternal rubella in the first trimester. Obviously the important prophylactic step had to be the administration of a vaccine to female children. Since isolation of the rubella virus (Parkman et al., 1962; Weller and Neva, 1962) and confirmation that the cultured virus causes clinical disease (Sever et al., 1962), strenuous efforts by several teams of investigators to develop such a vaccine were finally successful. The first five years' experience with a preventive program of immunization gives good reason to believe that the disease could now be eliminated (Krugman and Katz, 1974).

THERAPY. The treatment, both prophylactic and therapeutic, of bacterial endocarditis presents little problem beyond insistent propaganda in relation to the measures advised for prevention. Likewise, heart failure requires the usual measures with the proviso that patients with large left-to-right shunts should be operated upon after control if they fail to progress favorably. The intriguing method of closing the ductus with a Teflon plug at the time of cardiac catheterization has not yet received wide support (Porstmann et al., 1967, 1971).

Medical closure by noninvasive methods has included physical and pharmacologic methods.

(a) *Increased Ambient Oxygen Concentration.* The experimental reaction of the duct of newborn animals to alterations in arterial oxygen saturation led the authors to consider the use of high environmental oxygen in mature infants (but not in prematures) with frank patent ductus arteriosus at this age, but the variable response characterized by the following examples has dampened an initial enthusiasm.

One infant had gross congestive heart failure at nine days with a loud continuous murmur, single second heart sound, mild cyanosis at rest (marked on crying), liver 3 cm below right costal margin, and a blood pressure of 120/45 in the arm and 135/60 in the leg. The electrocardiogram revealed AQRS +150, right atrial hypertrophy, and combined ventricular hypertrophy (right greater than left), while the x-ray showed a huge heart. When the infant was placed in oxygen for one and a half hours before catheterization, the second heart sound became split. At catheterization aortic/pulmonary systolic pressure ratios were 82:50, a moderate left-to-right shunt was present, and the heart appeared smaller. In view of this response the infant was kept in 40 percent oxygen. The continuous murmur gradually decreased and disappeared six days later. At the age of five and a half months the infant weighed $18\frac{1}{2}$ lb, was clinically normal and had a normal chest film and electrocardiogram. Trial of such therapy in another infant with identical birth history and physical findings failed and eventually successful surgical obliteration of the duct was forced at the age of three weeks. In this patient, biopsy revealed that muscle was sparse in the duct wall and the pulmonary vascular bed was unusually mature. The explanation of these different responses may lie in the different action of duct muscle either because of predetermined anatomic alterations or because of the effects of metabolic disturbance on the normal action toward closure.

(b) *Prostaglandin Synthetase Inhibitors.* The use of prostaglandin synthetase inhibitors, especially indomethacin, to close the ductus arteriosus in premature infants is under trial. In ventilator-dependent infants with severe congestive heart failure secondary to a large ductus, indomethacin offers an often dramatically successful alternative to surgical ligation. When used, a transient but significant depression of urinary output occurs. It is not yet clear whether this results from decreased renal blood flow or from increased antidiuretic hormone production. Although permanent renal damage is unlikely, it remains to be proven that this never occurs. The use of indomethacin in the less sick infant in whom the ductus is not causing problems is much more controversial, and a few well-conducted clinical trials in selected centers are required before indomethacin can be accepted as an alternative to a policy of nonintervention in infants in whom eventual spontaneous closure can be anticipated.

Surgical Treatment. INDICATIONS. There are now few who doubt the importance of and necessity for surgery in the patent ductus arteriosus. Initially the criteria for closure of the patent ductus arteriosus were narrow, but in recent years they have broadened considerably. In uncomplicated cases operation may be advised after six months of age, certainly before the child starts school, although it may be performed safely throughout childhood. Ash and Fischer (1955) prefer to operate either before 24 months of age or after four years because of psychologic implications from hospitalization between two and four years. Krovetz and Warden (1962) found no difference between the surgical mortality in infants and older patients, but other experience has been different (Hara et al., 1962), and most surgeons would agree that overall mortality is slightly higher in infants than in older patients. Our experience at The Hospital for Sick Children (Trusler et al., 1968) clearly tells the story: 5 out of 60 babies operated on under the age of six months died though none of the 148 babies operated between 6 and 24 months died. Gross (1952) has discussed the problem relative to surgery in patients beyond this age range. The symptomatic infant group with large hearts requires operation as soon as the diagnosis is confirmed. The good results from such surgery (Gross, 1943; Wangensteen, 1947; Scott, 1950; Mustard, 1951) are now very clear. It is our belief that there should be no delay in returning these infants to a normal existence by means of surgery.

The difference of opinion about the necessity to intervene in the prematurely born infant, especially the baby with severe respiratory distress and deteriorating pulmonary function (Kitterman et al., 1972; Krovetz and Rowe, 1972), is becoming resolved. There is now better appreciation of early clinical evidence of the complication, and better techniques are available to assess shunt size. Fewer neonatologists are inclined today to persist with conservative and lengthy medical treatment in the face of a large left-to-right shunt not responding reasonably promptly to anticongestive therapy or minimal ventilatory support. Although very early closure has been favored by a few (Thibeault et al., 1975), most groups move to more direct attack on the ductus at a rather arbitrary stage following the development of congestive heart failure at or after trial of CPAP. The first step is usually to give prostaglandin synthetase inhibitors and, only if that regime fails, is it necessary to proceed to direct ligation. In either event, considerable care in pretreatment evaluation and excellent teamwork are essential to ensure a successful and incident-free pre- and posttreatment course.

There are no special problems associated with the decision to operate in individuals with isolated patent ductus arteriosus and hyperkinetic pulmonary hypertension apart from age, young infants under six months of age carrying a surgical risk higher than older babies or children. Normal hemodynamics are uniformly established as a result of surgery in this group.

By contrast, for patients with pulmonary hypertension and high pulmonary vascular resistance there are good reasons to pause and consider before a decision to operate is made. The basis for this view is that the long-term prognosis in Eisenmenger's syndrome, while hardly good, is at least superior to the prospect of perioperative death or to early demise from unrelieved congestive failure after removal of the escape mechanism provided by the septal defect (Clarkson et al., 1967) or presumably the ductus arteriosus. Such a course is inevitable at surgery for patients with pure right-to-left ductal shunt due to extremely high pulmonary vascular resistance. It is a distinct risk for patients with trivial shunts in either direction and may even occur when the shunt is only left-to-right.

More difficult is the situation where an individual has a left-to-right shunt that contributes 30 to 50 percent of his total pulmonary blood flow, where pressures in the two circuits are equalized, and where there is no arterial oxygen desaturation. The problem here is not the immediate survival but the late result. In these circumstances, Neutze (1965) found that he

was unable to predict the ultimate course. In five children operated at $2\frac{1}{2}$ to 7 years of age with ductus arteriosus the result was unsatisfactory in three patients: a relatively minor change in pulmonary vascular resistance occurring in one instance, and a progressive rise in pulmonary vascular resistance developing in the other two over periods of three to six years. In the remaining two patients, the pulmonary vascular resistance seven to ten years after operation had fallen from preoperative values of 15 units to between 3 and 5 units. Although there have been reported exceptions, it is usually true that a substantial fall in the pulmonary artery pressure measured at operation immediately after duct occlusion is a good prognostic sign and that an increase or unchanged pulmonary artery pressure or a trivial fall in the value are indicators of an eventually poor result. This generalization suggests there might be merit in attempting a temporary duct occlusion preoperatively. Thus in a hemodynamic situation of the type under discussion, Wisoff and associates (1966) utilized a balloon catheter occlusion technique and were able to accurately predict from pulmonary artery pressure reduction a good response to surgical division of a large ductus. Eighteen months later, catheterization of the heart in this patient showed a pulmonary artery pressure of 33/17 with a brachial artery pressure of 106/77.

It is the opinion of Kimball and McIlroy (1966), from careful examination of high vascular resistance cases, that patients with patent ductus arteriosus tolerated closure better than those with ventricular septal defect and similar degrees of pulmonary artery hypertension and increased pulmonary vascular resistance. They found that all cases that they had selected decreased pulmonary artery pressure and eventually their pulmonary vascular resistance after operation. The symptomatic improvement provided by the surgical treatment coupled with an avoidance postoperatively of pulmonary infection, exercise, and high altitude were regarded as important enough contributions to the disease that operation is recommended by them for all patients so long as there is net left-to-right shunt preoperatively. Such results of improvement, if not cure, are supported by data from other experience (Burchell, 1959).

It nevertheless should be apparent from these extremely limited data that there are serious difficulties in reaching consistently correct clinical decisions for the management of patients with patent ductus arteriosus and high pulmonary vascular resistance. The uncertainties of 1977 are not appreciably different from those that we faced in 1958 when the subject was first considered in this book. Our conclusions are that because of the grave doubts about long-term benefit it is still unwise to close the ductus of patients with high calculated pulmonary vascular resistance and pulmonary-to-systemic flow ratios of less than 2:1, except perhaps in infancy. The important provision is that there be a clinical picture concordant with these data. Such an approach covers the situation where cardiac catheterization data, because of undue sedation or other factors, reveals a picture of higher pulmonary vascular resistance than would be suspected on clinical grounds.

TYPE OF OPERATION. Gross and Hubbard (1939) reported the first ligation of a ductus arteriosus in August, 1938. Gross later changed his technique to one of division of the ductus (Gross, 1943) because of the recanalization of some early cases treated by ligation in continuity. A great number of operative reports supporting this technique have appeared in recent years.

Blalock (1946) suggested a modification of the ligation method known as suture ligation, which has been attended by good results (Scott, 1952; Mustard, 1955; Ash and Fischer, 1955). There are certain circumstances, e.g., a short, wide ductus, where division is preferable to suture ligation, according to Mustard (1955) and Sandblom and Ekström (1951). Bickford (1960) found that in 122 patients where the duct diameter at operation was not greater than 7 mm, recanalization occurred in less than 1 percent. On the other hand, in 106 patients where the diameter exceeded 7 mm, simple ligation resulted in incomplete closure in 16 percent. Groves and associates (1954) have found controlled hypotension in subjects with pulmonary hypertension or friable ductus to be a valuable adjunct to the operative technique.

IMMEDIATE RESULTS. Taylor and coworkers (1950), in studying 15 cases, showed that, upon closure of the ductus arteriosus, there were immediate increases in systemic systolic and diastolic pressure in every case. In our experience this increase may be sustained for several days and even reach alarming heights before returning to normal levels. In six of Taylor's cases, the pulmonary arterial pressures decreased immediately with closure of the ductus. Similar experiences have been reported by Grover and associates (1949) and Ekström (1952) even where the pulmonary pressure was as high as 90/40 mm, e.g., KLB 48, aged seven years (Ekström, 1952). Other investigators have shown the opposite result. Shephard (1954) reported two cases: one where the pulmonary pressure rose from 47/35 to 74/52 and another from 86/76 to 93/79. A more uniform rise seems to occur in severe pulmonary vascular disease (Bouchard et al., 1950). Even if an immediate fall in pulmonary pressure occurs in this type, it is not necessarily a good prognostic sign (Smith, 1954; Burchell, 1959). Patients with severe pulmonary vascular disease deteriorate immediately when the ductus is clamped.

In the uncomplicated case, closure of the ductus results in immediate disappearance of the continuous murmur. Gross (1952) and Ekström (1952) have

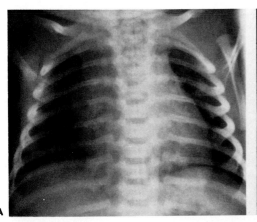
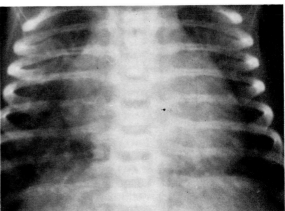
A   B

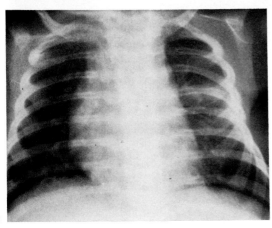
C

Figure 24-13. The chest films of R. H., a female neonate with patent ductus arteriosus.

   A. Aged one day: taken because of initial birth asphyxia. There was no respiratory distress apparent at this time.

   B. Aged two weeks: a portable film demonstrating considerable cardiomegaly.

   C. Aged three and a half weeks: three days after surgical division of the duct showing marked reduction in heart size.

commented on the striking diminution of activity and volume of the heart immediately after surgical closure of the ductus. The mortality at operation is low even when cases with associated defects, cases in failure, and cases with bacterial endocarditis are included. With division of the ductus, Gross (1952) reported an overall mortality rate of 2 percent in 482 cases. Using the suture ligation technique, Scott (1950) reports 2.5 percent mortality in 273 operations, Mustard (1955) 1.1 percent in 188 cases, and Ash and Fischer (1955) no mortality in 126 cases. Ekström reported from Sweden (1952), for both division and ligation, 3.5 percent mortality in 254 cases. Krovetz and Warden (1962) reported a mortality of 2 to 3 percent in 435 patients with isolated ductus. The mortality in 2929 operations in children under 14 years collected in a world survey by Waterman and associates (1956) was 2.3 percent. More recent reports from large children's hospitals confirm the low risk (Coggin et al., 1970; Panagopoulos et al., 1971).

Operative mortality (margin note)

LATE RESULTS In many patients with substandard physical development and a large shunt, considerable improvement may be expected in the year following surgery, but since other than cardiac factors frequently appear to influence the growth of these individuals, such satisfactory results cannot be predicted with great confidence. In those with retarded growth and small shunt, no hope can be held for any substantial gains from the preoperative percentile.

Those with large hearts may have an immediate decrease in size, or the heart size may merely remain stationary in relation to growth of the chest (Figure 24–13). Ekström (1952) showed a distinct reduction in heart volume in all cases, the most marked reduction occurring in those with the grossly abnormal preoperative values.

Electrocardiographic changes eventually revert to normal, provided there is no complicating defect or severe pulmonary hypertension. The speed with which this is accomplished varies inversely with the degree of abnormality established prior to operation.

EKG → normal p̄ op. (margin note)

The successful case has no continuous murmur in follow-up examination. About a fifth of the cases operated on at The Hospital for Sick Children had functional systolic murmurs noted during the follow-up. Two of the uncomplicated cases had a borderline organic systolic murmur without a thrill in the pulmonary area for which there was no obvious cause beyond a persistent dilatation of the pulmonary artery. In those patients in whom there is wide transmission of a residual systolic murmur to the lateral thorax and back, the possibility of pulmonary artery stenosis should be entertained, especially where a rubella history is known (Rowe, 1963). Mention has been made earlier of associated mitral regurgitation in some patients. Recurrence of the shunt develops occasionally when the surgical technique is other than duct division. Recurrence rates are very low (Scott, 1952), but the proponents of division feel even a low figure is too high a risk because of the inconvenience and danger attending a second operation. The list of people who regard ligation as obsolete seems to be getting larger (Jones, 1965; Marquis, 1968) but Dr. Porstmann may yet have the last word. Among 62 patients treated at catheterization with his plugging technique were several with recurrence after surgical ligation!

REFERENCES

Abbott, M. E.: *Atlas of Congenital Cardiac Disease.* American Heart Association, New York, 1936.

Adams, F. H.; Diehl, A.; Jorgens, J.; and Veasy, L. G.: Right heart catheterization in patent ductus arteriosus and aortic-pulmonary septal defect. *J. Pediatr.,* **40**:49, 1952.

Adams, F. H., and Forsyth, W. B.: The effect of surgery on the growth of patients with patent ductus arteriosus. *J. Pediatr.,* **39**:330, 1951.

Adams, F. H., and Linde, J.: Physiologic studies on the cardiovascular status of the normal newborn infant (with special reference to the ductus arteriosus). *J. Pediatr.,* **19**:431, 1957.

Allan, F. D.: An histological study of the nerves associated with the ductus arteriosus. *Anat. Rec.,* **139**:531, 1961.

Alzamora, V.; Rotta, A.; Gattilana, G.; Abugattas, R.; Rubio, C.; Bournonde, J.; Zapata, C.; Santa-Maria, E.; Binder, T.; Subiria, R.; Paredes, D.; Pando, B.; and Graham, G.: On the possible influence of great altitudes on the determination of certain cardiovascular anomalies. *Pediatrics,* **12**:259, 1953.

Amoroso, E. C.; Dawes, G. S.; and Mott, J. C.: Patency of the ductus arteriosus in the newborn calf and foal. *Br. Heart J.,* **20**:92, 1958.

Anderson, I. M., and Coles, H. M. T.: Patent ductus arteriosus with pulmonary hypertension. A review of nine cases including one with reversal of blood flow through the ductus. *Thorax,* **10**:338, 1955.

Anderson, R. C.: Causative factors underlying congenital heart malformations. I. Patent ductus arteriosus. *Pediatrics,* **14**:143, 1954.

Ash, R., and Fischer, D.: Manifestations and results of treatment of patent ductus arteriosus in infancy and childhood. An analysis of 138 cases. *Pediatrics,* **16**:695, 1955.

Auld, P. A.: Delayed closure of the ductus arteriosus. *J. Pediatr.,* **69**:61, 1966.

Bakker, P. M.: Morfogenese En Involutie Van De Ductus Arteriosus Bij Mens. (Thesis) *Den Haag,* Mouton and Co., 1962.

Barclay, A. E.; Barcroft, J.; Barron, D. H.; and Franklin, K. J.: Radiographic demonstration of circulation through the heart in adult and in fetus and identification of ductus arteriosus. *Am. J. Roentgenol.,* **47**:678, 1942.

Barclay, A. E.; Franklin, K. J.; and Prichard, M. M. L.: *The Foetal Circulation and Cardiovascular System, and Changes That They Undergo at Birth.* Blackwell Scientific Publications, Oxford, 1944.

Barnard, W. G.: Pathological changes in the wall of the ductus arteriosus. *St. Thomas's Hosp. Rep.* (2nd Series), **4**:72, 1939.

Bass, D. A. and Rowe, R. D.: Patent ductus arteriosus as a complicating factor in infants with other cardiac malformation. *Circulation,* **37–38 Suppl VI**:38, 1968.

Bauersfeld, S. R.; Adkins, P. C.; and Kent, E. M.: Patent ductus arteriosus in infancy. *J. Thorac. Surg.,* **33**:123, 1957.

Bayley, B. G.; Meyer, R. A.; Kaplan, S.; Ringenburg, W. E.; and Korfhagen, J.: The critically ill premature infant with patent ductus arteriosus and pulmonary disease—an echocardiographic assessment. *J. Pediatr.,* **86**:423, 1975.

Beck, W., Schrire, V.; Vogelpoel, L.; Nellen, M.; and Swanpoel, A.: Hemodynamic effects of amyl nitrite and phenylephrine on the normal human circulation and their relation to changes in cardiac murmurs. *Am. J. Cardiol.,* **8**:341, 1961.

Benn, J.: The prognosis of patent ductus arteriosus. *Br. Heart J.,* **9**:283, 1947.

Berdon, W. E.; Baker, D. H.; and James, L. S.: The ductus bump. *Am. J. Roentgenol.,* **95**:91, 1965.

Bickford, B. J.: Surgical aspects of patent ductus arteriosus. A review of 228 cases. *Arch. Dis. Child.,* **35**:92, 1960.

Bishop, R. C.: Delayed closure of the ductus arteriosus. *Am. Heart J.,* **44**:639, 1952.

Blalock, A.: Operative closure of the patent ductus arteriosus. *Surg. Gynecol. Obstet.,* **82**:113, 1946.

Bloom, K. R.; Rodriguez, L.; and Swan, E. M.: Echocardiographic evaluation of left to right shunt in ventricular septal defect and persistent ductus arteriosus. *Br. Heart J.*, **39**:260, 1977.

Bohn, H.: Ein wichtiges diagnostisches Phänomen sur Erkennung des offenen Ductus arteriosus Botalli. *Klin. Wschr.*, **17**:907, 1938.

Born, G. V. R.; Dawes, G. S.; Mott, J. C.; and Rennick, B. R.: The constriction of the ductus arteriosus caused by oxygen and by asphyxia in newborn lambs. *J. Physiol.*, **132**:304, 1956.

Bothwell, T. H.; Van Lingen, B.; Whidborne, J.; Kaye, J.; McGregor, M.; and Elliott, G. A.: Patent ductus arteriosus with partial reversal of the shunt. *Am. Heart J.*, **44**:360, 1952.

Bouchard, F.; Lason, R. L.; and Alvarez, V. R.: Huit cas de persistance du canal arteriel avec grande hypertension pulmonaire—dont quatre avec cyanose. 1st Congrès Mondial de Cardiologie, Paris, 1950.

Bouchard, F.; Lafont, H.; Gontard, F.; and Cornu, J. C.: Persistance du canal arterial et communication interventriculaire associe e: problemes de diagnostic. *Arch. Mal. Coeur*, **60**:1509, 1967.

Bromberger-Barnea, B.; Rowe, R. D.; and Bor, I.: Vascular tone in ductus arteriosus. *Circulation*, **32-II**:59, 1965.

Burchell, H. B.: Regression of pulmonary vascular hypertension after cure of intracardiac defects in pulmonary circulation. In Adams, W., and Veith, I. (eds.): *Pulmonary Circulation*. Grune & Stratton, Inc., New York, 1959.

Burchell, H. B.; Swan, H. J. C.; and Wood, E. H.: Demonstration of different effects on pulmonary and systemic arterial pressure by variation in oxygen content of inspired air in patients with patent ductus arteriosus and pulmonary hypertension. *Circulation*, **8**:681, 1953.

Burman, D.: Case report: familial patent ductus arteriosus. *Br. Heart J.*, **23**:603, 1961.

Burnard, E. D.: The cardiac murmur in relation to symptoms in the newborn. *Br. Med. J.*, **1**:134, 1959.

Burnell, R. H.; Joseph, M. C.; and Lees, M. H.: Progressive pulmonary hypertension in newborn infants. A report of two cases with no identifiable respiratory or cardiac disease. *Am. J. Dis. Child.*, **123**:167, 1972.

Campbell, M.: Patent ductus arteriosus and pulmonary hypertension. Some notes on prognosis. *Br. Heart J.*, **17**:511, 1955.

Campbell, M., and Hudson, R.: Patent ductus arteriosus with reversed shunt due to pulmonary hypertension. *Guy Hosp. Rep.*, **101**:26, 1951.

———: The disappearance of the continuous murmur of patent ductus arteriosus. *Guy Hosp. Rep.*, **101**:32, 1952.

———: Place of maternal rubella in the aetiology of congenital heart disease. *Br. Med. J.*, **1**:691, 1961.

Campbell, M.: Natural history of persistent ductus arteriosus. *Br. Heart J.*, **30**:4, 1968.

Cassels, D. E.: *The Ductus Arteriosus*. Charles C Thomas, Publisher, Springfield, Ill., 1973.

Chapman, C. B., and Robbins, S. L.: Patent ductus arteriosus with pulmonary vascular sclerosis and cyanosis. *Ann. Intern. Med.*, **21**:312, 1944.

Christie, A.: Normal closing time of the foramen ovale and the ductus arteriosus. *Am. J. Dis. Child.*, **40**:323, 1930.

Clarke, J. A.: An x-ray microscopic study of the vasa vasorum of the human ductus arteriosus. *J. Anat.*, **99**:527, 1965.

Clarkson, P. M.; Frye, R. L.; DuShane, J. W.; Wood, E. H.; and Weidman, W. H.: Prognosis in patients with ventricular septal defect and severe pulmonary vascular disease. (Abstr.) The Society for Pediatric Research, 37th annual meeting, Atlantic City, N.J., 1967, p. 9.

Clatworthy, H. W., and McDonald, V. G.: Optimum age for surgical closure of patent ductus arteriosus. *JAMA*, **167**:444, 1958.

Coceani, F., and Olley, P. M.: The response of the ductus arteriosus to prostaglandins. *Can. J. Physiol. Pharmacol.*, **51**:220, 1973.

Coceani, F., and Olley, P. M.: *Advances in Prostaglandin and Thromboxane Research*, Vol. 3. Raven Press, New York, 1977.

Coggin, C. J.; Parker, K. R.; and Keith, J. D.: Natural history of isolated patent ductus arteriosus and the effect of surgical correction: twenty years' experience at The Hospital for Sick Children, Toronto. *Canad. Med. Assoc. J.*, **102**:1, 1970.

Collela, C., Marino, B., and Reale, A.: Correlazioni tra le varizioni strutturali del dotto arterioso, polmonare durante la vita fetale e nel neonato: considerazioni sul meccanismo di chiusura del dotto arterioso. *Chir. Torac.*, **16**:477, 1963.

Cosh, J.: Patent ductus arteriosus with pulmonary hypertension. *Br. Heart J.*, **15**:423, 1953.

Cournand, A.: Recent observations on the dynamics of the pulmonary circulation. *Bull. N.Y. Acad. Med.*, **23**:27, 1947.

Crevasse, L. E., and Logue, R. B.: Atypical patent ductus arteriosus. The use of a vasopressor agent as a diagnostic aid. *Circulation*, **19**:332, 1959.

Cruickshank, B., and Marquis, R. M.: Spontaneous aneurysm of the ductus arteriosus. *Am. J. Med.*, **25**:140, 1958.

Cruze, K.; Elliott, L. P.; Schiebler, G. L.; and Wheat, M. W., Jr.: Unusual manifestations of patent ductus arteriosus in infancy. *Dis. Chest*, **43**:563, 1963.

Currarino, G., and Jackson, J. H., Jr.: Calcification of the ductus arteriosus and ligamentum Botalli. *Radiology*, **94**:139, 1970.

Dammann, J. F., Jr.; Berthrong, M.; and Bing, R. J.: Reverse ductus. A presentation of the syndrome of patent ductus arteriosus with pulmonary hypertension and a shunting of blood flow from pulmonary artery to aorta. *Bull. Hopkins Hosp.*, **92**:128, 1953.

Dammann, J. F., Jr., and Sell, C. G. R.: Patent ductus arteriosus in the absence of a continuous murmur. *Circulation*, **6**:110, 1952.

Danesino, V. L.; Reynolds, S. R. N.; and Rehman, I. H.: Comparative histological structure of the human ductus arteriosus according to topography, age and degree of constriction. *Anat. Rec.*, **121**:801, 1955.

Danilowicz, D.; Rudolph, A. M.; and Hoffman, J. I. E.: Delayed closure of the ductus arteriosus in premature infants. *Pediatrics*, **37**:74, 1966.

Dawes, G. S.; Mott, J. C.; and Widdicombe, J. C.: The patency of the ductus arteriosus in newborn lambs and its physiological consequences. *J. Physiol.*, **128**:361, 1955.

Dawes, G. S.; Mott, J. C.; Widdicombe, J. G.; and Wyatt, D. G.: Changes in the lungs of the newborn lamb. *J. Physiol.*, **121**:141, 1953.

Dawes, G. S.: Changes in the circulation at birth. In *The Heart and Circulation in the Newborn Infant*. Cassels, D. E. (Ed.). Grune and Stratton, New York, 1966, p. 77.

Deely, W. J.; Hagstrom, J. W. C.; and Engle, M. A.: Truncus insufficiency: common truncus arteriosus with regurgitant truncus valve. Report of four cases. *Am. Heart J.*, **65**:542, 1962.

Desligneres, S., and Larroche, J. Cl.: Ductus arteriosus. I. Anatomical development during the second half of gestation and its closure after birth. II. Histological study of a few cases of patent ductus arteriosus in infancy. *Biol. Neonate*, **16**:278, 1970.

Deverall, P. B., Lincoln, J. C. R., Aberdeen, E., Bonham-Carter, R. E. and Waterston, D. J.: Aorto-pulmonary window. *J. Thorac. Cardiovasc. Dis.*, **57**:479, 1969.

Dexter, L.: Right heart catheterization in congenital heart disease. *Mod. Med.*, **17**:92, 1949.

Dexter, L.; Dow, J. W.; Haynes, F. W.; Whittenberger, J. L.; Ferris, B. G.; Goodale, W. F.; and Hellems, H. K.: Studies of the pulmonary circulation in man at rest. Normal variations and the interrelations between increased pulmonary blood flow, elevated pulmonary arterial pressure and high pulmonary "capillary" pressures. *J. Clin. Invest.*, **29**:602, 1950.

Dexter, L.; Haynes, F. W.; Burwell, C. S.; Eppinger, E. C.; Sosman, M. C.; and Evans, J. M.: Studies of congenital heart disease. III. Venous catheterization as a diagnostic aid in patent ductus arteriosus, tetralogy of Fallot, ventricular septal defect and auricular septal defect. *J. Clin. Invest.*, **26**:561, 1947.

D'heer, H. A. H., and van Nieuwenhuizen, C. L. C.: Diagnosis of aortic septal defects. *Circulation*, **13**:58, 1956.

Donzelot, E., and D'Allaines, F.: *Traité des Cardiopathies Congénitales*. Masson & Cie, Paris, 1954.

Donzelot, E., and Heim de Balsac, R.: Essai de determination radiologique de la longeur du ligament et du canal arteriel. *Acta Cardiol.*, **3**:212, 1948.

DuShane, J. W., and Montgomery, C. E.: Patent ductus arteriosus with pulmonary hypertension and atypical clinical findings. *Proc. Mayo Clin.*, **23**:505, 1948.

Edwards, J. E., and Burchell, H. B.: Effects of pulmonary hypertension of the tracheobronchial tree. *Dis. Chest*, **38**:272, 1960.

Edwards, J. E.; Douglas, J. M.; Burchell, H. B.; and Christensen, N. A.: Pathology of the intrapulmonary arteries and arterioles in coarctation of the aorta associated with patent ductus arteriosus. *Am. Heart J.*, **38**:205, 1949.

Edmunds, L. H. Jr.; Gregory, G. A.; Heymann, M. A.; Kitterman, J. A.; Rudolph, A. M.; and Tooley, W. H.: Surgical closure of the ductus arteriosus in premature infants. *Circulation*, 48:856, 1973.

Ekström, G.: The surgical treatment of patent ductus arteriosus. A clinical study of 290 cases. *Acta Chir. Scand.*, Supp. 169, 1952.

Ekström, G.; Ekman, C. A.; and Möller, T.: Artificial ductus arteriosus in dog with secondary hypertension in the pulmonary artery. *Acta Chir. Scand.*, 102:296, 1951.

Elliott, L. P.; Ernst, R. W.; Anderson, R. C.; Lillehei, C. W.; and Adams, P., Jr.: Silent patent ductus arteriosus in association with ventricular septal defect. Clinical, hemodynamic, pathological and surgical observations in forty patients. *Am. J. Cardiol.*, 10:475, 1962.

Elliott, R. B., and Starling, M. B.: The effect of prostaglandin F_2, in the closure of the ductus arteriosus. *Prostaglandins*, 2:399, 1972.

Ellis, F. H., Jr; Kirklin, J. W.; Callaghan, J. A.; and Wood, E. H.: Patent ductus arteriosus with pulmonary hypertension. *J. Thorac. Surg.*, 31:268, 1956.

Engle, M. A.; Holswade, G. R.; Goldberg, H. P.; and Glenn, F.: Present problems pertaining to patency of the ductus arteriosus. I. Persistence of growth retardation after successful surgery. *Pediatrics*, 21:70, 1958.

Eppinger, E. C.; Burwell, C. S.; and Gross, R. E.: The effects of the patent ductus arteriosus on the circulation. *J. Clin. Invest.*, 20:127, 1941.

Evans, D. W., and Heath, D.: Disappearance of the continuous murmur in a case of patent ductus arteriosus. *Br. Heart J.*, 23:469, 1961.

Evans, J. R.; Rowe, R. D.; Downie, H. G.; and Rowsell, H. C.: Murmurs arising from ductus arteriosus in normal newborn swine. *Circ. Res.*, 12:85, 1963.

Everett, N. B., and Johnson, R. J.; A physiological and anatomical study of the closure of the ductus arteriosus in the dog. *Anat. Rec.*, 110:103, 1951.

Falcone, M. W.; Perloff, J. K.; and Roberts, W. C.: Aneurysm of the nonpatent ductus arteriosus. *Am. J. Cardiol.*, 29:422, 1972.

Fay, F. S.: Guinea pig ductus arteriosus I. Cellular and metabolic basis for oxygen sensitivity. *Am. J. Physiol.*, 221:470, 1971.

Fay, J. E., and Travill, A.: The "valve" of the ductus arteriosus—an enigma. *Can. Med. Assoc. J.*, 97:78, 1967.

Feldt, R. H.; Stickler, G. S.; and Weidman, W. H.: Growth of children with congenital heart disease. *Am. J. Dis. Child.*, 117:573, 1969.

Fleming, H. A., and Seal, R. M. E.: Staphylococcal infection following cardiac surgery. *Thorax*, 10:327, 1955.

Fowler, R. E. L., and Bevil, H. H.: Aneurysms of the sinuses of Valsalva. *Pediatrics*, 8:340, 1951.

Friedman, W. F.; Heymann, M. A.; and Rudolph, A. M.: Commentary: new thoughts on an old problem—patent ductus arteriosus in the premature. *J. Pediatr.* 90:338, 1977.

Friedman, W. F.; Hirschklau, M. J.; Printz, M. P.; Pitlick, P. T.; and Kirkpatrick, S. E.: Pharmacologic closure of patent ductus arteriosus in the premature infant. *N. Engl. J. Med.*, 295:526, 1976.

Gardiner, J. H., and Keith, J. D.: Prevalence of heart disease in Toronto children: 1948–1949. Cardiac registry. *Pediatrics*, 7:713, 1951.

Gennser, G., and Astedt, B.: Fibrinolytic activity in wall of human ductus arteriosus. *Experientia*, 27:679, 1971.

Gibson, G. A.: Persistence of the arterial duct and its diagnosis. *Edinburgh Med. J.*, 8:1, 1900.

Gilchrist, A. R.: Patent ductus arteriosus and its surgical treatment. *Br. Heart J.*, 7:1, 1945.

Gillman, R. G., and Burton, A. C.: Constriction of the neonatal aorta by raised oxygen tension. *Circ. Res.*, 19:755, 1966.

Girling, D. J., and Hallidie-Smith, K. A.: Persistent ductus arteriosus in ill and premature babies. *Arch. Dis. Child.*, 46:177, 1971.

Goldbloom, A.; Ferencz, C.; and Johnson, A. L.: The problem of differential diagnosis in infants with large hearts and increased blood flow to the lungs. *Am. J. Dis. Child.*, 86:4, 458, 1953.

Gray, I. R.: Paradoxical splitting of the second heart sound. *Br. Heart J.*, 18:21, 1956.

Gregg, N. M.: Congenital cataract following German measles in the mother. *Trans. Ophthal. Soc. Aust.*, 3:35, 1941.

Greig, H. W.; Anson, B. J.; McAfee, D. K.; and Kurth, L. E.: The ductus arteriosus and its ligamentous remnant in the adult. *Q. Bull. Northwest Univ. Med. Sch.*, 28:66, 1954.

Griswold, H. E.; Bing, R. J.; Handelsman, J. C.; Campbell, J. A.; and Le Brun, E.: Physiological studies in congenital heart disease. VII. Pulmonary arterial hypertension in congenital heart disease. *Bull. Hopkins Hosp.*, 84:76, 1949.

Gross, R. E.: Surgical therapy for the patent ductus arteriosus. *N. Y. J. Med.*, 43:1856, 1943.

—————: The patent ductus arteriosus. Observations on diagnosis and therapy in 525 surgically treated cases. *Am. J. Med.*, 12:472, 1952.

Gross, R. E., and Hubbard, J. P.; Surgical ligation of a patent ductus arteriosus. *JAMA*, 112:729, 1939.

Gross, R. E., and Longino, L. A.: The patent ductus arteriosus. Observations from 412 surgically treated cases. *Circulation*, 3:125, 1951.

Grover, R. F.; Swan, H., II; and Maaske, C. A.: Pressure changes in the pulmonary artery and aorta before and after ligation of the patent ductus arteriosus. *Fed. Proc.*, 8:63, 1949.

Groves, L. K.; Effler, D. B.; and Sones, F. M., Jr.: Controlled hypotension in the surgical treatment of certain cases of patent ductus arteriosus. Report of four cases. *Cleveland Clin. Quart.*, 21:169, 1954.

Gupta, J. M.; van Vliet, P. K. J.; Fisk, G. C.; and Wright, J. S.: Ductus ligation in respiratory distress syndrome. *J. Pediatr.*, 63:642, 1972.

Handler, J. J.: The foetal circulation and its changes at birth in some small laboratory animals. *J. Physiol.*, 133:202, 1956.

Hara, M.; Dungan, W. T.; Lincoln, B. M.; and McCutcheon, F. B.: Patent ductus arteriosus in early infancy. *Surgery*, 52:396, 1962.

Haring, O.; Luisada, A. O.; and Gasul, B. M.: Phonocardiography in patent ductus arteriosus. *Circulation*, 10:501, 1954.

Harris, P., and Heath, D.: *The Human Pulmonary Circulation*. E. & S. Livingstone Ltd., Edinburgh, 1962.

Hatcher, J. D.: Personal communication, 1960.

Heath, D.; Helmholz, H. F.; Burchell, H. B.; DuShane, J. W.; and Edwards, J. E.: Graded pulmonary vascular changes and hemodynamic findings in cases of atrial and ventricular septal defect and patent ductus arteriosus. *Circulation*, 18:1155, 1958a.

Heath, D.; Swan, H. J. C.; DuShane, J. W.; and Edwards, J. E.: The relation of medial thickness of small muscular pulmonary arteries to immediate postnatal survival in patients with ventricular septal defect or patent ductus arteriosus. *Thorax*, 13:267, 1958b.

Heiner, D. C., and Nadas, A. S.: Patent ductus arteriosus in association with pulmonic stenosis. A report of six cases. *Circulation*, 17:232, 1958.

Heymann, M. A.; Nies, A. S.; Rudolph, A. M.; and Melmon, K. I.: Role of bradykinin in neonatal circulatory changes. *Circulation*, 36:II:142, 1967.

Heymann, M. A., and Rudolph, A. M.: Control of the ductus arteriosus. *Physiol. Rev.*, 55:62, 1975.

Heymann, M. A.; Rudolph, A. M.; and Silverman, N. H.: Closure of the ductus arteriosus in premature infants by inhibition of prostaglandin synthesis. *N. Engl. J. Med.*, 295:530, 1976.

Hickam, J. B.: The pulmonary vascular resistance. *J. Clin. Invest.*, 28:788, 1949.

Hoffman, E.: Die Obliteration des Ductus arteriosus Botalli. *Langenbeck. Arch. Klin. Chir.*, 306:289, 1964.

Holman, E.: *Arteriovenous Aneurysm*. The Macmillan Co., New York, 1937.

Holman, E.; Gerbode, R.; and Purdy, A.: The patent ductus: a review of 75 cases with surgical treatment including an aneurysm of the ductus and one of the pulmonary artery. *J. Thorac. Surg.*, 25:111, 1953.

Holmes, R. L.: Some features of the ductus arteriosus. *J. Anat.*, 92:304, 1958.

Hornblad, P. Y.: Studies on closure of the ductus arteriosus III. Species differences in closure rate and morphology. *Cardiologia*, 51:262, 1967.

Hornblad, P. Y.: Embryological observations of the ductus arteriosus in the guinea pig, rabbit, rat and mouse. Studies on the closure of the ductus arteriosus. IV. *Acta Physiol. Scand.*, 76:49, 1969.

House, E. W., and Ederstrom, H. E.: Anatomical changes with age in the heart and ductus arteriosus in the dog after birth. *Anat. Rec.*, 160:289, 1968.

Hubbard, T. F., and Neis, D. D.: The sounds at the base of the heart in cases of patent ductus arteriosus. *Am. Heart J.* 59:807, 1960.

Hultgren, H.; Selzer, A.; Purdy, A.; Holman, E.; and Gerbode, F.: The syndrome of patent ductus arteriosus with pulmonary hypertension. *Circulation*, 8:15, 1953.

Hyrske, I.; Landtman, B.; Louhimo, I.; and Tuuteri, L.: Intermittent disappearance of the continuous murmur of patent ductus arteriosus. *Acta Paediatr. Scand.*, **54**:593, 1965.

Jager, B. V., and Wollenman, O. J., Jr.: An anatomical study of the closure of the ductus arteriosus. *Am. J. Pathol.*, **18**:595, 1942.

Jegier, W.; Blankenship, W.; Lind, J.; and Kitchen, A.: The changing circulatory pattern of the newborn infant studied by the indicator dilution technique. *Acta Paediatr.*, **53**:541, 1964.

Jegier, W.; Karn, G.; and Stern, L.: Operative treatment of patent ductus arteriosus complicating respiratory distress syndrome of the premature. *Can. Med. Assoc. J.*, **98**:105, 1968. ·

Johnson, R. E.; Wermer, P.; Kuschner, M.; and Cournand, A.: Intermittent reversal of flow in a case of patent ductus arteriosus. *Circulation*, **1**:1293, 1950.

Jones, J. C.: Twenty-five years experience with the surgery of patent ductus arteriosus. *J. Thorac. Cardiovasc. Surg.*, **50**:149, 1965.

Jones, R. W. A., and Pickering, D.: Persistent ductus arteriosus complicating the respiratory distress syndrome. *Arch. Dis. Child.*, **52**:274, 1977.

Jönsson, G.; Broden, B.; Hansson, H. G.; and Karnell, J.: Visualization of patent ductus arteriosus Botalli by means of thoracic aortography. *Acta Radiol.*, **30**:81, 1948.

Jose, A. D.; Ferencz, C.; Sheldon, H.; and Bahnson, H. T.: Progressive rise in pulmonary vascular resistance in a patient with patent ductus arteriosus: case report. *Bull. Hopkins Hosp.*, **108**:280, 1961.

Joyce, J. C., and O'Toole, S. P.: Congenital heart disease. Report on an unusually high incidence in one family. *Br. J. Med.*, **1**:1241, 1954.

Kato, H.; Oda, T.; Hirose, M.; Yoshizana, Y.; Uryu, K.; Oozono, I.; Honda, S.; Fukuda, H.; and Nagayama, T.: Intracardiac and external phonocardiographic study in infant with patent ductus arteriosus and pulmonary hypertension. *Jap. Circ. J.*, **32**:1571, 1968.

Keith, J. D., and Forsyth, C.: Aortography in infants. *Circulation*, **2**:907, 1950.

Keith, J. D.; Rowe, R. D.; and Vlad, P.: *Heart Disease in Infancy and Childhood*, 2nd ed. Macmillan Publishing Co., Inc., New York, 1967, p. 67.

Keith, T. R., and Sagarminaga, J.: Spontaneously disappearing mumur of patent ductus arteriosus. A case report. *Circulation*, **24**:1235, 1961.

Kelsey, J. R., Jr.; Gilmore, C. E.; and Edwards, J. E.: Bilateral ductus arteriosus representing persistence of each sixth aortic arch. *Arch. Pathol.*, **55**:154, 1953.

Kennedy, J. A., and Clark, S. L.: Observations on the physiological reactions of the ductus arteriosus. *Am. J. Physiol.*, **136**:140, 1942.

Keys, A., and Shapiro, M. J.: Patency of the ductus arteriosus in adults. *Am. Heart J.*, **25**:158, 1943.

Kidd, B. S. L.; Rose, V.; Collins, G.; Coggin, J; and Keith, J. D.: The haemodynamic spectrum of congenital left-to-right shunts in childhood. *Ann. R. C. Phys. Surg. (Can.)*, **21**:28, 1968.

Kilman, J. W.; Kakos, G. S.; Williams, T. E., Jr.; Craenen, J.; and Hosier, D. M.: Ligation of patent ductus arteriosus for persistent respiratory distress syndrome in premature infants. *J. Pediatr. Surg.*, **9**:277, 1974.

Kimball, K. G., and McIlroy, M. B.: Pulmonary hypertension in patients with congenital heart disease. Pre and postoperative hemodynamics, pulmonary function, and criteria for surgical closure of defects. *Am. J. Med.*, **41**:883, 1966.

Kitterman, J. A.; Edmunds, L. H., Jr.; Gregory, G. A.; Heymann, M. A.; Tooley, W. H.; and Rudolph, A. M.: Patent ductus arteriosus in premature infants: incidence, relation to pulmonary disease and management. *N. Engl. J. Med.*, **287**:47 3–7, 1972.

Kjellberg, S. R.; Mannheimer, E.; Rudhe, U.; and Jönsson, B.: *Diagnosis of Congenital Heart Disease*, 2nd ed. Year Book Publishers, Inc., Chicago, 1959, p. 531.

Kovalcik, V.: The response of the isolated ductus arteriosus to oxygen and anoxia. *J. Physiol.*, **169**:185, 1963.

Krovetz, L. J.; Lester, R. G.; and Warden, H. E.: The diagnosis of patent ductus arteriosus in infancy. *Dis. Chest*, **42**:241, 1962.

Krovetz, L. J., and Warden, H. E.: Patent ductus arteriosus. An analysis of 515 surgically proved cases. *Dis. Chest*, **42**:46, 1962.

Krovetz, L. J., and Gessner, I. H.: A new method utilizing indicator-dilution technics for estimation of left-to-right shunts in infants. *Circulation*, **32**:772, 1965.

Krovetz, L. J., and Rowe, R. D.: Patent ductus arteriosus,

prematurity and pulmonary disease. *N. Engl. J. Med.*, **287**:513, 1972.

Krugman, S., and Katz, S. L.: Rubella immunization: a five-year progress report. *N. Engl. J. Med.*, **290**:1375, 1974.

Laubry, C., and Pezzi, C.: *Traité des Maladies Congenitales du Coeur.* J. B. Bailliere & Fils, Paris, 1921.

Leachman, R. D.; De Franceschi, A.; Runge, Th. M.; and Cokkinos, D. V.: Frequency of pulmonary hypertension in patients of differing ages with atrial or ventricular septal defects and patent ductus arteriosus. *Acta Cardiol.*, **26**:480, 1971.

Leeds, S. E.: Effects of occlusion of experimental chronic patent ductus arteriosus on the cardiac output, pulse and blood pressure of dogs. *Am. J. Physiol.*, **139**:451, 1942.

Levine, S. H., and Harvey, W. P.: *Clinical Auscultation of the Heart.* W. B. Saunders Co., Philadelphia, 1949.

Levy, S. E., and Blalock, A.: Experimental observations on the effects of connecting by suture the main pulmonary artery to the systemic circulation. *J. Thorac. Surg.*, **8**:525, 1938.

Lewes, D.: The exercise test in patent ductus arteriosus. *Br. Heart J.*, **14**:357, 1952.

Lind, J., and Wegelius, C.: Human fetal circulation changes in the cardiovascular system at birth and disturbances in the post-natal closure of the foramen ovale and ductus arteriosus. *Cold Spring Harbor Symp., Quant. Biol.*, **19**:109, 1954.

Linde, L. M., and Adams, F. H.: Mitral insufficiency and pulmonary hypertension accompanying patent ductus arteriosus. Report of three cases. *Am. J. Cardiol.*, **3**:740, 1959.

Lowe, J. B.: Personal communication, 1963.

Lukas, D. S.; Araujo, J., and Steinberg, I.: The syndrome of patent ductus arteriosus with reversal of flow. *Am. J. Med.*, **17**:298, 1954.

Mancini, A. J.: A study of the angle formed by the ductus arteriosus with the descending thoracic aorta. *Anat. Rec.*, **109**:535, 1951.

Marcano, B., and Goldberg, S. J.: Patent ductus arteriosus: a correlation of electrocardiographic and physiologic information. *Am. J. Dis. Child.*, **117**:194, 1969.

Mark, H.: Jacobson, B.; and Young, D.: Coexistence of patent ductus arteriosus and congenital aortic valvular disease. *Circulation*, **17**:359, 1958.

Marquis, R. M., and Gilchrist, A. R.: The clinical syndrome of patent ductus arteriosus with pulmonary hypertension (Proc. Brit. Cardiac Soc.). *Br. Heart J.*, **17**:574, 1955.

McMurphy, D. M.; Heymann, M. A.; Rudolph, A. M.; and Melmon, K. L.: Developmental changes in constriction of the ductus arteriosus: Responses to oxygen and vasoactive agents in the isolated ductus arteriosus of the fetal lamb. *Pediatr. Res.*, **6**:231, 1972.

Mehrizi, A., and Drash, A.: Growth disturbance in congenital heart disease. *J. Pediatr.*, **61**:418, 1962.

Mitchell, S. C.: The ductus arteriosus in the neonatal period. *J. Pediatr.*, **51**:12, 1957.

Moghadam, A. N.; Khalil, E. F.; and Mattioli, L. F.: Intracardiac phonocardiography in the diagnosis of large patent ductus arteriosus in early infancy. *J. Pediatr.*, **67**:214, 1965.

Molnar, J. J.; Mesel, E.; Golinko, R. J.; and Rudolph, A. M.: Structure, histochemistry and physiology of ductus arteriosus in the dog. *J. Histochem. Cytochem.*, **10**:667, 1962.

Moss, A. J.; Emmanouilides, G. C.; Adams, F. H.; and Chuang, K.: Response of ductus arteriosus and pulmonary and systemic arterial pressure to changes in oxygen environment in newborn infants. *Pediatrics*, **33**:937, 1964.

Moss, A. J.; Emmanouilides, G.; and Duffie, E. R., Jr.: Closure of the ductus arteriosus in the newborn infant. *Pediatrics*, **32**:25, 1963.

Moss, A. J.; Emmanouilides, G. C.; Rettori, O.; Higashino, S. M.; and Adams, F. H.: Postnatal circulatory and metabolic adjustments in normal and distressed premature infants. *Biol. Neonate*, **8**:177, 1965.

Muir, D. C., and Brown, J. W.: Patent ductus arteriosus. *Arch. Dis. Child.*, **7**:291, 1932.

Murphy, D. A.; Outerbridge, E.; Stern, L.; Karn, G. M.; Jegier, W.; and Rosales, J.: Management of premature infants with patent ductus arteriosus. *J. Thorac. Cardiovasc. Surg.*, **67**:221, 1974.

Mustard, W. T.: Suture ligation of the patent ductus arteriosus in infancy. *Can. Med. Assoc. J.*, **64**:243, 1951.

———: Mortality in congenital cardiovascular surgery. *Can. Med. Assoc. J.*, **72**:740, 1955.

Myers, G. S.; Scannell, J. G.; Wyman, S. M.; Dimond, E. G.; and Hurst, J. W.: Atypical patent ductus arteriosus with absence of the usual aortic-pulmonary pressure gradient and of the characteristic murmur. *Am. Heart J.*, **41**:819, 1951.

Neal, W. A.; Bessinger, F. B., Jr.; Hunt, C. E.; and Lucas, R. V.: Patent ductus arteriosus complicating respiratory distress syndrome. *J. Pediatr.*, **86**:127, 1975.

Neill, C. A., and Mounsey, P.: Auscultation in patent ductus arteriosus with a description of two fistulae simulating patent ductus. *Br. Heart J.*, **20**:61, 1958.

Neutze, J. M.: Follow up of high resistance patients after shunt surgery. *N.Z. Med. J. Cardiac Supp.*, **64**:37, 1965.

Nora, J. J.; Gilliland, J. C.; Sommerville, R. J.; and McNamara, D. G.: Congenital heart disease in twins. *N. Engl. J. Med.*, **277**:568, 1967.

Ochsner, J. L.; Cooley, D. A.; McNamara, D. G.; and Kline, A.: Surgical treatment of cardiovascular anomalies in 300 infants younger than one year of age. *J. Thorac. Cardiovasc. Surg.*, **43**:182, 1962.

Olley, P. M.: Nonsurgical palliation of congenital heart malformations. *N. Engl. J. Med.*, **292**:1292, 1975.

Olley, P. M.: Personal communication, 1977.

Panagopoulos, Ph. G.; Tatooles, C. J.; Aberdeen, E.; Waterston, D. J.; and Bonham-Carter, R. E.: Patent ductus arteriosus in infants and children. A review of 936 operations (1946–69). *Thorax*, **26**:137, 1971.

Patterson, D. F.; Pyle, R. L.; Buchanan, J. W.; Trautvetter, E.; and Abt, D. A.: Hereditary patent ductus arteriosus and its sequelae in the dog. *Circ. Res.*, **29**:1, 1971.

Patterson, D. F.; Pyle, R. L.; and Buchanan, J. W.: Hereditary cardiovascular malformations of the dog. Proc. 4th Conf. on Clin. Delineation of Birth Defects Part XV Ed. Daniel Bergsma in *Birth Defects Orig. Art Series*, The National Foundation, N.Y., vol. 8, 1972, p. 160.

Penaloza, D.; Arias-Stella, J.; Sime, F.; Recavarren, S.; and Marticorena, E.: The heart and pulmonary circulation in children at high altitudes. Physiological anatomical and clinical observations. *Pediatrics*, **34**:568, 1964.

Polani, P. E., and Campbell, M.: Factors in the causation of persistent ductus arteriosus. *Ann. Hum. Genet.*, **24**:343, 1960.

Porstmann, W.; Wierny, L.; and Warnke, H.: Closure of persistent ductus arteriosus without thoracotomy. *German Med. Mon.*, **12**:259, 1967.

Porstmann, W.; Wierny, L.; Warnke, H.; Gerstberger, G.; and Romaniuk, P. A.: Catheter closure of patent ductus arteriosus. 62 cases treated without thoracotomy. *Radiol. Clin. North Am.*, **9**:203, 1971.

Powell, M. L.: Patent ductus arteriosus in premature infants. *Med. J. Aust.*, **2**:58, 1963.

Prec, K. J., and Cassels, D. E.: Dye dilution curves and cardiac output in newborn infants. *Circulation*, **11**:789, 1955.

Prec, K. J.; Cassels, D. E.; Rabinowitz, M.; and Moulder, P. V.: Cardiac failure and patency of the ductus arteriosus in early infancy. *J. Pediatr.*, **61**:843, 1962.

Pritchard, W. H.; Brofman, B. L.; and Hellerstein, W. K.: Clinical study in reversal of flow in patent ductus arteriosus. *J. Lab. Clin. Med.*, **36**:974, 1950.

Quiroga, C.: Partial persistence of the ductus arteriosus. *Acta Radiol.*, **55**:103, 1961.

Rausch, J.; Higgins, C.; Friedman, W.; and Goergen, T.: Evaluation of patent ductus arteriosus in preterm infants with respiratory distress. *Circulation*, **54**:(Suppl.) 11–39, 1976.

Ravin, A., and Darley, W.: Apical diastolic murmurs in patent ductus arteriosus. *Ann. Intern. Med.*, **33**:903, 1950.

Record, R. G., and McKeown, T.: Observations relating to the etiology of patent ductus arteriosus. *Br. Heart J.*, **15**:376, 1953.

Reis, R. L., and Anderson, R. P.: Constriction of the ductus arteriosus. Experimental observations in the newborn lamb. *J. Surg. Res.*, **4**:356, 1964.

Rees, S.: The chest radiograph in pulmonary hypertension with central shunt. *Br. J. Radiol.*, **41**:172, 1968.

Reinhold, J. D. L., and Nadas, A. S.: The role of auscultation in the diagnosis of congenital heart disease. A phonocardiographic study of children. *Am. Heart J.*, **47**:405, 1954.

Robertson, N. R. C.: Prolonged continuous positive airways pressure for pulmonary oedema due to persistent ductus arteriosus in the newborn. *Arch. Dis. Child.*, **49**:585, 1974.

Rose, V.; Hewitt, D.; and Milner, J.: Seasonal influences on the risk of cardiac malformation. Nature of the problem and some results

from a study of 10,077 cases. *Int. J. Epidemiol.*, **1**:235, 1972.

Ross, R. S.; Feder, F. P.; and Spencer, F. C.: Aneurysms of the previously ligated patent ductus arteriosus. *Circulation*, **23**:350, 1961.

Routier, D.: Remarques sur les signes d'auscultation dans la persistance du canal arteriel. *Arch. Mal. Coeur*, **30**:388, 1937.

Rowe, R. D.: Changes in the pulmonary hemodynamics of newborn infants. Essay in medicine, Royal College of Physicians of Canada, 1957.

Rowe, R. D.: In Oliver, T. K. Jr. (ed.): *Adaptation to Extrauterine Life: Report of the Thirty-first Ross Conference on Pediatric Research*. Ross Laboratories, Columbus, 1959, p. 36.

——: Maternal rubella and pulmonary artery stenosis. Report of eleven cases. *Pediatrics*, **32**:180, 1963.

Rowe, R. D., and James, L. S.: The normal pulmonary arterial pressure during the first year of life. *J. Pediatr.*, **51**:1, 1957.

Rowe, R. D., and Lowe, J. B.: Auscultation in the diagnosis of persistent ductus arteriosis in infancy: a study of 50 patients. *New. Zeal. Med. J.*, **63**:195, 1964.

Rowe, R. D.; Lowe, J. B.; and Barratt-Boyes, B. G.: Heart malformation in infancy. Initial experience from a cardiosurgical unit. *New. Zeal. Med. J.*, **60**:549, 1961.

Rowe, R. D., and Neill, C. A.: Patent ductus arteriosus in the first year of life: Factors influencing spontaneous closure. In *The Natural History and Progress in Treatment of Congenital Heart Defects*. Eds. Kidd, B. S. L., and Keith, J. D. Charles C Thomas, Publisher Springfield, Ill., 1971, p. 33.

Rudolph, A. M.; Drorbaugh, J. E.; Auld, P. A. M.; Rudolph, A. J.; Nadas, A. S.; Smith, C. A.; and Hubbell, J. P.: Studies on the circulation in the neonatal period. The circulation in the respiratory distress syndrome. *Pediatrics*, **27**:551, 1961.

Rutstein, D.; Nickerson, R. J.; and Heald, F. P.: Seasonal incidence of patent ductus arteriosus and maternal rubella. *Am. J. Dis. Child.*, **84**:199, 1952.

Saling, E.: Neue Untersuchungsergebnisse uber den Kreislauf des Kindes unmittelbar nach der Geburt. *Arch. Gynak.*, **194**:287, 1960.

Sandblom, P., and Ekström, G.: Surgical treatment of wide patent ductus arteriosus. *Acta Chir. Scand.*, **102**:167, 1951.

Sasahara, A. A.; Nadas, A. S.; Rudolph, A. M.; Wittenborg, M. H.; and Gross, R. E.: Ventricular septal defect with patent ductus arteriosus. A clinical and hemodynamic study. *Circulation*, **22**:254, 1960.

Sciacca, A., and Conderelli, M.: Involution of the ductus arteriosus. A morphological and experimental study with a critical review of the literature. *Bibl. Cardiol.*, No 10: 1–52, 1960.

Scott, H. W., Jr.: Closure of the patent ductus by suture ligation technique. *Surg. Gynecol. Obstet.*, **90**:91, 1950.

——: Surgical treatment of patent ductus arteriosus in childhood. *Surg. Clin. North Am.*, **32**:1299, 1952.

Scott, O., and Gearty, G. F.: Patent ductus arteriosus in infancy. *Arch. Dis. Child.*, **35**:465, 1960.

Sellors, T. H.: Surgery of the persistent ductus arteriosus. *Lancet*, **1**:615, 1945.

Sever, J. L.; Schiff, G. M.; and Traub, R. G.: Rubella virus. *JAMA*, **182**:663, 1962.

Shapiro, M. J.: Recent advances in surgical treatment of patent ductus arteriosus. *Mod. Concepts Cardiovasc. Dis.*, **16**:1, 1947.

Shephard, R. J.: Pulmonary arterial pressure in acyanotic congenital heart disease. *Br. Heart J.*, **16**:361, 1954.

Shepherd, J. J.; Werdinan, W. H.; Burke, E. C.; and Wood, E. H.: Hemodynamics in patent ductus arteriosus without a murmur. *Circulation*, **11**:404, 1955.

Siassi, B.; Emmanouilides, G. S.; Cleveland, R. J.; and Hirose, F.: Patent ductus arteriosus complicating prolonged assisted ventilation in respiratory distress syndrome. *J. Pediatr.*, **74**:11, 1969.

Siassi, B.; Goldberg, S. J.; Emmanouilides, G. C.; Hisashino, S. M.; and Lewis, E.: Persistent pulmonary vascular obstruction in newborn infants. *J. Pediatr.*, **78**:610, 1971.

Siegel, R. E.: Galen's experiments and observations on pulmonary blood flow and respiration. *Am. J. Cardiol.*, **10**:738, 1962.

Silva, D. G., and Ikeda, M.: Ultrastructural and acetylcholinesterase studies on the innervation of the ductus arteriosus, pulmonary trunk and aorta of the fetal lamb. *J. Ultrastruct. Res.*, **34**:358, 1971.

Silverman, N. H.; Lewis, A. B.; Heymann, M. A.; and Rudolph, A.

M.: Echocardiographic assessment of ductus arteriosus shunt in premature infants. *Circulation*, **50**:821, 1974.

Smith, G.: Patent ductus arteriosus with pulmonary hypertension and reversed shunt. *Br. Heart J.*, **16**:233, 1954.

Soulié, P.; Routier, D.; and Bernal, P.: Communication interventriculaire avec insuffisance aortique. *Arch. Mal. Coeur*, **42**:765, 1949.

Stevenson, J. G.: Fluid administration in the association of patent ductus arteriosus complicating respiratory distress syndrome. *J. Pediatr.*, **90**:257, 1977.

Storstein, O.; Humberfelt, S.; Müller, O.; and Rasmussen, H.: Studies in catheterization of the heart in cases of patent ductus Botalli. *Acta Med. Scand.*, **141**:419, 1952.

Stout, C., and Koehl, G.: Aortic embolism in a newborn infant. *Am. J. Dis. Child.*, **120**:74, 1970.

Swan, H. J. C.; Zapata-Diaz, J.; Burchell, H. B.; and Wood, E. H.: Pulmonary hypertension in congenital heart disease. *Am. J. Med.*, **16**:12, 1954.

Taussig, H. B.. In Heggesness, F. W. (ed.): *Congenital Heart Disease: Report of the 14th M and R Pediatric Research Conference*. M and R Laboratories, Columbus, 1954, p. 35.

————: *Congenital Malformations of the Heart. Vol II: Specific Malformations*. Harvard University Press, Cambridge, Mass., 1960, p. 492.

Taussig, H. B.; Bauersfeld, S. R.; and MacDonald, A. J.: Pulmonary hypertension with persistent patency of the ductus arteriosus. *Am. J. Dis. Child.*, **84**:496, 1952.

Taylor, B. E.; Pollack, A. A.; Burchell, H. B.; Clagett, O. T.; and Wood, E. H.: Studies of the pulmonary and systemic arterial pressure in cases of patent ductus arteriosus with special reference to effects of surgical closure. *J. Clin. Invest.*, **29**:745, 1950.

Thibeault, D. W.; Emmanouilides, G. C.; Nelson, P. J.; Lachman, R. S.; Rosengart, R. M.; and Oh, W.: Patent ductus arteriosus complicating the respiratory distress syndrome in preterm infants. *J. Pediatr.*, **86**:120, 1975.

Timpanelli, A. E., and Steinberg, I.: Calcification of the pulmonary artery in patent ductus arteriosus with reversal of blood flow. Report of four cases. *Am. J. Med.*, **30**:405, 1961.

Trusler, G. A.; Arayangkoon, P.; and Mustard, W. T.: Operative closure of isolated patent ductus arteriosus in the first two years of life. *Can. Med. Assoc. J.*, **99**:879, 1968.

Tutassaura, H.; Goldman, B.; Moes, C. A. F.; and Mustard, W. T.: Spontaneous aneurysm of the ductus arteriosus. *J. Thorac. Cardiovasc. Surg.*, **57**:180, 1969.

Umansky, R., and Hauck, A. J.: Factors in the growth of children

with patent ductus arteriosus. *Pediatrics*, **30**:540, 1962.

Usher, R. H.: Respiratory problems in newborn infants. *Postgrad. Med.*, **21**:44, 1962.

Walker, G. C., and Ellis, L. B.: The familial occurrence of congenital cardiac anomalies. *Proc. N. Engl. Heart Assoc.*, **41**:26, 1940–41.

Wallgren, G.; Hanson, J. S.; Tabakin, B. S.; Räihä, N.; and Vapaavouri, E.: Quantitative studies of the human neonatal circulation. V. Hemodynamic findings in premature infants with and without respiratory distress. *Acta Paediatr. Scand.* (Suppl.), **179**:71, 1967.

Wangensteen, O., quoted by Shapiro, M. J.: *Mod. Concepts Cardiovasc. Dis.*, **16**:1, 1947.

Waterman, D. H.; Samson, P. C.; and Bailey, C. P.: The surgery of patent ductus arteriosus; a report of the section on cardiovascular surgery. *Dis. Chest*, **29**:102, 1956.

Weller, T. H., and Neva, F. A.: Propagation in tissue culture of cytopathic agents from patients with rubella-like illness. *Proc. Soc. Exp. Biol Med.*, **3**:215, 1962.

Wennevold, A.: Intracardiac phonocardiography in the diagnosis of small patent ductus arteriosus with atypical murmur. *Acta Med. Scand.*, **183**:231, 1968.

White, P. D.: In Heggeness, F. W. (ed.): *Congenital Heart Disease: Report of the 14th M and R Pediatric Research Conference*. M and R Laboratories, Columbus, 1954, pp. 34 and 66.

Wilson, R. R.: Post-mortem observations on contraction of the human ductus arteriosus. *Br. Med. J.*, **1**:810, 1958.

Wood, P.: Congenital heart disease. *Br. Med. J.*, **2**:639, 693, 1950.

————: An appreciation of mitral stenosis. Part I. Clinical features. *Br. Med. J.*, **1**:1051, 1954.

Zachman, R. D.; Steinmetz, G. P.; Botham, R. J.; Graven, S. N.; and Ledbetter, M. K.: Incidence and treatment of the patent ductus arteriosus in the ill premature infant. *Am. Heart J.*, **87**:697, 1974.

Zapol, W. M.; Kolobow, T.; Doppman, J.; and Pierce, J. E.: Response of ductus arteriosus and pulmonary blood flow to blood oxygen tension in immersed lamb fetuses perfused through an artificial placenta. *J. Thorac. Cardiovasc. Surg.*, **61**:891, 1971.

Zetterqvist, P.: The etiology of patent ductus arteriosus. *Acta Paediatr. Scand.*, Suppl. **206**:42, 1970.

Zuberbuhler, J. F.; Lenox, C. C.; Park, S. C.; and Neches, W. H.: Continuous murmurs in the newborn. In Leon, D. F., and Shaver, J. A. (eds.): *Physiologic Principles of Heart Sounds and Murmurs*. American Heart Association Monograph No. 46. American heart Association, New York, 1975, p. 209.

25

Aortopulmonary Septal Defect

Richard D. Rowe

WHEN the embryo has a crown rump length of between 9 and 13 mm (Streeter's horizon XVI to XVII) the spiral aortopulmonary septum should fuse and finally separate the aorta from the pulmonary artery (van Mierop and Gessner, 1972). A failure of this process leaves a localized defect between the two great arteries just above their valve origins. The defect has been described at various times as an aorticopulmonary, aortopulmonary, or aortic septal defect, fenestration, fistula, or window. The term *partial truncus arteriosus* is not now usually employed.

The condition was first reported by Elliotson (1830–1831) and, though rare, is important since it can be corrected surgically. Maude Abbott (1936) reported ten among her collection of 1000 specimens, but less than 100 cases were reported in the reviews of Marquis (1968) and Neufeld and associates (1962). At The Hospital for Sick Children we have seen 23 examples among 15,104 patients with the congenital heart disease over the past 23 years. Thirty-three patients with aortopulmonary septal defect have been encountered at the Children's Hospital Medical Center in Boston (Nadas and Fyler, 1972), 17 at the University of Minnesota Hospitals (Blieden and Moller, 1974), and 9 at The Hospital for Sick Children, Great Ormond Street (Deverall et al., 1969).

Pathology

The defect consists of a round or oval communication of variable, but most often large, size. The defect lies between the left side of the ascending aorta and the right wall of the main pulmonary artery just anterior to the origin of the right main pulmonary artery branch (Neufeld et al., 1962). The condition is isolated in at least 50 percent of cases but associated cardiovascular anomalies are common. In our 23 patients, 14 were isolated examples, five had associated persistent ductus arteriosus (Morrow et al., 1962), and four had ventricular septal defects

(Tandon et al., 1974). Secundum atrial septal defects, interrupted aortic arch, coarctation of the aorta, subaortic stenosis, anomalous origin of the coronary arteries, pulmonary arteriovenous fistula, tetralogy of Fallot, origin of the right pulmonary artery from the aorta, and right aortic arch have been noted (Blieden and Moller, 1974). Ventricular hypertrophy is present (Downing, 1950), its degree and distribution being related to the size of the defect and the status of the lung vascular bed. Conversely, the histologic picture of the small vessels in the lung reasonably accurately reflects the size of the communication and the duration of a hemodynamic disturbance (Neufeld et al., 1962).

Cardiac Catheterization and Angiocardiography

Since the defect is most often large, the dynamics are similar to that of a large ventricular septal defect or patent ductus arteriosus. Within a few weeks or months of birth cardiac catheterization will show systemic pressure or levels nearly so in the right ventricle and pulmonary artery and a large left-to-right shunt at pulmonary arterial level. The aortic pulse pressure will be wide. By the end of infancy in patients with larger defects there will be evidence of high pulmonary vascular resistance (see Table 25–1). In the uncommon small communications, right ventricular and pulmonary arterial pressures are normal and left-to-right shunt by contrast is small.

Localization of the aorticopulmonary shunt to the proximal great artery level is possible by a variety of catheterization techniques. A catheter can be passed through the defect (though this is by no means always achieved) from either the venous or arterial sides and give an immediate indication of the presence of such a defect (D'heer and van Nieuwenhuizen, 1956). In one of our early cases the defect was not crossed but the ductus arteriosus was probed from the pulmonary artery. In reality the duct proved to be of trivial size

Table 25-1. PRINCIPAL SERIAL HEMODYNAMIC FINDINGS IN A GIRL WITH AN AORTOPULMONARY SEPTAL DEFECT STUDIED DURING INFANCY AND IN ADOLESCENCE*†

DATE OF STUDY	AGE	RA	RV	PA	PAW	QP/QS	SAO₂	BP
13.4.57	7 mo	1	65/0	65/30	11	3:1	95%	80/40
28.10.74	17 yr	0	100/5	100/55	2	1.4:1	92%	100/55

* In infancy patient had a large heart and other signs of a large left-to-right shunt. Operation was scheduled at age two years, but canceled when an unrelated bleeding disorder was detected. As an adolescent she had a small heart and clinical signs of pulmonary vascular disease.

† RA = right atrium; RV = right ventricle; PA = pulmonary artery; PAW = wedge pulmonary artery; Qp/Qs = pulmonary-to-systemic flow ratio; SaO₂ = arterial oxygen saturation; BP = blood pressure.

and the septal defect large. Localization of the shunt can be provided for most cases by recording indicator dilution curves from a systemic artery or the main pulmonary artery. After injection of dye into the ascending aorta, a large left-to-right shunt is recorded, whereas from the aortic arch the curve will be normal or show trivial disturbances of the downslope. Because of a number of questions that may still be unanswered by these methods aortography is a necessary part of the study.

Since the first reported examples of Gasul and associates (1951) and King and associates (1951), it has been apparent that angiography is essential to complete assessment. It has also been appreciated that because of marked dilution of contrast by massive shunting in most infant cases, there is a critical need for rapid film rates so that the precise site of the aortopulmonary shunt can be identified before the area is obliterated when contrast fills both vessels. Cineangiocardiography is of prime importance in achieving this objective. Less difficulty is encountered in the differential diagnosis when pulmonary vascular obstruction reduces the size of the left-to-right shunt (Figure 25–1). By showing two separate great arteries and a left-to-right shunt at proximal level, angiocardiography permits separation of patients with aortopulmonary septal defect from those with true

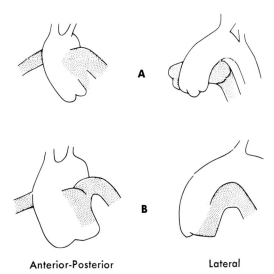

Figure 25-2. Diagrammatic representation of the frontal and lateral projections of the aortogram in (*A*) aortopulmonary septal defect and (*B*) truncus arteriosus. The important differentiation usually comes from the ability to distinguish two separate valve roots, so that high frame rates during angiography carry an advantage.

Anterior-Posterior   Lateral

truncus arteriosus (Figure 25–2) or patent ductus arteriosus. Other associated cardiovascular anomalies, e.g., ventricular septal defect, right aortic arch, or coarctation of the aorta, can be defined likewise in the usual manner by selective injections of contrast.

Clinical Features

In the *usual* case with a large defect tachypnea is an early sign during infancy. The patient is usually acyanotic at this age. Congestive heart failure is a common complication but is not invariable. Pulses are bounding. A murmur appears within a few weeks, which is most often nonspecific, short, and ejection in type along the left sternal border. Occasionally it may appear pansystolic or be loud. There is often an associated middiastolic murmur and occasionally pulmonary valve incompetence may be evident. The second heart sound is narrowly split and pulmonary valve closure is accentuated. In patients with high pulmonary vascular resistance mild cyanosis may be

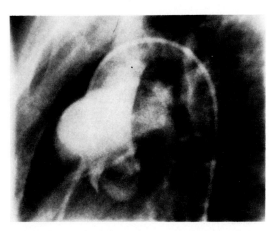

Figure 25-1. The lateral cineaortogram of a girl aged 17 years with a large aortopulmonary septal defect. The high pulmonary vascular instance in her particular case allows for easier demonstration of the aortic and pulmonary arterial roots.

seen, pulses are more likely to be normal, and there is frequently a short murmur, a loud pulmonary ejection sound, and a loud single heart sound.

In *occasional patients* (about 10 percent) with small defects there are no symptoms and the first sign will be the discovery of a heart murmur at routine examination. This murmur is continuous, and although it may appear lower in position than that usually encountered in patent ductus arteriosus, the murmur of aortopulmonary septal defect may be localized to the second left intercostal space (Gibson et al., 1950; Blieden and Moller, 1974). The second heart sound in these patients is normal, reflecting, with the continuous murmur, a normal or near-normal pulmonary arterial pressure.

Finally, *additional cardiovascular malformations* of significance may be masked by aortopulmonary septal defect as, for example, in the pulmonary stenosis of tetralogy of Fallot (Blieden and Moller, 1974) or anomalous coronary arteries (Burroughs et al., 1962), making further argument for detailed physiologic and angiocardiographic evaluation of such patients.

Radiologic Examination

The heart is slightly, moderately, or grossly enlarged, depending on the size of the defect and the state of the pulmonary vascular resistance. Figure 25-3 shows the heart size of a young boy with a small defect. With the more frequent larger defect the heart is bigger, the left atrium enlarged, and the lung vascularity markedly increased. The aortic knuckle is not enlarged (Blieden and Moller, 1974) and a right aorta is not uncommon, especially in patients with associated ventricular septal defect.

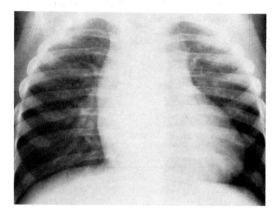

Figure 25-3. The chest x-ray of a boy aged 17 months with a small aortopulmonary septal defect. The Qp/Qs at cardiac catheterization was 2/1, and the pulmonary arterial pressures were normal. A continuous murmur was audible over the third left intercostal space anteriorly. Surgical confirmation of the diagnosis was obtained.

Electrocardiography

The electrocardiogram will be normal or show slight left ventricular hypertrophy in patients when the defect is small. In the more usual presentation varying degrees of frontal plane axis QRS and right ventricular hypertrophy, combined ventricular hypertrophy, or left ventricular heart hypertrophy will reflect the status of the pulmonary vascular bed (Figure 25-4).

Diagnosis

The diagnosis is not often easy. For the large defect the clinical picture is one of a large left-to-right shunt. The bounding pulses might suggest the diagnosis of *patent ductus arteriosus*, but we have never noted the abbreviated murmur so common with large ducts (Rowe and Lowe, 1964) to be present in these cases. The alternative of *truncus arteriosus* is unlikely because of the clear-cut splitting of the second heart sound in aortopulmonary septal defect.

Splitting of the second sound can, on occasion, occur in the truncus, and the characteristic ejection sound and right aortic arch of truncus can be found in aortopulmonary septal defect, so that the distinction between the two malformations is sometime quite fine. Echocardiography may detect two separate great vessel roots and so assists in this situation. *Ventricular septal defect* with a ductus or with aortic valvular regurgitation can be simulated by the aortopulmonary septal defect so that in the end the finding of an important left-to-right shunt with pulmonary hypertension means that further studies are necessary for diagnosis.

In the minority with small defects the chief danger is that the patient will be considered to have an isolated patent ductus arteriosus and referred for operation without confirmatory catheterization and angiocardiography. Because of the real rarity of aortopulmonary septal defect, especially in this form, our general approach to avoiding the error has been to submit for study any patient with apparent ductus arteriosus who shows even the slightest departure from the classic diagnostic features, e.g., atypical nature, duration, or position of the murmur, discordant features in the electrocardiogram or chest film. Admittedly there will be occasions when even with these precautions the malformation could be misdiagnosed as patent ductus arteriosus, but for most cardiologists the small risk is regarded as acceptable.

Prognosis

Earlier experience with the malformation suggested an unfavorable outlook. Death in infancy was from congestive heart failure, and late death resulted from pulmonary vascular obstruction, pneumonia,

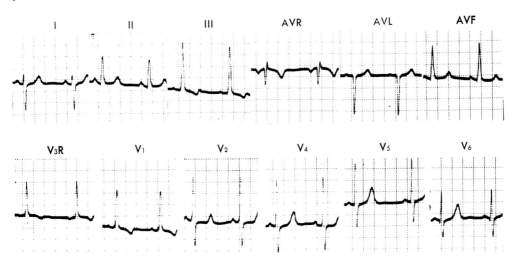

Figure 25-4. The electrocardiogram of a girl aged 17 years with a large aortopulmonary septal defect. The Qp/Qs at cardiac catheterization was 1.4/1, and the pulmonary arterial pressure was at systemic level. A pulmonary ejection click, short ejection systolic murmur, and markedly accentuated pulmonary valve closure sound were evident on auscultation.

or congestive heart failure (Downing, 1950). Diagnosis was often delayed and frequently discovered at operation or autopsy. Nowadays the diagnosis can be confidently reached at an early stage, and better medical and surgical therapy combined with improvement in postoperative care will almost certainly greatly improve the expectation of life for patients in the future.

Treatment

The treatment of choice is operative closure of the defect. Patients with small defects can be repaired electively after infancy. In those with large defects of complicating anomalies repair may well be necessary during infancy. In general, the timing of intervention can be decided in a way similar to the current approach for ventricular septal defect of large size; i.e., reasonably effective medical control of congestive failure allows deferral of the operation to the latter part of the first year of life, and failure to maintain good control argues for earlier surgery. The long-term outcome for nonoperated patients with large defects is bad (Blieden and Moller, 1974). The earlier techniques (Gross, 1952; Scott and Sabiston, 1953; Kirklin et al., 1955) employed ligation or division of the defect as is used with patent ductus arteriosus. After the introduction of cardiopulmonary bypass for repair of this malformation (Cooley et al., 1957), an approach through the pulmonary artery was suggested by Schumaker (1957) and later by Putman and Gross (1966), after which Wright and colleagues (1968) devised the transaortic closure method now in vogue (Deverall et al., 1969).

Hopefully the frustrating decisions for or against operation in patients with high pulmonary vascular resistance in aortopulmonary septal defect will soon

be a bad memory as the diagnostic and management decisions become properly confined to the first year or two of life.

REFERENCES

Abbott, M. E.: *Atlas of Congenital Cardiac Disease.* American Heart Association, New York, 1936.
Blieden, L. C., and Moller, J. H.: Aorticopulmonary septal defect. An experience with 17 patients. *Br. Heart J.,* **36**:630, 1974.
Burroughs, J. T.; Schmutzer, K. J.; Linder, F.; and Neuhaus, G.: Anomalous origin of the right coronary artery with aortico-pulmonary window and ventricular septal defect. Report of a case with complete operative correction. *J. Cardiovasc. Surg.,* **3**:142, 1962.
Cooley, D. A.; McNamara, D. G.; and Latson, J. R.: Aorticopulmonary septal defect: diagnosis and surgical treatment. *Surgery,* **42**:101, 1957.
Deverall, P. B.; Lincoln, J. C. F.; Aberdeen, E.; Bonham-Carter, R. E.; and Waterston, D. J.: Aortopulmonary window. *J. Thorac. Cardiovasc. Surg.,* **57**:479, 1959.
D'heer, H. A. H., and van Nieuwenhuizen, C. L. C.: Diagnosis of congenital aortic septal defects. Description of two cases and special emphasis on a new method which allows an accurate diagnosis by means of cardiac catheterization. *Circulation,* **13**:58, 1956.
Downing, D. F.: Congenital aortic septal defect. *Am. Heart J.,* **40**:285, 1950.
Elliotson, J.: Case of malformation of the pulmonary artery and aorta. *Lancet,* **1**:247, 1830–1831.
Fisher, E.; DuDrow, I. W.; Eckner, F. A. O.; and Hastreiter, A. R.: Aorticopulmonary septal defect and interrupted aortic arch: A diagnostic challenge. *Am. J. Cardiol.,* **34**:356, 1974.
Gasul, B. M.; Fell, E. H.; and Casas, R.: The diagnosis of aortic septal defects by retrograde aortography. *Circulation,* **4**:251, 1951.
Gibson, S.; Potts, W. J.; and Langewisch, W. H.: Aortic-pulmonary communication due to localized congenital defect of the aortic septum. *Pediatrics,* **6**:357, 1950.
Gross, R. E.: Surgical closure of an aortic septal defect. *Circulation,* **5**:858, 1952.
King, F. H.; Gordon, A.; Brahms, S.; Lasser, R.; and Bornn, R.: Aortic septal defect simulating patent ductus arteriosus. *J. Mount Sinai Hosp. N.Y.,* **17**:310, 1951.

Kirklin, J. W.; Ellis, F. H., Jr.; and Clagett, O. T.: Aortic-pulmonary septal defect. *Surg. Clin. North Am.*, **35**:975, 1955.

Marquis, R. M.: Aortopulmonary window. In *Paediatric Cardiology*. (Ed. Watson, H.). Lloyd-Luke, London, 1968, p. 286.

Morrow, A. G.; Greenfield, L. J.; and Braunwald, E.: Congenital aortopulmonary septal defect. Clinical and hemodynamic findings, surgical technic, and results of operative correction. *Circulation*, **25**:463, 1962.

Nadas, A. S., and Fyler, D.: *Pediatric Cardiology*, 3rd ed. W. B. Saunders Co., Philadelphia, 1972.

Neufeld, H. N.; Lester, R. G.; Adams, P., Jr.; Anderson, R. C.; Lillehei, C. W.; and Edwards, J. E.: Aorticopulmonary septal defect. *Am. J. Cardiol.*, **9**:12, 1962.

Putnam, T. C., and Gross, R. F.: Surgical management of aortopulmonary fenestration. *Surgery*, **59**:727, 1966.

Rowe, R. D., and Lowe, J. B.: Auscultation in the diagnosis of persistent ductus arteriosus in infancy: A study of 50 patients. *New Zeal. Med. J.*, **63**:195, 1964.

Schumaker, H. B.: In discussion of Cooley, D. A.; McNamara, D. G.; and Latson, J. R.: Aorticopulmonary septal defect. Diagnosis and surgical treatment. *Surgery*, **42**:101, 1957.

Scott, H. W., and Sabiston, D. C.: Surgical treatment for congenital aorticopulmonary fistula. *J. Thorac. Surg.*, **25**:26, 1953.

van Mierop, L. H. S., and Gessner, I. H.: Pathogenetic mechanisms in congenital cardiovascular malformations. In *Neonatal Heart Disease* (Eds., Friedman, W. F.; Lesch, M.; and Sonnenblick, E. H.). Grune & Stratton, New York, 1972, 1973 p. 1.

Tandon, R.; Da Silva, C. L.; Moller, J. H.; and Edwards, J. E.: Aorticopulmonary septal defect coexisting with ventricular septal defect. *Circulation*, **50**:188, 1974.

Wright, J. S.; Freeman, R. V.; and Johnston, J. B.: Aortopulmonary fenestration: A technique of surgical management. *J. Thorac. Cardiovasc. Surg.*, **55**:280, 1968.

26

Persistent Truncus Arteriosus

B. S. Langford Kidd

PERSISTENT truncus arteriosus is the name given to the condition in which all three circulations—the systemic, the pulmonary, and the coronary—arise from a single vessel leaving the base of the heart through a single valve.

Although first described over 100 years ago (Buchanan, 1864), its clinical recognition was not easy until recent introduction of valved conduits made surgical correction of the anomaly feasible (McGoon et al., 1968). Even now the diagnosis is often difficult, since truncus arteriosus may present in a variety of ways with no characteristic, definitive, and easily recognizable clinical, radiographic, or electrocardiographic signs to point toward the correct diagnosis.

Definition (i.e., a single trunk leaving the heart) separates this condition from aortic atresia, where there is one semilunar valve, but usually a hypoplastic ascending aorta gives rise to the coronary arteries and the brachiocephalic branches, which are perfused indirectly from the pulmonary artery through a ductus arteriosus. It also excludes pulmonary atresia for similar reasons, for here, although the perfusion of the lungs is from the aorta via a ductus or bronchial arteries, the pulmonary arteries do not arise from the common trunk. It also excludes aortopulmonary window, where there are two trunks arising from the base of the heart. Truncus arteriosus has also been termed common aortopulmonary trunk, truncus arteriosus communis, or persistent truncus arteriosus. However, for all practical purposes, truncus arteriosus has meaning, clarity, and brevity.

Following the first description of this anomaly milestones on the path to our present understanding were established by several studies. In 1942 Lev and Saphir classified truncus into complete, almost complete, and partial varieties. In 1949 Collett and Edwards in a classic paper reviewed 116 cases, developed strict diagnostic criteria, and proposed a division into five major anatomic types; this classification was "simplified" by Anderson and coworkers in 1957, and by Tandon and associates in 1963. In 1965 Van Praagh and Van Praagh studied 57 cases and presented a "new and simplified" anatomic classification, while Gasul and colleagues (1966) proposed both anatomic and functional classifications. The whole matter has recently been discussed in a dialogue between Edwards and Van Praagh (Edwards, 1976; Van Praagh, 1976).

Anatomic Features

Because the definitive diagnosis of truncus arteriosus is basically an angiographic one, the anatomic features of the anomaly are especially important. The basic feature is that one large trunk leaves the base of the heart due to a failure of the truncal septum to develop and separate the aorta from the pulmonary artery. This failure may be complete when the pulmonary artery branches arise directly from the trunk, or partial when there is a main pulmonary artery arising from the trunk.

The semilunar valve is commonly tricuspid. In Van Praagh and Van Praagh's 1965 series the valve was bicuspid in 7 percent and tricuspid in 67 percent, while 24 percent had four cusps. None had five or six leaflets. In the series of Bharati and coworkers (1974) one case was pentacuspid while the other proportions were nearly identical to Van Praagh's (tricuspid 68 percent, quadricuspid 25.3 percent, and bicuspid 6.7 percent). The valve cusps were usually of equal size, but one was sometimes larger than the others; in one-third of cases with a quadricuspid valve, the pulmonary leaflet was longer and taller than the others. Fairly often the cusps are thick and polyoid (Bharati et al., 1974) and appear to threaten the coronary ostia (Keith et al., 1958). Deely and coworkers (1963) reported deformed cusps in 4 of 42 cases and suggested that these valves could be incompetent. Roos (1935) suggested that these abnormal cusps, showing loose fibrous proliferation, with nodular formations along the valve margins (Feller, 1931) were the result of developmental arrest of local growth with persistence of fetal form. There is certainly little evidence of inflammatory change (Deely et al., 1963; Gelband et al., 1972). Truncal valve incompetence, present in seven of Gelband and associates' series of 12 infants, is presumably secondary to these changes.

The truncal valve overrides the ventricular septum and faces downward and slightly forward. The truncal valve circumference usually equals that of a normal semilunar valve and is never equal to the sum of the aortic and pulmonary valve rings.

The coronary ostia were abnormal in 49 percent of the Van Praagh and Van Praagh (1965) series, the most frequent variant being either right (19 percent) or left (5 percent) coronary arteries arising from the noncoronary cusp.

The ventricular septal defect is usually large and due principally to underdevelopment or virtual absence of the distal part of the pulmonary infundibulum. The defect does not have an upper border, lying as it does just underneath the truncal valve; the lower border is formed by the septal band in the proximal infundibulum. Thus, the defect is commonly very similar to that seen in tetralogy of Fallot (Van Praagh et al., 1970). However, in some cases the defect may be small (Rosenquist et al., 1976).

The truncal valve is in fibrous continuity with the mitral valve in all cases, and also with the tricuspid valve when the septal band is not well developed. Thus, there is no subtruncal conus.

There are two major variants in the anatomy of the pulmonary arteries seen in truncus arteriosus. In the first of these—the most frequent—the aortopulmonary septum is partly formed, so that while the main pulmonary artery is separate in its upper part, the septum is absent below so forming the common trunk. The distal main pulmonary artery gives rise to the right and left pulmonary arteries. In the second variant the aortopulmonary septum is entirely absent: there is no discrete main pulmonary artery, and both pulmonary arterial branches arise separately from the common trunk. In other, rarer, varieties, the right or left pulmonary artery may be absent, with the respective lung being supplied by collaterals. In all these types the primitive fourth arterial arch is well developed. However, in another rare variant, the fourth arch is poorly developed and the sixth arch predominates; this results in a small hypoplastic ascending aorta, or coarctation or atresia of the isthmus. In these cases there is a large persistent ductus arteriosus, which is continuous with the descending aorta (Van Praagh and Van Praagh, 1965).

The aortic arch was on the left in 58 percent of the series of Van Praagh and Van Praagh (1965) and on the right in 21 percent; it was interrupted or absent in 19 percent and unknown in 20 percent. At The Toronto Hospital for Sick Children in a series of 76 cases, 23 (31 percent) had a right aortic arch. This is the same as our experience in tetralogy of Fallot—also 31 percent with right aortic arch.

Associated Anomalies. Associated anomalies do occur, the commonest being persistent ductus arteriosus and coarctation of the aorta. Collett and Edwards (1949) reported single ventricle to occur in 25 percent of cases; however, more recently single

ventricle was not present in 57 autopsy cases of truncus arteriosus (Van Praagh and Van Praagh, 1965), nor was truncus found in 60 autopsy cases of single ventricle (Van Praagh et al., 1964). Multiple congenital noncardiovascular anomalies occur in about 20 percent of cases (Van Praagh and Van Praagh, 1965).

Hemitruncus. This is the name given to a very rare condition in which one pulmonary artery arises normally from the right ventricle while the other, usually supplying the lung opposite to the side of the aortic arch, arises from the ascending aorta. Whether this artery is an aberrant pulmonary artery or an aberrant systemic artery is not clear. If the artery arising from the aorta is small or pulmonary vascular resistance is high, hemitruncus may cause no symptoms and operative interference is not indicated. On the other hand, with low vascular resistance and a large artery, the lung may be overperfused and heart failure develops. In these cases banding of the artery, or even its implantation into the main pulmonary artery (using a graft), may be necessary.

Pseudotruncus. This is the name given by some authors to Collett and Edwards' type IV truncus, where the pulmonary circulation is supplied from the descending aorta. It will be discussed later.

Anatomic Classification

Collett and Edwards in a classic paper in 1949 described five types of truncus arteriosus (Figure 26–1).

Type I: A single pulmonary trunk and an ascending aorta arising from the common trunk.

Type II: The left and right pulmonary arteries arising close together from the posterior or dorsal wall of the truncus.

Type III: Right, left, or both pulmonary arteries arising independently from either side of the truncus.

Type IV: No pulmonary arteries and apparent absence of the sixth arterial arch, the lung being supplied by way of the bronchial arteries.

Type V: Aortopulmonary fenestration.

Other authors have taken issue with the inclusion of type IV as a variety of truncus (Anderson et al., 1957; Kjellberg et al., 1959; Van Praagh and Van Praagh, 1965; Keith et al., 1968). The difference of opinion is one of definition, and while some call this condition "pseudotruncus," it seems reasonable to conclude that type IV is not a variety of truncus as presently defined, since there is not a common trunk giving rise to the three circulations. Although in some cases there are small pulmonary arteries that may join in the midline, in others none can be identified at all. Thus, the single "trunk" in this case is really a solitary aorta, and the pulmonary portion of the truncus arteriosus is absent. McGoon, however, differentiates between type IV truncus and pulmonary arterial atresia

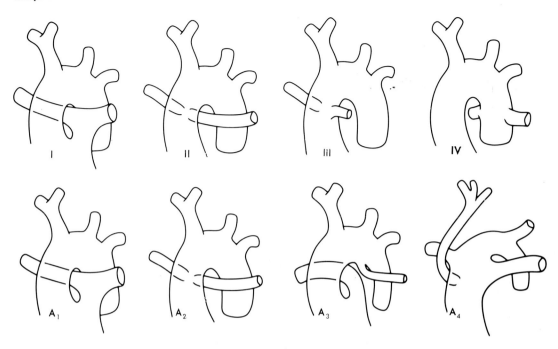

Figure 26-1. The types of persistent truncus arteriosus as described by Collett and Edwards (1949)(, *above*) and by Van Praagh and Van Praagh (1965)(*below.*)

(McGoon et al., 1970). In type IV truncus he includes those patients in whom only one major artery, arising from the descending aorta or arch, supplies each lung; pulmonary arterial atresia is defined in the case where two or more tortuous arteries arise from the descending aorta or arch and run a devious course to each lung. This separation is important from the surgical point of view since those cases with single vessels going to the lung can be offered repair using an external conduit (McGoon et al., 1968). However, from the semantic point of view, it is reasonable to drop the term "pseudotruncus" entirely and consider the type IV truncus of Collett and Edwards under the diagnostic heading of pulmonary outflow tract atresia with a ventricular septal defect, or tetralogy of Fallot with pulmonary atresia. Type V of Collett and Edwards, aortopulmonary window, would not be included today as truncus.

Anderson and coworkers (1957) proposed a modified "practical" classification in which "true truncus arteriosus" was divided into: type I—pulmonary arteries arising from the trunk proximal to the innominate arteries (the same as type I, II, and III of Collett and Edwards); type 2—absence of one pulmonary artery; type 3—absence of both pulmonary arteries; and type 4—partial truncus arteriosus (really aortopulmonary window). "Pseudotruncus" was divided into solitary aortic trunk with pulmonary atresia and solitary pulmonary trunk with aortic atresia. These last two are, by definition, not truncus. Aortopulmonary window, having two trunks arising from the heart by two semilunar valves, is similarly excluded. Tandon and

associates (1963) described a "clinical classification" where type 1 was the same as type I of Collett and Edwards and type 2 was included in their types II and III. They dropped types IV and V.

Van Praagh and Van Praagh (1965), based on an analysis of 57 cases, proposed the following classification : type A—those with a ventricular septal defect; and type B—those without (the latter being excessively rare, with only two specimens described). Type B, however, is probably not truncus, since with two semilunar valves, these two cases probably more closely resemble a variety of aortopulmonary window.

In Van Praagh's classification, type A (Figure 26–1) is subdivided into:

A1: Same as Collett and Edwards Type I.
A2: Same as Collett and Edwards Types II and III.
A3: Absence of one or the other pulmonary artery branches, the respective lung being supplied by collaterals or bronchial arteries, and "hemi-truncus."
A4: Poorly developed fourth arch with the aortic isthmus displaying hypoplasia, coarctation, atresia or absence, and with a large persistent ductus arteriosus.

The frequency of the various types in the Collett and Edwards and Van Praagh and Van Praagh series is shown in Table 26–1. Despite minor differences, it is clear that the types with either the main or both pulmonary artery branches arising from the common trunk comprise 80 to 90 percent of cases.

Table 26–1.   FREQUENCY OF TYPES OF TRUNCUS ARTERIOSUS

COLLETT AND EDWARDS (1949) n = 93	PERCENT	VAN PRAAGH AND VAN PRAAGH (1965) n = 57	PERCENT	CALDER ET AL. (1976) n = 100 PERCENT
Type I	48	Type A1	47	50
Type II	29	Type A2	28	21
		Indefinite (either A1 or A2)		9
Type III	11	Type A3	2	8
		Type A4	23	12
Type IV	12			
	——		——	——
	100		100	100

Physiologic Classification

The clinical picture and natural history of truncus arteriosus in infants and children are largely determined by the size of the pulmonary blood flow. This in turn depends on the pulmonary vascular resistance, or on any narrowing of the pulmonary arteries. From the hemodynamic point of view, cases of truncus arteriosus can be considered as:

Group 1: High pulmonary blood flow with low pulmonary vascular resistance. This is the common picture in infancy and is associated with congestive heart failure very resistant to medical treatment. Cyanosis is often not noted.

Group 2: Normal or only slightly increased pulmonary blood flow, commonly due to increasing pulmonary vascular resistance. These children do not have failure but are cyanosed on exertion.

Group 3: Low pulmonary blood flow. This may be due to (a) ostial narrowing or (b) progressive pulmonary vascular disease. Here cyanosis is marked.

Cases of types A1 and A2 of Van Praagh (Collett and Edwards types I, II, and III) will fall into group 1 early in infancy; since cases present in the first week or month, this suggests a more rapid than normal regression of the fetal pulmonary vasculature. The angulation possibly and any narrowing of the ostia certainly will play a part in slowing down the development of damage in the pulmonary vessel walls: if the child survives the initial high flow situation without protection of the pulmonary vasculature (either natural or acquired at surgery), pulmonary vascular disease will inevitably occur.

The high pulmonary blood flow in group 1 is responsible for the absence or mildness of cyanosis. There is a large pool of pulmonary venous blood returning to the left atrium and being ejected from the left ventricle into the common trunk. The right ventricle is also contracting to systemic pressure and ejecting the systemic venous return into the common trunk. The large ventricular septal defect allows free communication between left and right ventricles, and the resulting admixture of blood determines the depth of cyanosis.

Where the pulmonary blood flow is large, the volume overload on the heart is severe. Any coexisting insufficiency of the truncal valve will make matters worse, as a proportion of the ejected stroke volume regurgitates into the ventricles during diastole. Thus, congestive heart failure is common and as left atrial pressure rises, pulmonary edema and impairment of diffusion of oxygen from alveolus to capillary may cause desaturation of the pulmonary venous blood and increase cyanosis.

When pulmonary vascular resistance starts to climb in hemodynamic groups 2 and 3, the pulmonary venous return declines; although heart failure disappears, and the heart is smaller and the child "healthier," cyanosis will become more marked. Once pulmonary vascular resistance has risen to one-third to one-half systemic levels, this Eisenmenger reaction is probably progressive even though surgical correction—a high risk in these patients—may be successfully carried out.

Prevalence

Truncus arteriosus is a moderately rare condition: in the over 15,000 cases of congenital heart disease seen at The Hospital for Sick Children, truncus had a relative incidence of 0.7 percent. In smaller groups, for instance in children born between 1964 and 1968 and seen by us, its relative incidence was 0.82 percent. Looking at only those children born in the city of Toronto, its frequency is 1.10 percent. And for the general population, since there were 69,695 live births in the city during this period, its incidence is 1 in 11,616 live births or 0.086/1000.

Clinical Features

Children with truncus arteriosus present in the early weeks of life. Of 75 infants seen at The Hospital for Sick Children between 1948 and 1974, 20 (39 percent) were referred in the first week and 49 (65 percent) in the first month of life (Figure 26–2). By three months of age 91 percent had been referred. That it is a major defect with a poor prognosis is underlined by the age at death. Sixty-eight percent of the infants presenting early had died before reaching three months of age. In the series of Calder and associates (1976), the median age at death was five and a half weeks.

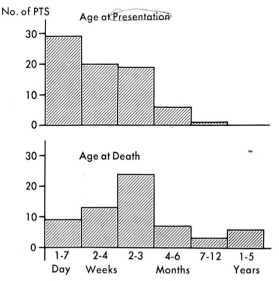

Figure 26-2. Age at presentation and age at death in 75 infants seen at The Hospital for Sick Children, Toronto.

The infants present in congestive heart failure, with or without an added chest infection. The overriding impression of these sick infants is that they have a large left-to-right shunt, since at this stage cyanosis is usually mild, and the clinical features are very similar to those of a child in heart failure due to a ventricular septal defect or a persistent ductus arteriosus. What mild cyanosis is present could be ascribed to pulmonary edema.

Failure to Thrive. Since the course of blood flow in this condition is never normal, difficulty usually dates from birth, and so failure to gain weight is a constant feature. Most infants have gained only a few grams over their birth weight.

Dyspnea. This is prominent because of congestive heart failure. It may take the form of simple tachypnea, with the rate increasing to 50 to 100 beats per minute; but as the condition persists with the addition of congestive heart failure due to excessive pulmonary blood flow, the lungs stiffen as compliance decreases, and breathing becomes labored. However, if the pulmonary blood flow is limited either by pulmonary ostial stenosis or by pulmonary vascular disease, dyspnea is not commonly seen.

Cyanosis. As indicated above, cyanosis in this condition is extremely variable and may be minimal or absent when the pulmonary blood flow is large. Where the pulmonary blood flow is nearly equal to systemic and heart failure is absent, it may be mild at rest, increasing on exertion or crying. However, where the pulmonary blood flow is low, cyanosis can be extremely marked, and accompanied in the older child by plethora, polycythemia, and finger clubbing. The severity of the cyanosis noted in The Hospital for Sick Children series is shown in Figure 26–3. In over one-half of the cases it was graded at 1 + or less when they were first seen in infancy.

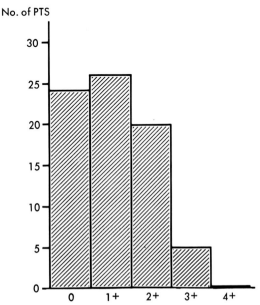

Figure 26-3. Depth of cyanosis noted in The Hospital for Sick Children series.

General Examination. The typical infant is obviously in congestive heart failure, with a hyperactive circulation and left-to-right shunting. The liver is enlarged and there are commonly rales in the chest. The peripheral pulses may be brisk and occasionally have been described as bounding, probably due in part to truncal valve incompetence (Gelband et al., 1972), but also to increased systemic run-off.

Heart Sounds. The first heart sound is usually reported as normal, and the second as loud and ringing. It might be expected that the second sound would invariably be described as single, but this is not the case (Table 26–2): in approximately one-half of cases the second sound has been reported as "closely split." Although this may reflect on the difficulties of accurate auscultation in the newborn period, in a proportion of cases the splitting has been documented by phonocardiography (Victorica et al., 1968). In these cases, either the cusps do not close synchronously, or the duplicated sound is set up by vibration in the arterial trunks.

Table 26–2. CHARACTERISTICS OF SECOND HEART SOUND

	SINGLE	SPLIT	UNSPECIFIED	TOTAL CASES
Tandon et al. (1963)	6	8	5	19
McNamara and Somerville (1968)	21	18	2	41
Calder et al. (1976)	42	38	20	100
Hospital for Sick Children, Toronto	30	34	10	74
Total	99	98	37	234

Ejection Clicks. A characteristic finding is a very prominent apical systolic ejection click heard in nearly every case.

Murmurs. Most patients are described as having systolic murmurs, if they live long enough. In some cases the murmur is described as pansystolic, harsh, and maximal in the third and fourth left intercostal spaces similar to a murmur arising from a ventricular septal defect. In others the murmur is described as ejection type, maximal at the left sternal border. A middiastolic murmur of relative mitral stenosis, maximal inside the apex, has also been reported in some cases. A continuous murmur is rarely reported, but an early diastolic murmur was heard in 36 percent of the series of Calder and coworkers (1976); however, in less than half of these was there angiographic or autopsy evidence of truncal insufficiency.

The Hospital for Sick Children's experience is illustrated in Figure 26–4. In 11 infants no murmur was heard and pansystolic and ejection murmurs were present in equal numbers. Early diastolic murmurs were noted less frequently than in Calder's 1976 series. In some children the systolic murmur is well conducted laterally and sounded similar to the murmur of pulmonary artery stenosis.

Victorica and colleagues (1968) reported a phonocardiographic study of 13 infants with truncus and confirmed the constant finding of an ejection click that did not vary with respiration. The ejection systolic murmur always ended before the second heart sound, which was wide in all cases (0.04 to 0.05 second). Four patients showed two discrete components of the second sound, which the authors believe was due to asynchronous tensing of the trunk and pulmonary arteries.

When a thrill was present, it was maximal at the lower left sternal edge, although occasionally also felt at the upper sternum or in the suprasternal notch.

Radiologic Examination

A consistent feature in the appearance of the cardiac shadow on x-ray is that it is large. Chest films in 60 infants taken at first presentation at The Hospital for Sick Children showed a cardiothoracic ratio of 55 percent or more in 56 cases and 64 percent

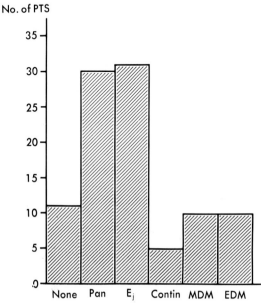

Figure 26-4. Types of murmurs heard in The Hospital for Sick Children series.

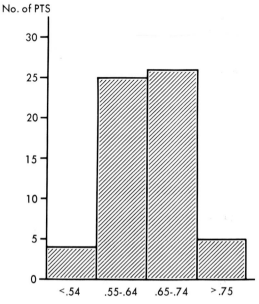

Figure 26-5. Cardiothoracic ratio on chest x-ray in The Hospital for Sick Children series.

or more in 31 cases (Figure 26–5). The mean was 65 percent and the range 52 to 88 percent. Tandon and associates (1963) reported 74 percent with "gross cardiomegaly," and McNamara and Somerville (1968), 84 percent with cardiothoracic ratios greater than 60 percent. Calder and coworkers (1976) reported cardiomegaly in all, with a median cardiothoracic ratio of 65 percent and a range of 51 to 81 percent. The cardiac outline has no specific shape. Both right and left ventricles are enlarged, and the pedicle usually appears narrow. Taussig (1947) described a sharp angulation of "shelf" on the left heart border below the pulmonary artery bay, but this is not a very common feature. Victorica and colleagues (1969) reported that in 11 of their 14 cases the cardiovascular silhouette resembled the "egg shape" commonly associated with complete transposition of the great arteries, but with the upper left border being straighter than in transposition.

Pulmonary plethora is marked, since the large majority of cases have increased pulmonary blood flow. Perhaps the most characteristic feature is a high origin of the pulmonary arteries. This may be seen on the right, but more typically on the left (Figure 26–6). A right aortic arch occurred in 31 percent of our cases, and the combination of pulmonary plethora and a right aortic arch should make one suspect truncus. However, it should be realized that there is extreme variability in the x-ray picture.

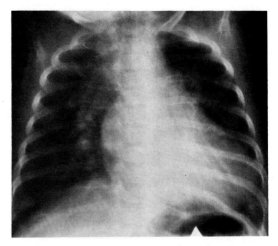

Figure 26-6. Chest x-ray in a patient with truncus arteriosus.

Echocardiography

Ultrasound is a new technique in the study of infants and children with congenital heart disease. In truncus arteriosus it is usually possible to record an echo that shows that the trunk overrides the ventricular septum. There is no anterior vessel, and no echoes arising from a pulmonary valve (Figure 26–7).

overriding trunk

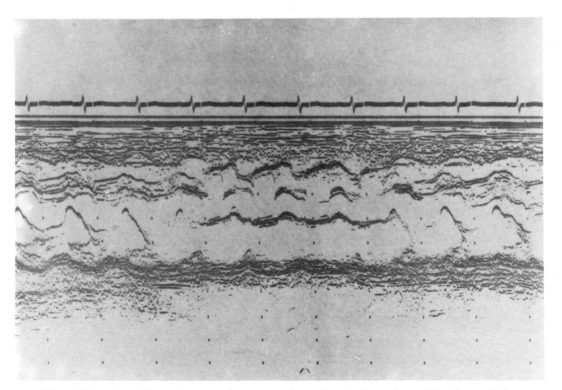

Figure 26-7. Echocardiogram in a case of truncus arteriosus, showing the trunk overriding the ventricular septum.

The absence of pulmonary valve echoes is what distinguishes the echocardiogram in truncus from that in tetralogy of Fallot (Chung et al., 1973), since the appearance of aortic overriding and absence of septal-aortic discontinuity are the same in each. Since the pulmonary valve echoes may be difficult to record, the failure to elicit them does not exclude tetralogy. The clinical picture will usually help here, since tetralogy is not a normal differential diagnosis for truncus in infancy. Shematek and colleagues (1977) have reported that cases of truncus have a large left atrium, compared to infants with tetralogy, and frequently (67 percent) have reduplications in the semilunar valve echoes.

Electrocardiography

In the series of 63 electrocardiograms available for analysis in this hospital, the mean QRS axis in the frontal plane varied between 0 and 240°, with a mean of 100° (Figure 26-8). The pattern of ventricular hypertrophy was also varied. As can be seen in Figure 26-9, while 14 percent had a normal ventricular loading pattern for their age, 15 percent had left and 35 percent right ventricular hypertrophy. In 36 percent combined ventricular hypertrophy was seen. Tandon and associates (1963) reported 79 percent with left or combined ventricular hypertrophy patterns, and McNamara and Somerville (1968), 71 percent with combined ventricular hypertrophy. Calder and coworkers (1976) reported combined hypertrophy in 45 percent, right in 20 percent and left in 20 percent. No specific electrocardiographic features have been identified. The vectorcardiogram is little different from those recorded in more simple lesions with the same degree of ventricular overload, and Victorica and associates (1968) reported

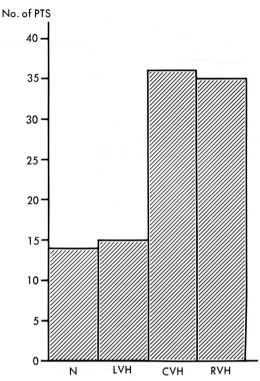

Figure 26-9. Ventricular hypertrophy pattern in The Hospital for Sick Children series.

combined ventricular hypertrophy in 70 percent of 14 cases.

▶Hemodynamics

Cardiac catheterization and angiocardiography are central to the diagnosis of this condition and good clear angiocardiograms are vital.

The venous catheter enters the right ventricle normally, and the pressure here is at systemic level. There is usually a step-up in oxygen saturation suggesting a ventricular septal defect. The catheter tip may pass easily out of the truncal valve, which may be in the position of the normal pulmonary artery. If difficulty is experienced, a Swan-Ganz catheter is often effective. When the catheter tip passes from the trunk into either the pulmonary artery branches or the aorta, two erroneous conclusions may be entertained:

1. That there is a ductus arteriosus and the catheter is passing from a normal pulmonary artery into the descending aorta, or

2. That there is an aortopulmonary window, and the catheter is passing through it into the ascending aorta and brachiocephalic branches. To make this clear, good angiograms are necessary. The oxygen saturation of the blood in the truncus is usually quite high, and in the 40 cases studied in infancy at The Hospital for Sick Children, while it varied between 44

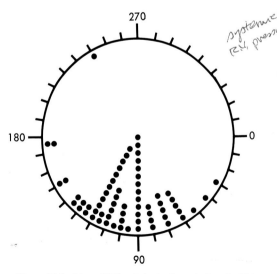

Figure 26-8. Mean QRS axis in the frontal plane in 63 cases of truncus arteriosus.

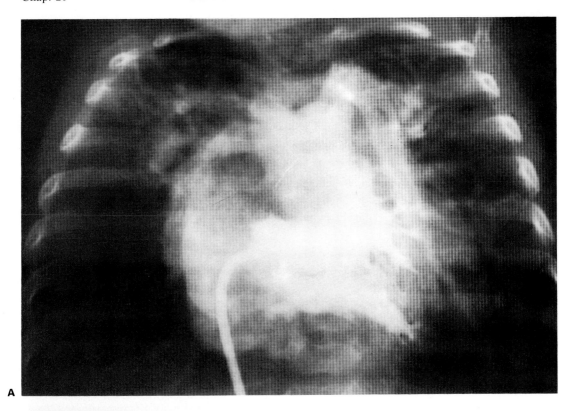

A

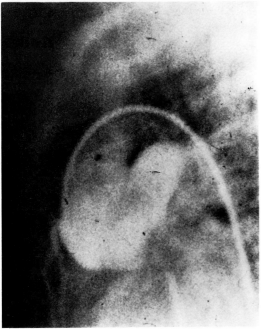

B

Figure 26-10. *A*. Selective ventricular angiocardiogram in a case of truncus arteriosus. *B*. Selective injection above the truncal valve.

and 93 percent, the mean was 83 percent. This would be compatible with the absence or mildness of clinical cyanosis.

The oxygen saturation in the pulmonary arteries is usually the same as that in the trunk but not invariably, as some streaming may occur. The pressure in the pulmonary artery branches is, in the majority of cases, equal to that in the trunk. Any significant gradient suggests either true or relative stenosis of the ostia. In cases in infancy, pulmonary capillary wedge as well as left ventricular end-diastolic and left atrial pressure is likely to be elevated

pulmonary hypertension

due to heart failure. Calculation of pulmonary blood flow shows that this is high in these cases, ranging from two to four times systemic, and that the calculated pulmonary vascular resistance is low. With time there is an inevitable development of pulmonary vascular disease: with the increase in pulmonary vascular resistance, pulmonary blood flow falls, and the systemic oxygen saturation is lower.

Angiocardiography

As indicated previously, this is the cornerstone of correct diagnosis in truncus arteriosus. In order to be certain of the anatomy, the injection should be made into the trunk and filmed in both anteroposterior and lateral projections. It may be necessary to pass a catheter retrogradely up an artery into the trunk to obtain the best injection. When this is done, the anatomy can be most clearly seen.

Ventricular injections will show dilated cavities communicating through a large ventricular septal defect lying just below the truncal valve, which overrides the ventricular septum. The truncal valve is usually of normal semilunar valve size. It sits in the normal position of the aortic valve in fibrous continuity with the mitral valve, since there is no conus intervening. The truncal valve, which is easily seen because it is thickened and may be polypoid, tends to face slightly anteriorly. This is a help in differentiating this condition from transposition, in which the aortic valve faces more forward; tetralogy of Fallot, where it faces straight down; and normal, where it faces more posteriorly (Calder et al., 1976). The origin of the main pulmonary artery from the posterior or left side of the trunk can usually be identified in the most common variety (Figure 26–10A). However, it is usually extremely difficult to tell even in the best angiograms whether or not there is a short main pulmonary artery (Figure 26–10B), or whether the branches are arising separately but close together. The clinical diagnosis often is "type 1½", and this point may only be resolved at surgery. The left pulmonary artery may arch higher than the right. The aortic arch is on the right in one-third of cases. Rarely either the right or left pulmonary arteries may be absent, the lung deriving its blood supply most often from bronchials. In some cases coarctation or aortic arch atresia may be identified.

Diagnosis

The usual presentation is of an infant in the first weeks of life who has failed to thrive from birth, and who has shown dyspnea. A murmur of doubtful significance has normally been heard, but cyanosis is an inconstant and variable feature.

On examination the infant is usually distressed with mild cyanosis. The pulses are present and may be brisk, the liver and the heart are enlarged, and there is usually an ejection systolic murmur and a well-marked ejection click. A middiastolic murmur may be heard, or an early diastolic murmur. The second sound is usually single but may be thick or split. The x-ray shows an enlarged heart with pulmonary plethora and the aortic arch may be on the right. The electrocardiogram shows combined, right, or left ventricular hypertrophy, with a frontal QRS axis of about $+100°$.

The initial assessment is usually of a large left-to-right shunt, caused by a large ventricular septal defect or a persistent ductus arteriosus. If the cyanosis is more marked, transposition of the great arteries with a ventricular septal defect may be considered. However, in ventricular septal defect and ductus, the second heart sound should be split; early diastolic murmurs are rare in transposition. Endocardial cushion defects show left-axis deviation on the electrocardiogram. Preductal coarctation of the aorta may be suspected since it is a common cause of heart failure in this age group. Aortic atresia or hypoplastic left heart syndrome would be excluded by the good peripheral pulses and the presence of increased left ventricular forces in the precordial electrocardiogram. In tricuspid atresia with transposition of the great arteries there are usually no right ventricular forces.

Helpful echocardiographic findings may be those of a single large great artery arising over the ventricular septum with reduplicated cusp echoes, no pulmonary artery echo, and a large left atrium.

The diagnosis will be made with certainty only from good angiograms. The most common error in the past has been confusion with ductus arteriosus and a ventricular septal defect, with or without coarctation of the aorta. Here, however, two great arteries arising from the heart should be seen. In aortopulmonary window, an aortic root injection may give the appearance of truncus. However, here again, a main pulmonary artery arising in front of the aorta and filling through the window should be seen in the lateral shot. In pulmonary atresia or aortic atresia, the atretic vessel can often be seen.

Prognosis

The prognosis in the past has been poor in this condition, and the median age at death in the series of Calder and coworkers (1976) was five weeks, ranging from nine hours to 14 years. The experience at The Hospital for Sick Children, Toronto, is illustrated in Figure 26–11. Only 36 percent of the children were still alive at three months, and only 22 percent (10 children) survived the first year. Death is usually from congestive heart failure, often with pneumonia associated.

Some cases do survive for longer periods and we have seen seven patients who are alive at over 20 years of age. They are all cyanosed and moderately limited and have no evidence of pulmonary vascular disease.

However, with the success of palliative procedures in infancy and corrective procedures in childhood the

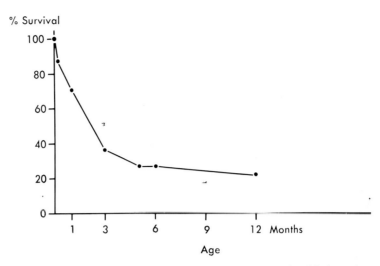

Figure 26-11. Graph of survival in cases seen at The Hospital for Sick Children.

prognosis will improve. It is likely, however, that in these children, truncal valve incompetence may be a major clinical problem (Deeley et al., 1963; Gelband et al., 1972).

Treatment

The initial treatment is of congestive heart failure and often of coincident chest infection. However, digoxin and diuretics rarely produce a significant improvement in those children with a very large pulmonary blood flow. Gelband and associates (1972) felt that truncal valve incompetence was an important hemodynamic feature of those cases with resistant heart failure, but this has not been our experience. However, early cardiac catheterization is indicated, and once the diagnosis has been made, the only hope for survival lies in surgery. Since children with truncus arteriosus with naturally occurring pulmonary artery stenosis tend to survive longer, surgical pulmonary artery banding is indicated (Smith et al., 1963; Heilbrunn et al., 1964; Kriedberg et al., 1964); banding will reduce the pulmonary blood flow, relieve the congestive heart failure, and protect the lungs from progressive pulmonary vascular disease. However, it is a procedure of considerable difficulty in a small and severely ill infant, and of the 15 infants with truncus in whom it has been attempted in The Hospital for Sick Children, only six have benefited from it, while nine have died. The success of this palliative procedure has become even more important with the development of a successful corrective operation. Following experiments in animals (Arai et al., 1965; Rastelli et al., 1967), McGoon and associates (1968) reported a successful case. The child was five and a half years old and had a gradient between the trunk and the pulmonary arteries of 42 to 53 mm of mercury. They detached the main pulmonary artery from the back of the truncus and then closed the ventricular septal defect so that the left ventricle alone ejected into the trunk, thus converting the trunk into an aorta. They

then attached an aortic homograft with its valve, proximally to a hole cut in the anterior surface of the right ventricle and distally to the distal main pulmonary artery stump (Figure 26–12). A similar

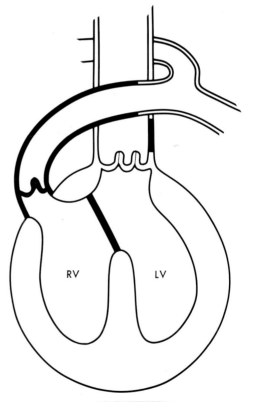

Figure 26-12. The Rastelli procedure for persistent truncus arteriosus. The pulmonary artery or arteries are removed from the trunk; the septal defect is closed so that the left ventricle alone ejects into the trunk, which thus becomes an aorta. A conduit—formerly an aortic homograft, but currently a valved dacron tube—is placed from the anterior right ventricular wall to the pulmonary arteries.

but unsuccessful attempt had previously been made by Cooley and Hallman (1966) using a Dacron tube and a prosthetic valve. Subsequent results with this procedure were encouraging (McGoon et al., 1970), but in the long term, calcification (which commonly occurs in pericardial grafts placed in the outflow tract of the right ventricle in tetralogy of Fallot) has been reported in the walls of this aortic homograft (McGoon et al., 1972). This has caused a switch to Dacron conduits with porcine (Hancock) valves. These do well.

As might be expected, the success of the operation depends in large part on the pulmonary vascular resistance. Where this is high, mortality is 60 percent, and where low, 17 percent (McGoon et al., 1970). The risk also seems high under five and over 12 years of age. Therefore, a prerequisite for this procedure is a low pulmonary vascular resistance, which will most likely occur where the pulmonary arteries are naturally narrow at their origin or where pulmonary artery banding has been successfully carried out. Midchildhood appears to be an ideal time (McGoon et al., 1973).

Because of the unrewarding results of palliation, Kirklin (1973) has suggested (on the basis of one successful case of his own and two of Barrett-Boyes) that definitive repair with the valved conduit should be carried out in the first year of life in patients who do not have ostial stenosis and have torrential pulmonary blood flow. He recognizes that the conduit may have to be replaced by a larger one at five to ten years of age, but believes this should be relatively easy. This has recently been carried out with success in a number of centers (Applebaum et al., 1976; Ebert et al., 1976; Singh et al., 1976; Sullivan et al., 1976).

In conclusion, truncus arteriosus is a potentially highly lethal, but rare, variety of congenital heart disease. The optimal plan of management for the common varieties of truncus at the present time is vigorous treatment of the congestive heart failure at presentation in infancy, followed shortly by accurate anatomic diagnosis by angiocardiography. Pulmonary artery banding is indicated for those children with large flow and high pressure in the pulmonary arteries, to be followed after the age of five years by the Rastelli procedure. Early definitive repair in infancy may become the treatment of choice.

REFERENCES

Anderson, R. C.; Obata, W.; and Lillehei, C. W.: Truncus arteriosus. Clinical study of 14 cases. *Circulation*, **16**:586, 1957.

Applebaum, A.; Bargeon, L. M., Jr.; Pacifico, A. D.; and Kirklin, J. W.: Surgical treatment of truncus arteriosus with emphasis on infants and small children. *J. Thorac. Cardiovasc. Surg.*, **71**:436, 1976.

Arai, T.; Tzzuki, Y.; Nogi, M.; Kurashige, K.; Koyanangi, H.; Nishida, H.; Ikeda, Y.; and Ichikawa, H.: Experimental study on bypass between the right ventricle and pulmonary artery, left ventricle and pulmonary artery, and left ventricle and aorta by means of homograft with valve. *Bull. Heart. Inst. Jap.*, **49**:62, 1965.

Bharati, S.; McAllister, H.; Rosenquist, G.; Miller, R.; Tatooles, C.;

and Lev, M.: The surgical anatomy of truncus arteriosus communis. *J. Thorac. Cardiovasc. Surg.*, **67**:501, 1974.

Buchanan, A.: Malformation of heart. Undivided truncus arteriosus. Heart otherwise double. *Trans. Pathol. Soc. Lond.*, **15**:89, 1864.

Calder, L.; Van Praagh, R.; Van Praagh, S.; Sears, W. P.; Corwin, P.; Levy, A.; Keith, J. D.; and Paul, M. H.: Truncus arteriosus communis. *Am. Heart J.*, **92**:23, 1976.

Collett, R. W., and Edwards, J. E.: Persistent truncus arteriosus: A classification according to anatomic types. *Surg. Clin. North Am.*, **29**:1245, 1949.

Cooley, D. A., and Hallman, G. L.: *Surgical Treatment of Congenital Heart Disease*. Lea & Febiger, Philadelphia, 1966.

Deeley, W. J.; Hagstrom, J. W. C.; and Engle, M. A.: Truncus insufficiency: Common truncus arteriosus with regurgitant truncus valve. *Am. Heart J.*, **65**:542, 1963.

Ebert, P. A.; Robinson, S. J.; Stanger, P.; and Engle, M. A.: Pulmonary artery conduits in infants younger than six months of age. *J. Thorac. Cardiovasc. Surg.*, **72**:351, 1976.

Edwards, J.: Persistent truncus arteriosus: A comment. *Am. Heart J.*, **92**:1, 1976.

Feller, A.: Zur Kenntnis der angeborene Herzkrankheiten; Truncus arteriosus communis persitens und seine formale Entstehung, *Virchows Arch. [Path. Anat.]*, **279**:869, 1931.

Gasul, B. M.; Arcilla, R. A.; and Lev, M.: *Heart Disease in Children. Diagnosis and Treatment*. J. B. Lippincott Co., Philadelphia, 1966.

Gelband, H.; Van Meter, S.; and Gersony, W. M: Truncal valve abnormalities in infants with persistent truncus arteriosus. A clinicopathological study. *Circulation*, **45**:397, 1972.

Heilbrunn, A.; Kittle, F.; and Deihl, A. M.: Pulmonary arterial banding in the treatment of truncus arteriosus. *Circulation*, Suppl., **29**:102, 1964.

Keith, J. D.; Rowe, R. D.; and Vlad, P.: *Heart Disease in Infancy and Childhood*. Macmillan Publishing Co., Inc., New York, 1958.

Keith, J. D.; Rowe, R. D.; and Vlad, P.: *Heart Disease in Infancy and Childhood*, 2nd ed. Macmillan Publishing Co., Inc., New York, 1968.

Kjellberg, S. R.; Mannheimer, E.; Rudhe, M.; and Jonsson, B.: *Diagnosis of Congenital Heart Disease*. Year Book Medical Publishers, Inc., Chicago, 1959, p. 330.

Kriedberg, M. B.; Fisher, J. H.; de Luca, F. G.; and Chernoff, H. L.: Pulmonary artery banding for persistent truncus arteriosus. *J. Pediatr.*, **64**:557, 1964.

Lev, M., and Saphir, O.: Truncus arteriosus communis persistens. *J. Pediatr.*, **20**:74, 1942.

McNamara, D. G., and Somerville, K. J.: Truncus arteriosus. In: *Heart Disease in Infants, Children and Adolescents*, A. J. Moss and F. H. Adams (eds.) Williams & Wilkins, Baltimore, 1968.

McGoon, D. C.; Rastelli, G. C.; and Ongley, P. A.: An operation for the correction of truncus arteriosus. *JAMA*, **205**:69, 1968.

McGoon, D. C.; Rastelli, G. C.; and Wallace, R. B.: Discontinuity between right ventricle and pulmonary artery. Surgical treatment. *Ann Surg.*, **172**:698, 1970.

McGoon, D. C.; Wallace, R. B.; and Danielson, G. K.: Homografts in reconstruction of congenital cardiac anomalies. Expanded operability in complex congenital heart disease. *Mayo Clin. Proc.*, **47**:101, 1972.

McGoon, D. C.; Wallace, R. B.; and Danielson, G. K.: The Rastelli operation. Its indications and results. *J. Thorac. Cardiovasc. Surg.*, **65**:865, 1973.

Rastelli, G. C.; Titus, J. L.; and McGoon, D. C.: Homograft of ascending aorta and aortic valve as a right ventricular outflow: An experimental approach to the repair of truncus arteriosus. *Arch. Surg.*, **95**:698, 1967.

Roos, A.: Persistent truncus arteriosus communis. *Am. J. Dis. Child.*, **50**:966, 1935.

Rosenquist, G. C.; Bharati, S.; McAllister, H. A.; and Lev, M.: Truncus arteriosus communis: Truncal valve anomalies associated with small conal or truncal septal defects. *Am. J. Cardiol.*, **37**:410, 1975.

Shematek, J.; Roland, J. M.; Kidd, B. S. L.; and Pieroni, D. R.: Truncal valve echoes in the differentiation of truncus arteriosus from tetralogy of Fallot. *Pediatr. Res.*, **11**:400, 1977.

Singh, A. K.; De Laval, M. R.; Pincott, J. R.; and Stark, J.: Pulmonary artery banding for truncus arteriosus in the first year of life. *Circulation*, **54**:(Suppl. III) 17, 1976.

Smith, G. W.; Thompson, W. M., Jr.: Dammann, J. F., Jr.; and Muller, W. H., Jr.: Use of the pulmonary artery banding procedure in treating type II truncus arteriosus. *Circulation,* **28**:807, 1963.

Sullivan, H.; Sulagman, R.; Replogle, R.; and Arulla, R.: Surgical correction of truncus arteriosus in infancy. *Am. J. Cardiol.,* **38**:113, 1976.

Tandon, R.; Hauck, A. J.; and Nadas, A. S.: Persistent truncus arteriosus: A clinical, hemodynamic and autopsy study of 19 cases. *Circulation,* **28**:1050, 1963.

Taussig, H. B.: Clinical and pathological findings in cases of truncus arteriosus in infancy. *Am. J. Med.,* **2**:26, 1947.

Van Praagh, R.: Classification of truncus arteriosus communis (TAC). *Am. Heart J.,* **92**:129, 1976.

Van Praagh, R.; Ongley, P. A.; and Swan, H. J. C.: Anatomic types of single and common ventricle in man. Morphologic and geometric aspects of 60 necropsied cases. *Am. J. Cardiol.,* **13**:367, 1964.

Van Praagh, R., and Van Praagh, S.: The anatomy of common aortico-pulmonary trunk (truncus arteriosus communis) and its embryological implication. A study of 57 necropsy cases. *Am. J. Cardiol.,* **16**:406, 1965.

Van Praagh, R.; Van Praagh, S.; Nebesar, R. A.; Muster, A. J.; Sinha, S. N.; and Paul, M. H.: Tetralogy of Fallot: Underdevelopment of the pulmonary infundibulum and its sequelae. *Am. J. Cardiol.,* **26**:25, 1970.

Victorica, B.; Gessner, I.; and Schiebler, G.: Phonocardiographic findings in persistent truncus arteriosus. *Br. Heart J.,* **30**:812, 1968.

Victorica, B. E.; Krovetz, L. J.; Elliott, L. P.; Van Mierop, L. H. S.; Bartley, T. D.; Gessner, I. H.; and Schiebler, G. L.: Persistent truncus arteriosus in infancy. *Am. Heart J.,* **77**:13, 1969.

27

Tetralogy of Fallot

Richard D. Rowe

T HE FIRST description of the anatomic defects now known as the tetralogy was made by the Dane, Nicholas Stensen (Willius, 1948), although it was Fallot, in a scholarly series of papers dated 1888, who separated the malformation from other types of *maladie bleue*. His name has become firmly associated with this congenital malformation. William Hunter (1784) reported a case in detail, and a number of autopsy descriptions are available in the medical literature of the nineteenth century.

Anatomy

Classically the tetralogy of Fallot consists of stenosis of the right ventricular outflow tract at one or more of various levels, a ventricular septal defect, right ventricular hypertrophy, and an aorta that straddles the septal defect at its origin.

Debate continues over what should properly be classified under the long-established title of the malformation. There are those who believe the only important clinical components of the malformation are ventricular septal defect and pulmonary stenosis, so that irrespective of the size or position of the ventricular communication or the degree of pulmonary stenosis, such patients are regarded as part of a clinical and hemodynamic spectrum of the malformation (McCord et al., 1957). Others prefer to confine the term *tetralogy of Fallot* to those with a large, specifically arranged ventricular communication with sufficient pulmonary stenosis to result in right-to-left shunting of blood. For this school the inclusion under tetralogy of Fallot of small ventricular defect with varying degrees of pulmonary stenosis or various-sized ventricular septal defects with trivial pulmonary stenosis is felt to be illogical. On the other hand, such a classification would exclude those patients with ventricular defects of the type classically observed in the frankly cyanotic tetralogy of Fallot in whom the development of hemodynamic and clinical evidence of infundibular stenosis is an acquired phenomenon (Gasul et al., 1957, Bécu et al., 1961) and would permit inclusion of patients with

subpulmonic ventricular septal defects (McGoon, 1971) or atrioventricularis communis (Lev et al., 1961; Fisher et al., 1975).

Definition has not yet been, and will not likely ever be, resolved to everyone's satisfaction. Our own view coincides with that proposed by Kirklin and Karp (1970): (1) the ventricular septal defect is large, (2) there is always anatomic abnormality of the pulmonary infundibulum (we would include angiographic evidence as well as operative), and (3) there is fibrous continuity of the aortic and mitral valves.

Primary Anatomic Considerations. VENTRICULAR SEPTAL DEFECT. The defect is large and only rarely will there be more than one. It is situated in the anterior part of the ventricular septum and, as usually described, frequently involves the membranous septum. The defect is confluent with the aortic ring and lies beneath the posterior part of the right and the anterior part of the posterior aortic cusp. Viewed from the right ventricle, the septal defect lies posterior to the crista between it and the anterior and medial leaflets of the tricuspid valve. Minor variations in the position of the defect occur (Lev and Eckner, 1964). The analysis of 112 specimens by Rosenquist and associates (1973) indicates that in almost two-thirds the ventricular defect is bounded posteriorly by muscle or a fibrous band possibly representing an inferior division of the embryonic infundibular septum that separates it from the membranous ventricular septum.

AORTIC RELATIONSHIP. An aortic root overriding or straddling the ventricular septal defect was part of the original description of the tetralogy. Classification of the degree of override was attempted from autopsy and angiographic means (Donzelot et al., 1949; Berri et al., 1952; Glover et al., 1952; Baffes et al., 1953; Brinton and Campbell, 1953; Johns et al., 1953; Kjellberg et al., 1959), but it was recognized by surgeons that such terminology was misleading in that reconstitution of the septal integrity by surgery without further plasty resulted in normal aortic–left ventricular relationships after repair. This concept of a normal aortic root position was not entirely accepted even by eminent pathologists (Lev, 1959;

Edwards, 1960; Goor et al., 1971), and difficulty naturally arose over patients who showed "extreme" dextroposition (Bahnson and Ziegler, 1950). The contributions of Van Praagh and Van Praagh (1965) to this problem have been widely accepted. For them a necessary part of tetralogy of Fallot is maintenance of normal fibrous continuity between the aortic and mitral valves. The aortic root is rotated to a variable degree so that the noncoronary cusp of the aortic valves lies more or less to the patient's right and more anterior than normally. Thus, whereas the anterior leaflet of the mitral valve is normally directly related to the noncoronary aortic cusp, in tetralogy of Fallot it has more continuity with the left aortic cusp. Posteriorly part of the noncoronary cusp is in relation to the ventricular defect as is the commissure between the noncoronary and the right aortic cusp somewhat more anteriorly (Kirklin and Karp, 1970).

For Goor and associates (1971) and Becker and associates (1975), on the other hand, the basic abnormality includes both conal malrotation and malseptation, which would place aortic dextroposition as a constant feature of the anomaly. They are inclined to view Fallot's tetralogy as part of a spectrum of ventricular septal defect and conal abnormality, which ranges from extreme tetralogy of Fallot with pulmonary atresia to simple ventricular septal defect, depending on the degree of anterior deviation of the conal septum.

PULMONARY STENOSIS. Few would now disagree with the view that an essential part of the complex of the tetralogy of Fallot lies in a disturbance of the right ventricular muscle bundle architecture and that therefore all patients with the tetralogy have narrowing of the infundibulum of some degree. In fact, some would go further and call the malformation the monology of Fallot (Van Praagh et al., 1970). For them the small size of the conus muscle made up by the parietal band and the adjacent free wall of the infundibulum are the primary cause of all other major parts of the malformation. Not all agree with this view (Goor et al., 1971; Becker et al., 1975).

The crista supraventricularis is rotated into a more vertical position. The septal band is hypertrophied, and the parietal band is deviated anteriorly away from the base of the tricuspid valve. The chordae that normally arise from adjacent portions of the anterior and septal leaflets of the tricuspid valve and insert into the ventricular septum at the papillary muscle to the conus are abnormally placed in the tetralogy of Fallot and are inserted usually at the lower edge of the ventricular septal defect. Thus the ventricular communication is located between the posteriorly displaced papillary muscle of the conus and the displaced crista. The degree of abnormality of the crista undoubtedly determines the size of the ostium infundibuli at birth and will determine whether or not the patient will exhibit pronounced cyanosis at that time (Lev, 1959; Edwards, 1960; Bécu et al., 1961).

Although the obstruction to pulmonary blood flow is primarily intracardiac and subvalvar, additional obstruction may occur at the pulmonary valve and

beyond. Earlier experiences from autopsy and operation reported different frequencies for the various sites of obstruction to pulmonary blood flow (Burke et al., 1951; Berri et al., 1952; Donzelot et al., 1952; Glover et al., 1952; Baffes et al., 1953; Brinton and Campbell, 1953; Brock et al., 1953; Johns et al., 1953; Hospital for Sick Children, Toronto, 1964). More pertinent are those recent papers that have examined the problem by relating the findings at open heart surgery to the anatomy visualized after selective right ventricular angiocardiography (Kirklin, 1968; McMyn, 1969; McGoon, 1971).

INFUNDIBULAR STENOSIS. Many different degrees and positions of the stenotic site within the outflow tract have been found, but there is general agreement that there are three major types of infundibular stenosis in this malformation.

Low Infundibular Stenosis (Figure 27–1). This is an obstruction at the ostium infundibulum that is associated with a large and well-developed infundibular chamber leading to a normally sized pulmonary valve ring, and usually a normal pulmonary valve. About 10 percent of such patients

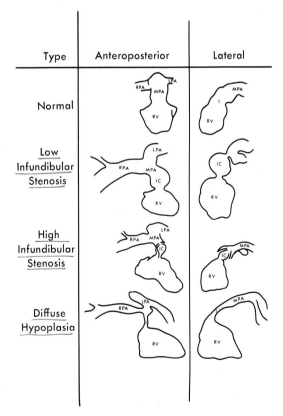

Figure 27-1. Diagrams from anteroposterior and lateral cineangiocardiograms of the various forms of infundibular stenosis in the tetralogy of Fallot (see pages 471, 472). To simplify, the aorta has not been drawn. *LPA,* left pulmonary artery; *RPA,* right pulmonary artery; *MPA,* main pulmonary artery; *I,* infundibulum; *IC,* infundibular chamber; *V,* pulmonary valve; *RV,* right ventricle.

have valvular stenosis. This type is the most common form of infundibular stenosis and probably accounts for as many as 40 percent of all operated cases.

High Infundibular Stenosis (Figure 27–1). In this situation the chamber above the obstruction is small and pulmonary valvular stenosis is common. Less commonly the valve is normal. High infundibular stenosis is present in about a third of all operated patients.

Diffuse Hypoplasia (Figure 27–1). In this form, the whole outflow tract of the right ventricle is considerably reduced in caliber and terminates in a small pulmonary valve ring. Pulmonary valvular stenosis occurs in about one-quarter of all such cases. It is the most serious form of obstruction in the average case because of the frequent need for extension of the repair beyond a simple operative resection (Kirklin, 1968).

McMyn (1969) describes an uncommon muscular form of stenosis that angiographically shows great mobility within the cardiac cycle and may correspond to the isolated valvular stenosis referred to by McGoon (1971).

VALVULAR STENOSIS. According to McMyn, (1969) more than 70 percent of patients with pulmonary valvar stenosis in the tetralogy have bicuspid pulmonary valve. The incidence of valvular stenosis is least in the patients with low infundibular stenosis and greatest in those with diffuse hypoplasia.

VALVULAR ATRESIA *(Figure 27–2)*. This represents the extreme form of obstruction at the valve. It may be present as a thin diaphragm occluding the ring but more commonly exists as a thick portion of ventricular wall with no obvious connection to pulmonary artery. In autopsy series pulmonary atresia of this type is present for approximately one-quarter of the specimens. Some patients with severe pulmonary stenosis but nevertheless documented passage between the right ventricle and pulmonary artery have been noted to acquire atresia at a previously stenotic site over the course of years. This has occurred most frequently in patients who have had satisfactory shunt procedures performed earlier in life and for whom selective angiocardiography prior to a latter corrected operation demonstrated the presence of pulmonary atresia (Fabricius et al., 1961). Roberts and coworkers (1969) reported such a change in four adult patients an average of 16 years after the initial shunt. Such atresia may develop in the infundibulum itself (Sabiston, 1964) as well as at the valve where calcification is an important component.

Absence of the pulmonary valve (Miller et al., 1962) is a bizarre form of abnormality where abortive valvular tissue is present at the junction of the sinus pocket wall in the pulmonary artery with the myocardium. Because of the inadequacy of the valvular tissue, pulmonary arteries beyond are aneurysmal in type. The valve ring is always very small and frequently there is associated infundibular stenosis. About one in every ten of these particular patients will have absence of the left pulmonary artery in addition. In general, absence of the pulmonary valve occurs in about 3 percent of any large series of patients with tetralogy of Fallot (Hospital for Sick Children, Toronto, 1967; Nagao et al., 1967).

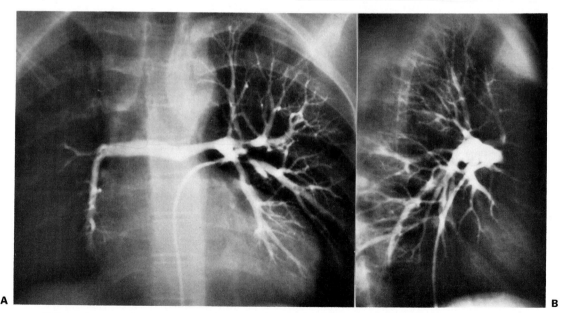

A   **B**

Figure 27-2. Pulmonary atresia in tetralogy of Fallot. Selective injection of a bronchial collateral vessel from the descending aorta clearly outlines in anteroposterior (*A*) and lateral (*B*) projections the state of the pulmonary arteries. The main pulmonary artery retains contrast because no blood is being ejected into it directly from the right ventricle; i.e., the valve is atretic. (Courtesy of Dr. R. I. White, Jr., The Johns Hopkins Hospital, Baltimore, Maryland.)

DISTAL PULMONARY TRACT⊕The remainder of the pulmonary tract, consisting of the main pulmonary artery and its major divisions, is most often underdeveloped to some degree⁄Two percent of the autopsied cases at The Hospital for Sick Children, Toronto, showed a fibrous cord, 82 percent were hypoplastic, and 16 percent were of apparently normal size⁄Even in the most severe cases with atresia of the valve there is usually a patent pulmonary arterial lumen. Arterial stenosis in the main trunk is most often due to shortening of the three edge of the cusps attached to the wall of the trunk at their commissure (Kirklin, 1968). The remaining pulmonary arterial stenoses encountered are usually of the central type, i.e., obstruction occurs in the distal portion of the main pulmonary artery and involves a segment extending into the origin of both main divisions (Figure 27–3). Few authors can provide any frequency figures for association of pulmonary arterial stenosis. In fact, it is unlikely that an accurate figure could be supplied from the operating table or in patients in whom large-film angiograms had not been obtained. Presumably significant pulmonary arterial stenosis was found in 3 patients of 161 reported by Nagao and colleagues (1967). McMyn (1969) simply refers to the fact that "coarctation of the branches is common." Others have reported a minimum incidence of pulmonary arterial stenosis in the range of between 11 and 23 percent (Bjork et al., 1963; Franch and Gay, 1963; Baum et al., 1964; Timoner et al., 1970). Gregoratos and associates (1965) reported four patients with unilateral left pulmonary stenosis, which they liken to the more severe absent left branch in tetralogy.

We have encountered a more diffuse form of pulmonary arterial stenosis in patients with rubella syndrome and tetralogy of Fallot (Rowe, 1972). Pulmonary arterial stenosis has also been noted in individuals with the Noonan syndrome and the tetralogy (Barratt-Boyes, 1968).

Single pulmonary artery is an interesting pulmonary artery variant of great clinical importance in the tetralogy of Fallot. Thomas (1941) reported one case in detail, and Blalock (1948) found 9 cases in 610 at operation or autopsy. Ross and Murphy (1949) described an autopsy with an absent left pulmonary artery and a vessel connecting the main pulmonary artery with the left subclavian artery. Nadas and associates (1953) reported four cases, including one autopsy, and reemphasized the clinical features allowing recognition before operation and autopsy. McKim and Wiglesworth (1954) described two

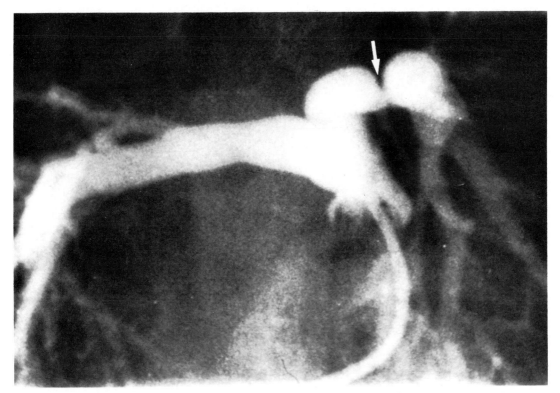

Figure 27-3. Selective "headup" pulmonary arteriogram in a four year old with severe tetralogy of Fallot. Notice that the main pulmonary artery is seen in its entire length and that the origins of both right and left main pulmonary artery branches are well visualized. The technique permits accurate assessment of obstruction within pulmonary artery branches. The *white arrow* points to a localized constriction in the midportion of the left pulmonary artery. (From Freedom, R. M., and Olley, P. M.: Pulmonary arteriography in congenital heart disease. *Catheterization & CV Diag.*, **2**:309, 1976.)

further postmortem-proved cases and two clinical cases of this type and discussed the embryologic aspects in detail. At The Hospital for Sick Children this type has been found 4 times in 128 autopsies. Absence of the right pulmonary artery in the tetralogy appears to occur rarely, if at all. Hemitruncus (right pulmonary artery from the ascending aorta), however, may be found on occasion.

Secondary Anatomic Considerations. A number of anomalies may be present in patients with tetralogy of Fallot anatomy that may be extravascular or acquired (Rowe and Uchida, 1961; Spear, 1964; Chrispin and Lillie, 1966; Celermajer et al., 1969). In

an earlier analysis of our autopsied patients the incidence of such anomalies was 20 percent. Of interest here are those additional anomalies that are cardiovascular in nature. A large number have been described (Blalock, 1948; Nagao et al., 1967; Rao et al., 1971) (Figure 27-4).

The right atrium is usually quite hypertrophied and the *tricuspid valve* shows varying degrees of mitralization (Lev, 1959). A *left superior vena cava* entering the coronary sinus has been found in 5 to 8 percent of patients (Nagao et al., 1967; Rao et al., 1971). We have encountered one patient with a left superior *vena cava connected to the left atrium.*

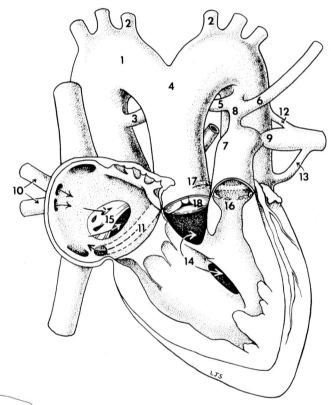

Figure 27-4. Associated cardiovascular anomalies reported in tetralogy of Fallot.
1, Right aortic arch.
2, Absent innominate artery (subclavian and carotid arteries arising separately).
3, Right aortic arch: left subclavian retroesophageal.
4, Double aortic arch (vascular ring).
5, Left aortic arch: right subclavian retroesophageal.
6, Patent ductus arteriosus arising from subclavian artery (not connected to aorta).
7, Unilateral absence of pulmonary artery.
8, Patent ductus arteriosus.
9, Pulmonary artery stenosis.
10, Partial anomalous pulmonary venous return with mitral atresia.
11, Persistent left superior vena cava.
12, Bronchial arteries entering pulmonary arteries.
13, Abdominal aorta to pulmonary artery connection.
14, Multiple ventricular septal defects.
15, Patent foramen ovale: atrial septal defect (secundum or primum).
16, Absent pulmonary valve.
17, Coronary artery anomalies.
18, Aortic valve with unequal-sized cusps or a small fourth cusp.
(Courtesy of Dr. G. C. Rosenquist, The Johns Hopkins Hospital, Baltimore.)

Partial anomalous pulmonary venous drainage is rare but has been reported (Blalock, 1948; Kjellberg et al., 1959). A variety of reports about *interatrial communications* exist. Edwards (1960) believes that patency of the foramen ovale is uncommon. Fallot (1888) reported 4 instances in 39 specimens, while Brinton and Campbell, (1953) reported 10 of their 25. In our previous examination of this question we found that two-thirds of our patients had an atrial defect but only 17 percent had "significant" openings. The exact proportion with atrial septal defects is obviously unclear, but the importance of the problem was recently stated by Levine and colleagues (1971) who showed that, among 50 patients after correction of the malformation, residual right-to-left shunts at atrial level were present in ten.

The pathway of the *bundle of His* in tetralogy patients has been examined in detail (Lev, 1959; Feldt et al., 1966). The main bundle is closely related to the posteroinferior margin of the defect. The right bundle, a direct continuation of the main, travels beneath the free margin of the inferior position of the defect. The fibers of the left anterior division are closely related to the first portion of the right bundle whereas the posterior division fibers arise more proximally from the main bundle.

The *right ventricle* is enlarged and hypertrophied while the *left ventricle* is usually normal. Real underdevelopment of the left ventricle appears rare (Nagao et al., 1967). We have observed in a few children a bilateral excess of ventricular muscle, which reduced the cavity sizes remarkably. The first few examples were seen in Polynesian infants but latterly we have encountered the same appearance in infants in the United States with the Noonan syndrome and the tetralogy. Though rare, the findings have practical significance in therapy as such babies respond poorly to shunt procedures. The presence of chronic myocardial ischemia in about one-third of young patients with the tetralogy dying after shunt procedures may likewise be a reason for the poor response to treatment (Tawes et al., 1969).

Anomalies of the *mitral valve* appear to be infrequent, mild, and not to affect prognosis. *Supravalvular mitral stenosis* (Hohn et al., 1968), *cor triatriatum* (Van Praagh et al., 1970), and *abnormal chordae* (Nagao et al., 1967) have been reported.

The *aortic valve* may also be abnormal either because of a bicuspid nature or because of valvular fusion (Glancy et al., 1968). Pressure differences across that valve and frank aortic regurgitation result in occasional patients presumably with this association. Examples of right coronary–noncoronary commissural deficiency with right coronary cusp prolapse into the ventricular septal defect have been reported (Van Praagh and McNamara, 1968).

CORONARY ARTERIES. Apart from changes in position of the coronary ostia due to counterclockwise rotation of the aortic root in tetralogy of Fallot (Lev, 1959; Goor et al., 1971), there tends to be an increase in vascular branching of the right coronary artery over the right ventricular outflow tract. In those with marked aortic dextroposition particularly, the possibility of there being a major vessel crossing the right ventricular outflow is increased. An anterior descending coronary artery ensuing from the right coronary artery has been found in 5 to 7 percent of autopsy material (Longenecker et al., 1961; Meng et al., 1965; Fellows et al., 1975). The incidence of this important anomaly is much less in surgical experience—1 in 168 consecutive repairs at the Johns Hopkins Hospital (Gott, personal communication), none in 161 operations (Nagao et al., 1967)—but prior knowledge of its presence is critical in surgical planning (Reemstsma et al., 1961). Single coronary arteries and origin of the right or left coronary artery from a pulmonary artery are even less commonly encountered (Friedman et al., 1960; Meng et al., 1965).

AORTIC ARCH. The aortic arch is right-sided and then usually right-descending, in 19 to 20 percent of patients (Corvisart, 1818; Blalock, 1948; Nagao et al., 1967; Rao et al., 1971). Among 40 patients studied by aortography, Rees and Somerville (1969) found the frequency of right aortic arch in those with pulmonary atresia to be twice that of subjects with pulmonary stenosis. In 85 autopsy specimens this difference has not been substantiated (Rao et al., 1971). Variations in aortic arch branching are not uncommon (Hospital for Sick Children, 1967; Blalock, 1948; Binet et al., 1966; Nagao et al., 1967). They include retroesophageal subclavian artery, aberrant or absent innominate artery, and rarely double aortic arch.

DUCTUS ARTERIOSUS. The duct may be present, normally closed, or absent. The incidence of patent ductus is only high during infancy and is therefore commonly seen with pulmonary atresia. There is a strong tendency for the duct to close eventually. Patency persisting beyond 15 months is unusual (Bass and Rowe, 1968) and is no higher than 2 percent in operative experience (Kirklin and Karp, 1970). An obliterated ductus that arose from the first portion of the left subclavian artery and connected to the pulmonary artery was found in three-quarters of the patients with right aortic arch operated upon by Blalock (1948). Partial persistence of the ductus (aortic end closed) is occasionally encountered. Agenesis of the ductus in tetralogy of Fallot and absent pulmonary valve may have a related pathogenesis (Thanopoulos et al., 1975).

OTHER COLLATERAL PATHWAYS. The bronchial arteries are usually increased in size and in older children and adolescents may provide a very substantial collateral channel for blood flow to the pulmonary arterial tree. These and even larger individual arteries from the aorta may enter the main pulmonary artery or one of its major divisions, though more often communication is with smaller pulmonary arteries.

The pulmonary vascular bed is not necessarily normal at birth. It most likely is normal patients with mild or only moderate degrees of pulmonary stenosis, but in those with more severe stenosis evidence from histologic observation indicates that the medial muscle mass of small pulmonary arteries is less than normal (Ferencz, 1960a; Naeye, 1961).

As the individual with the tetralogy ages, significant changes of the lung vascular bed become evident in the majority of cases. The small pulmonary vessels showed obstruction by thrombosis in 19 out of 21 patients examined at autopsy by Rich (1948). Best and Heath (1958) examined seven patients with cyanotic heart disease, five of whom had pulmonary stenosis with reduced pulmonary blood flow and severe polycythemia. In four of these five patients, thrombosis was found in 70 percent of small blood vessels examined, whereas in the cases with a higher pulmonary blood flow and a lesser degree of polycythemia, only 5 percent had such changes. The incidence of thrombotic lesions was noticeably high in the pulmonary veins as well as in the muscular pulmonary arteries.

In a very complete review of the problem by Ferencz (1960a), intrapulmonary thrombosis was seen in 24 of 33 patients with tetralogy of Fallot studied at postmortem. The lesions were variable in severity and recanalization was a frequent observation. Lesions were just as severe, if not more so, in the infant patients as in older ones, and there did appear to be some relationship between extensive pulmonary lesions and the clinical occurrence of cyanotic spells or cerebral thrombosis. By contrast, these thrombotic lesions were absent in the lungs of patients with tetralogy of Fallot who died more than one year after a shunt operation for that procedure, unless there had been clinical evidence to indicate a marked reduction in the volume of the left-to-right shunt through the anastomosis. Patients with a good clinical result from the operation dying of unrelated causes had normal lung vascular beds. In the same study, the lungs of patients who died in the first week in congestive heart failure following an anastomotic operation were found to show rupture of small pulmonary arteries with periarterial hemorrhage of varying degrees of severity, and in other patients dying later from pulmonary hypertension, the characteristic changes of medial hypertrophy were noted (Ferencz, 1960b).

Examination of the lung sections of 40 postmortem cases of tetralogy at The Hospital for Sick Children revealed the findings reported by Rich in a total of 30 percent: approximately 50 percent of the children over two years, and only 20 percent of those under the age of two years.

One histologic study of the pulmonary vascular bed in 28 cases of tetralogy of Fallot at Green Lane Hospital revealed thrombotic lesions in 16. In two patients the obstruction was sufficiently gross to have caused severe pulmonary hypertension, congestive heart failure, and death after surgical correction of the intracardiac defects (Windsor, 1962–1963). By contrast, among 61 patients in whom histologic examination of the pulmonary vascular bed was made, Kaplan (1972) was unable to demonstrate any correlation in those with changes with hematocrit level, the presence or absence of palliative shunt operations, or any particular clinical course.

In material obtained from lung biopsy Wagenvoort and coworkers (1967) demonstrated medial atrophy and intimal fibrosis secondary to thrombotic lesions in patients with tetralogy of Fallot more often than in others with pulmonary stenosis with intact ventricular septum.

Variation in the arrangement of elastic tissue in the main pulmonary artery of children with tetralogy of Fallot is consistent with the view that there is a group of patients in whom pulmonary stenosis develops after birth (Heath et al., 1959).

Etiology

As in most congenital heart defects, the actual cause of the arrested cardiac development in the tetralogy is unknown. In a few cases in the literature there has been a definite history of rubella in the first trimester of the particular pregnancy (Gibson and Lewis, 1952; Brinton and Campbell, 1953). Confirmed examples of the combination, usually manifested in most severe degrees of the malformation, have been noted in recent epidemics (Celermajer et al., 1969). The tetralogy also occurs in Down's syndrome and in the Noonan syndrome, although in each less frequently than other cardiac malformations. Polani and Campbell (1955) found 59 percent males in their cases. About 10 percent of our operated cases and 25 percent of the postmortem group had birth weights less than 2500 gm.

Frequency

Generally regarded as being the most important of the cyanotic malformations, the tetrad was found by Fallot (1888) to be responsible for 70 percent of all morbus caeruleus; Donzelot and D'Allaines (1954) and Mannheimer (1949) give figures of 67 percent and 52 percent, respectively. At The Hospital for Sick Children the tetralogy of Fallot has accounted for 9.7 percent of 15,104 patients with congenital heart malformation—the most frequent cyanotic malformation encountered and the second most frequent malformation in the entire group. In the Toronto Heart Registry (Gardiner and Keith, 1951; McLean and Keith, 1952) from birth to 15 years the number of cases of the tetralogy is equal to the number of all other cyanotic defects, and the tetralogy is the third most common defect in the total group. The risk of recurrence in sibs if there are no other affected first-degree relatives is about 3 percent (Nora et al., 1970).

Clinical Features

Cyanosis.   At some period in the first six months, cyanosis is noted in the vast majority of cases. In the postmortem group—presumably the most severe cases— cyanosis was noted in over 90 percent before six months of age, whereas in the operated and clinical cases about 75 percent became cyanosed in the same period. In the remainder cyanosis is delayed until the infant becomes more active. Taussig (1948) believes that this change occurs with closure of the ductus arteriosus during the latter part of the first year of life. An alternative explanation is that a moderate pulmonary stenosis converts to a severe degree of obstruction with the passage of time, thus reducing the pulmonary flow as the child grows (Gasul et al., 1957). In a very few, cyanosis is always minimal. Cold and exertion increase the degree of cyanosis. Clubbing is uncommon in the first six months and, for the most part, is related to severe degrees of cyanosis in children. Occasionally clubbing of moderate degree is present with minimal cyanosis and is very probably related to effort arterial oxygen desaturation.

Dyspnea. Dyspnea is prominent—at first with feeding or crying and later with walking. Paroxysmal dyspnea associated with marked cyanosis is common during infancy. Such "blue spells" may occur without warning, during infections or in the summer months but are most likely to occur around the time of breakfast and in the early evening hours. Although such incidents at first are of brief duration and irregular occurrence, they can become frequent and prolonged between 9 and 18 months. Seventy percent of our postmortem group in earlier years had "blue spells" in this period, and one-third of these were extremely severe. During the severe "blue spells," an infant may become unconscious and even develop serious paralysis. In the clinical cases reaching surgery, only 35 percent had "blue spells" of importance. Taussig (1948) has found a tendency to spontaneous improvement between 18 months and two years. This may possibly be due to development of collateral circulation. Nowadays the risks of permitting spells to recur are appreciated so that their appearance is an indication for major therapeutic moves.

The etiology of these "spells" is still unclear, but it is reasonably certain that they result from a periodic marked reduction of the already decreased blood flow to the lungs. During these episodes life is supported only by collateral blood flow to the lungs (Brock, 1957). Elegant clinical descriptions of the state were made by Fonó and Littmann (1957). These workers described disappearance of the systolic murmur, reduction in arterial oxygen saturation, reduction in pulmonary vascularity, and increased voltage of P wave with S-T segment depression in standard limb leads of the electrocardiogram during such spells. They considered that the developmental and morphologic appearance of muscle in the outflow tract of the right ventricle made it unusually susceptible to spasm and believed the most likely exciting stimulus to be reflex. These explanations gained support when others noted that during the "spells" an ejection systolic murmur ordinarily present and due to the infundibular stenosis

disappeared to return on recovery (Wood, 1958; Braudo and Zion, 1960). Documentation of changes in pulmonary artery and outflow tract pressure during such "spells" has been provided (Braudo and Zion, 1959; Johnson, 1961). The circumstances precipitating these spells have been so many and so varied that it has been difficult to envisage a common underlying factor. Johnson (1961) has suggested that release of norepinephrine (possible in most precipitating situations) by increasing myocardial contractile force might create a temporary complete obstruction in a previously markedly narrowed and hypertrophied right ventricular outflow tract. More recently a theory that satisfies the previously noted clinical features of the spell and at the same time provides a more acceptable physiologic basis for its origin has been devised (Morgan et al., 1965). In this view any situation that stimulates hyperpnea may precipitate an episode. Hyperpnea increases oxygen demands and cardiac output. Because the pulmonary blood flow is relatively fixed in the tetralogy, a lowered arterial oxygen saturation will result from the increased venoarterial shunt. The low arterial oxygen tension and pH as well as the higher CO_2 tension combine to stimulate the respiratory center to further hyperpnea, especially when respiratory control has been rendered normally sensitive by the benefit of sleep. A vicious cycle can then result to be broken only when respiratory responses are depressed by exhaustion, sedation, or general anesthesia. Rudolph and Danilowicz (1963) have indicated that some of these episodes in deeply cyanotic infants may be related to severe metabolic acidosis.

Approximately one-quarter of those patients with absent pulmonary valve will present as young infants with symptoms of severe airways obstruction due to bronchial compression (Bove et al., 1972).

Squatting. Closely allied to periodic dyspnea is the phenomenon of squatting, or squatting equivalents. William Hunter (1784) gave a good description of the now well-known postural changes that such subjects undertake. Infants prefer lying on one side hunched up like a fetus or in the knee-chest position. Older children avoid standing upright for long without movement of some sort or squat after effort. Oximetric studies show that the arterial oxygen saturation falls in these patients even on quiet standing. Squatting enables rapid return to previous levels or avoids any falls. Elastic bandages to the extremities or abdominal binders also may prevent the changes. Lurie (1953) has suggested that unfavorable postures, by reducing venous return, cause the returning venous blood to contain a lower concentration of oxygen. Thus, less saturated systemic venous blood mixing with saturated pulmonary venous blood results in an arterial mixture of lower saturation. Brotmacher (1957) deduced that squatting acutely angulated lower limb blood vessels and so reduced blood flow to the legs. An increase in cardiac output confined to the upper portion of the body resulted, and the arteriovenous oxygen difference was consequently lessened. Hypoxia to vital centers was thereby reduced. O'Donnell and McIlroy (1962) also found an increase in cardiac output, blood pressure, and arterial oxygen saturation with reduction of the right-to-left shunt in squatting. Since this effect was not observed with "squat-lying," they considered these developments to be due to a gravity effect on the circulation. Their interpretation is that the posture adopted shifts blood from the legs to the heart and lungs and so increases left ventricular output. The beneficial effect of this latter change is related to the anatomic and functional relationship of the ventricular septal defect to the aorta in tetralogy of Fallot, and these authors noted that such changes were not observed in pulmonary atresia, single ventricle with pulmonary stenosis, pulmonary stenosis with ventricular defects placed lower in the septum than in tetralogy of Fallot, or pulmonary stenosis with interatrial communication.

More recently Guntheroth and coworkers (1968) have shown that the flow of blood in the inferior vena cava is markedly decreased in a squatting-equivalent position. In their view the beneficial effects of squatting were that the posture (1) avoided syncope, (2) prevented blood of low oxygen saturation from the legs reaching the heart, so elevating arterial oxygen saturation even if the right-to-left shunt volume was unchanged, and (3) increased pulmonary blood flow through an increase in systemic vascular resistance.

Development.   Infants with the tetralogy usually gain weight slowly, over half of our postmortem group and about one-third of our clinical group behaving in this manner. Lund (1952), using the Wetzel grid, concluded that physique was never optimal and growth speed was slower than in the general population. Mehrizi and Drash (1962) found that almost two-thirds of their patients fell below the sixteenth percentile for height and weight. Moon face, regarded by Wood (1950) as strongly suggestive of pulmonary stenosis with normal aortic root, also occurs, though less frequently, in the tetrad. Mild thoracic deformities are common, some slight left precordial bulge being noticeable in older infants and children. Scoliosis, often advancing rapidly during adolescence, is much more common in cyanotic patients than in normal individuals (Luke and McDonnell, 1968; Jordan et al., 1972; Roth et al., 1973).

Cardiovascular Findings.   In the average case the apex beat is usually not displaced. Frequently tapping in character in children and adolescents, it is not noticeably abnormal in infants. Heart action as a whole is quiet.

The second heart sound in a pulmonary area varies in intensity. Although it may be reduced, it is most often loud and is only exceptionally split. Phonocardiograms show that the single second sound is due to aortic valve closure (Leatham, 1954). The delayed pulmonary valve closure sound is rarely heard but is often recorded phonocardiographically even in severe stenosis (Bousvaros, 1961; Tofler, 1963). In young infants with the atypical acyanotic form of the disorder the second sound may be entirely normal. A more obvious pulmonary valve closure sound in severe stenosis has been noted in older adult patients who have evidence of left ventricular hypertrophy. This peculiarity has been attributed to a lack of the usual cardiac rotation in such patients (Burch et al., 1964). An aortic ejection sound has been noted in cases with either very severe pulomary stenosis or pulmonary atresia (Vogelpoel and Schrire, 1955).

Some type of *cardiac murmur* was present in 75 percent of our autopsied cases and in all but 90 percent of the clinical group. *Absence of a murmur* is often accepted as indicating pulmonary atresia, but our observations show that there may also be no murmur when the obstruction is considerable but incomplete and at infundibular or valvular level or at both sites. By far the commonest type is a short, moderate-intensity ejection systolic murmur along the left sternal border that results from the infundibular stenosis. Three-fourths of such murmurs in our cases have been in the third and fourth left interspaces and one-fourth in the pulmonary area. The latter were frequently but not necessarily, related to valvular stenosis. The systolic murmur is accentuated within 15 seconds of administration of 0.25 to 0.5 mg phenylephrine (Vogelpoel et al., 1960). Intracardiac phonocardiography has shown a loud, diamond-shaped ejection systolic murmur in the pulmonary artery and a soft, delayed pulmonary valve closure sound 0.08 to 0.12 second after aortic valve closure (Feruglio and Gunton, 1960). In the rare case of a single pulmonary artery, the systolic murmur is often best heard on the side opposite the absent main branch. Because most frequently the left pulmonary artery is the vessel involved, the murmur is detected on the right of the sternum (Nadas et al., 1953). In the related absence of the pulmonary valve syndrome, a to-and-fro murmur is commonly heard, there being a systolic ejection murmur and an early diastolic murmur widely distributed over the chest. A *continuous murmur* in the pulmonary area occurred in 10 percent of our postmortem cases and rather less in the clinical cases. Of the former, pulmonary atresia was present in one-half and infundibular stenosis in the remainder. A softer, more widespread, continuous murmur usually means atresia with a marked collateral circulation through bronchial vessels. In infants, the pathologic evidence is that a patent ductus arteriosus is responsible for the continuous murmur and that increased blood flow through bronchial vessels is seldom responsible for its production. Nevertheless, even in infants, the diffuse, soft, continuous murmur usually can be proved by aortography to be due to bronchial arterial hypertrophy. Rather less than half of 22 patients with continuous murmur and pulmonary atresia investigated by Ongley and associates (1966) had a patent ductus arteriosus. Most of the remainder had other types of aortopulmonary collateral flow. In another study of 27 patients with continuous murmurs among 32 with pulmonary atresia and ventricular septal defect, Zutter and Somerville

(1971) found that when the murmur was localized below the left clavicle, its origin was always a patent ductus arteriosus, but that when there were additional sites involved, the origin was much more likely to be numerous large collateral vessels and not a ductus arteriosus. A continuous murmur over the right upper chest was uniformly associated with a right aortic arch and large collateral vessels to the right upper lobe. A *diastolic murmur* alone has been encountered only twice, and in each instance it appeared postoperatively. Soulié (1952) believed such a murmur is from a bicuspid aortic valve.

Thrills are not common in infancy and if present are faint.

Congestive heart failure never occurs in the classic form of this malformation during childhood; hence, findings of enlarged liver, gallop rhythm, and distended neck veins in cyanotic children before surgical intervention preclude the diagnosis of tetralogy. Exceptionally, in infants with anemia, subacute bacterial endocarditis (Bonham-Carter, 1958; Nadas and Hauck, 1960), or systemic hypertension (Holladay and Witham, 1957), or with anatomic variants such as absence of one pulmonary artery, absence of the pulmonary valve, or milder degrees of pulmonary stenosis, congestive heart failure may appear, and clinical improvement has been observed following digitalization (Rowe et al., 1955). Six congested African patients were described by Chesler and associates (1971), all under the age of 15 years. Each had severe stenosis and cyanosis, yet in the absence of anemia or infection had congestive failure and poor contractility with dilatation of the right ventricle. Autopsy showed subendocardial fibrosis.

Funduscopic examination shows distention of veins in the markedly cyanotic cases. The frequently dilated, tortuous retinal vessels and occasional papilledema seen in such patients correlate with low arterial oxygen saturation and high hematocrit levels are independent of age (Peterson and Rosenthal, 1972).

One clinical variant deserves special mention. These are infants with "atypical" tetralogy of Fallot presenting the clinical signs of ventricular septal defect of large size, frequent respiratory infections, rasping systolic murmur with thrill at the fourth left intercostal space, split second sound but reduced pulmonary component, and lack of cyanosis. The electrocardiogram shows combined ventricular hypertrophy with a QRS of about +90 degrees. The x-ray shows moderate cardiac enlargement with increased lung vascularity. In two out of five of our cases, a right aortic arch has been present. Cardiac catheterization reveals a large left-to-right shunt at ventricular level, a systemic systolic pressure level in the right ventricle, valvular pulmonary stenosis, normal pulmonary artery pressure, direct entry into the aorta from the right ventricle, and, usually, absence of any right-to-left shunt by arterial sampling, dye dilution studies, selective ether test, and angiocardiography. Only one (Rowe et al., 1955) of

the reported cases (Campbell, 1954; Moffitt et al., 1954; Sell et al., 1954) in this interesting group has come to autopsy. Even more important are related patients of the type originally reported by Gasul and colleagues (1957) and later amplified (Lynfield et al., 1961), where apparent transformation from simple ventricular septal defect without pulmonary stenosis to tetralogy of Fallot has occurred during infancy. There have been occasional examples of this change beyond the first decade (Bloomfield, 1964; Varghese et al., 1970), but most have been effected by age four years. A high incidence of this development in patients with ventricular septal defect, right aortic arch, and a narrow right ventricular outflow has been noted (Varghese et al., 1970). Tyrell and associates (1972) did not confirm a high incidence of right aortic arch but, using angiographic techniques, observed in the first study of such patients a large angle made by the outflow tract at the pulmonary valve level with the coronal plane ($>50°$), values similar to the established tetralogy and different from normal ($<50°$). Relative hypoplasia of the pulmonary valve ring was also present. In others the anatomy at operation or angiographically is not consistent with the tetralogy defect. In these the more common reason for development of increasing infundibular stenosis is an anomalous muscle bundle (Forster and Humphries, 1971). Rarely others develop a syndrome of very severe right ventricular hypertrophy due to increasing infundibular stenosis with reduction in size of the ventricular septal defect (Watson, 1971).

Radiologic Examination

Standard chest films provide useful information in diagnosis. The radiologic picture shows wide variation, and there can scarcely be said to be any typical cardiac contour. The most important constant findings are the normal or near-normal heart size and the reduction of lung vascular markings.

Contour. YOUNG INFANTS. In the anteroposterior view the contour is extremely variable, especially when the thymus contributes to the mediastinal opacity.

A tipped-up apex may be a pointer, but even this is found in some normal infants and, consequently, is of little real assistance in an individual case. Except in the extreme forms, the left cardiac border is normal at this age.

OLDER INFANTS AND CHILDREN. The appearances in older infants and children at x-ray become somewhat more stabilized. Examination of the x-ray contours in our postmortem-proved cases has shown that it is possible to visualize an infundibular chamber when this is large or moderate in size. Small chambers, however, do not contribute a bulge to the contour and cannot be distinguished from combined stenosis. On the basis of our autopsy controls, the clinical cases have been divided into four groups (Figure 27–5).

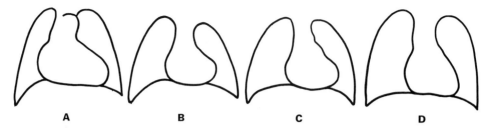

Figure 27-5. The common radiologic contours of the heart in tetralogy of Fallot. *A.* Pulmonary atresia, showing cardiac enlargement and large aortic knob. *B.* The classic contour, showing no cardiac enlargement, slight elevation of the apex, and a slight pulmonary bay. *C.* The contour of cases exhibiting an infundibular chamber. The characteristic of these is a bulge on the left middle arc of the cardiac border just below the position of the pulmonary artery. The apex is usually elevated as well, and the aortic knob may or may not be easily visible. Associated valvular stenosis cannot be excluded in this contour. *D.* The contour of cases with a right aortic arch. In these the left cardiac border is straight and the aortic knob may be seen on the right upper supracardiac border.

Those with right aortic arch (30 percent). Practically all have normal heart size, an aortic knob or sweep-up on the right (high) border, and no evidence of concavity on the left middle arc.

Those with infundibular chambers of moderate size (30 percent). These show a slight or distinct bulge along the lower left middle arc and may be easily confused with a slight pulmonary bulge. In this group the aortic knob is not necessarily prominent.

Those with a slight bay-shape in the left middle arc (30 percent). A few cases show this feature quite definitely, but the majority have minimal concavity. It is our impression that fluoroscopy shows the concavity better than the anteroposterior roentgenogram. The aortic knob is usually clearly evident.

Those with marked concavity of the left middle arc, large ascending aorta, and aortic knob (10 percent). These cases show at least moderate enlargement and usually represent the most severe types of the malformation, that is, pulmonary atresia.

A shelflike left lower border is evident in the anteroposterior view, and rotation to the left oblique position shows a projecting right ventricle and a large aortic sweep.

In the left anterior oblique view the pulmonary window is often very clear.

Rarely, gross cardiac enlargement is found. Diagnosis then is often impossible without further investigation.

Lung Vascularity. Study of the lung vascular markings, particularly at the hilus, permits an approximation of the amount of blood flow to the lungs.

Most cases appear to have normal or only slightly diminished vascular markings. Occasionally, dense hilar markings are seen in severe adolescent and adult cases, but these changes secondary to increase in bronchial flow to the lungs are rarely encountered in infants and children. Rib notching due to excessive collateral development in the intercostal arterial

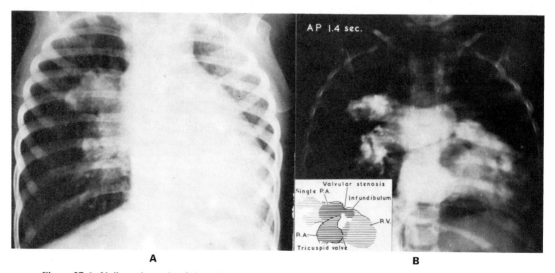

Figure 27-6. Unilateral atresia of the pulmonary artery in tetralogy of Fallot. The chest x-ray (*A*) and an anteroposterior frame from the venous angiocardiogram (*B*) of a patient with atresia of the left pulmonary artery, absence of the pulmonary valve, and a large ventricular septal defect. Only mild arterial oxygen desaturation was present because of the large pulmonary blood flow.

system is rare in children preoperatively except in patients with an absent, usually left, major branch of the pulmonary artery. Unilateral pulmonary artery atresia when associated with absent pulmonary valve gives rise to a tremendous increase in vascular markings in the opposite lung (Figure 27–6). Other patients with absence of the pulmonary valve show gross dilatation of the major pulmonary arteries with reduced peripheral lung vascular markings. Frequently in infancy signs of lung collapse or obstructive emphysema can be seen in this variant in addition (Bove et al., 1972; Pernot et al., 1972).

Sometimes the left pulmonary artery is visibly enlarged, and these cases almost invariably have a systolic murmur in the pulmonary area with associated valvular (dome) stenosis. Hypovascularity of the left upper lobe was seen in the chest films of approximately 20 percent of patients with cyanotic tetralogy examined by Wilson and Amplatz (1967). These authors suggest the appearance is due to a rotational effect on the heart in severe degrees of the malformation whereby the outflow jet of blood is directed more toward the right pulmonary artery. Differential blood flow within the lung in patients can be nicely confirmed by scanning techniques and is particularly valuable for pre- and postoperative assessment of complications or where there is severe chest deformity due to scoliosis (Haroutunian et al., 1969). Remarkable radiologic appearances are present in the previously mentioned atypical cases with increased pulmonary flow (Figures 27–7 and 27–8).

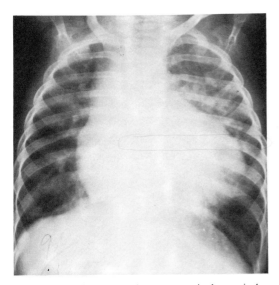

Figure 27-7. The radiologic appearance in the atypical tetralogy of infancy. Note the large heart and increased lung vascularity.

Barium swallow confirms the side of the aortic arch and may be performed quite safely in even severely ill infants. Barium will also reveal abnormalities of the aortic area branches such as a retroesophageal

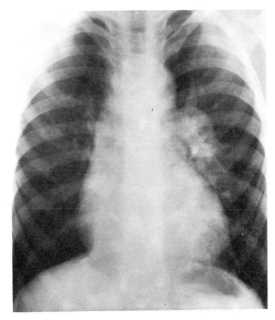

Figure 27-8. Tetralogy of Fallot with persistent ductus arteriosus. The chest x-ray of T. H. (471291) at seven years. Note the dilated left pulmonary artery.

subclavian vessel. In older cases enlarged bronchial arteries may indent the barium-filled esophagus.

Approximately 50 percent of patients with severe uncorrected cyanotic heart malformation between 12 and 29 years will be found osteoporotic, a change frequently, though not necessarily, accompanied by delayed skeletal maturation (White et al., 1971).

Electrocardiography

There is nothing specific about the electrocardiogram for the tetralogy of Fallot but the common findings are right-axis, deviation and right ventricular hypertrophy (Figure 27–9).

Axis QRS. Moderate to marked right-axis deviation (+120 to +210 degrees) is present in all except the "atypical" group with increased pulmonary flow. In such instances the axis is +60 to +90 degrees. In rare cases of pentalogy and the Noonan syndrome left-axis deviation has been recorded (Char et al., 1972; Gasul et al., 1949).

P Wave. Electrical evidence of right atrial hypertrophy is uncommon in childhood. None of our own cases under one year showed abnormally tall P waves, although we have seen this change in a few autopsy proven cases, and abnormal P waves were not common (1:10) even in the older children. Donzelot and associates (1951) and Joly and coworkers (1952) have shown a higher incidence (1:3 and 1:5, respectively) of right atrial hypertrophy in a series of older patients with the malformation. This appears to be one segment of the electrocardiogram that alters significantly with increasing age, as two-thirds of

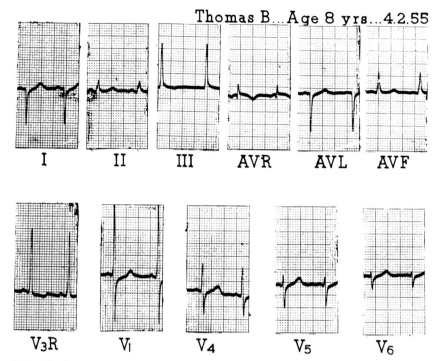

Figure 27-9. The electrocardiogram in tetralogy of Fallot. Right-axis deviation and moderate right ventricular hypertrophy. Transitional complex in V_1 to V_2.

adult patients have this abnormality (Higgins and Mulder, 1972).

QRS. LIMB LEADS. Horizontal electrical position is common. In aVR an abnormal R/Q ratio or height of R is frequent and was present in over 60 percent of our cases.

PRECORDIAL LEADS. Broadly speaking, the pattern of right ventricular hypertrophy with inverted R/S ratios (predominant R over the right precordium; predominant S over the left precordium) is found (Figure 27–9). The height of R in V_1 is not consistently as tall as in severe degrees of right ventricular hypertrophy but may increase slightly with age—a change probably related to changes in systemic pressure levels. Similarly the R wave not infrequently becomes the predominant portion of the complex in V_6 in older children.

The transitional complex commonly is situated in either V_1 or V_2. Marquis (1951) regards this as characteristic of the electrocardiogram, and we have found it to occur in about 40 percent of our cases. In the remainder the transitional zone may be normally placed or rotated to the left.

Incomplete right bundle branch block occurs in about 20 percent of cases, but a qR complex in the right precordium, so common in more severe degrees of right ventricular hypertrophy, is infrequent and does not necessarily hold the grave prognostic significance given it by Wood (1950). Complete right bundle branch block is common in adults (Higgins and Mulder, 1972).

Predominant left ventricular hypertrophy is extremely rare (Gasul et al., 1949; Ziegler, 1954; Hospital for Sick Children, 1955), but electrical evidence of associated left ventricular hypertrophy is not infrequent. This may occur without any associated anomalies. When a deep q is found in leads over the left precordium in the presence of right ventricular hypertrophy, left ventricular enlargement or hypertrophy of marked degree may be assumed. This type of tracing was seen in a Hospital for Sick Children patient whose autopsy revealed a left superior vena cava entering the left atrium, complicating the usual tetrad. Soulié (1952) believed that any evidence of left ventricular hypertrophy in the tetralogy is due to an associated patent ductus arteriosus. We have been able to confirm this opinion only once, in a child of three years. In ten patients with a mean age of 31 years, Burch and associates (1964) found well-developed left ventricular hypertrophy. All these patients had severe cyanosis and clubbing, and it is postulated that they probably had a large bronchial collateral supply to the lungs to account for the change.

Combined ventricular hypertrophy with predominant left-sided change is frequently found in the "atypical" cases with increased pulmonary blood flow.

T Wave. In adults or older children the electrocardiogram permits a definite statement about the degree of chamber hypertrophy, but in infants the problem has been much more complex because of the normal right ventricular dominance at this age. The important observation that the T wave in V_1 is only normally upright in the first 24 hours of life and thereafter constitutes evidence of abnormal right ventricular hypertrophy (Ziegler, 1954) has aided earlier recognition of the malformation in the young infant. Thus the usual case of tetrad in the younger age group exhibits an upright T in V_1 and only moderate right ventricular hypertrophy. It is probably fair to say that inversion of T in V_1 is never normal in infants with this malformation and, when present, merely indicates that the degree of right ventricular hypertrophy is more marked than usual.

The vectorcardiogram reflects these observations. The frontal plane vector is usually inscribed in a clockwise direction but occasionally is counterclockwise in cyanotic patients. The horizontal vector is more often clockwise and directed anteriorly and rightward (Khoury et al., 1965).

Blood Gases and Metabolic Changes

The ear oximeter has been found of use in studying the degree of arterial oxygen desaturation in cases of tetralogy of Fallot under varying conditions. The arterial oxygen desaturation present at rest in most cases increases slightly with standing alone and markedly with exercise. Some milder cases, clinically noncyanotic, may show a precipitous drop in arterial oxygen saturation during exercise. Although a considerable rise follows inhalation of 100 percent oxygen, the saturation seldom reaches 100 percent. Van Lingen and Whidborne (1952) believe that hyperventilation, while increasing the arterial oxygen desaturation in tetralogy, does not change the level in pulmonary stenosis with normal aortic root and venoarterial shunt. The effect of squatting has already been mentioned.

A number of investigators have sought to examine the influence of cyanotic congenital heart disease on acid-base balance in general and on myocardial behavior in particular. Early reports emphasized the remarkable body adaptation to this form of hypoxia (Talbott et al., 1941; Bing et al., 1948; Burchell et al., 1950). Morse and Cassels (1953) found arterial pH below normal range in about one-third of 60 cyanotic patients, there being a relationship between the degree of arterial unsaturation and this acidosis. Central blood lactate and pyruvate levels and lactate/pyruvate ratios in cyanotic patients were found inversely related to arterial oxygen tension (Green and Talner, 1964) suggesting that oxygen deficiency in the ranges examined does not influence the equilibrium between lactic and pyruvic acid. More recent work has failed to confirm an acidotic tendency in cyanotic patients or differences in the pattern of energy metabolism in the heart (Moffitt et al., 1970; Scheuer et al., 1970; White et al., 1972).

Under ordinary resting conditions the cyanotic patient with tetralogy of Fallot has a normal arterial pH and pCO_2. During hypoxic spells there is a profound drop in paO_2 and marked metabolic acidosis can develop rapidly (Talner and Ithuralde, 1970).

Blood Changes

Polycythemia is a common finding, and hemoglobin readings of over 20 gm per 100 ml of blood are not uncommon in severe cases. The hematocrit is abnormally high. Taussig (1948) believes that cases showing hemoglobin levels of 10 to 13 gm per 100 ml are in fact suffering from anemia. Rudolph and associates (1953) studied five patients with the tetrad who had such relative anemia. These patients were anorexic, poorly nourished, and had frequent "blue spells." These authors found that iron therapy increased the hemoglobin valves, raised the hematocrit, and resulted in clinical improvement and increased cyanosis. Where the hematocrit exceeded 70 percent, there was a return of symptoms, possibly due to increase in blood viscosity. The important aspect of fluidity of blood flow in polycythemic children has been further reviewed recently (Kontras et al., 1970).

Cassels and Morse (1947), Clay and associates (1951), and Verél (1961) studied blood volumes by a number of methods and found that, while the total blood volume and red cell volumes are increased, the plasma volume is reduced. Nelson and associates (1947) have found that the plasma volume was either normal or slightly increased. Detailed studies of the behavior of formed elements of the blood in the tetralogy have been made by Prader and Rossi (1950), and Rudolph and coworkers' (1953) paper includes an interesting study on the natural history of the erythrocyte count from birth to nine months in this malformation.

In addition to the question of polycythemia there have been considerable interest and concern over the hemorrhagic aspects of the cyanotic patient (Hartman, 1952). As Kaplan (1972) has observed, "in polycythemic patients there is a delicate balance between intravascular thrombosis and a bleeding diathesis." In a proportion of cyanotic patients and usually in some relation to the degree of polycythemia a variety of hemostatic disturbances can be demonstrated of which the most frequent seems to be an abnormality of platelet function (Ekert et al., 1970). The subject is still controversial, and although some authors believe low-grade intravascular coagulation to be the important factor responsible (Kompe and Sparrow, 1970), others have evidence to the contrary (Abildgaard and Schulman, 1968; Ekert et al., 1970; Maurer et al., 1972). The question is important especially for patients in whom correction by open heart methods is contemplated (Phillips et al., 1963). The debate over causation is matched by that over the need for routine evaluation of the common hemostatic factors prior to surgical intervention in these patients. For some (Ekert et al., 1970; Kaplan, 1972) an elaborate routine is instituted and

484　　　　　　　　　　　　　　　　　　　　SHUNTS

appropriate therapy undertaken before surgery. This includes suppression of accelerated fibrinolysis by intravenous epsilon aminocaproic acid and phlebotomy 48 hours preoperatively for thrombocytopenia. Others have abandoned the screening because so few patients with abnormal tests seem to develop bleeding problems. For them special attention to surgical hemostasis and, in the rare major bleeding diathesis, administration of fresh plasma with steroid therapy have appeared sufficient measures.

Echocardiography

The main variables in this malformation are the amount of pulmonary blood flow and the degree of aortic overriding. Unless there is increased flow because there is mild pulmonary stenosis or because of collateral sources of lung flow, the left atrial size is normal on the echocardiogram. Mitral-aortic valve continuity is a necessary finding for diagnosis, and most commonly overriding of the ventricular septum by the aorta can be visualized (Chung et al., 1973). The septal echo then does not become continuous with the anterior aortic wall echo and ends between the anterior and posterior aortic walls (Figure 27–10). This therefore provides an indication of the degree of aortic overriding. The more severe the pulmonary stenosis, the larger will be the aortic diameter. In very severe tetralogy it is difficult to visualize the pulmonary valve because of the marked hypoplasia and rotation of the right ventricular outflow tract. In less severe forms the pulmonary valve can be visualized.

Cardiac Catheterization and Angiocardiography

Bing and associates (1947) first confirmed the clinical and radiologic indications of reduced pulmonary blood flow and drew attention to the importance of collateral bronchial arterial flow in older children and adults with the tetralogy of Fallot. In the years that have followed more details have been added to this basic understanding of the hemodynamics in both the usual cyanotic patient and in the variants of the malformation. Little question surrounds the widely held proposition that since the ventricular septal defect is almost uniformly large, the hemodynamics of tetralogy of Fallot are related principally to the degree of right ventricular outflow obstruction. It is also apparent that the obstructive factor is a dynamic one likely to increase in degree with time particularly in infancy but also at a slower pace in the older individual. Even where there is atresia of the right ventricular outflow, the dynamics may still be affected through factors such as the volume of collateral lung blood flow, a change that may again be time-affected. The documentation of these hemodynamic changes has been made by cardiac catheterization but is in most cases a prelude (and to some incidental) to the more critically important angiocardiographic aspects used to gauge right ventricular outflow and pulmonary arterial anatomy.

Recent correlations of ventricular volume through angiocardiography and precise pressure measurements in the ventricular chambers have shown the

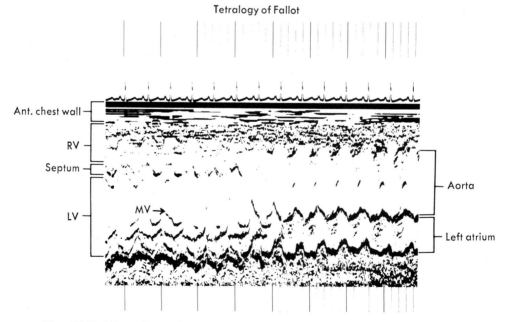

Figure 27-10. Echocardiogram in tetralogy of Fallot. Note right ventricular hypertrophy. A common finding is loss of the septal echo during the sweep just prior to visualizing the aortic root. *MV*, mitral valve; *RV*, right ventricle; *LV*, left ventricle.

complex nature of time-directional shunting between the two sides of the heart in more detail (Levin et al., 1966; Jarmakani et al., 1968). It is apparent from these studies that in the usual cyanotic form of the disorder the left ventricular pressure rise during isovolumic contraction precedes the right ventricular pressure rise, so that in this phase of the cardiac cycle a left-to-right shunt occurs. During ventricular ejection both ventricles eject into the aorta, while in isovolumic relaxation when the left ventricular pressure falls early as in the right, a right-to-left shunt occurs across the ventricular communication. Detailed attempts to quantify the shunts in tetralogy of Fallot from usual diagnostic catheterization techniques are an interesting but rather fruitless exercise. Statement of the net shunt magnitude in simple broad categories such as mild, moderate, or severe is probably all that can be justified from these crude data. Matters become more complicated when a true secundum atrial defect is present in addition, and most studies to date have simply identified the presence of such a defect. Of the various methods, vena caval injection of indocyanine green is probably the most accurate for the purpose. Likewise quantification of collateral flow is a complex matter and, even with detailed attention using perhaps unwarranted pursuit of the point, can scarcely be regarded as very accurate. One can, establish certain physiologic information about patients that is useful in the total assessment of the individual situation. Indicator dilution is certainly the most accurate assessment for right-to-left shunts, which in turn reflects the degree of obstruction to the right ventricular outflow tract. The arterial saturation may be a guide in the same direction, but it is not necessarily the most reliable indicator since an increase in pulmonary blood flow through collateral pathways may raise the arterial oxygen saturation substantially and thus mask the fact that the right-to-left shunt is really very large. With severe pulmonary stenosis the left-to-right shunt at the ventricular level is minimal by standard methods such as blood oxygen saturation sampling, though some obviously occurs, whereas with less severe outflow obstruction an obvious interventricular left-to-right shunt can be detected. For such patients the arterial oxygen saturation is usually higher and the right-to-left shunt by indicator dilution lower than in the more classic case.

The usual situation with cyanotic tetralogy of Fallot is that right atrial pressures are normal. A prominent atrial "a" wave is unusual in younger children but may develop in older patients and may therefore reflect increasing right ventricular hypertrophy and ventricular compliance change. The systolic pressure in the right ventricle is equivalent to that in the aorta, and the plateau of ejection visible on the pressure pulse resembles closely that seen in the left ventricle (Figure 27–11), factors that identify the importance and large size of the ventricular communication in the tetralogy of Fallot (Fineberg and Wiggers, 1936; Bouchard and Cornu, 1954). The

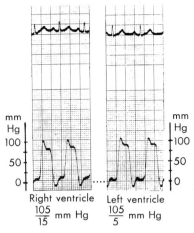

Figure 27-11. D.W., aged three years. The ventricular pressure pulses in tetralogy of Fallot. Note the similar appearances in each ventricle and the distinct ejection plateau in each instance.

pulmonary arterial pressure is low, and its level and form have a relationship to the severity of pulmonary stenosis. As a consequence, in severe stenosis at infundibular level the recognition of further distal obstruction (valvular, pulmonary arterial, or pulmonary vascular bed level) may be quite impossible from systolic pressure levels alone (Figure 27–12). Such restrictions again emphasize the importance of combining physiologic and angiographic and other measurements. Since the proximal level of obstruction is usually infundibular and only occasionally valvular, the differential pressure will necessarily most often be demonstrated at infundibular level. Artifact may be produced in this regard by use of catheters with multiple side holes for the pressure measurement. The best delineation of the level of obstruction from pressure change is obtained from catheters with a single side hole or two side holes very closely positioned several centimeters proximal to the catheter tip. These are better than the usual variety of intracardiac electrode catheters where there is close proximity of the holes to the tip. A small catheter size together with an electrode and a remote side hole position would be ideal for the purpose.

The passage of the catheter from the right ventricle into the aorta is almost inevitable in the tetralogy of Fallot. The position of entry and site of change of pressure pulse on withdrawal are characteristic of passage through a ventricular defect with a normal aortic root position.

Excellent indication of the magnitude of the right-to-left shunt is provided by sampling from the peripheral artery after the injection of green dye into the venae cavae or right atrium. The site of right-to-left shunting can be localized by injecting in turn into the pulmonary arteries, right ventricle, and right atrium (Swan and Wood, 1953). The precise determination of magnitude of left-to-right shunt using this technique because of the usual presence of a large left-to-right shunt in the tetralogy is more

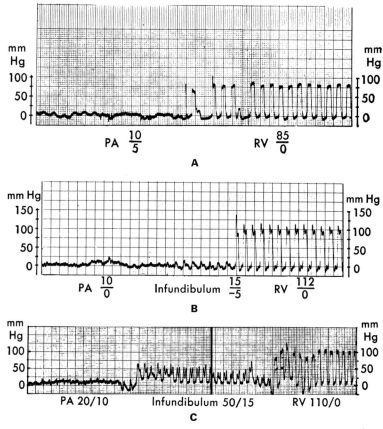

Figure 27-12. Cardiac catheterization in tetralogy of Fallot: the withdrawal tracing from pulmonary artery to right ventricle. *A.* Valvular stenosis. *B.* Infundibular stenosis. *C.* Combined valvular and infundibular stenosis.

uncertain and can be provided in only the broadest of terms. Aortic root injection can likewise detect only a large degree of collateral flow. As all who follow physiologic measurements in the catheterization laboratory know, a change from steady state, contrast material, and drugs can profoundly alter the magnitude and directions of shunting. Isoproterenol, for example, increases the right-to-left shunt and reduces the arterial oxygen saturation in the tetralogy (Cumming, 1970). Propranolol, in infants particularly, can abolish this response as well as the effect of exercise (Shah and Kidd, 1967).

Venous angiocardiography (Castellanos et al., 1938; Cooley et al., 1949; Donzelot et al., 1949; Campbell and Hills, 1950; Kreutzer et al., 1950; Dotter and Steinberg, 1951; Goodwin et al., 1953; Lowe, 1953; Hilario et al., 1954) has now been replaced entirely by selective angiocardiography (Jonsson et al., 1949; Kjellberg et al., 1959; Lester et al., 1965; McMyn, 1969). The debate over preference between serial biplane angiocardiograms and cine technique is coming to an end as the film resolution of the present cine method approaches that of the large-film procedure. Surgical interest lies in the nature of the pulmonary stenosis—its site and degree—the size of pulmonary ring and the main pulmonary artery

and the presence of pulmonary arterial stenosis or hypoplasia (Brandt, 1968). Additional questions that need to be clarified at study are whether there is a large ventricular septal defect or a single ventricle, whether there is mitral-aortic valve continuity, mitral valve abnormality, the coronary artery anatomy, and the source of any collateral pulmonary blood flow. The most useful and generally utilized views for right ventricular selective angiocardiograms are antero-posterior and lateral, though the septal defect is obviously better visualized with the patient in the left anterior oblique position. Other views may provide information to supplement after that obtained from the initial injection of contrast. Aortography has a position in the investigation of the tetralogy to an extent yet unclarified. In addition to its value in patients with collateral pulmonary blood flow, it can demonstrate the course of the right coronary artery and its conus branches more clearly than is usual from right ventricular angiocardiograms and so will identify major anomalies of critical surgical importance (White et al., 1972). Wedge arteriography (Windsor, 1962–1963; Castellanos et al., 1965) appears to be a useful method of assessing the anatomic state of the lung vascular bed in this malformation. In the search for abnormality in coronary artery branching or for extensive vascular bed thrombosis the question arises of the positive yield. Though the occurrence of coronary arterial abnormalities is probably only between 2 and 5 percent, the evidence is that a transvenous aortogram is a minor addition to the preoperative angiographic study, and the critical importance to outcome of knowledge of the presence of an anomalous coronary artery makes the case for routine study strong (Fellows et al., 1975). Major complications due to widespread lung arterial changes after open heart surgery are rare, but a reluctance to perform pulmonary wedge studies or obtaining them in a nonsystemic fashion has resulted in incomplete knowledge concerning their clinical value. Just as with the coronary anomaly, there is a need to define the candidates in whom the pulmonary arteriogram is likely to end in positive benefit to the patient.

The most difficult matters to be decided by angiocardiography are usually those involving the position of the aorta in relation to the left ventricular outflow or the true anatomy of the pulmonary arteries especially in patients with apparent absence of one branch (Porstmann et al., 1967; Wallsh et al., 1968) or in those with collateral flow supplying the lungs. Spurious forms of pulmonary atresia in very tight stenosis may be misinterpreted (Rockoff and Gilbert, 1965) but are not commonly missed. The recognition of pulmonary atresia where the only pathway to the lungs is through aortic branches is not difficult. The frequency of a frank or hidden pulmonary arterial tract in normal position and the point at which larger collateral vessels enter this system, if at all, have caused revival of old arguments. The pressure for definition has been intensified by the possibility, through a variety of grafting and prosthetic methods, of restoring the anatomic pathway from the right ventricle to the pulmonary arteries toward normal (Ross and Somerville, 1966; Barratt-Boyes, 1968; Kouchoukos et al., 1971; Kaplan 1972). It is this group of patients in whom aortography is critically important. The more selectively aortography is performed, the more likely it is that the anatomy will be accurately displayed (Chesler et al., 1970). The presence in such films of pulmonary arteries that meet in the midline is good evidence of pulmonary atresia with true functioning central pulmonary arteries—a potentially correctable arrangement. This appearance will frequently be seen in late films of patients with many small bronchial arteries supplying the lung and occasionally after selective injection of an aortic branch of patients who have larger vessels supplying other portions of the lung (Jefferson et al., 1972). It is in those patients with several large, seemingly unconnected vessels supplying different portions of each lung where the principal difficulties arise. Are these examples of absent sixth aortic arch (Stuckey et al., 1968) and, if so, can they be corrected or is the spectacular distribution of contrast to these larger vessels rendering invisible an underlying normal pulmonary arterial distribution? Significant efforts to provide definitive answers to these questions have emerged from the Leeds team (Macartney et al., 1973, 1974).

Three other variants have special features at angiocardiography. In *absence of the pulmonary valve* the most striking feature is an aneurysmal dilatation of the right and left pulmonary arteries with sharp narrowing distal to the secondary arterial branches. The valve ring in all cases is smaller than normal (Durnin et al., 1969), and an apparent dome shape or flat diaphragmatic form to the "valve" is visible (Harris et al., 1969; Macartney and Miller, 1970). Absence of the left pulmonary artery occasionally is associated (Durnin et al., 1969) (Figure 27–6).

The important information in patients with apparent tetralogy of Fallot and *suprasystemic right ventricular pressure* is whether there is indeed a small ventricular septal defect (Weis et al., 1961) or whether the defect is of usual size for the tetralogy but partially occluded through valvular tissue (Neufeld et al., 1960; Padmanabhan et al., 1971). The phasic variation of the obstructive element in the latter more usual situation should permit identification of the large defect size from a left ventricular contrast injection in the left anterior oblique projection. In addition, the right ventricular outflow tract anatomy is characteristic of the tetralogy. By contrast, no variation in the size could occur with a small ventricular septal defect, and the right ventricular outflow should in these cases appear more like that seen in pulmonary stenosis with normal aortic root.

The angiocardiographic appearances of the outflow tract and its angulation in *acyanotic forms* have been discussed earlier in this chapter.

Differential Diagnosis

The Newborn. For tetralogy of Fallot to produce serious symptoms in the newborn period is unusual. When *cyanosis* is prominent at this age, the prognosis is bad (Rowe and Mehrizi, 1968). Most such cases will not usually present before the second week after birth and will most often be in patients with severe infundibular stenosis or atresia where collateral flow may mask the problem initially. In any event, murmurs are often absent or, if present, continuous in these individuals. Transposition of the great arteries may confuse because of cyanosis, absence of a murmur, a single second heart sound, and right ventricular hypertrophy in the electrocardiograms. Cyanosis is usually more marked and early, and a careful review of the chest film should show some increase in lung vascular markings even if the cardiac silhouette is not typically egg-shaped in transposition in the first week of life. Other cyanotic malformations presenting at this age with reduced pulmonary blood flow such as tricuspid atresia or Ebstein's anomaly of the tricuspid valve are soon excluded by the characteristic electrocardiograms of left-axis deviation and left ventricular hypertrophy or right bundle branch block with large P waves, respectively. Pulmonary atresia with normal aortic root usually has a larger heart, frequently develops congestive heart failure, and there is a normal axis with left ventricular hypertrophy in the electrocardiogram. About one in eight patients with asplenia syndrome will die of hypoxia within 48 hours of delivery (Rowe and Mehrizi, 1968). Clinical recognition is aided by the detection of Howell-Jolly bodies. Other non-cardiac courses for cyanosis need exclusion in the first day or two of life.

Congestive failure has been present shortly after birth, but more often it develops within a few days of delivery in a proportion of patients with tetralogy of Fallot and absent pulmonary valves. The characteristic and loud to-and-fro murmur widely transmitted through the chest is diagnostic of this variant. Occasionally patients with pulmonary atresia or unilateral pulmonary atresia and large collateral flow may develop failure for a few days in the neonatal period.

Older Infants and Children. The *acyanotic* forms of tetralogy of Fallot are most often mistaken for isolated ventricular septal defect or isolated pulmonary stenosis depending upon the degree of outflow tract obstruction that is present. In patients with mild or no functional infundibular stenosis the physical signs and the x-ray and electrocardiographic appearances are perfectly compatible with a moderate-sized ventricular septal defect. The presence of right aortic arch in such patients should arouse clinical suspicion of the tetralogy. With moderate infundibular stenosis, which is the more common presentation of acyanotic tetralogy of Fallot, the murmur is usually long though often ejection in form, the second sound is normal, and the precordium is quiet. Again there is moderate right ventricular hypertrophy present in the electrocardiogram. Such patients can resemble those with a small ventricular septal defect, but the electrocardiogram of the acyanotic tetralogy invariably shows right ventricular hypertrophy. The signs more often appear consistent with isolated valve pulmonary stenosis. The murmur is usually lower along the left sternal border, however, and there is no ejection click as in valvular stenosis. Nevertheless this is sometimes a difficult differential diagnosis, and patients with equivocal findings warrant further investigation to make the rather important separation between the two malformations.

The *cyanotic malformations* likely to resemble more classic cyanotic forms of the tetralogy are many and may be divided into simple and complex forms.

SIMPLE   CYANOTIC   MALFORMATION. *Pulmonary Stenosis with Normal Aortic Root.* The severe form, the *grandes trilogies* of the French workers, rarely presents a problem in diagnosis. The onset of cyanosis is usually early, and in our experience squatting is exceptional. A prominent right ventricular heave along the left sternal border is present, and a harsh ejection systolic murmur in the second and third left intercostal spaces is accompanied by a thrill. Moon face is common, and there is usually a prominent "a" wave in the jugular venous

pulse. The heart is enlarged, and although the lung fields are clear, a pulmonary artery bulge is visible. The presence of right aortic arch should immediately question, while an electrocardiogram exhibiting extreme right ventricular hypertrophy should support, the diagnosis. Cardiac catheterization is of great help by localizing the shunt to atrial level and by showing a right ventricular pressure pulse unlike that of the left ventricle often with a level above systemic range. Angiocardiography reveals a wide right ventricular outflow tract and valvular stenosis with a contrast yet entering a dilated main pulmonary and left pulmonary artery.

It is interesting to note that in the pentalogy of Fallot, that is, Fallot plus atrial septal defect, the heart may function hemodynamically in some cases like tetrad and in other cases like severe pulmonary stenosis with normal aortic root and venoarterial shunt. Kjellberg and associates (1959) believe that a right-to-left interatrial shunt occurs in the pentalogy only when there is a severe pulmonary stenosis, a tricuspid valve deformity, or partial anomalous pulmonary venous drainage.

Severe Pulmonary Stenosis with "Small" Ventricular Septal Defect. This malformation (Hoffman et al., 1960; Weis et al., 1961) leads to profound cyanosis, prominent jugular "a" wave, right ventricular parasternal heave, usually a single second heart sound, and fairly severe right ventricular hypertrophy in the electrocardiogram. Radiologically the picture may resemble tetralogy of Fallot more than pulmonary stenosis with normal aortic root, which bears the closest clinical resemblance.

Pulmonary Stenosis and Ventricular Septal Defect with Hypoplastic Right Ventricle. This malformation has been described in detail by Williams and associates (1963). Cyanosis is common from birth or early infancy, large jugular "a" waves are visible in the neck, and there is a long, loud ejection systolic murmur maximal in the pulmonary area. The heart is slightly enlarged, and the radiologic appearance is not markedly different from that of tetralogy of Fallot. Features distinguishing such patients from those with pulmonary stenosis and interatrial shunt alone are the inactivity of the right ventricle to palpation along the left sternal border and little or no evidence of right ventricular hypertrophy in the electrocardiogram. This latter valuable clue is matched by the usually detectable paradoxic or reversed splitting of the second heart sound. The major shunt reversal does, in fact, occur at atrial level in these patients, and although they respond favorably initially to shunt procedures, in the end congestive heart failure appears and corrective surgery offers the only real help in these cases.

Anomalous Muscle Bundles in the Right Ventricle with Ventricular Septal Defect. The clinical picture may resemble tetralogy of Fallot and is very often confused with this lesion (Forster and Humphries, 1971). The obstruction, however, is in midright ventricle and is a consequence of muscle bands other than the parietal band. Since the appearance at ventriculotomy is bizarre, it is particularly important that the diagnosis be established preoperatively. This is best done from selective angiocardiograms into the right ventricle with the patient in the right anterior oblique position that show a wide slanting filling defect within the body of the ventricle (Fisher et al., 1971).

Tetralogy of Fallot with Unusual Electrocardiographic Signs. Occasional patients will present with unusual frontal plane axis QRS in the tetralogy. This is seen in the form of left-axis deviation, and it is probably always related to changes in conduction pathways of a primary or secondary nature. Examples are patients having tetralogy of Fallot with type B Wolff–Parkinson–White syndrome, patients with the Noonan syndrome, and those with congenital rubella. Confusion with tricuspid atresia is unlikely because right ventricular hypertrophy is always present in the tetralogy despite the unusual axis that may be associated on occasion.

COMPLEX CYANOTIC MALFORMATIONS. *Double-Outlet Right Ventricle.* Certain clinical differences may avoid confusion of the tetralogy of Fallot with double-outlet right ventricle with pulmonary stenosis. In this malformation squatting is uncommon, and the ejection systolic murmur is longer and harsher than in tetralogy of Fallot with comparable severity of cyanosis. Furthermore, the chest x-ray shows a larger heart, while the electrocardiogram reveals appreciable left ventricular potential in contrast to the tetralogy (Mehrizi, 1965). But there is no question that the clinical picture can be very similar to tetralogy of Fallot. Angiographic methods have been used to differentiate: the right ventricular selective angiocardiogram shows the aorta to be anteriorly placed in a lateral view, while the parietal band of the crista is missing in this projection and prominent in the anteroposterior frames (Dayem et al., 1967). If aortic-mitral discontinuity is present in either the echocardiogram (Chesler et al., 1971) or angiocardiogram (Baron, 1971), double-outlet right ventricle is most certainly present in suspected examples, but a clear distinction preoperatively is obviously not always possible (Lev et al., 1972) and the diagnosis may be evident for the first time in the operating theatre (Barratt-Boyes, 1968).

Complete Transposition of the Great Vessel with Pulmonary Stenosis. A proportion of these cases present a clinical picture identical with the tetrad, particularly in regard to cyanosis and clubbing, response at oximetry, electrocardiogram, small heart size, and reduced lung vascular markings. Cyanotic spells and squatting are less frequently seen than in the tetrad. An usual bulge high on the left border due to the aorta, or a convex left border with down-pointing apex, may allow recognition of the condition in some cases, but again selective angiocardiography is the critical investigation (Figure 27–13).

Single Ventricle with Pulmonary Stenosis. Although a number of patients have this combination of clinical signs and even chest x-rays much like those

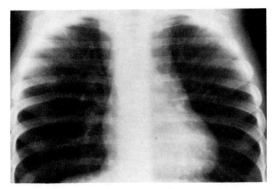

Figure 27-13. Differential diagnosis of tetralogy of Fallot. The chest x-ray of a cyanotic girl aged seven months. The heart size is normal, and there is reduced lung vascularity with a right aortic arch. Further study showed D-transposition of great arteries with a ventricular septal defect and severe subpulmonary stenosis.

seen in the tetralogy of Fallot, the radiologic contour of the heart and the electrocardiogram are often quite different in frank or subtle fashion. Echocardiography and, again, selective angiocardiography offer the best hope for accurate and important separation from the tetrad.

Asplenia Syndrome. This syndrome is more likely to create confusion with severe tetralogy of Fallot in smaller infants but should be considered in all cyanotic patients with reduced pulmonary blood flow. Plain x-rays may assist by showing ambiguous situs, a symmetric liver shadow, and central stomach or bilateral superior venae cavae. Howell-Jolly bodies in the blood smear or liver and splenic scans are most useful pointers to the diagnosis of the complex disorder.

Other. The atresia–truncus arteriosus dilemma has been referred to earlier. Rare conditions such as double-inlet left ventricle or mitral atresia with pulmonary stenosis have only in a few instances caused diagnostic confusion with the tetralogy. In older cases of tetralogy electrocardiograms may show certain differences in the electrocardiogram such as right bundle branch block or left ventricular hypertrophy and dense hilar vascularity due to the development of marked collateral circulation all of which can render clinical interpretation difficult and argue for detailed angiocardiography as the best means of diagnosis.

Course and Prognosis

Average Cases. The average case becomes progressively more cyanosed and dyspneic after the first six months. Many will have a period of "blue spells" in infancy, but a number escape without any such episodes; most emerge into childhood without having had serious difficulties. When a patient starts walking at a later age than normal children, he is more obviously disabled by his disease.

The dangerous first two years over, there appears to be an adaptation to the anoxia. The children are aware of their limitations, never require restriction of physical activity, and practically always adopt postural maneuvers such as squatting or lying to relieve any discomfort or dyspnea. At puberty there used to commence a progressive decline with increasing cyanosis and dyspnea, culminating in death at about the end of the second decade. There have been striking exceptions in the past, including the musician from Boston, reported by White and Sprague (1929), who was active until his death at 59 years, and recently reported survivors to the seventh decade (Bain, 1954; Bowie, 1961). Such cases should not be allowed to obscure the plain fact that the average age of survival is 12 years (Abbott, 1936), and that extremely few patients survive 20 years. Surgical advances may have altered this picture considerably.

Severe Cases. The severe cases have early cyanosis, feeding difficulties, and severe and prolonged "blue spells," often proceeding to cerebrovascular accidents. They frequently die from anoxia or attempted surgical relief at some period in the first year (Figure 27–14). It is noteworthy that of the 31 patients in this table who died during the first year of life, 15 had pulmonary atresia. If, to this number, surgical deaths with pulmonary atresia are added, it will be seen that of 53 patients with tetralogy of Fallot under one year of age, no less than 22 (42 percent) had pulmonary atresia at autopsy.

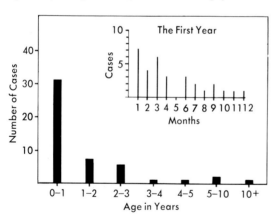

Figure 27-14. The age at death in 49 autopsy-proved cases of tetralogy of Fallot from The Hospital for Sick Children. Surgical deaths have been excluded.

Occasionally severe stenosis is associated with a large patent ductus arteriosus. These cases are not obviously cyanotic and therefore tend to present as the isolated form of the persistent ductus arteriosus. Such presentation is not uncommon in severe tetralogy in the rubella syndrome (Rowe, 1972). The major clue to the underlying defect is the existence of right ventricular hypertrophy in the electrocardiogram.

Cases with Increased Lung Vascularity. These cases constitute a small group. They may have markedly increased pulmonary blood flow or merely more than in the mild case of tetralogy of Fallot.

ATYPICAL TETRALOGY OF FALLOT. In infancy, forming the most marked example of this group, atypical tetralogy of Fallot resembles a large isolated ventricular septal defect, and cases may die from infection or heart failure. Extreme dystrophy is the rule. Those surviving infancy may continue to behave as if they have a noncyanotic lesion, but a number develop the more classic picture of tetralogy of Fallot with reduction of heart size and pulmonary vascularity associated with the onset of cyanosis and anoxic symptoms at the end of infancy.

CASES WITH A SINGLE PULMONARY ARTERY. These cases have unilateral pulmonary plethora. Most behave as an average case in regard to symptoms; but, where the pulmonary flow is truly excessive because of milder stenosis, cyanosis is delayed and the symptoms are more akin to the atypical tetrad of infancy.

CASES WITH LARGE PATENT DUCTUS ARTERIOSUS. These cases are not cyanotic and therefore tend to present as the isolated form of the persistent ductus arteriosus. The deception is all the more convincing when cardiac enlargement is present in addition to increased lung vascularity (see Figure 24–12) and the electrocardiogram shows combined ventricular hypertrophy with predominant left-sided involvement. Fortunately such large ducti are the exceptions, and for most cases the association of a patent ductus, while lessening the degree of cyanosis, fails to mask the underlying defect, which will be further suspected when the cardiac contour and electrocardiogram reveal the classic change.

CASES WITH ABSENT PULMONARY VALVE. The major point of interest in this group lies in the gross size of the pulmonary arteries. These aneurysmal structures frequently compress bronchi and may prove fatal on this account rather than from frank cardiac disability.

Complications

The final clinical incident in our fatal cases is shown in Table 27–1. Hypoxia is the basic reason for death in

Table 27-1. MODE OF DEATH IN 48 AUTOPSY-PROVED CASES OF TETRALOGY OF FALLOT. SURGICAL DEATHS HAVE BEEN EXCLUDED

FINAL CLINICAL INCIDENT	NUMBER OF CASES
Hypoxia	17
Infection	14
Thrombotic episode	5
Angiography or cardiac catheterization	4
Cerebral abscess	3
Congestive heart failure	2
Bacterial endocarditis	2
Heart block	1
Total	48

over three-fourths of the cases. One may reasonably assume that it is the prime factor in operative mortality and that extensive cerebral thrombosis is associated with hypoxia. More than one-third of the deaths were the result of infection.

Cerebrovascular Accidents. In a unique experience from the Harriet Lane Home Cardiac Clinic of over 1000 patients with tetralogy of Fallot, Clark found 4 percent with evidence of cerebrovascular accident (Tyler and Clark, 1957). Venous sinus thrombosis and arterial thrombosis or embolism may occur and explain some cases of this dreaded complication of the severely cyanotic infant patient. One of our patients with pulmonary atresia and tetralogy of Fallot died at age 11 months from widespread embolic episodes. An iliac straddle embolus, which had arisen from a mural thrombus on the left ventricle, caused gangrene of the lower limbs in this case. Martelle and Linde (1961), however, noted a more suggestive relationship between the development of hemiplegia and the presence of relative anemia than with high hematocrit levels. Such has been our own experience. In fact, specific occlusions are rarely found and most infarcts are probably anoxic in nature (Berthrong and Sabiston, 1951; Cohen, 1960).

Cerebral Abscess. This complication of the tetrad is very uncommon in the first two years of life. Among eight cyanotic patients with cerebral abscess (three deaths) representing rather more than one-quarter of cerebral abscess from all causes in the past ten years at The Hospital for Sick Children, four had tetralogy of Fallot (McGreal, 1962). All patients were over four years of age at the onset of symptoms. Headache (often localizing), fever, and lethargy were the common symptoms, frequently with fairly abrupt onset. Persistent vomiting and convulsions were late features, while an insidious onset or sudden hemiparesis was less common in our group of patients. No consistent microorganism was found responsible. Nine cases of tetralogy of Fallot among 13 patients with cerebral abscess and congenital heart disease over a recent 13-year period were reported by Matson and Salam (1961). Seven died. The 13 patients represented one-third of all cerebral abscesses in children during the same period.

Embolus from subacute bacterial endocarditis is practically never the cause of the abscess. A more likely explanation is that a small cerebral infarct becomes infected by one of what must be frequent, transient, systemic bacteremias in this malformation (Matson and Salam, 1961). All workers make a plea for prompt investigation of cerebral symptoms in cyanotic patients after infancy and the use of intensive antibiotic treatment with abscess aspiration. The excellent results that may attend a really vigorous approach to early diagnosis and treatment are attested to by a very low mortality, which has been reported by Clark (personal communication). In most reported experiences the results have been less satisfactory. In a 15- to 20-year follow-up of 779 patients who received a Blalock-Taussig anastomosis

for tetralogy of Fallot, Taussig and coworkers (1971) found 38 proven examples of brain abscess. In four patients multiple abscesses were present, and in each case symptoms had been present for more than a month before diagnosis. The outcome for this latter group was noted to be very poor, but in fact it often is so for even single brain abscesses. Twenty-five patients in Taussig's series were operated upon at several different institutions: 15 survived. The other 13 were found at autopsy so that the mortality in proven cases was over 60 percent in that series. The overall high mortality rate as well as the high incidence of sequelae in survivors in our view provides a major argument for proceeding with correction of the malformation at the earliest feasible age.

Subacute Bacterial Endocarditis. Abbott (1936) showed an incidence of 14 percent in the cyanotic cases. Taussig and associates (1951) found an incidence of 2 to 3 percent in 733 cases of tetralogy surviving the Blalock-Taussig procedure. Twenty-four patients among a group of 224 surviving 10 to 13 years after a Blalock-Taussig operation developed subacute bacterial endocarditis, and ten died (Taussig et al., 1962). Among 38 patients with congenital heart disease developing subacute endocarditis, Vogler and Doiney (1962) reported seven patients with tetralogy of Fallot. Four of these developed the infection after a Blalock-Taussig shunt. In a recent review of patients with tetralogy of Fallot followed 15 to 20 years after a Blalock-Taussig anastomosis, Taussig and associates (1971) reported 80 proven bouts of infective endocarditis in 71 patients and 41 reported but unconfirmed attacks. *Streptococcus viridans* was the causative organism in 43, *Staphylococcus* in 22. Sixteen of the seventy-one died including eight with staphylococcal infection. The mortality in the 112 patients of that study was 21 percent. Thus with time the number of patients involved increases, as one might predict. The mortality rate from this complication, on the other hand, though high, has lessened, presumably as a result of earlier diagnosis and more adequate treatment.

Tuberculosis. None of our cases died with tuberculosis. Fallot's original three cases all suffered from pulmonary tuberculosis, and many of the early reports of tetrad (even in infants) mentioned this infection. Brown (1950) believes there is an increased liability for the cyanotic case with pulmonary stenosis to develop phthisis and has reviewed the possible mechanisms in the light of recent knowledge concerning functional aspects of pulmonary circulation. The subject could be debated at great length, but in our experience pulmonary tuberculosis is no more likely to occur in cases of tetrad than in other children.

Sloan and associates (1954) have discussed the problem from the radiologic incidence in some 800 cases of pulmonary stenosis. They found that 2 percent had x-ray and clinical evidence of the infection. It was pointed out that experimental evidence shows that arterialization of blood in the pulmonary artery aggravates preexisting tuberculous lung lesions. They suggest measures at operation to avoid such potential hazard. Lung apical fibrosis simulating tuberculosis in patients with long-standing cyanosis should be considered before the infective label is applied (Haroutunian et al., 1972).

Congestive Heart Failure. This rare manifestation of tetralogy of Fallot in childhood groups occurs only under the circumstances mentioned earlier and never occurs in a classic case of the usual anatomy and fairly high hematocrit in childhood.

Pheochromocytoma. Among the five patients with cyanotic malformations of the heart and associated pheochromocytoma reported by Folger and associates (1964) were two with tetralogy of Fallot. The importance of this rare combination is emphasized by the death during the shunt operation in one subject who had no symptoms of the adrenal tumor.

Treatment

Until recently the treatment of the symptomatic infant with tetralogy of Fallot having spells was careful attention to feeding and iron intake, fluid balance, and the use of postures of advantage, morphine, and oxygen. The objective was to try to get such a patient through infancy after which time spontaneous improvement occurred (Taussig, 1948). Now the aim is to avoid recurrent hypoxic spells, an objective well founded by pathologic evidence of unexpected old infarcts in the brain of patients dying at surgery in decades gone by (Berthrong and Sabiston, 1951). There should be concern at the recurrence of episodes of severe hypoxia and acidosis in such infants (Rudolph and Danilowicz, 1963). The general explanation and management of spells and simple measures such as knee-chest position for the initial episode need to be disseminated. Those factors known to predispose to brain infarction in infants, notably relative anemia and dehydration, should be particularly cautioned against. But, as a general rule, the patient who starts to spell needs vigorous medical or surgical treatment. Two main drugs have been used for the acute spell: Morphine (Taussig, 1951) is a long-standing effective favorite in injected doses of 1 mg per 5 kg of body weight in combination with oxygen administration. More recently spells have been controlled extremely rapidly by the use of intravenous propranolol. In neonates and in some mostly acyanotic patients with spells propranolol may indeed be the treatment of choice for a period of months or even longer. In general, however, a failure to control spells completely should be an indication for surgical treatment. By acutely raising systemic resistance phenylephrine infusion has a beneficial effect on systemic arterial oxygen level and has been advocated as the medical treatment of choice for protracted spells (Nudel et al., 1976). There remains the question of treatment of developed cerebral thrombosis. Taussig (1951) advised venesection, intravenous glucose in water, and heparin, a therapy

also recommended by Kaplan (1972). Our own experience has not allowed us to be certain of the benefit of anticoagulant therapy. We tend to rely on general supportive measures as most patients improve rather quickly under any therapy. But the lessons should be clear. Surgical treatment is with few exceptions very important for the symptomatic infant, and what is now debatable is only whether the operation should be palliative or corrective at that age.

Types of Operation Available. PALLIATION. *The Blalock-Taussig Shunt (Blalock and Taussig, 1945).* As originally described this procedure consists of an anastomosis between a branch of the aorta and one of the pulmonary arteries. From the beginning this usually meant an anastomosis between the subclavian artery, less commonly the innominate artery, and the side of the left or right major pulmonary artery. The end-to-end anastomosis now is no longer employed. The end-to-side anastomosis is usually conducted on the side of the chest opposite to that where the aortic arch is situated since there is evidence that this "crossed" operation is more effective at least in young patients than an "uncrossed" procedure (same side as the aortic arch) (Taussig et al., 1971). The vertebral artery on the side of the anastomosis is now always ligated.

Potts' Operation (Potts et al., 1946). This procedure consists of a direct anastomosis between the descending aorta and the left pulmonary artery. A variety of other types of aortopulmonary shunt have been proposed and used over the years (Shumacker and Mandelbaum, 1962; Verney et al., 1962; Redo and Ecker, 1963), but the current favorite is that first described by Waterston (1962) in which the ascending aorta is anastomosed to the right pulmonary artery.

Pulmonary Valvulotomy and Infundibulectomy. These palliative measures are indirect and involve resection of infundibular muscle or valvulotomy by means of instruments passed through a small right ventricular incision (Brock, 1948; Sellors, 1948; Brock and Campbell, 1950; Brock, 1959).

The Vena Caval–Pulmonary Artery Operation (Carlon et al., 1951; Glenn, 1958; Bakuler and Kolesnikov, 1959). Generally known in North America as the Glenn procedure, this operation consists of an anastomosis of the superior vena cava to the distal end of the divided right pulmonary artery and has been utilized in the treatment of uncorrectable cyanotic malformations with pulmonary stenosis or atresia. The operation is now seldom if ever indicated in the tetralogy of Fallot since the advent of better approaches to the problem of pulmonary atresia.

Most palliative surgery is done under normothermic conditions, though some surgeons prefer a mild degree of hypothermia. Hyperbaric oxygenation is considered to offer additional advantage for the critically hypoxic patient (Bernhard et al., 1964).

CORRECTION. Closure of the ventricular septum by prosthetic patch, resection of the infundibular stenosis, and valvulotomy or relief of pulmonary arterial stenoses where indicated have become standard optimal treatment for the tetralogy of Fallot since the pioneering work of Lillehei (1955, 1956). Circulatory support during the operation is maintained by the technique of cardiopulmonary bypass even in very young infants where it may be combined with profound hypothermia. A variety of pumps, oxygenators, and methods of priming have been advocated. The open operation is fully described in the monograph of Kirklin and Karp (1970). Meticulous technique is essential in order that adequate closure of the ventricular defect be accomplished without damage to the conducting system of the heart, and for restoration of a normal-sized outflow to the right ventricle. Although in the average case of tetralogy of Fallot there is little problem to obtaining adequate relief of the infundibular obstruction, there are endless variants of the anatomy from the ostium infundibuli to the pulmonary artery bifurcation that can challenge the operator in his attempt to obtain an adequate reconstruction.

Selection of Patients and Timing of Surgery. Few would seriously debate the desirability of correction for tetralogy of Fallot. That should be the objective in every instance. Disagreement tends to arise only in regard to the age or size at which corrective surgery is performed and whether some preliminary palliative measure is likely to produce in the end a lower mortality and better result. Most surgeons would prefer to undertake immediate correction in patients about eight or nine years old when seen for the first time regardless of the nature of their obstruction. Obviously the best results occur in patients who are relatively mildly cyanotic or clinically acyanotic, and in those with low infundibular stenosis or where anomalous muscle bundles are creating the obstructive lesion. Patients with atresia particularly of the main pulmonary artery or of one major division carry an appreciably higher risk at time of correction and the ultimate outlook for these patients as well as for those who have absent pulmonary valve is less certain, though the brilliant surgical advances of the last decade have greatly altered the attitudes toward intervention in those situations.

An intermediate group of patients is composed of those who have high infundibular stenosis and a small pulmonary ring, often with a short, narrow main trunk of the pulmonary artery. Commonly there is pulmonary arterial stenosis in addition. These patients usually require some form of patch across the valve ring in order to accomplish a satisfactory relief of the outflow obstruction.

Obviously one of the more difficult decisions is in infants who are severely symptomatic because of periodic major blue spells or because of progressive cyanosis and polycythemia. It is here that surgical preferences differ. For some the answer lies in correction (Benson et al., 1962; Dobell et al., 1968; Woodson et al., 1969; Barratt-Boyes et al., 1971; Subramanian et al., 1971; Barratt-Boyes and Neutze, 1974; Castaneda et al., 1976). For others a pre-liminary shunting procedure is the wiser course (Aberdeen, 1971; Kirklin, 1971; Malm, 1971; Puga et al., 1972). There is no convincing evidence that the adequacy of repair is any less in infants surviving the correction when compared with comparable older subjects (Burnell et al., 1969; Sunderland et al., 1972). The main constraint over its use for the individual surgical team would appear to be the mortality rate from open heart surgery in a very young baby. When that rate approximates the 8 to 10 percent from correction of the malformation in older children and young adults, it is likely that palliative measures will become less widely used.

In general, then, the indication for surgical treatment is present in all patients with the tetralogy except those with no visible true pulmonary arteries. The timing of surgical treatment of whatever variety will have some variation, relating in part to anatomic factors, in part to the presence of a previous palliative shunt, and in part to the local surgical results. Those infants who suffer frequent and severe spells unrelated to anemia or who have faint murmurs when out of spells and for whom the use of propranolol is contraindicated or not effective, surgical treatment is clearly indicated. At present most units perform shunts in infancy and correct at that age only if the shunt fails. In early childhood the indications for operation are the presence of a rising hematocrit (greater than 65 percent) or hemoglobin (greater than 20 gm percent). For most of these open correction should be perfectly feasible.

How long the major repair of the malformation should be delayed in a particular patient in a particular unit is still controversial, but at present most surgeons take the view that about five years is an appropriate age for those whose clinical status permits a choice in the timing of operation (Kirklin and Karp, 1970; Puga et al., 1972).

Results of Treatment. PALLIATION. Since palliation is confined to the patients under the age of five at the present time and should not be performed in all patients, evaluation of the results should truly apply to the very young. Nowadays it is usual for a Waterston shunt to be provided for young infants and a Blalock-Taussig anastomosis on the site opposite the aortic arch in older infants and younger children. In the earliest efforts to palliate infants under a year of age, the mortality from the Blalock-Taussig procedure was 47 percent (Taussig et al., 1971), and although this figure has been improved over the years, the fact remains that there are no absolutely satisfactory palliative procedures for the very young. A fairly high operative risk exists for the patient with the tetralogy in newborns and patients under the age of six months regardless of the type of surgical procedure (Barratt-Boyes, 1968; Pickering et al., 1970; Aberdeen, 1971; Cole et al., 1971; Edmunds et al., 1971).

The principal risk to central shunt operations is the development of congestive heart failure and pulmonary vascular disease, while with the Blalock-Taussig procedure the more usual problem is that the anastomosis fails early or at a later phase due to thrombosis or narrowing at the site of anastomosis. Once the first six months are negotiated the shunt procedures carry a very much lower risk nowadays (Somerville et al., 1969; Pickering et al., 1971; Puga et al., 1972). Such individuals will proceed to corrective operation after the age of four. Because of a relatively short interval between shunt and correction the possibility of developing pulmonary vascular disease from a central shunt is now much less than formerly. For similar reasons other described late complications from shunting including infective endarteritis and subclavian steal syndrome are unlikely to occur (Fogler and Shah, 1965; Clarkson et al., 1967; Taussig et al., 1971). There is no appreciable evidence, except perhaps in the case of the Potts anastomosis, that the presence of a shunt influences the mortality at subsequent correction (Ebert and Sabiston, 1967; Azar et al., 1969; Gross et al., 1969).

results of shunts

With successful palliation by shunt cyanosis is strikingly relieved, and if clubbing is present it is lessened. Cyanosis may be present after exertion but squatting is rare. Hemoglobin and hematocrit values are reduced to normal or near-normal levels. Mehrizi and Drash (1962) found that two years after shunt operation the number of their patients below the sixteenth percentile for height and weight had halved from their preoperative figures. After aorticopulmonary anastomosis a continuous murmur is audible over the chest in the general region of the anastomosis. It is often not audible during the first few days of the postoperative period (particularly in the case of central shunt), but the presence of a good, loud shunt murmur is clear evidence that the anastomosis is likely to be successful. Some authorities recommend prompt shunt revision as the murmur disappears during the immediate postoperative period (Figure 27–15). After operation the heart size increases in the first month or so, a change that bears relation to the size of the shunt and usually reaches a period of stability within a few months. Cardiomegaly and congestive failure risk is likely to be greater in patients with central shunts than with the Blalock-Taussig operation where rather less than half of the cases develop increase in heart size. The anastomosed pulmonary artery may distend moderately, but progressive enlargement of the central pulmonary arteries following a Blalock-Taussig shunt is a reliable sign of developing pulmonary hypertension (Marr and White, 1972). The development of such pulmonary hypertension has been rare, occurring in less than 4 percent of 653 Blalock-Taussig operations reported by Taussig and associates (1971) (Figure 27–16). Six of the twenty-five involved had been described earlier (Leeds, 1958; Ross et al., 1958; McGaff et al., 1962; Folger and Otken, 1969). The proportion of patients developing pulmonary hypertension after shunt operations has been greater in those with large surgical communications, i.e., innominate or aorticopulmonary, than in a simple subclavian anastomosis (Daoud et al., 1966). The incidence of the complication

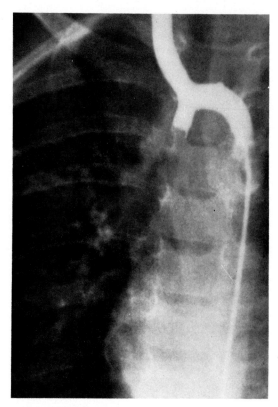

Figure 27-15. Acute occlusion of a Blalock-Taussig anastomosis. Selective angiogram from the innominate artery showing thrombosis in the right subclavian artery.

following a Potts anastomosis has been between 15 and 20 percent (Paul et al., 1961; Von Bernuth et al., 1970). By comparison a decline in shunt effectiveness over time has been a more significant problem with Blalock-Taussig shunts in the past. Just over half of 685 patients surviving a Blalock-Taussig shunt between 1945 and 1951 at the Johns Hopkins Hospital were living on their first anastomosis 15 years later. The majority of second operations were not performed till 10 to 12 years after the first, but 60 percent of infants originally operated upon under two years required a second procedure (Taussig et al., 1971). Unilateral rib notching may appear after a Blalock-Taussig operation because collateral channels develop to supply the affected areas following surgical interruption of the subclavian artery (Kent, 1953; Petersen, 1956). Hemoptysis has been described ten years after a Blalock-Taussig operation. It was related to an intercostal artery that became included in the lung vascular supply (Haroutunian and Neill, 1972). Gangrene of the arm has been reported rarely following a Blalock-Taussig operation (Lam, 1949; D'Allaines, 1950; Webb and Burford, 1952; Hanlon and Varco, 1953), including a one-year-old infant who developed demarcation in the left forearm by the third postoperative day. Mummification occurred, and an amputation was performed five weeks later. All examples probably

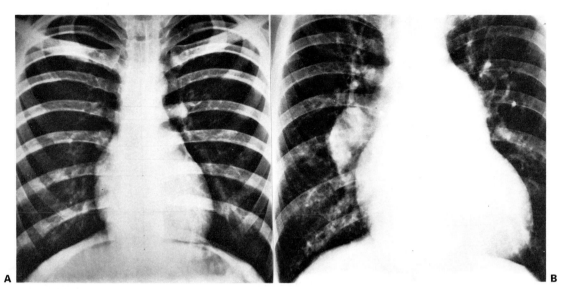

Figure 27-16. Pulmonary vascular disease following palliative surgery in tetralogy of Fallot. A man who had a Blalock-Taussig anastomosis at the age of 14 years. *A.* Preoperative chest x-ray. *B.* Chest x-ray at 39 years. The systolic pulmonary arterial pressure was at systemic level at this age. (Courtesy of Dr. R. I. White, Jr., The Johns Hopkins Hospital, Baltimore, Maryland.)

resulted from ligation of important collateral channels. Subclavian steal syndrome (Reivich et al., 1961), a form of basilar artery insufficiency, may occur after a Blalock-Taussig operation if the vertebral artery is not divided at the time of surgery. Not all patients with angiographic signs of "steal" have neurologic symptoms, so that age or other factors, possibly anatomic, act protectively in this situation. Clarkson and associates (1967) considered that symptoms were more likely to occur in patients with evidence of neurologic abnormalities preoperatively. Headache, visual disturbances, and syncope can appear in as short an interval as one year after operation, and such symptoms should immediately arouse suspicion of the complications. Aortography will support the diagnosis, and corrective surgery for the cardiac defect usually completely relieves the symptoms in childhood (Folger and Shah, 1965).

Minor Complication. A number of problems of a less serious nature may follow such operations. Horner's syndrome, diaphragmatic paralysis, vocal cord paralysis, hemothorax, and atelectesis have been noted.

Most operated cases are able to be up after several days and to undertake full activity within one to two months.

In 120 patients with tetralogy of Fallot treated by indirect infundibulectomy and valvulotomy Brock (1959) reported a 30 percent mortality in the first 27 cases and 7 percent in the next 93. The degree of clinical improvement was similar to that obtained from the shunt procedure. It is claimed that this operation not only improves the size of the outflow tract of the right ventricle but also enlarges the left ventricle gradually. If this is true, the chances of

eventual repair without major patching across the outflow should be enhanced by such preliminary palliation. Complications of the procedure are pulmonary hypertension from excessive left-to-right shunt and pulmonary valve regurgitation. The operation has not been adopted widely because it is technically more difficult to perform than a shunt, but good results have been achieved by a few groups in the United States (Lin et al., 1958; Weinberg et al., 1962; Taylor et al., 1963; Flege and Ehrenhaft, 1967).

CORRECTION. Results from this type of surgery have improved substantially over the last 15 years to the point where in several centers the risk rate is between 5 and 7 percent and in most centers is somewhere in the order of between 10 and 15 percent (Shumway et al., 1965; Goldman et al., 1966; Malm et al., 1966; Barratt-Boyes, 1968; Gotsman et al., 1969; Hawe et al., 1969; Kirklin and Karp, 1970). Clearly a number of factors influence the comparison of mortality between groups from different centers including the predominant age at surgery, the nature of case selection, and the surgical techniques. At The Hospital for Sick Children in Toronto between 1955 and 1968 232 patients underwent intracardiac repair for this malformation. When operative mortality was defined as death occurring within 30 days of surgery, the mortality in the first half of the series of 116 patients was 35 percent whereas in the second half, from 1965 onward, the mortality was 12 percent (Olley, 1971).

In survivors the patient first and foremost has normal arterial oxygen saturation, he is obviously pink, and the striking physical change is accompanied by rapid return to normal exercise tolerance and hemoglobin and hematocrit level. An important change that has not generally been appreciated and is most obvious in previously severely affected children has been an improvement in psyche and educational drive brought about by the repair. One has the suspicion that the reportedly high incidence of mental retardation in tetralogy of Fallot may be at least in part a consequence of hypoxia and may constitute a reversible situation. Abnormal cardiac physical signs usually remain. Of these, prominent jugular "a" waves and right ventricular lift for several months and a prominent systolic ejection murmur, diastolic murmur of pulmonary valvular regurgitation, and delayed pulmonary valve closure sounds are commonly encountered. The chest x-ray may show mild to moderate enlargement of the heart, and the electrocardiogram usually shows complete right bundle branch block.

complication at tet. repair The major complications that arise early in the postoperative period are bleeding (Kirklin and Karp, 1970), complete heart block (Lauer et al., 1960; Gomez et al., 1962), and respiratory difficulty of a variety of origins (Osborn, 1961). The problem with bleeding is usually identified by persistent drainage. It requires surgical exploration but then responds to simple measures at reentry. Only occasionally is it due to real disturbance of the clotting mechanisms. Immediately postoperatively patients with complete heart block need pacing support aided by the insertion of electrodes in myocardium before the chest is closed. The persistent complication is fortunately rare—not usually nowadays seen in more than 1 to 2 percent—but carries a very serious prognosis.

Another early problem is pulmonary edema, the cause of which is controversial. This complication requires the administration of diuretics and respiratory support, sometimes with the use of steroids in addition. Fortunately such developments are uncommon and nowadays appear to be better tolerated through improved therapy. Respiratory problems in general have been greatly assisted by the establishment of simpler ventilatory support such as is obtained with the positive end expiratory pressure technique of Gregory and associates (1971).

A further complication of the postoperative period that is common is some reduction in cardiac output. It is generally believed that this is related to the ventriculotomy, but it may also be associated with ischemia due to cross-clamping of the aorta (Kaplan, 1972). In any event, a good response of the heart to isoproterenol infusion is usual. Most centers in addition routinely support the myocardium by the administration of digoxin, which is begun during the latter part of the first postoperative 24-hour period.

Late postoperative complications include the postpericardiotomy syndrome and congestive failure secondary to residual ventricular shunt or to disturbed tricuspid valve function. This latter complication may be due to direct injury of the valve at the time of operation but is more often associated with residual outflow obstruction or severe pulmonary valve regurgitation in conjunction with poor right ventricular function. The latter is likely related

to infarction of the right ventricle from interference with myocardial blood supply.

It has recently become apparent that in addition to the dreaded complete heart block there may be more problems in store from the presence of complete right bundle branch block than had been supposed formerly. Complete right bundle branch block may be due to distal bundle damage related to the ventriculotomy incision (Gelband et al., 1971) or it may be from more proximal damage to the bundle during repair of the ventricular defect. In the latter circumstance the potential for damage to portions of the left fascicular system is real. In some instances (23 percent at The Hospital for Sick Children) there is a frank expression of damage to the left fascicle by the presence of left anterior hemiblock (Kulbertus et al., 1969; Rosenbaum et al., 1970; Downing et al., 1972; Godman et al., 1972; Wolff et al., 1972; Steeg et al., 1975; Sondheimer et al., 1976). (Figure 27–17). For these cases there is conflicting evidence concerning the subsequent risk of sudden death presumably due to the development of complete heart block but possibly from other arrhythmias. On the other hand, the prognosis for patients who had transient complete heart block, second degree heart block, or AV dissociation during surgery but not at the time of leaving the operating room is good, and the risk of recurrence is really very small in this group (Squarcia et al., 1971; Sondheimer et al., 1976). Localization of blocks by the analysis of His bundle electrograms can be superior to the routine electrocardiogram in predicting the course of patients who develop heart block (Anderson et al., 1972) and seems likely to become an important and necessary part of the postoperative evaluation of most if not all patients who have undergone corrective surgery.

One of the most difficult matters to assess indirectly over the long term is the state of hemodynamics after operation. Because residual murmurs and cardiac enlargement are usual and the electrocardiogram is always abnormal, physicians following their patients have tended to rely on the general well-being of the patient and the absence of congestive failure as indicative of good results. Most postoperative cardiac catheterization studies have been performed to examine specific aspects of postoperative hemodynamic behavior (Jarmakani et al., 1972), to assess patients in whom a suspicion of considerable abnormality of hemodynamic function has been suspected (Cornell et al., 1968) or in numbers that are not representative of the total operated group (Hallidie-Smith et al., 1967). In studies where an attempt has been made to evaluate all survivors of operative correction, residual defects have been found not infrequently (Malm et al., 1966; Barratt-Boyes, 1968; Gotsman et al., 1969; Levine et al., 1971). Residual left-to-right shunt through the ventricular septal defect has been found in 14 to 30 percent of such studies, and although most of these are small shunts, up to one-third may be sufficiently large to warrant reoperation. Residual pressure differences across the outflow tract of the right

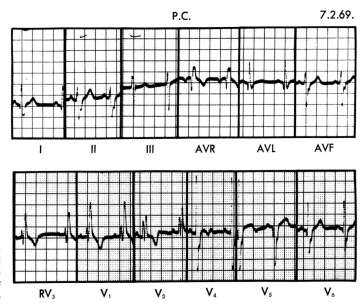

P.C.   7.2.69.

I   II   III   AVR   AVL   AVF

RV₃   V₁   V₂   V₄   V₅   V₆

Figure 27-17. The electrocardiogram in postoperative tetralogy of Fallot. An example of the complication of left anterior hemiblock in addition to the usual complete right bundle branch block.

ventricle have been shown present in between 12 and 25 percent of such patients. Pulmonary regurgitation is common and is inevitable in those patients in whom outflow patch insertion across the pulmonary annulus has been made. Even in these patients there seems to be no gross evidence of cardiac dysfunction over a decade later (Jones et al., 1972).

Additionally it has been noted that in about 20 percent of patients, most of whom have significant pulmonary regurgitation, a right-to-left shunt can be demonstrated at the atrial level. Embolic problems can result through a persistent patent formen ovale late in the postoperative period (Levine et al., 1971).

Left ventricular function is depressed in children with tetralogy of Fallot both before and after correction (Jarmakani et al., 1972). In a few instances with right ventricular systolic pressures at rest of more than 60 mm of mercury, exercise induced a rise in right ventricular end diastolic pressure coupled with a fall in stroke index indicating an abnormal myocardial response (Joransen and Moller, 1972). Most series emphasize that the clinical result is excellent to good in about 90 percent of the patients studied, and the long-term results to date bear out this optimistic attitude in large measure. The capacity to perform physical work on the bicycle ergometer at sub-maximal levels is surprisingly normal in many patients (Wessel et al., 1976). The description of residual abnormalities of the nature mentioned should not imply that the benefits from surgery are trivial, but it should remind us that together with other problems such as pulmonary arterial stenosis of mild degree, some outflow tract aneurysmal for-mation from patching (Figure 27–18), conduction defects of the type already mentioned, and intrapulmonary shunts as described by Moss and colleagues (1969), there are some uncertainties about the late outcome from correction. Patients with the correction should therefore be followed for life.

There are some particular categories of the malformation that bear emphasis in regard to the surgical treatment. Patients with pulmonary atresia still pose major surgical challenge. Many patients with this severe form of the malformation require treatment in infancy, and for them shunt operations improve rather fewer than those with reasonable outflow anatomy (Campbell, 1960). Part of this mortality is related to the presence of severe metabolic acidosis at the time newborn patients are taken to surgery (Aziz et al., 1975). The infusion of E-type prostaglandins dramatically improves the condition of such infants by increasing oxygenation through reopening of the ductus arteriosus (Olley et al., 1976). The Barrett operation and the Glenn procedure (Barrett and Daley, 1949; Young et al., 1963) have largely been replaced by a bolder and more ambitious attempt to correct the anomaly through the use of homograft aortic valve and aorta or a tubular prosthesis with a valve bridging the gap between the right ventricle and the major pulmonary artery divisions (Rastelli et al., 1965; Ross and Somerville, 1966; McGoon et al., 1968; Weldon et al., 1968; Wallace et al., 1969; Kouchoukos et al., 1971; McGoon, 1971; Brawley et al., 1972). Ligation or other means of closure (Zuberbuhler et al., 1974) of bronchial collateral vessels is a necessary additional step during repair. The pioneering efforts of the Mayo group in this area are of great importance. In suitable cases the operation can offer a completely different outlook for a malformation previously regarded as incurable. A similar approach to the problem of small annulus with severe stenosis or absent pulmonary valve may in the end be necessary (Cornel et al., 1971), but relatively simple measures such as closing the ventricular defect and patching across the narrow annulus in that situation have already produced a significant improvement in surgical results (Danielson et al., 1972; Jones et al., 1972).

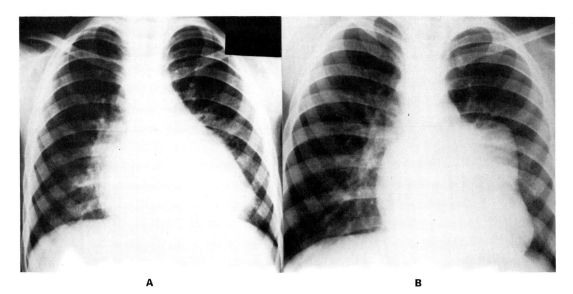

A   **B**

Figure 27-18. Aneurysm of the right ventricle. The chest x-rays of A.M. (550906) following correction of tetralogy of Fallot at age four years. A right ventricular outflow patch was inserted (*A*) soon after operation and (*B*) one year later. The right ventricular pressure was 35/3 and the pulmonary artery pressure 20/5. The appearance is unchanged in films up to 11 years.

A special problem exists for patients with absence of one major pulmonary artery division or for those patients with thrombosis in a major pulmonary artery following previous end-to-end anastomosis. The problem concerns the probability of pulmonary vascular disease existing in the single functioning vessel. Most surgical results have been rather discouraging, but recent experience in the correction of these variants has looked better (Mistrot et al., 1977). Occlusive disease of the pulmonary vascular bed apart from those cases with single pulmonary artery is believed to be excessively rare (Kirklin and Karp, 1970). The natural history of this potential problem remains to be described.

The status of the surgical achievement in tetralogy of Fallot has been aptly summarized by Bourland and McNamara (1970): "In our enthusiasm to secure patient and parent approval for operation we should not promise future gridiron glory; but we can anticipate a remarkable relief of symptoms sufficient for the patient to plan an education, a gainful occupation and a family life."

As with other forms of heart malformation, the ultimate psychologic health of the individual is not related to the original severity of the disease. It is reflected in the perception of the disorder harbored by the patient and those around him (Garson et al., 1974).

REFERENCES

Abbott, M. E.: *Atlas of Congenital Cardiac Disease.* American Heart Association, New York, 1936.

Aberdeen, E.: *The Willis B. Potts Memorial Symposium on Tetralogy of Fallot,* Chicago, Ill., 1971.

Abildgaard, C. F., and Schulman, I.: Absence of coagulation abnormalities in children with cyanotic congenital heart disease. *Lancet,* **2**: 660, 1968.

Anderson, P. A. W.; Rogers, M. C.; Cavent, R. C., Jr.; Jarmakani, J. M. M.; Jewett, P. H.; and Spach, M. S.: Reversible complete heart block following cardiac surgery. Analysis of His bundle electrograms. *Circulation,* **46**: 514, 1972.

Azar, H.; Hardesty, R. L.; Pontius, R. G.; Zuberbuhler, J. R.; and Bahnson, H. T.: A review of total correction in 200 cases of tetralogy of Fallot. *Arch. Surg.,* **99**: 281, 1969.

Aziz, K. U.; Olley, P. M.; Rowe, R. D.; Trusler, G. A.; and Mustard, W. T.: Survival after systemic to pulmonary arterial shunts in infants less than 30 days old with obstructive lesions of the right heart chambers. *Am. J. Cardiol.,* **36**: 479, 1975.

Baffes, T. G.; Johnson, F. R.; Potts, W. J.; and Gibson, S.: Anatomic variations in tetralogy of Fallot. *Am. Heart J.,* **46**: 657, 1953.

Bahnson, H. T., and Ziegler, R. F.: A consideration of the cases of death following operation for congenital heart disease of the cyanotic types. *Surg. Gynecol. Obstet.,* **90**: 60, 1950.

Bain, G. O.: Tetralogy of Fallot: survival to 70th year. *Arch. Pathol.,* **58**: 176, 1954.

Gakuler, A. N., and Kolesnikov, S. A.: Anastomosis of superior vena cava and pulmonary artery in the surgical treatment of certain congenital defects of the heart. *J. Thorac. Cardiovasc. Surg.,* **37**: 693, 1959.

Baron, M. G.: Radiologic notes in cardiology. Angiographic differentiation between tetralogy of Fallot and double outlet right ventricle. Relationship of the mitral and aortic valves. *Circulation,* **43**: 451, 1971.

Barratt-Boyes, B. G.: The surgery of tetralogy of Fallot, pulmonary atresia with ventricular septal defect and transposition of the great vessels. *Aust. Radiol.,* **12**: 311, 1968.

Barratt-Boyes, B. G., and Neutze, J. M.: Primary repair of tetralogy of Fallot in infancy using profound hypothermia with circulatory arrest and limited cardiopulmonary bypass. *Ann. Surg.,* **178**: 406, 1974.

Barratt-Boyes, B. G.; Simpson, M.; and Neutze, J. M.: Intracardiac surgery in neonates and infants using deep hypothermia with surface cooling and limited cardiopulmonary bypass. *Circulation,* Suppl. **33–34**: I–25, 1971.

Barrett, N. R., and Daley, R.: A method of increasing the lung blood supply in cyanotic congenital heart disease. *Br. Med. J.,* **1**: 699, 1949.

Bass, D. A., and Rowe, R. D.: Patent ductus arteriosus as a complicating factor in infants with other cardiac malformations. *Circulation,* **37–38** Suppl. VI: 38, 1968.

Baum, D.; Khoury, G. H.; Ongley, P. A.; Swan, H. J. C.; and Kincaid, O. W.: Congenital stenosis of the pulmonary artery branches. *Circulation*, 29:680, 1964.

Becker, A. E.; Connor, M.; and Anderson, R. H.: Tetralogy of Fallot: A morphometric and geometric study. *Am. J. Cardiol.*, 35:402, 1975.

Bécu, L.; Ikkos, D.; Ljungqvist, A.; and Rudhe, U.: Evolution of ventricular septal defect and pulmonary stenosis with left-to-right shunt into classic tetralogy of Fallot. *Am. J. Cardiol.*, 7:598, 1961.

Benson, P. F.; Joseph, M. C.; and Ross, D. N.: Total surgical correction of Fallot's tetralogy in the first year of life. *Lancet*, 2:326, 1962.

Bernhard, W. F.; Frittelli, G.; Tank, E. S.; and Carr, J. G.: Surgery under hyperbaric oxygenation in infants with congenital heart disease. *Circulation*, 29:Suppl. 91, 1964.

Berri, G. G.; Caprile, J. A.; and Kreutzer, R.: Anatomie de la tétrade de Fallot. *Arch. Mal. Coeur.*, 45:1082, 1952.

Berthrong, M., and Sabiston, D. C., Jr.: Cerebral lesions in congenital heart disease: review of autopsies in 162 cases. *Bull. Johns Hopkins Hosp.*, 89:384, 1951.

Best, P. V., and Heath, D.: Pulmonary thrombosis in cyanotic congenital heart disease without pulmonary hypertension. *J. Pathol. Bact.*, 75:281, 1958.

Bing, R. J.; Vandam, L. D.; and Gray, F. D.: Physiological studies in congenital heart disease. II. Results of preoperative studies in patients with tetralogy of Fallot. *Bull. Johns Hopkins Hosp.*, 80:121, 1947.

Bing, R. J.; Vandam, L. D.; Handelsman, J. C.; Campbell, J. A.; Spencer, R.; and Griswold, H. E.: Physiological studies in congenital heart disease. VI Adaptations to anoxia in congenital heart disease with cyanosis. *Bull. Johns Hopkins Hosp.*, 83:439, 1948.

Binet, J. P.; Carpentier, J.; Pottemain, M.; and Langlois, J.: Double aortic arch associated with tetralogy of Fallot in infants. *J. Thorac. Cardiovasc. Surg.*, 51:116, 1966.

Björk, V. O.; Lodin, H.; and Michaelsson, M.: Fallot's anomaly with peripheral pulmonary artery malformations. *J. Thorac. Cardiovasc. Surg.*, 45:764, 1963.

Blalock, A.: Surgical procedures employed and anatomical variations encountered in the treatment of congenital pulmonic stenosis. *Surg. Gynecol. Obstet.*, 87:385, 1948.

Blalock, A., and Taussig, H. B.: The surgical treatment of malformations of the heart in which there is pulmonary stenosis or pulmonary atresia. *JAMA*, 128:189, 1945.

Bloomfield, D. K.: The natural history of the ventricular septal defect in patients surviving infancy. *Circulation*, 29:914, 1964.

Bonham-Carter, R. E.: Anemia in tetralogy of Fallot. Symposium on congenital heart disease. *Br. Heart J.*, 20:279, 1958.

Bouchard, F., and Cornu, C.: Etude des courpes de pressions ventriculaire droite et artérielle pulmonaires dans les rétrécissements pulmonaires. *Arch. Mal. Coeur.* 47:417, 1954.

Bourland, B. J., and McNamara, D. G.: Tetralogy of Fallot: Natural course, indications for surgery and results of surgical treatment. *Cardiovasc. Clin.*, 2:195, 1970.

Bousvaros, G. A.: The pulmonary second sound in the tetralogy of Fallot. *Am. Heart J.*, 61:570, 1961.

Bove, E. L.; Shaher, R. M.; Alley, R.; and McKneally, M.: Tetralogy of Fallot with absent pulmonary valve and aneurysm of the pulmonary artery: Report of two cases presenting as obstructive lung disease. *J. Pediatr.*, 81:339, 1972.

Bowie, E. A.: Longevity in tetralogy of Fallot. Discussion of cases on patients surviving 40 years and presentation of two further cases. *Am. Heart J.*, 62:125, 1961.

Brandt, P. W. T.: The radiology of cyanotic congenital heart disease. *Aust. Radiol.*, 12:279, 1968.

Braudo, J. L., and Zion, M. M.: The cyanotic (syncopal) attack in Fallot's tetralogy. *Br. Med. J.*, 1:1323, 1959.

Brawley, R. K.; Gardner, T. J.; Donahoo, J. S.; Neill, C. A.; Rowe, R. D.; and Gott, V. L.: Late results after right ventricular outflow tract reconstruction with aortic root homografts. *J. Thorac. Cardiovasc. Surg.*, 64:314, 1972.

Brinton, W. D., and Campbell, M.: Necropsies in some congenital disease of the heart, mainly Fallot's tetralogy. *Br. Heart J.*, 15:335, 1953.

Bristow, J. D.; Menashe, V. D.; Griswold, H. E.; and Starr, A.: Total correction of tetralogy of Fallot. *Am. J. Cardiol.*, 8:358, 1961.

Brock, R. C.: Pulmonary valvulotomy for the relief of congenital pulmonary stenosis. *Br. Med. J.*, 1:1121, 1948.

———: *The Anatomy of Congenital Pulmonary Stenosis.* Cassell, London, 1957.

Brock, R. C., and Campbell, M.: Infundibular resection of dilatation for infundibular stenosis. *Br. Heart J.*, 12:403, 1950.

Brock, R. C.; Sellors, T. H.; and Hill, I. G. W.: Quoted by Brinton, W. D., and Campbell, M.: Necropsies in some congenital diseases of the heart, mainly Fallot's tetralogy. *Br. Heart J.*, 15:335, 1953.

Brotmacher, L.: Hemodynamic effects of squatting during repose. *Br. Heart J.*, 19:559, 1957.

Brown, J. W.: *Congenital Heart Disease.* Staple Press, Ltd., London, 1950.

Burch, G. E.; DePasquale, N. P.; and Phillips, J. H.: Tetralogy of Fallot associated with well developed left ventricular muscle mass and increased life span. *Am. J. Med.*, 36:54, 1964.

Burchell, H. B.; Taylor, B. E.; Knutson, J. R. B.; and Wood, E. H.: Circulatory adjustments to the hypoxemia of congenital heart disease of the cyanotic type. *Circulation*, 1:404, 1950.

Burke, E. C.; Kirklin, J. W.; and Edwards, J. E.: Sites of obstruction to pulmonary blood flow in tetralogy of Fallot, *Proc. Mayo Clin.*, 26:498, 1951.

Burnell, R. H.; Woodson, R. D.; Lees, M. H.; Bristow, J. D.; and Starr, A.: Results of correction of tetralogy of Fallot in children under four years of age. *J. Thorac. Cardiovasc. Surg.*, 57:153, 1969.

Campbell, M.: Simple pulmonary stenosis: pulmonary valvular stenosis with closed ventricular septum. *Br. Heart J.*, 16:273, 1954.

———: Results of surgical treatment for pulmonary atresia. *Br. Heart J.*, 22:527, 1960.

Campbell, M., and Hills, T. H.: Angiocardiography and cyanotic congenital heart disease. *Br. Heart J.*, 12:65, 1950.

Carlon, C. A.; Mondini, P. G.; and De Marchi, R.: Surgical treatment of some cardiovascular diseases (a new vascular anastomosis). *J. Internat. Coll. Surgeons*, 16:1, 1951.

Cassell, D. E., and Morse, M.: Blood volume in congenital heart disease. *J. Pediatr.*, 31:485, 1947.

Castaneda, A. R.; Williams, R. G.; Rosenthal, A.; and Sade, R. M.: Tetralogy of Fallot: primary repair in infancy. In Kidd, B. S. L., and Rowe, R. D. (eds.): *The Child with Congenital Heart Disease After Surgery.* Futura Publishing Co., Inc., Mount Kisco, N.Y., 1976, p. 63.

Castellanos, A.; Garcia, O.; Gonzalez, E.; Pereiras, R.; and Mercado, H.: The levoangiocardiogram in tetralogy of Fallot. *Radiology*, 75:774, 1960.

Castellanos, A.; Hernandez, F. A.; and Mercado, H. G.: Wedge pulmonary arteriography in congenital heart disease. *Radiology*, 85:838, 1965.

Castellanos, A.; Pereiras, R.; and Garcia, A.: L'Angiocardiographie chez l'infant. *Presse méd.*, 46:1747, 1938.

Celermajer, J. M.; Varghese, P. J.; and Rowe, R. D.: Cardiovascular lesions in rubella embryopaltry with special emphasis on pulmonary arterial disease. *Israel J. Med. Sci.*, 5:568, 1969.

Char, F.; Rodriquez-Fernandez, H. L.; Scott, C. I., Jr.; Borgaonker, D. S.; Bell, B. B.; and Rowe, R. D.: The Noonan syndrome—a clinical study of forty-five cases. The Fourth Conference on the Clinical delineation of birth defects. Part XV. In Dergsma, D. (ed.): *Birth Defects:* Orig. art. series., The National Foundation, N.Y. Vol. V, 1972, p. 110.

Chesler, E.; Beck, W.; and Schrire, V.: Selective catheterization of pulmonary or bronchial arteries in the preoperative assessment of pseudo-truncus arteriosus. *Am. J. Cardiol.*, 26:20, 1970.

Chesler, E.; Joffe, H. S.; Beck, W.; and Schrire, V.: Echocardiographic recognition of mitral-semilunar valve discontinuity. An aid to the diagnosis of origin of both great vessels from the right ventricle. *Circulation*, 43:725, 1971.

Chesler, E.; Joffe, H. S.; Beck, W.; and Schrire, V.: Tetralogy of Fallot and heart failure. *Am. Heart J.*, 81:321, 1971.

Chrispin, A. R., and Lillie, J. G.: The pyelogram following angiocardiography in children with congenital heart disease. *Proc. Roy. Soc. Med.*, 59:419, 1966.

Chung, K. J.; Nanda, N. D.; Manning, J. A.; and Gramiak, R.: Echocardiographic findings in tetralogy of Fallot. *Am. J. Cardiol.*, 31:126, 1973.

Clark, D. B.: Personal communication, 1964.

Clarkson, P. M.; Gomez, M. R.; Wallace, R. B.; and Weidman, W. H.: Central nervous system complications following Blalock-Taussig operation. *Pediatrics*, 39:18, 1967.

Clay, R. C.; Elliott, S. R., II; and Scott, H. W., Jr.: Changes in blood volume following operation for pulmonic stenosis: studies with Evans blue and radioactive phosphorous. *Bull. Johns Hopkins Hosp.*, **89**:337, 1951.

Cohen, M. M.: The central nervous system in congenital heart disease. *Neurology*, **10**:452, 1960.

Cole, R. B.; Muster, A. J.; Fixler, D. E.; and Paul, M. H.: Long term results of aortopulmonary anastomosis for tetralogy of Fallot. Morbidity and mortality 1946–1969. *Circulation*, **43**:263, 1971.

Cooley, R. N.; Bahnson, H. T.; and Hanlon, C. R.: Angiocardiography in congenital heart disease of the cyanotic type with pulmonic stenosis or atresia. *Radiology*, **52**:329, 1949.

Cornel, G.; Colokathis, B.; and Subramanian, S.: Heterograft valve implant in tetralogy with absent pulmonary valve. *Ann. Thorac. Surg.*, **11**:51, 1971.

Cornell, S. H.; Vlad, P.; and Ehrenhaft, J. L.: Angiographic and catheterization findings in patients with difficulties after total correction of tetralogy of Fallot. *Radiology*, **91**:321, 1968.

Corvisart, J. N.: *Essai sur les maladies et les lesions organiques du coeur et des gros vaisseaux ; extrait des lecons cliniques de ; publie sous ses yeux*, Vol. 36, 3rd ed., Mequignon-Marvis, Paris, 1818. Cited by Edwards (1960).

Cumming, G. R.: Editorial—Propranolol in tetralogy of Fallot. *Circulation*, **41**:13, 1970.

D'Allaines, F.: *Chirurgie du coeur*. Editions Scientifiques Francaises, Paris, 1950.

Danielson, G. K.; Stafford, E. F.; Mair, D. G.; and McGoon, D. C.: Tetralogy of Fallot with absent pulmonary valve: Surgical considerations and results. *Circulation*, **46**:Suppl. II–34, 1972.

Daoud, G.; Kaplan, S.; and Helmsworth, J. A.: Tetralogy of Fallot and pulmonary hypertension. *Am. J. Dis. Child.*, **111**:166, 1966.

Dayem, M. K. A.; Preger, L.; Goodwin, J. F.; and Steiner, R. E.: Double outlet right ventricle with pulmonary stenosis. *Br. Heart J.*, **29**:64, 1967.

Dobell, A. R. C.; Charrette, E. P.; and Chughtai, M. S.: Correction of tetralogy of Fallot in the young child. *J. Thorac. Cardiovasc. Surg.*, **55**:70, 1968.

Donzelot, E., and D'Allaines, F.: *Traité des Cardiopathies Congenitales*. Masson & Cie, Paris, 1954.

Donzelot, E.; D'Allaines, F.; Bubost, C.; Metianu, C.; Durant, M.; and Dunost, C.: Deductions chirurgicales tirées de l'étude de 54 pièces anatomiques de tetralogie de Fallot. *Sem. Hôp. Paris*, **28**:877, 1952.

Donzelot, E.; Emam-Zade, A. M.; Heim de Balsac, R.; Escalle, J. E.; and Antoine, M.: L'Angiocardiographie dans les maladies congenitales: techniques et resultats obtenus dans 74 cas. *Arch. Mal. Coeur*, **42**:35, 1949.

Donzelot, E.; Metianu, C.; Durand, M.; Cherchi, A.; and Vlad, P.: L'Electrocardiogramme dans la tetralogie de Fallot (étude de 100 cas). *Arch. Mal. Coeur*, **44**:97, 1951.

Dotter, C. T., and Steinberg, I.: *Angiocardiography* (Annals of Roentgenology, Vol. 20). Paul B. Hoeber, Inc., New York, 1951.

Downing, J. W., Jr.: Postsurgical left anterior hemiblock and right bundle branch block. *Br. Heart J.*, **34**:263, 1972.

Durnin, R. E.; Willner, R.; Virmani, S.; Lawrence, T. Y.; and Fyler, D. C.: Pulmonary regurgitation with ventricular septal defect and pulmonic stenosis—tetralogy of Fallot variant. *Am. J. Roentgenol.*, **106**:43, 1969.

Ebert, P. A., and Sabiston, D. C., Jr.: Surgical management of the tetralogy of Fallot: Influence of a previous systemic—pulmonary anastomosis on the results of open correction. *Ann. Surg.*, **165**:806, 1967.

Edmunds, L. H., Jr.; Fishman, N. H.; Heymann, M. A.; and Rudolph, A. M.: Anastomosis between aorta and right pulmonary artery (Waterston) in neonates. *N. Engl. J. Med.*, **284**:464, 1971.

Edwards, J. E.: Congenital malformations of the heart and great vessels. In Gould, S. E. (ed.): *Pathology of the Heart*, 2nd ed. Charles C Thomas, Publisher, Springfield, Ill., 1960, p. 317.

Ekert, H.; Gilchrist, G. S.; Stanton, R.; and Hammond, D.: Hemostasis in cyanotic congenital heart disease. *J. Pediatr.*, **76**:221, 1970.

Fabricius, J.; Hansen, P. F.; and Lindeneg, O.: Pulmonary atresia developing after a shunt operation for Fallot's tetralogy. *Br. Heart J.*, **23**:556, 1961.

Fallot, A.: Contribution a l'anatomie pathologique de la maladie bleue (cyanose cardiaque). *Marseille Méd.*, **25**:77, 138, 207, 270, 341, 403, 1888.

Feldt, R. H.; Du Shane, J. W.; and Titus J. L.: The anatomy of the

atrioventricular conduction system in ventricular septal defect and tetralogy of Fallot. Correlations with the electrocardiogram and vectorcardiogram. *Circulation*, **34**:774, 1966.

Fellows, K. E.; Freed, M. D.; Keane, J. F.; Van Praagh, R.; Bernhard, W. F.; and Castaneda, A. C.: Results of routine preoperative coronary angiography in tetralogy of Fallot. *Circulation*, **51**:561, 1975.

Ferencz, C.: The pulmonary vascular bed in tetralogy of Fallot. I. Changes associated with pulmonic stenosis. *Bull. Hopkins Hosp.*, **106**:81, 1960a.

———: The pulmonary vascular bed in tetralogy of Fallot. II. Changes following a systemic-pulmonary anastomosis. *Bull. Hopkins Hosp.*, **106**:100, 1960b.

Feruglio, G. A., and Gunton, R. W.: Intracardiac phonocardiography in ventricular septal defect. *Circulation*, **21**:49, 1960.

Fineberg, M. H., and Wiggers, C. J.; Compensation and failure of right ventricle. *Am. Heart J.*, **11**:255, 1936.

Fisher, C. H.; James, A. E.; Humphries, J. O.; Forsler, J.; and White, R. I., Jr.: Radiographic findings in anomalous muscle bundle of the right ventricle. *Radiology*, **101**:35, 1971.

Fisher, R. D.; Bone, D. K.; Rowe, R. D.; and Gott, V. L.: Complete atrioventricular canal associated with tetralogy of Fallot. *J. Thorac. Cardiovasc. Surg.*, **70**:265, 1975.

Flege, J. B., Jr., and Ehrenhaft, J. L.: Transventricular pulmonary valvotomy and infundibular resection for tetralogy of Fallot. *Dis. Chest*, **52**:727, 1967.

Folger, G. M., and Otken, L.: Pulmonary hypertension following Blalock-Taussig anastomosis: Report of a case with pulmonary arterial aneurysm, thrombosis and calcification. *Johns Hopkins Med. J.*, **125**:44, 1969.

Folger, G. M., Jr.; Roberts, W. C.; Mehrizi, A.; Shah, K. D.; Glancy, D. L.; Carpenter, C. C. J.; and Esterly, J. R.: Cyanotic malformations of the heart with pheochromocytoma. A report of five cases. *Circulation*, **29**:750, 1964.

Folger, G. M., and Shah, K. D.: Subclavian steal in patients with Blalock-Taussig anastomosis. *Circulation*, **31**:241, 1965.

Fonó, R., and Littmann, I.: *Die kongenitalen Fehler des Herzens und der grossen Gefässe*. Johann Ambrosius Barth, Leipzig, 1957, p. 196.

Forster, J. W., and Humphries, J. O.: Right ventricular anomalous muscle bundle. Clinical and laboratory presentation and natural history. *Circulation*, **43**:115, 1971.

Franch, R. H., and Gay, B. B., Jr.: Congenital stenosis of the pulmonary artery branches. A classification, with postmortem findings in two cases. *Am. J. Cardiol.*, **35**:512, 1963.

Freedom, R. M., and Olley, P. M.: Pulmonary arteriography in congenital heart disease. *Catheterization & CV Diag.*, **2**:309, 1976.

Friedman, S.; Ash, R.; Klein, D.; and Johnson, J.: Anomalous single coronary artery complicating ventriculotomy in a child with cyanotic congenital heart disease. *Am. Heart J.*, **59**:140, 1960.

Gardiner, J. H., and Keith, J. D.: Prevalence of heart disease in Toronto children, 1948–49. Cardiac Registry. *Pediatrics*, **7**:713, 1951.

Garson, A. Jr.; Williams, R. B., Jr.; and Reckless, J.: Long-term follow-up of patients with tetralogy of Fallot: Physical health and psychopathology. *J. Pediatr.*, **85**:429, 1974.

Gasul, B. M.; Dillon, R. F.; Vrla, V.; and Hait, G.: Ventricular septal defects: their natural transformation into those with infundibular stenosis or into the cyanotic or noncyanotic type of tetralogy of Fallot. *JAMA*, **164**:847, 1957.

Gelband, H.; Waldo, A. L.; Kaiser, G. A.; Bowman, F. O., Jr.; Malm, J. R.; and Hoffman, B. F.: Etiology of right bundle-branch block in patients undergoing total correction of tetralogy of Fallot. *Circulation*, **44**:1022, 1971.

Gibson, S., and Lewis, K. C.; Congenital heart disease following maternal rubella during pregnancy. *Am. J. Dis. Child.*, **83**:317, 1952.

Glancy, D. L.; Morrow, A. G.; and Roberts, W. C.: Malformations of the aortic valve in patients with the tetralogy of Fallot. *Am. Heart J.*, **76**:755, 1968.

Glenn, W. W. L.: Circulatory bypass of the right side of the heart IV. Shunt between superior vena cava and distal right pulmonary artery: Report of clinical application. *N. Engl. J. Med.*, **259**:117, 1958.

Glover, R. P.; Bailey, C. P.; O'Neill, T. J. E.; Downing, D. F.; and Wells, C. R. E.: The direct intracardiac relief of pulmonary stenosis in the tetralogy of Fallot. *J. Thorac. Surg.*, **23**:14, 1952.

Godman, M. J.; Roberts, N. K.; and Izukawa, T.: His bundle analysis of conduction disturbances following repair of ventricular septal defect and tetralogy of Fallot. *Circulation*, **46**: Suppl II-37, 1972.

Goldman, B. S.; Mustard, W. T.; and Trusler, G. S.: Total correction of tetralogy of Fallot. Review of ten years' experience. *Br. Heart J.*, **28**: 448, 1966.

Gomez, G.; Gonzalez, F.; Adams, P., Jr.; and Anderson, R. C.: Electrocardiographic findings after open-heart surgery in children. *Am. Heart J.*, **64**: 730, 1962.

Goodwin, J. F.; Steiner, R. E.; Mounsey, J. P. D.; MacGregor, A. G.; and Wayne, E. J.: A critical analysis of the clinical value of angiocardiography in congenital heart disease. *Br. J. Radiol.*, **26**: 161, 1953.

Goor, D. A.; Lillehei, C. W.; and Edwards, J. E.: Ventricular septal defects and pulmonic stenosis with and without dextroposition. *Chest*, **60**: 117, 1971.

Gott, V. L.: Personal communication.

Gotsman, M. S.; Beck, W.; Barnard, C. N.; O'Donovan, T. G.; and Schrire, V.: Results of repair of tetralogy of Fallot. *Circulation*, **40**: 803, 1969.

Greene, N. M., and Talner, N. S.: Blood lactate, pyruvate and lactate-pyruvate ratios in congenital heart disease. *N. Engl. J. Med.*, **270**: 1331, 1964.

Gregoratos, G.; Jones, R. C.; and Jahnke, E. J., Jr.: Unilateral peripheral pulmonic stenosis complicating tetralogy of Fallot: Diagnostic and therapeutic considerations. *J. Thorac. Cardiovasc. Surg.*, **50**: 202, 1965.

Gregory, G. A.; Kitterman, J. A.; Phibbs, R. H.; Tooley, W. H.; and Hamilton, W. K.: Treatment of the idiopathic respiratory-diseases syndrome with continuous positive airway pressure. *N. Engl. J. Med.*, **284**: 1333, 1971.

Gross, R. E.; Bernhard, W. F.; and Litwin, S. B.: Closure of Potts anastomosis in the total repair of tetralogy of Fallot. *J. Thorac. Cardiovasc. Surg.*, **57**: 72, 1969.

Guntheroth, W. G.; Morgan, B. C.; Mullins, G. S.; and Baum, D.: Venous return with knee-chest portion and squatting in tetralogy of Fallot. *Am. Heart J.*, **75**: 313, 1968.

Hallidie-Smith, K. A.; Dulake, M.; Wong, M.; Oakley, C. M.; and Goodwin, J. F.: Ventricular structure and function after radical correction of the tetralogy of Fallot. *Br. Heart J.*, **29**: 533, 1967.

Hanlon, M. H., and Varco, R. L., quoted by Kirklin, C. F., and Schafer, P. W.: Gangrene of the forearm after subclavian arterio-aortostomy for coarctation of the aorta. *Thorax*, **8**: 319, 1953.

Haroutunian, L. M.; Neill, C. A.; and Wagner, H. N., Jr.: Radioisotope scanning of the lung in cyanotic congenital heart disease. *Am. J. Cardiol.*, **23**: 387, 1969.

Haroutunian, L. M.; Neill, C. A.; and Dorst, J. P.: Pulmonary pseudofibrosis in cyanotic heart disease. A clinical syndrome mimicking tuberculosis in patients with extreme pneumonic stenosis. *Chest*, **62**: 587, 1972.

Haroutunian, L. M., and Neill, C. A.: Pulmonary complications of congenital heart disease: hemoptysis. *Am. Heart J.*, **84**: 540, 1972.

Harris, B. C.; Shaver, J. A.; Krovetz, F. W.; and Leonard, J. J.: Congenital pulmonary valvular insufficiency complicating tetralogy of Fallot. *Am. J. Cardiol.*, **23**: 864, 1969.

Hartman, R. C.: A hemorrhagic disorder occurring in a patient with cyanotic congenital heart disease. *Bull. Johns Hopkins Hosp.*, **91**: 49, 1952.

Hawe, A.; Rastelli, G. C.; Ritter, D. G.; Du Shane, J. W.; and McGoon, D. C.: Management of right ventricular outflow tract in severe tetralogy of Fallot. *Am. J. Cardiol.*, **23**: 118, 1969.

Heath, D.; Wood, E. H.; DuShane, J. W.; and Edwards, J. E.: The structure of the pulmonary trunk at different ages and in cases of pulmonary hypertension and pulmonary stenosis. *J. Pathol. Bact.*, **77**: 443, 1959.

Higgins, C. G., and Mulder, D. G.: Tetralogy of Fallot in the adult. *Am. J. Cardiol.*, **29**: 837, 1972.

Hilario, J.; Lind, J.; and Wegelius, C.: Rapid biplane angiocardiography in the tetralogy of Fallot. *Br. Heart J.*, **16**: 109, 1954.

Hoffman, J. I. E.; Rudolph, A. M.; Nadas, A. S.; and Gross, R. E.: Pulmonic stenosis, ventricular septal defect and right ventricular pressure above systemic level. *Circulation*, **22**: 405, 1960.

Hohn, A. R.; Jain, K. K.; and Tamer, D. M.: Supravalvular mitral stenosis in a patient with tetralogy of Fallot. *Am. J. Cardiol.*, **22**: 733, 1968.

Holladay, W. E., Jr., and Witham, A. C.: The tetralogy of Fallot: The

variability of its clinical manifestations. *Arch. Intern. Med.*, **100**: 400, 1957.

Hunter, W.: Three cases of malformation of the heart. *Medical Observations and Inquiries by a Society of Physicians in London*, **6**: 291, 1784.

Jarmakani, J. M. M.; Edwards, S. B.; Spach, M. S.; Canent, R. V.; Capp, M. P.; Hagan, M. J.; Barr, R. C.; and Jain, V.: Left ventricular pressure-volume characteristics in congenital heart disease. *Circulation*, **37**: 879, 1968.

Jarmakani, J. M. M.; Graham, T. P., Jr.; Canent, R. V., Jr.; and Jewett, P. H.: Left heart function in children with tetralogy of Fallot before and after palliative or corrective surgery. *Circulation*, **46**: 478, 1972.

Jefferson, K.; Rees, S.; and Somerville, J.: Systemic arterial supply to the lungs in pulmonary atresia and its relation to pulmonary artery development. *Br. Heart J.*, **34**: 418, 1972.

Johns, T. N. P.; Williams, G. R.; and Blalock, A.: The anatomy of pulmonary stenosis and atresia with comments on surgical therapy. *Surgery*, **33**: 161, 1953.

Johnson, A. M.: Norepinephrine and cyanotic attacks in Fallot's tetralogy. *Br. Heart J.*, **23**: 197, 1961.

Joly, F.; Folli, G.; and Carlotti, J.: Etude electrocardiographique comparee des triologies et tetralogies de Fallot. *Arch. Mal. Coeur*, **45**: 1108, 1952.

Jones, E. L.; Conti, C. R.; Neill, C. A.; Gott, V. L.; Brawley, R. K.; and Haller, J. A., Jr.: Long term evaluation of tetralogy patients with pulmonary valvular insufficiency resulting from outflow patch correction across the pulmonic annulus. *Circulation*, **46**: Suppl II-34, 1972.

Jönsson, G.; Brodén, B.; and Karnell, J.: Selective angiocardiography. *Acta Radiol.*, **32**: 486, 1949.

Joransen, J. A., and Moller, J. H.: Postoperative hemodynamic studies in tetralogy of Fallot. *Circulation*, **46**: II-98, 1972.

Jordan, C. E.; White, R. I., Jr.; Fischer, K. C.; Neill, C. A.; and Dorst, J. P.: The scoliosis of congenital heart disease. *Am. Heart J.*, **84**: 463, 1972.

Kaplan, S.: The treatment of tetralogy of Fallot. In *Progress in Cardiology*. Eds. Yu, P. N., and Goodwin, J. F. Lea & Febiger, Phila., 1972.

Kent, J. V.: Development of rib notching after surgical intervention in congenital heart disease with description of 2 cases. *Br. J. Radiol.*, **26**: 346, 1953.

Khoury, G. H.; Du Shane, J. W.; and Ongley, P. A.: The preoperative and postoperative vectorcardiogram in tetralogy of Fallot. *Circulation*, **31**: 85, 1965.

Kirklin, J. W.: Tetralogy of Fallot. Caldwell Lecture, 1967. *Am. J. Roentgenol.*, **102**: 253, 1968.

Kirklin, J. W., and Karp, R. G.: *The Tetralogy of Fallot. From a Surgical Standpoint.* W. B. Saunders Co., Philadelphia, 1970.

Kirklin, J. W.: In The Willis J. Potts Memorial Symposium on tetralogy of Fallot, Chicago, Ill., 1972.

Kjellberg, S. R.; Mannheimer, E.; Rudhe, U.; and Jönsson, B.: *Diagnosis of Congenital Heart Disease*, 2nd ed. Year Book Publishers, Inc., Chicago, 1959.

Kompe, D. M., and Sparrow, A. W.: Polycythemia in cyanotic congenital heart disease—a study of altered coagulation. *J. Pediatr.*, **76**: 231, 1970.

Kontras, S. B.; Bodenbender, J. G.; Craenen, J.; and Hosier, D. M.: Hyperviscosity in congenital heart disease. *J. Pediatr.*, **76**: 214, 1970.

Kouchoukos, N. T.; Barcia, A.; Bargeron, L. M.; and Kirklin, J. W.: Surgical treatment of congenital pulmonary atresia with ventricular septal defect. *J. Thorac. Cardiovasc. Surg.*, **61**: 70, 1971.

Kreutzer, R. O.; Caprile, J. A.; and Wessels, F. M.: Angiocardiography in heart disease in children. *Br. Heart J.*, **12**: 293, 1950.

Kulbertus, H. E.; Coyne, J. J.; and Hallidie-Smith, K. A.: Correction disturbances before and after surgical closure of ventricular Septal defect. *Am. Heart J.*, **77**: 123, 1969.

Lam, C.: The choice of side for approach in operations for pulmonic stenosis. *J. Thorac. Surg.*, **18**: 661, 1949.

Lauer, R. M.; Ongley, P. A.; Du Shane, J. W.; and Kirklin, J. W.: Heart block after repair of ventricular septal defect in children. *Circulation*, **22**: 526, 1960.

Leatham, A.: Splitting of the first and second heart sounds. *Lancet*, **2**: 607, 1954.

Leeds, S. E.: The tetralogy of Fallot in older persons up to the fifth decade. Results of subclavian-pulmonary anastomosis with a 5 to 10 year follow-up. *Am. J. Surg.*, **96**:234, 1958.

Lester, R. G.; Robinson, A. E.; and Osteen, R. T.: Tetralogy of Fallot. A detailed angiographic study. *Am. J. Roentgenol.*, **94**:92, 1965.

Lev, M.: The architecture of the conduction system in congenital heart disease. II. Tetralogy of Fallot. *Arch. Pathol.*, **67**:572, 1959.

Lev, M.: Pathology of congenital heart disease. In Luisada, A. A. (ed.): *Cardiology*, McGraw-Hill Book Co., Inc., New York, 1959, Vol. 3, pp. 6–16.

Lev, M.; Agustsson, M. H.; and Arcilla, R.: The pathologic anatomy of common atrioventricular orifice associated with tetralogy of Fallot. *Am. J. Clin. Pathol.*, **36**:408, 1961.

Lev, M.; Bharati, S.; Meng, L.; Libertson, R. R.; Paul, M. H.; and Idress, F.: A concept of double-outlet right ventricle. *J. Thorac. Cardiovasc. Surg.*, **64**:271, 1972.

Lev, M., and Eckner, F. A. O.: The pathologic anatomy of tetralogy of Fallot and its variations. *Dis. Chest*, **45**:251, 1964.

Levin, A. R.; Boineau, J. P.; Spach, M. S.; Canent, R. V., Jr.; Capp, M. P.; and Anderson, P. A. W.: Ventricular pressure-flow dynamics in tetralogy of Fallot. *Circulation*, **34**:4, 1966.

Levine, F. H.; Reis, R. L.; and Morrow, A. G.: Incidence and significance of patent foramen ovale after repair of tetralogy of Fallot. *Circulation*, **44**:II-191, 1971.

Lillehei, C. W.; Cohen, M.; Warden, H. E.; Read, R. C.; Aust, J. B.; DeWall, R. A.; and Varco, R. L.: Direct vision intracardiac surgical correction of the tetralogy of Fallot, pentalogy of Fallot and pulmonary atresia defects. Report of first ten cases. *Ann. Surg.*, **142**:418, 1955.

Lillehei, C. W.; DeWall, R. A.; Read, R. C.; Warden, H. E.; and Varco, R. L.: Direct vision intracardiac surgery in man using a simple disposable artificial oxygenator. *Dis. Chest*, **19**:1, 1956.

Lin, T. K.; Diehl, A. M.; and Kittle, C. F.: Hemodynamic complications in tetralogy of Fallot after pulmonary valvectomy or infundibulectomy (Brock procedure). *Am. Heart J.*, **55**:288, 1958.

Longenecker, C. G.; Reemtsma, K.; and Creech, O., Jr.: Anomalous coronary artery distribution associated with tetralogy of Fallot: a hazard in open cardiac repair. *J. Thorac. Cardiovasc. Surg.*, **42**:258, 1961.

Lowe, J. B.: The angiocardiogram in Fallot's tetralogy. *Br. Heart J.*, **15**:319, 1953.

Luke, M. J., and McDonnell, E. J.: Congenital heart disease and scoliosis. *J. Pediatr.*, **73**:725, 1968.

Lund, G. W.: Growth study of children with the tetralogy of Fallot. *J. Pediatr.*, **41**:572, 1952.

Lynfield, J.; Gasul, B. M.; Arcilla, R.; and Luam, L. L.: The natural history of ventricular septal defect in infancy and childhood. *Am. J. Med.*, **30**:357, 1961.

Macartney, F. J.; Deverall, P. B.; and Scott, O.: Haemodynamic characteristics of systemic arterial blood supply to the lungs. *Br. Heart J.*, **35**:28, 1973.

Macartney, F. J., and Miller, G. A. H.: Congenital absence of the pulmonary valve. *Br. Heart J.*, **32**:483, 1970.

Macartney, F. J.; Scott, O.; and Deverall, P. B. Haemodynamic and anatomical characteristics of pulmonary blood supply in pulmonary atresia with ventricular septal defect—including a case of persistent fifth aortic arch. *Br. Heart J.*, **36**:1049, 1974.

McCord, M. C.; Van Elk, J.; and Blount, S. G., Jr.: Tetralogy of Fallot. Clinical and hemodynamic spectrum of combined pulmonary stenosis and ventricular septal defect. *Circulation*, **16**:736, 1957.

McGaff, C. J.; Ross, R. S.; and Braunwald, E.: The development of elevated pulmonary vascular resistance in man following increased pulmonary blood flow from systemic-pulmonary anastomoses. *Am. J. Med.*, **33**:201, 1962.

McGoon, D. C.; Rastelli, G. C.; and Ongley, P. A.: An operation for the correction of truncus arteriosus. *JAMA*, **205**:69, 1968.

McGoon, D. C.: Intracardiac repair of tetralogy of Fallot. In *The Natural History and Progress in treatment of Congenital Heart Defects*. Eds. Kidd, B. S. L., and Keith, J. D. Charles C Thomas, Publisher, Springfield, Ill., 1971, p. 96.

McGreal, D. A.: Brain abscess in children. *Can. Med. Assoc. J.*, **86**:261, 1962.

McKim, J. S., and Wiglesworth, F. W.: Absence of the left pulmonary artery. A report of six cases with autopsy findings in three. *Am. Heart J.*, **47**:845, 1954.

McLean, J., and Keith, J. D.: Prevalence of heart disease in Toronto children, 1952–1953. Cardiac Registry, unpublished observations.

McMyn, J. K.: Tetralogy of Fallot. Angiocardiographic diagnosis compared with surgical findings. *Aust. Radiol.*, **13**:37, 1969.

Malm, J. R.: In The Willis J. Potts Memorial Symposium on tetralogy of Fallot. Chicago, Ill., 1971.

Malm, J. R.; Blumenthal, S.; Bowman, F. O., Jr.; Ellis, K.; Jameson, A. G.; Jesse, M. J.; and Yeoh, C. B.: Factors that modify hemodynamic results in total correction of tetralogy of Fallot. *J. Thorac. Cardiovasc. Surg.*, **52**:502, 1966.

Mannheimer, E.: *Morbus Caeruleus: an Analysis of 14 Cases of Congenital Heart Disease with Cyanosis.* By S. Eek et al. (Bibliotheca Cardiologica, Fasc. 4). Karger, Basel, 1949.

Marquis, R. M.: Unipolar electrocardiograms in pulmonary stenosis. *Br. Heart J.*, **13**:89, 1951.

Marr, K.; Giargiana, F. A.; and White, R. L., Jr.: Radiographic diagnosis of pulmonary hypertension following Blalock-Taussig shunts in patients with tetralogy of Fallot. *Radiology*, (Abstr.).**11b**:241, 1975.

Martelle, R. R., and Linde, L. M.: Cerebrovascular accidents in tetralogy of Fallot. *Am. J. Dis. Child.*, **101**:206, 1961.

Matson, D. D., and Salam, M.: Brain abscess in congenital heart disease. *Pediatrics*, **27**:772, 1961.

Maurer, H. M.; McCue, C. M.; Caul, J.; and Still, W. J. S.: Defective platelet aggregation in congenital heart disease. *Am. J. Cardiol.*, **29**:279, 1972.

Mehrizi, A.: Origin of both great vessels from the right ventricle. I. With pulmonic stenosis. Clinico-pathologic correlation in 18 autopsied cases. *Bull. Hopkins Hosp.*, **117**:75, 1965.

Mehrizi, A., and Drash, A.: Growth disturbance in congenital heart size. *J. Pediatr.*, **61**:418, 1962.

Meng, C. C. L.; Eckner, F. A. O.; and Lev, M.: Coronary artery distribution in tetralogy of Fallot. *Arch. Surg.*, **90**:363, 1965.

Miller, R. A.; Lev, M.; and Paul, M. H.: Congenital absence of the pulmonary valve. The clinical syndrome of tetralogy of Fallot with pulmonary regurgitation. *Circulation*, **26**:266, 1962.

Mistrot, J. J.; Bernhard, W. F.; Rosenthal, A.; and Castaneda, A. R.: Tetralogy of Fallot with a single pulmonary artery: operative repair. *Ann. Thorac. Surg.*, **23**:249, 1977.

Moffitt, E. A.; Rosevear, J. W.; and McGoon, D. C.: Myocardial metabolism in children having open heart surgery. *JAMA*, **211**:1518, 1970.

Moffitt, G. R., Jr.; Zinsser, H. F., Jr.; Kuo, P. T.; Johnson, J.; and Schnabel, T. G.: Pulmonary stenosis with left-to-right intracardiac shunts. *Am. J. Med.*, **16**:521, 1954.

Morgan, B. C.; Guntheroth, W. G.; and Mullins, R. S.: Physiologic studies of paroxysmal hyperpnea in cyanotic congenital heart disease. *Circulation*, **31**:70, 1965.

Morse, M., and Cassels, D. E.: Arterial blood gases and acid-base balance in cyanotic congenital heart disease. *J. Clin. Invest.*, **32**:837, 1953.

Moss, A. J.; Marcano, B.; Ruttenberg, H. D.; Desilets, D. T.; and Shapiro, B.: Intrapulmonary shunts in cyanotic congenital heart disease after surgical correction. *Am. J. Cardiol.*, **23**:818, 1969.

Nadas, A. S., and Hauck, A. J.: Pediatric aspects of congestive heart failure. *Circulation*, **21**:424, 1960.

Nadas, A. S.; Rosenbaum, H. D.; Wittenborg, M. H.; and Rudolph, A. M.: Tetralogy of Fallot with unilateral pulmonary atresia. *Circulation*, **8**:328, 1953.

Naeye, R. L.: Perinatal changes in the pulmonary vascular bed with stenosis and atresia of the pulmonic valve. *Am. Heart J.*, **61**:586, 1961.

Nagao, G. I.; Daoud, G. I.; McAdams, A. J.; Schwartz, D. C.; and Kaplan, S.: Cardiovascular anomalies associated with tetralogy of Fallot. *Am. J. Cardiol.*, **20**:206, 1967.

Nelson, W.; Mayerson, H. S.; Clark, J. H.; and Lyons, C.: Studies of blood volume in tetralogy of Fallot and in other types of congenital heart disease. *J. Clin. Invest.*, **16**:800, 1947.

Neufeld, H. N.; McGoon, D. C.; Du Shane, J. W.; and Edwards, J. E.: Tetralogy of Fallot with anomalous tricuspid valve simulating pulmonary stenosis with intact septum. *Circulation*, **22**:1083, 1960.

Nora, J. J.; McGill, C. W.; and McNamara, D. G.: Empiric risks in common and uncommon congenital heart lesions. *Teratology*, **3**:325, 1970.

Nudel, D. B.; Berman, M. A.; and Talner, N. S.: Effects of acutely increasing systemic vascular resistance on oxygen tension in tetralogy of Fallot. *Pediatrics*, **58**:248, 1976.

O'Donnell, T. V., and McIlroy, M. B.: The circulatory effects of squatting. *Am. Heart J.*, **64**:347, 1962.

Olley, P. M.: Follow-up of children treated with intracardiac repair for tetralogy of Fallot. In *The Natural History and Progress in Treatment of Congenital Heart Defects*. Eds. Kidd, B. S. L., and Keith, J. D., Charles, C Thomas, Publisher, Springfield, Ill., 1971, p. 195.

Olley, P. M.; Coceani, F.; and Bodach, E.: E-type prostaglandins: A new emergency therapy for certain cyanotic congenital heart malformations. *Circulation*, **53**:728, 1976.

Ongley, P. A.; Rahimtoola, S. H.; Kincaid, O. W.; and Kirklin, J. W.: Continuous murmur in tetralogy of Fallot and pulmonary atresia with ventricular septal defect. *Am. J. Cardiol.*, **18**:821, 1966.

Osborn, J. J.; Popper, R. W.; and Gerbode, F.: Pulmonary and cardiac function immediately after intracardiac surgery. Abstract 34th Scientific Sessions, A.H.A. *Circulation*, **24**:1010, 1961.

Padmanabhan, J.; Varghese, P. J.; Lloyd, S.; and Haller, J. A., Jr.: Tetralogy of Fallot with suprasystemic pressure in the right ventricle. A case report and review of the literature. *Am. Heart J.*, **82**:805, 1971.

Paul, M. H.; Miller, R. A.; and Potts, W. J.: Long term results of aortic-pulmonary anastomosis for tetralogy of Fallot. An analysis of the first 100 cases eleven to thirteen years after operation. *Circulation*, **23**:525, 1961.

Pernot, C.; Hoeffel, J. C.; Henry, M.; Worms, A. M.; Stehlin, H.; and Louis, J. P.: Radiological patterns of congenital absence of the pulmonary valve in infants. *Radiology*, **102**:619, 1972.

Petersen, O.: Rib-notching following the Blalock-Taussig operation. *Acta Radiol.*, **45**:308, 1956.

Peterson, R. A., and Rosenthal, A.: Retinopathy and papilledema in cyanotic congenital heart disease. *Pediatrics*, **49**:243, 1972.

Phillips, L. L.; Malm, J. R.; and Deterling, R. A., Jr.: Coagulation defects following extracorporeal circulation. *AMA Suppl.*, **157**:317, 1963.

Pickering, D.; Trusler, G. A.; Lipton, I.; and Keith, J. D.: Waterston anastomosis: comparison of results of operation before and after age 6 months. *Thorax*, **26**:457, 1971.

Polani, P. E., and Campbell, M.: An aetiological study of congenital heart disease. *Ann. Hum. Genet.*, **19**:209, 1955.

Porstmann, W.; El-Sallab, R. A.; and David, H.: Pseudo-aplasia of the right pulmonary artery associated with right-sided aortic arch. *Br. Heart J.*, **29**:527, 1967.

Potts, W. J.; Smith, S.; and Gibson, S.: Anastomosis of the aorta to a pulmonary artery. *JAMA*, **132**:627, 1946.

Prader, A., and Rossi, E.: Investigation of the cellular blood constituents in morbus caeruleus. *Helv. Paediatr. Acta*, **5**:159,172, 1950.

Puga, F. J.; Du Shane, J. W.; and McGoon, D. C.: Treatment of tetralogy of Fallot in children less than 4 years of age. *J. Thorac. Cardiovasc. Surg.*, **64**:247, 1972.

Rao, B. N. S.; Anderson, R. C.; and Edwards, J. E.: Anatomic variations in the tetralogy of Fallot. *Am. Heart J.*, **81**:361, 1971.

Rastelli, G. C.; Ongley, P. A.; Davis, G. D.; and Kirklin, J. W.: Surgical repair for pulmonary valve atresia with coronary artery–pulmonary artery fistula: Report of a case. *Mayo Clin. Proc.*, **40**:521, 1965.

Redo, S. F., and Ecker, R. R.: Intrapericardial aortico-pulmonary artery shunt. *Circulation*, **28**:520, 1963.

Reemtsma, K.; Longenecker, C. G.; and Creech, O.: Surgical anatomy of the coronary artery distribution in congenital heart disease. *Circulation*, **24**:782, 1961.

Rees, S., and Somerville, J.: Aortography in Fallot's tetralogy and variants. *Br. Heart J.*, **31**:146, 1969.

Reivich, M.; Holling, E. H.; Roberts, B.; and Toole, J. F.: Reversal of blood flow through the vertebral artery and its effect on cerebral circulation. *N. Engl. J. Med.*, **265**:879, 1961.

Rich, A. R.: A hitherto unrecognised rendency to the development of widespread pulmonary vascular obstruction in patients with congenital pulmonary stenosis (tetralogy of Fallot). *Bull. Johns Hopkins Hosp.*, **82**:389, 1948.

Roberts, W. C.; Friesinger, G. C.; Cohen, L. S.; Mason, D. T.; and Ross, R. S.: Acquired pulmonic atresia. Total obstruction to right ventricular outflow after systemic to pulmonary arterial anastomosis for cyanotic congenital cardiac disease. *Am. J. Cardiol.*, **24**:335, 1969.

Rockoff, S. D., and Gilbert, J.: Functional pulmonary atresia. A cause of angiocardiographic misinterpretation in tetralogy of Fallot. *Am. J. Roentgenol.*, **94**:85, 1965.

Rosenbaum, M. B.; Corrado, G.; Oliveri, R.; Castellanos, A., Jr.; and Elizari, M. V.: Right bundle branch block with left anterior hemiblock surgically induced in tetralogy of Fallot. Relation to the mechanism of electrocardiographic changes in endocardial cushion defects. *Am. J. Cardiol.*, **26**:12, 1970.

Rosenquist, G. C.; Sweeney, L. J.; Stemple, D. R.; Christianson, S. D.; and Rowe, R. D.: Ventricular septal defect in tetralogy of Fallot. *Am. J. Cardiol.*, **31**:749, 1973.

Ross, D. E., and Murphy, D. R.: Congenital malformation of the heart. *Can. Med. Assoc. J.*, **61**:114, 1949.

Ross, D. N., and Somerville, J.: Correction of pulmonary atresia with homograft aortic valve. *Lancet*, **2**:1446, 1966.

Ross, R. S.; Taussig, H. B.; and Evans, M. H.: Late hemodynamic complications of anastomotic surgery for treatment of the tetralogy of Fallot. *Circulation*, **18**:553, 1958.

Roth, A.; Rosenthal, A.; Hall, J. E.; and Mizel, M. D. Scoliosis and congenital heart disease. *Clin. Orthop. Rel. Res.*, **93**:95, 1973.

Rowe, R. D.: Cardiovascular disease in the rubella syndrome. *Cardiovasc. Clin.*, **4**:5, 1972.

Rowe, R. D., and Mehrizi, A.: *The Neonate with Congenital Heart Disease*. W. B. Saunders Co., Philadelphia, 1968.

Rowe, R. D., and Uchida, I. A.: Cardiac malformation in mongolism. A prospective study of 184 mongoloid children. *Am. J. Med.*, **31**:726, 1961.

Rowe, R. D.; Vlad, P.; and Keith, J. D.: Atypical tetralogy of Fallot: a noncyanotic form with increased lung vascularity. *Circulation*, **12**:230, 1955.

Rudolph, A. M., and Danilowicz, D.: Treatment of severe spell syndrome in congenital heart disease. *Pediatrics*, **32**:141, 1963.

Rudolph, A. M.; Nadas, A. S.; and Borges, W. H.: Haemotologic adjustments to cyanotic congenital heart disease. *Pediatrics*, **11**:454, 1953.

Sabiston, D. C., Jr.; Cornell, W. P.; Criley, J. M.; Neill, C. A.; Ross, R. S.; and Bahnson, H. T.: The diagnosis and surgical correction of total obstruction of the right ventricle. *J. Thorac. Cardiovasc. Surg.*, **48**:577, 1964.

Scheuer, J.; Shaver, J. A.; Kroetz, F. W.; and Leonard, J. J.: Myocardial metabolism in cyanotic congenital heart disease. *Cardiology*, **55**:193, 1970.

Sell, C. G. R.; Fowler, R. L.; Sailors, E.; Hyman, A. L.; Levy, L., II; and Ordway, N. K.: Physiological studies in cases of "Tetralogy of Fallot" with little or no overriding of the aorta. 2nd World Congress of Cardiology, Washington, D.C., 1954.

Sellors, T. H.: Surgery of pulmonary stenosis. A case in which the pulmonary valve was successfully divided. *Lancet*, **1**:988, 1948.

Shah, P. M., and Kidd, B. S. L.: Circulatory effects of propranolol in children with Fallot's tetralogy. *Am. J. Cardiol.*, **19**:653, 1967.

Shumacker, H. B., Jr., and Mandelbaum, L.: Ascending aortic-pulmonary artery shunts in cyanotic heart disease. *Surgery*, **52**:675, 1962.

Shumway, N. E.; Lower, R. R.; Hurley, E. J.; and Pillsbury, R. C.: Results of total surgical correction for Fallot's tetralogy. *Circulation*, **31 & 32**:I-57, 1965.

Sloan, R. D.; Hanlon, C. R.; and Scott, H. W., Jr.: Tuberculosis and congenital cyanotic heart disease. *Am. J. Med.*, **16**:528, 1954.

Somerville, J.; Yacoub, M.; Ross, D. N.; and Ross, K.: Aorta to right pulmonary artery anastomosis (Waterston's operation) for cyanotic heart disease. *Circulation*, **39**:593, 1969.

Sondheimer, H. M.; Izukawa, T.; Olley, P. M.; Trusler, G. A.; and Mustard, W. T.: Conduction disturbances after total correction of tetralogy of Fallot. *Am. Heart J.*, **92**:278, 1976.

Soulié, P.: *Cardiopathies Congenitales*. Exp. Scient. Franc., Paris, 1952.

Spear, G. S.: The glomerulus in cyanotic congenital heart disease and primary pulmonary hypertension. A review. *Nephron*, **1**:238, 1964.

Squarcia, U.; Merideth, J.; McGoon, D. C.; and Weidman, W. H.: Prognosis of transient atrioventricular conduction disturbances complicating open heart surgery for congenital heart defects. *Am. J. Cardiol.*, **28**:648, 1971.

Steeg, C. N.; Krongrad, E.; Devachi, F.; Bowman, F. O., Jr.; Malm, J. R.; and Gerson, W. M.: Postoperative left anterior hemiblock and right bundle branch block following repair of tetralogy of Fallot. Clinical and etiologic considerations. *Circulation*, 51:1026, 1975.

Stuckey, D.; Bowdler, J. D.; and Reye, R. D. K.: Absent sixth aortic arch: A form of pulmonary atresia. *Br. Heart J.*, 30:258, 1968.

Subramanian, S.; Wagner, H.; Vlad, P.; and Lambert, E. C.: Surface-induced deep hypothermia in cardiac surgery. *J. Pediatr. Surg.*, 6:612, 1971.

Sunderland, C. O.; Rosenberg, J. A.; Menashe, V. S.; Lees, M. H.; Bonchek, L. I.; and Starr, I.: Total correction of tetralogy of Fallot under two years of age. Postoperative hemodynamic evaluation. *Circulation*, 46:II-98, 1972.

Swan, H. J. C., and Wood, E. H.: Localisation of cardiac defects by dye-dilution curves recorded after injection of T-1824 at multiple sites in the heart and great vessels during cardiac catheterization. *Proc. Mayo Clin.*, 28:95, 1953.

Talbott, J. H.; Coombs, F. S.; Castleman, B.; Chamberlain, F. L.; Consolazio, W. V.; and White, P. D.: A record case of the tetralogy of Fallot, with comments on metabolic and pathologic studies. *Am. Heart J.*, 22:754, 1941.

Talner, N. S., and Ithuralde, M.: Biochemical and clinical studies of congestive heart failure in the newborn. *Proc. Assoc. Europ. Paediatr. Cardiol.*, 6:15, 1970.

Taussig, H. B.: Tetralogy of Fallot, especially the care of the cyanotic infant and child. *Pediatrics*, 1:307, 1948.

Taussig, H. B.; Crawford, H.; Pelargonio, S.; and Zacharioudakis, S.: Ten to thirteen year follow-up on patients after a Blalock-Taussig operation. *Circulation*, 25:630, 1962.

Taussig, H. B.; Crocetti, A.; Eshaghpour, E.; Keinonen, R.; Yap, K. N.; Bachman, D.; Momberger, N.; and Kirk, H.: Long-time observations on the Blalock-Taussig operation I. Results of the first operation. *Johns Hopkins Med. J.*, 129:243, 1971.

Taussig, H. B.; Crocetti, A.; Eshaghpour, E.; Keinonen, R.; Yap, K. N.; Bachman, D.; Momberger, N.; and Kirk, H.: Long-time observations on the Blalock-Taussig operation II. Second operations, frequency and results. *Johns Hopkins Med. J.*, 129:258, 1971.

Taussig, H. B.; Crocetti, A.; Eshaghpour, E.; Keinonen, R.; Yap, K. N.; Bachman, D.; Momberger, N.; and Kirk, H.: Long-time observations on the Blalock-Taussig operation III. Common complications. *Johns Hopkins Med. J.*, 129:274, 1971.

Taussig, H. B.; King, J. T.; Bauersfeld, S. R.; and Padvamati-Iyer, S.: Results of operation for pulmonary stenosis and atresia (report of 1000 cases). *Trans. Assoc. Am. Physicians*, 64:67, 1951.

Tawes, R. L., Jr.; Berry, C. L.; Aberdeen, E.; and Graham, G. R.: Myocardial ischemia in infants. Its role in three common congenital cardiac anomalies. *Ann. Thorac. Surg.*, 8:383, 1969.

Taylor, D. G.; Thornton, J. A.; Grainer, R. D.; and Verel, D.: Closed pulmonary valvotomy for the relief of Fallot's tetralogy in infancy. *J. Thorac. Cardiovasc. Surg.*, 46:77, 1963.

Thanopoulos, B.; Siassi, B.; and Emmanouilides. "Agenesis" of ductus arteriosus associated with the syndrome of tetralogy of Fallot and absent pulmonary valve. *Am. J. Cardiol.*, 35:173, 1975 (abstr.).

Thomas, H. W.: Congenital cardiac malformation. *J. Tech. Methods*, 21:58, 1941.

Timoner, M.; Fujioka, T.; Macrhz, R.; and De Court, L. V.: Estenoses de arterias pulmonaves. *Rev. Hosp. Clin. Fac. Med. S. Paulo*, 25:233, 1970.

Tofler, O. B.: The pulmonary component of the second heart sound in Fallot's tetralogy. *Br. Heart J.*, 25:509, 1963.

Tyler, H. R., and Clark, D. B.: Incidence of neurological complications in congenital heart disease. *Arch. Neurol. Psychiat.*, 77:17, 1957.

Tyrrell, M. J.; Kidd, B. S. L.; and Keith, J. D.: Diagnosis of tetralogy of Fallot in the acyanotic phase. *Circulation*, 42 (Suppl. III):113, 1970.

Van Lingen, B., and Whidborne, J.: Oximetry in congenital heart disease with special reference to the effects of voluntary hyperventilation. *Circulation*, 6:740, 1952.

Van Praagh, R., and McNamara. J. J.: Anatomic types of ventricular septal defect with aortic insufficiency. *Am. Heart J.*, 75:604, 1968.

Van Praagh, R., and Van Praagh, S.: The anatomy of common aortico pulmonary trunk (truncus arteriosus communis) and its embryological implications: A study of 57 necropsy cases. *Am. J. Cardiol.*, 16:406, 1965.

Van Praagh, R.; Van Praagh, S.; Nebesar, R. A.; Muster, A. J.; Siraha, S. N.; and Paul, M. H.: Tetralogy of Fallot: Under development of the pulmonary infundibulum and its sequelae. *Am. J. Cardiol.*, 26:25, 1970.

Varghese, P. J.; Allen, J. R.; Rosenquist, G. C.; and Rowe, R. D.: Natural history of ventricular septal defect with right sided aortic arch. *Br. Heart J.*, 32:537, 1970.

Verél, D.: Blood volume changes in cyanotic congenital heart disease and polycythemia rubra vera. *Circulation*, 23:749, 1961.

Verney, R. N.; Michaud, P.; Termet, H.; and Viard, H.: Intérêt de l'utilisation des anastomoses aorte-pulmonaire droite par prothèse artificielle dans certains cas de tétralogie de Fallot. *Arch. Mal Coeur*, 55:789, 1962.

Vogelpoel, L., and Schrire, V.: The role of auscultation in the differentiation of Fallot's tetralogy from severe pulmonary stenosis with intact ventricular septum and right to left intra-atrial shunt. *Circulation*, 11:714, 1955.

Vogelpoel, L.; Schrire, V.; Nellen, M.; and Swanepoel, A.: The use of phenylephrine in the differentiation of Fallot's tetralogy from pulmonary stenosis with intact ventricular septum. *Am. Heart J.*, 59:489, 1960.

Vogler, W. R., and Doiney, E. R.: Bacterial endocarditis in congenital heart disease. *Am. Heart J.*, 64:198, 1962.

Von Bernuth, G.; Ritter, D. G.; Schattenberg, T. T.; and Du Shane, J. W.: Severe pulmonary hypertension after Blalock-Taussig anastomosis in a patient with tetralogy of Fallot. *Chest*, 58:380, 1970.

Wagenvoort, C. A.; Nauta, J.; Van der Schaar, P. J.; Weeda, H. W. H.; and Wagenvoort, N.: Vascular changes in pulmonic stenosis and tetralogy of Fallot studied in lung biopsies. *Circulation*, 39:924, 1967.

Wallace, R. B.; Rastelli, G. C.; Ongley, P. A.; Titus, J. L.; and McGoon, D. C.: Complete repair of truncus arteriosus defects. *J. Thorac. Cardiovasc. Surg.*, 57:95, 1969.

Wallsh, E.; Reppert, E. H.; Doyle, E. F.; and Spencer, F. C.: "Absent" left pulmonary artery with tetralogy of Fallot. *J. Thorac. Cardiovasc. Surg.*, 55:333, 1968.

Waterston, D. J.: Léčeni Fallotovy tetralogie u děti? do jednoho yoku veku. *Rozh. Chir.*, 41:181, 1962.

Watson, H.: Acyanotic or atypical tetralogy of Fallot. In *The Natural History and Progress in Treatment of Congenital Heart Defects*. Eds. Kidd, B. S. L., and Keith, J. D., Charles C Thomas, Publisher, Springfield, Ill., 1971, p. 117.

Webb, W. R., and Burford, T. H.: Gangrene of the arm following use of the subclavian artery in a pulmono-systemic (Blalock) anastomosis. *J. Thorac. Surg.*, 23:1999, 1952.

Weinberg, M., Jr.; Bicoff, J. P.; Bucheleres, H. G.; Agustsson, M. H.; Behravesh, M; Andersen, J. H.; Fell, E. H.; and Gasul, B. M.: Pulmonary valvulotomy and infundibulotomy in infants. *J. Thorac. Cardiovasc. Surg.*, 44:433, 1962.

Weis, E.; Fridman, J.; and Shaffer, A. B.: Tetralogy of Fallot with small ventricular septal defect. *Acta Cardiol.*, 16:448, 1961.

Weldon, C. S.; Rowe, R. D.; and Gott, V. L.: Clinical experience with the use of aortic valve homografts for reconstruction of the pulmonary artery, pulmonary valve, and outflow portion of the right ventricle. *Circulation*, 37, 38:Suppl. II, 51, 1968.

Wessel, H. U.; Stout, R. L.; Guerrero, L.; and Paul, M. H.: Postoperative exercise studies in tetralogy of Fallot. In Kidd, B. S. L., and Rowe, R. D. (eds.): *The Child with Congenital Heart Disease After Surgery*. Futura Publishing Co., Inc., Mount Kisco, N.Y., 1976.

White, P. D., and Sprague, H. B.: The tetralogy of Fallot. Report of a case in a noted musician who lived until his sixtieth year. *JAMA*, 92:787, 1929.

White, R. D.; Moffitt, E. A.; Feldt, R. H.; and Ritter, D. G.: Myocardial metabolism in children with heart disease. *Anesth. Analg.*, 51:6, 1972.

White, R. I., Jr.; Jordan, C. E.; Fischer, K. C.; Dorst, J. P.; Nagy, J. M.; Garn, S. M.; and Neill, C. A.: Delayed skeletal growth and maturation in adolescent congenital heart disease. *Invest. Radiol.*, 6:326, 1971.

White, R. I., Jr.; Frech, R. S.; Castaneda, A.; and Amplatz, K.: The nature and significance of anomalous coronary arteries in tetralogy of Fallot. *Am. J. Roentgenol.*, 114:350, 1972.

Williams, J. C. P.; Barratt-Boyes, B. G.; and Lowe, J. B.: Underdeveloped right ventricle and pulmonary stenosis. *Am. J. Cardiol.*, 11:458, 1963.

Willius, F. A.: Cardiac clinics. CXXXIV. An unusually early description of the so-called tetralogy of Fallot. *Proc. Mayo Clin.*, **23**:316, 1948.

Wilson, W. J., and Amplatz, K.: Unequal vascularity in tetralogy of Fallot. *Am. J. Roentgenol.*, **100**:318, 1967.

Windsor, R. V. J.: Obstructive changes in the pulmonary arteries of Fallot's tetralogy. *Ann. Rep., Auckland (NZ) Med. Res. Foundation*, **15**:19, 1962–1963.

Wolff, G. S.; Rowland, T. W.; and Ellison, R. C.: Surgically induced right bundle-branch block with left anterior hemiblock. *Circulation*, **46**:587, 1972.

Wood, E. H., and Geraci, J. E.: Photoelectric determination of arterial oxygen saturation in man. *J. Lab. Clin. Med.*, **34**:387, 1949.

Wood, P.: Congenital heart disease. *Br. Med. J.*, **2**:639, 693, 1950.

———: Symposium on congenital heart disease. *Br. Heart J.*, **20**:282, 1958.

Woods, A.: The electrocardiogram in the tetralogy of Fallot. *Br. Heart J.*, **14**:193, 1950.

Woodson, R. D.; Burnell, R. H.; Herr, R. H.; Lees, M. H.; and Starr, A.: Surgical management of tetralogy of Fallot in children under age four. *Ann. Surg.*, **169**:257, 1969.

Young, W. G., Jr.; Sealy, W. C.; Houck, W. S., Jr.; Whalen, R. E.; Spach, M. S.; and Canent, R. V., Jr.; Superior vena cava—right pulmonary artery anastomosis in cyanotic heart disease. *Ann. Surg.*, **157**:894, 1963.

Ziegler, R. F.: Personal communication, 1954.

———: Some aspects of electrocardiography in infants and children with congenital heart disease. *Dis. Chest*, **25**:490, 1954.

Zuberbuhler, J. R.; Danker, E.; Zoltun, R.; Burkholder, J.; and Bahnson, H. T.: Tissue adhesive closure of aortic-pulmonary communications. *Am. Heart J.*, **88**:41, 1974.

Zutter, W., and Somerville, J.: Continuous murmur in pulmonary atresia with reference to aortography. *Br. Heart J.*, **33**:905, 1971.

28

Pulmonary Atresia with Normal Aortic Root

Robert M. Freedom and *John D. Keith*

PULMONARY atresia with normal aortic root (intact ventricular septum) has been recognized pathologically for many years (Hunter, 1783; Lordat, 1822; Hare, 1852–1853; Rokitansky, 1855; and others). Clinical interest is relatively recent (Novelo et al., 1951; Greenwold et al., 1956; Keith et al., 1958; Davignon et al., 1961; Benton et al., 1962; Elliott et al., 1963; Celermajer et al., 1968; Cole et al., 1968; Dhanavaravibul et al., 1970; Trusler et al., 1970; Bowman et al., 1971; Luckstead et al., 1972; Shams et al., 1971).

It is an uncommon anomaly, our 91 cases representing 1 percent of the total group of congenital cardiac malformations.

It is estimated that it occurs once in 70,000 children.

Pathology

The obstruction to the right ventricular outflow is complete (see Figure 28–1).

In the 75 anatomic specimens examined at The Hospital for Sick Children, Toronto, the atresia was found to assume several variants.

In the majority of cases (60 specimens) the pulmonary valve was an imperforate diaphragm. The three leaflets were completely fused, forming three well-defined raphae. The diameter of the valve ring exceeds 5 mm only rarely.

On two occasions the pulmonary valve was patent and bicuspid. The infundibulum was short and completely separated from the remainder of the right ventricle by a muscle mass (atresia of the bulbar ostium).

In three instances no valve structure could be identified and the pulmonary trunk was represented by a cord extending from the base of the heart to the bifurcation of the pulmonary artery. A similar case was reported by Kugel (1932).

Combined valvular and infundibular atresia has been described by several investigators (Peck and Wilson, 1949; Morgan et al., 1965; Dhanavaravibul et al., 1970; Moller et al., 1970; Shams et al., 1971;

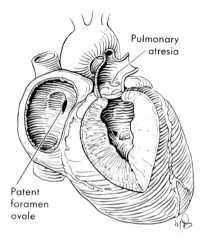

Figure 28-1. Atresia of the pulmonary valve. Visible are the open foramen ovale and the thick-walled ventricle with an underdeveloped chamber. Ductus arteriosus is patent.

Bowman et al., 1971; Freedom and Harrington, 1974). Aron and Edwards (1976) have studied the relationship between the right ventricular musculature and the pulmonary valve in normal patients and those with pulmonary valve atresia and intact ventricular septum. Their observations suggested that the muscle bundles of the right ventricle are closely related to the left and posterior pulmonary cusps in the normal. In the patient with pulmonary atresia and intact ventricular septum, there is hypertrophy of the muscle bundles related to the pulmonary cusps resulting in a narrow right ventricular infundibulum. Thus only a small segment of the atretic valve is in direct contact with the right ventricular cavity.

In a two-year-old boy with fully developed Ebstein malformation of the tricuspid valve, the large septal leaflet was attached to the septal surface of the right ventricle in a manner resulting in complete occlusion of the infundibulum. The pulmonary valve was tricuspid and normally formed, although both the valve ring and the pulmonary trunk were moderately hypoplastic.

Although there is a continuous spectrum of size of the *right ventricle*, with intermediate forms difficult to classify, grouping into a type with minute or small ventricle and one with normal or large right ventricle (Greenwold et al., 1956; Davignon et al., 1961) is both practical and important, since each category presents differentiating clinical and diagnostic features and significant surgical aspects.

In the majority of cases, the right ventricle is small but thick-walled. Edwards (1953) has likened it to a peach, the stone of which has been removed. As first described by Ogle (1896), the endocardium is commonly thick (up to 3 mm), white, and speckled (secondary fibroelastosis).

In occasional cases (case 2 of Taussig, 1947; Glaboff et al., 1950; Novelo et al., 1951; Davignon et al., 1961; one case at The Hospital for Sick Children) thrombotic material completely occludes this chamber.

We have found a normal size or large ventricle in only 15 percent of the 60 specimens examined. Endocardial fibrosis is less common.

The size of the *tricuspid valve* is proportionate to the size of the right ventricle (Van Praagh et al., 1976; Freedom et al., in press). With a normal or large right ventricle anatomic evidence of tricuspid regurgitation is obvious (short or absent chordae tendineae; thick, rolled, or redundant leaflets). Occasionally a fully developed Ebstein malformation is present (Kugel's case, 1932; Keith et al., 1958; Davignon et al., 1961; Schrire et al., 1961; Elliott et al., 1963).

When the right ventricle is small, malformations of the tricuspid valve seem equally frequent. The presence of low insertion of the septal leaflet (Ebstein-like malformation) and its frequency have been emphasized by Elliott and associates (1963). Regurgitation, even though less obvious anatomically, remains common. This is demonstrated almost invariably by right ventriculography.

Abnormal communications between the right ventricle and the coronary arteries have been reported by Grant (1926); Williams and associates (1951); Lauer and associates (1964). They represent embryonal intramyocardial spaces kept open by the elevated right ventricular pressures that communicate with the coronary artery. External examination of the heart will reveal at times a distended anterior descending branch and more often a subepicardial dimple situated at the lower region of the anterior interventricular groove. While such dimples were observed in approximately one-third of our specimens, the presence of anomalous connection between the right ventricular cavity and the coronary artery could be demonstrated anatomically or angiocardiographically in six cases only. For Davignon and associates (1961) they are a feature of the type with small right ventricular cavity. They may, however, occur with large cavity. Figure 28–7 (page 513) shows such an example. It has been suggested that these sinusoids may contribute to a right-sided

"circular shunt"; i.e., blood entering the blind right ventricle → intramyocardial sinusoids → coronary artery → coronary venous system → coronary sinus → right atrium → right ventricle. In addition, some of the right-to-left shunted blood returns to its chamber of origin through intracardial channels, bypassing the systemic capillary blood (Freedom and Harrington, 1974).

The *right atrium* is always enlarged, and the cases with large ventricular cavity and massive tricuspid regurgitation this chamber may reach aneurysmal proportions. Similarly, the left atrium may be larger than normal. This is the result of free blood flow from the right atrium when the interatrial communication is large.

The atrial septum is always patent but actual defects (foramen ovale type) occur in only 20 percent. The ductus arteriosus was found closed in 5 percent, probe-patent but snug in 55 percent, and widely patent in 40 percent. As a rule it closes early in life shutting off the only access to the pulmonary circuit.

Unusual Cases. Association of pulmonary atresia with a fully blown Ebstein malformation of the tricuspid valve occurred once and is also noted in several papers (Kugel, 1932; Schrire et al., 1961; Elliott et al., 1963). An additional case (already referred to) of this anomaly is of interest since the obstructive structure was the abnormal septal leaflet itself.

One case of dextrocardia with situs inversus and one of L-transposition of the great arteries ("corrected" transposition) were accompanied by pulmonary valve atresia and intact ventricular septum as the sole anomaly.

Hemodynamics

Two hemodynamic patterns emerge, depending on the size of the right ventricle and tricuspid valve.

With a minute tricuspid valve, right ventricular *inflow* obstruction exists: The right atrial blood is diverted almost in its entirety into the left atrium. Even though flow in and out of the ventricle is possible, overloading of this chamber does not occur. The outflow obstruction is insignificant. Its surgical relief will not appreciably diminish the atrial right-to-left shunt.

With a large tricuspid valve, the right ventricular *outflow* obstruction is dominant. Overloading of this chamber is manifest in the electrocardiogram, and surgical correction of the pulmonary valve will increase the forward flow and diminish the atrial shunt.

Obviously, intermediate forms are possible.

The first hemodynamic pattern is similar to that of tricuspid atresia; the second, to severe pulmonic stenosis.

If the tricuspid valve were competent, blood reaching the right ventricle would find no exit. Stasis thrombosis should occur, obliterating this chamber.

This may be the explanation for the few cases in which blood clots were found to fill the cavity (case 2 of Taussig, 1947; Glaboff et al., 1950; Novelo et al., 1951; two cases at The Hospital for Sick Children). In all other cases decompressing mechanisms were produced by either tricuspid regurgitation (whether the right ventricle was large or small) or cardioaortic fistulae draining blood via the coronary arteries into the aortic root. The latter phenomenon was observed in hearts with a small ventricle and also with large cavity when the tricuspid appeared competent (Figure 28–7, page 513). Pulmonary circulation is maintained by the ductus arteriosus. Survival is therefore a function of its patency.

Clinical Features

Cyanosis occurs commonly within the first few days of life and increases rapidly. The children with loud, continuous murmur may be acyanotic for several weeks after birth.

Tachypnea is an accompanying feature. Signs of cardiac failure (hepatomegaly, peripheral edema, apical gallop rhythm) are particularly common in the cases with large right ventricle and marked tricuspid regurgitation.

HEART MURMURS. In our series no murmurs could be heard in 23 percent of cases. Continuous murmurs were present in 32 percent, but they were loud only in half of them. In the remainder they were audible only on repeated examinations with the babies sleeping or under anesthesia. All patients older than two years had machinery murmurs.

Systolic murmurs were identified in 45 percent. These were usually faint and located either over the pulmonic and subclavian areas or at the left lower sternal border. The former are presumably of ductal origin while the latter are due to slight tricuspid regurgitation.

Nine patients had loud pansystolic murmurs with thrill at the lower sternum, some of them with preferential transmission toward the right chest. All had large hearts, large right ventricular cavity, and massive tricuspid regurgitation.

Electrocardiography

Tracings were available in 52 autopsied patients. In 16 of them follow-up recordings at variable intervals were made.

The initial electrocardiograms were interpreted with regard to axis deviation and atrial and ventricular overloading.

A left-axis deviation (+ 10 to − 30 degrees) was present in two newborn infants, but this shifted to + 60 and + 100 degrees within 24 hours. Right-axis deviation (+ 90 degrees or more) occurred in over half the patients.

Evidence of right atrial overloading was found in two-thirds but only seldom during the first week of life. No normal P waves were found beyond one month of age. Combined atrial enlargement was present in four patients, all older than four years. One

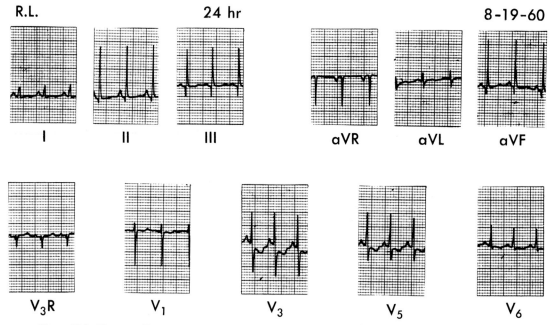

Figure 28-2. Electrocardiogram of a 24-hour-old baby girl who underwent pulmonary valvotomy when 56 hours old. Five years postoperatively the tracing remained virtually identical, even though she is free of murmurs, cyanosis, or exercise intolerance. A small right ventricular chamber was demonstrated by selective angiocardiography. (Courtesy of Dr. N. B. Thomson, Jr., Buffalo Children's Hospital, Buffalo.)

of them developed evidence of severe left atrial overloading following a Blalock-Taussig anastomosis.

In contrast to tricuspid atresia, the P-R interval and segment were short in only three cases.

Left ventricular overloading was present at the time of the initial examinations in 18 tracings (34 percent) (Figure 28–2). With two exceptions these were babies less than nine days old. The QRS axis ranged from +55 to +75 degrees, except the two instances of left-axis deviation mentioned above. Left ventricular dominance was indicated by rS complexes in leads V_3R and V_1, and R or qR complexes in V_5 or V_6. Inverted T waves in V_6 occurred in half of them. Both babies who survived beyond five months developed signs of associated right ventricular hypertrophy. One patient with a multiphasic QRS complex in V_6 (rsR′s′) had a typical Ebstein anomaly of the tricuspid valve.

Right ventricular overloading occurred in 18 patients (34 percent); 12 of these were less than 24 hours old. The survivors maintained their pattern of right ventricular overloading. The sole instance of acquired left ventricular hypertrophy occurred after an anastomotic procedure. All patients manifested right atrial overloading as well.

Evidence of right ventricular loading was supplied by QR, qR, or tall R waves in leads V_3R and V_1 and rS in leads V_5 and V_6. The two patients with multiphasic QRS (rsR′s′) had a fully developed Ebstein malformation of the tricuspid valve.

Combined ventricular overloading was present in 12 patients (25 percent) (Figure 28–3). The electrical axis varied between +65 and +90 degrees in all. P wave abnormalities occurred in one-half. Four patterns were discernible in the precordial leads: (a) QR, qR or Rs in V_3R, with rS in V_1 and V_2 and R or qR in V_6; (b) tall RS waves in V_3R or V_1 with Rs in V_6; (c) rS waves over the right precordium with tall RS waves in V_5 or V_6; (d) RS complexes across the chest. All these patients were under ten days of age.

Equivocal tracings were recorded four times (7 percent) when interpretation was questionable. In one patient evidence of marked right ventricular overloading became manifest at 13 months although the tracing appeared normal at four weeks.

A feature of significance was the frequency of progressive changes whenever the patients lived several weeks. The degree of right-axis deviation, right atrial overloading, and right ventricular hypertrophy increased, as a rule, as the babies grew older. On the other hand, tracings that appeared normal or showed left ventricular overloading in the neonatal period acquired signs of right ventricular hypertrophy on subsequent recordings.

Another feature of the group was the rarity of high-voltage QRS complexes in the precordial leads in babies younger than one year.

As pointed out by Greenwold and associates (1956) and Davignon and associates (1961), a correlation between right ventricular size and electrocardiographic findings exists in patients more than one week of age.

Our own cases confirmed the lack of correlation in the neonatal period, with the exception of the few who had gross right ventricular overloading and clinical evidence of tricuspid regurgitation. In the rest of the group a good correlation existed only at the two extremes of the spectrum. When pure left ventricular overloading was present, the right ventricular cavity

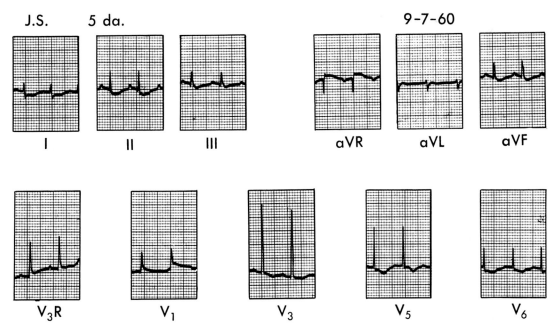

Figure 28-3. Electrocardiogram showing combined ventricular overloading in a five-day-old baby with pulmonary atresia and small right ventricular chamber.

was minute, while with gross right ventricular overloading, the cavity was large. Since intermediate forms are numerous, prediction on the basis of the electrocardiogram proved unreliable.

S-T–T wave segment abnormalities are not uncommon electrocardiographic findings in patients with pulmonary atresia and intact ventricular septum. Left ventricular strain patterns have been noted in a number of patients prior to performance of a systemic to pulmonary artery anastomosis (Schire et al., 1961; Celermajer et al., 1968). Elliott et al., 1963; Gamboa et al., 1966; It has been suggested that left ventricular ischemia might be related to the intramyocardial sinusoidal–coronary artery communications in those patients with severe right ventricular hypertension (Freedom and Harrington, 1974).

Radiologic Examination

Greenwold and coworkers (1956) have stressed that significant radiologic differences allow distinction of the two types. When the right ventricle is small, there is no cardiac enlargement and there may be convexity of the pulmonary artery segment. With a large right ventricle, the heart is markedly enlarged.

In our experience, the cases with large right ventricle most often have a markedly increased transverse diameter. One of them, however, had a cardiothoracic ratio of 0.55 at the age of two days, just prior to death. With a small right ventricle considerable variations occur. While no, or only slight, enlargement is the rule in the neonatal period (7 of 12 cases under ten days of age), marked cardiac enlargement (cardiothoracic ratios of 0.65 to 0.70)

was found in three babies during the first day of life. More constant is the fact that those babies who have only little or no enlargement at all will develop rapidly increasing hearts if they survive (Figure 28–4).

The cardiac silhouette is not characteristic (Figure 28–5). In young infants with small hearts the apex may be rounded and the pulmonary artery segment slightly concave if there is no interference from large thymic shadows. In older babies the right atrial segment becomes prominent and the pulmonary segment convex. Thus, while shortly after birth the cardiac contour may suggest or be compatible with tricuspid atresia, later in life it will more resemble that of pulmonary stenosis with normal aortic root. The progressive cardiac enlargement is more in keeping with the latter than with tricuspid atresia.

The pulmonary vasculature is decreased in all cases except those that have a large pulmonary blood supply through a patent ductus arteriosus. Since most cases have limited flow through the ductus, the study of the hilar shadows is important in reaching a clinical diagnosis.

Echocardiography

Echocardiography has proven useful in the diagnosis of pulmonary atresia and intact ventricular septum. In the majority of patients the right ventricular cavity will be small and its wall significantly hypertrophied. The tricuspid valve motion will often be impaired. The pulmonary root is small and often it is difficult to visualize. There will be aortic-mitral continuity with the left atrium and ventricle of normal size (Meyer and Kaplan, 1972; Chesler et al., 1970; Godman et al., 1974).

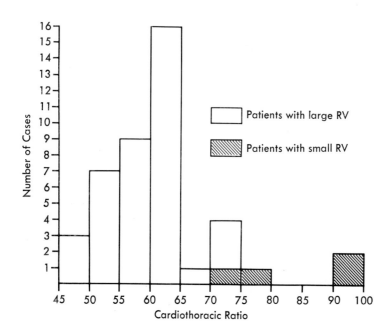

Figure 28-4. The distribution of the cardiothoracic ratios of 40 patients with small right ventricle and four with large right ventricle.

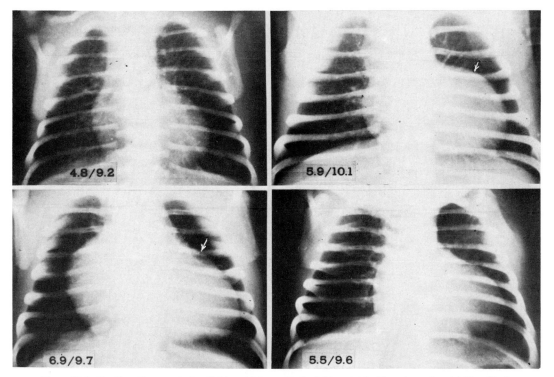

Figure 28-5. Cardiac silhouette in four babies with hypoplastic right ventricle. There is great variability of both heart size and configuration. The *arrow* points to the prominent left atrial appendage.

Angiocardiography

The venous angiocardiogram shows the "typical" filling sequence of tricuspid atresia. In some instances the right ventricle will fill adequately and the blind end of the infundibulum will show clearly. The pulmonary trunk and the valve opacify from the aorta through the ductus arteriosus. Other important features are the absence of aortic filling from the right ventricle and the absence of pulmonary artery opacification from the same chamber. The latter two findings will exclude a diagnosis of tetralogy of Fallot and pulmonary stenosis with normal aortic root.

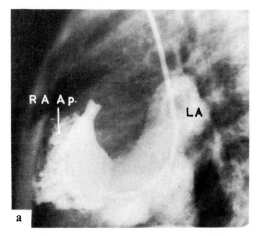
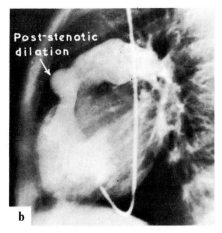

Figure 28-6. Right ventricular injections at nine years of age, before pulmonary valvotomy (*A*), and at 11 years (*B*), one year prior to death following exploratory thoracotomy. Atresia of the pulmonary valve, massive tricuspid regurgitation, and atrial right to left shunting are evident in *A*. Good filling of the pulmonary trunk and decreased tricuspid regurgitation are apparent in *B*. The size of the right ventricle has not increased even though systolic pressures dropped from 120 mm of mercury to 30 mm of mercury. There was no appreciable clinical improvement. (Courtesy of Dr. E. C. Lambert, Buffalo Children's Hospital, Buffalo.)

The selective angiocardiogram is preferred, and when performed from the right ventricle will demonstrate a right ventricle of small or large size, ending blindly at the level of the pulmonary valve (Figure 28–6) or infundibulum. No escape of contrast medium into the pulmonary artery will occur, but regurgitation into the right atrium is revealed. Thus, a selective angiocardiogram into the right ventricle is usually essential to delineate clearly the diagnosis and display the type of anatomy present.

The presence of right ventricular–aortic fistulae is best demonstrated by right ventricular injection in vivo (Figure 28–7). Communication with the coronary arteries is often best visualized in the lateral projection.

Although most reports suggest that the pulmonary atresia in patients with an intact ventricular septum is confined to the valvular area, both valvular and infundibular atresia is not uncommon. In order to precisely localize the site and length of obstruction, a double catheter technique was developed by Freedom and colleagues (1974). Simultaneous angiocardiography is performed with one catheter in the right ventricle and the other at the level of the ductus arteriosus in the neonate, and in the older patient with pulmonary atresia, one catheter is in the right ventricle and the other in the pulmonary artery via the systemic to pulmonary artery anastomosis. Biplane radiographs will allow accurate determination of the site and length of the atretic segment.

Among certain critically ill neonates having in common severe tricuspid regurgitation and subsystemic right ventricular pressures, selective right ventriculography may not distinguish those with anatomic from functional pulmonary atresia (Barr et al., 1974; Newfeld et al., 1967). With a normal pulmonary valve and infundibulum, functional obstruction in such patients results from a combination of massive tricuspid regurgitation and an elevated perinatal pulmonary vascular resistance. However, aortography has proven especially useful in this differential. Inspection of contrast material opposite the patent ductus arteriosus among patients with functional pulmonary atresia will usually demonstrate reflux of contrast across the patent pulmonary valve with subsequent opacification of right ventricle and atrium (Freedom et al., 1978).

Diagnosis

 early cyanosis

The diagnosis is suspected in babies who develop cyanosis shortly after birth, have reduced pulmonary vascular markings, and have an evolving electrocardiogram showing left ventricular loading with direct or indirect signs of right ventricular hypertrophy such as clockwise rotation, vertical or semivertical electrical position, right-axis deviation, and a qR pattern in V_3R.

There are at least six other conditions that are associated with cyanosis in the newborn and may have evidence of loading of left ventricle. These

DIFFERENTIAL include tricuspid atresia, tricuspid atresia with transposition of the great arteries, persistent truncus arteriosus, marked pulmonary stenosis with normal aortic root, common ventricle, and rarely simple transposition. While some of these may be excluded at times by echocardiography or by evidence of increased lung blood flow in the chest x-ray, frequently a selective angiocardiogram will be required.

The most common problem is to distinguish the anomaly from tricuspid atresia. In this latter malformation the heart remains normal in size or only slightly enlarged. The electrocardiographic pattern remains fixed from birth and usually shows both left-axis deviation with horizontal electrical position and left ventricular hypertrophy. There are no signs of associated right ventricular hypertrophy. When tricuspid atresia is associated with transposition of the great vessels and large pulmonary arteries (type II [c]), the electrocardiogram may be similar to that in pulmonary atresia with normal aortic root; however, the electrical position of the heart is usually horizontal rather than vertical as in pulmonary atresia. An x-ray of the chest is also helpful since it shows increased pulmonary vascular markings and a contour typical of transposition.

Critical pulmonary stenosis may be associated with hypoplasia of the right ventricle (Marquis, 1951; Joos et al., 1954; Soulie et al., 1956; Lauer et al., 1964; Freed et al., 1973). These patients may be extremely difficult to differentiate from those with pulmonary atresia and intact ventricular septum. The electrocardiograms and chest radiographs are quite similar. A harsh systolic ejection murmur is suggestive of pulmonary stenosis, but when tricuspid regurgitation dominates, the clinical differentiation may be impossible. Selective angiography should show continuity between the right ventricle and pulmonary artery, and the adequacy of the right ventricular sinus can be ascertained.

Transposition of the great vessels may occasionally show an electrocardiographic pattern similar to the common one of pulmonary atresia. However, the configurations of the heart and the findings of angiocardiography will differentiate the two anomalies.

The major diagnostic problem is to identify not only the anomaly under discussion but especially the subgroup having a small, normal, or large right ventricle since infants with such anatomy are susceptible to successful surgery. It is therefore important to do a selective angiogram into the right ventricle to show the chamber size and the level of obstruction, whether valvar, infundibular, or both.

Cardiac Catheterization

Physiologic data, although incomplete, were available in most of our patients and in some reported in the literature (Kjellberg et al., 1959; Paul and Lev, 1960; Davignon et al., 1961; Kiely et al., 1963). Right

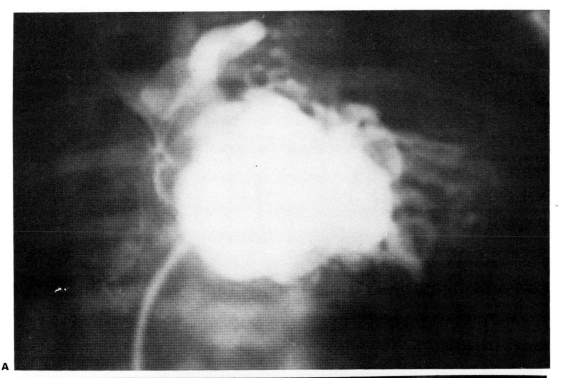

A

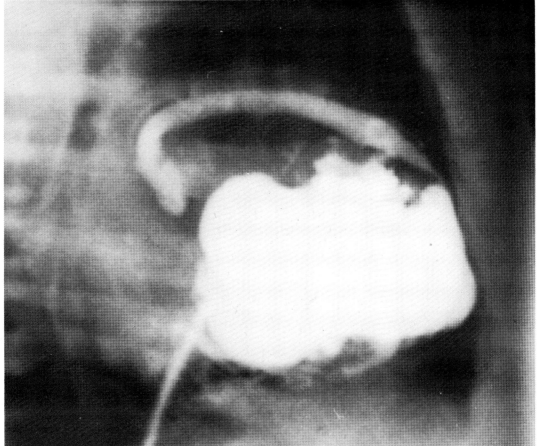

B

Figure 28-7. Right ventriculogram demonstrating a large sinusoid channel connecting the right ventricle to the aorta, in a case with large ventricular chamber and absent tricuspid regurgitation.

513

ventricular pressures were available in all, while left ventricular or systemic pressures were determined in many.

The right ventricular systolic pressure ranged from a low of 46 mm of mercury to a high of 155 mm of mercury. Only four times was it less than 100 mm of mercury. All pressure curves examined exhibited the triangular contour characteristic of outflow obstruction.

Eleven of fourteen patients had right ventricular pressures exceeding systemic values. Three of these had anomalous communications between the right ventricle and the coronary artery. The pressures were equal in the two ventricles in a 13-year-old boy with marked tricuspid regurgitation but without cardioaortic fistulae. The pulse contours were, however, quite dissimilar, suggesting the presence of an intact ventricular septum. In two instances the systemic pressures were significantly higher.

High ventricular end-diastolic pressures (over 10 mm of mercury) were recorded in some patients.

The atrial "a" waves and mean valves were invariably elevated. No atrial regurgitatant waves or end-diastolic pressure gradients were recorded across the tricuspid.

A massive atrial right-to-left shunt was invariable.

The systemic arterial saturation ranged from 21 to 79 percent.

Myocardial performance has been evaluated in only a small number of patients with pulmonary atresia and intact ventricular septum (Graham et al., 1974). Preoperative volume studies in eight of their patients demonstrates a diminutive right ventricle, with significant reduction of ejection fraction in most. The patient with severe tricuspid valve regurgitation has a large right ventricle, and the ejection fraction is close to normal. In three patients studied before and after successful valvotomy, the right ventricular end-diastolic volume has approached normal, with ejection fractions also in the normal range. However, these patients showed significant elevations of right ventricular end diastolic pressure and low volume measurements after valvotomy. These findings suggest impaired right ventricular distensibility.

Prognosis

Pulmonary atresia with intact ventricular septum has an exceedingly poor prognosis. The ages at death range from stillborn (Steiner, 1937) to 13 years (Lauer et al., 1964). One unusual case lived to age 20 years (Costa, 1930).

One-third of the cases have died by the end of the second week of life. Fifty percent are dead by the end of the first month. Longer survival is determined by the adequacy of the patent ductus arteriosus. The ages at death of 57 cases at The Hospital for Sick Children and the Buffalo Children's Hospital are shown in Figure 28–8.

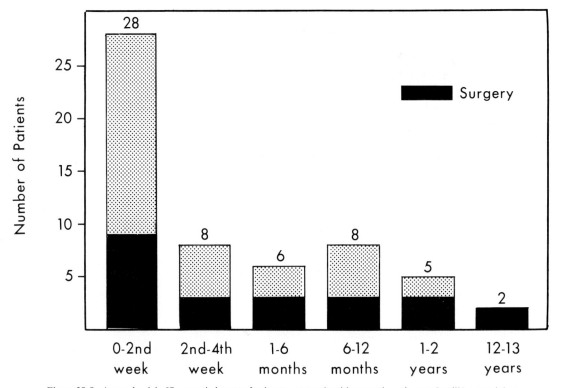

Figure 28-8. Age at death in 57 autopsied cases of pulmonary atresia with normal aortic root. It will be noted that the greatest mortality occurs in the first month of life.

Treatment

The mortality rate is very high in patients with pulmonary atresia and intact septum. Surgery must be performed early and type of procedure depends on the size of the right ventricle. If the infant has a large or normal-sized right ventricle (15 percent of cases), a pulmonary valvulotomy may be performed. If the infant has a small right ventricle, balloon septostomy should be done at the time of catheterization as soon as the diagnosis is established. Within a few hours the child may then be taken to the operating room where a Potts' anastomosis may be carried out followed by ligation of the patent ductus arteriosus to prevent flooding of the lungs. At The Hospital for Sick Children in Toronto in the last nine years, we have treated 26 patients with pulmonary atresia and intact septum this way and 20 are still alive and progressing moderately well.

Bowman and coworkers (1971) suggested that a patient with a small right ventricle should have a pulmonary valvulotomy as well as an aorto-pulmonary shunt at the initial operation, and Luckstead and associates (1972) recommended that a pulmonary valvulotomy be performed three or four months after the initial operation. There is some evidence to suggest that, in some cases of pulmonary atresia with small right ventricle, the ventricle can grow if a valvulotomy is done in early life.

In some instances short-term nonsurgical palliation of the patient with pulmonary atresia and intact ventricular septum can be accomplished. Survival of these patients depends on adequacy of the pulmonary blood flow, and, in the neonate, on patency of the ductus arteriosus. As the ductus constricts, progressive tissue hypoxia and acidosis occur, with concomitant clinical deterioration. Patency of the ductus arteriosus may be maintained by the use of prostaglandin E (Elliott et al., 1975; Olley et al., 1976; Heymann and Rudolph, 1977). The use of E-type prostaglandins in these patients is based on the observation that prostaglandins may relax the hypoxic fetal-lamb ductus arteriosus (Coceani and Olley, 1973).

Buffered formalin infiltration of the ductus arteriosus to maintain its patency has been used to ameliorate the decreased pulmonary blood flow in these patients. Rudolph and associates reported formalinization of a ductus arteriosus in a four-day-old with pulmonary atresia and intact ventricular septum in which the great vessel anatomy precluded the performance of a systemic to pulmonary artery anastomosis (1975).

Overall surgical results in this group of patients is disappointing (Trusler and Fowler, 1970; Shams et al., 1971; Parisi-Buckley et al., 1975). For the patient with diminutive right ventricle, severely stenotic tricuspid valve, and grossly underdeveloped and hypertensive right ventricle, initial palliation can be afforded by balloon septostomy, pulmonary valvotomy, and a systemic-pulmonary artery anas-

tomosis to augment pulmonary blood flow (Aziz et al., 1975). With rare exception, our experience has suggested that significant improvement in right ventricular dimensions is not achieved by these maneuvers, and the right ventricle remains hypertensive, with inflow and outflow obstruction. Rarely, significant improvement in right ventricular size is noted after such procedures (Graham et al., 1974; Rao et al., 1976).

At about six months of age, we have begun to recatheterize the patient with diminutive right ventricle who has obviously survived initial palliation. In those older patients with significant residual right ventricular ouflow tract obstruction, we have begun to perform an extensive infundibular resection, placing a patch across the pulmonary valve annulus. Unfortunately, although this may palliate or even cure severe pulmonary obstruction, the tricuspid valve is often so grossly stenotic with thick, shortened chordae tendineae and hypoplastic papillary muscles, that right ventricular filling is less than optimum. At the present time, the prognosis for those patients with diminutive right ventricle must be considered as guarded at best. Indeed, Rigby et al. (1977) have reported the successful application of this aggressive approach in a 32-hour-old newborn.

REFERENCES

Abbott, M. E.: New accessions in cardiac anomalies. I. Pulmonary atresia of inflammatory origin. *Bull. Intern. A. M. Museums*, **10**:111, 1924

————: *Atlas of Congenital Cardiac Disease*. American Heart Association, New York, 1936.

Abbott, M. E.; Lewis, D. S.; and Beattie, W. W.: Differential study of a case of pulmonary stenosis of inflammatory origin (ventricular septum closed) and two cases of (a) pulmonary stenosis and (b) pulmonary atresia of developmental origin with associated ventricular septal defect and death from paradoxical cerebral embolism. *Am. J. Med. Sci.*, **165**:636, 1923.

Abercrombie, J.: Congenital atresia of right ventricle; ductus arteriosus patent. *Trans. Path. Soc. Lond.*, **34**:78, 1883.

Alexander, W. S., and Green, H. C.: Coronary blood vessel arising from cardiac ventricle. Report of a case showing other cardiac anomalies. *Arch. Pathol.*, **53**:187, 1952.

Aziz, K. U.; Olley, P. M.; Rowe, R. D.; Trusler, G. A.; and Mustard, W. T.: Survival after systemic to pulmonary arterial shunts in infants less than 30 days old with obstructive lesions of the right heart chambers. *Am. J. Cardiol.*, **36**:479, 1975.

Barr, P. A.; Celermajer, J. M.; Bowdler, J. D.; and Cartmill, T. B.: Severe congenital tricuspid incompetence in the neonate. *Circulation*, **49**:962, 1974.

Bauer, D. deF., and Astbury, E.: Congenital cardiac disease. Bibliography of the 1,000 cases analysed in Maude Abbott's Atlas. With an index. *Am. Heart. J.*, **27**:688, 1944.

Benton, J. W., Jr.; Elliott, L. P.; Adams, P., Jr.; Anderson, R. C.; Hong, C. Y.; and Lester, R. G.: Pulmonary atresia and stenosis with intact ventricular septum. *Am J. Dis. Child.*, **104**:83, 1962.

Bifulco, E.; Mangiarddi, J. L.; and Sullivan, J. J., Jr.: Case report. Congenital pulmonary artery atresia with associated tricuspid hypoplasia. Report of two cases. *Am. J. Cardiol.*, **4**:401, 1959.

Bowman, F. O.; Malm, J. R.; Hayes, C. J.; Gersony, W. M.; and Ellis, K.: Pulmonary atresia with intact ventricular septum. *J. Thorac. Cardiovasc. Surg.*, **61**:85, 1971.

Buzzi, A.: Historical milestones. Description of congenital pulmonary atresia and tricuspid stenosis (Delmas, 1826). *Am. J. Cardiol.*, **4**:691, 1959.

Caddell, J. L.; and Whittemore, R.: Pulmonary atresia with dilated right ventricle. A case with congenital atrial flutter. *Am. J. Cardiol.*, **12**:254–62, 1963.

Campbell, M.: Results of surgical treatment for pulmonary atresia. *Br. Heart J.*, **22**:527, 1960.

Celermajer, J. M.; Bowler, J. D.; Gengos, D. C.; Cohen, D. G.; and Stuckey, D. S.: Pulmonary Valve fusion with intact ventricular septum. *Am. Heart J.*, **76**:452, 1968.

Chesler, E.; Joffe, H. S.; Vecht, R.; Beck, W.; and Schrire, V.: Ultrasound cardiography in single ventricle and the hypoplastic left and right heart syndromes. *Circulation*, **42**:123, 1970.

Chiche, P.: Etude anatomique et clinique des atresies tri-cuspidiennes. *Arch. Mal. Coeur*, **45**:980, 1952.

Coceani, F., and Olley, P.: The response of the ductus arteriosus to prostaglandins. *Can. J. Physiol. Pharmacol.*, **51**:220, 1973.

Cole, R. B.; Muster, A. J.; Lev, M., and Paul, M. H.: Pulmonary atresia with intact ventricular septum. *Am. J. Cardiol.*, **21**:23, 1968.

Collins, H. A.; Harbert, F. J.; Soltero, L. R.; McNamara, D. G.; and Cooley, D. A.: Cardiac surgery in the newborn. *Surgery*, **45**:506–19, 1959.

Cooley, D. A., and Hallman, G. L.: Cardiovascular surgery during the first year of life. Experience with 450 consecutive operations. *Am. J. Surg.*, **107**:474, 1964.

Costa, A.: Atresia congenita dell'ostio della pulmonare, con setto interventriculare chiuso e dotto di Botallo persistente in uomo di 20 anni. *Clin. Med. Ital.*, **61**:567, 1930.

Curl, S. W.: Two cases of congenital morbus cordis with atresia of the pulmonary artery and other defects. *Lancet*, **1**:87, 1905.

Davignon, A. L.; Greenwold, W. E.; DuShane, J. W.; and Edwards, J. E.: Congenital pulmonary atresia with intact ventricular septum: clinicopathologic correlation of two anatomic types. *Am. Heart J.*, **62**:591, 1961.

Dhanavaravibul, S.; Nora, J. J.; and McNamara, D. G.: Pulmonary valvular atresia with intact ventricular septum: Problems in diagnosis and results of treatment. *J. Pediatr.*, **77**:1010, 1970.

Edwards, J. E., in Gould, S. E. (ed.): *Pathology of the Heart*. Charles C. Thomas, Publisher, Springfield, Ill., 1953, p. 398.

Edwards, J. E.; Dry, T. J.; Parker, R. L.; Burchell, H. B.; Wood, E. H.; and Bulbulian, A. H.: *An Atlas of Congenital Anomalies of the Heart and Great Vessels*, 2nd ed. Charles C. Thomas, Publisher, Springfield, Ill., 1954, p. 93.

Edwards, J. E., and Gould, S. E.: *Pathology of the Heart*, ed. 2. Charles C. Thomas, Publisher, Springfield, Ill., 1959, p. 398.

Elliott, L. P.; Adams, P., Jr.; and Edwards, J. E.: Pulmonary atresia with intact ventricular septum. *Br. Heart J.*, **25**:489, 1963.

Elliott, R. B.; Starling, M. B.; and Neutze, J. M.: Medical manipulation of the ductus arteriosus. *Lancet*, **1**:140, 1975.

Fischer, L.: *Ein Fall von Kongenitaler Atresie des Konus der Arteria pulmonalis verbunden mit Trikuspidal Stenose und insuffizienz.* B. Georgi, Leipzig, 1904.

Freed, M. D.; Rosenthal, A.; Bernhard, W. F.; Litwin, S. B.; and Nadas, A. S.: Critical pulmonary stenosis with a diminutive right ventricle in neonates. *Circulation*, **48**:875, 1973.

Freedom, R. M.; Culham, G.; Moes, F.; Olley, P. M.; and Rowe, R. D.: The differentiation of functional from structural pulmonary atresia: The role of aortography. *Am. J. Cardiol.*, 1978 (In press).

Freedom, R. M., and Harrington, D. P.: Contributions of intramyocardial sinusoids in pulmonary atresia and intact ventricular septum to a right-sided circular shunt. *Br. Heart J.*, **36**:1061, 1974.

Freedom, R. M.; White, R. I., Jr.; Ho, C. S.; Gingell, R. L.; Hawker, R. E.; and Rowe, R. D.: Evaluation of patients with pulmonary atresia and intact ventricular septum by double catheter technique. *Am. J. Cardiol.*, **33**:892, 1974.

Gamboa, R.; Gersony, W. M.; Nadas, A. S.: The electrocardiogram in tricuspid atresia and pulmonary atresia with intact ventricular septum. *Circulation*, **34**:24, 1966.

Glaboff, J. J.; Gohmann, J. T.; and Little, J. A.: Atresia of the pulmonary artery with intact interventricular septum, *J. Pediatr.*, **37**:396, 1950.

Godman, M. J.; Tham, P.; and Kidd, B. S. L.: Echocardiography in the evaluation of the cyanotic newborn infant. *Br. Heart J.*, **36**:154, 1974.

Graham, T. P., Jr.; Bender, H. W.; Atwood, G. F.; et al.: Increase in right ventricular volume following valvulotomy for pulmonary

atresia or stenosis with intact ventricular septum. *Circulation*, II, **49–50**:69–79, 1974.

Grant, R. T.: Unusual anomaly of coronary vessels in malformed heart of child. *Heart*, **13**:273, 1926.

Greenwold, W. E.; Dushane, J. W.; Burchell, H. B.; Bruwer, A.; and Edwards, J. E.: Congenital pulmonary atresia with intact ventricular septum: two anatomic types. *Proc. 29th Sc. Sessions, Am. Heart A.*, (Oct.) 1956, p. 51, abstract.

Gross, P.: Concept of fetal endocarditis. A general review with report of an illustrative case. *Arch. Pathol.*, **31**:163, 1941.

Gueniot: *Gull. Soc. Anat. Paris*, 7(n.s.):159, 1862. Cited in Peacock (1869).

Guidici, C.; and Becu, L.: Case reports. Cardio-aortic fistula through anomalous coronary arteries. *Br. Heart J.*, **22**:729, 1960.

Hare, C. J.: Malformation of the heart. Complete closure of the orifice of the pulmonary artery. Very small foramen ovale. Cyanosis. *Trans. Path. Soc. Lond.*, **4**:81, 1852–1853.

Heymann, M. A., and Rudolph, A. M.: Ductus arteriosus dilatation by prostaglandin E, in infants with pulmonary atresia. *Pediatrics*, **59**:325, 1977.

Hunter, J.: *M. Observations & Enquiries*, **6**:291, 1783. Cited in Peacock (1869).

Jakubowitsch, A.: Ein Fall von congenitaler Atresie der Arteria pulmonalis. Beiträge zur Lehre von den angeborenen Erkrankungen der Herzens. Zurich, thesis published in 1897, p. 38.

Joos, H. A.; Yu, P. N.; Lovejoy, F. W., Jr.; Nye, R. E., Jr.; and Simpson, J. H.: Clinical and hemodynamic studies of congenital pulmonic stenosis with intact ventricular septum. *Am. J. Med.*, **17**:6, 1954.

Keith, A.: The Hunterian lectures on malformations of the heart. *Lancet*, **2**:359, 433, 519, 1909.

Keith, J. D.; Rowe, R. D.; and Vlad, P.: *Heart Disease in Infancy and Childhood*, 1st ed. Macmillan Publishing Co., Inc., New York, 1958.

Kieffer, S. A.; and Carey, L. S.: Radiological aspects of pulmonary atresia with intact ventricular septum. *Br. Heart J.*, **25**:655, 1963.

Kiely, B.; Morales, F.; and Rosenblum, D.: Pulmonary atresia with intact ventricular septum. *Pediatrics*, **32**:841, 1963.

Kjellberg, S. R.; Mannheimer, E.; Rudhe, U.; and Jonsson, B.: *Diagnosis of Congenital Heart Disease*, 2nd ed. Year Book Publishers, Inc., Chicago, 1959.

Kugel, M. A.: Congenital heart disease. A clinical and pathological study of two cases of truncus solitarius aorticus (pulmonary atresia). *Am. Heart J.*, **7**:262, 1932.

Lauer, R. M.; Fink, H. P.; Petry, E. L.; Dunn, M. I.; and Diehl, A. M.: Angiographic demonstration of intramyocardial sinusoids in pulmonary-valve atresia with intact ventricular septum and hypoplastic right ventricle. *N. Engl. J. Med.*, **271**:68, 1964.

Leo, H.: Über einen Fall von Entwicklungshemmung des Herzens. *Virchow Arch. Pathol. Anat.*, **103**:503, 1886.

Lordat (1822), in Gintrac, E.: *Observations et Recherches sur la Cyanose, ou Maladie Bleue*. J. Pinard, Paris, 1824, p. 201, obs. 53. Cited in Peacock (1869).

Lucas, R. C.: Heart from a case of cyanosis. Atresia of the pulmonary orifice; diminutive right ventricle; ventrical septum in the right auricle formed by an abnormally developed eustachian valve; interventricular septum complete; patent ductus arteriosus and foramen ovale. *Trans. Path. Soc. Lond.*, **26**:26, 1875.

Luckstead, E. F.; Mattioli, L.; Crosby, I. K.; Reed, W. A.; and Diehl, A. M.: Two-stage palliative surgical approach for pulmonary atresia with intact ventricular septum (type I). *Am. J. Cardiol.*, **29**:490, 1972.

Mangiardi, J. L.; Sullivan, J. J., Jr.; Bifulco, E.; and Lukash, L.: Congenital tricuspid stenosis with pulmonary atresia. Report of six cases. *Am. J. Cardiol.*, **11**:726, 1963.

Marquis, R. M.: Unipolar electrocardiography in pulmonary stenosis. *Br. Heart J.*, **13**:89, 1951.

Mautner, H.: Beiträge zur Entwicklungsmechanic, Pathologie und Klinik angeborener Herzfehler. *Jahrb. Kinderh.*, **96**:123, 1921.

Meyer, R. A., and Kaplan, S.: Echocardiography in the diagnosis of hypoplasia of the left or right ventricles in the neonate. *Circulation*, **46**:55, 1972.

Moller, J. H.; Girod, D.; Amplatz, K.; et al.: Pulmonary valvotomy in pulmonary atresia with hypoplastic right ventricle. *Surgery*, **68**:630, 1970.

Newfeld, E. A.; Cole, R. B.; and Paul, M. H.: Ebstein's

malformation of the tricuspid valve in the neonate. Functional and anatomic pulmonary outflow tract obstruction. *Am. J. Cardiol.*, **19**:727, 1967.

Norgan, B. C.; Stacy, G. S.; and Dillard, D. H.: Pulmonary valvular and infundibular atresia with intact ventricular septum. *Am. J. Cardiol.*, **16**:746, 1965.

Novelo, S.; Chait, L. O.; Zapata Diaz, J.; and Velazquez, T.: Atresia pulmonar y estenosis tricuspidea sin comunicación interventricular. *Arch. Inst. Cardiol. México*, **21**:325, 1951.

Ogle, C.: Atresia of the pulmonary artery. *Trans. Pathol. Soc. Lond.*, **47**:28, 1896.

Olley, P.: Nonsurgical palliation of congenital heart malformations. *N. Engl. J. Med.*, **292**:1292, 1975.

Olley, P. M.; Coceani, F.; and Bodach, E.: E-type prostaglandins. A new emergency therapy for certain cyanotic congenital heart malformations. *Circulation*, **53**:728, 1976.

Ollivier: *Bull Soc Anat Paris*, **6**(n.s.):320, 1861. Cited in Peacock (1869).

Parisi-Buckley, L.; Dooley, K. J.; and Fyler, D. C.: Pulmonary atresia and intact ventricular septum in New England. *Circulation*, **11** (51–52):225, 1975 (abst.).

Paul, M. H.; and Lev, M.: Tricuspid stenosis with pulmonary atresia. A cineangiographic-pathologic correlation. *Circulation*, **22**:198, 1960.

Peacock, T. B.: Malformation of the heart. Obliteration of the orifice of the pulmonary artery; open foramen ovale and ductus arteriosus; cyanosis. *Trans. Pathol. Soc. Lond.*, **15**:60, 1863–1864.

———: Malformation of the heart. Atresia of the orifice of the pulmonary artery; aorta communicating with both ventricles. *Trans. Pathol. Soc. Lond.*, **20**:61, 1869.

Peck, D. R., and Wilson, H. M.: Conventional roentgenography in the diagnosis of cardiovascular anomalies. *Radiology*, **53**:479, 1949.

Rao, P. S.; Liebman, J.; and Borkat, G.: Right ventricular growth in a case of pulmonary stenosis with intact ventricular septum and hypoplastic right ventricle. *Circulation*, **53**:389, 1976.

Rigby, M. L.; Silove, F. D.; Astley, R.; and Abrams, L. D.: Pulmonary atresia with intact ventricular septum. Open heart surgical correction at 32 hours. *Br. Heart J.*, **39**:573, 1977.

Rokitansky, C. F. von: *Wochenblatt Z Jahr*, **14**:225, 1855. Cited in Peacock (1869).

Rudolph, A. M.; Heymann, M. A.; Fishman, N.; and Lakier, J. B.: Formalin infiltration of the ductus arteriosus. A method for palliation of infants with selected congenital cardiac lesions. *N. Engl. J. Med.*, **292**:1263, 1975.

Schire, V.; Sutin, G. J.; and Barnard, C. N.: Organic and functional pulmonary atresia with intact ventricular septum. *Am. J. Cardiol.*, **8**:100, 1961.

Shams, A.; Fowler, R. S.; Trusler, G. A.; Keith, J. D.; and Mustard, W. T.: Pulmonary atresia with intact ventricular septum: Report of 50 cases. *Pediatrics*, **47**:370, 1971.

Soulié, P.; DiMatteo, J.; Vernant, P.; and Michaux, J.: L'hypertrophie ventriculaire gauche dans certaines triades de Fallot. *Arch. Mal. Coeur*, **49**:525, 1956.

Steiner, M. M.: Atresia of the pulmonary orifice with intact ventricular septum. *J. Pediatr.*, **10**:370, 1937.

Taussig, H. B.: *Congenital Malformations of the Heart.* The Commonwealth Fund, New York, 1947, p. 101.

Trusler, G. A.; and Fowler, R. S.: The surgical management of pulmonary atresia with intact ventricular septum and hypoplastic right ventricle. *J. Thorac. Cardiovasc. Surg.*, **59**:704, 1970.

Wagenvoort, C. A., and Edwards, J. E.: The pulmonary arterial tree in pulmonic atresia. *Arch. Pathol.*, **71**:646, 1961.

Wagner, L.: *Ein Fall von congenitaler Atresie der A. pulmonalis, congenataler mit Tricuspidalstenose, bei geschlossener Kammerscheidewand.* (Giessen) Darmstadt, 1889.

Williams, R. R.; Kent, G. B., Jr.; and Edwards, J. E.: Anomalous cardiac blood vessel communicating with the right ventricle: observations in a case of pulmonary atresia with an intact ventricular septum. *Arch. Pathol.*, **52**:480–87, 1951.

Zeigler, R. F., and Taber, R. E.: Diagnostic criteria and successful surgery in an operable form of complete pulmonary valve atresia (abstract). *Circulation*, **26**:807, 1962.

29

Tricuspid Atresia

Peter Vlad

Tricuspid atresia is a congenital anomaly of the cyanotic group in which the chief abnormality is an absence or imperforation of the tricuspid valve. It never appears as an isolated anomaly and is characterized by the association of four defects: (1) atresia of the tricuspid valve, (2) patency of the interatrial septum, (3) hyperplasia of the mitral valve and left ventricle, and (4) underdevelopment or absence of the right ventricle.

Tricuspid atresia is by far the most common type of nonfunctioning right ventricle but by no means the only one. Other conditions may be associated with underdevelopment of the right ventricle and atrioventricular valve. Pulmonary atresia with closed ventricular septum, overriding of the tricuspid valve

as seen in some cases of transposition of the great arteries, and primary tricuspid hypoplasia are such anomalies. They may be clinically mistaken for tricuspid atresia since the hemodynamics and, consequently, the roentgenologic and electrocardiographic findings are similar.

Prevalence

Tricuspid atresia has been found to occur in approximately 3 percent of congenital heart anomalies seen at postmortem (see Table 29–1) or clinically (see Table 29–2). Gardiner and Keith (1951) had two instances in 29 congenital cardiac deaths in the 1948–1949 Toronto Heart Registry, giving an

Table 29–1. INCIDENCE OF TRICUSPID ATRESIA IN POSTMORTEM CASES

AUTHOR	NUMBER OF AUTOPSIES	TRICUSPID ATRESIA	PERCENT
Abbott (1936)	1000	21	2.1
Gibson and Clifton (1938)	105	1	1.0
Edwards and Burchell (1949)	212	4	1.9
Sommers and Johnson (1951)	141	6	4.3
Donzelot and D'Allaines (1954)	95	5	5.3
Hospital for Sick Children, Toronto (1954)	574	29	5.1
Nadas and Fyler (1972)	1017	29	3
Total	3144	95	3.02

Table 29–2. INCIDENCE OF TRICUSPID ATRESIA IN CLINICAL CASES

AUTHOR	NUMBER OF CASES	TRICUSPID ATRESIA	PERCENT
Donzelot and D'Allaines (1954)	1100	33	3
Soulié (1952)	700	13	1.9
Mitchell et al. (1971)	457	5	1.2
Nadas and Fyler (1972)	10,624	115	1.08
Hospital for Sick Children, Toronto (1973)	10,535	139	1.32
Total	23,416	305	1.30

incidence of approximately one case in every 5000 births.

Embryology

According to Van Praagh (1973), tricuspid atresia is the result of an appropriate degree of malalignment of the ventricular septum relative to the atrioventricular canal. When the right ventricular sinus is absent, the ventricular septum is shifted to the right, obliterating the right atrioventricular orifice.

Rosenquist and coworkers' observation (1970) that the right atrial dimple (the presumed site of the atretic valve) transilluminates into the left ventricle regardless of anatomic type, size of the ventricular septum, or anatomy of the atrial septum supports this concept.

With a further degree of rightward shift, the tricuspid valve is spared and double-inlet left ventricle or common ventricle with right-sided outflow chamber results.

Van Praagh (1973) also pointed out that tricuspid atresia can occur with common atrioventricular canal and rarely with Ebstein's malformation of the tricuspid.

Anatomy

In the following paragraphs the features common to all tricuspid atresia will be reviewed, then the variations and the associated anomalies. This anatomic study is based on the review of 143 specimens, 51 of which were examined at The Hospital for Sick Children, Toronto.

Common Features. ATRESIA OF THE TRICUSPID ORIFICE. There is agenesis of this orifice. There is no connection whatever between the right atrium and right ventricle, and no valvular material can be identified on either gross or microscopic examination. An area of fibrosis or umbilication may be present on the floor of the atrium, and muscle fibers may radiate around it. Occasionally the atresia is of a membranous type. It is often associated with juxtaposition of the atrial appendages (Van Praagh, 1973). Minute valvular cusps may be present but are completely fused. Henriette (1861), Kelly (1868), Elster (1950), and Chiche (two cases) (1952) have reported the only five known cases of this type. Two of these had an additional pulmonary atresia (Elster, Chiche) and clotted blood into the right ventricle. This fact would suggest that the fusion of the tricuspid leaflets may be due to an acquired process that traps blood into the right ventricle. A similar phenomenon may be seen in the cases of pulmonary atresia with intact ventricular septum (second case of Taussig, 1936).

INTERATRIAL COMMUNICATION. The interatrial communication represents the only exit from the right atrium and is invariably present. It is usually a normal foramen ovale, and such was found in 66 percent of the group studied. The size of the patency is extremely variable, depending chiefly upon the age. It may be only slitlike, as is often the case with infants, or it may easily admit an index finger or a thumb in older patients. This structure plays a considerable role in the circulation and may represent the first obstacle in the way of the blood flow. Restrictive atrial communications, rarely, may be associated with an aneurysm of the fossa ovale. When large, this may produce mitral obstruction (Freedom and Rowe, 1976).

A defective interatrial septum is less frequent—its incidence is 33 percent both in the literature and in our own group. Again its dimensions are variable and may be as large as 25 by 30 mm (Schreiber, 1903). Such cases are more likely to survive for many years (cases of: Holmes [1824], 21 years; Schreiber [1903], 2½ years; Metianu et al. [1953], seven years). In the cases of Chapotot (1889) and Thomas (1941), in three patients of Metianu and associates (1953), and in one of ours there was complete absence of the interatrial septum.

THE MITRAL VALVE AND THE LEFT VENTRICLE. The mitral orifice is large, normally situated, and competent. Usually there are two leaflets, but an occasional case may have a tri- or multicuspid valve (Thomas, 1941; Ross, 1952; and three cases at The Hospital for Sick Children).

Overriding of the ventricular septum by the mitral orifice was encountered twice (once by Fragoyannis and Kardalinos [1962] and once by us).

The left ventricle is both enlarged and considerably hypertrophied. It forms most of the ventricular myocardium with its anterior, posterior, and diaphragmatic faces. The thickness of its walls may measure as much as 20 mm in older teen-agers (sixth case of Metianu et al., 1953) and 14 to 16 mm in small infants.

THE RIGHT VENTRICLE. This chamber is reduced in size and forms only a small portion of the ventricular myocardium. Its volume depends to a certain degree on the anatomic type, and in one of these, I(a) in Table 29–3 (page 520), gross examination of the specimen may fail to demonstrate its presence. However, most often it can be identified at the right upper aspect of the ventricular part when it extends medially to form a fourth or a third of the anterior face of the heart. Its anatomic structure is such that it is possible to distinguish several variants:

1. A minute, slitlike space with a thin endocardial lining, hidden within the right wall of the left ventricle. As noted by Edwards and Burchell (1949), in occasional cases only microscopic examination will allow its identification.

2. A moderate-sized chamber, with or without papillary muscles, appearing as a simple outpouching of the large left ventricle. A ventricular septal defect will allow free communication between the two ventricles.

3. More frequently the right ventricle has a capacity of a few milliliters only and has two

compartments. Cranially, there is a smooth, tubular chamber with thin endocardium, leading to the pulmonary artery and representing the infundibulum. Its diameter follows closely that of the pulmonary artery. The walls are 2 to 4 mm in thickness, but occasionally they may be thinner and then this segment may look, from the outside, like a mere prolongation of the pulmonary artery. Distally, there is a blunt muscular narrowing leading to the remnants of the inflow chamber, which is rough, lies on the lateral face of the ventricular mass, contains papillary muscles (the anterior one is readily identified) and trabeculae, and communicates with the left ventricle through a small ventricular septal defect.

4. On one occasion the sinus portion of the right ventricle was present in virtually normal size, extending below to the diaphragmatic surface of the heart. Its walls were thin, but the endocardium exhibited a marked degree of fibroelastosis, particularly in the region opposite the ventricular septal defect. The subpulmonary conus was of normal morphology.

5. The right ventricle was found to be the major chamber in a 2½-year-old boy with tricuspid atresia and solitus viscera, atria, and ventricles. The mitral valve overrode the crest of a displaced ventricular septum. While the left ventricle remained small, the right was large and gave off both great arteries. These features are similar to those reported by Fragoyannis and Kardalinos in their case. In addition, there was D-transposition of the great arteries with the aorta arising from a large infundibulum, the pulmonary valve was severely stenotic, and its outflow was compressed between the infundibular septum and the floor of the left atrium.

6. When L-transposition of the great arteries was associated with an L-bulboventricular loop, the dominant chamber was a left-sided right ventricle (morphologic), while the small chamber was a right-sided left ventricle. One such specimen existed in our series.

⑤ THE ATRIA. The right atrium and its appendages are constantly enlarged and thick-walled. The left is more variable but tends to enlarge, especially when a large interatrial communication allows free passage of the blood to this chamber.

Variations and Classification. A classification was first attempted by Kühne (1906), who distinguished two groups, with and without transposition of the great vessels. Wieland (1914) endorsed this classification and called them "simple" and "complicated," and Edwards and Burchell (1949) described two types in each group. We have amplified the latter to include eight types in all (Figure 29–1, Table 29–3).

TYPE I—WITHOUT TRANSPOSITION OF THE GREAT ARTERIES. Absence of transposition of the great vessels occurred in 99 of 143 anatomic cases (70 percent).

Type I(a)—Pulmonary Atresia, Closed Ventricular Septum, Virtual Absence of the Right Ventricular Chamber. Ten such cases have been encountered in our series: Taussig (1936), Roberts (1937), Elster (1950), Gasul et al. (1950), Guffau (1950), Abrams and Alway (1951), Chiche (two cases) (1952), Metianu et al. (1953), Hospital for Sick Children (1964).

The pulmonary artery is completely occluded, but the site of the atresia may vary. Valvular imperforation is more frequent than is the "cord" type. Raphae may be identified, and the pulmonary artery trunk is patent (Roberts, 1937; Elster, 1950; Chiche, 1952). Combined trunk and valve atresia has been reported twice (Taussig, 1936; Abrams and Alway, 1951).

The aorta is large and arises normally from the left ventricle. The ventricular septum is completely formed, and the right ventricle is reduced to a mere endocardial fold within the right upper portion of the ventricular myocardium. Its walls are thin. As shown by Edwards (1953), it is possible that certain cases reported as examples of single ventricle may be this type of tricuspid atresia. Microscopic sections of the

Table 29–3. RELATIVE FREQUENCY OF THE ANATOMIC TYPES—143 ANATOMIC SPECIMENS

	LITERATURE	HOSPITAL FOR SICK CHILDREN	TOTAL
I. Without transposition of the great arteries	61	38	99 (69%)
a. Pulmonary atresia	9	4	13
b. Pulmonary hypoplasia			
Small ventricular septal defect	43	30	73
c. No pulmonary hypoplasia			
Large ventricular septal defect	9	4	13
II. With D-transposition of the great arteries	31	9	40 (27%)
a. Pulmonary atresia	1	2	3
b. Pulmonary or subpulmonary stenosis	10	1	11
c. Large pulmonary artery	20	6	26
III. With L-transposition of the great arteries	—	4	4 (3%)
a. Pulmonary or subpulmonary stenosis	—	1	1
b. Subaortic stenosis	—	3	3

I Tricuspid Atresia With No Transposition (69 percent)

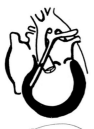 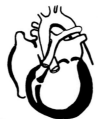 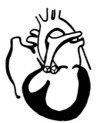

I (a) Pulmonary atresia

I (b) Pulmonary hypoplasia, small ventricular septal defect (*most common type*)

I (c) No pulmonary hypoplasia, large ventricular septal defect

II Tricuspid Atresia With D Transposition (27 percent)

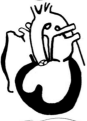 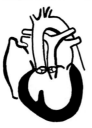 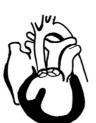

II (a) Pulmonary atresia

II (b) Pulmonary or subpulmonary stenosis

II (c) Large pulmonary artery

III Tricuspid Atresia With L Transposition (3 percent)

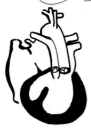 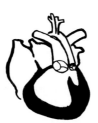

III (a) Pulmonary or subpulmonary stenosis

III (b) Subaortic stenosis

Figure 29-1. The anatomic classification of tricuspid atresia. The percentages indicate the relative frequency as found in 143 anatomic specimens.

subpulmonary region of the ventricle may be necessary to prove the presence of this endocardium-lined chamber.

The ductus arteriosus is patent and represents the only way through which the blood can reach the lungs. It is of small size and functionally inadequate, as proved by the severity of the symptoms at very early ages, the absence of a continuous murmur (five times in six cases with auscultatory data), and the poor life expectancy.

The bronchial arteries may carry some blood to the lungs, but they are not obvious at autopsy and are of negligible functional value. Life duration is short and averages two to three months. Pure, low infundibular atresia was seen twice at The Hospital for Sick Children. The pulmonary valve was fair-sized, patent, and bicuspid. There was a thin-walled, 15-mm-long infundibular chamber, and distally, but not communicating with it, an inflow chamber received blood from the large left ventricle through two ventricular septal defects. The ductus arteriosus was patent. Metianu and associates (1953) reported a case of combined infundibular and valvular atresia with patent pulmonary artery trunk, a good right ventricular cavity, and two ventricular defects.

In view of the recent observations that the ventricular septal defect may close spontaneously and that the infundibulum of the right ventricle may progressively become completely obstructed (see below), it appears certain that the hearts with a good-sized right ventricle, and with patent pulmonary valve and trunk, represent cases of acquired infundibular atresia with or without concomitant closure of the ventricular septal defect.

These patients are older in age and may develop large aortopulmonary collaterals. The disappearance of a previously loud systolic murmur may be the clinical clue that right ventricular patency has been lost.

Type I(b)—Pulmonary Hypoplasia with Subpulmonary Stenosis, Small Ventricular Septal Defect (Figure 29–2). This is the commonest type. There were 73 cases in this group, which represents 50 percent of all cases with tricuspid atresia, 70 percent of the type with no transposition of the great vessels.

The pulmonary artery is hypoplastic from its origin to its intrapulmonary branches. The valvular ring is narrower than normal but patent and of adequate size. In our cases its internal circumference varied between 5 and 27 mm, depending mainly on the age of the patients, and was about one-fourth to one-third that of the aorta. Apart from the case of Crocker (1879) where the disposition of the cusps achieved some degree of constriction, pulmonary valve stenosis was not encountered. Once (Kreutzer et al., 1954) the valve was reported to be absent.

A bicuspid valve is frequent. Fourteen of our thirty cases and almost one-half of the cases of Edwards and Burchell (1949) belonging to this group presented this feature. The cusps are fleshy and devoid of their normal transparency. However, there is neither fusion of the commissures nor reduction of the valvular diameter.

The right ventricle is of reduced size, and careful examination will reveal the presence of two compartments. Leading to the pulmonary valve is a tubular chamber 15 to 20 mm long. The diameter approximates closely that of the pulmonary artery. Its walls are relatively thin, normally between 2 and 5 mm; the endocardium is normal; and the cavity is smooth. It lies on the anterior face of the ventricular portion of the heart at its upper region and ascends obliquely from the right margin to the pulmonary valve. At its distal end there is a small orifice, the size of a pencil or less, situated terminally or subterminally. This structure represents the subpulmonary or infundibular stenosis and leads to the second compartment of the ventricle. The latter is flat on the lateral face of the ventricular myocardium, has a rough appearance, and contains rudimentary papillary muscles and trabeculae carneae. Its septal or medial face is the region where the ventricular septal defect opens.

In one case we found a persistent right ventricular sinus of virtually normal size.

The ventricular defect is usually of diminutive size. The largest ones in our group measured 9 by 3, 8 by 5, 7 by 4, and 7 by 3 mm. In the remaining 24 cases its largest diameter was under 5 mm.

Roberts and associates (1963) have shown that the defect may close spontaneously. Gallaher and Fyler (1967) reported three cases in which the clinical and angiocardiographic evidence indicated gradual decrease in size. It is, therefore, possible for a large defect in infancy to be found small at death. Rao (1977) estimates that spontaneous closure of the ventricular septal defect occurs in 38 percent of cases.

Occasionally two openings are present between the ventricles, as in the cases of Grayzel and Tennant (1934), Bellet and Steward (1933), and three seen at The Hospital for Sick Children.

The relationship between the two valvular orifices should also be noted. They are not situated in the same horizontal plane. The aortic valve may be as much as 15 mm below the level of the pulmonary valve. Consequently the ventricular septal defect is just below or only a few millimeters below the aortic valve, whereas, seen from the right ventricle, the whole length of this chamber is interposed between the pulmonary valve and the interventricular communication.

This relationship is different in types II and III where the origin of the two great arteries resides in the same horizontal plane.

A patent ductus arteriosus was present in 25 percent of the cases. It is usually small, admitting only a probe, and occurs most frequently in babies only a few months old. Rarely, its size is large enough to play a role in the pulmonary circulation. Once (Hübschmann, 1921) it lay on the right between the right branch of the pulmonary and the innominate arteries.

The pulmonary circulation in this type of tricuspid atresia is supplied by the left ventricle through the ventricular septal defect and thence the right ventricle and the pulmonary artery. Even though this vessel is always patent and most often of adequate size, there is reduced pulmonary flow. There are three possible responsible factors for this functional feature. First, the ventricular septal opening is of small size and represents an obstruction of the pulmonary pathways. Second, the subpulmonary stenosis is an important limiting factor of the flow to the lungs. And, finally, there is the diminutive right ventricle itself with its limited capacity. Furthermore, to these three anatomic obstructions a fourth dynamic one is added, i.e., the systolic contraction of the rudimentary ventricle and its stenosed infundibular area.

Whatever the cause, the degree of resulting anoxia is very severe, and death occurs early in life. The average life duration in cases of this type was found to be 11 months, even though occasional cases may live several years. (Eight were cases over one and one-half years, and the oldest was six years [Anderson and McKee, 1952].)

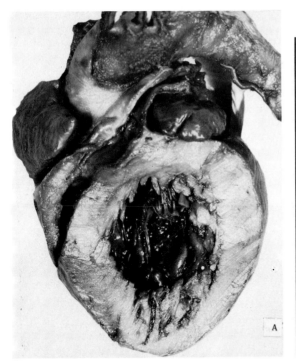
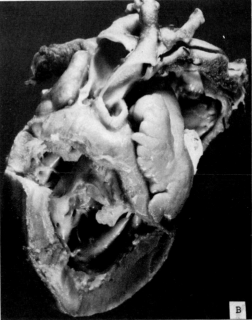
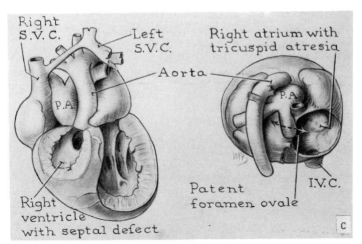

Figure 29-2. *A.* Ten-month-old female infant. <u>Marked cyanosis since birth</u>, occasional "blue spells," failure to thrive. Harsh systolic murmur, maximum at third and fourth left interspaces. Classic fluoroscopic appearance. ECG—left-axis deviation. No signs of congestive failure.

Autopsy: Tricuspid atresia—type I(b).

B and C. Poorly developed male infant, not cyanosed until three months old when admitted to the hospital with marked respiratory distress, gasping respirations, and slight generalized cyanosis.

Physical Examination: Short, faint systolic murmur, maximal in the third interspace; accentuated split second sound. Liver 5 cm below right costal margin; harsh cough; and fine, scattered rales bilaterally.

Fluoroscopy: Marked cardiac enlargement, narrow vascular pedicle with convex left border and pointing apex. Markedly increased pulmonary vascular markings. Cloudy opacity bilaterally, especially in hilar regions (see Figure 29-6).

Electrocardiogram: Slight right-axis deviation, vertical electrical position, signs of marked left ventricular hypertrophy in the precordial leads (see Figure 29-4).

Autopsy: Tricuspid atresia with *D*-transposition of the great vessels and large pulmonary artery (type II(c)).

Type I(c)—No Pulmonary Hypoplasia, Ventricular Septal Defect Opening into the Outflow Chamber of the Right Ventricle. Nineteen cases of this type have been reported: Holmes (1824), Chapotot (1889), Cooley et al. (1950), Sommers and Johnson (1951), Chiche (three cases) (1952), Astley et al. (1953), Metianu et al. (two cases) (1953), Carey and Edwards (1964), Gallaher and Fyler (three cases) (1967), Bohm et al. (1968), and Hospital for Sick Children.

The pulmonary artery and its valve are of the same size as the aorta or very close to it. In the three infants reported by Chiche (1952) the pulmonary artery was larger than the systemic artery, once twice its diameter.

The right ventricle remains small and relatively thin-walled.

The ventricular septal defect is of modest size but generally larger than in type I(b). Its high location will permit, in an occasional case, the pulmonary artery (case VII of Chiche, 1952) or the aorta (case III of Chiche) to override slightly the ventricular septum. The functional consequence of the greatest importance is that these cases have adequate or even increased pulmonary blood flow. The early death (one, two, and four months) of the cases with the pulmonary artery larger than the aorta (Chiche, 1952) would suggest that hemodynamically these cases are closer to the cases with transposition of the great vessels and may be clinically confused with them. Indeed, they present with little cyanosis, loud murmur, cardiomegaly, and signs of cardiac failure.

On the other hand, the remaining cases tended to have a balanced pulmonary circulation and lived an average of $11\frac{1}{2}$ years. The overall life expectancy in this type was eight years, but survival to 18, 21, 25, and 31 years was possible.

Associated defects are not frequent. One case (case VII of Chiche, 1952) had coarctation of the aorta.

It is possible, as demonstrated by Gallaher and Fyler (1967), Meng (1969), Marcano and associates (1969), and Rao and Sissman (1971), for the ventricular septal defect to decrease in size, occasionally within a few months after birth. These babies will then lose the manifestations of increased pulmonary flow and become hypoxic (as in type I[b]) requiring shunt operations.

Type II—With D-Transposition of the Great Arteries. Forty cases, or 27 percent, of the group reviewed had D-transposition of the great vessels. The relationship between the great arterial trunks was inverted, the aorta being the right anterior vessel, the pulmonary artery lying behind and to the left.

Complete transposition was present in 28 cases, the aorta arising entirely from the reduced right ventricle and the pulmonary artery from the large left ventricle.

Partial transposition was recorded 12 times and presented three possibilities: (1) both great vessels given off by the left ventricle (three cases) (Hedinger, 1915; Brinton and Campbell, 1953; Fragoyannis and Kardalinos, 1962); (2) both great vessels arising from the right ventricle (two cases) (Hospital for Sick

Children, 1964); (3) the pulmonary artery originating from the left ventricle, the aorta overriding the ventricular septum (six cases) (Manhoff and Howe, 1945; Cooley et al., 1950; Rogers et al., 1950; Metianu et al. [two cases], 1953; Hospital for Sick Children, 1964).

The configuration of the right ventricle and the appearance of the ventricular septal defect present a number of special features that are common to all types of tricuspid atresia with D-transposition of the great vessels.

The right ventricle tends to be larger than in type I, and its walls are thicker. In fact, they may have the same thickness as the left ventricle. The division into two compartments, which is constant in type I(b), is not present in this group. Its cavity is smooth and may look like a mere diverticular annex of the large left ventricle.

The ventricular septal defect is of considerable size and extends right to the aortic or pulmonary valve. Occasional cases may have complete absence of the interventricular septum.

The aortic and pulmonary valves are level, residing in the same horizontal plane.

Functionally this type of tricuspid atresia is much closer to common ventricles than the type with normal arterial relationship, with the exception of type I(c).

Type II(a)—Pulmonary Atresia, Aorta Arising from the Right Ventricle. Three cases of this type are known. Manhoff and Howe's case (1945) had a large transposed, but overriding aorta. The pulmonary artery lay behind and to the left and presented a cord atresia involving the valve and the main trunk up to the point of bifurcation. A wide patent ductus arteriosus supplied the pulmonary circulation.

At The Hospital for Sick Children there were two cases. The first was a two-day-old premature infant with dextrocardia and situs inversus. The aorta originated from the equivalent of the right ventricle and overrode the ventricular septum. The pulmonary artery was small (1 to 2 mm in diameter) but patent. The valve was completely occluded, and the ductus arteriosus was patent. The aortic arch and the descending aorta were on the right.

In the second case (13 days old) the aorta was not overriding, the pulmonary artery trunk was patent (5 mm in diameter), and its valve had a membrane obstruction with two identifiable raphae. There was a long patent ductus arteriosus, and the left subclavian artery originated from the descending aorta. A persistent left superior vena cava was also found.

Type II(b)—Pulmonary or Subpulmonary Stenosis, Aorta Off the Right Ventricle, Pulmonary Artery Off the Left Ventricle [Type II(a) of Edwards and Burchell, 1949]. Instances of this type were reported by Gelpke (1883), Hedinger (1915), Hübschmann (1921), Cooley et al. (1950), Rogers et al. (1950), and Metianu and associates (1953), each of whom had two cases.

A large, high ventricular septal defect is present and may allow the aorta to override the septum, as in the cases of Metianu and associates (1953), Rogers and coworkers (1950), and Cooley and associates (1950). As described by Edwards (1953), this large interventricular communication is limited superiorly by a muscular ridge that lies at the right of the transposed pulmonary artery and descends obliquely to end in the posterior wall of the smaller ventricular chamber. Inferiorly, a second muscular ridge is the muscular part of the septum ventriculorum.

The pulmonary stenosis is of three types:

1. Dome stenosis of the pulmonary valve (eighth case of Cooley et al., 1950).
2. Subpulmonary stenosis is more frequent (cases of Metianu et al., 1953; Rogers et al., 1950). Immediately below the pulmonary valve there is a narrow tract formed to the right by the crista supraventricularis and to the left by the anterior leaflet of the mitral valve. A fibrous bridge extends between the two.
3. Combined stenosis (one case of Metianu et al., 1953) with valve stenosis and narrow subpulmonary tract.

The pulmonary valve may be bicuspid and the trunk of the pulmonary artery hypoplastic (one case of Cooley et al., 1950; one case of Metianu et al., 1953) or of normal size (Rogers et al., 1950).

Large bronchial arteries were recorded in Rogers and associates' case. Cooley and coworkers' case had, in addition, the pulmonary veins entering the right atrium.

A feature that occurs occasionally in complex anomalies and may be encountered in this type of tricuspid atresia is juxtaposition of the atrial appendages (Dixon, 1954). These two structures lie along each other on the left of the great vessels and protrude anteriorly at the base of the heart. Such observations have been reported by Hübschmann (1921), Rogers and associates (1950), and Metianu and associates (1953).

Because of the restricted pulmonary flow this anomaly is tolerated as well as type I(c). The age at death was 56 years in Hedinger's case, 27 years in Gelpke's, 12 years in Rogers' case, and eight and seven years in Metianu's cases.

The average life duration in nine cases (excluding Hedinger's case) was seven years and four months.

Type II(c)—Large Pulmonary Artery [Type II(b) of Edwards and Burchell, 1949] (Figure 29–1), page 521). This possibility is more frequent than the previous one. There are 20 case reports in the literature (Sieveking, 1854; Kelly, 1868; Robertson, 1911; Wason, 1934; Eisenberg and Gibson, 1941; Robinson and Howard, 1948; Dickson and Jones, 1948; Edwards and Burchell, 1949; Sokolow and Edgar, 1950; Kroop, 1951; Chiche [two cases], 1952; Ross, 1952; Brinton and Campbell, 1953; Marder et al., 1953; Astley et al., 1953; Dunsky, 1947; Macafee and Patterson [three cases], 1961) and six from The Hospital for Sick Children.

Here the pulmonary artery is large, and its diameter may be two to four times that of the aorta. This latter vessel may thus be relatively hypoplastic. Bicuspid pulmonary valves may be encountered, but they are not as frequent as in type I(b).

An association of coarctation of the aorta was noted eight times (Chiche [case IX], 1952; Dickson and Jones, 1948; Kroop, 1951; Sokolow and Edgar, 1950; Brinton and Campbell, 1953; Marder et al., 1953; Macafee and Patterson [case 3], 1961; Hospital for Sick Children) and seems to be more frequent than in any other type of tricuspid atresia. Similarly, the ductus arteriosus is patent in half the cases (Marcano et al., 1969).

Other additional anomalies are infrequent. Kroop's case had a persistent left superior vena cava entering the left atrium. In one of the cases observed at The Hospital for Sick Children a large left superior vena cava drained into the coronary sinus after receiving the left upper pulmonary vein. An aneurysm of the membranous septum occurred in another of our cases.

According to Gasul and associates (1950), cases with this anomaly may have reduction of the systemic flow consequent to the presence of infundibular (subaortic) stenosis of the right ventricle or of a small ventricular septal defect. Donzelot and D'Allaines (1954) and Taussig (1947) mention the possible existence of aortic atresia with systemic circulation maintained through a large patent ductus arteriosus. One such example is reported by Polanco and Powell (1955) in a case of isolated dextrocardia.

Far from being a favorable condition, the excessive pulmonary blood flow that is present in this type will lead to heart failure and death in infancy. The average life expectancy was found to be three months, if one excludes the six-year-old boy of Macafee and Patterson (1961).

TYPE III—WITH L-TRANSPOSITION OF THE GREAT ARTERIES. Although it seems probable that some of the cases with transposition reported previously are of this variety, it was found impossible to identify them with certainty from the description in the literature. We have found four such specimens. All occurred in individuals with visceroatrial situs solitus and left-sided hearts. In three, the classic arterial relationship was accompanied by D-type bulbo-ventricular loop (no ventricular inversion), and, therefore, the hypoplastic ventricle was a small right-sided right ventricle, and the atretic valve was a right-sided tricuspid. Subaortic stenosis with aortic hypoplasia (but no coarctation of the aorta) occurred twice, while subpulmonic stenosis with a tricuspid valve occurred once.

Once, the major ventricle was a left-sided right ventricle (L-type bulboventricular loop) and the patent valve, therefore, a left-sided tricuspid. Both great arteries arose from the large ventricle, and there was significant subaortic stenosis with severe hypoplasia of the aortic arch and preductal coarctation.

Hemodynamics

Whatever the anatomic type, the intracardiac circulation is the same in all. The absence of communication between the right atrium and ventricle will necessarily result in a massive right-to-left shunt at atrial level and will always be accompanied by desaturation of the peripheral arterial blood. The patency of the interatrial septum is the only way blood can reach the systemic circuit. The left atrium becomes the mixing chamber and the left ventricle is the only propelling ventricle maintaining, directly or indirectly, both pulmonary and systemic circulations. Such obligatory atrial shunts occur in other instances of hypoplastic right heart (e.g., pulmonary atresia with intact ventricular septum, primary hypoplasia of the right ventricle) and in total anomalous pulmonary venous return.

The *pulmonary circulation* is tenuously maintained by a patent ductus arteriosus in the cases with pulmonary atresia, and by the ventricular septal defect via the right ventricle in those with normally related great arteries. A small defect or an obstructed right ventricle results in a decreased pulmonary flow. When transposition is present, the pulmonary circulation is supplied directly by the left ventricle. A small ventricular septal defect (subaortic stenosis) may then interfere with the systemic circulation. This phenomenon may be responsible for the associated aortic arch anomalies encountered in type II(c) (hypoplastic ascending aorta or aortic arch, coarctation of the aorta, patent ductus arteriosus).

As is the case in other congenital anomalies of the heart (e.g., ventricular septal defect, transposition of the great arteries, tetralogy of Fallot), the hemodynamics of tricuspid atresia may change through the patient's life-span since the intracardiac anatomy itself may undergo progressive modifications. The atrial communication may diminish in size (Bargeron et al., 1972) producing an increased obstruction to right atrial outflow. The ventricular septal defect may decrease or close completely (Roberts et al., 1963; Gallaher and Fyler, 1967; Meng, 1969; Rao and Sissman, 1971; Bargeron et al., 1972; Shaher et al., 1973; Rao, 1977) transforming a state of pulmonary plethora with cardiac failure into a situation of decreased pulmonary flow with hypoxia, or progressively diminishing an already decreased pulmonary flow. Spontaneous diminution of the ventricular septal defect has also been reported in cases with transposition of the great arteries (Rao, 1977). The right ventricular outflow may progressively occlude even to the point of producing atresia of the infundibulum (Gabriele, 1969; Bargeron et al., 1972). A patent ductus arteriosus may close, eliminating the only route of blood to the lung in babies with pulmonary atresia. Finally, when forward flow to the lungs ceases as the result of infundibular occlusion or closure of a ventricular septal defect, aortic-pulmonary collaterals may take over their perfusion (Bargeron et al., 1972).

The surgical procedures performed on these patients will themselves have effects with physiologic and anatomic consequences. Examples are the development of obstructive pulmonary vascular disease and the acquisition of unilateral pulmonary artery branch occlusion following Potts-Smith or Waterston arterial shunts.

Patients with large ventricular septal defects, even with normally related great arteries, may have pulmonary hypertension of systemic range.

Obstructive pulmonary vascular disease may develop with large ventricular defect and pulmonary hypertension (types I[c], II[c]) and may be found occasionally in those with subpulmonic obstruction. Presumably this develops prior to spontaneous closure of the ventricular septal defect or of the right ventricular infundibulum, or as the result of pulmonary thromboses secondary to severely obstructed pulmonary artery inflow. It may occur in *either* lung, following Glenn anastomosis and after excessive arterial shunts.

Clinical Features

Cyanosis. Since the majority of cases have severely decreased pulmonary flow, cyanosis tends to be severe and progressive. A minority of patients (12 to 15 percent) will be acyanotic when first seen in infancy. They represent cases with increased pulmonary blood flow (types I[c] and II[c]).

The time of onset is an index of degree of pulmonary obstruction and, therefore, has prognostic value. When cyanosis was present during the neonatal period, 80 percent of untreated babies were dead before six months of age and had an average life-span of five months. When it appeared after one month of age, the average age at death was over four years.

When a patient acquires subpulmonic obstruction or when the ventricular septal defect closes, the transition from an acyanotic state to severe hypoxia may rapidly take place over a period of a few months.

Clubbing. Clubbing of the fingers is almost constant in the patients over two years of age. It may develop as early as three or four months after birth.

Squatting. According to Chiche (1952) and Metianu and associates (1953), squatting is frequent. This may be so in older patients, but we failed to see this phenomenon or its equivalents in our cases. Only 1 of 14 patients in the walking age squatted.

Dyspnea. Dyspnea or exercise intolerance is part of the hypoxia picture. It is a frequent feature, and in babies becomes striking with crying and feeding. In the cases with transposition of the great vessels it may be dramatic and accompanied by coughing or gasping respirations.

Signs of Venous Congestion. Distention of the neck veins with visible pulsations is accepted by Astley and associates (1953) as a valuable diagnostic sign. In infants, however, this finding is rather exceptional.

The liver is most often palpable but not enlarged. Significant hepatic enlargement (more than 1.5 cm below the costal margin) was recorded in the cases with large pulmonary flow (type I[c], II[c] and III). Two other instances belonged to the "common" type, and they were the only ones with liver pulsations. In this respect our experience is in agreement with that of Wittenborg and associates (1951).

According to Taussig, "a pulsating liver of normal size combined with the absence of right ventricular enlargement is presumptive evidence of tricuspid atresia and a well-formed auricular septum with a relatively small defect."* Of our two cases with this phenomenon, one had a small defect measuring 4 by 6 mm and the second a large foramen ovale measuring 16 by 14 mm.

Pulmonary Second Sound. The pulmonary second sound is pure in the cases with reduced pulmonary blood flow and thus becomes a helpful diagnostic sign. Splitting may occur with pulmonary plethora.

Murmurs. Analysis of 49 cases reveals the following findings:

1. Precordial murmurs were absent in 18 percent. Faint, soft systolic murmurs occurred in 30 percent. Loud, harsh murmurs occurred in 50 percent. An accompanying thrill was palpable in 18 percent only.

A continuous murmur in the pulmonary area, other than that occurring after an anastomotic operation, was present once.

A pulmonary diastolic murmur accompanied a harsh systolic murmur in a child at the age of two years but disappeared a year later.

2. Loud murmurs were present more frequently in survivors over one year of age, but they were also heard in infants. Only three children of this group died of natural death, and the average life duration was six years and two months.

Absence of murmurs was rare in cases that survived the first year of life. Only four were over 12 months of age, whereas 17 were under this age. The mortality rate in this group was 87 percent; the average life expectancy, 7½ months.

3. The loud murmurs were of the ejection type, and their maximal intensity was at the lower left sternal border. Presumably they originate at the ventricular defect. In three instances they were better heard in the second left interspace. These cases were proved angiocardiographically to have transposition of the great arteries with pulmonic stenosis. Two cases had loud, stenotic murmurs and thrill over the aortic area and anatomically had subaortic stenosis.

4. Correlation with the underlying anatomic types allows the following generalizations. With transposition and pulmonic (type II [b]) or subaortic stenosis (type III [c]) characteristic murmurs tend to be present. Apical middiastolic rumbles are most common with transposition and large pulmonary

flow and in the occasional case with large ventricular septal defect and absence of transposition. Ductal murmurs favor the presence of pulmonary atresia even though, occasionally, they will be heard in babies with type I (b). Low sternal murmurs are usually associated with type I (b) provided the ventricular defect is not minute.

5. The disappearance of an apical middiastolic rumble indicates spontaneous diminution of the ventricular septal defect in a case without transposition. The diminution or disappearance of a systolic murmur reflects a decreasing pulmonary flow either by progressive right ventricular outflow obstruction or by closing of the ventricular septal defect.

Signs of Heart Failure. Hepatomegaly, pitting edema, pulmonary congestion or pulmonary edema, and engorgement of the neck veins were invariably present when transposition of the great vessels was associated with large pulmonary arteries, but may occur in absence of transposition (type I[c]). A gallop rhythm was heard on occasion.

In the cases with moderate or diminished pulmonary flow, signs of failure were exceptional and seen in older patients, especially those who survive beyond their twenties. Postoperatively, if the size of the aorticopulmonary shunt exceeds a critical level, the excessive pulmonary flow and the consequently increased left atrial blood volume may tend to close the foramen ovale, thus reducing the atrial right-to-left shunt. In this manner the anastomotic operation will increase the burden of the right atrium, already overloaded. The resultant venous congestion may produce the full-blown picture of congestive heart failure.

Electrocardiography

In 1921, in an era when no electrocardiograms in cases of tricuspid atresia had been published, Laubry and Pezzi predicted that this type of examination should show a normal or left preponderance pattern. They also sensed the diagnostic significance of this finding. Rihl and associates (1929) were the first to publish a tracing showing left-axis deviation and thus confirmed this impression.

Taussig (1936) stressed the great diagnostic value of the presence of left-axis deviation in a cyanotic infant and felt that this is always suggestive of tricuspid atresia or marked hypoplasia of the tricuspid valve. Brown (1936) noted that a normal or left-axis deviation may be recorded at any age. Edwards and Burchell (1949) and Donzelot and associates (1950) confirmed this impression and emphasized that left-axis deviation may be present in cyanotic anomalies other than tricuspid atresia. The subject has been investigated by Brink and Neill (1955), Cabrera and associates (1961), Gamboa and coworkers (1966), Guller and colleagues (1969), Folger and coworkers (1969), Marcano and associates (1969), Davachi and colleagues (1970),

---

* Taussig, H. B.: *Congenital Malformations of the Heart.* The Commonwealth Fund, New York, 1947, p. 83.

Ellison and Restieux (1972), and others. Attempts have been made to correlate the electrocardiographic and vectorcardiographic appearance with the underlying anatomic arrangement and with hemodynamic characteristics. These efforts have yielded observations of a general order but no specific relationships.

QRS Axis. LEFT-AXIS DEVIATION. An axis situated between 0° and −90° is the common finding. This was found to occur in 81 to 88 percent of the cases (Brink and Neill, 1955; Keith et al., 1967; Gamboa et al., 1966). It is associated with a superior, counterclockwise frontal vector loop. In its electrogenesis, Guller, DuShane, and Titus (1969) implicated an abnormality of the conduction system. Their histologic studies demonstrate an abnormally early origin of the left bundle with marked elongation of the right, suggesting an abnormal sequence of myocardial activation. This may also be responsible for the relatively short P-R segment found with some frequency.

In general, a left superior axis occurs in the common anatomic type (I[b]) and when transposition coexists with decreased pulmonary blood flow (II[b]). In both instances the right ventricular size tends to be small.

NO AXIS DEVIATION. An electrical axis situated between 0° and +90° has been encountered in 7 percent of cases. It is associated with an inferior, counterclockwise, or figure-of-eight frontal vector loop. Anatomically, it is found more frequently but not exclusively in cases with transposition of the great arteries and usually but not necessarily in those with increased pulmonary flow.

RIGHT-AXIS DEVIATION. This was reported in sporadic cases (Dickson and Jones, 1948; Chiche, 1952; Astley et al., 1953; Kreutzer et al., 1954; Sullivan and Mangiardi, 1958). We found it in 4 percent of our cases. Until recently we believed that this will occur only when a large pulmonary flow is associated with transposition of the great arteries (types II[c] and III[b]), hence a relatively large right ventricle. In two cases, both without transposition or restriction of lung flow (I[c]), the right ventricle was sufficiently large to inscribe an electrical axis beyond +90°. One of these cases was a newborn infant who at six weeks developed cardiac failure and had measured systemic pulmonary artery hypertension. By eight months of age he became hypoxic, developed pulmonary oligemia, the loud precordial murmur faded, and the electrical axis shifted to the left. This sequence is that of spontaneous occlusion of a large ventricular septal defect with concomitant right ventricular regression.

Precordial Leads. The precordial leads show the normal adult progression of the QRS and the T waves. This left ventricular dominance is in itself abnormal in babies and children indicating left ventricular hypertrophy or overloading. Quantitative criteria for left ventricular hypertrophy (abnormally deep S waves over the right or abnormally tall R waves over the left precordium) may also be present. Inverted T waves in V_5 and V_6 occur in 40 to 50 percent of cases, and all anatomic types. Vectorcardiographically the horizontal loop is inscribed counterclockwise, leftward, and posteriorly. Sizable R waves in V_1 or V_2, terminal rightward forces, and anteriorly directed LMSV (leftward maximal spacial vector) reflect the presence of a relatively large right ventricle (Ellison and Restieux, 1972) as occurs with a large ventricular septal defect with or without transposition. Incidentally, these cases may have increased pulmonary flow.

Evidence of right ventricular hypertrophy (Figure 29–5) occurs in no more than 1 percent and seems to be associated with anatomic arrangements that are

R.R. 2 mo. ♂10.9.52.

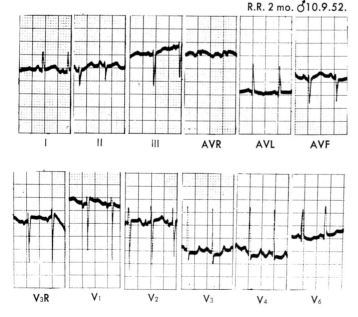

Figure 29-3. Typical electrocardiogram in tricuspid atresia. Infant, aged two months.
Autopsy: Tricuspid atresia, type I(b). Wide, patent foramen ovale with normally developed valvular flap. Small (4 × 3 mm) ventricular septal defect. Small right ventricle with tubular infundibulum leading to a hypoplastic pulmonary artery. Bicuspid, nonstenosed pulmonary valve. Closed ductus arteriosus. Gross right atrial and left ventricular hypertrophy.

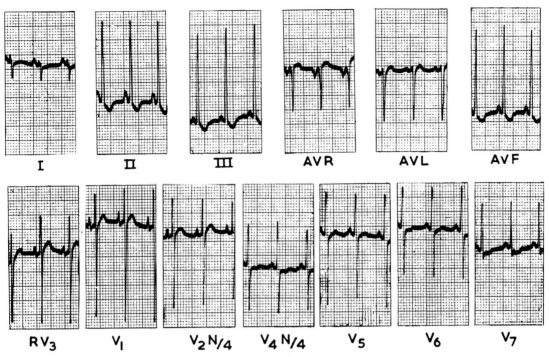

Figure 29-4. The electrocardiogram of a male infant three months of age. History and anatomic findings given in Figure 29-2B; roentgenogram reproduced in Figure 29-6B.

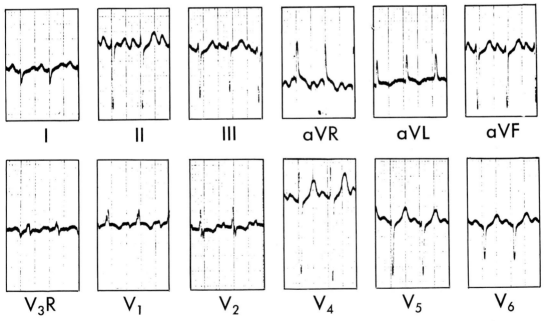

Figure 29-5. The electrocardiogram of a two-and-one-half-year-old boy. QRS axis at −130 degrees. Right ventricular overloading. No left ventricular hypertrophy.

Autopsy: Tricuspid atresia with *D*-transposition of the great arteries. The atrial septum is normally formed, with a foramen ovale defect. The infundibular septum is shifted to the right, forming a wide subaortic outflow and a severely obstructed subpulmonary infundibulum. The left atrioventricular valve (mitral) overrides a leftward-displaced ventricular septum. The left ventricle is small, while the right is large. There is a large ventricular septal defect.

more complex than usual. Absence of evidence of left ventricular hypertrophy occurred in cases of Kroop (1950), Chiche (1952), Kreutzer and coworkers (1954), Guller (1969), and Nadas and Fyler (1972).

P-R Segment. A true Wolff–Parkinson–White syndrome occurred only once in our series, although a relatively short P-R interval was found in about half the tracings.

P Wave. Abnormally high P waves are frequent in infants. Its height does not correlate well with atrial pressure or with the size of the atrial septal defect.

Evidence of combined atrial hypertrophy (tall, notched, and/or wide P waves) is frequent (81 percent in the Gamboa et al. [1966] series) in patients beyond infancy and older ages.

Radiologic Examination

Heart Size. Essentially this is a function of pulmonary flow. When it is *diminished*, as is the case in most patients, the heart size remains normal (77 percent had a cardiothoracic ratio under 0.55). Occasionally, marked cardiomegaly is present (5 percent had cardiothoracic ratios above 0.65). The heart size tends to remain the same throughout life. After shunt procedures, a slight degree of enlargement is common. Marked enlargement follows excessive shunts.

When the anatomic arrangement leads to *increased pulmonary flow* (types I[c], II [c], and III [b]), marked cardiac enlargement is present (average cardiothoracic ratio of 0.74). The increase in size is rapidly progressive, as are all other signs of cardiac failure.

Decrease in heart size will occur when a large ventricular septal defect closes or when subpulmonic obstruction develops.

Configuration of the Cardiac Outline. The roentgen appearance of the heart presents several variants.

"CHARACTERISTIC" APPEARANCE OF TRICUSPID ATRESIA (Figure 29–6A) (Taussig 1936). In the posteroanterior projection the right border is flattened and does not extend beyond the spinal shadow. Its lower segment may even be concave and limited distally by a slight bulging due to right atrial or inferior vena caval distention; the left border presents a tall, blunt lower arc, forming an apex high above the diaphragm; above it there is a concave middle arc due to the angular junction of the descending aorta with the lower segment; the vascular pedicle is rather narrow.

In the left anterior oblique view the anterior border of the heart is straight, far behind the chest wall, and does not protrude in front of the aortic plane. Its superior segment may be prominent and the inferior one concave; the posterior border overlaps the vertebral column and clears it only with a marked degree of rotation or in the lateral view; the vascular pedicle may remain narrow (especially in the cases with pulmonary atresia), and the "pulmonary window" is clear.

"COEUR EN SABOT" APPEARANCE (Witten-

borg et al., 1951). Here the apex is less blunt and high, the concavity of the left middle segment is more prominent, and the right border may be convex and prominent. In the left anterior oblique view the anterior border is normally convex, sometimes flatter than usual. The posterior border is prominent.

The similarity with some cases of tetralogy of Fallot is striking. According to Astley and associates (1953), in the left anterior oblique projection a moderate posterior projection that involves not only the lower (left ventricular) segment but also the upper (left atrial) segment is a reliable differentiating feature.

"TRANSPOSITION OF THE GREAT VESSELS" APPEARANCE (Figure 29–6B). If transposition of the great arteries with pulmonary plethora is present, the cardiac contour takes the characteristic "egg shape"; the pedicle is narrow, and the left border is convex with the apex pointing downward and out. Roentgenologic differentiation between transposition of the great vessels with and without tricuspid atresia is impossible. As Taussig (1947) pointed out, terminally the condition resembles a complete transposition of the great vessels more closely than a nonfunctioning right ventricle with tricuspid atresia.

In the cases with L-transposition (type III), the left upper cardiac border is formed by the ascending aorta (Figure 29–6C).

VARIABLE, NONSPECIFIC APPEARANCE. Frequently the cardiac contour does not fit either of the previously described appearances. The apex may not be elevated or rounded. The left middle segment may be full or even slightly bulging. Further variations and sometimes complete distortion of the cardiac appearance are encountered in cases complicated by dextrocardia.

In the left anterior oblique projection the heart may be "ball-shaped" (Elster, 1950).

NORMAL CONTOURS. Finally, occasional cases have contours entirely within normal limits. These variants seem to be more frequent in the patients with adequate pulmonary flow.

Pulmonary Vascular Markings. Sixty-two percent of all cases of tricuspid atresia have deficient pulmonary circulation. This explains the high frequency of the roentgenologic signs of pulmonary oligemia. The pulmonary vascular markings are markedly reduced, and in small infants it may be impossible to identify any hilar shadowing. The lung fields are clear, and this becomes a striking finding when one examines an infant under the fluoroscope. In older cases the extensive development of bronchial collaterals may alter the clarity of the lung fields. Numerous small circular or peppery shadows will be present throughout, extending far to the periphery. No definite branch of the pulmonary artery can be delineated, even though the hilar regions may present a cloudy opacity (Campbell and Gardner, 1950; Chiche, 1952). Normal pulmonary vascularity was present in ten instances that had nonspecific contours with some fullness of the left middle segment. They are believed to belong to the anatomic types I(c) and II(b).

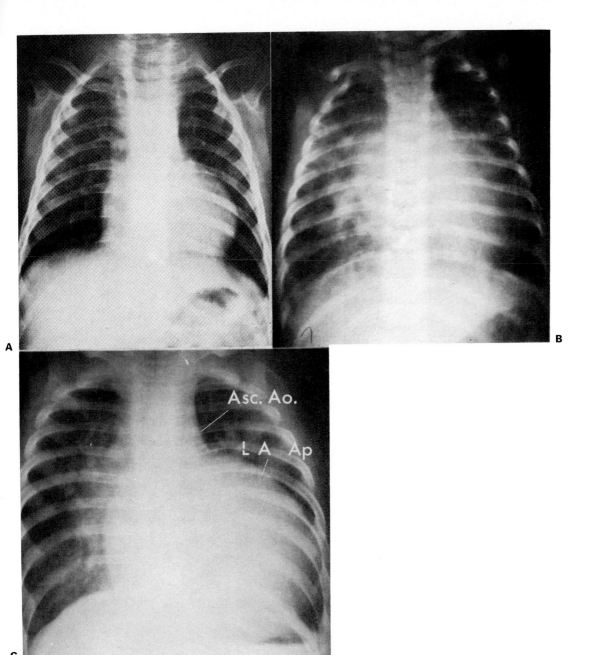

Figure 29-6. *A.* Frontal roentgenogram of an infant aged nine months.

Slight generalized cyanosis noticed at birth, becoming marked at rest at six months. Paroxysmal episodes of cyanosis at six months, very severe and frequent over the last month of life. Marked dyspnea at rest. Slight clubbing of the fingernails.

Fluoroscopy: The typical cardiac contour of tricuspid atresia: straight right border; round, high-arched apex; concave left middle arch. Clear lung fields with scanty hilar markings.

Autopsy: Revealed tricuspid atresia (type I[b]).

B. Chest plate of an infant with tricuspid atresia with transposition of the great vessels and large pulmonary artery. Radiologic findings are diagnostic for transposition of the great vessels: narrow vascular pedicle, prominent right border, convex left cardiac border with pointing apex, marked pulmonary congestion.

The diagnosis of tricuspid atresia cannot be made on the basis of radiologic signs. The slight degree of cyanosis of late onset along with electrocardiographic signs of left ventricular hypertrophy are suggestive evidence. Angiocardiography will show the typical sequence of tricuspid atresia and will visualize the arterial relationships.

C. Chest x-ray of the same patient as in Figure 29-8. Marked cardiac enlargement and increased pulmonary vasculature. The left cardiac border is formed by the ascending aorta, the huge left atrial appendage, and the left ventricle.

531

Increased pulmonary vascularity occurs under four circumstances:

1. In cases with atresia of the pulmonary artery if a large ductus arteriosus is patent. In one of our cases slight prominence of the pulmonary vasculature was associated with the presence of a continuous murmur and very slight cyanosis. The infant died at the age of 11 months, shortly after his continuous murmur became inaudible, and the autopsy revealed the presence of infundibular atresia with a ductus arteriosus undergoing obliteration.

2. In cases with a normal-sized pulmonary artery with large ventricular septal defects and no transposition of the great vessels.

3. In patients who have had a successful systemic-pulmonary anastomosis.

4. In the presence of transposition of the great vessels with large pulmonary artery. The pulmonary artery trunk itself is not visible in the anteroposterior projection, but its branches are considerably enlarged and may be traced out to the periphery of the lungs. In addition to this, diffuse, cloudy opacity of the hilar regions and right upper lobe may produce a typical pulmonary edema pattern, which occurs early in life in the terminal stages of the disease.

Aortic Arch. A right aortic arch may be visualized by barium swallow. Instances of this association have been published by Guffau (1950), Wittenborg and coworkers (1951), Sommers and Johnson (1951), and Marder and colleagues (1953). Its incidence is less high than in tetralogy of Fallot. In the present series we have had eight such cases (8 percent) in the absence of dextrocardia. Even though infrequent, detection of an aortic indentation on the right side of the esophagus does not rule out the diagnosis of tricuspid atresia. Most of the cases with right aortic arch belonged to type I(b), but they may occur in patients with transposition of the great vessels (Figure 29-7).

Other X-ray Findings. Distention of the superior vena cava is not infrequent. According to Taussig (1947), its presence—as the presence of a prominent right border—is due to difficulty in expelling the blood from the right atrium in the cases with small atrial communications.

The presence of a dilated inferior vena cava was noted by Castellanos, Garcia, and Gonzáles (1960). Kieffer and Carey (1963) pointed out that this finding was present in six of seven angiocardiograms with tricuspid atresia and none of 11 angiocardiograms of proven pulmonary atresia with intact ventricular septum.

Left atrial enlargement, so frequent in anatomic specimens, is only occasionally demonstrated by conventional roentgenology in the cases with pulmonary ischemia. Astley and associates (1953), who first noted this phenomenon, feel that the presence of such signs is constant in the cases with pulmonary plethora. Our cases with transposition of the great vessels and pulmonary congestion conformed to this rule.

Asynchronous pulsation of the anterior and posterior borders of the heart has been described as a fluoroscopic sign of tricuspid atresia (Snow, 1952). However, its value is in doubt since it is inconstant and difficult to detect at any age, especially in children.

Angiocardiography

The angiocardiographic features of tricuspid atresia have been well established since the publications of Campbell and Hills (1950) and Cooley and associates (1950), who demonstrated the two chief diagnostic signs, i.e., the typical sequence of opacification of the heart chambers and the constant presence of the area of nonopacification cast by the right ventricle.

Cooley and associates (1950) also emphasized that valuable additional information, such as the size of the atrial septal defect and the anatomic position of the great arteries, can be obtained with this method. Marder and associates (1953), reviewing the data obtained with conventional roentgenography and angiocardiography, admitted the superiority of the latter as a diagnostic method but concluded that conventional roentgenology is more reliable in the detection and assessment of pulmonary flow.

Improved techniques and selective injections greatly increased the reliability of this method. Angiocardiography remains the method of choice both as a diagnostic and as a confirmatory test and needs to be performed, as a minimum, from both the right atrium and the left ventricle.

Typical "Sequence of Tricuspid Atresia." The contrast material will invariably fill the heart chambers in the same sequence: right atrium, left atrium, left ventricle, and thence the great arteries (Figure 29-7B). Even though typical for tricuspid atresia, this order of filling is not pathognomonic. The same sequence will be encountered in pulmonary atresia with intact ventricular septum and other types of tricuspid hypoplasia. Moreover occasional severe cases of pulmonary stenosis with patent foramen ovale and instances of pentalogy of Fallot (tetralogy plus atrial septal defect) have the same dynamics. Mehrizi and colleagues (1964) reported the same sequence in cases of total anomalous pulmonary venous return to the coronary sinus, when the angiocardiograms were obtained from the superior vena cava. This "typical" phenomenon is, therefore, highly suggestive but not diagnostic in itself.

The frontal plane angiogram is by far superior in demonstrating the phenomenon.

Nonopacification of the Right Ventricle. As repeatedly noted, the left ventricle fills earlier than the right. In the frontal view this will result in the presence of a clear triangular zone with the base on the diaphragm and the two sides limited by the right atrium or the inferior vena cava on the right and by the left ventricle on the left ("right ventricular window" of Campbell and Hills, 1950).

This triangular notch may fill on later plates.

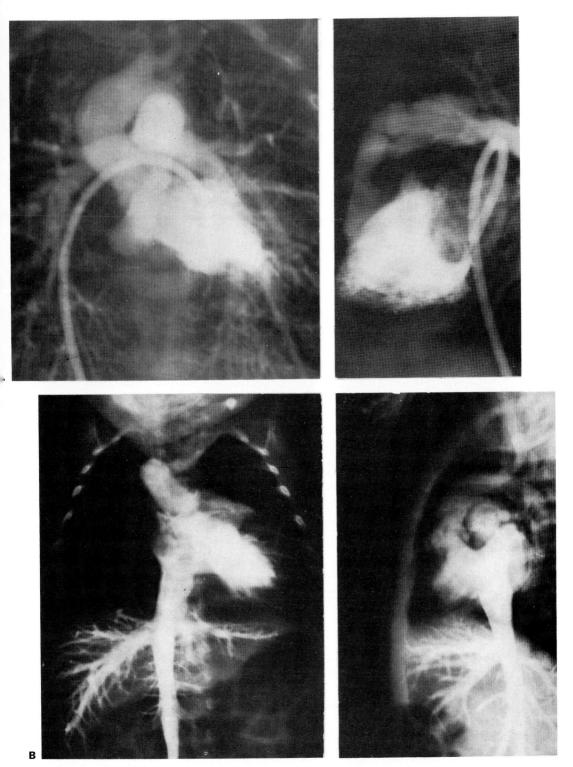

B

Figure 29-7. *A*. Selective angiocardiogram taken from the left ventricle. In the anteroposterior view the right ventricle appears as a small diverticulum filling from the left ventricle. The pulmonary artery fills passively before opening of the aortic valve. In the lateral view a distinct narrowing in the subpulmonary region occurs in ventricular systole. The aorta and pulmonary artery are normally interrelated. *B*. Typical "sequence of tricuspid atresia" in a case associated with transposition of the great vessels and pulmonary stenosis (type II[b]), and right aortic arch. Note the marked hepatic reflux, the "right ventricular window," and the patent ductus arteriosus.

533

Right Atrial Dimple. When a right atrial injection is made in the right anterior oblique projection, the dimple may be visualized on the floor of the right atrium.

Atrial Septal Defect. This may be outlined and its size evaluated in the left anterior oblique view.

Ebstein Anomaly. When produced by an Ebstein anomaly, tricuspid atresia shows a diagnostic angiocardiographic appearance: a blind smooth pouch (the atrialized right ventricle) extends downward from the floor of the right atrium (Van Praagh et al., 1971). On left ventricular injections this pouch remains nonopaque, while the outflow region of ventricle opacifies via the ventricular septal defect.

The Great Arteries. The origin of the great arterial trunks is clearly demonstrated in the lateral projection.

In the absence of transposition the aorta arises well behind the anterior border of the heart. It then arches upward and forward to form the aortic arch. The pulmonary artery may fill simultaneously from a point situated in front of the aortic valve (in type I [c] with a large ventricular septal defect and normal pulmonary artery) or late after the systemic trunk. The latter possibility occurs in the type I(b) where the great vessels are supplied by the left ventricle through a small ventricular septal defect. Visualization of the rudimentary ventricle and pulmonary artery requires left ventricular injections.

When the arteries are transposed, the aorta is placed at the anterior border of the heart (lateral projection) and its valve is high in position. The frontal projection will identify the type of transposition. Figure 29–7 is an example of D-type, Figure 29–8 of L-type.

The presence of pulmonary stenosis may be directly shown or assumed on indirect criteria (Marder et al., 1953): delayed appearance of radiopaque material in the pulmonary circuit, small caliber of the opacified pulmonary arteries, and nonopacification of the pulmonary artery branches.

The sequence of filling of the great arterial trunks is reversed in the anatomic type II(c) where the large pulmonary artery fills first, directly from the left ventricle, and the aorta later from the right ventricle.

Diagnosis

The characteristic features of tricuspid atresia usually permit a diagnosis without extensive investigation. These include cyanosis, associated with left-axis deviation in the electrocardiogram and a left ventricular hypertrophy pattern in the precordial leads. The cardiac contour frequently presents a somewhat flattened right atrium, a normal or slight increase in heart size, and a blunt apex with a concavity or lack of prominence of the pulmonary artery area. Pulmonary vasculature is diminished except when there is associated transposition of the

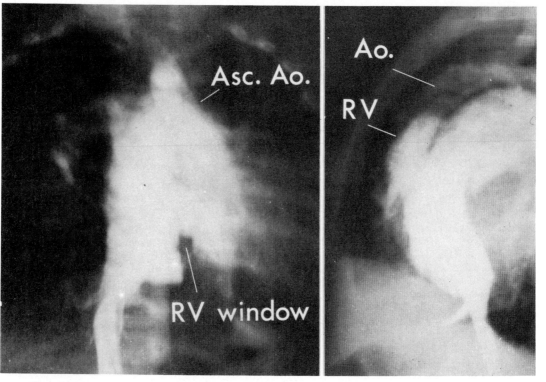

Figure 29-8. L-Transposition of the great arteries: the small aorta is left-anterior, the large pulmonary artery right-posterior. A large ventricular septal defect leads to a small right ventricle (lateral view).

great arteries or a large ventricular septal defect. These two complications occur in only one-fourth of the total group. When the clinical findings do not permit a diagnosis, echocardiography may be of assistance. It will demonstrate a small right ventricle and large left ventricle containing the mitral valve and absence of the tricuspid valve. This is particularly significant in the newborn baby where the right atrioventricular valve is commonly easy to locate. Angiocardiography will clarify the picture by showing the right atrial dimple, easy filling of the left atrium and left ventricle, a large left ventricle, a small right ventricle filling in retrograde fashion from the left, and some hypoplasia of the pulmonary artery.

Differential Diagnosis. The differential diagnosis should include all cyanotic anomalies with left-axis deviation and/or left ventricular overloading. Some of these are the following: pulmonary atresia with normal aortic root; severe pulmonic stenosis with tricuspid and right ventricular hypoplasia; primary hypoplasia of the right ventricle and tricuspid valve (without pulmonic stenosis); cyanotic forms of common atrioventricular canal and ostium primum atrial defect (high pulmonary resistance, pulmonic stenosis); right ventricular origin of both great arteries (double-outlet right ventricle); common ventricle; transposition of the great arteries; truncus arteriosus; left atrial drainage of the left superior and/or inferior vena cava; Eisenmenger's complex; tetralogy of Fallot with atrial septal defect (pentalogy); Ebstein's anomaly with type B Wolff–Parkinson–White syndrome; pulmonary arteriovenous fistula; and asplenia syndrome.

When there is increased lung flow, the following need to be considered: ventricular septal defect, common ventricle, common atrioventricular canal, transposition of the great arteries, and double-outlet right ventricle. Differentiation necessitates cardiac catheterization and angiocardiography.

Differentiation of Anatomic Types. The clinical electrocardiographic, and x-ray findings, supplemented by angiocardiography, will allow clarification of most of the anatomic details.

TYPE I(B)—PULMONARY HYPOPLASIA, tinuous murmur in a severely cyanotic infant or young child highly favors this type. There are transparent lung fields and a narrow vascular pedicle in both frontal and left anterior oblique views. Left ventriculography will demonstrate the absence of a ventricular septal defect and opacification of small pulmonary arteries by way of a ductus arteriosus.

TYPE I(B)—PULMONARY HYPOPLASIA, SMALL VENTRICULAR SEPTAL DEFECT. Infants with this anatomic type have marked early cyanosis and increasingly frequent "blue spells." Roentgenologically (fluoroscopically) they tend to have the typical findings, with scanty hilar shadows and the usual signs of right ventricular hypoplasia with left ventricular enlargement. In the angiocardiogram the great vessels are normally interrelated, but the pulmonary artery is small and fills late and poorly. Contract injection into the left ventricle will

show the small right ventricular chamber leading into the pulmonary artery.

TYPE I(C)—NO PULMONARY HYPOPLASIA, LARGE VENTRICULAR SEPTAL DEFECT. This anatomic type should be suspected in children a few years old and in teen-agers with late onset of the symptoms. The vascular markings may be slightly reduced, normal, or even slightly increased. The angiocardiogram shows the great vessels arising in the normal situation, and the pulmonary artery filling adequately through a ventricular septal defect.

TYPE II(A)—D-TRANSPOSITION OF THE GREAT ARTERIES AND PULMONARY ATRESIA. Infants with this anatomic type have severe anoxia and classical roentgenologic findings. The lateral-projection angiocardiogram shows the aorta arising high at the base in an extreme anterior position. The ascending aorta is in continuation with the anterior cardiac border. The pulmonary arteries are poorly filled by way of a ductus arteriosus.

TYPE II(B)—D-TRANSPOSITION OF THE GREAT ARTERIES AND PULMONARY OR SUB-PULMONARY STENOSIS. Older children or young adults with moderate symptoms of very late onset are of this type. There is a harsh systolic murmur with thrill in the pulmonary area. Diffuse multiple nodular shadows of bronchial collateral circulation may be present on chest plates. The lateral angiocardiogram shows the great arteries in transposed position. Stenosis of the pulmonary valve or subvalvular area may be visualized.

TYPE II(C)—D-TRANSPOSITION OF THE GREAT ARTERIES AND LARGE PULMONARY ARTERY. This type is difficult to differentiate from complete transposition of the great vessels without tricuspid atresia since roentgenologically they may be identical, and, furthermore, occasional cases of transposition of the arterial trunks have left-axis deviation with left ventricular hypertrophy. However, some of the cases have a cardiac contour of tricuspid atresia. In this case the size of the heart is gradually enlarging, and there is excessive lung blood flow. The cyanosis is minimal, sometimes not detected clinically, and of late onset when the patient is in failure. In complete transposition without tricuspid atresia, cyanosis occurs very early and precedes the signs of failure by weeks or months.

TYPE III—L-TRANSPOSITION OF THE GREAT ARTERIES. This is essentially an angiocardiographic finding but may be suspected occasionally by the presence of the ascending aorta forming the left upper border of the cardiac silhouette or by the presence of auscultatory findings of aortic obstruction.

Prognosis

Tricuspid atresia is one of the most serious congenital cardiac anomalies. As previously recorded by many writers, its prognosis is very poor. Although the cases of Holmes (1824; case lived 21 years), Cooley and coworkers (1950; 25 years), Gelpke

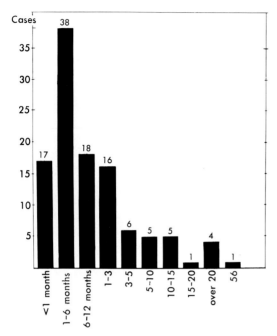

Figure 29-9. The age at death of 111 autopsy-proved cases of tricuspid atresia of all anatomic types. It will be noted that 49.5 percent of the cases were under six months of age; 66 percent died by the end of the first year of life; only 10 percent survived over ten years. The total figure includes the cases examined at The Hospital for Sick Children as well as reports from the literature.

(1883; 27 years), Geraci and associates (1948; alive at 35 years), and Hedinger (1915; 56 years) survived beyond adolescence, they represent the exception to the rule.

A review of the age at death in 111 cases (Figure 29–9) disclosed that almost one-half of all (49.5 percent) died before the age of six months. At one year of age 66 percent were dead and at ten years 90 percent. Only 11 cases, or 10 percent, survived over the age of ten years.

The prognosis depends to a certain extent on the various anatomic types and, obviously, on the *degree* of the resultant hemodynamic disorder.

When pulmonary atresia was present (types I[a] and II[a]), the average life expectancy was two and two-thirds months. The presence of a patent ductus arteriosus producing a continuous murmur may allow survival for some time longer, but there is no evidence that its normal obliterative tendency is altered. On the other hand, even when present, it does not seem to delay anoxic death for long.

Where large pulmonary arteries were present in cases with transposition of the great vessels, the average duration of life was three months. The excessive flow to the lungs may alter the clinical picture but not the poor outlook.

The cases with the "common" type of tricuspid atresia (Type I[b]) lived an average of 11 months.

In the anatomic type I(c) pulmonary-systemic balance is more likely to be achieved, and for this

reason it becomes compatible with a longer life. The life expectancy was found to be eight years even though a few cases had excessive blood flow to the lungs and died early in infancy. Since the ventricular septal defect may close, at times within a few months, hypoxic manifestations may occur in an unpredictable manner.

Finally, the best-tolerated anatomic combination seems to be that with transposition of the great vessels and pulmonary or subpulmonary stenosis (type II[b]). Here the life duration averaged seven years and four months after exclusion of the oldest case of tricuspid atresia on record (56 years in Hedinger's case).

In conclusion, the presence of loud systolic murmurs (especially when accompanied by thrills), the later occurrence of cyanosis, the presence of some—but not exaggerated—pulmonary vascular markings, and the demonstration of pulmonary stenosis in cases with transposition would represent signs of relatively good prognosis.

Cyanosis with onset during the first weeks or months of life, the absence of loud murmurs, and signs of poor or excessive pulmonary blood flow portend an early demise. A continuous murmur heard in infancy does not justify optimism.

Treatment

Surgical Management. Tricuspid atresia is an uncorrectable anomaly; hence, only surgical palliation is possible. Its purpose is (1) to increase the pulmonary flow when this is deficient, (2) to remove intracardiac barriers that interfere with free flow of blood (the atrial septum), and (3) to diminish lung flow when it is excessive.

Amelioration of pulmonary flow is achieved by one of the classic shunt procedures (Blalock-Taussig, Potts-Smith, Waterston) or cavopulmonary anastomosis (Glenn). Optimal age for surgery seems to be between five and ten years, but relatively few patients reach this age. Consequently, surgical treatment must frequently be performed during the first year of life. Temporization is possible only in the few babies with no or few symptoms and in occasional preschool children. A continuous murmur in a child several years old may represent a contraindication. In infants it does not, since the patent ductus commonly occludes in a rapid and unpredictable manner, causing severe aggravation of the hypoxic symptoms.

The operative mortality is in inverse relation to the age of the patients: it is extreme in infancy, when it may exceed 50 percent, and decreases with age, to reach a minimum of 7 percent between five and seven years. The number of persistently good results increases with age at operation, to reach a maximum between five and ten years.

Riker, Potts, and associates (1963) summarized their experience with shunt procedures in 80 cases at the Children's Memorial Hospital in Chicago as follows: Immediate mortality 18 percent, late mortality 26 percent; of the 56 percent who survived a few years after surgery, an excellent result occurred in 16 percent, a good result in 66 percent, fair in 8, and poor in 10 percent. Postoperative deaths were due to cardiac failure (oversized opening, excessive enlargement of the anastomosis due to body growth) and infections.

With Blalock-Taussig anastomoses the incidence of postoperative cardiac failure is significantly smaller. On the other hand, because of the smaller size of the shunt, the number of good results will be somewhat reduced. Spectacular results with such procedures in babies two days to eight months old were obtained by Cooley, who reports a survival rate of 81 percent (Ochsner et al., 1962; Cooley and Hallman, 1964).

Superior vena cava–pulmonary artery anastomosis (Figure 29–10), as proposed by Glenn and Patino (1958), has been considered to be the method of choice for right ventricular bypass. Glenn pointed out that in order for this to be successful the size of the pulmonary artery needs to be no less than half the diameter of the superior vena cava. While the mortality with this operation has been satisfactory (14 percent) in patients over the age of two years, in babies it proved to be prohibitive. Glenn, Browne, and Whittemore (1966) recorded a mortality of 95 percent in infants under one month. Edwards and Bargeron (1968) attributed the poor results to cerebral edema and hypovolemic shock, both related to superior caval obstructions. After introducion of a method of delayed ligation of the azygos vein, in order to allow temporary decompression of the superior vena cava

system, and utilization of fluid replacement by monitoring right atrial pressure, the procedure became applicable to infants as well (8.6 percent mortality).

The long-range results are in a substantial number of cases disappointing. Bargeron and associates (1972) found that 10 of 34 patients followed for up to nine years deteriorated sufficiently to require further palliation. The basic physiologic disorder was a progressively diminishing pulmonary flow, consequent to one or more anatomic causes, as follows: (1) Collateral vessels from the superior to the inferior vena cava allowing the blood to bypass the right lung. Most often they were acquired late after the operation. (2) Spontaneous closure of the right ventricular outflow tract or of the ventricular septal defect. Under these circumstances the left lung may become perfused by aortopulmonary collaterals. (3) Obstruction at the atrial level requiring atrial septostomy. (4) Superior vena cava obstruction produced by obstructive vascular disease of the right lung or by stenosis of the Glenn anastomosis. (5) Severe obstructive pulmonary vascular disease of the *left* lung occurred in two cases in which the ventricular septal defect or the subpulmonic conus occluded completely. It precluded blood flow through an arterial shunt to the left lung. They concluded that the disappearance of a previously loud murmur represents an indication for an immediate shunting procedure to the left lung. The development of pulmonary arteriovenous shunts has been reported by McFaul and associates (1976).

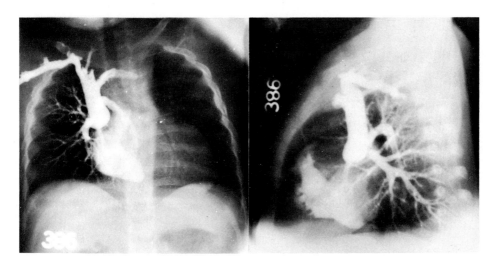

Figure 29-10. Manual injection of contrast into an antecubital vein, six months following a cavopulmonary anastomosis. Azygos reflux and flow into the right atrium through a small persistent opening to the right atrium.

Four-year-old girl at death who had a short-lived, slight degree of improvement following a Potts-Smith anastomosis at the age of nine months. Cavopulmonary anastomosis was performed at 20 months. This was followed by marked improvement, but also by a full-blown picture of S.V.C. obstruction: distended neck veins, marked edema of face and neck, extensive petechiae over face, neck, and upper chest. Over the following three years there were recurrent edema of the face and eyelids with hepatomegaly and severe progression of cyanosis and shortness of breath.

Repeat studies (two years postoperatively) showed the presence of high superior caval pressures (mean of 19 mm of mercury), normal right atrial pressures (mean of 7 mm of mercury), marked dilatation of the azygos vein, and canalization of a previously nonexistent left superior vena cava with drainage into the coronary sinus.

It appears certain that other patients with Glenn shunts will follow the same fate during the second postoperative decade.

More recently (1971) Fontan and Baudet and Kreutzer and associates offered, independently, a new operative approach, consisting of diverting all the right atrial blood into the pulmonary trunk and closing the atrial communication. In the Fontan operation a Glenn anastomosis is performed first, the proximal end of the right pulmonary artery is anastomosed by way of a homograft valve to the right atrium, the proximal end of the pulmonary trunk is ligated, and the atrial septal defect is closed. A second homograft valve is inserted in the inferior vena cava to prevent regurgitation. Kreutzer does not require a previous Glenn procedure. A valved conduit connects the right atrial appendage to the distal cut end of the pulmonary trunk. The atrial septal defect is partially closed, although he intends to close it completely in future cases. Both procedures require a good-size pulmonary artery and a heart sufficiently large to allow utilization of homograft valves. According to Fontan and to Kreutzer, the patients may not have pulmonary hypertension since the blood flow to the lungs depends on the limited pumping ability of the right atrium, hence its application only to the cases with pulmonic stenosis (types I[b] and II[b]). It is entirely conceivable, however, that the procedures may also apply to patients with increased pulmonary flow, provided the pulmonary vascular resistance is not elevated. At the time of this writing the experience with these operations is limited, although it is quite apparent that they represent an excellent method of correction hypoxia, inasmuch as they abolish all right-to-left shunts. An increasing number of technical variants and other approaches using valved conduit operations are being offered and require evaluation (Henry and Danielson, 1974; Henry et al., 1974; Gago et al., 1976).

Removal of the atrial septum (Blalock-Hanlon procedure) in combination with a shunt procedure tends to reduce the operative mortality and the incidence of postoperative cardiac failure. It is indicated when the clinical findings point to the presence of a small patent foramen ovale (pulsating neck veins, pulsating liver, tall P waves in the electrocardiogram, large right atrium by x-ray, significant pressure gradient between the two atria). In symptomatic infants the statistical probability favors a small patent foramen ovale.

A large atrial communication can effectively be achieved by balloon atrial septostomy in infants (Rashkind et al., 1967, 1969) and occasionally in older babies (Lenox and Zuberbuhler, 1970).

When tricuspid atresia is accompanied by excessive pulmonary flow, banding of the pulmonary artery (Muller-Dammann procedure) is the method of controlling cardiac failure. Ochsner and associates (1962) refer to four such instances with no surgical mortality and no further evidence of failure.

The procedure is to be avoided when transposition is absent, inasmuch as the ventricular septal defect of

babies may diminish spontaneously. The Toronto experience and policies regarding the surgical management are reviewed by Williams et al. (1976).

Our own general philosophy regarding the surgical approach to patients with tricuspid atresia is as follows:

1. The hypoxic *infant* undergoes a balloon atrial septostomy and a Waterston or other appropriate anastomosis at the earliest possible time.

When the pulmonary circulation depends exclusively on a patent ductus arteriosus, an anastomotic procedure is carried out and the ductus is ligated if necessary.

The infant in cardiac failure, as the result of increased pulmonary flow, is managed medically as much as possible. Pulmonary artery banding is performed if decongestive measures fail, as is likely when transposition of the great arteries is present. In this category of patients abnormalities of the aortic arch (e.g., patent ductus arteriosus, coarctation of the aorta) need to be sought and appropriately handled at early ages.

2. In the symptomatic *child*, a Blalock-Taussig shunt is preferred. Atrial septectomy is performed in conjunction with this if there are signs of right atrial outflow obstruction, or subsequent to the shunt, if manifestations of cardiac failure develop.

3. The older child or the *adolescent* with progressive symptoms, increasing hematocrit, or with decrease or disappearance of a previously loud murmur is a candidate for a Fontan or Kreutzer operation, provided the anatomic arrangement is favorable and the pulmonary resistance is estimated to be normal. Under unfavorable circumstances, an arterial shunt is urgently indicated.

REFERENCES

Abbott, M. E.: *Atlas of Congenital Cardiac Disease*. American Heart Association, New York, 1936.

Abrams, H. L., and Alway, R. H.: Tricuspid atresia. *Pediatrics*, **7**:660, 1951.

Alexander, F., and White, P. D.: Four important congenital cardiac conditions causing cyanosis to be differentiated from the tetralogy of Fallot: tricuspid atresia, Eisenmenger's complex, transposition of the great vessels and single ventricle. *Ann. Intern. Med.*, **27**:64, 1947.

Anderson, R. C.; Lillehei, C. W.; and Lester, R. G.: Corrected transposition of the great vessels of the heart. *Pediatrics*, **20**:626, 1957.

Anderson, R. M., and McKee, E. E.: Congenital tricuspid atresia. *Am. Heart J.*, **43**:761, 1952.

Astley, R.; Oldham, J. S.; and Parsons, C.: Congenital tricuspid atresia. *Br. Heart J.*, **15**:287, 1953.

Bakulev, A. N., and Kolesnikov, S. A.: Anastomosis of superior vena cava and pulmonary artery in the surgical treatment of certain congenital defects of the heart. *J. Thorac. Surg.*, **37**:693, 1959.

Bargeron, L. M.; Karp, R. B.; Barcia, A.; Kirklin, J. W.; Hunt, D.; and Deverall, P. B.: Late deterioration of patients after superior vena cava to right pulmonary artery anastomosis. *Am. J. Cardiol.*, **30**:211, 1972.

Bellet, S., and Stewart, H. L.: Congenital heart disease. Atresia of tricuspid orifice. *Am. J. Dis. Child.*, **45**:1247, 1933.

Birkhead, N. C., and Wood, E. H.: The diagnosis of tricuspid atresia. *Proc. Mayo Clin.*, **32**:506, 1957.

Blackford, L. M., and Hoppe, D.: Functionally two-chambered heart. *Am. J. Dis. Child.*, **41**:1110, 1931.

Blount, S. G., Jr.; Ferencz, C.; Friedlich, A.; Mudd, J. G.; Carroll, D. G.; and Bing, R. J.: Physiological studies in congenital heart disease. XII. The circulatory dynamics in patients with tricuspid atresia. *Bull. Hopkins Hosp.*, **89**:153, 1951.

Blumenthal, S.; Brahms, S. A.; and Sussman, M. L.: Symposium on congenital heart disease; tricuspid atresia with transposition of the great vessels successfully treated by surgery. *J. Mount Sinai Hosp. N.Y.*, **17**:328, 1951.

Bohm, R.; Schmidt, K. H.; Gunther, K. H.; and Plass, R.: Tricuspid atresia and ventricular septal defect in a 31 year old woman. *Cardiologia*, **53**:11, 1968.

Breslich, P. J.: Congenital atresia of the tricuspid orifice. *Trans. Chicago Pathol. Soc.*, **13**:307, 1930.

Brink, A. J., and Neill, C. A.: The electrocardiogram in congenital heart disease, with special reference to left axis deviation. *Circulation*, **12**:604, 1955.

Brinton, W. D., and Campbell, M.: Necropsies in some congenital diseases of the heart, mainly Fallot's tetralogy. *Br. Heart J.*, **15**:335, 1953.

Brock, R.: Tricuspid atresia: A step toward corrective treatment. *J. Thorac. Cardiovasc. Surg.*, **47**:20, 1964.

Brown, J. W.: Congenital tricuspid atresia, *Arch. Dis. Child.*, **11**:275, 1936.

Brown, J. W.; Heath, D.; and Morris, T. L.: Tricuspid atresia. *Br. Heart J.*, **18**:499, 1956.

Cabrera, E.; Hernández, Y.; and Morales, D.: Vectocardiograma de la atresia tricuspidea. *Arch. Cardiol. Mexico*, **31**:587, 1961.

Campbell, M.: The frequency of different types of congenital heart disease. *Br. Heart J.*, **15**:462, 1953.

———: Tricuspid atresia and its prognosis with and without surgical treatment. *Br. Heart J.*, **23**:699, 1961.

Campbell, M., and Gardner, F. E.: Radiological features of enlarged bronchial arteries. *Br. Heart J.*, **12**:183, 1950.

Campbell, M., and Hills, T. H.: Angiocardiography in cyanotic congenital heart disease. *Br. Heart J.*, **12**:65, 1950.

Canent, R. V.; Spach, M. S.; and Young, W. G.: Cardiopulmonary dynamics in patients with anastomosis of the superior vena cava to the right pulmonary artery. *Circulation*, **36**:47, 1964.

Carey, L. S., and Edwards, J. E.: Tricuspid atresia: Report of a case without transposition or pulmonary stenosis. *Am. J. Roentgenol.*, **91**:321, 1964.

Carlon, C. A.; Mondini, P. G.; and Demarchi, R.: Sulle modalita per realizzare l' anastomosi fra la vena cava superiore e il ramo destro della arteria polmonare. *G. Ital. Chir.*, **6**:11, 1950.

Castellanos, A.; García, O.; and Gonzáles, E.: Atresia tricuspidea en la infancia. Su diagnostico angiocardiographico. *Radiol Panama*, **11**:21, 1960.

Chapotot: Sur un cas de malformation congénitale du coeur, sans cyanose. *Lyon Méd.*, **62**:424, 1889.

Chiche, P.: Etude anatomique et clinique des atrésies tri-cuspidiennes. *Arch. Mal. Coeur*, **44**:981, 1952.

Cooley, D. A., and Hallman, G. L.: Surgery during the first year of life for cardiovascular anomalies: a review of 500 consecutive operations. *J. Cardiovasc. Surg.*, **5**:584, 1964.

Cooley, R. N.; Sloan, R. D.; Hanlon, C. R.; and Bahnson, H. T.: Angiocardiography in congenital heart disease of cyanotic type. II. Observations on tricuspid stenosis or atresia with hypoplasia of right ventricle. *Radiology*, **54**:848, 1950.

Crocker, H. R.: Case of congenital malformation of the heart. *Trans. Pathol. Soc. Lond.*, **30**:276, 1879.

Cumming, G. R.; Ferguson, C. C.; Briggs, J. N.; and Brownell, E. G.: Tricuspid atresia. Treatment by superior vena cava—pulmonary artery anastomosis. *J. Thorac. Cardiovasc. Surg.*, **40**:31, 1960.

Davachi, F.; Lucas, R. V.; and Holler, J. H.: The electrocardiogram and vectorcardiogram in tricuspid atresia. Correlation with pathologic anatomy. *Am. J. Cardiol.*, **25**:18, 1970.

Deverall, P. B.; Lincoln, J. C. R.; Aberdeen, E.; Bonham-Carter, R. E.; and Waterston, D. J.: Surgical management of tricuspid atresia. *Thorax*, **24**:239, 1969.

Dick, M.; Fyler, D. C.; and Nadas, A. S.: Tricuspid atresia. Clinical course in 101 patients. *Am. J. Cardiol.*, **36**:327, 1975.

Dickson, R. W., and Jones, J. P.: Congenital heart block in an infant with associated multiple congenital cardiac malformations. *Am. J. Dis. Child.*, **75**:81, 1948.

Dixon, A. St. J.: Juxtaposition of the atrial appendages: two cases of an unusual congenital cardiac deformity. *Br. Heart J.*, **16**:153, 1954.

Dobner (Aschaffenburg): Zur Kasuistik der Missbildungen des Herzens. Congenitale stenose des Conus der Pulmonarterie. Defect in der Scheidewand der Kammern und Vorkammern. Offenes Foramen ovale. Atresie des Ostium venosum dextrum und Verkummerung des rechten Ventrikels. Tod durch Lungentuber-culose im elften Lebensjahre. *Wien. Med. W. Wschr.*, *603*, 1872.

Donzelot, E., and D'Allaines, F.: *Traité des Cardiopathies Congenitales.* Masson & Cie, Paris, 1954.

Donzelot, E.; Durand, M.; Metianu, C.; and Vlad, P.: L'Axe electrique normal ou devié à gauche dans les cardiopathies congénitales cyanogènes. Etude de 29 cas personnels. Interet diagnostique. *Arch. Mal. Coeur;* **43**:577, 1950.

Dunsky, I.: Tricuspid atresia, hypoplastic transposed aorta and associated defects of a triocular heart. *Arch. Pathol.*, **43**:412, 1947.

Edwards, J. E.: Congenital malformations of the heart and great vessels. In Gould, S. E. (ed.): *Pathology of the Heart.* Charles C. Thomas, Publisher, Springfield, Ill., 1953.

Edwards, J. E., and Burchell, H. B.: Congenital tricuspid atresia: a classification. *Med. Clin. North Am.*, **33**:1177, 1949.

Edwards, W. S., and Bargeron, L. M., Jr.: Superior vena cava to pulmonary artery shunt for tricuspid atresia in an infant. *Surgery*, **49**:205, 1961.

Edwards, W. S., and Bargeron, L. M., Jr.: The superiority of the Glenn operation for tricuspid atresia in infancy and childhood. *J. Thorac. Cardiovasc. Surg.*, **55**:60, 1968.

Eisenberg, G., and Gibson, S.: Congenital heart disease and the electrocardiogram. *J. Pediatr.*, **19**:452, 1941.

Ellison, R. C., and Restieaux, N. J.: *Vectorcardiography in Congenital Heart Disease.* W. B. Saunders Co., Philadelphia, 1972.

Elster, S. K.: Congenital atresia of pulmonary and tricuspid valves. *Am. J. Dis. Child.*, **79**:692, 1950.

Farnsworth, P. B.; Ehlers, K. H.; Levin, A. R.; Ho, E.; and Engle, M. A. E.: Clinical spectrum of tricuspid atresia: Diagnostic and surgical applications. *Circulation*, **36**:Suppl. 2:106, 1967.

Ferber, R. H.: Zur Pathologie der Herzkrankheiten im fruhesten Kindesalter. *Arch. Heilkunde.*, **7**:423, 1866.

Folger, G. M.; Witham, A. C.; and Ellison, R. G.: Tricuspid atresia with transposition of the great vessels. *J. Pediatr.*, **74**:946, 1969.

Fontan, F., and Baudet, E.: Surgical repair of tricuspid atresia. *Thorax*, **26**:240, 1971.

Fontan, F.; Maunico, F. B.; Baudet, E.; et al.: "Correction" de l'atrésie tricuspidienne: rapport de deux cas "corrigés" par l'utilization d'une technique chirurgicale nouvelle. *Ann. Chir. Thorac. Cardiovasc.*, **10**:39, 1971.

Fontan, F.: In *Heart Disease in Infancy. Diagnosis and Surgical Treatment.* B. G. Barrat-Boyes, J. M. Neutze, and E. A. Harris, Eds. Churchill Livingstone, London, 1973, p. 247.

Fragoyannis, S., and Kardalinos, A.: Transposition of the great vessels, both arising from the left ventricle (juxtaposition of pulmonary artery). Tricuspid atresia, atrial septal defect and ventricular septal defect. *Am. J. Cardiol.*, **10**:601, 1962.

Freedom, R. M., and Rowe, R. D.: Aneurysm of the atrial septum in tricuspid atresia. Diagnosis during life and therapy. *Am. J. Cardiol.*, **38**:265, 1976.

Gabriele, O. F.: Progressive obstruction of pulmonary blood flow in tricuspid atresia. *J. Thorac. Cardiovasc. Surg.*, **59**:447, 1970.

Gago, O.; Salles, C. A.; Stern, A. M.; Spooner, E.; Brandt, R. L.; and Morris, J. E.: A different approach for the total correction of tricuspid atresia. *J. Thorac. Cardiovasc. Surg.*, **72**:209, 1976.

Gallaher, M. E., and Fyler, D. C.: Observations on changing hemodynamics in tricuspid atresia without associated transpo-sition of the great vessels. *Circulation*, **35**:381, 1967.

Gamboa, R.; Gersony, N. M.; and Nadas, A. S.: The electrocardiogram in tricuspid atresia and pulmonary atresia with intact ventricular septum. *Circulation*, **34**:24, 1966.

Gardiner, J. H., and Keith, J. D.: Prevalence of heart disease in Toronto children. 1948–1949 Cardiac Registry. *Pediatrics*, **7**:713, 1951.

Gasul, B. M.; Fell, E. H.; Marino, J. J.; and Davis, C. B.: Tricuspid atresia. Report of two cases of young infants with successful operation. *Am. J. Dis. Child.*, **78**:16, 1949.

Gasul, B. M.; Fell, E. H.; Mavrelis, W.; and Casas, R.: Diagnosis of tricuspid atresia or stenosis in infants: based upon a study of 10 cases. *Pediatrics*, **6**:862, 1950.

Gasul, B. M.; Weinberg, M., Jr.; Luan, L. L.; Fell, E. H.; and Bicoff, I.: Superior vena cava—right main pulmonary artery anastomosis. *JAMA*, 171:1797, 1959.

Gelpke: Seltener Fall von angeborenen Herzfehler. Inaugural-dissertation, Basel, 1883.

Geraci, J.; Dry, T.; and Burchell, H.: Atrial septal defect and probable tricuspid atresia in adults. *Proc. Mayo Clin.*, 23:510, 1948.

Gibson, S., and Clifton, W. M.: Congenital heart disease. A clinical and postmortem study of one hundred and five cases. *Am. J. Dis. Child.*, 55:761, 1938.

Glenn, W. W. L., and Patino, J. F.: Circulatory by-pass of the right heart. I. Preliminary observations on the direct delivery of vena cava blood in the pulmonary arterial circulation. *Yale J. Biol. Med.*, 27:147, 1954.

Glenn, W. W. L.: Circulatory by-pass of the right side of the heart. IV. Shunt between superior vena cava and distal right pulmonary artery—report of clinical application. *N. Engl. J. Med.*, 259:117, 1958.

Glenn, W. W. L.; Browne, M.; and Whittemore, R.: *Heart and Circulation in Newborn and Infant.* Grune & Stanton, Inc., New York, 1966, p. 348.

Goodwin, J. F.; Steiner, R. E.: Mounsey, J. P. D.; MacGregor, A. G.; and Wayne, E. J.: A critical analysis of the clinical value of angiocardiography in congenital heart disease. *Br. Heart J.*, 26:161, 1953.

Grayzel, D. M.; and Tennant, R.: Congenital atresia of the tricuspid orifice and anomalous origins of the coronary arteries from the pulmonary artery. *Am. J. Pathol.*, 10:791, 1934.

Guffau, G.: Tricuspid atresia and right ventricular hypoplasia, *Rev. Chilena Pediatr.*, 21:266, 1950. Abstracted in *Am. J. Dis. Child.*, 87:88, 1954.

Guller, B.; Titus, J. L.; and DuShane, J. W.: Electrocardiographic diagnosis of malformations associated with tricuspid atresia: Correlation with morphologic features. *Am. Heart J.*, 78:180, 1969.

Guller, B.; DuShane, J. W.; and Titus, J. L.: The atrioventricular conduction system in two cases of tricuspid atresia. *Circulation*, 40:217, 1969.

Guller, B.; Kincaid, O. W.; Ritter, D. G.; et al.: Angiocardiographic findings in tricuspid atresia: Correlation with hemodynamic and morphologic featues. *Radiology*, 93:531, 1969.

Guller, B.; Ritter, D. G.; and Kincaid, O. W.: Tricuspid atresia with pulmonary atresia and total anomalous pulmonary venous connection to the right superior vena cava. *Mayo Clin. Proc.*, 47:105, 1972.

Hedinger, E.: Transposition der grossen Gefässe bei rudimentarer linker Herzkammer bei einer 56 jährigen Frau. *Z. Allg. Pathol.*, 26:529, 1915.

Henriette: Rapport au sujet d'une note de M. le docteur Henriette sur un cas de cyanose generale, liée à un vice congenitale du coeur, par M. Van Kempen. *Gaz. Méd. Paris*, 16:618, 1861.

Henry, J. N., and Danielson, G. K.: Successful "correction" of tricuspid atresia. Results of a detailed anatomical study. *Surg. Form*, 25:163, 1974.

Henry, J. N.; Devlo, R. O. E.; Ritter, D. G.; Mair, D. D.; Davis, G. D.; and Danielson, G. K.: Tricuspid atresia. Successful surgical "correction" in two patients using porcine xenograft valves. *Mayo Clin. Proc.*, 49:803, 1974.

Hess, J. H.: Congenital atresia of the right auriculo-ventricular orifice with complete absence of tricuspid valve. *Am. J. Dis. Child.*, 13:167, 1917.

Holder, E. C., and Pick, J.: Congenital heart disease: Atresia of the tricuspid orifice, hypoplasia of the right ventricle, septal defects and patent ductus arteriosus. *J. Tech. Methods*, 19:135, 1939.

Holmes, *Edinburgh M. & Clin. Tr.*, 1:252, 1824.

Hübschmann, P.: Zwei Fälle Von Seltener Herzmissbeildung sogenannter Tricuspidalverschluss). *Verh. Deutsch. Ges. Pathol.*, 18:174, 1921.

Iliffe, W.: Peculiarity of structure of heart: no tricuspid orifice. *Med. Times*, 2:456, 1867.

Jönsson, G.; Broden, B.; and Karnell, J.: Selective angiocardiography. *Acta Radiol.*, 32:486, 1949.

Jordan, J. C., and Saunders, C. A.: Tricuspid atresia with prolonged survival. A report of two cases with a review of the world literature. *Am. J. Cardiol.*, 18:112, 1966.

Just-Viera, J. O.; Rivé-Mora, E.; Altieri, P. L.; et al.: Tricuspid

atresia and the hypoplastic right ventricular complex: Complete correction for long-term survival. *Surg. Forum*, 22:165, 1971.

Kelly, C.: Malformation of the heart in a case of cyanosis. *Trans. Pathol., Soc. Lond.*, 19:1851, 1868.

Kettler, L.: Eine besonders gearteter Fall von Transposition der grossen Gefässe, *Arch. Pathol. Anat.*, 287:10, 1932.

Kieffer, S. A., and Carey, L. S.: Tricuspid atresia with normal aortic root. Roentgen-anatomic correlation. *Radiology*, 80:605, 1963.

Kreutzer, G.; Bono, H.; Galindez, E.; DePalma, C.; and Laura, J. P.: An operation for the correction of tricuspid atresia. Am. College of Surgeons, Atlantic City, Oct., Nov., 1971.

Kreutzer, G.; Galindez, E.; Bono, H.; DePalma, C.; and Laura, J. P.: An operation for the correction of tricuspid atresia. *J. Thorac. Cardiovasc. Surg.*, 66:613, 1973.

Kreutzer, R.; Caprile, J. A.; Berre, G. G.; and Becu, L. M.: L'Electrocardiogramme dans l'atrésie tricuspidienne. *Arch. Mal. Coeur*, 47:113, 1954.

Kreysig: *Krankheiten des Herzens*, Berlin, 1817, Vol. 3, p. 104. Cited in Schreiber (1903).

Kroop, I. G.: Congenital tricuspid atresia. *Am. Heart J.*, 41:549, 1951.

Kroop, I. G., and Grishman, A.: The variability of the electrocardiogram in congenital tricuspid atresia. *J. Pediatr.*, 37:231, 1950.

Kühne, M.: Über zwei Fälle kongenitaler Atresie des Ostium venosum dextrum. *Jahresb. Kinderh.*, 63:225, 1906.

Kyger, E. R.; Reul, G. J., Jr.; Sandiford, F. M.; Wukash, D. C.; Hallman, G. L.; and Cooley, D. A.: Surgical palliation of tricuspid atresia. *Circulation*, 52:685, 1975.

Lambert, E. C.; Macmanus, J. E.; and Paine, J. R.: Indications for and results of cardiac surgery in infants. *N.Y. J. Med.*, 55:2471, 1955.

Laubry, C., and Pezzi, C.: *Traité des Maladies Congénitales du Coeur.* Baillière Fils, Paris, 1921.

Leininger, C. R., and Gibson, S.: Observations on 26 infants under one year of age operated on for tetralogy of Fallot or tricuspid atresia. *Pediatrics*, 7:341, 1952.

Lenox, C. C., and Zuberbuhler, J. R.: Balloon septostomy in tricuspid atresia after infancy. *Am. J. Cardiol.*, 25:723, 1970.

Lev, M., and Saphir, O.: Transposition of the large vessels. *J. Tech. Methods*, 17:126, 1937.

Levy, R. J., and Rosenquist, G. C.: Anatomical variations in tricuspid atresia: Report of two cases with previously undescribed lesions. *Hopkins Med. J.*, 126:1970.

Lind, J., and Wegelius, C.: Angiocardiographic studies in children. In Levine, S. Z. (ed.): *Advances in Pediatrics.* Year Book Publishers, Inc., Chicago, Vol. 5, 1952.

Macafee, C. A. J., and Patterson, G. C.: Congenital tricuspid atresia with transposition of the great vessels. *Br. Heart J.*, 23:308, 1961.

Manhoff, L. J., and Howe, J. S.: Congenital heart disease: tricuspid atresia and mitral atresia associated with transposition of the great vessels. *Am. Heart J.*, 29:90, 1945.

Marcano, B. A.; Riemenschneider, T. A.; Ruttenberg, H. D.; Goldberg, S. J.; and Gyepes, M.: Tricuspid atresia with increased pulmonary blood flow. An analysis of 13 cases. *Circulation*, 40:399, 1969.

Marder, S. H.; Seaman, W. B.; and Scott, W. G.: Roentgenologic considerations in the diagnosis of congenital tricuspid atresia. *Radiology*, 61:174, 1953.

McFaul, R. C.; Tajik, A. J.; Mair, D. D.; Danielson, G. K.; and Seward, J. B.: Development of pulmonary arteriovenous shunt after superior vena cava–right pulmonary artery (Glenn) anastomosis. *Circulation*, 54:(Suppl. II) 101, 1976.

Mehrizi, A.; Dekker, A.; and Ottesen, O. E.: Angiocardiographic feature of total anomalous venous return to coronary sinus simulating tricuspid atresia or stenosis. *J. Pediatr.*, 65:615, 1964.

Meng, C. C.: Spontaneous closure of ventricular septal defect in tricuspid atresia. *J. Pediatr.*, 75:697, 1969.

Metianu, C.; Durand, M.; Collado-Madera, S.; and Guillemot, R.: Atresie tricuspidienne: presentation de 6 cas verifiés anatomiquement. *Bull. Scient. Roumain*, 3:67, 1963.

Meyer, R. A., and Kaplan, S.: Echocardiography in the diagnosis of hypoplasia of the left or right ventricle in the neonate. *Circulation*, 46:55, 1972.

Miller, R. A.; Pahlajani, D.; Serratto, M.; et al.: Clinical studies after Fontan's operation for tricuspid atresia. *Am. J. Cardiol.*, 33:157, 1974.

Mitchell, S. C.; Korones, S. B.; and Berendes, H. W.: Congenital heart disease in 56,109 births. Incidence and natural history. *Circulation*, **43**:323, 1971.

Murphy, G. R., and Bleyer, L. F.: Atresia of the tricuspid orifice. *Am. J. Dis. Child.*, **46**:351, 1933.

Nadas, A. S., and Fyler, D. C.: *Pediatric Cardiology*, 3rd ed. W. B. Saunders Co., Philadelphia, 1972.

Neill, C. A., and Brink, A. J.: Left axis deviation in tricuspid atresia and single ventricle. The electrocardiogram in 36 autopsied cases. *Circulation*, **12**:612, 1955.

Nuland, S. B.; Glenn, W. W. L.; and Guilfoil, P. H.: Circulatory bypass of the right heart. III. Some observations on long term survivors. *Surgery*, **43**:184, 1958.

Ochsner, J. L.; Cooley, D. A.; McNamara, D. G.; and Kline, A.: Surgical treatment of cardiovascular anomalies in 300 infants younger than one year of age. *J. Thorac. Cardiovasc. Surg.*, **43**:182, 1962.

Polanco, G. B., and Powell, A. M.: Unusual combination of cardiac anomalies in a case of isolated dextrocardia. *Am. Heart J.*, **49**:102, 1955.

Pujatti, G.; Lise, M.; and Morea, M.: Septal and arterial shunts in tricuspid atresia. *Lancet*, **2**:1311, 1967.

Rao, P. S.: Natural history of the ventricular septal defect in tricuspid atresia and its surgical implications. *Br. Heart J.*, **39**:276, 1977.

Rao, P. S., and Sissman, N. J.: Spontaneous closure of physiologically advantageous ventricular septal defects. *Circulation*, **43**:83, 1971.

Rao, P. S.; Jue, K. L.; Isabel-Jones, J.; and Ruttenberg, H. D.: Ebstein's malformation of the tricuspid valve with atresia. Differentiation from isolated tricuspid atresia. *Am. J. Cardiol.*, **32**:1004, 1973.

Rashkind, W.; Friedman, S.; Waldhausen, J. A.; and Miller, W. W.: Management of tricuspid atresia in infancy: Use of balloon catheter atrial septostomy followed by ascending aorta to right pulmonary artery anastomosis. *Circulation*, **36**, Suppl. 2:217, 1967.

Rashkind, W.; Waldhausen, J.; Miller, W.; and Friedman, S.: Palliative treatment in tricuspid atresia. Combined balloon atrioseptostomy and surgical alteration of pulmonary blood flow. *J. Thorac. Cardiovasc. Surg.*, **57**:812, 1969.

Rihl, J.; Terplan, K.; and Weiss, F.: Über einen Fall von Agenesie der Tricuspidalklappe. *Med. Klin.*, **25**:1543, 1929.

Riker, W. L., and Miller, R.: The diagnosis and treatment of tricuspid atresia. *Surgery*, **38**:886, 1955.

————: The diagnosis and treatment of tricuspid atresia. *J. Thorac. Cardiovasc. Surg.*, **45**:886, 1963.

Riker, W. L.; Potts, W. J.; Grana, L.; Miller, R. A.; and Lev, M.: Tricuspid atresia or stenosis complexes. A surgical and pathologic analysis. *J. Thorac. Cardiovasc. Surg.*, **45**:423, 1963.

Roberts, J. T.: A case of congenital pulmonary and tricuspid atresia with right ventricular hypoplasia. *J. Tech. Methods*, **17**:97, 1937.

Roberts, W. C.; Morrow, A. G.; Mason, D. T.; and Braunwald, E.: Spontaneous closure of ventricular septal defect: Anatomic proof in an adult with tricuspid atresia. *Circulation*, **27**:90, 1963.

Robertson, J. I.: Congenital abnormality of the heart: a case of cor triloculare biatriatum. *Lancet*, **1**:872, 1911.

Robinson, A., and Howard, J. E.: Atresia of the tricuspid valve with transposition of the great vessels. *Am. J. Dis. Child.*, **75**:575, 1948.

Rogers, H. M.; Cordes, J. H.; and Edwards, J. E.: Congenital tricuspid atresia in a boy twelve years of age. *Am. J. Dis. Child.*, **80**:427, 1950.

Rosenquist, G. C.; Levy, R. J.; and Rowe, R. D.: Right atrial-left ventricular relationships in tricuspid atresia—position of the presumed site of the atretic valve as determined by transillumination. *Am. Heart J.*, **80**:493, 1970.

Ross, C. F.: A case of tricuspid atresia with transposition of the great vessels. *Arch. Dis. Child.*, **27**:89, 1952.

Ross, D. N., and Somerville, J.: Surgical correction of tricuspid atresia. *Lancet*, **1**:845, 1973.

Rowe, R. D., and Mehrizi, A.: *The Neonate with Congenital Heart Disease*. W. B. Saunders Co., Philadelphia, 1968.

Schlichter, J.; Hellerstein, H. K.; and Katz, L. N.: Aneurysm of the heart: a correlative study of one hundred and two proved cases. *Medicine*, **33**:43, 1954.

Schreiber, E.: Ein Fall von angeborener Missbildung des Herzens. *Arch. Pathol. Anat.*, **173**:387, 1903.

Shaher, R.; Farina, M.; and Kausel, H.: Spontaneous closure of ventricular septal defect. Tricuspid atresia following Waterston's anastomosis. *N.Y. State J. Med.*, **73**:455, 1973.

Shumacker, H. B., Jr., and Glover, J.: Tricuspid atresia with special reference to shunt procedures. *J. Cardiovasc. Surg.*, **2**:2, 1961.

Sieveking, E. H.: Congenital malformation of the heart. Absence of the right auriculo-ventricular orifice, patulous foramen ovale, defective interventricular septum. *Trans. Pathol. Soc. Lond.*, **5**:97, 1854.

Singh, S. P.; Astley, R.; and Parsons, C. G.: Hemodynamic effects of balloon septostomy in tricuspid atresia. *Br. Med. J.*, **1**:225, 1968.

Snow, P. J. D.: Tricuspid atresia: a new radioscopic sign. *Br. Heart J.*, **14**:387, 1952.

Sokolow, M., and Edgar, A. L.: A study of the V leads in congenital heart disease, with particular reference to ventricular hypertrophy and its diagnostic value. *Am. Heart J.*, **40**:232, 1950.

Soloff, L. A.: Congenital aortic atresia: report of the first case with left axis deviation. *Am. Heart J.*, **37**:123, 1949.

Sommers, S. C., and Johnson, J. M.: Congenital tricuspid atresia. *Am. Heart J.*, **41**:130, 1951.

Soulié, P.: *Cardiopathies Congenitales*. Exp. Scient. Franc., Paris, 1952.

Stanford, W.; Armstrong, R. G.; Cline, R. E.; and King, T. D.: Right atrium-pulmonary artery allograft for correction of tricuspid atresia. *J. Thorac. Cardiovasc. Surg.*, **66**:105, 1973.

Subramanian, S.; Carr, I.; Waterston, D. J.; and Bonham-Carter, R. E.: Palliative surgery in tricuspid atresia. Forty-two cases. *Circulation*, **32**:977, 1965.

Sullivan, J. J., and Mangiardi, J. L.: Tricuspid atresia with right axis deviation: case report and review. *Am. Heart J.*, **55**:450, 1958.

Swan, H.; Maresh, G. J.; and Fisher, G. R.: Criteria of operability in tricuspid stenosis. *J. Pediatr.*, **35**:604, 1949.

Taussig, H. B.: The clinical and pathological findings in congenital malformations of the heart due to defective development of the right ventricle associated with tricuspid atresia or hypoplasia. *Bull. Hopkins Hosp.*, **59**:435, 1936.

————: *Congenital Malformations of the Heart*. II. Specific Malformations. The Commonwealth Fund, New York, 1960.

Taussig, H. B.; Keinonen, R.; Momberger, N.; and Kirk, H.: Long term observations of the Blalock-Taussig operation. IV. Tricuspid atresia. *Johns Hopkins Med. J.*, **132**:135, 1973.

Thomas, H. M.: Congenital cardiac malformations. *Bull. Int. A. M. Museums*, **21**:58, 1941.

Valleix, F. L. I.: *Bull. Soc. Anat. Paris*, p. 253, 1834.

Van Praagh, R.; Ando, M.; and Dungan, W. T.: Anatomic types of tricuspid atresia: Clinical and developmental implications. *Circulation*, **44**:suppl. 2:115, 1971.

Van Praagh, R.; In B. G. Barratt-Boyes, J. M. Neutze, and E. A. Harris (eds.): *Heart Disease in Infancy. Diagnosis and Surgical Treatment*. Churchill Livingstone, London, 1973, p. 246.

Walker, W. R.; Sbokos, C. G.; and Lennox, S. C.: Correction of tricuspid atresia. *Br. Heart J.*, **37**:282, 1975.

Wason, J.: Absence of tricuspid orifice with transposition of great vessels and pulmonary artery forming descending aorta through patent ductus. *J. Tech. Methods*, **13**:106, 1934.

Waterston, D. J.: Treatment of Fallot's tetralogy in children under one year of age. *Rozhl. Clin.*, **41**:183, 1962.

Wieland, E.: Zur Klinik und Morphologie der angeborenen Tricuspidalatresie. *Jahresb. Kinderh.*, **79**:1914.

Williams, W. G.; Rubis, L.; Trusler, G. A.; and Mustard, W. T.: Palliation of tricuspid atresia: Potts-Smith, Glenn and Blalock-Taussig shunts. *Arch. Surg.*, **110**:1383, 1975.

Williams, W. G.; Rubis, L.; Fowler, R. S.; Rao, M. K.; Trusler, G. A.; and Mustard, W. T.: Tricuspid atresia: results of treatment in 160 children. *Am. J. Cardiol.*, **38**:235, 1976.

Wittenborg, M. H.; Neuhauser, E. B. D.; and Sprunt, W. H.: Roentgenographic findings on congenital tricuspid atresia with hypoplasia of the right ventricle. *Am. J. Roentgenol.*, **64**:712, 1951.

Ziegler, R. F.: Symposium on cardiovascular diseases: clinical cardiac catherization in infants and children. *Pediatr. Clin. North Am.*, **1**:93, 1954.

CHAPTER

30

Aortic Atresia

Robert M. Freedom

ONE OF the earliest descriptions of aortic atresia was written by Dilg in the year 1883. By 1890, Martens was able to collect references to 27 cases, and, by 1950, Monie and de Pape had assembled 27 more. The characteristic arrangement of defects, as shown in Figure 30–1, consists of marked underdevelopment of the whole left side of the heart, including the aorta, aortic valve, left ventricle, and left atrium. In contradistinction, the right side of the heart is grossly enlarged, with a large right atrium, larged right ventricle, and widely patent ductus arteriosus, which delivers blood into the aorta. It is obvious that the burden of the circulation falls on the right ventricle and that the left is essentially nonfunctional.

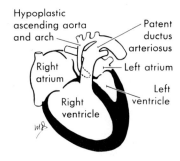

Figure 30-1. Characteristic arrangement of defects in aortic atresia.

Pathology

There are several variations in degree of underdevelopment in the left heart and aorta, yet each fits into the same clinical and pathologic picture. All of our cases showed hypoplasia of the aorta. Though small, the ascending aorta was always patent. This might be expected since the coronary vessels arise from the base of the aorta, and, if they are not supplied with blood, the heart ceases to function and the baby dies early in fetal life.

The right atrium is always enlarged and dilated, and the left atrium is always small. The atria communicate by a patent foramen ovale or modest atrial septal defect (76 percent of cases) or a large atrial septal defect or common ventricle (17 percent of cases), and 6 percent of these have an intact septum. The latter may be associated with a patent mitral valve, or a ventricular septal defect, or a communication between the left atrium and the coronary sinus, or some anomalous pulmonary vein drainage, but occasionally there is no communication demonstrable between the pulmonary venous return and the right side of the heart (Watson et al., 1960).

Beckman and associates (1975) recently reviewed alternate pathways to pulmonary venous flow in left-sided obstructive lesions. Left ventricular myocardial sinusoids that can be demonstrated anatomically in patients with aortic atresia provide egress for blood from the blind left ventricle.

These sinusoids communicate with myocardial veins, ramifications of coronary arteries, or directly into myocardial capillaries. From either of these sites, blood would ultimately be delivered to the right ventricle via the coronary sinus and right atrium.

The tricuspid valve is large and the mitral valve is always small. Twenty percent of cases have mitral atresia. The left ventricle is tiny and thick-walled and nestles in the upper portion of the ventricular mass. Its wall thickness is 7 mm.

The right ventricle is consistently large and dilated. In no instance did we find a case of transposition of the great vessels with this anomaly, and the pulmonary artery is always large and normally branched, but the aorta begins blindly at the base of the heart. The aortic valve most commonly consists of a domelike structure with the coronary arteries originating in a normal manner just above it. The ascending aorta is hypoplastic and averages 5 mm in circumference. In all cases there is a very large patent ductus arteriosus continuing smoothly into the descending aorta. On the posterior wall of the aorta immediately proximal to its junction with the ductus there is almost invariably a ridge 2 mm high and similar to that seen in coarctation of the aorta.

Examination of the lungs, both microscopic and gross, reveals marked engorgement of the pulmonary capillaries with some edema and fluid in the ovale and often areas of atelectasis with or without hemorrhage.

Fifty percent of the cases had an associated endocardial fibroelastosis of the left ventricle. This occurred only in cases that had a patent mitral valve; it never appeared when there was complete atresia of that structure. It appears a necessary requirement, therefore, to have the left ventricle communicate with the left atrium and be bathed by circulating blood in order to produce endocardial fibroelastosis in this type of case.

Rarely, aortic atresia will occur with a normal-sized left ventricle and mitral apparatus (Freedom et al., 1975; Pellegrino and Thiene, 1976; Roberts et al., 1976; Freedom et al., 1977b). We have now examined seven hearts with aortic atresia, ventricular septal defect, and normally developed left ventricle. Invariably, a large ventricular septal defect is present. Conal-type ventricular defects were evident in five; membranous defect in one; and a complete atrioventricular canal defect in a single patient. The conal defects were a manifestation of either conal deformity, similar to the so-called "supracristal" defect, or conoventricular malalignment. Subaortic atresia in the patient with conal defect resulted from a combination of leftward deviation of the conal septum and a continuation of the curvature of the heart tube itself, the so-called ventriculoinfundibular fold. Maladherent anterior leaflet of the common atrioventricular valve obliterated the subaortic vestibule in the patient with complete common atrioventricular canal. In this regard, Silverberg (1965) has reported the coexistence of aortic atresia with endocardial cushion defect, but, in his patient, there was marked hypoplasia of the left ventricle.

In the patients studied in this institution, and from the reports in the literature, the ascending aorta is severely hypoplastic, with both membranous and subvalvular aortic atresia, despite a normally developed left ventricle. Except in the one patient with atrioventricular canal, the mitral valve has been normal, although aortic and mitral atresia, large ventricular defect, and normal left ventricle have been documented in one patient (Roberts et al., 1976). The epicardial distribution of the coronary arteries in the patient with aortic atresia and normal left ventricle would suggest a normally developed left ventricle. Indeed, this has recently been stressed in the aortography of aortic atresia (Freedom et al., 1977a).

Pathophysiology

The length of survival is dependent on the presence or absence of four anatomic defects. (1) An atrial septal defect will allow decompression of the left atrium and promote mixing. Krovetz and associates (1970) determined that the lowest arterial oxygen saturations occurred in those with closed foramen ovales. (2) A large patent ductus arteriosus will allow

sufficient aortic blood flow to perfuse the myocardium and the tissues. The presence of a catheter in the ductus may cause sufficient reduction in flow to lead to collapse. (3) A large ventricular septal defect is unusual (12/172), but when present helps to decompress the left ventricle and left atrium and allows better mixing. This defect was present in one patient who survived to 3.5 years without surgery but in their patient, the left ventricle was hypoplastic (Moodie et al. (1972). (4) A degree of narrowing of the pulmonary artery branches (beyond the PDA) will prolong life, by reducing the pulmonary blood flow and subsequent left atrial hypertension in the phase when pulmonary vascular resistance begins to decrease in the newborn.

In a typical case of aortic valve atresia the blood from the lungs returns to the left atrium and then crosses through the foramen ovale to the right atrium. This mixture of pulmonary to systemic venous blood enters the right ventricle and is propelled out by way of the pulmonary artery partly to the lungs and partly through the patent ductus into the descending and ascending aorta. In this way the head and neck and arms are supplied as well as the ascending aorta and coronary arteries in a retrograde fashion; since the whole circulation depends on the right atrium and right ventricle, they are dilated and hypertrophied, and there is a systemic level of systolic pressure in the right ventricle and pulmonary artery branches. The cyanosis is due to a mixing of the oxygenated venous blood returning from the lung with the systemic venous blood in the right atrium. The dyspnea is related to the pulmonary congestion and edema, partly due to obstruction in the left atrial chamber and also due to heart failure, which is invariably present at some stage of the baby's illness. The heart failure is due to the additional load of the circulation thrust on the right ventricle after delivery since the general systemic circulation plus the pulmonary circulation is supplied by the right ventricle. If the obstruction at the foramen ovale level is minor and the strength in the right ventricle is maintained, these babies have only a minor degree of cyanosis. However, as pulmonary edema increases and failure of the ventricular muscle becomes progressive, cyanosis of the lips and fingernails deepens steadily.

Heart failure occurs early as a rule, an average of two and a half days after birth. The liver is enlarged 3 cm or more below the right costal margin, rales may appear in the chest, occasionally pitting edema is visible in the extremities, and the spleen is often palpable.

Prevalence

Congenital aortic atresia is not a rare anomaly and is probably somewhat more common than is realized since all cases die in the first few weeks or months of life, and the vast majority are buried undiagnosed. At The Hospital for Sick Children, Toronto, it has been found 80 times in 15 years and accounts for 1.2 percent of the total. Familial aortic atresia has been reported (Rao et al., 1969).

This anomaly is associated with a very short life. Most cases do not survive the first month: 25 percent of cases dying in the first month from congenital heart disease have aortic atresia. Abbott's estimate (1936) of an average length of life of four days has generally been borne out by cases subsequently reported in the literature. The age at death in our group is seen in Figure 30–2.

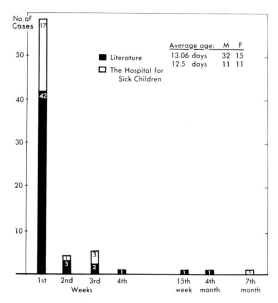

Figure 30-2. Age at death in aortic atresia.

Clinical Features

The chief presenting feature of this type of defect is the appearance of signs of heart failure in the first week or two of life. Dyspnea is commonly present from the first few days of life, with respiratory rates varying from 60 to 120 per minute. The liver enlarges progressively because of the excessive load on the right ventricle.

Cyanosis eventually becomes apparent. During the first day or two of life it may be minimal, and occasionally it may be insufficient to attract attention in the nursery. In 30 percent of our cases it was apparent to the attending staff on the first day of life; in 35 percent it appeared on the second day of life; and in a further 35 percent it appeared at varying intervals up to 14 days. In one case the cyanosis was not noted until three weeks of age. The arterial oxygen level may vary from 40–50 percent to 80–90 percent. The most hypoxic patients have severe restriction at atrial level with hemorrhagic pulmonary edema. Most of our patients have arterial oxygen saturation in room air in the 70s and 80s.

These oxygen levels indicate minor or moderate degrees of cyanosis. Most frequently the babies appear an unhealthy, slightly gray color with a cyanotic tinge to the lips. They are not as blue as in transposition of the great vessels, tricuspid atresia, or pulmonary atresia.

Since most of these infants are in some distress when first seen, they invariably have a tachycardia of approximately 150 per minute. The heart sounds are clear-cut, but as the baby's condition deteriorates they become fainter. A constant pulmonary ejection click is audible in some patients. This click probably results from the dilated main pulmonary artery. The second heart sound is single. Among our 38 infants, 40 percent had heart murmur and 60 percent had none. There was no characteristic location of the murmur; some were in the pulmonary area and others down the left border of the sternum. In one case, the murmur was localized at the apex. Those cases of aortic atresia associated with ventricular septal defects usually had a well-heard systolic murmur in the fourth left interspace near the sternum. However, ventricular septal defects were present in three cases only. Occasionally a continuous murmur may be heard due to flow through the foramen ovale (Ross et al., 1963; Rowe, 1963).

Characteristically, all pulses are feeble, including the carotids. Indeed, in the patient with aortic atresia and severe ductal constriction, all the pulses may be palpably imperceptible. However, prior to significant narrowing of the ductus arteriosus, the femoral pulses may be palpable, but usually their amplitude is reduced when compared to normal.

Radiologic Examination

The heart shadow is usually enlarged to both right and left. There is a full left border and a rounded apex, which is slightly raised. There is usually a wide great-vessel area and a full, slightly bulging right atrium. The hilar shadows are increased and congested. This shadowing may at times be better shown by x-ray than under the fluoroscope since some degree of atelectasis may be present, which diminishes the clarity of the outline of the hilar areas. Only rarely does the heart appear within normal limits for size. There was slight enlargement in one-fourth of our cases, moderate enlargement in one-half, and gross enlargement in another fourth. A significant number of patients will show distinctive pulmonary venous congestion.

Electrocardiography

In our cases the electrocardiogram frequently showed certain features that were suggestively diagnostic when they occurred in the first week or two of life and were associated with the clinical signs of dyspnea and cyanosis.

All tracings showed evidence of right ventricular hypertrophy. This at times took the form of abnormally high voltage, but in many instances it was evident only in the R/S ratio in V_1 or in a prolonged activation over the right precordium. The T waves

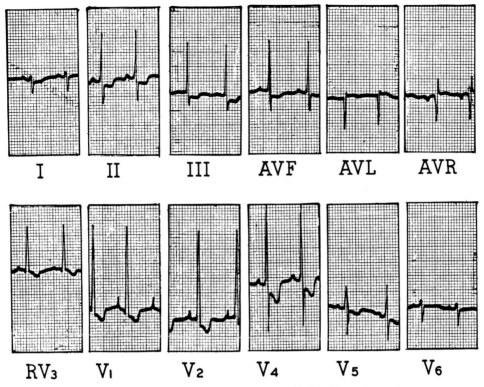

I   II   III   AVF   AVL   AVR

RV₃   V₁   V₂   V₄   V₅   V₆

Figure 30-3. Electrocardiogram of a five-day-old girl with aortic atresia.

were upright in V_1 in 80 percent. This was associated with inverted T waves in V_5 or V_6 in two-thirds of the cases. In the other one-third the T waves were either flat or upright over the left precordium. The T wave changes may result, in part, from subendocardial ischemia. Perfusion of the coronary arteries depends on patency of the ductus arteriosus. With ductal constriction, coronary perfusion pressure will fall, resulting in progressive subendocardial ischemia. A qR pattern of rather marked right ventricular hypertrophy was present in 40 percent. The electrical axis varied from +95 to +180 degrees. The electrical position was usually horizontal. The P-R interval varied from 0.10 to 0.16 second. The range of P_2 was from 1.0 to 3.5 mm in height, with an average of 2.0 mm.

An example is shown in Figure 30–3. This electrocardiogram at five days shows right hypertrophy with a high R/S ratio in V_1, inverted T waves in V_1 to V_5, and upright T waves in V_6. There is a qR pattern in V_1.

A small number of patients with aortic atresia will demonstrate electrocardiographic evidence of left ventricular hypertrophy (Strong et al., 1970). The genesis of this pattern is not clear.

Angiocardiography

Angiocardiography offers a direct method of diagnosis that reveals much of the pathology. Figure 30–4 shows a venous angiogram (A) on a baby suffering from this condition at two months of age and an aortogram (B) on the same baby. The aortogram shows the hypoplastic aorta filling in retrograde fashion and demonstrates the coronary vessels arising from the base. A large patent ductus can be seen partly outlined. In the venous angiogram a huge right ventricle and a large pulmonary artery with large, congested hilar vessels are evident. The pulmonary artery overshadows the aorta. This baby died subsequently at seven months of age. Although retrograde filling of the diminutive ascending aorta may be achieved by right ventricular or pulmonary artery angiography, visualization of the ascending aorta may occasionally be inadequate. Retrograde aortography via the umbilical artery or right axillary artery will nicely demonstrate the diminutive ascending aorta and coronary arteries. Usually, contrast material will remain in the aortic sinuses and coronary arteries for a longer time than normal, confirming the retrograde (ductal) perfusion of the aortic root.

The angiocardiographic appearance of the aortic root, sinuses of Valsalva, and the caliber of the ascending aorta may show considerable variation (Freedom et al., 1975). In some patients, the size of the aortic root will approach the normal. Selective aortography in the aortic root can also demonstrate coronary artery–cameral fistulous communications.

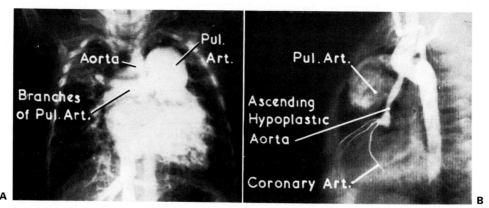

Figure 30-4. Aortic atresia. Baby died at seven months of age. *A.* Venous angiogram on this baby at two months of age. *B.* Aortogram on the same baby.

Diagnosis

Aortic atresia is the most common cause of heart failure in the newborn. Therefore, the diagnosis is readily suspected in an infant who develops heart failure coupled with slight cyanosis in the first week of life. An enlarged heart and an electrocardiographic pattern of marked right ventricular hypertrophy with strain help to complete the diagnostic picture. In doubtful cases the anomaly can be shown best by an aortogram.

Differential Diagnosis

In the differential diagnosis, one should exclude critical aortic stenosis, with or without endocardial fibroelastosis, neonatal myocarditis, mitral atresia with normal aortic root and inadequate atrial communication, coarctation syndromes, aortic arch interruption, and total anomalous pulmonary venous return with obstruction. Rarely should one consider simple transposition of the great arteries. The heart in D-transposition often has a characteristic shape, and pulmonary overcirculation is less conspicuous than in the patient with aortic atresia. Similarly, radiographic evidence of pulmonary venous congestion is most uncommon in the patient with D-transposition of the great arteries and intact ventricular septum.

The patient with critical aortic stenosis, or severe endocardial fibroelastosis, or myocarditis may all show signs of severe congestive heart failure with poor peripheral perfusion. The neonate with critical aortic stenosis may present with an insignificant heart murmur, no aortic click, and evidence of poor peripheral perfusion. The electrocardiogram of the patient with critical aortic stenosis may show left ventricular hypertrophy with strain, but severe right ventricular hypertrophy is not uncommonly found. The neonate with myocarditis may have an identical clinical presentation, although a maternal history of infection or evidence of viremia in the infant may suggest the diagnosis of myocarditis. The electrocardiogram may show low voltages and ST-T segment changes consistent with myocarditis. The patient with severe endocardial fibroelastosis may occasionally present in severe heart failure early in the first week of life. The electrocardiogram may show striking voltage criteria of left ventricular hypertrophy with strain. Finally, it should be stressed that there is a continuum of abnormalities starting with aortic and mitral atresia, but including critical aortic stenosis with varying degrees of left ventricular hypoplasia, endocardial fibroelastosis, and mitral valve abnormalities. One can usually easily exclude tetralogy of Fallot, tricuspid or pulmonary atresia, and single ventricle with pulmonary stenosis by the absence of pulmonary plethora and the usually more severe cyanosis that occurs with severe pulmonary outflow obstruction.

The patient with obstructed total anomalous pulmonary venous return, usually infradiaphragmatic, will often show severe tachypnea, dyspnea, pulmonary edema, and severe congestive heart failure. These infants usually show intense cyanosis, and the heart size is frequently normal in contrast to the patient with aortic atresia who is usually only mildly cyanosed, and whose heart is at least moderately enlarged. The electrocardiograms in both conditions may show marked right ventricular hypertrophy, with a qR pattern in the right precordial leads.

The patient with coarctation syndrome or aortic arch interruption may present with findings of severe congestive heart failure. Not infrequently, the pulse discrepancy between upper and lower extremities may not become apparent until the congestive heart failure is treated. Careful measurement of the upper and lower extremity blood pressures by Doppler should always be performed. Furthermore, survival of the patient with aortic arch interruption usually depends on patency of the ductus arteriosus. As those patients frequently have associated intracardiac defects, the patient with aortic arch interruption and aortic atresia may have a very similar presenting findings.

Ultrasonography has proven most helpful in the diagnosis of aortic atresia. The pertinent echocardiographic findings include a diminutive aortic root, abnormal mitral excursion and motion, small left atrium and left ventricule. In contrast, the right ventricle and anterior root (pulmonary artery) are larger than normal (Meyer and Kaplan, 1972).

Cardiac catheterization will show a large left-to-right shunt at atrial level. In the absence of hemorrhagic pulmonary edema, left atrial blood will often be nearly fully saturated, with a systemic saturation between 65 to 90 degrees, reflecting obligatory mixing at right atrial level. Right ventricular and pulmonary artery systolic pressures will be equal to or greater than systemic pressure. Not infrequently, a pressure gradient can be measured across the ductus, consistent with ductal narrowing. Passage of the catheter across the narrow ductus arteriosus may be associated with bradycardia and/or ventricular fibrillation or asystole as coronary blood flow may be compromised. A significant pressure gradient across the atrial septum is often found, confirming the presence of a restrictive atrial communication. Selective aortography will demonstrate the diminutive ascending aorta and coronary arterial circulation. Left atrial angiography will usually reveal extreme mitral stenosis or atresia, with opacification of the right atrium and right ventricle via the left-to-right atrial shunt. Very rarely, selective left atrial injection will sequentially opacify a large left atrium, left ventricle, and the pulmonary artery via a ventricular septal defect. Thus, the angiographic demonstration of aortic atresia usually, but not always, indicates severe hypoplasia of the left heart chambers and mitral apparatus. As mentioned earlier, aortic atresia with a diminutive ascending aorta can exist with a normally developed left ventricle. Visualization of the coronary arteries is important to the assessment of ventricular size, and both anteroposterior and lateral or oblique projections are necessary to assess the relative distributions of the anterior descending and circumflex coronary arteries. Recently, Rosengart and his colleagues (1976) have advocated single-film retrograde umbilical aortography with the diagnosis of the hypoplastic left-heart syndrome. If performed only in the anteroposterior projection, one could not adequately assess the epicardial distribution of the coronary arteries, hence, left ventricular dimension.

A careful and selective cardiac catheter will differentiate between those lesions that can be treated by surgery (critical aortic stenosis, certain types of aortic arch interruptions, etc.) and those for which only medical therapy is indicated.

Prognosis

The prognosis is uniformly poor. These infants usually die in the first week of life. As is shown in Figure 30–2, a few survive longer and may occasionally live up to seven months of age. Such exceptions are rare.

The longest survivor in the literature was 3.5 years (Moodie et al., 1972). The longest survival at The

Hospital for Sick Children, Toronto, has been one and one-half years.

Treatment

Successful surgical therapy would seem difficult to achieve since the aorta and left ventricle are so hypoplastic. Enlarging the opening in the atrial septum might improve the circulation slightly but could not be expected to help significantly.

Supportive therapy with oxygen and digitalis is of very limited benefit and is chiefly indicated while the diagnosis is in doubt. Until the diagnosis of aortic atresia and the hypoplastic left-heart syndrome is confirmed, either by cardiac catheterization and angiocardiography or by echocardiography, the intra-arterial administration of E-type prostaglandins may be of value in maintenance of patency of the ductus arteriosus (Olley et al., 1976).

Theoretically, if an adequate opening was made between the two atria and a banding of both right and left pulmonary arteries was carried out so that there was an adequate blood flow to the lungs and the pressure was reduced so that the pulmonary edema and congestion were eliminated, the heart might carry on in the same manner as a single ventricle. Recently Cayler and associates (1970) have suggested an aortopulmonary shunt in addition to the above. This makes for a feasible if complicated total procedure carrying a high risk and uncertain late benefits. Most centers including our own presently regard the usual form of the malformation as inoperable (Doty and Knott, 1977).

REFERENCES

Abbott, M. E.: *Atlas of Congenital Cardiac Disease*, American Heart Association, New York, 1936, p. 48.

Anderson, N. A., and Sano, M. E.: Aortic atresia with hypoplasia of left ventricle. *Am. J. Dis. Child.*, **62**:629, 1941.

Beckman, C. B.; Moller, J. H.; and Edwards, J. E.: Alternate pathways to pulmonary venous flow in leftsided obstructive anomalies. *Circulation*, **52**:509, 1975.

Cayler, G. G.; Smeloff, E. A.; and Miller, G. E., Jr.: Surgical palliation of hypoplastic left side of the heart. *N. Engl. J. Med.*, **282**:780, 1970.

Dilg, J.: Ein Beitrag zur Kenntniss seltener, Herzanomalien im Anschluss an einen Fall von angeborner linksseitiger Conusstenose. *Arch. Pathol. Anat.*, **91**:193, 1883.

Doty, D. B., and Knott, H. W.: Hypoplastic left heart syndrome. Experience with an operation to establish functionally normal circulation. *J. Thorac. Cardiovasc. Surg.*, **74**:624, 1977.

DuShane, J. W.: Clinico-pathologic correlation of some less common cyanotic congenital cardiac defects in infants. *Med. Clin. North Am.*, **32**:879, 1948.

Evans, W.: Congenital stenosis (coarctation), atresia, and interruption of the aortic arch. Study of 28 cases. *Q. J. Med.*, **2**:1, 1933.

Freedom, R. M.; Culham, J. A. G.; Moes, C. A. F.; and Harrington, D.: Selective aortic root angiography in the hypoplastic left heart syndrome. *Eur. J. Cardiol.*, **4**:25, 1976.

Freedom, R. M.; Culham, J. A. G.; and Rowe, R. D.: Aortic atresia with normal left ventricle: distinctive angiocardiographic findings. *Cathet. Cardiovasc. Diag.*, 1977.

Freedom, R. M.; Dische, M. R.; and Rowe, R. D.: Conal anatomy in aortic atresia, ventricular septal defect, and normally developed left ventricle. *Am. Heart J.*, **94**:689, 1977.

Freedom, R. M.; Williams, W. G.; Dische, M. R.; and Rowe, R. D.: Anatomic variants in aortic atresia: Potential candidates for ventriculo-aortic reconstitution. *Br. Heart J.*, **38**:821, 1976.

Friedman, S.; Murphy, L.; and Ash, R.: Aortic atresia with hypoplasia of the left heart and aortic arch. *J. Pediatr.*, **38**:354, 1951.

Gauss, H.: Congenital obliteration of the aorta. *Am. J. Dis. Child.*, **12**:606, 1916.

Krovetz, L. J.; Rowe, R. D.; and Scheibler, G. L.: Hemodynamics of aortic valve atresia. *Circulation*, **42**:953, 1970.

Lev, M., and Killian, S. T.: Hypoplasia of the aorta without transposition, with electrocardiographic and histopathologic studies of the conduction system. *Am. Heart J.*, **24**:794, 1942.

Lippincott, S.: Congenital atresia of the aortic valve without septal defect. *Am. Heart J.*, **17**:502, 1939.

Martens, G.: Zwei Fälle von Aortenatresie. *Arch. Pathol. Anat.*, **121**:322, 1890.

Meyer, R. A., and Kaplan, S. Echocardiography in the diagnosis of hypoplasia of the left or right ventricle in the neonate. *Circulation*, **46**:55, 1972.

Monie, I. W., and de Pape, A. D. J.: Congenital aortic atresia: Report of one case with analysis of 26 similar reported cases. *Am. Heart J.*, **40**:595, 1950.

Moodie, D. S.; Gallen, W. J.; and Friedberg, D. Z.: Congenital Aortic Atresia. Report of long survival and some speculations about surgical approaches. *J. Thorac. Cardiovasc. Surg.*, **63**:726, 1972.

Olley, P. M.; Coceani, F.; and Bodach, E.: E-type prostaglandins. A new emergency therapy for certain cyanotic congenital heart malformations. *Circulation*, **58**:731, 1976.

Pellegrino, P. A., and Thiene, G.: Aortic valve atresia with a normally developed left ventricle. *Chest*, **65**:1, 1976.

Philpott, N.: Congenital atresia of the aortic ring. *Ann. Intern. Med.*, **2**:422, 1928.

Rao, S. S.; Gootman, N.; and Platt, N.: Familial aortic atresia.

Report of a case of aortic atresia in siblings. *Am. J. Dis. Child.*, **118**:919, 1969.

Roberts, J. T.: Case of congenital aortic atresia, with hypoplasia of ascending aorta, normal origin of coronary arteries, left ventricular hypoplasia, and mitral stenosis. *Am. Heart J.*, **12**:448, 1936.

Roberts, W. C.; Perrly, L. W.; Chandra, R. S.; Myers, G. E.; Shapiro, S. R.; and Scott, L. P.: Aortic valve atresia: a new classification based on necropsy study of 73 cases. *Am. J. Cardiol.*, **37**:753, 1976.

Rosengart, R.; Jarmakani, J. M.; and Emmanouilides, G. C.: Single film retrograde umbilical aortography in the diagnosis of hypoplastic left heart syndrome. *Circulation*, **51**:345, 1976.

Ross, J., Jr.; Braunwald, E.; Mason, D. T.; Braunwald, N. S.; and Morrow, A. G.: Interatrial communication and left atrial hypertension. A cause of continuous murmur. *Circulation*, **28**:853, 1963.

Rowe, R. D.: Personal communication, 1963.

Silberberg, B.: Coexistent aortic and mitral atresia associated with persistent common atrioventricular canal. *Am. J. Cardiol.*, **16**:754, 1965.

Strong, W. B.; Liebman, J.; and Perrin, E.: Hypoplastic left ventricle syndrome. Electrocardiographic evidence of left ventricular hypertrophy. *Am. J. Dis. Child.*, **120**:511, 1970.

Taussig, H. B.: *Congenital Malformations of the Heart*. The Commonwealth Fund, New York, 1947, p. 177.

Walker, R., and Klinck, G. H.: Congenital aortic and mitral atresia. *Am. Heart J.*, **24**:752, 1942.

Watson, D. G.; Rowe, R. D.; Conen, P. E.; and Duckworth, J. W.: Mitral atresia with normal aortic valve. Report of 11 cases and review of the literature. *Pediatrics*, **25**:450, 1960.

Wesson, H., and Beaver, D. C.: Congenital atresia of the aortic orifice. *J. Tech. Methods*, **14**:86, 1935.

Wiglesworth, F. W.: A case of congenital aortic atresia with unusual hyperplasia of the endocardial elastic tissue of the left auricle and ventricle. *J. Tech. Methods*, **15**:153, 1936.

CHAPTER

31

Congenital Mitral Atresia

John D. Keith

T HE TERM "mitral atresia with normal aortic valve" has been chosen to describe this group of cases of congenital heart disease. The mitral valve is absent, and there is no opening between the left atrium and either ventricle. In fact, the whole left side of the heart is underdeveloped, associated with a small left atrium and a small or absent left ventricle. These hearts function as if they had but one ventricle. Atresia of the mitral valve is often coupled with atresia or extreme stenosis of the aortic valve, or with marked hypoplasia of the ascending aorta. However, such cases have different clinical and physiologic features; therefore, this chapter will be confined to cases with a normal aortic valve and an ascending aorta of good caliber.

Incidence

Abbott (1936) noted five instances of mitral atresia in her analysis of 1000 necropsies of patients with congenital heart disease, of which only two fully satisfied the criteria of this report. Edwards and Rodgers (1947) noted five cases of mitral atresia in the collection from the Mayo Clinic of 212 specimens with major cardiovascular malformations. Other authors also indicate the rarity of mitral atresia, even as compared to other valvular atresias.

Watson and associates (1960) collected 11 cases at The Hospital for Sick Children and 41 from the literature, making a total of 52 cases. Twenty-two were males and 30 females.

Embryology

Odgers (1939) has shown that the left lateral atrioventricular endocardial cushion forms the posterior cusp of the mitral valve, that the ventral and dorsal atrioventricular endocardial cushions, which fuse in the midline, form both the anterior cusp of the mitral valve and the medial cusp of the tricuspid valve,

and the right lateral atrioventricular endocardial cushion continuous with the right bulbar ridge forms both the posterior and anterior cusps of the tricuspid valve. This occurs while the embryo is six to seven weeks old. Later the cushion tissue is invaded by ventricular muscle, which is then replaced by collagen. It is suggested that in mitral atresia the left lateral cushion and the central cushion fuse at this stage or earlier, thus failing to produce a valve. The associated defects are probably secondary to the resultant changes in blood flow, although some may result from the same insult to the embryo which produced the mitral atresia.

Friedman and associates (1955) consider that hypoplasia of the left heart is a basic development anomaly which is uniformly associated with stenosis or atresia of the mitral and/or aortic valves. If this hypothesis is accepted, the etiologic factor involved would be the fact that a rudimentary left atrium is unable to produce sufficient blood flow to lead to the normal development of the mitral half of the atrioventricular canal. This leads to its obliteration by the atrioventricular cushions. The left ventricle, having thus been deprived of its normal blood flow, then fails to develop, which in turn will lead to diminished aortic blood flow and possible stenosis of the aortic valve or coarctation of the aorta, unless sufficient blood flow reaches this vessel through the interventricular foramen.

The high incidence of patent ductus arteriosus and preductal coarctation of the aorta might be related to reduced aortic flow in the absence of a normally functioning left ventricle. It is noteworthy that no cases with pulmonary stenosis had coarctation or interruption of the aorta.

On the basis of the cases studied and the available evidence, it would seem that mitral atresia is the basic defect, and that once this has occurred there is no stimulus for the left ventricle to develop. It is also responsible for the diversion of the inferior vena caval flow through the tricuspid valve with, therefore, a reduced flow into the left atrium and rudimentary development of this chamber.

Pathology

There is, of course, no mitral valve structure, although there is often a dimple or shallow depression in the floor of the left atrium. Although the atretic mitral valve is usually represented by a dimple, we have seen examples of membranous mitral atresia. In such instances, the valve leaflets are fused and are not patent, but there are primitive elements of apparatus. In addition, mitral atresia has been observed in some patients with atrioventricular canal defects and grossly underdeveloped left ventricle (see below). The left atrium is small, although its walls are often thick and hypertrophied. A few cases have endocardial fibroelastosis of the left atrium. The right atrium is always large. The two atria usually communicated via a patent foramen ovale (two-thirds of cases) or other atrial septal defect (one-third of cases). The septum may be intact occasionally. One such case had a levoatrial cardinal vein, another had an opening between the left atrium and the coronary sinus, but in three infants there was no demonstrable communication between the pulmonary venous return and the right side of the heart (Watson et al., 1960; Lucas et al., 1962; Shone and Edwards, 1964; Beckman et al., 1975).

Anomalies of the venous return are frequent. A persistent left superior vena cava was present in many. Various forms of total anomalous pulmonary venous return are seen. Minor anomalies of the course of the systemic and pulmonary veins to their correct atria are common (Shone and Edwards, 1964; Beckman et al., 1975; Macartney et al., 1976).

The tricuspid valve is large but normal. The right ventricle is always large and thick-walled. In one-quarter of the cases no left ventricle is seen. When the left ventricle is present, it usually communicates with the right via a ventricular septal defect, usually small and high. The left ventricle is of normal size in only a rare instance, being small or rudimentary in the others.

There may be pulmonary atresia, pulmonary stenosis, and bicuspid or otherwise malformed, but not stenosed, pulmonary valves. Frequently the great vessels are transposed or the aorta is dextraposed (Eliot et al., 1965; Cabrera et al., 1974; Glancy and Roberts, 1976; Moreno et al., 1976). The coronary arteries are usually normal. The right aortic arch and right descending aorta may occur.

The ductus arteriosus is patent in 80 percent of cases. Coarctation of the aorta may be present.

Rarely, mitral atresia may be associated with straddling tricuspid valve (Rosenquist, 1974). Mitral atresia has also been observed in patients with endocardial cushion defect and underdeveloped left ventricle. The mitral valve is primitive, and the common atrioventricular valve communicates predominantly with the right ventricle. There is often subaortic stenosis, and rarely atresia in this situation, resulting from the maladherent anterior leaflet (Macartney et al., 1976).

Pathophysiology

In a typical case of mitral atresia with normal aortic valve, the blood returns from the lungs to the left atrium, crosses to the right atrium where it mixes with the systemic venous return, and passes into the (right) ventricle and out both the aorta and pulmonary artery. The potential sites of obstruction are between the lungs and the right atrium (usually at the atrial septum), in the pulmonary outflow, and at the aortic isthmus. The ventricular septal defect is a site of obstruction since it is the only mode of entrance of circulation into the left ventricle.

Since it is chiefly the right heart chambers that accept and propel both the systemic and pulmonary venous returns, the right atrium and ventricle are always enlarged and hypertrophied. The constant finding at necropsy of a small left atrium might be explained by the frequent presence of associated malformations tending to decrease the volume of pulmonary venous return to that chamber (e.g., pulmonary stenosis or anomalous pulmonary venous drainage), except that even in cases where the anatomy might favor enlargement of the left atrium, it is still relatively hypoplastic.

These hearts function similarly to those with a single ventricle. There is a systemic level of systolic pressure in the right ventricle and, in the absence of pulmonary stenosis, in the pulmonary arteries as well. The left atrial exit is often inadequate, and back pressure may be produced in the pulmonary veins. These two factors tend to produce pulmonary congestion. Diminution in the pulmonary flow, due either to this congestion or to pulmonary stenosis, has been cited as the cause of the cyanosis, but it seems more reasonable to attribute the cyanosis to the obligatory mixing of the venous returns in the right atrium.

Clinical Features

History. Most infants with this anomaly developed persistent cyanosis during the first week of life, while others were not noted to become cyanosed until as late as seven months of age, and some were never continuously blue. The cyanosis was usually worse on crying or feeding, and cyanotic episodes were only sometimes relieved by oxygen or morphine. Rapid, labored, or irregular breathing was reported in two-thirds of the cases. Failure to gain was frequent among those who survived the first weeks of life and was noted in a number. Other symptoms were irritability, lethargy, difficulty in feeding, cardiac irregularities, fainting spells, and convulsions. Three of the children who lived more than one year developed definite exercise intolerance.

Physical Examination. The physical findings of cyanosis, dyspnea, and physical retardation are common. A few of the older children may have a precordial bulge and digital clubbing. Definite murmurs have been noted in one-third; five of these had pulmonary stenosis with characteristic murmur, and this bore no obvious relationship to any specific cardiac defect. The second sound in the pulmonic area is usually described as accentuated. Splitting of the second sound, if present, was close. Blood pressure determinations may indicate coarctation of the aorta. Congestive heart failure is frequent.

Ross and associates (1963) described three cases of mitral stenosis and one of mitral atresia with continuous murmurs due to a small interatrial opening and left atrial hypertension. The differentiation of this murmur from that caused by a systemic arterial shunt can be made by attention to three points. First, the continuous murmur they described was localized to the lower sternal border and was usually louder on the right than the left. Second, the murmur increased in intensity with inspiration, and, third, there was a marked reduction or complete abolition of the murmur by the Valsalva maneuver. The presence of a continuous murmur due to this cause has been confirmed by Rowe (1963) in some infants with aortic or mitral atresia whose pulmonary venous return is forced through a foramen ovale in a reverse direction.

Oximetry

A number of our cases were studied by ear oximetry. Eight-five percent showed definite arterial oxygen desaturation at rest. The majority showed a definite drop in saturation on crying or exercise.

Radiologic Examination

Ninety-five percent had cardiac enlargement, but there was no apparent relationship between the degree of enlargement and the type of associated defects. The cardiothoracic ratio ranges from 0.47 to 0.67, with an average of 0.58. Often the roentgenogram suggests enlargement of one or both right heart chambers. The apex is frequently tipped up and the pulmonary artery often prominent. Sometimes the presence of an "egg shape" or a narrow base suggested transposition of the great vessels. More commonly, the heart may be described as globular. We noted only one case with the left atrium enlarged. The pulmonary vascularity is increased when pulmonary stenosis is not present.

Electrocardiography

Electrocardiographic data show the P waves are peaked, ranging in height from 1.5 to 7 mm, and averaging 3.5 mm. The ÂQRS averaged +140 degrees but was normal in one case and leftward on rare occasions. Most cases have a horizontal or semihorizontal position and clockwise rotation. One-quarter of the patients have Q waves in the right precordial leads; occasionally there may be bilateral

Q waves. Right ventricular hypertrophy according to our criteria was noted in all infants seen at The Hospital for Sick Children with electrocardiograms and in those reported in the literature. There was left ventricular hypertrophy in the case described by Megevand and coworkers (1953). The T waves are usually upright in V_1.

Echocardiography

Absence of the mitral valve echo, or marked thickening with minimal amplitude of the mitral excursion in concert with a small left ventricle, is consistent with mitral atresia (Lundstrom, 1972). These echographic features of mitral atresia may also be observed in patients with mitral atresia and single ventricle, double-outlet right ventricle, and other forms of complex heart malformations.

Angiocardiography

Angiocardiograms in cases diagnosed as mitral atresia are described by Kjellberg and associates (1955), Gasul and associates (1957), and Watson and coworkers (1960). Venous angiocardiograms show a large right atrium and ventricle and yield some other information but tend to be unsatisfactory because of dilution and because of the large right chambers obscure the rest of the heart. The preferred procedure to demonstrate mitral atresia would be a selective study and with injection of contrast material into the left atrium.

Angiocardiography should also demonstrate such associated malformations as transposition of the great vessels and pulmonary stenosis and may outline the small left ventricle or may suggest single ventricle.

Cardiac Catheterization

Catheter studies show a pronounced rise in oxygen saturation between the vena caval and right atrial samples, with little further rise. There were relatively high pressures with large "a" waves in the right atrium and systemic level of systolic pressure in the right ventricle (60 mm of mercury or more). The pressures may be similar in both atria, but the oxygen saturation in the left atrium is significantly higher. In one case the descending aorta was entered through a ductus arteriosus, and the systolic pressure and oxygen saturation there were almost the same as in the right ventricle and pulmonary artery.

Differential Diagnosis

Infants and children with mitral atresia exhibit slight to moderate cyanosis and dyspnea, failure to thrive, second heart sounds in the pulmonary area, which are usually accentuated, and single and nonspecific murmurs. Congestive heart failure is frequent and coarctation not uncommon. This means that, on the basis of history and physical examination, this malformation closely mimics a number of common congenital cardiac defects.

Two investigations, namely a roentgenogram of the chest and an electrocardiogram, will assist in a preliminary narrowing of the possibilities.

Roentgenographically, where there is obviously increased pulmonary blood flow, the chief malformations likely to confuse are isolated preductal coarctation of the aorta, aortic atresia or severe stenosis, transposition of the great vessels, truncus arteriosus, corrected transposition of the great vessels with a ventricular septal defect, and total anomalies of the pulmonary venous return. The roentgenographic appearance of pulmonary congestion, rather than increased flow, does not exclude mitral atresia but would favor malformations such as congenital mitral stenosis, contracted endocardial fibroelastosis, cor triatiatum, and total anomalous pulmonary venous return of the infradiaphragmatic variety. Roentgenographic evidence of reduced pulmonary blood flow, in the case of mitral atresia with pulmonary stenosis, may be confused with pulmonary atresia or stenosis with normal aortic root, tetralogy of Fallot, and single ventricle or transposition of the great vessels with pulmonary stenosis.

One fairly consistent feature of the electrocardiogram in mitral atresia is a qR pattern in the right precordial leads. While this feature is not specific, it should provide a very useful diagnostic aid since it is rare in the malformations already considered in the differential diagnosis with the exclusion of aortic atresia, total anomalous pulmonary venous drainage, single ventricle with pulmonary stenosis, corrected transposition with ventricular septal defect, and isolated pulmonary stenosis. Rarely, cardiac rhabdomyoma may simulate mitral atresia (Mair et al., 1977).

Cardiac catheterization and angiocardiography are necessary for final clarification. Aortic atresia, single ventricle, and total anomalous pulmonary venous return at the cardiac level often reveal identical catheterization data. Right ventricular angiocardiography is frankly misleading, but selective injection of contrast media into the left atrium should provide the necessary confirmation of an atretic mitral valve.

Treatment

Clearly, medical management of this malformation will not be attended by conspicuous success. Enlargement of the atrial septal defect has been suggested in patients with restrictive atrial communication. Balloon septostomy may achieve this in the early weeks of life. Park and his associates (1975, 1976) have reported nonsurgical atrial septostomy using a blade catheter in a 7-week-old with mitral atresia, double-outlet right ventricle, and a very restrictive atrial defect. At present the importance of the defect lies in its differentiation from potentially operable lesions and in giving an accurate prognosis to the parents of affected infants. The patient with mitral atresia and pulmonary stenosis may be benefited by augmenting pulmonary blood flow by construction of a systemic-to-pulmonary artery anastomosis. If left atrial pressure is elevated, however, because of a restrictive atrial communication, the surgical anastomosis may not function (Friedman et al., 1976). In such an instance, surgical atrial septectomy or septostomy should be combined with a systemic-to-pulmonary artery anastomosis. In the patient with mitral atresia, unobstructed systemic blood supply, and normal pulmonary artery pressure (i.e., from pulmonary stenosis or pulmonary arterial banding), one could theoretically divert pulmonary venous return into the tricuspid valve, and route systemic venous blood to the distal pulmonary artery, ligating the proximal pulmonary artery. This would bring systemic blood to the lungs, and the patient's own tricuspid valve would serve as the patient's "systemic atrioventricular valve." To our knowledge this approach has not been successfully used through mid-1977.

REFERENCES

Abbott, M. E.: *Atlas of Congenital Cardiac Disease.* American Heart Association, New York, 1936, p. 50.

Abrams, H. L.: Persistence of fetal ductus function after birth. *Circulation,* **18**:206, 1958.

Beckman, C. B.; Moller, J. H.; and Edwards, J. E.: Alternate pathways to pulmonary venous flow in left-sided obstructive anomalies. *Circulation,* **52**:509, 1975.

Bergman, W., and Morales, O.: A rare form of congenital heart disease. *Acta Paediatr.,* **35**:364, 1948.

Brockman, H. L.: Congenital mitral atresia, transposition of the great vessels and congenital aortic coarctation. *Am. Heart J.,* **40**:301, 1950.

Cabrera, A.; Azcuna, J. I.; and Bilbao, F.: Single primitive ventricle with D-transposition of the great vessels and atresia of the left A.V. valve. *Am. Heart J.,* **88**:225, 1974.

Campbell, M.; Reynolds, G.; and Trounce, J. R.: Six cases of single ventricle with pulmonary stenosis. *Guy Hosp. Rep.,* **102**:99, 1953.

Conn, J. J.; Clark, T. E.; and Kissane, R. W.: Cor triloculare. *Am. J. Med.,* **8**:187, 1950.

Dudzus, M.: Über Cor triloculare biatriatum mit Atresia des linken venosen. *Arch. Pathol. Anat.,* **237**:32, 1922.

Durie, B., and Wyndham, N. R.: Description of two human specimens with congenital absence of the spleen, abnormal arrangements of the great vessels, abnormal cardiac cavities, and other congenital defects. *Med. J. Aust.,* **2**:174, 1942.

Edwards, J. E.: In Gould, S. E. (ed.): *Pathology of the Heart.* Charles C Thomas, Publisher, Springfield, Ill., 1953, p. 386.

Edwards, J. E., and Dushane, J. W.: Thoracic venous anomalies: 1. Vascular connections of the left atrium and the left innominate vein (laevo-atrio-cardinal vein) associated with mitral atresia in premature closure of the foramen ovale. *Arch. Pathol.,* **49**:517, 1950.

Edwards, J. E., and Rodgers, H. M.: Atresia of the orifice of the mitral valve. *J. Tech. Methods,* **27**:62, 1947.

Eliot, R. S.; Shone, J. D.; Kanjab, V. I.; Ruttenberg, H. D.; Carey, L. S.; and Edwards, J. E.: Mitral atresia: A study of 32 cases. *Am. Heart J.,* **70**:6, 1965.

Evans, W.: Congenital stenosis (coarctation), atresia, and interruption of the aortic arch. *Q. J. Med.,* **2**:1, 1933.

Friedman, S.; Edmunds, L. H.; Saraclar, M.; and Weinstein, E. M.: Mitral atresia with premature closure of foramen ovale. A rare hemodynamic cause for failure of Blalock-Taussig anastomosis to relieve inadequate pulmonary blood flow. *J. Thorac. Cardiovasc. Surg.*, **71**:117, 1976.

Friedman, S.; Murphy, L.; and Ash, R.: Congenital mitral atresia with hypoplastic non-functioning left heart. *Am. J. Dis. Child.*, **90**:176, 1955.

Gasul, B.; Hait, G.; Dillon, R. F.; and Fell, E. H.: *The Salient Points and the Value of Venous Angiography in the Diagnosis of the Cyanotic Types of Congenital Malformations of the Heart.* Charles C Thomas, Publisher, Springfield, Ill., 1957, pp. 50, 72.

Glancy, D. L., and Roberts, W. C.: Congenital obstructive lesions involving the major pulmonary veins, left atrium, or mitral valve: A clinical, laboratory, and morphological survey. *Cathet. Cardiovasc. Diag.*, **2**:215, 1976.

Harris, J. S., and Farber, S.: Transposition of the great cardiac vessels with special reference to the phylogenetic theory of Spitzer. *Arch. Pathol.*, **28**:427, 1939.

Hollman, A.: Personal communication re case noted in Electrocardiographic diagnosis of right ventricular hypertrophy in infancy and childhood. *Br. Heart J.*, **20**:129, 1958.

Hu, C. H.: Congenital malformation of heart with anomalous insertion of pulmonary veins, absence of spleen, situs inversus of abdominal viscera and other development errors. *Am. J. Pathol.*, **5**:389, 1929.

Ivemark, B. I.: Implications of agenesis of the spleen in the pathogenesis of conotruncus anomalies in childhood. *Acta Paediatr.*, **44**:Suppl. 104, 1955, p. 110.

Jost, J.: *Zur Casuistik der Angeborenen Fehler des linken Herzens.* Giessen, 1896, p. 27.

Keith, J. D.; Rowe, R. D.; and Vlad, P.: *Heart Disease in Infancy and Childhood.* Macmillan Publishing Co., Inc., New York, 1958, pp. 38, 43.

Kintner, E. P.: Congenital malformation of the heart: interruption of the aortic arch, mitral valve orifice atresia, and persistent left superior vena cava. *Lab. Invest.*, **2**:388, 1953.

Kjellberg, S. R.; Mannheimer, E.; Rudhe, U.; and Jonnson, B.: *Diagnosis of Congenital Heart Disease.* Year Book Publishers, Inc., Chicago, 1955, p. 571.

Kleinerman, J.; Yang, W-M.; Hackel, D. B.; and Kaufman, N.: Absence of the transverse aortic arch. *Arch. Pathol.*, **65**:490, 1958.

Krumbhaar, E. B.: A congenital cardiac anomaly: atresia of the mitral orifice and separation of the left auricle and ventricle, with appended case of absent left ventricle. *J. Mount. Sinai Hosp. N.Y.*, **8**:737, 1942.

Lam, C. R.; Knights, E. M.; and Ziegler, R. F.: Combined mitral and pulmonary atresia. *Am. Heart J.*, **46**:314, 1953.

Large, H. L.: Congenital mitral atresia; report of 2 cases. *Am. J. Med. Sci.*, **219**:268, 1950.

Lawrence, T. W. P., and Nabarro, D.: A case of congenital malformation of the heart, with abnormalities of abdominal viscera: absence of spleen, absence of hepatic section of inferior cava. *J. Anat. Physiol.*, **36**:63, 1901.

Lucas, R. V., Jr.; Lester, R. G.; Lillehei, C. W.; and Edwards, J. E.: Mitral atresia with levoatrial cardinal vein. A form of congenital pulmonary venous obstruction. *Am. J. Cardiol.*, **9**:607, 1962.

Lundstrom, N. R.: Ultrasound-cardiographic studies of the mitral valve in young infants with mitral atresia and mitral stenosis, hypoplasia of the left ventricle and cor triatriatum. *Circulation*, **45**:324, 1972.

Macartney, F. J.; Bain, H. H.; Ionescu, M. I.; Deverall, P. B.; and Scott, O.: Angiocardiographic/pathologic correlations in congenital mitral valve anomalies. *Eur. J. Cardiol.*, **4**:191, 1976.

McIntosh, C. A.: Cor biatriatum triloculare. *Am. Heart J.*, **1**:735, 1926.

Mair, D. D.; Titus, J. L.; Davis, G. D.; and Ritter, D. G.: Cardiac rhabdomyoma simulating mitral atresia. *Chest*, **71**:102, 1977.

Manhoff, L. J., and Howe, J. S.: Congenital heart disease: tricuspid atresia and mitral atresia associated with transposition of the great vessels. *Am. Heart J.*, **29**:90, 1945.

Megevand, R. P.; Paul, R. N.; and Parker, J.: Single ventricle with diminutive outlet chamber associated with coarctation of the aorta and other cardiac anomalies. *J. Pediatr.*, **43**:687, 1953.

Moenckeberg, J. G.: In Henke, F., and Lubarsch, O.: *Handbuch der Speziellen Pathologischen Anatomie und Histologie*, Springer, Berlin, 1924, Vol. 2, p. 124. Quoted by Scriba.

Moreno, F.; Quero, M.; and Diaz, L. P.: Mitral atresia with normal aortic valve. A study of eighteen cases and a review of the literature. *Circulation*, **53**:1004, 1976.

Nihoyannopoulos, J.; Zannos, L.; Oeconomou-Mavrou, C.; and Statherou, E.: Report of a case with congenital absence of the spleen and levocardia. *J. Clin. Pathol.*, **9**:323, 1956.

Noonan, J., and Nadas, A. S.: The hypoplastic left heart syndrome. *Pediatr. Clin. North Am.*, November, 1958, p. 1029.

Odgers, P. N. B.: The development of the atrio-ventricular valves in man. *J. Anat.*, **73**:643, 1939.

Park, S. C.; Neches, W. H.; Zuberbuhler, J. R.; Lenox, C. C.; and Zoltan, R. A.: Successful non-surgical atrial septostomy by blade catheter. *Circulation* (Suppl. II), **53, 54**:169, 1976 (abstr.).

Park, S. C.; Zuberbuhler, J. R.; Neches, W. H.; Lenox, C. C.; and Zoltan, R. A.: A new atrial septostomy technique. *Cathet. Cardiovasc. Diag.*, **1**:195, 1975.

Potter, E. L.: *Pathology of the Fetus and Newborn.* Year Book Publishers, Inc., Chicago, 1952, p. 225.

Putschar, W. J. G., and Manion, W. C.: Congenital absence of the spleen and associated anomalies. *Am. J. Clin. Pathol.*, **26**:429, 1956.

Rosen, L.; Bowden, D. H.; and Uchida, I.: Structural changes in the pulmonary arteries in the first year of life. *Arch. Pathol.*, **63**:316, 1957.

Rosenquist, G. C.: Over-riding right atrioventricular valve in association with mitral atresia. *Am. Heart. J.*, **87**:26, 1974.

Ross, J., Jr.; Braunwald, E.; Mason, D. T.; Braunwald, N. S.; and Morrow, A. G.: Interatrial communication and left atrial hypertension. A cause of continuous murmur. *Circulation*, **28**:853, 1963.

Rossi, E.: Herzkrankheiten im Sauglingsalter. Georg Thieme Verlag, Stuttgart, 1954, p. 149.

Rowe, R. D.: Personal communication, 1963.

Schwanen, H.: Zwei seltene Herzmisbildungen. *Ztschr. Geburt. Gynak.*, **106**:416, 1932.

Scriba, K.: Ueber die angeborene Atresie des Mitral- und Tricuspidalostimums. *Zentrabl. Allg. Pathol.*, **67**:353, 1937.

Shone, J. D., and Edwards, J. E.: Mitral atresia with pulmonary venous anomalies. *Br. Heart J.*, **26**:241, 1964.

Spolverini, L. M., and Barbieri, D.: Ueber die angeborenen Herzfehler. *Jahrb. Kinderh.*, **6**:472, 1902.

Taussig, H. B.: *Congenital Malformations of the Heart.* The Commonwealth Fund, New York, 1947, p. 295.

Teller, W. M.: Congenital mitral atresia. *Am. Heart J.*, **56**:304, 1958.

Theremin, E.: *Affections Congenitales du Coeur.* Asselin et Houzeau, Paris, 1895, p. 161.

Vega, E. G.: Corazon monoventricular, triatrial (?) por agenesia mitral y ventricular izquierda. *Rev. Cubana Pediatr.*, **28**:545, 1956.

Voussure, G.; Zylberszac, S.; and Pele, S.: Atresie mitrale et ventricule unique. *Acta Cardiol.*, **11**:185, 1956.

Watson, D. G.; Rowe, R. D.; Conen, P. E.; and Duckworth, J. W.: Mitral atresia with normal aortic valve. Report of 11 cases and review of the literature. *Pediatrics*, **25**:450, 1960.

32

Anomalies of Venous Return

Richard D. Rowe

ANOMALIES OF SYSTEMIC VENOUS RETURN

PERSISTENCE OF THE LEFT SUPERIOR VENA CAVA

Frequency

THE EXACT frequency of all the different types of persistent left superior vena cava is unknown, but it is believed to be found once in every 350 autopsies and once in every 200 of the general population (Steinberg et al., 1953). In patients with congenital heart disease a persistent left superior vena cava has been noted in between 3 and 5 percent (Campbell and Deuchar, 1954; Fraser et al., 1961; Cha and Khoury, 1972).

Pathologic Anatomy

In all varieties of a persistent left superior vena cava the anomaly can be considered the result of a failure to atrophy of the left anterior cardinal vein below the origin of the brachiocephalic vein. Thus, after a union of the left jugular and left subclavian veins, a left superior vena cava descends vertically in the thorax to the left of the spine. The anatomy of the proximal connection of the persistent left superior vena cava varies, there being several possible arrangements.

Group (a): Proximal Connection of the Left Superior Vena Cava to the Coronary Sinus. This is by far the most frequent type. The anomaly is most often an isolated one (Beattie, 1931; Abbott, 1936; McManus, 1941; Friedlich et al., 1950), in which case there is no functional disturbance. Winter (1954) found this to be the case in 60 percent of 174 cases in the literature. The right superior vena cava is usually present but may be absent (Beattie, 1931; Karnegis et al., 1964) and in 40 percent there is a communication between the venae cavae (Winter, 1954). Associated defects are being more commonly seen and recorded since the advent of accessory studies in congenital

heart disease. These are chiefly atrial septal defects and partial anomalies of pulmonary venous return (Winter, 1954; Miller et al., 1955; Fraser et al., 1961) but have included almost every known cardiac malformation. Association with anomalies of the inferior vena cava has also been reported (Campbell and Deuchar, 1954).

Group (b): Proximal Connection of the Left Superior Vena Cava to the Left Atrium. Much less commonly the persistent left superior vena cava communicates directly with the left atrium. This has been found as an isolated anomaly (Davis et al., 1959; Tuchman et al., 1956; Sherafat et al., 1971). The condition may exist with or without a right superior vena cava attached normally to the right atrium (Taybi et al., 1965). Other cases have been described all of which were associated with complicating anomalies (Diaz et al., 1949; Feindt and Hauch, 1953; Gasul et al., 1953; Friedlich et al., 1950; Peel et al., 1956). One autopsy-proved case of tetralogy of Fallot complicated by this variant was encountered at The Hospital for Sick Children, Toronto. In a further two cases (Mankin and Burchell, 1953; Odman, 1953), one or several pulmonary veins entered the left superior vena cava distal to its connection with the left atrium. The former case was different from others in that, although most of the blood from the left superior vena cava drained into the left atrium, the left superior vena cava was actually connected to the coronary sinus, a communication existing between the sinus and the left atrium. A case of McCotter (1916) had a similar arrangement to that of Mankin and Burchell except that there were no accompanying anomalies of the pulmonary veins. The child described by Sherafat and colleagues (1971) presented at the age of five years with cerebral abscess. There were mild cyanosis and clubbing associated with a left dominant electrocardiogram. The left superior vena cava was large and tortuous and was repaired. Although this form of connection is usually associated with mild cyanosis, in some there may be no arterial oxygen desaturation (Meadows and Sharp, 1965).

Group (c); No Proximal Communication of the Left Superior Vena Cava. UNION OF LEFT SUPERIOR VENA CAVA AND PULMONARY VEINS. In both partial (left) and total anomalous pulmonary venous drainage, the pulmonary veins may unite and enter a persistent left superior vena cava that has a connection with the systemic venous circulation at the left innominate vein only. This variant is described in more detail under the section on anomalous pulmonary venous drainage.

LEFT SUPERIOR VENA CAVA ASSOCIATED WITH ATRESIA OF THE OSTIUM OF THE CORONARY SINUS. Several cases of this malformation were collected by Edwards (1953). Venous blood from the heart, under these circumstances, reaches the right atrium indirectly through the left superior vena cava, left innominate vein, and right superior vena cava. A variant of this anomaly exists where the atretic right atrial ostium of the coronary sinus is associated with a venous connection into the left atrium. Atresia of the coronary sinus can also occur without a persistent left superior vena cava and in such cases the coronary sinus communicates with the left atrium. Other anomalies are usually present (Falcone and Roberts, 1972).

Diagnosis

There are no specific physical or electrocardiographic signs permitting unequivocal recognition in any variety, although about one-third of the patients with left superior vena cava draining into the coronary sinus and congenital intracardiac defect show left-axis deviation of the P wave between +15 degrees and +340 degrees (Momma and Linde, 1969).

Abnormal left jugular pulsation has been a physical feature that can be the first clue to the presence of a persistent left superior vena cava (Colman, 1967). A probably X-linked recessive form of Pierre-Robin's syndrome with left superior vena cava and atrial defect has been described (Gorlin, 1970). In any of the three groups mentioned above, in x-rays of the chest a vertical venous shadow is often, but not invariably, visible along the left border of the supracardiac portion of the mediastinum. This sign is almost always absent in infant cases and is most obvious after the first six months of life in the case of group (c) with total anomalous venous drainage into a left superior vena cava.

Nuclear angiography would appear to offer a useful method for confirming these arrangements.

During cardiac catheterization from a left antecubital vein, the catheter enters a left superior vena cava and right heart via the coronary sinus in most cases of group (a) (Figure 32–1), or the left atrium and left ventricle in cases of group (b). In the latter group cardiac catheterization is not without

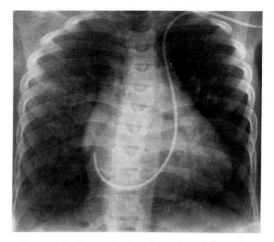

Figure 32-1. Demonstration of a persistent left superior vena cava connected to the coronary sinus. The patient had an isolated atrial septal defect. The cardiac catheter has entered the right atrium from an antecubital vein through the left superior vena cava and coronary sinus.

danger; for example, the case of Peel and associates (1956) terminated in death during the procedure, whereas in a case at The Hospital for Sick Children shock developed after the procedure. The catheter may also be passed into the left superior vena cava and pulmonary veins in group (c) cases. In complicated cases angiocardiography usually provides the most definitive information (Castellanos et al., 1944; Diaz et al., 1949). With the venous technique from the left arm, the presence or absence of cross communication between the venae cavae is established and the subsequent course of the contrast permits a statement of the type of left superior vena cava and associated malformations. It may be necessary to perform studies from the right arm as well. Selective angiocardiography is not, therefore, the method of choice initially, particularly in the complicated cases.

Treatment

In the majority of patients in group (a) no treatment is necessary for the persistent channel. In an isolated case of group (b) cure may be accomplished by simple ligation of the left superior vena cava provided that a superior vena cava exists on the right. Alternatively, anastomosis of the anomalous vessel to the right atrium may be performed. Even complicated cases of this type may be greatly improved by ligation of the left superior vena cava (Diaz et al., 1949; Feindt and Hauch, 1953). The available surgical measures for left superior vena cava of certain cases of group (c) are outlined in the section on anomalous pulmonary venous drainage. Finally, in an occasional case, surgery for an associated defect may be obstructed by the presence of a left superior vena cava. It is unwise to ligate the vessel unless preliminary investigation has clarified its connections. Occlusion of the vessel at operation has long been the method of evaluation (Frank and Maloney, 1968), but the occlusion of a left superior vena cava by a balloon catheter allows evaluation of the collateral arrangements through pressure and angiographic methods for patients with a variety of major malformations where such details are essential for correct surgical management (Freed et al., 1973).

DRAINAGE OF THE RIGHT SUPERIOR VENA CAVA TO THE LEFT ATRIUM

This variant is considered to be a developmental defect of the sinus venosus and, although rare, seems more frequent than either isolated drainage of the left superior vena cava to the left atrium or of an inferior vena cava to the left atrium. Three patients between two and ten years of age have been reported (Wood, 1956; Kirsch et al., 1961; Braudo et al., 1968), one of these being a three-year-old child investigated and treated for this malformation at The Hospital for Sick Children (Figure 32–2). All the children with the anomaly have been cyanotic and showed clubbing, but the degree of these signs has varied. The electrocardiogram, likewise, has ranged from normal to distinct left ventricular hypertrophy, while the heart size on x-ray has usually been normal. In our case the right jugular vein was grossly distended by crying, and the arterial oxygen saturation in this patient fell from 81 to 63 percent during such effort. Indicator dilution curves from the superior and inferior vena cava together with contrast injection established the diagnosis. Nuclear angiocardiography has been a useful diagnostic tool (Park et al., 1973).

Successful surgical repair was achieved in the case of Kirsch and associates (1961) and in our patient

(Braudo et al., 1968). In the latter case two pulmonary veins from the right lung were seen to enter a varicose superior vena cava at the time of surgery.

ABSENCE OF THE INFERIOR VENA CAVA (ANOMALOUS INFERIOR VENA CAVA WITH AZYGOS CONTINUATION)

Frequency

The frequency of this venous anomaly is difficult to estimate. Stackelberg and associates (1952) found it twice in 100 angiocardiograms from the malleolar vein. Anderson and associates (1961), in a comprehensive review of the topic, reported that the anomaly occurred in 0.6 percent of their patients with congenital heart disease and were able to collect 26 previous reports to add to 15 personal cases.

Pathologic Anatomy

Normally the azygos vein communicates with either the right renal vein or the inferior vena cava. In the latter type during cardiac catheterization in infant cases, the right atrium may very rarely be entered by both routes. In the true anomaly, however, the inferior vena cava becomes continuous with the lower portion of the azygos system, losing all connection with the inferior portion of the heart. In such cases the only course for blood from the lower extremities into the right atrium is through the azygos vein and the superior vena cava. The anomaly is a failure to fuse of the hepatic and prerenal segments of the inferior vena cava together with a persistence of either the right lumbar azygos or left lumbar hemiazygos veins. In about 50 percent of cases the malformation occurs in

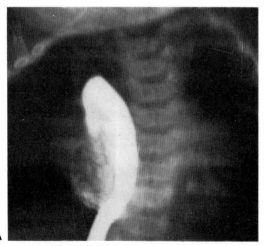

A

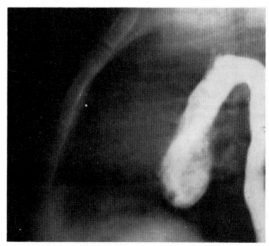

B

Figure 32-2. Absence of the proximal portion of the inferior vena cava. Venous angiocardiogram from the saphenous vein showing contrast entering the right atrium from the superior vena cava after having traversed the azygos vein.

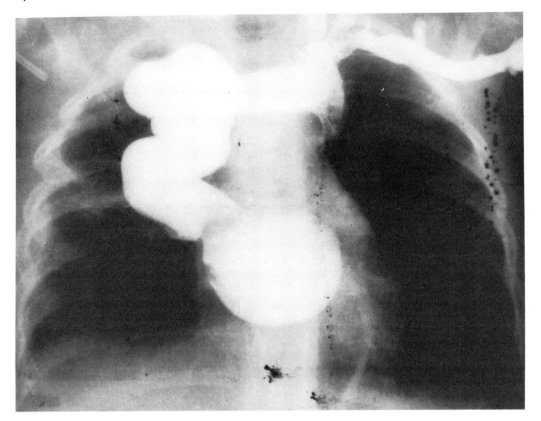

Figure 32-3. Connection of a right superior vena cava to the left atrium. Angiographic appearance in a three-year-old child from The Hospital for Sick Children (Braudo et al., 1968).

association with a combination of dextrocardia or levocardia, cor biloculare, and pulmonary atresia (Taussig, 1947; Campbell et al., 1952; Anderson et al., 1955; Hospital for Sick Children, 1956). The remaining cases are accompanied by less severe defects either of the septal variety (Stackelberg et al., 1952; Downing, 1953) or of the pulmonary veins (Levinson et al., 1953). We have encountered the rather unusual complex of levocardia and secundum atrial septal defect with azygos continuation of the inferior vena cava. Very rarely the anomaly may be an isolated one (Stackelberg et al., 1952). Over half the cases have other venous anomalies, of which a persistent left superior vena cava is the chief. The hepatic veins enter separately into the right atrium, but in cases associated with levocardia they may enter the left atrium. It is probable that many of the reported cases with this malformation were examples of the polysplenia syndrome (Freedom and Ellison, 1973).

Diagnosis

The anomaly by itself is, of course, benign, but in the cyanotic cases its presence is a sure sign of a complicated intracardiac defect.

On plain x-ray films, as has been shown by Downing (1953), there is a characteristic rounded density in the superior mediastinum projecting to the right at the level of the normal junction of the superior vena cava and right atrium. A more frequent sign of azygous continuation, especially in cyanotic patients with abnormalities of the abdominal situs, is absence of the inferior vena caval shadow on an adequate lateral chest film (Heller et al., 1971). It has been stressed by O'Reilly and Grollman (1976) that the presence of a caval shadow does not exclude the diagnosis of absent inferior vena cava because the cranial component of the hepatic segment may show as inferior vena cava in the lateral film. Pleural reflections, parenchymal densities, and even some normal individuals may explain absence of the inferior vena cava line shadow in individuals with normal attachment.

The majority of patients with azygous continuation as part of complex congenital heart malformations such as in polysplenia will have leftward and superior P wave axes (Freedom and Ellison, 1973).

Cardiac catheterization from the groin may be confusing until the tip enters the superior vena cava and right atrium via the azygos vein. Manipulation further than the right ventricle is difficult by this inferior approach unless Swan-Ganz flotation balloon catheters are employed (Kelly et al., 1971). The condition may be missed entirely if catheterization or angiocardiography is performed from an arm vein. A venous angiocardiogram from the leg produces a characteristic appearance (Figure 32–3), a similar appearance being evident with radionuclide venography (Freedom and Treves, 1973).

Treatment and Prognosis

There is no specific treatment, the prognosis being that of the associated intracardiac anomaly.

INFERIOR VENA CAVA ENTERING A LEFT ATRIUM

A few patients have been described where the inferior vena cava enters the left atrium instead of the right (Gardner and Cole, 1955; Gautam, 1968; Kim et al., 1971). Although there is debate about the authenticity of the defect, survival into adult life is usually described. Cyanosis from birth is to be expected but varies in degree. The electrocardiogram shows normal axis of the QRS with marked left ventricular hypertrophy. The importance of this anomaly, though it is rare, lies in the fact that it may be satisfactorily demonstrated with modern techniques and that surgical correction is possible. Two patients described by Taybi and associates (1965) each showed an anomalous left inferior vena cava with left azygos continuation to a left superior vena cava and left atrium. Both patients had a common atrium as part of their congenital heart malformation and one had polysplenia.

LEVOATRIOCARDINAL VEIN

Edwards and DuShane (1950) introduced the term "levoatriocardinal vein" to describe communications between the left atrium and a systemic vein other than through a left superior vena cava or coronary sinus. In these cases the anomalous vessel arises from the dorsal aspect of the left atrium near the entrance of a pulmonary vein and ascends dorsal to the bronchus and pulmonary artery on the side on which it originates. The condition is probably due to a failure to atrophy of early connections of pulmonary venous elements with the cardinal veins.

In the several cases reported, the most striking feature has been the association with atrioventricular valve atresia. The case of McIntosh (1926) was one of mitral atresia with a closed foramen ovale in which the vessel communicated with the superior vena cava on the right. That of Edwards and DuShane (1950) was an identical intracardiac anomaly in which the anomalous vein connected with the left innominate vein. Another case of Harris and associates (1927) was one of transposition of the great vessels in which the vein joined the right internal jugular vein.

Lambert (1959) has reported catheterization data from a five-month-old infant whose major lesion was hypoplasia of the left heart coupled with the above type of anomalous vein.

The two patients described by Taybi and associates (1965) had mitral or tricuspid valve atresia.

ANOMALIES OF PULMONARY VENOUS RETURN

WHERE pulmonary veins, instead of entering the left atrium, join the right atrium or its tributaries, the malformation is referred to as anomalous pulmonary venous drainage. Edwards (1953) prefers "anomalous pulmonary venous connection" as an anatomic term.

The first report of anomalous pulmonary venous drainage was that of a case of the partial anomaly described by Winslow in 1739. A seven-day-old infant with pulmonary venous drainage into the superior vena cava and cor biloculare (Wilson, 1798) was the first reported case of the complete anomaly. The first description of complete anomalous pulmonary venous drainage unassociated with other serious defects was that of Friedlowski (1868). Since the important paper of Brody (1942) an increasing volume of reports on the pathologic and clinical aspects of anomalous pulmonary venous drainage has appeared in the medical literature. The subject may be classified into the partial or complete anomaly with a further subdivision into complicated or uncomplicated forms, depending upon the presence or absence of major intracardiac defects. The embryologic basis for such anomalies has been described (Neill, 1956) and is discussed in Chapter 8.

PARTIAL ANOMALOUS PULMONARY VENOUS DRAINAGE—COMPLICATED FORM

Pathology

In the complicated form of the partial anomaly a variety of associated intracardiac defects has been described. Most common of these, from both pathologic reports and operative experience, is atrial septal defect. Anatomically, the defect is most often high and posteriorly placed in the atrial septum. Next most frequent are the complex defects such as tetralogy of Fallot, tricuspid atresia, and single ventricle, followed by ventricular septal defect and, more rarely, patent ductus arteriosus, in that order. With rare exceptions the drainage anomaly is confined to the right-sided pulmonary veins. Most commonly, the site of insertion of the anomalous veins is directly into right atrium. Somewhat less frequently the superior vena cava, coronary sinus, and inferior vena cava are sites of entry.

Frequency

The association of partial anomalous pulmonary venous drainage with other intracardiac defects is not uncommon but is frequently not recognized clinically, particularly in the more complex anomalies. Previously demonstration of this association was confined to occasional cases where the cardiac catheter entered the anomalous vein at study, where indicator dilution studies had been performed, by angiocardiography, or at autopsy. Corrective operative techniques, however, have enabled surgeons to show that about 15 percent of cases with atrial septal defects, for example, have pulmonary veins connected to either the right atrium or superior vena cava (Lewis et al., 1955; Ellis and Kirklin, 1955). The proportion of patients in relatively large series of atrial septal defect with superior caval complex is about 6 percent (Bedford, 1960; Evans et al., 1961). The terms "sinus venosus" (Brock and Ross, 1959) and "superior caval defect" have been used interchangeably for this particular type of atrial communication.

Clinical Features

The presence of partial anomalous pulmonary venous drainage will not necessarily ameliorate the symptoms of complicated cyanotic defects. On the other hand, it sometimes increases the symptoms associated with an *atrial septal defect.* Cases of this particular combination may occasionally cause diagnostic problems in symptomatic infant cases. More frequently the association is compatible with a longer life, and cases reported among older children and adults have had rather minor, if any, symptoms. Eventually symptoms of fatigue, exertional dyspnea, and, finally, congestive heart failure may develop. In both children and adults the clinical picture cannot usually allow differentiation from that of the isolated atrial septal defect (McCormack et al., 1960). Mankin and Burchell (1953), on the other hand, have suggested that the more impressive the clinical picture and the more evidence of right heart enlargement, the greater is the possibility of the combined lesion.

There is no specific physique associated with the anomaly, although growth retardation has been observed (Mehrizi and Drash, 1962). The growth behavior following operation has also been studied (Mehrizi et al., 1966).

A right ventricular lift and hyperdynamic precordium are evident physical signs, while auscultation invariably reveals accentuation of pulmonary valve closure in infants with pulmonary hypertension. In others, the usual fixed splitting of the second heart sound is present. Murmurs are variable, but there is usually an ejection systolic murmur of moderate intensity in the pulmonic area and a tricuspid middiastolic flow murmur along the lower left sternal border. A pulmonary diastolic murmur may also be evident when flows are large. Thrills are uncommon in infants but have been reported in older patients.

Electrocardiography

The electrocardiogram of the symptomatic infant most often reveals evidence of right ventricular hypertrophy. Otherwise the usual incomplete bundle branch block characteristic of isolated atrial septal defects is found.

Radiologic Examination

The cardiothoracic ratio and lung vascularity are most often increased. The left atrium is not enlarged. Only rarely is it possible to identify partial anomalous pulmonary venous drainage to the superior vena cava by inspection of the plain chest film.

Cardiac Catheterization

Cardiac catheterization provides evidence of a left-to-right shunt at atrial level. The pulmonary artery pressure is almost invariably elevated, but the magnitude of this change varies considerably, and often after infancy the pulmonary artery pressure level is not greatly in excess of the normal. The atrial septal defect will be probed directly by the catheter, and pulmonary veins connected to the superior vena cava may similarly be entered from that vessel. Insertion of the catheter into the right pulmonary veins from an atrium is an unsatisfactory method of demonstrating whether the veins are anomalously connected. Adding to the difficulty in children is the fact that the foramen ovale may be patent, and an incorrect assumption of atrial septal defect may be made when the catheter is passed into the left heart. These difficulties may be overcome simply if one or more of several further points are examined. After dye is injected into a suspected anomalously draining pulmonary vein, if the dilution pattern revealed by systemic arterial sampling is similar to that obtained after injection into either the superior vena cava or inferior vena cava, then that pulmonary vein must drain into the right atrium or its tributaries (Swan et al., 1953). In patients with the more frequent problem of superior caval atrial defect, the rise in oxygen saturation in blood samples begins in the superior vena cava, the catheter enters the right superior pulmonary vein in the characteristic position from the superior vena cava, and the high position of the atrial

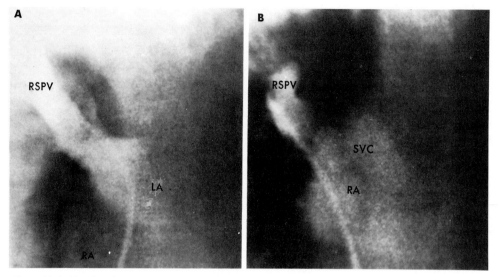

Figure 32-4. Identification of abnormally connected right pulmonary veins to the right atrium. In the normal situation (*A*) a horizontal superior margin to the atrium identifies the roof of that chamber. In the abnormal connection (*B*) there is an irregular margin rather than a roof at atrial level because of rapid dilution of the contrast entering the right atrium principally by superior venal caval blood.

defect is confirmed by the presence of a small right-to-left shunt in systemic arterial dilution patterns following injections into the superior vena cava but not from the inferior caval injections. These findings are opposite to those that are demonstrated in centrally placed secundum atrial defects (Swan et al., 1957). We have found when using the inferior approach to the heart that the high position of the catheter on crossing the atrial septum is helpful in confirming the superior caval complex. Anatomic, as well as functional, information about a particular pulmonary vein is best obtained, however, by cineangiography after injection of contrast material into the pulmonary vein with the patient in the frontal position (Folger et al., 1966) (Figure 32–4).

Angiocardiography

Simple venous angiocardiography is not helpful in this particular combination of malformations, but selective angiocardiography from the left atrium or pulmonary vein (as above) is of considerable help in confirming both the position and size of the atrial communication as well as the presence of anomalously draining pulmonary veins. In the more frequent superior caval–type defect, contrast injection to the left atrium with the patient in the left anterior oblique view shows a broad jet of contrast passing superiorly and posteriorly into the right atrium and superior vena cava—a striking contrast to the anterior midatrial of contrast seen in secundum atrial defects after left atrial injections. Left ventricular contrast injection will reveal prolapsed mitral valve leaflets in the same proportion of patients as simple secundum atrial defect.

Treatment

Since the combination of atrial septal defect with partial anomalous pulmonary venous drainage may produce symptoms at an earlier age than either the isolated atrial septal defect or partial anomalous pulmonary venous drainage separately, some patients will require operative repair at an earlier age than usual. With the increasing use of cineangiography and indicator dilution techniques, the diagnosis of the combination may be made preoperatively with some assurance. Where extracorporeal circulation is employed for the operation, the differentiation between isolated atrial defects and defects with anomalous pulmonary venous drainage has little practical importance, but if the patient is young it is important that the anatomic details be known ahead of time.

The indications for surgery are congestive failure or other serious symptoms with cardiac enlargement in the younger child or the presence of a significant shunt in older patients.

While techniques established earlier (Neptune et al., 1953; Ellis and Kirklin, 1955; Lewis et al., 1955; Bedford et al., 1957) have been used successfully in large numbers of patients, in some, where at least one of the anomalous pulmonary veins has ended relatively high in the superior vena cava, late complications may be encountered (Friedli et al., 1972). Despite the use of gussets, varying degrees of obstruction to the superior vena cava and the residual defects in the partition have been noted. A number of ingenious surgical techniques have been proposed to avoid these developments (Robicsek et al., 1969; Puig-Massana et al., 1972). Our own results have been more satisfactory in that superior vena caval obstruction was not found in any of the 25 long-term evaluations.

PARTIAL ANOMALOUS PULMONARY VENOUS DRAINAGE—ISOLATED FORM

Pathology

In the isolated form of the partial anomaly, by definition, no other major intracardiac anomaly is present. The foramen ovale, however, may be patent without interfering with this concept. The pulmonary veins affected are again chiefly those from the right lung, but in about one-third of the cases the left pulmonary veins are involved. The site of connection of the anomalous veins varies but for the right pulmonary veins is most commonly to the superior vena cava. This is the arrangement in half the cases, the remainder inserting into right atrium, inferior vena cava, superior vena cava plus right atrium, azygos vein, and coronary sinus, in that order of frequency (Moes et al., 1966). The pathologic features of partial anomalous pulmonary venous drainage to the inferior vena cava associated with hypoplasia of the right lung were described originally by Park (1912–1913) and have been reviewed by several authors (Neill et al., 1960; Ferencz, 1961; Kittle and Crockett, 1962). In cases with anomalous drainage of the left pulmonary veins, at least 85 percent communicate with the left innominate vein by a left superior vena cava unconnected to the coronary sinus. Rarely, a left pulmonary vein has been attached to the left subclavian vein or coronary sinus.

In the isolated anomaly there may be no obvious pathology in the heart itself at autopsy. Evidence of the extra load on the right heart and pulmonary circuit may be seen in older cases by right atrial and right ventricular dilatation and hypertrophy. The pulmonary artery then is larger than normal. The foramen ovale may be open or closed. The cause of death may be congestive heart failure. A case is rarely seen with the pulmonary veins entering a common sinus that communicates with each atrium. Though anatomically, therefore, the partial form, it may behave clinically as a complete anomaly, and in this extremely uncommon type the right atrium and right ventricle are grossly hypertrophied and dilated, the left heart being relatively underdeveloped. The behavior of the heart in life and the degree of right atrial and right ventricular hypertrophy and dilatation at autopsy are not strictly related to the anatomic degree of abnormal pulmonary venous connection that may be found. More important is the amount of blood flowing to the lung segments that are drained by the pulmonary veins concerned.

Frequency

It has been estimated that about 1 in every 200 routine autopsies shows partial anomalous pul-

monary venous drainage (Hughes and Rumore, 1944; Healey, 1952). A familial occurrence has been noted (Neill et al., 1960; Ferencz, 1961; Kittle and Crockett, 1962).

Clinical Features

Whether or not symptoms appear in a patient with isolated, partial anomalous pulmonary venous drainage is governed basically by the proportion of pulmonary blood flow that is rerouted to the right atrium or its tributaries by the anomalous pulmonary venous return. On the basis of either the age at death or shunt calculations obtained by examining cross-sectional areas of the anomalously draining pulmonary veins, a number of investigators have concluded that decompensation does not develop if less than 50 percent of the pulmonary venous blood drains into the right heart (Brody, 1942; Hughes and Rumore, 1944; Compere and Forsyth, 1944; and Muir, 1953). Other reports have shown that symptoms may appear in relatively young adults and that congestive heart failure may overtake the patient at an older age when 50 percent or more of the pulmonary venous return enters the right heart. Generally speaking, this latter degree of the anomaly carries a prognosis comparable to atrial septal defect, which means that symptoms almost always develop at some time in adult life. The variability of the age at onset of symptoms and the fact that some never have any symptoms and others at cardiac catheterization at a time of marked disability have shown pulmonary hypertension support the importance of other factors in addition to the anatomy. The possibility of differing proportions of pulmonary blood flow to affected segments and the response of the individual pulmonary vasculature to a prolonged increase in pulmonary blood flow explain the variation in the clinical picture of cases with identical degrees of partial anomalous pulmonary venous drainage.

There will be no symptoms at any time in those with anomalous drainage of only one pulmonary vein. This is exemplified by a case aged 66 years described by Muir (1953). The clinical picture with a greater proportion of anomalous pulmonary venous drainage shows considerable variation. There may be no symptoms whatsoever even in adults. Such a case is described in an 86-year-old man reported by Dean and Fox (1928). Symptoms are virtually unknown in childhood in this variety of the malformation. Half the cases with the scimitar syndrome have no symptoms and half have exertional dyspnea, probably related to pulmonary, rather than cardiac, difficulties. Two infants reported by Mortenson and Lindstrom (1971) with scimitar syndrome developed congestive heart failure at the age of nine days and $7\frac{1}{2}$ months, respectively. One had severe pulmonary hypertension but neither had pulmonary vascular obstruction from histologic examination of the removed right lung. A few cases develop fatigue and slight exertional dyspnea in early adult life (Geraci and Kirklin, 1953; Cooley and Mahaffey, 1955). In others at this age the condition is discovered after routine physical examination or upon x-ray of the chest. A minority develop severe symptoms at this time. The advanced picture of dyspnea, cyanosis, and congestive heart failure usually does not appear until late adult life (Storstein and Tveten, 1954).

Splitting of the second heart sound, unlike atrial septal defect, is normal in its response during inspiration and expiration. The splitting may be normal but may also on occasion be quite wide. For this latter reason, there may be difficulty at auscultation in distinguishing the anomaly from atrial septal defect in a few patients. The important point is that in atrial septal defect inspiration delays aortic valve closure because the left-to-right shunt across the atrial communication is decreased in that phase of respiration (Shafter, 1960; Frye et al., 1962). Normally, and in isolated partial anomalous pulmonary venous return as well, aortic valve closure is earlier during inspiration than it is in expiration. The second sound splitting therefore moves with respiratory change in partial anomalous pulmonary venous drainage so long as the atrial septum is intact. There may be no murmur, a systolic murmur in the pulmonary area, or a harsh, diffuse systolic murmur with thrill over the precordium. Middiastolic murmurs and continuous murmurs have been encountered. Congestive heart failure is usually a very late phenomenon. The reduction in flow across the mitral valve in patients with acquired mitral stenosis and congenital partial anomalous pulmonary venous drainage alters the physical signs of the mitral lesion significantly and may cause problems in diagnosis (Varnauskas et al., 1963; and Wassermil and Hoffman, 1962). To our knowledge, this association has not been reported in children.

Electrocardiography

A normal tracing or one with incomplete right bundle branch block is the rule in childhood. The electrocardiographic findings characteristic of total anomalous pulmonary venous drainage are not a feature of the partial form, and the tracings more often resemble those of simple atrial septal defect. Normal tracings are likely due to anomalous drainage of a single vein or, where the whole of one lung is drained by anomalous veins, to reduction of blood flow to that lung because of associated hypoplasia of that organ. Atrial and right ventricular hypertrophy may be present in older cases exhibiting pulmonary hypertension. An abnormally long P-R interval has been described.

Radiologic Examination

The heart is usually of normal size or only slightly enlarged. Gross enlargement is a rare and late finding. The pulmonary artery segment may be more prominent than usual and the lung vascularity either normal or slightly increased. Hilar dance is unusual in the lesser degrees of the anomaly. A rather prominent right atrium may suggest the presence of this anomaly on occasion. In a chest x-ray, when a broad crescentic vessel lies close to the right atrium and, following the curve of this chamber's border, descends to the level of the diaphragm, one can conclude that the right pulmonary veins are draining to the inferior vena cava. This characteristic appearance has been described by Dotter and associates (1949), Grishman and coworkers (1949), Snellen and Albers (1952), and Bruwer (1953). Approximately half of the reported cases with this complex have shown some degree of dextroversion of the heart. The apt term "scimitar syndrome" has been applied to the unique appearances of this condition (Neill et al., 1960). (Figure 32–5). Appearances classic for this syndrome have been reported where the anatomy of the right pulmonary vein, though unusual, was that of normal connection to the left atrium (Blake et al., 1965; Morgan et al., 1971). Where the pulmonary veins from the right side enter the superior vena cava, there may be some distension of this channel in the plain film. Similarly, an opacification in the film on the left supracardiac border, produced by pulmonary veins from the left lung draining into the innominate vein, may provide a clue to the underlying anatomy. No distinctive or pathognomonic pattern is evident in those cases with partial anomalous pulmonary venous drainage into the right atrium or coronary sinus. Occasionally tomography has been of help in demonstrating these abnormal connections (Dalith and Neufeld, 1960).

Bruwer (1953) and Ferencz (1961) have pointed out that the disparity in size of the hemithoraces frequently seen in partial anomalous pulmonary venous drainage is not uncommonly the result of associated hypogenesis and sequestration of part of the right lung. In such cases the left pulmonary artery may be more prominent than the right main branch.

Cardiac Catheterization

In isolated anomalous pulmonary venous drainage, conclusive demonstration of the anomalously draining vein is provided by direct insertion of the cardiac catheter when connection exists with the innominate vein, the superior vena cava, or the inferior vena cava. A number of authors have concluded that there is an anomalous drainage when the catheter has entered a pulmonary vein from an atrial chamber that has been presumed to be the right. Although this is frequently a correct assumption, it is not acceptable as final proof of an anomalous drainage since the position of the catheter entering the right pulmonary vein through a foramen ovale, atrial septal defect, or directly from the right atrium is indistinguishable. Consequently, some other method of confirmation should be used when possible. Of these the most conclusive is cineangiography.

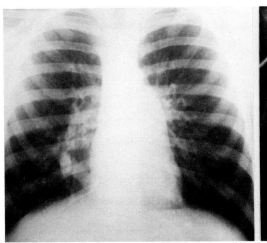 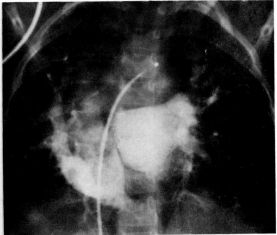

A   B

Figure 32-5. X-ray in the scimitar syndrome. *A.* The chest film of a girl of five years with a pulmonary vein visible at the right cardiophrenic angle. *B.* The pulmonary venous phase following injection of contrast into the main pulmonary artery of an eight-year-old girl. Veins from the right lung drain into the inferior vena cava, while those from the left lung drain normally into the left atrium. The interatrial septum is seen intact and is visible in this anteroposterior projection because of the cardiac rotation associated with hypoplasia of the right lung.

Indirect evidence of anomalous pulmonary venous drainage is provided by rise in blood oxygen saturation encountered on sampling the innominate vein, superior vena cava, inferior vena cava, or right atrium, depending upon the site of insertion of the anomalous vein. Warnings of the misinterpretation that may be made of the normal variations in oxygen saturation in the venous tributaries of the right heart have been voiced in a paper by Johansson (1961). When this rise is evident in the right atrium, the only information that it supplies is that there is a left-to-right shunt at that level. The possible causes of this shunt are several. A relatively small-volume shunt is more suggestive evidence of partial anomalous pulmonary venous drainage than is a large-volume shunt, which suggests the presence of atrial septal defect. The most consistently accurate information appears to have come from the use of indicator dilution techniques (Swan et al., 1953). From injection of dye into both right and left pulmonary arteries or into the anomalous vein itself, it is possible to make an accurate statement concerning the drainage of the pulmonary venous return of each lung or of a particular pulmonary vein, and quantitation with these techniques gives an accurate indication of the amount of flow that passes through each lung. Especially is this feasible in the scimitar syndrome, where it has been found that approximately a quarter of the total pulmonary blood flow goes through the right lung (Fiandra et al., 1962). Occasionally the proportion may be considerably higher (Frye et al., 1962).

Pressures in the right heart and pulmonary circuit may be entirely normal. In older cases, particularly those with symptoms from the anomaly, there is frequently associated moderate pulmonary hypertension.

Angiocardiography

In the partial form of anomalous pulmonary venous drainage without associated defects, angiocardiography affords real help in diagnosis. Very convincing angiocardiograms have been shown in cases where the right pulmonary veins drain into the inferior vena cava (Dotter et al., 1949; Grishman et al., 1949; Snellen and Albers, 1952; Findlay and Maier, 1951; Arvidsson, 1954). Slightly better clarity is obtained from selective injection of the contrast medium into the pulmonary artery (Figure 32–5). This latter technique may also reveal insertion into other areas in other types of the anomaly. Kjellberg and associates (1959) have injected contrast into the anomalously draining pulmonary vein directly and have shown, for example, that the vein connects only with the right atrium. Cineangiocardiography has been more satisfactory than other techniques (Folger et al., 1966).

Diagnosis

Cases with isolated anomalous drainage of a single pulmonary vein may present no features allowing recognition and will, if seen at a younger age, be described as having a normal heart. For practical purposes this is not a serious error.

In those with a larger proportion of the pulmonary venous return entering the right atrium or its tributaries, the main diagnostic problem is that of an atrial septal defect. In a patient with other physical findings suggesting atrial septal defect—hyperdynamic heart, right ventricular lift, modest ejection systolic murmur and moderate accentuation of pulmonary valve closure, diastolic overloading of the right ventricle in the electrocardiogram, and cardiomegaly with plethora on chest x-ray—yet with normal splitting of the second sound, the possibility of isolated partial anomalous pulmonary venous drainage should be entertained. Confirmation of the diagnosis, except in the type with connection to the inferior vena cava, frequently rests on the result of the hemodynamic studies. Indicator dilution techniques are helpful, but selective angiography into the left atrium or pulmonary artery and into individual pulmonary veins assists materially. Calculation of the shunt volume will aid in the decision for surgery in doubtful cases.

Treatment

Since it is now possible to be reasonably certain about the anatomic arrangements preoperatively through detailed catheterization and angiographic studies, the surgical approach is straightforward. The early experiences of Kirklin and associates (1953, 1956), Cooley and Mahaffey (1955), and Lewis and associates (1955) with partial anomalous pulmonary venous drainage from either lung have been amplified by others (Frye et al., 1962). Though in the scimitar syndrome lobectomy or pneumonectomy may be needed more often, restoration to normal pulmonary venous drainage can be offered those few with large shunts (Törnvall et al., 1961; Sanger et al., 1963). Recent modifications of this method of repair have been described using an intra-atrial pericardial conduit (Murphy et al., 1971).

TOTAL ANOMALOUS PULMONARY VENOUS DRAINAGE

Pathology

Complicated Form. In the complicated form of the total anomaly a variety of associated intracardiac defects have been described. Cor biloculare, single ventricle, transposition of the great vessels, truncus arteriosus, ventricular septal defect, and gross systemic venous anomalies have been demonstrated. Patients with tetralogy of Fallot or with tricuspid atresia have also been reported (Cooley et al., 1950; Guller et al., 1972; Muster et al., 1973). If one includes cases with asplenia, long survival is uncommon. The oldest case, reported by Michaelsohn (1920), was a male dying at 21 years with complete anomalous pulmonary venous drainage into the left superior vena cava with associated situs inversus and cor biloculare. In 25 percent of these cases, the pulmonary veins communicated with the right heart through connections below the diaphragm, and in 10 percent the connection was directly into the right atrium. The remainder inserted into either the superior vena cava or the left superior vena cava or had multiple insertions of which one was usually the superior vena cava and the other either the innominate vein, the

portal vein, or the inferior vena cava. Less common sites of insertion were into the right innominate, left gastric, hepatic, or azygos veins and the sinus venosus (Darling et al., 1957).

Recently, Delisle and associates (1976), in assessing an experience with 35 autopsies of this type, found that two-thirds had heterotaxy and that within that group obstructed veins occurred in about half the cases, frequently being masked by associated pulmonary atresia. In most cases, whether heterotaxy was present or not, a very complex intracardiac anomaly existed.

Isolated Form. In the isolated form of the complete anomaly, the site of insertion of the anomalous veins has considerable practical importance. Snellen and Albers (1952) first suspected that the total anomalous pulmonary venous drainage into a left superior vena cava would prove to be more common in clinical practice than had been formerly suspected. Publications since have supported the contention of Keith and associates (1954) that the commonest variety is where all four pulmonary veins drain into the left innominate vein through a left superior vena cava (Table 32–1) (Gott et al., 1956; Dowling et al., 1957; Burroughs and Edwards, 1960; Bonham-Carter et al., 1969; Gathman and Nadas, 1970). Almost half the cases are accounted for by this anatomy. Next most common appears to be drainage of all four pulmonary veins into the coronary sinus, followed rather closely by infradiaphragmatic connections and drainage into the right atrium and superior vena cava. The first instance of total anomalous pulmonary venous drainage into the inferior vena cava directly was published by Gott and associates (1956). The same authors described total anomalous pulmonary venous drainage with insertion into two widely separated sites. Anatomic studies of cases of total anomalous pulmonary venous drainage unassociated with other cardiac malformations have been made by Darling and associates (1957), Burroughs and Edwards (1960), and Blake and associates (1965). The classification of Darling and associates has become the one most widely used and divides the level of anomalous venous insertion into four groups:

Group I—Supracardiac
Group II—Cardiac
Group III—Infracardiac
Group IV—Mixed

Their classification has been used in Table 32–1. Apart from the uncommon case in group IV, where insertion of pulmonary veins is at more than one level, there is some variation within the other groups as to the anatomic detail of drainage into a particular level. Most commonly all four pulmonary veins unite to form single, large, sinus-like channel which then joins the systemic circulation at the particular level. This is usual where there is total anomalous pulmonary venous drainage into the left superior vena cava, right superior vena cava, or below the diaphragm. Two or

Table 32–1. LEVEL AND SITE OF CONNECTION FOR 180 PROVEN CASES (AUTOPSY OR OPERATION) OF TOTAL ANOMALOUS PULMONARY VENOUS DRAINAGE WITHOUT ASSOCIATED MAJOR INTRACARDIAC DEFECTS AT THE HOSPITAL FOR SICK CHILDREN (1950–1973)

GROUP	LEVEL	NO. IN GROUP	PERCENT OF TOTAL
I	Supracardiac	85	47
II	Cardiac	55	30
III	Infracardiac	32	18
IV	Mixed	8	5
	Totals	180	100

more points of connection at the same level have been recorded in cases of complete anomalous pulmonary venous drainage both of the type draining into the superior vena cava and of that draining into the right atrium, but this arrangement is uncommon (Keith et al., 1954; Darling et al., 1957; Burroughs and Kirklin, 1956; Burroughs and Edwards, 1960). By contrast, connection of the pulmonary vein to the right atrium by two orifices rather than by one or four (Scott and Welch, 1965) was reported by Blake and associates (1965). Connection to the superior vena cava may occur at or below the point of azygos vein entry. The mixed type of connection accounts for between 5 and 10 percent of most large series. In this group connection pairing to left superior vena cava and coronary sinus and to the right and left superior venal cavae are the most frequently encountered (Hospital for Sick Children series; Bonham-Carter et al., 1969; Gathman and Nadas, 1970). It is now evident that many variations of the arrangements at any one level of connection can occur (Blake et al., 1965; Trinkle et al., 1968; Moes et al., 1966).

Earlier descriptions of the anomaly were colored by the striking pulmonary venous obstruction that was evident in type-III malformation. It has since become apparent that pulmonary venous obstruction may also occur in other types of the disorder. This may occur either because the orifice of the anomalous connecting vein is small at the site of insertion into the right side or because the connecting vein is obstructed at some point in its course prior to the site of connection to the systemic circuit. Again, although most examples fit rather simply into this description, there is some variation in the anatomy, and some cases with obstruction have quite bizarre anatomic arrangements for the return of the pulmonary venous blood (Blake et al., 1965; Moes et al., 1966; Shadravan et al., 1971).

A number of workers have emphasized the importance of examining, during the course of routine autopsies, for anomalies of the pulmonary venous return immediately after the pericardium has been opened. Unless a methodical routine of examining for pulmonary venous return is made in every instance, it is our experience that cases of all groups except group I may be missed during the initial stages of dissection. The important practical point is that where total anomalous pulmonary venous drainage exists, the heart can be lifted upward and forward on its vascular pedicle because the left atrium is not anchored as it normally is by the pulmonary veins.

Details of the changes in size of the vessels and chambers in autopsied cases have been provided by Keith and associates (1954) and Darling and associates (1957). The appearance of the heart on opening the chest is uniform in all types except group III where the anomaly of drainage is below the diaphragm. In the other groups the right atrium and right ventricle are strikingly enlarged and dilated, having five times the capacity of the corresponding left chambers, which by comparison are underdeveloped. Although left ventricular mass is normal, the cavity is compromised by severe septal displacement which, with a reduced left heart inflow, probably contributes to the low systemic output in these patients (Bove et al., 1975). Although the thickness of the right ventricular wall does not differ greatly from the left, the hypertrophy of the former chamber is masked to a great extent by the extreme dilatation present. In all cases there is an interatrial communication that is in many fatal cases due to a patent foramen ovale (73 percent of our cases) but may be due to the presence of a large secundum atrial septal defect (27 percent). The ductus arteriosus is patent in approximately 25 percent of the cases, the remainder having only bare probe patency or being closed. The general dilatation of the right heart is shared by the pulmonary artery. The internal circumference of this vessel usually is one and one-half times that of the aorta. The tricuspid valve ring is also considerably larger than the mitral. Darling and associates (1957) observed that only one-third of their cases had a significant medial fibrous intimal thickening of the intrapulmonary arteries, but marked changes were consistently present in cases with pulmonary venous obstruction (Falsetti et al., 1964; Samuelson et al., 1970). The case of Levy and associates (1954) with extreme pulmonary arteriolar changes during the first year of life in the absence of pulmonary venous obstruction is exceptional (Ferencz et al., 1971). A pathologic finding of considerable importance in clinical terms is the subendocardial infarction that is found in many cases during infancy at autopsy affecting right ventricular papillary muscles (Kangos et al., 1969).

Frequency

Accurate figures of the frequency of total anomalous pulmonary venous drainage unassociated with major intracardiac defects are not available. Maude Abbott (1936) found 1 case in her 1000 postmortems of congenital heart disease. Darling and coworkers (1957) reported 16 cases, or 2 percent of all autopsied cases of congenital heart disease, at the Boston Children's Hospital in the past 25 years. In our overall experience with 15,104 patients, seen within a 20-year period, the frequency of total anomalous pulmonary venous drainage was 1.3 percent of all cardiac malformations. In the experience at the Great Ormond Street Hospital, London, total anomalous pulmonary venous return accounted for 6 percent of 1000 autopsies in congenital heart disease (Bonham-Carter et al., 1969). Although the sex incidence has been equal (Bonham-Carter et al., 1969) or has shown a male predominance (Gathman and Nadas, 1970; Jensen and Blount, 1971), the numbers upon which these conclusions have been based were small—61, 52 and 27 patients, respectively. In the 180 patients from The Hospital for Sick Children (Figure 32–1) there were 112 males and 68 females. This male predominance was unequivocal for all varieties except that of type IV where the number was too small to be certain of this relationship.

Hemodynamics

In the isolated form, oxygenated blood returning from the lungs enters the right atrium directly or indirectly, usually by means of a single common pulmonary vein at one of the four stated levels. Thus pulmonary venous blood with high oxygen saturation mixes in the right atrium with systemic venous blood of lower saturation. A variable proportion of both streams then passes from the right atrium both through a defect in the atrial septum (patent foramen ovale or true atrial septal defect) to the left heart and aorta and through the tricuspid valve to the right ventricle and pulmonary artery. The factors influencing this alteration in hemodynamics are discussed under the heading of cardiac catheterization. As a generalization, however, it may be said that, subject to these varying influences, the oxygen saturation of blood in the heart and systemic arteries is approximately the same.

Clinical Features

Complicated Form. In those cases complicated by major intracardiac anomalies, life expectancy is often prolonged by the presence of anomalous pulmonary venous drainage, which acts as a natural partial correction. Such was the situation in a personal case with a boy aged 11 years who had considerable disability with marked cyanosis from birth. He died during cardiac catheterization, and at autopsy he showed complete transposition of the great vessels, pulmonary stenosis, atrioventricularis communis, and complete anomalous pulmonary venous drainage into the left superior vena cava and was almost certainly an example of the complex cardiac disorder associated with congenital asplenia. There are reports of survivors beyond infancy with tricuspid atresia (Guller et al., 1972; Cooley et al., 1950), and although in some cases the anomaly may preclude natural survival during the first year, recent surgical accomplishments indicate potential for assistance at any age (Barratt-Boyes et al., 1972; Sapsford et al., 1972).

Isolated Form. The clinical picture in the types unassociated with major intracardiac defects is determined by four variables: (1) The level of pulmonary arteriolar resistance and the tone of the ductus arteriosus, i.e., factors that govern the pulmonary blood flow. (2) The degree of pulmonary venous obstruction, i.e., the presence or absence of anatomic obstruction at the connecting site, within the pulmonary vein or from external compression of the anomalous vein; or relative pulmonary venous obstruction associated with torrential pulmonary blood flow. (3) The nature of the atrial communication, i.e., whether there is a foramen ovale defect or a true secundum atrial communication. (4) The state of the right ventricular myocardium, i.e., whether or not there is infarction.

It is difficult to classify every patient within these categories for some will show the influence of several variables. It is also true that the overwhelming majority of patients present with symptoms during infancy, but it is probably fair to say that clinical presentation occurs in three main forms: (1) the infant with low pulmonary vascular resistance and huge pulmonary blood flow, a small-to-moderate foramen ovale flap deficiency, and without organic pulmonary venous obstruction but with degrees of subendocardial infarction of right ventricular muscle; (2) the infant with pulmonary venous obstruction; and (3) the asymptomatic or mildly symptomatic older child or adult with normal pulmonary vascular resistance, a large atrial communication of the true secundum type, and no pulmonary venous obstruction.

The birth weight of patients is within the usual range. Familial association has been reported (Paz et al., 1971; Gathman and Nadas, 1970; Kaufman et al., 1973), as has an association with malformation syndromes (Gathman and Nadas, 1970).

The Infant with High Pulmonary Blood Flow. The earliest sign encountered in symptomatic infants is tachypnea and cyanosis. Cyanosis is not infrequently more obvious in the perinatal period, and though it may persist, it tends to diminish or even clear in about half of those where documentation is available from birth. In the majority, a muddy discoloration of equivocal cyanosis is more usual at rest and is frequently not recognized by parents or physicians. More obvious cyanosis or intense cyanosis, though it can be seen at a late stage in these patients, is most often an indication that pulmonary venous obstruction coexists. Clubbing is consequently rare in this variety.

Tachypnea, on the other hand, is always present and a sign of great importance especially early in life. In the first-born, the grandmother usually notices this sign when the infant is brought home from the hospital. Where previous children have been born, the mother will notice the breathing to be obviously different from the siblings at the same age. At this stage cyanosis is often absent, the infant does not look ill, and the complaint may easily be disregarded unless the malformation is kept in mind. Over the next few weeks or months the infant fails to gain satisfactorily and may become dusky intermittently. Frequent changes of formula are an invariable notation in the histories of these patients. This situation may continue indefinitely until either a heart murmur is detected, distinct cyanosis or gross dyspnea appears, or the failure to thrive demands further investigation.

Failure to thrive is invariable and is reflected early in those with large pulmonary blood flow. Striking dystrophy is present after the first month or two. The precise time of presentation varies greatly but nowadays about 90 percent may be recognized as having heart disease in the first month of life—as many as one-third on the first day, about a third during the first month of life, and another third at a postnatal check-up during the second month. Because a specific diagnosis may not be appreciated, referral to centers tends to be delayed for some months in as many as half the patients. Inevitably the liver becomes enlarged, the precordium bulging, the heart obviously overactive, and a gallop rhythm and cardiac murmurs develop. These signs of right heart overload and failure are present in almost half the patients by one month of age. Congestive heart failure in the first week, though uncommon, certainly can occur and is not necessarily associated with pulmonary venous obstruction. It may be secondary to an unusually rapid decline of pulmonary vascular resistance in some patients (Rowe and Mehrizi, 1968). It is found in about 60 percent of patients overall (Bonham-Carter et al., 1969).

The first sound is very loud. The second sound is often closely split, and whether or not the splitting is fixed at this age is debated. For some it is common (Lowe, 1965; Bonham-Carter et al., 1969) even in infants and for others it is rare (Gathman and Nadas, 1970). Our experience is more in line with that of Lowe (1965) and Bonham-Carter and associates (1969). Third heart sounds are common. A soft systolic ejection murmur along the left sternal border has been described as the common murmur present. About a third of the patients have no obvious murmur, but a blowing early systolic murmur along the lower left

sternal murmur that has characteristics of tricuspid regurgitation (Keith et al., 1954) is becoming increasingly recognized as a feature of the disorder even in the perinatal period. More commonly this murmur appears later and may be transient but often increases in intensity and duration with time. Loud regurgitant murmurs of this sort carry a very serious prognosis because they indicate major sub-endocardial damage of right ventricular muscle and appreciable interference with the tricuspid valve apparatus. A middiastolic murmur of tricuspid origin is common and said to be more frequent in patients who have less than severe pulmonary hypertension (Gathman and Nadas, 1970). A continuous murmur secondary to turbulence along the anomalous venous channel or at its connecting site has been noted in cases with pulmonary venous obstruction. This murmur is also present occasionally where no pulmonary venous obstruction occurs either from autopsy or from angiographic evidence in our experience and that of Jensen and Blount (1971). It is most likely that a relative if not an anatomic obstruction associated with the very high flow through the channel accounts for these cases. We have not detected a continuous murmur due to a patent ductus arteriosus with left-to-right shunt in the infant cases where that association occurs in approximately 25 percent.

About one-third of symptomatic infants have the clinical and radiologic picture during life of pulmonary venous obstruction (Hospital for Sick Children series; Bonham-Carter et al., 1969). In our group, 80 percent had group-III (infradiaphragmatic) connection to the systemic venous circuit (Johnson et al., 1958; Lucas et al., 1961). All our group-III cases had this picture, and it is rare to find it otherwise (Ainger, 1962). The remaining 20 percent of our group were equally divided between connections to the right superior vena cava and to the left superior vena cava. Ultimately the cause for the different clinical behavior of these cases lies in the difficulty of egress of pulmonary venous blood from the lungs into the systemic circuit. Where pulmonary venous attachment occurs below the diaphragm, this is probably most often due to postnatal reduction in caliber of the ductus venosus. Of the supracardiac level connections, those to the right superior vena cava seem to have an unusually small orifice at the actual site of the connection, and the same explanation may also apply to connections of the left superior vena cava to the left innominate vein (Hauck et al., 1960; Kauffman et al., 1962; Hastreiter et al., 1962). In the left-sided type, however, stenotic areas in the left superior vena cava in association with compression of this vein between the left pulmonary artery and the left main bronchus—the hemodynamic vise—are the more usual explanation (Elliott and Edwards, 1962). Cases with coronary sinus connection are not exempt from having pulmonary venous obstruction but the association is uncommon. When it occurs, the impediment to flow seems to be within the pulmonary veins prior to entry into the coronary sinus itself (Gathman and Nadas, 1970).

Patients with pulmonary venous obstruction of whatever site have a brief and stormy life characterized by early-appearing and intense cyanosis, frequently worsened during feeding (Lucas et al., 1961). Marked dyspnea is a feature, and the liver is usually enlarged. Murmurs are absent or, if present, inconspicuous. The patients appear to die from pulmonary edema or anoxia.

Symptoms in most patients surviving into adult life have been slight, mild exertional dyspnea being the chief complaint. Although this may have been noted from a relatively early age, few of these patients develop significant disability until the third decade. It is likely that this course is due to the presence of a large atrial communication, lack of pulmonary venous obstruction, an ideal maturation of the pulmonary vascular bed in relation to the increased flow and near-perfect balance of those variables, the mismatch of which frequently results in deterioration of the subject in infancy. Long-term survivors have not experienced congestive failure as younger persons and behave more like patients with simple secundum atrial defect (Burchell, 1956; Bonham-Carter et al., 1969; Jensen and Blount, 1971). A survivor to 46 years has been reported (Jensen and Blount, 1971).

Electrocardiography

Detailed reports of the electrocardiogram in children with this malformation have been published previously (Keith et al., 1954). The tracings follow a relatively uniform pattern. Most often there is a moderate right-axis deviation in the order of $+130$ degrees. P waves are abnormally tall and peaked in either precordial or standard leads, or both. This is a change that is progressive after birth and is evident in serial tracings. The change becomes obvious for most patients between one and three months of age (Gathman and Nadas, 1970).

The ventricular complex indicates right ventricular hypertrophy of marked degree, a tall R wave in V_1 and little or no S wave in the same leads, and a low R wave and deep S wave in V_5 and V_6. Approximately two-thirds of the cases have shown an R wave exceeding 5 mm in aVR. The most striking feature about the electrocardiogram is the frequent presence of a q wave in the right precordial leads (Figure 32-6). Gathman and Nadas (1970) found such a pattern in 30 of 75 cases. In those patients in infancy where qR pattern is not evident, there is a similar pattern of r s R[1] in the right chest leads. These observations were confirmed by DuShane (1956), but others have found fewer with changes of this type (Gessner et al., 1964; Jensen and Blount, 1971) and do not feel the sign helpful in diagnosis. Our experience has been restated more recently by Rowe and Mehrizi (1968), and we continue to regard this electrical indication of a large right atrium (Sodi-Pallares, 1956) and probably indirectly also of papillary muscle infarction (Kangos et al., 1969) as an important and practical clue to diagnosis. Complete right bundle branch block and type B Wolff-Parkinson-White syndrome have been

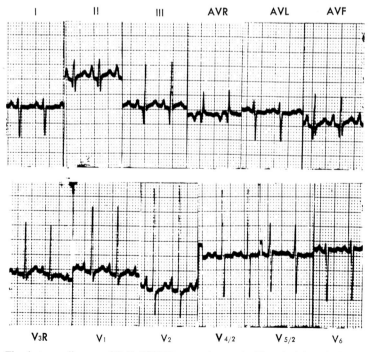

Figure 32-6. The electrocardiogram of D. F. (303877) at age six months. There is right-axis deviation with right atrial and right ventricular hypertrophy. Note the qR pattern in right chest leads. The diagnosis confirmed at autopsy was total anomalous pulmonary venous return into the coronary sinus.

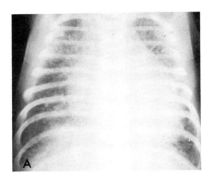

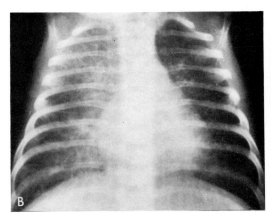
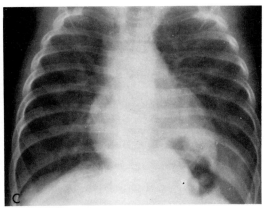

Figure 32-7. The chest x-ray in total anomalous pulmonary venous drainage with pulmonary venous obstruction. *A.* B. H., 19 days, who died of hypoxia at 20 days. Connection to the systemic circuit was through a small orifice in the right superior vena cava! *B.* D. C., a male infant aged 34 days with autopsy-proved total anomalous venous return to the portal vein. *C.* B. H., 8½ months, who died two months after attempts at surgical correction. The pulmonary venous connection was through a small orifice into an otherwise normal azygos vein.

encountered (Gathman and Nadas, 1970), but right ventricular hypertrophy with clockwise horizontal vectorial loop is the usual situation. In the first two weeks of life, the T wave in the precordial leads is upright and becomes inverted with increasing age. After this brief period the T wave is inverted regularly in RV_3 and V_1. With increasing evidence of right ventricular strain, the negativity of this wave is extended across to the left chest. About half of the cases have shown T wave inversion in leads II, III, and aVF. These signs most likely reflect ischemic change.

In the experience with infants there has been no significant difference in electrocardiograms obtained from either those patients with low or high pulmonary artery pressure, those with atrial septal defect or patent foramen ovale, or those with high or low blood oxygen saturations in a systemic artery, but in those with left-to-right shunts through a patent ductus arteriosus we have noted the presence of biventricular hypertrophy on occasion. Burchell (1956) has shown a close correlation between the degree of right ventricular dominance and the pulmonary artery pressure in adult cases. Those older patients with a normal pulmonary artery pressure had incomplete right bundle branch block in the precordial leads, while those with severe pulmonary hypertension

showed an extreme right ventricular hypertrophy pattern.

Radiologic Examination

In the least common group of the malformation—patients with pulmonary venous obstruction—the heart is usually, though not always, normal in size (Figure 32–7; Figure 32–10B). The lung vascularity is rarely unremarkable in these cases, but characteristically the lung fields show a fluffy opacification due to pulmonary venous congestion (Harris et al., 1960). The presence of Kerley B lines is a helpful sign of pulmonary venous obstruction, especially in newborns where noncardiac disorders may mimic the radiologic picture of pulmonary venous congestion (Robinson et al., 1969). All other types have increased lung vascularity, and the majority have a moderate degree of heart enlargement. It is our opinion that many ill infants without frank pulmonary venous obstruction show a mixed appearance in chest films with increased flow and venous congestion combined. These may be cases with relative obstruction due to high pulmonary venous flow. Progressive cardiac enlargement often

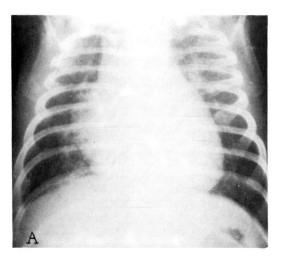 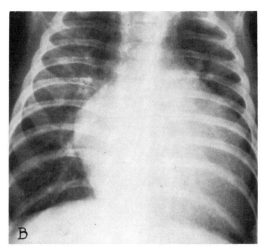

Figure 32-8. Increase in cardiac size with age in total anomalous pulmonary venous drainage. The x-rays of S. V., a patient with connection into a left superior vena cava, who died of congestive heart failure at nine weeks of age. There was no evidence of pulmonary venous obstruction (arterial oxygen saturation, 87 percent). *A.* 14 days, C.T.R. 0.63. *B.* Nine weeks, C.T.R. 0.70.

occurs in the first few months of life (Keith et al., 1954, Figure 32–8). The right ventricular enlargement, particularly of the outflow tract of the right ventricle, frequently obscures the pulmonary dilatation noticeable at operation and autopsy. This appearance of the left cardiac border gives rise to what has been described as a characteristic "boxlike" contour (Gott et al., 1956) (Figure 32–9).

This contour has certainly been present in a large number of cases of this malformation, but we have also found it in patients with other defects, particularly atrioventricularis communis, partial anomalous pulmonary venous drainage with atrial septal defect, and atrial septal defect plus ventricular septal defect. The aorta is always left-sided and is

usually small. A localized indentation of the anterior aspect of the barium-filled esophagus just above the diaphragm in lateral films has been described as an additional characteristic of the infradiaphragmatic variety of connection but it is not specific and occasionally is seen in other forms (Eisen and Elliott, 1968). Likewise a more major deviation posteriorly of the barium-filled esophagus is not infrequently seen in the coronary sinus form of the anomaly but in most cases no abnormality is recognizable from the barium swallow.

Apart from these general features, various authors have ascribed apparently specific cardiac contours for the differing anatomic types of the malformation. The only really convincing one is that which is present

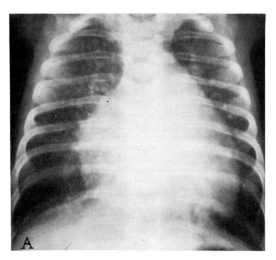 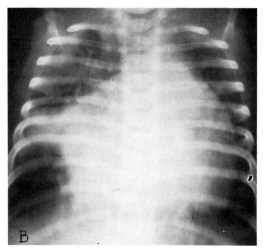

Figure 32-9. The radiologic appearance of total anomalous pulmonary venous drainage at cardiac level. *A.* M. W., two months, who died in congestive failure at two and one-half months. Autopsy-proved connection into the right atrium. *B.* M. B., three months, who died at that age of congestive failure. Autopsy-proved connection into the coronary sinus.

when all pulmonary veins drain into the innominate vein via a persistent left superior vena cava (Figure 32–10*D*). The dilatation of the left superior vena cava, left innominate vein, and right superior vena cava then produces a rounded supracardiac shadow, which with the rest of the heart results in a "figure-of-eight" or "snowman" appearance. It was first described by Snellen and Albers (1952) and has been confirmed by several subsequent authors. The contour takes some time to develop, occasionally but not usually being evident before the age of four months (Figure 32–10*A, C*). Bruwer (1956) has illustrated the differential diagnosis of this appearance, which may be simulated in the expiratory chest film of normal children, in partial anomalous pulmonary venous drainage into a left superior vena cava, and by mediastinal neoplasms. We have also seen a similar appearance in some infants with a large thymus and, after the development of congestive failure, in a case of severe pulmonary stenosis with

normal aortic root with associated persistent left superior vena cava draining into the coronary sinus. A sign in very young infants, heralding a later more classic "snowman," is a density anterior to the trachea in the lateral chest film (Weaver et al., 1976).

Snellen and Albers (1952) also drew attention to a peculiarly high bulge of the right atrium in the anteroposterior films of a personal case and one of Taussig (1947) where all pulmonary veins entered the coronary sinus. This appearance is not invariable and has been observed in proved cases with drainage of all pulmonary veins directly into the right atrium or the left superior vena cava (Figures 32–9*A* and 32–10*C*).

When all pulmonary veins drain into the right superior vena cava, there may be a bulge of this structure (Bruwer, 1956). Infant cases usually do not show this sign, and occasionally a unilaterally visible right superior vena cava may be misleading (Figure 32–10*C*). Unilateral emphysema from compression of the left main bronchus between a left vertical vein

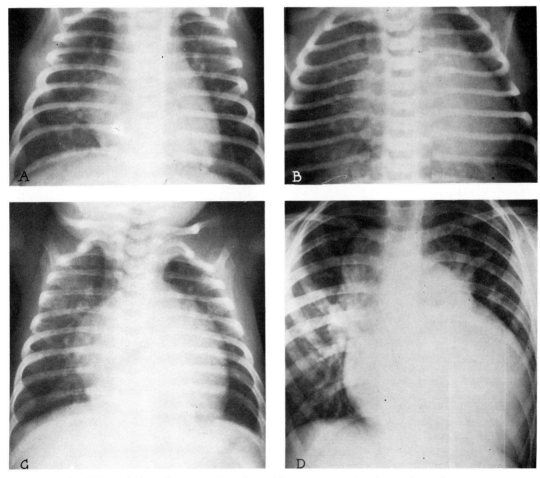

Figure 32-10. The variable cardiac contour in patients with autopsy-proved total anomalous pulmonary venous drainage into a left superior vena cava. *A.* S. V., five days. Note relatively normal shape and slight increase in pulmonary vascularity. This patient died of congestive failure at nine weeks. *B.* W. L., aged eight days. Death on the day of x-ray was to hypoxia. Note signs of pulmonary venous obstruction. *C.* K. D., eight weeks. Died following venous angiocardiography at eight weeks. Note "boxlike" contour. *D.* B. P., four years. Died at surgical correction 7½ years. Note classic figure-of-eight silhouette.

and the left pulmonary artery occurs rarely (Sulayman et al., 1975).

Echocardiography

Total anomalous pulmonary venous return produces marked right ventricular volume overload. A large right ventricular chamber with abnormal septal motion has therefore been described in this condition (Tajik et al., 1972). In our experience normal septal motion in the presence of associated pulmonary hypertension is also seen (Diamond et al., 1971).

The left atrial dimension may be minute (Glaser, 1972). The left ventricular mitral valve and aortic measurements are usually at the lower limits of normal for the age of that patient (Meyer and Kaplan, 1973). The common pulmonary venous channel may be identified behind the left atrial posterior wall (Pacquet and Gutgesell, 1975).

The above features combined with the clinical findings permit accurate identification of this malformation.

Cardiac Catheterization

Many reports of cardiac catheterization in groups of patients with isolated, complete anomalous pulmonary venous drainage have now been published (Friedlich et al., 1950; Snellen and Albers, 1952; Levinson et al., 1953; Gardner and Oram, 1953; Keith et al., 1954; Gott et al., 1956; Swan et al., 1956; Bonham-Carter et al., 1969; Gathman and Nadas, 1970; El-Said et al., 1972). Data of diagnostic significance have emerged from examination of blood oxygen saturation values, exploration with the catheter tip, and examination of pulmonary arterial pressure.

Blood Oxygen Saturations. The level of insertion of the pulmonary veins can be established by noting the site at which high blood oxygen saturation is obtained. Such changes are found in the left innominate vein in cases of drainage into a persistent left superior vena cava, in the superior vena cava in cases of drainage into that vessel, in the right atrium in those with drainage directly into this chamber or through the coronary sinus, and in the hepatic veins or inferior vena cava in infradiaphragmatic types. The detection of high oxygen tension and saturation in blood from the hepatic vein at a time when the descending aortic blood has low values is almost pathognomonic for total anomalous pulmonary venous return below the diaphragm and is easily established through cord sampling at birth.

It was noted by Taussig (1947) that the oxygen saturation of blood in the right atrium was high in all variants and could be identical with that in the systemic circuit. In all types of the anomaly, all blood from both pulmonary and systemic circulations returns to the right atrium. In the majority, most of the blood then passes through the tricuspid valve to the right ventricle and pulmonary artery. Provided the pulmonary resistance is low, there will then be a very much greater flow of blood through the lung than through the systemic circuit. As a consequence, a great quantity of highly saturated blood from the lung returns to mix with a lesser quantity of desaturated systemic venous blood. Thus the oxygen saturation of blood in the right atrium and systemic arteries remains high as long as the high pulmonary blood flow is maintained. If, on the other hand, the pulmonary resistance is increased, the pulmonary blood flow becomes reduced and a smaller volume of highly saturated blood returns from the lung to the right atrium. The oxygen saturation of blood in the right atrium and systemic arteries then becomes relatively low. Swan and associates (1956) have recently shown that low pulmonary vascular resistance is found in cases with high arterial oxygen saturation and high vascular resistance in cases with low arterial oxygen saturation. Likewise, in 15 infant cases at The Hospital for Sick Children the critical systemic arterial oxygen saturation was 80 percent, above and below which level the pulmonary artery pressure was only moderately or severely elevated respectively. In all infants, the average systemic arterial oxygen saturation was 81 percent.

Pressures. Mean right atrial pressure values for patients dying in infancy were higher than those surviving longer and correlated with the higher levels of pulmonary artery pressure in nonsurvivors (Serratto et al., 1967), but mean right atrial pressures were found by Gathman and Nadas (1970) to be unrelated to pulmonary arterial pressure levels.

The pulmonary artery pressure of patients with this malformation has been studied in two main age periods. In the infant group, exemplified by the patients under one year examined at The Hospital for Sick Children, pulmonary hypertension has been found in nearly all cases. About half have shown a systolic pressure in the pulmonary artery equaling or approximating systemic systolic levels, whereas the remainder have exhibited a more moderate pulmonary hypertension. A normal pressure has been the exception, and, in the group as a whole, severe symptoms have been prominent. By contrast, many cases first detected and studied at an older age have shown normal or only slightly elevated pulmonary artery pressures although marked pulmonary hypertension has been found in at least half the patients examined after the age of 20 years.

In the presence of pulmonary venous obstruction, pressure differences across the obstructed point within the pulmonary vein have been observed to range as high as 30 to 66 mm of mercury (Behrendt et al., 1972).

Exploration with the Catheter. It is usually possible, by manipulation with the catheter tip, to pass into the anomalous pulmonary veins attached to the left innominate vein through a persistent left superior vena cava (Whitaker, 1954). In our experience this is more easily performed when the left innominate vein is approached from below, through the femoral vein. Entry into the left pulmonary veins in such cases is not conclusive evidence of a total drainage anomaly, and to confirm the latter arrangement it is necessary to pass the catheter into the right as well as the left thorax.

Where pulmonary veins connect with the superior vena cava, entry with the catheter may be made when the anomalous vessels are approached from above through an arm vein. A similar problem arises as to whether this is a total or partial drainage anomaly when only one pulmonary vein or two pulmonary veins are catheterized. If the left pulmonary veins as well can be entered from the superior vena cava, the evidence is strong for a total anomaly.

There have been no reports to date of direct catheter entry into the common pulmonary vein when all pulmonary veins drain into the inferior vena cava.

If all pulmonary veins connect to the right atrium or coronary sinus, it is possible to enter the anomalous channels directly from the right atrium. As it is not usually possible to be certain that the catheter has not first entered the left atrium, little is gained from the mere entry of catheter into the vein. Under these circumstances use of indicator dilution techniques or cineangiography has a special value.

Indicator Dilution. The arterial curve following injection of Evans blue dye into a peripheral vein has been reported by Nicholson and associates (1951) and Keith and coworkers (1954). The indicator dilution illustrated a short appearance time with a double dip characteristic of right-to-left shunt and a prolonged disappearance time, or produced a flattened curve where the shunt patterns were obscured. These studies have been confirmed and refined by subsequent reports from Burroughs and Kirklin (1956), Swan and associates (1956), and Samet and associates (1963), using selective injection of indicators.

Angiocardiography

Adequate selective injection of contrast into the main pulmonary artery usually results in good visualization of all four pulmonary veins and the resultant connection to the systemic circuit. It is particularly true in cases of total anomalous pulmonary venous return to the left superior vena cava (Figure 32–11). It is often true for mixed connections (Kjellberg et al., 1959; Rowe et al., 1956). It is further possible to determine the actual site of

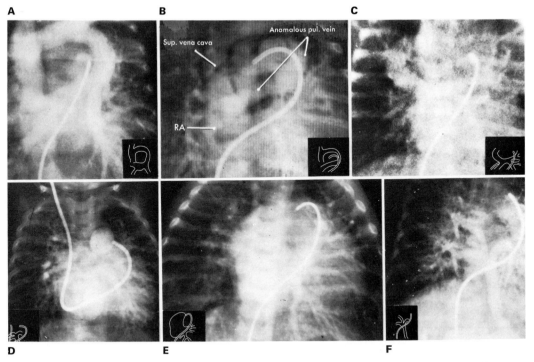

Figure 32-11. The angiocardiogram in total anomalous pulmonary venous return: the pulmonary venous phase after contrast injection into the main pulmonary artery in infants with autopsy or operative confirmation of the particular variety of the isolated anomaly. *A.* The classic appearance of unobstructed connection to the left innominate vein through a left superior vena cava. *B.* A narrowed segment (rather higher than the usual hemodynamic vise) near the systemic venous connection. *C.* Connection into the terminal portion of the azygos vein. *D.* The characteristic "egg" over the spine seen with connection to the coronary sinus. *E.* Diffuse atrial opacification with contrast seen when pulmonary veins drain directly into the atrium (three orifices in this instance). *F.* Infradiaphragmatic drainage to the portal vein. (Courtesy of Dr. C. Ho.)

connection in patients in whom the pulmonary venous drainage is at cardiac level (Rowe et al., 1961). In those with coronary sinus connection a characteristic egg-shaped structure appears discretely within the right atrium (Figure 32–11).

On the contrary, in patients in whom pulmonary veins connect directly to the right atrium, contrast fills this structure more diffusely. The appearances of total anomalous pulmonary venous return to the superior vena cava either directly or through the azygos communication can usually be distinguished (Moes et al., 1966) (Figure 32–11). Most difficulty arises with those patients having severe pulmonary venous obstruction. The angiographic appearances in such patients with infradiaphragmatic connections were first demonstrated by Johnson and coworkers (1958) and have since been elaborated (Lucas et al., 1961, 1972). An important feature in these cases is that opacification of the portal system and accumulation of contrast in the liver vessels is usually not evident for 10 to 12 seconds after the injection. In all examples there is real merit to selective pulmonary venous injection especially where the pulmonary artery injection has not clarified the anatomy beyond all doubt. These efforts, however, may require special techniques or even be unsuccessful because of the small orifices for entry coupled with the high velocity of flow through the orifice.

Diagnosis

Because in the early stages there is frequently no cyanosis or heart murmur, failure to gain weight may be the presenting symptom in the young infant case. Unless attention is paid to tachypnea, precordial bulging, and mild cyanosis on crying, the diagnosis may be delayed for several months. By this stage more obvious signs will have appeared, such as heart murmurs, cyanosis, or congestive heart failure; investigation will have been advised for the failure to thrive; or admission to hospital with respiratory infection and "pneumonia" may have occurred.

Once a cardiac basis for the symptoms is recognized, the diagnosis of complete anomalous pulmonary venous drainage unassociated with major defects is made on the combination of a general dystrophic appearance, equivocal or mild cyanosis, the absence or a nonspecificity of murmurs, and cardiac enlargement with increased lung vascularity and electrocardiographic appearances—particularly the evidence in right precordial leads of a qR pattern indicating right atrial hypertrophy and right ventricular hypertrophy. The exception to this general picture occurs in those patients with pulmonary venous obstruction, typically in infradiaphragmatic type of insertion of the anomalous pulmonary veins, where there is intense cyanosis from birth, a comparatively normal heart size, and death by the age of three months from anoxia or congestive failure.

In newborn infants, a clinical picture closely similar to that of complete anomalous pulmonary venous drainage is presented by infants with aortic and/or mitral atresia. The very early age at which these patients develop a congestive heart failure and an abnormal qR pattern in the electrocardiogram usually permits their differentiation from cases of the venous malformation who develop such signs at a later period. Other malformations causing difficulty in differentiation at this age are congenital mitral stenosis, cor triatriatum, and individual stenosis of pulmonary veins (Shone et al., 1962; Tingelstad et al., 1969), lymphangiectasis (France and Brown, 1971), transient tachypnea of the newborn (Kuhn et al., 1969), and transient myocardial ischemia (Rowe and Hoffman, 1972).

Ostium primum defects of the atrial septum produce a large heart and sometimes heart failure in infancy, and the clinical picture again may be similar to that of the pulmonary venous drainage anomaly. The electrocardiogram shows left-axis deviation and some evidence of left ventricular hypertrophy and the left atrium is often found enlarged (Blount et al., 1956), features never seen in patients with complete anomalous pulmonary venous drainage.

It is extremely rare for simple secundum defects of the atrial septum to produce such a severe clinical picture in early infancy, but atrial septal defects associated with anomalous insertion of the right pulmonary veins may be very difficult to separate from the complete pulmonary venous drainage anomaly on clinical grounds alone.

Complete transposition of the great vessels is easily excluded by the more obvious cyanosis from an early age and a characteristic egg-shaped heart enlargement at x-ray.

Occasionally cases of large ventricular septal defect or patent ductus arteriosus with pulmonary hypertension may mimic the disorder.

In older patients the clinical syndrome closely resembles isolated atrial septal defect.

A few means exist whereby the different types of complete anomalous pulmonary venous drainage may be differentiated. In rather less than one-fourth of the cases of a persistent left superior vena caval type of drainage anomaly, a continuous murmur will be audible in the pulmonary area, and this sign is an extremely helpful one when present. Most assistance is, however, obtained from the chest x-ray. In the left superior vena caval type of drainage, a "figure-of-eight" contour is present in the chest film after the first few months of life. Conditions simulating this appearance have already been described. The insertion of pulmonary veins at cardiac level frequently gives a peculiar high angulation to the upper right border of the right atrium in the first few months of life.

The echocardiogram seems to be a most promising tool for the affected infant patient and already holds a clear superiority in excluding many of the disorders that may mimic total anomalous pulmonary venous return at this age.

Cardiac catheterization, selective dye studies, and selective angiocardiography from the pulmonary artery provide the best means of confirming and refining the clinical diagnosis.

Prognosis

Examination of the natural history of the disease shows that over 80 percent of the cases die in infancy (Figure 32–12) (Keith et al., 1954; Darling et al., 1957). The mere fact that an infant case is discovered with serious symptoms indicates a poor outlook. The worst prognosis exists in those cases with insertion of the anomalous channel at infradiaphragmatic level or other types of pulmonary venous obstruction. They invariably die in the first few weeks or months of life. Cases with vein connections at other levels are most likely to die in the first year of life from congestive heart failure. A small proportion of them survives into adult life and may have only mild symptoms by the third decade (Snellen and Albers, 1952; Gardner and Oram, 1953; Miller and Pollack, 1954; Bruce and Hagen, 1954; Gott et al., 1956; Swan et al., 1956). Nevertheless, the overall picture of life expectancy is a grim one and survival beyond infancy is the exception. Obviously the later the onset of symptoms, the better is the prognosis. It would appear that the degree of mixing of the pulmonary and systemic venous blood in the right atrium and the presence of an atrial septal defect are the most important factors governing survival. There have been conflicting reports about the state of the atrial communication and prognosis. Empirically, it can be assumed that in the absence of pulmonary venous obstruction a large atrial septal defect will enhance patient survival by permitting easy egress of mixed venous blood to the systemic circulation. Burroughs and Edwards (1960)

and others (Seratto et al., 1967) demonstrated this relationship in pathologic material while experience from angiographic data shows an earlier appearance of serious symptoms with smaller atrial communications (Faulkner, 1968). The finding of substantial atrial defect in asymptomatic older children with a malformation and the reported response to balloon atrial septostomy (Miller et al., 1967; Seratto et al., 1968; Mullins et al., 1972) or open atrial septectomy (Berman et al., 1972) all support this view. The debate is due to a few exceptions with large atrial septal defects who die of progressive congestive failure relatively early in infancy and in whom anatomic pulmonary venous obstruction can be excluded as well as in the poor response of others to balloon atrial septostomy later proven to be adequate. An overall assessment must concur with the general thesis that a large atrial septal defect benefits the patient but that other factors can negate its benefit and lead to early demise of the patient not treated surgically. These factors are anatomic pulmonary venous obstruction, early development of unusually low pulmonary vascular resistance or prolonged retention of high pulmonary vascular resistance, and the development of right ventricular myocardial infarctions (Kangos et al., 1969). Data obtained from the hemodynamic study of older patients show that a low pulmonary artery pressure with a high flow is coupled with a high systemic arterial oxygen content and favors survival (Swan et al., 1956).

Treatment

Indications. A fairly serious problem exists for the great majority of patients with this malformation who present with severe symptoms in early infancy.

balloon septostomy in Total veins

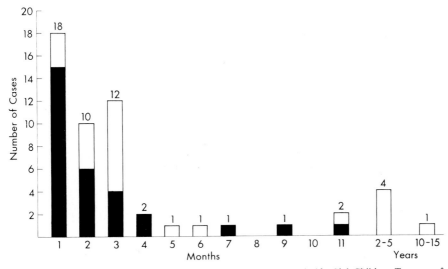

Figure 32-12. The age at death in 53 autopsy-proved cases from The Hospital for Sick Children, Toronto, of total anomalous pulmonary venous drainage unassociated with major intracardiac defects. The clear portion of each column represents surgical deaths.

Management for them in most instances must be surgical. That is unequivocally the case in the presence of organic pulmonary venous obstruction. The patient with frank pulmonary venous obstruction cannot be relieved by either anticongestive measures or septostomy since pulmonary venous congestion and high pulmonary venous pressure are straight mechanical problems. Unless this can be relieved surgically, the clinical course will be progressively downhill with death in early infancy. In the most urgent cases of all, those with infradiaphragmatic connection, rapid deterioration before recognition or surgical action can be instituted has taken a heavy toll. A great majority have died and there are barely a dozen reports of successful correction (Sloan et al., 1962; Cooley and Balas, 1962; Woodwark et al., 1963; Jegier et al., 1967; Llewellyn et al., 1968; Mustard et al., 1968; Mody et al., 1969; Joffe et al., 1971A; Barratt-Boyes et al., 1972). The results using profound hypothermia at Green Lane Hospital have been outstanding. Their four patients, aged five, six, and eight days and three months, respectively, all survived correction (Barratt-Boyes et al., 1972). Survival in even premature infants has been reported (Sparrow et al., 1976). Obstruction at cardiac or supracardiac levels has recently been reviewed by Joffe and associates (1971B). Of 55 reported cases, 64 percent has the obstruction at the left superior vena cava, 25 percent in the right superior vena cava or azygous connection, and fewer than 10 percent involved only either right atrial or coronary sinus connections. Here again, even though the decline of this group is not usually so rapid as in the infradiaphragmatic variety, only seven patients have been reported as successfully corrected since the first account in a 20-month-old child (Venables et al., 1964).

There is considerable debate as to whether the same policy is required for those patients in chronic congestive heart failure without frank pulmonary venous obstruction. There is no real question of the natural history of the disease in these severely affected infants—most will die. For the few survivors the serious impact on infant and parents of the major physical and psychologic growth failure and repeated hospitalization during a stormy first year should give pause to all advocates of purely temporizing medical therapy. There is still room for argument, however, on management of the seriously ill young infant with high flow without frank pulmonary venous obstruction, because it is in this group that benefit from creation of an atrial defect by balloon atrial septostomy has been claimed (Miller et al., 1967; Seratto et al., 1968; Mullins et al., 1972). The majority of infants in these reports lacked significant interatrial pressure differences before septostomy and arterial oxygen saturation was usually unchanged by the procedure. Yet a distinct clinical and hemodynamic improvement occurred in almost 75 percent of these patients for periods lasting up to two years. In some of those who do not improve balloon atrial septostomy may not have produced an adequate defect, possibly because the foramen flap was thick and tough. For

these a later septectomy during the first year may carry less risk than full correction (Berman et al., 1972). Not all centers have had such favorable responses in patients after balloon septostomy and these groups tend to proceed fairly rapidly to correction. Although there can be little doubt that the procedure does not assist all patients, the number of failures and the data allowing judgment on whether or not the septostomy produced a larger opening are not available. Surgical observations by Behrendt and associates (1972) show interatrial communication with a diameter between 4 and 7 mm at correction in infants under the age of one year and would explain why for some patients septostomy fails to improve matters. Until these questions are fully clarified the recommendations of El-Said and associates (1972) for infants with total anomalous pulmonary venous return without pulmonary venous obstruction seem appropriate for most centers: at the time of diagnostic cardiac catheterization balloon atrial septostomy should be performed on all patients. This procedure should be followed by intensive anticongestive measures. Surgical correction can be deferred in those responding favorably until at least the latter part of the first year of life or until the survival of correction for very young infants in a particular center approximates results obtained in older patients. Failure to obtain unequivocal improvement within a short period after these medical measures is an indication for correction.

For the relatively few patients with particular balancing factors that permit an asymptomatic course through childhood and whose signs are more like those of atrial septal defect there are no particular problems in management. The decision for them is simply that total correction should be performed electively after infancy. Their surgical mortality should properly be low—in the order of 5 percent—unless there is late onset of pulmonary vascular obstruction (Williams et al., 1968; Gomes et al., 1970).

Techniques. The principles underlying surgical treatment are based upon the work of Brantigan (1947), Gerbode and Hultgren (1950), and Muller (1951). They involve anastomosis of the common pulmonary vein to the left atrium, obliteration of the connection between the common pulmonary vein and the systemic venous system, and closure of the interatrial communication. In more recent years some refinements of or variations on older techniques (Cooley and Oschner, 1957; Mustard et al., 1962; Williams et al., 1964; Thompson, 1965; Roe, 1970; Van Praagh et al., 1972; Kawashima et al., 1973) and newer supportive measures (Dillard et al., 1967; Gregory et al., 1971) have been added to the operation. Each approach has its advocates but most support has passed to a method involving median sternotomy, mobilization of pericardial attachments, closure of the ductus arteriosus in infants under the age of four months, direct and wide anastomosis of the common pulmonary venous sinus to the left atrium, and closure of the foramen through a left atrial incision (Kirklin, 1973). Some find that spontaneous closure of the foramen ovale will occur later and so leave that structure alone during the operation (Mustard et al., 1968; Silove et al., 1972). Special considerations apply to patients with mixed connections (Gomes et al., 1970; Klint et al., 1972; Neligan et al., 1972). A technique involving anastomosis of the common pulmonary vein to both atria and construction of a pericardial conduit across the floor of the fossa ovalis has been successfully applied to patients with extremely small left atria (Goor et al., 1976).

Results.   Early reports of corrective procedures for these malformations were not encouraging (Burroughs and Kirklin, 1956; Gott et al., 1956; Mustard and Dolan, 1957). The mortality in the past decade has been extremely high for the young patient—up to 90 percent in the first year of life—and, even though improved recently, is still in general much higher than one would hope to see. The hospital mortality for infants under the age of six months is around 50 percent in most centers. Concern over the high death rate in babies is reflected by an increasing emphasis being placed on the young infant by those working in the field (Thompson, 1965; Mustard et al., 1968; Llewellyn, 1968; Leachman et al., 1969; Gomes et al., 1970; Gersony et al., 1971; Barratt-Boyes et al., 1971, 1973; Behrendt et al., 1972; El-Said et al., 1972). Attempts to define those factors most influencing operative mortality in recent years have been made by several groups (Leachman et all., 1969; Gomes et al., 1970; El-Said, 1972; Behrendt et al., 1972 and Kirklin, 1973). In all analyses age at operation appeared as the most important factor, a point between three and six months being critical and below which survival was uncommon. Pulmonary hypertension also carries prognostic importance. In an earlier edition of this book we reported a major difference in pulmonary arterial/systemic arterial systolic pressure ratios: 0.46 in survivors as opposed to 0.95 in fatal cases. Behrendt and associates (1972) found that few patients with preoperative pulmonary arterial/systemic arterial pressure ratios greater than 0.75 survived surgery. This would imply that the highest mortality exists for patients with pulmonary venous obstruction. By contrast, El-Said and associates (1972) could find no correlation between mortality and pressure ratios or pulmonary venous obstruction. For them, operation under six months of

age, connection to the right superior vena cava or azygous system regardless of age, and failure to offer maximum anticongestive care preoperatively were major contributing factors to operative death. Recent reports from The Hospital for Sick Children, Great Ormond Street, have been rather more encouraging with regard to the struggle for success in corrective operations for infants less than the age of three months (Breckenbridge et al., 1973; de Laval et al., 1973).

The battle over whether the left ventricle is too small to accept the new dynamics after repair is almost over. About one-third of patients have left ventricular end-diastolic volumes less than 67 percent of normal, but overall there appears little difference in patients with total anomalous pulmonary venous return from normals (Graham et al., 1972). A wide anastomosis and enlargement of the small left atrium together with careful monitoring of left atrial pressure post-operatively seem important goals to achieve at and after operation (Kirklin, 1973). The role of profound hypothermia in overcoming the age barrier is uncertain. There can be no question that this method can provide the best results for newborn and young infants with the most severe presentations (Thompson, 1965; Barratt-Boyes et al., 1973), which would argue that in some unknown fashion cardio-pulmonary perfusion techniques of the type used with normothermia are responsible in large measure for the poor results in the very young. While better perfusion techniques may eventually replace deep hypothermia, this latter method presently offers the best approach, especially in view of the growing belief that patients should be operated upon after diagnosis not only in cases with pulmonary venous obstruction but in all others as well, unless a dramatic improvement follows the performance of balloon atrial septostomy. This approach aims to restore circulatory pathways to normal before the cumulative effects of gross pulmonary congestion from relative pulmonary venous obstruction, of right ventricular ischemia, and of growth failure are exerted.

Progress has certainly been made in the surgical treatment of this malformation but we are hardly yet in a position to claim a success story (Engle, 1972). Long-term results in survivors are usually excellent, in both general clinical and hemodynamic terms (Williams et al., 1968; Gomes et al., 1971; Herdorf et al., 1974).

COR TRIATRIATUM (TRIATRIAL HEART, STENOSIS OF THE COMMON PULMONARY VEIN)

THIS rare malformation consists of an accessory chamber that lies within the left atrium and receives the pulmonary veins. There is still a difference of opinion about the embryogenesis. An earlier concept that the chamber resulted from an abnormal septum primum (Borst, 1905) has given way to the view that the abnormality is a failure of incorporation of the embryonic common pulmonary vein into the left

atrium (Griffith, 1903; Palmer, 1930; Pfennig, 1941; Loeffler, 1949; Edwards et al., 1951). The critical analysis and review of Van Praagh and Corsini (1969) concludes that cor triatriatum results from entrapment of the left atrial ostium of the common pulmonary vein by that tissue of the right horn of the sinus venosus from which the septum primum develops. This entrapment leads to failure of the common pulmonary vein to be incorporated into the left atrium during the fifth week of fetal life.

Since the original description by Church (1868), there have been approximately 100 cases reported. The malformation is rare, being the least common bar one (less than 0.1 percent) in 15,104 cases of congenital heart malformation seen at The Hospital for Sick Children between 1950 and 1972. The malformation is usually relatively "pure" but in about one in four patients the atrial malformation is associated with cyanotic congenital heart disease of a complex nature (Hospital for Sick Children; Van Praagh and Corsini, 1969).

Pathology

The accessory chamber lies posteriosuperiorly and medial in relation to the remainder of the left atrium and is in contact with the upper portion of the atrial septum. Its superior aspect is entered by the pulmonary veins, while inferiorly the chamber funnels to communicate with the body of the left atrium, the left atrial appendage, and the mitral valve (Figure 32–13). In the majority of cases this communication is a single, rigid, sometimes calcified orifice between 2 and 5 mm in diameter. In some cases it is wide (over 10 mm in diameter), whereas in two reported cases there was no communication at all between the two chambers (Stoeber, 1908; Tannenberg, 1930). In addition to the usual diaphragmatic type, Marin-Garcia and associates (1975) have

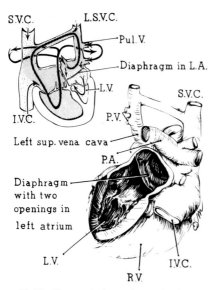

Figure 32-13. The anatomic specimen of a three-year-old boy with a triatrial heart who died of acute pulmonary edema after a long history of dyspnea and progressive exercise intolerance. The dividing diaphragm has two openings (2 × 2 and 2 × 4 mm). A left superior vena cava connects the accessory chamber to the left innominate vein and receives the left pulmonary veins.

described hourglass and tubular-shaped types of the malformation where there is constriction but no membrane within the left atrium. Microscopically the diaphragm consists of endocardium, connective tissue, some elastic tissue, and, occasionally, muscle fibers. The atrial septum is closed in half the cases. According to the concept of Van Praagh and Corsini, a septum primum is continuous with the atrial diaphragm and, therefore, the foramen ovale must always open into the ventral chamber. These authors believe that apparent exceptions are due to abnormal openings between the pulmonary venous chamber and the right sinus horn portion of the right atrium.

Associated anomalies of the pulmonary veins have occurred (Edwards et al., 1951; Becu et al., 1955; Hospital for Sick Children). In two of our cases the left pulmonary veins joined the left superior vena cava connecting the "chamber" with the left innominate vein, while in a third case there was a separate anomalous drainage of the left superior pulmonary vein to the left superior vena cava, which was connected to the left innominate vein. Four examples exist where tetralogy of Fallot was the complicating defect (Preisz, 1890; Hospital for Sick Children; Nagao et al., 1967; Van Praagh and Corsini, 1969). Examples have also been reported of tricuspid atresia and D-transposition of the great arteries (Hospital for Sick Children). The functional consequences of this lesion seen at autopsy are pulmonary congestion of marked degree and considerable hypertrophy and dilatation of the right atrium and right ventricle. The mitral valve is normal.

It is usual to see moderate medial hypertrophy of small muscular pulmonary arteries and arterioles in this condition and occasional cases may show more severe change with intimal involvement.

Reports of fibrous band in the left atrium (Fowler, 1882; Goforth, 1926; McNamara et al., 1947) may represent lesser degrees of the malformation.

Hemodynamics

The presence of a stenotic exit from the accessory chamber in the left atrium produces obstruction to pulmonary venous outflow, pulmonary congestion, pulmonary and right heart hypertension, and eventual right heart failure. The degree of this depends entirely on the size of the ostium.

Clinical Features

The time of onset of symptoms varies with the degree of stenosis at the exit of the accessory chamber. In those with a small ostium symptoms nearly always appear during infancy. Most of the reported cases appeared normal at birth. Obvious dyspnea appeared during the first few months of life. Sometimes persistent cough was a prominent feature (Wolfe et al., 1968; Park et al., 1972). These signs or difficulty with feeding and failure to thrive often bring patients into medical hands. Hemoptysis has been reported once (Brickman et al., 1970) but anemia is quite common and probably secondary to pulmonary hemorrhage (Breck and Harper, 1973). Pulmonary edema may be the first indication of heart disease (Vineberg and Gialloretto, 1956; Hospital for Sick Children).

Where there is a larger ostium, the onset of dyspnea may be delayed. In some patients exertional dyspnea during childhood is not disabling and the onset of frank congestive heart failure may be delayed until early adult life. In those with a very large ostium lengthy survival without symptoms is possible (Loeffler, 1949). The evidence from reported cases is that probably 50 percent are in the category of larger ostia but most of these are still important during childhood and only a relatively small number reach adult life.

The physical examination in symptomatic infants shows a dystrophic appearance, dyspnea, absence of central cyanosis, and basal lung rales. Liver enlargement is frequent in the infant cases, and edema accompanies this sign of congestive heart failure in older children and adult cases. In a ten-month-old girl at The Hospital for Sick Children, facial edema was so marked as to suggest a nephritic basis.

The second heart sound is always accentuated and is usually narrowly split. A modest ejection systolic murmur and occasionally a regurgitant systolic murmur are maximal at the xiphisternum or apex and present in about half the cases. Diastolic murmurs, usually the result of regurgitation, have been reported in children as well as adults (Miller et al., 1964). A continuous murmur, when present, is most often due to extreme obstruction within the chamber and to a very high differential pressure across the ostium. A left-to-right shunt from a patent ductus arteriosus is a much less likely possibility. A presystolic murmur has been noted only once (Borst, 1965).

Radiologic Examination

Slight to moderate cardiac enlargement is the rule (Figure 32–14). One case with absence of the pericardium had cardiomegaly and displacement of the heart to the left side. A heart of normal size may be present in adult patients. Right ventricular enlargement is visible in oblique views. The pulmonary artery segment shows a distinct bulge, while the central lung vasculature though increased does not pulsate. Evidence of pulmonary venous congestion is usual. The butterfly-wing distribution of vascular markings characteristic of acute pulmonary edema was seen in a three-month-old patient at The Hospital for Sick Children.

The left atrial appendage may be prominent (van der Horst and Gotsman, 1971), but left atrial enlargement is not to be expected in this malformation and gross deviation of the barium-filled esophagus is unusual. Nevertheless, apparent enlargement of the left atrium detected in this way was

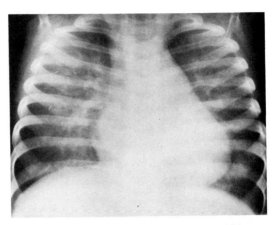

Figure 32-14. The chest x-ray of a 12-month-old boy, H. S. C. (517753) with cor triatriatum. There are cardiomegaly and pulmonary venous congestion. There was moderate pulmonary hypertension at cardiac catheterization. The pulmonary arterial wedge pressure was 20 mm of mercury.

noted in Case 3 of Jegier and associates (1963). Miller and associates (1964) also reported evidence of left atrial enlargement in their three cases.

Electrocardiography

The picture is uniform (Figure 32–15). ÂQRS is oriented rightward and usually lies between +120 and +160 degrees. P waves are peaked and, if not excessively tall, at least suggest right atrial hypertrophy. Precordial leads most commonly show extreme right ventricular hypertrophy with a qR pattern in right chest leads, deep T inversion over the right-sided leads, and occasionally T inversion even in II, III, and AVF (Hospital for Sick Children; Wolfe et al., 1968; Wilson et al., 1971; Park et al., 1972). These findings of right atrial enlargement and extreme right ventricular hypertrophy and even of right ventricular ischemia might be predicted from the very nature of the pathologic anatomy. It is also likely that the size of the ostium in the accessory chamber bears a direct relationship to the degree of disturbance revealed in the electrocardiogram, in which case adults with larger ostia presumably would show more moderate degrees of right ventricular hypertrophy or, in rare cases, even no abnormality of the tracing.

Cardiac Catheterization

At catheterization, moderate to marked right ventricular and pulmonary arterial hypertension has been recorded. Characteristic is the finding of a high pulmonary artery wedge pressure in both children and adults. The range of mean values of this measurement has lain between 16 and 40 mm of mercury. The orifice size can be predicted fairly closely from data obtained at cardiac catheterization

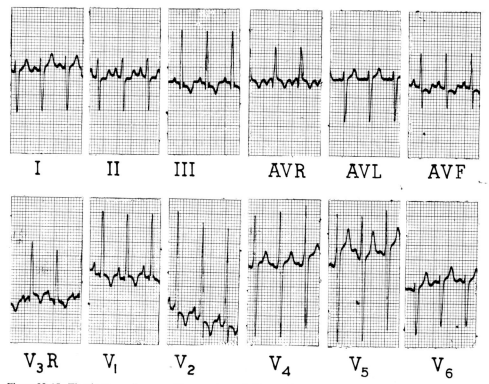

Figure 32-15. The electrocardiogram of the case shown in Figure 32-13. Marked right-axis deviation with signs of right atrial hypertrophy and right ventricular strain.

(Pedersen and Therkelsen, 1954; Jegier et al., 1963).

If the catheter can, in addition, be inserted through a patent foramen ovale and a normal left atrial pressure is obtained, the diagnosis of cor triatriatum is certain. Unfortunately, it would theoretically be possible to do this in only 30 percent of the patients because of the condition of the foramen ovale. The diagnosis is not necessarily excluded by the finding of a high atrial pressure on the left side since abnormal connections exist between the right atrium and the accessory chamber in a proportion of patients.

When anomalies of pulmonary venous drainage are associated, a rise in oxygen saturation in blood sampled from the point of right-sided drainage of the anomalous vessel will be obtained in addition to the previous findings.

Angiocardiography

The possibility that angiocardiography might confirm the diagnosis was suggested by Kjellberg and associates (1959) in one case each of divided right atrium and constriction of the right superior pulmonary vein. A clear demonstration by selective angiocardiography from the main pulmonary artery is possible in the complete left atrial malformation, the intra-atrial diaphragm being seen as a slanting, thin, linear filling defect within the left atrium (Miller et al., 1964). The filling defect is visible in the

anteroposterior view is an oblique line passing from the supralateral to an inferomedial position (Figure 32–16). It is occasionally almost vertical and exhibits little movement (LaSalle et al., 1963; Park et al., 1972; van der Horst and Gotsman, 1971). In older patients it may be possible to manipulate the injecting catheter retrogradely into the accessory chamber (van der Horst and Gotsman, 1971) (Figure 32–16).

Diagnosis

Severe Cases. These infants fail to thrive and become dyspneic in the first few months of life. Gross cyanosis is rarely seen, but peripheral cyanosis due to failure may exist. A systolic murmur may be present, or there may be no murmur. Evidence of pulmonary congestion, cardiac enlargement, and frequently acute heart failure is found, marked right ventricular hypertrophy in the electrocardiogram completing the preliminary findings. Cardiac catheterization narrows the differential diagnosis principally by the detection of a high pulmonary artery wedge pressure. This finding has particular significance when radiologic examination has failed to show left atrial enlargement.

The presence of a heart murmur in the patient is a helpful indication of an underlying cardiac basis, but if no murmur is present the cause of symptoms may be masked for several months. Failure to thrive may lead to an initial diagnosis of inadequate feeding, malformations of the genitourinary or gastrointestinal tract, or metabolic diseases of various types. Similarly, the pulmonary congestion with respiratory distress, though frequently associated with heart failure, has in the past been interpreted as a consequence of parenchymal disease of the lung (Brickman et al., 1970).

The chest x-ray, by revealing cardiac enlargement and hilar congestion, should provide a clue to the cardiac origin of the symptoms. Once it is clear that heart disease is present, further studies are essential for elucidation of the defect. It is now becoming clear that echocardiography offers a major opportunity to reduce the list of diagnostic possibilities at this stage (Lundstrom, 1972; Nimura et al., 1974; Gibson et al., 1974; Pacquet and Gutgesell, 1975).

Various septal defects or combinations thereof, such as atrial septal defect, ventricular septal defect, patent ductus arteriosus, with pulmonary hypertension, when in severe failure may, on occasion, show physical signs and electrocardiographic as well

as radiologic features that are compatible with cor triatriatum. Cardiac catheterization, however, usually clarifies the diagnosis readily. In this study, the key feature that specifically excludes the malformation of the cor triatriatum is the demonstration of a wedge pulmonary artery pressure that is either normal or only modestly elevated. There should hardly ever be confusion with idiopathic or primary pulmonary hypertension in the differential diagnosis but again a normal wedge pressure measurement is present in that state. More difficulty arises in distinguishing cor triatriatum from those other malformations that produce an elevated wedge pulmonary arterial pressure. Several such conditions can mimic the triatrial disorder:

1. COMPLETE ANOMALOUS PULMONARY VENOUS DRAINAGE WITH PULMONARY VENOUS OBSTRUCTION. This defect has a very similar, clinical, radiologic, and electrocardiographic picture. In isolated cor triatriatum, cardiac catheterization, besides showing a high pulmonary artery wedge pressure, fails to demonstrate shunts in either

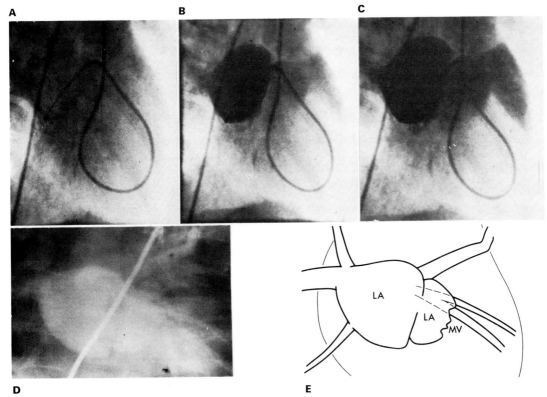

Figure 32-16. Selected frames from 35-mm cine film. *Top,* 45-degree right anterior oblique projection showing the retrograde arterial catheter (*A*) passing through the left anterior mitral valve and lower left atrium into the posterior chamber, (*B*) contrast filling the dorsal chamber with delay in emptying, and (*C*) late filling of the true left atrium. Studies in a 12-year-old girl reproduced with permission of the authors (Van der Horst, R. L., and Gotsman. M. S.: Cor triatriatum: angiographic diagnosis by retrograde catheterization of the dorsal accessory chamber. *Br. J. Radiol.,* **44**:273, 1971). *D.* Anteroposterior projection with schematic diagram (*E*) of the levophase following pulmonary arterial injection of contrast in a 12-month-old boy whose chest x-ray is shown in Figure 32-14. The abnormal septum was excised shortly afterward. At age seven years the data from cardiac catheterization were normal.

direction and so excludes the venous anomaly. However, one in seven cases with cor triatriatum is associated with partial anomalous pulmonary venous drainage, which will be evident on cardiac catheterization. In these cases the important hemodynamic features allowing correct diagnosis of the underlying triatrial heart are the high pulmonary artery wedge pressure and a normal arterial oxygen saturation in the presence of a high pulmonary artery pressure. Even then the diagnostic problem may be a complicated one: One three-year-old boy at The Hospital for Sick Children with the clinical and hemodynamic pictures of complete anomalous pulmonary venous drainage was diagnosed after cardiac catheterization (pulmonary wedge: 18 mm of mercury) and selective angiocardiography as a case of partial anomalous pulmonary venous drainage and cor triatriatum. At operation a high pulmonary venous pressure was confirmed but no accessory chamber was found. At autopsy the pulmonary veins collected into a retrocardiac common vein that communicated with each atrium through a very small ostium (3 by 3 mm).

2. CONGENITAL STENOSIS OF INDIVIDUAL PULMONARY VEINS. A score of examples of this entity have shown a clinical picture of failure to thrive, modest cyanosis, nonspecific systolic murmur, marked right ventricular hypertrophy in the electrocardiogram, and chest films with pulmonary venous obstruction. Survival beyond the first year is unusual (Edwards, 1960; Shone, 1962). The veins are either hyperplastic or stenotic close to their point of connection to the left atrium. A few cases have been diagnosed before death and one, at least, has been successfully corrected (Kawashima et al., 1971; Park et al., 1974).

3. ATRESIA OF THE COMMON PULMONARY VEIN. Seven cases of complete atresia of the common pulmonary vein have been reported in association with normally related ventricles and great arteries but with foramen ovale patency and the patent ductus arteriosus (Lucas et al., 1962; Levine et al., 1967; Rywlin and Fojaco, 1968; Hawker et al., 1972). Three other cases have had a small accessory pulmonary vein that was an inadequate compensation and the clinical course has been similar to the complete atresia (Hastreiter et al., 1962; Hauck et al., 1960; Folger and Mody, 1974). The presentation is one of an early onset of cyanosis, tachycardia, and dyspnea with x-rays and electrocardiograms characteristic of severe pulmonary venous obstruction. Death usually occurs during the first month of life but the condition is operable.

4. SUPRAVALVULAR STENOSING RING OF THE LEFT ATRIUM. This condition (Manubens et al., 1960) consists of a thick circular ridge immediately above the mitral valve. It appears to be an almost total partitioning of the left atrium but its relationship and embryogenesis vis-à-vis cor triatriatum are uncertain. The reported cases have been associated with other malformations, particularly ventricular septal defect or patent ductus arteriosus, and consequently have

presented serious diagnostic difficulties during life. We have encountered a patient with the isolated lesion in whom marked pulmonary hypertension was present, the left atrium was equivocally enlarged at barium swallow, and there was gross cardiomegaly. An electrocardiogram, normal six months before death, showed gross right atrial and right ventricular hypertrophy at the final admission at the age of four years. Cardiac catheterization confirmed the presence of severe pulmonary hypertension and cineangiocardiography from the pulmonary artery showed slight delay in contrast clearing from the right atrium (Mehrizi et al., 1965). Other cases have been reported (Rao et al., 1969).

5. CONGENITAL MITRAL STENOSIS. This condition can produce identical findings but a presystolic murmur and the presence of an opening snap, together with considerable enlargement of the left atrium and findings at echocardiography, may appreciably assist the differentiation.

6. TUMORS OF THE LEFT ATRIUM. This condition can conceivably produce similar clinical features but filling defects revealed by echocardiography or angiocardiography probably offer most help in the diagnostic problem.

7. ENDOCARDIAL FIBROELASTOSIS AND SEVERE VALVULAR AORTIC STENOSIS. These conditions usually can be excluded because of the electrocardiogram. Although an exceptional case of endocardial fibroelastosis may show marked right ventricular hypertrophy (Vlad et al., 1955), the vast majority of cases of both conditions show extreme left ventricular hypertrophy, a type of tracing never seen in cor triatriatum. Marked left atrial enlargement, commonly present in endocardial fibroelastosis and severe aortic stenosis, is not encountered in triatrial heart. Echocardiography assists.

8. HYPOPLASTIC LEFT HEART MALFORMATIONS. Both mitral atresia with a normal aortic valve (Edwards, 1960) and the more common form of aortic atresia, with or without mitral atresia, have on occasion shown features that are virtually identical to those of cor triatriatum. The differential problem can always be resolved by adequate studies, but in general the extremely early presentation of the more common form of hypoplastic left heart disorder makes the likelihood of confusion remote, since cor triatriatum is not a disease that causes death usually within the first few days of life.

Less Severe Cases. Patients not developing serious symptoms until adult life pose slightly different problems in diagnosis.

The dyspnea, cough, pulmonary congestion, and radiologic signs may be confused with lung disease such as tuberculosis (Vineberg and Gialloreto, 1956). A cardiac basis for the symptoms is more usually recognized since both systolic and diastolic murmurs are a feature of the older cases. The diagnosis then rapidly becomes one involving left heart obstructive lesions of which mitral stenosis is the chief.

In a particular patient of either group of severity, even after all techniques have been explored, the combined data may merely narrow the diagnosis to an obstructive left heart lesion, in which case only surgical exploration can establish the answer.

Prognosis

The outlook in these patients is governed entirely by the size of the ostium leading from the accessory chamber of the left atrium. If this is nonexistent or if the ostium is less than 3 mm in diameter, death will occur in infancy from heart failure—the result of severe pulmonary congestion and hypertension. This was the case in approximately 50 percent of reported cases. With ostial diameters in the order of 5 to 7 mm, the life-span is unpredictable though clearly shortened. With a diameter over 7 mm, the duration of life is longer and this larger orifice may be compatible with quite lengthy survival. The fact remains that about 80 percent of patients with cor triatriatum have died before the age of 20 years.

The successful operative treatment of adult cases (Vineberg and Gialloreto, 1956; Lewis et al., 1956; Barrett and Hickie, 1957; Lam, 1958) followed by excellent results in children (Anderson and Varco, 1961; Jegier et al., 1963; Miller et al., 1964; Perry et al., 1967; Ahn et al., 1968; Wolfe et al., 1968; Park et al., 1972; van der Horst and Gotsman, 1971) should mean that the prognosis will be radically altered provided the cases reach a cardiac surgeon. Some 23 successful operations have already been reported. Since the majority of patients present symptoms in childhood, the responsibility for diagnosis, and consequent improvement in prognosis, rests with the family practitioner and pediatrician.

Treatment

Beyond intensive digitalization for those patients in congestive heart failure, there is no place for delay in the investigation and surgical treatment of these children. With the diagnosis confirmed or narrowed to the possibilities mentioned, surgical exploration is indicated. The fear that severe pulmonary vascular disease might lead to incomplete cure has not been confirmed. On the contrary, an adequate fall in pulmonary artery pressure within a few months of the operation is the general rule (Anderson and Varco, 1961; Jegier et al., 1963; Miller et al., 1964) even though challenge by exercise may reveal residual· increases in pulmonary vascular resistance (Wolfe et al., 1968).

REFERENCES

Anomalies of Venous Return

Abbott, M. E.: *Atlas of Congenital Cardiac Disease.* American Heart Association, New York, 1936.

Ainger, L. E.: Infradiaphragmatic anomalous pulmonary venous connection. Report of an unusual case. *Am. J. Dis. Child.,* **104**:662, 1962.

Anderson, R. C.; Adams, P., Jr.; and Burke, B. · Anomalous inferior vena cava with azygos continuation (infrahepatic interruption of the inferior vena cava). Report of 15 cases. *J. Pediatr.,* **59**:370, 1961.

Anderson, R. C.; Heilig, W.; Novick, R.; and Jarvis, C.: Anomalous inferior vena cava with azygos drainage: so-called absence of the inferior vena cava. *Am. Heart J.,* **49**:318, 1955.

Arvidsson, H.: Anomalous pulmonary vein entering the inferior vena cava examined by selective angiocardiography. *Acta Radiol.,* **41**:156, 1954.

Barratt-Boyes, B. G.; Simpson, M.; and Neutze, J. M.: Intracardiac surgery in neonates and infants using deep hypothermia with surface cooling and limited cardiopulmonary bypass. *Circulation,* Suppl. **43**:25, 1971.

Barratt-Boyes, B. G.; Nichols, T. T.; Brandt, P. W. T.; and Neutze, J. M.: Aortic arch interruptions associated with patent ductus arteriosus, ventricular septal defect and total anomalous pulmonary venous connection. Total correction in an 8-day-old infant by means of profound hypothermia and limited cardiopulmonary bypass. *J. Thorac. Cardiovasc. Surg.,* **63**:367, 1972.

Barratt-Boyes, B. G.: Complete correction of cardiovascular malformations in the first two years of life using profound hypothermia. *Heart Disease in Infancy, Diagnosis and Management.* Proceedings of the Second International Symposium. Churchill Livingstone, London, 1973, p. 25.

Beattie, J.: The importance of anomalies of the superior vena cava in man. *Can. Med. Assoc., J.,* **25**:281, 1931.

Bedford, D. E.: The anatomical types of atrial septal defect. *Am. J. Cardiol.,* **6**:568, 1960.

Bedford, D. E.; Sellors, T. H.; Somerville, W.; Belcher, J. R.; and Besterman, E. M. M.: Atrial septal defect and its surgical treatment. *Lancet,* **1**:1255, 1957.

Behrendt, D. M.; Aberdeen, E.; Waterston, D. J.; and Bonham-Carter, R. E.: Total anomalous pulmonary venous drainage in infants. Clinical and hemodynamic findings, methods and results of operation in 37 cases. *Circulation,* **46**:347, 1972.

Berman, M. A.; Fishbone, G.; and Stansel, H. C., Jr.: Total anomalous pulmonary venous return with obstruction at the foramen ovale. Successful palliation by open atrial septectomy. *Am. J. Surg.,* **124**:679, 1972.

Blake, H. A.; Hall, R. J.; and Manion, W. C.: Anomalous Pulmonary Venous Return. *Circulation,* **32**:406, 1965.

Blount, S. G., Jr.; Balchum, O. J.; and Gensini, G.: The persistent ostium primum atrial septal defect. *Circulation,* **13**:499, 1956.

Bonham-Carter, R. E.; Capriles, M.; and Noe, Y.: Total anomalous pulmonary venous drainage. A clinical and anatomical study of 75 children. *Br. Heart J.,* **31**:45, 1969.

Bove, K. E.; Geiser, E. A.; and Meyer, R. A.: The left ventricle in anomalous pulmonary venous return. Morphometric analysis of 36 fatal cases in infancy. *Arch. Pathol.,* **99**:522, 1975.

Brantigan, O. C.: Anomalies of the pulmonary veins: their surgical significance. *Surg. Gynecol. Obstet.,* **84**:653, 1947.

Braudo, M.; Beanlands, D. S.; and Trusler, G.: Anomalous drainage of the right superior vena cava into the left atrium. *Can. Med. J.,* **99**:715, 1968.

Breckenridge, I. M.; de Laval, M.; Stark, J.; and Waterston, D. J.: Correction of total anomalous pulmonary venous drainage in infancy. *J. Thorac. Cardiovasc. Surg.,* **66**:447, 1973.

Brock, R., and Ross, D. N.: The sinus venosus type of atrial septal defect. *Guy Hosp. Rep.,* **108**:291, 1959.

Brody, H.: Drainage of the pulmonary veins into the right side of the heart. *Arch. Pathol.,* **33**:221, 1942.

Bruce, R. A., and Hagen, J. M. V.: Anomaly of total pulmonary venous connection: report of a case with survival for 31 years. *Am. Heart J.,* **47**:785, 1954.

Bruwer, A.: Roentgenologic findings in anomalous pulmonary venous connection. *Proc. Mayo Clin.,* **28**:480, 1953.

——: Roentgenologic findings in total anomalous pulmonary venous connection. *Proc. Mayo Clin.,* **31**:171, 1956.

Burchell, H. B.: Total anomalous pulmonary venous drainage: clinical and physiologic patterns. *Proc. Mayo Clin.,* **31**:161, 1956.

Burroughs, J. T., and Edwards, J. E.: Total anomalous pulmonary venous connection. *Am. Heart J.,* **59**:913, 1960.

Burroughs, J. J., and Kirklin, J. W.: Complete surgical correction of total anomalous venous connection: report of three cases. *Proc. Mayo Clin.,* **31**:182, 1956.

Campbell, M., and Deuchar, D. C.: The left-sided superior vena cava. *Br. Heart J.,* **16**:423, 1954.

Campbell, M.; Gardner, F.; and Reynolds, G.: Cor biloculare. *Br. Heart J.,* **14**:317, 1952.

Castellanos, A.; Pereiras, R.; and Garcia-Lopez, A.: Anomalies de les venas cavas en las cardiopatias congenitas. Prim. Cong. Soc. Inter-Amer. Cardiol., Mexico, 1944.

Cha, E. M., and Khoury, G. H.: Persistent left superior vena cava. Radiologic and clinical significance. *Radiology,* **103**:375, 1972.

Colman, A. L.: Diagnosis of left superior vena cava by clinical inspection: a new physical sign. *Am. Heart J.,* **73**:115, 1967.

Compere, D. E., and Forsyth, H. F.: Anomalous pulmonary veins: report of case. *J. Thorac. Surg.,* **13**:63, 1944.

Cooley, D. A., and Balas, P. E.: Total anomalous pulmonary venous drainage into inferior vena cava: report of a successful surgical correction. *Surgery,* **51**:798, 1962.

Cooley, D. A., and Mahaffey, D. E.: Anomalous pulmonary venous drainage of entire left lung: report of a case with surgical correction. *Ann. Surg.,* **142**:986, 1955.

Cooley, D. A., and Ochsner, A., Jr.: Correction of total anomalous pulmonary venous drainage. *Surgery,* **42**:1014, 1957.

Cooley, R. N.; Sloan, R. D.; Hanlon, R. C.; et al.: Angiocardiography in congenital heart disease of cyanotic type II. Observations of tricuspid stenosis or atresia with hypoplasia of the right ventricle. *Radiology,* **54**:848, 1950.

Dalith, F., and Neufeld, H.: Radiological diagnosis of anomalous pulmonary venous connection: a tomographic study. *Radiology,* **74**:1, 1960.

Darling, R. C.; Rothney, W. B.; and Craig, J. M.: Total pulmonary venous drainage into the right side of the heart; report of 17 autopsied cases not associated with other major cardiovascular anomalies. *Lab. Invest.,* **6**:44, 1957.

Davis, W. H.; Jordaan, F. R.; and Snyman, H. W.: Persistent left superior vena cava drainage into the left atrium as an isolated anomaly. *Am. Heart J.,* **57**:616, 1959.

Dean, J. C., and Fox, G. W. (1928): Cited by Brody (1942).

de Laval, M.; Stark, J.; and Waterston, D. J.: Mixed type of total anomalous pulmonary venous drainage. Surgical correction in 3 infants. *Ann. Thorac. Surg.,* **16**:464, 1973.

Delisle, G.; Ando, M.; Calder, A. L.; Zuberbuhler, J. R.; Rochenmacher, S.; Alday, L. E.; Mangino, O.; Van Praagh, S.; and Van Praagh, R.: Total anomalous pulmonary venous connection: Report of 93 autopsied cases with emphasis on diagnostic and surgical considerations. *Am. Heart J.,* **91**:99, 1976.

Diamond, M. D.; Dillon, J. C.; Haine, C. L.; Chang, S.; and Feigenbaum, H.: Echocardiographic features of atrial septal defect. *Circulation,* **43**:129, 1971.

Diaz, A.; Castellanos, A.; and Garcia, O.: Espectacular mejoria de un caso de "pentalogia" solamente con la seccion de la vena cava superior izquierda persistente. *Arch. Inst. Cardiol. México,* **19**:314, 1949.

Dillard, D. H.; Mohri, H.; Hessel, E. A.; Anderson, H. N.; Nelson, R. J.; Crawford, E. W.; et al.: Correction of total anomalous pulmonary venous drainage in infancy utilizing deep hypothermia with total circulatory arrest. *Circulation,* **35**:105, 1967.

Dotter, C. T.; Hardisty, N. M.; and Steinberg, I.: Anomalous right pulmonary vein entering the inferior vena cava. *Am. J. Med. Sci.,* **218**:31, 1949.

Downing, D. F.: Absence of the inferior vena cava. *Pediatrics,* **12**:675, 1953.

DuShane, J. W.: Total anomalous pulmonary venous connection: clinical aspects. *Proc. Mayo Clin.,* **31**:167, 1956.

Edwards, J. E.: Congenital malformations of the heart and great vessels, in Gould, S. E. (ed.): *Pathology of the Heart.* Charles C Thomas, Publisher, Springfield, Ill., 1953, Chap. 5, p. 266.

Edwards, J. E., and DuShane, J. W.: Thoracic venous anomalies. I. Vascular connection between the left atrium and the left innominate vein (laevoatriocardinal vein) associated with mitral atresia and premature closure of the foramen ovale (case 1). II. Pulmonary veins draining wholly into the ductus venosus (case 2). *Arch. Pathol.,* **49**:517, 1950.

Eisen, S., and Elliott, L. P.: A plain film signs of total anomalous pulmonary venous connection below the diaphragm. *Am. J. Roentgenol.,* **102**:372, 1968.

Elliott, L. P., and Edwards, J. E.: The problem of pulmonary venous obstruction in total anomalous pulmonary venous connection to the left innominate vein. *Circulation,* **25**:913, 1962.

Ellis, F. H., Jr., and Kirklin, J. W.: Anomalous pulmonary venous connections. *Surg. Clin. North Am.,* **35**:997, 1955.

El-Said, G.; Mullins, C. E.; and McNamara, D. G.: Management of total anomalous pulmonary venous return. *Circulation,* **45**:1240, 1972.

Engle, M. A.: Total anomalous pulmonary venous drainage. Success story at last. *Circulation,* **46**:209, 1972.

Evans, J. R.; Rowe, R. D.; and Keith, J. D.: The clinical diagnosis of atrial septal defect in children. *Am. J. Med.,* **30**:345, 1961.

Falcone, M. W., and Roberts, W. C.: Atresia of the right atrial ostium of the coronary sinus unassociated with persistence of the left superior vena cava: a clinicopathologic study of four adult patients. *Am. Heart J.,* **83**:604, 1972.

Falsetti, H. L.; Naeye, R. L.; Tabakin, B. S.; and Hanson, J. S.: Uncomplicated total anomalous pulmonary venous return below the diaphragm. Report of a case. *Dis. Chest,* **46**:102, 1964.

Faulkner, S. L.: Unpublished observations, 1968.

Feindt, H. R., and Hauch, H. J.: Über drei fälle von doppelter oberer hohlvene (Beitrag zur Diagnostik dieser Kongenitalen missbildung). *Z. Kreislaufforsch.,* **42**:53, 1953.

Ferencz, C.: Review article: congenital abnormalities of pulmonary vessels and their relation to malformations of the lung. *Pediatrics,* **28**:993, 1961.

Ferencz, C.; Greco, J. M.; and Libi-Sylora, M.: Variability of Pulmonary Vascular Disease in Certain Malformations of the Heart; in *The Natural History and Progress in Treatment of Congenital Heart Defects.* Eds. Kidd, B. S. L., and Keith, J. D. Charles C Thomas, Publisher, Springfield, Ill., 1971, p. 300.

Fiandra, O.; Barcia, A.; Cortes, R.; and Stanham, J.: Partial anomalous pulmonary venous drainage into the inferior vena cava. *Acta Radiol.,* **57**:301, 1962.

Findlay, C. W., Jr., and Maier, H. C.: Anomalies of the pulmonary vessels and their surgical significance. *Surgery,* **29**:604, 1951.

Folger, G. M., Jr.; Rowe, R. D.; and Criley, J. M.: Partial anomalous drainage of right pulmonary veins from normally connected pulmonary veins. Cineangiographic differentiation. *South. Med. J.,* **59**:389, 1966.

France, N. E., and Brown, R. J. K.: Congenital pulmonary lymphangiectasis. Report of 11 examples with special reference to cardiovascular findings. *Arch. Dis. Child.,* **46**:528, 1971.

Frank, C. G., and Maloney, J. V., Jr.: Surgical significance of congenital anomalies of the coronary sinus. *J. Cardiovasc. Surg.,* **9**:420, 1968.

Fraser, R. S.; Dvorkin, J.; Rossall, R. E.; and Eidem, R.: Left superior vena cava. A review of associated congenital heart lesions, catheterization data and roentgenologic findings. *Am. J. Med.,* **31**:711, 1961.

Freed, M. D.; Rosenthal, A.; and Bernhard, W. F.: Balloon occlusion of a persistent left superior vena cava in the preoperative evaluation of systemic venous return. *J. Thorac. Cardiovasc. Surg.,* **65**:835, 1973.

Freedom, R. M., and Ellison, R. C.: Coronary sinus rhythm in the polysplenia syndrome. *Chest,* **63**:952, 1973.

Freedom, R. M., and Treves, S.: Splenic scintigraphy and radionuclide venography in the heterotaxy syndrome. *Radiology,* **107**:382, 1973.

Friedli, B.; Guerin, R.; Davignon, A.; Fouron, J. C.; and Stanley, P.: Surgical treatment of partial anomalous pulmonary venous drainage: A long-term follow-up study. *Circulation,* **45**:159, 1972.

Friedlich, A.; Bing, R. J.; and Blount, S. G.: Physiological studies in congenital heart disease. IX. Circulatory dynamics in the anomalies of venous return including pulmonary arteriovenous fistula. *Bull. Hopkins, Hosp.,* **86**:20, 1950.

Friedlowsky, A. (1868): Cited by Brody (1942).

Frye, R. L.; Marshall, H. W.; Kincaid, O. W.; and Burchell, H. B.: Anomalous pulmonary venous drainage of the right lung into the inferior vena cava. *Br. Heart J.,* **24**:696, 1962.

Gardner, F., and Oram, S.: Persistent left superior vena cava draining the pulmonary veins. *Br. Heart J.,* **15**:305, 1953.

Gardner, D. L., and Cole, L.: Long survival with inferior vena cava draining into left atrium. *Br. Heart J.,* **17**:93, 1955.

Gasul, B. M.; Weiss, H.; Fell, E. H.; Dillon, R. F.; Fisher, D. L.; and Marienfeld, C. J.: Angiocardiography in congenital heart disease correlated with clinical and autopsy findings. *Am. J. Dis. Child.,* **85**:404, 1953.

Gathman, G. E., and Nadas, A. S.: Total anomalous pulmonary

venous connection. Clinical and physiologic observations of 75 pediatric patients. *Circulation,* 42:143, 1970.

Gautam, H. P.: Left atrial inferior vena cava with atrial septal defect. *J. Thorac. Cardiovasc. Surg.,* 55:827, 1968.

Geraci, J. E., and Kirklin, J. W.: Transplantation of left anomalous pulmonary vein to left atrium: report of a case. *Proc. Mayo Clin.,* 28:472, 1953.

Gerbode, F., and Hultgren, H.: Observations on experimental atriovenous anastomoses with particular reference to congenital anomalies of the venous return to the heart and to cyanosis. *Surgery,* 28:235, 1950.

Gersony, W. M.; Bowman, F. O.; Steeg, C. N.; Hayes, C. J.; Jesse, M. J.; and Malm, J. R.: Management of total pulmonary venous drainage in early infancy. *Circulation,* 43, Suppl. I:19, 1971.

Gessner, I. H.; Krovetz, L. J.; Wheat, M. W., Jr.; Shanklin, D. R.; and Schiebler, G. L.: Total anomalous pulmonary venous connection. Electro-vector cardiographic hemodynamic and anatomic correlations in 11 cases. *Am. Heart J.,* 68:459, 1964.

Glaser, J.: The differential diagnosis of total anomalous pulmonary venous drainage in infancy by echocardiography. Amer. Acad. Pediat. Annual meeting, Program abstr., 1972.

Gomes, M. M. R.; Feldt, R. H.; McGoon, D. C.; and Danielson, G. K.: Total anomalous pulmonary venous connection. Surgical considerations and results of operation. *J. Thorac. Cardiovasc. Surg.,* 60:116, 1970.

Gomes, M. M. R.; Feldt, R. H.; McGoon, D. C.; and Danielson, G. K.: Long-term results following correction of total anomalous pulmonary venous connection. *J. Thorac. Cardiovasc. Surg.,* 61:253, 1971.

Goor, D. A.; Yellin, A.; Frand, M.; Smolinsky, A.; and Neufeld, H. N.: The operative problem of small left atrium in total anomalous pulmonary venous correction: report of 5 patients. *Ann. Thorac. Surg.,* 22:245, 1976.

Gorlin, R. J.; Cervenka, J.; Anderson, R. C.; Sauk, J. J.; and Bevis, W. D.: Robin's Syndrome. A probably x-linked recessive subvariety exhibiting persistence of left superior vena cava and atrial septal defect. *Am. J. Dis. Child.,* 119:176, 1970.

Gott, V. L.; Lester, R. G.; Lillehei, C. W.; and Varco, R. L.: Total anomalous pulmonary return. An analysis of thirty cases. *Circulation,* 13:543, 1956.

Graham, T. P., Jr.; Jarmakani, J. M.; and Canent, R. V., Jr.: Left heart volume characteristics with a right ventricular volume overload. Total anomalous pulmonary venous connection and large atrial septal defect. *Circulation,* 45:389, 1972.

Gregory, G. A.; Kitterman, J. A.; Phibbs, R. H.; Tooley, W. H.; and Hamilton, W. K.: Treatment of the idiopathic respiratory-distress syndrome with continuous positive airway pressure. *N. Engl. J. Med.,* 284:1333, 1971.

Grishman, A.; Poppel, M. H.: Simpson, R. S.; and Sussman, M. L.: The roentgenographic and angiocardiographic aspects of (1) aberrant insertion of pulmonary veins associated with interatrial septal defect and (2) congenital arteriovenous aneurysm of the lung. *Am. J. Roentgenol.,* 62:500, 1949.

Guller, B.; Ritter, D. G.; and Kincaid, O. W.: Tricuspid atresia with pulmonary atresia and total anomalous pulmonary venous connection to the right superior vena cava. *Mayo Clin. Proc.,* 47:105, 1972.

Harris, H. A.; Gray, S. H.; and Whitney, C.: The heart of a child aged 22 months presenting an anomalous vein from the pulmonary auricle to the right internal jugular vein, transposition of the great vessels and left superior vena cava. *Anat. Rec.,* 36:31, 1927.

Harris, C. B. C.; Neuhauser, E. B. D.; and Giedion, A.: Total anomalous pulmonary venous return below the diaphragm. Roentgen appearances in three patients diagnosed during life. *Am. J. Roentgen,* 84:436, 1960.

Hastreiter, A. R.; Paul, M. H.; Molthan, M. E.; and Miller, R. A.: Total anomalous pulmonary venous connection with severe pulmonary venous obstruction. A clinical entity. *Circulation,* 25:916, 1962.

Hauck, A. J.; Rudolph, A. M.; and Nadas, A. S.: Pulmonary venous obstruction in infants with anomalous pulmonary venous drainage. *Am. J. Dis. Child.,* 100:744, 1960.

Healey, J. E., Jr.: An anatomic survey of anomalous pulmonary veins: their clinical significance. *J. Thorac. Surg.,* 23:433, 1952.

Heller, R. M.; Dorst, J. P.; James, A. E.; and Rowe, R. D.: A useful sign in the recognition of Azygos continuation of the inferior vena cava. *Radiology,* 101:519, 1971.

Hordof, A. J.; Hayes, C. J.; Bowman, F. O., Jr.; Malm, J. R.; and Gersony, W. M.: Hemodynamic assessment of total anomalous pulmonary venous connection (TAPVC) following correction during infancy. *Am. J. Cardiol.,* 33:144, 1974.

Hughes, C. W., and Rumore, P. C.: Anomalous pulmonary veins. *Arch. Pathol.,* 37:364, 1944.

Jegier, W.; Charrette, E.; and Dobell, A. R. C.: Infradiaphragmatic anomalous pulmonary venous drainage. Normal hemodynamics following operation in infancy. *Circulation,* 35:396, 1967.

Jensen, J. B., and Blount, S. G., Jr.: Total anomalous pulmonary venous return. A review and report of the oldest surviving patient. *Am. Heart J.,* 82:387, 1971.

Joffe, H. S.; O'Donovan, T. G.; Glaun, B. P.; Chesler, E.; and Schrire, V.: Subdiaphragmatic total anomalous pulmonary venous drainage; report of a successful surgical correction. *Am. Heart J.,* 81:250, 1971.(A)

Joffe, H. S.; Chesler, E.; O'Donovan, T. G.; and Schrire, V.: Successful correction of supradiaphragmatic total anomalous pulmonary venous drainage with obstruction in a 3-month-old infant. *J. Thorac. Cardiovasc. Surg.,* 62:238, 1971(b).

Johannson, B. W.: Oxygen saturation of the blood in different parts of the central venous system. Its importance for the diagnosis of anomalous pulmonary veins. *Acta. Med. Scand.,* 170:287, 1961.

Johnson, A. L.; Wiglesworth, F. W.; Denbar, J. S.; Siddoo, S.; and Grajo, M.: Infradiaphragmatic total anomalous pulmonary venous connection. *Circulation,* 17:340, 1958.

Kangos, J. J.; Ferrer, M. I.; Franciosi, R. A.; Blanc, W. A.; and Blumenthal, S.: Electrocardiographic changes associated with papillary muscle infarction in congenital heart disease. *Am. J. Cardiol.,* 23:801, 1969.

Karnegis, J. N.; Winchell, P.; and Edwards, J. E.: Persistent left superior vena cava, fibrous remnant of the right superior vena cava and ventricular septal defect. *Am. J. Cardiol.,* 14:573, 1964.

Kauffman, S. L.; Ores, C. N.; and Anderson, P. H.: Two cases of total anomalous pulmonary venous return of the supracardiac type with stenosis simulating infradiaphragmatic drainage. *Circulation,* 25:376, 1962.

Kaufman, R. L.; Boynton, R. C.; Hartmann, H. F.; Morgan, B. C.; and McAlister, W. H.: Family studies in congenital heart diseases III: Total anomalous pulmonary venous connection in two sisters and their female maternal first cousin. In *Birth Defects: Original Article Series,* Vol. 8:5. The National Foundation, New York, 1973, p. 88.

Kawashima, V.; Nakano, S.; Matsuda, H.; Miyamoto, T.; and Manabe, H.: Successful correction of total anomalous pulmonary venous drainage with a new surgical technique. *J. Thorac. Cardiovasc. Surg.,* 66:959, 1973.

Keith, J. D.; Rowe, R. D.; Vlad, P.; and O'Hanley, J. H.: Complete anomalous pulmonary venous drainage. *Am. J. Med.,* 16:23, 1954.

Kelly, D. T.; Krovetz, L. J.; and Rowe, R. D.: Double-lumen flotation catheter for use in complex congenital cardiac anomalies. *Circulation,* 44:910, 1971.

Kim, Y. S.; Serratto, M.; Long, D. M.; and Hastreiter, A. R.: Left atrial inferior vena cava with atrial septal defect. *Ann. Surg.,* II:165, 1971.

Kirklin, J. W.; Swan, H. J. C.; Wood, E. H.; Burchell, H. B.; and Edwards, J. E.: Anatomic, physiologic and surgical considerations in repair of interatrial communications in man. *J. Thorac. Surg.,* 29:37, 1955.

Kirklin, J. W.; Ellis, F. H., Jr.; and Wood, E. H.: Treatment of anomalous pulmonary venous connections in association with interatrial communications. *Surgery,* 39:389, 1956.

Kirklin, J. W.: Total anomalous pulmonary venous connection. Surgical treatment for total anomalous pulmonary venous connection in infancy. Heart Disease in Infancy, Proceedings of the Second International Symposium, 1973, vol. 89.

Kirsch, W. M.; Carlsson, E.; and Hartmann, A. F., Jr.: A case of anomalous drainage of the superior vena cava into the left atrium. *J. Thorac. Cardiovasc. Surg.,* 41:550, 1961.

Kittle, C. F., and Crockett, J. E.: Vena cava bronchovascular syndrome—a triad of anomalies involving the right lung. Anomalous pulmonary vein, abnormal bronchi and systemic pulmonary arteries. *Ann. Surg.,* 156:222, 1962.

Kjellberg, S. R.; Mannheimer, E.; Rudhe, U.; and Jönsson, B.: *Diagnosis of Congenital Heart Disease.* Year Book Publishers, Inc., Chicago, 1959.

Klint, R.; Weldon, C.; Hartmann, A., Jr.; Schad, N., et al.:

Mixed-type total anomalous pulmonary venous drainage. *J. Thorac. Cardiovasc. Surg.*, **63**:164, 1972.

Kuhn, J. P.; Fletcher, B. D.; and DeLemos, R. A.: Roentgen findings in transient tachypnea of the newborn. *Radiology*, **92**:751, 1969.

Lambert, E. C.: In Zimmerman, H. A. (ed.): *Intravascular Catheterization.* Charles C Thomas, Publisher, Springfield, Ill., 1959, p. 225.

Leachman, R. D.; Cooley, D. A.; Hallman, G. L.; Simpson, J. W.; and Dear, W. E.: Total anomalous pulmonary venous return. Correlation of hemodynamic observations and surgical mortality in 58 cases. *Ann. Thorac. Surg.*, **7**:5, 1969.

Levinson, D. C.; Griffith, G. C.; Cosby, R. S.; Zinn, W. J.; Jacobson, G.; Dimitroff, S. P.; and Oblath, R. W.: Transposed pulmonary veins. A correlation of clinical and cardiac catheterization data. *Am. J. Med.*, **15**:143, 1953.

Levy, A. M.; Naeye, R. L.; Tabakior, B. S.; and Hanson, J. S.: Far-advanced internal proliferation and severe pulmonary hypertension secondary to total anomalous pulmonary venous drainage. *Am. J. Cardiol.*, **16**:280, 1965.

Lewis, F. J.; Taufic, M.; Varco, R. L.; and Niazi, S.: The surgical anatomy of atrial septal defects: experiences with repair under direct vision. *Ann. Surg.*, **142**:401, 1955.

Llewellyn, M. A.; Cullum, P. A.; Thomas, J. B.; and Anderson, I. M.: Infracardiac total anomalous pulmonary venous drainage. *Br. Med. J.*, **3**:35, 1968.

Lowe, J. B.: Total anomalous pulmonary venous connection in infancy. *N.Z. Med. J.* (Cardiac Suppl.), **64**:15, 1965.

Lucas, R. V., Jr.; Adams, P., Jr.; Anderson, R. C.; Varco, R. L.; Edwards, J. E.; and Lester, R. G.: Total anomalous pulmonary venous connection to the portal venous system: a cause of pulmonary venous obstruction. *Am. J. Roentgenol.*, **86**:561, 1961.

Lucas, R. V., Jr.: Congenital causes of pulmonary venous obstruction. *Cardiovasc. Clin.*, **4**:19, 1972.

Mankin, H. T., and Burchell, H. B.: Clinical considerations in partial anomalous pulmonary venous connections: report of two unusual cases. *Proc. Mayo Clin.*, **28**:463, 1953.

McCormack, R. J. M.; Marquis, R. M.; Julien, D. G.; and Griffiths, H. W. C.: Partial anomalous pulmonary venous drainage to its surgical correction. *Scot. Med. J.*, **5**:367, 1960.

McCotter, R. E.: Three cases of persistence of the left superior vena cava. *Anat. Rec.*, **10**:371, 1916.

McIntosh, C. A.: Cor biatriatum triloculare. *Am. Heart J.*, **1**:735, 1926.

McManus, J. F.: A case in which both pulmonary veins emptied into a persistent left superior vena cava. *Can. Med. Assoc. J.*, **45**:261, 1941.

Meadows, W. C., and Sharp, J. T.: Persistent left superior vena cava draining into the left atrium without arterial oxygen unsaturation. *Am. J. Cardiol.*, **16**:273, 1965.

Mehrizi, A., and Drash, A.: Growth disturbance in congenital heart disease. *J. Pediatr.*, **61**:418, 1962.

Mehrizi, A.; Drash, A.; and Davis, M.: Growth retardation in congenital heart disease. II. Ventricular septal defect, atrial septal defect and aortic stenosis: growth following surgical correction. Unpublished observations, 1966.

Meyer, R. A., and Kaplan, S.: Noninvasive techniques in pediatric cardiovascular disease. *Circulation*, **15**:341, 1973.

Michaelsohn, A. (1920): Cited by Hughes and Rumore (1944).

Miller, G.; Inmon, T. W.; and Pollock, B. E.: Persistent left superior vena cava. *Am. Heart J.*, **49**:267, 1955.

Miller, G., and Pollack, B. F.: Total anomalous pulmonary venous drainage. *Am. Heart J.*, **49**:127, 1954.

Miller, W. W.; Rashkind, W. J.; Miller, R. A.; Hastreiter, A. R.; et al.: Total anomalous pulmonary venous return, effective palliation of critically ill infants by balloon atrial septostomy. *Circulation*, **36**, Suppl II:189, 1967.

Mody, M. R.; Gallen, W. J.; and Lepley, D.: Total anomalous pulmonary venous drainage below the diaphragm. *Am. J. Cardiol.*, **24**:575, 1969.

Moes, C. A. F.; Fowler, R. S.; and Trusler, G. A.: Total anomalous pulmonary venous drainage into the azygos vein. *Am. J. Roentgenol.*, **98**:378, 1966.

Momma, K., and Linde, L. M.: Abnormal rhythms associated with persistent left superior vena cava. *Pediatr. Res.*, **3**:210, 1969.

Morgan, J. R., and Forker, A. D.: Syndrome of hypoplasia of the right lung and dextroposition of the heart; "scimitar sign" with normal pulmonary venous drainage. *Circulation*, **43**:27, 1971.

Mortensson, S. W., and Lundstrom, N. R.: Broncho-pulmonary vascular malformation syndrome causing left heart failure during infancy. *Acta Radiol.*, **11**:449, 1971.

Muir, A. R.: Anomalous pulmonary venous drainage. *Thorax*, **8**:65, 1953.

Muller, W. H., Jr.: The surgical treatment of transposition of the pulmonary veins. *Ann. Surg.*, **134**:683, 1951.

Mullins, C. E.; El-Said, G.; Neches, W. H.; et al.: Balloon atrial septostomy: A temporary palliative procedure for total anomalous pulmonary venous return. Amer. Acad. Pediat. Ann. meeting, Program abstract, 1972.

Murphy, J. W.; Kerr, A. R.; and Kirklin, J. W.: Intracardiac repair for anomalous pulmonary venous connection of right lung to inferior vena cava. *Ann. Thorac. Surg.*, **11**:38, 1971.

Mustard, W. T., and Dolan, F. G.: Surgical treatment of total anomalous pulmonary venous drainage. *Ann. Surg.*, **145**:379, 1957.

Mustard, W. T.; Keith, J. D.; and Trusler, G. A.: Two-stage correction for total anomalous pulmonary venous drainage in childhood. *J. Thorac. Cardiovasc. Surg.*, **44**:477, 1962.

Mustard, W. T.; Keon, W. J.; and Trusler, G. A.: II Transposition of the lesser veins (total anomalous pulmonary venous drainage). *Progr. Cardiovasc. Dis.*, **11**:145, 1968.

Muster, A. J.; Paul, M. H.; and Kikaidoh, H.: Tetralogy of Fallot associated with total anomalous pulmonary venous drainage. *Chest*, **64**:323, 1973.

Neill, C. A.: Development of the pulmonary veins with reference to the embryology of anomalies of pulmonary venous return. *Pediatrics*, **18**:880, 1956.

Neill, C. A.; Ferencz, C.; Sabiston, D. C.; and Sheldon, H.: The familiar occurrence of hypoplastic right lung with systemic arterial blood supply and venous drainage "Scimitar" syndrome. *Bull. Hopkins Hosp.*, **107**:1, 1960.

Nelligan, M. C.; O'Malley, E.; and Blake, S.: Correction of type IV (mixed level) total anomalous pulmonary venous drainage. *Thorax*, **27**:219, 1972.

Neptune, W. B.; Bailey, C. P.; and Goldberg, H.: Surgical correction of atrial septal defects associated with transposition of pulmonary veins. *J. Thorac. Surg.*, **25**:623, 1953.

Nicholson, J. W.; Burchell, H. B.; and Wood, E. H.: A method for the continuous recording of Evans blue dye curves in arterial blood. *J. Lab. Clin. Med.*, **37**:353, 1951.

Odman, R.: A persistent left superior vena cava communicating with the left atrium and pulmonary vein. *Acta Radiol.*, **40**:554, 1953.

O'Reilly, R. J., and Grollman, J. H., Jr.: The lateral chest film as an unreliable indicator of azygos continuation of the inferior vena cava. *Circulation*, **53**:891, 1976.

Pacquet, M., and Gutgesell, H.: Echocardiographic features of total anomalous pulmonary venous connection. *Circulation*, **51**:599, 1975.

Park, E. A.: Defective development of the right lung, due to anomalous development of the right pulmonary artery and vein, accompanied by dislocation of the heart simulating dextrocardia. *Proc. N.Y. Pathol. Soc.*, **12**:88, 1912–1913.

Park, H. M.; Smith, E. T.; and Silberstein, E. B.: Isolated right superior vena cava draining into left atrium diagnosed by radionuclide angiocardiography. *J. Nucl. Med.*, **14**:240, 1973.

Paz, J. E., and Castella, E. E.: Familial total anomalous pulmonary venous return. *J. Med. Genet.*, **8**:312, 1971.

Peel, A. A. F.; Blum, K.; Kelly, J. C. C.; and Semple, T.: Anomalous pulmonary and systemic venous drainage. *Thorax*, **11**:119, 1956.

Puig-Massana, M.; Murtra, M.; and Revuelta, J. M.: A new technique in the correction of partial anomalous pulmonary venous drainage. *J. Thorac. Cardiovasc. Surg.*, **64**:108, 1972.

Robicsek, F.; Sanger, P. W.; and Daugherty, H. K.: Surgical treatment of partial anomalous pulmonary venous return into the superior vena cava. A technical modification. *Ann. Surg.*, **169**:305, 1969.

Robinson, A. E.; Chen, J. T. T.; Bradford, W. D.; and Lester, R. G.: Kerley B lines in total anomalous pulmonary venous connection below the diaphragm (type II.) *Am. J. Cardiol.*, **24**:436, 1969.

Roe, B. B.: Posterior approach to correction of total anomalous pulmonary venous return. Further experience. *J. Thorac. Cardiovasc. Surg.*, **59**:748, 1970.

Rowe, R. D.; Glass, I. H.; and Keith, J. D.: Total anomalous pulmonary venous drainage at cardiac level. Angiocardiographic differentiation. *Circulation*, **23**:77, 1961.

Rowe, R. D., and Hoffman, T.: Transient myocardial ischemia of the newborn: a form of severe distress in term infants. *J. Pediatr.*, 81:243, 1972.

Rowe, R. D., and Mehrizi, A.: *The Neonate with Congenital Heart Disease.* W. B. Saunders, Philadelphia, 1968.

Rowe, R. D.; Vlad, P.; and Keith, J. D.: Selective angiocardiography in infants and children. *Radiology*, 66:344, 1956.

Samet, P.; Bernstein, W. H.; and Jacobs, W.: Indicator dilution curves in complicated atrial septal defects. *Am. J. Cardiol.*, 11:513, 1963.

Samuelson, A.; Becker, A. E.; and Wagenvoort, C. A.; A morphomatic study of pulmonary veins in normal infants and infants with congenital heart disease. *Arch. Pathol.*, 90:112, 1970.

Sanger, P. W.; Taylor, F. H.; and Robicsek, R.: The "Scimitar syndrome." Diagnosis and treatment. *Arch. Surg.*, 86:580, 1963.

Sapsford, R. N.; Aberdeen, E.; Watson, D. A.; and Crew, A. D.: Transposed great arteries combined with totally anomalous pulmonary veins. A report of a successful correction. *J. Thorac. Cardiovasc. Surg.*, 63:360, 1972.

Scott, L. P., III, and Welch, C. C.: Factors influencing survival in total anomalous pulmonary venous drainage in-infants. *Am. J. Cardiol.*, 16:286, 1965.

Serratto, M.; Bucheleres, H. G.; Arevalo, F.; Hastreiter, A.; and Muller, R. A.: Total anomalous pulmonary venous connection without obstruction. Hemodynamic and prognostic importance of foramen ovale size. *Circulation*, 36:232, 1967.

Serratto, M.; Bucheleres, H. G.; Bicoff, P.; Miller, R. A.; and Hastreiter, A. R.: Palliative balloon atrial septostomy for total anomalous pulmonary venous connection in infancy. *J. Pediatr.*, 73:734, 1968.

Shadravan, I.; Baucum, R.; Fowler, R. L.; Villadeigo, R.; and Puyau, R.: Obstructed anomalous pulmonary venous return. *Am. Heart J.*, 82:232, 1971.

Shafter, H. A.: Splitting of the second heart sound. *Am. J. Cardiol.*, 6:1013, 1960.

Sherafat, M.; Friedman, S.; and Waldhausen, J. A.: Persistent left superior vena cava draining into the left atrium with absent right superior vena cava. *Ann. Thorac. Surg.*, 11:160, 1971.

Shone, J. D.; Amplatz, K.; Anderson, R. C.; Adams, P., Jr.; and Edwards, J. E.: Congenital stenosis of individual pulmonary veins. *Circulation*, 26:574, 1962.

Silove, E. D.; Behrendt, D. M.; Aberdeen, E.; and Bonham-Carter, R. E.: Total anomalous pulmonary venous drainage II. Spontaneous functional closure of interatrial communication after surgical correction in infancy. *Circulation*, 46:351, 1972.

Sloan, H.; Mackenzie, J.; Morris, J. D.; Stern, A.; and Sigmann, J.: Open-heart surgery in infancy. *J. Thorac. Cardiovasc. Surg.*, 444:459, 1962.

Snellen, H. A., and Albers, F. H.: The clinical diagnosis of anomalous pulmonary venous drainage. *Circulation*, 6:801, 1952.

Sodi-Pallares, D.; Calder, R. M.: The Precordial Leads, Right Ventricular Hypertrophy. In, *New Bases of Electrocardiography.* C. V. Mosby Co., St. Louis, 1956, p. 236.

Somerville, J.: Hypernatremia-special problems with angiocardiography in total anomalous pulmonary venous drainage. *Br. Heart J.*, 32:320, 1970.

Sparrow, A. W.; Mohan, K.; and Gonzalez-Lavin, L.: Successful correction of a total anomalous pulmonary venous connection in a 2.5 kilogram premature neonate. *Am. J. Cardiol.*, 37:108, 1976.

Stackelberg, B.; Lind, J.: and Wegelius, C.: Absence of inferior vena cava diagnosed by angiocardiography. *Cardiologia*, 21:583, 1952.

Steinberg, I.; Dubilier, W.; and Lukas, D.: Persistence of left superior vena cava. *Chest*, 24:479, 1953.

Storstein, O., and Tveten, H.: Anomalous drainage of pulmonary veins from the right lung to the superior vena cava with patent foramen ovale as the cause of congestive heart failure in a 68 year old man. *Acta Med. Scand.*, 148:77, 1954.

Sulayman, R.; Thilenius, O.; Replogle, R.; and Arcilla, R. A.: Unilateral emphysema in total anomalous pulmonary venous return. *J. Pediatr.*, 87:433, 1975.

Swan, H. J. C.; Burchell, H. B.; and Wood, E. H.: Differential diagnosis at cardiac catheterization of anomalous pulmonary venous drainage related to atrial septal defects or abnormal venous connections. *Proc. Mayo Clin.*, 28:452, 1953.

Swan, H. J. C.; Kirklin, J. W.; Becu, L. M.; and Wood, E. H.: Anomalous connection of right pulmonary veins to superior vena cava with interatrial communications. *Circulation*, 16:54, 1957.

Swan, H. J. C.; Toscano-Barboza, E.; and Wood, E. H.: Hemodynamic findings in total anomalous pulmonary venous drainage. *Proc. Mayo Clin.*, 31:177, 1956.

Tajik, A. J.; Gau, G. T.; and Schattenberg, T. T.: Echocardiogram in total anomalous pulmonary venous drainage. Report of case. *Mayo Clin. Proc.*, 47:247, 1972.

Taussig, H. B.: *Congenital Malformations of the Heart.* The Commonwealth Fund, New York, 1947.

Taybi, H.; Kurlander, G. J.; Lurie, P. R.; and Campbell, J. A.: Anomalous Systemic venous connection to the left atrium or to a pulmonary vein. *Am. J. Roentgenol.*, 94:62, 1965.

Thomson, N. B., Jr.: Complete repair of total anomalous pulmonary venous drainage in infancy. *Am. J. Surg.*, 109:788, 1965.

Tingelstad, J. B.; Aterman, K.; and Lambert, E. C.: Pulmonary venous obstruction. Report of a case mimicking primary pulmonary hypertension, with a review of the literature. *Am. J. Dis. Child.*, 117:219, 1969.

Törnvall, S. S.; Jackson, K. H.; Alvayay, J. C.; Vargas, A. C.; Koch, W.; and Zarate, E.: Anomalous drainage of the pulmonary veins into the inferior vena cava. *J. Thorac. Cardiovasc. Surg.*, 42:413, 1961.

Trinkle, J. K.; Danielson, G. K.; Noonan, J. A.; and Stephens, C.: Infradiaphragmatic total anomalous pulmonary venous return. *Ann. Thorac. Surg.*, 5:55, 1968.

Tuchman, H.; Brown, J. F.; Huston, J. H.; Weinstein, A. B.; Rowe, G. G.; and Crumpton, C. W.: Superior vena cava draining into left atrium. Another cause for left ventricular hypertrophy with cyanotic congenital heart disease. *Am. J. Med.*, 21:481, 1956.

Van Praagh, R.; Harken, A. H.; Delisle, G.; Ando, M.; and Gross, R. E.: Total anomalous pulmonary venous drainage to the coronary sinus. *J. Thorac. Cardiovasc. Surg.*, 64:132, 1972.

Varnauskas, E.; Forsberg, S. A.; Paulin, S.; and Bjure, J.: The syndrome of anomalous pulmonary venous drainage with enlarged left atrium reflecting mitral stenosis. *Am. J. Med.*, 35:577, 1963.

Venables, A. W.; Campbell, P. E.; and Westlake, G. W.: Total anomalous pulmonary venous drainage with unusual features. *Br. Heart J.*, 26:129, 1964.

Wassermil, M., and Hoffman, M. S.: Partial anomalous pulmonary venous drainage associated with mitral stenosis with an intact atrial septum. A distinctive hemodynamic syndrome. *Am. J. Cardiol.*, 10:894, 1962.

Weaver, M. D.; Chen, J. T. T.; Anderson, P. A. W.; and Lester, R. G.: Total anomalous pulmonary venous connection to left vertical vein. A plain-film sign useful in early diagnosis. *Radiology*, 118:679, 1976.

Whitaker, W.: Total pulmonary venous drainage through a persistent left superior vena cava. *Br. Heart J.*, 16:177, 1954.

Williams, G. R.; Richardson, W. R.; and Campbell, G. S.: Repair of total anomalous pulmonary venous drainage in infants. *J. Thorac. Cardiovasc. Surg.*, 47:199, 1964.

Williams, G. R.; Thompson, W. M., Jr.; Garrett, D. H.; and Greenfield, L. J.: Surgical management of total anomalous pulmonary venous drainage via left ventricle anomalous trunk. *J. Cardiovasc. Surg.*, 9:470, 1968.

Wilson, J.: A description of a very unusual formation of the human heart. *Phil. Trans. Roy. Soc. London*, 88:346, 1798.

Winslow: *Mém Acad Roy Sc*, 1739, Cited by Brody (1942).

Winter, F. S.: Persistent left superior vena cava: survey of world literature and report of 30 additional cases. *Angiology*, 5:90, 1954.

Woodwark, G. M.; Vince, D. J.; and Ashmore, P. G.: Total anomalous pulmonary venous return to the portal vein. Report of a case of successful surgical treatment. *J. Thorac. Cardiovasc. Surg.*, 45:662, 1963.

Cor Triatriatum

Ahn, C.; Hosier, D. M.; and Sirak, H. D.: Cor triatriatum. A case report and review of other operatic cases. *J. Thorac. Cardiovasc. Surg.*, 56:177, 1968.

Anderson, R. C., and Varco, R. L.: Cor triatriatum. Successful diagnosis and surgical correction in a three year old girl. *Am. J. Cardiol.*, 7:436, 1961.

Barrett, N. R., and Hickie, J. B.: Cor triatriatum. *Thorax*, 12:24, 1957.

Becu, L. M.; Tauxe, W. N.; DuShane, J. W.; and Edwards, J. E.: Anomalous connection of pulmonary veins with normal pulmonary venous drainage. Report of a case with pulmonary venous stenosis and cor triatriatum. *Arch. Pathol.*, **59**:563, 1955.

Borst, M.: Ein cor triatriatum. *Zbl. Pathol.*, **16**:812, 1905.

Breck, J. M., and Harper, J. J.: Anemia, fever, and cardiac failure. Clinicopathological conference. *J. Pediatr.*, **83**:136, 1973.

Brickman, R. D.; Wilson, L.; Zuberbuhler, J. R.; and Bahnson, H. T.: Cor Triatriatum. Clinical presentation and operatic treatment. *J. Thorac. Cardiovasc. Surg.*, **60**:523, 1970.

Church, W. S.: Congenital malformation of heart; abnormal septum in the left auricle. *Trans. Pathol. Soc. London*, **19**:188, 1868.

Dubin, I. N.; Hollinshead, W. H.; and Durham, N. C.: Congenitally insufficient tricuspid valve accompanied by an anomalous septum in the right atrium. *Arch. Pathol.*, **38**:225, 1944.

Edwards, J. E.: Congenital malformations of the heart and great vessels. In Gould, S. E. (ed.): *Pathology of the Heart*. Charles C Thomas, Publisher, Springfield, Ill., 1953.

————: Congenital stenosis of pulmonary veins. Pathologic and developmental considerations. *Lab. Invest.*, **9**:46, 1960.

Edwards, J. E.; DuShane, J. W.; Alcott, D. L.; and Burchell, H. B.: Thoracic venous anomalies. II. Atresia of the common pulmonary vein, the pulmonary veins draining wholly into the superior vena cava (case 3). IV. Stenosis of the common pulmonary vein (cor triatriatum) (case 4). *Arch. Pathol.*, **51**:446, 1951.

Fowler, J. K.: Membranous band in the left auricle. *Trans. Pathol. Soc. London*, **33**:77, 1882.

Goforth, J. L.: Unique heart anomaly: free fibrous cord passing through three heart chambers to the aorta. *JAMA*, **86**:1612, 1926.

Gombert, H.: Beiträge zur pathologie der vochofssheidewand des herzens. *Beitr. Pathol. Anat.*, **91**:483, 1933.

Griffith, T. W.: Note on a second example of division of the cavity of the left auricle into two compartments by a fibrous band. *J. Anat. Physiol.*, **37**:255, 1903.

Folger, G. M., Jr., and Mody, G. T.: Atresia of the common pulmonary vein: report of one case. *Pediatrics*, **54**:62, 1974.

Gibson, D. G.; Honey, M.; and Lennox, S. C.: Cor triatriatum. Diagnosis by echocardiography. *Br. Heart J.*, **36**:835, 1974.

Hauck, A. J.; Rudolph, A. M.; and Nadas, A. S.: Pulmonary venous obstruction in infants with anomalous pulmonary venous drainage. *Am. J. Dis. Child.*, **100**:744, 1960 (abstr.).

Hastreiter, A. R.; Paul, M. H.; Molthan, M. E.; and Miller, R. A.: Total anomalous pulmonary venous correction with severe pulmonary venous obstruction. A clinical entity. *Circulation*, **35**:916, 1962.

Hawker, R. E.; Celermajer, J. M.; Gengos, D. C.; Cartmill, T. B.; and Bowdler, J. D.: Common pulmonary vein atresia. Premortem diagnosis in two infants. *Circulation*, **46**:368, 1972.

Jegier, W.; Gibbons, J. E.; and Wiglesworth, F. W.: Cor triatriatum: clinical, hemodynamic and pathological studies: surgical correction in early life. *Pediatrics*, **31**:255, 1963.

Kawashima, Y.; Ueda, T.; Naito, Y.; Morikawa, E.; and Manabe, H.: Stenosis of pulmonary veins. Report of a patient corrected surgically. *Ann. Thorac. Surg.*, **12**:196, 1971.

Kjellberg, S. R.; Mannheimer, R. E.; Rudhe, U.; and Jönsson, B.: *Diagnosis of Congenital Heart Disease*: Year Book Publishers, Inc., Chicago, 1959.

Lam, C. R.: Aspects of cardiac surgery. *Mod. Med.*, **26**:134, 1958.

LaSalle, R.; Ethier, M.; Stanley, P.; and Davignon, A.: Cor triatriatum. Report of a case with emphasis on cineangiocardiography. *Can. Med. Assoc. J.*, **89**:616, 1963.

Levine, M. A.; Moller, J. H.; Amplatz, K.; and Edwards, J. E.: Atresia of the common pulmonary vein. Case report and differential diagnosis. *Am. J. Roentgenol.*, **100**:322, 1967.

Lewis, F. J.; Varco, R. L.; Faufic, M.; and Niazi, A.: Direct vision repair of triatrial heart and total anomalous pulmonary venous drainage. *Surg. Gynecol. Obstet.*, **102**:713, 1956.

Loeffler, E.: Unusual malformation of the left atrium pulmonary sinus. *Arch. Pathol.*, **48**:371, 1949.

Lucas, R. V., Jr.; Woolfrey, B. F.; Anderson, R. C.; Lester, R. G.; and Edwards, J. E.: Atresia of the common pulmonary vein. *Pediatrics*, **29**:729, 1962.

Lundstrom, N.-R.: Ultrasound cardiographic studies of the mitral valve region in young infants with mitral atresia, mitral stenosis, hypoplasia of the left ventricle, and cor triatriatum. *Circulation*, **45**:324, 1972.

McNamara, W. L.; Baker, L. A.; and Costich, K.: Asymptomatic congenital anomaly of the heart: congenital muscular cord bridging walls of auricle above center of mitral valve. *Am. Heart J.*, **34**:288, 1947.

Manubens, R.; Krovetz, L. J.; and Adams, P. R., Jr.: Supravalvular stenosing ring of the left atrium. *Am. Heart J.*, **60**:286, 1960.

Marin-Garcia, J.; Tandon, R.; Lucas, R. V., Jr.; and Edwards, J. E.: Cor triatriatum: Study of 20 cases, *Am. J. Cardiol.*, **35**:59, 1975.

Mehrizi, A.; Hutchins, G. M.; Wilson, E. F.; Breckenbridge, J. C.; and Rowe, R. D.: Supravalvular mitral stenosis. *J. Pediatr.*, **67**:1141, 1965.

Miller, G. A. H.; Ongley, P. A.; Anderson, M. W.; Kincaid, O. W.; and Swan, H. J. C.: Cor triatriatum. Hemodynamic and angiographic diagnosis. *Am. Heart J.*, **68**:298, 1964.

Nagao, G. I.; Daoud, G. I.; McAdams, A. J.; Schwartz, D. C.; and Kaplan, S.: Cardiovascular anomalies associated with tetralogy of Fallot. *Am. J. Cardiol.*, **20**:206, 1967.

Nimura, Y.; Matsumoto, M.; Beppu, S.; Matsuo, H.; Sakakibara, H.; and Abe, H.: Noninvasive preoperative diagnosis of cor triatriatum with ultrasonocardiotomogram and conventional echocardiogram. *Am. Heart J.*, **88**:240, 1974.

Palmer, R. G.: Cardiac anomaly (so-called double left auricle). *Am. Heart J.*, **6**:230, 1930.

Park, M. K.; Ricketts, H. J.; and Guntheroth, W. G.: Cor triatriatum, an operable form of pulmonary hypertension. *Am. J. Dis. Child.*, **123**:501, 1972.

Park, S. C.; Neches, W. H.; Lenox, C. C.; Zuberbuhler, J. R.; Siewers, R. D.; and Bahnson, H. T.: Diagnosis and surgical treatment of bilateral pulmonary vein stenosis. *J. Thorac. Cardiovasc. Surg.*, **67**:755, 1974.

Pedersen, A., and Therkelsen, F.: Cor triatriatum: a rare malformation of the heart probably amenable to surgery. *Am. Heart J.*, **47**:676, 1954.

Perry, L. W.; Scott, L. P., III; and McClenathan, J. E.: Cor triatriatum: Preoperative diagnosis and successful surgical repair in a small infant. *J. Pediatr.*, **71**:840, 1967.

Pfennig, E.: Anomale Septumbildung in linken Vorhof des menschlichen Herzens. *Virchow. Arch. Pathol. Anat.*, **307**:579, 1941.

Preisz, H.: Beiträge zur Lehre von den angeborenen Herzanomalien. *Beitr. Pathol. Anat.*, **7**:245, 1890.

Rao, B. N. S.; Anderson, R. C.; Lucas, R. V., Jr.; Castaneda, A.; Ibarra-Perez, C.; Korns, M. E.; and Edwards, J. E.: Supravalvular stenosing ring of the left atrium. *Am. Heart J.*, **77**:538, 1969.

Rowe, R. D., and James, L. S.: The pattern of response of pulmonary and systemic arterial pressures in newborn and older infants to short periods of hypoxia. *J. Pediatr.*, **51**:5, 1957.

Rywlin, A. M., and Fojaco, R. M.: Congenital pulmonary lymphangectasis associated with a blind common pulmonary vein. *Pediatr.*, **41**:931, 1968.

Shone, J. D.; Amplatz, K.; Anderson, R. C.; Adams, P., Jr.; and Edwards, J. E.: Congenital stenosis of individual pulmonary veins. *Circulations*, **26**:574, 1962.

Sternberg, C.: Beitrage zur Herzpathologie. *Verh. Deutsch. Ges. Pathol.*, **16**:253, 1913.

Stoeber, H.: Ein weiterer Fall von cor triatriatum mit eigenartig gekreuzten mundung der lungenvenen *Virchow. Arch. Pathol. Anat.*, **193**:252, 1908.

Tannenberg, J.: Pathogenese einer seltenen Herzmissbildung. *Klin. Wchr.*, **9**:1473, 1930.

Van der Horst, R. L., and Gotsman, M. S.: Cor triatriatum: Angiographic diagnosis by retrograde catheterization of the dorsal accessory chamber. *Br. J. Radiol.*, **44**:273, 1971.

Van Praagh, R., and Corsini, I.: Cor triatriatum: Pathologic anatomy and a consideration of morphogenesis based on 13 postmortem cases and a study of normal development of the pulmonary vein and atrial septum in 83 human embryos. *Am. Heart J.*, **78**:379, 1969.

Vineberg, A., and Gialloreto, O.: Report of a successful operation for stenosis of common pulmonary vein (cor triatriatum). *Can. Med. Assoc. J.*, **74**:719, 1956.

Vlad, P.; Rowe, R. D.; and Keith, J. D.: The electrocardiogram in primary endocardial fibroelastosis. *Br. Heart J.*, **17**:189, 1955.

Wilson, J. W.; Graham, T. P.; Gehweiler, J. A.; and Canent, R. V.: Cor triatriatum with intact subdividing diaphragm and partial anomalous pulmonary venous connection to the proximal left atrial chamber (an unreported type). *Pediatrics*, **47**:745, 1971.

Wolfe, R. R.; Ruttenberg, H. D.; Desilets, D. T.; and Mulder, D. E.: Cor triatriatum. Total correction in an infant. *J. Thorac. Cardiovasc. Surg.*, **56**:114, 1968.

SECTION

B

CONOTRUNCAL MALPOSITIONS

CHAPTER

33

Complete Transposition of the Great Arteries

B. S. Langford Kidd

COMPLETE transposition of the great arteries is the congenital cardiac defect that has attracted the most attention over the past decade. This has been not only because it is a fairly common defect, representing 9 percent of all cases seen at The Hospital for Sick Children, Toronto, but also because of the striking innovations in treatment (Mustard, 1964; Rashkind and Miller, 1966) that have so changed the prognosis for children born with this disorder. Before these advances, 95 percent of these children died before reaching their second birthday. Now nearly 70 to 80 percent may survive.

Following descriptions by Steno (1672), Baillie (1797), Langstaff (1811), and Farre (1814), transposition of the great arteries was first categorized in a systematic manner by von Rokitansky in 1875. He described two forms, anomalous and corrected. Vierodt, in a classification in 1898 that was to be echoed in 1915 by Maude Abbott, described partial, corrected, and complete forms. Spitzer in 1923 described four degrees of transposition: (1) riding aorta; (2) simple, with only the aorta transposed (double-outlet right ventricle); (3) crossed, with both vessels transposed; and (4) mixed. Harris and Farber (1939) recognized that the three segments of the heart (atria, ventricles, and great arteries) could be either right- or left-sided and described eight transpositions

(Figure 33–1). In 1956 Cardell proposed a physiologic differentiation and described physiologically corrected—in which pulmonary venous blood was ejected into the aorta—and physiologically uncorrected forms. When this concept is applied to Harris and Farber's classifications, types II, III, IV, and VII are physiologically corrected. On the other hand, types II, IV, VI, and VIII are anatomically corrected in that the aorta arises from the left ventricle, and these, using strict criteria, are not transpositions at all.

Only types I and V are neither anatomically nor physiologically corrected, and so are called "complete." When the term "corrected" is unqualified in common usage, it means "physiologically corrected," and describes types III and VII. However, it should be realized that the physiologic correction refers only to the route of the blood through the heart, since it is very rare to find a patient with this condition who does not have an associated malformation—ventricular septal defect, single ventricle, or pulmonary stenosis.

The question of nomenclature has been difficult. Abbott (1927), Lev (1937, 1953), and Edwards (1960) defined transposition as an alteration in the position of the two great vessels relative to the ventricles of the heart or to each other at their origin. This definition is somewhat loose and would embrace such entities as

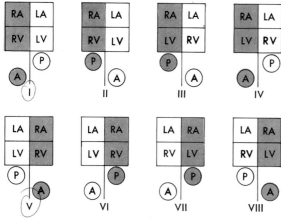

Figure 33-1. The eight transpositions of Harris and Farber (1939). *RA + LA, RV + LV,* right and left atria and ventricles. *A,* Aorta. *P.* Pulmonary artery. Shaded chambers contain desaturated blood.

590

tetralogy of Fallot, double-outlet right ventricle, and persistent truncus arteriosus. Cardell (1956) and Shaher (1964) defined transposition as a reversal of the anteroposterior relationship of the aorta and pulmonary artery. Goor and Edwards (1973) also proposed that the term "transposition" refers only to the mutual interrelationships of the semilunar valves, regardless of their ventricular origin.

In 1964, however, Van Praagh and associates stated that it was the relationship between the mitral and the aortic valves that was central to the transposition question. Grant (1962) had suggested that in transposition there was a shift in the orientation of the fibroplastic continuum, which normally holds the aortic part of the truncus in fibrous continuity with the mitral part of the atrioventricular canal. In transposition, he stated, it held the pulmonic part of the truncus in continuity with the mitral ring. So Van Praagh in his definition (1967) emphasized the loss of mitral-aortic continuity, the presence of a subaortic conus, and the loss of the subpulmonary conus. He recognized two types of transposition, D- (for dextro-) transposition, when the aorta was to the right of the pulmonary artery ("complete transposition"), and L- (for levo-) transposition, when the aorta was to the left of the pulmonary artery ("corrected transposition"). He felt at that time that D-transposition was transposition in a D-loop (the normal type of ventricular looping) and that L-transposition was transposition with an L-ventricular loop. This "loop rule" has not proved particularly useful, since in as many as 17 percent of cases of complete or D-transposition, the aortic valve is actually situated to the left of the pulmonary valve (Carr et al., 1968). This raises the whole question of the external frame of reference (which Van Praagh discusses fully in Chapter 36), since the condition is obviously the same (complete transposition) whether or not the great arteries are a centimeter to the left or right or straight anteroposterior.

More recently, however, Van Praagh advocated a return to a strict and even more limited definition than that of Abbott (1927). While stating that a subaortic conus and mitral-pulmonary continuity were present in 92 of 100 unselected cases of transposition (Van Praagh et al., 1971; Van Praagh, 1971), he now defines transposition as the condition in which both great arteries are "placed across" the ventricular septum and arise over the wrong ventricles. For other positional anomalies of the great arteries (double-outlet right and left ventricles, Chapter 35; type C single ventricle, Chapter 23; and anatomically corrected transposition, Chapter 34), he used the term "malposition" (Janeway, 1877; Robertson, 1913).

While this discussion has continued, the hemodynamics in transposition were clarified by Bing and his colleagues (Campbell et al., 1949) and four clinical groupings defined by Noonan and associates (1960). Following the contributions to the surgery for transposition of such workers as Blalock and Hanlon (1950), Baffes (1956), Edwards and Bargeron (1965), Albert (1955), Merendino (1957), Kay and Cross

(1957), Senning (1959), and Mustard (1964), the understanding of the physiology and management of the circulatory problems in children with transposition has improved immensely.

Definition, Embryology and Anatomy

In this chapter, it is not intended to enter into the controversy of transposition definitions and semantics. Since the last edition of this text, this has been extensively set out in the writings of Van Praagh (1966, 1971, and Chapter 36 of this book), by Van Mierop (1963a, 1963b, 1963c, 1970, 1971), by De La Cruz (1956), and by Goor and Edwards (1973), and has been reviewed in Shaher's book on the subject (1973). As Rashkind (1971) has pointed out, these polemics do little to clarify the hemodynamic disorder, which is what the physiologically oriented clinician is concerned with, although they may be of major importance to the more anatomically oriented surgeon (Kirklin, 1973).

In this chapter the clinical features common to children with this malformation will be described. Also, a description of the present-day management of these children will be given and, finally, an account of what we may expect to find postoperatively.

The condition "complete transposition of the great arteries" is that in which the right ventricle gives rise to the aorta and the left ventricle, the pulmonary artery. The atria and ventricles are usually in situs solitus, and not inverted. The aorta is usually anteriorly situated and to the right of the pulmonary artery, which is posterior and to the left (Figure 33-2).

There are a number of embryologic theories as to the morphogenesis of complete transposition, which

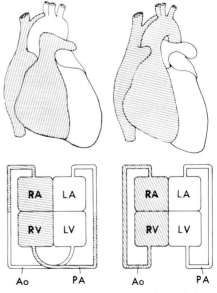

Figure 33-2. The normal heart and circulation are contrasted with those in complete transposition of the great arteries. Conventions as in Figure 33-1.

are discussed in the references cited above. The two most preponderant are, first the differential conal development theory. This was originally proposed by Sir Arthur Keith (1909) as the differential conal absorption theory and was supported by Lev and Saphir (1937) and Goor and Edwards (1973). Other evidence, however, suggests that there is probably differential conal growth as well as resorption (De La Cruz and Da Rocha, 1956; Grant, 1962; and DeVries and Sanders, 1962). Whichever is most important, this theory holds that in the normal, the different rates of growth and/or resorption of the subsemilunar conuses result in the subpulmonary conus bringing the pulmonary artery round anteriorly and to the left, while the loss of the subaortic conus allows the aorta to sink posteriorly and to the right. In transposition, however, the subaortic conus either grows or is not resorbed. Thus the aorta remains high, anterior, and to the right, while the subpulmonary conus is lost, and the pulmonary artery is low, posterior, and to the left. The second major explanation is the straight aorticopulmonary septum theory (De La Cruz and Da Rocha, 1956; Van Mierop, 1970). This theory holds that truncal ridges 2 and 4 rather than ridges 1 and 3, fuse to form the septum. This results in a nontwisting of the great arteries and so an anterior aorta. It does not, however, explain the relationship of the coronary arteries or the associated conal abnormalities (Goor and Edwards, 1973).

The condition is called "complete transposition" to differentiate it from "corrected transposition" (see Chapter 34) in which the transposition is corrected by ventricular inversion. Using the segmental approach to diagnosis (see Chapter 36), complete transposition occurs most commonly in a solitus individual with solitus atria, solitus ventricles, and D-transposed great arteries (S-D-D). In the inversus individual the same hemodynamic condition is represented by inversus atria, inversus ventricles, and L-transposed arteries (I-L-L). In either case, the course of the circulation is right atrium–right ventricle–aorta–

body–systemic veins–right atrium as one circulation, and left atrium–left ventricle–pulmonary artery–lungs–pulmonary veins–left atrium as the other (Figure 33–2). These two circulations, in parallel instead of in series, are obviously incompatible with life unless there is mixing, which can take place at atrial, ventricular, or great artery level.

Mixing at the atrial level, prior to any intervention, takes place across the foramen ovale, which may be functionally imperfect. The septum, however, limits shunting at this level, and unless this opening is improved, the small volume of blood shunted is not compatible with life. Rarely there is an atrial septal defect of the secundum variety, and when this is large, mixing may be good. This is compatible with improved prognosis.

Shunting at the ventricular level is via a ventricular septal defect, which is present in 40 percent of cases (Figure 33–3) (Kidd et al., 1971). The ventricular septal defect in transposition is most often in the usual position for ventricular septal defects—that is, in the membranous septum. This represented 55 percent in the series reported by Shaher (1973); 12 percent were situated more anteriorly, within the muscle bundles of the crista, while 13 percent were ventricular septal defects of the atrioventricular canal type, with the defect extending posteriorly to the junction of the mitral and tricuspid valves. Three of these eight cases had anomalies of the atrioventricular valves. Thirteen percent had defects in the muscular septum, and in 7 percent the defects were multiple. Spontaneous closure of a ventricular septal defect in complete transposition was documented in one case from The Hospital for Sick Children (Shaher et al., 1965).

Shunting at the great artery level occurs mostly via the ductus arteriosus (which is usually widely patent in most postmortem series in which the patient has died early). The proportion in which it persists decreases as age increases.

The other possible site of shunting at great artery level is via the bronchial circulation. The bronchial

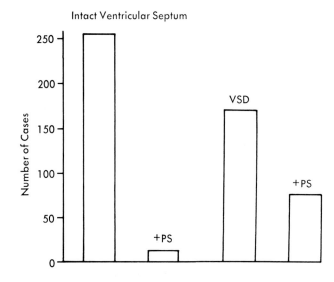

Figure 33-3. Number of patients seen of four groups of complete transposition. *VSD,* Ventricular septal defect. *PS,* Pulmonary stenosis.

arteries play a large part in supplying the lungs in conditions where there is pulmonary hypoperfusion, such as tetralogy of Fallot and pulmonary atresia (Chapters 27 and 28). It is not clear to what extent these may function in transposition without pulmonary stenosis. Folse and associates (1961) reported large bronchials in a case with transposition and pulmonary hypertension, and Cudkowicz and Armstrong (1952) demonstrated an extensive bronchial circulation in another case by injection techniques. However, despite this evidence and the forebodings of Burchell (1966), in our experience it is uncommon to see significant opacification of the lungs or extensive collateral shunting in an aortogram in patients with transposition without very severe pulmonary stenosis.

Pulmonary stenosis in transposition is a common associated malformation, occurring in 6 percent of cases with an intact septum and in 31 percent of those with a ventricular septal defect (Figure 33–3). This is very similar to the percentages found by Liebman and associates (1969), which were 4 percent and 28 percent, respectively. The nature of the obstruction in a small postmortem series of some of these patients was examined by Shaher and associates (1967). They found that when the ventricular septum was intact, the commonest cause of obstruction to left ventricular outflow was a bulging of the septum into the outflow tract, which they felt was acquired. When there was a ventricular septal defect, pulmonary valve stenosis was present in all cases, although 63 percent had a bulging septum and three had subvalvular fibromuscular tunnels in addition.

Coronary Arteries. This has been studied in three large series (Rowlett, 1962; Elliott et al., 1963; Shaher and Puddu, 1966) and the most common pattern is that in which the coronaries resemble the normal. The left coronary artery arises from the left sinus and divides into: the left anterior descending artery, which courses down the anterior interventricular sulcus toward the apex, and the left circumflex, which runs round to the left. In 70 percent of these cases the circumflex branch runs in front of the left ventricular outflow tract and so could interfere with attempts at surgical relief of pulmonary stenosis in this area. The right coronary artery arises from the posterior sinus. This variety is two to three times as frequent as the next most common variant, in which the coronary arteries arise from the left and posterior sinuses as before, but the circumflex artery takes its origin from the right coronary instead of the left. Other variations are very rare.

Other associated anomalies are rare, occurring in less than 10 percent (Liebman et al., 1969). The most common is right aortic arch, and the second, coarctation of the aorta. Rarely the right ventricle may be hypoplastic (Riemenschneider et al., 1968).

Physiology

In complete transposition, there are two separate circulations in parallel, rather than in series—a situation obviously incompatible with life. If there is not a communication between these two circuits the fully oxygenated blood that returns from the lungs is ejected again into the pulmonary arteries without giving up any oxygen, and the reduced blood returning from the body is ejected again into the aorta without gaining any.

The total blood flow in each of the two circuits is variable, may be large, and can vary independently. The volume of the blood exchanged between the two circulations is usually small in comparison. It is this small volume shunt that is the true physiologic circulation in transposition. As Rudolph (1974) points out, the systemic circulation (since it is largely the systemic venous return being ejected into the aorta) could be considered as the physiologic right-to-left shunt; and similarly the pulmonary blood flow (largely coming from the pulmonary veins and being ejected via the pulmonary artery) could be considered the physiologic left-to-right shunt. However, in this chapter the term "shunt" will be used in its anatomic sense, as the volume of blood crossing the anatomic septum, rather than in its physiologic sense.

In this frame of reference, then, the right-to-left shunt is that volume of blood which, returning to the right atrium, crosses the septum and is ejected into the pulmonary artery. This was termed the "effective pulmonary blood flow" by Bing and associates (Campbell et al., 1949). In transposition, this right-to-left shunt must be balanced by an equal and opposite left-to-right shunt which, returning to the left atrium, is ejected into the aorta (the effective systemic blood flow) (Figure 33–4). If these two volumes are not equal over any period of time, one circulation will become overfilled and the other depleted of blood. To give an idea of the dimensions of the various flows, in The Hospital for Sick Children experience, the pulmonary blood flow varied between 5 to 20 L/min/m^2, the systemic between 5 to 10 L/min/m^2, and the volume shunted (the effective flow) usually varied from 0.7 to 1.5 L/min/m^2 (Shaher and Kidd, 1966; Kidd and Mustard, 1966; Kidd et al., 1971).

Flow calculation in complete transposition of the great arteries is fraught with difficulties. Since the arteriovenous oxygen difference across the lungs is small, minor variations in technique and the unavoidable errors of oxygen measurement assume critical importance. Added to this is the difficulty in obtaining a representative pulmonary artery blood sample. It is now fairly simple to enter the pulmonary artery in this condition using either a preformed catheter or a Swan-Ganz balloon catheter; however, it is likely that there is some immeasurable admixture, distal to the sampling point, from the bronchial circulation that will tend to reduce the pulmonary artery oxygen saturation and so the calculated pulmonary blood flow. These difficulties in calculating pulmonary blood flow make the important calculation of pulmonary vascular resistance—the predictor of operability—hazardous.

The physiology of the circulation of a child with transposition during fetal life is not greatly disturbed.

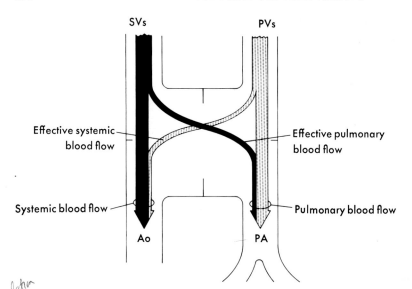

Figure 33-4. Diagram of the circulation and shunts in complete transposition. Explanation in text.

fetal circulation
c transposition

There will be a reversal of the normal situation, in which the more oxygenated blood, returning via the umbilical vein to the inferior vena cava, crosses to the left atrium and perfuses the upper part of the body via the left ventricle and ascending aorta. In transposition this blood will cross to eject through the pulmonary artery and, via the ductus, perfuse the lower part of the body, while the less oxygenated superior vena cava blood will perfuse the upper segment. This circulatory disturbance does not appear to be deleterious, since there is no evidence of an undue preponderance of transposition cases in fetal deaths, and most cases of transposition are born with normal or slightly increased birth weights (Liebman et al., 1969).

After birth the ductus remains patent for a variable period of time. This allows for some mixing between the two circulations and will be associated with persistence of high pressure in the pulmonary circulation. When the ventricular septum is intact and the ductus starts to close, the pulmonary artery pressure drops toward normal (Tynan, 1972) and hypoxia and acidosis become more marked. When, however, there is a ventricular septal defect, the pulmonary artery pressure remains high (Noonan, 1960; Shaher and Kidd, 1966, 1969; Kidd et al., 1971; Mair et al., 1971), and these are the patients who are especially at risk of pulmonary vascular disease.

It might be expected that in the early weeks of life, as pulmonary vascular resistance continues to fall, pulmonary blood flow would increase. However, hemodynamic calculations (Tynan, 1972), and angiocardiographic measurements of left ventricular volume, and calculations of systolic outputs from it (Graham et al., 1971) have demonstrated no such correlation with age. There is, however, a wide scatter of values in these modes of estimation, and the explanation of this unexpected finding may lie more in the inexactness of the techniques of measure-

ment than in the physiology of the pulmonary circulation.

Classification

The clinical classification of complete transposition of the great arteries is commonly made on the basis of the presence or absence of communication between the two circulations at ventricular level, and on the presence or absence of pulmonary outflow obstruction. Thus Noonan and associates (1960) described type I with an intact ventricular septum; type II with a ventricular septal defect; 2a with pulmonic stenosis; type 2b with pulmonary vascular obstruction; and type 2c with large pulmonary blood flow. Van Praagh and associates (1967) spoke of group 1 with intact septum, group 2 with ventricular septal defect, and group 3 with ventricular septal defect and pulmonary stenosis. Kidd and associates (1971) defined four groups:

Group 1: With intact ventricular septum
Group 2: With intact ventricular septum and pulmonary stenosis
Group 3: With ventricular septal defect
Group 4: With ventricular septal defect and pulmonary stenosis

The incidence of these subgroups in The Hospital for Sick Children series is illustrated in Figure 33-3.

Rowe and Mehrizi (1968) described three major hemodynamic groups; those with inadequate communication between the two circulations (mainly the group with intact ventricular septum); those with adequate communication (mainly the group with ventricular septal defects); and those with obstruction to pulmonary blood flow. To surgeons there are two main divisions: simple transposition (those with an intact ventricular septum) and complex transposition (those with a ventricular septal defect, pulmonary stenosis, or both).

Prevalence

Complete transposition of the great arteries represents 9 percent of the total clinical cases of congenital heart disease seen at The Hospital for Sick Children—an incidence of about 1 in 4000 live births. Liebman and associates (1969), in an excellent study of life and death in transposition, estimate a frequency of 1 in 4500 live births. The male/female sex ratio was 1.8:1, varying in the assorted subgroups between 1.5:1 in transposition with intact ventricular septum to 2.5:1 in transposition with a ventricular septal defect. There was an increased incidence of maternal diabetes, which has been suggested as 11.4 times as frequent in this condition as in the general population. This has also been noted by Rowe and Mehrizi (1968) and Mitchell and associates (1971). Infants of diabetic mothers are known to be large (Miller 1945), and Mehrizi and Drash (1961) had suggested that infants with transposition of the great arteries were also large at birth. However, in The Hospital for Sick Children series, the mean birth weight was 3354.7 gm with a standard deviation of 581.4 gm; it did not differ between subgroups and was not significantly different from that of a control series (3322.7 gm). This confirms the findings of Liebman and associates (1969).

The incidence of complete transposition in any neonatal series depends on the nature of the series. For instance, in autopsy series between 1927 and 1965, transposition ranged between first and third (and 10 percent and 27 percent of the total) as a leading cause of death due to congenital cardiovascular malfunction under one month of age. In a clinical series of 100 consecutive newborns with heart malformations seen at Green Lane Hospital, New Zealand, it rated second, with 14 percent (Rowe and Mehrizi, 1968). At The Hospital for Sick Children, Toronto, in 1973, transposition represented 20 percent of newborns undergoing cardiac catheterization in the first month of life and 30 percent of those catheterized in the first week.

Clinical Features

The typical presentation of a patient with complete transposition of the great arteries is in the newborn period. In a consecutive series of 404 infants seen at The Hospital for Sick Children between 1948 and 1968, the ages of presentation at the Cardiac Center are as illustrated in Figure 33–5. They have been split into two main groups: those with and without ventricular septal defects. Those with an intact ventricular septum presented earlier—47.5 percent in the first seven days of life and 74.5 percent within the first month—while among those with a ventricular septal defect, only 13.5 percent had presented in the first week, 43.5 percent in the first month, and 78.5 percent by the end of the third month.

There are three main clinical syndromes of presentation in the newborn period:

Group 1: Hypoxia and acidosis
Group 2: Congestive heart failure
Group 3: Pulmonary oligemia

Group 1. This group with hypoxia and acidosis are those who have inadequate communication between the two circulations. The ventricular septum is either intact, or if there is a ventricular septal defect, it is very small. These babies are noted shortly after birth to be cyanosed and distressed. Placing the baby in oxygen does not help—the baby becomes more distressed, and a typical blood gas analysis in pH 7.0

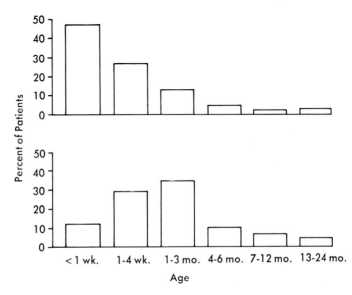

Figure 33-5. Age at presentation of (*above*) infants with complete transposition and intact ventricular septum, and (*below*) infants with complete transposition and a ventricular septal defect.

with PCO_2 35 mm of mercury and PO_2 25 mm of mercury. When the hyperoxic test is administered, following ten minutes of breathing 100 percent oxygen, the PO_2 shows either no change or a rise of 1 to 2 mm of mercury. On physical examination the baby appears well-nourished and of a good size; he is cyanosed and distressed with tachycardia and tachypnea. The pulses are good and blood pressures normal. The apex beat is not displaced, and on auscultation the first heart sound is normal and the second either single or very narrowly split. There is usually a faint nonspecific ejection systolic murmur, though this may be absent. There are no clicks or other added sounds. If observation is continued, the distress gets worse, and signs of congestive failure appear, with enlargement of the liver below the costal margin. Repeat blood gas may show pH 6.8 units, PCO_2 25 mm of mercury, and PO_2 19 mm of mercury.

Group 2. In this group (which corresponds roughly with those patients with transposition and a large ventricular septal defect), the cyanosis and acidosis are not so marked since there is better opportunity for mixing between the two circulations. These children do not present quite as early, on the average, as the children with an intact ventricular septum (Figure 33–5). The picture is often one of respiratory distress, congestive heart failure, and cyanosis, which may not be noticeable at first in some cases, but becomes more obvious with time. Rarely differential cyanosis is noted with more cyanosis in the face and upper extremities than in the lower. This indicates that a persistent ductus arteriosus is perfusing the lower extremities and should always raise the question of a coexisting coarctation of the aorta or an interrupted aortic arch.

On physical examination, these group 2 babies appear large and well-nourished. The clinical impression is mainly that of respiratory distress with marked tachypnea and tachycardia. There is often indrawing and the liver is felt 3 to 4 cm below the left costal margin. The cyanosis may be mild or marked. The pulses are usually present and forceful. The precordium is hyperactive with a right ventricular lift. The first heart sound is normal and the second either single or closely split. There is usually a harsh pansystolic or long ejection systolic murmur, best heard at the lower left sternal border. Diastolic murmurs are rare. Even though the ductus arteriosus can be demonstrated at aortography to be persistent in nearly every case of transposition of the great arteries seen early in life, it is very uncommon to hear a continuous ductus murmur or even a late systolic murmur spilling over into diastole.

Blood gases in these patients indicate a lesser degree of disturbance with an arterial PO_2 between 30 to 40 mm of mercury and oxygen saturation to match. PCO_2 is usually normal or slightly reduced, and the pH, 7.30 to 7.40. Oxygen breathing improves the PO_2 only 3 to 5 mm of mercury. If observation is continued, the congestive heart failure continues to be severe and resistant to medical management.

Pulmonary edema is common, and chest infections supervene. Cyanosis becomes more severe.

Group 3. The third clinical group are those who correspond roughly to the anatomic group of patients with obstruction to left ventricular outflow or pulmonary stenosis. They present much later than the other groups: heart failure is rare, and cyanosis, though present, may be mild. Before the era of successful intervention in this condition, these patients represented the majority of those who survived infancy.

The clinical presentation is usually that of a murmur and cyanosis, usually in the first three months of life. The degree of cyanosis is variable and often is worse on crying. Heart failure is extremely rare. On physical examination the child is not distressed and may be moderately cyanosed. The pulses are good, and the liver is not enlarged. The precordium is quiet, although there may be left or right ventricular impulses. The first heart sound is normal, and the second is single. There is usually a harsh ejection systolic murmur at the upper left sternal border, considerably harsher than the usual soft murmur that is quite common in transposition. Occasionally the pulmonary stenosis may be more severe, and the patient may present in severe cyanosis at around the end of the first week of life. There are severe hypoxia and acidosis, without heart failure. The sudden deterioration in these children is almost certainly due to the closure of the ductus arteriosus, which, in the face of critical pulmonary stenosis, has been perfusing the pulmonary circulation.

In all these clinical groupings, it is important to check the femoral pulses because of the possibility of associated problems in the aortic arch such as interruption or a coarctation of the aorta.

Radiologic Examination

The chest x-ray has been valuable in diagnosing complete transposition of the great arteries since Fanconi in 1932 described the narrow vascular pedicle at the base of the heart and attributed it to the course of the aorta in front of and parallel to the pulmonary artery. He also described the progressive enlargement of the heart over a period of months. Taussig (1938) pointed out that the narrowness of the vascular pedicle seen in the anteroposterior view disappeared when the child was rotated into the oblique position, and that a characteristic that separated these children from those with other causes of persistent cyanosis (such as tetralogy of Fallot) was the presence of vascular markings that were either normal or increased rather than diminished (Keith et al., 1953).

It is important to emphasize, however, that in the first few days of life when it is of vital importance to make a rapid and correct diagnosis, the cardiac silhouette is often not characteristic (Gallagher et al., 1966) (Figure 33–6). The heart may be of normal size,

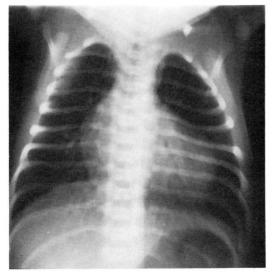

Figure 33-6. Chest x-ray of a newborn with complete transposition.

and the pulmonary vascularity may be normal, especially when the ventricular septum is intact. However, in 29 percent of Shaher's (1973) series, the heart was characteristically "egg-shaped" even on the first day of life. The "egg" lies obliquely on its side, with the narrow end at the cardiac apex, the shoulder where the pulmonary artery would be in the normal, and the "top of the egg" at the upper right atrium.

In the second group, with a ventricular septal defect and good mixing, the cardiac shadow is usually enlarged with both ventricles involved (Figure 33-7). The narrow superior pedicle and absence of a large main pulmonary artery shadow are characteristic. However, the right and left pulmonary arteries are usually clearly seen, and the pulmonary vascular

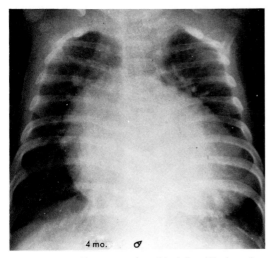

4 mo.   ♂

Figure 33-7. Chest x-ray of an older infant. The heart is enlarged and typically egg-shaped.

markings are increased. Pulmonary edema may be present (Carey and Elliott, 1964).

With increasing age, even in the intact ventricular septum group, the heart increases in size, the shape becomes more characteristic, and hilar vascularity becomes more obviously increased.

In the group with pulmonary stenosis the picture may be confused with tetralogy of Fallot, in that in both the lung fields are oligemic, and the heart is small. It is often very difficult to differentiate them on the chest film, although the convex-upward border to the empty pulmonary artery bay, rather than the concave upward one typical of the "boot-shaped" heart in tetralogy, may be helpful.

Echocardiography

This relatively new technique is of especial value in the diagnosis of the sick cyanotic neonate. In transposition of the great arteries we have found that the mitral and tricuspid valves are easily located and have normal excursion (Godman et al., 1974). The ventricular septum is normal, as are the right and left ventricular cavities. There is continuity between the mitral valve apparatus and the posterior border of the posterior great artery (the pulmonary artery in this case) and the septum and its anterior border.

There are a number of techniques for defining the relationship of the great arteries. Gramiak and associates (1973) proposed that the relative positions of these vessels was helpful. In the normal, the anterior artery (the pulmonary artery) is to the left, and the posterior artery is more medial. In complete transposition, however, the anterior artery (the aorta) is located by angling the transducer more medially, and the posterior is more lateral. The diagnostic accuracy of this test depends on the aorta being at the right, which is often, but not always, true (see the "loop rule," Chapter 36).

Another useful finding is the simultaneous visualization of both great arteries at the same transducer position, which is common in transposition where the great arteries are more anteroposterior to each other and run a parallel course (Dillon et al., 1973) (Figure 33-8). Third, the posterior semilunar valve (the pulmonary valve) opens earlier and closes later than the anterior one, the reverse of normal (Hirshfeld et al., 1974).

Even more recently, the use of multicrystal devices or sector scanning shows promise in contributing further to noninvasive diagnosis.

Electrocardiography

The electrocardiograms and vectorcardiograms in complete transposition of the great arteries have been extensively reviewed by Noonan and associates (1960), Elliott and associates (1963), Shaher and Deucher (1966), and Khoury and associates (1967). It is felt that they reflect the physiology of the two circulations as well as the anatomy of the transposition and the associated septal defects or pulmonary stenosis.

The rhythm in complete transposition is, in the great majority, sinus rhythm. The P-R interval is normal, and atrioventricular block in the absence of intervention is rare.

The ventricular electrocardiogram in the newborn with transposition usually falls into the normal limits for a baby of this age: in other words, a normal right ventricular hypertrophy, with a rightward QRS axis in the frontal plane, usually 90 to 120°, and dominant rightward forces in the precordial leads. However, in transposition this pattern persists, instead of regressing to the left as that of the normal newborn will (Figure 33–9).

Infants in group 2 with ventricular septal defects have a higher incidence of combined ventricular hypertrophy, reflecting the systemic pressure in the left ventricle. In the series of Elliott and associates (1963), isolated right ventricular hypertrophy in the electrocardiogram was seen in 81 percent of patients with small communications (at atrial level or very small ventricular septal defects), and biventricular hypertrophy in 80 percent of those with large

communications. This finding is supported by the vector loops reported by Khoury and associates (1967) that showed combined ventricular hypertrophy in 80 percent of children with transposition and ventricular septal defects. The finding of pure right ventricular hypertrophy in cases of transposition and pulmonary vascular obstruction (Van Praagh et al., 1966) had not been confirmed (Ellison and Restieaux, 1972).

In the follow-up of children with transposition it is important to know if the left ventricular pressure is high, since in the absence of pulmonary stenosis, this implies pulmonary hypertension and the risk of progressive pulmonary vascular disease. This has been studied by Mair and associates (1970) and Restieaux and associates (1972), who found that the vector provided more useful information than the electrocardiogram (because the left ventricular forces are canceled early by the inevitably increased right ventricular voltages). Combining the direction of the QRS loop in the horizontal plane with the left maximal spatial voltages, a prediction of left ventricular pressure could be made. If the horizontal loop was counterclockwise or initially counterclockwise and figure-of-eight and the left maximal spatial

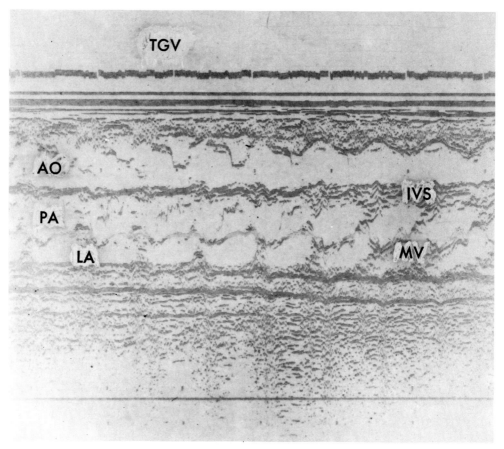

Figure 33-8. Echocardiogram in a patient with complete transposition. Both aortic and pulmonary valves are seen in the same transducer position.

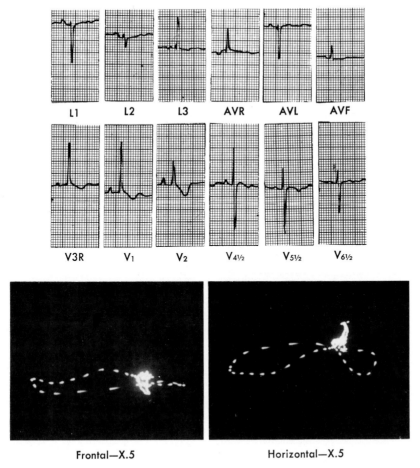

L1   L2   L3   AVR   AVL   AVF

V3R   V₁   V₂   V₄½   V₅½   V₆½

Frontal—X.5   Horizontal—X.5

Figure 33-9. Electrocardiogram and vector loops from a child with complete transposition and an intact ventricular septum.

voltage was more than 1.8 mV, this indicated that the left ventricular pressure was at or near systemic level, provided the hematocrit was not too high.

A diminution of right ventricular forces in a case of transposition should always alert one to the possibility of hypoplastic right ventricle (Riemenschneider et al., 1968).

Cardiac Catheterization

Diagnostic cardiac catheterization is usually carried out in the newborn period with three purposes: (1) to confirm the diagnosis of transposition, (2) to determine the associated lesions—the most common being ventricular septal defect, pulmonary stenosis, persistent ductus arteriosus, and coarctation, and (3) to carry out balloon atrial septostomy.

If the diagnosis of transposition is considered in a newborn, entry to the venous circulation should be through a vein large enough to subsequently admit a balloon catheter for atrial septostomy. Although this can be done percutaneously (see Chapter 6), this requires manipulation and dilatation of the vein, and thus the venous cutdown route is preferred in our department in these patients. The incision in the right groin is made just below the inguinal ligament, and the saphenous vein, saphenous bulb, and femoral vein are located (Mullins et al., 1972). If possible, the catheter is introduced through the saphenous vein or bulb; failing this, through the femoral vein *distal* to the saphenofemoral junction, leaving the saphenous vein intact. This is, in our view, preferable to the very proximal site preferred by Rashkind (Rashkind and Miller, 1968). Using the femoral vein above the inguinal ligament makes the situation much more difficult if the vein tears and the bleeding upper end retracts into the pelvis, and it almost certainly causes thrombosis of the entire venous system at this level, which makes subsequent percutaneous catheterization almost impossible.

The diagnostic procedure is rapidly carried out. Very desaturated blood is found in the right atrium, and when the catheter passes into the right ventricle, it has a systolic pressure at systemic level. The catheter can usually be passed upward into the aorta, which is also desaturated. If there is no ventricular septal defect, there may be no step-up in oxygen saturation from the superior vena caval sample to the aortic sample, or a very small step-up.

The feat of entering the aorta from the right ventricle does not, of itself, make the diagnosis of complete transposition, since this could happen in tetralogy of Fallot, double-outlet right ventricle, single ventricle, or truncus arteriosus. So the catheter should next be passed into the left atrium and pulmonary veins. These are usually fully saturated, and the left atrial pressure is often 3–6 mm of mercury higher than that in the right. The catheter should then be advanced to the left ventricle, which contains only very slightly desaturated blood. The left ventricular pressure is always systemic when there is a ventricular septal defect, and may vary from systemic in the newborn period to less than one-half systemic in the closed ventricular septum group. If pulmonary stenosis is excluded, the level of the left ventricular pressure in the intact septum group depends on whether or not a ductus is present (Shaher and Kidd, 1968), and on the patient's age, since the pressure falls with time as pulmonary vascular resistance regresses (Tynan, 1972; Kidd, 1976).

It is not our practice to attempt to pass a catheter into the pulmonary artery in newborns with transposition, since this prolongs the study and is not necessary for the initial diagnosis. It is necessary to do this, however, at subsequent hemodynamic assessments, and many techniques for accomplishing this have been elaborated (Carr and Wells, 1966; Celermajer et al., 1970; Pickering et al., 1971). The technique we employ currently is to use a Swan-Ganz catheter, inflate the balloon in the left atrium, and allow it to float in through the mitral valve and out the pulmonary artery.

At the initial study it is our practice to take three cineangiograms using the biplane facility. One shot is made in the right ventricle, one in the left ventricle,

and a third in the ascending aorta to ascertain the presence or absence of a persistent ductus or coarctation.

Angiocardiography

Selective angiocardiograms in transposition of the great arteries should be carried out in both ventricles, in both anteroposterior and lateral projections. The lateral projection is usually in the plane of the ventricular septum, which in complete transposition is much more in the frontal plane, rather than in the oblique plane as in the normal, or in the sagittal plane as in congenitally corrected transposition. The classic findings in transposition were first defined by Castellanos and associates (1938, 1950) as filling of the aorta following an injection into the right ventricle. The right ventricular angiogram usually shows a chamber situated in the normal position, with a well-trabeculated sinus portion and hypertrophied wall. Above it is a smooth-walled infundibulum or conus, which gives rise to a high and anteriorly situated aortic valve. This valve is usually situated to the right of the pulmonary artery, but may be in front of it, or to the left (Carr et al., 1968) (Figure 33–10). The aorta courses back and in the vast majority of cases descends on the left. Right aortic arch does occur, but is rare.

If there is ventricular septal defect, the left ventricle and pulmonary artery will opacify from the right ventricular injection, and the size and position of the ventricular septal defect will be seen (Figure 33–11). Very rarely the right ventricle is hypoplastic (Riemenschneider et al., 1968).

The left ventricular injection, carried out through a catheter, which crosses the atrial septum and the mitral valve, shows a chamber of normal size and left ventricular configuration lying behind the right ventricle (Figure 33–12). It gives rise to the pulmonary

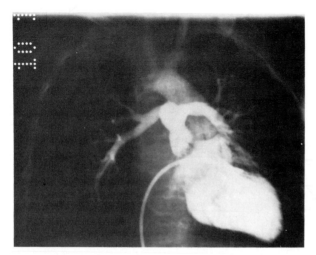
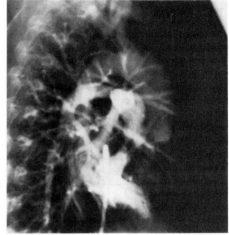

Figure 33-10. Left ventricular injection in a case of complete transposition with left ventricular outflow tract obstruction and a ventricular septal defect. Note that, although this is complete transposition, the aorta is actually to the left of the pulmonary artery.

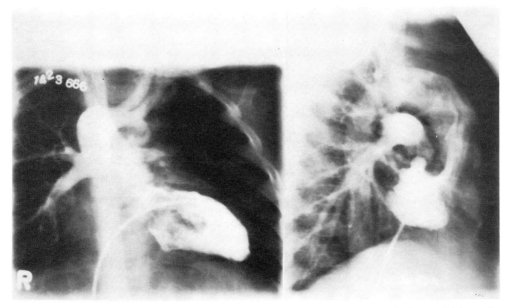

Figure 33-11. Left ventricular injection in a child with complete transposition and a ventricular septal defect and pulmonary stenosis. The right ventricle and anterior aorta fill through the ventricular septal defect.

artery, and the pulmonary valve is low and posterior compared to the aortic valve. The ventricular septum in complete transposition is characteristically bowed backward (Figure 33–10), and the left ventricular outflow tract sweeps around this convexity, which can present significant obstruction (Shaher et al., 1967).

The distribution of blood flow to the lungs in transposition is of interest. There is uneven distribution favoring the right lung, which can be so severe as to suggest left pulmonary artery thrombosis or stenosis. It appears, however, that this predominance of flow to the right lung—which can be

demonstrated angiographically (Muster et al., 1976) and using radioisotopes (Vidne et al., 1976)—is likely due to morphologic and hydraulic factors. The inclination of the left ventricular outflow tract and the main pulmonary artery is normally to the right, and with time favors the development of this uneven distribution, for it is not present in the newborn (Muster et al., 1976). It persists following the Mustard procedure (Morgan et al., 1972; Vidne et al., 1976).

The main pulmonary artery is usually normal in size, although in some cases it may be aneurysmally dilated (Aziz et al., 1976). The left ventriculogram will

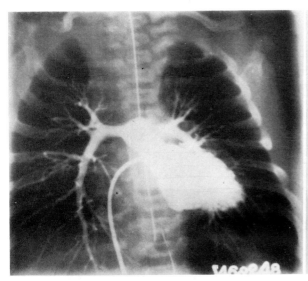
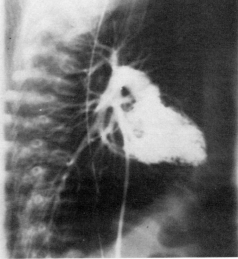

Figure 33-12. Left ventricular injection in a child with complete transposition. The pulmonary artery is posterior, and the ventricular septum is intact.

also demonstrate the site and nature of any pulmonary stenosis, which may be valvular or subvalvular (Shaher et al., 1967).

The diagnostic study should conclude with an aortogram to define the state of the ductus arteriosus and whether or not there is a coarctation or other aortic arch anomaly.

Diagnosis

The diagnosis of complete transposition of the great arteries is first of all facilitated by the knowledge that this condition is a frequent cause of cyanosis, respiratory distress, and heart failure in the newborn. With this suspicion in mind, the clinical findings and a negative hyperoxic test, together with a chest x-ray (which does not show a small heart with underperfused lungs and may show the typical egg-shaped heart), an electrocardiogram (which is normal or rightward), and an echocardiogram (which excludes single ventricle, truncus, and hypoplastic right heart and may be characteristic of transposition), make the suspicion almost a certainty. Definitive diagnosis is by angiocardiography and should be followed immediately in all cases by balloon atrial septostomy.

Balloon Atrial Septostomy

Before this procedure was introduced by Rashkind and Miller (1966), as mentioned earlier, the prognosis of newborns with transposition was poor (Van Praagh et al., 1966). The surgical approach to this problem was to improve mixing by removal of the atrial septum (Blalock and Hanlon, 1950). However, while this procedure was beneficial in older children and resulted in improved survival (Venables, 1966; Deverall et al., 1969), in younger children, particularly those under two weeks old, the survival was still poor. The common cause of death was hemorrhagic edema of the right lung (Cornell et al., 1966), probably caused by the clamping of the right pulmonary veins during excision of the atrial septum. Even open atrial septectomy had a survival rate of only 17 percent under two weeks of age (Trusler, 1964).

The technique introduced by Edwards and Bargeron (1965) had somewhat better results early in life. In this technique the atrial septum is moved to the left, so that the right pulmonary veins are in the right atrium, and the foramen ovale is dilated. This procedure does not cause pulmonary problems, and a survival rate of 90 percent in 18 babies with transposition was reported (Trusler and Kidd, 1969).

In the balloon septostomy procedure (Rashkind and Miller, 1966), a catheter with a latex-balloon at the tip is passed up the inferior vena cava into the right atrium and maneuvered across the atrial septum via the foramen ovale into the left atrium. Its position in the left atrium is verified by a number of methods. If it is a double-lumen catheter, a pressure tracing or

blood sample will verify its position. If it is a single-lumen catheter, passing the tip into a pulmonary vein indicates that the catheter is in the left atrium rather than the right ventricle. If the balloon is slightly distended with fluid, a damped pressure tracing can be recorded. The other method is to inspect the catheter position in the lateral view, either by using the biplane mode or by moving the child onto his side. If the catheter passes posteriorly, it is in the left atrium; if anteriorly, it is in the right ventricle. These precautions are necessary since it is obviously important to tear the atrial septum rather than the tricuspid valve. When one is satisfied that the catheter tip is in the left atrium, the balloon is inflated with 1.5 to 3.0 ml of dilute contrast material and the balloon is withdrawn forcibly down into the inferior vena cava by a sharp rapid tug of limited excursion (Figure 33–13).

The operator often has a sensation of tearing as the balloon crosses the septum, which is usually when the balloon is near the mouth of the inferior vena cava. The procedure is repeated two or three times to ensure the optimal opening, but it is the first tug that is important, since unless this is abrupt, the result will be a stretching of the flap of the foramen and temporary instead of permanent improvement in mixing.

The immediate results of this procedure are an improvement in oxygen saturation (Figure 33–14), improvement of the metabolic acidosis, and an abolition of the pressure gradient between left and right atria (Figure 33–15). The resulting opening between the two atria (Figure 33–16) is usually 12 by 15 mm in size (Rashkind, 1971; Paul, 1971), and the torn "valve" tissue folds back and disappears with time.

The complications of this procedure at The Hospital for Sick Children have been remarkably few. Occasionally a balloon will burst, and then most often the latex remains attached to the catheter and can be withdrawn. Rarely, however, portions have remained in the circulation and in one instance had to be surgically removed from the iliac bifurcation.

Rashkind balloon atrial septostomy should be carried out on all cases of transposition at the time of initial catheterization in the newborn period. Although Rashkind and others (Rashkind and Miller, 1968; Neches et al., 1972) advocate its use in older infants and children, we have found repeated attempts often ineffectual in infants over three months of age. There are obviously other applications for this technique: for example, in the hypoplastic right or left heart syndrome and in total anomalous pulmonary venous drainage, where life depends on the circulation crossing the atrial septum (Rashkind and Miller, 1968, and Chapters 28–32 of this text).

Clinical Course and Management

The clinical results of balloon atrial septostomy are now generally very good, although at first the hospital mortality varied between 15 and 27 percent (Singh et

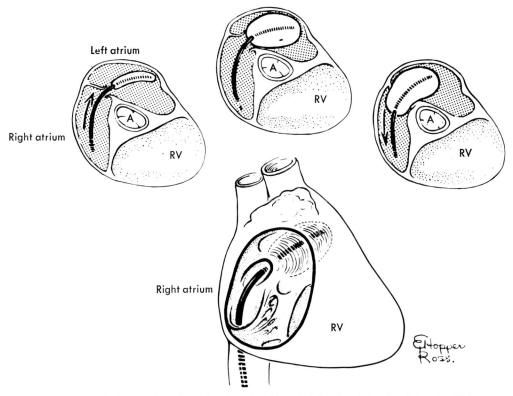

Figure 33-13. The balloon on the catheter tip is introduced into the left atrium, inflated, and sharply withdrawn.

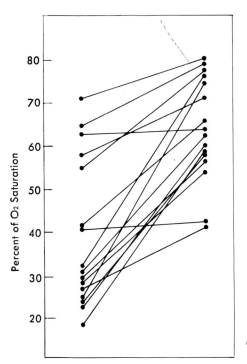

Figure 33-14. Changes in oxygen saturation after balloon atrial septostomy. Note that there was little improvement in the oxygen saturation if this was already good, as in cases with a ventricular septal defect.

al., 1969; Venables, 1970; Tynan, 1971; Rashkind, 1971; Clarkson, 1972). In one multicenter study the results were not as good (Parisi and Fyler, 1973). In a series of patients with balloon atrial septostomy at The Hospital for Sick Children in 1969–1970 the hospital mortality was 8 percent (Hawker and Kidd, 1972).

The usual course for the infant with transposition and a successful septostomy is to maintain normal acid-base balance and PO_2 of around 40 mm of mercury. On occasion an infant who has had an apparently successful septostomy will remain hypoxic immediately, and the oxygen saturation will not start to improve for one to two days (Rashkind, 1971). In another group the hypoxia persists, and we have not found that surgical septectomy will improve the situation, which is presumably due to poor mixing. It is possible that an increased volume of total pulmonary blood flow, either per se (Tynan, 1972; Mair and Ritter, 1974) or by creating turbulence and so better mixing (Clarkson et al., 1976a), is necessary for good oxygen saturation in these children, or it may be that the poor mixing is due to problems with ventricular compliance.

Cerebrovascular accidents have been a problem in the hypoxic infants with transposition. The incidence of thrombotic episodes has varied between 17 and 24 percent (see Table 33-1). Cottrill and Kaplan (1971) in a study of the pathology of cerebrovascular accidents in young children with transposition and tetralogy

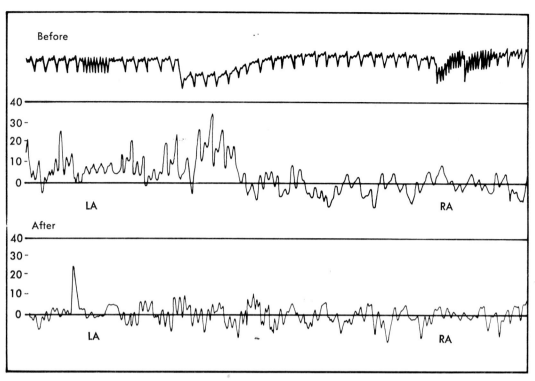

Figure 33-15. Changes in the pressure tracing on withdrawal from left to right atrium before and after septostomy.

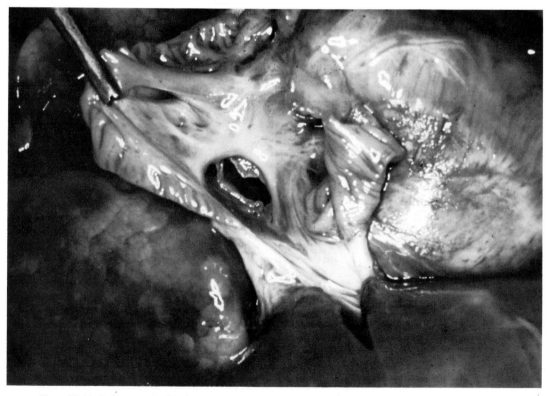

Figure 33-16. A photograph of the foramen ovale with the torn "valve." This child died at surgery for ligation of a large persistent ductus arteriosus three days after septostomy.

found that the predominant lesion (19 of 29 cases) was thrombosis in veins and dural sinuses rather than in the arteries.

Table 33-1.   INCIDENCE OF CEREBRAL THROMBOSIS IN COMPLETE TRANSPOSITION OF THE GREAT ARTERIES

	PERCENT
Tyler and Clark (1957)	11
Rashkind (1971)	17
Paul (1971)	7
Hawker and Kidd (1972)	8
Phornphutkul et al. (1973)	2.4

The conventional wisdom concerning the cause of these episodes is that they are caused by hypoxia and polycythemia, this latter giving a raised hematocrit and increased blood viscosity. However, thrombosis can occur in very young infants before the polycythemia develops; and, later on, while the oxygen tension and oxygen saturation of the arterial blood are low, in the child who has developed compensatory polycythemia, the arterial oxygen content and so the oxygen delivery to the brain is often normal. Further, Phornphutkul et al. (1972) noted that in their series the mean corpuscular hemoglobin concentration was lower in the cases that developed cerebral thromboses. This would support the contention of Martelle and Linde (1961) that relative anemia may be an important etiologic factor.

Whatever the cause, the incidence of this complication seems to be lower in 1976 than it was in 1966, which may or may not be due to earlier intervention, either further palliation or total correction (Clarkson et al., 1972). None of The Hospital for Sick Children cases had very high hemoglobins or hematocrits, and it seems likely that these episodes are more often related to febrile illnesses and dehydration, or interventions such as cardiac catheterization and angiography, venesection (Parsons et al., 1971), or surgery. In some instances, there is no obvious antecedent factor.

Whenever a child who has done well initially starts to deteriorate with increasing cyanosis and rising hematocrit, the question is whether further palliation is required. Formerly, when it was felt that the optimal age for the Mustard procedure was about two years, further palliation was frequent and was carried out in between 30 to 50 percent of cases (Kidd, 1976). The actual procedure was sometimes repeat balloon septostomy (Rashkind, 1971; Neches et al., 1972), while other series utilized either the procedure described by Blalock and Hanlon (1950) or that of Edwards and Bargeron (1965). In recent years, however, the age for elective total repair has advanced downwards, and surgical palliation is now more or less confined to (1) cases of simple transposition, where there is inadequate septostomy and the baby is under two months of age, and (2) cases where the anatomy is complex and it is desired to postpone

corrective surgery to a later date (Kidd, 1976). Significant pulmonary stenosis is of course an indication for systemic-pulmonary anastomosis, usually by a Blalock–Taussig shunt. Occasionally it may be necessary to resect a coarctation or ligate a persistent ductus arteriosus.

Plauth and associates (1970) reported follow-up cardiac catheterization on 65 patients who had been followed for between two months and 11 years. They reported that spontaneous closure of ventricular septal defects occurred in about 20 percent of cases, while natural and iatrogenic atrial septal defects persisted. Pulmonary stenosis was more frequent at restudy, and pulmonary vascular obstructive disease developed even in patients with intact ventricular septum at an average age of nine years, although one case was documented as early as $2\frac{1}{2}$ years of age.

Pulmonary Vascular Disease

The question of progressive pulmonary vascular disease in complete transposition of the great arteries has been a subject of concern. There is no doubt that there is an increased incidence of pulmonary vascular disease in this condition over what is found in other cyanotic and noncyanotic congenital heart disease (Ferencz, 1966; Wagenvoort, 1968; Viles et al., 1969; Ferencz et al., 1971; Shaher, 1973; Newfeld et al., 1974), and the general finding is that pulmonary vascular disease was almost universal and severe when there was a ventricular septal defect and was, except in rare instances, mild when the ventricular septum was intact (Kidd, 1976). Recently, in addition to Plauth and associates (1970), Lakier and associates (1975) have reported pulmonary vascular obstruction in 5 of 29 cases of transposition with an intact septum. Clarkson and associates (1976a) suggest that the rarity of postmortem findings of pulmonary vascular disease of the higher Heath and Edwards (1958) grades may be due to the fact that in the postmortem series mentioned above, the intact septum group died mostly in the first three months of life and so did not live long enough to develop more severe vascular obstructive disease. Pulmonary stenosis and pulmonary artery banding did not always prevent the advance of this complication (Plauth et al., 1970; Clarkson et al., 1976a), and progression has been reported in a few cases even subsequent to the Mustard procedure (Newfeld et al., 1974; Mair et al., 1974; Rosengart et al., 1975).

The ultimate aim of the clinician in this regard is to assess the severity of pulmonary vascular obstruction during life. This is not easy (Mair et al., 1971; Lakier et al., 1975) because of the difficulties in quantitating pulmonary blood flow, as discussed in the "Physiology" section. Another variable is the viscosity of the blood, which may be greatly increased in cyanosed patients with high hematocrits in this condition (Hoffman, 1972).

These, among other factors, have caused most centers to bring the elective age for Mustard

optimum age for Mustard I – 2 yrs.

procedure down from that originally recommended by Mustard and associates (1964)—about two years of age—into the first year of life.

Corrective Surgery

The surgical correction of complete transposition of the great arteries had been an objective for many years. Early attempts had been at the arterial end, and Mustard and associates (1954) reported attempts to retranspose the aorta and pulmonary arteries using monkey lungs as a biologic oxygenator. The approach to the venous solution to the problem was pioneered by Baffes (1956), who shunted the inferior vena cava to the left atrium and the right pulmonary veins to the right atrium. Albert (1954) suggested an intracardiac baffle, and Merendino and associates (1957) carried out two such "venous transposition" procedures using an Ivelon prosthesis. It appeared that the circulation was corrected, but neither patient survived. Senning (1959) also designed an operation at the venous end, but it was not until Mustard (1964) that a procedure was described which was generally successful (Mustard et al., 1964; Aberdeen et al., 1965; Cooley et al., 1966; Dillard et al., 1969; Danielson et al., 1971; Breckenridge et al., 1972; Clarkson et al., 1972; Champsaur et al., 1973).

The Mustard procedure consists of removing the atrial septum and replacing it with a baffle or wall made of pericardium which, placed around the superior and inferior venae cavae, directs the blood from these vessels to the mitral valve and allows the pulmonary venous blood to travel to the tricuspid valve (Figure 33–17). This operation in general works well (Kidd and Mustard, 1966), although it is not without problems, including some, such as postoperative baffle leaks (Kidd and Mustard, 1966; Rodriquez-Fernandez, 1972), which are usually very minor. Others are more important. *venous obstruction* Obstruction of venous return at the baffle may affect either the pulmonary or systemic veins. Obstruction of the pulmonary venous return is due to suturing too near the pulmonary veins or to ballooning of the baffle because it is too large (Mustard, 1971). Caval obstruction has been very common when Dacron is used for the baffle (Stafford and McGoon, 1973; Stark et al., 1976; Venables et al., 1974) but is less common with pericardium.

arrhythmias Arrhythmias have been a major problem postoperatively in most series, and suturing too close to the sinoatrial or atrioventricular nodes and division of the internodal tracts have been implicated (El Said et al., 1972; Rodriquez-Fernandez et al., 1972; Gillette, 1974; Ebert et al., 1974; Clarkson et al., 1976b). Some arrhythmias may develop late after surgery and may be a cause of sudden death in postoperative cases. Most arrhythmias are of the supraventricular type with tachy- and brady-arrhythmias suggestive of the sick sinus syndrome. Junctional rhythm is common (Trusler et al., 1976; Varghese and Roland, 1976).

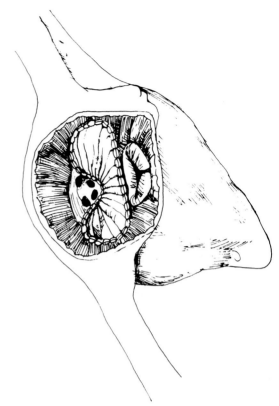

Figure 33-17. Mustard's operation. A pericardial baffle channels the caval blood to the mitral valve, while the pulmonary venous blood flows to the tricuspid valve. Thus venous transposition physiologically corrects the arterial transposition.

(1) A major concern has been whether the right ventricle can maintain good ventricular function as the systemic ventricle over a prolonged period of time. The successful clinical course of many patients suggests that this may be so. Few patients have gone into right ventricular failure, and assessment of right ventricular function by calculation of contractility indices (Godman et al., 1976) has suggested that the right ventricle functions in many patients at the level of contractility of a normal left ventricle. Jarmakani and Canent (1973) and Graham and associates (1975), however, have found depressed ejection fractions measured angiographically in all patients both before and after the Mustard procedure. Although good correlation usually exists between peak velocity of the contractile element and the ejection fraction, they do measure events at different times of the cardiac cycle (peak velocity of contraction being before ejection begins), and they can vary independently (Kreyanbuhl et al., 1968).

(2) Another possible critical factor in the long-term switching of ventricular function is the question of perfusion of the right ventricular myocardium by the coronary arteries. We calculated systolic and diastolic pressure time indices as an index of subendocardial supply and demand (Buckberg et al., 1972) in 36

patients (including some both before and after a Mustard correction) and found that the supply/demand ratio was 0.73 ± 0.173, a figure lower than that recorded from normal children for the left ventricle (Freedom et al., 1974). Patchy areas of ischemic necrosis in the right ventricular myocardium have been reported in pathologic specimens (Astley and Parsons, 1952; Campbell and Hudson, 1958; Noonan et al., 1960; Shaher, 1962).

Postoperative tricuspid regurgitation was described by Waldhausen and associates (1971) and by Tynan and associates (1972), but this has not been a common problem, occurring most often when there is a ventricular septal defect and the repair has been through the tricuspid valve (Godman et al., 1976). Considering complex transposition, now, if a ventricular septal defect is also present it must be repaired. This makes the operation technically more difficult, because the approach to the defect may be either through the delicate and important tricuspid valve or via an incision in the systemic ventricle (McGoon, 1972). The other complicating factor in these cases is the high incidence of pulmonary hypertension (Kidd, 1976), unless there is pulmonary stenosis or there has been a pulmonary artery banding.

The baneful effect of pulmonary vascular disease on operative mortality is well-known (Mustard et al., 1964; Mair et al., 1974). The realization of this fact means that either pulmonary artery banding—which does not always retard pulmonary vascular disease (Clarkson et al., 1976a)—must be carried out in early infancy or repair should be carried out in the first year of life.

For the patient with transposition and a ventricular septal defect in whom the pulmonary vascular resistance had already risen, Lindesmith and associates (1972) proposed the (palliative) Mustard procedure. They reported that these patients were considerably symptomatically improved if the intra-atrial baffle was inserted, but the ventricular septal defect left alone. This approach has recently been reviewed by Lindesmith and associates (1975) and by the Mayo Clinic group (Mair et al., 1976), and it is clear that these patients undergo considerable improvement, both of arterial oxygen saturation and of hemoglobin concentration and hematocrit and that this improvement is more than a simple switching of aortic and pulmonary artery saturation (Mair et al., 1976). Although the follow-up on these patients is short as yet, it could be expected that the pulmonary vascular disease might advance more slowly than when transposition was present. Patients with simple ventricular septal defects and advanced pulmonary vascular disease may lead fairly normal lives, at least into young adulthood (Clarkson et al., 1968; Hallidie-Smith, 1972). The presence of congenital pulmonary stenosis tends to protect the pulmonay vasculature from progressive pulmonary vascular obstructive disease. However, the left ventricular outflow tract is poorly situated for access for successful relief of the obstruction. Although this can be attempted through the pulmonary artery or through the ventricular septal defect from the right ventricle, the difficulty of these procedures, and the higher operative mortality, have encouraged the use of a Rastelli-type operation for this condition. Here, while the ventricular septal defect is repaired so that the left ventricle ejects into the aorta, the pulmonary artery is detached from the left ventricle and attached to the anterior aspect of the right ventricle via a Dacron-valved conduit (Rastelli et al., 1969).

Conclusion

In conclusion, the outlook for children with transposition of the great arteries has improved over the past decade. Whereas formerly 95 percent mortality before two years of age was found (Van Praagh et al., 1967), it is now possible to maintain a 10 to 20 percent mortality (Kidd, 1976).

This can be achieved by, first, a balloon septostomy in early infancy for all cases of transposition.

If the child has transposition with an intact ventricular septum, and the result of septostomy is good, total correction can be postponed to 10 to 12 months. If, however, the result is not good and cyanosis increases, total correction can be carried out at around four to six months. For trouble earlier than three months, we recommend a Blalock-Hanlon procedure, and then a Mustard procedure at around 12 months.

In group 2, where there is a significant ventricular septal defect, the choice is between a Mustard repair and patch closure of the defect at four to six months, or an Edwards procedure and pulmonary artery banding at about three months with postponement of debanding, defect closure, and Mustard repair until around 24 months.

If the child is first seen with pulmonary vascular obstructive disease, a palliative Mustard procedure can be carried out, leaving the septal defect alone. This will improve cyanosis and symptomatology and convert a transposition with an Eisenmenger reaction into a straightforward Eisenmenger syndrome.

When there is transposition, a ventricular septal defect, and pulmonary stenosis, if the situation is well-balanced, observation until four to five years of age is indicated, because these children do well. However, if the pulmonary stenosis is severe, there is an option between a systemic-pulmonary Blalock-Taussig shunt or complete repair, either by a Mustard intra-atrial baffle, ventricular septal defect closure, and widening of the left ventricular outflow tract, or a Rastelli-type operation.

As pointed out by McGoon (1972), these operations are not corrective and carry long-term problems of some severity. The search for alternative solutions still continues, and improved techniques for dealing with the coronary arteries have prompted a return to great artery switching procedures (Mustard et al., 1954). A small number of cases have been treated in this way at a few centers, with some survivors (Jatene et al., 1975; Ross et al., 1976; Yacoub et al., 1976). This procedure may hold greater long-term promise; it is, however, too early yet to say. One thing, however, is clear, that the prognosis for infants with complete transposition of the great arteries has improved dramatically over the past decade.

REFERENCES

Abbott, M. E.: Congenital heart disease. In: Osler and McCrae's *Modern Medicine*. Lea & Febiger, Philadelphia, 1927.

Aberdeen, E.; Waterston, D. J.; Carr, I.; Graham, G.; Bonham-Carter, R. E.; and Subramanian, S.: Successful "correction" of transposed great arteries by Mustard's operation. *Lancet*, 1:1233, 1965.

Albert, H. M.: Surgical correction of transposition of the great vessels. *Surg. Forum*, 5:74, 1955.

Astley, R., and Parsons, C.: Complete transposition of the great arteries. *Br. Heart J.*, 14:13, 1952.

Aziz, K. V.; Nanton, M. A.; Kidd, B. S. L.; Moes, C. A. F.; and Rowe, R. D.: Variations in the size and distensibility of the pulmonary arteries in d-transposition of the great arteries. *Am. J. Cardiol.*, 38:452, 1976.

Baffes, T. G.: A new method for surgical correction of transposition of the aorta and pulmonary artery. *Surg. Gynecol. Obstet.*, 102:227, 1956.

Baillie, M.: *The Morbid Anatomy of Some of the Most Important Parts of the Human Body*, 2nd ed. Johnson and Nicol, London, 1797, p. 38.

Blalock, A., and Hanlon, C. R.: The surgical treatment of complete transposition of the aorta and pulmonary artery. *Surg. Gynecol. Obstet.*, 90:1, 1950.

Breckenridge, I. M.; Stark, J.; Oelert, H.; Graham, G. R.; Bonham-Carter, R. E.; and Waterston, D. J.: Mustard's operation for transposition of the great arteries: Review of 200 cases. *Lancet*, 1:1140, 1972.

Buckberg, G. D.; Fixler, D. C.; Archie, J. P.; and Hoffman, I. E.: Experimental subendocardial ischemia in dogs with normal coronary arteries. *Circ. Res.*, 30:67, 1972.

Burchell, H. G.: Some hemodynamic problems in transposition of the great vessels. *Circulation*, 33:181, 1966.

Campbell, J. A.; Bing, R. J.; Handelsman, J. C.; Groswold, H. E.; and Hammond, M.: Physiological studies in congenital heart disease. VIII. The physiological findings in two patients with complete transposition of the great vessels. *Johns Hopkins Hosp. Bull.*, 84:269, 1949.

Campbell, P. M., and Hudson, R. E. B.: A case of Taussig-Bing transposition with survival for 34 years. *Guys Hosp. Rep.*, 107:14, 1958.

Cardell, B. S.: Corrected transposition of the great vessels. *Br. Heart J.*, 18:186, 1956.

Carey, L. S., and Elliott, L. P.: Complete transposition of the great vessels. Roentgenographic findings. *Am. J. Roentgenol.*, 91:529, 1964.

Carr, I.; Tynan, M.; Aberdeen, E.; Bonham-Carter, R. E.; Graham, G.; and Waterston, D. J.: Predictive accuracy of the "loop rule" in 109 children with classical complete transposition of the great arteries (TGA). *Circulation*, 38:VI-52, 1968 (abstr.).

Castellanos, A.; Pereiras, R.; and Garcia, A.: L'angiocardiographie chez l'enfant. *Presse Med.*, 46:1474, 1938.

Castellanos, A.; Pereiras, R.; and Garcia, A.: Angiocardiography: Anatomico-roentgenological forms of the transposition of the great vessels. *Am. J. Roentgenol.*, 64:255, 1950.

Champsaur, G. L.; Sokol, D. M.; Trusler, G. A.; and Mustard, W. T.: Repair of transposition of the great arteries in 123 pediatric patients. *Circulation*, 48:1032, 1973.

Clarkson, P. M.; Barratt-Boyes, B. G.; Neutze, J. M.; and Lowe, J. B.: Results over a ten-year period of palliation followed by corrective surgery for complete transposition of the great arteries. *Circulation*, 45:1251, 1972.

Clarkson, P. M.; Frye, R. L.; DuShane, J. W.; Burchell, H. B.; Wood, E. H.; and Weidman, W. H.: Prognosis for patients with ventricular septal defect and severe pulmonary vascular obstructive disease. *Circulation*, 38:129, 1968.

Clarkson, P. M.; Neutze, J. M.; Barratt-Boyes, B. G.; and Brandt, P. W. T.: Late postoperative hemodynamic results and cineangiocardiographic findings after Mustard atrial baffle repair for transposition of the great arteries. *Circulation*, 53:525, 1976(a).

Clarkson, P. M.; Barratt-Boyes, B. G.; and Neutze, J. M.: Late dysrhythmias and disturbances of conduction following Mustard operation for complete transposition of the great arteries. *Circulation*, 53:519, 1976(b).

Clarkson, P. M.; Neutze, J. M.; Wardill, J. C.; and Barratt-Boyes, B. G.: The pulmonary vascular bed in patients with complete transposition of the great arteries. *Circulation*, 53:539, 1976(c).

Cooley, D. A.; Hallman, G. L.; Bloodwell, R. D.; and Leachman, R. D.: Two-stage surgical treatment of complete transposition of the great vessels. *Arch. Surg.*, 93:704, 1966.

Cottrill, C. M., and Kaplan, S.: Cerebral vascular accidents in cyanotic congenital heart disease. *Circulation* (Suppl. II) 43,44:95, 1971.

Cudkowicz, L., and Armstrong, J. B.: Injection of the bronchial circulation in a case of transposition. *Br. Heart J.*, 14:374, 1952.

Danielson, G. K.; Mair, D. D.; Ongley, P. A.; Wallace, R. B.; and McGoon, D. W.: Repair of transposition of the great arteries by transposition of venous return. *J. Thorac. Cardiovasc. Surg.*, 61:96, 1971.

De La Cruz, M. V., and Da Rocha, J. P.: An ontogenetic theory for the explanation of congenital malformations involving the truncus and conus. *Am. Heart J.*, 51:782, 1956.

Deverall, P. B.; Tynan, M. J.; Carr, I.; Panagopoulos, P.; Aberdeen, E.; Bonham-Carter, R. E.; and Waterston, D. J.: Palliative surgery in children with transposition of the great arteries. *J. Thorac. Cardiovasc. Surg.*, 58:721, 1969.

De Vries, P. A., and Saunders, J. B. de C. M.: Development of the ventricles and a spiral outflow tract in the human heart. A contribution to the development of the human heart from age group IX to age group XV. Carnegie Inst Washington Publ 621; *Contrib. Embryol.*, 37:87, 1962.

Dillard, D. H.; Mohri, H.; Merendino, K. A.; Morgan, B. C.; Baum, D.; and Crawford, E. W.: Total surgical correction of transposition of the great arteries in children less than six months of age. *Surg. Gynecol. Obstet.*, 129:1258, 1969.

Dillon, J. C.; Feigenbaum, H.; Konecke, L. L.; Keutel, J.; Hurwitz, R. A.; Davis, R. H.; and Chang, S.: Echocardiographic manifestations of D-transposition of the great vessels. *Am. J. Cardiol.*, 32:74, 1973.

Edwards, J. E.: Congenital malformations of the heart and great vessels. In *Pathology of the Heart* (S. E. Gould, ed.), 2nd ed. Charles C Thomas, Publisher, Springfield, Ill., 1960, pp. 354.

Edwards, W. S., and Bargeron, L. M., Jr.: More effective palliation of transposition of the great arteries. *J. Thorac. Cardiovasc. Surg.*, 49:790, 1965.

Elliott, L. P.; Neufeld, H. N.; Anderson, R. C.; Adams, P.; and Edwards, J. E.: Complete transposition of the great vessels. *Circulation*, 32:1105, 1963.

Elliott, L. P.; Anderson, R. C.; Tuna, N.; Adams, P. Jr.; and Neufeld, H. N.: Complete transposition of the great vessels. II. An electrocardiographic analysis. *Circulation*, 32:1118, 1963.

Ellison, C., and Restieaux, N.: *Vectorcardiography in Congenital Heart Disease*. W. B. Saunders, Philadelphia, 1972.

El-Said, G.; Rosenberg, H. S.; Mullins, C. S.; Hallman, G.; Cooley, D. A.; and McNamara, D. G.: Dysrhythmias after Mustard's operation for transposition of the great arteries. *Am. J. Cardiol.*, 30:526, 1972.

Farre, J. R.: *Pathological Researches*. Essay I. On Malformations of the Human Heart: Illustrated by Numerous Cases, and Five Plates Containing Fourteen Figures; and Preceded by Some Observations on the Method of Improving the Diagnostic Part of Medicine. Longman, Hurst, Rees, Orme, and Brown, London, 1814, p. 28.

Ferencz, C.: Transposition of the great vessels: Pathophysiological consideration based upon a study of the lungs. *Circulation*, 33:661, 1960.

Ferencz, C.; Greco, J. M.; and Libi-SyLora, M.: Variability of pulmonary vascular disease in certain malformations of the heart. In: *The Natural History and Progress in Treatment of Congenital Heart Defects*. B. S. L. Kidd and J. D. Keith, eds. Charles C Thomas, Publisher, Springfield, Ill., 1971.

Folse, R.; Roberts, W. C.; and Cornell, W. P.: Increased bronchial collateral circulation in a patient with transposition of the great vessels and pulmonary hypertension. *Am. J. Cardiol.*, **8**:282, 1961.

Freedom, R. F.; Williams, G. J.; Olley, P. M.; and Kidd, B. S. L.: Pressure time indices in D-transposition of the great arteries. *Circulation*, **51**:1167, 1975.

Gallaher, M. E.; Fyler, D. C.; and Lindesmith, G. G.: Transposition with intact ventricular septum: its diagnosis and management in the small infant. *Am. J. Dis. Child.*, **111**:248, 1966.

Gillette, P. C.; El-Said, G. M.; Sivarajan, N.; Mullins, C. E.; Williams, R. L.; and McNamara, D. G.: Electrophysiological abnormalities after Mustard's operation for transposition of the great arteries. *Br. Heart J.*, **36**:186, 1974.

Godman, M. J.; Friedli, B.; Pasternac, A.; Kidd, B. S. L.; Trusler, G. Z.; and Mustard, W. T.: Hemodynamic studies in children four to ten years after the Mustard operation for transposition of the great arteries. *Circulation*, **53**:532, 1976.

Godman, M. J.; Tham, P.; and Kidd, B. S. L.: Echocardiography in the evaluation of the cyanotic newborn infant. *Br. Heart J.*, **36**:154, 1974.

Goor, D. A., and Edwards, J. E.: The spectrum of transposition of the great arteries with specific reference to developmental anatomy of the conus. *Circulation*, **48**:406, 1968.

Graham, T. P., Jr.; Atwood, G. F.; Boucek, R. J.; Boerth, R. C.; and Nelson, J. H.: Right heart volume characteristics in transposition of the great arteries. *Circulation*, **51**:881, 1975.

Gramiak, R.; Chung, K. J.; Nanda, N.; and Manning, J.: Echocardiographic diagnosis of transposition of the great vessels. *Radiology*, **106**:187, 1973.

Grant, R.: The morphogenesis of transposition of the great vessels. *Circulation*, **36**:819, 1962.

Hallidie-Smith, K. A.; Edwards, R. E.; Wilson, R.; and Zeidifard, E.: Long-term cardiorespiratory assessment after surgical closure of ventricular septal defect in childhood. *Br. Heart J.*, **37**:553, 1975.

Harris, J. S., and Farber, S.: Transposition of the great cardiac vessels with special reference to the phylogenetic theory of Spitzer. *Arch. Pathol.*, **28**:427, 1939.

Hawker, R. E., and Kidd, B. S. L.: The modified natural history of transposition of the great arteries. Its influence on the timing of the Mustard procedure. *Can. Med. Assoc. J.*, **107**:644, 1972. (abstr.).

Heath, D., and Edwards, J. E.: Pathology of hypertensive pulmonary vascular disease: A description of six grades of structural changes in the pulmonary arteries with special reference to congenital cardiac septal defects. *Circulation*, **18**:533, 1958.

Hirschfeld, S.; Meyer, R. A.; and Kaplan, S.: Non-invasive right and left systolic time intervals by echocardiography. *Pediatr. Res.*, **8**:350, 1974.

Hoffman, J. I. E.: Diagnosis and treatment of pulmonary vascular disease. *Birth Defects*, **8**:9, 1972.

Janeway, E. G.: Malposition of the aorta and pulmonary artery—thrombus in heart and cerebral emoblism—death from intestinal hemorrhage. *Med. Rec.*, **12**:811, 1877.

Jarmakani, J. M. M., and Canent, R. V.: Pre- and post-operative right ventricular function in children with transposition of the great vessels. *Circulation*, **48** (suppl. IV):IV-23, 1973.

Jatene, A. D.; Fontes, V. F.; Paulista, P. P.; et al.: Successful anatomic correction of transposition of the great vessels. A preliminary report. *Arq. Bras. Cardiol.*, **28**:461, 1975.

Kay, E. B., and Cross, F. S.: Surgical treatment of transposition of the great vessels. *Surgery*, **38**:712, 1955.

Keith, A.: The Hunterian lectures on malformations of the heart. *Lancet*, **2**:359, 453, 519, 1909.

Keith, J. D.; Rowe, R. D.; and Vlad, P.: *Heart Disease in Infancy and Childhood*, 1st ed. Macmillan Publishing Co., Inc., New York, 1953.

Keith, J. D.; Neill, C. A.; Vlad, P.; Rowe, R. D.; and Chute, A. L.: Transposition of the great vessels. *Circulation*, **17**:830, 1953.

Khoury, G. H.; Shaher, R. M.; and Fowler, R. S.: The vectorcardiogram in complete transposition of the great vessels: Analysis of fifty cases. *Circulation*, **35**:178, 1967.

Kidd, L., and Mustard, W. T.: Hemodynamic effects of a totally corrective procedure in transposition of the great vessels. *Circulation*, **33** + **34**(suppl. I): I-28, 1966.

Kidd, B. S. L.; Tyrell, M. J.; and Pickering, D.: Transposition 1969. In: *The Natural History and Progress in Treatment of Congenital*

Heart Defects, B. S. L. Kidd and J. D. Keith (eds.). Charles C Thomas, Publisher, Springfield, Ill., 1971.

Kidd, B. S. L.: The fate of children with transposition of the great arteries following balloon atrial septostomy. In: *The Child with Congenital Heart Disease After Surgery*, B. S. L. Kidd and R. D. Rowe (eds.). Futura Publishers, New York, 1976.

Kirklin, J. W.: Evaluating the results of cardiac surgery. *Circulation*, **48**:323, 1973.

Krayenbuehl, H. P.; Bussmann, W. D.; Turina, M.; and Luthy, E.: Is the ejection fraction an index of myocardial contractility? *Cardiologia*, **53**:1, 1968.

Lakier, J. B.; Stanger, P.; Heymann, M. A.; Hoffman, J. I. E.; and Rudolph, A. M.: Early onset of pulmonary vascular obstruction in patients with aortopulmonary transposition and intact ventricular septum. *Circulation*, **51**:875, 1975.

Langstaff; Case of a singular mal-formation of the heart. *Lond. Med. Rev.*, **4**:88, 1811.

Lev, M., and Saphir, O.: Transposition of the large vessels. *J. Tech. Methods*, **17**:126, 1937.

Lev, M.: *Autopsy Diagnosis of Congenitally Malformed Hearts*. Charles C Thomas, Publishers, Springfield, Ill., 1953, p. 13.

Liebman, J.; Cullum, L.; and Belloc, N. B.: Natural history of transposition of the great arteries. Anatomy and birth and death characteristic. *Circulation*, **40**:237, 1969.

Lindesmith, G. G.; Stiles, Q. R.; Tucker, B. L.; Gallaher, M. E.; Stanton, R. E.; and Meyer, B. W.: The Mustard operation as a palliative procedure. *J. Thorac. Cardiovasc. Surg.*, **63**:75, 1972.

Lindesmith, G. G.; Meyer, B. W.; Stanton, R. E.; Gallaher, M. E.; Stiles, Q. R.; and Jones, J. C.: Surgical treatment of transposition of the great vessels. *Ann. Thorac. Surg.*, **8**:12, 1969.

Mair, D. D.; Macartney, F. J.; Weidman, W. H.; Ritter, D. G.; Ongley, P. A.; and Smith, R. E.: The vectorcardiogram in complete transposition of the great arteries. Correlation with anatomic and haemodynamic findings and calculated left ventricular mass. *J. Electrocardiol.*, **3**:217, 1970.

Mair, D. D.; Ritter, D. G.; Ongley, P. A.; and Helmholz, H. F., Jr.: Hemodynamics and evaluation for surgery of patients with complete transposition of the great arteries and ventricular septal defect. *Am. J. Cardiol.*, **28**:623, 1971.

Mair, D. D.; Macartney, F. J.; Weidman, W. H.; Ritter, D. G.; Ongley, P. A.; and Smith, R. E.: The vectorcardiogram in complete transposition of the great arteries: an attempt at correlation with anatomic and hemodynamic findings and left ventricular mass. In: *Vectorcardiography*, 2nd ed., Hoffman, I. (ed.). North-Holland Publishing Company, Amsterdam, pp. 610–23, 1971.

Mair, D. D., and Ritter, D. G.: Factors influencing intercirculatory mixing in patients with complete transposition of the great vessels. *Am. J. Cardiol.*, **30**:653, 1972.

Mair, D. D.; Danielson, G. K.; Wallace, R. B.; and McGoon, D. W.: Long term follow-up of Mustard operation survivors. *Circulation*, **50**:11(Suppl. II), 1974.

Mair, D. D.; Ritter, D. G.; Danielson, G. K.; Wallace, R. B.; and McGoon, D. C.: The palliative Mustard operation: Rationale and results. *Am. J. Cardiol.*, **37**:762, 1976.

Martelle, R. R., and Linde, L. M.: Cerebrovascular accidents in tetralogy of Fallot. *Am. J. Dis. Child.*, **101**:95, 1961.

Merendino, K. A.; Jesseph, J. E.; Herron, P. W.; Thomas, G. I.; and Vetto, R. R.: Interatrial venous transposition; a one-stage intracardiac operation for the conversion of complete transposition of the aorta and pulmonary artery to corrected transposition. *Surgery*, **42**:898, 1957.

Miller, H. C.: Cardiac hypertrophy and extramedullary erythropoiesis in newborn infants of prediabetic mothers. *Am. J. Med. Sci.*, **209**:447, 1945.

Mitchell, S. C.; Sellmann, A. H.; Westphal, M. C.; and Park, J.: Etiologic correlates in a study of congenital heart disease in 56,109 births. *Am. J. Cardiol.*, **28**:653, 1971.

Morgan, J. R.; Miller, B. L.; Daicoff, G. R.; and Andrews, E. J.: Hemodynamic and angiographic evaluation after Mustard procedure for transposition of the great arteries. *J. Thorac. Cardiovasc. Surg.*, **64**:879, 1972.

Mullins, C. E.; Neches, W. H.; and McNamara, D. G.: The infant with transposition of the great arteries, 1. Cardiac catheterization protocol. *Am. Heart J.*, **84**:597, 1972.

Mustard, W. T.; Chute, A. L.; Keith, J. D.; Sirek, A.; Rowe, R. D.;

and Vlad, P.: A surgical approach to transposition of the great vessels with extracorporeal circuit. *Surgery*, **36**:39, 1954.

Mustard, W. T.: Successful two-stage correction of transposition of the great vessels. *Pediatr. Surg.*, **55**:469, 1964.

Mustard, W. T.; Keith, J. D.; Trusler, G. A.; Fowler, R.; and Kidd, L.: The surgical management of transposition of the great vessels. *J. Thorac. Cardiovasc. Surg.*, **48**:953, 1964.

Muster, A. J.; Paul, M. H.; Van Grondelle, A.; and Conway, J. J.: Abnormal distribution of the pulmonary blood flow between the two lungs in transposition of the great arteries. In: *The Child with Congenital Heart Disease After Surgery*, Eds. B. S. L. Kidd and R. D. Rowe. Futura Publishers, New York, 1976.

Neches, W. H.; Mullins, C. E.; and McNamara, D. G.: The infant with transposition of the great arteries II. Results of balloon atrial septostomy. *Am. Heart J.*, **84**:603, 1972.

Newfeld, E. A.; Paul, M. H.; Muster, A. J.; and Idriss, F. S.: Pulmonary vascular disease in complete transposition of the great arteries: A study of 200 patients. *Am. J. Cardiol.*, **34**:75, 1974.

Noonan, J. A.; Nadas, A. S.; Rudolph, A. M.; and Harriss, G. B. C.: Transposition of the great arteries: A correlation of clinical, physiologic and autopsy data. *N. Engl. J. Med.*, **263**:592, 1960.

Parisi, L., and Fyler, D. C.: Management of transposition of the great arteries in New England. *Am. J. Cardiol.*, **31**:151, 1973 (abstr.).

Parsons, C. G.; Astley, R.; Burrows, F. G. O.; and Singh, S. P.: Transposition of the great arteries: a study of 65 infants followed for 1 to 4 years after balloon septostomy. *Br. Heart J.*, **33**:725, 1971.

Paul, M. H.: Transposition of the great arteries: Physiologic data. In: *The Natural History and Progress in Treatment of Congenital Heart Defects*, B. S. L. Kidd and J. D. Keith (eds.). Charles C Thomas, Publisher, Springfield, Ill., 1971.

Phornphutkul, C.; Rosenthal, A.; Nadas, A. S.; and Berenberg, W.: Cerebrovascular accidents in infants and children with cyanotic congenital heart disease. *Am. J. Cardiol.*, **32**:329, 1973.

Plauth, W. H., Jr.; Nadas, A. S.; Bernhard, W. F.; and Fyler, D. C.: Changing hemodynamics in patients with transposition of the great arteries. *Circulation*, **42**:131, 1970.

Rashkind, W. J., and Miller, W. M.: Creation of an atrial septal defect without thoracotomy: A palliative approach to complete transposition of the great arteries. *JAMA*, **196**:992, 1966.

Rashkind, W. J.: Balloon atrial septostomy for transposition of the great arteries: technique and follow up. In: *The Natural History and Progress in Treatment of Congenital Heart Defects*, B. S. L. Kidd and J. D. Keith (eds.). Charles C Thomas, Publisher, Springfield, Ill., 1971.

Rashkind, W. J.: Transposition of the great arteries. In: *The Pediatric Clinics of North America*, Vol. 18, *Pediatric Cardiology*, S. Kaplan (ed.). W. B. Saunders Company, Philadelphia, 1971.

Rastelli, G. C.; McGoon, D. C.; and Wallace, R. B.: Anatomic correction of the great arteries with ventricular septal defect and subpulmonary stenosis. *J. Thorac. Cardiovasc. Surg.*, **58**:545, 1969.

Restieaux, N. J.; Ellison, R. C.; Albers, W. H.; and Nadas, A. S.: The Frank electrocardiogram in complete transposition of the great arteries: Its use in assessment of left ventricular pressure. *Am. Heart J.*, **83**:219, 1972.

Riemenschneider, T. A.; Vincent, W. R.; Ruttenberg, H. D.; and Desilets, D. T.: Transposition of the great vessels with hypoplasia of the right ventricle. *Circulation*, **38**:386, 1968.

Robertson, M. I.: The comparative anatomy of the bulbus cordis with special reference to abnormal position of the great vessels in the human heart. *J. Pathol. Bacteriol.*, **18**:191, 1913.

Rosengart, R.; Fishbein, M.; and Emmanouilides, G. C.: Progressive pulmonary vascular disease after surgical correction (Mustard procedure) of transposition of great arteries with intact ventricular septum. *Am. J. Cardiol.*, **35**:107, 1975.

Ross, D.; Rickards, A.; and Somerville, J.: Transposition of the great arteries: Logical anatomical arterial correction. *Br. Med. J.*, **1**:1109, 1976.

Rudolph, A. M.: *Congenital Disease of the Heart*. Year Book Medical Publishers, Inc., Chicago, 1974.

Senning, A.: Surgical correction of transposition of the great arteries. *Surgery*, **45**:966, 1959.

Shaher, R. M.: The haemodynamics of complete transposition of the great vessels. *Br. Heart J.*, **26**:343, 1964.

Shaher, R. M.; Fowler, R. S.; Kidd, B. S. L.; Moes, C. A. F.; and Keith, J. E.: Spontaneous closure of a ventricular septal defect in a case of complete transposition of the great vessels. *Can. Med. Assoc. J.*, **93**:1037, 1965.

Shaher, R. M., and Deuchar, D. C.: The electrocardiogram in complete transposition of the great vessels. *Br. Heart J.*, **28**:265, 1966.

Shaher, R. M., and Kidd, L.: Hemodynamics of complete transposition of the great vessels before and after the creation of an atrial septal defect. *Circulation*, Suppl. I: **33 & 34**:I-3, 1966.

Shaher, R. M., and Puddu, G. D.: Coronary arterial anatomy in complete transposition of the great vessels. *Am. J. Cardiol.*, **17**:355, 1966.

Shaher, R. M., and Kidd, L.: Effect of ventricular septal defect and patent ductus arteriosus on left ventricular pressure in complete transposition of the great vessels. *Circulation*, **37**:232, 1968.

Shaher, R. M.: *Complete Transposition of the Great Arteries*. Academic Press, New York and London, 1973.

Singh, S. P.; Astley, R., and Burrows, F. G. O.: Balloon septostomy for transposition of the great arteries. *Br. Heart J.*, **31**:722, 1969.

Spitzer, A.: The architecture of normal and malformed hearts. *Virchow. Arch. Pathol. Anat.*, **243**:81, 1932.

Stenonis, N.: Acta Hofmensa 71 (obs. 3), 1671. (Cited by Brown, J. W.: *Congenital Heart Disease*. Staples Press, London, 1959.

Taussig, H. B.: Complete transposition of the great vessels. *Am. Heart J.*, **16**:728, 1938.

Trusler, G. A.; Mustard, W. T.; and Fowler, R. S.: The role of surgery in the treatment of transposition of the great vessels. *Can. Med. Assoc. J.*, **91**:1096, 1964.

Trusler, G. A., and Kidd, B. S. L.: Surgical palliation in complete transposition of the great vessels. Experience with Edwards procedure. *Can. J. Surg.*, **12**:83, 1969.

Trusler, G. A.; Mulholland, H. C.; Takeuchi, Y.; Kidd, B. S. L.; and Mustard, W. T.: Long term results of intra-atrial repair of transposition of the great arteries. In Julio C. Davila (ed.): *Second Henry Ford Hospital International Symposium on Cardiac Surgery*. Appleton-Century-Crofts, New York, 1977, p. 368.

Tyler, H. R., and Clark, D. B.: Cerebrovascular accidents in patients with congenital heart disease. *A.M.A. Arch. Neurol. Psychiat.*, **77**:483, 1957.

Tynan, M.: Survival of infants with transposition of great arteries after balloon atrial septostomy. *Lancet*, **1**:621, 1971.

Tynan, M.: Transposition of the great arteries: Changes in the circulation after birth. *Circulation*, **46**:809, 1972.

Tynan, M.; Aberdeen, E.; and Stark, J.: Tricuspid incompetence after the Mustard operation for transposition of the great arteries. *Circulation*, **45**:13, 1972.

Van Mierop, H. S.; Alley, R. D.; Kausel, H. W.; and Stranahan, A.: Pathogenesis of transposition complexes. 1. Embryology of the ventricles and great arteries. *Am. J. Cardiol.*, **12**:216, 1963a.

Van Mierop, L. H. S., and Wiglesworth, F. W.: Pathogenesis of transposition complexes. 2. Anomalies due to faulty transfer of the posterior great artery. *Am. J. Cardiol.*, **12**:226, 1963b.

Van Mierop, L. H. S., and Wiglesworth, F. W.: Pathogenesis of transposition complexes. 3. True transposition of the great vessels. *Am. J. Cardiol.*, **12**:233, 1963c.

Van Mierop, L. H. S.: Pathology and pathogenesis of common cardiac malformations. *Cardiovasc. Clin.*, **2**:27, 1970.

Van Mierop, L. H. S.: Transposition of the great arteries. I. Clarification or further confusion? *Am. J. Cardiol.*, **28**:735, 1971.

Van Praagh, R.; Van Praagh, S.; Vlad, P.; and Keith, J. D.: Anatomic types of congenital dextrocardia. Diagnostic and embryologic implications. *Am. J. Cardiol.*, **13**:510, 1964.

Van Praagh, R.; Vlad, P.; and Keith, J. D.: Complete transposition of the great arteries. In: *Heart Disease in Infancy and Childhood*, 2nd ed. Keith, J. D.; Rowe, R. D.; and Vlad, P. (eds.). Macmillan Publishing Co., Inc., New York, 1967, pp. 682.

Van Praagh, R.: Transposition of the great arteries. II. Transposition clarified. *Am J. Cardiol.*, **28**:739, 1971.

Van Praagh, R.; Perez-Trevino, C.; Lopez-Cuellar, M.; Baker, F. W.; Zuberbuehler, J. R.; Quero, M.; Perez, V. M.; Moreno, V.; and Van Praagh, S.: Transposition of the great arteries with posterior aorta, anterior pulmonary artery, subpulmonary conus and fibrous continuity between aortic and atrioventricular valves. *Am. J. Cardiol.*, **28**:621, 1971.

Venables, A. W.: Complete transposition of the great vessels in infancy with reference to palliative surgery. *Br. Heart J.*, **28**:335, 1966.

——— Balloon atrial septostomy in complete transposition of the great arteries in infancy. *Br. Heart J.*, **32**:61, 1970.

Vidne, B. A.; Duszynski, D.; and Subramanian, S.: Pulmonary blood flow distribution in transposition of the great arteries. *Am. J. Cardiol.*, **38**:62, 1976.

Viles, P. H.; Ongley, P. A.; and Titus, J. L.: The spectrum of pulmonary vascular disease in transposition of the great arteries. *Circulation*, **40**:31, 1969.

Wagenvoort, C. A.; Nauta, J.; Van Der Schaar, P. J.; Weeda, H. W. H.; and Wagenvoort, N.: The pulmonary vasculature in complete transposition of the great vessels, judged from lung biopsies. *Circulation*, **38**:746, 1968.

Waldhausen, J. A.; Pierce, W. S.; Park, C. S.; Rashkind, W. J.; and Friedman, S.: Physiologic correction of transposition of the great arteries. *Circulation*, **43**:738, 1971.

Yacoub, M. H.; Radley-Smith, R.; and Hilton, C. J.: Anatomical correction of complete transposition of great arteries and ventricular septal defect in infancy. *Br. Med. J.*, **1**:1112, 1976.

34

Congenitally Corrected Transposition of
the Great Arteries

B. S. Langford Kidd

ALTHOUGH the term "congenitally corrected transposition of the great arteries" has been described as a "triple whammy" meaning virtually nothing to anybody but congenital heart buffs (Van Praagh, 1970), this unwieldy title describes a well-defined group of patients who have recognizable characteristics in common, who present with similar clinical syndromes, and who together pose diagnostic and therapeutic problems related to their disordered cardiac anatomy. The term was introduced by von Rokitansky, who in 1875 described the hearts of two infants, stating that "the transposition of the great vessels was corrected by the position of the ventricular septum." It is now recognized that it is ventricular inversion that "corrects" the transposition of the great arteries, with the result that the course of the circulation resembles the normal—with the systemic venous return going to the lungs and the pulmonary venous return passing out by the aorta to the body.

To grasp the terminology in widespread use today to describe the cardiac chambers, it is important to understand that the adjectives "right" and "left" describe not only relative position or "sidedness" but also, more importantly, the morphologic identity of the chamber (Lev, 1954). Thus, the right atrium receives the systemic venous return and has a limbus and fossa ovalis on its septal surface. The right ventricle has a tricuspid atrioventricular valve, and its cavity has a coarsely trabeculated wall, divided by the crista supraventricularis into a sinus or body and a conus or outflow tract. The left atrium features the pulmonary venous return and the septum primum, and the left ventricle has a bicuspid atrioventricular valve, no conus, and a finely trabeculated wall. These definitions apply whether the particular chamber is on its usual side or not. The atria and the ventricles, therefore, have a definite identity and can be described as being "solitus," or on their usual side, or "inversus" when there is inversion or right-left reversal.

In congenitally corrected transposition of the great arteries, "transposition" means that the great arteries are "transposed" across the ventricular septum; the aorta arises above the morphologically right ventricle, and the pulmonary artery arises above the morphologically left ventricle. However, there is also ventricular inversion, which means that the right ventricle giving rise to the aorta is left-sided and receives its blood from the left atrium and pulmonary veins, while the left ventricle giving rise to the pulmonary artery is right-sided and receives its blood from the right atrium and systemic veins. Thus, there is physiologic correction of the course of the blood flow, which goes right atrium–left ventricle–pulmonary artery–lungs–left atrium–right ventricle–aorta–body (Figure 34–1). Unfortunately, however, nearly all the patients have other lesions as well, and the "correction" is very far from perfect. Ventricular septal defect, single ventricle, pulmonary stenosis, left atrioventricular valve regurgitation, and conduction disturbances are the most commonly associated defects.

Following the initial description by von Rokitansky (1875), important contributions to our understanding of this condition are those by Spitzer (1923), Walmsley (1931), Harris and Farber (1939), Lev (1953), Cardell (1956), Schiebler and associates (1961), and Van Praagh and Van Praagh (1966).

Anatomic Features

The heart in corrected transposition shows the aorta arising anteriorly and to the left, while the pulmonary artery is situated to the right and posterior. However, as with all complex congenital lesions in which there are positional anomalies, it is wise to define the situation in terms of each of the three cardiac segments—atria, ventricles, and great arteries.

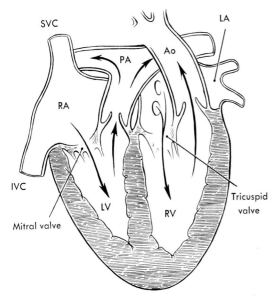

Figure 34-1. Diagram of the circulation in congenitally corrected transposition of the great arteries. Note that the great arteries are transposed, i.e., arise from their incorrect ventricles, but that the ventricles are inverted, so correcting the circulation.

The atria in corrected transposition are in situs solitus in 95 percent of cases (Bjarke and Kidd, 1976). This means that the atria are in their usual relationship with the left atrium to the left and the right atrium to its right. In virtually every case of congenital heart disease the stomach is on the same side as the left atrium; this situation is, therefore, usually described as visceroatrial situs solitus. The ventricles, however, are inverted, with the right ventricle on the left and the left ventricle on the right. The relationship of the ventricles is determined by the direction of looping of the primitive heart tube between the twenty-third and twenty-fifth day of embryonic life. The heart tube is fixed at both ends, and with continued longitudinal growth of its midportion, it bends or loops; it usually does this anteriorly and to the right—a D-(or dextro) loop. The proximal part of the tube (which is going to become the left ventricle) is therefore situated behind and to the left of the more distal or bulbus cordis portion (which is destined to become the right ventricle), lying anteriorly and to the right.

However, when the bulboventricular loop swings to the left— an L (levo) loop—this embryologic defect means that the proximal, left ventricular portion will lie on the right and the distal, right ventricular portion on the left (de la Cruz et al., 1959). As the atrial portion of the heart is "anchored" and linked with visceral situs, this abnormal looping does not affect atrial position, but results in a discordance between atria and ventricles. While there is visceroatrial situs solitus, there is ventricular situs inversus.

It should be noted that the L-looping would be the usual situation in a situs inversus individual—a person in whom all the viscera have undergone right-left reversal, creating a "mirror-image" situation. In these people, an L-loop would not produce atrioventricular discordance, since both atria and ventricles would be in situs inversus. In the inversus individual discordance is produced by a D-loop, and in fact, this was the basis for the corrected transposition in 5 percent of the 101 cases seen at The Hospital for Sick Children, Toronto (Bjarke and Kidd, 1976).

Considering the third cardiac segment—the great arteries—these are transposed. That is, they lie on the "unusual" side of the ventricular septum. In the usual situation the concordant D-loop of the ventricles is associated with a D-position of the great arteries, the aortic valve being to the right of the pulmonary valve. The great arteries may be either normally situated—with the aortic valve posterior, to the right, and over the left ventricle—or transposed—with the aortic valve anterior, to the right, and over the right ventricle. Similarly, in the situs inversus person, the concordant L-loop is associated with L-position of the great arteries—either normal, with the aortic valve to the left and posterior—or transposed—with the aortic valve to the left and anterior. These two concordant varieties of transposition are "complete."

When there is a discordant cardiac loop (either an L-loop with visceroatrial situs solitus or a D-loop with visceroatrial situs inversus), the great arteries are usually in the transposed position. The exceptions to this rule, isolated ventricular inversion, are very rare (Van Praagh and Van Praagh, 1966). So, in summary, in the common variety of corrected transposition (with visceroatrial situs solitus and an L-loop giving ventricular situs inversus), there is L-transposition of the great arteries, with the aortic valve lying anteriorly and to the left above the left-sided right ventricle, and the pulmonary valve posterior and to the right above the right-sided left ventricle. In the rare variety with visceroatrial situs inversus and a D-loop, the aorta arises anteriorly and to the right over a right-sided right ventricle and the pulmonary artery posteriorly and to the left over a left-sided left ventricle. That there is a true transposition in all these cases is confirmed by the presence of a subaortic conus and by the loss of mitral-aortic continuity (Van Praagh, 1971).

Isolated ventricular inversion is the name given to the extremely rare situation where the ventricles are inverted but the great arteries are not transposed. There are probably three cases in the literature (Ratner et al., 1921; Lev and Rowlatt, 1961 [case 10]; Van Praagh and Van Praagh, 1966). In the last case, seen at this hospital, a four-month-old child was diagnosed at angiography as having situs solitus of the viscera and atria, ventricular inversion, and two ventricular septal defects. The aorta arose low and posteriorly from the morphologically left ventricle and the pulmonary artery high and anteriorly from the morphologically right ventricle. At postmortem following pulmonary artery banding, the left ventricle was confirmed as being on the right, but since there was mitral-aortic fibrous continuity with the aorta over the left ventricle, and since the conus was over the left-sided right ventricle under the pulmonary artery, there was no transposition. However, the heart functioned in the mode of complete transposition, as the effect of the atrioventricular discordance was not "corrected" by ventriculo-arterial malalignment as it is in congenitally corrected transposition.

Another very rare condition is *anatomically corrected transposition of the great arteries* (Harris and Farber, 1939). Van Praagh and Van Praagh (1967) described three cases and suggested that this condition may arise when the "loop rule" (Van Praagh et al., 1964) is broken. This rule states that if the aorta is to the right of the pulmonary artery, there is likely to be a ventricular D-loop and so the left ventricle will be on the left; but if the aorta is on the left, there is an L-loop with the left ventricle inverted and so on the right.

In these three cases there was a D-loop and L-transposition in two and an L-loop and D-transposition in one. There was a combined conus, no mitral-aortic continuity, and the aorta arose anterior to the pulmonary valve in all. The first type have both anatomic and physiologic correction since the aorta arose over the left-sided left ventricle, and the pulmonary artery over a right-sided right ventricle. In the second type there is anatomic, but no physiologic correction, since there was ventricular inversion but D-transposition. However, because in all three the great arteries arose above the morphologically appropriate ventricle, this condition should be called "anatomically corrected malposition" since the arteries are not transposed across the ventricular septum (Van Praagh et al., 1971). Recently, Kirklin and associates (1973) described operating on three of these children for ventricular septal defect and pulmonary stenosis. The children all had the first type of malformation, and Kirklin and associates, in the course of defining a surgical classification of the basic cardiac malformations, proposed confining the term "anatomically corrected malposition" to this type, since both the atrioventricular and ventriculoarterial relationships are concordant but the aorta is malposed and on the left; the second type they would term "isolated ventricular inversion with D-transposition of the aorta." Anderson and associates (1975) speak of "concordant" or "discordant" anatomically corrected malposition of the great arteries, which is both clearer and more comprehensive.

There are three results of ventricular inversion in corrected transposition of the great arteries that have considerable clinical importance. The first is that the atrioventricular valve and its valve apparatus goes along with its ventricle; the left atrioventricular valve is therefore tricuspid. Clinically, this valve is incompetent in so many patients with corrected transposition that it has been suggested that left atrioventricular regurgitation should be considered a

basic part of the pathologic entity (Schiebler et al., 1961). An Ebstein's malformation of this left-sided tricuspid valve is found in a proportion of cases (Schiebler et al., 1961; Van Mierop et al., 1961). The fact that the right atrioventricular valve is the bicuspid mitral valve means that the cavity of the venous left ventricle contains the large papillary muscles attached to it, and this makes a surgical approach to a ventricular septal defect (conventionally through the pulmonary or right ventricle) difficult (Figure 34–2).

The second consequence of the ventricular inversion is that the coronary arteries are also inverted (Walmsley, 1931; Cardell, 1956). This means that the anterior descending coronary artery, which usually arises from the left coronary artery and runs down the interventricular sulcus in corrected transposition, arises from the right side (Figure 34–3) and passes over the pulmonary outflow tract to run down the front of the heart. This also poses surgical difficulties.

The third consequence is that the conducting system is inverted (Walmsley, 1931; Lev et al., 1963). The bundle of His has a longer course from the atrioventricular node across the upper part of the ventricular septum than in the normal (Yater et al.,

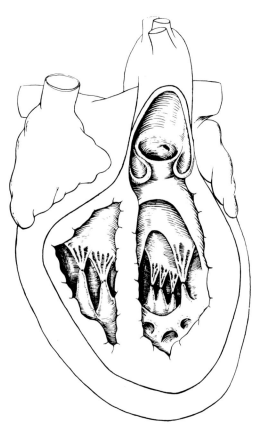

Figure 34-2. The ventricular inversion means that the pulmonary ventricle contains the large papillary muscles associated with the mitral valve.

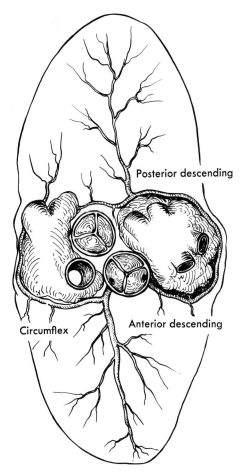

Figure 34-3. Diagram of the course of the coronary arteries, which are inverted in corrected transposition.

1933). The left bundle, with its anterior and posterior radiations, lies on the right side of the septum, while the right bundle branch runs in its normal manner along the septal band to the moderator band, but in the left side of the septum (Figure 34–4). This long course of the bundle of His may well explain why there is a very high incidence of heart block, occurring both spontaneously and as a result of surgery.

Associated Lesions

Only 1 percent of cases with corrected transposition of the great arteries have "normal" hearts. All the rest have valvular stenosis, regurgitation or atresia, intracardiac shunts, or conduction disturbances that upset normal physiology and are either lethal or necessitate palliative or corrective surgery.

Of the 101 cases seen at The Hospital for Sick Children, Toronto, with adequate information for accurate diagnosis of corrected transposition and of the associated anomalies, 96 were of the usual type, with visceroatrial situs solitus, ventricular inversion, and L-transposition of the great arteries. Five cases

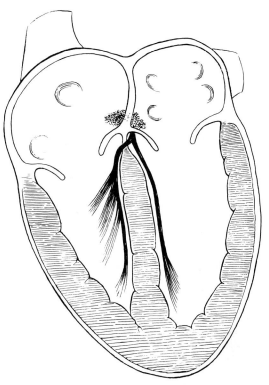

Figure 34-4. Diagram of the conducting system in corrected transposition, which is inverted.

had visceroatrial situs inversus, a D-loop of the ventricles, and D-transposition. The high incidence of positional anomalies of the heart within the chest in corrected transposition has been noted by Loosekoot (1967), and in our series was present in 17 percent: 11 children had dextrocardia and six mesocardia.

Pulmonary stenosis was the most common associated lesion, occurring in 53 percent of the cases. It was present in roughly half of the cases in each subgroup (Figure 34–5) whether they had a ventricular septal defect, a single ventricle, or an intact ventricular septum. The pulmonary stenosis may be valvular or subvalvular with a membranous or fibrous ring (Cardell, 1956; Levy et al., 1963). In our series, the obstruction was valvular in 16 patients, subvalvular in ten, combined in ten, and not specified in nine. Eight patients had pulmonary atresia. Other varieties of pulmonary stenosis have been described including some due to "parachute" or other deformities of the right-sided mitral valve (Todd et al., 1963).

Ventricular septal defect is common among the cases reported and occurred in 44 percent of our group. The defects vary in size, but are usually large (Berry et al., 1964). They generally lie just below the pulmonary valve, but may have a sheet of membranous septum between them and the valve (Scheibler et al., 1961).

Single ventricle was present in 40 percent of our cases. All these cases had the most common variety, a single left ventricle (Van Praagh et al., 1964). There

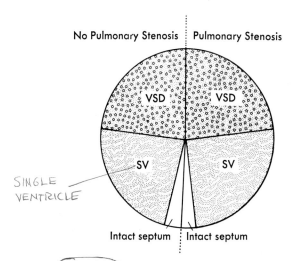

SINGLE VENTRICLE

Figure 34-5. Major associated defects in corrected transposition. (Reproduced from Bjarke, B., and Kidd, B. S. L.: Congenitally corrected transposition of the great arteries. A clinical study of 101 cases. *Acta Paediatr. Scand.*, **65**:153, 1976.)

was a large, morphologically left single ventricle, which gave rise to the transposed pulmonary artery. This ventricle communicated with a rudimentary outflow chamber (the right ventricular infundibulum), which, lying to the left and anteriorly, gave rise to the transposed aorta. Single ventricle was found in 42 percent of the large series of Friedberg and Nadas (1970), and although the cases of single ventricle are not included in the series of two other groups (Schiebler et al., 1961; Ruttenberg et al., 1966), there are good embryologic and semantic reasons for their inclusion.

Only 14 children in our series had an intact ventricular septum, and this is a similar incidence to that in the literature (Table 34–1).

Schiebler and associates (1961) remarked on the high frequency of malformation of the left

atrioventricular valve. The authors reported that the valve was deformed in 11 of their 13 autopsied cases. In seven of these the deformity was of the Ebstein pattern with attachment to varying degrees of the basal part of the septal and posterior cusps to the ventricular wall. There is also usually chordal shortening and malinsertion. In our clinical series, an abnormal left atrioventricular valve was found in 21 percent. This figure, representing only angiographically proven instances, may be slightly low. Friedberg and Nadas (1970) reported 14 of 60 cases had left atrioventricular regurgitation and a further six cases had stenosis or atresia. In 1967 Loosekoot collected 202 cases of corrected transposition from the literature: 70 of these had definite left atrioventricular valve abnormalities, and 20 had an Ebstein's type of malformation.

Other associated lesions have also been reported, and in our series atrial septal defect (12 cases), persistent ductus arteriosus (11 cases), and coarctation of the aorta (six cases) were those most frequently found.

Prevalence

Among 10,535 cases of congenital heart disease diagnosed at The Hospital for Sick Children, there are 101 cases of corrected transposition—an incidence of 0.90 percent. Using an incidence figure for congenital heart disease in the general population of 0.8 percent, this would give an incidence for corrected transposition of 0.0077 percent, or 1 in 13,000 live births. This figure is likely to be an underestimate of the true incidence since it is very likely that a number of patients with corrected transposition are not diagnosed as such, especially those without associated heart malformations. For instance, mild or moderate left atrioventricular valve insufficiency may be diagnosed as being rheumatic in origin, or an

Table 34–1. ASSOCIATED DEFECTS IN 310 CASES OF CORRECTED TRANSPOSITION OF THE GREAT ARTERIES FROM THE LITERATURE

	SINGLE VENTRICLE		VENTRICULAR SEPTAL DEFECT		INTACT SEPTUM		
	Without PS	*With PS*	*Without PS*	*With PS*	*Without PS*	*With PS*	L-AV INCOMP
Anderson et al (1957)	3	0	8	1	2	3	—
Kernan (1958)	0	0	3	0	0	0	1
Schiebler et al. (1961)	—	—	18	6	7	2	11
Lev and Rowlett (1961)	—	—	2	3	3	0	7
Ellis et al. (1962)	0	2	13	11	4	0	6
Honey (1963)	2	0	3	3	2	0	2
Berry et al. (1964)	1	0	6	4	2	0	6
Ruttenberg et al. (1966)	—	—	15	18	2	3	—
Friedberg and Nadas (1970)	12	13	18	13	3	1	14
Bjarke and Kidd (1976)	21	19	20	24	7	7	21
	39	34	106	83	32	16	68

isolated congenital lesion, while conduction disturbances may be ascribed to other causes.

There was a male sex preponderance, with a male to female ratio of 1.35:1.

In this series there were 237 siblings of the 101 propositi. Six of these had congenital heart disease, all in three families. Two siblings had complete or D-transposition of the great arteries, two had ventricular septal defects, and two were "blue babies." Mitchell (1971) has described an apparent association between maternal diabetes and transposition, and of this series four children had diabetic mothers, and two had diabetic fathers.

Clinical Features

The presentation and clinical course of children with corrected transposition are largely determined by the associated defects. There are thus three clinical groupings. First, the left-to-right shunt group will include all those children with ventricular septal defect or single ventricle without significant obstruction to pulmonary blood flow. Cyanosis will be the prominent feature in the second clinical group, with right-to-left shunting and a reduction in pulmonary blood flow due to pulmonary stenosis. The third and smallest clinical group are those with an intact ventricular septum. They will have either the murmur of left atrioventricular valve incompetence or an arrhythmia; rarely no abnormalities may be detected.

The age at presentation of 101 cases at our cardiac center is illustrated in Figure 34–6. Most cases presented in infancy with only 18 appearing after the first birthday. Within the first year, 48 percent were referred in the first three months and 35 percent from three months to one year. Those with no pulmonary obstruction presented earlier than those with pulmonary stenosis. The cardinal presenting signs were murmurs in 46 percent of our cases, cyanosis in 59 percent, heart failure in 11 percent, and failure to thrive in 6 percent (Figure 34–7). In only two children was an arrhythmia alone the reason for referral.

In the patients without obstruction to pulmonary blood flow, the histories were of breathlessness, fatigue, failure to thrive, frequent chest infections, and congestive heart failure. Eight out of nine similar patients described by Shem-Tov and associates (1970) were also mildly cyanosed. On the other hand, cyanosis was prominent and present from birth in those children with significant obstruction to pulmonary blood flow. Cyanotic spells can occur. Growth retardation and dyspnea were also common. In our series of 101 cases, 54 percent were or became cyanosed, and 25 percent were in congestive heart failure at some point.

The physical findings in these two groups are again those dictated by the associated lesions. The large left-to-right shunt group have a hyperdynamic precordium with a precordial bulge and cardiac enlargement, while in those cases with pulmonary stenosis the heart is quieter. There are three auscultatory points of some interest due to the positions of the cardiac chambers. First, the murmur of left atrioventricular valve incompetence is often maximal in the fourth interspace near the sternum rather than at the apex. This is due to the fact that the two ventricles lie side by side in corrected transposition, with the ventricular septum in the sagittal plane rather than in the left anterior oblique plane; the murmur is conducted to the chest wall medial to the apex. This murmur may, therefore, mask or be confused with the typical pansystolic murmur of a ventricular septal defect.

Second, the murmur of pulmonary stenosis, though often heard well in the pulmonary area, may

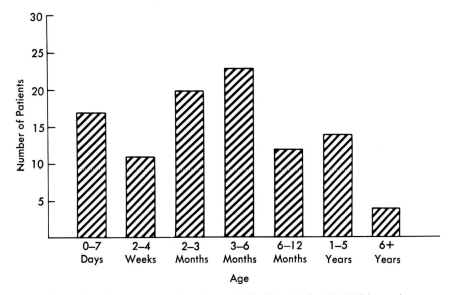

Figure 34-6. Age at presentation of cases in The Hospital for Sick Children series.

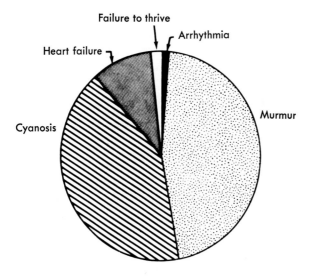

Figure 34-7. Major presenting sign or symptom in The Hospital for Sick Children series.

be maximal lower down on the left side (Anderson et al., 1957) or indeed may be louder in the aortic area. This is because the pulmonary valve is displaced posteriorly and inferiorly in this condition. A right parasternal systolic ejection murmur may give rise to the erroneous diagnosis of aortic stenosis rather than pulmonary stenosis (Honey, 1963).

The third auscultatory anomaly that has been described in corrected transposition is a single, loud, and often palpable, second heart sound to the left of the sternum (Gasul et al., 1959). This sound arises from the aortic valve, which lies anteriorly, close to the chest wall. It may be necessary to auscultate more rightward to hear the contribution of the distant pulmonary valve. This physical finding may, if misinterpreted, suggest the diagnosis of pulmonary hypertension (Caulfield et al., 1967).

However, we, as well as Honey (1963) and Friedberg and Nadas (1970), have found this last sign less constant than has been suggested. The quality of the second sound was noted in 87 of our cases and in only 47 (53 percent) was it called "single." Thirty-seven of these patients had pulmonary stenosis. Thus 70 percent of the cases with pulmonary stenosis had a single second sound, and 21 percent of those without. Sixty percent of cases where it was noted were considered to have a second sound of normal intensity.

Kraus and associates (1969) reported that in 10 of 13 patients with corrected transposition in which both right and left precordial pulsations could be recorded, the right-sided ventricle contracted before the left-sided ventricle. This is the opposite of the normal situation, where the electromechanical intervals over the left ventricle are shorter than those over the right. This physical sign is due to inversion of the ventricles and their conducting systems.

The high incidence of dysrhythmias in corrected transposition has been noted by many workers (Cardell, 1956; Anderson et al., 1957; Schiebler et al., 1961; Berry et al., 1964; Rotem et al., 1965), and the abnormal inverted course of the conducting system has been held responsible for this. About 8 to 20 percent of patients will have bradycardia due to complete heart block (Bjarke and Kidd, 1976; Friedberg and Nadas, 1970; Schiebler et al., 1961). A further analysis of the conduction disturbances in this condition is found in the Electrocardiography section.

Radiologic Examination

Abnormalities in the chest x-ray plain film may point to the diagnosis of corrected transposition of the great arteries even when no hint has been picked up on routine physical examination. However, it would be unwise to rely on this too heavily, since, particularly in cases with minimal or no associated anomalies, the chest radiograph can be entirely normal.

The three basic abnormal findings are:

1. The presence of a gently sloping ascending aortic shadow in the upper left cardiac silhouette.

2. The absence of any main pulmonary artery shadow when the physical findings suggest a large left-to-right shunt.

3. Positional anomalies such as dextrocardia with situs solitus, mesocardia, or levocardia with situs inversus.

While the disordered anatomy is central to the radiographic findings, the associated malformations again play a large part in molding the final result. Thus, if there is a closed ventricular septum, there is often only mild cardiac enlargement or none at all (Figure 34–8). If, however, left atrioventricular valve regurgitation becomes more marked, left atrial and systemic ventricular enlargement will result and some pulmonary venous engorgement (Schiebler et al., 1961) (Figure 34–9). The finding of Kerley's B lines helps to confirm this cause of pulmonary engorgement (Honey, 1963).

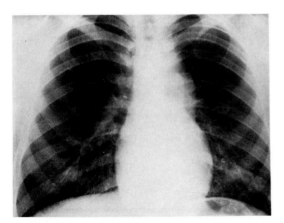

Figure 34-8. Straight x-ray in a case of corrected transposition with a prominent left-sided ascending aorta.

When there is large left-to-right shunting (as with ventricular septal defect or single ventricle without pulmonary stenosis), there is often considerable cardiomegaly and pulmonary plethora. However, because of the narrow, more anteroposterior aortic arching, the vascular pedicle at the base of the heart may remain narrow (Honey, 1961; Becu et al., 1955; Lester et al., 1960; Beck et al., 1961) in this way resembling complete or D-transposition of the great arteries. Of significance, however, is the non-appearance of the large main or left pulmonary artery, which one would expect with a large left-to-right shunt (Anderson et al., 1957). So, when the clinical diagnosis of ventricular septal defect or similar lesion with large pulmonary blood flow and pulmonary hypertension is made, and the pulmonary artery shadow is not prominent, corrected transposition should spring to mind.

In some cases the medially placed main pulmonary artery may compress the barium-filled esophagus posteriorly (Anderson et al., 1957; Lester et al., 1960; Schiebler et al., 1961) although this is not consistent (Shem-Tov et al., 1971). The right pulmonary artery emerges high and has a "waterfall" appearance. Ellis and associates (1962) and Carey and Ruttenberg (1964) report that in one-half of their cases with this unobstructed variety of corrected transposition, they could not note any prominence of the upper left cardiovascular silhouette due to the ascending aorta. This is presumably due to the smaller aorta when the left-to-right shunt is large.

When there is a right-to-left shunt, as in the cases with an associated ventricular septal defect and pulmonary stenosis, the pulmonary blood flow is reduced, so that the heart size is often normal and the lung fields oligemic. In these cases the aorta is large and frequently visible as a convex, or at least straight, opacity running on a slope up to the usual position of the aortic knuckle (Anderson et al., 1957; Lester et al., 1960; Ellis et al., 1962). This is very characteristic of this condition, although such structures as an

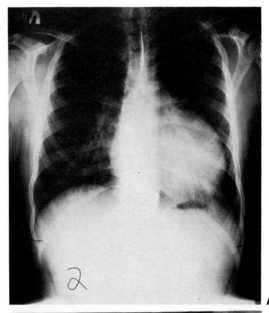

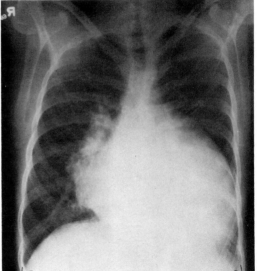

Figure 34-9. *A* and *B*. Progressive enlargement of the heart at a four-year interval in a boy with corrected transposition and increasing left atrioventricular valve regurgitation.

enlarged thymus, anomalous veins, and a right aortic arch may simulate it (Ellis et al., 1962).

When there are positional anomalies, the suspicion of corrected transposition should be kept in mind. In dextrocardia with situs inversus, a D-bulbo-ventricular loop, giving ventricular inversion, and D-transposition, the situation is exactly the "mirror image" of the situs solitus, L-loop and L-transposition. The prominent ascending aorta will be to the right. When, however, there is dextrocardia with situs solitus, and an L-loop giving ventricular inversion, and L-transposition, while the ventricles may be in the right chest, the ascending aorta will be at the left upper cardiac shadow.

Echocardiography

The abnormal anteroposterior plane of the ventricular septum in this condition makes it difficult to record echocardiographically. Those patients with a ventricular septal defect may therefore resemble single ventricle (Meyer and Kaplan, 1973) both clinically and echocardiographically. The anterior root (aorta) is found to the left of the posterior root (pulmonary artery). Systolic time intervals must therefore be used to determine the identity of the vessels (Solinger et al., 1974; Hirschfeld et al., 1975). Pulmonary-mitral continuity can be demonstrated (Meyer et al., 1974). Abnormalities of the systemic (tricuspid) valve may be recorded.

Electrocardiography

Just as the plain chest film can alert the clinician to the possibility of corrected transposition, so, too, the electrocardiogram can be helpful in this regard. While there are two major characteristics "typical" of corrected transposition, here again their presence and their recognition are affected by the associated malformations.

The two features are (1) a very frequent occurrence of arrhythmias and (2) the abnormal direction of the initial phases of ventricular depolarization. These are both probably due to the disordered anatomy of the conducting system as described in 1931 by Walmsley and later by Yater (1933) and Lev and associates (1963). The atrioventricular node lies above and to the left of the central fibrous body that joins the mitral and tricuspid valves; from there the bundle of His passes downward and to the left eventually emerging on the right (left ventricular) side at the summit of the ventricular septum. Here it travels beneath the pars membranacea and then gives off the right bundle on the left side, which passes down along its usual course to the moderator band. On the right side of the septum the bundle gives off anterior and posterior fascicles, which spread over the right-sided left ventricle. Walmsley (1931) states in a footnote to his paper that fibrosis of the main stem associated with its longer course through the fibrous tissue at the base of the ventricles was the cause of heart block in the case he described—a 35-year-old man who had a heart rate of 40 per minute for ten years.

As noted above, conduction abnormalities are frequent, and complete heart block (Anderson et al., 1957; Schiebler et al., 1961), partial heart block (Cumming, 1962; Rotem and Hultgren, 1965; Cardell, 1956; Walker et al., 1958), Wolff-Parkinson-White syndrome (Schiebler et al., 1961), and atrial dysrhythmias (Honey, 1963) have been described. In our series, 17 patients had atrioventricular block of varying degrees (Table 34–2). Eight of them had

complete heart block—in five it was complete when the child was first seen, and the remaining three had long P-R intervals or 2:1 block preceding the onset of complete heart block. Three cases of paroxysmal tachycardia occurred; three patients had Wolff-Parkinson-White syndrome, first-degree heart block, and a normal ECG between attacks, respectively.

Table 34–2. INCIDENCE OF CONDUCTION ABNORMALITIES IN 101 HOSPITAL FOR SICK CHILDREN CASES

AV block	
1°	7
2°	2
3°	8
AV dissociation	1
Junctional dysrhythmias	
Nodal rhythm	1
Wandering pacemaker	3
Paroxysmal tachycardia	3
Atrial fibrillation-flutter	3
Ventricular extrasystoles	2
Supraventricular extrasystoles	2

We were unable to find any correlation between the presence, duration, and type of arrhythmias and any of the associated cardiac lesions. Two of our cases had complete heart block diagnosed in utero, and in some cases in the literature, onset has been late (Walmsley, 1931). These findings are similar to those of Anderson and associates (1957), Berry and associates (1964), and Schiebler and associates (1961). Friedberg and Nadas (1970) recently reported that 17 percent of their series had first-degree atrioventricular block, 3 percent had second degree, and 12 percent complete heart block, a slightly higher incidence than we found.

The second important and remarkable electrocardiographic finding in corrected transposition of the great arteries is the abnormal direction of the initial ventricular depolarization. Normally, with a normal bundle of His and without ventricular inversion, the initial depolarization is of the ventricular septum, proceeding from left to right. This sequence of depolarization accounts for the Q waves seen in the left precordial leads of the standard electrocardiogram. In corrected transposition, however (as was first pointed out by Anderson and associates in 1957), the initial depolarization of the septum proceeds in the opposite direction—from right to left. This results in Q waves in the right precordial chest leads, and no Q waves over the left chest (Figure 34–10).

Ruttenberg and associates (1966) published an excellent review of both electrocardiograms and vectorcardiograms in 30 cases of corrected transposition with the cardiac apex on the correct side; for, as might be expected, when there is dextrocardia or other positional anomaly, the electrocardiogram varies widely. However, in this restricted series there

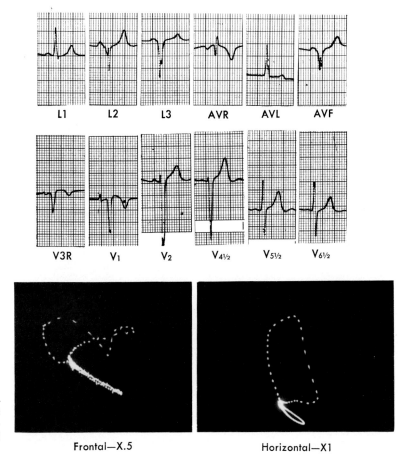

Figure 34-10. Electrocardiogram and vectorcardiogram in a child with corrected transposition. Note the abnormal initial electrical focus.

Frontal—X.5   Horizontal—X1

were no Q waves over the left chest in any instance. This was true whether there was pulmonary stenosis or a considerable left-to-right shunt. The vector loop had a straight efferent limb but moved anteriorly and superiorly in most cases. Ellison and Restieux (1972) reported that in 22 cases an anterior leftward direction to the initial vector was present whether there was right or left ventricular hypertrophy. Shem-Tov and associates (1971) noted that the Q wave rule in corrected transposition did not hold in cases where there is right atrioventricular valve atresia or a persistent atrioventricular canal.

Patients with large left-to-right shunts tend to show "left" ventricular hypertrophy (tall R waves in V_6) or combined ventricular hypertrophy, with large RS complexes in the midprecordium, and tall R waves in V_1 or V_4R and V_6 (Ruttenberg et al., 1966). Where there was pulmonary stenosis, tall R waves in V_1 or V_4R indicating "right" ventricular hypertrophy were more common. Shem-Tov and associates (1971) reported that the main QRS axis in the frontal plane was less than $+100°$ in the cases without obstruction to pulmonary blood flow, but more than $+100°$ when pulmonary stenosis was present.

Ellison and Restieux (1972) found the left maximal spatial voltage useful in assessing severity of left atrioventricular valve regurgitation and the right maximal spatial voltage in assessing the severity of pulmonary stenosis.

It is clear, therefore, that, used intelligently, the electrocardiogram can be of considerable value not only in diagnosing corrected transposition, but in assessing the severity of the associated lesions. Where there are positional anomalies, however (although Shem-Tov and associates in 1971 found the electrocardiogram useful in diagnosing atrial situs), it is very difficult to be sure of the ventricular position using the electrocardiogram alone.

Hemodynamics

Although, as indicated above, the diagnosis of corrected transposition may be suspected on clinical grounds, and the suspicion may be strongly supported on the basis of the x-ray and the electrocardiogram, the cornerstone of diagnosis is cardiac catheterization and good clear angiograms.

When the ventricular septum is intact, the pressures and saturations throughout the right heart may be normal; however, the first catheterization confirmation of the diagnosis is when the catheter tip (usually with considerable difficulty and much maneuvering) passes from the ventricle into the pulmonary artery and is found to lie in a much more medial position than usual. If there is significant left atrioventricular valve regurgitation, the pulmonary capillary wedge pressure may be elevated, with tall V waves and a sharp Y descent.

Since, however, 85 to 90 percent of cases have either a ventricular septal defect or a single ventricle, there is usually a large step-up in oxygen saturation as soon as the ventricle is entered. The pressures in the pulmonary artery and venous ventricles are also usually elevated often to systemic outflow levels, and it is important to obtain good wedge and pulmonary artery pressures, as calculation of total and arteriolar pulmonary vascular resistances will play a large part in determining the feasibility of corrective surgery.

When there is a low pulmonary artery pressure, the pulmonary stenosis may be either valvular or subvalvular. It may be possible to enter the aorta through a ventricular septal defect, which will then be found to lie over the upper left cardiac border.

When there is a single ventricle present, there may be considerable fluctuation in oxygen saturation in the ventricular cavity with only small movements of the catheter tip, as streaming occurs. It may be difficult to advance the catheter tip through the bulboventricular foramen into the small right ventricular outflow chamber and into the aorta. In 7 percent of Friedberg and Nadas's cases there was obstruction to aortic outflow ("subaortic stenosis") at the site of this communication.

The left ventricle and left atrium, entered either across the atrial septum or retrogradely from the aorta, are usually at full saturation. If the left atrioventricular valve regurgitation is severe, the left ventricular end-diastolic and left atrial pressures may be elevated. The left atrial pressure pulse may show v waves as high as 30 mm of mercury.

A hazard of cardiac catheterization is the occurrence of arrhythmias. In 42 of the 142 catheterizations carried out on patients with corrected transposition in our laboratories, the operator reported more arrhythmias than he would usually encounter. Only seven, however, needed treatment: five cases of supraventricular tachycardia, one case of atrial flutter, and a fatal case of ventricular tachycardia in a seven-month-old baby in 1959.

Angiocardiography

This technique provides the definitive answer in cases of corrected transposition, outlining the ventricles and great arteries, and demonstrating their positions and relationships.

In corrected transposition, the ventricles tend to lie side by side, with the septum in the sagittal plane rather than the right anterior–left posterior relationship of the normal oblique septum. An injection into the right-sided ventricle will show it to have the characteristics of a left ventricle, in that it is smooth-walled and has a broad waist and narrow tail, like a plump carrot (Figure 34–11*A*). From it, the contrast

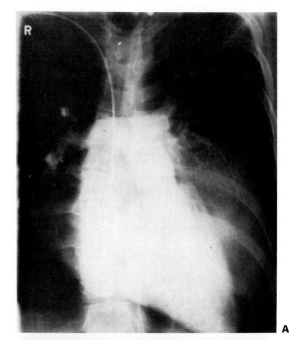

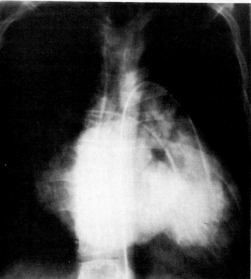

Figure 34-11. *A.* An injection in the right-sided left ventricle of the boy whose chest radiographs are shown in Figure 34-9. Note the medial position of the pulmonary artery. *B.* Injection into the left-sided right ventricle. This child had gross left atrioventricular valve incompetence, and the dye outlines the giant left atrium as well as the aorta.

will outline a main pulmonary artery that lies centrally in the chest over the spine, much more medially than usual. In the lateral view the ventricle comes out to the anterior chest wall. Its outflow tract, however, is seen to incline backward, and the pulmonary valve is low and posterior.

Injection into the systemic arterial left-sided right ventricle shows it to be lying beside the left ventricle in the anteroposterior projection. It is usually more spherical and shows the trabeculations typical of a right ventricle. The aortic valve is high on the left side, and the ascending aorta forms an opacity that runs upwards forming the upper left cardiovascular shadow. It arches back and descends on the same side of the spine, giving a very narrow appearance of the aortic arch in this view. The lateral projection shows this ventricle to overlie the other ventricle. However, its outflow tract shows a subaortic conus and passes anteriorly, giving rise to the aortic valve and aorta high and to the front (Figure 34–12).

With dextrocardia and situs solitus the appearances are very similar to those described, but with the ventricles more in the right chest; the aorta continues to form the upper left cardiac border. With situs inversus, a D-loop, and D-transposition, the situation is the "mirror image" of the solitus.

The associated lesions will, of course, be visible in the angiograms; pulmonary stenosis will often be clearly seen and the level of the narrowing noted (Figure 34–13). The size of the ventricular septal defect can be seen following injection into the ventricle that is giving the predominant shunt, either right-to-left or left-to-right. The severity of the left atrioventricular valve incompetence is assessed by injection into the arterial ventricle (Figure 34–11*B*).

To determine whether single ventricle is present or not, rapid injection of a bolus of dye into the ventricle is necessary. It will usually show the typical picture of a large single left ventricle that gives rise to the pulmonary artery, lying medially and posteriorly, and may or may not show pulmonary stenosis. The contrast also passes through a defect, the bulboventricular foramen, situated to the left and anteriorly into a chamber that is the right ventricular infundibulum in an inverted position. This chamber is always small, but may be very small and restrictive, causing a pressure gradient between the main ventricle and the aorta. It forms a small wedge-shaped chamber that lies anteriorly, superiorly, and to the left and gives rise to a high, anterior, and leftward aortic valve.

To be sure that it is a single ventricle, injections into the ventricle reached through both the right and left atrioventricular valves are often necessary. Accurate definition of the outflow chamber may require injection through a retrograde aortic catheter with the tip just below the aortic valve.

The abnormal inverted coronary artery anatomy may be distinguished on ventricular or aortic injection.

Diagnosis

The diagnosis of corrected transposition of the great arteries is often difficult and depends in the final analysis on good angiograms.

In children with large left-to-right shunts presenting with breathlessness and heart failure, the murmurs and heart sounds may not be helpful. The x-ray may or may not show the aortic shadow at the upper left cardiovascular silhouette; but, on the other hand, will *not* show a large pulmonary artery. The presence of Q waves in the right chest and their absence on the left may be the best precatheterization aid to diagnosis.

Children with a right-to-left shunt and pulmonary stenosis tend to simulate tetralogy of Fallot. However, the prominent aortic shadow on the upper left in these cases, together with the electrocardiographic signs, will suggest corrected transposition.

The presence of a ventricular septum, the point of differentiation between those cases with a ventricular septal defect and those with single ventricle, must be demonstrated by angiogram. Isolated mitral regurgitation presents a diagnostic problem, especially in an older patient, and although the presence of conduction disturbances, the x-ray, and the electrocardiogram may be helpful, cardiac catheterization may be required to make the diagnosis.

Finally, there are an unknown number of patients with "normal" hearts and no associated malformation. Here again the diagnosis is angiographic.

It is also worth noting that there is a high incidence of corrected transposition when the heart is in an abnormal position. So when there is situs solitus and dextrocardia, or situs inversus and levocardia (that is, when the position of the heart does not match the situs), a discordant ventricular loop should be suspected. Although isolated ventricular discordance

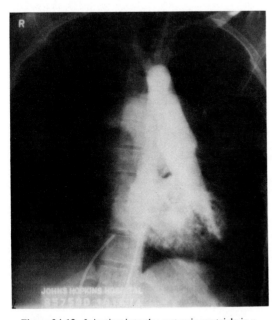

Figure 34-12. Injection into the systemic ventricle in a case of corrected transposition and a ventricular septal defect. Note the subaortic conus, the high aortic valve, the course of the ascending aorta on the upper left cardiac border, and the faint filling of the medially placed pulmonary artery.

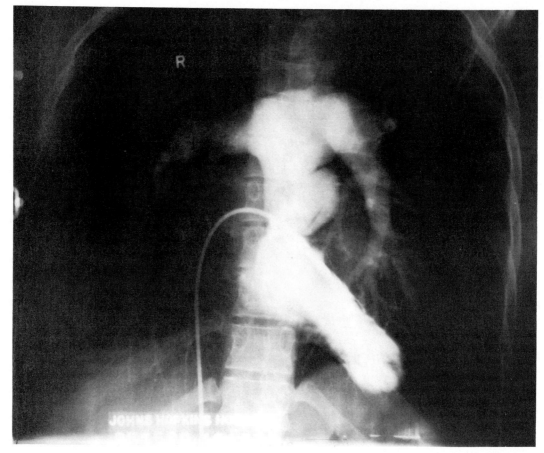

Figure 34-13. Injection into the right-sided left ventricle: a child with corrected transposition, no ventricular septal defect, and pulmonary stenosis.

does occur, corrected transposition is much more common in this situation.

Prognosis

Prognosis is extremely varied in corrected transposition and depends largely on the associated malformations. Cases with severe hemodynamic disturbances such as ventricular septal defect or single ventricle, or with severe pulmonary stenosis, may not survive infancy without palliative surgery. On the other hand, patients with mild left atrioventricular incompetence or "normal" hearts may have no circulatory disturbances for many years. Often it is a conduction disturbance that brings them to the notice of a physician.

In our series of 101 cases, the follow-up ranges from one month to 26 years with a mean of 6.7 years. The mean age of the survivors is 9.8 years (four months to 27 years). Twenty-five patients have died, but most of the deaths (18) occurred before the age of one year. Four of the seven later deaths were surgical. While no patient with an intact ventricular septum has died in this series, of those with a ventricular septal defect or single ventricle, 10 of 46 (22 percent) with pulmonary stenosis and 15 of 41 (37 percent) without have died. Friedberg and Nadas (1970) in a similar series found 16 deaths out of 60 (27 percent). However, only 31 percent of their deaths were in the first year of life.

In our series, heart failure was felt to be the major contributory factor in most of the deaths (Table 34-3).

Table 34-3. DEATH IN CONGENITAL CORRECTED TRANSPOSITION OF THE GREAT ARTERIES

MAJOR FACTOR	UNDER 1 YEAR	OVER 1 YEAR
Heart failure	10	1
Hypoxia	3	1
	(+CHF in 2)	(+CHF in 3)
	(+hypoxia in 2)	(+hypoxia in 1)
Surgery	4	4
	Hypoxia 2	Hypoxia 1
Catheterization	1	0
Total	18	7
Associated with arrhythmias	3	4

The patients who are alive are well and carrying on fairly normal lives, with some limitations of exercise tolerance. How long this will continue is impossible to say until longer follow-up is available. Progressive pulmonary vascular disease has been reported in a small proportion of cases by Friedberg and Nadas (1970). The long-term view depends on two factors:

1. Will conduction disturbances develop in many of these patients with time?
2. How will the left-sided right ventricle support the systemic circulation over many years?

Corrected transposition is in one sense a natural experiment that, from the ventricular viewpoint, models closely the end result of total correction of complete or D-transposition of the great arteries by the Mustard procedure. In both these situations a ventricle not "ideally suited" to the development of high intraventricular pressure (Rushmer, 1970) is called upon to support a normal cardiac output at systemic pressure for a normal lifetime.

The papers of Cumming (1962) and Rotem and Hultgren (1965) reviewing corrected transposition without associated anomalies suggest that these patients may have a normal life-span, but with some impairment of cardiac function. Heart block may occur suddenly after the age of 20 and be life-threatening; however, today pacemakers and valve replacement may improve the outlook in these cases. Nagle and associates (1971) and Dodek and Neill (1972) have reported cases of 45-and 60-year-old men with angina and congestive heart failure due to this lesion. Benchimol and Sundararajan (1971) suggest that although the oldest recorded patient was 73 years of age (Lieberson et al., 1969), a normal life-span is unlikely though theoretically possible.

Only time and further follow-up will provide the answers to these questions.

Treatment

Medical treatment in corrected transposition is really confined to the management of congestive heart failure, usually arising from large left-to-right shunts in infancy. Conventional therapy with digoxin and diuretics will help in the initial attack. However, the improvement may not be lasting, and recourse to surgery will become necessary.

Palliation of this situation consists largely of pulmonary artery banding; this reduces pulmonary blood flow and lowers the pressure in the peripheral pulmonary arteries. This will probably be the definitive treatment for those children with single ventricle and unobstructed pulmonary circulation. However, when there is a ventricular septal defect, corrective surgery is feasible. The risks of this have been previously discussed. The coronary arteries limit the ventriculotomy, the presence of large muscle bundles in the right-sided ventricle interferes with access, and the long course of the bundle of His makes heart block a fairly frequent postoperative complication (Anderson et al., 1957; El-Sayed et al.,

1962). All these factors tend to place the operative mortality rate around 40 percent (El-Sayed et al., 1962; Hallman et al., 1967; Friedberg and Nadas, 1962; Kidd and Bjarke, 1976). Of our eight cases operated on through a right-sided transventricular approach, four died: one with a myocardial infarct, two with arrhythmias, and one because he had an unexpected single ventricle. Of the four survivors, three have first-degree heart block and one, junctional rhythm. All have bundle branch block patterns.

Approach via the venous atrium does avoid the coronary arteries, but access to the ventricular septal defect or pulmonary valve is difficult and one of the mitral cusps has to be removed to allow a reasonable view. In one of our cases this resulted in residual valve incompetence.

For many of these reasons, access to the ventricular septum through a left-sided ventriculotomy has appeal, and this has been utilized with encouraging results (Berry et al., 1964; Kay et al., 1965; Hallman et al., 1967; Kidd et al., 1972).

For the cyanotic patients, if cyanosis is severe or spells are occurring, palliation is by a systemic-pulmonary anastomosis. We have found this necessary in 25 of 46 children with single ventricle or ventricular septal defect and pulmonary stenosis. Seventeen of these were Blalock-Taussig anastomoses, and eight were Pott's anastomoses. These last include one surgical death and two late deaths. One Glenn caval-pulmonary artery anastomosis has been carried out.

Correction is theoretically possible for those patients with a ventricular septal defect and pulmonary stenosis. The obstruction may be confined to the valve, but there is often subvalve obstruction as well (Friedberg and Nadas, 1970; Bjarke and Kidd, 1976). Access to this area is very difficult with a right-sided ventriculotomy or through the right atrium, as well as through a left-sided ventriculotomy.

Progress in the surgical management of single ventricle (see Chapter 23) has brought the possibility of surgical correction for cases of corrected transposition and single ventricle. McGoon et al. (1976) have recently reported that this subgroup of single ventricle, those with L-transposition and an outflow chamber, have better results than others at the time of surgery. Since this surgery is best carried out at a later age (over three years at least), palliation in infancy will certainly be required as a first step.

Isolated left atrioventricular valve incompetence can be treated by valve replacement (King et al., 1964; Puyau et al., 1964). Haiderer and associates (1971) recommended left atrial approach to this area.

Complete heart block may require insertion of a pacemaker.

Thus, surgery in these patients is directed at the associated life-threatening lesions and is very risky. The ideal course to follow with any particular child with this anomaly is therefore ill-defined, and recommendations for long-term management will only emerge as the natural history of this condition and of the patients treated medically and surgically becomes clear.

REFERENCES

Anderson, R. C.; Lillehei, C. W.; and Lester, R. G.: Corrected transposition of the great vessels of the heart: A review of 17 cases. *Pediatrics*, **20**:626, 1957.

Anderson, R. H.; Becker, A. E.; Loosekoot, T. G.; and Gerlis, L. M.: Anatomically corrected malposition of the great arteries. *Br. Heart J.*, **37**:993, 1975.

Becu, L. M.; Swan, H. J. C.; DuShane, J. W.; and Edwards, J. E.: Ebstein malformation of the left atrioventricular valve in corrected transposition of the great vessels with ventricular septal defect. *Proc. Mayo Clin.*, **30**:483, 1955.

Benchimol, A.; Tio, S.; and Sundararajan, V.: Congenital corrected transposition of the great vessels in a 58-year-old man. *Chest*, **59**:634, 1971.

Berry, B. W.; Roberts, W. C.; Morrow, A. G.; and Braunwald, E.: Corrected transposition of the aorta and pulmonary trunk. *Am. J. Med.*, **36**:35, 1964.

Bjarke, B. B., and Kidd, B. S. L.: Congenitally corrected transposition of the great arteries. A clinical study of 101 cases. *Acta Paediatr. Scand.*, **65**:153, 1976.

Cardell, B. S.: Corrected transposition of the great vessels. *Br. Heart J.*, **18**:186, 1956.

Carey, L. S., and Ruttenberg, H. D.: Roentgenographic features of congenital corrected transposition of the great vessels. A comparative study of 33 cases with a roentgenographic classification based on the associated malformations and hemodynamic states. *Am. J. Roentgenol.*, **92**:623, 1964.

Caulfield, W. H.; Bostock, B.; and Perloff, J. K.: Corrected transposition of the great vessels with isolated pulmonic stenosis: The paradox of pulmonic stenosis with physical signs of pulmonary hypertension. *Am. J. Cardiol.*, **19**:285, 1967.

Cumming, G. R.: Congenital corrected transposition of the great vessels without associated intracardiac anomalies. A clinical, hemodynamic and angiographic study. *Am. J. Cardiol.*, **10**:605, 1962.

De La Cruz, M. U.; Anselmi, G.; Cisneros, F.; Reinhold, M.; Portillo, B.; and Espino-Vela, J.: An embryological explanation for the corrected transportation of the great vessels. *Am. Heart J.*, **57**:104, 1959.

Dodek, T. P.; Cheitlin, M. D.; and McCarty, R. J.: Corrected transposition of the great arteries masquerading as coronary artery disease. *Am. J. Cardiol.*, **30**:910, 1972.

Ellis, K.; Morgan, B. C.; Blumenthal, S.; and Andersen, D. H.: Congenitally corrected transposition of the great vessels. *Radiology*, **79**:35, 1962.

Ellison, R. C., and Restieux, N. J.: *Vectorcardiography in Congenital Heart Disease*. W. B. Saunders, Philadelphia, 1972, p. 146.

El-Sayed, H., et al.: Corrected transposition of the great vessels: Surgical repair of associated defects. *J. Thorac. Cardiovasc. Surg.*, **44**:443, 1962.

Friedberg, D. Z., and Nadas, A. S.: Clinical profile of patients with congenital corrected transposition of the great arteries. *N. Engl. J. Med.*, **282**:19, 1970.

Gasul, B. M.; Graettinger, J. S.; and Bucheleres, G.: Corrected transposition of the great vessels: Demonstration of a new phonocardiographic sign of this malformation. *J. Pediatr.*, **55**:180, 1959.

Haiderer, O.; Bahler, R.; Carson, P.; and Kennedy, J. H.: Congenital corrected transposition of the great vessels. Surgical treatment of associated incompetence of the systemic atrioventricular valve. *J. Thorac. Cardiovasc. Surg.*, **61**:933, 1971.

Hallman, G. L.; Gill, S. F.; and Bloodwell, R. D.: Surgical treatment of cardiac defects associated with corrected transposition of the great vessels. *Circulation* (Suppl. I) **35, 36**:133, 1967.

Harris, J. S., and Farber, S.: Transposition of the great cardiac vessels with special reference to the phylogenetic theory of Spitzer. *Arch. Pathol.*, **28**:427, 1939.

Hirschfeld, S.; Meyer, R.; Schwartz, D. C.; Korfhagen, J.; and Kaplan, S.: Measurement of right and left systolic time intervals by echocardiography. *Circulation*, **51**:304, 1975.

Honey, M.: The diagnosis of corrected transposition of the great vessels. *Br. Heart J.*, **25**:313, 1963.

King, H.; Kilman, J. W.; Petry, E. L.; and Shumacker, H., Jr.: Surgical correction of "mitral" incompetence in corrected transposition of the great vessels. *J. Thorac. Cardiovasc. Surg.*, **47**:769, 1964.

Kirklin, J. W.; Pacifico, A. D.; Bargeron, L. M., Jr.; and Soto, B.: Cardiac repair in anatomically corrected malposition of the great arteries. *Circulation*, **48**:153, 1973. Kraus, Y.; Yahini, J. H.; Shem-Tov, A.; and Neufeld, H. N.: Precordial pulsations in corrected transposition of the great vessels. Diagnostic value of the electro-mechanical interval. *Am. J. Cardiol.*, **23**:684, 1969.

Lester, G. R.; Andersen, R. C.; Amplatz, K.; and Adams, P.: Roentgenologic diagnosis of congenitally corrected transposition of the great vessels. *Am. J. Roentgenol.*, **83**:985, 1960.

Lev, M.: Pathologic diagnosis of positional variations in cardiac chambers in congenital heart disease. *Lab. Invest.*, **3**:71, 1954.

Lev, M.: The pathologic anatomy of cardiac complexes associated with transposition of arterial trunks. *Lab. Invest.*, **2**:296, 1953.

Lev, M.; Licata, R. H.; and May, R. C.: The conduction system in mixed levocardia with ventricular inversion (corrected transposition). *Circulation*, **28**:323, 1963.

Lev, M., and Rowlatt, U. F.: The pathologic anatomy of mixed levocardia. A review of 13 cases of atrial or ventricular inversion with or without corrected transposition. *Am. J. Cardiol.*, **8**:263, 1961.

Levy, M. J.; Lillehei, C. W.; Elliott, L. P.; Carey, L. S.; Adams, P., Jr.; and Edwards, J. E.: Accessor valvular tissue causing subpulmonary stenosis in corrected transposition of great vessels. *Circulation*, **27**:494, 1963.

Lieberson, A. D.; Schumacker, R.; Childress, R. H.; and Genovese, P. D.: Corrected transposition of the great vessels in a 73 year old man. *Circulation*, **39**:96, 1969.

Loosekoot, G.: *Gecorrideerde Transposities*. Thesis, Scheltema and Holkema, Amsterdam, 1967.

Meyer, R. A., and Kaplan, S.: Noninvasive techniques in pediatric cardiovascular disease. *Prog. Cardiovasc. Dis.*, **15**:341, 1973.

Meyer, R. A.; Schwartz, D. C.; Covitz, W.; and Kaplan, S.: Echocardiographic assessment of cardiac malposition. *Am. J. Cardiol.*, **33**:896, 1974.

McGoon, D. C.; Marcelletti, C.; Danielson, G. K.; Wallace, R. B.; Ritter, D. G.; and Maloney, J. D.: The problem of correcting single and common ventricle. *Circulation*, **54**:(Suppl. II), 101, 1976.

Mitchell, S. C.; Korones, S. B.; and Berendes, H. W.: Congenital heart disease in 56,109 births. Incidence and natural history. *Circulation*, **43**:232, 1971.

Nagle, J. P.; Cheitlin, M. D.; and McCarty, R. J.: Corrected transposition of the great vessels without associated anomalies: Report of a case with congestive failure at 45. *Chest*, **60**:367, 1971.

Puyau, F. A.; Little, J. A.; and Collins, H. A.: Mitral valve prosthesis in childhood. *Am. J. Dis. Child.*, **108**:651, 1964.

Ratner, B.; Abbott, M. E.; and Beattie, W. W.: Rare cardiac anomaly. Cor triloculare biventriculare in mirror-picture dextrocardia with persistent omphalo-mesenteric bay, right aortic arch and pulmonary artery forming descending aorta. *Am. J. Dis. Child.*, **22**:508, 1921.

Rokitansky, K. F.: *Die Defekte der Scheidewande des Herzens*. Braumuller, Vienna, 1875, pp. 81–86.

Rotem, C. E., and Hultgren, H. N.: Corrected transposition of the great vessels without associated defects. *Am. Heart J.*, **70**:305, 1965.

Rushmer, R. F.: *Cardiovascular Dynamics*. W. B. Saunders, Philadelphia, 1970.

Ruttenberg, H. D.; Elliot, L. P.; Anderson, R. C.; Adams, P.; and Tuna, N.: Congenital corrected transposition of the great vessels, correlation of electrocardiograms and vectorcardiograms with associated cardiac malformations and hemodynamic states. *Am. J. Cardiol.*, **17**:339, 1966.

Schiebler, G. L.; Edwards, J. E.; Burchell, H. B.; DuShane, J. W.; Ongley, P. A.; and Wood, E. H.: Congenital corrected transposition of the great vessels. *Pediatrics*, **27**:851, 1961.

Shem-Tov, A.; Deutsch, V.; Yahini, J. H.; Kraus, Y.; and Neufeld, H. N.: Corrected transposition of the great arteries. A modified approach to the clinical diagnosis in 30 cases. *Am. J. Cardiol.*, **27**:99, 1971.

Solinger, R.; Elbl, F.; and Minhas, K.: Deductive echocardiographic analysis in infants with congenital heart disease. *Circulation*, **50**:1072, 1974.

Spitzer, A.: Uber den Bauplan des normalen und missbildeten Herzens: Bersuch einer phylogentischen Theorie. *Virchow. Arch. Pathol. Anat.*, **243**:81, 1923.

Todd, D. B.; Anderson, R. C.; and Edwards, J. E.: Inverted malformations in corrected transposition of the great vessels. *Circulation*, **32**:298, 1965.

Van Mierop, L. H. S.; Alley, R. D.; Kansel, H. W.; and Stranahan, A.: Pathogenesis of transposition complexes. I. Embryology of the ventricles and great arteries. *Am. J. Cardiol.*, **12**:216, 1963.

Van Praagh, R.: What is congenitally corrected transposition? *N. Engl. J. Med.*, **282**:1097, 1970.

Van Praagh, R.; Ongley, P. A.; and Swan, H. J. C.: Anatomic types of single of common ventricle in man. Morphologic and geometric aspects of 60 necropsied cases. *Am. J. Cardiol.*, **13**:367, 1964.

Van Praagh, R.; Perez-Trevino, C.; and Lopez-Cuellar, M.: Transposition of the great arteries with posterior aorta, anterior pulmonary artery, subpulmonary conus and fibrous continuity between aortic and atrioventricular valves. *Am. J. Cardiol.*, **28**:631, 1971.

Van Praagh, R., and Van Praagh, S.: Anatomically corrected transposition of the great arteries. *Br. Heart J.*, **29**:112, 1967.

Van Praagh, R., and Van Praagh, S.: Isolated ventricular inversion. A consideration of the morphogenesis, definition and diagnosis of nontransposed and transposed great arteries. *Am. J. Cardiol.*, **17**:395, 1966.

Van Praagh, R.; Vlad, P.; and Keith, J. D.: Anatomic types of congenital dextrocardia. Diagnostic and embryologic implications. *Am. J. Cardiol.*, **13**:510, 1964.

Walker, W. J.; Cooley, D. A.; McNamara, D. G.; and Moser, R. H.: Corrected transposition of the great vessels, atrioventricular heart block, and ventricular septal defect. A clinical triad. *Circulation*, **17**:249, 1958.

Walmsley, T.: Transposition of the ventricles and the arterial stems. *J. Anat.*, **65**:528, 1931.

Yater, W. M.; Lyon, J. A.; and McNabb, P. E.: Congenital heart block: Review and report of the second case of complete heart block studied by serial sections through the conduction system. *JAMA*, **100**:1831, 1933.

35

Double-Outlet Right Ventricle

Henry M. Sondheimer, Robert M. Freedom, and *Peter M. Olley*

DOUBLE-OUTLET right ventricle identifies a diverse group of rare cardiac malformations that share the common feature that both the aorta and the pulmonary artery arise primarily from the morphologic right ventricle. The term "double-outlet right ventricle" was first suggested by Witham (1957) when he reviewed four hearts—one with a subaortic ventricular septal defect (VSD) and no pulmonic stenosis, one with a subpulmonic VSD and no pulmonic stenosis, one with subaortic VSD and pulmonic stenosis, and one with a subaortic VSD and pulmonary atresia—and noted the basic similarities in all of them. Interest in this lesion was further increased when surgical correction was successfully attempted in the same year for a child with double-outlet right ventricle and a subaortic VSD without pulmonic stenosis (Kirklin, 1957; Kirklin et al., 1964). Pathologic series began to appear from several centers, and the anatomy of double-outlet right ventricle with its associated cardiac and noncardiac lesions began to be clarified. (Neufeld et al., 1961a; Neufeld et al., 1961b; Neufeld et al., 1962; Mehrizi, 1965; Venables and Campbell, 1966.)

Anatomy

Double-outlet right ventricle has been defined as that situation in which there are two ventricles and two great vessels, with all of one great vessel and more than half of the second great vessel arising from the right ventricle (Lev et al., 1972). When the pulmonary artery overrides the interventricular septum there may be mitral-pulmonic valve continuity, but when the aorta overrides the interventricular septum there should be no mitral-aortic continuity. Double-outlet right ventricle is characterized by the relationship of the great arteries to the ventricular septal defect and the presence or absence of valve or subvalvular pulmonic stenosis. The patient with a subaortic ventricular septal defect without pulmonic stenosis will frequently have streaming of oxygenated left ventricular blood into the aorta and remain acyanotic until pulmonary vascular disease develops (Figure

35–1*A*). These children, therefore, resemble patients with a large ventricular septal defect and normal great vessels (Engle et al., 1963). However, a patient with a subpulmonic VSD and no pulmonic stenosis, the Taussig-Bing malformation, will have streaming of the left ventricular blood into the pulmonary artery while systemic venous return is largely directed to the aorta causing cyanosis from birth (Figure 35–1*B*), with a higher oxygen saturation in the pulmonary artery than in the aorta (Taussig and Bing, 1949; Sridaroment et al., 1976). Clinically these children resemble patients with D-transposition of the great vessels and a ventricular septal defect as they are both cyanotic and develop early congestive heart failure. A third group of patients have a VSD that is doubly committed to the two great vessels (Figure 35–1*C*) (Lev et al., 1972; Zamora et al., 1975). The VSD can be "uncommitted," at a distance from either great vessel (Figure 35–1*D*). Finally, there may be no VSD with the only outlet of blood from the left heart being across the atrial septum (Edwards et al., 1952; MacMahon and Lipa, 1964).

One severe complication of double-outlet right ventricle is spontaneous diminution in size of the VSD. As the VSD represents the source of egress of blood from the left ventricle in this condition, restriction in its size leads to increasing clinical symptomatology (Serratto et al., 1967; Lavoie et al., 1971).

Patients with double-outlet right ventricle and a subaortic VSD have pulmonic stenosis more often than not. Sixty-four of one hundred and five patients (61 percent) with double-outlet right ventricle and subaortic VSD had pulmonic stenosis in the accumulated series at the Mayo Clinic, Johns Hopkins Hospital, The Hektoen Institute, and the University of Minnesota (Neufeld et al., 1961; Mehrizi, 1965; Lev et al., 1972; and Zamora et al., 1975). The clinical series at The Hospital for Sick Children, Toronto, in the past 20 years (Table 35–1) also shows that 61 percent, 28 of 46, of the patients with subaortic VSD had pulmonic stenosis (Sondheimer et al., 1977). These patients resemble clinically patients with tetralogy of Fallot (Figure 35–1*E*).

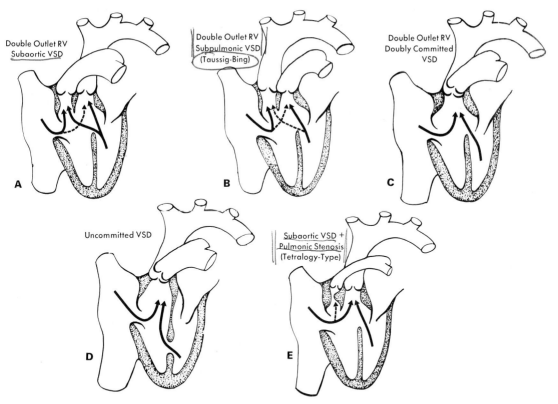

Figure 35-1. (A) Diagrammatic representation of double-outlet right ventricle with subaortic VSD and no pulmonic stenosis. Most of the left ventricular output is directed to the aorta with most of the systemic venous return directed to the pulmonary artery, so that cyanosis is rarely a finding prior to the development of pulmonary vascular disease.

(B) Diagrammatic representation of double-outlet right ventricle with subpulmonic VSD and no pulmonic stenosis. Most of the left ventricular output is directed to the pulmonary artery with most of the systemic venous return directed to the aorta. Cyanosis is almost always found, and the oxygen saturation in the pulmonary artery is usually higher than in the aorta.

(C) Diagrammatic representation of double-outlet right ventricle with a doubly committed VSD. The streaming of left ventricular blood will be toward both great vessels so that the oxygen saturation in the aorta and pulmonary artery will be approximately equal. The presence of cyanosis or congestive heart failure will depend on the volume of pulmonary blood flow, determined in infancy by the presence or absence of pulmonic stenosis.

(D) Diagrammatic representation of double-outlet right ventricle with an uncommitted VSD. The VSD is low in the interventricular septum and distant from either great vessel. Complete mixing of systemic, venous, and left ventricular blood will occur in the right ventricle, and there will be equal oxygen saturations in the aorta and pulmonary artery. The presence of cyanosis or congestive heart failure will again depend on the pulmonary blood flow.

(E) Diagrammatic representation of double-outlet right ventricle with subaortic VSD and pulmonic stenosis. Although most of the left ventricular output is directed toward the aorta, with the aortic oxygen saturation higher than the pulmonary artery saturation, the decreased pulmonary blood flow reduces left ventricular return and leads to early cyanosis, as in tetralogy of Fallot.

Pulmonic stenosis is reported in 4 of the 27 patients with double-outlet right ventricle and subpulmonic VSD in Lev's series but was not seen in Zamora's nine cases or in the clinical series of 26 cases at The Hospital for Sick Children.

The aorta and pulmonary artery in double-outlet left ventricle typically have bilateral conus with similar valve heights (Figure 35–2). The aorta is usually to the left of the pulmonary artery, or D-malposed (Van Praagh 1973). However, a small group of patients have L-malposition with the aorta to the left of the pulmonary artery (Lincoln et al.,

1975; Van Praagh et al., 1975). These patients have all had valve or subvalvar pulmonic stenosis, and their repair is complicated by the right coronary artery crossing anterior to the pulmonary artery.

In addition to pulmonic stenosis, left-sided obstructive lesions, specifically aortic coarctation and interruption, subaortic and aortic valve stenosis, and mitral stenosis and atresia, are quite common in double-outlet right ventricle. (Lev and Bharati, 1973). We found 11 cases of aortic coarctation or interruption in 80 cases of double-outlet right ventricle in our clinical series (Table 35–2). Eight of

Table 35–1. DOUBLE-OUTLET RIGHT VENTRICLE

Hospital for Sick Children 1956–1975*

87 Patients
- 80 Primary referrals
  - 26 Subpulmonic VSD (Taussig-Bing)
  - 18 Subaortic VSD
  - 28 Subaortic VSD + Pulmonic stenosis
  - 8 Uncommitted VSD
- 7 Secondary referrals

* There were 87 patients with double-outlet right ventricle seen at The Hospital for Sick Children born in the 20 years from 1956 through 1975. Seven were referred for corrective surgery after primary care at other centers. The breakdown of the 80 patients referred for their primary care is shown. The group with uncommitted VSD includes one child whose VSD was closed.

Table 35–2. DOUBLE-OUTLET RIGHT VENTRICLE PLUS COARCTATION*

TYPE OF DORV	ALIVE	DEAD
Subpulmonic VSD	1	7
Subaortic VSD	1	2 (1 interrupted arch)
Subaortic VSD + PS	—	—
Uncommitted VSD	—	—

* Of the 80 patients with double-outlet right ventricle, ten had coarctation of the aorta and one had an interrupted aortic arch. Coarctation was not seen in the 28 patients with double-outlet right ventricle, subaortic VSD, and pulmonic stenosis. The most frequent association was with subpulmonic VSD, and the prognosis for this combination is very poor.

these patients had the Taussig-Bing malformation. Seven of these eight children with both the Taussig-Bing malformation and coarctation of the aorta died before four months of age, though this difficult combination can be successfully treated (Wedemeyer et al., 1970). Mitral valve disease was found in ten cases of double-outlet right ventricle without pulmonic stenosis (Table 35–3). The mitral disease was fatal in each case, though in two patients with the Taussig-Bing malformation the stenotic or straddling mitral valve was unrecognized until the time of attempted total correction.

Table 35–3. DOUBLE-OUTLET RIGHT VENTRICLE PLUS MITRAL VALVE DISEASE*

TYPE OF DORV	ATRESIA	STENOSIS	STRADDLING
Subpulmonic VSD	1	1	2
Subaortic VSD	4	1	—
Subaortic VSD + PS	—	—	—
Uncommitted VSD	1	—	—

* Severe mitral abnormalities have been found in ten cases. None of these patients is still alive. Mitral abnormalities were not found in the 28 patients with double-outlet right ventricle, subaortic VSD, and pulmonic stenosis.

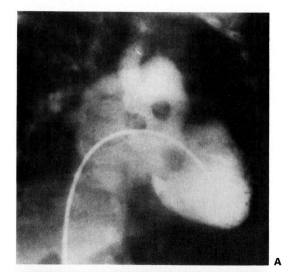

A

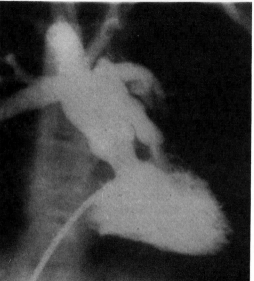

B

Figure 35-2. *A.* Left ventricular angiogram (AP) in a three-month-old child with double-outlet right ventricle, subaortic VSD, and no pulmonic stenosis. Note the conus beneath and between the semilunar valves and the distance from the mitral valve to aortic or pulmonic valve.

B. Right ventricular angiogram (AP) in a five-year-old child with double-outlet right ventricle, subaortic VSD, and pulmonic stenosis. Note the bilateral conus, although the anatomy is similar to Tetralogy of Fallot. At surgical correction she was found to have a 15-mm gap between the mitral and aortic valves.

None of our 28 patients with double-outlet right ventricle with subaortic VSD and pulmonic stenosis had aortic coarctation or mitral valve disease. Lev and his associates (1972) had 35 such patients without mitral or aortic disease, whereas Zamora, Moller, and Edwards (1975) did have one patient with subaortic VSD and pulmonic stenosis who had mitral atresia.

Other cardiac lesions can be seen with double-outlet right ventricle, including endocardial cushion defects (Sridaromont et al., 1975), asplenia, polysplenia, and total anomalous pulmonary venous return.

Embryology

Pathologically, double-outlet right ventricle forms part of a continuum of abnormalities beginning with tetralogy of Fallot and proceeding through double-outlet right ventricle with subaortic VSD, double-outlet right ventricle with subpulmonic VSD, to D-transposition of the great vessels with a ventricular septal defect (Lev et al., 1972). In tetralogy of Fallot there is mitral aortic continuity and only subpulmonic conus (Van Praagh, 1973). In double-outlet right ventricle with subaortic VSD there is bilateral conus and aortic-mitral continuity is lost, but the amount of subaortic conus may be quite small. In the Taussig-Bing malformation the amount of subaortic conus is increased while the amount of subpulmonic conus is diminished (Van Praagh, 1968). Subaortic stenosis may result from the increased subaortic conus. In D-transposition of the great vessels with VSD there is typically only a subaortic conus while mitral-pulmonic valve continuity is present (Van Praagh, 1973; Goor and Edwards, 1973).

Embryologic support for this thesis of a continuum is provided by the recent work of Goor, Dische, and Lillehei (1972) and Anderson and his associates (1974a). Each group has reviewed embryologic hearts from horizons 15 through 22 of Streeter. At horizon 15 the entire truncus overlies the primitive right ventricle with the anlage of the aortic valve to the right of the anlage of the pulmonic valve. There are three critical events in normal development in the next few days of embryologic life—counterclockwise inversion of the distal conus (viewed from below), which carries the future aortic valve posteriorly and to the left; Leftward shift of the conoventricular junction allowing the aortic conus to override the left ventricle instead of the right; and an unequal absorption of conus from beneath the semilunar valves so that some subpulmonic conus remains but there is no residual subaortic conus and mitral-aortic continuity is established. Both groups agree on these critical events though Anderson and his associates (1974a) suggest that conal absorption may be partially causative to inversion of the distal conus, rather than following it.

Hearts with double-outlet right ventricle maintain the early relationship of both semilunar valves above the right ventricle with a rightward aortic valve because of failure of conoventricular shift and absence of inversion of the distal conus (Goor and Edwards, 1973; Anderson et al., 1974b). There is absorption of some conus bilaterally but there is residual conus below each semilunar valve. In situations where there is more subpulmonic conus the VSD tends to be subaortic, and when there is more subaortic conus the VSD tends to be subpulmonic.

In hearts with double-outlet right ventricle and L-malposition of the aorta, there has presumably been clockwise rather than counterclockwise inversion of the distal conus, leading to the aortic valve being leftward and anterior to the pulmonic valve at the end of cardiac development (Goor and Edwards, 1973).

Goor and Edwards in 1972 presented a "bulbo-ventricular heart" that they felt showed failure of absorption of conus as well as lack of conal inversion and failure of conoventricular shift (Goor and Edwards, 1972). This resulted in double-outlet right ventricle of a very primitive variety. We have recently seen what we believe is a similar heart in a child with pulmonic stenosis who was palliated at three days of age by a Blalock-Taussig anastomosis. Our patient did not have the asplenia syndrome.

Clinical Features

The clinical presentation of patients with double-outlet right ventricle is primarily dependent on the relationship of the VSD to the great vessels, the presence or absence of pulmonic stenosis, and the presence or absence of associated cardiac lesions such as coarctation of the aorta, mitral valve disease, or endocardial cushion defects. Clinically patients may resemble those with a large VSD, those with tetralogy of Fallot, or those with complete transposition of the great arteries and a VSD. We have recently reviewed the patients with double-outlet right ventricle presenting at The Hospital for Sick Children over a 20-year-period, 1956–1975 (Sondheimer et al., 1977). Twenty-six of these children had subpulmonic VSD without pulmonic stenosis, 18 had subaortic VSD without pulmonic stenosis, and 28 had subaortic VSD with pulmonic stenosis (Table 35–1). Eight had uncommitted, doubly committed, or (in one case) an absent VSD. Fifty-seven of eighty (71 percent) were male.

The patients with subpulmonic VSD presented at one day to 14 months of age with 18 of 26 presenting before two months of age (Figure 35–3). Presenting symptoms were cyanosis in 11 cases, congestive heart failure in two cases, and both cyanosis and congestive heart failure in 13 cases. Physical findings usually indicated cardiomegaly, pulmonary hypertension, and a loud pansystolic murmur of a VSD with a thrill. Cyanosis was almost always present. Chest x-ray showed cardiomegaly, increased pulmonary vascularity, and a prominent pulmonary artery segment. Twenty-four of twenty-five with levocardia had a left aortic arch. Only 1 of 26 had dextrocardia, and this child also had a left aortic arch. The electrocardiogram showed right-axis deviation in most cases. An RSR pattern was frequently seen but only one patient presented with right bundle branch block. These children had a high frequency of aortic coarctation, eight cases, and mitral valve disease, four cases (Tables 35–2 and 35–3). Two children had

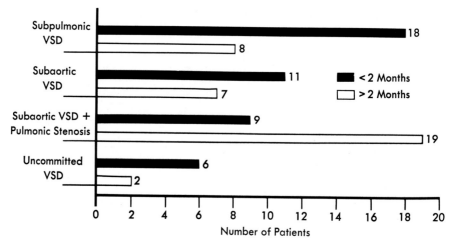

Figure 35-3. The age of referral of the 80 primary cases of double-outlet right ventricle seen at The Hospital for Sick Children. Patients with subpulmonic VSD tended to present more frequently in infancy, whereas patients with subaortic VSD and pulmonic stenosis were more likely to present after two months of age.

subaortic stenosis. Fourteen of twenty-six had no significant cardiac or noncardiac congenital malformation besides their double-outlet right ventricle.

Diagnosis in double-outlet right ventricle with subpulmonic VSD is dependent on complete hemodynamic and angiographic evaluation. Angio-grams must be performed in both ventricles to define the VSD and its relationship to the great vessels and should also be performed in the aorta to rule out coarctation and coronary artery abnormalities, and in the pulmonary artery to visualize pulmonary venous return and the mitral valve.

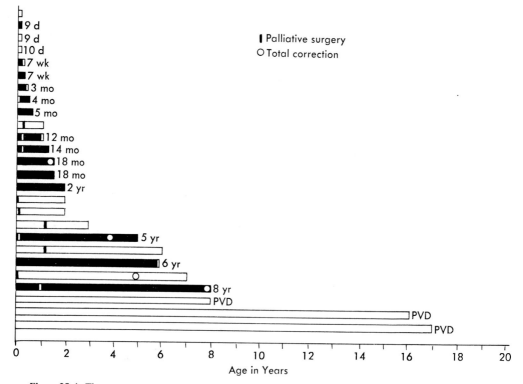

Figure 35-4. The current age or age at death of the 26 patients with double-outlet right ventricle, subpulmonic VSD, and no pulmonic stenosis. Surviving patients are represented by open bars, and children who have died have their age of death entered. Nine of the twenty-six died before one year of age. There had been many palliative operations, but only four attempts at total correction with only one current survivor. The three oldest survivors have pulmonary vascular disease.

The combination of double-outlet right ventricle with subpulmonic VSD and coarctation was fatal in seven of eight cases by four months of age. Overall we have had only nine survivors (35 percent) of the 26 patients with double-outlet right ventricle and subpulmonic VSD from this 20-year review. Of these only one has been corrected, three have pulmonary vascular disease, and five are currently palliated with pulmonary artery banding and awaiting further surgery (Figure 35–4).

The patients with double-outlet right ventricle and subaortic VSD without pulmonic stenosis presented at one day to 11 months of age. Clinically they appear very similar to patients with large ventricular septal defects and systemic pressure in the right ventricle and pulmonary artery. Physical findings are those of a large left-to-right shunt at ventricular level with pulmonary hypertension. Chest x-ray showed cardiomegaly, increased pulmonary vascularity, and an enlarged pulmonary artery segment. One of sixteen patients with levocardia had a right aortic arch as well as one of two with dextrocardia. It was suggested at one time that the diagnosis in these patients could be suspected prior to catheterization by the electrocardiogram (Neufeld et al., 1961), but we would agree with later reports that this is probably not so (Engle et al., 1963; Krongrad et al., 1972) as only 1 of our 18 patients had left-axis deviation with a counterclockwise frontal loop at the time of presentation. Echocardiography has been helpful in the precatheterization diagnosis in recent years (Chesler et al., 1971; French and Popp, 1975). The finding of aortic-mitral discontinuity on echo, or at least a variance in the depth of these structures with the posterior aortic root significantly anterior to the mitral valve in the presence of moderately severe aortic override of the interventricular septum, suggests double-outlet right ventricle (Figure 35–5). Five of the eighteen patients with double-outlet ventricle, subaortic VSD, and no pulmonic stenosis had significant mitral valve disease (Table 35–3) that contributed directly to their death. Nine of these eighteen patients had no significant cardiac or noncardiac malformation besides their double-outlet right ventricle. Overall (Figure 35–6) 9 of these 18 patients are alive—three have been corrected after pulmonary artery banding in infancy, three have been banded and are awaiting correction, two have pulmonary vascular disease, and one infant is awaiting primary correction. The prognosis in this group is therefore better than in the patients with double-outlet right ventricle and subpulmonic VSD.

The patients with double-outlet right ventricle with subaortic VSD and pulmonic stenosis have the best prognosis of any group. They are protected from pulmonary vascular disease by their pulmonic stenosis and present at a later age with 19 of 28 presenting after two months (Figure 35–3). Their course is uncomplicated by coarctation of the aorta or mitral valve disease (Tables 35–2 and 35–3) and they are clinically very similar to patients with tetralogy of Fallot. They presented with cyanosis and only slightly enlarged hearts. Pulmonary vascularity on chest x-ray tended to be normal to decreased depending on

Double Outlet RV

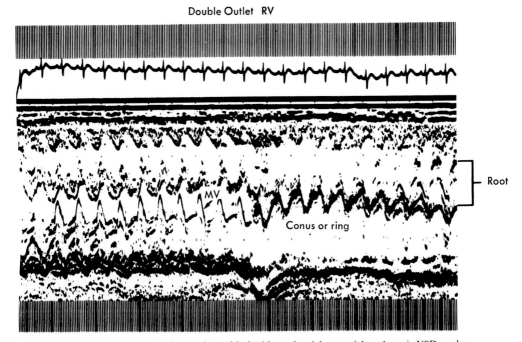

Figure 35-5. Echocardiographic walk in a patient with double-outlet right ventricle, subaortic VSD, and no pulmonic stenosis. There is marked septal override with the aortic root originating primarily from the right ventricle. In going from the anterior mitral leaflet (*MV*) to the posterior aortic wall there is a clear change in depth, implying anatomic discontinuity.

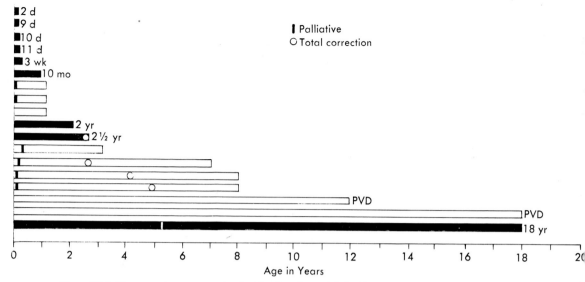

Figure 35-6. The current age or age at death of the 18 patients with double-outlet right ventricle, subaortic VSD, and no pulmonic stenosis. Survivors are represented by open bars. Six children died before one year of age; four have had attempted total correction with three survivors. The two oldest survivors have pulmonary vascular disease.

the degree of pulmonic stenosis. Mirowski, Mehrizi, and Taussig (1963) reported a high incidence of complete right bundle branch block in this condition, but we observed complete right bundle branch block in only 1 of 28 cases. Precatheterization diagnosis has been difficult prior to echocardiography and has been dependent on angiocardiography for differentiation from tetralogy of Fallot (Cheng, 1962; Hallerman et al., 1970a and 1970b; Baron, 1971). Seven of twenty-three patients (30 percent) with double-outlet right ventricle, pulmonic stenosis, and levocardia had a right aortic arch. Of four with dextrocardia, one had a right aortic arch; and the one patient with mesocardia and this combination had a right aortic arch. Thirteen of these twenty-eight patients had no significant cardiac or noncardiac malformations besides their double-outlet right ventricle. The clinical course of these patients (Figure 35–7) has been better than of the groups without pulmonic stenosis. Twenty-one of twenty-eight (75 percent) are alive—seven have been corrected, 12 have been palliated, and two are unoperated. Of the seven deaths only one has been subsequent to attempted total correction.

Of the eight patients with uncommitted, doubly committed, or absent VSD, three are alive, four are dead, and one has been lost to follow-up. The three survivors were all banded in infancy. Six of the eight patients in this small group presented before two months of age (Figure 35–3).

Rogers, Hagstrom, and Engle (1965) reported seven cases of double-outlet right ventricle in children with trisomy-18. None of our 80 patients has been shown to have trisomy-18, but one child with subaortic VSD and pulmonic stenosis did have 13–15 trisomy. This child died at four days of age. There have been no other chromosomal abnormalities.

Double-outlet right ventricle has been reported in patients with the asplenia and polysplenia syndromes (Rose et al., 1975). Three of our patients had the asplenia syndrome; two died at 7 and 15 months of age, respectively. One of these was the only patient with total anomalous pulmonary venous return in this series. One three-year-old with asplenia, double-outlet right ventricle, subaortic VSD, and pulmonic stenosis is still alive after a Blalock-Taussig anastomosis. Two of our patients had the polysplenia syndrome. One died at home at four years of age after a Blalock-Taussig shunt. One three-year-old with an uncommitted VSD is alive, having been banded at 13 months of age.

Although double-outlet right ventricle is usually seen in patients with levocardia, D-ventricular loop, and D-malposed aorta (Van Praagh, 1973), situs inversus with both atrioventricular concordance (ILL) and atrioventricular discordance (IDD) has been reported. Sixty-nine of our eighty patients had levocardia, situs solitus, D-ventricular loop, and D-malposition of the great vessels. One child with subaortic VSD and pulmonic stenosis had SDL anatomy with an L-malposed aorta. Nine patients had dextrocardia and one patient had mesocardia. Seven patients had situs inversus. Of these, six had atrioventricular concordance and one had atrio-ventricular discordance.

Endocardial cushion defect is a severe complication when associated with double-outlet right ventricle (Sridaromont et al., 1975). Five of our patients had endocardial cushion defects.

Double-outlet right ventricle with straddling mitral valve is a rare combination first reported by Tandon, Moller, and Edwards (1973). Two of our patients with double-outlet right ventricle and subpulmonic VSD

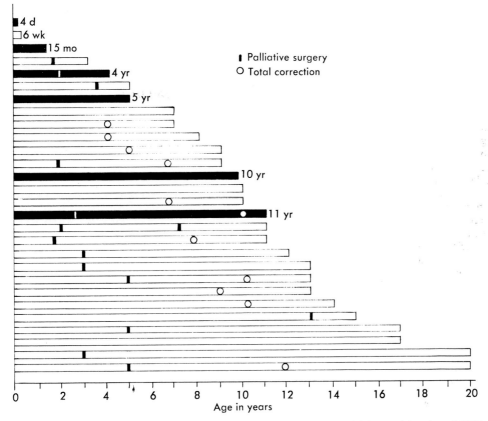

Figure 35-7. The current age or age at death of the 28 patients with double-outlet right ventricle, subaortic VSD, and pulmonic stenosis. The 21 survivors are represented by open bars. The overall prognosis is clearly better than for those with double-outlet right ventricle without pulmonic stenosis.

had biventricular insertion of the mitral valve and both died, one during attempted total correction.

Surgery

Total correction of double-outlet right ventricle was first performed by Kirklin in May, 1957, when he operated on two children on successive days who had double-outlet right ventricle with subaortic VSD without pulmonic stenosis. One of these two patients survived. Kirklin recognized the anatomy in each case and placed a tunnel of synthetic material to direct the flow from the left ventricle to the aorta (Kirklin, 1957; Kirklin et al., 1964). It was critical that the VSD not be closed, which would completely block egress of blood from the left ventricle (Redo et al., 1963). Correction of patients with double-outlet right ventricle with subaortic VSD and pulmonic stenosis was also attempted in 1957 but was not performed successfully by the Mayo Clinic group until 1961 (Kirklin et al., 1964). The most recent reviews of the large surgical experience with double-outlet right ventricle with subaortic VSD at the Mayo Clinic showed a 22 percent mortality in patients without pulmonic stenosis and a 32 percent mortality in patients

with pulmonic stenosis (Gomes et al., 1971a and 1971b).

Correction of double-outlet right ventricle with obstructive VSD was first reported by Mason and his associates (1969). They correctly anticipated the location of the His bundle in double-outlet right ventricle and enlarged the VSD by resecting a portion of the fibrous rim anterior to the mitral valve.

Surgical correction of double-outlet right ventricle with subpulmonic VSD was first reported by use of an intraventricular tunnel from the VSD to the aorta (Thompson, 1967; Patrick and McGoon, 1968). However, it was soon found to be simpler in most cases to direct the left ventricular blood to the pulmonary artery at the time of the VSD closure and then perform an atrial baffle operation to redirect venous inflow (Hightower et al., 1969). This now appears to be the procedure of choice. Repair of double-outlet right ventricle with a subaortic VSD, pulmonic stenosis, and L-malposition of the aorta has been recorded occasionally (Lincoln, 1972; Danielson et al., 1972; Lincoln et al., 1975). This lesion has the added difficulty of the fact that the right coronary artery crosses anteriorly to the pulmonary outflow tract making relief of the pulmonic stenosis more difficult.

Kiser and his associates (1968) reported the repair of three patients with double-outlet right ventricle, situs solitus, and atrioventricular discordance (SLL). Two of the three survived. Stewart and his associates (1976) reported the successful repair of a single patient with double-outlet right ventricle, situs inversus, and atrioventricular concordance (ILL). One girl with the same anatomy was corrected at The Hospital for Sick Children by Dr. William Mustard in 1968.

Singh, Letsky, and Stark (1976) reported transient hemolysis after correction of double-outlet right ventricle. Their patient improved spontaneously after six weeks, and they hypothesized that his symptoms began to clear as the endothelialization of his Dacron patch became complete.

There can be no question that great improvement in the overall outlook for patients with double-outlet right ventricle has occurred since the institution of "corrective" procedures for these malformations. Current management of the infant with double-outlet right ventricle is now directed to palliation in anticipation of corrective surgery or, in an occasional patient, to primary repair of his difficult cardiac lesion.

REFERENCES

Anderson, R. H.; Wilkinson, J. L.; Arnold, R.; and Lubkiewicz, K.: Morphogenesis of bulboventricular malformations I. Consideration of embrygenesis in the normal heart. *Br. Heart J.*, **36**:242, 1974a.

Anderson, R. H.; Wilkinson, J. L.; Arnold, R.; Becker, A. E.; and Lubkiewicz, K.: Morphogenesis of bulboventricular malformations II. Observations on malformed hearts. *Br. Heart J.*, **36**:948, 1974b.

Baron, M. G.: Radiologic notes in cardiology, angiographic differentiation between tetralogy of Fallot and double-outlet right ventricle, relationship of the mitral and aortic valves. *Circulation*, **43**:451, 1971.

Cheng, T. O.: Double outlet right ventricle, diagnosis during life. *Am. J. Med.*, **32**:637, 1962.

Chesler, E.; Joffe, H. S.; Beck, W.; and Schrire, V.: Echocardiographic recognition of mitral-semilunar valve discontinuity, an aid to the diagnosis of origin of both great vessels from the right ventricle. *Circulation*, **43**:725, 1971.

Danielson, G. K.; Ritter, D. G.; Coleman, H. N., III; and Du Shane, J. W.: Successful repair of double-outlet right ventricle with transposition of the great arteries (aorta anterior and to the left), pulmonary stenosis, and subaortic ventricular septal defect. *J. Thorac. Cardiovasc. Surg.*, **63**:741, 1972.

Edwards, J. E.; James, J. W.; and DuShane, J. W.: Congenital malformation of the heart, origin of transposed great vessels from the right ventricle associated with atresia of the left ventricular outlet, double orifice of the mitral valve, and single coronary artery. *Lab. Invest.*, **1**:197, 1952.

Engle, M. A.; Steinberg, I.; Lukas, D. S.; and Goldberg, H. P.: Acyanotic ventricular septal defect with both great vessels from the right ventricle. *Am. Heart J.*, **66**:755, 1963.

French, J. W., and Popp, R.: Variability of echocardiographic discontinuity in double outlet right ventricle and truncus arteriosus. *Circulation*, **51**:848, 1975.

Gomes, M. M. R.; Weidman, W. H.; McGoon, D. C.; and Danielson, G. K.: Double-outlet right ventricle without pulmonic stenosis, surgical considerations and results of operation. *Circulation*, **43–44**:Suppl. I–31, 1971a.

Gomes, M. M. R.; Weidman, W. H.; McGoon, D. C.; and Danielson, G. K.: Double-outlet right ventricle with pulmonic stenosis, surgical considerations and results of operation. *Circulation*, **43**:889, 1971b.

Goor, D. A.; Dische, R.; and Lillehei, C. W.: The conotruncus I. Its normal inversion and conus absorption. *Circulation*, **46**:375, 1972.

Goor, D. A., and Edwards, J. E.: The conotruncus II. Report of a case showing persistent aortic conus and lack of inversion of the truncus (a bulboventricular heart). *Circulation*, **46**:385, 1972.

Goor, D. A., and Edwards, J. E.: The spectrum of transposition of the great arteries with specific reference to developmental anatomy of the conus. *Circulation*, **48**:406, 1973.

Hallerman, F. J.; Kincaid, O. W.; Ritter, D. G.; Ongley, P. A.; and Titus, J. L.: Angiocardiographic and anatomic findings in origin of both great arteries from the right ventricle. *Am. J. Roentgenol. Radium Ther. Nucl. Med.*, **109**:51, 1970a.

Hallerman, F. J.; Kincaid, O. W.; Ritter, D. G.; and Titus, J. L.: Mitral-semilunar valve relationships in the angiography of cardiac malformations. *Radiology*, **94**:63, 1970b.

Hightower, B. M.; Barcia, A.; Bargeron, L. M.; and Kirklin, J. W.: Double-outlet right ventricle with transposed great arteries and subpulmonary ventricular septal defect. The Taussig-Bing malformation. *Circulation*, **39–40**:Suppl. I–207, 1969.

Kirklin, J. W.: Personal correspondence to R. D. Rowe, 1957.

Kirklin, J. W.; Harp, R. A.; and McGoon, D. C.: Surgical treatment of origin of both vessels from right ventricle, including cases of pulmonary stenosis. *J. Thorac. Cardiovasc. Surg.*, **48**:1026, 1964.

Kiser, J. C.; Ongley, P. A.; Kirklin, J. W.; Clarkson, P. M.; and McGoon, D. C.: Surgical treatment of dextrocardia with inversion of ventricles and double-outlet right ventricle. *J. Thorac. Cardiovasc. Surg.*, **55**:6, 1968.

Krongrad, E.; Ritter, D. G.; Weidman, W. H.; and DuShane, J. E.: Hemodynamic and anatomic correlation of electrocardiogram in double-outlet right ventricle. *Circulation*, **46**:995, 1972.

Lavoie, R.; Sestier, F.; Gilbert, G.; Chameides, L.; Van Praagh, R.; and Grondin, P.: Double outlet right ventricle with left ventricular outflow tract obstruction due to small ventricular septal defect. *Am. Heart J.*, **82**:290, 1971.

Lev, M., and Bharati, S.: Double outlet right ventricle, association with other cardiovascular anomalies. *Arch. Pathol.*, **95**:117, 1973.

Lev, M.; Bharati, S.; Meng, C. C. L.; Liberthson, R. R.; Paul, M. H.; and Idriss, F.: A concept of double-outlet right ventricle. *J. Thorac. Cardiovasc. Surg.*, **64**:271, 1972.

Lincoln, C.: Total correction of d-loop double-outlet right ventricle with bilateral conus, l-transposition, and pulmonic stenosis. *J. Thorac. Cardiovasc. Surg.*, **64**:435, 1972.

Lincoln, C.; Anderson, R. H.; Shinebourne, E. A.; English, T. A. H.; and Wilkinson, J. L.: Double outlet right ventricle with l-malposition of the aorta. *Br. Heart J.*, **37**:453, 1975.

MacMahon, H. E., and Lipa, M.: Double-outlet right ventricle with intact interventricular septum. *Circulation*, **30**:745, 1964.

Mason, D. T.; Morrow, A. G.; Elkins, R. C.; and Friedman, W. F.: Origin of both great vessels from the right ventricle associated with severe obstruction to left ventricular outflow. *Am. J. Cardiol.*, **24**:118, 1969.

Mehrizi, A.: The origin of both great vessels from the right ventricle, I. With pulmonic stenosis, II. Without pulmonic stenosis. *Johns Hopkins Hosp. Bull.*, **117**:75, 1965.

Mirowski, M.; Mehrizi, A.; and Taussig, H. B.: The electrocardiogram in patients with both great vessels arising from the right ventricle combined with pulmonic stenosis. *Circulation*, **28**:1116, 1963.

Neufeld, H. N.; DuShane, J. W.; Wood, E. H.; Kirklin, J. W.; and Edwards, J. E.: Origin of both great vessels from the right ventricle, I. Without pulmonary stenosis. *Circulation*, **23**:399, 1961a.

Neufeld, H. N.; DuShane, J. W.; and Edwards, J. E.: Origin of both great vessels from the right ventricle II. With pulmonary stenosis. *Circulation*, **23**:603, 1961b.

Neufeld, H. N.; Lucas, R. V., Jr.; Lester, R. G.; Adams, P., Jr.; Anderson, R. C.; and Edwards, J. E.: Origin of both great vessels from the right ventricle without pulmonary stenosis. *Br. Heart J.*, **24**:393, 1962.

Patrick, D. L., and McGoon, D. C.: An operation for double-outlet right ventricle with transposition of the great arteries. *J. Cardiovasc. Surg.*, **9**:537, 1968.

Redo, S. F.; Engle, M. A.; Holswade, G. R.; and Goldberg, H. P.: Operative correction of ventricular septal defect with origin of both great vessels from the right ventricle. *J. Thorac. Cardiovasc. Surg.*, **45**:526, 1963.

Rogers, T. R.; Hagstrom, J. W. C.; and Engle, M. A.: Origin of both great vessels from the right ventricle with the trisomy-18 syndrome. *Circulation*, **32**:802, 1965.

Rose, V.; Izukawa, T.; and Moes, C. A. F.: Syndromes of asplenia and polysplenia. A review of cardiac and non-cardiac malformations in 60 cases with special reference to diagnosis and prognosis. *Br. Heart J.*, **37**:840, 1975.

Serratto, M.; Arevalo, F.; Goldman, E. J.; Hastreiter, A.; and Miller, R. A.: Obstructive ventricular septal defect in double outlet right ventricle. *Am. J. Cardiol.*, **19**:457, 1967.

Singh, A.; Letsky, E. A.; and Stark, J.: Hemolysis following correction of double outlet right ventricle. *J. Thorac. Cardiovasc. Surg.*, **71**:226, 1976.

Sondheimer, H. M.; Freedom, R. M.; and Olley, P. M.: Double outlet right ventricle: Clinical spectrum and prognosis. *Am. J. Cardiol.*, **39**:709, 1977.

Sridaromont, S.; Feldt, R. H.; Ritter, D. G.; Davis, G. D.; and Edwards, J. E.: Double outlet right ventricle (DORV): Hemodynamic and anatomic correlations. *Am. J. Cardiol.*, **38**:85, 1976.

Sridaromont, S.; Feldt, R. H.; Ritter, D. G.; Davis, G. D.; McGoon, D. C.; and Edwards, J. E.: Double-outlet right ventricle associated with persistent common atrioventricular canal. *Circulation*, **52**:933, 1975.

Stewart, S.; Farnham, J. D.; Schreiner, B.; and Manning, J.: Complete correction of double outlet right ventricle with situs inversus, l-loop, and l-malposition (I.L.L.) with subaortic VSD and pulmonary stenosis. *J. Thorac. Cardiovasc. Surg.*, **71**:129, 1976.

Tandon, R.; Moller, J. H.; and Edwards, J. E.: Communication of mitral valve with both ventricles associated with double outlet right ventricle. *Circulation*, **48**:994, 1973.

Taussig, H. B., and Bing, R. J.: Complete transposition of the aorta and a levoposition of the pulmonary artery: Clinical, physiological, and pathological findings. *Am. Heart J.*, **37**:551, 1949.

Thomson, N. B., Jr.: Complete repair of Taussig-Bing abnormality. *Ann. Thorac. Surg.*, **4**:420, 1967.

Van Praagh, R.: What is the Taussig-Bing malformation? *Circulation*, **38**:445, 1968.

Van Praagh, R.: Conotruncal malformations. In *Heart Disease in Infancy: Diagnosis and Surgical Treatment*. Eds. B. G. Barratt-Boyes; J. M. Neutze; and E. A. Harris. Churchill Livingstone, Edinburgh and London, 1973, pp. 141–88.

Van Praagh, R.; Perez-Trevino, C.; Reynolds, J. L.; Moes, C. A. F.; Keith, J. D.; Roy, D. L.; Belcourt, C.; Weinberg, P. M.; and Parisi, L. F.: Double outlet right ventricle S. D. L. with subaortic ventricular septal defect and pulmonary stenosis. *Am. J. Cardiol.*, **35**:42, 1975.

Venables, A. W., and Campbell, P. E.: Double outlet right ventricle. A review of 16 cases with 10 necropsy specimens. *Br. Heart J.*, **28**:461, 1966.

Wedemeyer, A. L.; Lucas, R. V., Jr.; and Castaneda, A. R.: Taussig-Bing malformation, coarctation of the aorta, and reversed patent ductus arteriosus: Operative correction in an infant. *Circulation*, **42**:1021, 1970.

Witham, A. C.: Double outlet right ventricle. A partial transposition complex. *Am. Heart J.*, **53**:928, 1957.

Zamora, R.; Moller, J. H.; and Edwards, J. E.: Double-outlet right ventricle, anatomic types and associated anomalies. *Chest*, **68**:672, 1975.

CHAPTER

36

Dextrocardia, Mesocardia, and Levocardia: The Segmental Approach to Diagnosis in Congenital Heart Disease

Richard Van Praagh and *Peter Vlad*

DEXTROCARDIA

DEXTROCARDIA is defined literally as a right-sided heart.

Right-sided hearts have long fascinated man. Aristotle (384–322 B.C.) observed situs inversus in animals. Fabricius reported the first case of dextrocardia in man in 1606. Another case was reported by Severinus in 1643. Riolanus reported two more cases, one of which occurred in the French queen, Marie de Medici (1573–1642) (Manchester and White, 1938). However, it soon became evident that dextrocardia was not confined to royalty; as Peacock noted in 1866, dextrocardia was also reported from Paris in 1650 in the man who was executed for the murder of the Duke of Beaufort.

The first of many classifications of dextrocardia was proposed in 1749 by Sénac, who divided right-sided hearts into two types, congenital and acquired.

Although initially diagnosed only at autopsy, dextrocardia began to be recognized in life during the early 1800s because of the improvement of percussion and auscultation. Following the advent of the x-ray and the electrocardiogram, it could be said in 1924 that the diagnosis of the presence of a right-sided heart "has become comparatively easy" (Jones, 1924). The development of cardiac catheterization and angiocardiography during and following World War II (1939–1945) made accurate intracardiac diagnosis possible in right-sided hearts. The simultaneous invention of palliative surgery for congenital heart disease, followed by corrective surgery, made diagnostic accuracy essential. In this century, many have contributed to the present understanding of dextrocardia, and the growth of this understanding may be traced in detail through the references listed at the end of this chapter.

Segmental Approach to Diagnosis

From the diagnostic standpoint, it may be said that there are three major cardiac segments (developmental units, or "building blocks" of the heart):

1. *The visceroatrial situs* (locations of the viscera and the atria).

2. *The ventricular loop* (locations of the ventricles).

3. *The conotruncus* (locations of the infundibulum and great arteries).

The general idea of the segmental approach to diagnosis in congenital heart disease is the following:

1. One diagnoses the anatomic type of each of the three major cardiac segments.

2. Mentally, one puts the three major segments together. This is the segmental combination or set of {atria, ventricles, great arteries}.

3. One then searches for associated malformations within each of the major segments, and between them. In terms of set theory of the "new" mathematics, associated anomalies may be regarded as subsets that occur within each segmental set.

4. Then one assesses the function or physiologic resultants of the system (segmental combination and associated malformations).

5. Finally, one assesses therapeutic options, both medical and surgical.

The foregoing, in essence, is the clinical problem posed by congenital heart disease. The segmental method constitutes points 1 and 2 above.

The segmental approach to diagnosis is independent of cardiac position, because it rests on basic developmental and anatomic principles. Consequently, this approach applies to normally located hearts (levocardia in situs solitus), as well as to

638

abnormally located hearts such as dextrocardia, mesocardia, isolated levocardia, the malpositions associated with pericardial defects, and the various types of ectopia cordis (Van Praagh, 1968).

In the segmental approach to diagnosis, reference is made to the three *major* cardiac segments. Why major? Because in fact there are at least eight cardiac segments, or independent developmental units, composing the heart:

1. *The sinus venosus.* This forms the venous portion of the morphologically right atrium (RA)—the superior and inferior venae cavae, coronary sinus, right and left venous valves, inferior limbic band, and septum primum (Van Praagh and Corsini, 1969).

2. *The primitive atrium.* This forms the muscular part of both atria—the right and left atrial appendages (with characteristic musculi pectinati), and septum secundum, i.e., the superior limbic band.

3. *The common pulmonary vein.* This forms the right and left pulmonary veins and the smooth dorsal wall of the left atrium between the pulmonary veins.

4. *The atrioventricular canal.* The endocardial cushions of the AV canal form the tricuspid and mitral valves and the canal septum.

5. *The ventricle* of the bulboventricular loop forms the morphologically left ventricle (LV).

6. *The proximal bulbus cordis* of the bulbo-ventricular loop gives rise to the morphologically right ventricle (RV).

7. *The distal bulbus cordis* forms the conus arteriosus or infundibulum.

8. *The truncus arteriosus* gives rise to the ascending aorta and main pulmonary artery (Streeter, 1942, 1945, 1948, 1951; Neill, 1956, Lewis and Abbott, 1915 and 1916; de la Cruz and da Rocha, 1956; de la Cruz et al., 1959; Van Mierop et al., 1963).

To facilitate diagnostic accuracy, however, the foregoing eight cardiac segments may be simplified by combination into *three major cardiac segments* (Van Praagh et al., 1964 and 1965; Van Praagh, 1972): (1) the visceroatrial situs; (2) the ventricular loop; and (3) the conotruncus: the atria, ventricles, and great arteries, respectively.

Atrial Localization: Types of Visceroatrial Situs

There are three main types of visceroatrial situs (Figure 36–1):

1. Situs solitus (solitus = usual or ordinary, hence normal).

2. Situs inversus, a mirror image of normal.

3. Situs ambiguus (Van Mierop et al., 1970), the ambiguous situs that is typical of the syndromes of asplenia and polysplenia (Ivemark, 1955), but that can occur with a normal spleen (Freedom, 1971; Niibori et al., 1971).

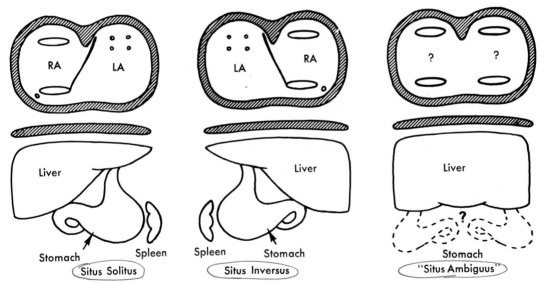

Figure 36-1. The visceroatrial concordances for atrial localization. The type of visceral situs and the type of atrial situs almost always are the same. The three types of visceroatrial situs are situs solitus (usual, ordinary, customary, hence normal); situs inversus, apparent mirror-image of situs solitus; and situs ambiguus, often associated with the asplenia and polysplenia syndromes, but occasionally with a normally formed spleen, in which both the type of visceral situs and the type of atrial situs are anatomically uncertain or indeterminate. Note the symmetric liver shadow of situs ambiguus and the absence of the spleen. Note also that septum primum, the flap valve of the foramen ovale, is shown as a direct upward extension of the left wall of the inferior vena cava, septum primum being the major component of the left venous valve. Probably the single most reliable indicator of the location of the morphologically right atrium (*RA*) is the location of the inferior vena cava. *LA.* Morphologically left atrium. (Modified from Van Praagh, R.: The segmental approach to diagnosis in congenital heart disease. In Bergsma, D. [ed.]: Part XV, "The Cardiovascular System." Baltimore: Williams & Wilkins for the National Foundation–March of Dimes *BD:OAS* VIII[5], 1972.)

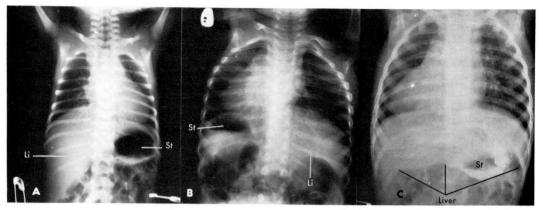

Figure 36-2. Posteroanterior chest roentograms for atrial localization. *A.* Situs solitus. *B.* Situs inversus. *C.* Situs ambiguus with asplenia. In all three, the type of visceral situs and the type of atrial situs were the same: both normal in *A*, both inverted in *B*, and both anatomically uncertain in *C*. *Li.* Liver shadow. *St.* Stomach bubble. (Reproduced from Van Praagh, R.: The segmental approach to diagnosis in congenital heart disease. In Bergsma, D. [ed.]: Part XV. "The Cardiovascular System." Baltimore: Williams & Wilkins for The National Foundation–March of Dimes, *BD:OAS* VIII[5], 1972.)

From the diagnostic standpoint, the type of visceral situs and the type of atrial situs almost always are the same (Figure 36–1): both in situs solitus, both in situs inversus, or both ambiguous. These are *the visceroatrial concordances.* In the plain chest x-ray (Figure 36–2), the locations of the liver shadow and stomach bubble usually indicate the atrial locations with accuracy:

1. Right-sided liver shadow and left-sided stomach bubble indicate situs solitus of the viscera and atria (Figure 36–2*A*).

2. Left-sided liver shadow and right-sided stomach bubble indicate situs inversus of the viscera and atria (Figure 36–2*B*).

3. An abnormally symmetric liver shadow and a shifting stomach bubble (that can be left-sided, midline, or right-sided, because of a common gastrointestinal mesentery) should suggest asplenia. Although the liver often is symmetric in asplenia, it can resemble the liver in situs solitus or in situs inversus. "Bilateral right-sidedness" is characteristic of asplenia (Stanger et al., 1968); this is regarded as a helpful mnemonic, not as a basic biologic truth. One often can see the air bronchogram, particularly in films taken with high kilovoltage (KV). Hence, the right-and left-sided air bronchograms both have the appearance of a right air bronchogram, because of the presence of an eparterial bronchus bilaterally. (*Epi* is a Greek word meaning upon, or over. The bronchus to the right upper lobe normally is upon, or passes over, the right pulmonary artery. Hence, the right upper lobe bronchus is eparterial—upon or over the right pulmonary artery.) In polysplenia, "bilateral left-sidedness" is typical (Stanger et al., 1968); again, this is regarded merely as a useful mnemonic. Normally, the left main stem bronchus passes beneath the left pulmonary artery. The left bronchus is hyparterial. (*Hypo* is a Greek word meaning under. Hypo + arteria = hyparterial.) Normally there is no

eparterial branch of the left bronchus. Thus, in high KV films, patients with polysplenia often have left air bronchograms bilaterally—hyparterial bronchi bilaterally. They appear long and "swaybacked" (concave superiorly), very different from right bronchi that give off an eparterial branch early (Van Mierop et al., 1970).

Thus, concerning atrial localization, plain chest x-rays (Figure 36–2) provide three clues: (1) liver shadow, (2) stomach bubble, and (3) air bronchogram.

Visceroatrial Discordance. Although visceroatrial concordance is the rule (Figures 36–1 and 36–2), visceroatrial discordance does occur rarely, as was first demonstrated angiocardiographically by Hastreiter and Rodriguez-Coronel (1968). The inferior vena cava (IVC) drains into the contralateral morphologically right atrium (RA) by switching sides at the level of the liver. Both possibilities have been documented (Hastreiter and Rodriguez-Coronel, 1968):

1. *Situs solitus of the abdominal viscera with situs inversus of the atria.* The IVC is right-sided within the abdomen, switches from right to left at the liver, and drains into the left-sided RA.

2. *Situs inversus of the abdominal viscera with situs solitus of the atria.* The IVC is left-sided within the abdomen and switches from left to right at the liver to drain into the right-sided RA.

Isolated atrial inversion is a newly recognized entity reported by Clarkson, Brandt, Barratt-Boyes, and Neutze (1972). It also exemplifies visceroatrial discordance: the viscera are in situs solitus; the atria are in situs inversus; the ventricles are in situs solitus; and the great arteries are normally interrelated. Since the cavae and aorta both are left-sided, while the pulmonary veins and artery both are right-sided, the systemic and pulmonary circulations are in parallel, as in transposition of the great arteries, rather than in

ASPLENIA

POLYSPLENIA

series, as occurs normally. This first known case of isolated atrial inversion was successfully corrected by a Mustard procedure.

IVC-RA Concordance. Despite their viscero-atrial discordance, the aforementioned rare cases all demonstrate IVC-RA concordance. When present, the IVC almost always returns to the RA, even if it has to switch sides to do so. Convincing reports of the IVC returning to the morphologically left atrium (LA) are very rare. We are aware of only two such cases that seem definite (Gardner and Cole, 1955; Gautam, 1968). Thus, for atrial localization, the IVC is an exceedingly reliable diagnostic marker of RA (de la Cruz et al., 1962). By contrast, the superior vena cava (SVC) is of little help in atrial localization because it may open into either atrium.

In the asplenia syndrome, Freedom (1971) suggested that the IVC may be a reliable indicator of the basic type of visceroatrial situs. If this concept is substantiated by further study, then situs ambiguus would lose much of its ambiguity. It would become a partial or heterotaxic form of situs solitus or situs inversus, depending on the location of the IVC. Hence, there may well be only two basic types of visceroatrial situs (solitus and inversus), rather than three, as Figure 36–1 suggests.

When the IVC is absent, can the visceroatrial situs be diagnosed accurately? When the suprarenal-to-

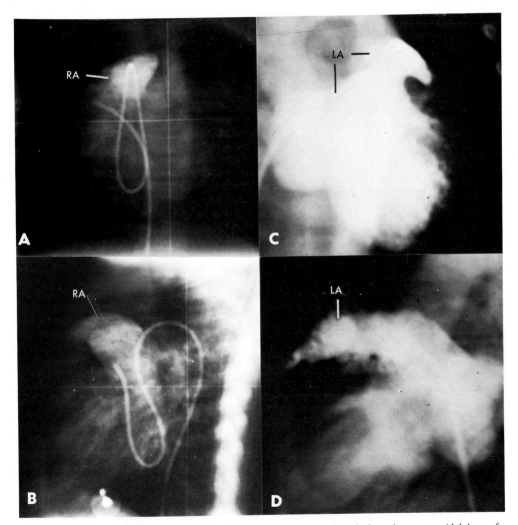

Figure 36-3. Angiocardiographic appearance of atrial appendages. The broad triangular or pyramidal shape of the right atrial appendage (*RA*) is very different from the long, relatively thin, tubular appearance of the left atrial appendage (*LA*). *A* and *C* are posteroanterior projections; *B* and *D* are left lateral projections. In *A* and *C* the catheter course describes the candy cane or shepherd's crook course of an azygos extension to the superior vena cava, indicating absence of the suprarenal-to-subhepatic segment of the inferior vena cava (so-called absence of the inferior vena cava). (Reproduced from Van Praagh, R.: The segmental approach to diagnosis in congenital heart disease. In Bergsma, D. [ed.]: Part XV, "The Cardiovascular System." Baltimore: Williams & Wilkins for The National Foundation–March of Dimes, *BD:OAS* VIII[5], 1972.)

subhepatic segment of the IVC is absent, and is associated with an azygos extension to the SVC, Leachman and associates (1973) have stated that the side of the azygos extension appears to correspond to the location of the IVC, thereby indicating the type of visceroatrial situs: solitus if right-sided and inversus if left-sided. We have the same impression, although we have not made a systematic study of this question. In addition to the laterality of the azygos extension in so-called absence of the IVC, it is noteworthy that the hepatic segment of the IVC is *not* absent in this condition. Hence the hepatic IVC, visualized by reflux of contrast following venous or selective right atrial angiocardiography, can be utilized in atrial localization.

There are at least three other good methods of atrial localization: (1) electrocardiographic; (2) angiocardiographic; and (3) surgical inspection.

The electrocardiographic method of atrial localization depends on the spatial axis of the P waves. We have found this to be reliable except when supraventricular arrhythmias coexist. When the P waves suggest situs inversus (negative P wave in lead I, etc.), one should also think of the asplenia syndrome. In asplenia, there is a high incidence of bilateral superior venae cavae, presumably with bilateral sinoatrial (SA) nodes (Van Mierop et al., 1964). The frequent similarity of the P waves in asplenia and in situs inversus appears to reflect the high incidence of left SVC and left SA node in asplenia. When the chest x-ray suggests one type of visceroatrial situs and the P waves suggest the other type, this dichotomy should suggest the possibility of asplenia or polysplenia.

The angiocardiographic method of atrial localization utilizes not only the cavae and the pulmonary veins, but also the shape of the atrial appendages, which usually is distinctive and different. The right atrial appendage is relatively large, broad, and pyramidal (Figure 36–3*A* and *B*). By contrast, the left atrial appendage is relatively small, narrow, and tubular—like the map of Central America, or a pointing finger (Figure 3*C* and *D*). These characteristic differences in the shape of RA and LA reflect differences in the degree of incorporation of the appendage into the body (main cavity) of the atrium. In the RA, the appendage is incorporated into the cavity to a major degree; hence the large, broad, pyramidal shape of the RA appendage. In the LA, the appendage is incorporated minimally—almost not at all—into the body of the atrium; hence the

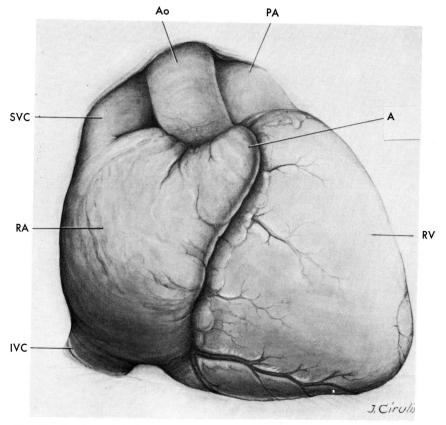

Figure 36-4. Exterior of morphologically right atrium (*RA*). Because the right atrial appendage (*RAA*) is well incorporated into the cavity or body of the RA, the shape of the RA is triangular or pyramidal, very different from that of the left atrial appendage. *SVC*, Superior vena cava; *IVC*, inferior vena cava; *RV*, morphologically right ventricle; *PA*, main pulmonary artery; *Ao*, aorta.

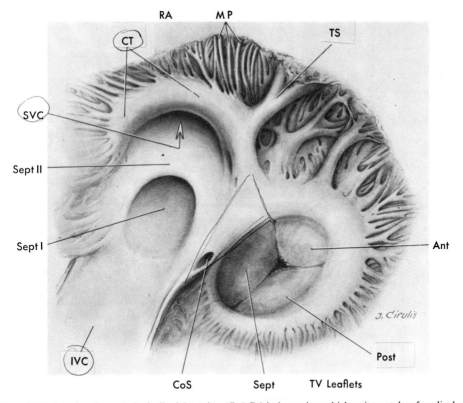

Figure 36-5. Interior of morphologically right atrium (*RA*). RA is that atrium which on its septal surface displays septum secundum (*Sept II*), also known as the superior limbic band. The inferior vena cava (*IVC*) is a highly reliable diagnostic marker of RA. The superior vena cava (*SVC*) also normally returns to the RA, but is not as diagnostically reliable as the IVC, because the SVC can drain directly into the morphologically left atrium. The coronary sinus (*CoS*) is also noteworthy. SVC, IVC, and CoS are the main structures of the venous component (sinus venosus part) of RA. Septum primum (*Sept I*) is the major component of the left venous valve (Van Praagh et al., 1969). It is directly continuous with the left wall of the IVC. The remnant of the so-called left venous valve demarcates Sept I from the IVC. The left venous valve mechanism is bifid, being composed of the small demarcating remnant known as the left venous valve, and Sept I. Since Sept I is a venous valve, it can readily be torn by balloon atrial septostomy. It grows upward and opens to the left of Sept II, for hemodynamic reasons. Sept I is the "door" opening into the LA, permitting right-to-left shunting, but preventing left-to-right shunting. Sept II is the "door jam," the crista dividens of the prenatal circulation in which the oxygenated placental venous blood returns up the IVC and divides into the via sinistra supplying the left heart and brain, and into the via dextra supplying the right heart and lower body through the ductus arteriosus. The crista terminalis (*CT*) is the muscular ridge lying immediately lateral to the entry of SVC. The crista terminalis on the inside corresponds to the sulcus terminalis or sinoatrial sulcus on the outside of RA, where the sinoatrial node is located. The crista terminalis is a terminal crest in the sense that it demarcates the termination of the smooth venous portion of the right atrium medially (sinus venosus component) from the muscular right atrial appendage laterally (derived from the primitive atrium). Note the musculi pectinati (*MP*). Pectinate means comblike. These characteristic muscles of the right atrial appendage do not crisscross, but tend to be quite parallel, like the teeth of a comb, or like a cock's comb. The tinea sagittalis (*TS*), which means sagittal worm, gives the right atrium its characteristic external shape superiorly. The leaflets of the tricuspid valve (*TV*) are anterior (*Ant*), posterior (*Post*), and septal (*Sept*).

small, narrow, tubular shape of the LA appendage.

Surgical inspection permits accurate atrial localization. As soon as the pericardium is open, a glance at the external shape of the appendages usually is sufficient to ascertain which is which (Figures 36–4 and 36–6). If both appendages are relatively large, broad, and pyramidal ("bilateral right-sidedness"), asplenia probably is present.

Atrial septal surface morphologies also can be utilized at open heart surgery:

RA is that atrium which on its septal surface displays septum secundum (the superior limbic band) (Figures 36–5 and 36–28).

LA is that atrium which on its septal surface displays septum primum, the flap valve of the foramen ovale (Figures 36–7 and 36–22).

Thus, as is shown in Figure 36–1, septum primum lies to the left of septum secundum in situs solitus, to the right of septum secundum in situs inversus, and in asplenia the septum primum is often poorly

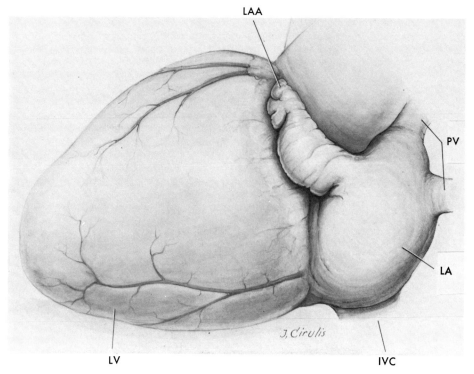

Figure 36-6. External appearance of morphologically left atrium (*LA*). The left atrial appendage (*LAA*) is relatively long and thin and tubular because it is poorly incorporated into the cavity or body of the LA. The inferior vena cava (*IVC*) opens partly into LA, in the sense that it overrides septum secundum, facilitating the via sinistra—the entry of oxygenated blood from the placenta into the left heart and thence to the brain. *PV*, Left pulmonary veins.

lateralized relative to septum secundum, or deficient; hence, situs ambiguus.

In summary, the methods of atrial localization are:

1. The visceroatrial concordances (chest x-ray, Figures 36–1 and 36–2).

2. IVC-RA concordance (catheter course, Figure 36–3, or venous angiocardiography).

3. Atrial shapes (angiocardiography, Figure 36–3, or inspection at surgery, Figures 36–4 and 36–6).

4. P waves of the electrocardiogram (Figures 36–21, 36–24, and 36–27).

5. Atrial septal surface morphologies (Figures 36–5, 36–7, 36–22, and 36–28) and the relationship between septum primum and septum secundum (Figures 36–1, 36–5, and 36–7, open heart surgery and pathology).

From the diagnostic standpoint, probably the most reliable and practical method of atrial localization is by IVC-RA concordance. However, in a given case, we often use several of the aforementioned methods.

Ventricular Localization: Types of Ventricular Loop

The precardiac mesoderm of the *cardiogenic crescent* (Figure 36–8A) migrates cephalically and medially to form the *straight cardiac tube* (Figure 36–8B). Normally, the straight tube bends to the right forming a *D-loop* (Figure 36–8C); *dextro* or D = right. Abnormally, the straight tube bends to the left forming an *L-loop* (Figure 36–8D); *levo* or L = left.

D-Loop formation places the proximal bulbus cordis (future RV) to the right of the ventricle (future LV) of the bulboventricular loop, resulting in normally interrelated ventricles (Figure 36–9). L-Loop formation places the proximal bulbus cordis (future RV) to the left of the ventricle (future LV) of the bulboventricular loop, resulting in ventricular inversion (Figure 36–9).

Ventricular D-loop and L-loop thus are defined as RV right-sided and as RV left-sided, respectively (Figures 36–8 and 36–9).

The mechanism underlying D-loop formation has been clarified by Manasek and associates (1971), who concluded that loop formation is due to a change in the shape of the myocardial cells. This change in cell shape depends on myofibril formation. The myofibrils appear to function as a cytoskeleton, controlling the shape of the cardiac myocytes. This protein-dependent (myofibril-dependent) change in cell shape is reflected at the organ level as D-loop formation.

Possible mechanisms of D-loop formation that have been disproved include:

1. Limitation of space within the pericardial sac: This idea has long been discredited by the observation that the heart loops if grown in vitro (explanted), with no limitation of space whatever (Bacon, 1945).

2. Embryonic hemodynamics, or flow molding: Manasek and associates (1971) found (on the suggestion of Dr. Grier Monroe) that culturing chick embryos in a high K$^+$ medium, completely inhibiting the heartbeat, did not prevent looping. D-Loop formation occurred in an apparently entirely normal fashion in the potassium-arrested embryonic chick heart.

3. Differential cell growth, left side greater than right: This concept was disproved by colchicine (Manasek et al., 1971). Arrest of mitosis by colchicine did not influence D-loop formation.

Only by disrupting cardiac myofibril formation with cytochalasin B were Manasek and associates (1971) able to prevent cardiac loop formation. When cytochalasin B was washed out, then D-looping occurred normally. When cytochalasin B was reintroduced, the embryonic heart unlooped! And when this compound was again washed out, the heart relooped! Manasek's elegant experiments, utilizing a variety of techniques (light microscopy, polarizing microscopy, electron microscopy, the scanning

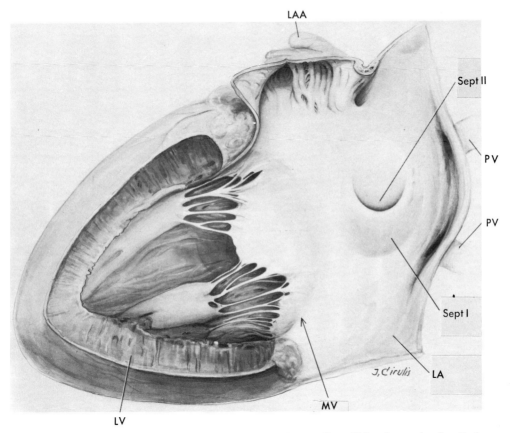

Figure 36-7. Interior of morphologically left atrium (*LA*). LA is that atrium which on its septal surface displays septum primum (*Sept I*), the flap valve of the foramen ovale, which is the major component of the left venous valve. Note that Sept I faces superiorly. The foramen ovale is the oval opening between septum secundum (*Sept II*) above and Sept I below. Note that Sept I is oriented like a sailor's hammock as seen from the left atrial aspect. Septum primum is often shown in diagrams as though it resembled a new moon. The appearance is obtained by making the ventricular apex point straight down. This remarkable misorientation of the heart, the "apex-pointing-at-the-toes syndrome," appears to have been one of the factors leading to the erroneous notion that septum primum grows downward from the dorsal and superior aspects of the atrial wall in order to occlude ostium primum. However, ostium primum is occluded not by septum primum, but by endocardial cushion tissue of the atrioventricular canal. Hence, an accurate understanding of the orientation of Sept I is important. The left atrial appendage (*LAA*) takes little part in the formation of the left atrial cavity. The pulmonary veins (*PV*) normally return to the LA. Note also the inflow aspect of the mitral valve (*MV*), in particular the deep anterior leaflet of the mitral valve (the "door") and the much shallower posterior leaflet of the mitral valve (the "door jam"), the upper and lower commissures and papillary muscles (anterolateral and posteromedial, respectively), the normal interpapillary muscle distance, and the well-formed interchordal spaces. However, the morphology of an atrioventricular valve corresponds to the ventricle of entry, the left ventricle (*LV*), rather than to the atrium of exit (*LA*). Hence, it is not intended to suggest that the MV is an essential morphologic characteristic of the LA.

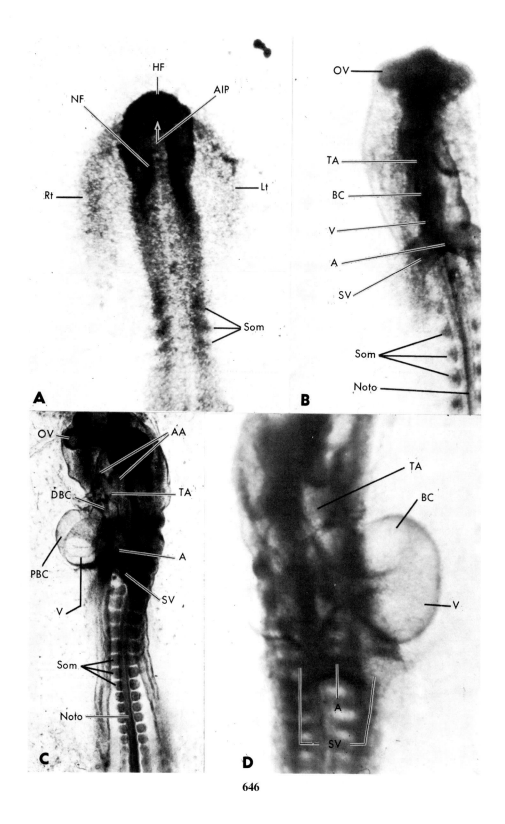

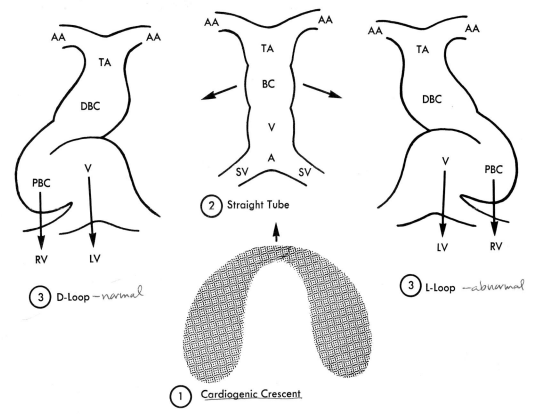

Figure 36-9. The three major stages in cardiac loop formation: (*1*) the cardiogenic crescent stage; (*2*) the straight tube stage; and (*3*) the cardiac loop stage, normally to the right (D-loop) or abnormally to the left (L-loop). *AA*, Arterial arches; *TA*, truncus arteriosus; *DBC*, distal bulbus cordis; *PBC*, proximal bulbus cordis; *V*, ventricle; *A*, atrium; *SV*, sinus venosus. (Modified from Van Praagh, R.: The segmental approach to diagnosis in congenital heart disease. In Bergsma, D. [ed.]: Part XV, "The Cardiovascular System." Baltimore: Williams & Wilkins for The National Foundation–March of Dimes, *BD:OAS* VIII [5] 1972.)

electron microscope, and the analysis of cell orientations by computer) all appear to support the aforementioned interpretation.

Since protein (e.g., myofibril) formation is now known to be under genetic control, this being part of the fascinating DNA-RNA story well summarized by one of its discoverers, Watson (1965), we think that we may be seeing the first glimpse of the long-sought bridge between the gene, on the one hand, and the *morphogenesis of organs*, on the other. Cell shape change, depending on cytoskeletons of various protein types, may well prove to be at least one of the mechanisms of widespread importance linking the genome to organic morphogenesis.

Figure 36-8. Stages in cardiac loop formation, explanted chick embryos viewed from the ventral aspect.

A. Cardiogenic crescent composed of left (*Lt*) and right (*Rt*) halves of precardiac mesoderm that are continuous across the midline, resembling an upside-down horseshoe. *HF*, Head fold; *AIP*, anterior intestinal portal; *NF*, neural fold; *Som*, somites.

B. Straight tube stage. *TA*, Truncus arteriosus; *BC*, bulbus cordis; *V*, ventricle; *A*, atrium; *SV*, sinus venosus; *OV*, optic vesicle; *Noto*, notochord.

C. D-loop. The proximal bulbus cordis (*PBC*) lies to the right of the ventricle (*V*) of the bulboventricular loop; due to looping of the straight heart tube to the right (*dextro*, or D). PBC will give rise to RV, and V will give rise to LV. Thus, D-loop formation results in normally interrelated ventricles, RV lying to the right of LV. Sinus venosus (*SV*) leads into the atrium (*A*). The distal bulbus cordis (*DBC*), which forms the infundibulum or conus, leads to the truncus arteriosus (*TA*), from which the aorta and pulmonary artery form, and TA leads to the arterial arches (*AA*).

D. L-loop. Looping or folding of the straight heart tube to the left (*levo*, or L) is believed to result in ventricular inversion, because the bulbus cordis (*BC*), from which RV develops, comes to lie to the left of the ventricle (*V*), from which the LV develops. Other abbreviations as previously.

(Reproduced from Van Praagh, R.: The segmental approach to diagnosis in congenital heart disease. In Bergsma, D. [ed.]: Part XV, "The Cardiovascular System." Baltimore: Williams & Wilkins for The National Foundation–March of Dimes, *BD:OAS* VIII[5], 1972.)

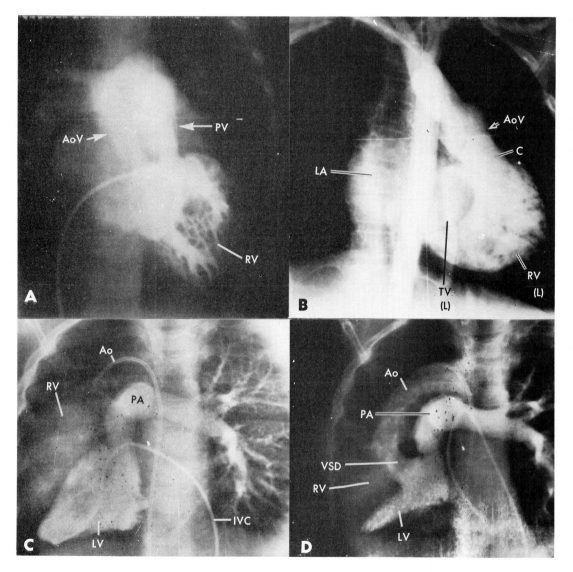

Figure 36-10. Angiocardiographic features of morphologically right ventricle, (*RV*) and of morphologically left ventricle (*LV*).

A. Note the coarsely trabeculated, globular RV in this case of the Taussig-Bing malformation. The aortic valve (*AoV*) and pulmonary valve (*PV*) are at approximately the same height and are side by side, as is indicated by the shadow of the conal septum (parietal band) that runs approximately sagittally separating the aortic and pulmonary outflow tracts.

B. Corrected transposition in situs solitus, with selective injection into the left-sided morphologically right ventricle, RV (L). The globular configuration (shape) and the coarse trabeculation are evident. The conus (*C*) beneath the L-transposed aortic valve (*AoV*) and the left-sided tricuspid valve, TV (L), are noteworthy. Considerable regurgitation is occurring through the left-sided TV into the left atrium (*LA*), indicating tricuspid regurgitation, left-sided. The catheter is not through the tricuspid valve orifice, this selective injection having been made through a retrograde arterial catheter passed through the AoV.

C. Corrected transposition in situs inversus. A venous catheter has been passed up the left-sided inferior vena cava (*IVC*) and into the left-sided ventricle, which displays a foot-shaped configuration in diastole and a smooth or relatively untrabeculated appearance, highly characteristic of the morphologically left ventricle (*LV*). The transposed pulmonary artery (*PA*) arises from the LV. By exclusion the right-sided ventricle must be the morphologically right ventricle (*RV*) and a retrograde arterial catheter marks the course of the D-transposed aorta (*Ao*) and indicates the presence of a right aortic arch, not surprising in situs inversus.

D. Same case as in C. Note the systolic appearance of LV that resembles a beaver's tail. The ventricular septal defect (*VSD*) and the stenotic subpulmonary conus beneath the pulmonary valve are clearly visualized. All of these angiocardiograms are in the posteroanterior projection.

(*A* and *B* reproduced from Van Praagh, R.: The segmental approach to diagnosis in congenital heart disease.

Methods of ventricular localization may be summarized as follows:

1. Ventricular angiocardiography.
2. Electrocardiographic interpretation.
3. Deductions based on the arteries.

Selective biventricular angiocardiography is (assuming excellent technique) the best method of ventricular localization. Direct visualization of the distinctive and different internal morphologies of RV (Figure 36–10*A* and *B*) and of LV (Figure 36–10*C* and *D*) is, we believe, the most reliable method of identifying the ventricles. RV is globular in shape (Figure 36–10*A* and *B*), whereas LV is foot-shaped in diastole (Figure 36–10*C*) and tail-shaped in systole (Figure 36–10*D*). RV is coarsely trabeculated (Figure 36–10*A* and *B*), whereas LV is finely trabeculated or nontrabeculated (Figure 36–10*C* and *D*). Often one can see the moderator band of RV, dividing the apex into an inflow tract apex behind the moderator band, and an outflow tract apex in front of the moderator band; this is most clearly seen in two-chambered RV (anomalous muscle bundles RV).

However, it must be added that ventricular hypertrophy, hypoplasia, and unaccustomed locations (as in dextrocardia and the other cardiac malpositions) may result in confusing variations from the aforementioned typical configurations (shapes) and patterns of trabeculation. For example, LV may appear coarsely trabeculated if viewed from its apex towards its base, because of the large papillary muscles arising from the left ventricular free wall that can be visualized in this unaccustomed projection.

The electrocardiographic method of ventricular localization of Sodi-Pallares and associates (1959) and Portillo and associates (1959) is based on the morphologies of the unipolar QRS complexes, which in turn are related to the sequence of ventricular activation. We think that this method, while interesting and useful, is not as reliable as the angiocardiographic methods mentioned above, and to follow. Nonetheless, the paper by Portillo and associates (1959) merits careful study, we think. Although an understandably unpopular view among radiologists, we think that difficult angiocardiograms should be studied with the electrocardiogram (ECG) in hand. One should ask the question, "Which ventricle is *that*?" both of the angiocardiogram and of the ECG. In terms of ventricular localization, the ECG often is more helpful after the angiocardiogram than before it. In difficult cases, the ECG and the angio should be studied *together* (rather than examining each in isolation, often by different physicians). Examples of the ECG method of ventricular localization will be given subsequently. Abnormalities of ventricular conduction make the electrocardiographic method of ventricular localization unreliable.

The arterial method of ventricular localization depends on the angiocardiographic demonstration of the relationship between the aortic and pulmonary valves, and on the origin and distribution of the coronary arteries (Figure 36–11).

The loop rule (Van Praagh et al., 1964) summarizes the usual relationships between the great arteries and the ventricles (Figure 36–11):

1. The usual or solitus type of normally related great arteries, D-transposition, and D-malposition of the great arteries (transposed or malposed aortic valve to the right—*dextro* or D—relative to the transposed or malposed pulmonary valve) usually are associated with a D-loop (RV right-sided).

2. The inverted or mirror-image type of normally related great arteries, L-transposition, and L-malposition of the great arteries (transposed or malposed aortic valve to the left—*levo* or L—relative to the transposed or malposed pulmonary valve) usually are associated with an L-loop (RV left-sided).

Hence, the loop rule (Figure 36–11) is a summary of the usual arterioventricular relations, which may be summarized informally as follows:

1. The usual type of normal relationship between the great arteries, the usual type of transposition, and the usual type of malposition of the great arteries are associated in the majority of cases with normally interrelated ventricles.

2. The inverted type of normally related great arteries, inverted (L-) transposition, and inverted malposition of the great arteries are associated in the majority of cases with inverted ventricles.

It should be noted parenthetically that *malposition of the great arteries* indicates an abnormal relationship between the great arteries, but in which the great arteries are not transposed. They are malposed. Examples of malposition of the great arteries include double-outlet right ventricle, double-outlet left ventricle, and the anatomically corrected relationship. In none of these malpositions of the great arteries is transposition present: the aorta does not originate above the morphologically right ventricle, and the pulmonary artery does not also arise above the morphologically left ventricle. Thus, although transposition of the great arteries is not present in these conditions in any literally accurate sense, nonetheless the great arteries certainly are malposed. Transposition could be regarded as a type of malposition of the great arteries. However, when transposition is present, it is customary to call it that. The term and concept of malposition of the great arteries make it possible to use the term and concept of transposition of the great arteries accurately.

Exceptions to the loop rule are quite common. This is to be expected because the loop rule is merely a statement of the usual. Any unusual type of arterial-to-ventricular relationship is thus likely to be an

---

[*Legend continued from facing page.*]
In Bergsma, D. [ed.]: Part XV, "The Cardiovascular System." Baltimore: Williams & Wilkins for The National Foundation–March of Dimes, *BD: OAS* VIII[5], 1972. *C* and *D* reproduced from Van Praagh, R., et al.: Diagnosis of the anatomic types of congenital dextrocardia. *Am. J. Cardiol.*, **15**:234, 1965.)

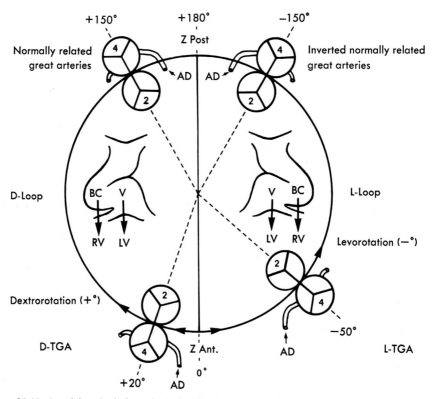

Figure 36-11. Arterial method of ventricular localization. The semilunar interrelationship, plus the origin and distribution of the coronary arteries, demonstrated angiocardiographically, can be very helpful in ventricular localization. Normally related great arteries and D-transposition of the great arteries (D-TGA) usually are associated with a ventricular D-loop (RV right-sided). Inverted normally related great arteries and L-transposition of the great arteries (L-TGA) usually are associated with a ventricular L-loop (RV left-sided). This statement of the usual arterial-to-ventricular relationships is known as the *loop rule*. The anterior descending coronary artery (*AD*) arises from the left coronary artery with a D-loop, both with normally related great arteries and with D-TGA, and from the right coronary artery with an L-loop, both with inverted normally related great arteries with L-TGA. Thus the origin of AD from the left or right coronary artery can be very helpful in ventricular localization. Also, the distribution of the coronary arteries over the epicardial surface of RV and LV is highly characteristic and therefore diagnostically useful. (Modified from Van Praagh, R.: The segmental approach to diagnosis in congenital heart disease. In Bergsma, D. [ed.]: Part XV, "The Cardiovascular System." Baltimore: Williams & Wilkins for The National Foundation–March of Dimes, *BD:OAS* VIII[5], 1972.)

exception to the loop rule. Perhaps any statement of the usual, such as the loop rule, needs no defence. However, Carr and associates (1968) have stated that there are so many exceptions that this "rule" is not helpful. One of the points that they were making is that selective biventricular angiocardiography is the best way of identifying the ventricles and is highly desirable in complex congenital heart disease. We have always agreed with that. The purpose of the loop rule has been to help identify the ventricles when selective ventriculography is, for any reason, less than clear-cut. We all know that even in the best of institutions, there are plenty of angiocardiograms that are difficult to interpret with certainty in terms of ventricular configuration and trabeculation. So the loop rule is designed to facilitate ventricular localization in such "problem cases."

How good (or bad) is the loop rule? Exceptions to

the loop rule have occurred with the following frequencies:

1. In dextrocardia, an anatomic study 4 percent (2/51 cases) (Van Praagh et al., 1964).

2. In single ventricle, an anatomic study, 8 percent (5/60 cases) (Van Praagh et al., 1964).

3. In complete D-transposition, an angiocardiographic study, 17 percent (19/109 cases) (Carr et al., 1968).

4. In transposition of the great arteries as a whole, not confined to complete D-transposition only, 6 percent (7/114 cases) (Barcia et al., 1967) and 9 percent (6/70 cases) (Guerin et al., 1970). The accuracy of the loop rule in angiocardiographic studies of transposition of the great arteries (TGA) is summarized in somewhat greater detail in Table 36–1.

Hence, the incidence of incorrect prediction plus nonprediction of the locations of RV and LV by the

Table 36-1. ACCURACY OF THE LOOP RULE

AUTHORS	CORRECT		INCORRECT		EQUIVOCAL‡	
	No.	*Percent*	*No.*	*Percent*	*No.*	*Percent*
Carr et al. (1968)*	75/109	69	19/109	17	15/109	14
Guerin et al. (1970)†	41/70	58	6/70	9	23/70	33

* TGA in D-loop only.
† TGA in D-and L-loops.
‡ Equivocal = *A*-TGA, aortic valve directly anterior to pulmonary valve, hence loop rule nonpredictive.

loop rule proved to be much higher than is desirable (Table 36-1): 31 percent (Carr et al., 1968) and 42 percent (Guerin et al., 1970).

The coronary arteries can significantly improve the accuracy of the arterial method of ventricular localization. With a D-loop, the coronary arteries are not inverted, whereas with an L-loop they are. For example, with a D-loop, the anterior descending coronary artery arises from the *left* coronary, both with normally related great arteries and with D-transposition (Figure 36-11). But with an L-loop, the anterior descending originates from the *right* coronary artery, both with inverted normally related great arteries and with L-transposition (Figure

36-11). Given good coronary visualization (which is unusual except with aortic root injection or with selective coronary arteriography), the distribution of the coronary arteries is very helpful in localizing the ventricles: the preventricular branches, and particularly the marginal branch, are very characteristic of RV (Figure 36-12); and the diagonals to the large anterolateral and posteromedial papillary muscle groups are very characteristic of LV (Figure 36-14).

It has been our experience repeatedly, in difficult cases, that the coronaries solve the problem of which ventricle is which. For example, let us say, there is a case of dextrocardia with situs solitus of the viscera and atria. The aorta arises from the left border of the

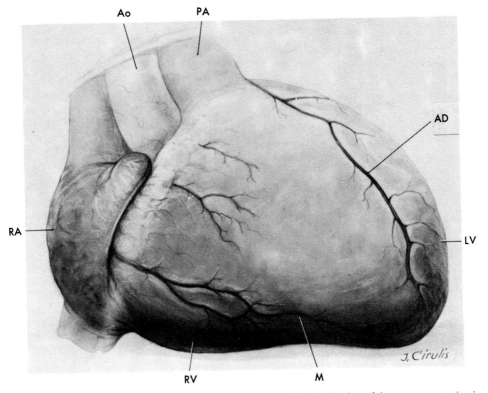

Figure 36-12. Exterior of morphologically right ventricle (*RV*). The distribution of the coronary arteries, in particular the marginal branch (*M*) of the right coronary artery, is very highly characteristic of RV. The conal and preventricular branches are also characteristic. *Ao*, Aorta; *PA*, pulmonary artery; *AD*, anterior descending coronary artery; *RA*, morphologically right atrium; *LV*, morphologically left ventricle.

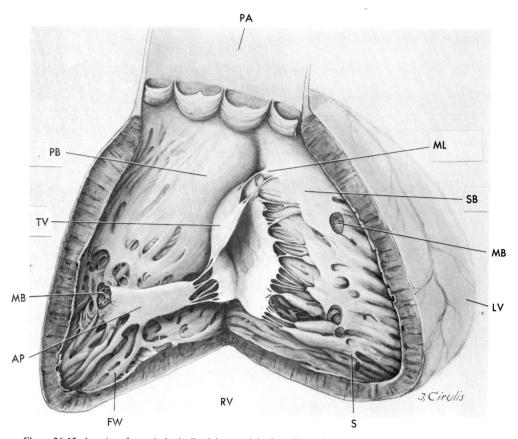

Figure 36-13. Interior of morphologically right ventricle (*RV*). The trabeculae carneae (fleshy ridges) of RV are relatively coarse, few, and straight, compared with those of the LV. The right ventricular papillary muscles are relatively small; they obscure the interior of the right ventricular free wall to a minor degree, making right ventriculotomy readily possible; and they arise from both the free wall (*FW*) and septal surfaces (*S*). The anterolateral papillary muscle group (*AP*), the papillary muscle of the conus, or muscle of Lancisi (*ML*) or muscle of Luschka, and the chordal insertions from the septal leaflet of the tricuspid valve (*TV*) into the septal band (*SB*) are noteworthy. The moderator band (*MB*) conveys the right bundle branch and spans the right ventricular cavity from the septal band to the superior aspect of the anterolateral papillary muscle. The tricuspid leaflets vary in number from two to four, but are all of approximately the same depth, although the anterior leaflet is usually somewhat deeper than the others. The tricuspid valve is an inflow valve only. The right ventricular outflow tract normally is formed by the parietal band (*PB*) and by the SB. The PB forms a crista supraventricularis (supraventricular crest), which normally separates the three pulmonary valve leaflets from the tricuspid valve leaflets. The right bundle branch of the ventricular conduction system runs along the inferior surface of the septal band and across the moderator band to reach the anterolateral papillary muscle on the right ventricular free wall. This right bundle branch is a superior radiation. In the right ventricle there is no inferior radiation. The distribution of the ventricular conduction system corresponds to that of the large papillary muscle groups, and in the right ventricle there is only one papillary muscle group of any size, namely the anterolateral (*AP*). The right ventricle normally is supplied mainly by one coronary artery only, the right coronary artery. Essentially all of the aforementioned features are different when one compares RV with LV. Note the "suture" or demarcation between the parietal band and the septal band, accurately indicating that the parietal and septal bands are two different conal structures, rather than two different parts of one structure, the crista supraventricularis as it is classically defined. Only the parietal band forms a supraventricular crest, the septal band being an integral part of the right ventricular septal surface anterosuperiorly. The parietal and septal bands separate or dissociate at this demarcation or "suture," in many forms of congenital heart disease (tetralogy, truncus, transposition, double-outlet RV and LV). The infundibulum, which means funnel, or the conus, which means cone, is regarded as an independent part of the heart, not an intrinsic or inseparable part of the morphologically right ventricle. Normally, of course, the infundibulum (parietal band, septal band, and related subsemilunar conal free wall) is related to the RV. The true right ventricle is regarded as the right ventricular sinus body or inflow tract, that portion lying below the septal and moderator bands—that part which is absent in single left ventricle with an infundibular outlet chamber. This is the true RV from a developmental standpoint. From an anatomic standpoint, however, it is customary to regard the infundibulum as a part of the RV because this normally is the case. In terms of definitive postnatal anatomy, it is of interest to note that there really are two right ventricular apices, as anomalous muscle bundles of the right ventricle illustrate. The apex of the true RV, of the right

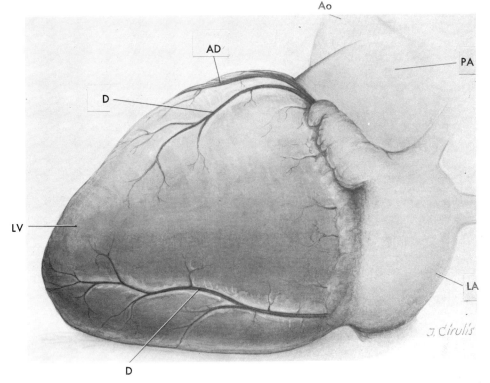

Figure 36-14. Exterior appearance of the morphologically left ventricle (*LV*). The diagonals (*D*) to the upper and lower papillary muscle groups (the anterolateral and posteromedial papillary muscles) are very highly characteristic of LV and are thus of assistance in ventricular localization. Other abbreviations as previously.

heart, to the left of the pulmonary artery, which is stenotic. Both great arteries originate above the left-sided ventricle. There is an unresolved debate concerning which ventricle is which. Neither ventricle has a clear-cut and absolutely definite configuration or trabeculation. The semilunar interrelationship (loop rule) suggests an L-loop. But some think that the left-sided ventricle is just too smooth to be an RV (and everyone knows that the loop rule isn't always right!).

Let us suppose that you are asked to see the case. You can see exactly why everyone has assumed this or that position (D-loop or L-loop). Then you see the coronaries light up on the cine, or you spot them on the large films. The anterior descending comes from the *right* coronary artery. Then you see that the

circumflex branch is right-sided. The coronary *origins* and *distributions* are definitely inverted. Problem solved: L-loop, definitely.

When the aortic valve is—or appears to be—directly in front of the pulmonary valve, and the ventricular architecture is debatable, again the coronary origins and distributions solve the problem, in our experience. Hence, we are sure that most of the equivocal cases listed in Table 36–1 can readily be resolved by the coronary arteries.

However, the coronary method of ventricular identification is not 100 percent reliable; but then, very few things are! The *origins* of the coronary arteries occasionally may not indicate the type of ventricular loop correctly. For example, in double-outlet right ventricle with situs solitus of the viscera

<hr>

[*Legend continued from facing page.*]
ventricular inflow tract, lies inferior and posterior to the septal and moderator band. The outflow tract apex, the apex of the infundibulum, lies anterior and superior to the moderator band. Speaking anatomically, these two right ventricular apices are well seen and are clearly separated in anomalous muscle bundles of the right ventricle, i.e., in two-chambered RV produced by a high and obstructive moderator band. It may well be that the true RV (the inflow tract posteroinferior to the septal and moderator bands) is a conal specialization, a right ventricular outpouching that was one of the adaptations associated with the development of air breathing. Although the parietal band may dissociate widely from the septal band and right ventricle, at the "suture" or demarcation shown between these two structures in the normal heart, it is interesting that the septal band never dissociates from the RV, to the best of our knowledge. The true RV is the sinus or body that outpouches below the septal band. Hence, the distinction between conal and right ventricular structures, while customary, may in a phylogenetic sense be far from sharp, if, as seems likely, the right ventricular sinus is a conal specialization.

and atria, ventricular D-loop, and L-malposition of the great arteries, the anterior descending coronary artery can arise from the right coronary artery (instead of from the left coronary artery as is usual with a D-loop). Even the *distributions* of the coronary arteries can defy interpretation as, for example, in some cases of single (common) ventricle. Nonetheless, the coronary method of ventricular localization is very useful. In difficult cases, we *combine all available methods* of ventricular identification. When this is done, almost always a confident diagnostic consensus emerges.

The arterial method of localizing the ventricles thus involves two main considerations (Figure 36–11):

1. The relationships between the great arteries at the semilunar valves.

2. The origins and distributions of the coronary arteries.

The echocardiographic method of ventricular

identification has been pioneered by Solinger, Elbl, and Minhas (1974). These workers have applied the segmental approach to the diagnosis of congenital heart disease to echocardiography. For example, when the aortic valve lies to the right of the pulmonary valve, one usually is dealing with a ventricular D-loop (Figure 36–11). The aortic valve is to the right and posterior with normally related great arteries, to the right and side-by-side with tetralogy of Fallot and double-outlet right ventricle, and to the right and anterior with D-transposition. Thus, both normally and abnormally, the aorta is usually right-sided with a D-loop (Figure 36–11). Conversely, the aortic valve usually is left-sided with an L-loop (Figure 36–11): posterior and to the left with the inverted type of normally related great arteries, side-by-side and to the left with tetralogy and double-outlet right ventricle (left-sided), and anterior and to the left with L-transposition.

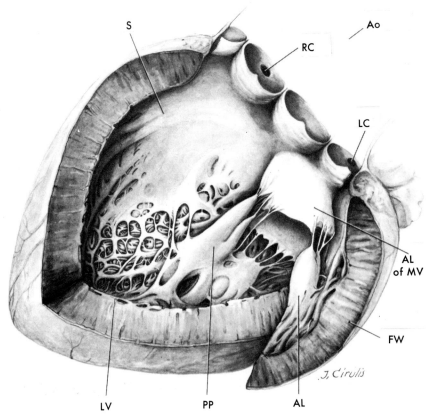

Figure 36-15. Interior of morphologically left ventricle (*LV*). The superior septal surface (*S*) is smooth, whereas the inferior septal surface displays a lattice-like mesh of numerous, fine, oblique trabeculae carneae. The anterolateral (*AL*) and posteromedial papillary muscle groups (*PP*) are large, originate only from the left ventricular free wall (*FW*), and obscure the interior of this free wall to a major degree, making left ventriculotomy difficult except at the apex or high paraseptally. The absence of a muscular subaortic infundibulum or conus permits direct fibrous continuity between the aortic leaflets and the anterior leaflet (*AL*) of the mitral valve (*MV*). The commissure separating the noncoronary and left coronary (*LC*) aortic leaflets is directly above the middle of the anterior leaflet of the mitral valve. The commissure between the noncoronary and right coronary (*RC*) aortic leaflets lies directly above the pars membranacea septi. The superior and inferior radiations of the left bundle can often be seen faintly as they course over the smooth portion of the left ventricular septal surface toward the upper and lower papillary muscle groups, respectively.

When the aortic valve is to the right of the pulmonary valve, be the semilunar interrelationship normal or abnormal, this may be called a *D-conotruncus* (indicating that the aortic valve is to the right or *dextro* relative to the pulmonary valve).

When the aortic valve is to the left of the pulmonary valve, be the semilunar interrelationship normal or abnormal, this may be called an *L-conotruncus* (indicating that the aortic valve is to the left or *levo* relative to the pulmonary valve).

The tricuspid valve's septal leaflet normally does not separate far from the right ventricular septal surface because the septal leaflet of the tricuspid valve is attached to the right ventricular septal surface (Figure 36–13). By contrast, the septal or medial leaflet of the mitral valve does separate widely from the left ventricular septal surface because, normally, the septal leaflet of the mitral valve does not attach to

the left ventricular septal surface (Figure 36–15). These differences can be elicited echocardiographically. Also, semilunar-atrioventricular contiguity or separation can be appreciated echocardiographically. Since the diameter of the pulmonary artery is normally somewhat greater than that of the aorta, and since the component of the second heart sound associated with pulmonary valve closure usually follows the component associated with aortic valve closure, it may be possible echocardiographically to determine which great artery is which. Then, if one demonstrates aortic-mitral contiguity, normally related great arteries is probable (Figure 36–16*A* and *B*). If one finds pulmonary-mitral contiguity, then transposition (D- or L-) is probable (Figure 36–16*C* and *D*). If one finds semilunar-atrioventricular discontiguity—wide separation—then a bilateral conus (Figure 36–*E* and

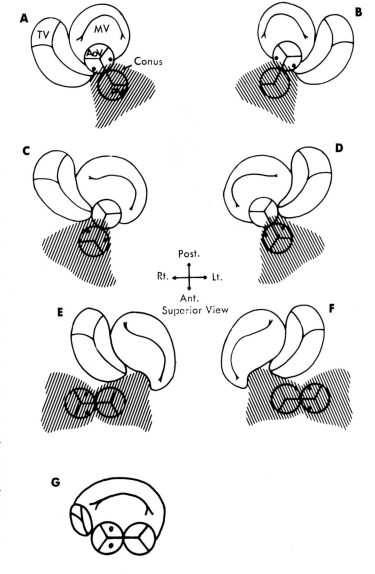

Figure 36-16. Anatomic types of conus or infundibulum. The conal or infundibular muscle is indicated by crosshatching. The normal subpulmonary conus with normally related great arteries, both with the D-loop (*A*) and with the L-loop (*B*), prevents fibrous continuity between the pulmonary valve (*PV*) and the tricuspid valve (*TV*) and mitral valve (*MV*). The normal absence of subaortic conal musculature permits fibrous continuity between the aortic valve (*AoV*) and the anterior leaflet of the mitral valve and with the tricuspid valve by way of the pars membranacea septi. The subaortic conus, with absence of subpulmonary muscular conus, is characteristic of typical transpositions both with the D-loop (*C*) and with the L-loop (*D*). The subaortic conal musculature prevents aortic-atrioventricular fibrous continuity and the absence of subpulmonary conal muscle permits pulmonary-mitral direct fibrous continuity. The bilateral conus beneath both the aortic valve and the pulmonary valve prevents semilunar-atrioventricular fibrous continuity and is shown both with the D-loop (*E*) and with the L-loop (*F*). In *G*, absence of subsemilunar conal musculature permits fibrous continuity between both the aortic and the pulmonary valve and the atrioventricular valves as in the case of double-outlet left ventricle with intact interventricular septum of Paul and associates (1970). Absence of subsemilunar conal musculature has not as yet been found with an L-loop.

F) with double-outlet right ventricle would bear serious consideration. If one were to demonstrate aortic-mitral and pulmonary-mitral contiguity (Figure 36–16*G*), then double-outlet left ventricle would merit careful consideration.

At the present time, echocardiography is becoming more and more reliable as experience accrues and equipment improves. However, echocardiography is still far from being highly reliable. Echocardiography is nonetheless a very important noninvasive form of investigation. At present, echo is a valuable adjunct to cardiac catheterization and angiocardiography. In complex congenital heart disease, angiocardiography remains our diagnostic Supreme Court—the court of last appeal. But echocardiography is becoming more and more helpful in many ways, not only in making the diagnosis, but also in follow-up.

In summary, the principal methods of localizing the ventricles are:

1. Selective ventriculography.
2. The arterial method (the various semilunar interrelationships, and the origins and courses of the coronary arteries).
3. Deductive electrocardiography.
4. Deductive echocardiography.

The accuracy of the various angiocardiographic methods of ventricular localization depends on a variety of factors that includes: (1) the technical quality of the angiocardiograms; (2) the sites of injection; and (3) one's understanding of ventricular anatomy. Although enormously important, nothing further will be said here concerning angiocardiographic technique. The interested reader should consult experts in angiocardiography such as Dr. Alberto Barcia (1972). Regarding sites of injection, selective injections into both ventricles should be routine. If one does this, then one's incidence of unpleasant, often left-sided surprises at operation will be reduced. Concerning ventricular anatomy, the reader is invited to study Figures 36–12 to 36–15 with care. Later on, these drawings are supplemented by photographs (Figures 36–22, 36–25, and 36–28).

Types of Conotruncus

The conotruncus (infundibulum and great arteries) may be classified in terms of the location of the muscular conus or infundibulum into four major anatomic types (Figure 36–16):

1. Subpulmonary.
2. Subaortic.
3. Bilateral (subaortic and subpulmonary).
4. Absent or rudimentary (virtually no muscular conus beneath either great artery).

The four anatomic types of conus, and the various conotruncal malformations now known to be associated with each, are summarized in Figure 36–17. This material has been presented in detail elsewhere (Van Praagh, 1973); in the interests of brevity, the following is a résumé only.

The Subpulmonary Conus. Subpulmonary conal musculature, without a muscular subaortic conus, prevents pulmonary-atrioventricular fibrous continuity and permits aortic-mitral fibrous continuity (Figures 36–16 and 36–17). The subpulmonary conus (Figure 36–17) is associated with *normally related great arteries* in situs solitus and in situs inversus.

Underdevelopment of the subpulmonary conus appears to result in the *tetralogy of Fallot* (Van Praagh et al., 1970) (Figure 36–17).

Atresia of the subpulmonary conus plus a truncal septal defect is believed to result in *truncus arteriosus communis* (Van Praagh and Van Praagh, 1965) (Figure 36–17).

Hypoplasia and leftward displacement of the conal septum (parietal band or crista supraventricularis), producing subaortic narrowing, often is present with *interruption of the aortic arch* (Van Praagh et al., 1971).

Isolated ventricular inversion (Van Praagh and Van Praagh, 1966) is situs solitus of viscera and atria, a ventricular L-loop, and the solitus type of normally related great arteries. *Isolated ventricular noninversion* (Espino-Vela et al., 1970) is situs inversus of the viscera and atria, a ventricular D-loop, and the inverted type of normally related great arteries. Both isolated ventricular inversion and isolated ventricular noninversion have normally related great arteries and hence have a subpulmonary conus with aortic-mitral fibrous continuity (Figures 36–17 and 36–18).

These two entities constitute *isolated ventricular discordance*: isolated ventricular inversion in situs solitus, and isolated ventricular noninversion in situs inversus (Figure 36–18).

Since isolated ventricular discordance is characterized by a subpulmonary conus and normally related great arteries (relative to the ventricles, ventricular septum, and atrioventricular canal), it is therefore not surprising that isolated ventricular discordance is subject to all the woes that the subpulmonary conus is heir to, namely, pulmonary infundibular stenosis, or atresia, and a ventricular septal defect ("tetralogy of Fallot").

From the physiologic standpoint, isolated ventricular discordance functions like complete (physiologically uncorrected) transposition of the great arteries (Figure 36–18), and surgically should be treated as such. Cases with pulmonary outflow tract stenosis or atresia and ventricular septal defect should be treated surgically like transposition with pulmonary stenosis or atresia and ventricular septal defect.

It should be added that de la Cruz and her colleagues (Espino-Vela et al., 1970) prefer somewhat longer designations. Instead of speaking of isolated ventricular noninversion (which appeals to us because it is clear and brief), de la Cruz prefers the longer designation, ventricular inversion without transposition of the great vessels in situs inversus. Her abbreviation for this situation is: ventricular inversion in situs inversus. In other words, when the morphologically right ventricle is right-sided and the morphologically left-ventricle is left-sided in a patient

Conotruncal Correlations

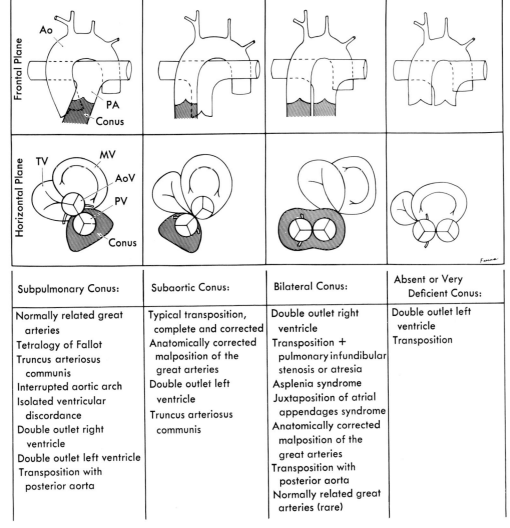

Subpulmonary Conus:	Subaortic Conus:	Bilateral Conus:	Absent or Very Deficient Conus:
Normally related great arteries Tetralogy of Fallot Truncus arteriosus communis Interrupted aortic arch Isolated ventricular discordance Double outlet right ventricle Double outlet left ventricle Transposition with posterior aorta	Typical transposition, complete and corrected Anatomically corrected malposition of the great arteries Double outlet left ventricle Truncus arteriosus communis	Double outlet right ventricle Transposition + pulmonary infundibular stenosis or atresia Asplenia syndrome Juxtaposition of atrial appendages syndrome Anatomically corrected malposition of the great arteries Transposition with posterior aorta Normally related great arteries (rare)	Double outlet left ventricle Transposition

Figure 36-17. What types of conus are associated with what types of relationships between the great arteries and between the great arteries and the ventricles? This figure summarizes all the presently known conotruncal correlations.

with situs inversus of the viscera and atria, de la Cruz calls this ventricular inversion for situs inversus. The difficulty is that other observers say: No. The ventricles are not inverted, whereas the atria and great arteries are inverted (Figure 36–18). We prefer to speak of isolated ventricular noninversion rather than isolated ventricular inversion in situs inversus because the former is briefer and we think clearer. However, we also think that de la Cruz's terminology is perfectly acceptable because it is accurate. This and other terminologies are included here because we think it is helpful to be familiar with as many of these "languages" as possible.

A rare form of *TGA with a posterior aorta* can have a very short subpulmonary conus, with or without

pulmonary stenosis (Van Praagh et al., 1971) (Figure 36–18).

Double-outlet left ventricle of the "tetralogy type" (Kerr et al., 1971) also has a very short and stenotic subpulmonary conus and a subaortic VSD (Figure 36–18).

The Subaortic Conus. The presence of subaortic conal musculature prevents aortic-atrioventricular fibrous continuity and permits pulmonary-mitral fibrous continuity (Figures 36–16 and 36–17).

Typical TGA, complete and corrected, in both types of situs, has a subaortic conus, without subpulmonary conus (Figure 36–18).

Anatomically corrected malposition of the great arteries (Van Praagh and Van Praagh, 1966; Van

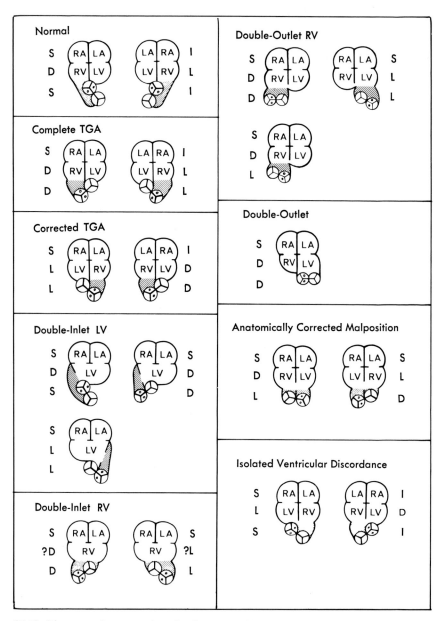

Figure 36-18. Diagrammatic presentation of various types of human heart, i.e., segmental combinations and interrelations. Asplenia and some types of single ventricle have been omitted. Also omitted is isolated atrial inversion: situs solitus of the viscera, situs inversus of the atria, D-loop, and normally related great arteries, i.e. {S, I, D, S} (Clarkson et al., 1972; see Table 36-2).

Praagh et al., 1971) also can have a subaortic conus only. We have studied such a case with situs solitus, D-loop, L-malposition of the great arteries, and VSD (Figure 36–18).

The Bilateral Conus. The presence of conal musculature beneath both the aortic and pulmonary valves prevents any semilunar-atrioventricular fibrous continuity (Figures 36–16 and 36–17).

A bilateral conus occurs with *TGA* with pulmonary infundibular stenosis or atresia and VSD. Occasionally, a bilateral conus occurs with TGA, VSD, but without pulmonary stenosis (PS) (Figure 36–18).

Double-outlet right ventricle (DORV) typically has a bilateral conus; e.g., the Taussig-Bing malformation (Taussig and Bing, 1949; Van Praagh, 1968).

The asplenia syndrome (Ivemark, 1955) often has a bilateral conus with pulmonary infundibular stenosis or atresia. DORV is the rule in asplenia, not TGA (aorta from RV, pulmonary artery from LV) (Figure 36–17).

The juxtaposition of the atrial appendages syndrome (Melhuish and Van Praagh, 1968) has a bilateral conus in the majority of cases, often with pulmonary outflow tract obstruction (Figure 36–17).

Anatomically corrected malposition of the great arteries (Van Praagh and Van Praagh, 1967) usually has a bilateral conus (Figure 36–17).

Normally related great arteries rarely can have a bilateral conus. We have studied a case with a well-developed subpulmonary conus and a very slim band of subaortic conal musculature, 1 mm wide (Van Praagh, 1972). Although this very small amount of subaortic conal musculature did not prevent an essentially normal type of aortic-mitral approximation, nonetheless it did result in aortic-mitral fibrous discontinuity (Figure 36–17).

The Absent Conus. Conal muscle can rarely be absent, or rudimentary, beneath both semilunar valves, as in the remarkable case of double-outlet left ventricle of Paul and associates (1970) (Figures 36–16 to 36–18). "Absent" conus does not mean that the conus was totally absent. Rather, it means that there was no conus beneath the semilunar valves. For example, in Paul's case, the conus was blind (atretic) and related only to the RV, the ventricular septum was intact, and both great arteries arose entirely above the LV. Thus, the conus was absent beneath the great arteries, but some conal musculature was present above the RV. Rarely, the subsemilunar conus may be sufficiently deficient in *TGA* to permit not only pulmonary-mitral fibrous continuity, but also aortic-tricuspid fibrous continuity.

The aforementioned conal anatomy can be well visualized angiocardiographically. Moreover, conal development (growth, lack of growth, and absorption) is considered to be a factor of prime importance in the morphogenesis of normally and abnormally related great arteries (Keith, 1909; Van Praagh and Van Praagh, 1966; Goor et al., 1972).

Segmental Combinations (Sets)

Since we have considered each of the three major cardiac segments (visceroatrial situs, ventricular loop, and conotruncus), we are now in a position to put the segments together—to consider the known segmental combinations and interrelations (Figure 36–18).

The combinations of visceroatrial situs, ventricular loop, and conotruncus that make up the various types of normal and abnormal human heart constitute different segmental sets. Consideration of these sets is greatly facilitated (simplified and abbreviated) by the use of symbols.

Segmental Symbols and Words. (Melhuish and Van Praagh, 1968; Van Praagh, 1972). The three types of visceroatrial situs may be represented as follows: solitus = S; inversus = I; and ambiguus or asplenia = A.

The types of ventricular loop may be symbolized as follows: D-loop = D; L-loop = L; uncertain or indeterminate type of loop = X (X standing for the unknown).

The types of relationship between the semilunar valves of the great arteries may be abbreviated as follows: solitus normal = S; D-transposition or D-malposition = D; L-transposition or L-malposition = L; transposition or malposition in which the aortic valve is directly anterior to the pulmonary valve = A; and the inverted normal relation between the great arteries = I.

Listing the segments in the direction of blood flow—situs, loop, arteries—the segmental set of the solitus normal heart (Figure 36–18) is {S,D,S}. The inverted normal heart is {I,L,I}. Complete TGA in situs solitus is {S,D,D}. Complete TGA in situs inversus is {I,L,L}. Corrected transposition in situs solitus is {S,L,L}. Corrected transposition in situs inversus is {I,D,D}, and so on.

However, in classic complete transposition of the great arteries, the aortic valve can lie somewhat to the *left* of the pulmonary valve, as occurred in 17 percent of the cases of Carr and associates (1968). Is this an L-transposition? Yes. Wouldn't it invite confusion with classic corrected transposition to call it an L-transposition? No, not if one mentions the segmental combination as well: transposition {S,D,L}. Transposition of the {S,D,L} type is perfectly clear.

In designations of the various types of congenital heart disease (Figure 36–18), the *words* indicate the relationships that exist between the cardiac segments. Examples include transposition of the great arteries (meaning that the aorta arises above RV and that the pulmonary artery originates above LV), double-inlet left ventricle, double-inlet right ventricle, double-outlet right ventricle, double-outlet left ventricle, etc. The *symbols* indicate the spatial orientations of the cardiac segments. For example, the segmental combination {S,D,D} occurs in several different situations (Figure 36–18): transposition, double-inlet left ventricle, double-inlet right ventricle, double-outlet right ventricle, and double-outlet left ventricle. These words indicate the abnormal relationships that exist between adjacent cardiac segments, while the symbols specify the spatial orientations of the cardiac segments.

Words can indicate not only the relationships between adjacent segments, but even the relationships that exist among all three segments. In the term *complete transposition of the great arteries*, the word *transposition* specifies the relationship between the conotruncus and the ventricular loop: aorta arising above RV and pulmonary artery originating above LV. *Complete* indicates the relationship between the conotruncus and the visceroatrial situs, complete meaning physiologically uncorrected (Figure 36–18): caval blood going to the aorta and pulmonary venous blood going to the pulmonary artery. There are two types of complete transposition, as the symbols indicate (Figure 36–18): {S,D,D} and {I,L,L}.

Similarly, in the term *corrected transposition of the great arteries*, the word *transposition* specifies the arterioventricular relationship, which is the same as in complete transposition (above). However, the word *corrected* specifies the physiologically corrected relationship between the conotruncus and the visceroatrial situs (Figure 36–18): caval blood to the pulmonary artery and pulmonary venous blood to the aorta (lack of associated anomalies permitting!). There are two types of corrected transposition, as the symbols indicate (Figure 36–18): {S,L,L} and {I,D,D}.

Summary. In the designations of the various types of congenital heart disease (Figure 36–18), the words indicate the segmental interrelationships and the symbols indicate the segmental spatial orientations.

The External Frame of Reference Problem

It is not entirely satisfactory to attempt to describe and classify the positional variations of the ventricles and great arteries in terms of *fixed external* spatial coordinates such as anterior, posterior, right, and left. The only entirely satisfactory frame of reference is the *internal* one: which atrium connects with which ventricle, and which ventricle connects with which great artery? (The physiologists have known this for years!)

The insistence that TGA be defined as an anterior aorta and a posterior pulmonary artery suggests a lack of understanding of what may be called the external frame of reference problem. In the D- and L-terminology, the external frame of reference is the Z axis, which is the sagittal plane projected on the horizontal plane. In the definition of TGA as an anterior aorta, the external frame of reference that is being used is the X axis, which is the frontal plane projected on the horizontal plane. Biologically, both external frames of reference are similarly unbasic. In TGA, the biologically basic considerations are the anatomy and embryology of the conotruncus, not the semilunar interrelationship relative to the X axis (or the Z axis) in the horizontal plane. This understanding is particularly relevant to dextrocardia because it is not rare for TGA to have a posterior aorta, apparently secondary to the cardiac malposition, as occurred in 11 percent (4/36) of personally studied cases (Van Praagh et al., 1964).

Another example is given to emphasize the current importance of the external frame-of-reference problem. In the *Taussig-Bing malformation*, the semilunar valves can lie side-by-side, as in the original case (Taussig and Bing, 1949). Recent experience, however, suggests that it may be more usual for the aorta to lie somewhat anteriorly to the pulmonary artery in this anomaly (Hightower et al., 1969); thus, Taussig-Bing = double-outlet RV, bilateral conus, and subpulmonary VSD. It has been advocated that when the abnormally located aorta does not lie anteriorly to the pulmonary artery, i.e., when the abnormally located aortic valve is beside or posterior to the pulmonary valve, a special designation should be used: partial distortion (de la Cruz and da Rocha, 1956). Within this approach, some Taussig-Bings are

partial distortions (side-by-side semilunar valves), while others are transpositions (anterior aorta). Since the conotruncal anatomy is exceedingly similar in both (bilateral conus, etc.), calling some Taussig-Bing malformations by one designation and others by a different designation seems to us to be artificial and unbasic. This is another example of the problems associated with external frames of reference. The basic biologic considerations in the Taussig-Bing malformation are considered to be the anatomy and embryology of the conotruncus (and the ventricles), not the spatial orientation of the semilunar valves relative to the frontal plane.

In the Taussig-Bing malformation, the great arteries may accurately be described as displaying *D-malposition* (Van Praagh et al., 1971). "Malposition" is used in the interests of accuracy. "Transposition of the great arteries" is not used, because both great arteries are not transposed (*trans* = across and *ponere* = to place) relative to the ventricular septum; only the aorta is transposed. Double outlets (RV and LV) are *partial transpositions*, literally (accurately) speaking. Since there are two types of partial transposition, double-outlet right ventricle and double-outlet left ventricle, we do not use the term partial transposition. Instead, we use the more specific designations double-outlet right ventricle and double-outlet left ventricle.

The term "transposition of the aorta and pulmonary artery" was introduced by Farre in 1814 in his description of the third known case. By "transposition" Farre meant that the aorta arose from the RV and the pulmonary artery originated from the LV. Relative to the suggestion that TGA be defined as an anterior aorta and a posterior pulmonary artery (Van Mierop, 1971), perhaps it should be added that Farre did not even mention the anteroposterior relationship between the great arteries; nor did Baillie (1797) who described the first case; nor did Langstaff (1811) who published the second case. All of these early authors were struck by the fact that the aorta arose from the RV and the pulmonary artery originated from the LV, this being what Farre meant by his term "transposition."

Hence, our suggestion (Van Praagh et al., 1971) that TGA be used to mean origin of the aorta from the RV and origin of the pulmonary artery from the LV is consistent with both the literal meaning and the original usage of this term. The suggestion (Angelini and Leachman, 1972) that we have introduced an entirely new definition of TGA is thus not correct. This erroneous impression was reached before our recent rediscovery of the early history of TGA, summarized above.* Thus, the definition of transposition of the great arteries as origin of the aorta above the RV and origin of the pulmonary artery above the LV is hardly original, this definition being consistent

---

* We would like to acknowledge with gratitude the assistance of Mr. Richard Wolfe, Rare Book Librarian, Countway Library, Harvard Medical School.

both with the original usage (Farre, 1814) and with the basic meaning (*trans, ponere*) of this term.

Moreover, from the practical standpoint, it is not satisfactory to define TGA as an anterior aorta, not only because TGA can have side-by-side great arteries or a posterior aorta, but also because an anterior aorta often also occurs with double-outlet right ventricle, double-outlet left ventricle, and anatomically corrected malposition of the great arteries. Consequently, although an anterior aorta should certainly suggest the possibility of TGA, it is important to appreciate that it is not a highly reliable sign of TGA because of the existence of false positives and false negatives.

For the sake of understanding, it is very important that each of the anatomic and embryologic types of TGA be carefully distinguished from the others. In terms of conal morphology, there are four different anatomic types of conal malformation that can be associated with TGA, accurately defined (Van Praagh et al., 1971):

1. Subaortic conus, with pulmonary-mitral fibrous continuity (common type, 92 percent).
2. Subaortic and subpulmonary (bilateral) conus, without semilunar-atrioventricular fibrous continuity (uncommon type, 8 percent).
3. Subpulmonary conus, with aortic-mitral fibrous continuity (rare, much less than 1 percent).
4. Bilaterally deficient conus, with aortic-tricuspid and pulmonary-mitral fibrous continuity (rare, much less than 1 percent).

These are four different malformations, despite the similarity of their arterioventricular relationships, and despite the fact that all may be called TGA.

Since there are at least four different anomalies now called TGA, some workers would like to separate these anomalies from each other by calling each by a different name. Only typical TGA would be called transposition. The other three anomalies would be called something else. The problem is to find other names that most workers would agree to, and use. We think that a more practical solution is to distinguish the various anatomic types of TGA, rather than trying to insist on different names for each type.

Precisely this situation pertained in dextrocardia. An effort was made to distinguish the various types of right-sided heart by calling each by a different name (e.g., dextrocardia, dextroversion, dextrorotation, dextroposition, etc.). This was not a success in part because different individuals and different schools used the same terms differently. Merely describing the various anatomic types, rather than using different special names, has proved helpful in dextrocardia. A similar approach to TGA seems indicated.

It must be appreciated clearly that one of the major problems associated with TGA is *the concept itself*. Unfortunately, TGA, even when used accurately, is not one entity (as everyone wishes it were!). It is at least four different entities. Why? Because of the concept—the basic meaning—of transposition of the great arteries. Transposition is one type of arterioventricular *relationship*. But unfortunately, it

is *not* just one *anatomic entity* (type of malformation). In the transposition *concept*, one set of variables (conotruncal malformations) is described and classified in terms of a second set of variables (the ventricles and ventricular septum, which are assumed to be normal, but in fact may not be). *Solving for one variable in terms of a second* would be a cardinal sin in mathematics or logic. But we do this for the best of clinical and physiologic reasons in TGA—because the arterioventricular relations are so important.

Still, this approach remains not entirely satisfactory. *One must also solve for the variable conotruncal malformations, in terms of the conotruncus itself.* Only by clearly separating *the various anatomic types of TGA* can the weakness of the concept be overcome. The weakness of the concept is that while TGA specifies one general type of arterioventricular relationship, it turns out that there are at least four anatomically and embryologically different entities that can have a transposed type of arterioventricular relationship.

Once the foregoing is widely appreciated, much of the controversy concerning TGA will disappear. The solution is not to argue whether this or that entity is, or is not, a type of TGA. Rather, we think the solution is to define precisely the anatomic type of conotruncal malformation with which one is concerned. Then one may also apply whatever type of relationships term (TGA, DORV, DOLV, anatomically corrected malposition) that accurately describes the associated arterioventricular relationship. But as one is applying the relationships term, one knows full well that there are several different anatomic entities that display each of the abnormal types of arterioventricular relationship. One knows that each of these abnormal relationships is a broad, heterogenous category. Not just TGA. So are the double-outlets RV and LV.

Nonetheless, one diagnoses the arterioventricular *relationship* as accurately as possible, just as one diagnoses the conotruncal *malformation* as precisely as possible.

The relationship diagnosis, and the malformation diagnosis, are two different but interrelated diagnoses. Consider the following example of two hearts. One has complete D-TGA with subaortic conus and intact ventricular septum. The other has complete D-TGA with bilateral conus, VSD, and pulmonary stenosis. In this example, both hearts have the same arterioventricular *relationship diagnosis* (D-TGA). But the *malformation diagnosis* is very different (subaortic conus, versus bilateral conus, VSD, and PS).

One of the important sources of the controversy concerning the definition of TGA is apparent failure to distinguish between the relationship diagnosis and the malformation diagnosis; i.e., it is widely assumed that they are synonymous. It is hoped that the example of double-outlet RV will help to make this distinction clear. Double-outlet right ventricle obviously is a relationship diagnosis, composed of several different anatomic entities (Neufeld et al., 1961, 1962). The same clearly is also true of TGA. The

Table 36–2. HOW MANY TYPES OF HUMAN HEART ARE THERE?

TYPES OF HEART	SITUS SOLITUS	SITUS INVERSUS
1. Normal	{S,D,S}	{I,L,I}
2. Complete transposition of the great arteries	{S,D,D}	{I,L,L}
3. Corrected transposition of the great arteries	{S,L,L}	{I,D,D}
4. Double-inlet LV (single LV with infundibular outlet chamber)	{S,D,S} {S,D,D} {S,L,L}	
5. Double-inlet RV (single RV)	{S,D,D} {S,L,L}	
6. Double-outlet RV	{S,D,D} {S,D,L} {S,L,L}	{I,L,L} {I,L,D} {I,D,D}
7. Double-outlet LV	{S,D,D} {S,D,L}	
8. Anatomically corrected malposition of the great arteries	{S,D,L} {S,L,D}	{I,D,L}
9. Isolated ventricular discordance	{S,L,S}	{I,D,I}
10. Isolated atrial inversion	{S,I,D,S}*	

* {S,I,D,S} indicates situs solitus of the viscera, situs inversus of the atria, ventricular D-loop, and the solitus type of normal relationship between the great arteries.

definition of TGA is considered in greater detail subsequently (see dextrocardia with corrected transposition in situs inversus, {I,D,D}).

How many types of human heart are there? By "types of heart," what is usually meant in this context is: *segmental combinations and interrelations* (Table 36–2) (Van Praagh, 1972).

Are there only ten different types of human heart (Table 36–2)? No doubt there are more. Only entities we are sure exist are mentioned in Table 36–2. Asplenia was omitted because it seems likely that situs ambiguus represents a heterotaxic form either of situs solitus or of situs inversus (Freedom, 1971). However, a third column could be added to Table 36–2, if desired. This kind of case may be symbolized as follows: {A(I),L,L} meaning situs ambiguus (basically situs inversus), L-loop, L-TGA. The basic type of visceroatrial situs may be considered to be situs solitus when the inferior vena cava is right-sided, and situs inversus when the inferior vena cava is left-sided (Freedom, 1971). Also omitted from Table 36–2 are associated anomalies such as septal defects or valvular malformations, because such associated anomalies are irrelevant to the segmental combinations and interrelations ("types of heart").

More important than the completeness of Table 36–2 is the idea of viewing complex congenital heart disease in terms of segmental combinations and interrelations, and the concept of diagnosing any heart, no matter how complex, in a step-by-step manner, segment by segment.

Now we are in a position to apply the segmental method of diagnosis to any patient with congenital heart disease, including the cardiac malpositions.

Findings in Dextrocardia

The findings in 51 personally studied autopsied cases of congenital dextrocardia are summarized in Table 36–3 and Figure 36–19 (Van Praagh et al., 1964).

The order of frequency of the various types of dextrocardia was (Table 36–3):

1. The commonest type of dextrocardia was the normal heart (30 percent). Interestingly, the solitus normal {S,D,S} exceeded the inverted normal {I,L,I} (classic mirror-image dextrocardia), 18 percent versus 12 percent, respectively.

2. Corrected TGA was second in frequency, 28 percent: {S,L,L} = 22 percent and {I,D,D} = 6 percent.

3. Third in frequency was single (common) ventricle, 20 percent. These ten cases were as follows:

a. Absence of the sinus or body of RV, resulting in a single LV with an infundibular outlet chamber, i.e., type A (Van Praagh et al., 1964), in six cases: {S,L,L} = 3, {I,L,L} = 1, {A,L,L} = 2.

b. Absence of the LV (type B) was the only form of single (common) ventricle not represented in this series.

c. Absence or marked underdevelopment of the ventricular septum (type C) occurred in two cases: {S,X,D} = 2.

d. Absence of morphologically identifiable RV, LV, and ventricular septum (type D), i.e., an abnormally differentiated or undifferentiated bulboventricular loop, was found in two cases: {A,D,D} = 1 and {A,L,L} = 1. (The sidedness of the

**Table 36–3. ANATOMIC TYPES OF CONGENITAL DEXTROCARDIA
IN 51 AUTOPSIED CASES***

TYPES OF HEART	SEGMENTAL SETS	NO. OF CASES	PERCENT OF SERIES
1. Normal heart	{S,D,S}	9	18
2. Inverted normal heart	{I,L,I}	6	12
3. Complete transposition in situs solitus	{S,D,D}	0	0
4. Complete transposition in situs inversus	{I,L,L}	6	12
5. Corrected transposition in situs solitus	{S,L,L}	12	22
6. Corrected transposition in situs inversus	{I,D,D}	3	6
7. Single (common) ventricle†		10	20
8. Asplenia	{A,D,D}	2	4
	{A,L,L}	3	6

* Data from Van Praagh et al. (1964).
† For greater detail concerning the types of single ventricle found in this series, please see text.

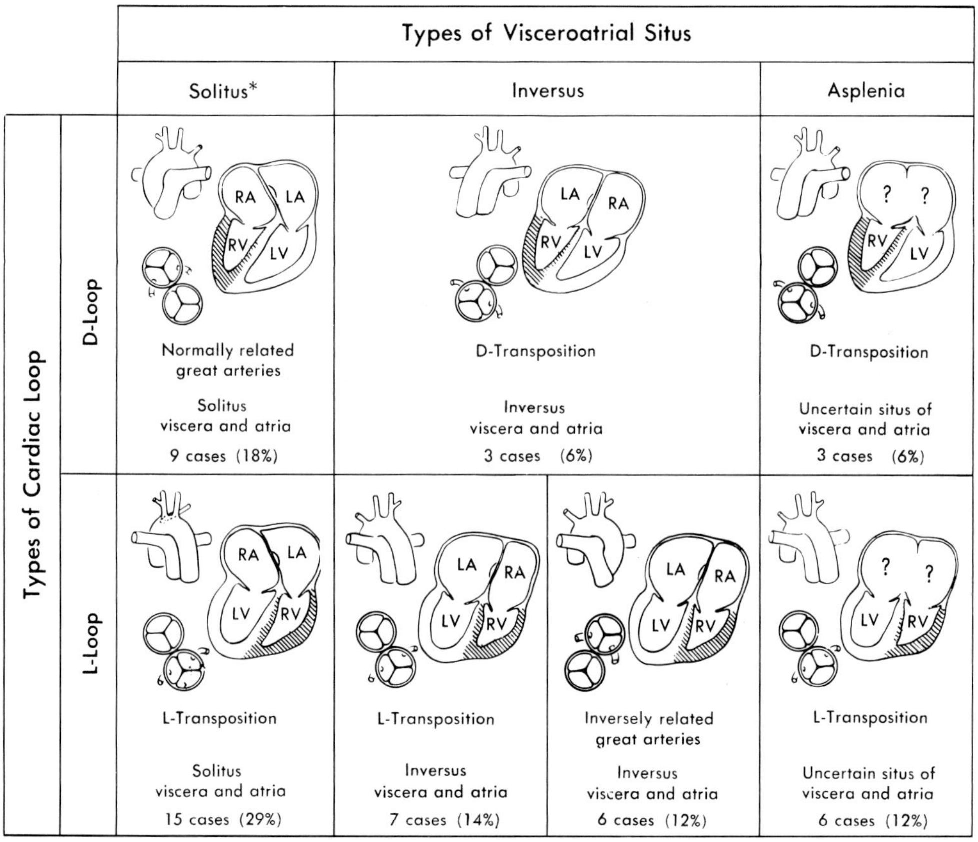

*Two cases of common ventricle (Type C) with situs solitus and d-transposition are not shown, because
the type of cardiac loop was indeterminate. The ventricular apex was pointed posteriorly in both.

Figure 36-19. Diagrammatic summary of 51 autopsy-proved cases of dextrocardia, presented in terms of the types of visceroatrial situs, the types of ventricular loop, and the types of semilunar interrelationship that were found. (Reproduced from Van Praagh, R., et al.: Anatomic types of dextrocardia. Diagnostic and embryologic implications. *Am. J. Cardiol.*, **13**:510, 1964.)

infundibulum and aorta was presumed to indicate the orientation, D- or L-, of the ventricular loop.)

4. Close behind single ventricle in frequency was asplenia, 18 percent. Two ventricles were present in five cases, {A,D,D} = 2 and {A,L,L} = 3. Single (common) ventricle occurred in four cases of asplenia, {A,L,L} = 3 and {A,D,D} = 1.

5. The least frequent type of dextrocardia in this series was complete TGA (with two ventricles and one spleen), 12 percent {S,D,D} = 0 and {I,L,L} = 12 percent.

Associated malformations must be omitted here, despite their obvious importance, in the interests of brevity. (Please see Table II, Van Praagh et al., 1964.)

Notably absent from this series were tetralogy of Fallot, truncus arteriosus communis, and the rarer segmental combinations such as isolated ventricular discordance, {S,L,S} and {I,D,I}, and anatomically corrected malposition, {S,D,L} and {S,L,D}.

Tetralogy of Fallot appears to be quite rare in dextrocardia, but it has been reliably reported by de la Cruz and associates (1962), Lev and associates (1968), and Morgan and associates (1972).

Truncus arteriosus communis appears to be very rare in dextrocardia. In a personal study of 57 autopsied cases of truncus (Van Praagh and Van Praagh, 1965), none had dextrocardia, and we are not aware of any reported case of typical truncus in a right-sided heart.

Anatomically corrected malposition of the great arteries has been reported with dextrocardia; Case 1 is {S,D,L} (Van Praagh and Van Praagh, 1967).

In the juxtaposition of the atrial appendages syndrome (Melhuish and Van Praagh, 1968), the frequency of dextrocardia was found to be approximately twice as high as in a control series of transpositions without juxtaposition of the atrial appendages, 22 percent compared with 12 percent,

respectively. Thus, there is a tendency toward dextrocardia in the juxtaposition of the atrial appendages syndrome.

Other Studies. In 1968, Lev and associates reported the pathologic anatomy in 41 cases of congenital dextrocardia (Table 36–4).

Perusal of these data is of interest in several respects:

1. The high frequency of the polysplenia syndrome (29 percent) and the asplenia syndrome (20 percent), splenic dysgenesis comprising almost half this series (49 percent).

2. The high frequency of corrected transposition, {S,L,L} = 22 percent,

3. The lower frequencies of normally related great arteries, {S,D,S} = 7 percent and {I,L,I} = 10 percent, and of complete transposition, {S,D,D} = 5 percent and {I,L,L} = 2 percent.

Lev and associates (1968) reported one case of *tetralogy of Fallot in mirror-image dextrocardia,* {I,L,I}.

Regarding ventricular localization, Lev and associates emphasized several diagnostically helpful points:

1. The value of the anterior descending coronary artery, as above (Figure 36–11).

2. The course of the pulmonary artery when the great arteries are not transposed (explained below).

3. The course of the aorta when the great arteries are transposed (explained below).

When the great arteries are not transposed and a D-loop is present, the pulmonary artery (PA) almost always runs posteriorly and *leftward,* passing to the left of the ascending aorta (Ao) (Figure 36–22). This course of the PA to the left of the ascending Ao reflects the normal (noninverted) twist of the truncus, and a normally formed truncus strongly suggests the

**Table 36–4.   ANATOMIC TYPES OF CONGENITAL DEXTROCARDIA
IN LEV'S 41 AUTOPSIED CASES***

TYPES OF HEART	SEGMENTAL SETS	NO. OF CASES	PERCENT OF SERIES
1. Normal heart	{S,D,S}	3	7
2. Inverted normal heart	{I,L,I}	4	10
3. Complete transposition in situs solitus	{S,D,D}	2	5
4. Complete transposition in situs inversus	{I,L,L}	1	2
5. Corrected transposition in situs solitus	{S,L,L}	8	20
6. Corrected transposition in situs inversus	{I,D,D}	0	0
7. Single ventricle (type A)	{S,L,L}	1	2
8. Double-outlet right ventricle	{S,D,D}	1	2
	{I,L,L}	1	2
9. Polysplenia		12	29
10. Asplenia		8	20

* Percentages reduced to nearest whole number. This table is based on Table 1 of Lev et al. (1968). Segmental sets in polysplenia and asplenia not given since they are incompletely reported. For associated malformations, please see original paper.

coexistence of a normal ventricular D-loop (RV right-sided) (Figures 36–9 and 36–11). When a normally related PA runs posteriorly and *rightward*, passing to the right of the ascending Ao, this reflects the inverted normal twist of the truncus, and a mirror-image normal truncus suggests the strong probability that a mirror-image ventricular L-loop (RV left-sided) also coexists (Figures 36–9 and 36–11).

When the great arteries are transposed, the convexity of the ascending aorta usually is directed rightward with a D-loop (Figure 36–28) and leftward with an L-loop (Figure 36–25), which also may be helpful in ventricular localization.

Lev's terminology and classification of the dextrocardias (1968) are:

1. *Dextroversion* = the normal type of heart {S,D,S} and complete transposition {S,D,D}.

2. *Presumptive dextroversion* = the same as (1) above, except that the classification of the atria as being in situs solitus (S) is not certain, usually because of the coexistence of asplenia or polysplenia.

3. *Mirror-image dextrocardia* = the inverted normal type of heart {I,L,I} and complete transposition in situs inversus {I,L,L}.

4. *Presumptive mirror-image dextrocardia* is the same as (3) above, except that situs inversus of the atria is anatomically uncertain, usually because of coexistence of the asplenia or polysplenia syndromes and the abnormal atrial septal morphologies associated therewith.

5. *Mixed dextrocardia* indicates ventriculoatrial discordance, as in corrected transposition {S,L,L} and {I,D,D}, isolated ventricular inversion {S,L,S}, isolated ventricular noninversion {I,D,I}, and anatomically corrected malposition {S,L,D} (Figure 36–18).

6. *Dextrocardia, type undetermined,* indicates that the atria and/or ventricles cannot be identified morphologically.

The foregoing classification and terminology are presented here because much of the older literature is couched in this kind of special dextrocardia nomenclature, which the interested reader will want to be able to understand.

Thus, Lev's classification of dextrocardia (1968) essentially boils down to three main types: (1) dextroversion, i.e., the normal heart in the right chest; (2) mirror-image dextrocardia, i.e., the inverted normal heart; and (3) mixed dextrocardia, i.e., hearts with ventriculoatrial discordance. There are three other types in which all of the cardiac chambers are not identified morphologically.

However, if one classifies Lev's findings in ordinary terminology (Table 36–4), instead of in his special dextrocardia terminology, one finds that there are ten different types of right-sided heart, not three (or six). Why this discrepancy? If one compares Lev's classification (1968) with Table 36–4, one will note that Lev's classification omits the great arteries. It should be added that Lev's classification of dextrocardia is a good example of the classic type of classification of dextrocardia. There are many older classifications of dextrocardia that are quite like Lev's, and typically, they omit the great arteries. We think that a satisfactory classification of dextrocardia cannot omit the great arteries; they are too important to be ignored.

We think that special dextrocardia terminologies should be phased out because they are unnecessary, confusing, and hence undesirable. Different authors have used these same special terms with very different meanings, "dextroversion" being a noteworthy example of confused usage (Paltauf, 1901; Schmidt and Korth, 1954; Korth and Schmidt, 1954; Grant, 1958; Arcilla and Gasul, 1961; Cooley and Billig, 1963; Lev et al., 1968). Ordinary terms are considered preferable to special ones because virtually everyone understands what the ordinary terms mean.

Double-Outlet Right Ventricle. Hallerman and associates (1970) published an angiocardiographic and anatomic study of DORV, and of their 34 cases with two ventricles and a VSD, seven had dextrocardia (20 percent). There were three segmental combinations, or types of heart, in these seven dextrocardias with DORV: (1) {S.L.L} in five patients; (2) {S.L.D} in one; and (3) {I,L,L} in one. All seven had pulmonary outflow tract stenosis.

Anatomic Types of Dextrocardia. If one combines the findings of Van Praagh and associates (1964) and Lev and associates (1968), a general picture of the pathologic anatomy of congenital dextrocardia emerges, based on 92 postmortem cases (Table 36–5).

Since the asplenia and polysplenia syndromes (Ivemark, 1955; Forde and Finby, 1961; Lucas et al., 1962) together comprise the single largest group (32 percent) in this combined series of 92 cases (Table 36–5), *when one thinks of dextrocardia, one should think of asplenia and polysplenia,* and of the complex congenital heart disease that typifies these syndromes. Particularly important from the surgical standpoint in asplenia and polysplenia are: common atrioventricular canal, usually complete, with or without mitral or tricuspid stenosis or atresia; single or common ventricle; double-outlet right ventricle, or transposition of the great arteries, with pulmonary outflow tract stenosis or atresia; common atrium; bilateral superior venae cavae; interruption of the inferior vena cava with azygos extension to a superior vena cava, typical of polysplenia, but not of asplenia; total anomalous pulmonary venous drainage, often (but certainly not always) subdiaphragmatic with obstruction, frequent in asplenia; ipsilateral pulmonary venous drainage (right-sided pulmonary veins connecting with right-sided atrium, and left-sided pulmonary veins connecting with left-sided atrium, frequent in polysplenia).

In view of the complexity of the congenital heart disease usually associated with the asplenia syndrome, and often (but less frequently) associated with the polysplenia syndrome, such cases have to be assessed very carefully, even for palliative (shunt) surgery. Total anomalous pulmonary venous connection with obstruction may become evident only following a shunt procedure, when pulmonary edema

**Table 36–5.   ANATOMIC TYPES OF CONGENITAL DEXTROCARDIA
BASED ON 92 POSTMORTEM CASES**

TYPES OF HEART	SEGMENTAL SETS	NO. OF CASES	PERCENT OF SERIES
1. Normal heart	{S,D,S}	12	13
2. Inverted normal heart	{I.L.I}	10	11
3. Complete transposition	{S,D,D}	2	2
2. Complete transposition in situs inversus	{I.L.L}	8	9
5. Corrected transposition	{S,L,L}	23	25
6. Corrected transposition in situs inversus	{I,D,D}	3	3
7. Single (common) ventricle	{S,X,D}	2	2
	{S,L,L}	1	1
8. Double-outlet right ventricle	{S,D,D}	1	1
	{I,L,L}	1	1
9. Asplenia and polysplenia syndromes		29	32

develops in association with the radiologic picture of pulmonary venous obstruction (the "butterfly" pattern in the plain PA chest x-ray). Thus from the surgical standpoint, despite the great recent advances, the asplenia and polysplenia syndromes remain unsolved therapeutic challenges. In dextrocardia, asplenia and polysplenia should never be forgotten. Indeed, they should be excluded specifically. Particularly helpful in the diagnosis of these syndromes are: the symmetric liver shadow (Figure 36–2), shifting stomach bubble, bilateral right air bronchograms (asplenia), bilateral left air bronchograms (polysplenia), Howell-Jolly bodies, splenic scan, and the splenic artery on angiocardiography. For more specific anatomic data concerning dysplenia and its subgroups (asplenia, polysplenia, and accessory spleen), please see Isolated Levocardia (Table 36–7).

Kartagener's Syndrome. The triad of situs inversus totalis, paranasal sinusitis, and bronchiectasis was described in 1933 by Kartagener. This syndrome, which was not recognized in our necropsy series, typically occurs in individuals with mirror-image dextrocardia {I,L,I} and functionally normal hearts. Bronchiectasis occurs in as many as 25 percent of patients with situs inversus, but probably in less than 0.5 percent of the general patient population (Logan et al., 1965). This bronchiectasis is 50 to 100 times commoner in situs inversus than in situs solitus. The oldest known patient with this syndrome is a 72-year-old farmer's wife, suggesting that with reasonable medical supervision, this syndrome may be compatible with a full life-span (Miller and Divertie, 1972).

Why bronchiectasis? It is currently thought that there may well be a congenital anatomic and hence functional defect of the mucociliary epithelium (Miller and Divertie, 1972). The cilia do not move or beat in a normal fashion. Clearing of the tracheobronchial tree is thought to depend largely on coughing, rather than on ciliary action.

A recent exciting discovery may well explain the defective or absent ciliary action in the respiratory epithelium of patients with Kartagener's syndrome. Afzelius and associates (1975) have discovered a lack of dynein arms in the tails of immotile spermatozoa in two brothers, both of whom have chronic sinusitis and bronchiectasis, and one of whom has situs inversus totalis—Kartagener's syndrome. The dynein arms are responsible for flagellar motion of human sperm tails. Absence of dynein arms is thought to result in immotile sperm, leading to infertility, despite the fact that the number, oxygen consumption, and lactic acid production of the spermatozoa are normal. However, the exciting inference relative to Kartagener's syndrome is that a similar lack of dynein arms in the cilia of the respiratory epithelium could lead to immotile respiratory cilia, thereby setting the stage for the development of bronchiectasis. Whether or not this in fact is the case is presently unknown, but it looks as though we are at long last on the verge of a basic understanding of the bronchiectasis part of Kartagener's syndrome. Are such patients also infertile? This has not been a recognized part of Kartagener's syndrome, but the findings of Afzelius and associates (1975) suggest that this might well be the case. This too merits further investigation.

What about the situs inversus totalis part of Kartagener's triad? Situs inversus totalis has long been believed to be due to a single recessive autosomal gene (Cockayne, 1938). As Torgersen (1949) pointed out, "Situs inversus is no simple alternative to the normal situs. It is the most complicated among anomalies, concerning not only the situs, but all details of structure." Ig A, thymic and lymphatic tissues, and skin test responsiveness have all been found to be normal in situs inversus totalis (Miller and Divertie, 1972). The foregoing, then, has been the generally accepted understanding of situs inversus totalis, namely, that it is due to an autosomal recessive gene.

However, an exciting new light has recently been shed on this problem by Layton (1976). Based on his experiments with an inbred strain of mice that has a high incidence of situs inversus totalis (never more than 50 percent), Layton has concluded that situs solitus is due to the presence of a dominant gene that normally controls visceral situs. But when this dominant gene for situs solitus is absent, then the visceral situs is determined *in a random fashion*: it may be situs solitus, situs inversus, or a mixture of the two (situs ambiguus). Layton's observations may explain not only situs inversus, but situs ambiguus that typically is associated with congenital asplenia and polysplenia. This author states: "It is hypothesized that the normal allele at the *iv* locus exhibits complete dominance and controls normal visceral asymmetry. Absence of this control allows the sense of visceral asymmetry to be determined in a random fashion. This hypothesis appears to apply to the inheritance of situs inversus in man and also to the experimental production of situs inversus."

Thus, Layton's hypothesis (which is well supported by much experimental data) is that situs inversus and situs ambiguus both are the randomly occurring results of absence of the dominant gene for situs solitus (the normal allele at the *iv* locus). Referable to the findings of Afzelius and associates (1975) concerning immotile spermatozoa with and without situs inversus, Layton's mice with situs inversus do not suffer from infertility. What proportion of patients with Kartagener's syndrome have immotile sperm and resulting infertility remains to be established.

In summary, the new clues to the understanding of Kartagener's syndrome are:

1. The bronchiectasis may well be secondary to immotility of the respiratory cilia, which in turn may be due to absence of the protein dynein that is necessary to normal ciliary motion. Infertility due to immotile sperm that lack dynein in their tails (Afzelius et al., 1975) may be an unrecognized component of Kartagener's syndrome. Further studies of the respiratory cilia and of the prevalence of infertility in Kartagener's syndrome are needed.

2. New data (Layton, 1976) indicate that situs inversus totalis is due to absence of the dominant gene for situs solitus, the normal allele at the *iv* locus. Absence of this dominant gene results in development of situs that is random: it may be situs solitus, or situs inversus, or situs ambiguus. Hence, this one genotype appears to explain several different phenotypes.

Clinical Features and Diagnosis

Several illustrative, autopsy-proved cases will now be presented to demonstrate the segmental approach to diagnosis in congenital dextrocardia. It will also be seen that these cases are of interest per se.

Dextrocardia with a Normal Type of Heart {S,D,S}. TYPE OF VISCEROATRIAL SITUS. The chest x-ray (Figure 36–20*A*) shows a right-sided liver shadow and a left-sided stomach bubble, suggesting that this is dextrocardia with situs solitus of the viscera and atria (isolated dextrocardia). The electrocardiogram (Figure 36–21) also suggests situs solitus of the atria, the spatial $\hat{A}P$ being oriented anteriorly, inferiorly, and leftward. The presence of situs solitus (S) is confirmed by the right-sided location of the inferior vena caval catheter (Figure 36–20*B*).

TYPE OF VENTRICULAR LOOP. Electrocardiographically (Figure 36–21), the RS complexes from V_8R to V_2 correctly suggest the presence of a large, right-sided RV (Portillo et al., 1959). The qrS complexes from V_3 to V_5 accurately suggest that the LV is left-sided (Portillo et al., 1959). Angiocardiographically, the right-sided ventricle (Figure 36–20*B* and *C*) appears globular in shape and more coarsely trabeculated than does the left-sided ventricle, suggesting that RV is right-sided and LV is left-sided: D-loop (D). This is confirmed by the presence of normally related great arteries.

TYPE OF CONOTRUNCUS. The conotruncus is normal, as stated above. The pulmonary valve is anterior and superior, reflecting the presence of a subpulmonary conus. The aortic valve is posterior and inferior, reflecting absence of a muscular subaortic conus. The pulmonary valve is anterior, superior, and to the *right*, relative to the aortic valve, which is posterior, inferior, and to the *left*. Thus, the semilunar valves do not display a semilunar relationship that is entirely typical of the solitus normal (Figure 36–11). The pulmonary valve should be anterior, superior, and to the *left* (Figure 36–11), not anterior, superior, and to the *right* (Figure 36–20), as in fact is the case, apparently secondary to the pivoting of the heart into the right hemithorax. Note that the main pulmonary artery (Figure 36–20*B*) passes to the *left* of the ascending aorta (Figure 36–20*D*). This is a solitus normal type of conotruncus. In an inverted normal type of conotruncus, the main pulmonary artery passes to the *right* of the ascending aorta. Hence, in this case, despite the somewhat atypical semilunar interrelationship secondary to the dextrocardia, it is clear that we are dealing with a solitus normal type of conotruncus that may be symbolized as S.

TYPE OF SEGMENTAL SET {S,D,S}. This briefly and conveniently indicates: situs solitus of the viscera and atria (S), ventricular D-loop (D), and the solitus normal type of relationship between the great arteries (S), i.e., a normal type of heart.

Autopsy confirmed the foregoing. Figure 36–22 illustrates many of the features of normal cardiac morphology mentioned previously.

ASSOCIATED MALFORMATIONS. The hemivertebrae seen through the stomach bubble (Figure 36–20*A*) should suggest the possibility that this dextrocardia is secondary to hypoplasia or aplasia of the right lung. The frequent coexistence of hemivertebrae and pulmonary hypoplasia or aplasia was stressed by Caffee (1945). Note the hypoplasia of the right pulmonary artery (Figure 36–20*B*). This

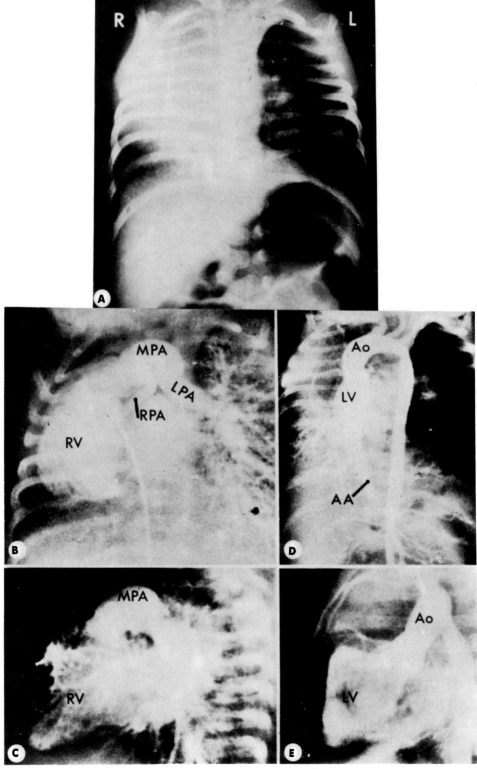

hypoplastic, unilobed right lung also received an anomalous systemic artery from the descending thoracic aorta (Figure 36–20D). The right upper pulmonary veins connected to the superior vena cava and the right lower pulmonary veins connected to the inferior vena cava.

The aortic arch severely compressed the trachea anteriorly: note the anteriorly indented air shadow behind the aortic arch in Figure 36–20E. Respiratory distress with marked stridor resulted. Due to severe hypoplasia of the right lung, this normal heart was right-sided and quite posterior. The normal left aortic arch (Figure 36–20D) severely compressed the trachea anteriorly as the aortic arch passed from the right to the left side. The stridor was relieved by aortopexy (fixing the aorta anteriorly to the sternum). Unfortunately, the sutures used to perform the aortopexy gave way. The aorta returned to its previous posterior location, compressing the trachea. The patient was strangled by his normal aortic arch before reoperation could be performed.

Thus, a normal aortic arch mimicked a tight vascular ring because of hypoplasia of the right lung and its positional sequelae: the heart came to lie in the right hemithorax, posteriorly; hence the trachea was compressed as the aorta passed from right to left. *Severe anterior tracheal compression is not a well-known sequela of hypoplasia of the right lung.* Normally, the left aortic arch does not pass from right to left, in the frontal plane, immediately anterior to the trachea, as occurred in this case. Normally, the left aortic arch lies anteriorly and to the left of the trachea, the aorta running in a semisagittal direction over the left main stem bronchus—not in the frontal plane from right to left, immediately anterior to the trachea, as in this case. *Severe tracheal compression can occur without a vascular ring.*

Hence, this was a lung problem, not a heart problem.

DIAGNOSIS. Dextrocardia secondary to hypoplasia of the right lung, with anomalous systemic arterial supply, and anomalous right pulmonary venous drainage to superior and inferior venae cavae, with a normal heart in the right chest {S,D,S}.

Dextrocardia with Corrected Transposition {S,L,L}. TYPE OF VISCEROATRIAL SITUS. Situs solitus (S), as is indicated by the liver shadow and stomach bubble in the plain chest x-ray (Figure 36–23A), the P waves of the electrocardiogram

(Figure 36–24), and the location of the inferior vena cava (catheter, Figure 36–23B).

TYPE OF VENTRICULAR LOOP. Electrocardiographically (Figure 36–24), in V_6R and V_5R, rsR complexes are inscribed, erroneously suggesting that RV may be right-sided. In V_6, a qRs complex is seen, inaccurately suggesting that LV may be left-sided. Lead aVR displays an RS morphology, very unusual for normally interrelated ventricles; this might suggest that perhaps the ventricles are *not* normally interrelated. Perhaps the ventricles are inverted? Hence, we think that it is fair to say that the electrocardiographic evidence concerning ventricular localization in this case is not entirely clear-cut and straightforward. For most observers, it is too subtle, i.e., confusing and misleading.

Angiocardiographically, however, L-TGA is present (Figure 36–23B–E). This suggests that an L-loop is probable (Figure 36–11). This is corroborated by relatively smooth appearance of the right-sided ventricle (Figure 36–23B and D). Hence, it is concluded that an L-loop (L) is present.

TYPE OF CONOTRUNCUS: L-TGA (L) with a subaortic conus, indicated by the high location of the aortic valve, without a subpulmonary conus, indicated by the low position of the pulmonary valve (Figure 36–23B–E).

TYPE OF SEGMENTAL SET: {S,L,L}. This briefly indicates: situs solitus of the viscera and atria (S), ventricular L-loop (L), and L-transposition of the great arteries (L), i.e., classic corrected transposition.

Corrected L-TGA is one of the commonest forms of dextrocardia, apparently for two reasons: (1) Situs solitus is the commonest form of visceroatrial situs; and (2) L-loops belong in the right chest (as in mirror-image dextrocardia).

Autopsy confirmed the foregoing (Figure 36–25). In the exterior view of the heart, note that the anterior descending coronary artery arises from the right coronary artery. The right-sided ventricle displays the morphology typical of LV, while the left-sided ventricle has a morphology entirely characteristic of RV. The subaortic muscular conus widely separates the L-transposed aortic valve from the left-sided tricuspid valve. The absence of subpulmonary conal musculature permits fibrous continuity between the pulmonary valve and the right-sided mitral valve.

ASSOCIATED MALFORMATIONS. A subpulmonary VSD (Figure 36–25) permitted a large

---

Figure 36–20. Chest x-ray and selective right ventricular angiocardiogram in dextrocardia with situs solitus, D-loop, and normally related great arteries {S, D, S}. *A* is the plain posteroanterior chest roentgenogram; *B* and *C* are simultaneous posteroanterior and left lateral projections, respectively, of a selective injection into the right-sided RV; *D* and *E* are simultaneous posteroanterior and left lateral projections, respectively, of the levophase. This normal heart is in the right chest secondary to hypoplasia of the right lung. In *A*, note the hemivertebrae seen through the stomach bubble. In *B*, the right-sided location of the inferior vena caval catheter and the hypoplasia of the right pulmonary artery (*RPA*) are noteworthy. In *D*, note the anomalous artery (*AA*) arising from the celiac axis and passing through the diaphragm to supply the lower portion of the right lung. In *E*, the air shadow in the trachea indicates that the aortic arch is indenting the trachea anteriorly. *B* and *D* are posteroanterior projections, and *C* and *E* are simultaneous left lateral projections, respectively. (Reproduced from Van Praagh, R., et al.: Diagnosis of the anatomic types of congenital dextrocardia. *Am. J. Cardiol.*, **15**:234, 1965.)

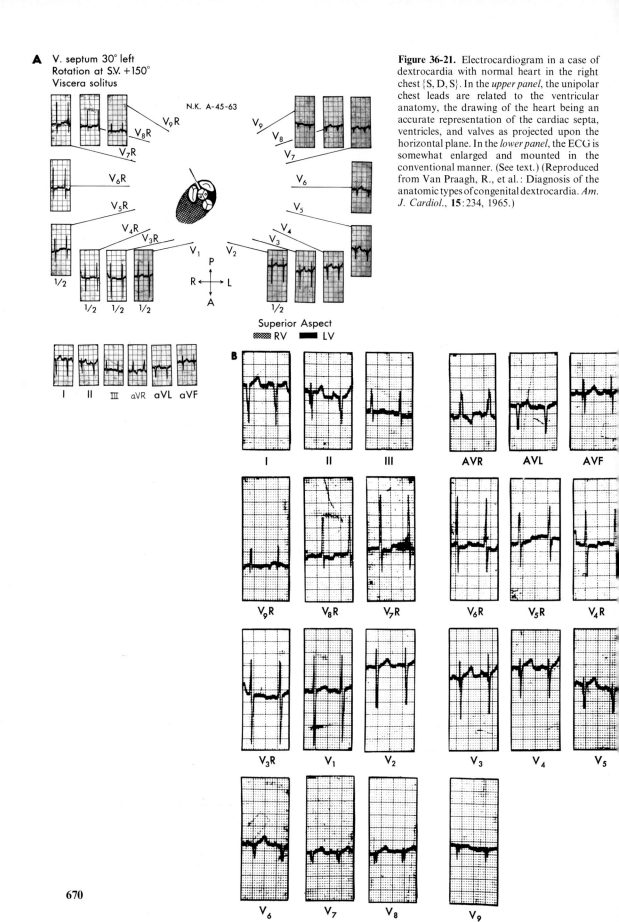

A V. septum 30° left
Rotation at S.V. +150°
Viscera solitus

N.K. A-45-63

Superior Aspect
▨ RV   ▮ LV

Figure 36-21. Electrocardiogram in a case of dextrocardia with normal heart in the right chest {S, D, S}. In the *upper panel*, the unipolar chest leads are related to the ventricular anatomy, the drawing of the heart being an accurate representation of the cardiac septa, ventricles, and valves as projected upon the horizontal plane. In the *lower panel*, the ECG is somewhat enlarged and mounted in the conventional manner. (See text.) (Reproduced from Van Praagh, R., et al.: Diagnosis of the anatomic types of congenital dextrocardia. *Am. J. Cardiol.*, **15**:234, 1965.)

left-to-right shunt leading to increased pulmonary vascularity (Figure 36–23A) and the clinical picture of congestive heart failure.

DIAGNOSIS. Dextrocardia with corrected L-TGA {S,L,L}, VSD, and congestive heart failure.

Dextrocardia with Corrected Transposition in Situs Inversus {I,D,D}. TYPE OF VISCEROATRIAL SITUS. Situs inversus (I), as is suggested by the right-sided stomach bubble and left-sided liver shadow (Figure 36–26A), the P waves of the electrocardiogram (Figure 36–27), and as is confirmed by the left-sided inferior vena cava (catheter position, Figure 36–26B).

TYPE OF VENTRICULAR LOOP: D-Loop (D). Although the electrocardiographic evidence concerning ventricular localization is not entirely clear, in our opinion (Figure 36–27), the angio-cardiographic findings permit diagnostic certainty. The left-sided and anterior ventricle is clearly LV, its configuration and trabeculation in diastole (Figure 36–26B) and systole (Figure 36–26D) being unmis-

takable. By exclusion, the right-sided and posterior ventricle, which is less well visualized, must be RV.

TYPE OF CONOTRUNCUS: D-TGA (D). The high location of the aortic valve reflects the presence of a subaortic conus, and the presence of a stenotic subpulmonary conus is seen beneath the pulmonary valve in Figure 36–26C. Hence, a bilateral (subaortic and subpulmonary) conus is present. Note that the ascending aorta is somewhat posterior to the pulmonary valve (Figure 36–26C and D).

Does the posterior aorta indicate that TGA is not present? No, it does not. TGA definitely *is* present (autopsy-proved). But, it may be objected, there is a right aortic arch (Figure 36–26B). The patient is cyanotic and clubbed. There is a VSD (Figure 36–26D) with pulmonary infundibular and valvular stenosis (Figure 36–26C). The aorta is a bit posterior to the pulmonary artery. Why isn't this tetralogy of Fallot? Because the pulmonary artery is related to the LV and the aorta is related to the RV, the aorta being far removed from the mitral valve.

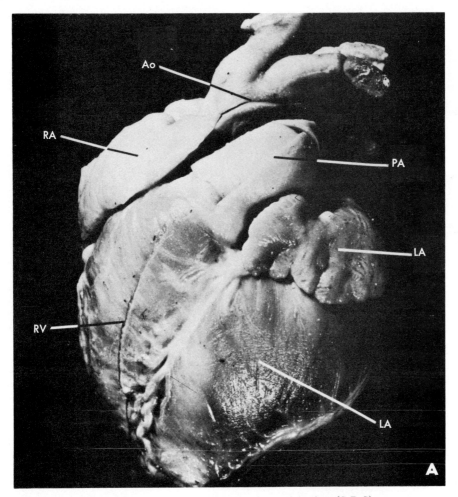

Figure 36-22. Anatomy of dextrocardia with normal heart in the right chest {S, D, S}.
    In the exterior view (A), the ventricular apex is seen to point rightward, and the cardiac chambers and great arteries accurately appear to be normally interrelated.

[Figure and legend continued overleaf.]

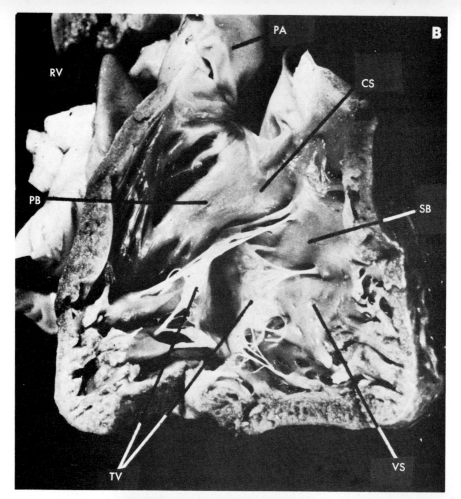

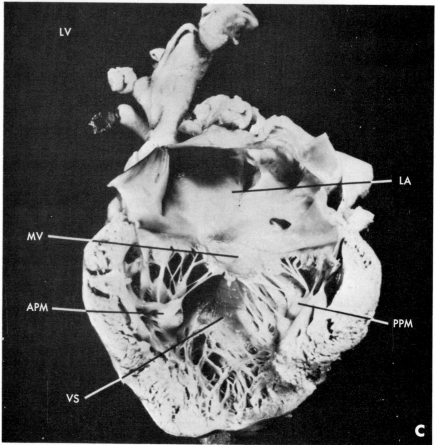

TGA is the rule with a discordant ventricular loop (when the ventricles do not correspond to the atria). In this case, there is a discordant D-loop in situs inversus. (In situs inversus, there "should" be a concordant L-loop.) Tetralogy of Fallot has aortic-mitral fibrous continuity and is a variant of normally related great arteries, not TGA (Van Praagh et al., 1970). Thus, when the ventricular loop is discordant, tetralogy of Fallot and any other variant of normally related great arteries is improbable, TGA being the rule. However, ventricular discordance with normally related great arteries does occur rarely, i.e., isolated ventricular discordance (Figure 36–18). However, in the present case, the great arteries obviously are not related normally to these discordant D-loop ventricles (Figure 36–26B–E).

TGA with a posterior aorta is not rare in dextrocardia, this being found in 4 of our 36 autopsied cases (11 percent) (Van Praagh et al., 1964). This is merely another illustration of abnormal spatial relationships secondary to the cardiac malposition, referred to above as *the external frame of reference problem*. The unsatisfactory external frame of reference in this instance is the frontal plane, or the X axis projected on the horizontal plane, which is used to judge anteroposterior semilunar interrelationships. If the ventricles are oriented normally relative to the type of loop that is present (D), i.e., if the ventricular apex is pointed leftward as should be the case with D-loops, then the transposed aortic valve becomes anterior. The semilunar relationship becomes typical of TGA when the ventricular malposition is "corrected" in this way. Hence, the atypical semilunar interrelationship—TGA with a posterior aorta—is considered to be secondary to the ventricular malposition. The posterior aorta in this type of case appears to have nothing to do with the type of conotruncal malformation that is present.

Hence, to insist that TGA is not present in this type of case because the aorta is posterior indicates a lack of understanding of the *external* coordinates (anterior-posterior, and right-left) that we often use for convenience. One should not forget that these external coordinates *are* merely conveniences. Only the *internal* relationships are entirely reliable, i.e., incapable of being artifacted by cardiac malposition.

It must be added that it is possible for TGA to be present with a posterior aorta, *without* cardiac malposition. However, this is rare and these cases are *not* typical transpositions (Van Praagh et al., 1971):

1. There is a short subpulmonary muscular conus and no subaortic muscular conus. Hence, there is no pulmonary-atrioventricular fibrous continuity and there is aortic-atrioventricular fibrous continuity. This malformation is very different from typical TGA (subaortic muscular conus, with no subpulmonary muscular conus).

2. There is a bilateral conus, the subpulmonary component being better developed than the subaortic component (Van Praagh, 1971). This too is different from typical TGA, but it is closer.

Does typical TGA (subaortic conus only), with normally located ventricles, ever have a posterior aorta? No, not to the best of our present knowledge. This is why some excellent authorities such as de la Cruz (1956) and Van Mierop (1971) believe that TGA may be defined as an anterior aorta and a posterior pulmonary artery. This definition adequately covers the typical case.

However, ventricular malpositions do occur. Transposition variants also occur, as above. We are certain that *typical* TGA (subaortic muscular conus with pulmonary-mitral fibrous continuity) can have a posterior aorta if ventricular malposition coexists. This is why, when faced with cases that did not fit the aforementioned definition of anteroposterior reversal of the great arteries, we searched for a definition of TGA that would truly define, one that would not have a lot of troublesome exceptions—a definition that had to be correct. Finally, we realized that the literal meaning of the concept (*trans* = across and *ponere* = to place) could hardly be wrong. There could not be any exception to a literally accurate definition (aorta from RV, pulmonary artery from LV)—by definition! Subsequently, we were pleased to discover that this was exactly what the inventor of the term, Dr. John Farre, had meant in the first place (1814).

How good does a definition have to be? Must there be no exceptions whatever? If some exceptions are permissible, how many? Indeed, what is the definition of definition? *These questions are basic to the controversy concerning the definition of TGA and apply directly to dextrocardia;* hence these problems are considered briefly here.

The concept of definition is probably as old as language itself. Definitions have always been essential to science. For example, they were necessary for Thales (640–548 B.C.) and Pythagoras (567–497 B.C.), the inventors of deductive geometry (Terry, 1964).

Figure 36-22 B and C.

The opened right ventricle (*RV*) and pulmonary artery (*PA*) show (*B*) the conal septum of crista supraventricularis (*CS*), which extends onto the right ventricular free wall forming a parietal band (*PB*), the septal band (*SB*), the "suture" or demarcation between PB and SB, the leaflets of the tricuspid valve (*TV*), and the coarsely trabeculated right ventricular septal surface (*VS*).

The opened left atrium (*LA*), mitral valve (*MV*), and left ventricle (*LV*) show (*C*) the anterolateral papillary muscle group (*APM*) and the posteromedial papillary muscle group (*PPM*), the smooth superior left ventricular septal surface, and the numerous, fine, oblique trabeculations of the left ventricular septal surface as one progresses toward the apex and about the base of the papillary muscles.

(Reproduced from Van Praagh, R., et al.: Anatomic types of dextrocardia. Diagnostic and embryologic implications. *Am. J. Cardiol.*, **13**:510, 1964.)

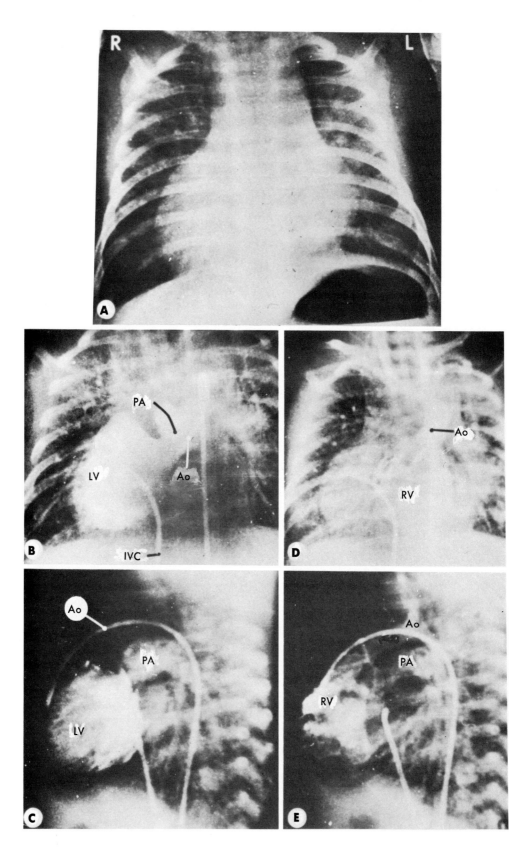

Aristotle (384–322 B.C.), the inventor of logic, thought that *the principle of contradiction* is basic: "It is impossible that the same quality should both belong and not belong to the same thing." Aristotle stated that this primary principle is "the source of all other axioms." The principle of contradiction is the basis of the mathematical method that Aristotle called *reductio ad absurdum* (Terry, 1964).

After a hiatus of more than 2000 years, the English logician and mathematician, George Boole (1815–1864) translated the principle of contradiction into simple algebra, this being the starting point of *symbolic logic (Boolean algebra).*

Here is an example of how Boole's algebra translates words into mathematics (from Terry, 1964). In Figure 36–29:

1. Let 1 represent the universe of all living beings.
2. Let x be the class of all living beings who are men.
3. Then $1 - x$ is the class of all living beings who are not men.
4. Then $(x)(1 - x)$ is the class of all living beings who are at the same time both men and nonmen.
5. Since there are *no* such beings, their number is 0. (One is not supposed to mention missing links, such as *Australopithecus*, at this point! The assumption that there are no genuinely transitional forms seems to be the weakness of the principle of contradiction.)
6. The formula representing the principle of contradiction, the basic formula of symbolic logic, is:

$$(x)(1 - x) = 0$$

No point can be both inside the circle and outside the circle at the same time (Figure 26–29). (It is assumed that there are no points, representing beings, who are *on* the circle, neither inside nor outside.)

To apply the principle of contradiction to the definition of TGA (Figure 36–29):

1. Let 1 represent all congenital heart disease.
2. Let x be the class of all transpositions of the great arteries.
3. Then $1 - x$ is the class of all congenital heart disease that is non-TGA.
4. Thus $(x)(1 - x)$ is the class of all congenital heart disease that is at the same time both transposition and nontransposition.
5. The principle of contradiction assumes that there are *no* such cases; hence their number is 0.
6. $(x)(1 - x) = 0$ states that there are no cases that are at the same time TGA and non-TGA.

Thus, a satisfactory definition (represented by the circle, Figure 36–29) of TGA (represented by x,

Figure 36–29) should completely separate TGA (x) from non-TGA ($1 - x$).

To define basically means to limit (*de + finire*), as the circle does in Figure 36–29.

To summarize, how good does a definition have to be? Ideally, in accord with the principle of contradiction, there should be no exceptions. This must be our goal.

Now to return to our case:

This case (Figure 36–26) does not satisfy Van Mierop's definition (1971) of TGA because of the posterior aorta. For the same reason, de la Cruz (1956) would not call this a case of transposition of the great arteries; instead she would invoke a special term, partial distortion in orthoposition. In fact, however, TGA really *is* present. Even the semilunar interrelationship becomes typical, with an anterior aorta, if the ventricular malposition is "corrected" by pointing the apex of this D-loop leftward, as it "should" point, instead of abnormally to the right, as it does point. This kind of case is a transposition, functions as a transposition, and above all should be treated surgically as a transposition.

SEGMENTAL COMBINATION: {I,D,D}. This briefly indicates: situs inversus of the viscera and atria, ventricular D-loop, and D-transposition of the great arteries. This combination adds up to corrected transposition in situs inversus.

Autopsy confirmed the foregoing (Figure 36–28). In addition, note that the RV is small-chambered. The tricuspid valve overrides the ventricular septum. This results in a VSD of the AV-canal type (RV view), without a common atrioventricular canal. On the left side, a typical RA opens into a typical LV (ventriculoatrial discordance).

ASSOCIATED MALFORMATIONS. Pulmonary stenosis, infundibular and valvular; VSD of the AV-canal type; small-chambered RV; overriding tricuspid valve; right aortic arch.

DIAGNOSIS. Dextrocardia with corrected D–TGA {I,D,D}, and the aforementioned associated malformations.

TRANSPOSITION TERMINOLOGY. It is noteworthy that "complete" and "corrected" indicate the situs, while "D" and "L" indicate the semilunar interrelationship. For example, there is complete D-TGA and complete L-TGA; these are {S,D,D} and {I,L,L}, respectively. And there is corrected L-TGA and corrected D-TGA; these are {S,L,L} and {I,D,D}, respectively. Thus, combining the words (complete and corrected) with the symbols (D and L) permits designations of appealing clarity and brevity.

Figure 36-23. Chest x-ray and angiocardiogram in dextrocardia with corrected transposition in situs solitus {S, L, L}. *A* is a plain posteroanterior chest roentgenogram; *B* and *C* are simultaneous posteroanterior and left lateral projections, respectively, of a selective injection into the right-sided LV; *D* and *E* are simultaneous posteroanterior and left lateral projections, respectively, of a selective injection through a retrograde aortic catheter into the left-sided RV. In *A* the normally located liver shadow and stomach bubble suggest situs solitus of the viscera and atria, which is confirmed in *B* by the right-sided location of the inferior vena caval catheter (*IVC*). The aorta (*Ao*) originates anteriorly and to the left of the pulmonary artery (*PA*). L-Transposition of the great arteries accurately suggests that an L-loop is present with a morphologically right ventricle (*RV*) being left-sided and with a morphologically left ventricle (*LV*) being right-sided. (Reproduced from Van Praagh, R., et al.: Diagnosis of the anatomic types of congenital dextrocardia. *Am. J. Cardiol.*, **15**:234, 1965.)

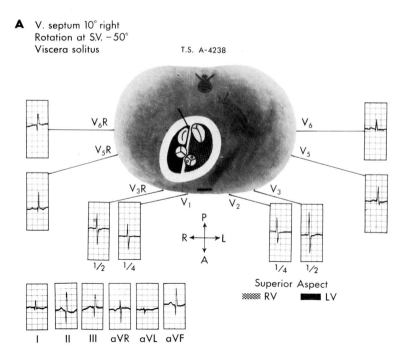

A V. septum 10° right
Rotation at S.V. −50°
Viscera solitus

T.S. A-4238

V₆R

V₅R

V₃R

V₁   V₂

V₆

V₅

V₃

P

R ←→ L

A

1/2   1/4   1/4   1/2

Superior Aspect
▨▨▨ RV   ■■■ LV

I   II   III   aVR   aVL   aVF

Figure 36-24. Electrocardiogram in dextrocardia with corrected transposition in situs solitus {S, L, L}. In the *upper panel*, the unipolar chest leads are related to the cardiac chambers as projected upon the horizontal plane; see heart diagram within thorax. In the *lower panel* the ECG is somewhat enlarged and mounted conventionally (see text). (Reproduced from Van Praagh, R., et al.: Diagnosis of the anatomic types of congenital dextrocardia. *Am. J. Cardiol.*, **15**:234, 1965.)

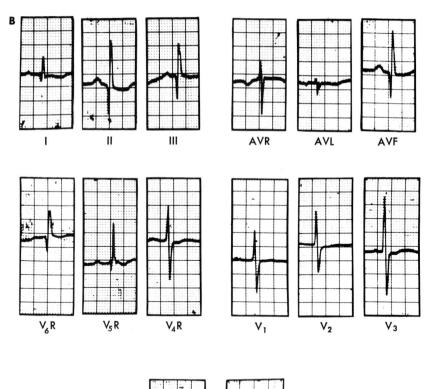

B

I   II   III   AVR   AVL   AVF

V₆R   V₅R   V₄R   V₁   V₂   V₃

V₅   V₆

Conclusions

Dextrocardia should be ignored, insofar as possible; i.e., one should approach the diagnosis of a right-sided heart just as one would that of a left-sided heart, using a step-by-step (segment-by-segment) and morphologic approach. Special approaches, special terminologies, and special classifications should be avoided in the interest of clarity, and because they are unnecessary. Nothing should be "corrected" for dextrocardia: chest x-rays, electrocardiograms, or angiocardiograms. This artifacts the data that should be used for chamber localization. This applies particularly to dextrocardia with complex congenital heart disease. If, however, one is certain that one is dealing with mirror-image-dextrocardia with inversion *both* of the atria and of the ventricles, then "correction" of the electrocardiogram by reversal of the arm and precordial leads may assist interpretation. But if the atria and ventricles both are

not inverted, then such "correction" is confusing, rather than helpful.

The "through-a-looking-glass-darkly" approach —replete with imaginary mirrors, spits, and hinges—should be dispensed with. It is suggested that the looking-glass world of so much of the dextrocardia literature should be abandoned because it is both unnecessary and confusing. In the operating room, reality must be faced as it is. Otherwise, like Perseus slaying Medusa, one must operate while looking in a mirror!

In the past, dextrocardia has been regarded as a "different world" compared with left-sided hearts. This is simply not the case. It's the same old play, with most of the familiar characters that we are all used to. Only the stage is different (right-sided, instead of left-sided), and this does not matter. Even in the best of cardiology departments, dextrocardia used to be a *bête noire*. Customarily confident cardiologists, faced with a case of dextrocardia, would turn ashen and mutter, "I'll never be able to figure out where

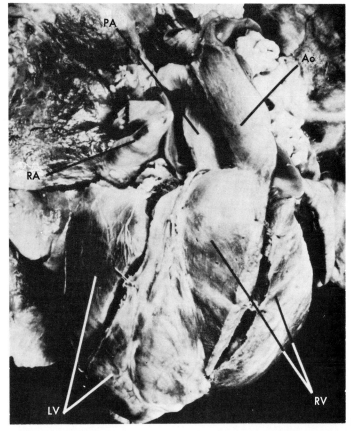

Figure 36-25. Anatomy of dextrocardia with corrected transposition in situs solitus {S, L, L}.

In the external view (*A*), note the rightward orientation of the ventricular apex indicating dextrocardia; the curved external surface of the morphologically right ventricle (*RV*), which is left-sided; the relatively flat external surface of the morphologically left ventricle (*LV*), which is right-sided; the transposed aorta (*Ao*), which is anterior and to the left of the transposed pulmonary artery (*PA*); the anterior descending coronary artery arising from the right coronary artery; and the broad, pyramidal appendage of the morphologically right atrium, which is right sided (*RA*).

[*Figure and legend continued overleaf.*]

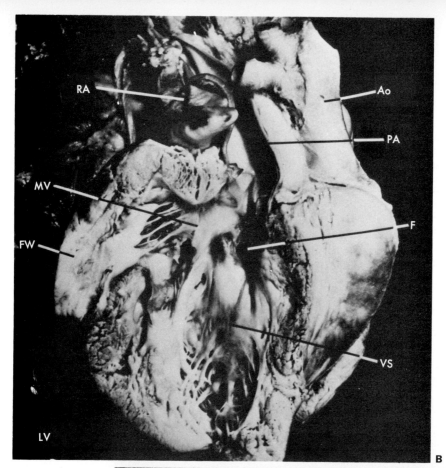

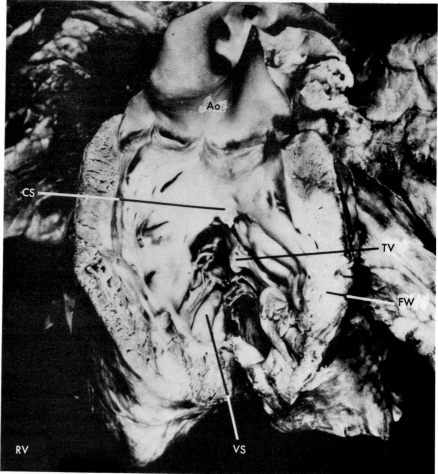

anything is!" Quite seriously, the segmental approach to diagnosis should make this a thing of the past.

Jaunty general surgeons, about to fix a tracheoesophageal fistula in an infant with dextrocardia (which may well be secondary to aspiration and atelectasis of the right lung), would become uncharacteristically unnerved. Should one do a right or a left thoracotomy? The argument, while peering at the chest x-rays, would run somewhat as follows:

"Since dextrocardia is present, there's likely to be a right aortic arch. I wish I could really see the arch on these films, but I can't! To avoid the aortic arch, we'd better do a left thoracotomy."

Wrong! The side of the aortic arch usually correlates with the type of visceroatrial situs, not with the location of the heart in the thorax. A left arch is usual in situs solitus and a right arch is to be anticipated in situs inversus, no matter where the heart is. Since the infant with the TE fistula has situs solitus, a left aortic arch is very probable, despite the presence of dextrocardia. Hence, a right thoracotomy would be preferable. It should be added that a high KV chest x-ray usually spoils this diagnostic game, because then one frequently *can* see the aortic arch.

The location of the heart within the thorax (dextrocardia, mesocardia, or levocardia) is not a basic biologic consideration. But the type of visceroatrial situs is basic; all asymmetric viscera normally conform to the type of situs. Remember that in quadrupeds, the heart is midline within a deep thorax; i.e., mesocardia is normal in many quadrupeds. It seems that one of the liabilities associated with man's assumption of an outright posture (in addition to low back pain!) is anteroposterior flattening of the thorax, making cardiac lateralization to the left or right a desirable secondary adaptation.

Dextrocardia has inspired separate languages, separate classifications, and unusual diagnostic approaches. *It is this dextrocardia mystique that must be eliminated,* because it is mainly this—the special terms, classifications, and approaches–that have made dextrocardia a difficult and intimidating problem. The anatomy per se of dextrocardia is no different from that of left-sided congenital heart disease (Tables 36–3 to 36–5). Dextrocardia is *not* a different world when analyzed in basic terms: situs, loop, and conotruncus (Figures 36–1, 36–9, 36–17, and 36–18).

Hence, it is urged that special cardiac malposition terminologies, classifications, and approaches be abandoned because they are unnecessary, and they obstruct (rather than assist) understanding. Ordinary terms and approaches are entirely adequate, this being a major theme of the present chapter.

In addition to giving rise to special terminologies and classifications, dextrocardia has even inspired poetry, of a sort, with which we may conclude this section. The following fragment was attributed to the printer's devil and appeared at the end of Professor Allen Thompson's paper more than a century ago (quoted by Stevenson, 1937):

Once nature a change in man's fabric to try,
His stomach and vitals set entirely awry;
To the left of his belly the liver was found,
And his heart to the right—but all otherwise sound.
Such hodge-podge of structure would hinder, you'd
* think,*
The due courses of blood, of meat, and of drink:
But, strange to relate, they most fitly proceeded
Exactly the way that for health was most needed.
It has often been said of the just and the kind,
That the heart in the right place you're quite sure to
* find;*
And as to our case, I should like to be told,
If this great moral law was still likely to hold.

MESOCARDIA

MESOCARDIA indicates that the heart is located in approximately the middle of the thorax; i.e., the heart lies predominantly neither to the right, nor to the left, in the plain posteroanterior chest roentgenogram.

Mesocardia is derived from two Greek words: *meso* = middle, and *kardia* = heart.

The literature on mesocardia is curiously sparse. Thus, it is fortunate indeed that Lev and associates

---

Figure 36-25 B and C.

In the view of the opened morphologically left ventricle (*LV*), which is right-sided (*B*), note the smooth superior septal surface (*VS*), the numerous, fine, oblique trabeculae carneae of the apical portion of the left ventricular septal surface, the relatively large papillary muscles that arise exclusively from the left ventricular free wall (*FW*), obscuring the interior of the left ventricular free wall to a major degree and making left ventriculotomy difficult except at the apex and high paraseptally, the subpulmonary ventricular septal defect (*F*), the transposed pulmonary artery (*PA*), and the direct fibrous continuity between the pulmonary valve and the anterior leaflet of the mitral valve (*MV*), permitted by absence of subpulmonary conal musculature.

In the view of the opened morphologically right ventricle (*RV*), which is left-sided (*C*), and the L-transposed aorta (*Ao*), note the coarse right ventricular trabeculae carneae both of the septal surface (*VS*) and of the free wall surface (*FW*), and the wide separation of the transposed aortic valve from the left-sided tricuspid valve (*TV*) by the well-developed subaortic crista supraventricularis (*CS*).

(Reproduced from Van Praagh, R., et al.: Anatomic types of dextrocardia. Diagnostic and embryologic implications. *Am. J. Cardiol.,* **13**:510, 1964.)

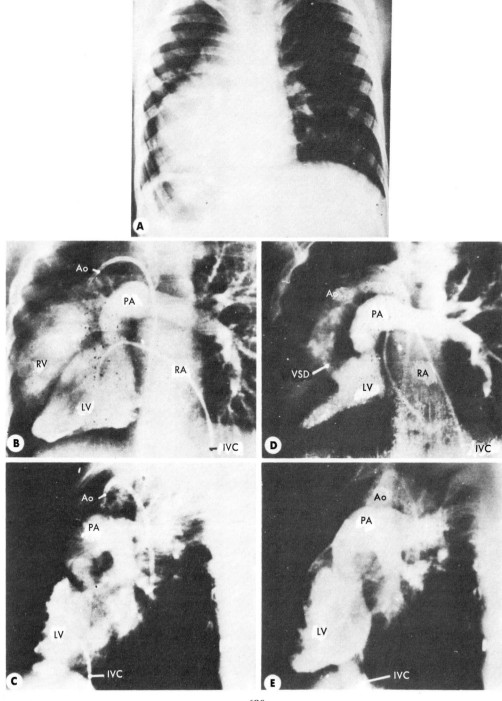

(1971) have written a paper on this subject. Lev defines mesocardia as "that condition in which the longitudinal axis of the heart lies in the mid-sagittal plane, with the heart possessing no distinct apex, and this is due to an inherent development of the heart." The ventricles appear flattened frontally, as though the interventricular septum pressed against the sternum and then the ventricles expanded outward on each side of the sternum, instead of the ventricular

apex elongating itself unopposed into either the left or right hemithorax. (We do not know if such mechanical factors really play a role in the formation of these blunt, apexless ventricles; the foregoing is merely what the external appearance suggests as a possible explanation.)

An attempt is made to summarize Lev's findings and to present them in ordinary terminology in Table 36–6.

Table 36–6. PATHOLOGIC ANATOMY OF MESOCARDIA: 13 CASES*

TYPES OF HEART	SEGMENTAL SETS	NO. OF CASES	PERCENT OF SERIES
Normal type of heart with Tricuspid stenosis (1) Common AV canal (1) ASD, VSD, PDA (1) ASD 1, polysplenia (1)	{S,D,S}	4	31
Probably normal type of heart with Common atrium Common AV canal Pulmonary stenosis } (1) Complete AV block Accessory spleen	{S,D,S}	1	8
Complete transposition Single ventricle (1)	{S,D,D}	2	15
Double-outlet RV with Common AV canal } Accessory spleen } (1)	{S,D,D}	1	8
Corrected transposition Tricuspid stenosis (lt-sided) (1) Ebstein's anomaly (2) (1 Ebstein's with accessory spleen)	{S,L,L}	3	23
Double-outlet RV, lt-sided, with Common AV canal, PS, and accessory spleen	{S,L,L}	1	8
Corrected transposition in Situs inversus with ASD II and ASD I	{I,D,D}	1	8

* Based on Table 1 of Lev et al., (1971). ASD = atrial septal defect; ASD II = secundum type of atrial septal defect; ASD I = ostium primum type of atrial septal defect; AV = atrioventricular; PDA = patent ductus arteriosus; VSD = ventricular septal defect. Percentages rounded off to nearest whole number.

Figure 36–26. Chest x-ray and angiocardiography in dextrocardia with corrected transposition in situs inversus {I, D, D}. *A* is a plain posteroanterior chest roentgenogram; *B* and *C* are simultaneous posteroanterior and left lateral projections, respectively, of a selective injection into the left-sided LV during diastole, while *D* and *E* are simultaneous posteroanterior and left lateral projections, respectively, during systole. In *A*, the right-sided stomach bubble and the left-sided liver shadow accurately suggest situs inversus of the viscera and atria, as is confirmed in *B* by the left-sided location of the inferior vena caval catheter (*IVC*). The morphologically right atrium (*RA*) is left-sided. D-transposition of the great arteries is present (*B* to *E*), the aorta (*Ao*) lying to the right of the pulmonary artery (*PA*). In the lateral projections (*C* and *E*), it is seen that the Ao is mildly but distinctly posterior to the PA. Since the PA originates above the morphologically left ventricle (*LV*) and since the Ao originates above the morphologically right ventricle (*RV*), transposition of the great arteries is definitely present. Thus, this is transposition of the great arteries with a posterior aorta. If the ventricles are oriented in a direction normal for a D-loop, the apex pointing leftward, then the transposed aorta becomes as anterior as one usually sees with transposition of the great arteries. Hence, the posterior location of the aorta in this transposition is regarded as secondary to the cardiac malposition. In *D*, the ventricular septal defect (*VSD*) is well seen and stenotic subpulmonary conal musculature is also visualized. There is a bilateral conus, not only subaortic but also subpulmonary, with pulmonary stenosis (infundibular and valvular). In *B* and *D*, the diastolic and systolic pictures of LV are well seen. The presence of a right aortic arch is also noteworthy, this being consistent with situs inversus of the viscera and atria. The sidedness of the aortic arch correlates best with the type of visceroatrial situs, not with the left- or right-sided location of the heart. Dextrocardia does not necessarily suggest that a right aortic arch will be present, whereas situs inversus does. (Reproduced from Van Praagh, R., et al.: Diagnosis of the anatomic types of congenital dextrocardia. *Am. J. Cardiol.*, **15**:234, 1965.)

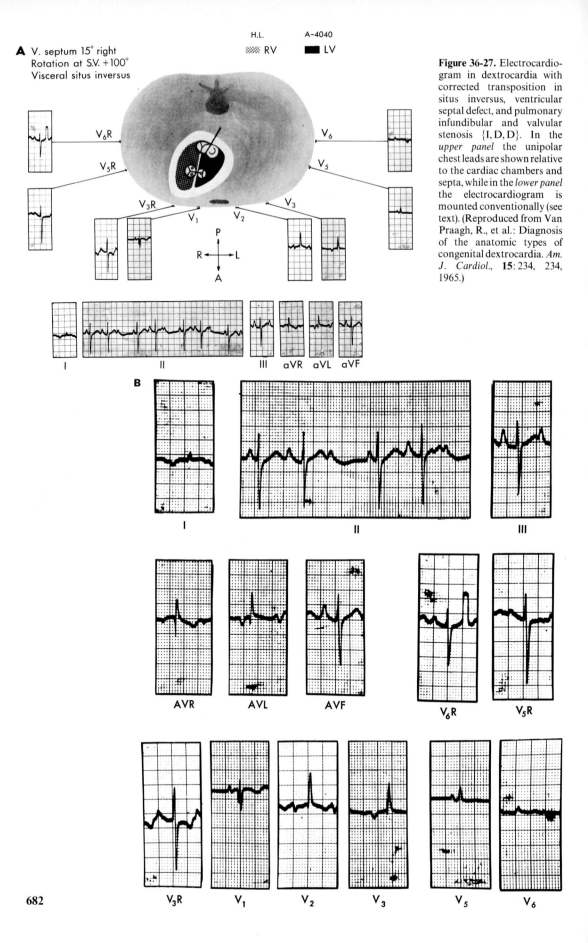

A V. septum 15° right
Rotation at S.V. +100°
Visceral situs inversus

H.L.   A-4040
░░ RV   ■ LV

V₆R

V₅R

V₃R
V₁   V₂

V₆

V₅

V₃

P
R —— L
A

I   II   III   aVR   aVL   aVF

B

I   II   III

AVR   AVL   AVF   V₆R   V₅R

V₃R   V₁   V₂   V₃   V₅   V₆

Figure 36-27. Electrocardiogram in dextrocardia with corrected transposition in situs inversus, ventricular septal defect, and pulmonary infundibular and valvular stenosis {I, D, D}. In the *upper panel* the unipolar chest leads are shown relative to the cardiac chambers and septa, while in the *lower panel* the electrocardiogram is mounted conventionally (see text). (Reproduced from Van Praagh, R., et al.: Diagnosis of the anatomic types of congenital dextrocardia. *Am. J. Cardiol.*, **15**: 234, 234, 1965.)

Table 36–7. MALFORMATIONS ASSOCIATED WITH LEVOCARDIA, VISCERAL HETEROTAXY, AND SPLENIC DYSGENESIS*

MALFORMATIONS	ASPLENIA (10 CASES)	POLYSPLENIA (4 CASES)	ACCESSORY SPLEEN (9 CASES)
Lungs			
Bilaterally quadrilobed	2		
Bilaterally trilobed	6	1	2
Bilaterally bilobed	1	2	2
Solitus		1	5
Inversus	1		
IVC			
Right-sided	7	2	2
Left-sided	3		3
Absent		1	4
Not stated		1	
SVC			
Bilateral	6	1	4
Right only	4	1	2
Left only		2	3
Pulmonary veins			
Normal	1	1 (CT)	6
TAPVC	8	3	
Ipsilateral*	1		3
AV valves			
Normal			2
T At and cleft MV	1		
Common AV canal	8	3	6
Mitral stenosis			1
Mitral atresia		1	
Not stated	1		
Ventricles			
Normally formed	8	4	9
Single (common) V	2		
Great arteries			
Normally related	3	3	3
Double-outlet RV		1	2
Truncus, atypical	1		
D-Transposition	4		4
L-Transposition	2		
Outflow tracts			
No obstruction	3	1	
Pulmonary stenosis	3	1	2
Pulmonary atresia	4		4
Aortic stenosis		1	1
Coarctation of aorta		1	3

* Based on Table 1 of Liberthson et al. (1973). Cardiac segments are not tabulated since these data were not completely reported. Ipsilateral pulmonary veins means that right-sided pulmonary veins drain to right-sided atrium or to right side of common atrium, while left-sided pulmonary veins connect to left-sided atrium or to left side of common atrium. *Abbreviations:* AV = atrioventricular; CT = cor triatriatum; MV = mitral valve; RV = morphologically right ventricle; TAPVC = totally anomalous pulmonary venous connection; T At = tricuspid atresia; V = ventricle.

Polysplenia is widely supposed to be characterized by bilaterally bilobed lungs ("bilateral left-sidedness"). In this small group of four cases, half showed the expected pattern, but half did not. Again, "bilateral left-sidedness" is a helpful mnemonic, but other patterns are also to be anticipated (Table 36–7).

In patients with accessory spleen, the majority (5/9) had a normal bronchial pattern, but bilaterally trilobed patterns (2/9) and bilaterally bilobed patterns (2/9) also occurred.

3. *Regarding the inferior vena cava* (IVC), in asplenia it was more often right-sided (7/10) than left-sided (3/10), again suggesting that many of these cases have partial situs solitus, not partial situs inversus.

In polysplenia, the suprarenal-to-subhepatic segment of the IVC is widely thought to be frequently absent. Hence, it is interesting that of these four cases, the IVC was absent in only one case. But the IVC was absent in 4/9 cases with accessory spleen. Hence, in this study, absence of the IVC occurred both with polysplenia and with accessory spleen, but was typical of neither (a minority in both groups).

4. *Concerning the pulmonary veins*, total anomalous pulmonary venous connection was, unsurprisingly, found to be the rule with asplenia (8/10 cases, Table 36–7). Ipsilateral pulmonary veins (right veins to right-sided atrium, and left veins to left-sided atrium) are often regarded as typical of polysplenia, and this indeed pertained in three of these four cases. However, ipsilateral pulmonary veins also occurred with asplenia (1/10) and with accessory spleen (3/9 cases, Table 36–7).

Ipsilateral pulmonary veins pose an interesting and difficult surgical problem, which we think is surgically solvable in the following way. The anatomic findings suggest that it should be possible to construct a Y-shaped pericardial baffle that would lead the pulmonary venous blood to the systemic ventricle. The caval blood would flow in front of the baffle and would enter the pulmonary ventricle. This operation would be a "reverse Mustard," i.e., constructing an interatrial conduit for the pulmonary venous return, instead of for the systemic venous return (as in the Mustard procedure).

5. *Regarding the atrioventricular valves*, common atrioventricular canal predominated in all three dysplenic groups: asplenia (8/10 cases), polysplenia (3/4), and accessory spleen (6/9 patients).

6. *Single (common) ventricle* was found only with asplenia (2/10 cases).

7. *Concerning relationships between the great arteries*, a normal relationship was infrequent with asplenia (3/10), the rule with polysplenia (3/4), and a minority with accessory spleen (3/9 cases). Transposition predominated with asplenia (6/10 cases) and occurred in almost half the patients with accessory spleen (4/9 cases).

8. *Regarding outflow tract obstruction (stenosis or atresia)*, pulmonary outflow tract obstruction predominated with asplenia (7/10 cases) and accessory spleen (6/9 cases), but was the exception with polysplenia (1/4 cases, Table 36–7).

Treatment and Prognosis

The treatment and prognosis in the cardiac malpositions are essentially similar to those of normally located hearts, everything depending on the malformation, its severity, early and accurate diagnosis, and surgical expertise. One of the most important bases of successful surgery is a good understanding of the anatomy. With a median sternotomy, the presence of dextrocardia does not matter.

In 1963, Cooley and Billig reported what they believed were the first surgical repairs, in dextrocardia, of atrial septal defect, ventricular septal defect, and tetralogy of Fallot. Kay and associates (1965) reported VSD closure through a left-sided ventriculotomy. This appears to have been a right ventriculotomy, left-sided, in a classic corrected transposition {S,L,L}, with VSD. In 1968, Kiser and associates reported the brilliant surgical correction of dextrocardia {S,L,L} with double-outlet RV, VSD, and PS. This paper merits careful study. A most important step in their operation was extensive resection of the obstructive subpulmonary conal musculature. The stenotic pulmonary valve ring was incised in a vertical direction posteriorly, and then was sewn together in a horizontal direction, to reduce the pulmonary annular stenosis. Finally, the VSD patch was sutured to the left of the pulmonary valve, thereby separating the pulmonary and systemic circulations.

Conduction System

An understanding of the conduction system and the intraoperative use of the probe to identify the His bundle are as important in the surgery of the cardiac malpositions as in the surgery of normally located hearts. Titus (1973) has published two papers concerning the normal anatomy of the conduction system that may be regarded as a "base line." *Normally* (Figure 36–30), the His bundle arises from a posterior atrioventricular node, just in front of the coronary sinus. The His bundle then passes anteriorly and superiorly toward the superior commissure of the tricuspid valve. Here it dives or penetrates, running beneath the membranous septum (Figure 36–30). If a ventricular septal defect is present, the His bundle runs along its lower rim. This normal course of the His bundle had been known for many years, based on the work of Lev (1957 and 1968) and many others.

In 1963, Lev, Licata, and May published a study of the conduction system in classic corrected transposition {S,L,L}, which they studied by serial sections and wax plate reconstruction. They found that the conduction system was inverted, with a prolonged course of the His bundle. In other words, the His bundle arose from an essentially normally located (posterior) AV node and pursued the expected course, except for being inverted, which was anticipated because of the inversion of the ventricles. Hence, the conduction system in this one case of classic corrected transposition was found to be a mirror image of the normal conduction system.

However, later in the same year (1963), Lev, Fielding, and Zaeske published another study of the conduction system in corrected transposition {S,L,L} in an infant with congenital complete heart block. They found that the normal (posterior) AV node ended blindly, not giving rise to the His bundle. An accessory (anterior) AV node was found in the anterior right atrial free wall where it joined the atrial septum anteriorly. This anterior AV node gave rise to a very thin AV bundle that reached the morphologically left ventricle (right-sided) by passing between the annuli of the right-sided mitral and pulmonary valves. This tenuous His bundle ran *above* the ventricular septal defect and then bifurcated into inverted left and right bundle branches. However, the significance of these observations was not appreciated for a decade.

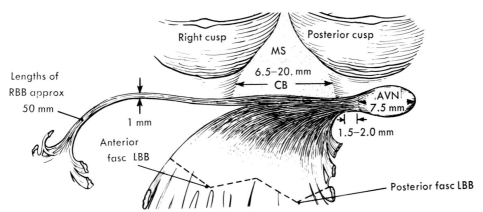

Figure 36-30. Normal atrioventricular conduction system. This is a schematic representation of the normal adult AV conduction system, viewed from the left ventricular aspect. Normally, the His bundle passes beneath the membranous septum (*MS*), and if a membranous type of ventricular septal defect is present, the AV bundle runs along the inferior and posterior margin of the VSD. Note the measurements of the various parts of the adult AV conduction system, in mm. *AVN*, Atrioventricular node; *CB*, common bundle; *fasc*, fascicle; *LBB*, left bundle branch; *RBB*, right bundle branch. (Reproduced from Titus, J. L.: Normal anatomy of the human cardiac conduction system. *Mayo Clin. Proc.*, **48**:24, 1973.)

In 1973 and 1974, Anderson and his colleagues focused attention on the conduction system in corrected transposition {S,L,L}. In a histopathologic study of 11 cases, the His bundle ran from an *anterior* AV node (Figure 36–31*A*). This anterior AV node was located in the anterior wall of the right atrium, adjacent to the atrial septum, and just behind and to the right of the pulmonary valve (Figure 36–31*A*). From this anterior and superior AV node, the His bundle passed between the mitral valve to the right and the pulmonary valve to the left (Figure 36–31*A* and *B*). In other words, when one looks at the right-sided LV and pulmonary artery from the right side (Figure 36–31), the His bundle runs *in front of* the pulmonary annulus. More precisely, the His bundle is to the right, or lateral, relative to the pulmonary annulus (Figure 36–31). Then the His bundle proceeds downward into the right-sided LV. When a ventricular septal defect (VSD) is present, the His bundle continues downward into the right-sided LV by running along *the upper rim*—the superior and anterior margin—of the VSD (Figure 36–32), instead of running along the lower rim—the inferior and posterior margin—of the VSD, as in the normal type of heart with a concordant D-loop. In one of Anderson's 11 cases, the normal posterior AV node also connected with the ventricles, as in the case of Lev, Licata, and May (1963).

The great surgical importance of the work of Anderson and his colleagues was immediately appreciated and was confirmed by electrophysiologic identification of the His bundle in the operating room (Kupersmith et al., 1974; Waldo et al., 1975). This meant that in a case of L-TGA {S,L,L} with ventricular septal defect and pulmonary stenosis, one cannot relieve the pulmonary stenosis by excising myocardium of the stenotic "roof" of the pulmonary outflow tract—because the His bundle runs in the roof of the outflow tract, just below the pulmonary valve. Instead of myocardial resection in this area, it currently is considered preferable to run a Rastelli type of external valved conduit from the right-sided LV to the pulmonary artery, in order to bypass the pulmonary outflow tract stenosis. In this way one hopes to avoid the development of complete AV block, even though one knows that there is a relatively high frequency of AV block that develops in L-TGA spontaneously.

Since *single ventricle* can now be corrected surgically (Edie et al., 1973; Ionescu et al., 1973; Arai et al., 1973; Danielson et al., 1974), an understanding of the conduction system in single (common) ventricle has now become essential, and this has been provided by several different groups (Jones et al., 1973; Anderson et al., 1974; Bharati and Lev, 1975; Maloney et al., 1975).

In single LV with an infundibular outlet chamber, the His bundle typically arises from an anterior AV node and penetrates to the right of the transposed pulmonary valve. Then, where does the His bundle run? Does it run in the superior and anterior rim of the bulboventricular foramen, similar to typical corrected transposition (Figures 36–31 and 36–32)? Or does it run in the posterior and inferior rim of the defect, similar to its location in the normal heart (Figure 36–30)? Or does the His bundle run behind the bulboventricular foramen—posterior or dorsal to the defect? Published and unpublished data vary.

Briefly, we think that if the bulboventricular foramen is located quite far anteriorly, as it often is in single LV, then the His bundle will usually pass behind and below the bulboventricular foramen in its descent to reach the left ventricular septal surface. When the bulboventricular foramen is quite anterior, the His bundle passes close to its posterior and inferior quadrant, both in D- and L-loops. Hence, if surgical

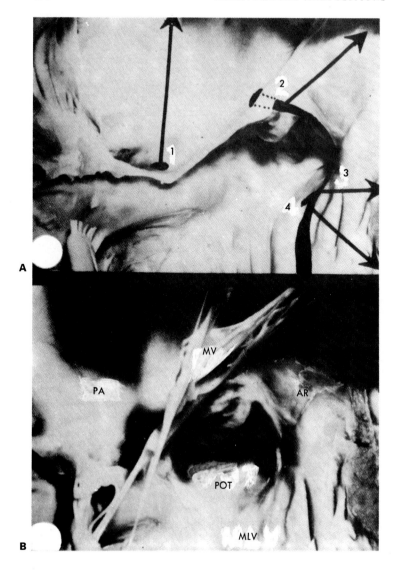

A

B

Figure 36-31. His bundle in corrected transposition {S, L, L}. Study *B* first, for orientation, and then *A*. These are right lateral views of the morphologically right atrium (*RA*), the right-sided mitral valve (*MV*), the right-sided morphologically left ventricle (*MLV*), the right-sided pulmonary outflow tract (*POT*) and pulmonary valve, and the anterior recess (*AR*) in front of the pulmonary outflow tract. In *B*, the mitral valve is present. In *A*, the deep septal leaflet of the mitral valve has been removed in order to expose the AV conduction system more clearly. The His bundle (AV bundle) is drawn in using a heavy black line. The black dot at *1* is the location of the normal posterior AV node, which is just in front of the coronary sinus. This posterior AV node is hypoplastic and gives rise to no His bundle. The black dot at *2* indicates the location of the anterior AV node that does give rise to the His bundle (black line). Tracing the course of the His bundle, note that it first pierces the fibrous tissue between the mitral valve to the right and the pulmonary valve to the left. This fibrous tissue is often called the central fibrous body and this portion of the His bundle is called the penetrating portion, which is represented by dotted lines in *A*. When the His bundle emerges from the central fibrous body, it runs around the right or lateral margin of the pulmonary valve. Then the bundle heads inferiorly (at *3*, in *A*) and runs toward the left ventricular septal surface, where it bifurcates into the left and right bundle branches (at *4*, in *A*). (Reproduced from Anderson, R. H.; Becker, A. E.; Arnold, R.; and Wilkinson, J. L.: The conducting tissues in congenitally corrected transposition. *Circulation*, **50**:911, 1974.)

enlargement of such a bulboventricular foramen is necessary—because the foramen is (or has progressively become) obstructively small, resulting in a form of muscular subaortic stenosis—the surgical enlargement should be carried out in the anterior and superior quadrants of the bulboventricular foramen.

However, if the bulboventricular foramen is quite posterior relative to the pulmonary annulus and the entry of the His bundle into the ventricular portion of the heart, then the His bundle may pass along the superior and anterior margins of the bulboventricular foramen in order to reach the left ventricular septal surface. If surgical enlargement of such a foramen is necessary, it should be done in the inferior and posterior quadrants of the bulboventricular foramen.

Thus, the variable accounts of the course of the His bundle in single LV with infundibular outlet chamber may well be understandable in terms of the variable

location of the bulboventricular foramen relative to the entry of the His bundle into the ventricular portion of the heart: if the His enters well behind the foramen, then the His runs behind and below the foramen; but if the His enters more or less above the foramen, then the bundle may well run above and in front of the foramen in order to reach the left ventricular septal surface.

In view of our present ignorance concerning the variations in the course of the His bundle relative to the bulboventricular foramen in single LV with infundibular outlet chamber, we think that intraoperative electrophysiologic mapping of the course of the His bundle is highly desirable in this anomaly in order to avoid surgically induced heart block.

Since mapping cannot be done during hypothermic arrest, such cases may be begun utilizing conventional, normothermic cardiopulmonary bypass.

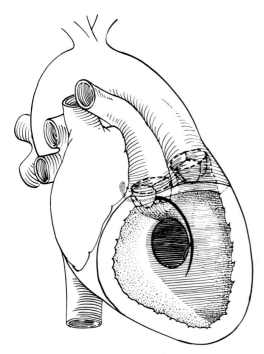

Figure 36-32. The His bundle in corrected transposition {S, L, L}. Arising from an anterior AV node, the His bundle penetrates between the mitral annulus to the right and the pulmonary annulus to the left. Then the His bundle runs around the right lateral aspect of the pulmonary valve. At this point it heads inferiorly and runs along the superior and anterior margins of the ventricular septal defect. This is the opposite of normal. Normally, the His bundle runs along the inferior and posterior margins of a VSD. (Reproduced from Maloney, J. D.; Ritter, D. G.; McGoon, D. C.; and Danielson, G. K.: Identification of the conduction system in corrected transposition and common ventricle at operation. *Mayo Clin. Proc.*, **50**: 387, 1975.)

After mapping has been completed, hypothermic arrest may then be accomplished, when desired, by core cooling, without the usual form of surface cooling by ice packs.

In other words, a principle that may well have widespread applicability in the surgical repair of congenital heart disease in infants and young children appears to be: map first at normal temperature; then cool and correct.

The course of the conduction system in *single (common) ventricle without an infundibular outlet chamber* appears to be highly variable and unpredictable (Anderson, personal communication). The His bundle may pass to the right of the right AV valve in order to reach the single (common) ventricle. In such cases, intraoperative mapping of the conduction system during normothermic bypass also is strongly indicated. In such cases, one should avoid cutting what may appear to be a free-running tendon because this "tendon" can be the His bundle (Anderson, personal communication).

In corrected transposition in situs inversus {*I,D,D*}, Drs. Macdonald Dick and Aldo Castaneda of the Children's Hospital Medical Center in Boston found electrophysiologically at open heart surgery in one patient that the His bundle ran in *the inferior and posterior margin* of the ventricular septal defect (Dick et al., 1977).

Is it possible to understand these variable locations of the His bundle in congenital heart disease? Briefly, it looks as though the conduction system is where it must be in order to make contact with the ventricles. In other words, if there is significant malalignment between the ventricular septum and the atrial septum, there is no way that the normally located posterior AV node can make contact with the displaced interventricular septum. However, the anterior AV node can make contact with the ventricles, because it is close both to the conal septum and to the anterior portion of the interventricular septum, no matter how displaced the ventricular septum may be posteriorly. Hence, in situations characterized by displacement of the interventricular septum relative to the atrial septum, the normal posterior AV node is often hypoplastic, and the His bundle contacts the ventricles via the anterior AV node. This situation—an anterior AV node giving rise to the His bundle—was first described by Monckeberg (1913).

Thus, much has recently been learned concerning the origin and course of the His bundle in various types of congenital heart disease that is highly relevant to the avoidance of heart block when surgical repair is undertaken.

Antibiotic Prophylaxis for Asplenia

This is another recent therapeutic advance that is highly relevant to the cardiac malpositions (Tables 36–5 and 36–6). It has been our experience that successfully palliated survivors of the asplenia syndrome can die in less than 24 hours from fulminating pneumococcal septicemia. In a review of our patients with congenital asplenia, Waldman and associates (1977) found that these individuals have a greatly increased risk of infection by encapsulated bacteria: *Klebsiellae* or *E. coli* in the young infant, and *Pneumococcus* or *H. influenzae* in infants six months of age or older. In view of the prevalence of pneumococcal and *H. influenzae* sepsis in patients with congenital asplenia, we now recommend continuous antibiotic prophylaxis for asplenic children and adults as follows: amoxicillin, 25 mg/kg/day, divided into two doses, the maximum being 1 gm/day; or ampicillin, 50 mg/kg/day, divided into four doses, the maximum being 2 gm/day. The advantage of the newer and hence less familiar amoxicillin as compared with the more familiar ampicillin is the b.i.d. dosage schedule in the former, compared with the q.i.d. dosage schedule in the latter. We suggest that antibiotic prophylaxis be commenced upon diagnosis of the asplenia syndrome and that it be continued indefinitely.

Conclusions

The central themes of this chapter are two:

1. That patients with cardiac malpositions should be approached diagnostically just like patients with normally positioned hearts—step-by-step, segment-by-segment.

2. That a good understanding of the pathologic anatomy of congenital heart disease is basic to accurate diagnosis and successful surgery.

REFERENCES

Dextrocardia

Abbott, M. E., and Moffatt, W.: Mirror-picture dextrocardia, complicated by mitral aplasia and pulmonary hypoplasia, with great hypertrophy of the transposed "right" chambers, *Can. Med. Assoc. J.*, **20**:611, 1929.

Abbott, M. E.: *Atlas of Congenital Cardiac Disease*. American Heart Association, New York, 1936, p. 58.

Abbott, G. A., and Russek, H. I.: Calcareous aortic stenosis in a case of dextrocardia with situs inversus. *Am. J. Med. Sci.*, **204**:516, 1942.

Abrahamson, L.: Four cases of congenital dextrocardia, including a case with sino-auricular block. *Q. J. Med.*, **18**:335, 1924–25.

Adams, R., and Churchill, E. D.: Situs inversus, sinusitis, bronchiectasis. *J. Thorac. Surg.*, **7**:206, 1937.

Afzelius, B. A.; Eliasson, R.; Johnsen, Ø.; and Lindholmer, C.: Lack of dynein arms in immotile human speramatozoa. *J. Cell. Biol.*, **66**:225, 1975.

Anderson, R. C.; Lillehei, C. W.; and Lester, R. G.: Corrected transposition of the great vessels of the heart: A review of 17 cases. *Pediatrics*, **20**:626, 1957.

Anderson, R. H.; Arnold, R.; and Jones, R. S.: D-bulboventricular loop with l-transposition in situs inversus. *Circulation*, **46**:173, 1972.

Anderson, R. H.; Arnold, R.; and Wilkinson, J. L.: The conducting system in congenitally corrected transposition. *Lancet*, **1**:1286, 1973.

Anderson, R. H.; Becker, A. E.; Arnold, R.; and Wilkinson, J. L.: The conducting tissues in congenitally corrected transposition. *Circulation*, **50**:911, 1974.

Anderson, R. H.; Arnold, R.; Thapar, M. K.; Jones, R. S.; and Hamilton, D. I.: Cardiac specialized tissue in hearts with an apparently single ventricular chamber (double inlet left ventricle). *Am. J. Cardiol.*, **33**:95, 1974.

Angelini, P., and Leachman, R.: Anterior pulmonary artery from the left ventricle: revolution or restoration? *Circulation*, **46**:II–97, 1972 (abst.).

Arai, T.; Ando, M.; Takao, A.; and Sakakibara, S.: Intracardiac repair for single or common ventricle: creation of a straight artificial septum. *Bull. Heart Inst. Japan*, **14**:81, 1972–1973.

Arcilla, R. A., and Gasul, B. M.: Congenital dextrocardia. Clinical angiocardiographic and autopsy studies on 50 patients. *J. Pediatr.*, **58**:39, 1961.

Arén, P.: A case of isolated congenital dextrocardia. *Acta Med. Scand.*, **128**:179, 1947.

Aristotle, cited by Lineback, P. E.: An extraordinary case of situs inversus viscerum totalis. *JAMA*, **75**:1775, 1920.

Ayres, S. M., and Steinberg, I.: Dextrorotation of the heart. An angiocardiographic study of forty-one cases. *Circulation*, **27**:268, 1963.

Bacon, R. L.: Self-differentiation and induction in the heart of amblystoma. *J. Exp. Zool.*, **98**:87, 1945.

Baillie, M.: *The Morbid Anatomy of Some of the Most Important Parts of the Human Body*, 2nd ed. Johnson and Nicol, London, 1797, p. 38.

Barcia, A.: Coronary angiography techniques and new areas of investigation. *Horizons in Cardiology, Texas Heart Institute, Third Annual Symposium*, June 1–3, 1972, p. 24.

Barcia, A.; Kincaid, O.; Davis, G. D.; Kirklin, J. W.; and Ongley, P.

A.: Transposition of the great arteries, an angiocardiographic study. *Am. J. Roentgenol.*, **100**:249, 1967.

Bharati, S., and Lev, M.: The course of the conduction system in single ventricle with inverted (l-) loop and inverted (l-) transposition. *Circulation*, **51**:723, 1975.

Belaisch, G., and Nouaille, J.: Les dextrocardies chez l'enfant. Essai de classification. *Arch. Franc. Pediatr.*, **26**:679, 1969.

Billig, D. M.; Hallman, G. L.; Bloodwell, R. D.; and Cooley, D. A.: Surgical treatment of cardiac defects associated with variations in cardiac position. *J. Thorac. Cardiovasc. Surg.*, **55**:80, 1968.

Burchell, H. B., and Pugh, D. H.: Uncomplicated isolated dextrocardia ("dextroversio cordis" type). *Am. Heart J.*, **44**:196, 1952.

Caffey, J.: *Pediatric X-Ray Diagnosis*. Year Book Publishers, Inc., Chicago, 1945, p. 229.

Campbell, M., and Reynolds, G.: The significance of the direction of the P wave in dextrocardia and isolated laevocardia. *Br. Heart J.*, **14**:481, 1952.

Campbell, M., and Deuchar, D. C.: Dextrocardia and isolated laevocardia. I. Isolated laevocardia. *Br. Heart J.*, **27**:69, 1965.

Campbell, M., and Deuchar, D. C.: Dextrocardia and isolated laevocardia. II. Situs inversus and isolated dextrocardia. *Br. Heart J.*, **28**:472, 1966.

Capon, N. B., and Chamberlain, E. N.: A case of true dextrocardia. *Lancet*, **208**:918, 1925.

Carr, I.; Tynan, M.; Aberdeen, E.; Bonham-Carter, R. E.; Graham, G.; and Waterston, D. J.: Predictive accuracy of the "loop rule" in 109 children with classical complete transposition of the great arteries (TGA) *Circulation*, **38**:VI–52, 1968 (abstr.).

Chapman, C. B., and Gibbons, T.: New aids in the diagnosis of dextrocardia. *Am. Heart J.*, **39**:507, 1950.

Clarkson, P. M.; Brandt, P. W. T.; Barratt-Boyes, B. G.; and Neutze, J. M.: "Isolated atrial inversion". Visceral situs solitus, visceroatrial discordance, discordant ventricular d-loop without transposition, dextrocardia: diagnosis and surgical correction. *Am. J. Cardiol.*, **29**:877, 1972.

Clerc, A., and Bobrie, J.: Réflexions sur un cas de dextrocardie pure. *Arch. Mal. Coeur*, **11**:145, 1918.

Cockayne, E. A.: The genetics of transposition of the viscera. *Q. J. Med.*, **7**:479, 1938.

Cooley, D. A., and Billig, D. M.: Surgical repair of congenital cardiac lesions in mirror image dextrocardia with situs inversus totalis. *Am. J. Cardiol.*, **11**:518, 1963.

Crawford, J. H., and Warren, C. F.: Coronary thrombosis in a case of congenital dextrocardia with situs inversus. *Am. Heart J.*, **15**:240, 1938.

Dalcq, A.: Sur les opérations susceptibles de provoquer l'inversion du situs viscerum chez les anoures. *Acta Anat.*, **4**:100, 1947.

Danielson, G. K.; Giuliani, E. R.; and Ritter, D. G.: Successful repair of common atrium associated with complete atrioventricular canal. *J. Thorac. Cardiovasc. Surg.*, **67**:152, 1974.

Daves, M. L., and Pryor, R.: Cardiac positions, a primer. *Am. Heart J.*, **79**:408, 1970.

De la Cruz, M. V., and da Rocha, J. P.: An ontogenetic theory for the explanation of congenital malformations involving the truncus and conus. *Am. Heart J.*, **51**:782, 1956.

De la Cruz, M. V.; Anselmi, G.; Cisneros, F.; Reinhold, M.; Portillo, B.; and Espino-Vela, J.: An embryologic explanation for the corrected transposition of the great vessels: additional description of the main anatomic features of this malformation and its varieties. *Am. Heart J.*, **57**:104, 1959.

De la Cruz, M. V.; Polansky, B. J.; and Navarro-Lopez, F.: The diagnosis of corrected transposition of the great vessels. *Br. Heart J.*, **24**:483, 1962.

De la Cruz, M. V.; Espino-Vela, J.; Attie, F.; and Muñoz, C. L.: Embryologic theory for ventricular inversions and their classification. *Am. Heart J.*, **73**:777, 1967.

De la Cruz, M. V.; Anselmi, G.; Muños-Castellanos, L.; Nadel-Ginard, B.; and Muñoz-Armas, S.: Systematization and embryological and anatomical study of mirror-image dextrocardias, dextroversions, and laevoversions. *Br. Heart J.*, **33**:841, 1971.

De la Cruz, M. V., and Nadal-Ginard, B.: Rules for the diagnosis of visceral situs, truncoconal morphologies, and ventricular inversions. *Am. Heart J.*, **84**:19, 1972.

Dick, M.; Van Praagh, R.; Rudd, M.; Folkerth, T.; and Castaneda, A. R.: Electrophysiologic delineation of the specialized atrioventricular conduction system in two patients with corrected transposition of the great arteries in situs inversus (I,D,D). *Circulation*, 55:896, 1977.

Edie, R. N.; Ellis, K.; Gersony, W. M.; Krongrad, E.; Bowman, F. O.; and Malm, J. R.: Surgical repair of single ventricle. *J. Thorac. Cardiovasc. Surg.*, 66:350, 1973.

Fabricius, cited by Cleveland, M.: Situs inversus viscerum; anatomic study. *Arch. Surg.*, 13:343, 1926.

Farre, J. R.: *Pathological Researches. Essay I. On Malformations of the Human Heart: Illustrated by Numerous Cases, and Five Plates, Containing Fourteen Figures; and Preceded by Some Observations on the Method of Improving the Diagnostic Part of Medicine.* Longman, Hurst, Rees, Orme and Brown, London, 1814, p. 28.

Foggie, W. E.: Congenital dextrocardia. Cor triloculare biventriculare. *Edinburgh Med. J.*, 5:428, 1910.

Forde, W. J., and Finby, N.: Roentgenographic features of asplenia, a tetralogic syndrome of visceral symmetry. *Am. J. Roentgenol.*, 86:523, 1961.

Freedom, R. M.: The heterotaxy syndrome. *Circulation*, 44:II–115, 1971 (abstr.).

Garvin, J. A.: Dextrocardia with pulmonary artery arising from the aorta. *Am. J. Dis. Child.*, 34:133, 1927.

Goor, D. A.; Dische, R.; and Lillehei, C. W.: The conotruncus. I. Its normal inversion and conus absorption. *Circulation*, 46:375, 1972.

Goor, D. A., and Edwards, J. E.: The transition from double outlet right ventricle to complete transposition, a pathologic study. *Am. J. Cardiol.*, 29:267, 1972 (abstr.).

Grant, R. P.: The syndrome of dextroversion of the heart. *Circulation*, 18:25, 1958.

Grollman, J. H.: Ontogenetic method of classifying cardiac position. *Am. J. Roentgenol.*, 100:564, 1967.

Gubbay, E. R.: Isolated congenital dextrocardia. *Am. Heart J.*, 50:356, 1955.

Guerin, R.; Soto, B.; Karp, R. B.; Kirklin, J. W.; and Barcia, A.: Transposition of the great arteries. Determination of the position of the great arteries in conventional chest roentgenograms. *Am. J. Roentgenol.*, 110:747, 1970.

Hallerman, F. J.; Kincaid, O. W.; Ritter, D. G.; Ongley, P. A.; and Titus, J. L.: Angiocardiographic and anatomic findings in origin of both great arteries from the right ventricle. *Am. J. Roentgenol.*, 109:51, 1970.

Hastreiter, A. R., and Rodriguez-Coronel, A.: Discordant situs of thoracic and abdominal viscera. *Am. J. Cardiol.*, 22:111, 1968.

Heim de Balsac, R.; Metianu, C.; and Emam-Zadé, A. M.: *Traité Des Cardiopathies Congenitales.* Masson et Cie., Paris, 1954, p. 1034.

Hightower, B. M.; Barcia, A.; Bargeron, L. M.; and Kirklin, J. W.: Double-outlet right ventricle with transposed great arteries and subpulmonary ventricular septal defect. The Taussig-Bing malformation. *Circulation*, 39:1–207, 1969.

Ionescu, M. I.; Macartney, F. G.; and Wooler, G. H.: Intracardiac repair of single ventricle with pulmonary stenosis. *J. Thorac. Cardiovasc. Surg.*, 65:602, 1973.

Ivemark, B.: Implications of agenesis of the spleen on the pathogenesis of conotruncus anomalies in childhood. *Acta Pediatr. Scand.*, 44:590 and Suppl. 104, 1955.

Jaubert de Beaujeu, A., and Benmussa: Deux cas de dextrocardie isolée. *Arch. Mal Coeur*, 32:141, 1939.

Jones, H. W.: Types of dextrocardia. *Br. Med. J.*, 1:147, 1924.

Jones, R. S.; Anderson, R. H.; Arnold, R.; Thapar, M.; and Hamilton, D.: Study of specialized conducting tissue in cases of single ventricle. *Br. Heart J.*, 35:554, 1973.

Kartagener, M.: Zur pathogenese der Bronchiektasien. I. Mitteilung: Bronchiektasien bei Situs viscerum inversus. *Beitr. Klin. Erforsch. Tuberk. Lungenkr.*, 83:489, 1933.

Katsuhara, K.; Kawamoto, S.: Wakabayashi, T.; and Belsky, J. L.: Situs inversus totalis and Kartagener's syndrome in a Japanese population. *Chest*, 61:56, 1972.

Kay, E. B.; Rodriguez, P.; and Zimmerman, H. A.: Surgery for ventricular septal defect in dextroversion through a left ventriculotomy. *Am. J. Cardiol.*, 15:267, 1965.

Keith, A.: The Hunterian lectures on malformations of the heart. Lecture II. *Lancet*, p. 433, Aug. 14, 1909.

Kerr, A. R.; Barcia, A.; Bargeron, L. M.; and Kirklin, J. W.: Double-outlet left ventricle with ventricular septal defect and pulmonary stenosis: Report of surgical repair. *Am. Heart J.*, 81:688, 1971.

Kiser, J. C.; Ongley, P. A.; Kirklin, J. W.; Clarkson, P. M.; and McGoon, D. C.: Surgical treatment of dextrocardia with inversion of ventricles and double-outlet right ventricle. *J. Thorac. Cardiovasc. Surg.*, 55:6, 1968.

Korth, C., and Schmidt, J.: Dextroversio cordis. *Arch. Kreislaufforsch.*, 20:167, 1954.

Kossman, C. E.: Galvanometric potentials of the extremities and of the thorax in congenital dextrocardia. *Am. Heart J.*, 20:322, 1940.

Kupersmith, J.; Krongrad, E.; Gersony, W. M.; and Bowman, F. O.: Electrophysiologic identification of the specialized conduction system in corrected transposition of the great arteries. *Circulation*, 50:795, 1974.

Lake, K., and Sharma, O. P.: Kartagener's syndrome and deafmutism: an unusual association. *Chest*, 64:661, 1973.

Langstaff: Case of a singular mal-formation of the heart. *London Med. Rev.*, 4:88, 1811.

Lansing, A. M., and Scofield, E. L. W.: Mitral valvotomy in a patient with dextrocardia and situs inversus. *Chest*, 66:580, 1974.

Laubry, C., and Pezzi, C.: *Traité des Maladies Congénitales du Coeur.* J. B. Baillière et Fils, Paris, 1921, p. 268.

Layton, W. M.: Random determination of a developmental process: Reversal of normal visceral asymmetry in the mouse. *J. Hered.*, 67:336, 1976.

Leachman, R. D.; Cokkinos, D. V.; and Zamalloa, O.: Discordance of the suprahepatic inferior vena cava and right atrium from liver situs. Report of 2 cases with dextrocardia and clinical implications. *Chest*, 63:926, 1973.

Lev, M.: *Autopsy Diagnosis of Congenitally Malformed Hearts.* Charles C Thomas, Publisher, Springfield, Ill., 1953, p. 13.

Lev, M.: The conduction system in the human heart. *Military Med.*, 120:262, 1957.

Lev, M.; Liberthson, R. R.; Eckner, F. A. O.; and Arcilla, R. A.: Pathologic anatomy of dextrocardia and its clinical implications. *Circulation*, 37:979, 1968.

Lev, M.; Licata, R. H.; and May, R. C.: The conduction system in mixed levocardia with ventricular inversion (corrected transposition). *Circulation*, 28:232, 1963.

Lev, M.; Fielding, R. T.; and Zaeske, D.: Mixed levocardia with ventricular inversion (corrected transposition) with complete atrioventricular block. A histopathologic study of the conduction system. *Am. J. Cardiol.*, 12:875, 1963.

Lev, M.: Conduction system in congenital heart disease. *Am. J. Cardiol.*, 21:619, 1968.

Levin, P. D.; Faber, L. P.; and Carleton, R. A.: Cardiac herniation after pneumonectomy. *J. Thorac. Cardiovasc. Surg.*, 61:104, 1971.

LeWald, L. T.: Complete transposition of the viscera. A report of twenty-nine cases with remarks on etiology. *JAMA*, 84:261, 1925.

Lewis, F. T., and Abbott, M. E.: Reversed torsion of the human heart. *Anat. Rec.*, 9:103, 1915.

Lewis, F. T., and Abbott, M. E.: Reversed torsion of the ventricular band of the embryonic heart in the explanation of certain forms of cardiac anomaly. *Bull. Int. A. M. Museums*, 6:111, 1916.

Lichtman, S. S.: Isolated congenital dextrocardia. *Arch. Int. Med.*, 48:683, 1931.

Logan, W. D.; Abbott, O. A.; and Hatcher, C. R.: Kartagener's triad. *Dis. Chest*, 48:613, 1965.

Lowe, C. R., and McKeown, T.: An investigation of dextrocardia with and without transposition of abdominal viscera with a report of a case in one monozygotic twin. *Am. Eugen.*, 18:267, 1954.

Lucas, R. V.; Neufeld, H. N.; Lester, R. G.; and Edwards, J. E.: The symmetrical liver as a roentgen sign of asplenia. *Circulation*, 25:973, 1962.

Maloney, J. D.; Ritter, D. G.; McGoon, D. C.; and Danielson, G. K.: Identification of the conduction system in corrected transposition and common ventricle at operation. *Mayo Clin. Proc.*, 50:387, 1975.

Manasek, F.; Burnside, M. B.; and Van Praagh, R.: Heart looping and fibril formation. *Circulation*, 44:II-116, 1971 (abstr.).

Manchester, B., and White, P. D.: Dextrocardia with situs inversus complicated by hypertensive coronary heart disease. *Am. Heart J.*, 15:493, 1938.

Meyer, P.: Dextrocardie pure congénitale sans inversion des cavités cardiaques. *Arch. Mal. Coeur*, 30:971, 1937.

Mayer, R. A.; Schwartz, D. C.; Covitz, W.; and Kaplan, S.: Echocardiographic assessment of cardiac malposition. *Am. J. Cardiol.*, 33:896, 1974.

Miller, R. D., and Divertie, M. B.: Kartagener's syndrome. *Chest*, **62**:130, 1972.

Miller, B. L.; Medrano, G. A.; and Sodi-Pallares, D.; Vectorcardiogram in dextrocardia, dextroversion and dextroposition. *Am. J. Cardiol.*, **21**:830, 1968.

Mirowski, M.; Neill, C. A.; and Taussig, H. B.: Left atrial ectopic rhythm in mirror-image dextrocardia and in normally placed malformed hearts. Report of twelve cases with "dome and dart" P waves. *Circulaton*, **27**:864, 1963.

Moffett, R. D., and Neuhof, S.: Congenital dextrocardia with patent interventricular septum, with fluoroscopic and electrocardiographic examination. *Am. J. Dis. Child.*, **10**:1, 1915.

Momma, K., and Linde, E. M.: Cardiac rhythms in dextrocardia. *Am. J. Cardiol.*, **25**:420, 1970.

Monckenberg, J. G.: Zur entwicklungsgeschichte des atrioventrikularsystems. *Verhandl. deutsch Pathol., Gesellsch.*, **16**:228, 1913.

Morgan, J. R.; Forker, A. D.; and Trummer, M. J.: Left aortic arch and right superior vena cava in mirror-image dextrocardia with tetralogy. *Chest*, **61**:92, 1972.

Nadas, A. S., and Fyler, D. C.: *Pediatric Cardiology*, 3rd ed., W. B. Saunders Company, Philadelphia, 1972, p. 656.

Nakata, H.; Nakagawa, E.; Mihara, K.; Tokunaga, M.; Moirita, K.; and Koga, I.: Dextrocardia, small right hemithorax, and abnormal pulmonary vessel. *Chest*, **68**:359, 1975.

Nazarian, M.; Currarino, G.; Webb, W. R.; Willis, K.; Kiphart, R. J.; and Wilson, H. E.: Accessory diaphragm. Report of a case with complete physiological evaluation and surgical correction. *J. Thorac. Cardiovasc. Surg.*, **61**:293, 1971.

Neill, C. A.: Development of the pulmonary veins, with reference to the embryology of anomalies of pulmonary venous return. *Pediatrics*, **18**:880, 1956.

Neufeld, H. N.; Du Shane, J. W.; Wood, E.; Kirklin, J. W.; and Edwards, J. E.: Origin of both great vessels from the right ventricle. I. Without pulmonary stenosis. *Circulation*, **23**:399, 1961.

Neufeld, H. N.; DuShane, J. W.; and Edwards, J. E.: Origin of both great vessels from the right ventricle. II. With pulmonary stenosis. *Circulation*, **23**:603, 1961.

Neufeld, H. N.; Lucas, R. V.; Lester, R. G.; Adams, P.; Anderson, R. C.; and Edwards, J. E.: Origin of both great vessels from the right ventricle without pulmonary stenosis. *Br. Heart J.*, **24**:393, 1962.

Niibori, S.; Ando, M.; Takao, A.; and Sakakibara, S.: Viscero-atrial heterotaxic syndrome. *Bull. Heart Inst. Japan*, **13**:72, 1971.

Olsen, A. M.: Bronchiectasis in dextrocardia; observations on etiology of bronchiectasis. *Am. Rev. Tuberc.*, **47**:435, 1943.

Owen, S. A.: A case of complete transposition of the viscera, associated with mitral stenosis, including a description of electrocardiographic tracings. *Heart*, **3**:113, 1911-12.

Paltauf, R.: Dextrocardie und dextroversio cordis. *Wien. klin. Wchnschr.*, **14**:1032, 1901.

Parsons-Smith, B.: A note on dextrocardia, complete and incomplete, with four illustrative cases. *Lancet*, **197**(2):1076, 1919.

Paul, M. H.; Sinha, S. N.; Muster, A. J.; Cole, R. B.; and Van Praagh, R.: Double outlet left ventricle. Report of an autopsy case with an intact ventricular septum and consideration of its developmental implications. *Circulation*, **41**:129, 1970.

Peacock, T. B.: *On Malformations of the Human Heart etc with Original Cases and Illustrations*, 2nd ed. John Churchill and Sons, London, 1866, p. 1.

Portillo, B.; Anselmi, G.; Sodi-Pallares, D.; and Medrano, G. H.: Importance of the unipolar leads in the diagnosis of dextrocardias, levocardias, dextropositions and dextrorotations. *Am. Heart J.*, **57**:396, 1959.

Potts, P. H., and Ashman, R.: A case of dextrocardia with right (functional left) ventricular predominance, ventricular ectopic beats, and retrograde conduction. *Am. Heart J.*, **2**:152, 1926.

Ptashkin, D.; Stein, E.; and Warbasse, J. R.: Congenital dextrocardia with anterior wall myocardia infarction. *Am. Heart J.*, **74**:263, 1967.

Ratner, B.; Abbott, M. E.; and Beattie, W. W.: Cor triloculare biventriculare in mirror-picture dextrocardia with persistent omphalo-mesenteric bay, right aortic arch and pulmonary artery forming descending aorta. *Am. J. Dis. Child.*, **22**:508, 1921.

Reinberg, S. A., and Mandelstam, M. E.: On the various types of dextrocardia and their diagnostics. *Radiology*, **11**:240, 1928.

Reisman, H. A.: Dextrocardia in children. *Ann. Int. Med.*, **10**(1):200, 1936.

Richardson, J. S.: Chest leads in congenital and acquired dextrocardia. *Br. Heart J.*, **4**:80, 1942.

Riolanus, cited by Upson, W. O.: Transposed viscera. *Am. J. Roentgenol.*, **8**:385, 1921.

Rösler, H. Beiträge zur Lehre von den angebornenen Herzfehlern. VI. Uber die angeborene isolierte rechtslage des Herzens. *Wien. Arch. inn. Med.*, **19**:505, 1930.

Ruskin, A.; Tarnower, H.; Lattin, B.; and Robb, G. P.: Isolated dextrocardia, with diodrast studies. *Am. Heart J.*, **25**:116, 1943.

Schmidt, J., and Korth, C.: Die Klink der dextrokardien. *Arch. Kreislaufforsch.*, **21**:188, 1954.

Schmutzer, K. J., and Linde, L. M.: Situs inversus totalis associated with complex cardiovascular anomalies. *Am. Heart J.*, **56**:761, 1958.

Sénac: *Traité de la Structure du Coeur, de son Action, et de ses Maladies*, Paris, 1749.

Severinus, cited by Cleveland, M.: Situs inversus viscerum; anatomic study. *Arch. Surg.*, **13**:343, 1926.

Shah, K. D.; Neill, C. A.; Wagner, H. N.; and Taussig, H. B.: Radioisotope scanning of the liver and spleen in dextrocardia and in situs inversus with levocardia. *Circulation*, **29**:231, 1964.

Shaher, R. M.; Duckworth, J. W.; Khoury, G. H.; and Moes, C. A. F.: The significance of the atrial situs in the diagnosis of positional anomalies of the heart. I. Anatomic and embryologic considerations. *Am. Heart J.*, **73**:32, 1967.

Shaher, R. M.; Moes, C. A. F.; and Khoury, G. H.: The significance of the atrial situs in the diagnosis of positional anomalies of the heart. II. An angiocardiographic study of 29 patients. *Am. Heart J.*, **73**:41, 1967.

Shepard, E. M., and Stewart, H. J.: Interpretation of the electrocardiogram, dextrocardia with situs inversus. *Am. Heart J.*, **36**:55, 1948.

Silberstein, A. G., and Steinberg, I.: Case report. Contrast cardiovascular study of a patient with rheumatic mitral valvular disease and dextrocardia with complete situs inversus. *N. Y. State J. Med.*, **43**(2):1755, 1943.

Sodi-Pallares, D.; Bisteni, A.; Fishleder, B. L.; and Medrano, G. A.: Importance of the unipolar morphologies in the interpretation of the electrocardiogram: the theoretical basis of the unipolar morphologies and its correlation with vectorial analysis, with cardiac activation and with the potential variations at the epicardial surface of the heart. *Am. Heart J.*, **57**:590, 1959.

Solinger, R.; Elbl, F.; and Minhas, K.: Deductive echocardiographic analysis in infants with congenital heart disease. *Circulation*, **50**:1072, 1974.

Soulié, P.: *Cardiopathies Congénitales*. Expansion Scientifique Française, Paris, 1952, p. 260.

Squarcia, U.; Ritter, D. G.; and Kincaid, O. W.: Dextrocardia: Angiocardiographic study and classification. *Am. J. Cardiol.*, **32**:965, 1973.

Stanger, P.; Benassi, R. C.; Korns, M. E.; Jue, K. L.; and Edwards, J. E.: Diagrammatic portrayal of variations in cardiac structure. Reference to transposition, dextrocardia and the concept of four normal hearts. *Circulation*, **37**:Suppl. 4, 1968.

Steinberg, M. F.; Grishman, A.; and Sussman, M. L.: Angiocardiography in congenital heart disease. I. Dextrocardia. *Am. J. Roentgenol.*, **48**:141, 1942.

Stevenson, D. S.: Isolated uncomplicated dextrocardia. *Q. J. Med.*, **6**:395, 1937.

Streeter, G. L.: Developmental horizons in human embryos. Description of age group XI, 13 to 20 somites, and age group XII, 21 to 29 somites. *Carnegie Inst., Washington, D.C., Contrib. Embryology*, **30**:211, 1942.

Streeter, G. L.: Developmental horizons in human embryos. Description of age group XIII, embryos about 4 or 5 millimeters long, and age group XIV, period of indentation of the lens vesicle. *Carnegie Inst., Washington, D.C., Contrib. Embryology*, **31**:27, 1945.

Streeter, G. L.: Developmental horizons in human embryos. Description of age groups XV, XVI, XVII, and XVIII, being the third issue of a survey of the Carnegie Collection. *Carnegie Inst., Washington, D.C., Contrib. Embryology*, **32**:133, 1948.

Streeter, G. L.: Developmental horizons in human embryos. Description of age groups XIX, XX, XXI, XXII, and XXIII, being the fifth issue of a survey of the Carnegie Collection. *Carnegie Inst., Washington, D.C., Contrib. Embryology*, **34**:165, 1951.

Taussig, H. B.: *Congenital Malformations of the Heart. Volume II: Specific Malformations.* Harvard University Press, Cambridge, Mass., 1960, p. 963.

Taussig, H. B., and Bing, R. J.: Complete transposition of the aorta and a levoposition of the pulmonary artery. *Am. Heart J.*, **37**:551, 1949.

Terry, L.: *The Mathmen.* McGraw-Hill Book Company, New York, 1964.

Titus, J. L.: Normal anatomy of the human cardiac conduction system. *Mayo Clin. Proc.*, **48**:24, 1973.

Titus, J. L.: Anatomy of the conduction system. *Circulation*, **47**:170, 1973.

Torgersen, J.: Genetic factors in visceral asymmetry and in the development and pathologic changes of lungs, heart and abdominal organs. *Arch. Pathol.*, **47**:566, 1949.

Torner-Soler, M.; Balaguer-Vintro, I.; and Carrasco-Azemar, J.: Cardiac dextroposition: hypoplasia of the right pulmonary artery with right venous pulmonary drainage into the inferior vena cava. *Am. Heart J.*, **56**:675, 1958.

Van Mierop, L. H. S.; Alley, R. D.; Kansel, H. W.; and Stranahan, A.: Pathogenesis of transposition complexes. I. Embryology of the ventricles and great arteries. *Am. J. Cardiol.*, **12**:216, 1963.

Van Mierop, L. H. S.; Patterson, P. R.; and Reynolds, R. W.: Two cases of congenital asplenia with isomerism of the cardiac atria and the sinoatrial nodes. *Am. J. Cardiol.*, **13**:407, 1964.

Van Mierop, L. H. S.; Eisen, S.; and Schiebler, G. L.: The radiographic appearance of the tracheobronchial tree as an indicator of visceral situs. *Am. J. Cardiol.*, **26**:432, 1970.

Van Mierop, L. H. S.: Transposition of the great arteries. I. Clarification or further confusion? *Am. J. Cardiol.*, **28**:735, 1971.

Van Praagh, R.; Ongley, P. A.; and Swan, H. J. C.: Anatomic types of single or common ventricle in man: Morphologic and geometric aspects of 60 necropsied cases. *Am. J. Cardiol.*, **13**:367, 1964.

Van Praagh, R.; Van Praagh, S.; Vlad, P.; and Keith, J. D.: Anatomic types of congenital dextrocardia. Diagnostic and embryologic implications. *Am. J. Cardiol.*, **13**:510, 1964.

—————: Diagnosis of the anatomic types of congenital dextrocardia. *Am. J. Cardiol.*, **15**:234, 1965.

Van Praagh, R., and Van Praagh, S.: The anatomy of common aortico-pulmonary trunk (truncus arteriosus communis) and its embryologic implications. A study of 57 necropsied cases. *Am. J. Cardiol.*, **16**:406, 1965.

Van Praagh, R., and Van Praagh, S.: Anatomically corrected transposition of the great arteries. *Br. Heart J.*, **24**:112, 1967.

Van Praagh, R.: Malposition of the heart. In *Heart Disease in Infants, Children and Adolescents*, A. J. Moss and F. H. Adams (eds.). Williams & Wilkins Co., Baltimore, 1968, p. 602.

Van Praagh, R.: What is the Taussig-Bing malformation? *Circulation*, **44**:445, 1968.

Van Praagh, R., and Corsini, I.: Cor triatriatum: Pathologic anatomy and a consideration of morphogenesis based on 13 postmortem cases and a study of normal development of the pulmonary vein and atrial septum in 83 human embryos. *Am. Heart J.*, **78**:379, 1969.

Van Praagh, R.; Van Praagh, S.; Nebesar, R. A.; Muster, A. J.; Sinha, S. N.; and Paul, M. H.: Tetralogy of Fallot: underdevelopment of the pulmonary infundibulum and its sequelae. Report of a case with cor triatriatum and pulmonary sequestration. *Am. J. Cardiol.*, **26**:25, 1970.

Van Praagh, R.; Pérez-Treviño, C.; López-Cuellar, M.; Baker, F.; and Van Praagh, S.: Transposition of the great arteries with posterior aorta, anterior pulmonary artery, subpulmonary conus

and fibrous continuity between aortic and atrioventricular valves. *Am. J. Cardiol.*, **28**:621, 1971.

Van Praagh, R.: Transposition of the great arteries. II. Transposition clarified. *Am. J. Cardiol.*, **28**:739, 1971.

Van Praagh, R.; Bernhard, W. F.; Rosenthal, A.; Parisi, L. F.; and Fyler, D. C.: Interrupted aortic arch: surgical treatment. *Am. J. Cardiol.*, **27**:200, 1971.

Van Praagh, R.: The segmental approach to diagnosis in congenital heart disease. *Birth Defects: Original Article Series*, **8**:4, 1972.

Van Praagh, R.: Conotruncal malformations. In Barratt-Boyes, B. G.; Neutze, J. M.; and Harris, E. A. *Heart Disease in Infancy.* (eds.): Churchill and Livingstone, Edinburgh, 1973, p. 141.

Van Praagh, R.: Les malformations conotroncales. *Coeur, Numéro Spécial:* 15, 1973.

Van Praagh, R.: Dextrocardia—classify it as it really is. *Am. J. Cardiol.*, **34**:382, 1974.

Vaquez, H., and Donzelot: Dextrocardie et dextroversion. *Presse Méd.*, **28**:41, 1920.

Waldo, A. L.; Pacifico, A. D.; Bargeron, L. M.; James, T. N.; and Kirklin, J. W.: Electrophysiological delineation of the specialized A-V conduction system in patients with corrected transposition of the great vessels and ventricular septal defect. *Circulation*, **52**:435, 1975.

Waller, A. D.: On the electromotive changes connected with the beat of the mammalian heart, and of the human heart in particular. *Phil. Trans. Roy. Soc. Lond.*, **180**:169, 1889.

Watson, J. D.: *Molecular Biology of the Gene.* W. A. Benjamin, Inc., New York, 1965.

Welsh, R. A., and Felson, B.: Uncomplicated dextroversion of the heart. *Radiology*, **66**:24, 1956.

Willius, F. A.: Congenital dextrocardia. *Am. J. Med. Sc.*, **157**:485, 1919.

Willius, F. A.: Congenital dextrocardia with situs transversus complicated by hypertensive heart disease; electrocardiographic changes. *Am. Heart J.*, **7**:110, 1931.

Wynn-Williams, N.: Bronchiectasis: A study centered on Bedford and its environs. *Br. Med. J.*, **1**:1194, 1953.

Zelikovsky, A.; Vidne, B.; and Levy, M. J.: Mirror-image dextrocardia in situs inversus and coarctation of the aorta. *Chest*, **66**:297, 1974.

Mesocardia and Levocardia

Attie, F.; Malpartida, F.; Poveda, J. J.; Testelli, M. R.; and Espino Vela, J.: Acyanotic levoversion in situs inversus. *Chest*, **64**:668, 1973.

Ferencz, C.: Visceral heterotaxy with malformed heart. Similar findings in a child and a puppy. *Anat. Rec.*, **149**:229, 1964.

Keith, J. D.; Rowe, R. D.; and Vlad, P.: *Heart Disease in Infancy and Childhood*, 1st ed. Macmillan Publishing Co. Inc., New York, 1958, p. 557.

Lev, M.; Liberthson, R. R.; Golden, J. G.; Eckner, F. A. O.; and Arcilla, R. A.: The pathologic anatomy of mesocardia. *Am. J. Cardiol.*, **28**:428, 1971.

Liberthson, R. R.; Hastreiter, A. R.; Sinha, S. N.; Bharati, S.; Novak, G. M.; and Lev, M.: Levocardia with visceral heterotaxy—isolated levocardia: pathologic anatomy and its clinical implications. *Am. Heart J.*, **85**:40, 1973.

Nakajima, K.; Kudo, T.; Yokoyama, M.; Nogi, M.; Konno, S.; and Takao, A.: Levocardia and situs inversus. Anatomical and clinical investigations, with special reference to new classification. *Respir. Circ.*, **18**:765, 1970.

Waldman, J. D.; Rosenthal, A.; Smith, A. L.; Shurin, S.; and Nadas, A. S.: Sepsis in congenital asplenia. *J. Pediatr.*, **90**:555, 1977.

OBSTRUCTIONS, REGURGITATIONS, AND OTHER MALFORMATIONS

37

Aortic Stenosis: Valvular, Subaortic, and Supravalvular

Peter M. Olley, Kenneth R. Bloom, and *Richard D. Rowe*

AORTIC stenosis in its various forms has been found in 7 percent of more than 15,000 patients with heart disease seen at The Hospital for Sick Children. Since over 1 percent of the population has a bicuspid aortic valve, the potential number of candidates for aortic valve stenosis is obviously larger than these clinical figures would suggest. Clinically recognizable aortic stenosis, however, is the sixth most frequent malformation encountered in a regional hospital practice. Of this large group approximately 83 percent have valvular stenosis and 9 percent have discrete (fibrous or fibromuscular) subaortic stenosis. Full clinical descriptions of supravalvular aortic stenosis and muscular subaortic stenosis in children have emerged comparatively recently. These two conditions form a much smaller proportion of aortic stenosis in the young and by contrast with the other forms seldom show signs of obstructive heart disease early in infancy.

In this chapter we shall deal with the subject in three sections:

1. Valvular aortic and discrete subaortic stenosis.
2. Muscular subaortic stenosis.
3. Supravalvular aortic stenosis.

VALVULAR AORTIC AND DISCRETE SUBAORTIC STENOSIS
Peter M. Olley

VALVE stenosis is the commonest cause of left ventricular obstruction in both children and adults. Stenosis may be present at birth or may be acquired by fibrosis and calcification of a congenitally malformed but originally nonobstructive aortic valve. Rheumatic aortic stenosis is exceedingly uncommon in children but occurs in adults.

Pathology

Several types of congenitally abnormal valves have been described (Edwards, 1958, 1965; Roberts, 1969, 1970). Unicuspid valves have either a central orifice without lateral attachments to the aortic wall or an eccentric orifice with one lateral attachment to the aortic wall at the level of the orifice. In the former there is no commissure and the valve forms a simple dome resembling the type of semilunar valve often seen in pulmonary stenosis. The eccentric orifice unicuspid valve has a single commissure. Most frequently seen is the bicuspid aortic valve in which the cusps are arranged either to the left and right with anterior and posterior commissures or the cusps are positioned anterior and posterior with left and right commissures. A third raphe or false commissure is usually present. Such bicuspid valves open less completely than a normal tricuspid valve and coapt less well in diastole. Occasionally a tricuspid aortic valve is seen with marked disparity in cusp size, which may lead to fibrosis and calcification and ultimately to stenosis. Quadricuspid aortic valves usually function normally but on rare occasions develop stenosis.

Valves with fewer cusps are more likely to be stenotic, and Edwards (1958) has emphasized that unicuspid valves are stenotic from birth and are the most frequent finding in infants dying from congenital aortic valve stenosis. Bicuspid and abnormal tricuspid valves may be nonobstructive at birth but thicken and calcify in response to hemodynamic stress and eventually become stenotic. In an autopsy series of 168 patients, aged 15 to 65

698

years, with isolated aortic stenosis studied by Roberts (1970), 59 (35 percent) had tricuspid aortic valves, while among 27 patients over 65 years old 25 (93 percent) were tricuspid. Among the 15-to-65 age group about half the patients had additional mitral valve thickening suggesting an additional rheumatic etiology. The origin of the aortic stenosis in the other patients was unclear but could have resulted from abnormal blood flow patterns through a structurally malformed, although tricuspid, valve leading to progressive fibrosis and ultimate stenosis (Figure 37–1).

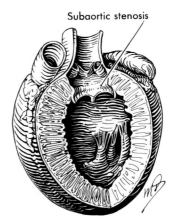

Subaortic stenosis

Figure 37-2. Subaortic fibrous ring type of stenosis immediately below the aortic valve. Enlarged, thickened left ventricle.

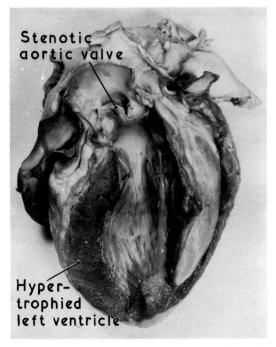

Stenotic aortic valve

Hyper-trophied left ventricle

Figure 37-1. J. O'H. Died at three years of age of cerebral embolus secondary to subacute bacterial endocarditis. Aortic stenosis and hypertrophied left ventricle are shown.

Discrete subaortic stenosis may take several forms. Kelly and associates (1972) described two main types. Type I consists of a thin discrete membrane lying immediately beneath the aortic valve (Figure 37–2), while type II is situated about 1 cm below the valve and embodies a fibromuscular ring that narrows the outflow tract and may encroach on the anterior leaflet of the mitral valve. Occasionally a fibromuscular tunnel narrows the left ventricular outflow tract for several centimeters. This latter deformity was present in 9 of 33 patients described by Reis and associates (1971) but was found in only 3 of the 51 children studied by Newfeld and associates (1976).

First described by Chevers in 1842, discrete subaortic stenosis accounts for approximately one-tenth of all cases of aortic stenosis in childhood. Roberts (1973) has emphasized that acquired lesions of the aortic valve are common in patients with

subaortic stenosis due to jet lesions causing thickening and fibrosis of the valve leaflets. Consequently the aortic valve often becomes incompetent in these patients. Discrete subaortic stenosis has traditionally been attributed to incomplete atrophy of the bulbus cordis (Keith, 1924); however, Van Praagh and associates (1970) have suggested that it may result from maldevelopment of the endocardial cushion tissue of the atrioventricular canal that usually forms the anterior leaflet of the mitral valve.

Subaortic stenosis may also occur in lesions of the mitral valve such as accessory valvular tissue or the abnormal insertion of a normal or cleft mitral valve leaflet to the interventricular septum (Sellers et al., 1964). Finally, subaortic stenosis may occur as part of an endocardial cushion defect or be caused by an obstructive bulboventricular canal septal defect in single ventricle complexes.

Significant obstruction to left ventricular ejection in the absence of aortic regurgitation leads to concentric hypertrophy of the left ventricle with little dilatation. The thickened ventricle offers more resistance to filling, and even when compensated left ventricular end diastolic pressure rises. Corresponding elevations in left atrial, pulmonary artery, and right ventricular pressures occur, and both the left atrium and right ventricle may enlarge and hypertrophy. Occasionally marked myocardial fibrosis limited to the left ventricle also develops (Marquis and Logan, 1955). Poststenotic dilatation of the ascending aorta frequently accompanies aortic valve stenosis. According to Roach (1963), this dilatation results from a localized increase in aortic wall distensibility. Turbulent blood flow creates vibrations that damage the elastic fibers and break down the links between collagen fibers in the aortic wall.

In infants aortic stenosis may be associated with left ventricular hypoplasia and endocardial fibroelastosis; the abnormal left ventricle offers considerable obstruction to inflow from the left atrium, which

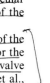

E.F.E.

may enlarge, stretching the foramen ovale, leading to left-to-right shunting at atrial level. Under these conditions the diagnosis of aortic stenosis may be difficult.

Hypoplasia of the aorta is rare but sometimes, as in the case described by Richter (1953), the aortic valve ring itself is smaller than normal and accompanied by relatively little cusp thickening.

Cook and associates (1947) described a rare form of acquired aortic valve stenosis complicating xanthoma tuberosum hypercholesteremia in which the stenosis was due to xanthomatous infiltration of the valve.

Aortic valve calcification is rare before the age of 15 years.

Clinical Features

Most children with congenital aortic stenosis are asymptomatic and grow and develop normally. The discovery of a heart murmur is the usual reason for referral. Although the clinical findings of both valve and discrete subvalve stenosis have much in common, there are features that may permit their differentiation at the bedside. More difficult at times is the clinical estimation of the severity of the obstruction. The manifestations of aortic stenosis also vary considerably in different age groups.

Table 37–1 summarizes the clinical findings of 300 patients with congenital aortic stenosis at The Hospital for Sick Children and the Toronto General Hospital, during childhood and up to the age of 30. It will be noted that dyspnea and heart failure are common during the first year of life, occurring in three-quarters of the cases that presented with signs and symptoms in that period. Between one and five years signs or symptoms of any sort are rarely noted. After the age of five years and before 15 years, dyspnea and syncope are found with increasing frequency, but the incidence still does not exceed 10 percent of the cases with aortic stenosis in the pediatric age group. Angina is a relatively rare finding in childhood. Most children with this anomaly appear to be normal from external appearance, and only a few have a sallow complexion such as is reported in adult life. As a rule, the growth curves show normal height and weight of these children for their age (Kjellberg, 1958), but a few of them are appreciably underweight (Marquis and Logan, 1955). The principal symptoms in the late teens and young adult life are dyspnea, syncope, and chest pain. Heart failure is more likely to occur when the aortic stenosis is associated with some other heart lesion such as endocardial fibroelastosis or patent ductus arteriosus. Thus, the majority of the patients with symptoms are either under one or over ten years of age. With the exception of the babies in the first year of life, it is important to remember that 70 percent of the pediatric age group with this condition are entirely asymptomatic.

The first heart sound is usually normal in all forms of left ventricular outflow tract obstruction. The characteristic murmur corresponds in time to left ventricular ejection and therefore begins shortly after S_1. Typically it is diamond-shaped with a crescendo-decrescendo quality and ends before aortic valve closure (Figure 37–3). The murmur is usually well heard over most of the precordium but in children is maximal in the aortic area and is well conducted into

Table 37–1. CLINICAL FINDINGS IN 300 PATIENTS WITH CONGENITAL AORTIC STENOSIS AT VARIOUS AGE GROUPS*†

AGE IN YEARS	0–1	13 MO.–4 YR.	5–9	10–14	15–20	21–30	TOTAL
NO. OF PATIENTS	24	38	84	101	39	14	300
SYMPTOMS AND SIGNS							
Dyspnea	18	1	6	14	19	13	71
Syncope	0	1	4	12	11	6	34
Angina	0	0	2	4	7	5	18
Heart failure	18	2	0	0	2	3	25
Systolic thrill	1	34	71	90	32	11	239
Ejection click	6	23	53	57	15	4	158
LV impulse	1	6	35	54	24	14	134
Pulse pressure 25 mm Hg or less	2	17	31	43	17	4	114
ELECTROCARDIOGRAM							
LVH	10	16	48	67	26	12	179
RVH	10	3	0	0	0	0	13
X-RAY							
CTR > 50%	18	23	30	38	9	4	122
Poststenotic dilatation	0	1	14	22	12	4	53

* Peckham, G. B.; Keith, J. D.; and Evans, J. R.: *Can. Med. Assoc. J.*, **91**:639, 1964.
† Both valvular and subaortic fibrous ring types are included together in these figures.

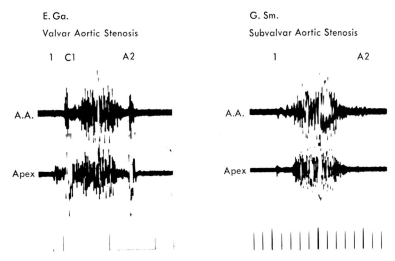

Figure 37-3. A comparison of the sounds and murmurs in aortic valvular stenosis and subvalvular aortic ring stenosis.

The tracing of aortic valve stenosis, in E. Ga., shows a relatively faint first heart sound, a well-heard systolic click, an ejection-type systolic murmur, and a clearly demonstrable aortic second sound.

On the other hand, in the patient G. Sm. with subvalvular aortic stenosis, although the first sound was faint, there was no audible systolic click, and the aortic valve closure showed minimal vibrations at both the aortic area and the apex, which would obviously be inaudible with the stethoscope.

These findings are frequently helpful in differentiating between these two types of aortic stenosis. (Courtesy of Dr. C. M. Oakley, Postgraduate Medical School, Hammersmith, London, England.)

the neck, especially the right side. In infants and patients under five the murmur may be maximal at the left sternal border and out toward the apex. Bargeron and associates (1954) found that 20 percent of adults with aortic stenosis had a systolic murmur that was confined to the apical region. Predictions of the severity of obstruction do not correlate well with the configuration or length of the murmur, but in children at least the intensity of the murmur is fairly useful in predicting the aortic valve gradient (Ellison et al., Joint Study on the Natural History of Congenital Heart Disease, 1976). This relationship between loud ejection systolic murmurs and severe stenosis was first observed in adult patients (Braunwald et al., 1963).

In nearly all infants and children with aortic valve stenosis the ejection systolic murmur is preceded by an ejection click that coincides with sudden arrest of ascent of the domed stenotic valve when its elastic limits are met. This abrupt deceleration of the oncoming column of blood causes a high-frequency vibration recognized as an ejection click (Shaver et al., 1975). This sound is best heard at the apex and down the left sternal border and does not vary with respiration. Absence of a click in a patient with congenital aortic valve stenosis is rare but implies an immobile valve. Though gross calcification explains this development in adults, in infants and young children the reason is an excessive degree of thickening of valve cusps. In contrast with valve stenosis, audible ejection sounds are infrequent in discrete subvalve lesions and therefore the absence of such a sound favors localization of the obstruction to below the valve.

Left ventricular ejection is usually prolonged in all forms of aortic stenosis resulting in delayed aortic valve closure with consequent alteration in the second heart sound, which may exhibit abnormally narrow splitting, become single, or its components may become reversed with P_2 preceding A_2. This latter feature is often difficult to appreciate on auscultation because A_2 may be diminished in intensity and P_2 obscured by the murmur. A palpable thrill in the aortic area is present in most children with severe valve or discrete subvalve stenosis, and early diastolic murmurs due to associated aortic regurgitation are relatively common with both levels of obstruction. In the Joint Study on the Natural History of Congenital Heart Disease postoperative cardiac catheterization showed that about 16 percent of the operated patients still had or had redeveloped critical stenosis. Only 14 percent of the children and 1/15 infants were considered to have excellent results. One may conclude that aortic valvotomy is a palliative procedure that may reduce the gradient for a period of years but that eventually further surgery may be necessary in many of the patients. Unlike valve and supravalve stenosis, subvalve stenosis may be associated with an apical middiastolic rumble due to obstruction to left ventricular filling by encroachment of the anterior mitral cusp on the mitral valve orifice as well as on the left ventricular outflow tract. Rheumatic heart disease must be excluded in such patients. An audible S_4 may be heard in any form of severe left ventricular outflow obstruction.

Left ventricular hypertrophy may be appreciated on palpation but the heart is not significantly enlarged

need addition surgery p̄ valvotomy

unless there is moderate aortic regurgitation or left ventricular failure ensues. In the event of failure, especially in infants, the murmurs often become much softer or disappear altogether.

The characteristic changes in the arterial pulse described in adults with aortic stenosis, which include a slow rate of rise, a sustained peak, and a gradual descent, occur less frequently in children who may have normal brachial pulses in the presence of severe obstruction. Examination of the carotid pulses may improve the clinical assessment.

Noninvasive Assessment of Aortic Stenosis

Radiologic Examination. The chest film is occasionally helpful in evaluating patients with suspected aortic stenosis but especially in older children with significant obstruction may be completely normal. Infants with aortic stenosis and heart failure have cardiomegaly and pulmonary edema (see Figures 37–4 and 37–5). Older children without failure may show some left ventricular and left atrial enlargement when the narrowing is severe. Dilatation of the ascending aorta seen as a double shadow on the upper right border of the heart occurs in a large percentage of cases with valve stenosis but is rarely seen in association with subvalve stenosis. Fifty percent of cases of valvular stenosis have a moderate or marked degree of enlargement or dilatation, 25 percent slight, and in 25 percent the aorta is normal.

Calcification of the aortic valve cusps is a rare occurrence under the age of 15 years but has been recorded occasionally in the latter part of the

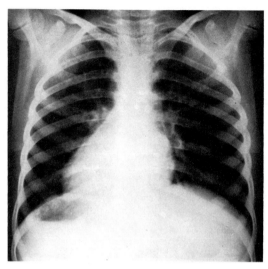

Figure 37-5. G. A., aged seven years. Slight cardiac enlargement. Good exercise tolerance. Died suddenly at 13 years of age playing rugby football. Severe aortic stenosis was confirmed at postmortem.

pediatric age group. In adults it occurs with increasing frequency with advancing years from about 25 percent in the third decade of life to the vast majority of cases over 45 years of age. Calcification is best appreciated in its early stages at fluoroscopy.

Electrocardiography and Vectorcardiography. Although the standard electrocardiogram is usually abnormal in patients with severe obstruction, exceptions have been reported (Reynolds et al., 1960) and a normal tracing cannot be relied on to exclude severe obstruction. Increased left ventricular voltages with a widened angle between the mean QRS and T vectors to greater than 100° in the frontal plane often occur in more severe stenosis, but the most significant abnormality is the pattern of left ventricular strain with S-T depression and T wave inversion in leads V_{5-6} (Figure 37–6). At times these changes may be seen in patients with mild stenosis. However, it should be emphasized that one cannot rely heavily on the resting electrocardiogram to assess the severity of aortic stenosis.

Attempts to incorporate the electrocardiogram with other signs of the disorder have been made with the objective of improving clinical estimates of severity from the electrocardiogram alone. For valvular aortic stenosis the Joint Study on the Natural History of Congenital Heart Defects (Ellison et al., 1976) tried to define those patients with small pressure gradients, hoping to avoid cardiac catherization for such patients. In this study flattened or inverted T waves in V_6 were found to be inconsistent with mild disease. The final criterion based on a multivariate analysis involved only the intensity of the systolic murmur, the presence or absence of an early diastolic murmur, and the voltages of the Q and R waves in lead V_6. The LV-aortic systolic gradient (mm of mercury) could be predicted from 13 (murmur score on 0–6

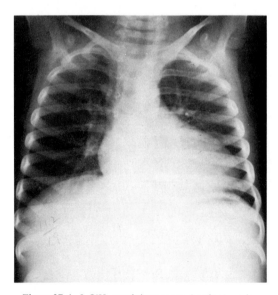

Figure 37-4. J. O'H., aged three years. Aortic stenosis. See postmortem specimen in Figure 37-1. Harsh systolic murmur maximum in third and fourth left interspaces near sternum. Enlarged heart shadow shown above.

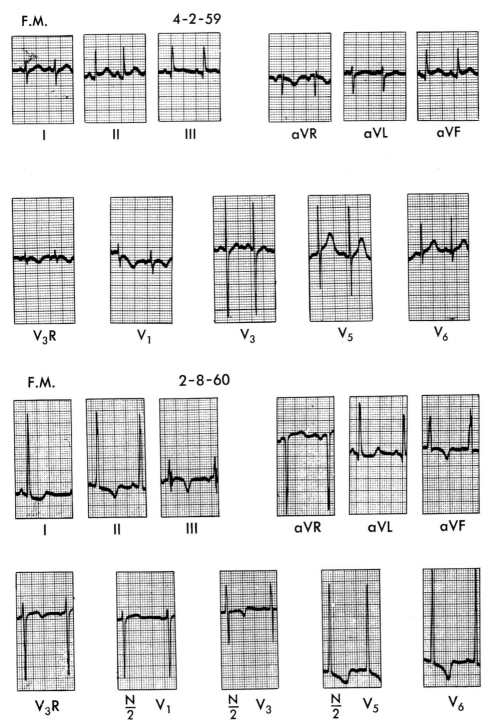

Figure 37-6. Subaortic fibrous stenosis. Case F. M. At age eight years she was asymptomatic with normal electrocardiogram (4-2-59). At age nine years she developed syncopal attacks and electrocardiogram (2-8-60) showed left ventricular hypertrophy with strain. Left heart catheterization showed L.V. body 320/24, ascending aorta, 100/80 gradient 220 mm of mercury. Angiogram showed small chamber below valve.

scale, reduced by 1 in presence of an early diastolic murmur) $+ R_{V6} - 6(QV_6) - 9$. However, 6 of 161 of the patients with an estimated gradient of less than 45 mm of mercury proved at catheterization to have gradients of 80 mm of mercury or more.

Left ventricular hypertrophy in the vectorcardiogram results in an abnormal shift of the mean spatial QRS posteriorly, superiorly, and to the left with an increase in maximal QRS forces and a widened QRS-T angle.

Hugenholtz and Gamboa (1964) have demonstrated that, by using the vectorcardiogram and measuring the sum of selected spatial vectors, one may obtain an excellent correlation with the left ventricular peak pressure. The selected vectors consist of the maximum spatial vector plus the vector occurring 0.01 second before and 0.01 and 0.02 second after the maximum spatial vector. When the sum of these vectors added up to less than 4 mV, the left ventricular peak systolic pressure was always less than 120 mm of mercury. When they came to 7 or 8 mV, the pressure was in the neighborhood of 200 mm of mercury.

Fowler (1965), after evaluating the repolarization wave, found that ST-T wave changes were very useful in predicting the severity of the aortic stenosis provided the frontal axis of QRS was +45 or greater. The following features indicated severe stenosis with a peak systolic gradient of over 50 mm of mercury: (1) a frontal axis of the T wave superior to +15 degrees; thus, an axis of +10, zero, or -10 would be consistent with severe stenosis; (2) the sum of the frontal and horizontal QRS T angles greater than 100 degrees; and (3) an R/T ratio in V_5 or V_6 of greater than 10. If any one of these criteria was positive, there was an 80 to 90 percent chance that the peak systolic gradient between left ventricle and aorta was over 50 mm of mercury. More recently Reeve and associates (1966) have cast some doubt on the usefulness of the vectorcardiogram in assessing the severity of congenital aortic stenosis.

EXERCISE ELECTROCARDIOGRAM. Because of these difficulties Halloran (1971) examined the exercise ECG in 31 children with aortic stenosis aged 8 to 18 years. Of 15 patients with gradients exceeding 50 mm of mercury only one patient had S-T depression exceeding 2 mm in V_5 at rest. On exercise, however, 14/15 developed such changes. In contrast, of the 16 patients with gradients under 50 only one had a positive exercise test. Undoubtedly carefully supervised exercise electrocardiograms can be of great value in assessing the severity of aortic stenosis and the need for further investigation.

Echocardiography. Ultrasound recordings are able to differentiate between the normal and the abnormal aortic valve. Nanda and associates (1974) described the echocardiographic features of bicuspid aortic valves, which included eccentricity of aortic valve closure and multilayered diastolic echoes in the aortic root. These findings were confirmed in nonobstructed valves by Radford and associates (1976). They also noted that in the presence of a

ventricular septal defect or tetralogy of Fallot eccentric closure of the aortic leaflets proved an unreliable sign of a bicuspid aortic valve. Other studies have reported the use of ultrasound to detect aortic valve pathology (Gramiak and Shah, 1970; Feizi et al., 1974). Bennett and associates (1975) used echocardiographic left ventricular dimensions to assess the degree of obstruction in a group of adult patients with aortic stenosis. In patients with good left ventricular function peak systolic pressure in the left ventricle was estimated from the ratio of end-systolic wall thickness over end-systolic cavity dimension multiplied by 225. By subtracting the measured systolic pressure (taken by sphygmomanometer) an aortic valve gradient was obtained and compared with the gradient measured at catheterization. The r value of the correlation between the estimated and measured gradient was 0.87. The method proved suitable for patients with coexistent mitral valve disease or aortic regurgitation. It was unreliable for patients with poor left ventricular function. Blackwood and associates (1976) have obtained good correlation with this method in children with valvar, subvalvar, or supravalvar obstruction. A conversion factor of 237 was used in the under-20-years age group.

The echocardiographic features of discrete subaortic stenosis have been described (Popp et al., 1974; Davis et al., 1974). Suggestive although not diagnostic features include aortic valve closure in early systole with persistent valve closure throughout the remainder of systole, coarse fluttering of the leaflets, and absence of asymmetric septal hypertrophy. Subaortic stenosis produced by a long muscular narrowing ("tunnel") of the left ventricular outflow tract may be appreciated by a narrowing of the left ventricular outflow tract seen on the echocardiographic sweep from left ventricle to aortic root (Figure 37-7). Premature aortic valve leaflet closure was also seen in this patient.

Weyman and associates (1976) found that cross-sectional echocardiography improved the accuracy of localizing the left ventricular outflow tract obstruction.

Pulse Wave Analysis and Systolic Time Intervals. The characteristic arterial pulse in aortic valve stenosis has stimulated many attempts to correlate the aortic valve gradient or calculated orifice size with components of the arterial pulse. Bonner and associates (1973) studied a group of adults with aortic stenosis and showed that ejection time index, maximum rate of rise of carotid pulse, and the timing of the peak of the systolic murmur best correlated with the severity of obstruction. Lyle and associates (1971) found that the slope of the first two-thirds of systolic upstroke in the carotids also correlated well with the gradient in adults. These studies confirmed earlier reports of the value of these parameters in adults (Mason et al., 1964; Arani and Carleton, 1967). Unfortunately there have been few studies of the predictive value of these measurements in children. Hawker and associates (1974) were unable

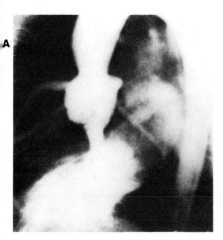

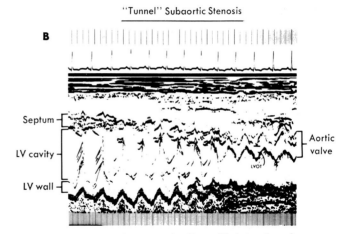

Figure 37-7. Cineangiogram and echocardiogram from patient with a long muscular ("tunnel") obstruction of the left ventricular outflow tract (*LVOT*). Note narrowing of the LVOT. *LV* = Left ventricle.

to correlate any of several central and peripheral pulse characteristics with either aortic valve gradient or its calculated area. They postulated that in children the pulse wave form is considerably modified by the healthy compliant arteries and is therefore valueless in assessing aortic stenosis severity.

Ibraham and associates (1973) found a significant inverse relationship between the pressure gradient and isovolumic contraction time in adult patients with aortic valve stenosis. The ratio of left ventricular ejection time to isovolumic contraction time also correlated well.

While fairly useful in adults, measurements derived from external pulse recordings and phonocardiograms are of less predictive value in children.

Conclusion. As no noninvasive procedure is absolutely reliable, there seems little question that patients with clinical findings suggesting aortic stenosis require cardiac catheterization for complete evaluation of their problem. Room for debate as to the timing of such studies in asymptomatic patients with a normal electrocardiogram certainly exists, but undoubtedly every patient who shows left ventricular hypertrophy and/or strain should be catheterized without undue delay while any patients with dyspnea, syncope, or angina should be studied regardless of the electrocardiographic findings.

Cardiac Catheterization and Selective Angiography

Even in severe aortic valve stenosis it is usually possible to pass a catheter retrogradely across the aortic valve to the left ventricle. In infants when this is not feasible, the procedure may be carried out by passing a catheter across the foramen ovale, the left atrium, into the left ventricle, and taking pressures and performing a selective angiogram in that site (see Figure 37–8). If the foramen ovale cannot be passed, a transseptal catheter may be inserted. The retrograde technique is more satisfactory because direct readings

of various portions of the left ventricle can be readily achieved and a withdrawal tracing into the aorta may clearly show the site of the stenosis and more accurately portray the peak systolic gradient between the left ventricle and the aorta. It also may reveal, at times, associated lesions and one may assess the aortic valve insufficiency if present.

Angiography is extremely useful in aortic stenosis to delineate the level and anatomy of the obstruction. Left ventricular injections will outline the chamber, the thickness of the left ventricular wall, and the presence of mitral regurgitation. Aortic root injections demonstrate clearly the mobility of the aortic valve, the orifice position and size, the size of the valve ring, and the presence or absence of poststenotic dilatation.

Diagnosis

▶ **Differentiation of Valvular from Subvalvular Ring Stenosis.** There are several reasons for differentiating between these two types of stenosis. The subvalvular ring was considered previously less severe by Spencer and associates (1960). More recently Braunwald and others (1964) have found no difference in severity. The subvalvular ring is considerably less common, but when present, one may hope to treat it more completely than the valvular type since the surgeon can at times end up with a normal valve. This is a theoretic rather than a practical difference since the surgeon as a rule finds this anomaly more difficult to deal with than the valvular type.

Braunwald found the sex ratio, male to female, to be 5.8/1 in aortic valvular stenosis, while in the subvalvular type it was 1.9/1. A diastolic murmur has been reported to be more common in the subaortic variety (Taussig, 1960; Braunwald et al., 1964). More recently Hohn and associates (1965) found no difference in the incidence of this murmur in the various subdivisions of aortic stenosis in children.

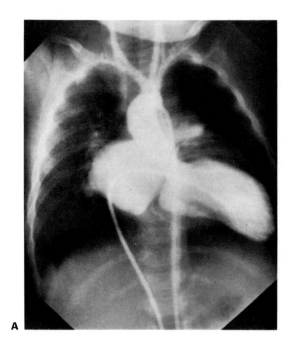

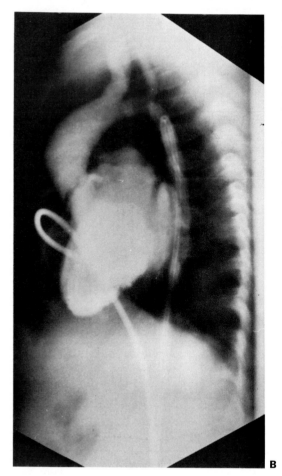

Valvular Ao. Stenosis

DP 6 mos

LV
170/8

Ao.
78/48

−240

mmHG

−0

Figure 37-8. D. P., aged six months. Left ventricular injection demonstrating valvular aortic stenosis and mitral regurgitation. *A.* Anteroposterior view. *B.* Lateral view. *C.* Pressure tracing left ventricle and aorta.

The presence of an ejection sound or click is a useful differentiating sign between the two sites of obstruction; if this is carefully listened for, 90 to 100 percent of the valvular type are found to have such a sound, and it occurs rarely if ever in persons with a subvalvular ring (Vogel, 1965). The x-ray rarely shows much dilatation of the ascending aorta in subvalvular stenosis. This sign is frequently present in the valvular type.

Middiastolic murmurs are more common in the subvalvular ring type.

It is obvious from the above that the differentiation is sufficiently difficult by clinical means that a left heart catheter study is required to identify the precise site of the lesion. A careful and slow withdrawal of the catheter in the area of the valve as well as an angiogram is usually necessary.

However, the presence of supravalvular aortic stenosis may be suspected in a child with a systolic murmur in the aortic area almost invariably accompanied by a thrill with unequal pulses at the wrist, who is mentally retarded and has characteristic facies, with or without defective teeth or strabismus. An electrocardiogram commonly shows left ventricular hypertrophy but may show right and left ventricular loading combined. A cardiac catheterization of both the right and left sides of the heart is essential for adequate study.

If the facies and mental retardation are absent, a loud aortic systolic murmur with unequal radial pulses is suggestive of supravalvular aortic stenosis. ▷Muscular subaortic stenosis, however, is characterized by a late appearance of the murmur several years after birth as a rule. The murmur frequently is best heard at the apex and is often associated with a middiastolic murmur. Typically there is a rapid upstroke of the pulse at the wrist or in the carotid artery. The heart may be enlarged, but the aorta is rather small in the x-ray. The electrocardiogram may show Q waves in the left precordium and not uncommonly a delta wave. At cardiac catheterization the site of the obstruction may be outlined both by catheter and by angiogram, and there is a characteristic response to ectopic beats.

Pulmonary valve stenosis may at times give a murmur that is somewhat similar to that of aortic stenosis over the upper end of the sternum. It also may be accompanied in the milder forms by a systolic click, but in pulmonary stenosis the click is usually louder and the cardiac impulse is related to the right ventricle rather than the left. The pulmonary component of the second sound is fainter in pulmonary stenosis. The electrocardiogram shows evidence of right ventricular hypertrophy, and, of course, in severe cases there may be cyanosis. Cardiac catheterization will differentiate this from aortic stenosis.

A small ventricular septal defect has a harsh systolic murmur heard best over the third and fourth left interspaces, which may be of the ejection type and is commonly accompanied by a thrill. Unfortunately, similar findings may occur in aortic stenosis, making the differential diagnosis difficult in early life. Later, in aortic stenosis the murmur shifts to the appropriate aortic area and the diagnosis is usually clarified. However, the presence of a systolic click, dilatation of the aorta, a murmur that is also well heard in the aortic area, T wave changes suggesting left ventricular strain, hilar shadows that are within normal limits—all favor a diagnosis of aortic stenosis. If any doubt exists, a cardiac catheterization should be carried out.

When aortic stenosis occurs with patent ductus arteriosus, coarctation of the aorta, pulmonary stenosis, ventricular septal defect, interrupted aortic arch, and tricuspid stenosis, one may then have the signs of both the aortic valve lesion and the other associated defect as well. When more than one lesion is suspected, it is well to carry out adequate cardiac catheterization and angiocardiographic studies to clearly define the lesions present.

Prognosis and Natural History

Several factors influence the prognosis in valvular stenosis or discrete subaortic stenosis. These include the site of the stenosis, the severity, the presence or absence of associated defects, the presence or absence of congestive heart failure, the occurrence of infective endocarditis, angina, or syncope, and finally the response to surgery.

Congestive heart failure occurred in 8 percent of 300 patients with congenital aortic stenosis between birth and 30 years. The majority of these (18 of 25) developed it in the first year of life. Only two, or approximately 1 percent, of the total occurred between the ages of 1 and 15 years. Five occurred between 15 and 20. Similar figures are reported by Hohn and associates (1965) who also found that the majority of their cases occurred in infancy. They report three cases that were in congestive heart failure in the first two or three months of life and had survived and were doing well four to seven years later. After the age of two years, only 2 percent of their children with aortic stenosis had congestive heart failure. However, in the adult group (over the age of 15) approximately 25 percent developed congestive heart failure at some time.

Mortality. Those who die with congestive heart failure in the first year of life in our experience frequently have evidence of endocardial fibroelastosis involving the left ventricle, the aortic valve, and, as a rule, the mitral valve to some degree. In this latter group when the aortic stenosis is measured, the degree of narrowing is approximately 50 percent of the aortic ring itself, whereas those dying without endocardial fibroelastosis have a tighter stenosis, approximating 30 percent or less of the aortic ring. Thus, it seems likely that infants who succumb in the first year of life with a combination of aortic stenosis and endocardial fibroelastosis die of the combined lesion, since neither the endocardial fibroelastosis nor the aortic stenosis may be sufficient to be lethal when isolated (Manning et al., 1964). Subaortic ring stenosis does not appear to be a cause of cardiac failure or death in infancy.

Among those with a fatal outcome in the first year of life, the electrocardiogram is abnormal, the heart is enlarged, and a murmur is usually heard. The electrocardiogram characteristically shows left ventricular hypertrophy with strain, but may simply show the combined hypertrophy pattern, or on occasion right ventricular hypertrophy alone. Right bundle branch block may occasionally produce this latter pattern. In such cases special studies are required to clearly delineate the diagnosis.

Sudden death has been reported in aortic stenosis by various authors to range from 4 to 18 percent (Marquis and Logan, 1955; Wood, 1956; Nadas, 1962; Hohn, 1965). In a recent review of sudden unexpected death from cardiovascular causes in children in which a total of 226 sudden deaths in children were analyzed, aortic stenosis accounted for 17 percent of the total and therefore was the commonest cause of sudden death among patients who had had no previous surgery (33 of 186, 18 percent) (Lambert et al., 1974).

In our group of 300 patients (Peckham et al., 1964) there were only four sudden deaths (approximately 1 to 2 percent). In all four patients the clinical criteria for severe aortic stenosis were present. Glew and associates (1969) analyzed eight incidents of sudden death due to aortic stenosis with an incidence of 1 percent. Sudden death from aortic stenosis in childhood between the ages of 1 and 15 years appears to be relatively uncommon and occurs in less than 2 percent of patients, and the risk is confined to those patients with severe aortic stenosis. Such patients may, however, be asymptomatic and have normal resting electrocardiograms. Clinical and cardiac catheter studies should make it possible in most instances to identify children who are likely to have this occur and have them operated on as a prophylactic measure. These deaths may occur in either valvular or subvalvular fibrous obstruction.

As was indicated above, deaths in the pediatric age group are most common in the first year of life, usually associated with congestive heart failure and endocardial fibroelastosis. Prompt treatment with digitalis, oxygen, and other supportive measures may help these infants, but a cardiac catheter study is probably required in order to identify those who have sufficient aortic stenosis to warrant valvular surgery. Because of the combined presence of valvular disease and endocardial fibroelastosis, and frequently some evidence of mitral valve involvement, the mortality is likely to remain high in this special group.

Aortic regurgitation, as identified by an early diastolic murmur, occurs eventually in at least 20 percent of patients over one year of age (Peckham, 1964). There is a distinct tendency for this finding to increase with increasing age. We have not found any correlation between the presence or absence of aortic regurgitation and the severity of the aortic stenosis, although occasionally the onset of infective endocarditis has resulted in the appearance of increase of a diastolic murmur and a wider pulse pressure. Hohn and coworkers (1965) have shown that the incidence of aortic regurgitation is essentially the same in valvular aortic stenosis and subvalvular ring stenosis. They report a 25 to 30 percent incidence in each category. Their data also show that aortic regurgitation can occur in the supravalvular type as well as in persons with subaortic muscular stenosis.

Infective endocarditis has not been a major problem in our experience in aortic stenosis. It occurred six times in our 300 patients; all recovered but two. Since aortic valve surgery has become more widespread, the risk of infective endocarditis at such times has increased. One of our cases occurred in the postoperative period. One patient who subsequently died developed marked aortic insufficiency with widening of the pulse pressure and congestive heart failure. This event has been reported sporadically in the past (Wood, 1958). The Joint Study on the Natural History of Congenital Heart Disease found that infective endocarditis was more commonly a complication of valvular aortic stenosis than it was of pulmonary valvular stenosis.

Syncope occurred in 11 percent in the Toronto series. It did not occur in the first year of life. It occurred once between the ages of 13 months and four years, four times between five and nine years, and 12 times between 10 and 14 years, obviously increasing with age. As a rule, syncope occurs in the cases with a marked gradient between the left ventricle and aorta, usually considerably over 50 mm of mercury. However, it can occur occasionally in patients with a gradient of less than 50 mm of mercury. This sign is of sufficient import that it provides a good indication for cardiac surgery. As a general rule, the patients with syncope have electrocardiographic evidence of left ventricular hypertrophy, often with strain, and the majority have cardiac enlargement on radiologic examination. Hohn and associates (1965) suggest that the cause of syncope in those with gradients of less than 50 mm of mercury may be low cardiac output, since three of their seven cases had high arteriovenous oxygen differences.

Angina is a relatively infrequent symptom in infancy and childhood, occurring in only 2.5 percent of our children with evidence of aortic stenosis. However, it has been reported in approximately 22 percent of adults between the ages of 15 and 30 years, and it appeared in a curve of increasing frequency after the age of 30. Many parents say that their children have pain in the chest, but on careful questioning it is quite clear that it is not angina and is not related to the heart. It is easier to evaluate this symptom in the adult age group since the evidence can be dissected in greater detail by cross-examination of the patient. After questioning a child, if one is convinced that angina with effort does occur, this symptom increases the seriousness of the prognosis. It may occur with a normal or abnormal electrocardiogram; it may occur occasionally with a gradient of less than 15 mm of mercury. At times it occurs in association with syncope, and the two together are clear indications for surgery since sudden death may occur if nothing is done.

Calcific aortic valve stenosis on a bicuspid valve may develop in older children but is much more common in the adult age group. Perforation or destruction of the aortic valve by infective endocarditis may precipitate fatal congestive heart failure, and either direct surgery on the valve or replacement with a prosthetic valve may be indicated urgently.

The natural history of aortic stenosis in children has been somewhat clarified by several recent serial hemodynamic studies. Friedman, Modlinger, and Morgan (1971) concluded from a retrospective study of nine patients that a progressive increase in severity was relatively common. Cohen, Friedman, and Braunwald (1972) performed repeat catheterizations at a mean of seven years after the initial study in 15 patients all originally asymptomatic. Twelve showed increased severity of the obstruction. In a similar study El-Said and associates (1972) concluded that aortic stenosis was a progressive disease and that the increased gradient with time was due to increased flow across the fixed stenotic area, the increased flow being due to the normal increase in cardiac output with growth. They also concluded that progression was more marked in patients with discrete subvalve or supravalve stenosis. Mody and Mody (1975) confirmed these findings, and in their study 7 of 13 patients with originally mild gradients progressed to surgical significance. Hurwitz (1973) found little change in patients with mild stenosis but progression in the more severe group. Serial cardiac catheterization of 294 patients in the Joint Study on the Natural History of Congenital Heart Disease showed that while pressure gradients were unchanged at final examination in just over half the patients, there was a significant gradient increase in almost one-third, some even with trivial obstruction initially. A decrease in the gradient was most unusual. It is safest to conclude that aortic stenosis is a progressive condition, even when originally mild, and that such patients should be followed closely. Symptoms and an abnormal electrocardiogram at rest or on exercise are firm indications for investigation. Asymptomatic patients with normal electrocardiographic findings both at rest and on exercise will almost certainly have gradients of less than 50 mm of mercury.

Treatment

Aortic valvotomy in childhood can only be considered a palliative procedure. The primary indication for operation is the presence of severe obstruction. A peak systolic gradient exceeding 75 mm of mercury in association with a normal cardiac output or an effective aortic orifice less than 0.5 sq cm/sq meter of body surface area represents severe or critical obstruction to left ventricular outflow (Friedman and Pappelbaum, 1971). Surgery should be recommended for critical stenosis or in the presence of symptoms or left ventricular strain with gradients in the 50-mm-of-mercury range. If there are no symptoms and a gradient of less than 50 mm of mercury, the child should be followed over a period of several years with a reexamination, including radiology and electrocardiogram, once a year. If symptoms develop or if there is an advance in the electrocardiographic finding, a repeat left heart catheterization is required; then the need for operation may be reviewed in the light of such findings.

Surgery should be considered urgent for patients with critical aortic stenosis because they may die suddenly. Until successful operation they should be limited from all strenuous activity. Patients with gradients between 25 to 50 mm of mercury who are asymptomatic and who have a normal exercise electrocardiogram can be allowed all physical activities with the exception of organized competitive sports, while patients with gradients less than 25 need not be restricted. However, it is important to review the history and findings at least once a year so that any progression of the lesion may be identified. Since the aortic valve may be the seat of bacterial infection, these children should have the usual preventive measures at the time of tonsillectomy, oral surgery, or dental extractions.

The operation utilizes total cardiopulmonary bypass. The ascending aorta is occluded below the innominate artery and incised above the aortic valve. In this way, both the valve stenosis and subaortic ring stenosis may be dealt with. There are several variations of the former, including a bicuspid valve with a portion of the commissures attached and a reduction in the size of the lumen. There may be three cusps with varying degrees of obstruction. Sometimes one cusp is small and underdeveloped, the lumen being protected in diastole by the other two cusps, which may not be adequate.

If the surgeon incises the commissures too deeply, insufficiency may result, or if a defective cusp is incised, it may not be adequate in diastole. When the whole valve consists of one cusp, incision may result in serious aortic insufficiency and congestive heart failure. Such cases may need replacement of the valve with a prosthesis (Kirklin, 1962). [*handwritten: unicusp valve needs replacement*]

A good result is achieved when the peak systolic gradient between the left ventricle and the aorta is reduced to less than 20 mm of mercury. If it is between 20 and 50 mm of mercury, the result is only fair, and if it is greater than 50, the result is poor. When the texture of the valve and the arrangements of the cusps are such that after surgery the valve approximates the normal mobility and shape, the result over the years is likely to be excellent. If the valve cusps are excessively distorted, thickened, or difficult to deal with surgically, the stenosis may not be susceptible to adequate repair. In certain cases it may be necessary to go in a second time at a later date and replace the valve with a prosthetic one.

Including all ages, the overall early mortality for aortic valvotomy is around 6 percent (Ellis et al., 1962; Putnam et al., 1964; Cooley et al., 1965). Conkle and associates (1973) reported on their experience with 38 patients aged 1 to 21 years with no operative deaths and reduction of the peak systolic gradient in all patients (32) studied postoperatively.

The subaortic ring stenosis may cause difficulty if it is attached to the aortic valve cusps or if it is deeply adherent to the aortic cusp and the mitral valve. The technique must then be to excise the ring stenosis without damaging the other structures. This can be achieved in many cases, and then one has an excellent result because the aortic valve functions normally. At times the surgical treatment may be very hazardous because of the intimate relationship of the stenotic ring with the mitral or aortic valve or conduction system. The reduction in gradient across the obstruction has not proved as consistent as with the valvular stenosis. [*handwritten: subaortic stenosis*]

In reviewing their experience with discrete subaortic stenosis, Kelly and associates (1972) reported good surgical results for patients with type I, the thin discrete membrane, but much poorer results from type II in which the ring is thicker associated with muscular hypertrophy and possible encroachment on the anterior leaflet of the mitral valve. Aortic incompetence may develop or increase after surgery for both types of discrete subaortic stenosis. Newfeld and associates (1976) reported an operative mortality of 5 percent in a series of 40 patients operated on. Seventeen of the survivors were restudied by cardiac catheterization one to eight years after surgery. Nine of these patients had gradients greater than 50 mm of mercury reflecting either inadequate resection or proliferation of the previously resected subvalvular fibrous tissue.

A second operation may be thus required in many patients as they progress into adult life because of the occurrence of restenosis. On past experience this is likely to be a relatively common development. Another problem is the child with a relatively mild aortic valve stenosis. There is little knowledge on how many will develop progressive narrowing of the valve opening and require operation in later life. Early operation appears contraindicated at the present, but further investigation and experience are needed in this area. There is still room for considerable improvement in the techniques of handling these forms of congenital heart disease, but the remarkable progress in the past suggests we can be optimistic in the future.

Management of Infants with Aortic Stenosis in the First Year of Life. The infants who present with signs and symptoms in the first year of life are usually critically ill with congestive heart failure. The majority have a systolic murmur in the aortic area, but occasionally it is heard over the left precordium or may even be absent. There is frequently a striking contrast between the forceful cardiac impulse and the relatively small amplitude of the arterial pulse. Electrocardiogram shows left ventricular hypertrophy or left ventricular and right ventricular hypertrophy combined, or occasionally right ventricular hypertrophy alone. When left ventricular hypertrophy is present, the strain pattern of T wave flattening or inversion in V_6 is commonly present.

The diagnosis may be suspected by the above considerations, but cardiac catheterization is required to confirm it and to determine the degree of obstruction. If the gradient between the left ventricle and the aorta is less than 30 or 40 mm of mercury, valvotomy may not benefit the infant. However, if the gradient is greater, surgery is certainly indicated. When one is dealing with the lower gradients associated with heart failure, it is highly probable that the aortic valve lesion is associated with endocardial fibroelastosis. In such cases the prompt and prolonged administration of digitalis is indicated, with whatever other supportive measures are required.

The special problems of isolated aortic stenosis during infancy have been the subject of two recent reviews (Lakier et al., 1974; Keene et al., 1975).

MUSCULAR SUBAORTIC STENOSIS
Kenneth R. Bloom

Synonyms

Synonyms include idiopathic hypertrophic subaortic stenosis (IHSS), hypertrophic obstructive cardiomyopathy (HOCM), asymmetric septal hypertrophy (ASH), obstructive cardiomyopathy (OCM), functional subaortic stenosis, familial hypertrophic subaortic stenosis, functional obstruction of the left ventricle, and others. This plethora of nomenclature is a tribute to the large degree of mystery that has surrounded this disease since its original description.

Background

In 1907 Schmincke described hypertrophy of the muscular wall of the left ventricular outflow tract and postulated a type of obstruction that could lead to further hypertrophy of the left ventricle. Bernheim in 1910 referred to left ventricular hypertrophy that caused enlargement of the septum, which in turn protruded into the right ventricle. Davies in 1952 described similar pathology in several members of a family, some of whom had died suddenly. Brock brought the subject into open discussion by his observations in 1957. This was followed by the presentation by Teare in 1958 on asymmetric hypertrophy of the left ventricle. The practical importance of diagnosing this form of left ventricular outflow obstruction prior to surgery was stressed by Morrow and Braunwald (1959). Successful surgical relief of the obstruction was reported by Goodwin and coworkers (1960) who also defined many of the clinical features of this condition. Many detailed reviews have been published (Frank and Braunwald, 1968; Wolstenholme and O'Connor, 1971; Wigle et al., 1973; Goodwin, 1974; and Maron et al., 1976).

Definition

McKinney (1974) describes the typical patient with this disease as having massive asymmetric hypertrophy of the septal portion of the outflow tract of the left ventricle and diffuse hypertrophy of the ventricular walls. There are many exceptions to this oversimplification.

Etiology

The familial nature of this disease has always been recognized. Originally, the diagnosis depended on cardiac catheterization and therefore the vast majority of patients were symptomatic. Some obviously did have family histories, but there were apparently two groups, spontaneous (65 to 75 percent) and familial (25 to 35 percent). The availability of echocardiography as a reliable noninvasive method of making the diagnosis has changed this concept. Clark and coworkers (1973), using asymmetric septal hypertrophy as the disease marker, concluded that this disease was transmitted as an autosomal dominant trait with a high degree of penetrance in nearly all patients. Chromosomes are normal. Shah (1975) added a note of caution to this concept, as using asymmetric septal hypertrophy as the sole marker for the disease may result in overdiagnosis. Further investigation is required. Hypertension may coexist and its place in the etiology is uncertain (Hamby et al., 1971). The place of catecholamines is similarly controversial.

Association with Other Congenital Abnormalities

This disease may occasionally complicate other cardiac anomalies (Somerville and McDonald, 1968; Parker et al., 1969; Shem-Tov et al., 1971). These associated abnormalities are commonly forms of fixed left ventricular outflow tract obstruction, but atrial septal defects, endocardial cushion defects, pulmonary stenosis, and dextrocardia have also been described in this combination. Asymmetric septal hypertrophy and dynamic obstruction occur, but it is probable that this hypertrophy is secondary to the abnormal afterload on the ventricle rather than a separate genetically determined disease entity (Bloom et al., 1975; and Maron et al., 1975). Both these authors showed normal hypertrophy patterns in the coexistent disease, as opposed to the disorganized pattern in the familial form. In addition, relatives of the affected patients with other anatomic heart disease were found to be normal by Maron and his coworkers (1975).

The association of the morphologic and functional features of muscular subaortic stenosis with infiltrative disease, particularly Pompe's disease (Ehlers et al., 1962; Hohn et al., 1965), and in infants of diabetic mothers (Gutgesell et al., 1976) has been documented. An association has been noted with Friedrich's ataxia (Gach et al., 1971). Polani and Moynahan (1972) described a syndrome of multiple symmetric lentigines, obstructive cardiomyopathy, growth retardation, and intellectual impairment. A genetically triggered abnormality of neural crest elements was postulated. Subclinical skeletal muscle dysfunction, usually generalized, was present in 65 percent of patients studied with electromyography by Meerschwam and Hootmans (1970). Progressive muscular dystrophy was diagnosed in relatives of two of their patients.

Incidence

The advent of echocardiography has shown that this disease is far more widespread than originally thought.

It has been documented in all age groups from newborns onward. Males appeared to predominate in the initial analyses, but both sexes are probably equally affected (Clark et al., 1973).

Some races are rarely affected, particularly Black Africans and American Negroes (Wolstenholme and O'Connor, 1971).

Pathology

Roberts (1973) tabulated the following gross anatomic features (Figure 37–9):

1. Disproportionate hypertrophy of the ventricular septum.
2. Small or normal-sized left and right ventricular cavities.
3. Endocardial mural plaque in the left ventricular outflow tract.
4. Thickened mitral valve leaflets.
5. Dilated left and right atria.
6. Hypertrophied free walls of all four cardiac chambers.
7. Normal or near-normal aortic valve cusps.
8. Normal-sized ascending aorta.

The major histologic abnormalities are disorganization of muscle cell bundles and abnormal orientation of myofibrils and myofilaments of individual muscle cells. The hypertrophied myocardial cells are thick and short with bizarre nuclei. A perinuclear halo appears to be due to accumulations of glycogen (Van Noorden et al., 1971). These authors were unable to confirm either increased nerve fibers or an increased noradrenaline content in the myocardium. An increased amount of fibrous tissue is present.

The myocardium is variously affected and not all changes are always present (Maron et al., 1974). The right ventricle may be more severely affected than the left (Barr et al., 1973). Some hearts may not show asymmetric septal hypertrophy (Roberts, 1973) although this may have been present at an earlier stage of the disease.

Asymmetric septal hypertrophy itself is not unique to muscular subaortic stenosis and may accompany a variety of congenital heart diseases (Maron et al., 1975).

Pathophysiology

The abnormal septal hypertrophy frequently displaces the anterior mitral valve leaflet (Figure 37–9). The papillary muscles and chordal alignment of the mitral valve mechanism are also affected. Myofibril disorganization results in an abnormal pattern of contraction. The narrowing of the left ventricular outflow tract by the abnormal systolic anterior motion of the anterior mitral valve leaflet results in an afterload being imposed on the left ventricle late in the ejection phase. This differs from other forms of obstruction. Falikov and coworkers (1976) have documented two patients in whom the

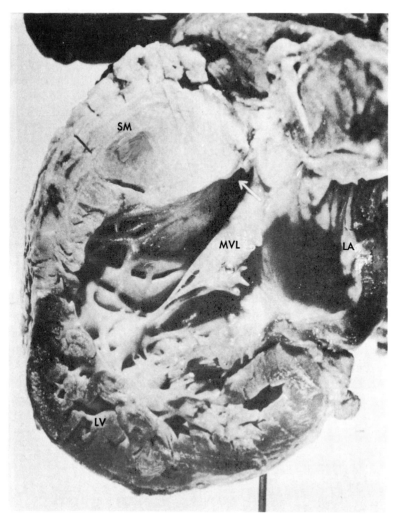

Figure 37-9. Postmortem heart specimen. The septal mass (*SM*) involving the upper half of the ventricular system is shown bulging into the left ventricular outflow tract anteriorly below the aortic valve (*arrow*). The posterior aspect of the outflow tract is formed by the anterior leaflet of the mitral valve (*MVL*). The thickened free wall of the left ventricle (*LV*) and the left atrial cavity (*LA*) are also shown.

dynamic obstruction was at midventricular level. The disease is a dynamic one and obstruction may both develop (Williams, 1973) and regress, with progressive advance and deterioration of the disease (Goodwin, 1974). Mitral regurgitation frequently occurs and its severity is related to the severity of the outflow obstruction (Wigle et al., 1969).

Clinical Features

Symptoms. Patients with this disease may be totally asymptomatic, or they may be completely crippled. The usual age of presentation is in the third to the fourth decade.

Exertional dyspnea, fatigue, angina pectoris, and dizziness on standing are common. Syncope and palpitations secondary to arrhythmias may be noted. Symptoms of congestive heart failure with edema and orthopnea occur as the disease progresses.

Physical Examination. The physical findings vary with the state of the disease and degree of obstruction.

The peripheral pulses have a rapid upstroke with a bimodal flow pattern. Boughner and coworkers (1975) confirmed this flow pattern in patients with outflow obstruction using Doppler techniques. The apical beat is forceful and frequently double in that the atrial contraction produces a palpable presystolic expansion wave. The auscultatory features have been evaluated by Nellen (1971), Tucker (1975), and their coworkers. The first heart sound is normal apart from an occasional prolongation of the interval measured from the Q wave on the electrocardiogram to the first major component of the first heart sound. Systolic clicks do occur rarely and may be intermittent and early. A delayed onset systolic murmur (Figure 37–10) is present in virtually all patients and is maximally audible at the lower left sternal border inside the apex. This murmur typically decreases in intensity on squatting and increases when the patient stands. Amyl nitrite increases the intensity, and phenylephrine or methoxamine will decrease it. The second heart sound varies from wide splitting of its components to complete reversal. Complete or partial reversal is related to a greater degree of outflow obstruction and is probably a result of the

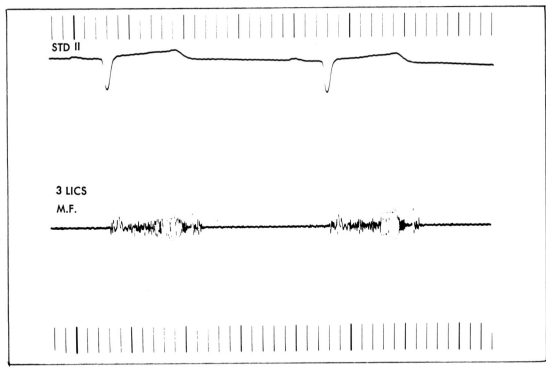

Figure 37-10. Phonocardiogram showing late accentuating systolic murmur in 7-month child with muscular subaortic stenosis. No demonstrable gradient or mitral regurgitation at catheter. $LICS$ = left intercostal space; $M.F.$ = medium frequency.

prolongation of the left ventricular ejection time (Wigle et al., 1967). A middiastolic murmur that may be either left-or right-sided in origin is frequently present. An early diastolic murmur that may be due to minimal aortic regurgitation is rare.

Electrocardiography

This is almost always abnormal and is therefore helpful in the evaluation. A progression of changes is seen over several years' observation (Figure 37–11). The electrical axis is usually between 0 and +90 degrees. Frank and Braunwald (1968) found it to be between 0 and −90 degrees in 30 percent of patients.

Some features of the Wolff–Parkinson–White syndrome, notably a short atrioventricular conduction time and a delta wave, are frequently seen. Braudo and coworkers (1964) described a pattern of deep Q waves with normal or small R waves over the left precordium (Figure 37–11). These Q waves are probably due to septal hypertrophy. Over a period of years several cases subsequently developed tall R waves and a decrease in size or absence of the Q wave, thus leading to the typical pattern of left ventricular hypertrophy. It is believed that this series of events indicates primary hypertrophy of the septum with a subsequent progressive increase in the thickness of the free wall of the left ventricle as obstruction develops.

In many children the T wave over the left precordium is upright initially but tends to flatten or become depressed and inverted over a period of several years. Patterns suggestive of myocardial infarction possibly due to myocardial fibrosis may be present. Normal sinus rhythm is usually present in childhood. Ectopic beats and atrial fibrillation occur in about a third of patients.

P wave abnormalities usually showing atrial hypertrophy are seen in about 50 percent of patients. This usually indicates more advanced disease (Frank and Braunwald, 1968).

Radiologic Examination

The heart size is either normal or only slightly enlarged in approximately 60 percent of patients. The others have moderate-to-marked enlargement (Frank and Braunwald, 1968). Occasionally massive cardiomegaly occurs in symptomatic infants (Maron et al., 1975). A marked left ventricular gradient may occur with little or no increase in heart size, although the left ventricle may appear enlarged in the left anterior oblique view. Braunwald and coworkers (1964) conclude that the left atrium is larger in the patients who were markedly symptomatic. The ascending aorta is normal in shape and appearance. The right ventricle and atrium may be enlarged. The hilar shadows and the pulmonary vascularity are

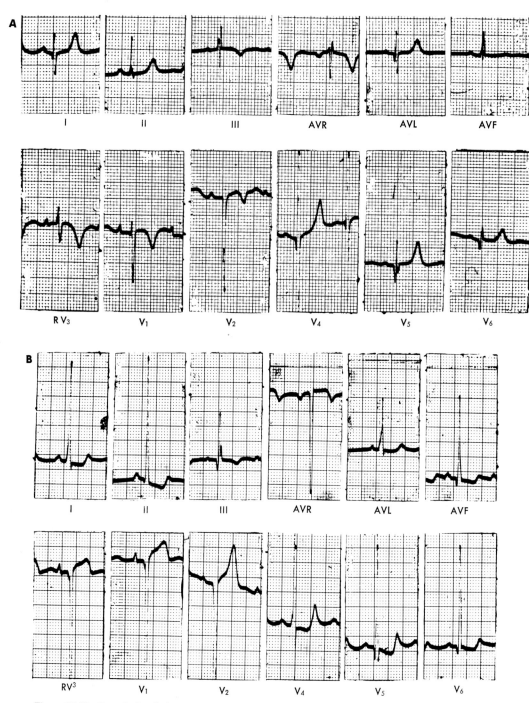

Figure 37-11. Case C. A., died at seven years with subaortic muscular stenosis. At 3 years and 11 months electrocardiogram (*A*) showed deep Q wave in V_6 due to septal hypertrophy. Later this was overshadowed by hypertrophy of the free wall of left ventricle leading to a tall R wave in V_7 at six years (*B*).

within normal limits. Serial x-rays may show progressive enlargement over several years.

Echocardiography

Since Moreyra and his coworkers (1969) first commented on the use of this technique in this disease, its widespread application is changing concepts of incidence and etiology (Shah et al., 1969; Henry et al., 1973; and Clark et al., 1973).

The echocardiographic features are (Figure 37–12):

1. Asymmetric septal hypertrophy with a ratio of septum to LV wall of 1.3 or greater when measured at the true minor axis.
2. Diminished left septal surface excursion.
3. Abnormal systolic anterior motion of the anterior mitral valve leaflet not necessarily implying obstruction.
4. Premature systolic aortic valve leaflet closure when obstruction to the left ventricular outflow is present.

All features are not always present (Rossen et al., 1974). They may be simulated by other diseases (Rees et al., 1976). In particular, asymmetric septal hypertrophy has been shown to occur in other conditions unrelated to muscular subaortic stenosis (Goodman et al., 1974; and Larter et al., 1976).

Echocardiography also has important use in the detection of the asymptomatic relatives of affected patients (Clark et al., 1973) and the repeated follow-up of the individual patient with regard to both the pathogenesis of the disease and the effects of treatment (Shah et al., 1972). It is of great practical importance in diagnosing coexistent dynamic and fixed left ventricular outflow tract obstruction (Chung et al., 1974; and Bloom et al., 1975).

Myocardial Imaging

The use of myocardial perfusion scanning following the intravenous administration of thallium 201 has been shown by Bulkley and coworkers (1975) to provide another noninvasive method of evaluating this condition. The addition of a gated cardiac pool scan using technetium 99 M electrolytically labeled human serum albumen, allows confirmation of the shape of the interventricular septum as a negative image. An analysis of regional myocardial wall motion and systolic cavity obliteration can be made (Bulkley et al., 1975).

Cardiac Catheterization

Gradients may be demonstrated across both the left and right ventricular outflow tracts (Figure

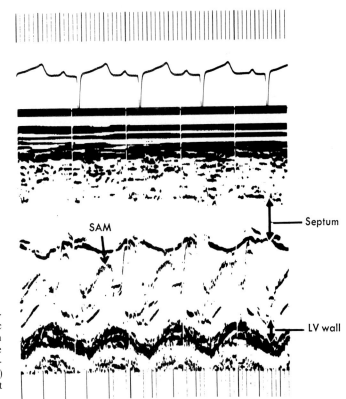

Figure 37-12. Echocardiogram of seven-month-old child with muscular subaortic stenosis. Note systolic anterior motion (*SAM*) of anterior mitral valve leaflet. There is marked disproportionate septal thickening as compared to the left ventricular (*LV*) wall. No gradient was demonstrated at catheterization.

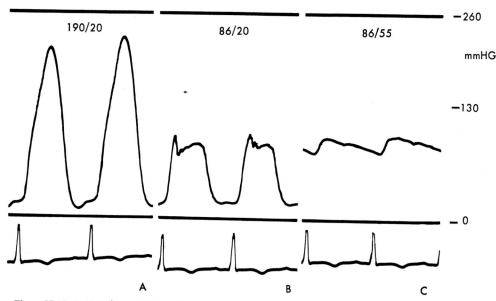

Figure 37-13. R. C., 10½ years. Subaortic muscular stenosis. Marked elevation of systolic pressure in body of left ventricle (*A*), markedly decreased in outflow area (*B*) between marked muscular contraction of body of left ventricle and aortic valve. Aortic pressure tracing (*C*) shows small pulse pressure associated with rapid rise of upstroke.

37–13). The high probability of catheter entrapment in a small hypertrophied ventricular chamber has led to controversy as to the presence of a gradient in some situations (Criley et al., 1965). Wigle and coworkers (1967) have stressed the importance of localizing the obstruction to the left ventricular inflow tract and distinguishing this from the high pressures obtained when the tip of the catheter is embedded in the myocardium. Falikov and coworkers (1976), however, have shown a gradient at midventricular level without catheter entrapment.

The gradient across the left ventricular outflow tract may be evoked or reduced by the use of drugs and maneuvers. In general, an increase in the afterload on the left ventricle, a decrease in contractility, or an increase in end-diastolic volume will tend to reduce the gradient; the gradient is worsened by a reduction in afterload or increase in contractility (Table 37–2). These effects can be assessed at cardiac catheterization.

Cineangiography

The diagnosis is usually based on the clinical, noninvasive, and hemodynamic data.

Good angiographic visualization of the septum can be made with diagnostic accuracy by utilizing the technique of biventricular cineangiography (Redwood et al., 1974; Moes et al., 1964).

The other features of abnormal mitral valve motion, irregular muscular hypertrophy, a small cavity, mitral regurgitation, and dilated coronary arteries may all be appreciated by left ventriculography (Figure 37–14) and aortography.

Table 37–2.   METHODS OF VARYING THE GRADIENT

DRUG OR MANEUVER	MAIN HEMODYNAMIC EFFECT	EFFECT ON GRADIENT
Isoproterenol	↑ Contractility ↓ Afterload ↓ Volume	Marked ↑
Digitalis glycosides	↑ Contractility	↑
Amyl nitrite	↓ Afterload	↑
Nitroglycerin	↓ Afterload	↑
Valsalva maneuver (strain phase)	↓ Volume ↓ Afterload (probable)	↑
Post extrasystolic beat	↑ Volume ↑ Contractility	↑
α-Adrenergic stimulation	↑ Afterload	↓
β-Adrenergic blockade	↓ Contractility	↓
Infusion of volume expanders	↑ Volume	↓

Differential Diagnosis

It is important both to distinguish this condition from fixed left ventricular outflow obstruction and to recognize the occasional coexistence of the two forms.

In addition, primary mitral valve disease, usually incompetence, but occasionally stenosis, ventricular septal defect, and ischemic heart disease, usually with papillary muscle dysfunction, can simulate some of the features.

Adequate clinical, noninvasive, and catheterization techniques can enable the diagnosis to be made with accuracy.

Treatment

The most effective method of permanently relieving significant obstruction is surgery. This usually takes the form of ventriculomyotomy or myomectomy. The abnormal systolic anterior motion of the anterior mitral valve leaflet as seen on the echocardiogram is frequently abolished (Shah et al., 1972). This relief of obstruction has been shown to be associated with a lower incidence of sudden death than in those patients with obstruction who are treated only with β-blocking drugs. (Shah et al., 1974). These results must be interpreted with caution. A bias exists, as patients with no outflow obstruction were excluded (Goodwin, 1974). However, it is possible that relief of obstruction may slow the progress of this disease. Cooley and his coworkers (1973) proposed prosthetic replacement of the mitral valve as an alternative form of therapy. This has not received wide acceptance, and further evaluation of this in the long term is required. Propranolol is the β blocker most widely evaluated in the drug treatment of the obstructed form of this disease. The experience of Stenson and coworkers (1973) and many others is that propranolol results in an initial improvement that may last some months, but that symptoms and gradients return.

The drug treatment of the nonobstructed patients or those with labile obstruction is primarily β blockade, usually propranolol. Those with labile obstruction show the most benefit. Seven of ten of this group of patients in Wigle and coworkers' series (1974) showed complete relief of symptoms, with the other three showing improvement.

Neither the long-term prognosis nor the risk of sudden death appears to be appreciably influenced by the use of propranolol. However, because of the initial favorable response, a clinical trial of this drug seems indicated in symptomatic patients.

Complications

As the disease progresses, the clinical course may be altered by many complicating factors. These are atrial fibrillation, either paroxysmal or sustained; systemic and pulmonary emboli; bacterial endocarditis; and

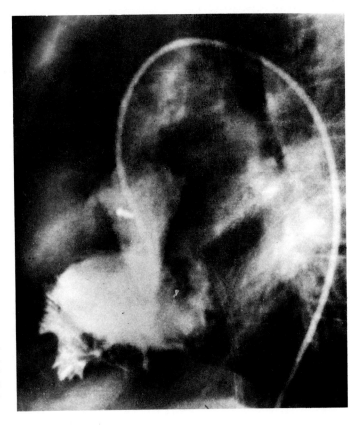

Figure 37-14. Left ventricular angiocardiogram showing narrowing of the subvalvular region. The ventricular chamber extends well forward with an indentation adjacent to the somewhat narrowed segment.

progressive cardiac dilatation with the onset of severe congestive heart failure.

These complications are treated on their merits with digitalis and anticoagulants being used as required.

Prognosis

The clinical course of 119 patients has been reviewed by Hardarson and coworkers (1973). They found that the average age of onset of symptoms was 28 years. The average duration of symptoms before death was nine years. Sudden death tended to be more common in the younger patients and children. Five out of seventeen children died suddenly. Sudden death probably results from ventricular fibrillation or, rarely, asystole. It is related neither to the functional class of the patient nor to activity (Maron et al., 1976).

The estimated mortality is about 15 percent of patients at five years and 35 percent at ten years. The prognosis seems unaltered by either drugs or surgery.

The prognosis of the totally asymptomatic relatives of affected patients whose only detectable pathology is an abnormal echocardiogram remains unknown at this time.

SUPRAVALVULAR AORTIC STENOSIS
Richard D. Rowe

CHEVERS (1842) was the first to describe a congenital constriction of the aortic lumen just above the aortic valve in close proximity to the attachment of the commissures. It was not until 1930 that the term "supravalvular aortic stenosis" was introduced by Mencarelli (1930) after he had made a detailed study of the morbid anatomy. Almost 30 more years passed before the literature on clinical and hemodynamic aspects of the disorder was reviewed by Denie and Verheugt (1958) and Morrow and associates (1959). A major increase in interest in the malformation in the early 1960s occurred when patients with an expanded syndrome of supravalvular aortic stenosis with characteristic facies, mental retardation, and other abnormalities were related to some disturbance of calcium metabolism (Black and Bonham-Carter, 1963). Surgical relief of supravalvular aortic stenosis began about the same time. Over the past decade publication of a number of small series of cases or individual case reports has contributed further to the clinical picture and shown a wide spectrum of the disorder.

Pathology

Supravalvular aortic stenosis is a narrowing in the ascending aorta of variable degree and by definition is localized just above the sinuses of Valsalva. Early autopsy descriptions emphasize bands or fibrous membranes with a central orifice stretching across a normal-sized aortic lumen, but numerous more recent descriptions of the pathologic anatomy identify the bands to be nonobstructive. A true fibrous membrane with central orifice is uncommon and forms probably no more than 10 percent of all types of the obstruction. There are in fact two main appearances (Figure 37–15): an hourglass narrowing of the aorta, which occurs in 66 percent of the patients, and a diffuse narrowing of the aortic lumen beginning just above the aortic sinuses and extending throughout the ascending aorta, which has been seen in over 20 percent (Denie and Verheugt, 1958; Morrow et al., 1959; Neufeld et al., 1961; Petersen et al., 1965; Rastelli et al., 1966).

The histologic appearance described by Perou (1961) is that of an angulation and unfolding of the aortic wall with a focal disorganization of the media at that point capped by a zone of intimal thickening or hypertrophy showing some degenerative changes with calcification.

There are good reasons to believe that the two gross pathologic forms described are only a reflection of differing degrees of generalized involvement of the whole of the aortic wall. The diffuse "hypoplasia" presents with a smaller aortic lumen than the more localized variety because the intimal changes are so extensive in the former (Beuren, 1972). There is a trend toward more frequent stenosis of the origin of aortic arch branches in the hypoplastic form, which would also support this view (Antia et al., 1967). If this is correct, it follows that with rare exception most patients with supravalvular aortic stenosis fit into a spectrum of a generalized disease of conducting arteries rather than into the narrower problem of a localized aortic abnormality such as one sees in coarctation of the aorta (Rowe, 1972).

A number of other observations about the disease add strength to this argument. Beuren and associates (1964) and Antia and associates (1967) showed that pulmonary arterial stenosis is frequently associated with supravalvular aortic stenosis. The wall of the pulmonary arteries is usually thickened in a manner similar to that observed in the aorta. As with the aorta, stenosis may be localized to a stress point such as the pulmonary artery bifurcation, it may appear as numerous distal obstructions of intrapulmonary segments of the vessels, or there may be a generalized hypoplasia of the pulmonary arteries. This variable expression again may be related to the severity of the generalized pulmonary arterial wall disease in any particular patient.

The aortic valve cusps are thickened in about a third of the specimens. Bicuspid aortic valves are probably not more frequently observed than in the population at large, a striking contrast with the situation for classic coarctation of the aorta. The upper margin of the aortic cusps may be adherent to the aortic wall at the stenotic site (about 20 percent) and may rarely involve the coronary ostium (Roberts, 1973). The coronary arteries may be quite normal but more often they are large, dilated, and tortuous. The vessels are thick-walled and the intima also is thickened or shows atherosclerotic patches. Occasionally there is narrowing of a coronary artery just beyond its ostium (Figure 37–15A). It is uncertain whether the smaller coronary vessels are abnormal in this condition, but certainly patchy fibrosis of the left ventricle sometimes with calcification has been reported, and angina appears frequently in older patients even when the coronary orifices are found unobstructed at operation (Underhill et al., 1971). Left ventricular hypertrophy is very often present and usually so in those with severe stenosis. Right ventricular hypertrophy, when present, reflects the severity of an associated pulmonary arterial and/or valvular stenosis.

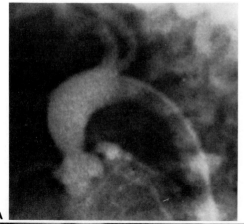

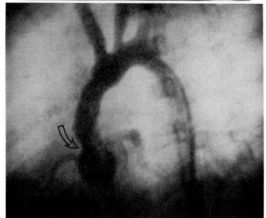

Figure 37-15. The hourglass (*A*) and hypoplastic (*B*) forms of supravalvular aortic stenosis. Aortograms in the left anterior oblique position. (See also Figure 41-10, page 799.)

There have been occasional reports of true cardiac malformation associated with supravalvular aortic stenosis but the association is not particularly common: ventricular septal defect, atrial septal defect, and subaortic stenosis (Beuren, 1972; Jones and Smith, 1975; Keane et al., 1976). All other associated vascular defects—pulmonary and aortic valve stenosis, aortic valve regurgitation, coarctation of the aorta, patent ductus arteriosus, aortic aneurysm, hypoplastic descending aorta, carotid, renal, and mesenteric arterial stenoses—could be secondary either to the major supravalvular obstruction in the aorta or pulmonary artery or to the basic vessel wall abnormality. Coarctation of the aorta does seem to occur relatively commonly as an association of supravalvular aortic stenosis (Bliddal et al., 1969), and an angiographic appearance of forme fruste of coarctation is frequently seen (Beuren, 1972), which might suggest that the supravalvular aortic stenosis could have origins prenatally and minimally reduce fetal blood flow in the ascending aorta (Hutchins, 1971). Mitral regurgitation has been reported on several occasions. Beuren (1972) noted that five of his patients had mitral regurgitation, one with a calcified mitral annulus. Mitral stenosis has also been noted (Driscoll et al., 1974). Most of these observations have been in patients with abnormal facies and a probable hypercalcemic background, but the numbers are too few to be sure that this feature is confined to that subgroup of patients (Vazquez et al., 1968). We have encountered an example of mitral regurgitation in a patient with abnormal facies without supravalvular aortic stenosis or pulmonary artery stenosis but with hypoplasia of the aorta (Char and Rowe, 1972). Others have documented that a frequent abnormality is prolapse of the mitral apparatus with thick collagenous changes in the valve at autopsy (Becker et al., 1972).

Incidence and Pathogenesis

At The Hospital for Sick Children, Toronto, 19 patients with supravalvular aortic stenosis have been observed among 15,104 cases of heart disease. In the supravalvular aortic stenosis series of Beuren (1972), Antia and associates (1966), and Kurlander and associates (1966), approximately one-third of the patients had the extended syndrome with abnormal facies and mental retardation. This first group is the one where there is strong circumstantial evidence of a fetal disturbance in calcium storage and postnatal expression of idiopathic hypercalcemia. That case is based on the important evidence of Black and Bonham-Carter (1963) who related the abnormal facies in older children with the aortic disorder to the facies of children seen in an epidemic of idiopathic hypercalcemia in the United Kingdom at an earlier time when milk formulae were heavily fortified with vitamin D. Beuren (1972) attributed the high number of cases of this form of the disease in Northern Germany to the "stoss" dose of vitamin D given to pregnant women in that area at that time. Hooft and associates (1963) and Garcia and associates (1964) documented hypercalcemia in infants with supravalvular aortic stenosis, while Coleman (1965) and Friedman and Roberts (1966) proved that vitamin D administered in high doses to pregnant animals could cross the placenta and produce hypercalcemia in the offspring. The experimentally produced aortic abnormalities had similarities to those of supravalvular aortic stenosis in man. Other evidence to relate disturbance of calcium metabolism with the disorder in humans has been summarized in a major review by Seelig (1969). Only the most tenuous evidence of an excess of vitamin D intake has been shown for the mothers of most cases of supravalve aortic stenosis, however, and even where high doses have been documented as in Germany and England, only a fraction of the infants in those areas seem to have been affected. An increased sensitivity to vitamin D on the part of the mother or child could be considered a cause (Cooke, 1968). Evidence from skeletal and dental x-rays suggests that children with eventual supravalvular aortic stenosis can have major abnormalities of calcium homeostasis during fetal life. Whether this is due to excessive intake or to absorption of vitamin D before and during the pregnancy of some mothers or to a failure of regulatory mechanisms for blood calcium in pregnancy or some combination is uncertain. There are some difficulties about relating supravalvular

aortic stenosis to hypercalcemia because documented cases of hypercalcemia exist with abnormal facies but no supravalvular aortic disease (Wiltse et al., 1966).

Because hypercalcemia is seldom demonstrated in infancy for patients who later have supravalvular aortic stenosis and because only one-third of the patients with "elfin" facies were found to have supravalvular aortic stenosis, Jones and Smith (1975) think it unlikely that the disorder is one of calcium homeostasis, prefer to call the disorder "Williams elfin facies syndrome," and consider it a sporadic occurrence of unknown etiology.

The *second group* of supravalvular aortic stenosis is one occurring in individuals who have a normal facies and normal mentality. This group is regarded by most workers as sporadic in nature and unrelated, even remotely, to a disturbance of calcium metabolism.

The *third group* is a smaller one with familial aggregation of patients (McCue et al., 1968). It is believed to be transmitted through an autosomal dominant mechanism with variable expression.

Our work (Antia et al., 1967) and that of Beuren (1972) suggest that all three groups are the eventual consequence of disturbed calcium metabolism in fetal or postnatal life.

Clinical Features

The birth weights of patients with supravalvular stenosis are usually within the lower normal range.

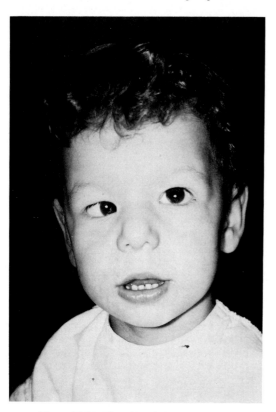 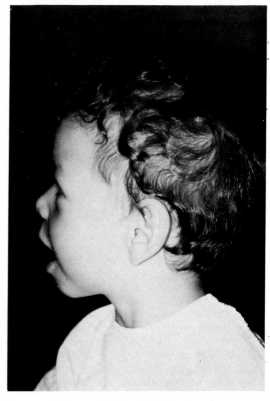

Figure 37-16. The "elfin" facies seen in many patients with supravalvular aortic stenosis. G. B. at two years.

Postnatal feeding problems and a slow weight gain during infancy are relatively common observations. Though later development may be apparently quite normal, many patients show growth retardation. Cardiac symptoms are rare in infancy or early childhood. In older children with severe supravalvular aortic stenosis, dyspnea with exertion, syncope, or angina pectoris may occur (Keane et al., 1976).

The most striking physical sign is the facies of those patients with the syndrome described by Williams and associates (1961) and by Beuren (1972) (Figure 37–16). This facial appearance, described as "elfin" in infancy, becomes coarser and more clearly recognized in the older child. There is periorbital fullness, epicanthal folds, anteverted nares, long philtrum, and thick lips with an open mouth (Jones and Smith, 1975). There is usually a marked difference between the facial appearance of affected subjects and their sibs. In this group of patients mental retardation with a discordant extroverted personality is characteristic. Minor skeletal abnormalities, strabismus, and inguinal hernia are also frequently seen.

The sporadic and familial cases without abnormal facies do not appear to have the above features, although extensive testing can reveal subtle impairment of intelligence and other evidence to support a similar though less extensive damage to body systems other than the cardiovascular system (Antia et al., 1967).

The cardiac signs of supravalvular aortic stenosis, on the other hand, are quite uniform in all three groups when present: there is an ejection systolic murmur that is maximal in the aortic area and is conducted strikingly into the carotid vessels. The murmur is three to four of six intensity grades in children and will usually have been detected some time during the first year. A thrill is always present in the suprasternal notch, even when the murmur is of the lower order of intensity. Aortic clicks are not encountered but aortic closure sounds are often accentuated. An early diastolic murmur is not usually heard, despite the fact that angiographic evidence commonly reveals aortic valve regurgitation.

An additional softer ejection systolic murmur may be heard peripherally over the lung, suggesting the presence of an associated pulmonary arterial stenosis, but it is sometimes difficult to recognize this murmur as having a separate origin from the louder aortic one. For the same reasons the murmurs due to an associated coarctation of the aorta or to mitral regurgitation may be difficult to recognize with certainty.

The arterial pulse is more prominent in the right arm and systolic blood pressure is higher there than in the left arm, a result of the high-velocity jet of blood from the aortic obstruction being preferentially directed into the innominate artery—Coanda effect (French and Guntheroth, 1970; Goldstein and Epstein, 1970). Excessive tortuosity of retinal and cerebral vessels was described in a 12-year-old patient by Fay and colleagues (1966).

A host of other studies including chromosomal analyses, rectal biopsies, and blood calcium levels in patients with supravalvular stenosis, particularly in those with the extended syndrome, have been reported normal (Jones and Smith, 1975). Early appearances of secondary sex characteristics in girls with the abnormal facies led Beuren (1972) to believe that a vitamin D estrogenic effect might be responsible.

Electrocardiography

The precordial leads of the standard electrocardiogram in patients with supravalvular aortic stenosis can be normal, although more usually they show left ventricular hypertrophy. The change is more striking in older subjects, reflecting the general tendency for the effect of aortic obstruction to increase slowly with age. Occasionally there is right ventricular hypertrophy, particularly when there is associated pulmonary arterial or pulmonary valvular stenosis of severe degree. In a study of 26 patients with supravalvular aortic stenosis between 20 months and 30 years of age a spectrum of electrocardiographic change was found comparable to that for patients with valvular aortic stenosis of varying degree. Left ventricular hypertrophy, wide QRS-T angles in the frontal plane, or a strain pattern tended to separate patients with severe from those with mild stenosis, but there were numerous exceptions (Maron and Sissman, 1971). The characteristic of vectorcardiograms of eight patients examined by Gaum and associates (1972) was a horizontal plane QRS loop showing the maximum vector directed to the right and posteriorly suggesting the presence of left ventricular hypertrophy or left posterior hemiblock.

Because of the interest in the relationship between supravalvular aortic stenosis and idiopathic hypercalcemia of infancy, the electrocardiogram in the clinical phase of hypercalcemia has importance. An abnormally broad, notched, and tall T wave was found in the standard and left chest leads of over 90 percent of patients with infantile hypercalcemia by Coleman (1965). Although this effect was noted to persist longer than the elevation of serum calcium, it has not been commented on in the records of those children with supravalvular aortic stenosis who have had the expanded syndrome suggesting a previous abnormality of calcium metabolism.

Radiologic Examination

Most chest x-rays of patients with supravalvular aortic stenosis show hearts of normal size, only a third to a quarter showing any degree of cardiomegaly and then of relatively slight degree (Antia et al., 1967; Kurlander et al., 1966).

Of those with evidence of cardiac enlargement the left ventricle is most often the recognizable chamber affected, and only when .there is very severe pulmonary arterial stenosis with relatively mild supravalvular aortic stenosis is there usually right ventricular enlargement. Although some patients with the hourglass form of the obstruction may show mild-to-moderate dilatation in the ascending aorta (Figure 37–15A), other patients in the same subgroup and those with the hypoplastic form of the obstruction do not show this change and have a small aortic knob (Kupic and Abrams, 1966). The usual density just superior to the right atrium and to the right of the midline in these patients may be deficient as a result of the small, relatively medially placed ascending aorta (Kurlander et al., 1966). Lung vascular markings are usually normal despite the presence of an associated pulmonary artery stenosis. Osteosclerosis is seen in the film of infant patients with idiopathic hypercalcemia (Figure 37–17).

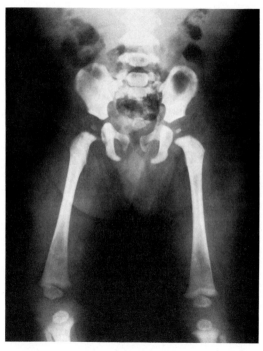

Figure 37-17. X-ray of the lower body of an infant aged nine months with documented idiopathic hypercalcemia and supravalvular aortic stenosis showing osteosclerosis particularly evident at the femoral metaphases.

Echocardiography

The echocardiogram can be a useful confirmatory study of the site of obstruction in this disorder (Usher et al., 1974). Bolen and associates (1975) and Nasrallah and Nihill (1975) both demonstrated a decrease in aortic dimensions at the level of the ascending aorta when contrasted with the level of the aortic leaflet. There is, however, an underestimate of the severity of narrowing by this method.

Cardiac Catheterization and Angiocardiography

The severity of supravalvular aortic stenosis can be confirmed by retrograde left heart catheterization. Peak systolic pressure gradients across the stenosis have ranged from as low as 10 mm of mercury (Maron and Sissman, 1971) to as high as 191 mm of mercury (Keane et al., 1976). Serial catheterization studies at intervals up to nine years do not suggest that any increase in the pressure gradient is common but rather large changes may occasionally occur in the follow-up of younger children (Keane et al., 1976). The concept of a diffuse nature of the arterial lesion in supravalvular aortic stenosis gains support from the finding that the normal amplification of the arterial pressure pulse as it proceeds along the aorta to the periphery may be abolished in the patient with expanded hypercalcemic syndrome (Krovetz, quoted by Rowe, 1972).

Aortography and angiocardiography are the methods of choice for anatomic definition of the disorder. It is now essential to do extensive mapping of the conducting arteries in such patients. Adequate right ventricular and aortic root contrast injection in a number of different projections are necessary to ensure detailed visualization of the main pulmonary artery and its major branches, left ventricular size and function, deformity in the ascending aorta, the aortic valve, the coronary arteries, and other aortic and branch vessel origins. The hourglass and hypoplastic forms of supravalvular aortic stenosis are well displayed from the ascending aortic injection (Figure 37–15). The length of the segment of obstruction varied from 0.5 to 3.0 cm in a review of reported angiograms conducted by Kupic and Abrams (1966). The angiographic assessment of severity in these 69 cases was mild for 21 percent, moderate for 56 percent, and severe for 17 percent. The aortic size in that report was thought to be normal in 60 percent, hypoplastic in 30 percent, and dilated in 10 percent. Ottesen and associates (1966) found evidence of aortic valve incompetence in 10 of 15 patients with supravalvular aortic stenosis. The coronary arteries in all studies have been dilated and tortuous. Stenoses distal to the origin of a major coronary artery have been less commonly observed. On the other hand, stenoses at the origin of the carotid, subclavian, mesenteric, and celiac axis arteries have been observed in between a third and a half of recent studies (Kurlander et al., 1966; Ottesen et al., 1966) (Figure 37–19). Coarctation of the aorta was encountered in 15 percent of one series of 24 patients (Kurlander et al., 1966) and the relatively frequent mild narrowing of the thoracic aorta in that region has previously been referred to. Hypoplasia of the descending aorta has been the subject of comment (Ottesen et al., 1966) though more difficult to quantify. There are insufficient data to decide whether the generalized abnormality of the systemic arterial wall is at more risk for injury and thrombosis after percutaneous

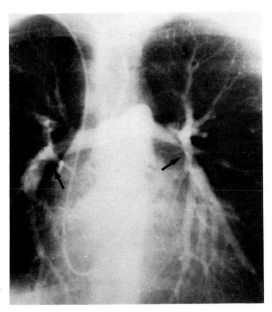

Figure 37-18. Pulmonary arterial stenosis of the peripheral type. Right ventricular angiocardiogram in a patient with supravalvular aortic stenosis. (See also Figure 41-10, page 799.)

femoral artery entry for these mapping procedures.

Pulmonary arterial stenosis may be of the bifurcation type or peripheral in form (Figure 37–18). The exact proportion of patients with supravalvular aortic stenosis who have pulmonary arterial stenosis is uncertain but it is at least 50 percent and probably closer to three-quarters of patients. The pulmonary arterial stenosis may take the form of bifurcation type or be more peripheral in nature. The latter form may be more common, but gradation from one to the other, as with the aortic lesion, is likely to be a matter of degree of wall involvement rather than a distinctly different form of the disorder.

The original report of Williams and associates (1961) did not assess pulmonary artery pressure or perform arteriograms in the pulmonary circuit of their patients and there is a paucity of data on the state of the pulmonary arteries in young patients with the disorder. Our impression is that pulmonary artery stenosis is seldom severe in young children, whereas supravalvular aortic stenosis can be. In the youngest infant we have studied (Garcia et al., 1964) the pulmonary artery stenosis was bifurcation in type and very mild. He had an hourglass aortic constriction of moderately severe degree (Figure 37–15A). Petersen and associates (1965) noted that where there was localized hourglass deformity in the aorta, other areas of stenosis, such as in the aortic arch vessels, had the same type of localized obstruction. The finding of localized obstruction in the pulmonary arterial system in our case may be a reflection of that expected change. There may be another explanation. In a disorder such as hypercalcemia where the basic involvement of conducting vessel walls could be

expected to be uniform, the expression of the disease would likely be influenced by postnatal hemodynamics. Especially if the metabolic effect became manifest in early infancy when the pulmonary artery pressure is relatively low, pulmonary arterial stenosis might be slower to develop (Varghese et al., 1969). One might then predict that the aortic lesion would in general be more severe and the pulmonary vascular abnormality would take considerably longer to evolve. The comparative severity of pulmonary arterial as opposed to systemic arterial lesions of idiopathic hypercalcemia in the young is the reverse of the situation found in congenital rubella although paradoxic variations in both types have been reported (Vince, 1970; Rowe et al., 1974).

Prognosis

There is some angiographic and clinical evidence to suggest the severity of supravalvular aortic stenosis is not related to the presence or absence of abnormal facies or the expanded form of the lesion (Kurlander et al., 1966; Wiltse et al., 1966). To add to the difficulties of prognosis, infants with both mild and severe forms of hypercalcemia in infancy have been found *not* to have evidence of supravalvular aortic

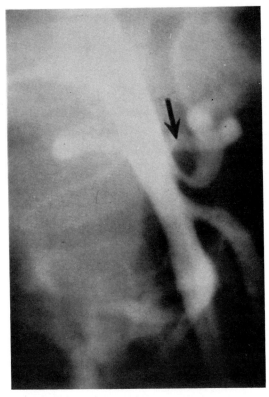

Figure 37-19. Right lateral projection showing aortic hypoplasia and stenosis of the superior and mesenteric arteries in a patient aged seven years who had documented idiopathic hypercalcemia during infancy.

stenosis in later life, but there has been little systematic follow-up in all forms of the vascular disorder. At another extreme, in 26 adults between 16 and 70 years of age with supravalvular aortic stenosis, of whom five had abnormal facies, Pansegrau and associates (1973) found angina and congestive heart failure to be common presenting symptoms. Sudden death was also encountered in this group, and one of the two patients documented by Williams and associates (1961) who had operative treatment for the stenosis died unexpectedly a few years later. An autopsy showed excellent relief of the obstruction, a very thick left ventricular myocardium, and patchy myocardial fibrosis. Aortic aneurysms, aortic dissection, and infective endocarditis are included among the late complications (Roberts, 1973). Of the 68 patients reviewed by Petersen and associates (1965) 27 had died. Fifteen of the deaths were connected with surgical intervention, and of the remaining 12 patients, six had died unexpectedly, four of congestive heart failure and two of causes apparently unrelated.

Treatment

Since the exact mechanism by which patients with the expanded syndrome of Williams and associates (1961) and Beuren (1972) suffer deranged calcium and vitamin D metabolism is unknown, preventive measures are difficult. Possibly the simplest preventive measure for limiting infantile hypercalcemia would be to ensure that no pregnant woman receives more than the recommended amounts of either vitamin D or calcium in her daily diet, and vitamin D intake during pregnancy should be continuously and carefully supervised. Early detection and appropriate therapy are probably the most important elements in lessening the damage caused by infantile hypercalcemia, but even the severe cases are sometimes difficult to diagnose. In the presence of failure to thrive, irritability, hypotonia, poor appetite, and vomiting, particularly if there is no ready explanation for the symptoms, serial serum calcium determinations and suitable x-rays may be desirable (Cooke, 1968).

Successful surgical correction of supravalvular aortic stenosis was first conducted in 1956 and reported by McGoon and colleagues (1961). Operative intervention for severe supravalvular aortic stenosis is now widely practiced (Williams et al., 1961; Starr et al., 1961; Hara et al., 1962; Morrow et al., 1963; Cooley et al., 1965; Cornell et al., 1966; Rastelli et al., 1966; Robicsek et al., 1970). Though resection of a membrane and excision of an aortic section have both been employed, the currently favored technique for the common hourglass type of deformity is that which McGoon and associates originally employed—aortotomy with insertion of a large prosthetic gusset. In the most recent series excellent immediate results have been obtained in children with discrete hourglass deformity (Weisz et al., 1976). It is well recognized that the diffuse form of supravalvular aortic stenosis is much less amenable to

surgical repair and carries such a high risk at operation that a left ventricular-aortic bypass shunt that diverts most of the left ventricular output into the descending thoracic aorta is now being recommended (Keane et al., 1976).

REFERENCES

Valvular Aortic and Discrete Subaoric Stenosis

Arani, D. T., and Carleton, R. A.: Assessment of aortic valvular stenosis from the aortic pressure pulse. *Circulation*, **36**:30, 1967.

Bargeron, J.; Abelmann, W. H.; Vazquez-Milan, H.; and Ellis, L. B.: Aortic stenosis: clinical manifestations and course of the disease. Review of one hundred proved cases. *Arch. Int. Med.*, **94**:911, 1954.

Bennett, D. H.; Evans, D. W.; and Raj, M. V. J.: Echocardiographic left ventricular dimensions in pressure and volume overload. Their use in assessing aortic stenosis. *Br. Heart J.*, **37**:971, 1975.

Blackwood, R. A.; Bloom, K. R.; and Williams, C. M.: Echocardiographic prediction of left ventricular pressure in children. *Ultrasound in Medicine*, **IIIA**:197, 1976.

Blackwood, R. A.; Bloom, K. R.; and Williams, C. M.: Aortic stenosis in children: Experience with echocardiographic prediction of severity. *Circulation* (in press), 1978.

Bonner, A. J. Jr.; Sacks, H. N.; and Tavel, M. E.: Assessing the severity of aortic stenosis by phonocardiography and external carotid pulse recordings. *Circulation*, **48**:239, 1973.

Braunwald, E.; Roberts, W. C.; Goldblatt, A.; Aygen, M. M.; Rockoff, S. D.; and Gilbert, J. W.: Aortic stenosis: physiological, pathological and clinical concepts. *Ann. Int. Med.*, **58**:494, 1963.

Chevers, N.: Observations on diseases of the orifice and valves of the aorta. *Guy's Hosp. Rep.*, **387**:1842.

Chiariello, L.; Agosti, J.; Vlad, P.; and Subramanian, S.: Congenital aortic stenosis: Experience with 43 patients. *J. Thorac. Cardiovasc. Surg.*, **72**:182, 1976.

Cohen, L. S.; Friedman, W. F.; and Braunwald, E.: Natural history of Mild Congenital Aortic Stenosis Elucidated by Serial Hemodynamic studies. *Am. J. Cardiol.*, **30**:1, 1972.

Conkle, D. M.; Jones, M.; and Morrow, A. G.: Treatment of congenital aortic stenosis; An evaluation of the late results of aortic valvotomy. *Arch. Surg.*, **107**:649, 1973.

Cook, C. D.; Smith, H. L.; Giesen, C. W.; and Berdez, G. L.: Xanthoma tuberosum, aortic stenosis, coronary sclerosis and angina pectoris. Report of a case in a boy thirteen years of age. *Am. J. Dis. Child.*, **73**:326, 1947.

Cooley, D. A.; Beall, A. C.; Hallman, G. L.; and Bricker, D. L.: Obstructive lesions of the left ventricular outflow tract. Surgical treatment. *Circulation*, **31**:612, 1965.

Davis, R. H.; Feigenbaum, H.; Chang, S.; Konecke, L. L.; and Dillon, J. C.: Echocardiographic manifestation of Discrete Subaortic stenosis. *Am. J. Cardiol.*, **33**:277, 1974.

Edwards, J. E.: Pathologic aspects of cardiac valvular insufficiencies. *Arch. Surg.*, **77**:634, 1958.

Edwards, J. E.: Pathology of left ventricular outflow obstruction, *Circulation*, **31**:586, 1965.

Ellis, F. H.; Ongley, P. A.; and Kirklin, J. W.: Results of surgical treatment for congenital aortic stenosis. *Circulation*, **25**:29, 1962.

Ellison, R. S.; Wagner, H. R.; Weidman, W. H.; and Miettinen, O. S.: Congenital valvular aortic stenosis: Clinical detection of small pressure gradient. Joint Study on the Natural History of Congenital Heart Defects. *Am. J. Cardiol.*, **37**:757, 1976.

El-Said, G.; Galioto, F. M.; Mullins, C. E.; and McNamara, D. G.: Natural hemodynamic history of congenital aortic stenosis in childhood. *Am. J. Cardiol.*, **30**:6, 1972.

Feizi, O.; Symons, C.; and Yacoub, M.: Echocardiography of the aortic valve. *Br. Heart J.*, **36**:341, 1974.

Fowler, R. S.: Ventricular repolarization in congenital aortic stenosis. *Am. Heart J.*, **70**:603, 1965.

Friedman, W. F.; Modlinger, J.; and Morgan, J. R.: Serial hemodynamic observations in asymptomatic children with valvar aortic stenosis. *Circulation*, **43**:91, 1971.

Friedman, W. F., and Pappelbaum, S. J.: Indications for Hemodynamic Evaluation and Surgery in Congenital Aortic Stenosis. *Pediatr. Clin. North Am.*, **18**:1207, 1971.

Glew, R. H.; Varghese, P. J.; Krovetz, L. J.; Dorst, J. P.; and Rowe, R. D.: Sudden death and congenital aortic stenosis. A review of eight cases with an evaluation of premonitory clinical features. *Am. Heart J.*, **78**:615, 1969.

Gramiak, R., and Shah, P. M.: Echocardiography of the normal and diseased aortic valve. *Radiology*, **96**:1, 1970.

Halloran, K. H.: The telemetered exercise electrocardiogram in congenital aortic stenos)s. *Pediatrics*, **47**:31, 1971.

Hawker, R. E.; Seara, C. A.; and Krovetz, L. J.: Distalward Modification of the arterial pulse wave in children with clinical aortic stenosis. *Circulation*, **50**:181, 1974.

Hohn, A. P.; Van Praagh, S.; Moore, D.; Vlad, P.; and Lambert, E. C.: Aortic stenosis. *Circulation*, **32**:1114, 1965.

Hugenholtz, P. G., and Gamboa, R.: Effect of chronically increased ventricular pressure on the electrical forces of the heart. *Circulation*, **30**:511, 1964.

Hurwitz, R. A.: Valvar aortic stenosis in childhood: Clinical and hemodynamic history. *J. Pediatr.*, **82**:228, 1973.

Ibrahim, M.; M.; Siliem, M.; Delahaye, J. P.; and Froment, R.: Systolic time intervals in valvular aortic stenosis and idiopathic hypertrophic subaortic stenosis. *Br. Heart J.*, **35**:276, 1973.

Keene, J. F.; Bernhard, W. F.; and Nadas, A. S.: Aortic stenosis surgery in infancy. *Circulation*, **52**:1138, 1975.

Keith, A.: Schorstein Lecture on the fate of the bulbus cordis in the human heart. *Lancet*, **2**:1267, 1924.

Kelly, D. T.; Wulfsberg, B. A.; and Rowe, R. D.: Discrete Subaortic stenosis. *Circulation*, **46**:309, 1972.

Kirklin, J. W.: Factors in improved morbidity and mortality rates after total aortic valve replacement. *Surg. Clin. North Am.*, **42**:1537, 1962.

Kjellberg, S. R.; Mannheimer, E.; Rudhe, V.; and Johnson, B.: *Diagnosis of Congenital Heart Disease*, 2nd ed., Year Book Publishers, Inc. Chicago, 1958.

Lakier, J. B.; Lewis, A. B.; Heymann, M. A.; Stanger, P.; Hoffman, J. I. E.; and Rudolph, A. M.: Isolated aortic stenosis in the Neonate. Natural history and hemodynamic considerations. *Circulation*, **50**:801, 1974.

Lambert, E. C.; Menon, V. A.; Wagner, H. R.; and Vlad, P.: Sudden unexpected death from Cardiovascular disease in children. *Am. J. Cardiol.*, **34**:89, 1974.

Lyle, D. P.; Bancroft, W. H.; Tucker, M.; and Eddleman, E. E., Jr.: Slopes of the carotid pulse wave in normal subjects, aortic valvular diseases and hypertrophic subaortic stenosis. *Circulation*, **43**:374, 1971.

Manning, J. A.; Sellers, F. J.; Bynum, R. S.; and Keith, J. D.: The medical management of clinical endocardial fibroelastosis. *Circulation*, **24**:60, 1964.

Marquis, R. M., and Logan, A.: Congenital aortic stenosis and its surgical treatment. *Br. Heart J.*, **17**:373, 1955.

Mason, D. T.; Braunwald, E.; Ross, J., Jr.; and Morrow, A. G.: Diagnostic value of the first and second derivatives of the arterial pressure pulse in aortic valve disease and in hypertrophic subaortic stenosis. *Circulation*, **30**:90, 1964.

Mody, M. R., and Mody, G. T.: Serial hemodynamic measurements in congenital valvular and subvalvular aortic stenosis. *Am. Heart J.*, **89**:(2), 137, 1975.

Nadas, A. S.; Hauwaert, L. V.; Hauck, A. J.; and Gross, R. E.: Combined aortic and pulmonic stenosis. *Circulation*, **25**:346, 1962.

Nanda, N. C.; Gramiak, R.; Manning, J.; Mahoney, E. B.; Lipchik, E. C.; and Deweese, J. A.: Echocardiographic recognition of the congenital bicuspid aortic valve. *Circulation*, **49**:870, 1974.

Newfeld, E. A.; Muster, A. J.; Paul, M. H.; Idriss, F. S.; and Riker, W. L.: Discrete Subvalvular aortic stenosis in childhood. Study of 51 patients. *Am. J. Cardiol.*, **38**:53, 1976.

Peckham, G. B.; Keith, J. D.; and Evans, J. R.: Congenital aortic stenosis: Some observations on the natural history and clinical assessment. *Can. Med. Assoc. J.*, **91**:639, 1964.

Popp, R. L.; Silverman, J. F.; French, J. W.; Stinson, E. B.; and Harrison, D. C.: Echocardiographic findings in discrete subvalvular aortic stenosis. *Circulation*, **49**:226, 1974.

Putman, T. C.; Harris, P. D.; Bernard, W. F.; and Gross, R. E.: The surgical management of congenital aortic stenosis. *J. Thorac. Cardiovasc. Surg.*, **48**:540, 1964.

Radford, D. J.; Bloom, K. R.; Izukawa, T.; Moes, C. F.; and Rowe, R. D.: Echocardiographic assessment of bicuspid aortic valves. Angiographic and Pathological correlates. *Circulation*, **53**:80, 1976.

Reeve, R.; Kawamata, K.; and Selzer, A.: Reliability of

vectorcardiography in assessing the severity of congenital aortic stenosis. *Circulation*, **34**:92, 1966.

Reis, R. L.; Peterson, L. M.; Mason, D. T.; Simon, A. L.; and Morrow, A. G.: Congenital fixed subvalvular aortic stenosis: An anatomical classification and correlations with operative results. *Circulation*, **43**:Suppl. 1: 1–11, 1971.

Reynolds, J. L.; Nadas, A. S.; Rudolph, A. M.; and Gross, R. E.: Critical congenital aortic stenosis with minimal electro-cardiographic changes: A report on two siblings. *N. Engl. J. Med.*, **262**:276, 1960.

Roberts, W. C.: Pathologic aspects of Valvular and subvalvular (discrete and diffuse) aortic stenosis. In Kidd, B. S. L., and Keith, J. D. (eds.): *The Natural History and Progress in Treatment of Congenital Heart Defects*. Charles C Thomas, Publisher, Springfield, Ill. 1969.

Roberts, W. C.: The structure of the aortic valve in clinically isolated aortic stenosis. An autopsy study of 162 patients over 15 years of age. *Circulation*, **42**:91, 1970.

Roberts, W. C.: The congenitally bicuspid aortic valve: A study of 85 autopsy cases. *Am. J. Cardiol.*, **26**:72, 1970.

Roberts, W. C.: Valvular, subvalvular and supravalvular aortic stenosis: Morphologic features. *Cardiovasc. Clin.*, **5**:97, 1973.

Sellers, R. D.; Lillehei, C. W.; and Edwards, J. E.: Subaortic stenosis caused by anomalies of the atrial ventricular valve. *J. Thorac. Cardiovasc. Surg.*, **48**:289, 1964.

Shaver, J. A.; Griff, F. W.; and Leonard, J. J.: Ejection sounds of left-sided origin. In American Heart Association Monograph Number 46. *Physiologic Principles of Heart Sounds and Murmurs*.

Spencer, F. C.; Neill, C. A.; Sand, L.; and Bahnson, H. T.: Anatomical variations in 46 patients with congenital aortic stenosis. *Am. Surg.*, **26**:204, 1960.

Taussig, H. B.: *Congenital Malformations of the Heart*, 2nd ed., Harvard University Press, Cambridge, Mass., 1960, Vol. II, p. 835.

Van Praagh, R.; Corwin, R. D.; Dahlquist, E. H., Jr.; Freedom, R. M.; Matteoli, L.; and Nebesar, R. A.: Tetralogy of Fallot with severe left ventricular outflow tract obstruction due to anomalous attachment of the mitral valve to the ventricular septum. *Am. J. Cardiol.*, **26**:93, 1970.

Vogel, J. H., and Blount, S. G., Jr.: Clinical evaluation in localizing level of obstruction to outflow from left ventricle, importance of early systolic ejection clock. *Am. J. Cardiol.*, **15**:782, 1965.

Weyman, A. E.; Feigenbaum, H.; Jurwitz, R. A.; Girod, D. A.; Dillon, J. C.; and Chang, S.: Localisation of left ventricular outflow obstruction by crosssectional echocardiography. *Am. J. Med.*, **60**:33, 1976.

Wood, P.: *Diseases of the Heart and Circulation*. Eyre & Spottiswoode, Ltd., London, 1956.

Muscular Subaortic Stenosis

Barr, P. A.; Celermajer, J. M.; Bowdler, J. D.; and Cartmill, T. B.: Idiopathic hypertrophic obstructive cardiomyopathy causing severe right ventricular outflow tract obstruction in infancy. *Br. Heart J.*, **35**:1109, 1973.

Bernheim, P. I.: De l'asystolie veineuse dans l'hypertrophie du coeur gauche par stenose concomitante du ventricule droit. *Rev. med.*, **30**:785, 1910.

Bloom, K. R.; Meyer, R. A.; Bove, K. E.; and Kaplan, S.: The association of fixed and dynamic left ventricular outflow obstruction, *Am. Heart J.*, **89**:586, 1975.

Boughner, D. R.; Schuld, R. L.; and Persaud, J. A.: Hypertrophic obstructive cardiomyopathy—Assessment by echocardiographic and Doppler ultrasound techniques. *Br. Heart J.*, **37**:917, 1975.

Braudo, M.; Wigle, E. D.; and Keith, J. D.: A distinctive electrocardiogram in muscular subaortic stenosis. *Am. J. Cardiol.*, **13**:98, 1964 (abstr.).

Braunwald, E.; Lambrew, C. T.; Rockoff, S. D.; Ross, J., Jr.; and Morrow, A. G.: Idiopathic hypertrophic subaortic stenosis: Description of the disease based on an analysis of 64 patients. *Circulation*, **29** (Suppl. 4):1, 1964.

Brock, R.: Functional obstruction of the left ventricle (acquired aortic subvalvular stenosis). *Guy Hosp. Rep.*, **106**:221, 1957.

Bulkley, B. H.; Rouleau, J.; Strauss, H. W.; and Pitt, B.: Idiopathic hypertrophic subaortic stenosis: Detection by thallium 201 myocardial perfusion imaging. *N. Engl. J. Med.*, **293**:1113, 1975.

Chung, K. J.; Manning, J. A.; and Gramiak, R.: Echocardiography in Coexisting hypertrophic subaortic stenosis and fixed left ventricular outflow obstruction. *Circulation*, **49**:673, 1974.

Clark, C. E.; Henry, W. L.; and Epstein, S. E.: Familial prevalence and genetic transmission of Idiopathic hypertrophic subaortic stenosis. *N. Engl. J. Med.*, **289**:709, 1973.

Cooley, D. A.; Leachman, R. D.; and Wukash, D. C.: Diffuse muscular subaortic stenosis: Surgical treatment, *Am. J. Cardiol.*, **31**:1, 1973.

Criley, J. M.; Lewis, K. B.; White, R. I., Jr.; and Ross, R. S.: Pressure gradients without obstruction—A new concept of "hypertrophic subaortic stenosis." *Circulation*, **32**:71, 1965.

Davies, L. G.: A familial heart disease. *Br. Heart J.*, **14**:206, 1952.

Ehlers, K. H.; Hagstrom, J. W. C.; Lukas, D. S.; Redo, S. F.; and Engle, M. A.: Glycogen-storage disease of the myocardium with obstruction to left ventricular outflow. *Circulation*, **25**:96, 1962.

Falikov, R. E.; Resnekov, L.; Bharati, S.; and Lev, M.: Mid ventricular obstruction: A variant of obstructive cardio-myopathy. *Am. J. Cardiol.*, **37**:432, 1976.

Frank, S., and Braunwald, E.: Idiopathic hypertrophic subaortic stenosis: Clinical analysis of 126 patients with emphasis on natural history. *Circulation*, **37**:759, 1968.

Gach, J. V.; Andriange, M.; and Franck, G.: Hypertrophic obstructive cardiomyopathy and Friedrich's ataxia. *Am. J. Cardiol.*, **27**:436, 1971.

Goodman, D. J.; Harrison, D. C.; and Popp, R. L.: Echocardiographic features of primary pulmonary hypertension. *Am. J. Cardiol.*, **33**:438, 1974.

Goodwin, J. F.: The congestive and hypertrophic cardio-myopathies—A decade of study. *Lancet*, **1**:733, 1970.

Goodwin, J. F.: Prospects and predictions for the cardiomyopathies. *Circulation*, **50**:210, 1974.

Goodwin, J. F.; Hollman, A.; Cleland, W. P.; and Teare, D.: Obstructive cardiomyopathy simulating aortic stenosis. *Br. Heart J.*, **22**:403, 1960.

Gutgesell, H. P.; Mullins, C. E.; Gillette, P. C.; Speer, M.; Rudolph, A. J.; and McNamara, D. G.: Transient hypertrophic subaortic stenosis in infants of diabetic mothers. *J. Pediatr.*, **89**:120, 1976.

Hamby, R. I.; Roberts, G. S.; and Meron, J. M.: Hypertension and hypertrophic subaortic stenosis. *Am. J. Med.*, **51**:474, 1971.

Hardarson, T.; de la Calzada, C. S.; Curiel, R.; and Goodwin, J. F.: Prognosis and mortality of hypertrophic obstructive cardio-myopathy. *Lancet*, **2**:1462, 1973.

Henry, W. L.; Clark, E. C.; and Epstein, S. E.: Asymmetric septal hypertrophy. Echocardiographic identification of the patho-gnomonic anatomic abnormality of IHSS. *Circulation*, **47**:225, 1973.

Hohn, A. R.; Lowe, C. U.; Sokal, J. E.; and Lambert, E. C.: Cardiac problems in the glycogenoses with specific reference to Pompe's disease. *Pediatrics*, **35**:313, 1965.

Larter, W. E.; Allen, H. D.; Sahn, D. J.; and Goldberg, S. J.: The asymmetrically hypertrophied septum. Further differentiation of its causes. *Circulation*, **53**:19, 1976.

Maron, B. J.; Edwards, J. E.; Ferrans, V. J.; Clark, C. E.; Lebowitz, E. A.; Henry, W. L.; and Epstein, S. E.: Congenital heart malformations associated with disproportionate ventricular septal thickening, *Circulation*, **52**:926, 1975.

Maron, B. J.; Ferrans, V. J.; Henry, W. L.; Clark, C. E.; Redwood, D. R.; Roberts, W. C.; Morrow, A. G.; and Epstein, S. E.: Differences in distribution of myocardial abnormalities in patients with obstructive and nonobstructive asymmetric septal hyper-trophy (ASH), Light and electron microscopic findings. *Circulation*, **50**:436, 1974.

Maron, B. J.; Henry, W. L.; Clark, C. E.; Redwood, D. R.; Roberts, W. C.; and Epstein, S. E.: Asymmetric septal hypertrophy in childhood, *Circulation*, **53**:1976.

McKinney, B.: In *Pathology of the Cardiomyopathies*. Butterworth, London, 1974, p. 48.

Meerschwam, I. S., and Hootmans, W. J. M.: Electromyographic findings in hypertrophic obstructive cardiomyopathy. *Pathol. Microbiol. (Basel)*, **35**:86, 1970.

Moes, C. A.; Peckham, G. B.; and Keith, J. D.: Idiopathic hypertrophy of the interventricular septum causing muscular subaortic stenosis in children. *Radiology*, **83**:283, 1964.

Moreyra, E.; Klein, J. J.; Shimada, H.; and Segal, B. L.: Idiopathic hypertrophic subaortic stenosis diagnosed by reflected ul-trasound. *Am. J. Cardiol.*, **23**:32, 1969.

Morrow, A. G., and Braunwald, E.: Functional aortic stenosis. *Circulation*, **21**:181, 1959.

Nellen, M.; Beck, W.; Vogelpoel, L.; and Schrine, V.: Auscultatory phenomena in hypertrophic obstructive cardiomyopathy. Ciba

Study Group No. 37. Wolstenholme and O'Connor (ed)., J. & A. Churchill, London, 1971, p. 77.

Parker, D. P.; Kaplan, M. A.; and Connolly, J. E.: Coexistent aortic valvular and functional hypertrophic subaortic stenosis. *Am. J. Cardiol.*, **24**:307, 1969.

Polani, P. E., and Moynhan, E. J.: Progressive cardiomyopathic lentiginosis. *Q. J. Med., New Series*, **41**:205, 1972.

Redwood, D. R.; Scherer, J. L.; and Epstein, S. E.: Biventricular cineangiography in the evaluation of patients with asymmetric septal hypertrophy. *Circulation*, **49**:1116, 1974.

Rees, A.; Elbl, F.; Minhas, K.; and Solinger, R.: Echocardiographic evidence of outflow tract obstruction in Pompe's disease. *Am. J. Cardiol.*, **37**:1103, 1976.

Roberts, W. C.: Valvular, subvalvular and supravalvular aortic stenosis: Morphologic features. In Edwards, J. E. (ed.): *Clinical Pathological Correlations 2.* F. A. Davis, Philadelphia, 1973, p. 119.

Rossen, R. M.; Goodman, D. J.; Ingham, R. E.; and Popp, R. L.: Echocardiographic criteria in the diagnosis of idiopathic hypertrophic subaortic stenosis. *Circulation*, **50**:747, 1974.

Schmincke, A.: Ueber linkseitige musculose conusstenosen. *Deutsch Med. Wochnschr.*, **33**:2082, 1907.

Shah, P. M.: IHSS-HOCM-MSS-ASH (Editorial). *Circulation*, **51**:577, 1975.

Shah, P. M.; Adelman, A. G.; Wigle, E. D.; Gobel, F. L.; Burchell, H. B.; Hardarson, T.; Curiel, R.; de la Calzada, C.; Oakley, C. M.; and Goodwin, J. F.: The natural (and unnatural) history of hypertrophic obstructive cardiomyopathy. A multicentre study. *Circ. Res.*, **34**:35 Suppl. II–179, 1974.

Shah, P. M.; Gramiak, R.; and Kramer, D. H.: Ultrasound localization of left ventricular outflow obstruction in hypertrophic obstructive cardiomyopathy. *Circulation*, **40**:3, 1969.

Shah, P. M.; Gramiak, R.; Adelman, A. G.; and Wigle, E. D.: Echocardiographic assessment of the effects of surgery and propranolol on the dynamics of outflow obstruction in hypertrophic subaortic stenosis. *Circulation*, **45**:516, 1972.

Shem-Tov, A.; Deutsch, V.; Yahini, J. H.; and Neufeld, H. M.: Cardiomyopathy associated with congenital heart disease. *Br. Heart J.*, **33**:782, 1971.

Somerville, J., and McDonald, L.: Congenital anomalies in the heart with hypertrophic cardiomyopathy. *Br. Heart J.*, **30**:713, 1968.

Stenson, R. E.; Flamm, M. D., Jr.; Harrison, D. C.; and Hancock, E. W.: Hypertrophic subaortic stenosis. Clinical and hemodynamic effects of long-term propranolol therapy. *Am. J. Cardiol.*, **31**:763, 1973.

Teare, D.: Asymmetrical hypertrophy of the heart in young adults. *Br. Heart J.*, **20**:1, 1958.

Tucker, R. B. K.; Zion, M. M.; Pocock, W. A.; and Barlow, J. B.: Auscultatory features of hypertrophic obstructive cardio-myopathy. A study of 90 patients. *S. African Med. J.*, **49**:179, 1975.

Van Noorden, S.; Olsen, E. G. J.; and Pearse, A. G. E.: Hypertrophic obstructive cardiomyopathy, a histological, histochemical, and ultrastructural study of biopsy material. *Cardiovasc. Res.*, **5**:118, 1971.

Wigle, E. D.; Adelman, A. G.; Auger, P.; and Marquis, Y.: Mitral regurgitation in muscular subaortic stenosis. *Am. J. Cardiol.*, **24**:698, 1969.

Wigle, E. D.; Adelman, A. G.; and Felderhof, C. H.: Medical and surgical treatment of the cardiomyopathies. *Circ. Res.*, **34**:35, Suppl. II–1974.

Wigle, E. D.; Auger, P.; and Marquis, Y.: Muscular subaortic stenosis—The direct relation between the intraventricular pressure difference and the left ventricular ejection time. *Circulation*, **36**:36, 1967.

Wigle, E. D.; Feldeshof, C. H.; Silver, M. D.; and Adelman, A. G.: Hypertrophic obstructive cardiomyopathy. In Fowler, N. O. (ed.): *Myocardial Disease.* Grune and Stratton, 1973, p. 297.

Williams, R. G.; Ellison, R. C.; and Nadas, A. S.: Development of left ventricular outflow obstruction in idiopathic hypertrophic subaortic stenosis. *N. Engl. J. Med.*, **288**:868, 1973.

Wolstenholme, G. E. W., and O'Connor, M.: *Hypertrophic Obstructive Cardiomyopathy.* Ciba Foundation Study Group No. 37. J. & A. Churchill, London, 1971.

Supravalvular Aortic Stenosis

Antia, A. U.; Wiltse, H. E.; Rowe, R. D.; Pitt, E. L.; Levin, S.; Ottesen, O. E.; and Cooke, R. E.: Pathogenesis of the supravalvular aortic stenosis syndrome. *J. Pediatr.*, **71**:431, 1967.

Becker, A. E.; Becker, M. J.; and Edwards, J. E.: Mitral valvular abnormalities associated with supravalvular aortic stenosis. Observations in 3 cases. *Am. J. Cardiol.*, **29**:90, 1972.

Beuren, A. J.; Schulze, G.; Eberle, P.; Harmjanz, D.; and Apitz, A.: The syndrome of supravalvular aortic stenosis, peripheral pulmonary stenosis, mental retardation and similar facial appearance. *Am. J. Cardiol.*, **13**:471, 1964.

Beuren, A. J.: Supravalvular aortic stenosis: A complex syndrome with and without mental retardation. In *Birth Defects: Original Article Series* 8: No. 5. The National Foundation—March of Dimes, Williams & Wilkins Co., Baltimore, 1972, p. 45.

Black, J. A., and Bonham-Carter, R. E.: Association between aortic stenosis peripheral pulmonary stenosis, mental retardation, and similar facial appearance. *Lancet*, **2**:745, 1963.

Bliddal, J.; Dupont, B.; Melchior, J. C.; and Ottesen, O. E.: Case report. Coarctation of the aorta with multiple anomalies in idiopathic hypercalcemia of infancy. *Acta Pediatr.*, **58**:652, 1969.

Bolen, J. L.; Popp, R. L.; and French, J. W.: Echocardiographic features of supravalvular aortic stenosis. *Circulation*, **52**:817, 1975.

Char, F., and Rowe, R. D.: Infantile hypercalcemia syndrome with mitral regurgitation and hypoplasia of aorta. In *Birth Defects: Original Article Series 8:* No. 5. The National Foundation—March of Dimes, Williams & Wilkins Co., Baltimore, 1972, p. 258.

Chevers, N.: A collection of facts illustrative of the morbid conditions of the pulmonary artery as bearing on the treatment of cardiac and pulmonary diseese. *London Med. Gaz.*, **38**:1846.

Cooke, R. E.: Infantile hypercalcemia and vitamin D. *Hosp. Pract.*, **3**:87, 1968.

Cooley, D. A.; Beall, A. C., Jr.; Hallman, G. L.; and Bricker, D. L.: Obstructive lesions of the left ventricular outflow tract. Surgical treatment. *Circulation*, **31**:612, 1965.

Cornell, W. P.; Elkins, R. C.; Criley, J. M.; and Sabiston, D. C., Jr.: Supravalvular aortic stenosis. *J. Thorac. Cardiovasc. Surg.*, **51**:484, 1966.

Denie, J. J., and Verheugt, A. P.: Supravalvular aortic stenosis. *Circulation*, **18**:902, 1958.

Driscoll, D. J.; Friedberg, D. Z.; and Gallen, W. J.: Idiopathic hypercalcemic syndrome with mitral stenosis. *Wis. Med. J.*, **73**:S115, 1974.

Faye, J. E.; Lynn, R. B.; and Partington, M. W.: Supravalvular aortic stenosis, mental retardation and a characteristic facies. *Can. Med. Assoc. J.*, **94**:295, 1966.

Fraser, D.; Kidd, B. S. L.; Kooh, S. W.; and Paunier, L.: A new look at infantile hypercalcemia. Pediatr. Clin. North Am., **13**:503, 1966.

French, J. W., and Guntheroth, W. G.: An explanation of asymmetric upper extremity blood pressures in supravalvular aortic stenosis. The Coanda effect. *Circulation*, **42**:31, 1970.

Friedman, W. F., and Roberts, W. D.: Vitamin D and the supravalvular aortic stenosis syndrome. The transplacental effects of vitamin D on the aorta of the rabbit. *Circulation*, **34**:77, 1966.

Garcia, R. E.; Friedman, W. F.; Kaback, M. M.; and Rowe, R. D.: Idiopathic hypercalcemia and supravalvular aortic stenosis. Documentation of a new syndrome. *N. Engl. J. Med.*, **271**:117, 1964.

Gaum, W. E.; Chou, Te-C.; and Kaplan, S.: The vectorcardiogram and electrocardiogram in supraventricular aortic stenosis and coarctation of the aorta. *Am. Heart J.*, **84**:620, 1972.

Goldstein, R. E., and Epstein, S. E.: Mechanism of elevated innominate artery pressures in supravalvular aortic stenosis. *Circulation*, **42**:23, 1970.

Hara, M.; Dugan, T.; and Lincoln, B.: Supravalvular aortic stenosis. Report of successful excision and aortic re-anastomosis. *J. Thorac. Cardiovasc. Surg.*, **43**:212, 1962.

Hooft, C.; Vermassen, A.; and Blancquaert, A.: Observations concerning the evolution of the chronic form of idiopathic hypercalcemia in children. *Helvet. paediatr. acta*, **18**:138, 1963.

Hutchins, G. M.: Coarctation of the aorta explained as a branch point of the ductus arteriosus. *Am. J. Pathol.*, **63**:203, 1971.

Jones, K. L., and Smith, D. W.: The Williams elfin facies syndrome. A new perspective. *J. Pediatr.*, **86**:718, 1975.

Keane, J. F.; Fellows, K. E.; LaFarge, C. G.; Nadas, A. S.; and Bernhard, W. F.: The surgical management of discrete and diffuse supravalvar aortic stenosis. *Circulation*, **54**:112, 1976.

Krovetz, L. J.: Unpublished observations. Quoted by Rowe, R. D.

(1972).

Kupic, E. A., and Abrams, H. L.: Supravalvular aortic stenosis. *Am. J. Roentgenol.*, **98**:822, 1966.

Kurlander, G. J.; Petry, E. L.; Taybi, H.; Lurie, P. R.; and Campbell, J. A.: Supravalvar aortic stenosis. Roentgen analysis of twenty-seven cases. *Am. J. Roentgenol.*, **98**:782, 1966.

McCue, C. M.; Spicuzza, T. T.; Robertson, L. W.; and Mauck, H. P., Jr.: Familial supravalvular aortic stenosis. *J. Pediatr.*, **73**:889, 1968.

McGoon, D. C.; Mankin, H. T.; Vlad, P.; and Kirklin, J. W.: The surgical treatment of supravalvular aortic stenosis. *J. Thorac. Cardiovasc. Surg.*, **41**:125, 1961.

Maron, B. J., and Sissman, N. J.: The electrocardiogram in supravalvular aortic stenosis. *Am. Heart J.*, **82**:300, 1971.

Mencarelli, L.: Stenosi supravalolare aortica and annelo. *Arch. Ital. Anat. Istol. Pat.*, **1**:829, 1930.

Morrow, A. G.; Waldhausen, J. A.; Peters, R. L.; Bloodwell, R. D.; and Braunwald, E.: Supravalvular aortic stenosis, *Circulation*, **20**:1003, 1959.

Nasrallah, A. T., and Nihill, M.: Supravalvular aortic stenosis. Echocardiographic features. *Br. Heart J.*, **37**:662, 1975.

Neufeld, H. N.; Wagenvoort, C. A.; Burchell, H. B.; and Edwards, J. E.: Idiopathic atrial fibrillation. *Am. J. Cardiol.*, **8**:193, 1961.

Ottesen, O. E.; Antia, A. U.; and Rowe, R. D.: Peripheral vascular anomalies associated with the supravalvular aortic stenosis syndrome. *Radiology*, **86**:430, 1966.

Pansegrau, D. G.; Kioshos, J. M.; Durnin, R. E.; and Kroetz, F. R.: Supravalvular aortic stenosis in adults. *Am. J. Cardiol.*, **31**:635, 1973.

Perou, M. L.: Congenital supravalvular aortic stenosis. A morphological study with attempt at classification. *Arch. Pathol.*, **71**:453, 1961.

Peterson, T. A.; Todd, D. B.; and Edwards, J. E.: Supravalvular aortic stenosis. *J. Thorac. Cardiovasc. Surg.*, **50**:734, 1965.

Rastelli, G. B.; McGoon, D. C.; Ongley, P. A.; Mankin, H. T.; and Kirklin, J. W.: Surgical treatment of supravalvular aortic stenosis. Report of 16 cases and review of the literature. *J. Thorac. Cardiovasc. Surg.*, **51**:873, 1966.

Roberts, W. C.: Valvular, subvalvular, and supravalvular aortic stenosis: Morphologic features. In *Clinical Pathologic Correlations 2 Cardiovascular Clinics*, Vol. 5, No. 1., F. A. Davis Company, Philadelphia, 1973, p. 98.

Robicsek, F.; Sanger, P. W.; Dougherty, H. K.; and Saucer, P.; Surgical treatment of hypoplasia of the ascending aorta. *Vasc. Surg.*, **4**:1, 1970.

Rowe, R. D.: Stenosis of conducting arteries in infants and children. In *Birth Defects: Original Article Series*, **8**: (No. 5): 69, 1972.

Rowe, R. D.; Kelly, D. T.; McCue, C.; and Ottesen, O.: Unusual distribution of vascular damage as sequelae of idiopathic hypercalcemia and congenital rubella syndrome. In *Birth Defects: Original Article Series*, **10**: (No. 4), 361, 1974.

Seelig, M. S.: Vitamin D and cardiovascular, renal and brain damage in infancy and childhood. *Ann. N.Y. Acad. Sci.*, **147**:539, 1969.

Starr, A.; Dotter, C.; and Groswold, H.: Supravalvular aortic stenosis: Diagnosis and treatment. *J. Thorac Cardiovasc. Surg.*, **41**:134, 1961.

Underhill, W. L.; Tredway, J. B.; D'Angelo, G. J.; and Baay, J. E. W.: Familial supravalvular aortic stenosis. Comments on the mechanisms of angina pectoris. *Am. J. Cardiol.*, **27**:560, 1971.

Usher, B. W.; Goulden, D.; and Murgo, J. P.: Echocardiographic detection of supravalvular aortic stenosis. *Circulation*, **49**:1257, 1974.

Varghese, P. J.; Izukawa, T.; and Rowe, R. D.: Supravalvular aortic stenosis as part of rubella syndrome, with discussion of pathogenesis. *Br. Heart J.*, **31**:59, 1969.

Vazquez, A. M.; Zuberbuhler, J. R.; and Kenny, F. M.: Mitral insufficiency in association with the syndrome of idiopathic hypercalcemia of infancy. *J. Pediatr.*, **73**:907, 1968.

Vince, D. J.: The role of rubella in the etiology of supravalvular aortic stenosis. *Can. Med. Assoc. J.*, **103**:1157, 1970.

Weisz, D.; Hartmann, A. F., Jr.; and Waldon, C. S.: Results of surgery for congenital supravalvular aortic stenosis. *Am. J. Cardiol.*, **37**:73, 1976.

Williams, J. C. P.; Barratt-Boyes, B. G.; and Lowe, J. B.: Supravalvular aortic stenosis. *Circulation*, **24**:1311, 1961.

Wiltse, H. E.; Goldbloom, R. B.; Antia, A. U.; Ottesen, O. E.; Rowe, R. D.; and Cooke, R. E.: Infantile hypercalcemia syndrome in twins. *N. Engl. J. Med.*, **275**:1157, 1966.

38

Bicuspid Aortic Valve

John D. Keith

I N 1886 Osler presented evidence that the bicuspid aortic valve was a relatively common finding at autopsy, more frequent than other congenital heart defects. Earlier in the medical literature, Paget (1844) had called attention to the fact that it was liable to be the seat of infection or deteriorating change. In 1846, Lloyd recognized a bicuspid aortic valve in a baby dying early in life and the valve was apparently otherwise normal. The major contributions to our knowledge of the natural history of the bicuspid aortic valve have been in the 20- to 80-year age group. Lewis and Grant (1923) noted how frequently the aortic stenosis was associated with the bicuspid aortic valve. Campbell and Kauntz (1953) studied the prevalence of calcification in aortic stenosis, including the bicuspid anomaly.

For many years, aortic stenosis was considered to be the site of rheumatic infection, whether the valve was bicuspid or not. Roberts (1969) has clearly shown that rheumatic fever is rarely the cause of this pathology. This has led to more accurate assessment of the bicuspid aortic valve and its course through life, as well as the complications that it may initiate or develop with the passage of time.

In summary, the complications that may occur include a gradual thickening of the valve cusps over many years, leading in some cases to stenosis and/or calcification. Some valves become incompetent; many are the site of infective endocarditis. The bicuspid valve is characteristically associated with specific congenital heart malformations in many instances, such as coarctation of the aorta, ventricular septal defect, aortic regurgitation, or endocardial fibroelastosis.

Anatomy

Both Osler (1886) and Lewis and Grant (1923) presented detailed anatomic descriptions of this anomaly. More recently, Roberts (1970) examined the aortic valves in 85 cases in which the anatomy of the valve showed it to be bicuspid. The arrangement of the cusps and the presence or absence of raphe was

recognizable in about 59 instances. In 28 of the 59 patients, one cusp was located anteriorly and the other posteriorly. The commissures were thus positioned to right and left. In each of the 28 patients, both coronaries arose in front of the anterior cusp. A raphe occurred in 16 of the 28 and was always located in the anterior cusp and identified with the coronary arteries.

In 31 of the patients, the cusps were situated to the right and left with the commissures pointing anteriorly and posteriorly. With this anatomy the right coronary arose from behind the right cusp and the left coronary from behind the left cusp. A raphe was present in 14 of the 31 patients and was always positioned in the right sinus of Valsalva.

Raphes were observed in 30 of the 59 hearts, in which they could adequately be identified; however, Roberts suggests that they were more common than these figures indicate, since 10 of the 13 patients with normally functioning valves had raphes present. When heavy deposits of calcium existed, the raphe could not be dissected with clarity. The recognition of raphe is rarely difficult in infancy or childhood. However, the problem arises in the older age groups when aortic stenosis and marked valve distortion occur. In trying to decide whether there are three cusps, there may be a fusion of two of the three cusps, making a three-cusp valve indistinguishable from a bicuspid aortic valve with a raphe.

Osler in 1886 listed the characteristics of a congenitally bicuspid aortic valve as follows:

1. The raphe is located where normally the true commissure would be between the left and right anterior aortic valve cusps.

2. The length of the free margin of the cusp containing no raphe is slightly shorter (by an average of 12 percent) than the length of the margin of the cusp containing a raphe.

3. The free border of the raphe or "conjoint cusp" is straight or curled and free of nodular thickenings indicative of corpora arantii.

4. The border of an attachment of the raphe cusp as viewed from the ventricular aspect presents the contour either of a single semilunar cusp or of a

shallow groove suggestive of junction of two cusps. (5) The raphe may be located on the aortic wall alone or may extend onto the valve cusp for variable distances, but in either case it usually divides the sinus of Valsalva into equal-sized units.

Waller and coworkers (1973) have investigated the anatomy and histology of the bicuspid aortic valve and identified two dominant types: one is the classic type described above, with a low ridge or raphe along the aortic aspect of the attached cusp; in the other, which is also of congenital origin, a ridge protrudes from the aorta and appears as a tall raphe, the upper edge corresponding to the level of the aortic cusps. They refer to the attachment at the ridge end of the bicuspid valve to the aorta as a commissural mound. It may extend toward the center of the aorta lumen. At first glance the ridge has the appearance of a raphe, but Waller and associates (1973) have clearly demonstrated distinct differences. Such cases are included under the category of congenital bicuspid aortic valve since they function as a two-cusp valve even though they may have three sinus pockets.

Bacon and Matthews (1959) reviewed data on 48 specimens of bicuspid aortic valve. All of those over 50 years of age showed thickening of the valve cusps, and the majority also had evidence of calcification. Between the ages of 20 to 49 were five cases that showed thickening of the valve. Their series included two cases between 10 and 19, only one of which had thickening of the aortic valve cusps. However, the authors do record nodularity of the cusps in several examples of the earlier age groups, when they in fact did not record any true thickening.

At The Hospital for Sick Children in Toronto (see Figure 38–1), out of our 140 cases of bicuspid aortic valve, we had three in the age group between 10 and 20, all of whom showed some thickening of the valve. In the cases between five and ten a few showed very slight nodularity, but below five all of the valves appeared normal except for the bicuspid arrangement. Of course, in the presence of the congenital aortic stenosis thickening and narrowing of the valve occurred from birth. This latter group is considered separately.

Incidence as an Isolated Defect

The high incidence of bicuspid aortic valve has been recognized since 1886 when Osler reported that 1.2 percent of 800 routine autopsies revealed this anomaly. This figure excluded eight cases of infective endocarditis. Such exclusion appears legitimate since infective endocarditis was a common event at that time, and when it occurred, the patient usually died in the hospital after a lengthy illness, thus increasing the ratio in routine autopsies.

Roberts (1970) reports finding 13 aortic bicuspid valves in 1440 routine postmortems on adults (0.9 percent). All had thickened but normally functioning cusps. More recently Silver (1973) examined 1057 adult hearts at consecutive autopsies and found ten

with bicuspid aortic valve (1 percent). In addition there were three with infective endocarditis and two with associated congenital defects of the heart (coarctation of aorta).

Izukawa and Keith found seven bicuspid aortic valves as an isolated cardiac anomaly in 550 consecutive autopsies in infants and children without other cardiac defects, giving an incidence of 1.3 percent (see Table 38–1).

Table 38–1. INCIDENCE OF ISOLATED BICUSPID VALVES

	NUMBER OF AUTOPSIES	NUMBER OF BICUSPID AORTIC VALVES	PERCENT
Osler (1886)	800	10	1.2
Roberts (1970)	1440	13	0.9
Silver (1973)	1057	10	1.0
Izukawa and Keith (1973)	550	7	1.3

The significance of the high prevalence of this apparently benign anomaly can be better understood when it is realized that over a lifetime a variety of complications may be initiated by it. These include:

1. Progressive thickening of the cusps.
2. Bacterial endocarditis.
3. Aortic stenosis.
4. Calcification stenosis.
5. Aortic valve regurgitation.
6. With other congenital heart defects.

Almost all cases coming to autopsy in adult life present evidence of thickening of the aortic cusps. In childhood they are usually thin and filmy, as in the normal aortic tricuspid valve.

Edwards (1961) in an editorial reviewed the relationship of structure and function of the bicuspid aortic valve. He points out that the normal tricuspid aortic valve has sufficient length of tissue to allow it to open completely and close completely with each heartbeat.

The bicuspid aortic valve may have equal or unequal cusps, and Edwards (1961) stresses the fact that unless the leaflets were of extra length, the valve would be somewhat stenotic, since the cusps would not open as completely as the tricuspid variety. Since 13 percent of ventricular septal defects and over 50 percent of cases of isolated coarctation of the aorta have bicuspid aortic valve. If the valve interferes with the flow of blood, there should be either a gradient across it, or a murmur, or both. Since one rarely finds systolic murmur in the aortic area, with either ventricular septal defects or coarctation of the aorta, one can only conclude that the bicuspid aortic valve is not stenotic or obstructed in childhood but may

[handwritten margin note: 30% to 50% of coarc. have bicuspid A.V.]

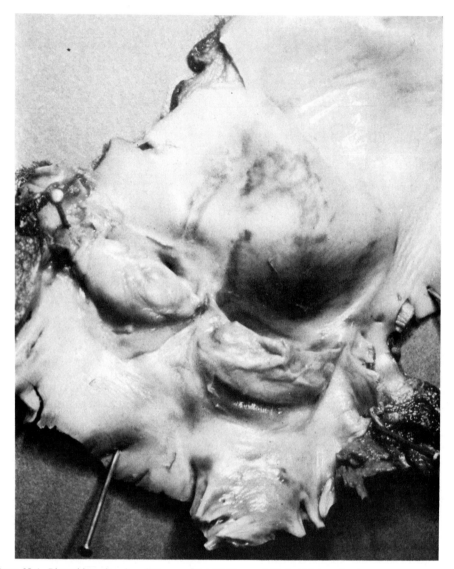

Figure 38-1. Bicuspid aortic valve of 15-year-old child. Note wrinkled, slightly redundant cusps. Lipid stain in the aorta is more prominent beyond one cusp.

become so gradually in adult life when it frequently thickens and may calcify.

Edwards points out that when there is a cusp of extra length it may prolapse, causing aortic regurgitation or, if there is not regurgitation, the somewhat collapsed aortic valve may be traumatized in such a way as to initiate thickening. Whether this is the cause or not, the valves do in fact thicken appreciably after the age of 20.

The valves of the veins throughout the body are bicuspid, but remain competent. The pulmonary valve may also be bicuspid, but there is no evidence that it becomes regurgitant unless there is pulmonary hypertension or a congenital anomaly apart from the bicuspid anatomy.

An uncomplicated bicuspid aortic valve is rarely regurgitant in childhood unless it is a developmentally redundant valve or there is a significant systemic hypertension present, as in coarctation of the aorta. When the coarctation is corrected (if it is done early in childhood), the diastolic murmur frequently disappears. That may not be related to the number of cusps.

Bicuspid Aortic Valve and Aortic Stenosis

Aortic stenosis is the fifth most common congenital heart defect in the pediatric age group. In the heart registry at The Toronto Hospital for Sick Children 720 cases of congenital valvar stenosis have been identified by clinical, hemodynamic, or postmortem studies. The incidence of a bicuspid valve among them is unknown since most of them are alive. Hohn (1968) found the valve to be bicuspid in 50 percent of 22 cases of congenital aortic stenosis. This is supported by the data of Roberts (1970), who also found a prevalence of 50 percent among 105 cases. The autopsy series at The Toronto Hospital for Sick Children includes 23 instances of valvar aortic stenosis. Four, or 17.4 percent, had a bicuspid aortic valve. Since most of the autopsies in this latter group were in infants in the first year of life, the data are not comparable with those from the two other groups mentioned above. A summary of the data at The Hospital for Sick Children appears in Table 38–2.

Table 38–2. AORTIC VALVE

	TOTAL	BICUSPID
Vascular ring	13	0
Aortic stenosis		
Supravalvular	0	
Subvalvular	12	1 (8.3%)
Valvular	23	4 (17.4%)
Complicated	49	11 (22.4%)
Total	84	16 (19%)

Roberts (1970) has pointed out that the natural history of the bicuspid aortic valve is unknown. However, data are slowly accumulating that may permit further insight into the prognosis of individuals with this anomaly. The available evidence suggests that little or no change in function occurs in the first 20 years of life, but slight irregular thickening may occur. After that some degree of thickening of the cusps is usually present, but the valve continues to be functionally normal. Most infants and young children have shown no thickening of the two valve cusps. However, in two cases in the teen-age group some slight thickening had appeared and lipid stains demonstrated a patchy increase in Sudan III uptake in areas related to the altered hemodynamics. This includes not only the valve but also the portion of the aorta adjacent to the valve.

Campbell (1968) has assembled information bearing on this problem and presented curves that estimate the age-related incidence of calcific stenosis in various types of aortic valvar disease (congenital, acquired, bicuspid, tricuspid). (See Figure 38–2.) The rate of calcification is much greater in the bicuspid than the normal tricuspid valve and occurs at an earlier age. This is particularly so when the underlying defect is congenital aortic stenosis. From 20 to 40 years of age most cases of congenital aortic stenosis acquire some calcareous deposits. These develop more slowly and at a later period (40 to 60 years) when the basic defect is a functionally normal bicuspid aortic valve. Campbell's data indicate that the normal tricuspid aortic valve may exhibit calcification, but when it occurs its appearance is at later milestones (50 to 75 years). He estimates that by age 60 eight times as many bicuspid valves are calcified as in the normal tricuspid variety. (See Figure 38–2.)

Bicuspid Aortic Valve and Infective Endocarditis

Thirty-seven years after Osler's observations Lewis and Grant (1923) reviewed the incidence of bacterial endocarditis among adults with bicuspid aortic

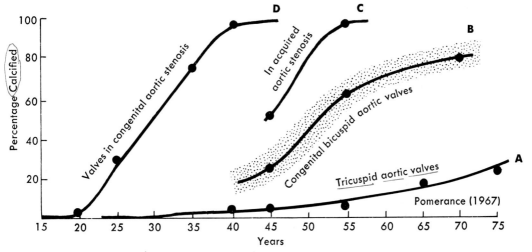

Figure 38-2. Calcific aortic stenosis and congenital bicuspid aortic valves, incidence of calcification with increasing age. *A.* In normal aortic valve with three cusps. (Based on 865 cases of Pomerance, 1967.) *B.* In congenital bicuspid aortic valves the shaded area defines the probable limits of accuracy. *C.* In the aortic valves of acquired aortic stenosis. (*B* and *C* are based mainly on Wauchope, 1928, and Bacon and Mathews, 1959.) *D.* In the valves of congenital aortic stenosis. (Based mainly on Campbell, 1968, and Baker and Somerville, 1964.) (Reproduced from Campbell, M.: Calcific aortic stenosis and congenital bicuspid aortic valves. *Br. Heart J.,* **30**: 606, 1968.)

Table 38–3. BICUSPID AORTIC VALVE, 85 CASES*

	NUMBER	AGE	INFECTIVE ENDOCARDITIS
Aortic stenosis	61	16–79 (49)	5
Aortic regurgitation (pure)	11	15–55 (31)	8
Functionally normal valve	13	23–59 (95)	0
	72% Male	28% Female	

* Data from Roberts (1970).

valves. They considered 23 percent an underestimate of this association. Wauchope (1928) found infective endocarditis in approximately 13 percent of 52 cases. More recently Roberts (1970) reported 85 cases of bicuspid aortic valves, 15 percent having had infective endocarditis; all of the latter had evidence of aortic valve disease, either stenosis or regurgitation. Roberts's findings are summarized in Table 38–3.

Silver (1973) found three cases of infective endocarditis among 13 bicuspid valves. These were encountered in 1057 autopsies over a three-year period. Thus there is only one case of infective endocarditis on a bicuspid aortic valve coming to autopsy per year in a hospital (Toronto General Hospital) of 1200 beds serving a population of approximately 1,000,000. Since there is good evidence that 1 in 100 in the population has a bicuspid aortic valve, there should be 10,000 people with this anomaly in each million people. Obviously only a small fraction of them end up with infective endocarditis. (The majority could be cured medically.)

The association with coarctation of the aorta accounts for 45 percent of all the bicuspid aortic valves in our autopsy series among 1785 congenital heart defects. The ventricular septal defect is second with 30 percent; aortic stenosis is third with 11 percent; endocardial fibroelastosis is fourth with 10 percent; endocardial cushion defects fifth with 8 percent. Thus, these five defects account for 74 percent of the total (Table 38–4).

There are a variety of other congenital heart defects associated with a bicuspid aortic valve but at an incidence that is at or only slightly above that of

normal children. For example, in 125 children with tetralogy of Fallot only one had a bicuspid aortic valve, an incidence of 0.8 percent. In Toronto General Hospital the incidence was slightly higher with 7 out of 304 cases, or 2.3 percent.

It is interesting to speculate on the etiologic relationship between bicuspid aortic valve and various congenital heart defects. When there is a major flow shunted through the aortic valve, as in tetralogy of Fallot, it is associated with a low or normal incidence of bicuspid aortic valve (0.8 percent). Hutchins (1972) suggests that coarctation of the aorta is the result of a slightly obstructed aortic valve, which leads to an increased ductal flow in the fetus and thus to the development at the junction of the ductus and aorta of a branch site that later becomes a coarcted aorta. The anatomy of the coarctation does certainly suggest this, but the etiologic relation proposed by Hutchins does not appear to be borne out by our findings since such a defect as total anomalous pulmonary vein drainage, which has a low aortic flow, has not been associated with a bicuspid aortic valve in any of our 86 cases (Table 38–5).

Table 38–5. COARCTATION OF AORTA AND BICUSPID AORTIC VALVE, HOSPITAL FOR SICK CHILDREN AUTOPSY DATA

COARCTATION OF AORTA	TOTAL	BICUSPID AORTIC VALVE
Isolated	13	7 (54%)
With PDA	56	23 (41%)
With VSD	16	4 (25%)
With VSD and PDA	46	14 (30.5%)
With EFE	9	3 (33.3%)
With EFE and PDA	3	1 (14.9%)
Totals	217	63 (29%)

Bicuspid Aortic Valve and Dissecting Aneurysm

Gore (1953) drew attention to the fact that dissecting aneurysms that cause death under the age of 40 frequently had other associated congenital

Table 38–4. BICUSPID AORTIC VALVE IN ASSOCIATION WITH OTHER CONGENITAL HEART DEFECTS, HOSPITAL FOR SICK CHILDREN, AUTOPSY DATA

DEFECTS	TOTAL NO.	BICUSPID AORTIC VALVE	PERCENT
Coarctation of aorta	217	63	29.0
Inter. aortic arch	22	6	27.2
Aortic stenosis	84	16	19.0
Primary endocard. fibroelastosis	50	9	18.0
VSD (isolated)	151	20	13.3
Endocard. cush. defect	99	8	8.1

anomalies present. Nine of thirty-two cases had a bicuspid aortic valve. This association occurred whether the aneurysm was due to an elastic type of medial degeneration or a muscle type (only one of the nine cases with bicuspid valve had coarctation of the aorta).

The Perinatal Mortality Survey (1958) revealed 5 of 22 cases of anencephaly as having a bicuspid aortic valve.

Bicuspid Aortic Valve and Coarctation of the Aorta and Aortic Stenosis

Since the bicuspid aortic valve occurs in approximately a third of the cases of coarctation of the aorta, and aortic valvar stenosis is a common development in adult life when bicuspid aortic valve is present, one would expect an increase in the association of these three abnormalities with the passage of time.

Smith and Matthews (1955) assembled 27 cases in which coarctation and aortic stenosis coexisted; 20 of the 27 had aortic bicuspid valves, an incidence of 74 percent. This is twice the prevalence of bicuspid aortic valve ordinarily found in coarctation of the aorta.

Fowler (1970), at The Hospital for Sick Children, Toronto, in analyzing 700 cases of aortic valvar stenosis found 31 had a combination of coarctation of the aorta and aortic stenosis. However, these were children who were born with congenital aortic stenosis and not a lesion that developed at a later age.

Now that so many cases of coarctation of the aorta have been successfully resected, it is of increasing significance to know whether or not there is a progressive development of thickening stenosis or calcification of the aortic valve in the third, fourth, or fifth decade of life. Since it is not feasible to do aortic angiograms on all of these cases, the diagnosis or possibility of aortic valve or stenosis should be considered if a murmur is present to the right of the sternum and is gradually increasing in intensity over the years.

Endocardial fibroelastosis is well recognized as a secondary phenomenon of several congenital heart defects, particularly severe aortic stenosis in early life, aortic atresia or mitral atresia, coarctation of the aorta, and congenital mitral regurgitation.

As a primary phenomenon it has been considered by some as a myocardopathy or a myocarditis. This is discussed elsewhere (see Chapter 52). However, the finding of an incidence of 18 percent of aortic bicuspid valves in 50 primary cases contributes additional evidence that endocardial fibroelastosis is a congenital abnormality of the heart (see Table 38–6).

Ventricular Septal Defect

In the uncomplicated cases of ventricular septal defect coming to autopsy, 13.3 percent of 151 had a

Table 38–6.
ENDOCARDIAL FIBROELASTOSIS AND BICUSPID AORTIC VALVE CONTRASTED WITH VENTRICULAR SEPTAL DEFECT, HOSPITAL FOR SICK CHILDREN AUTOPSY DATA

	TOTAL	AORTIC VALVE BICUSPID
Endocardial fibroelastosis		
Primary	50	9 (18.0%)
Secondary	76	5 (6.6%)
Totals	126	14 (11.1%)
Ventricular septal defect		
Uncomplicated	151	20 (13.3%)
Complicated	290	22 (7.6%)
Totals	441	42 (9.5%)

bicuspid aortic valve. If such an incidence is present in the usual patient seen in office practice with classic signs of the septal opening, it suggests that a number may eventually develop one or more of the complications that revolve around a bicuspid aortic valve.

Clinical Identifications

The bicuspid aortic valve can now be identified during life in the majority of patients with this anomaly by echocardiography. Edler and colleagues (1961) originally obtained ultrasonic signals from the aortic valve cusps. Gramiak and Shah (1968) first described an adequate method of studying the aortic root by echocardiography and were able to identify the anatomic components. Nanda and coworkers (1974) have used the method to study 21 patients with bicuspid aortic valve proved either at operation or by angiocardiography. Their findings were compared with cases of known tricuspid aortic valves. In the latter, when the valve was in the closed position the echo was in the center of the aortic lumen. In contrast, the valve cusps in the bicuspid group in diastole were eccentric. An index of one-half of the aortic lumen over the minimum distance of the diastolic cusp echo to the aortic wall was 1 to 1.25 with tricuspid valve, while the range was 1.5 to 5.6 in the presence of a bicuspid aortic valve. This suggests that the bicuspid aortic valve has one cusp smaller than the other, which is often the case. However, even when the cusps appear to be equal, shifting the echo recorder slightly produced an eccentric tracing, which does not occur with a similar maneuver in the presence of a tricuspid valve. Such an index apparently is not significantly affected by valvotomy in aortic stenosis.

A bicuspid aortic valve is characteristically redundant and thus folds and unfolds in diastole and systole, which, as pointed out by Nanda (1974), may account for beat-to-beat variation in the ultrasonic beam.

Radford and associates (1976) recorded echocardiograms in 89 patients whose aortic valves had been adequately defined by selective angiography or assessed surgically or at autopsy. The eccentricity index (EI) referred to above was measured at the onset of diastole. There were 31 patients with known bicuspid aortic valves. Twenty-three, or 75 percent of the 31, had an abnormal EI of 1.3 or greater. All of the patients with nonobstructed tricuspid aortic valves had central echoes. Multilayered diastolic echoes were frequently found in patients with bicuspid aortic valves but were also seen in two patients with known tricuspid aortic valves.

Of the 21 patients with a ventricular septal defect only one had a definite bicuspid aortic valve, but six had an abnormal eccentricity index. This positive sign appeared to be related to the presence of a high membraneous ventricular septal defect or at times associated with aortic valve prolapse. Radford and coworkers thus demonstrated that in the absence of a ventricular septal defect an eccentricity index of 1.3 or greater is good evidence of a bicuspid aortic valve. However, they also showed that a bicuspid valve may be present when the EI is within normal limits.

One of the most useful studies recently presented is that of Leatham and colleagues (1975) from St. George's Hospital, London, England. They reported 45 cases followed for 5 to 20 years. None had aortic stenosis initially. They were suspected and identified by physical signs, which were confirmed ultimately at surgery, autopsy, or echocardiography. The most characteristic clinical finding was an ejection sound, which occurred 0.1 to 0.16 second after the Q wave of the electrocardiogram. This was recognized by a stethoscope or a sound recording. This ejection sound followed the mitral valve closure by 0.04 to 0.1 second and therefore was considered to be associated with opening of the aortic valve (first reported by Wood, 1956).

The echocardiogram showed a diastolic closure line that was eccentric and/or associated with multiple echoes. Leatham and associates point out that when the transducer was aligned with the apex there was a dome aortic valve appearance that appeared and disappeared with diastole and systole.

Over the period of prolonged follow-up there were no deaths related to the aortic valve, although 8 percent died of unrelated causes. Four percent developed definite aortic stenosis, 8 percent had mild stenosis, 6 percent had mild aortic regurgitation, 8 percent became the site of bacterial endocarditis but recovered with treatment, and 62 percent were unchanged over the long period.

Thus if one includes the 8 percent with mild stenosis and the 6 percent with mild aortic regurgitation with the 62 percent unchanged, one may reach the conclusion that 76 percent have continued to lead a functionally normal life over this period of 5 to 25 years. Since echocardiography has become a routine tool in the investigation of minimal or questionable cardiac sounds or murmurs, a large number of cases of bicuspid aortic valves are being identified in healthy individuals. It may prove that the vast majority of these, i.e., more than 77 percent will continue to live functionally normal lives.

The majority of children with a bicuspid aortic valve have not developed an audible ejection click in the pediatric age group. A faint systolic murmur in the aortic area with or without a widely split first sound may make one suspect the diagnosis.

In summary, the bicuspid aortic valve occurs in approximately 1 percent of the population. In Canada and the United States on the basis of known incidence figures there should be 2½ million people with this defect. The prevalence of significant complications related to this underlying anomaly must be exceedingly low since only a small percentage of the total 2¼ million end up in the autopsy room or on the operating table. The majority appear to have a functionally normal valve although it is usually thickened by the time adult life is reached.

Maron and coworkers (1973) reviewed 171 patients who had coarctation of the aorta and had been followed for an average of 20 years to age 40. About 25 percent had signs of aortic valve disease, though there were documented cases of bacterial endocarditis. One would suspect that approximately 50 percent of this group had a bicuspid aortic valve associated with the coarctation.

REFERENCES

Bacon, A. P. C., and Matthews, M. B.: Congenital bicuspid aortic valves and the etiology of isolated valvular stenosis. Q. J. Med., 28:545, 1959.
Baker, C., and Somerville, J.: Results of surgical treatment of aortic stenosis. Br. Med. J., 1:197, 1964.
Campbell, M., and Kauntz, R.: Congenital aortic valvular stenosis. Br. Heart J., 15:179, 1953.
Campbell, M.: The natural history of congenital aortic stenosis. Br. Heart J., 30:514, 1968.
Campbell, M.: Calcific aortic stenosis and congenital bicuspid aortic valves. Br. Heart J., 30:606, 1968.
Edler, I.; Gustafson, A.; Karlefors, T.; Christensson, B.: Mitral and aortic valve movement recorded by an ultrasonic echo method. An experimental study. Acta. Med. Scand., 170:(Suppl. 370), 67, 1961.
Edwards, J. E.: The congenital bicuspid aortic valve. Circulation, 23:485, 1961.
Fowler, R. S.: Sudden Death in Aortic Stenosis in Childhood. Presented at the 6th World Congress of Cardiology, London, Sept., 1970.
Gore, I.: Dissecting aneurysms of the aorta in persons under forty years of age. Arch. Pathol. 55:1, 1953.
Gramiak, R., and Shah, P. M.: Echocardiography of the aortic root. Invest. Radiol., 3:356, 1968.
Grant, R. T.; Wood, J. E.; and Jones, T. D.: Heart valve irregularities in relation to subacute bacterial endocarditis. Heart, 14:247, 1928.
Hohn, A. R.; Von Praagh, S.; Moore, A. A. D.: Vlad, P.; and Lambert, E. C.: Aortic stenosis. Circulation, 32:4, 1965.
Hohn, A. R.; Tingelstad, J. B.; Israel, R.; et al.: Intrapulmonary shunts in congestive heart disease. Am. J. Dis. Child., 115:202, 1968.
Hutchins, G. M.: Coarctation of the aorta as a branch-point of the ductus arteriosus. Am. J. Pathol., 63:203, 1971.
Izukawa, T., and Keith, J. D.: Unpublished observations, 1973.
Leatham, A.; Mills, P.; Leech, G.; and Davies, M.: Diagnosis and prognosis of bicuspid non-stenotic aortic valve. Br. Heart J., 37:781, 1975 (Abstr.).
Lewis, D. S.; Beattie, W. W.; and Abbott, M. E.: Differential study of case of pulmonary stenosis of inflammatory origin. Am. J. Med. Sci., 165:636, 1923.

Lewis, T., and Grant, R. T.: Observations relating to subacute infective endocarditis, notes on normal structure of aortic valve, bicuspid aortic valves of congenital origin; bicuspid aortic valves in subacute infective endocardits. *Heart*, **10**:20, 1923,

Lloyd: Aortic valvular disease. *Trans. Pathol. Soc. Lond.*, **1**:40, 1846–1848.

Maron, B. J.; Humphries, J. O'N.; Rowe, R. D.; and Mellits, E. D.: Prognosis of surgically corrected coarctation of the aorta. A 20-year postoperative appraisal. *Circulation*, **47**:119, 1973.

Mithcell, S. C.; Korones, S. B.; and Berendes, H. W.: Congenital heart disease in 56, 109 births. *Circulation*, **43**:323, 1971.

Nanda, N. C.; Gramiak, R.; Manning, J.; Mahoney, E. B.; Lipchik, E. O.; and DeWeese, J. A.: Echocardiographic recognition of the congenital bicuspid aortic valve. *Circulation*, **49**:370, 1974.

Osler, W.: The bicuspid condition of the aortic valves. *Trans. Assoc. Am. Physicians*, **2**:185, 1886.

Paget, J.: On Obstructions of the branches of the pulmonary artery. *Trans. Roy. Med. Chir. Soc., London*, **27**:162, 1844.

Peacock, T. B.: *On Malformations of the Human Heart*, 2nd ed. J. Churchill & Sons, London, 1866.

Pomerance, A.: Personal communication, 1967. Cited in Campbell, M., 1968.

Radford, D. J.; Bloom, K. R.; Izukawa, T.; Moës, C. A. F.; and Rowe, R. D.: Echocardiographic assessment of bicuspid aortic valves. Angiographic and pathological correlates. *Circulation*, **53**:80, 1976.

Roberts, W. C., and Elliott, L. P.: Lesions complicating a congenitally bicuspid aortic valve. Anatomic and radiographic features. *Radiol. Clin. North Am.*, **6**:409, 1968.

Roberts, W. C.: Anomalous left ventricular band. An unemphasized cause of a precordial musical murmur. *Am. J. Cardiol.*, **23**:735, 1969.

Roberts, W. C.; Friesinger, C. C.; Cohen, L. S.; et al.: Acquired pulmonic atresia. Total obstruction of right ventricular outflow after systemic to pulmonary arterial anastomoses for cyanotic congenital cardiac disease. *Am. J. Cardiol.*, **24**:335, 1969.

Roberts, W. C.: Anatomically isolated aortic valvular disease: The case against its being of rheumatic etiology. *Am. J. Med.*, **49**:151, 1970.

Roberts, W. C.: The congenital bicuspid aortic valve: A study of 85 autopsy patients. *Am. J. Cardiol.*, **26**:72, 1970.

Roberts, W. C.: The structure of the aortic valve in clinically isolated aortic stenosis. An autopsy study of 162 patients over 15 years of age. *Circulation*, **42**:91, 1970.

Rose, V.: Live births, City of Toronto. Personal communication, 1971.

Silver, M.: Bicuspid aortic valve as an isolated defect. Personal communication, 1973.

Smith, D. E., and Matthews, B.: Aortic valvular stenosis with coarctation of the aorta. With special reference to the development of aortic stenosis upon congenital bicuspid valve. *Br. Heart J.*, **17**:198, 1955.

Waller, B. F., et al.: Bicuspid aortic valve. Comparison of congenital and acquired types. *Circulation*, **48**:1140, 1973.

Wauchope, G. M.: The clinical importance of variations in the number of cusps forming the aortic and pulmonary valves. *Q. J. Med.*, **21**:383, 1928.

Wood, P.: *Disease of the Heart and Circulation*. Eyre and Spotiswood, London, 1956.

CHAPTER

39

Coarctation of the Aorta

John D. Keith

I N THE year 1760, Morgagni performed a postmortem on a monk and drew attention to a constriction of the aorta a short distance from the heart. Later, many cases were reported in the literature during the nineteenth century. In 1903, Bonnet divided coarctation of the aorta into two main groups, infantile and adult. In the former the coarctation lies above the ductus arteriosus and may be localized or diffuse narrowing; in the latter the constriction is just below the entrance of the ductus and is commonly localized. In general, this is a useful classification, but occasionally it may be difficult to decide into which group a particular case fits since anatomically the coarctation may stride the entrance of the ductus arteriosus. When the ductus arteriosus is attached above the constriction, it is referred to as a *postductal coarctation*; when it enters below the constriction, it is referred to as a *preductal coarctation*. This requires further division depending on whether the ductus is open or closed (see Figure 39–1).

Prevalence

The frequency of coarctation of the aorta at postmortem is indicated by a review of eight references * in the literature. It occurred 46 times in 70,850 autopsies, which gives an incidence of 1 in 1540. Sloan and Cooley (1953) found that it occurred once in every 500 autopsies. It has not been discovered clinically with this frequency. In the Toronto Cardiac Registry during 1969 it occurred in 1 of every 4000 children between the ages of birth and 15 years and was eighth in order of frequency among congenital heart defects. Perlman (1944) found it occurred once in every 10,000 army recruits. Approximately 5 percent of the cases of congenital heart disease at The Hospital for Sick Children, Toronto, have coarctation of the aorta. (See Figure 1–3, page 4.)

Other Anomalies Occurring with Coarctation

Since the major number of deaths from coarctation of the aorta occur in the first year of life, the incidence of the major associated anomalies is most clearly shown when related to that age group (see Table

---

* Lochte, Fawcette, Jaffe and Sternberg, Meixner, Hansteen, Ophuls—cited by Blackford (1928) and Evans (1933).

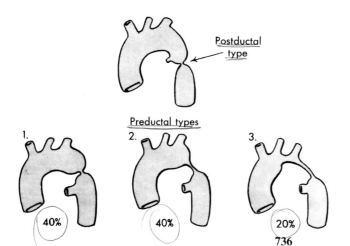

Figure 39-1. Coarctation of the aorta.

39–1.　A patent ductus arteriosus is the most commonly associated defect, occurring in 64 percent of cases presenting in the first year of life. Besides the infants studied at autopsy, this figure includes those in whom the patent ductus was recognized only at operation or by angiocardiogram. A clinically discernible continuous murmur was uncommon in this age group. If only the postmortem cases are considered, the incidence of the patent ductus rises to 95 percent. This is true because the majority of deaths were in the first two months of life. Ventricular septal defect is found in 32 percent, transposition of the great vessels in 10 percent, and atrial septal defect in 6.5 percent. Thus, isolated coarctation of the aorta is found in only 18 percent of infants presenting with signs or symptoms in the first year of life (Glass et al., 1960; Malm and Blumenthal, 1963; Tawes and associates, 1969; Sinha and associates, 1969; Becker et al., 1970). Apart from bicuspid aortic valve which is commonly associated, frank aortic valve disease is often expressed in patients after coarctectomy (Jacobson et al., 1953; Maron et al., 1973; Simon and Zloto, 1974). Varying degrees of mitral valve disease may be almost as frequent (Rosenquist, 1974), but frank mitral stenosis or regurgitation is probably together not apparent in more than 10 percent (Easthope et al., 1969; Freed et al., 1974; Simon and Zloto, 1974). The place of echocardiography in the diagnosis of these additional anomalies is now well appreciated (Scovil et al., 1976).

Other less commonly associated anomalies include hypoplasia of the aortic valve, partial anomalous pulmonary vein drainage into the right atrium, anomalous right subclavian artery above and below the coarcted segment, arteriovenous fistulae of the internal mammary artery, left superior vena cava into the coronary sinus, and complete heart block.

Apart from transposition of the great vessels, the cyanotic group of congenital heart anomalies is rarely found with coarctation of the aorta. The association with endocardial fibroelastosis has been reported a number of times; 4 percent of the patients at The Hospital for Sick Children in the pediatric age group with coarctation of the aorta also had endocardial fibroelastosis.

Campbell and Polani (1961) found Turner's syndrome in 2 percent of their series of 151 adults and children. Other congenital anomalies such as hypospadias, club foot, and mental and ocular defects appeared to occur sporadically. They conclude that there is a higher incidence of other major cardiac malformation than one would expect by chance (8 percent). A similar percentage was recorded by Lang and Nadas (1956).

A most difficult group of associated diseases is found in the first week or two of life and is composed of such conditions as prematurity, respiratory distress syndrome, sepsis, atelectasis, tracheoesophageal fistula, pneumonia, and heart failure. Their presence often misleads one from recognizing

Table 39–1. COARCTATION OF AORTA UNDER ONE YEAR (SEEN FIRST UNDER ONE YEAR), TOTAL 358

SITE	COARC. ISOLATED*†	PDA COARC.	PDA VSD COARC.	PDA ASD COARC.	TGV PDA VSD COARC.	VSD COARC.	PDA VSD ASD COARC.	TGV PDA VSD ASD COARC.	TGV VSD ASD COARC.	TGV VSD COARC.
Preductal	12(3)	65(28)	48(16)	11(0)	9(2)	0(0)	6(0)	4(2)	2(0)	2
Postductal	73(65)	20(13)	0(2)	4(0)	4(2)	7(4)	0(0)	0(1)	0(0)	1
Not defined	22(19)	1(0)	0(2)	0(0)	2(1)	0(5)	0(0)	1(0)	0(3)	2
Juxtaductal	(1)									
Total	108(88)	86(41)	52(20)	15(0)	15(5)	12(9)	6(0)	6(3)	5(3)	5

SITE	TGV COARC.	VSD ASD COARC.	ASD COARC.	COMMON AV CANAL PDA COARC.	SINGLE ATRIUM PDA COARC.	COMMON AV CANAL PUL. STEN. COARC.	TGV PDA ASD COARC.	TGV ASD COARC.	MISC.
Preductal	1	4(0)	0(1)	2	1	1	1(0)	0	10‡
Postductal	0	0(0)	1(0)	0	0	0	0(0)	0	2‡
Not defined	3	0(0)	0(0)	0	0	0	0(0)	1	20§
Juxtaductal									
Total	4	4(0)	2(1)	2	1	1	1(0)	1	32

* Survival is indicated by parentheses.
† Coarc. = coarctation; PDA = patent ductus arteriosus; VSD = ventricular septal defect; ASD = atrial septal defect; TGV = transposition of the great vessels.
‡ Patency of ductus not defined at necropsy.
§ All died but no necropsy was obtained and investigations were incomplete.

the associated diagnosis of coarctation of the aorta. The noncardiac condition is likely to be the prime cause of death in this age group. Malm and Blumenthal (1963) found one or more of these diseases in 25 percent of cases of coarctation dying in the first week of life.

Etiology

At one time the skodaic hypothesis was favored as an explanation of the etiology of coarctation of the aorta. In this view the coarctation is due to an overgrowth of the tissue that normally closes the ductus. For several reasons, which have been well reviewed by Edwards and coworkers (1948), this view appears untenable in the majority of cases. Although tissue similar to that present in the ductus arteriosus is found in the coarcted segment, the narrowing, whether localized or diffuse, is considered a developmental defect, as in other forms of congenital heart disease (Balis et al., 1966). However, this subject has been investigated extensively by Gilman (1966) with experimental work in various animals and demonstrated that there can be a localized reactive constriction of the aorta in this area following birth. He further postulates that in humans such constriction may be subsequently followed by hyperplasia and lead to permanent narrowing.

More recently, Hutchins (1971) initiated the concept that the position of the coarcted segment opposite the aortic end of the ductus arteriosus suggests it arises as a branch point of that channel. In this view the patient with coarctation should have a ductal blood flow which exceeds aortic flow during early development. The idea has since been expanded by Rudolph and associates (1972).

Talner and Berman (1975) point out that ductal constriction begins at the pulmonary artery end and initially this minimizes the effect of the Porlecier aortic shelf (or coarctation) and permits sufficient flow to transmit pressure to femoral pulsations. During the first or second week after birth when the aortic end of the ductus completes its constriction, the aortic flow and pressure are reduced and the femoral pulses become diminished or absent. It is therefore suggested that femoral pulses be rechecked one and two weeks after birth if any suspicion of coarctation of the aorta exists, particularly if there is evidence of heart failure.

Infectious agents such as German measles have not appeared to play any part in the development of a coarcted aorta. Hereditary factors are nonexistent or minimal; maternal age and birth order have no significance. Campbell and Polani (1961) have reviewed the influence of these and related factors.

Sex Incidence

Most reports in the literature indicate that coarctation is more prevalent in males than females.

Campbell and Polani (1961) put the ratio at two to one.

Familial Occurrence

The familial occurrence of coarctation is exceedingly rare. Klemola (1939) reported two cases in the same family—a father and a son. Taylor and Pollock (1953) reported three instances in one family—a mother, a son, and a daughter.

Pathology

The constriction may be above or below the insertion of the ductus arteriosus or precisely at the ductus. One can divide them into two functional groups, postductal and preductal.

Postductal Type—Adult. In the postductal type, or adult type, of coarctation there is a localized constriction, almost amounting to a diaphragm, with the aorta reduced in size rather abruptly at the site of the narrowing, and below the constriction the aorta broadens out again rapidly to a diameter that is usually greater than the aorta above the constriction. The constriction itself has an internal diameter varying between 0.5 and 2 mm as a rule, but occasionally there is no opening at all. Rarely there is complete interruption or absence of the aortic arch (see Figure 39–1).

Edwards and associates (1948) pointed out that histologically the site of the coarctation is characterized by a localized medial thickening on which is superimposed new intimal tissue. They also demonstrated the presence of a jet lesion on the wall of the aorta just distal to the coarctation. In the postductal type, the left ventricle is usually hypertrophied at postmortem. An associated finding of interest is the presence of a bicuspid aortic valve in approximately 50 percent of the uncomplicated cases. In our present investigations we reviewed the postmortem findings in the group of preductal coarctation (see Table 39–1) and found 25 percent of this group had a bicuspid aortic valve.

In adults, patients with coarctation of the aorta die of rupture of the aorta, intracranial hemorrhage, heart failure, subacute bacterial endocarditis, and dissecting aneurysms. However, in infancy and childhood nearly all the deaths that occur are due to either heart failure or some associated cardiac anomaly.

Preductal Type—Infantile. In the preductal, or infantile, type where coarctation of the aorta is above the entrance of the ductus arteriosus, the ductus is usually found to be patent in early life. Clagett and coworkers (1954) found a closed ductus inserted below the coarctation in 16 percent of cases coming to operation in adult life. The ductus fills from whichever vessel has the higher pressure, or when the pressures are similar, the filling is toward the circulation with the lower resistance. The pressure may be higher in the aorta than the pulmonary artery. Since the pressure and the peripheral resistance via the descending aorta are usually higher than those in the pulmonary artery, one may usually expect the flow of blood to be from the aorta to the pulmonary artery. The authors have had an opportunity to study this both by aortogram and venous angiogram as well as by cardiac catheterization (see Figure 39–11, page 750). In this illustration there is contrast medium passing from the aorta through the coarctation into the descending aorta and then following the pulmonary artery and its branches; thus the flow is toward the lung fields. This is the most common pattern encountered. In many instances, however, the flow to the lung fields is sufficient to raise the pulmonary pressure to systemic levels, and then the direction of the flow will depend on the differential between pulmonary and peripheral systemic vascular resistance. At The Hospital for Sick Children cardiac catheterization was carried out on many cases of a preductal infantile type, the descending aorta being entered with the catheter. In all but one instance the peripheral resistance from the systemic circulation was greater than that of the pulmonary. This usually results in bidirectional flow, into the descending aorta from the right ventricle in the early part of each systole and in the latter part predominantly toward the lung fields. Even when there is absence of the aortic isthmus, and the descending aorta must clearly depend on the right ventricle to perfuse it, it was found in one such case studied that the peripheral resistance was higher below the coarctation than in the pulmonary vascular tree. Thus, while the right ventricle pumped into both descending aorta and pulmonary artery, the chief flow was through the lung fields.

There were three general types of preductal coarctation (Figure 39–1):

1. A localized constriction just above the entrance of the ductus. This type occurred in 40 percent of cases.

2. A diffuse narrowing extending the length of the isthmus from the entrance of the ductus up to the left subclavian artery. This type occurred in 40 percent of cases.

3. A narrowing that includes not only the isthmus but extends further into the aortic arch. Twenty percent of our cases fell into this group.

On review of the postmortem findings, it was found that there was considerable difference in the location and extent of the narrowing and that this varied with the associated defects. The presence of associated major defects was related in some degree to the type of coarctation. In group 1 there were only 16 percent with major associated anomalies. In group 2 there were 28 percent with other major defects. In group 3, on the other hand, there were 80 percent with major defects. Thus, if the coarctation is a localized one, further cardiac anomalies are least common. If the coarcted segment is a long one, associated anomalies such as transposition of the great vessels, atrio-ventricularis communis, ventricular septal defect, and common ventricle are much more commonly found. With complete interruption of the aortic arch 80 percent were found to have ventricular septal defect (Everts-Suarez and Carson, 1959).

Collateral Circulation.   In 1837, Michel first drew attention to collaterals in coarctation of the aorta and pointed out that they communicated between the arteries of the upper part of the body above the coarctation and those below. The dilated and tortuous collateral vessels are chiefly from the subclavian artery and its branches. The intercostals, the internal mammaries, the muscular phrenic, the superior epigastric, the transverse cervical, the scapular group, and the lateral thoracic all participate in channeling a more adequate blood flow to the lower part of the body. The anterior spinal artery also participates in this. The visible evidence of these dilated tortuous collateral vessels is present in some x-rays showing notching of the ribs due to the continuous pressure of the intercostals against the posterior and inferior aspects of the rib. Superficially, the scapular vessels may sometimes be seen winding in a sinuous fashion beneath the skin of the back and pulsating visibly. In some instances of coarctation of the aorta, dilated tortuous collaterals may be demonstrated by angiocardiography in the first few weeks or months of life.

In the past it was considered probable that, in the preductal type with the ductus entering the descending aorta below the coarctation, the baby did not have an opportunity to develop collaterals before the birth and thus after birth faced a gradual closing of the ductus, leading to early failure and death. The evidence is rather against this hypothesis for the following reasons:

1. Collaterals can be demonstrated by angiocardiography in most infants with preductal coarctation, and deaths are due to the association with other defects rather than due to the coarctation alone. It should also be remembered that survival in preductal coarctation is not uncommon (Clagett et al., 1954).

2. Many deaths occur in infants whose ducti have remained widely patent, and 80 percent of our cases with heart failure in the first year of life had a patent ductus. This is especially true for the preductal type.

3. The collateral circulation can be demonstrated to occur in cases of the preductal type with a widely open ductus (the ductus was patent in 95 percent of those who died). Collaterals were demonstrated by angiocardiography in early weeks of life.

4. Collateral circulation is always readily available in infancy; for example, one can cut the subclavian artery or the femoral with impunity and an excellent collateral circulation opens up promptly. Page (1940) in his experiments on coarctation in dogs was unable to maintain hypertension above the artificial constriction because of the promptly developing collaterals.

5. Hypertension in the preductal type with the ductus opening below the coarctation appears to be of approximately the same order as in other forms of coarctation (see Figure 39–5, page 745). The blood

pressure in the legs in the postductal coarctation is essentially the same as in the other group. This was demonstrated in five of our cases and in two of Calodney and Carson's (1950) where blood pressure readings in the leg were available. If the pressure is elevated above the constriction before birth, one might expect collaterals to open up in both the preductal and postductal types.

6. The higher mortality in the preductal type appears to be related to the more frequent presence of associated defects, whether they be of the cyanotic type or the noncyanotic variety, such as patent ductus arteriosus.

The difference in mortality between the preductal and postductal group can be explained on the basis of the presence of associated heart anomalies. Forty percent of the preductal type have significant defects apart from the patent ductus; 14 percent of the postductal type have associated defects (usually ventricular septal defects). Thus the difference in mortality of 30 percent can be explained on this basis.

Cause of Hypertension. There are two opposing views concerning the cause of hypertension in coarctation of the aorta: renal hypothesis and mechanical hypothesis.

Goldblatt and coworkers (1939) showed that a hypertension occurred in 24 hours after producing artificial constriction of the aorta just above the renal arteries in a dog. He thus demonstrated a renal factor operating to produce a delayed hypertension when the blood supply to the kidney was impaired. The application of this hypothesis to the production of hypertension in coarctation of the aorta has been advocated by Steele (1941), Page (1940), Scott and Bahnson (1951), and others.

Scott and coworkers (1954) have recently presented excellent experimental evidence of the operation of the renal mechanism in coarctation of the aorta by producing a constriction of the aorta in dogs who had one kidney grafted into the neck. This was followed by hypertension above the constriction over several weeks. The removal of the kidney remaining below the coarctation was followed by a reduction in the hypertension to normal levels.

A study of arterioles above and below the coarctation by Painter and associates (1952) showed a similar degree of hypertrophy of the media, thus giving indirect support for the renal hypothesis.

On the other hand, the mechanical hypothesis, which was first suggested by Blumgart and coworkers (1931), has been supported by Gupta and Wiggers (1951) and by Bing and associates (1948). In acute experiments in animals, Gupta and Wiggers demonstrated that a constriction of the aortic lumen of more than 50 percent is followed by an immediate rise in systolic pressure above the constriction and a fall below it. They concluded that hypertension is explicable on the basis of a mechanical factor rather than a renal one. They point out that besides an increased resistance above the constriction, there is a reduced capacity and distensibility of the aortic

chamber into which the left ventricle empties with each systole.

In our studies of infants we have found that there is hypertension above and hypotension below the coarctation from the first few days of life in the majority of infants with this anomaly. The pressure differential has been demonstrated in infants at five days of age in our series and at ten days of age in Calodney and Carson's (1950). In our cases and in those of Calodney and Carson, hypertension was noted to occur in both the preductal and postductal types in early life. In some of the preductal type, the ductus may be widely patent and may at times carry a large blood flow into the descending aorta and to the kidneys. Such cases would appear to diminish the importance of a renal factor. The fact that such blood may be only two-thirds saturated with oxygen does not alter this conclusion.

Page and coworkers (1959) have suggested that the altered renal pulse wave that occurs below a coarcted segment of the aorta may be responsible for the hypertension. Kirkendall and associates (1959) have examined the mechanism of the altered hypertension and have recently shown (1959) no renal hemodynamic abnormalities of significance in the cases that were not in congestive heart failure. The renal vascular resistance was similar to that in normotensive individuals. Renal blood flow and plasma clearance showed no evidence of renal ischemia. There was a sharp difference between patients in the coarctation group and those suffering from essential hypertension. These authors concluded that generalized arterial constriction is not characteristic of patients with coarctation and the hypertension of the upper part of the body is not caused by a circulating humoral vasoconstrictor, as is postulated in primary renal hypertension or, as is sometimes demonstrated in coarctation of the aorta, in laboratory animals.

The evidence of either a renal mechanism or a mechanical one, or both, is substantiated to some degree by studies on experimental animals. The presence of a mechanical factor would seem incontrovertible in both man and experimental animal studies and the renal component would appear proved in experimental animals by the brilliant work of Scott and Bahnson (1951). However, when applied to man, such abnormal renal physiology has yet to be clearly shown. The relief of obstruction by a corrective surgical anastomosis causes an immediate drop in blood pressure in the upper circulatory compartment. This points to a mechanical component. The subsequent further fall in blood pressure in the upper extremities, which extends over months or years, may be related to circulatory readjustments that would include: (1) a gradual expansion of the hypoplastic aorta below the coarcted area, (2) a regression of a decreased elasticity of the arteries in the upper part of the body that has resulted from prolonged hypertension, and (3) the effects of the suture line at the site of the repair. This may have left some narrowing of the aorta of a moderate degree that would not alter the blood pressure under normal conditions, but with the other factors it may play some part in maintaining a pressure somewhat above the normal level.

The evidence of a mechanical component and a renal component appears significant on both sides, suggesting that several factors are operating in coarctation of the aorta to produce hypertension. It may be that the renal factor plays a part in adult life, but the evidence is strongly against a renal component playing a significant role in infancy.

POSTDUCTAL COARCTATION—ADULT TYPE, OVER ONE YEAR OF AGE

Clinical Features

Children over one year of age with coarctation of the aorta usually have no symptoms, and the defect is identified incidentally during the examination for some other reason.

The presenting complaint in most cases is the finding of a heart murmur or systolic hypertension on routine examination by the family physician or the school doctor. This was the case in 95 percent over one year of age in our series. Five percent of this age group had dyspnea with signs of heart failure.

The age when first seen by a physician varied from 1 to 15 years, the majority of cases being recognized as having coarctation when they were four to five years of age.

These children usually look healthy and well to the examining physician. They are perhaps a little thinner than the average; they are rarely obese. There is commonly a visible pulsation in the sternal notch; this is a characteristic finding and should make one suspect coarctation of the aorta immediately. Pulsating collateral vessels are rarely seen in childhood, but in a few of our cases we have noted them around the scapular areas.

Blood Pressure. The most diagnostic finding is hypertension in the arm and hypotension in the legs. Figure 39-2 shows the systolic blood pressure readings of children over one year of age. The systolic pressure varied from 110 to 220 in the arm, and averaged 140 to 145 mm of mercury. The systolic pressure in the leg was invariably lower; in many cases it was not obtainable; in those where a reading was obtainable, it varied from 60 to 100. The femoral arteries were usually not palpable in this group, being felt in only one-fourth of the cases.

Heart Murmurs. A heart murmur was heard in all our cases over one year of age with one exception. The usual murmur was a moderate systolic one heard down the left sternal border. It was often well transmitted to the back or to the apex. It was less harsh and less widely transmitted than murmurs that are due to pulmonary stenosis or a ventricular septal defect. None of our cases had a thrill associated with the murmur. In 25 percent the point of maximum intensity was in the first left interspace, in 50 percent it was in the second and third left interspaces, and in 25 percent in the third and fourth left interspaces. Although the murmur is far from diagnostic, there is something suggestive about it that sets it apart from other murmurs in congenital heart disease. This type of murmur coupled with a pulsating sternal notch is a highly suggestive combination.

Electrocardiography

The chief point of interest in the electrocardiogram in the postductal type of coarctation of the aorta is evidence of presence or absence of ventricular hypertrophy. Electrocardiograms with precordial leads were available in 135 cases in this group. The findings are shown in Figure 39-2. It will be seen that the majority showed evidence of left ventricular hypertrophy. Only 12 percent were within normal limits. Thus, a much higher percentage than has been noted in the past have evidence of left ventricular hypertrophy when precordial leads are available.

When an associated ventricular septal defect occurs with coarctation, the combination may lead to pulmonary vascular obstruction (Eisenmenger's complex). A similar process may accompany a patent

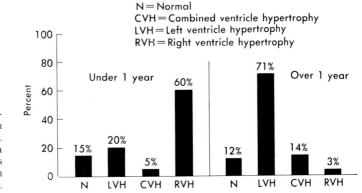

Figure 39-2. Electrocardiographic patterns in coarctation of the aorta are shown over one year and under one year of age. The vast majority under one year have a right ventricular loading pattern, whereas those over one year show a pattern indicating overloading of the left ventricle.

N = Normal
CVH = Combined ventricle hypertrophy
LVH = Left ventricle hypertrophy
RVH = Right ventricle hypertrophy

ductus with coarctation. In both instances one may find a right ventricular hypertrophy or loading pattern in the electrocardiogram.

Radiologic Examination

Heart Size. The heart was found to be within normal limits for size in 45 percent, grossly enlarged in 5 percent, and slightly to moderately enlarged in 50 percent. Postmortem studies always show some increase in thickness of the left ventricle when coarctation is present. In spite of such hypertrophy, no clinical enlargement may be evident in nearly half the cases.

The shape of the heart will vary. The left border is usually full or bulging and the apex protruding out and downward. Under the fluoroscope in the left anterior position, enlargement of the left ventricle is commonly evident. When associated defects are present, such as a ventricular septal defect, patent ductus arteriosus, or mitral insufficiency, the heart is larger than the average case of coarctation of the aorta.

After operation there is little change in heart size in those who have had no previous enlargement. However, in those in whom the heart was considerably enlarged, a dramatic decrease occasionally occurred in the succeeding months.

Other Information. As well as an estimation of heart size, the radiograph offers further information. There may be notching of the ribs present, which is readily identified by x-ray. This was present in one-third of our group over one year of age, the youngest case being five years of age.[*] Such tortuous loops are shown in an angiogram, Figure 39-3. One may occasionally see dilated ascending aorta or evidence of a hypoplastic arch. In some cases there may be a visible indentation at the site of the coarctation, especially in the left anterior oblique view, producing the so-called "E" sign. There may be an alteration of the contour of the barium-filled esophagus that corresponds with the level of the aortic arch and another wider indentation at the site of the poststenotic dilation of the aorta. The latter is well illustrated in Figure 39-4, which shows angiogram and a barium swallow combined. A conspicuous feature in many cases is the prominence with pulsation of the upper left border of the heart just above where one would expect to find the aortic knob; this slight bulge is due to the left subclavian artery and can usually be seen pulsating briskly. Its upward course can be recognized as it proceeds toward the left arm.

---

[*] *Causes of rib notching:*
Arterial: Coarctation of the aorta, thrombosis of abdominal aorta, Blalock-Taussig operation, tetralogy of Fallot, Ebstein's malformation, unilateral absence of pulmonary artery.
Venous: Superior vena caval obstruction.
Arteriovenous: Intercostal arteriovenous fistula, pulmonary arteriovenous fistula.
Other: Hyperparathyroidism, intercostal neurinoma, idiopathic.

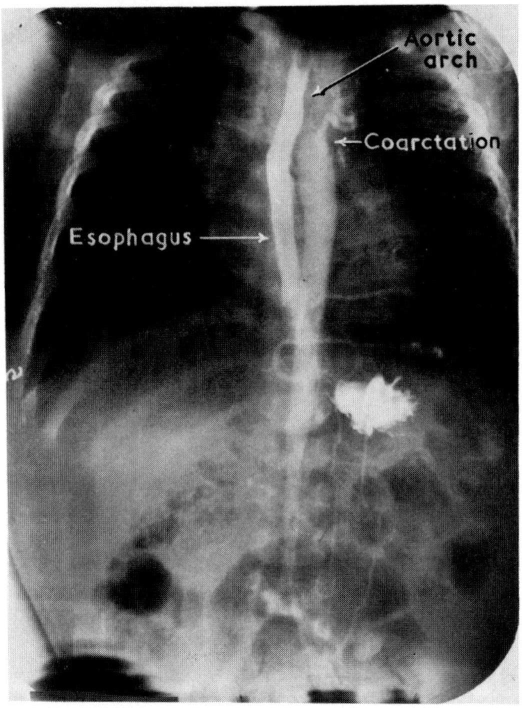

Figure 39-3. D. T., aged 14 months. During the performance of an angiogram this baby regurgitated some barium that had been in the stomach previously and revealed the slight displacement of the esophagus due to poststenotic dilatation of the aorta.

Angiocardiography

An aortogram will reveal the aortic arch and the coarctation in a very lucid fashion. If the ductus is patent and the flow is from the aorta into the ductus, this may also be readily visualized by this method. The collateral circulation can be well shown, particularly the internal mammary and the branches arising from the left subclavian and communicating with the intercostal vessels. Associated defects are best demonstrated by the combination of cardiac catheterization and selective angiocardiography.

Diagnosis

The diagnosis is rarely difficult to make in this age group over one year since the absence of femoral pulsations or the presence of weak femoral pulsations provides an identifying clue. The blood pressures then confirm this finding and demonstrate a hypertension in the arm and hypotension in the leg. None of the other causes of hypertension in childhood demonstrate hypotension in the leg (a rare female patient will have underdevelopment or hypoplasia of the aortic tree below the level of the heart—such children may have weak femoral pulsations [Schuster and Gross, 1962]). It is perhaps worth reiterating that most children with coarctation of the aorta in this age group have a marked pulsation in the sternal notch. A

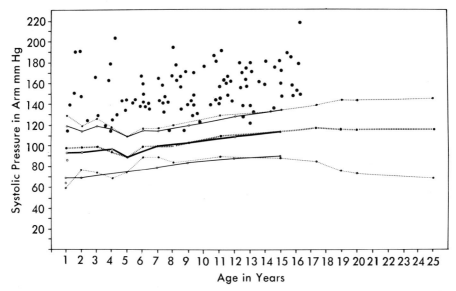

Figure 39-4. Systolic arm pressures before operation in 123 children whose coarctation was resected after one year are plotted against age. The mean and ± standard-deviation lines represent values from normal population as described in the text.

diagnostic problem is more likely to arise in connection with associated anomalies. The most common defect is a patent ductus, which is found in 20 percent of this age group. As a general rule, a continuous murmur in the pulmonary area identifies its presence, but a continuous murmur may be lacking and yet an aortogram or operation may reveal the patency of the ductus. On rare occasions there is pulmonary hypertension of a degree that reverses the flow through the ductus, and one will find a lower oxygen content in the blood to the legs than to the arms. Cyanosis may be noted in the toes but not in the fingers.

The left subclavian artery may occasionally arise from the aorta below the coarctation. The blood pressure in the left arm will then be relatively low, while hypertension is noted in the right arm. Atresia of the left subclavian artery may occur, in which case no pulse or blood pressure will be obtainable on the left. An interesting diagnostic problem is presented when a patient is discovered to have pulses absent in all four extremities. This clinical picture is due to coarctation of the aorta of the type just described plus an aberrant right subclavian taking its origin from the aorta below the constriction. The diagnosis may be suspected by the absent pulses, especially when accompanied by some of the radiologic signs of coarctation. The electrocardiogram may show left ventricular hypertrophy. An aortogram is rarely needed to confirm the diagnosis.

Complications

A number of complications, mainly affecting the systemic arteries, can develop during the clinical course of adult type coarctation of the aorta.

Vascular complications in coarctation of the aorta are rare in infancy and childhood. Cerebral hemorrhage, cerebral thrombosis, ruptured aorta, and necrotizing arteritis have all been described (Landtman and Tuuteri, 1959; Perez-Alvarez and Oudkerk, 1955; Hurt and Hanbury, 1957). Reifenstein's series of 104 cases contains only three patients with intercranial hemorrhage or ruptured aorta under 20 years of age as compared with seven times that number in the over-20 age group. Shearer and associates (1970) have summarized the literature with cerebrovascular accident and recorded 35 cases under the age of 20 years. Two-thirds of them were over the age of ten when the cerebrovascular accident occurred and only 10 percent (three cases) were under the age of five. The blood pressure was recorded in a minority of cases but in each case was always over 140 mm of mercury. The autopsy data suggest that the hemiplegia of cerebrovascular accident was due to rupture of an intercerebral vessel or aneurysm and was rarely caused by thrombosis or embolism.

At The Hospital for Sick Children, Toronto, we have had 762 cases of coarctation of the aorta with only two instances of cerebrovascular accident, one aged five years and the other three weeks. The blood pressure in the infant was 200/100.

Infective endarteritis near the site of the coarcted segment is rarely encountered in children but is a dreaded complication because it may be complicated by rupture. The organism involved is usually staphylococcus. Endocarditis of the aortic valve is a particular dread because the valve is so often abnormal in coarctation. It is therefore very important to ensure that protective antibiotic cover be provided at times of risk even when the coarctation is apparently entirely relieved by surgery.

Aortic regurgitation usually develops because of an underlying bicuspid aortic valve and can be recognized sometimes before clinical signs become evident by diastolic mitral valve flutter on an echocardiogram (Scovil et al., 1976).

Other complications, including premature coronary arterial disease and unexpected death, are a reminder that small vessels may also be significantly affected in coarctation of the aorta (Vlodaver and Neufeld, 1968; Maron et al., 1973; Simon and Zloto, 1974).

Treatment

Schuster and Gross (1962) performed 487 surgical repairs of coarctation of the aorta with a mortality of 4.1 percent and a morbidity rate among the survivors of 4 percent. These data apply to the age group over one year and chiefly to the group between the ages of 8 and 20 years. Others have reported a varying operative death rate depending on the presence or absence of complications. Bailey and associates (1957), summarizing the operative literature, found an average mortality of 8.6 percent in 1601 cases.

Improving techniques are indicated by the fact that the operative mortality has been lower in the past five years than previously. It is lowest in the 5-to-15-year age group. It is lower when the patients with associated lesions are eliminated; thus, if one includes only the patients with pure or isolated coarctation of the aorta in Gross's data, without any complicating lesions, the mortality is only 1.6 percent. This is a remarkable record and supports his contention that the resection is more safely done after the first year of life and before the age when aneurysms and arteriosclerotic lesions become common. In a recent review the mortality in patients after the first year was 2 percent (Luidesmith et al., 1971).

The postoperative blood pressure levels reported by Schuster and Gross at the time of follow-up indicated that 60 percent had systolic pressures less than 131 mm of mercury. Thirty-six percent had levels between 131 and 150, and 4 percent were over 150 mm of mercury. These levels need to be related to age to be accurately interpreted, but since the largest number of patients were treated between 10 and 25 years and the follow-up is an average of five years, one can only conclude that this is a satisfactory response even though the mean level is above average.

Although he prefers direct union of the two aortic segments, Gross recommends grafts under special circumstances and over the years has inserted 70 homografts (14.3 percent). His indications for such homografts include the presence of a long aortic segment, an inadequate caliber of the upper aortic segment, the resection of an aneurysm, and the presence of certain technical complications. Fortunately, it is rarely necessary to insert a graft in the

child since the special circumstances referred to above occur infrequently and the young aorta is more pliable and more readily freed, permitting it to bridge the gap when the coarcted segments have been removed. Homografts not uncommonly lead to calcification of the insert in one-third to one-half of the cases in the next five to ten years (Schuster and Gross, 1962). An alternative method is to bridge the gap with a prosthesis of Dacron or Teflon, and this is recommended by several experienced surgeons (Foster et al., 1965; Foster et al., 1960; Edwards and Lyons, 1958; and Harrison, 1959).

In the past it has been considered that the site of anastomosis may not grow with the child if it is performed in the first five or ten years of life. Experimental studies indicate that there is usually satisfactory growth in anastomoses in young animals when following them through to maturity (Moss et al., 1959), but in some instances the growth may be lagging after two or three years (Sauvage and Harkins, 1952). There is good clinical evidence that the anastomosis grows with the child, and the majority of our cases operated after the first year of life have had a satisfactory drop in systemic pressure following surgery, and this has been maintained over the follow-up period of three to ten years (see Figures 39–4 and 39–5).

Nanton and Olley (1976) have reviewed the blood pressure recordings on 190 patients operated on at The Hospital for Sick Children between 1 and 15 years of age and found 45 cases (or 24 percent) had some evidence of postoperative hypertension. These included 17 patients with diastolic hypertension alone, 20 with systolic hypertension alone, and eight with both. It is difficult to predict whether this pattern will be maintained on into adult life with further long-term follow-up studies. They also showed there was a more satisfactory drop in pressure if the patients were operated on between four and six years compared to 10 to 15 years.

If the child is well and active, and free from complicating defects, it appears suitable to wait until he reaches the age of four or five years before proceeding with surgical correction. However, if any special reason presents itself earlier, one should not hesitate to operate immediately. There are certain commanding circumstances that lead to early surgery. These include the cases that have congestive heart failure during the waiting period, or who have an associated defect that may be producing irreversible pulmonary vascular changes or jeopardizing life. There is little doubt that a child of three or four years of age with chronic heart failure should have the aortic constriction removed.

Children who have a large ventricular septal defect may develop irreversible changes in the pulmonary arteries. These children should have surgery before the pulmonary hypertension becomes irreversible, especially if there is evidence of progressive increase in pulmonary vascular resistance. When there is an associated patency of the ductus, it is preferable to

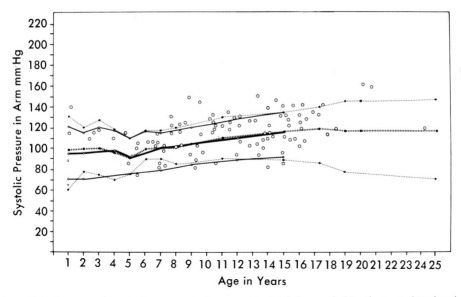

Figure 39-5. Postoperative systolic pressures in the arms, at the last follow-up, in 95 patients are plotted against age in the same way as in Figure 39-4. Eighty percent of patients have pressures within the normal limits.

operate on the ductus and the coarctation together, since the second operation is made more difficult by the matted tissues that surround the previously dissected site. A small patent ductus with little or no enlargement of the heart and no evidence of pulmonary hypertension might well be left until five years of age. Catheterization will be required prior to operation in order to properly evaluate the pulmonary vascular system. Where there is associated rheumatic heart disease with mitral insufficiency, mitral stenosis, or aortic insufficiency, the association with coarctation of the aorta is harmful. Such patients should be carefully studied and, when indicated, the lesions corrected.

Postoperative paraplegia has been observed by Bing and associates (1945) once, Gross (1953) twice, and Beattie and coworkers (1953) once; and it has occurred twice in our series. It appears to be primarily

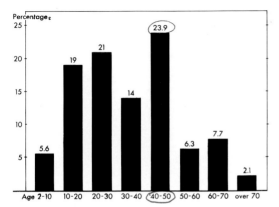

Figure 39-6. Postductal coarctation of the aorta. Percentage of deaths per decade of age. (Data from Reifenstein et al. [1947] and Bauer and Astbury [1944].)

due to a thrombosis of the spinal artery. The reason for this complication is not clear, but it may be associated with prolonged occlusion of the aorta or the necessity of tying numerous collateral vessels. It is a major catastrophe, since the patient is much worse off than before the operation. Pontius and associates (1954) have shown experimentally that hypothermia will greatly reduce the incidence of paraplegia following the temporary occlusion of the aorta in animals. When prolonged occlusion of the aorta appears necessary, hypothermia should be used as an adjunct in such cases.

From the physician's standpoint one must consider each case on its own merit, regarding the need, risks, and benefits of operation. The mortality is relatively low in the hands of a skilled surgeon, and all patients have some relief of their hypertension. The mortality without operation increases with each decade, as is shown in Figure 59-6. An appreciable number of cases die in the second decade of life, but death between one and ten years has become very uncommon in recent years in children supervised by their physician.

Maron and associates (1973) presented a 20-year postoperative appraisal of 240 patients followed after surgical correction for coarctation of the aorta at the Johns Hopkins Hospital. The mean age at operation was 20 years and varied from 2 to 40 years. Forty-two percent had no change or had an increased blood pressure over the preoperative value. This less favorable result compared with that found in children was undoubtedly related in part to the late mean age at operation. It is also important to recognize that there was a high incidence of late postoperative complications such as congestive heart failure, cerebral vascular hemorrhage, and sudden death from cardiovascular disease. Aortic regurgitation and bacterial endocarditis, while they did occur occasionally, were uncommon complications.

Thus, operation in childhood appears safe, and the result is usually good. It would seem, therefore, that most cases of coarctation should be operated on at some time. The optimum period is four to six years of age, since by that time the aorta is large enough to carry out the technical procedures; there is good elasticity at that age; and, most important, the lumen is large enough to provide an adequate blood flow to lower the hypertension and carry an adequate blood flow to the lower extremities for the rest of the patient's life.

In the third decade or later, the aorta is less elastic, and very slow atherosclerosis, aneurysms, and aortic insufficiency are more frequently encountered, bleeding from the collaterals is more common and more difficult to control, and the operation is, therefore, more risky.

Moes and coworkers (1964) point out that the aorta has a diameter at eight years of age that is 72 percent of the adult diameter. Restenosis occasionally occurs after operation in the first year of life. It is a relatively rare occurrence if the operation is carried out after the first year or two of life. Thus, a case can be made for operating on children before the age of seven, preferably at four, five, or six, on the basis that they may develop hemiplegia. Twenty years ago repair of the coarctation was usually undertaken between 10 and 12 years of age. This age has been dropping steadily and the majority of surgeons now seem to prefer to do it somewhere between four and eight years. The risk of a cerebrovascular accident is not great, probably less than 1 percent of children over two. Other indications for early surgery include the possibility of congestive heart failure, sudden increase in size of the heart or significant sustained rise in degree of systemic hypertension, or the association of some other congenital heart defect that would make it imperative that one or both lesions be treated early. The risk of these complications is much higher if the coarctation is not recognized until adult life (Maron, 1973).

Postoperative Complications. Postoperative paradoxic hypertension was first reported in a fatal case by Sealy (1953). Since then the problem has been widely recognized and frequently associated with abdominal pain. Three types of postoperative blood pressure response have been noted by Sealy and associates (1957). Their first was a reactive hypertension that occurred after an initial drop and rose to a peak within 36 hours of surgical correction. Approximately one-sixth of Sealy's cases fell into this category. The second type was more delayed and lasted longer—usually subsiding in one to three weeks. Nearly one-half of his cases responded in this manner. It was from this group that abdominal pain was more likely to arise. The remaining one-half of patients showed no postoperative hypertension.

Postoperative abdominal pain has been recorded so commonly that a special category may be made for such cases. Ring and Lewis (1956) report 28 percent of their patients, and Sealy 20 percent, had this symptom following surgical correction of the aortic anomaly. It should be pointed out that 16 percent of patients with

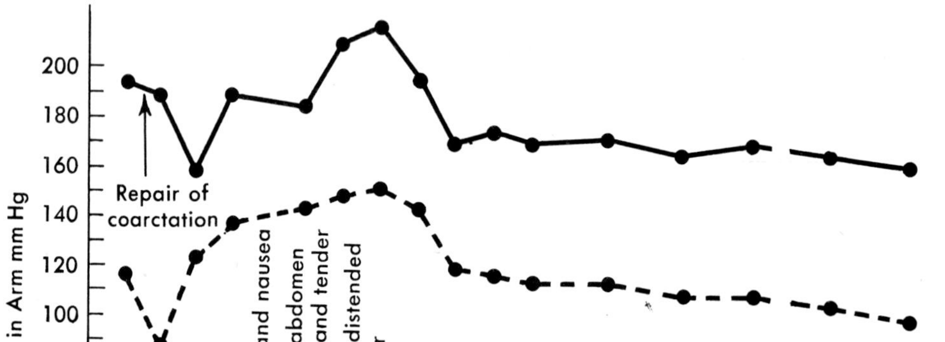

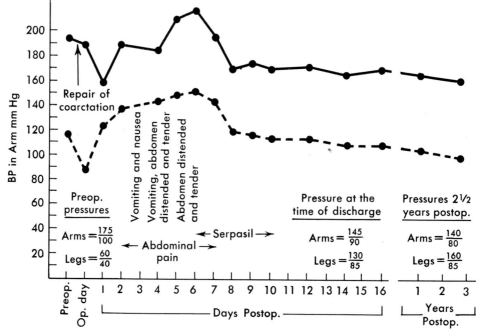

Figure 39-7. Postoperative course in 8½-year-old boy, J. P. Note that the pressures came down to near-normal level immediately after surgery, and after about 48 hours he had a secondary rise in blood pressure associated with acute abdominal symptoms. Blood pressure was extremely labile during this period.

patent ductus arteriosus have been reported to have abdominal pain following surgery (March et al., 1960). However, in coarctation intestinal vascular involvement may occur in varying degrees of severity, sometimes producing only a mild pain in the abdomen during the first week following operation and lasting a day or two, or a more severe pain associated with abdominal rigidity and lasting a week or more. Usually the milder attacks subside with heat and sedation and use of such drugs as reserpine or hydralazine hydrochloride, but occasionally the episodes are severe enough to warrant a laparotomy. At such times a hyperemic segment of bowel is recognized, and in some cases the surgeon can identify necrotizing arteritis with areas requiring bowel excision (Ring and Lewis, 1956; Sealy et al., 1957). Although the mechanism of such lesions cannot be precisely recognized, it is clearly a development of the postoperative period and is associated with hypertension. There is initial flooding of the lower part of the body that appears to cause a blood vessel reaction that may be traumatic. Hyperactive adrenal glands and vascular spasm have been suggested as possible causative factors (Srouji and Trusler, 1965). The majority of patients are not harmed by the new circulatory dynamics, but a number do react unfavorably and demand special attention in the postoperative period. We have only had one case with signs sufficient to warrant a laparotomy. Hyperemia was found and the patient's incision closed again. The labile blood pressure in a child with postoperative abdominal pain is shown in Figure 39–7.

These findings suggest, as Sealy has already indicated, that the temporary hypertension developing in the postoperative period may be due to reflexes from pressure set at a high level before operation, with the mechanism continuing after relief of the obstruction. With the tension in the aortic wall reduced, the receptors may react in a variety of ways and may require a prolonged period of readjustment (March et al., 1960). March and associates reported, however, that 74 percent of their patients had blood pressures within two standard deviations of normal after an average follow-up period of four years. Similar satisfactory results are shown in Figure 39–5, from The Toronto Hospital for Sick Children.

COARCTATION OF THE AORTA— UNDER ONE YEAR OF AGE

SINCE more than half of the cases of coarctation of the aorta present with signs or symptoms in the first year of life, it is obvious that this age group constitutes the chief problem from the point of view of both diagnosis and therapy.

Our experience in the last 25 years has been that two-thirds of the cases seen in the first year of life have the preductal type. The incidence of the various types, based on data obtained at postmortem and operation and by clinical findings, is shown in Table 39–1. The preductal type usually presents signs and symptoms in the first six weeks of life, whereas, although the postductal type may develop signs during that period they appear later in the majority of cases.

The early appearance of heart failure and the higher mortality in the preductal type appear to be related to the frequent presence of associated heart anomalies chiefly of the noncyanotic group. This includes, particularly, the patent ductus arteriosus. Coarctation of the aorta is the second leading cause of heart failure in infancy and childhood. See also Sinha and associates (1969) and Tawes and associates (1969).

The problem of the future is better realized when one reviews the data for infants, children, and adults over the past 20 years. There were, each year, twice as many deaths in the first year of life among infants with coarctation of the aorta as there were in all the children and adults over one year of age during the same interval (see Figure 39–8).

Clinical Features

The signs and symptoms in the preductal and postductal types are similar, with the exception that cyanosis may occur at times in the former group while it is rare in the latter. Since the two types are clinically similar in the first year of life they will be discussed together.

Approximately 80 percent are referred with a history of recent onset of dyspnea, some as early as 48 hours after birth (Marks et al., 1953). The rest are brought to the doctor because of the discovery of a heart murmur or, occasionally, for some unrelated pediatric problem that leads to further investigation and diagnosis.

Cyanosis. In the postductal group cyanosis was uncommon except as a terminal event in those who died. On the other hand, in the preductal group cyanosis had been present from birth intermittently in 20 percent of the cases that got into difficulty in the first two months of life (Glass et al., 1960). In the latter group, all had severe associated congenital heart defects, such as transposition of the great vessels or common ventricle. In babies with preductal coarctation with other major defects, a minor degree of cyanosis or ashen color may be present when there is marked respiratory distress or heart failure.

Heart Murmurs. In half of the cases no murmur was heard. These were, in most instances, the younger infants who died early. In some cases a faint systolic murmur was at first concealed by crying or stressful breathing but was heard later on subsequent examination. When the murmur was present, it was maximum between the second and third left interspaces in the majority, but might also be heard in the pulmonary area or between the third and fourth left interspaces, and occasionally at the apex in 10 percent. When the murmur was maximum in the third

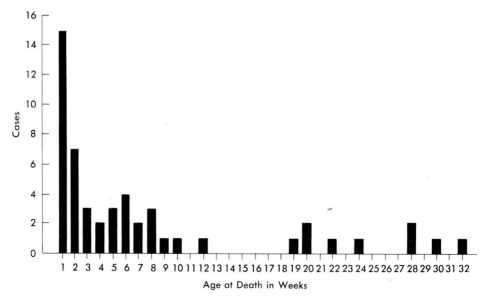

Figure 39-8. Shows the age of death in the patients with coarctation who died in the first year of life. The largest number die in the first week.

and fourth left interspaces and accompanied by a thrill, it was not uncommonly due to an associated patent interventricular septum. A large percentage of those with heart failure had a patent ductus arteriosus in spite of the fact that no murmur was heard.

Signs of Heart Failure. Heart failure was present in 70 percent of those babies whose coarctation was discovered in the first year of life. Dyspnea was a constant symptom with respiratory rates from 40 to 120 per minute. All had some enlargement of the liver, frequently three to four fingerbreadths down from the costal margin in a line between the umbilicus and the right nipple. Slightly edematous skin markings were commonly found, but frank edema was rare. Rales in the chest were heard occasionally, and in a few very severe cases there was pulmonary edema. The heart was always enlarged to some degree, but the size varied considerably and was usually dependent on the rapidity with which failure developed in the first few weeks or months after birth. Those whose failure was slowly progressive and untreated had larger hearts than those whose signs appeared suddenly.

Blood Pressure. The femoral arteries were not palpable in two-thirds of the cases, whether or not a preductal type of coarctation was present. Arm systolic blood pressure readings varied from 70 to 180 mm of mercury, being lower when congestive heart failure supervened. Systolic pressures in both arm and leg were of essentially the same order whether the ductus was opening below or above the coarctation, but slightly higher readings were obtained in the postductal group. The blood pressure by direct-reading intra-arterial needle is shown in a five-day-old baby in Figure 39–9.

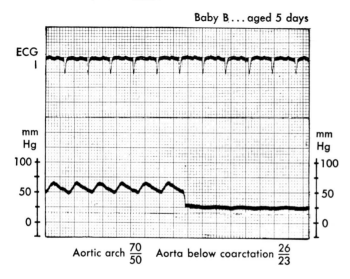

Figure 39-9. Coarctation of the aorta—preductal type. Direct intra-arterial pressure recordings.

The blood pressure was always higher in the arm than in the leg, but when marked failure was present, the blood pressure in the upper extremities fell to the normal range and gave a similar reading to that found in the leg. With the administration of digitalis and other supportive therapy, the pressure then rose again in the arm and the differential became evident.

Electrocardiography

A summary of the electrocardiographic findings under one year of age in relation to ventricular hypertrophy is shown in Figure 39–3. In the preductal type in the first two months of life, right ventricular hypertrophy is invariably present if the ductus remains open. In one case at two months of age, the ductus was closed and the electrocardiogram showed left ventricular hypertrophy. In the postductal group, although right ventricular hypertrophy dominates in the first two months, either a normal or left ventricular hypertrophy curve may be found. Thus, the presence of right ventricular hypertrophy does not differentiate between these two anatomic types, but the presence of left ventricular hypertrophy or a normal curve indicates that one is dealing with either a postductal type or preductal type with a closed ductus.

In our postductal type followed into the second year of life, all cases showed the appearance of left ventricular hypertrophy pattern developing between six months and a year. In the preductal group if the ductus remained widely patent and there was pulmonary hypertension present from this or other causes, the right ventricular pattern persisted. A similar finding is reported by Lang and Nadas (1956). When a marked left heart strain pattern appears with inverted T waves over the left precordium, the association of coarctation with endocardial fibroelastosis should be suspected.

Radiologic Examination

The cardiac outline of the heart of an infant with coarctation is shown in Figure 39–10. There is almost invariably enlargement of the heart, but the outline may vary considerably. In most cases there is a somewhat full left border of the heart, sometimes associated with a raised apex; in others the apex is blunt and pointing slightly down. There is no significant difference between the two groups except that the hearts appear somewhat larger in the postductal type since most of these patients have survived longer (Garman et al., 1965).

In the postductal type it will be noted that patient R. McC. (Figure 39–10) showed enlargement of the heart over a period of one month. The first x-ray, taken at ten days of age, shows the heart at the upper limits of normal; at one month of age it nearly fills the chest.

Both the hilar shadows and the lung fields are congested if heart failure is present. If there is a large patent ductus, the hilar shadows are congested and may be pulsating. In infants useful information can often be obtained from a barium swallow. This will frequently reveal an indentation of the left aortic arch and beneath it a secondary indentation due to a poststenotic dilatation of the aorta immediately below the coarctation. Thus a general displacement of the aorta to the right is not an uncommon finding in babies with this anomaly. An esophagram with an associated aortogram shows this clearly (see Figure 39–4).

An aortogram will readily reveal the whole area of the aorta or the great vessels arising from it, the coarctation and the descending aorta, and collateral circulation (see Figure 39–11). Thus the degree and extent of the coarctation as well as its position can be accurately appraised by the surgeon.

This procedure may differentiate between the postductal type and the preductal type. Diffuse

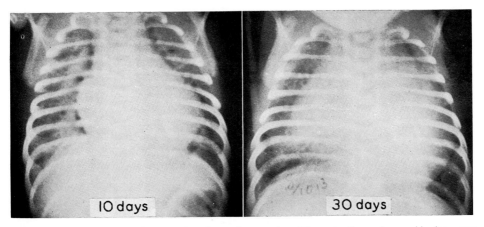

Figure 39-10. R. Mc., aged ten days. Postductal type of coarctation of the aorta. X-rays show rapid enlargement of the heart over a period of 20 days, associated with development of heart failure.

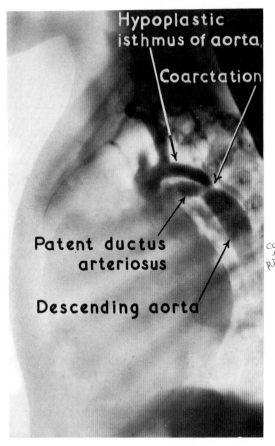

Figure 39-11. Preductal type of coarctation with patent ductus arteriosus, the ductus filling in retrograde fashion with the aorta beyond the coarctation.

hypoplasia of the aortic arch will be readily evident if present and is strong evidence in favor of the preductal type. If the ductus is filled from the arch above the coarctation, it will clearly be a postductal, or adult, pattern. If the ductus fills from the descending aorta below the coarctation, it will obviously be a preductal, or infantile, type. If no filling occurs above or below, one cannot rule out the preductal type. The ductus may be carrying the blood in reverse flow from pulmonary artery to aorta, or the pressure in the pulmonary artery and arch may be sufficiently similar so that the contrast medium will not move from one vessel to the other.

Diagnosis

The diagnosis should be suspected in any baby with a heart murmur, any baby with dyspnea or who shows signs of heart failure, or an infant who has evidence of cyanotic congenital heart disease. Thus, every infant with signs or symptoms referable to the heart should be examined for evidence of coarctation of the aorta. When coarctation of the aorta is present, the femoral pulsations are usually faint or absent, and blood

pressure will be higher in the arms than in the legs except where there is marked failure. Here the pressures may be the same but the usual hypertension will reappear above the constriction once the failure has been combated. One should be particularly suspicious of signs of heart failure developing in the first three months of life. Marks and associates (1953) recognized a case at two days of age by the presence of dyspnea and a defect in the aortic knob shown in the x-ray of the heart.

The electrocardiogram may show right or left ventricular hypertrophy or a normal tracing. The x-ray will usually show some enlargement of the heart, which is generalized and commonly associated with congestion either of the hilar areas or in the lung fields. An aortogram will clearly confirm the diagnosis.

In patients with coarctation of the aorta coming to operation or necropsy within the first six months of life, the ductus arteriosus is almost invariably patent. This was noted in the present series with a frequency of 95 percent. Others have noted this association with similar frequency. Calodney and Carson (1950) found a patent ductus in 19 of 21 infants and children who came to necropsy under 20 months of age. The figures are different in adult life among patients with coarctation. Dry et al. (1953) noted that 10 percent of their series of cases, chiefly adults, had a patent ductus. March et al. (1960) found 14 percent in those over one year of age. Mustard et al. (1955) found an incidence of patent ductus of 20 percent in children after the first year. Returning to the first year of life, Glass et al. (1960), from postmortem data, found an incidence in 95 percent of patent ductus arteriosus, and the overall incidence in the first year of life was 60 percent. It is apparent, therefore, that one should consider the ductus likely to be open and functioning in the first few months of life, even though the majority of patients will not have a continuous murmur audible. See also Tawes and associates (1969).

Another feature of the early weeks or months of life is the incidence of the preductal, or infantile, type of coarctation of the aorta with the ductus entering below the coarctation. Ninety percent of the patients who were examined at autopsy had this arrangement and only 10 percent had the postductal, or adult, type. After one leaves the pediatric age group, the reverse is found. Eighty-four percent of groups studied at operation by investigators at the Mayo Clinic by Clagett and associates (1954) had a postductal type, and only 13 percent were preductal. In 3 percent the site of entrance of the ductus could be determined. The high mortality in the first year of life is brought about by the early heart failure which appears to be due to the combined effects of the hypertension and an associated left-to-right shunt. Two-fifths of the cases examined at this center had lesions other than patent ductus arteriosus when seen in the first year of life. These include ventricular septal defect, 33 percent; transposition of the great vessels, 18 percent; and atrial septal defect, 60 percent. A somewhat similar incidence was reported by Calodney and Carson (1950) and Tawes and associates (1969).

The combination of a patent ductus arteriosus and a preductal coarctation is apparently much more serious than when a postductal coarctation is present. During the early hours or days of life there may well be a venous oxygen content of the blood in the region of the patent ductus, which would minimize the effect of oxygen on closing the ductus. A wide patency of the ductus will flood the lung fields and maintain a high pressure in the pulmonary vascular tree. The major flow through the ductus may be toward the peripheral lung fields or it may be through the ductus toward the systemic circulation. It will be in both directions at the same time if the pressures are similar, as is frequently the case in preductal coarctation with a patent ductus.

Many cases of coarctation of the aorta will be diagnosed with increasing frequency if the condition is kept in mind during the examination of infants in the first few weeks of life, since it is one of the most common causes of heart failure in the newborn period. In many instances the diagnosis will be made in the newborn nursery if palpation of the femoral arteries is part of the routine examination of newborn infants in distress. Confirmation can be made then by determining the blood pressures in the arms and legs. Few cases are missed in this way.

In differentiating between preductal and postductal coarctation, the following points are useful. If the failure occurs in the first month of life, it is more likely to be the preductal type. If left ventricular hypertrophy appears in the electrocardiogram, one is more likely to be dealing with the postductal type. A diffuse hypoplasia of the aortic arch suggests a preductal type. An aortogram may occasionally reveal a ductus opening into the descending aorta when a preductal type is present and may at times clearly reveal the ductus opening into the aorta above the coarctation when a postductal type is present. When the ductus is not patent, there is no necessity to differentiate between the two since they are then functionally the same. To be able to differentiate between preductal and postductal coarctations may be of questionable value. It is helpful in deciding the urgency for corrective surgery since the preductal type appears to have a much poorer prognosis and may require prompt treatment.

Treatment

Many surgeons have demonstrated the competence with which the technical procedure of an anastomosis can be performed in infants with coarctation of the aorta. These include Gross (1953), Kirklin and associates (1952), Baronofsky and Adams (1954), Mustard and associates (1955), Tawes and associates (1969), Hallman and associates (1967), and Sinha and associates (1969). When the coarcted segment is localized, it is relatively simple to remove it and join the two ends of the aorta together. On the other hand, when there is a hypoplastic arch that gives off the left subclavian and left common carotid, the narrowing may at times extend back to the anomalous artery and correction is more of a problem. Mustard and associates (1955) have shown in infants that the aorta can be mobilized under such circumstances and the hypoplastic and the coarcted portion removed. When the upper portion of the hypoplastic segment is cut on a bias, it will approximate in size that of the descending aorta to which it is joined. A gusset of prosthetic material, pericardium, or section of the left subclavian artery has recently been used to widen the narrow segment in these babies with success (Waldhausen and Nahrwold, 1966; Reul et al., 1974).

In spite of the fact that the anastomotic procedure is technically quite feasible in infants, the operative mortality remains relatively high in the first year of life. Most of this mortality occurs in patients in the first few months of life and reaches its peak in the newborn period. The affected patients are those with atrial or ventricular defects, patent ductus arteriosus, or even more complex cases, and they frequently have narrowed arch and isthmic segments as well as the localized constriction. Recently substantial improvement in mortality has been achieved with better

Table 39–2. MORTALITY IN SURGICAL TREATMENT OF COARCTATION OF THE AORTA IN THE FIRST YEAR OF LIFE

		NUMBER OF CASES OPERATED ON	SURGICAL MORTALITY, %
Mathey et al.	1954	5	20
Adams et al.	1955	8	25
Lester and Margalis	1957	20	40
Kempton and Waterson	1957	4	25
Mortensen et al.	1959	8	0
Morris et al.	1960	19	10
Behrer	1960	17	47
Glass et al.	1960	34	41
Malm and Blumenthal	1963	12	50
Tawes et al.	1968	333	45
Pelletier et al.	1969	31	29
Champsaur et al.	1972	86	32
Connors et al.	1975	18	17

anticongestive measures and postoperative support, especially assisted ventilation. The surgical mortality in various centers where operation has been carried out in the first year of life is shown in Table 39–2.

As Tawes and coworkers (1968) point out, the surgical mortality in the first year of life is meaningless unless it is subdivided on the basis of age at operation, since the risk is chiefly in the first few weeks or months.

AGE AT SURGERY*	TAWES ET AL. (1968) SURGICAL MORTALITY %
0–6 weeks	67
6 weeks–3 months	43
3 months–6 months	27
6 months–1 year	4.5

* Tawes et al. (1968)

At The Hospital for Sick Children, Champsaur (1972) reported similar figures as follows: 0–6 weeks—41%; 6 weeks–3 months—23%; 3 months–6 months—0%; and 6 months–1 year—16%.

In all who survived the operation, the heart failure was promptly relieved. Marked clinical improvement occurred with increased weight gain and a return to general good health. The blood pressures done repeatedly in the years following surgery have returned to and remained at a satisfactory level in the majority of cases.

The blood pressures postoperatively are shown in Figure 39–12. It will be noted that a few months to ten years after operation over half had a systolic pressure in the right arm of 110 mm of mercury or less; a few had a pressure between 110 and 130 mm; only two had a pressure over 130 mm.

Subsequently, Eshagpour and Olley (1972) reviewed these cases at a mean of five years postoperatively. Only six had isolated coarctation of the aorta initially. Many had associated patent ductus arteriosus or a ventricular septal defect or both. Forty-one percent had upper limb systolic pressures exceeding the normal by 2 standard deviations when examined an average of five years later. Those that were considered to be associated with a substantiated diagnosis of recoarctation of the aorta totaled 16 percent.

Figure 39–8 reveals the short life of infants who developed congestive heart failure in the neonatal period. This covers approximately ten years, and when the incidence is compared with that in later life, it is clear that there are more deaths each year among infants with coarctation of the aorta in the first year of life than in all other years of life combined, children and adults included. Thus this neonatal period constitutes our greatest challenge in dealing with this anomaly.

It has been pointed out by Lang and Nadas (1956), Whittemore (1955), Engle (1956), and others that with medical care and continuous use of digitalis some of these babies can be tided over the critical period of early infancy, making operation unnecessary in the first year of life. This raises the question as to which cases should be treated medically and which cases treated surgically.

The babies who show signs and symptoms of congestive heart failure in the first year of life may be divided into several subgroups. Less than a third of them are straightforward cases of coarctation of the postductal, or adult, type. These are the cases that are being treated medically by Lang and Nadas, Whittemore, Engle, and others with success. The

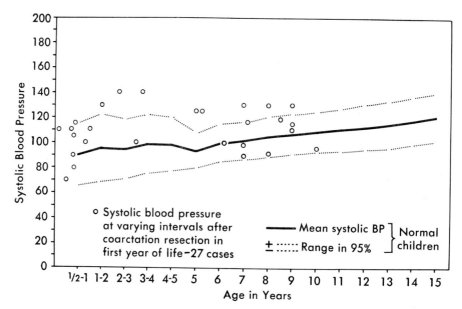

Figure 39-12. Postoperative systolic blood pressure readings in a group of 27 infants when coarctation was resected in the first year of life. Blood pressure readings at various intervals after corrective surgery.

onset of failure is usually after the first month or two of life.

▷The preductal type, as a rule, comprises a more complicated category. Here a patent ductus arteriosus also occurs in the majority, throwing an additional load on the right ventricle, especially in those cases who have a pressure in the pulmonary artery that approaches systemic and those who may have a reversal of blood flow through the ductus. Other cardiac anomalies are commonly found in this group, most particularly the ventricular septal defect, but also atrial septal defect, atrioventricularis communis, single ventricle, transposition of the great vessels, and tetralogy of Fallot. At present the evidence from many centers indicates that many such infants are short-lived and do not respond to medical therapy. Few have the benefit of surgery. Among our cases that have died, the age at death in the first year of life of all types is shown in Figure 39–8.

Our first newborn treated surgically was admitted to the hospital in severe failure at 12 days of age. After a few hours he appeared practically moribund in spite of oxygen, digitalis, etc. The diagnosis was coarctation. Operation was carried out at midnight as an emergency procedure; the circulation was so poor that the incision failed to bleed when the operation was started. A preductal type of coarctation was removed, anastomosis completed, and the baby survived. Recoarctation required a second operation at age 15 years.

It is helpful to divide infants with coarctation into three groups when considering the special problem of selection of cases for surgery.

GROUP I. In group I there are those who have been found to have coarctation incidentally during an examination. In these the heart may show some degree of enlargement, but there is no evidence of failure. Such babies will, in most instances, develop naturally and can be operated on at the optimum time.

GROUP II. Group II includes those babies who develop heart failure after the first two months of life and have no evidence of associated defects. If they are not too desperately ill when first seen, they will respond well to digitalis, and in many instances will not require surgery until later in life at a more optimum time. Such cases should be carried on digitalis for several months until it is no longer required.

If these infants do not respond adequately to digitalis, surgical resection should be carried out promptly (see Figure 39–13).

GROUP III. Infants with coarctation who develop congestive heart failure in the first two months of life usually have associated defects, whether it be patent ductus arteriosus or some other lesion. When they go into failure at such an early age, the majority die whether digitalis is given or not. There is a high mortality with surgery but it is less than with medical therapy alone. The earlier in life the infant goes into failure, the less likely he is to survive. Many will improve temporarily with digitalis and

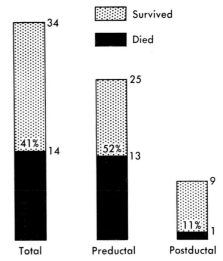

Figure 39-13. The operative mortality for infants under one year of age is shown. The preductal type has a much higher death rate than the postductal type.

then progress to a fatal outcome over a few days. ▷Infants with coarctation of the aorta and in congestive heart failure in the first month or six weeks of life are best treated with digitalis as soon as the diagnosis is made. The baby may be digitalized over a period of 8 to 12 hours. Oxygen, and furosemide may be used as indicated. Such babies will often improve considerably with such therapy and, if operated on during this stage of improvement, will survive. The ductus is closed at the same time that the coarctation is resected. A ventricular septal defect may be left unattended, repaired, or palliated by pulmonary artery banding, varying upon its size and the local surgical experience. Moderate to small defects, regardless of shunt size, can probably be given medical trial after coarctectomy, as many become smaller over time (Neches et al., 1977).

If endocardial fibroelastosis accompanies the coarctation, as indicated by inverted T waves in precordial lead V_6 and a positive mumps antigen skin test, prompt surgery is usually required.

Prognosis

In the past, without digitalis 60 percent of the postductal type of infants who developed signs or symptoms in the first year of life died, as did 90 percent of those with the preductal type. The more frequent association with serious cardiac defects mediates against the preductal type.

However, with the prompt early use of digitalis, this mortality can be greatly reduced and, in those who do not respond to digitalis, surgery will offer successful correction in the majority. Thus, the prognosis in the future should be good. There should be relatively few deaths among those with simple coarctation of the aorta. When it is complicated by serious cyanotic-producing congenital heart anomalies, the mortality will continue to be high unless the complicating defect is one that can be corrected at the same time as the coarctation.

Recurrent Coarctation of the Aorta or Restenosis of Coarctation of the Aorta

d'Abreu and Parsons (1956) reported examples of restenosis occurring after the usual end-to-end anastomosis performed to correct coarctation of the aorta. Infants who had been successfully treated were found to have excellent pulsation of femoral arteries, but within a period of a few months or a few years, the pulses disappeared in the legs and a tightly coarcted narrowing of the aorta could be demonstrated by aortography. Similar findings have been reported by Khoury and Hawes (1968), Ibarra-Perez and associates (1969), and Hallman and coworkers (1967). The restenosis has been attributed to various causes: (1) inadequate repair of the initial operation, (2) failure of growth of the anastomosis when performed in a small child, or (3) restenosis in the region of the original suture line, due to either fibrosis,

thrombosis, or granuloma. Finally, (4) Mulder and Linde (1959) have suggested that there is residual ductal tissue in the aorta well above and below the actual site of the coarctation, so that unless this is removed, reactive hyperplasia may occur after adequate correction and result in restenosis.

Khoury and Hawes described 9 of 25 infants who showed technically successful coarctation where operation was followed by development of restenosis. Cerilli and Lauridsen (1965) described six patients, 5 to 24 years of age, in whom reoperation for recurrent coarctation was necessary. Parsons and Astley (1966) reported immediate and delayed restenosis in ten patients, five of whom were under one year of age and five over eighty years of age at the time of operation.

Eshaghpour and Olley (1972) and Connors and associates (1975) have shown a relatively high incidence of recoarctation of the aorta, 16 to 33 percent in the infant group. This need not inhibit the decision for surgery early in life if the baby is in failure or his survival endangered. However, it does point to the importance of avoiding operation in infancy if it is not necessary. The appropriate time appears to be around five years of age.

COARCTATION OF THE ABDOMINAL AORTA

COARCTATION of the abdominal aorta is an uncommon lesion that, in spite of its rarity, needs to be considered each time one finds an elevated systemic blood pressure, particularly if there is evidence of an associated renal involvement.

This type of defect was first described by Quain in 1847 and later by Power in 1861, but it appears to have a different origin from that of a thoracic coarctation, since a variety of etiologic factors may lead to its evolution. These include (1) a fusion error in the development of the paired dorsal aortae, (2) a form of primary aortitis, (3) nonspecific aortitis, (4) infantile hypercalcemia, (5) rubella, (6) von Recklinghausen's disease, (7) pulseless disease, (8) certain infectious diseases, and (9) periaortic fibrosis.

Incidence

Onat (1969) puts the incidence at autopsy at 1:62 (500 postmortems). Sloan and Cooley, in 1953, estimated that abdominal coarctation occurs in about 2 percent of all types of coarctations. At The Hospital for Sick Children, we have seen 762 cases of coarctation of the aorta in the upper thoracic area of the isthmus but at the same time we have only seen four cases of abdominal coarctation. Sloan and Cooley (1953) found that female-to-male relationship was approximately 2:1. In a Japanese study by Daymond and Kamura (1964) the relationship was approximately three females to one male, and a similar female preponderance was reported by Sen and associates

(1963) and by DeBakey and associates (1967). However, Onat found the proportion was 33 females to 29 males in a study involving Caucasians in Turkey.

The type of narrowing may be circumscribed as in thoracic aorta and this occurs in approximately two-thirds of the cases. The other third have a diffused hypoplasia sometimes covering several centimeters. One or both renal arteries are involved in approximately two-thirds of the cases. Other cardiovascular lesions may occur simultaneously; these include aortic valvar stenosis, mitral regurgitation, pulmonary artery stenosis, and coarctation of the isthmus. A bicuspid aortic valve is seen in approximately 30 percent of the cases with coarctation in the thoracic aorta but so far has not been reported in abdominal coarctation. This, in itself, suggests the two types have different origins.

Diagnosis

The accurate diagnosis depends on showing by angiocardiography the abdominal aorta and renal arteries. Since it is impractical or undesirable to do such studies routinely in all cases of coarctation of the aorta, it is important to select certain signs that will aid in suggesting that one should look for narrowing below the diaphragm. Thus, following the identification of a gradient difference between the blood pressure in arm and leg, particular attention should be paid to the following: (1) a bruit over the abdomen or lumbar areas, (2) evidence of associated renal disease, (3) heart failure, particularly in the presence of coarctation in children after the age of one year, (4) unusually high blood pressure in the arms, e.g., over 180 mm of mercury, (5) a barium swallow that fails to show the E sign in the area of the aortic arch, and (6) notching isolated to the lower ribs is a suspicious sign of abdominal coarctation, as is the presence of any renal abnormality.

Symptoms are usually mild in infancy and childhood, although occasional headache, weakness, and even heart failure may occur. The latter has been reported in 16 percent of cases, chiefly in the early childhood years but can occur rarely in infancy. In thoracic coarctation it is very common to have heart failure in the infant age group, but it is rare to have this occur after one year of age.

Surgical Management

Coarctation of the abdominal aorta usually requires corrective surgery. There is no urgency for such procedure in childhood unless congestive heart failure is present or the blood pressure is excessively high.

No one center has been able to treat any large number of such cases surgically but a modest surgical experience has developed in recent years in dealing with this problem. Fifty-three patients have been reported as having some operation for correction of this anomaly. Most of these have had relief of their hypertension. Thirty-seven had a satisfactory drop in blood pressure; 15 had minimal or insignificant drop in pressure; and six have died postoperatively of congestive heart failure.

Surgery may involve one or more procedures; either a simple resection of a localized coarcted area or, at times, a graft, either a homograft or prosthetic, may be required if there is a prolonged hypoplastic aortic segment. If there is renal artery involvement, as is frequently the case, the surgeon must be prepared to deal with such pathology, by either a graft or bypass technique. DeBakey in 1967 recommended a bypass or repair of the renal artery if there is a gradient between the aorta and the renal artery. At times the visceral arteries may be hypoplastic and narrowed and may require bypass connection to deal adequately with the patient. The multiplicity of problems involved are reviewed and summarized by Schurch and associates (1975), although they are approaching from the type that includes neurofibromatosis.

PSEUDOCOARCTATION OF THE AORTA

PSEUDOCOARCTATION of the aortic arch was first described by three authors independently, including Steinberg, Robb, and Souders and associates, all in 1951. It has been defined as an elongation and kinking of the aortic isthmus that differs from true coarctation of the aorta by the absence of significant narrowing of the lumen. The subject has been well reviewed by Dungan and associates (1970), Kavanagh-Gray (1970), Steinberg and associates (1969), and Hoeffel and colleagues (1975). There have been 90 cases reported in the literature to date, many of them with excellent angiograms showing the pseudocoarcted area of kinking. The characteristic appearance is that of a long aortic arch elevated slightly toward the head and toward the left with a kink occurring at the aortic isthmus distal to the origin of the left subclavian. There is little or no obstruction at this point, but as a rule a murmur is audible, either due to the kinking or due to an associated congenital anomaly of the heart. The blood pressures are found to be normal in arm and leg, although minor differences have been reported.

There is no collateral circulation, such as is found in true coarctation of the aorta. The heart size is usually normal unless there is associated heart defect. There is a wide, high aortic arch in the anteroposterior film of the chest with a bulge usually recognizable in the left upper border of the mediastinum due to a dilated portion of the aorta above the kink. At times this bulge is sufficient to be referred to as an aneurysm and has been mistakenly diagnosed as a tumor until angiocardiography demonstrated its true origin. The majority of cases reported in the literature to date were identified in adult life but a number have been recognized in childhood, the youngest being a two-month-old boy reported by Kavanagh-Gray (1970).

With the clinical signs indicated above, the diagnosis may be suspected but angiocardiography is necessary to confirm it and is best done in the AP and in the right posterior oblique projection.

The prognosis is usually good. A few deaths have been reported but usually these are related to the associated anomalies rather than to the pseudocoarctation itself. There have been a number of patients reported to have died of an aneurysm in the aorta in their thirties and forties.

Bicuspid aortic valve has been noted to be associated with this lesion, as has been aortic stenosis, subaortic stenosis, corrected transposition, ventricular septal defect, infundibular stenosis, patent ductus, fibroelastosis, and aneurysm of the aortic sinuses.

It is believed by some that the ligamentum ductus may contribute to the kinking, and at times there may be some advantage to be gained from severing the ligamentum if there is a difference to the blood pressure in the arm and the leg. Surgery in limited cases has been recommended by Gay and Young (1969).

INTERRUPTED AORTIC ARCH + 80% V.S.D

THIS anomaly has been subdivided by Celoria and Patton into three types.

Type A: Interruption of the aortic arch distal to the left subclavian artery. This type comprised 42 percent of the cases reviewed by Van Praagh (1971). *Type B:* The interruption occurs between the left common carotid artery and the left subclavian artery. It occurs in 53 percent of the overall group. *Type C:* Interruption of the aortic arch proximal to the left carotid artery. It is found in only 5 percent of the total.

most common

Eighty percent of such infants have an associated ventricular septal defect. Other anomalies may occur as well.

In the series reported by Van Praagh (1971), this lesion accounted for 4 percent of the deaths in neonates dying of congenital heart disease.

The hemodynamic effect of the interrupted arch is similar to severe coarctation of the aorta with the presence of a patent ductus. The lower aorta arises from the pulmonary artery as a continuation of a patent ductus. The frequent presence of a ventricular septal defect further complicates the clinical and therapeutic picture.

The surgeons prefer to do as complete a repair as possible, joining two ends of the aorta and eliminating the patent ductus (Trusler and Izukawa, 1975). A variety of other procedures have been reported in dealing with this lesion. Murphy (1971, 1973), Tyson and associates (1970), Barratt-Boyes and associates (1972). These include (1) a graft, and (2) turning down subclavian artery into descending aorta.

REFERENCES

Coarctation of the Thoracic Aorta

Acevedo, R. E.; Thilenius, O. G.; Moulder, P. V.; and Cassels, D. E.: Kinking of the aorta (pseudocoarctation) with coarctation. *Am. J. Cardiol.*, 21:442, 1968.

Adams, P., Jr.; Keele, M.; and Baronofsky, I. D.: Coarctation of aorta in infants. *J. Lancet*, 75:66, 1955.

Alderson, J. D.: Single coronary artery, and dissecting aneurysm of ascending aorta following resection of coarctation of aorta. *Thorax*, 27:90, 1972.

Bahn, R. C.; Edwards, J. E.; and Du Shane, J. W.: Coarctation of the aorta as a cause of death in early infancy. *Pediatrics*, 8:192, 1951.

Bahnson, H. T.: Coarctation of the aorta and anomalies of the aortic arch. *Surg. Clin. North Am.*, 32:1313, 1952.

Bailey, C. P.: Report of the section on cardiovascular surgery, American College of Chest Physicians, On the surgical treatment of coarctation of the aorta. *Dis. Chest*, 31:468, 1957.

———: Morphogenesis of human aortic coarctation. *Exp. Mol. Pathol.*, 6:25, 1967.

Balis, J. U.; Chan, A. S.; and Conen, P. E.: Lathyrogenic injury to foetal rat aorta and post-natal repair. *Exp. Mol. Pathol.*, 5:396, 1966.

Baronofsky, I. D., and Adams, P., Jr.: Resection of an aortic coarctation in a two week old infant. *Ann. Surg.*, 139:494, 1954.

Barratt-Boyes, B. G.; Nicholls, T. T.; Brandt, P. W. T.; and Neutze, J. M.: Aortic arch interruption associated with patent ductus arteriosus, ventricular septal defect, and total anomalous pulmonary venous connection. *J. Thorac. Cardiovasc. Surg.*, 63:367, 1972.

Bauer, D. de F., and Astbury, E. C.: Congenital cardiac disease: bibliography of the 1,000 cases analyzed in Maude Abbott's Atlas, with an index. *Am. Heart J.*, 27:688, 1944.

Beattie, E. J.; Nolan, J.; and Howe, J. S.: Paralysis following surgical correction of coarctation of the aorta. *Surgery*, 33:754, 1953.

Becker, A. E.; Becker, M. J.; and Edwards, J. E.: Anomalies associated with coarctation of aorta. Particular reference to infancy. *Circulation*, 41:1067, 1970.

Behrer, M. R.; Peterson, F. D.; and Goldring, D.: Coarctation of the aorta and associated patent ductus arteriosus. II. Postoperative studies of infants. *J. Pediatr.*, 56:246, 1960.

Bellet, S., and Gelfand, D.: Coarctation of the aorta: rupture through a "jet lesion" distal to the point of coarctation. *Arch. Intern. Med.*, 90:266, 1952.

Benson, C. D.; Mustard, W. T.; Ravitch, M. M.; Snyder, W. M.; and Welch, K. J.: *Pediatric Surgery*, vol. 1. Year Book Publishers, Inc., Chicago, 1962, p. 419.

Bing, R. J.; Handelsman, J. C.; Campbell, J. A.; Griswold, H. E.; and Blalock, A.: The surgical treatment and the physiopathology of coarctation of the aorta. *Ann. Surg.*, 128:803, 1948.

Blackford, L. M.: Coarctation of the aorta. *Arch. Intern. Med.*, 41:702, 1928.

Blalock, A., and Park, E. A.: The surgical treatment of experimental coarctation of the aorta. *Ann. Surg.*, 119:445, 1944.

Bliddal, J.; Dupont, B.; Melchior, J. C.; and Ottesen, O. E.: Coarctation of the aorta with multiple artery anomalies in idiopathic hypercalcemia of infancy. *Acta Paediatr. Scand.*, 58:632, 1969.

Blumgart, H. L.; Lawrence, J. S.; and Ernstene, A. C.: The dynamics of the circulation in coarctation (stenosis of the isthmus) of the aorta of the adult type, relation to essential hypertension. *Arch. Intern. Med.*, 47:806, 1931.

Bonnet, L. M.: Sur la lésion dite stenose congénitale de l'aorte dans la région de l'isthme. *Rev. Méd. Paris*, 23:108, 255, 335, 418, 481, 1903.

Boyd, D. P.: Surgical treatment of coarctation of the aorta in the adult. *Am. Surg.*, 20:1246, 1954.

Bramwell, C.: Coarctation of the aorta: II. Clinical features. *Br. Heart J.*, 9:100, 1947.

Brown, G. E., Jr.; Clagett, O. T.; Burchell, H. B.; and Wood, E. H.: Preoperative and postoperative studies of intraradial and intrafemoral pressures in patients with coarctation of the aorta. *Proc. Mayo Clin.*, 23:352, 1948.

Bruwer, A., and Pugh, D. G.: A neglected roentgenological sign of coarctation of the aorta. *Proc. Mayo Clin.*, 27:377, 1952.

Bull, C.; Hoeksem, A. T.; Duckworth, J. W. A.; and Mustard, W. T.: An experimental study of the growth of arterial anastomoses. *Can. J. Surg.*, 6:383, 1963.

Busch, F.: Roentgen examination in coarctation of the aorta. *Acta Radiol.*, 37:216, 1951.

Calodney, M. M., and Carson, M. J.: Coarctation of the aorta in early infancy. *J. Pediat.*, 37:46, 1950.

Campbell, M., and Baylis, J. H.: Course and prognosis of coarctation of the aorta. *Br. Heart J.*, 18:475, 1956.

Campbell, M., and Cardell, B. S.: A case of Eisenmenger's complex with coarctation of the aorta. *Guy Hosp. Rep.*, 102:327, 1953.

Campbell, M., and Polani, P. E.: The etiology of coarctation of the aorta. *Lancet*, 1:463, 1961.

Campbell, M., and Suzman, S.: Coarctation of the aorta. *Br. Heart J.*, 9:185, 1947.

Celoria, G. C., and Patton, R. B.: Congenital absence of the aortic arch. *Am. Heart J.*, 58:407, 1959.

Cerilli, J. L., and Laurisden, P.: Reoperation for coarctation of the aorta. *Acta Chir. Scand.* 129:391, 1965.

Champsaur, G.: Personal communication, 1972.

Christensen, N. A.: Coarctation of the aorta: historical review. *Proc. Mayo Clin.*, 23:322, 1948.

Christensen, N. A., and Hines, E. A., Jr.: Clinical features in coarctation of the aorta: a review of 96 cases. *Proc. Mayo Clin.*, 23:339, 1948.

Clagett, O. T.: The surgical treatment of coarctation of the aorta. *Proc. Mayo Clin.*, 23:359, 1948.

Clagett, O. T., and DuShane, J. W.: Diagnosis and management of coarctation of the aorta in children. *Pediatr. Clin. North Am.*, Feb., 1954, p. 173.

Clagett, O. T.; Kirklin, J. W.; and Edwards, J. E.: Anatomic variations and pathologic changes in coarctation of the aorta: a study of 124 cases. *Surg. Gynecol. Obstet.*, 98:103, 1954.

Clatworthy, H. W., Jr.; Sako, Y.; Chisholm, T. C.; Culmer, C.; and Varco, R. L.: Thoracic aortic coarctation. Its experimental production in dogs, with special reference to technical methods capable of inducing significant intraluminal stenosis. *Surgery*, 28:245, 1950.

Cleland, W. P.; Counihan, T. B.; Goodwin, J. F.; and Steiner, R. E.: Coarctation of the aorta. *Br. Med. J.*, 2:379, 1956.

Connors, J. P.; Hartmann, A. F.; and Weldon, C. S.: Considerations in the surgical management of infantile coarctation of aorta. *Am. J. Cardiol.*, 36:489, 1975.

Counihan, T. B.: Changes in the blood pressure following resection of coarctation of the aortic arch. *Clin. Sci.*, 15:149, 1956.

Crafoord, C., and Nylin, G.: Congenital coarctation of aorta and its surgical tteatment. *J. Thorac. Surg.*, 14:347, 1945.

Culbertson, J. W.; Eckstein, J. W.; Kirkendall, W. M.; and Bedell, G. N.: General hemodynamics and splanchnic circulation in patients with coarctation of the aorta. *J. Clin. Invest.*, 36:1537, 1957.

d'Abreu, A. L., and Parsons, C.: Surgical treatment of children with coarctation of the aorta. *Br. Med. J.*, 2:390, 1956.

De Grott, J. W. C., and Hartog, H. A. P.: Indications for operation of coarctation of the aorta in children. *Arch. Chir. Neerl.*, 5:329, 1953.

Deterling, R. A., Jr.: Resection of an acquired coarctation of the low thoracic aorta and replacement with a preserved vessel graft. *J. Thorac. Surg.*, 2:290, 1953.

Donnan, F. de S., and Beck, D.: Subarachnoid haemorrhage and hypertension in a case of coarctation of the aorta. *Arch. Middlesex Hosp.*, 4:144, 1954.

Dotter, C. T.; Steinberg, I.; and Catalano, D.: Roentgenologic aspects of coarctation of the aorta. *N. Y. J. Med.*, 58:182, 1953.

Dotter, C. T., and Steinberg, I.: *Angiocardiography*. Paul B. Hoeber, Inc., New York, 1951, p. 181.

Dry, T. J.; Clagett, O. T.; Saxon, R. F.; Pugh, D. G.; and Edwards, J. E.: Double aortic arch associated with coarctation of the aorta: surgically treated patient. *Dis. Chest*, 23:36, 1953.

Dubilier, W.; Taylor, T. L.; and Steinberg, I.: Aortic sinus aneurysm associated with coarctation of the aorta. *Am. J. Roentgenol.*, 73:10, 1955.

Dungan, W. T.; Char. F.; Gerald. B. E.; and Campberg. S. G.: Pseudocoarctation of the aorta in childhood. *Am. J. Dis. Child.*, 119:401, 1970.

Easthope, R. N.; Tawes, R. L., Jr.; Bonham-Carter, R. E.; Aberdeen, E.; and Waterston, D. J.: Congenital mitral valve disease associated with coarctation of the aorta. *Am. Heart. J.*, 77:743, 1969.

Edwards, J. E.; Christensen, N. A.; Clagett, O. T.; and McDonald, J. R.: Pathologic considerations in coarctation of the aorta. *Proc. Mayo Clin.*, 23:324, 1948.

Edwards, J. E.; Clagett, O. T.; Drake, R. L.; and Christensen, N. A.: The collateral circulation in coarctation of the aorta. *Proc. Mayo Clin.*, 23:333, 1948.

Edwards, J. E.; Douglas, J. M.; Burchell, H. B.; and Christensen, N. A.: Pathology of intrapulmonary arteries and arterioles in coarctation of aorta associated with patent ductus arteriosus. *Am. Heart J.*, 38:205, 1949.

Edwards, W. S., and Lyons, C.: Three years' experience with peripheral arterial grafts of crimped nylon and teflon. *Surgery*, 107:62, 1958.

Engle, M. A.: Personal communication, 1956.

Eshaghpour, E., and Olley, P. M.: Recoarctation of the aorta following coarctectomy in the first year of life. A follow-up study. *J. Pediatr.*, 80:809–14, 1972.

Evans, W.: Congenital stenosis (coarctation), atresia, and interruption of the aortic arch (a study of twenty-eight cases). *Q. J. Med.*, 2:1, 1933.

Everts-Suarez, E. A., and Carson, C. P.: The triad of congenital absence of the aortic arch (isthmus aortae). Patent ductus arteriosus and interventricular septal defect—a trilogy. *Ann. Surg.*, 150:153, 1959.

Figley, M. M.: Accessory roentgen signs of coarctation of the aorta. *Radiology*, 62:671, 1954.

Foster, J. H.; Collins, H. A.; Jacobs, J. K.; and Scott, H. W., Jr.: Long term follow-up of homografts used in the treatment of coarctation of the aorta. *J. Cardiovasc. Surg.*, 6:111, 1965.

Foster, J. H.; Ekman, C.; and Scott, H. W., Jr.: Late behavior of vascular substitutes: three to five year follow-up of arterial homografts and synthetic prostheses in experimental animals. *Ann. Surg.*, 151:867, 1960.

Freed. M. D.; Keane. J. R.; Van Praagh, R.; Castaneda. A. R.; Bernhard. W. F.; and Nadas. A. S.: Coarctation of the aorta with congenital mitral regurgitation. *Circulation*. 49:1175, 1974.

Furman, R. H.; Kennedy, J. A.; and Daniel, R. A.: Coarctation of the aorta complicated by dissecting aneurysm in pregnancy: report of a case with survival studied by arteriography. *Am. Heart J.*, 43:765, 1952.

Gaertner, R. A., and Blalock, A.: Experimental coarctation of the ascending aorta. *Surgery*, 40:712, 1956.

Gammelgaard, A., and Friis-Hansen, B.: Acute abdominal reaction following operation for coarctation of the aorta. *Acta Chir. Scand.*, 119:361, 1960.

Garman, J. E.; Hinson, R. E.; and Eyler, W. R.: Coarctation of the aorta in infancy: Detection on chest radiographs. *Radiology*, 85:418, 1965.

Gay, W. A., and Young, W. G.: Pseudocoarctation of the aorta, a reappraisal. *J. Thorac. Cardiovasc. Surg.*, 58:739, 1969.

Gerbode, F.: The use of the enlarged left subclavian artery to overcome defects associated with complicated coarctation of the aorta. *Surgery*, 37:58, 1955.

Gerbode, F., and Hultgren, H.: A method of producing coarctation of the aorta in the growing animal. *Surgery*, 29:441, 1951.

Gerbode, F.; Purdy, A.; Alway, R.; Piel, G.; and Da Costa, A.: Surgical treatment of the aorta in infancy. *Am. J. Surg.*, 89:1138, 1955.

Gillman, R. G., and Burton, A. C.: Constriction of the neonatal aorta by raised oxygen tension. *Circ. Res.*, 19:755, 1966.

Glass, I. H.; Mustard, W. T.; and Keith, J. D.: Coarctation of the aorta in infants. *Pediatrics*, 26:109, 1960.

Glenn, F., and O'Sullivan, W. D.: Coarctation of the aorta. *Ann. Surg.*, 136:770, 1952.

Goldblatt, H.: Experimental renal hypertension. *Am. J. Med.*, 4:100, 1948.

Goldblatt, H.; Kahn, J. R.; and Hanzal, R. F.: IX. The effect on blood pressure of constriction of the abdominal aorta above and below the site of origin of both main renal arteries. *J. Exp. Med.*, 69:649, 1939.

Goldblatt, H.; Lynch, J.; Hanzal, R. F.; and Summerville, W. W.: Studies on experimental hypertension. I. The production of persistent elevation of systolic blood pressure by means of renal ischemia. *J. Exp. Med.*, 59:347, 1934.

Gonzalez-Cerna, J. L.; Villavicencio, L.; Molina, B.; and Bessudo, L.: Nonspecific obliterative aortitis in children. *Ann. Thorac. Surg.*, 4:193, 1967.

Gross, R. E.: Coarctation of the aorta: surgical treatment of one hundred cases. *Circulation*, 1:41, 1950.

———: Coarctation of the aorta. *Circulation*, 7:757, 1953.

Gross, R. E., and Hufnagel, C. A.: Coarctation of the aorta: experimental studies regarding its surgical correction. *N. Engl. J. Med.*, 233:287, 1945.

Grotts, B. F.: Coarctation of the aorta in a child. *US Armed Forces Med. J.*, 3:585, 1952.

Groves, L. K., and Effler, D. B.: Problems, in the surgical management of coarctation of the aorta. *J. Thorac. Cardiovasc. Surg.*, 39:60, 1960.

Gupta, T. C., and Wiggers, C. J.: Basic hemodynamic changes produced by aortic coarctation of different degrees. *Circulation*, 3:17, 1951.

Hagstrom, J. W. C., and Steinberg, I.: Pathologic lesion in pseudocoarctation of arch of aorta. (abstr.) *Circulation*, 26:726, 1962.

Hallman, G. L.; Yasher, J. L.; Bloodwell, R. D.; and Colley, D. A.: Surgical correction of coarctation of the aorta in the first year of life. *Ann. Thorac. Surg.*, 4:106, 1967.

Harrison, J. H.: Synthetic materials as vascular prostheses. Long term studies on grafts of nylon, dacron, orlon, and teflon replacing large blood vessels. *Surg. Gynecol. Obstet.*, 108:433, 1959.

Hoeffel, J. C.; Henry, M.; Mentre, B.; Louis, J. P.; and Pernot, C.:

Pseudocoarctation or congenital kinking of the aorta: radiological considerations. *Am. Heart J.*, **89**:428, 1975.

Huang, T. T.; Wolma, F. J.; and Tyson, K. R.: Coarctation of the abdominal aorta. *Am. J. Surg.*, **120**:598, 1970.

Hurt, R. L., and Hanbury, W. J.: Intestinal vascular lesions simulating polyarteritis nodosa after resection of coarctation of the aorta. *Thorax*, **12**:258, 1957.

Hurwitt, E. S., and Altman, S. F.: Observations on the growth of aortic anastomoses in puppies: II. Comparative effects of silk and catgut sutures on the growth of vascular anastomoses. *Angiology*, **5**:27, 1954.

Hurwitt, E. S., and Brahms, S. A.: Observations on growth of aortic anastomoses in puppies. *An.. Surg.*, **133**:200, 1951.

Hurwitt, E. S., and Rosenblatt, M. A.: Observations on the growth of aortic anastomoses in puppies. III. Use of absorbable gelatin sponge (Gelfoam) in relation to growth. *Arch. Surg.*, **70**:491, 1955.

Hutchins, G. M.: Coarctation of the aorta as a branch-point of the ductus arteriosus. *Am. J. Pathol.*, **63**:203, 1971.

Ibarra-Perez, C.; Castaneda, A. R.; et al.: Re-coarctation of the aorta. Nineteen year clinical experience. *Am. J. Cardiol.*, **23**:778, 1969.

Jacobson, G.; Cosby, R. S.; Griffith, G. C.; and Meyer, B. W.: Valvular stenosis as a cause of death in surgically treated coarctation of the aorta. *Am. Heart J.*, **45**:889, 1953.

Johnson, A. L.; Ferencz, C.; Wiglesworth, F. W.; and McRae, D. L.: Coarctation of the aorta complicated by patency of the ductus arteriosus. *Circulation*, **4**:242, 1951.

Jones, M. D., and Steinbach, H. L.: Coarctation of the aorta with regression of rib notching following surgery. Report of a case. *Radiology*, **63**:248, 1954.

Kavanagh-Gray, D., and Chiu, P.: Kinking of the aorta (pseudocoarctation). *Can. Med. Assoc. J.*, **103**:717, 1970.

Keefer, E.; Glen, F.; and Dotter, C.: Resection and end-to-end anastomosis of thoracic aorta in puppies; two and three quarter year follow-up. *Ann. Surg.*, **134**:969, 1951.

Kempton, J. J., and Waterston, D. J.: Coarctation of aorta presenting as cardiac failure in early infancy. *Br. Med. J.*, **2**:442, 1957.

Khoury, G. H., and Hawes, C. R.: Recurrent coarctation of the aorta in infancy and childhood. *J. Pediatr.*, **72**:801, 1968.

Kirkendall, W. M.; Culbertson, J. W.; and Eckstein, J. W.: Renal hemodynamics in patients with coarctation of the aorta. *J. Lab. Clin. Med.*, **53**:6, 1959.

Kirklin, J. W.; Burchell, H. B.; Pugh, D. G.; Burke, E. C.; and Mills, S. D.: Surgical treatment of coarctation of the aorta in a ten week old infant: report of a case. *Circulation*, **6**:411, 1952.

Kittle, C. F., and Schafer, P. W.: Gangrene of the forearm after subclavin arterioaortostomy for coarctation of the aorta. *Thorax*, **8**:319, 1953.

Klemola, E.: Ueber familiäres Aufteten von Isthmusstenose der Aorta. *Acta Med. Scand.*, **98**:355, 1939.

Kondo, B.; Winsor, T.; Raulston, B. O.; and Kuroiwa, D.: Congenital coarctation of the abdominal aorta: a theoretically reversible type of cardiac disease. *Am. Heart J.*, **39**:306, 1950.

Landtman, B., and Tuuteri, L.: Vascular complications in coarctation of the aorta. *Acta Paediatr.*, **48**:329, 1959.

Lang, H. T., and Nadas, A. S.: Coarctation of the aorta with congestive heart failure in infancy—medical treatment. *Pediatrics*, **17**:45, 1956.

Lavin, N.; Mehta, S.; Liberson, M.; and Pouget, J. M.: Pseudo-coarctation of the aorta: An unusual variant with coarctation. *Am. J. Cardiol.*, **24**:584, 1969.

Leading article: Coarctation of the aorta. *Lancet*, **2**:867, 1953.

Lester, R. G.; Margulis, A. R.; and Nice, C. M., Jr.: Roentgenographic evaluation of coarctation of the aorta in infants. *JAMA*, **163**:1022, 1957.

Little, R. C.: The etiology of hypertension in coarctation of the aorta. *South. Med. J.*, **46**:911, 1953.

Luidesmith, G. G.; Stanton, R. E.; Stiles, Q. R.; Meyer, B. W.; and Jones, J. C.: Coarctation of the thoracic aorta. Current review. *Ann. Thorac. Surg.*, **11**:482, 1971.

Lyons, H. A.: Coarctation of the aorta. *U.S. Armed Forces Med. J.*, **5**:47, 1954.

McGregor, M., and Medalie, M.: Coarctation of the aorta. *Br. Heart J.*, **14**:531, 1952.

Malm, J. R., and Blumenthal, S.: Observations on coarctation of the aorta in infants. *Arch. Surg.*, **86**:96, 1963.

March, H. W.; Hultgren, H. W.; and Gerbode, F.: Immediate and remote effects of resection on the hypertension in coarctation of the aorta. *Br. Heart J.*, **22**:361, 1960.

Marks, D. N.; Shapiro, R. S.; and Joseph, L. G.: Roentgenographic diagnosis of coarctation of the aorta in a two-day old infant. *J. Pediatr.*, **43**:453, 1953.

Maron, B. J.; O'Neal Humphries, J.; Rowe, R. D.; and Mellits, E. D.: Prognosis of surgically corrected coarctation of the aorta: A 20-year postoperative appraisal. *Circulation*, **47**:119, 1973.

Master, A. M.; Dublin, L. I.; and Marks, H. H.: Normal blood pressure range and its clinical implications. *JAMA*, **143**:1464, 1950.

Mathey, J., et al.: Traitement chirurgical de la stenose isthmique de l'aorte chez le nourrisson. *Mem. Acad. Chir.*, **80**:89, 1954.

Moes, C. A.; Peckham, G. B.; and Keith, J. D.: Idiopathic hypertrophy of the interventricular septum causing muscular subaortic stenosis in children. *Radiology*, **83**:283, 1964.

Morris, G. C.; Cooley, D. A.; DeBakey, M. E.; and Crawford, E. S.: Coarctation of the aorta with particular emphasis upon improved techniques of surgical repair. *J. Thorac. Surg.*, **40**:705, 1960.

Mortensen, J. D.; Cutler, P. R.; Rummel, W. R.; and Veasy, L. G.: Management of coarctation of the aorta in infancy. *J. Thorac. Surg.*, **37**:502, 1959.

Moss, A. J.; Adams, F. H.; O'Loughlin, B. H.; and Dixon, W. J.: The growth of the normal aorta and of the anastomotic site in infants following surgical resection of coarctation of the aorta. *Circulation*, **19**:338, 1959.

Mulder, D. G., and Linde, L. M.: Recurrent coarctation of the aorta in infancy. *Am. Surg.*, **25**:908, 1959.

Murphy, D. A.; Collins, G.; and Dobell, A. R. C.: Surgical correction of type A congenital aortic arch interruption. *Ann. Thorac. Surg.*, **11**:593, 1971.

Murphy, D. A.; Lemire, G. G.; Tessler, L.; and Dunn, G. L.: Correction of type B aortic arch interruption with ventricular and atrial septal defects in a three day old infant. *J. Thorac. Cardiovasc. Surg.*, **65**:882, 1973.

Murray, G.: Surgical treatment of coarctation of the aorta. *Can. Med. Assoc. J.*, **62**:241, 1950.

Mustard, W. T.; Rowe, R. D.; Keith, J. D.; and Sirek, A.: Coarctation of the aorta with special reference to the first year of life. *Ann. Surg.*, **141**:429, 1955.

Nadas, A. S.: *Pediatric Cardiology*. W. B. Saunders Company, Philadelphia, 1957.

Nanton, M. A., and Olley, P.: Residual hypertension after coarctectomy in children. *Am. J. Cardiol.*, **47**:769, 1976.

Neches, W. H.; Park, S. C.; Lenox, C. C.; Zuberbuhler, J. R.; Siewers, R. D.; and Hardesty, R. L.: Coarctation of the aorta with ventricular septal defect. *Circulation*, **55**:189, 1977.

Olney, M. B., and Stephens, H. B.: Coarctation of the aorta in children. *J. Pediatr.*, **37**:639, 1950.

Onat, T., and Zeren, E.: Coarctation of the abdominal aorta. Review of 91 cases. *Cardiology*, **54**:140, 1969.

O'Rourke, M. F., and Cartmill, T. B.: Influence of aortic coarctation on pulsatile hemodynamics in the proximal aorta. *Circulation*, **44**:281, 1971.

O'Sullivan, W. D.: Atresia of the subclavian artery associated with coarctectomy in children. *Am. J. Cardiol.*, **47**:769, 1976.

Page, I. H.: The effect of chronic constriction of the aorta on arterial blood pressure in dogs: an attempt to produce coarctation of the aorta. *Am. Heart J.*, **19**:218, 1940.

Page, I. H.; Dustan, H. P.; and Poutasse, E. F.: Mechanisms, diagnosis and treatment of hypertension of renal vascular origin. *Ann. Intern. Med.*, **51**:196, 1959.

Painter, R. C.; Hines, E. A., and Edwards, J. E.: Measurement of arterioles in coarctation of the aorta. *Circulation*, **6**:727, 1952.

Parsons, C. G., and Astley, R.: Recurrence of aortic coarctation after operation in childhood. *Br. Med. J.*, **1**:573, 1966.

Pelletier, C.; Davignon, A.; F-Ethier, M.; and Stanley, P.: Coarctation of the aorta in infancy. *J. Thorac. Cardiovasc. Surg.*, **57**:171, 1969.

Perez-Alvarez, J. J., and Oudkerk, S.: Necrotizing arteriolitis of the abdominal organs as a postoperative complication following correction of coarctation of the aorta. *Surgery*, **37**:833, 1955.

Perlman, L.: Coarctation of the aorta: clinical and roentgenological analysis of 13 cases. *Am. Heart J.*, **28**:24, 1944.

Polani, P. E.; Hunter, W. F.; and Lennox, B.: Chromosomal sex in Turner's syndrome with coarctation of the aorta. *Lancet*, **2**:210, 1954.

Pontius, R. G.; Brockman, H. L.; Hardy, E. G.; Cooley, D. A.; and

DeBakey, M. E.: The use of hypothermia in the prevention of paraplegia following temporary aortic occlusion: experimental observations. *Surgery*, 36:33, 1954.

Potts, W. J.: Technic of resection of coarctation of the aorta with aid of new instruments. *Ann. Surg.*, 131:466, 1950.

Power, J. H.: Observations on disease of the aortic valves producing both con-constriction of the aortic orifice and regurgitation through it into the left ventricle, accompanied with abnormal enlargement of the two internal mammary arteries and atrophy of the abdominal aorta and its iliac branches. *Dublin Q. J. Med.*, 32:314, 1861.

Pritchard, J. A.: Coarctation of the aorta and pregnancy. *Obstet. Gynecol. Surv.*, 8:775, 1953.

Pugh, D. G.: The value of roentgenologic diagnosis in coarctation of the aorta. *Proc. Mayo Clin.*, 23:343, 1948.

Rathi, L., and Keith, J. D.: Post-operative blood pressures in coarctation of the aorta, *Br. Heart J.*, 26:671, 1964.

Reifenstein, G. H.; Levine, S. A.; and Gross, R. E.: Coarctation of the aorta; a review of 104 autopsied cases of the "adult type," 2 years of age or older. *Am. Heart J.*, 33:146, 1947.

Reul, G. J.; Kabbani, S. S.; Sandiferd, F. M.; Wukasch, D. C.; and Cooley, D. A.: Repair of coarctation of the thoracic aorta by patch graft aortoplasty. *J. Thorac. Cardiovasc. Surg.*, 68:696, 1974.

Rhodes, P. H., and Durbin, E.: Coarctation of the aorta in childhood: review of the literature and report of three cases. *Am. J. Dis. Child.*, 64:1073, 1942.

Riemenschneider, T. A.; Emmanouilides, G. C.; Hirose, F.; and Linde, L. M.: Coarctation of the abdominal aorta in children: report of three cases and review of the literature. *Pediatrics*, 44:716, 1969.

Ring, D. M., and Lewis, F. J.: Abdominal pain following surgical correction of coarctation of the aorta: a syndrome. *J. Thorac. Surg.*, 31:718, 1956.

Robb, G. P.: Atlas of angiocardiography prepared for the American Registry of Pathology, A.F.I.P., National Research Council, Washington, D.C., 1951.

Robbins, L. L., and Wyman, S. M.: Coarctation of the thoracic aorta: signs demonstrable by conventional roentgenography. *N. Engl. J. Med.*, 248:747, 1953.

Robicsek, F.; Mullen, D. C.; and Daughterty, H. K.: Aortic aneurysms involving the origin of the renal arteries: A simple solution to a complicated problem. *Surgery*, 70:425, 1971.

Rogers, H. M.; Rudolph, C. C.; and Cordes, J. H., Jr.: Coarctation of the aorta in infancy: report of two cases with death from left ventricular failure. *Am. J. Med.*, 13:805, 1952.

Rosenberg, H. S.: Coarctation of the aorta. Morphology and pathogenic considerations. In Rosenberg, H. S., and Bolande, R. P. (eds.): *Perspectives in Pediatric Pathology.* Year Book Publishers, Inc., Chicago, 1973, page 339.

Rosenquist, G.: Congenital mitral valve disease associated with coarctation of the aorta. A spectrum that includes parachute deformity of the mitral valve. *Circulation*, 49:985, 1974.

Rosenthal, L.: Coarctation of the aorta and pregnancy: report of five cases. *Br. Med. J.*, 1:16, 1955.

Rudolph, A. M.; Heymann, M. A.; and Spitznas, U.: Hemodynamic considerations in the development of narrowing of the aorta. *Am. J. Cardiol.*, 39:514, 1972.

Sauvage, L. R., and Harkins, H. N.: Growth of vascular anastomoses: experimental study of influence of suture type and suture method with note on certain mechanical factors involved. *Bull. Hopkins Hosp.*, 91:276, 1952.

Schenk, W. G.; Menno, A. D.; and Martin, J. W.: Hemodynamics of experimental coarctation of the aorta. *Ann. Surg.*, 153:163, 1961.

Schroeder, H. A., and Olsen, N. S.: Pressor substances in arterial hypertension. II. Demonstration of pherentasin, a vasoactive material procured from blood. *J. Exp. Med.*, 92:545, 1950.

Schuster, S. R., and Gross, R. E.: Surgery for coarctation of the aorta. A review of 500 cases. *J. Thorac. Cardiovasc. Surg.*, 43:54, 1962.

Scott, H. W., Jr.: and Bahnson, H. T.: Evidence for a renal factor in the hypertension of experimental coarctation of the aorta. *Surgery*, 30:206, 1951.

Scott, H. W., Jr.; Collins, H. A.; Langa, A. M.; and Olsen, N. S.: Additional observations concerning the physiology of the hypertension associated with experimental coarctation of the aorta *Surgery*, 36:445, 1954.

Scovil, J. A.; Nanda, N. C.; Gross, C. M.; Lombardi, A. C.; Gramiak, R.; Lipchik, E. O.; and Manning, J. A.:

Echocardiographic studies of abnormalities associated with coarctation of the aorta. *Circulation*, 53:953, 1976.

Sealy, W. C.: Indications for surgical treatment of coarctation of the aorta. *Surg. Gynecol. Obstet.*, 97:301, 1953.

Sealy, W. C.; De Maria, W.; and Harris, J.: Studies of the development and nature of the hypertension in experimental coarctation of the aorta. *Surg. Gynecol. Obstet.*, 90:193, 1950.

Sealy, W. C.; Harris, J. S.; Young, W. G.; and Galloway, H. A.: Paradoxical hypertension following resection of coarctation of aorta. *Surgery*, 42:135, 1957.

Sen, P. K.; Kinare, S. G.; Engineer, S. D.; and Parulhar, G. B.: The middle aortic syndrome. *Br. Heart J.*, 25:610, 1963.

Shackleton, J.; Jones, R. S.; and Hamilton, D.: Preductal coarctation in the newborn period. Relief of coarctation utilising L. subclavian onlay graft. *Eur. J. Cardiol.*, 3:376, 1975.

Shearer, W. T.; Rutman, J. Y.; Weinberg, W. A.; and Goldring, D.: Coarctation of the aorta and cerebrovascular accident: A proposal for early corrective surgery. *J. Pediatr.*, 77:1004, 1970.

Shumacker, H. B., Jr.: Use of the subclavian artery in the surgical treatment of coarctation of the aorta. *Surg. Gynecol., Obstet.*, 93:491, 1951.

Simon, A. B., and Zloto, A. E.: Coarctation of the aorta. Longitudinal assessment of operated patients. *Circulation*, 50:456, 1974.

Sinha, S. N.; Kardatzke, M. L.; Cole, R. B.; et al.: Coarctation of the aorta in infancy. *Circulation*, 40:385, 1969.

Sloan, R. D., and Cooley, R. N.: Coarctation of the aorta: the roentgenologic aspects of one hundred and twenty-five surgically confirmed cases. *Radiology*, 61:701, 1953.

Smyth, P. T., and Edwards, J. E.: Pseudocoarctation, kinking or buckling of the aorta. *Circulation*, 46:1027, 1972.

Solomon, N. H., and King, H.: Coarctation of the aorta in the newborn: two cases diagnosed clinically,. *Am. Pract.*, 3:706, 1952.

Souders, C. R.; Pearson, C. M.; and Adams, H. D.: An aortic deformity simulating mediastinal tumor: a subclinical form of coarctation. *Dis. Chest*, 20:35, 1951.

Srouji, M. N., and Trusler, G. A.: Paradoxical hypertension and the abdominal pain syndrome following resection of coarctation of the aorta. *Can. Med. Assoc. J.*, 92:412, 1965.

Stansel, H. C., and Newbold, R.: Recurrent coarctation of the aorta. *Ann. Thorac. Surg.*, 11:380, 1971.

Stauffer, H. M., and Rigler, L. G.: Dilatation and pulsation of the left subclavian artery in the roentgen-ray diagnosis of coarctation of the aorta: roentgenkymographic studies in thirteen cases. *Circulation*, 1:294, 1950.

Steele, J. M.: Evidence for general distribution of peripheral resistance in coarctation of the aorta: report of three cases. *J. Clin. Invest.*, 20:473, 1941.

Steinberg, I.; Engle, M. A.; Holswade, G. R.; and Hagstrom, J. W. C.: Pseudocoarctation of the aorta associated with congenital heart disease. Report of ten cases. *Am. J. Roentgenol.*, 106:1, 1969.

Talner, N. S., and Berman, M. A.: Postnatal development of obstruction in coarctation of the aorta: Role of the ductus arteriosus. *Pediatrics*, 56:4, 1975.

Tawes, R. L., Jr.; Berry, C. L.; and Aberdeen, E.: Congenital bicuspid aortic valves associated with coarctation of the aorta in children. *Br. Heart J.*, 31:127, 1969.

Taylor, R. R., and Pollock, B. E.: Coarctation of the aorta in three members of a family. *Am. Heart J.*, 45:470, 1953.

Taylor, S. H., and Donald, K. W.: Circulatory studies at rest and during exercise in coarctation of the aorta before and after operation. *Br. Heart J.*, 22:117, 1960.

Thorner, M. C.; Griffith, G. C.; and Carter, R. A.: Rib notching in coarctation of the aorta in children. *Ann. Western Med. Surg.*, 6:675, 1952.

Tonelli, L.; Baisi, F.; and Malizia, E.: Pre- and post-operative renal function in coarctation of the aorta and its relationship to the genesis of hypertension. *Acta Med. Scand.*, 148:35, 1954.

Trusler, G. A., and Izukawa, T.: Interrupted aortic arch and ventricular septal defect. *J. Thorac. Cardiovasc. Surg.*, 69:1, 1975.

Tyson, K. R. T.; Harris, L. C.; and Nghiem, Q. X.: Repair of aortic arch interruption in the neonate. *Surgery*, 67:1006, 1970.

Van Buchem, F. S. P.; Homan, B. P.; Dingemanse, E.; and Huis. In t'Veld, L. D.: Endocrine disturbances in coarctation of the aorta. *Acta Med. Scand.*, 143:399, 1952.

Van Praagh, R.; Bernhard, W. P.; Rosenthal, A.; Parisi, L. F.; and Flyer, D. C.: Interrupted aortic arch: Surgical treatment. *Am. J. Cardiol.*, 27:200, 1971.

Vlodaver, Z.; and Neufeld, H. N.: The coronary arteries in coarctation of the aorta. *Circulation*, **37**:449, 1968.

Vulliamy, D. G.: Turner's syndrome with coarctation of the aorta. *Proc. Roy. Soc. Med.*, **46**:279, 1953.

Wakim, K. G.; Slaughter, O.; and Clagett, O. T.: Studies on the blood flow in the extremities in cases of coarctation of tha aorta: determinations before and after excision of the coarctate region. *Proc. Mayo Clin.*, **23**:347, 1948.

Waldhausen, J. A., and Nahrwold, D. L.: Repair of coarctation of the aorta with a subclavian flap. *J. Thorac. Cardiovasc. Surg.*, **51**:532, 1966.

Walker, G. L., and Stanfield, T. F.: Retinal changes associated with coarctation of the aorta. *Tr. Am. Ophthal. Soc.*, **50**:407, 1952.

Walker, R. M., and Haxton, H.: The surgical treatment of coarctation of the aorta. *Br. J. Surg.*, **42**:26, 1954.

Whittemore, R.: Personal communication, 1955.

Ziegler, R. F.: The genesis and importance of the electrocardiogram in coarctation of the aorta. *Circulation*, **9**:371, 1954.

Coarctation of the Abdominal Aorta

Bahnson, H. T.; Cooley, R. N.; and Sloan, R. D.: Coarctation of the aorta at unusual sites. Report of two cases with angiocardiographic and operative findings. *Am. Heart J.*, **38**:905, 1949.

Baird, R. J.; Labrosse, C. J.; and Evans, J. R.: Coarctation of the abdominal aorta. *Dis. Chest*, **48**:517, 1965.

Bjork, V. O., and Intonti, F.: Coarctation of abdominal aorta with right renal artery stenosis. *Ann. Surg.*, **160**:54, 1964.

Bliddal, J.; Dupont, B.; Melchior, J. C.; and Ottensen, O. E.: Coarctation of the aorta with multiple artery anomalies in idiopathic hypercalcemia of infancy. *Acta Paediatr. Scand.*, **58**:632–37, 1969.

Daimon, S., and Kitamura, K.: Coarctation of the abdominal aorta. *Jap. Heart J.*, **5**:562, 1964.

Danaraj, T. J.; Wong, H. O.; and Thomas, A.: Primary arteritis of aorta causing renal artery stenosis and hypertension. *Br. J. Med.*, **25**:153, 1963.

DeBakey, M. E.; Garrett, H. E.; Howell, J. F.; and Morris, G. C.: Coarctation of the abdominal aorta with renal arterial stenosis: Surgical considerations. *Ann. Surg.*, **165**:83, 1967.

Doberneck, R. C., and Varco, R. L.: Congenital coarctation of the abdominal aorta. *J. Lancet*, **88**:143, 1968.

Emmanouilides, G. C., and Hoy, R. C.: Transumbilical aortography and selective aortography in newborn infants. *Pediatrics*, **39**:337, 1967.

Gerbasi, F. S.; Kibler, R. S.; and Margileth, A. M.: Coarctation of the abdominal aorta. *J. Pediatr.*, **52**:191, 1952.

Glenn, F.; Keefer, E. B. C.; Speer, D. S.; and Dotter, C. T.: Coarctation of the lower thoracic and abdominal aorta immediately proximal to the celiac axis. *Surg. Gynecol. Obstet.*, **94**:561, 1952.

Gonzaley-Corna, J. L.; Villavicencio, L.; Moline, B.; and Bessudo, L.: Nonspecific obliterative aortitis in children. *Ann. Thorac. Surg.*, **4**:193, 1967.

Huang, T. T.; Wolma, F. J.; and Tyson, K. R.: Coarctation of the abdominal aorta, etiologic considerations in surgical management. *Am. J. Surg.*, **120**:598, 1970.

Kondo, B.; Winsor, T.; Raujston, B. O.; and Kurouva, D.: Congenital coarctation of the abdominal aorta. *Am. Heart J.*, **39**:309, 1950.

Loggie, J. M. H.: Hypertension in children and adolescents, I. Causes and diagnostic studies. *J. Pediatr.*, **74**:331, 1969.

Morris, G. C.; DeBakey, M. E.; Cooley, D. A.; and Crawford, E. S.: Subisthmic aortic stenosis and occlusive disease. *Arch. Surg.*, **80**:87, 1960.

Onat, T., and Zeren, E.: Coarctation of the abdominal aorta, Review of 91 cases. *Cardiologia*, **54**:140–57, 1969.

Quain, R.: Partial coarctation of the abdominal aorta. *Trans. Path. Soc. (London)*, **1**:244, 1847.

Robicsek, F.; Sanger, P. W.; and Daugherty, H. K.: Coarctation of the abdominal aorta diagnosed by aortography. *Ann. Surg.*, **162**:227, 1964.

Schmidt, D. M., and Rambo, O. N., Jr.: Segmental intimal hyperplasia of the abdominal aorta and renal arteries producing hypertension in an infant. *Am. J. Clin. Pathol.*, **44**:546, 1965.

Schurch, W.; Messerli, F. H.; Genest, J.; Lefebvre, R.; Roy, P.; Cartier, P.; and Rojo-Ortega, J. M.: Arterial hypertension and neurofibromatosis: Renal artery stenosis and coarctation of abdominal artery. *Can. Med. Assoc. J.*, **113**:879, 1975.

Siassi, B.; Klyman, G.; and Emmanouilides, G. C.: Hypoplasia of the abdominal aorta associated with the rubella syndrome. *Am. J. Dis. Child.*, **120**:476, 1970.

Sloan, R. D., and Cooley, R. N.: Coarctation of the aorta. Roentgenologic aspects of one hundred and twenty-five surgically confirmed cases. *Radiology*, **61**:701, 1953.

Wiltse, H. E.; Goldbloom, R. B.; Antia, A. U.; Ottesen, O. E.; Rowe, R. D.; and Cooke, R. E.: Infantile hypercalcemia syndrome in twins. *N. Engl. J. Med.*, **275**:1157, 1966.

40

Pulmonary Stenosis with Normal Aortic Root

Richard D. Rowe

THIS malformation was first described by Morgagni in 1761, but it was Fallot who separated seven cyanotic examples of the disorder from 39 cases of the tetralogy and described a morbid "trilogy," a term still used, particularly by French workers. Variations in the clinical picture, resulting both from differing degrees of the pulmonary stenosis and from shunts through associated septal defects or abnormal arteriovenous communications, are now well recognized. The need for a term more inclusive than pure pulmonary stenosis, isolated or uncomplicated pulmonary stenosis, or pulmonary stenosis with intact septa or patent foramen ovale became apparent. Abrahams and Wood (1951) used the term "pulmonary stenosis with normal aortic root." Under this heading these authors included simple pulmonary stenosis, pulmonary stenosis with arteriovenous shunt, and pulmonary stenosis with venoarterial shunt. Further subdivisions include the notation of valvular or infundibular stenosis and mild, moderate, or severe degree of stenosis. While this classification is possibly the most descriptive and useful so far suggested, and one to which we have adhered over the years, it still has imperfections. The more generally accepted term seems to be pulmonary stenosis "with intact ventricular septum." That of course carries no merit over "normal aortic root" because it excludes patients with small to moderate-sized ventricular defects, but the general semantic problem is now so well recognized that there is seldom confusion over different reports on the subject.

Prevalence

Postmortem studies in congenital heart disease have suggested in the past that pulmonary stenosis with normal aortic root is rare (Abbott, 1936). In recent years, however, clinical reports have indicated that the malformation is responsible for about 10 percent of congenital heart disease. Abrahams and Wood (1951) found an incidence of 11.6 percent of 689 cases, and Campbell (1954) found 10 percent of

1130 cases of congenital heart disease. At The Hospital for Sick Children, Toronto, 1471 cases (9.9 percent) of pulmonary stenosis with normal aortic root have been observed in a total of 15,104 patients with congenital heart disease from birth to 15 years. At the Children's Hospital Medical Center in Boston the corresponding proportion was 7.5 percent (Nadas and Fyler, 1972). Different seasonal peaks of birth rate have been found for patients with pulmonary stenosis in Ontario (Rose et al., 1972), males peaking in the fall, females in the spring.

In an examination of the sibs of 125 patients with pulmonary stenosis, Campbell (1962) found that 2.2 percent had a cardiac malformation, usually pulmonary stenosis, while in the data of Nora and associates (1970) the probability of recurrence in siblings of pulmonary stenosis was 2.9 percent. In one unidentical twin pair seen in the neonatal period at Green Lane Hospital, one member was found to have moderate pulmonary stenosis of the simple type. The other died of pulmonary atresia with hypoplastic right ventricle. Angiographically confirmed valvular stenosis of mild and moderate severity has been reported in father and daughter, respectively (McCarron and Perloff, 1974), and familial pulmonary stenosis has been discussed in some detail recently by Klinge and Laursen (1975).

Anatomy

Obstruction to Pulmonary Blood Flow.

VALVULAR STENOSIS. In the severe form (see Figure 40–1) there is a fusion of cusps to form a dome projecting within the pulmonary artery. The dome has a small central perforation, 1 to 3 mm in diameter, at its apex. Eccentric position of the orifice may occur. Three raphae extend from the central perforation along the superior surface of the dome to the wall of the pulmonary trunk. In many cases only the peripheral portions of the raphae are distinctly visible. These linear elevations probably represent the point at which valve fusion has occurred. Occasionally four raphae are visible (Selzer et al.,

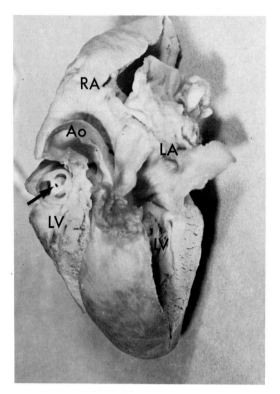

Figure 40-1. The pulmonary valve in critically severe pulmonary stenosis with normal aortic root. The heart of a one-day-old infant. There is a pinhole orifice to the pulmonary valve, which has three raphes (*arrow*). Note the marked hypertrophy of the right atrium (*RA*). *Ao* = aorta; *LA* = left atrium; *LV* = left ventricle.

INFUNDIBULAR STENOSIS. Abbott (1936) reported two specimens with infundibular stenosis among 1000 autopsies of congenital heart malformation. One was a boy of 14 years with two minute orifices at the lower bulbar portion of the right ventricle. In clinical reports the incidence has been higher—approximately 10 percent in the combined experiences of Abrahams and Wood (1951), Campbell (1954), Kjellberg and associates (1959), and Brock (1961). Of the 1471 patients with pulmonary stenosis and intact ventricular septum seen at The Hospital for Sick Children over the past 23 years, only 40 (2.7 percent) had isolated infundibular pulmonary stenosis. Among 228 patients with pulmonary stenosis and intact ventricular septum, Zaret and Conti (1973) found only three cases (1.3 percent) with pure infundibular stenosis. While it is possible that infundibular stenosis may be truly isolated and congenital, there is now increasing evidence that many such cases are a development secondarily in association with ventricular septal defect that later closes (Watson et al., 1969; case records of the Massachusetts General Hospital, 1969; Brock, 1961; Gamble and Nadas, 1965; and Zaret and Conti, 1973).

COMBINED VALVULAR AND INFUNDIBULAR STENOSIS. This form is even less frequent than the infundibular type. It is, however, comparatively common to find a reduction in size of the infundibulum in association with severe valvular stenosis due to marked muscle hypertrophy, particularly in the anterior wall and crista region of the right ventricle. Some degree of endocardial fibroelastosis in the infundibulum may accompany this hypertrophy. These changes may result in significant infundibular obstruction, particularly in older cases.

Right Ventricle. Although the right ventricle is usually normal in the architectural sense in this malformation (Lev, 1959), muscular hypertrophy is present in varying degree. The cavity size appears relatively reduced in angiocardiograms and at autopsy in cases with severe stenosis. It is sometimes difficult to declare a borderline between this reduction of the right ventricular size due to muscular hypertrophy and that of true underdevelopment of the right ventricle with pulmonary stenosis. The latter (Findlay, 1879; Wood, 1942; Chiche, 1952; Astley et al., 1953; Brown et al., 1956; Kjellberg et al., 1959; Taussig, 1960; Williams et al., 1963; Freed et al., 1973) seems to be a distinctly separate malformation with a diminutive right ventricle, hypoplasia of the tricuspid orifice, pulmonary stenosis, and atrial septal defect where the ventricle contains unusually dense fine trabeculae filling the apex of the chamber and the outflow tract. This arrangement suggests that the embryonic spongy mesenchymatous tissue normally present in the ventricle during its development has failed to absorb (see Chapter 8).

Myocardial infarcts were found by Franciosi and Blanc (1968) in the absence of coronary artery disease in eight of nine patients with pulmonary stenosis

1949; Edwards, 1953). A bicuspid pulmonary valve was found at autopsy in 20 percent of our cases, but the incidence of abnormal cusp number for the majority of patients with pulmonary stenosis is not known. Calcification of the pulmonary valve is rare and confined to patients with moderate or severe stenosis (Gabriele and Scatliff, 1970; Rodriguez et al., 1972). An association with infective endocarditis has been suggested by Dinsmore and associates (1966).

In moderate stenosis peripheral fusion only occurs, the central portion of each cusp remaining free. The resultant orifice is then much larger than in the severe form (Soulié et al., 1953).

While most patients with pulmonary valve stenosis have valve thickening of some degree, a small proportion, about 10 to 15 percent of patients, has been shown to have exceptionally thick leaflets—so-called dysplastic valves (Koretzky et al., 1969; Jeffrey et al., 1972). Three cusps are present but there is little if any fusion of these mucoid leaflets, and obstruction to flow results from the combination of sheer bulk of the valve tissue and a rather small pulmonary valve annulus. We have found that most patients with the Noonan syndrome and even trivial pulmonary stenosis have dysplastic valves (Rodriguez–Fernandez et al., 1972).

coming to autopsy. These changes were found in subendocardial regions of the free wall and in the papillary muscles of the right ventricle of patients dying with severe stenosis and marked right ventricular hypertrophy. Clinical evidence in newborns with severe pulmonary stenosis argues strongly that right ventricular ischemia is more frequent than had been supposed in younger age groups. An extreme example with massive septal and right ventricular infarction in a 12-year-old patient with a right ventricular systemic pressure of 100 mm of mercury has been reported (Dimond and Lin, 1954).

Pulmonary Artery. The pulmonary artery almost always shows poststenotic dilatation, the circumference of the trunk exceeding that of the aorta. There are several exceptions to the rule. One of these is in severe infundibular stenosis where hypoplasia of the pulmonary arteries is usual. In very young infants with severe valvular stenosis the pulmonary trunk does not always exhibit poststenotic dilatation, although this has often developed within a few months after birth and may later become marked. A further exception is noted in cases of pulmonary valvular stenosis complicated by the presence of central pulmonary arterial stenoses, where the main pulmonary artery is smaller than the major branches. Moderate degrees of infundibular stenosis, by comparison, are associated with considerable pulmonary dilatation. These observations have suggested an inverse relationship between the severity of stenosis and degree of pulmonary artery dilatation (Ayres and Lukas, 1960; Rudhe et al., 1962). Boughner and Roach (1971) have shown in elegant experiments that vibrations induced by murmurs produce dilatation of arterial walls under conditions that are related to both age of the vessel and the frequency range contained in the murmur. These experimental findings may explain the individual variation in poststenotic dilatation and the inconstant relationship of the latter to the severity of stenosis.

Right Atrium. The right atrium shows changes, the character of which depends on the severity and type of malformation. In severe stenosis right atrial hypertrophy is usual, the wall sometimes reaching an astonishing degree of change with marked thickening and trabeculation. An anomaly dividing the right atrium into two chambers has been described (Dubin et al., 1944; Gombert, 1933; Sternberg, 1913; Kjellberg et al. 1959; Folger, 1968; Hansing et al., 1972). The coronary sinus opens into the medial chamber, which in turn opens into the tricuspid orifice. The smaller lateral chamber receives both venae cavae and the appendage and opens into the medial chamber through a relatively wide orifice. In our experience the latter malformation, not uncommonly seen in the autopsies of severe pulmonary stenosis with normal aortic root, produces no functional disturbance. The tricuspid orifice is most often normal, although functionally it may be narrowed. About one in five specimens will have the tricuspid ring distinctly reduced in size. Such change

varies in degree from a truly stenotic valve ring to a mildly hypoplastic form.

Septa. Whether the pulmonary stenosis is severe or moderate, the atrial septum may be completely closed. Probe or wide patency of the foramen ovale occurs in about three-fourths of the autopsied cases. A wide defect of this septum is more commonly seen accompanying the moderate form than the severe form of stenosis. The ventricular septum is closed in most cases of severe stenosis, but ventricular septal defects occur. Of 12 patients with severe infundibular stenosis without obvious shunt and with right ventricular systolic pressures ranging between 82 and 170 mm of mercury, small muscular ventricular defects were found at operation in seven (Slade, 1963). In moderate pulmonary stenosis the detection of ventricular defects is made simpler by blood sampling or indicator dilution methods.

In normal hearts the membranous portion of the ventricular septum below the aortic valve is flush with the muscular part. In over two-thirds of all cases with severe pulmonary stenosis with normal aortic root, at any age and with either valvular or infundibular obstruction, the upper one-third of the muscular septum bulges convexly into the cavity of the left ventricle, obscuring in part the membranous septum when viewed from that side. In many this results in some reduction in the width of the outflow tract of the left ventricle. It is not to be expected that cases with moderate stenosis would show this change.

Cirrhosis of Liver. Campbell (1954) drew attention to the marked cardiac cirrhosis commonly present in fatal adult cases. Such advanced changes are not seen in the young, although minor alterations in liver architecture such as central lobular atrophy or marked congestion may be seen in liver sections of infant autopsies. Two of our fatal cases (aged six and seven years) showed early fibrotic changes.

Aorta and Left Ventricle. By definition the aorta arises usually from the outflow tract of the left ventricle and is normal in size in the majority of cases. Occasionally it is obviously dilated. Among 20 autopsied cases we found no instance of bicuspid aortic valve (Izukawa and Keith, unpublished observation). The aortic arch branching is normal but right aortic arch with right descending aorta in this malformation is extremely rare. Our own experience still does not include an example of this combination. It may be that the combination is confined to patients with infundibular stenosis and previous ventricular septal defect. Occasionally the ductus arteriosus is patent. Increase in size and number of branches of the bronchial arteries has been demonstrated in older patients but is not a feature in the young. When the cavity of the left ventricle is examined in specimens, it is found to be of generous size. The wall may show some hypertrophy, but only when there is severe stenosis, especially in cases with marked right-to-left shunt between the atria with hypoplastic right ventricle, is there usually marked hypertrophy of the left ventricular wall. Even then it seldom approaches the thickness of the right ventricle. Parachute mitral valve has been reported in association (Glancy et al., 1971).

Widespread Cardiovascular Disease. Bécu and colleagues (1976) have recently drawn attention to myocardial dysplasia and necrosis, coronary arterial occlusions, and higgledy-piggledy aortic wall histology in 25 unoperated patients at autopsy. They found similar abnormalities in 14 of another 53 patients who had undergone surgical treatment for severe pulmonary valve stenosis, some of whom died. In the survivors, hypertrophic cardiomyopathy was a feature. Most of the affected patients were infants and apparently only one case was considered to have the Noonan syndrome. Since characteristically the additional disease was associated with a thick, poorly mobile pulmonary valve and other congenital stigmata, there may still be some relationship to that syndrome.

Hemodynamics

Severe Stenosis. Owing to the minute orifice through which blood is propelled into the pulmonary artery, there is an elevation of the right ventricular pressure behind the obstruction. The degree of this elevation has a direct relationship to the severity or "tightness" of the stenosis and frequently exceeds the systemic levels in systole. All other effects are the result of this simple fact. The right ventricle hypertrophies concentrically and enormously, as does the right atrium. The end result is right heart failure and death. In the presence of an associated patent foramen ovale there may be right-to-left shunt of variable magnitude causing cyanosis of corresponding severity. A fairly large shunt of this type is usual in even moderate degrees of pulmonary stenosis when the right ventricle is underdeveloped (Williams et al., 1963) and often persists after relief of more severe pulmonary stenosis if attempts were not made to enlarge the right ventricular cavity at operation.

Mild-to-Moderate Stenosis. Where the obstruction to pulmonary blood flow is less important, only mild-to-moderate elevations of right ventricular pressure result. The systolic values never reach systemic levels in this form. The right ventricular hypertrophy is correspondingly moderate. Even when defects of the atrial and ventricular septa are present, the direction of the resultant shunt will be left to right and rarely in the reverse direction. Cyanosis, therefore, is not usually found in this type, and the right heart strain is never severe enough to cause heart failure and death in childhood.

Clinical Features

From a clinical viewpoint pulmonary stenosis with normal aortic root is best described as either mild-to-moderate or severe. In our experience the two grades are of equal frequency.

Mild-to-Moderate Stenosis. A major clinical feature is the lack of cyanosis at any stage. The physical development is usually normal except in those with arteriovenous shunts who may be moderately dystrophic. Dyspnea with effort is reportedly rare and was claimed in about one-third of our cases. In these it was never marked and in most was equivocal. Squatting never occurs. Familial occurrence has been reported (Coblentz and Mathivat, 1952).

The jugular venous pulse is normal, and there are no signs of heart failure. There may be some precordial bulge in cases with arteriovenous shunt, but the physique is most often normal, moon face being rare (20 percent). The apex beat is unremarkable, although a few will show a tapping right ventricular-type apical impulse (Abrahams and Wood, 1951). Those with a ventricular septal defect may have a left ventricular-type apical thrust.

An ejection systolic murmur is always present. The murmur varies in length and intensity but usually is moderately loud and ends before aortic valve closure.

It has been appreciated for many years that in mild stenosis the systolic murmur is relatively soft and short, whereas in more severe degrees of stenosis the murmur is louder and longer (Leatham and Weitzman, 1957), a relationship that has also been shown for aortic valve stenosis (Braunwald et al., 1963). But unlike the situation in aortic stenosis there is in pulmonary stenosis a positive correlation between the level of right ventricular systole pressure and the position in systole where the murmur peaks: the more severe the stenosis, the later in systole the peaking (Vogelpoel and Schrire, 1960; Gamboa et al., 1964). The murmur increases in duration and intensity after the inhalation of amyl nitrate (Vogelpoel et al., 1959). The murmur is usually maximal in the second left intercostal space. Patients with moderate infundibular or combined stenosis with or without arteriovenous shunts exhibit murmurs either in the second left intercostal space or the third or fourth left intercostal space in about equal proportions. In valvular stenosis, whether associated or not with arteriovenous shunt, the murmur is maximal in the second left intercostal space. Thus the finding of a murmur in the fourth left intercostal space is very suggestive of infundibular stenosis, but this type of obstruction cannot be excluded if the murmur is higher. The intensity is most often about grade 3. A thrill is unusual. In trivial obstructions the murmur is fainter. A mid diastolic murmur may be heard at the apex of those cases with moderate stenosis accompanied by a large-volume left-to-right shunt.

A high-pitched ejection sound or systolic click, loudest in expiration in the second and third left intercostal spaces, is heard in trivial and moderate stenosis and is frequently confused with wide splitting of the first sound in this area (Leatham, 1954).

The click is related to sudden doming of the pulmonary valve as seen on cineangiocardiograms and results from the opening motion of the valve being checked (Hultgren et al., 1969). An inverse relationship between severity and the Q-click interval

late cyanosis

on the phonocardiogram has been found (Gamboa et al., 1964). Important correlations of respiratory changes in the click to different hemodynamics in variable degrees of the stenosis have been made. Hultgren and associates (1969) found from such analysis in 16 patients that when the diastolic pressure in the pulmonary arteries consistently exceeded the right ventricular end-diastolic pressure, a click was present in all phases of the respiratory cycle. On the other hand, if on inspiration the right ventricular end-diastolic pressure exceeded the diastolic pressure in the pulmonary artery no click will be recorded. These observations have recently been strengthened by echocardiographic evidence (Weyman et al., 1974). The second heart sound in the pulmonary area is most often distinctly split in children and is of normal intensity. In a few cases the sound of pulmonary valve closure is reduced as well as delayed. The closer the case approaches the upper range of severity within this group, the less likely is splitting to be detected and the fainter the pulmonic component of the sound becomes. This correlation between degree of stenosis and width of splitting of the second heart sound in the pulmonary area has been demonstrated by Leatham and Weitzman (1957) using phonocardiographic and right ventricular pressure measurements. Occasionally the second heart sound is widely split and fixed in the presence of an intact atrial septum in patients with mild stenosis. Where this occurs there is usually marked poststenotic dilatation and presumably deficiency in vessel recoil plays a role (Schrire and Vogelpoel, 1962; Singh, 1970).

Blood pressure and peripheral pulses are usually normal.

Severe Stenosis. In this group symptoms are a feature, but a proportion (25 percent) will have none. The most impressive sign is the generalized cyanosis seen in those with venoarterial shunts (Currens et al., 1945; Engle and Taussig, 1950). The degree of cyanosis depends to a large extent on the volume of the shunt passing through a patent foramen ovale. Some severe cases with patent foramen ovale have no shunt, some show minute shunt insufficient to produce clinical cyanosis at rest or with exercise, some show cyanosis only with exercise, and some are cyanosed at rest. A central right-to-left shunt was present in two-thirds of our cases of this severe form. The shunt was exhibited as clinical cyanosis at rest or on exercise and was confirmed by oximetry or by the selective indicator injection at cardiac catheterization. Only 15 percent of the cases were moderately or markedly cyanosed, and 20 percent had clubbing of the fingers. This suggests that, in childhood at least, obvious cyanosis and clubbing are rather uncommon but that small-volume venoarterial shunts are frequent. It might be that with progressive age the size of this shunt increases in some of these patients, who will then become more obviously cyanosed. Campbell (1954) found that of 44 cyanotic patients with pulmonary stenosis with normal aortic root some 10 percent were cyanosed at birth, and a total of 25 percent were cyanosed by four years of age, the remainder becoming cyanotic well after that age. The average age of onset of cyanosis in the total group was 14.4 years. At The Hospital for Sick Children, one-quarter were cyanosed from birth, half by one year of age, and a total of two-thirds by five years.

In the simple form of severe stenosis no central cyanosis occurs, but peripheral cyanosis has been reported (Shephard, 1955; Campbell, 1954).

Some limitation of exercise tolerance is noted in the majority of cases. All the cyanosed cases are affected by exertional dyspnea, but many of the simple cases, even those with extreme stenosis, claim no disability. In infants and young children with congestive heart failure dyspnea is, of course, a striking feature. Characteristic of the severe form in infancy, and commonly a grave prognostic sign in infants, is periodic dyspnea unassociated with congestive failure. We still have not seen a single example of squatting after exertion in proved pulmonary stenosis with normal aortic root. Abrahams and Wood (1951) reported one instance in 18 cases; Campbell (1954), 20 percent of 31 cases—one proved at autopsy; and Donzelot and D'Allaines (1954), 30 percent. Personal cases with the clinical findings of this malformation, slight cyanosis and squatting with effort, have been found, after further detailed accessory studies, to have tetralogy of Fallot. Consequently, we accept the diagnosis with a considerable degree of caution in the presence of squatting.

In older cases episodes of fainting and precordial pain are not uncommon (Abrahams and Wood, 1951; Campbell, 1954; Lasser and Genkins, 1957), and even sudden death has been reported (Marquis, 1951). One $3\frac{1}{2}$-year-old child reported by Dimond and Lin (1954), after attacks of epigastric pain on effort relieved by rest, died following sustained chest pain from infarction of the right ventricular wall and ventricular septum. Although many episodes of this type are undoubtedly the result of coronary insufficiency, occasional cases may be encountered where the symptoms are the result of an alteration in cardiac rate. One of our cases who exhibited the Wolff-Parkinson-White syndrome was subject to attacks of paroxysmal atrial tachycardia.

The physique is usually normal. Wasted infants are not seen. Moon face (Wood, 1950) is common—about half of our cases—but neither invariable nor pathognomonic.

Increased amplitude of "a" waves in the jugular venous pulse is nearly always visible in the severe forms of pulmonary stenosis with normal aortic root. Many cases have giant "a" waves that are extremely obvious. Careful inspection of the neck veins after appropriate positioning of the patient will enable this sign to be demonstrated even in infant patients.

Enlargement of the liver with pulsation in the absence of frank failure is uncommon. A few cases will exhibit this sign in association with the giant "a" waves in the neck, but it is by no means a constant accompaniment of the severe forms even in infancy. Again, when present it is certain evidence of very severe stenosis.

↑ "a" waves

The apex beat is tapping in character. A distinct right ventricular heave over the sternal border is notable in the majority. Abrahams and Wood (1951) attached great importance to this sign, which is not a feature in the moderate cases or in the tetralogy of Fallot. Their observations were subsequently quantified for children (Schmidt and Craige, 1965). A thrill in the pulmonic area extended to the suprasternal notch and the left carotid, or both carotid arteries, is almost constant. In small infants a thrill may be absent.

The systolic murmur is loud, harsh, and long, and in most instances, as 90 percent of the stenoses are of valvular type, it will be heard maximally in the second left intercostal space. In severe stenosis the peak intensity of the murmur occurs later in systole than one sees in milder forms of obstruction (Vogelpoel and Schrire, 1960; Gamboa et al., 1964). Patients with infundibular stenosis may show a murmur maximal in the third or fourth left intercostal space (Abrahams and Wood, 1951; Mannheimer and Jönsson, 1954). But these generalizations are not always true. Occasionally the murmur of valvular stenosis is maximal in the first left intercostal space. Two of our autopsied cases of valvular pulmonary stenosis showed murmurs maximal in the third or fourth left intercostal space, whereas two verified cases of infundibular stenosis had murmurs that were loudest in the second left intercostal space. Similarly in five children with proved infundibular stenosis, Slade (1963) found the long systolic murmur to be maximal in the second left intercostal space in four instances. It is generally true also that the murmurs of severe stenosis are loud. Although Dimond and Lin (1954) found no relationship between the intensity of the murmur and the severity of the stenosis as judged by the height of the right ventricular pressure, Mannheimer and Jönsson (1954) believe that correlation is possible. In an analysis at The Hospital for Sick Children of ten infants dying with severe pulmonary stenosis with normal aortic root, six had very loud, harsh, systolic murmurs of grade-4 to -5 intensity with a thrill, whereas four had grade-3 murmurs without thrill. The youngest infant, in congestive heart failure 12 hours after birth, was noted to have a loud continuous murmur in the pulmonary area for 24 hours which was replaced by a grade-5 systolic murmur with thrill until death at 59 hours. Thus, whereas a minority of infants may have murmurs less intense than those of older patients, none has insignificant murmurs. These findings compare well with those obtained in older children.

There is sometimes difficulty in making clinical estimates of the severity of pulmonary valve obstruction in patients with the Noonan syndrome. It is likely that this problem relates to the presence of the dysplastic valve, which must influence the behavior of the second sound. The redundancy of valve tissue also can be expected to abolish the ejection click as happens in the stiff valve of calcific aortic stenosis. Another area where the murmur may be atypical is in some neonates with very severe stenosis who present with massive tricuspid regurgitation (see Figure 40–8, page 777). In these patients there is a loud pansystolic murmur at the lower left sternal border and often no murmur in the pulmonary area.

Diastolic murmurs are rare and occur only after distortion of the pulmonic valve ring or cusps by complications such as progressive poststenotic dilatation of the pulmonary artery (Dimond and Lin, 1954) or infective endocarditis (Abrahams and Wood, 1951).

A continuous murmur is found in the presence of an associated patent ductus arteriosus.

Phonocardiography reveals that the aortic component of the second sound in this area is obscured in the systolic murmur, and that pulmonary valve closure, when recorded, has a low amplitude and occurs 0.06 to 0.10 second after aortic valve closure. This wide degree of splitting of the second sound, not appreciable clinically, is regarded as being due to prolonged ventricular systole (Leatham, 1952; Mannheimer and Jönsson, 1954). Fixed splitting may occur (Schrire and Vogelpoel, 1962).

The pulmonary ejection sound in severe stenosis cannot be separated clinically from the first heart sound in the pulmonary area, although simultaneous phonocardiograms from mitral and pulmonary areas suggest its presence (Leatham, 1952). Gamboa and associates (1964) have found a combination of the q-ejection click interval, q-peak magnitude of the murmur, and semilunar valve closure interval to be more useful than any individual sign in estimating the severity of right ventricular hypertension in pulmonary stenosis. One important diagnostic feature in patients with hypoplastic right ventricle is the paradoxic reverse splitting of the second heart sound encountered in that variant (Williams et al., 1963).

Electrocardiography

Consistent, though distinctly different, electrical events characterize the different grades of pulmonary stenosis with normal aortic root.

Mild-to-Moderate Stenosis. In cases of pulmonary stenosis proven by cardiac catheterization to have slight or moderate elevation of right ventricular pressure, a normal electrocardiogram has been reported (Abrahams and Wood, 1951; Soulie et al., 1953; Dimond and Lin, 1954). In a series of 85 patients with pulmonary valvular stenosis and right ventricular systolic pressures less than 80 mm of mercury, Levine and Blumenthal (1965) found 65 percent had either normal electrocardiograms or equivocal signs of right heart overload. We have seen normal tracings with patients having right ventricular systolic pressures as high as 65 mm of mercury, but with the exception of those patients with quite-trivial-severity stenosis there is usually some evidence of right ventricular overload (Figures 40–2 to 40–4). Both Fowler (1968) and Ellison and Restieaux (1972) have shown that QRS conduction delay is characteristic of mild-severity stenosis. Complete right bundle

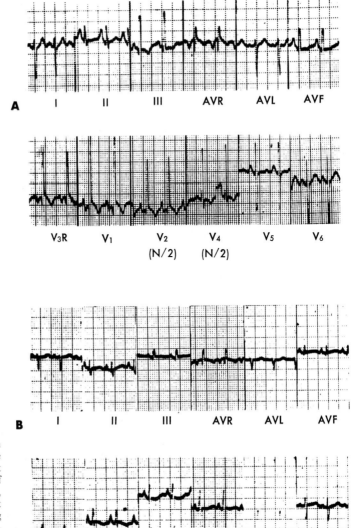

Figure 40-2. The electrocardiogram in severe valvular pulmonary stenosis. *A.* The tracing from a 16-month-old girl with a right ventricular pressure at 160/20 mm of mercury. There are right-axis deviation, right atrial hypertrophy, and severe right ventricular hypertrophy. *B.* The tracing from a 16-day-old boy with autopsy-proved, critically severe valvular pulmonary stenosis. There are right-axis deviation, right atrial hypertrophy, and right ventricular hypertrophy.

branch block was found in 4 percent of 100 patients with pulmonary stenosis by the latter authors and all four had mild obstruction at the pulmonary valve. The joint study of the natural history of congenital heart disease data (Ellison and Miettinen, 1974) documented that in the 20 percent of 539 nonoperated patients with isolated pulmonary stenosis and an RSR[1] pattern in V[1] the stenosis was less severe than in patients with corresponding "pure" R in V$_1$.

In patients with moderately severe stenosis there tends to be some right-axis deviation and inversion of R/S ratio in V$_1$. P waves are usually normal and the T wave direction in lead V$_1$ is variable, about half the patients having inversion of the T and half having a positive T. These signs of right ventricular hypertrophy, so well termed "discrete" by French workers,

may be quite similar to many cases of tetralogy of Fallot (Soulié et al., 1953). The right maximum spatial vector increases in proportion to the increase in right ventricular pressure giving a correlation coefficient of 0.73 (Ellison and Restieaux, 1972). Similar degrees of correlation can be obtained from combining elements of the scalar electrocardiogram (Fowler and Keith, 1968).

Severe Stenosis. No normal tracings have been reported in this group. On the contrary, much more striking electrocardiographic evidence of right ventricular hypertrophy is to be expected in these cases. These facts were noted by Campbell and Brock (1955), Marquis (1951), and Soulié and associates (1951) in comparative descriptions of the electrical events in tetralogy of Fallot and severe pulmonary

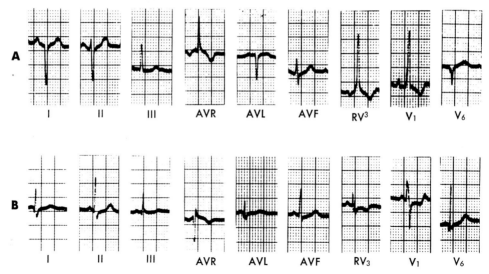

Figure 40-3. The electrocardiogram in simple pulmonary valve stenosis. *A.* A child with severe stenosis where the right ventricular systolic pressure was 103 mm of mercury. There are right-axis deviation and marked right ventricular hypertrophy. The frontal QRS-T angle is 105 degrees. *B.* A child with mild stenosis where the right ventricular systolic pressure was 42 mm of mercury. There is a normal QRS frontal axis, and the frontal QRS-T angle is 0 degree.

stenosis with normal aortic root. Soulié and associates (1951) found that the characteristic features were extreme right-axis deviation, abnormally tall, peaked P waves, inverted R/S ratios in V_1 and V_6, deep inversion of T wave in leads II and III, and precordial leads as far to the left as V_4. These findings applied to severe cases both with and without venoarterial shunt but were invariably in those with the shunt. In our cases the Â QRS was further rightward, and the R/S ratio in V_1 was invariably inverted when contrasted with the tracings of patients with mild-to-moderate severity stenosis (Figures 40–2 and 40–3A). The R wave in V_1 was in excess of 28 mm in 60 percent of cases. Similarly, P waves were abnormal in 75 percent of our severe cases, and in 50 percent a qR pattern was present, especially in

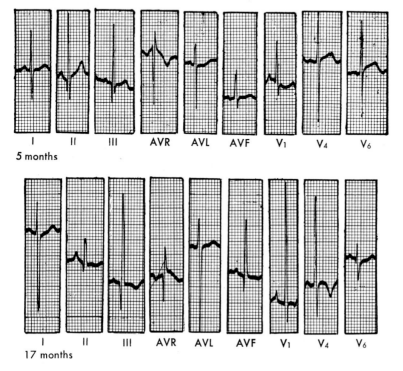

5 months

17 months

Figure 40-4. The electrocardiogram in pulmonary valvular stenosis. Change from moderate right ventricular hypertrophy to right atrial and severe right ventricular hypertrophy in an infant boy in the space of one year.

patients with a venoarterial shunt. Not only is this sign strongly indicative of severe right ventricular hypertrophy but it may be related to subendocardial ischemia and infarction of papillary muscles in the right ventricle in severe stenosis (Franciosi and Blanc, 1968). In our patients the presence of an upright T in V_1 with right ventricular pressures in excess of 100 mm of mercury was uncommon, most patients showing deep T wave inversion at this stage. In two-thirds of our patients this sign was evident in leads as far to the left as V_4 and often went as far as V_5 or V_6.

Unusual Features. Occasional cases in infancy, particularly in the newborn period, show Â QRS between +30 and 60 degrees and have evidence of pure left ventricular hypertrophy often with right atrial overload (Mustard et al., 1960). Although the postoperative course of these babies was such as to exclude a severe degree of right ventricular underdevelopment, it would appear reasonably certain that they had variants of this malformation. In the older cases reported by Williams and coworkers (1963) one of the clues to this lay in the presence in the electrocardiogram of more left ventricular potentials than would be expected in simple severe pulmonary stenosis. Occasionally left-axis deviation or superiorly oriented frontal plane loop will be encountered in patients with pulmonary stenosis. Six infants and children with a frontal plane Â QRS between +270 and +320 degrees reported by Stoermer and associates (1968) were considered to be have to a conduction anomaly of the left bundle. Ellison and Restieaux (1972) found that 7 percent of their patients had a counterclockwise superior loop. The relationship of this conduction anomaly to the presence of associated anomalies such as the Noonan syndrome is not entirely clear from either report. For Ellison and Restieaux (1972) the relationship between the right maximum spatial vector in the vectorcardiogram and the right ventricular pressure was essentially the same in those patients with left-axis deviation as for those with an inferiorly placed frontal loop.

Electrocardiographic Correlations. CHANGES WITH AGE. The moderate type of right ventricular hypertrophy seen in moderate stenosis is characteristically not changed throughout life. It is never found that a minimal right ventricular hypertrophy becomes marked in this type. A few young infant cases with moderate right ventricular hypertrophy in the electrocardiogram may develop changes to severe right ventricular hypertrophy within a year or so (Figure 40–4). This does not mean necessarily that a moderate stenosis has "tightened" but more likely that a severe stenosis has produced an elevation in right ventricular pressure from the increase in cardiac output necessitated by growth. On the other hand, in severe stenosis there may be no change with age, at least in childhood. For example, one of our patients followed from two months to six years showed an axis of +110 degrees, a qR pattern in V_1 with an R of 33 mm in height, and deep inversion as far as V_2 with P waves 4 mm and peaked. It is more common,

however, for the severe cases to show slowly progressive changes with age. The axis of QRS seldom changes significantly, although infants frequently have a rather low order of right-axis deviation in the first few months. The P wave may be abnormally tall early, but it is more frequently found that this change increases over the years. For example, one infant with a P of 2.5 mm at two weeks had an increase to 4 mm in height over the first two years. Similarly the height of R in V_1, which may be distinctly abnormal from an early age, may show further increase over the years. For example, one child aged three years had an R in V_1 of 19 mm that had increased to 31 mm by five years. In the same way either a qR pattern in V_1 may appear during childhood or the q may increase in size. The precordial T wave may change in two ways: deep inversion of T may extend from V_3 or V_4 to V_6; or, if the wave remains stationary, it may become deeper. One of our children at four years had deep T inversion as far as V_2 that extended to V_5 by eight years. It will occasionally be seen in cases with considerable venoarterial shunt that q waves appear in the left chest, thus suggesting a degree of left ventricular hypertrophy or dilatation. A few severe infant cases have shown moderate left ventricular hypertrophy in the electrocardiogram.

HEMODYNAMIC RELATIONSHIPS. P wave: Generally speaking, high right atrial pressures are associated with abnormally tall P waves, but in our group one-fourth of those with abnormal P waves had a mean right atrial pressure under 6 mm. P waves were abnormal and indicative of right atrial hypertrophy in one-quarter of the cases with a right ventricular systolic pressure under 100 mm of mercury of Cayler and associates (1958) but in only 6 percent of a similar series of Scherlis and associates (1963).

qR in V_1: In a similar way this pattern is frequently, but not necessarily, associated with a mean right atrial pressure of more than 8 mm.

R in V_1: None of our catheterized cases with a right ventricular pressure less than 100 mm of mercury had an R in V_1 exceeding 28 mm, and all except one had an R in V_1 between 4 and 25 mm. However, for any given pressure the height of R in V_1 was extremely variable. For example, with a right ventricular pressure of 75 mm in systole, the height of R in V_1 ranged from 4 to 28 mm. In the severe form about half the cases with a right ventricular pressure over 100 mm had an R in V_1 exceeding 30 mm. Nevertheless, a correlation between increasing height of R in V_1 and increasing level of right ventricular pressure is statistically significant.

Thus where the R exceeds 30 mm, severe stenosis is certainly present and a systolic pressure in the right ventricle of at least 150 mm will always be found on cardiac catheterization. In those cases with severe stenosis and a high right ventricular pressure but a low R in V_1, there will be found, with rare exception, T wave inversion in the right precordial leads extending at least as far as V_4, which offers the clue to interpretation. Scherlis and associates (1963) also found a reasonably good correlation of the voltage of

R in V_1 and right ventricular pressure, but Bentivoglio and coworkers (1960) rejected the relationship between these two variables because 22 of 36 of their patients with a right ventricular systolic pressure of 100 mm or more had an R in V_1 of less than 20 mm. In a more detailed consideration of this problem, it has been found that R in V_1 correlates better with valve area than with the pressure gradient across the valve, while the mean axis QRS correlates best with pressure gradient (Bassingthwaighte et al., 1963).

In a study of the electrocardiograms of 136 children with pulmonary stenosis from birth to 15 years at The Hospital for Sick Children, Fowler and Keith (1968) found good correlation of severity with RV_1 plus SV_6, RV_1 alone, and QRS Triangle. Considered simultaneously, the most useful indicators of right ventricular pressure were RV_1, frontal plane Â QRS, QRS-T angle, and R/S in V_1. These authors felt that such scalar measurements were almost as useful as the corrected orthogonal leads in predicting severity (Figure 40–3). When RV_1 is more than 35 mm, frontal plane QRS-T angle is 180 degrees, there is no S wave in V_1, and the R in V_1 is more than 30 mm, a valvotomy is required. When RV_1 is more than 15 mm, the frontal plane Â QRS is more than 90 degrees, and the QRS-T angle is greater than 60 degrees, a catheterization is required to establish the severity.

T wave: In our group no cases with a right ventricular pressure less than 100 mm of mercury in systole showed deep T wave inversion to V_4, whereas when the pressure exceeded 100 mm in systole in the right ventricle almost two-thirds of the cases had deep T inversion as far as V_4.

A variety of analyses have been applied to the Frank vectorcardiogram to improve hemodynamic correlations (Gamboa et al., 1966; Witham et al., 1968; Rasmussen and Sørland, 1973; Guller et al., 1974). Because conduction delay in the right or left bundle interferes with the assessment, modifications of prediction equations become necessary in patients who have such tracings (Fowler, 1968; Rasmussen and Sørland, 1973; Ellison and Miettinen, 1974).

DIAGNOSTIC IMPORTANCE. In the severe forms of pulmonary stenosis with normal aortic root the electrocardiogram is very characteristic in its exhibition of severe right ventricular and right atrial hypertrophy. It can at once be distinguished from that seen in tetralogy of Fallot, which never reaches the same degree of right ventricular hypertrophy. Furthermore, right atrial hypertrophy is much less commonly seen in the tetrad, especially in children. By comparison, the moderate forms of pulmonary stenosis with normal aortic root have electrocardiograms that are, in many instances, strikingly similar to those obtained in tetralogy of Fallot. This differentiation is particularly useful in a group of cases with tetralogy of Fallot and valvular stenosis who may mimic very closely the physical signs of pulmonary stenosis with normal aortic root. We have never encountered a cyanotic case of pulmonary

stenosis with normal aortic root with moderate right ventricular hypertrophy.

PROGNOSTIC IMPORTANCE. In those cases of the severe form where there is a marked right ventricular hypertrophy and perhaps right atrial hypertrophy, a progressive inversion of T wave from a position in the midprecordium to as far as V_6, over the course of a short period of time, is very suggestive of a serious outcome unless the stenosis is relieved by surgery (Marquis, 1951; Johnson and Johnson, 1952). Most observers are agreed that a progression of the T inversion in a short interval is an indication for surgery. Less unanimity has been shown on the significance of a stationary and rather deep T inversion. It is generally believed, with good reason, that this indicates a severe degree of right ventricular hypertrophy and strain.

Of 31 cyanotic patients (Campbell, 1954) six had P-R intervals of 0.21 to 0.31 second, and these patients had all died by the time of reporting. However, this sign signifying a serious prognosis is not necessarily grave, for two other noncyanotic cases have done well. It was seen in one of seven severe cases described by Marquis (1951) and was not a finding in our fatal cases. Arrhythmias encountered both pre- and postoperatively in children treated by Deverall and associates (1970) were associated with a profile of cyanosis, very high right ventricular pressure, and gross right ventricular hypertrophy prior to operation. This suggested the possibility that myocardial ischemia might be the underlying cause for such disturbances.

Radiologic Examination

The roentgenologic features of pulmonary stenosis with normal aortic root have been well reviewed (Blount et al., 1954; Dow et al., 1950; Greene et al., 1949; Healey et al., 1949; Kjellberg et al., 1959; Lucas and Moller, 1970).

Cardiac Contour and Size. The cardiac contour may be normal and the right border not suggestive of right atrial enlargement, except in a proportion of severe cases or in moderate cases with atrial septal defect and left-to-right shunt. The apex is usually down-pointing and rounded, and only occasionally is there a tipped-up apex.

Cases of mild-to-moderate stenosis usually show no cardiac enlargement unless there is an associated arteriovenous shunt, but cases with severe stenosis frequently have large hearts, about 50 percent having a cardiothoracic ratio in excess of 0.55. Those cases of the severe form in which enlargement is encountered in most instances will have this change at a very early age (Figure 40–5). Tricuspid regurgitation undoubtedly contributes to right atrial enlargement and the overall cardiomegaly in these patients. Progressive change in size over the years is rare but can occur. We have had examples followed from infancy, in which this was noted, and others have been reported (Johnson and Johnson, 1952; Gibson, 1954).

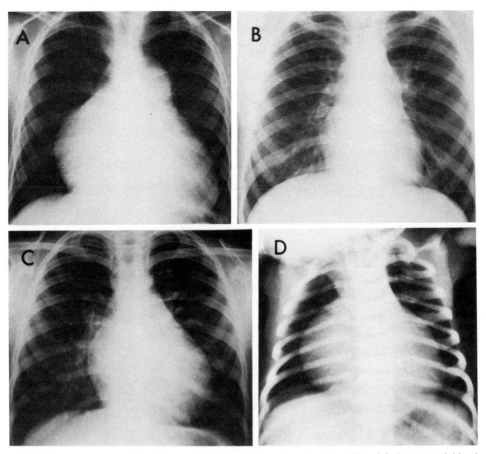

Figure 40-5. The chest x-ray in pulmonary stenosis. *A.* Severe stenosis with right-to-left shunt at atrial level. Cardiomegaly with main pulmonary artery bulge and reduced lung vascularity in a boy with a right ventricular pressure of 150/20 mm of mercury. *B.* Severe stenosis without shunts: normal heart size and lung vascularity with prominent main pulmonary artery in a girl with a right ventricular pressure of 200/15 mm of mercury. *C.* Moderate stenosis with left-to-right atrial shunt: slight cardiomegaly with increased lung vascularity in a girl with a right ventricular pressure of 100/10 mm of mercury. *D.* Severe stenosis in the newborn: the cardiomegaly is largely due to a large right atrium associated with tricuspid regurgitation (see Figure 40-8*A*).

A distinctive feature of the cardiac contour is a pulmonary artery bulge present in 90 percent of cases. In the majority this takes the form of a moderate bulge and in less than 5 percent it is aneurysmal during childhood. An increase in size of the main left pulmonary artery branch in contrast with the normal size of the right pulmonary artery is characteristic of the anomaly (Gay and Franch, 1960). These findings are quite uncharacteristic of isolated infundibular stenosis.

Right ventricular enlargement and forward projection are most obvious in the lateral chest film. Marked anterior bulging of the right ventricle in this view is confined to patients with considerable cardiac enlargement. In others, right ventricular hypertrophy may be reflected in the spinal overlapping of the left ventricle. Occasionally, in infundibular stenosis, a chamber may be visualized in the anteroposterior view.

The barium swallow will confirm the aorta to be usually of normal size and to have an arch that is left-sided. In our experience, any case with right aortic arch and right descending aorta, in which a diagnosis of pulmonary stenosis with normal aortic root has been entertained, has later been shown to be a case of tetralogy of Fallot with valvular stenosis but other experiences have been reported at variance with this (Campbell, 1954; Gamble and Nadas, 1965). Retroesophageal vessels, such as aberrant origin of the right subclavian artery, revealed by this method so frequently in the tetralogy of Fallot, are not encountered in pulmonary stenosis with normal aortic root. Left atrial enlargement is uncommon except in the occasional patient with associated ventricular septal defect where slight enlargement of this chamber may be seen.

Lung Vascular Markings. In chest films, lung vascularity is usually normal, regardless of the severity of the stenosis, unless there is venoarterial shunting. Then, lung vascularity is reduced. Where the lung vascular markings are increased patients will be shown to have arterial venous shunts from an atrial septal defect or from a ventricular septal defect, associated with moderate degrees of pulmonary stenosis.

Echocardiography

Gramiak and colleagues (1972) were the first to note that the echocardiogram in pulmonary stenosis showed the posterior leaflet of the pulmonary valve moving to its open position earlier than expected during atrial systole. These observations were a natural outcome of the demonstration provided by Hultgren and associates (1969) that a positive gradient exists at end-diastole across the pulmonary valve in pulmonary stenosis being present in both phases of respiration as the stenosis becomes moderately severe. The concept was expanded by Weyman and colleagues (1974) who determined that moderate-to-severe pulmonary stenosis was likely to be present when the posterior leaflet motion in late ventricular diastole, i.e., after atrial systole, was exaggerated above the normal. Milder stenosis showed normal motion of the leaflet. Goldberg and associates (1975) found exceptions and inconsistencies that they attributed to the effects of valve morphology in their subjects though they do not mention whether any had dysplastic valves. They suggested increased right ventricular wall thickness as an additional diagnostic aid in severe cases. Left ventricular hypertrophy, present in about one-quarter of all patients with the Noonan syndrome (Nora et al., 1975) and possibly in other forms (Bécu et al., 1976), lends itself to detection by this technique, especially since its presence may be unsuspected clinically in many patients. Further experience is necessary to clarify the role of echocardiography in severity assessment for this malformation.

Cardiac Catheterization

The important early studies through cardiac catheterization of adults and children with pulmonary stenosis demonstrated the pressure difference between the right ventricle and the main pulmonary artery, the level of that obstruction as defined by pressure changes in tracings obtained during withdrawal of the catheter from the main pulmonary artery to the right ventricle, characteristics of right ventricular and right atrial pressure pulses, and the presence of associated anomalies (Pollock et al., 1948; Greene et al., 1949; Cournand et al., 1949; Dow et al., 1950; Abrahams and Wood, 1951; Adams et al., 1951; Larsson et al., 1951; Maraist et al., 1951; Soulié et al., 1951; Bing et al., 1954).

Although the pressure difference across the pulmonary valve still remains a very important method of assessing severity, emphasis in the laboratory in more recent years for patients with the pure form of the disorder has rather moved to attempts to incorporate and define the influence of flow in this assessment, to examine methods of determining right ventricular myocardial function, and to utilize the application of cineangiocardiography for anatomic evaluation of the right ventricle and the pulmonary stenosis itself.

Pressures. When a catheter is withdrawn from the pulmonary artery to the right ventricle, a continuous pressure record will reveal the degree of obstruction by the pressure difference across the valve and frequently the site of obstruction from the position of the pressure change and the nature of the alteration in the pressure tracing (Figure 40–6).

In valvular stenosis of severe degree there is obliteration of the usual pressure pulse in the pulmonary artery branches and extremely low mean values are found. On entering the main pulmonary artery, distortion of the pressure record with large negative deflections is fairly constant. This is due to turbulence set up by the jet of blood entering the pulmonary artery with each ventricular systole and is maximal just distal to the pulmonary valve. The moment the catheter enters the right ventricle, an abrupt rise in systolic pressure occurs. Much the same situation exists in mild-to-moderate valvular stenosis, except that the pulmonary artery pressure pulse is then preserved and the level of pulmonary artery pressure is higher than in patients with severe stenosis. The actual level of right ventricular pressure used to distinguish mild-to-moderate from severe obstruction is arbitrary and often selected at a level above which patients should undergo valvotomy. For most groups, this is between 70 and 80 mm of mercury.

Changes in pressure at lower or both valvular and lower levels in the right ventricle usually indicate infundibular or combined stenosis. It is possible, through the use of electrode catheters or catheters with a single pressure sampling orifice some distance from the tip, to define rather precisely the site or sites of pulmonary stenosis. Because abrupt catheter movement or use of multiple whole catheters can lead to inaccuracies in withdrawal tracing assessments, most groups now rely on angiography to clarify the site of obstruction, rather than placing emphasis on the pressure measurements.

Similarly, while it is of interest to observe the abnormal form of the right ventricular pressure pulse (Bouchard and Cornu, 1954; Harris, 1955) (Figure 40–6) in all types of pulmonary stenosis with normal aortic root, this feature is much less important in the assessment today.

The right atrial pressure curve shows giant "a" waves in virtually all severe cases and in none of the mild or moderate obstructions. A slow rate of the "y" descent with a consequently shallow or absent "y" trough in the atrial pulse of patients with severe muscular infundibular obstruction secondary to valvular stenosis and a normal "y" descent and trough in those with insignificant obstruction have proved helpful diagnostic points in the hands of Vogelpoel and associates (1964).

Pressure/Flow Relationships. What has attracted considerable attention is the complex relationship

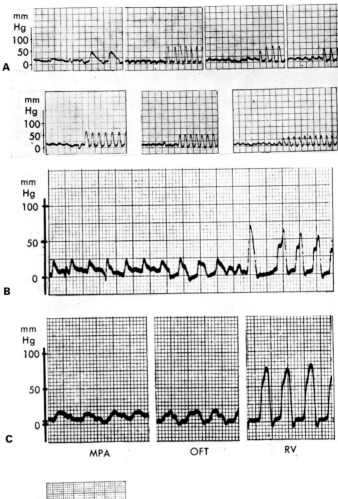

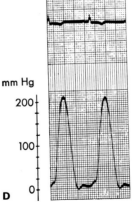

Figure 40-6. Pressure tracings taken during withdrawal of an end-hole catheter from the main pulmonary artery to the right ventricle in patients with pulmonary stenosis and an intact ventricular septum. *A.* Tracings from seven patients with mild pulmonary stenosis. The right ventricular pressure pulse is triangular and does not show the normal ejection plateau. *B and C.* Tracings from two patients with infundibular stenosis. The pressure pulse from the body of the right shows a slanting "plateau of ejection", and the pressure difference occurs below the level of the pulmonary valve. *D.* The symmetric pointed appearance to the right ventricular pressure pulse in severe valvular pulmonary stenosis.

between pressure, flow, and myocardial function in pulmonary stenosis. Since the initial publication that attempted to relate measured pressures across the valve orifice with flow through the area of the orifice (Gorlin and Gorlin, 1951), there has been enthusiasm for the calculation (Campbell, 1960; Bassingthwaighte et al., 1963; Hugenholtz et al., 1963; Rudolph, 1974). For these authors the accuracy of the measurement appeared good. It was recognized

that small pressure gradients existed across the valve until the orifice area was reduced to less than 1 sq cm. These investigations led to the suggestion that patients with valve areas in the range of 0.8 sq cm should undergo surgical treatment. They also had attraction to explaining why minimal surgical incision of the valve in severe cases can produce decided clinical improvement. The matter has been discussed again very fully recently (Rudolph, 1974).

Others have preferred to invoke the concept of pulmonary valvular resistance, recognizing the problems of measurement of area inherent in the hydraulic formulations (Moller and Adams, 1966). Recent analyses by the U.S. Joint Study of the Natural History of Congenital Heart Disease have looked specifically at the problem and particularly at the influence of a variety of factors on the peak systolic pressure difference across the pulmonary valve. The most important correlation appears to be with heart rate. Once the pressure gradient is adjusted for heart rate, there is no statistically added value from including the cardiac output itself (Mittinen and Rees, 1977). Obviously, the questions raised are very important, and further examination may eventually lead to an acceptable, practical, and less complex manner by which severity of the disorder can be measured from the ingredients obtained at cardiac catheterization.

This interest in the dynamics of pulmonary stenosis has been reflected in a growing literature on the result of exercise on the pressure-flow characteristics of individuals with this malformation, especially in patients with evidence of mild-to-moderate severity at rest. While standard submaximal exercise techniques in the catherization laboratory have been successful in adults (Lewis et al., 1964; Howitt, 1966), these methods have been feasible only for older children (Moller et al., 1972; Stone et al., 1974). Pediatricians have turned to alternatives for the very young such as the infusion of isoproterenol (Moss and Duffiie, 1963; Brodsky et al., 1970) or glucagon (Dimich et al., 1972). Others have turned from the invasive technique to the response of maximal effort (Goldberg et al., 1969) or of submaximal level of exercise (Bar-Or and Shephard, 1971; Godfrey, 1974) in the exercise laboratory.

The findings from studies of this sort have been that in adults with pulmonary stenosis who have resting right ventricular pressures in the order of 90 mm of mercury or less the normal response of the cardiac output to submaximal exercise occurs, but the cardiac output and stroke volume are lower at rest and on exercise where the right ventricular pressure is above that particular value. For children similar findings have been noted, the more severe degrees of pulmonary stenosis being associated with fixed or lower stroke volume, elevated right ventricular end-diastolic pressure, and suboptimal responses of cardiac output to exercise. These changes clearly are a reflection of altered right ventricular compliance. The important difference in the young as opposed to older individuals with these data is that within one year of pulmonary valvotomy, cardiac catheterization will show a decrease in right ventricular end-diastolic pressure and improvement in the stroke response to exercise. This implies that resolution of muscular hypertrophy is responsible for the improvement in children, whereas myocardial fibrosis explains the failure of the myocardial response to exercise to improve after operation in adults (Stone et al., 1974). In the experience of Dimich and associates (1972) the

effect of glucagon closely simulates moderate exercise, but most authors agree that isoproterenol does not increase the cardiac output to the same degree as is achieved with exercise for a given heart rate. The result is that isoproterenol infusions tend to indicate a more severe degree of stenosis than might actually be present. As a result of a consistent correlation for peak gradients with each technique at cardiac catheterization, a regression equation can be generated. Its use allows reasonably accurate prediction of the exercise valvular gradient from the data obtained during isoproterenol infusion (Truccone et al., 1977).

Two related aspects of assessment of stenosis severity deserve mention here. They are the attempts to measure valve orifice size by angiocardiography (Puyau et al., 1968) and measurement of right ventricular volume in the resting state (Graham et al., 1973; Arcilla et al., 1971). To date these latter methods have not proved particularly useful in clinical practice though they offer useful adjuncts to other methods of assessing natural history of the disorder.

Shunts. VENOARTERIAL SHUNT. Obvious right-to-left shunts will be evident by the presence of clinical cyanosis, by some arterial oxygen desaturation in those with smaller shunts, or by indicator dilution curves showing varying degrees of early appearance of the indicator in systemic curves following injection in the venae cavae. Almost always the requirement before such a shunt will be present is the presence of both severe obstruction at the pulmonary valve and an atrial communication of either widely stretched foramen type or true secundum atrial defect. Very rarely there is a minute ventricular septal defect present, and the shunt may then be detected only at the time of right ventricular injection of contrast material. Detailed pressure flow assessment of atrial shunts and severe pulmonary stenosis with intact ventricular septum by Levin and associates (1970) showed a right-to-left atrial pressure differential in ventricular diastole with a left-to-right atrial pressure differential throughout ventricular systole.

ARTERIOVENOUS SHUNT. Oxygen analysis will localize an arteriovenous shunt, if present, to atrial or ventricular level in the moderate forms, or to the pulmonary artery in all degrees of stenosis (Cournand et al., 1949; Taylor and DuShane, 1950; Wood, 1950; Abrahams and Wood, 1951; Deuchar and Zak, 1952; Broadbent et al., 1953; Campbell, 1954; Disenhouse et al., 1954; Magidson et al., 1954; Moffit et al., 1954; Rudolph et al., 1954; Eldridge and Hultgren, 1955; Hubbard and Koszewski, 1956). Detection of smaller-volume arteriovenous shunts is materially assisted by the use of the hydrogen electrode or by indicator dilution techniques, particularly using the two-catheter method. Passage of the catheter across the atrial septum is not by itself evidence of a shunt but is helpful corroboration of the site of the shunt when its presence has been demonstrated in other ways (Swan et al., 1953, 1954).

There is still debate as to how much gradient across the pulmonary valve may occur when there is a left-to-right shunt yet an anatomically normal pulmonary valve or infundibulum. The problem is most often encountered in patients with atrial septal communications. In 13 such patients from The Hospital for Sick Children, the systolic pressure gradient across the pulmonary valve ranged between 20 and 77 mm of mercury (Evans et al., 1961). The right ventricular pressure pulse was symmetric in form with a pointed peak in each instance, and the left-to-right shunt was of moderate size. In six of these patients, where the systolic pressure gradient exceeded 50 mm of mercury, surgical relief of the stenosis was performed. In the remaining seven, the systolic pressure gradient was reduced though not eliminated by closure of the atrial communication, and the surgeon noted a persistent thrill in the pulmonary artery in four.

Angiocardiography

The technique of choice is selective cineangiocardiography. The standard method involves right ventricular contrast injection with biplane, anteroposterior, and lateral projections. When examination of the main pulmonary artery bifurcation segments is indicated, an angled technique gives superior viewing of the area in question. Contrast usually provides a reasonably good indication of right ventricular cavity size and an appreciation of the tricuspid valve orifice and the dynamic changes in the right ventricular outflow. Information is also provided on the thickness and mobility of the valve and its orifice size (Figure 40–7). A jet of contrast is seen most often passing anteriorly in the pulmonary artery to strike the anterosuperior aspect of the main trunk. Poststenotic dilatation is visible. If pulmonary artery stenosis is present, this is usually clearly visualized for the right pulmonary artery by the classic projection but can be much more satisfactorily shown with angled views. Apart from poststenotic dilatation, which is unrelated to the severity of obstruction (D'Cruz et al., 1964), the above features generally tend to be more marked with increasing severity of obstruction. Thus more marked reduction in the right ventricular cavity size, more striking reduction in the right ventricular outflow tract in systole, a thicker and less mobile pulmonary valve, and a smaller jet size are characteristic of severe stenosis. In newborn babies with papillary muscle dysfunction, tricuspid regurgitation may be quite severe (Figure 40–8).

The levophase is often useful in determining the presence and site of any left-to-right shunting, particularly at atrial level, and may show abnormality of the left ventricular musculature in patients with the Noonan's syndrome (Ehlers et al., 1972). In that condition the dysplastic pulmonary valve (Jeffrey et al., 1972) is extremely common (Rodriguez-Fernandez et al., 1972).

On the basis of ventricular volume studies, Nakazawa and associates (1976) have shown that right and left ventricular function is normal in patients with isolated valvular pulmonary stenosis, but that when a major right-to-left atrial shunt is present, ventricular function is depressed to a variable degree. They recommend volume studies for full assessment of the latter group.

Diagnosis

Simple Pulmonary Stenosis. Pulmonary stenosis of this type can be recognized in a noncyanotic individual of normal physique who may or may not have fatigue and dyspnea with exertion and who has a pulmonary ejection click and an ejection systolic murmur between grade 3 and 6 in intensity, with or without a thrill, maximum in the second left intercostal space. The pulmonary component of the second heart sound may be normal, reduced and delayed, or absent. A right ventricular lift and abnormally prominent jugular "a" wave will be seen if the stenosis is moderate or severe. Except in very severe cases the heart size is normal though a prominent pulmonary artery bulge is usually present. The electrocardiogram may be normal or show varying degrees of right ventricular hypertrophy. The diagnosis is seldom difficult in severe or moderately severe degrees of the malformation when the clinical signs and accessory studies have been assembled. Principal difficulties in diagnosis arise in the variable clinical features of newborns with critically severe pulmonary stenosis, patients with the Noonan's syndrome, and patients with mild forms of the stenosis.

IDIOPATHIC DILATATION OF THE PULMONARY ARTERY. There is still debate over whether this condition represents a mild form of pulmonary stenosis or is truly a congenital abnormality of the pulmonary artery alone. The right ventricular pressure is normal on physiologic study. Clinically, such patients have a pulmonary artery lift, a loud pulmonary ejection click, and wide splitting of the second heart sound. The distinguishing point from significant pulmonary stenosis is that pulmonary valve closure is usually loud and early diastolic murmurs can be detected in up to 80 percent of patients. Radiologically the pulmonary artery segment is very prominent. The electrocardiogram is frequently normal but may show right ventricular hypertrophy or a variety of conduction disturbances (Ramsay et al., 1967).

STRAIGHT BACK SYNDROME. This condition (Daty et al., 1956; Rawlings, 1960; DeLeon et al., 1965; Tampas and Lurie, 1968) may mimic mild pulmonary stenosis by virtue of a normal second heart sound and an ejection systolic murmur of between grade 2 and 3/6 intensity in the pulmonary area. It is usually unassociated with a click. The presence of a pectus excavatum deformity together

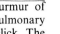

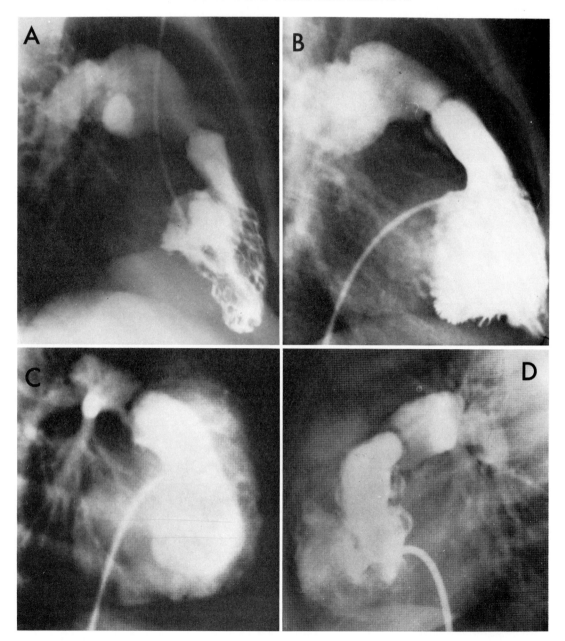

Figure 40-7. Selective right ventricular angiocardiograms in pulmonary valve stenosis. Lateral views in systole. *A.* Moderately narrow jet through a thickened, domed, pulmonary valve; poststenotic dilatation of the pulmonary trunk. Right ventricular pressure 128/2 mm of mercury. Boy, aged 11 years. *B.* Wide jet through a thickened, domed pulmonary valve; poststenotic dilatation of the pulmonary trunk. Right ventricular pressure 32/0 mm of mercury. Boy, aged four years. *C.* Critically severe stenosis of a thick pulmonary valve with massive tricuspid regurgitation and no poststenotic dilatation of the pulmonary trunk (see Figure 40-5D). Right ventricular pressure exceeded systemic level. Boy, aged 16 days. *D.* Narrow jet through a thickened, domed pulmonary valve with moderate poststenotic dilatation of the pulmonary trunk. Right ventricular pressure 160/20 mm of mercury. Girl, aged 16 months.

with a narrow anteroposterior diameter of the chest is helpful in bringing the possibility to mind.

SECONDUM ATRIAL SEPTAL DEFECT. The classic large flow atrial defect is easy to differentiate from mild pulmonary stenosis, but cases with small

defect where the pulmonary to systemic flow ratio is less than 2.0 may show wide but variable splitting of the second heart sound, no middiastolic murmur, a normal heart size, and a modest increase or normal lung vascular markings. These cases may be extremely difficult to distinguish and in fact may not certainly be differentiated sometimes until indicator dilution studies have been performed or cardiac catheterization undertaken. The echocardiogram may be very useful, since the right ventricle is almost always enlarged in small atrial defects of this sort.

MITRAL VALVE PROLAPSE. Occasional examples of this disorder will have a click and murmur audible maximally in the pulmonary area, possibly because transmission of the transients and the mitral regurgitation is directed toward the left atrial appendage (see Chap. 43).

PULMONARY ARTERIAL STENOSIS. This disorder is commonly associated with mild pulmonary valve stenosis, and the physical signs are frequently similar. In the bilateral form of the disease the most useful clue to the associated arterial anomaly lies in the wide transmission of the systolic murmur to the axillae and to the back. Other help may exist when there is a rubella background, a history of sibs with pulmonary stenosis, or the presence of intrahepatic biliary dysgenesis (Greenwood et al., 1976).

CONGENITAL ABSENCE OF THE PULMONARY VALVE. This condition can produce the physical signs and radiologic features and electrocardiophic evidence of severe pulmonary stenosis. What distinguishes this malformation from the simpler valvular obstruction is the presence of an early diastolic murmur. Such a to-and-fro murmur in the presence of signs of severe pulmonary stenosis is almost pathognomonic. Heart failure is common in the first few months of life (Ito et al., 1961), and secondary compression effects of the aneurysmal dilatation of pulmonary artery branches can produce severe respiratory dysfunction. Milder degrees of the malformation can be better tolerated.

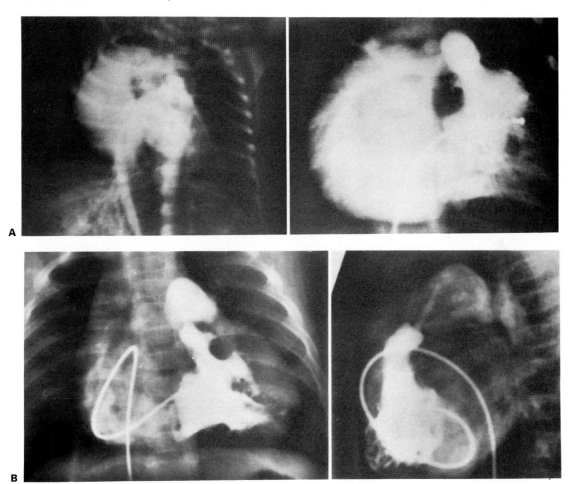

Figure 40-8. Angiocardiograms in the newly born. *A. Left*, venous angiocardiogram of an infant aged 14 hours. There was gross congestive failure. At autopsy ventricular size was equal, and there were gross right atrial dilatation and a minute orifice in the stenotic pulmonary valve. *Right*, selective right ventricular angiocardiograms in an infant aged 16 days. There is massive tricuspid regurgitation present, which was abolished by valvotomy. *B.* An infant aged four weeks with critically severe valvular pulmonary stenosis and patent foramen ovale. Anteroposterior and lateral views at the time of a selective right ventricular angiocardiogram. The right ventricular pressure was 160/10 mm of mercury. (Courtesy of Dr. R. M. Freedom, The Hospital for Sick Children, Toronto.)

AORTIC VALVE STENOSIS. Although the physical signs of valvular aortic stenosis in older children are unlikely to be confused with pulmonary stenosis, this distinction is not always so clear in young infants because the murmur of the left-sided lesion can occasionally be confined to the left sternal border and the electrocardiogram may show signs of right ventricular dominance rather than left ventricular overload. Furthermore, though the aortic ejection click is characteristically apical in position and uninfluenced by respiration, these features may be less conclusive in young infants where respirations will be faster and transmission of the pulmonary ejection sound is much wider than in older children and adults.

VENTRICULAR SEPTAL DEFECT. Some infant patients with pulmonary stenosis have a rather low position of the systolic murmur along the left sternal border, and this may occasionally lead to confusion with ventricular septal defects of small size. The phonocardiogram often assists (Mannheimer and Jönsson, 1954), but small ventricular defects of the type most likely to confuse may produce a diamond-shaped systolic murmur (Van der Hauwaert and Nadas, 1961). In diagnostic problems of this type the administration of amyl nitrite will reduce the length and intensity of the murmur of ventricular defect but will intensify the murmur of pulmonary stenosis (Vogelpoel et al., 1961). The murmur of aneurysmal transformation of the ventricular septal defect, which has late systolic accentuation (Pieroni et al., 1971), is sometimes confused with the infundibular stenosis of acyanotic tetralogy of Fallot but is seldom the cause of misdiagnosis of pulmonary valvular obstruction.

COMBINED PULMONARY AND AORTIC STENOSIS. This rare association may occur as either valvular stenosis alone, infundibular and subaortic stenosis in combination, or both valvular and subvalvular obstruction (Beard et al., 1957; Horlick and Merriman, 1957; Sissman et al., 1959; and Neufeld et al., 1960). In some cases, the clinical findings of pulmonary stenosis obscured those of the aortic lesion, while in others, the aortic situation constituted the major presentation and the pulmonary stenosis was found in the course of investigation. Appropriately the electrocardiograms of the reported cases have shown variation from left-axis deviation with left ventricular hypertrophy through combined ventricular hypertrophy to right ventricular hypertrophy alone. Four of the five cases from the above series died, and three of these were under four months of age. Successful surgical treatment in an older patient has been reported (Beard et al., 1957).

PULMONARY STENOSIS SECONDARY TO OTHER DISEASE. *Left Ventricular Myocardial Disease.* Myocarditis, glucogen storage disease, and obstructive muscle disease of the left ventricle have been noted to produce infundibular stenosis in some patients (Grosse-Brockhoff and Loogen, 1962; Ehlers et al., 1962; Goodwin, 1964; Barr et al., 1973).

Tumors. The clinical and hemodynamic picture of patients with right ventricular or pulmonary valve myxomata may closely resemble that of severe isolated pulmonary stenosis (Gottsegen et al., 1963; Catton et al., 1963). Neurofibromatosis has been reported to result in infundibular stenosis (Pung et al., 1955; Rosenquist et al., 1970) or valvular stenosis (Kaufman et al., 1972). Pulmonary stenosis in other disorders of pigmentation has been described, e.g., the little leopard syndrome (Gorlin et al., 1969; Pickering, 1971; Sommerville and Bonham-Carter, 1972) in association with infundibular stenosis due to a right-sided hypertrophic muscular disease; the syndrome of pulmonary stenosis, café-au-lait pigmentation, and dull intelligence has been reported by Watson (1967).

The Noonan's Syndrome (Noonan and Ehmke, 1963). About half the cases have congenital heart malformation and most of these have pulmonary stenosis (Nora et al., 1970). Characteristic facial features and other phenotypic stigmata should be the clue to the association. The fact that those with pulmonary stenosis very frequently have dysplastic pulmonary valves (Rodriguez-Fernandez et al., 1972) leads to problems in diagnosis and in the assessment of obstruction severity on the basis of the physical signs. Ejection clicks are frequently absent, the electrocardiogram may show left-axis deviation, and there is occasionally a paradoxically low intensity of the systolic murmur where the obstruction is severe. Hypertrophic disease of the left ventricle occurs in a proportion of patients (Ehlers et al., 1972; Phornphutkul et al., 1973), possibly in as many as 25 percent (Nora et al., 1975). It is often, but not necessarily, associated with pulmonary stenosis or other cardiac anomaly. Thus heart disorder in the Noonan syndrome is hardly that of simple pulmonary stenosis (Char et al., 1972; Caralis et al., 1974). Such patients demand a very thorough investigation for this reason and because the disease is transmitted as a dominant.

Carcinoid Cardiovascular Disease. This disease may be associated with pulmonary stenosis. Patients develop abdominal pain, diarrhea, weight loss, and paroxysms of flushing. The physical examination reveals facial telangiectasis, wheezing, liver enlargement, and an organic murmur over the pulmonary or xiphisternal areas. Radiologic and electrocardiographic evidence of right ventricular hypertrophy of variable severity is found. Cardiac catheterization or angiocardiography has confirmed the presence of pulmonary stenosis (McKusick 1956; Thorson et al., 1954). Death occurs from cardiac failure. Autopsy shows a carcinoid of the small bowel with liver metastases and pulmonary or tricuspid valvular stenosis. It is believed that the cardiovascular phenomena are related to the excretion by the tumor cells of excessive amounts of serotonin.

The majority of patients are middle-aged, but, although no children have died of the disease, symptoms first developed at the age of six years in one patient dying at 19 (Thorson et al., 1954).

Pulmonary Stenoses with Arteriovenous Shunt. These stenoses are always moderate in degree. Symptoms are more frequent. Cyanosis is absent. The murmur and thrill are either in the pulmonary area from the valvular stenosis or low along the left sternal border from the associated ventricular defect or infundibular stenosis. The second sound may be closely or widely split, and the apex beat may be tapping or thrusting. Fluoroscopically some enlargement is the rule, a pulmonary artery bulge is visible, and the lung vascularity appears slightly increased. The electrocardiogram most often shows moderate right ventricular hypertrophy or incomplete right bundle branch block. Although one may suspect the association of defects, and experience helps in this regard, proof is lacking until cardiac catheterization has been performed. The commonest error clinically is to label such cases as either isolated ventricular septal defect or simple pulmonary stenosis. In this situation *isolated atrial septal defect* may usually be excluded by the fact that in such patients the second heart sound is not only widely split but fixed in this regard with changes in respiration. Furthermore, the pulmonary valve closure sound is usually somewhat accentuated.

Pulmonary Stenosis with Venoarterial Shunt. In its classic form this defect has effort dyspnea but no squatting. There is slight to marked cyanosis and clubbing. Moon face is often present. A long, harsh systolic thrill in the pulmonary area with an absent or single reduced second pulmonic sound is found. Giant "a" waves are seen in the neck veins, and the liver may be enlarged and firm. Occasional infant cases develop congestive failure or suffer severe anoxic spells. Fluoroscopy reveals moderate to gross cardiac enlargement, distinct pulmonary artery bulge, down-pointing apex, and reduced lung vascularity. The electrocardiogram contains evidence of extreme right ventricular hypertrophy and most often right atrial hypertrophy. Cardiac catheterization indicates a pointed right ventricular pressure pulse exceeding systemic levels in systole and a low pulmonary artery pressure. The venoarterial shunt is localized to the atrial level.

TETRALOGY OF FALLOT. With valvular stenosis or infundibular stenosis with a large chamber, tetralogy of Fallot is differentiated by the history of squatting, the loud, though single, second heart sound, and, apart from exceptional cases, the absence of "a" waves in the jugular pulse. An important, though not invariable, feature at x-ray is the normal heart size. The apex is more often up-tilted and not down-pointing. A pulmonary artery bulge (or chamber bulge) may occur (Rowe et al., 1955). Most helpful in the presence of cyanosis is the only moderate right ventricular hypertrophy on the electrocardiogram of tetralogy of Fallot—a feature never seen in cyanotic cases of pulmonary stenosis with normal aortic root. Cardiac catheterization needs only a right ventricular pressure pulse for differential diagnosis of these two conditions. This, in the tetrad, has a plateau, whereas in pulmonary

stenosis with normal aortic root of this variety it is rounded, symmetric, and greater than systemic level in systole. Severe pulmonary stenosis with a smaller ventricular defect may lead to confusion by showing clinical, radiologic, and sometimes angiographic signs of tetralogy.

TRANSPOSITION OF THE GREAT ARTERIES. Confusion of cyanotic pulmonary stenosis with intact ventricular septum in the usual forms of D-transposition of the great arteries is not common, but in transposition with pulmonary stenosis and more complex intracardiac anatomy, especially where there is L-transposition, the difficulty is occasionally very real. Likewise, patients with D-transposition and ventricular defect with pulmonary vascular obstruction and bulging pulmonary artery segment commonly create diagnostic difficulties radiologically, but here the low-grade intensity of the systolic murmur would be incompatible with the severity of cyanosis for pulmonary stenosis with intact ventricular septum and a right-to-left atrial shunt.

RIGHT HEART HYPOPLASIA. Although left-axis deviation and left ventricular hypertrophy differentiate tricuspid atresia from other types of pulmonary stenosis, occasionally a newborn infant with cyanosis, no significant murmur, a large heart, and reduced lung vascularity, with left ventricular hypertrophy, will be found not to have pulmonary atresia and hypoplastic left ventricle but critically severe pulmonary valvular stenosis with a normal-sized right ventricle (Mustard et al., 1960; Freed et al., 1973). Often those findings are of course indicative of pulmonary atresia or critically severe pulmonary stenosis with hypoplastic right ventricle. Rarely isolated right ventricular hypoplasia without pulmonary stenosis will present in precisely the same manner (Okin et al., 1969). In older infants and children with small right ventricle and pulmonary stenosis, paradoxic splitting of the second sound may be a helpful point in diagnosis (Williams et al., 1963).

EBSTEIN'S DISEASE. Ebstein's disease of the tricuspid valve frequently produces a cyanotic infant or child with a systolic murmur of moderate intensity situated over the sternum or apex, a grossly enlarged heart with absence of pulmonary artery bulge, and reduced lung vascularity. The electrocardiogram provides the major clue to differentiation, for it almost always shows reduced voltage and complete right bundle branch block, a finding rarely seen in adult cases of severe pulmonary stenosis with normal aortic root but never encountered in infants or children.

PULMONARY VASCULAR DISORDERS. Occasional term infants of this group raise problems in diagnosis by mimicking cyanotic congenital heart disease. The heart may be enlarged; the electrocardiogram not infrequently shows moderate right ventricular hypertrophy in an abnormal degree after the first 24 hours; and there is frequently a tricuspid regurgitant systolic murmur, a right ventricular lift along the left sternal border, and there may be a prominent "a" wave in the jugular venous pulse. The main differentiating points from pulmonary stenosis lie in the character of the second heart sound. The pulmonary valve closure is usually very notable and the splitting of the second heart sound is often narrow. These signs of course suggest pulmonary hypertension, and the current terminology for that disorder, though varied, reflects that fact.

PULMONARY VASCULAR OBSTRUCTION. Primary pulmonary hypertension may be associated with cyanosis from a venoarterial atrial shunt, extreme right ventricular hypertrophy in the electrocardiogram, and reduced lung vascular markings. The absence of a murmur and the presence of a loud click and a closely split or single second heart sound help indicate the real cause for the pulmonary bulge and right heart hypertension.

Ventricular defect of the Eisenmenger type having major right-to-left shunt for the same reasons should seldom be confused with pulmonary stenosis with right-to-left shunt.

Assessment of Severity

When the diagnosis has been reached on clinical grounds, an important next step is to determine the degree of severity of the stenosis. The widely accepted standard upon which this judgment is made rests with the resting pressure difference across the pulmonary valve and/or the peak systolic right ventricular pressure level. There is not uniform agreement about what level is "mild" and what level is "severe," but convenient cutoff points for mild stenosis are differential pressure of less than 50 mm of mercury and a right ventricular peak systolic pressure of less than 70 mm of mercury and for severe stenosis a differential pressure of 80 mm of mercury and a peak right ventricular systolic pressure of more than 100 mm of mercury. This leaves an intermediate category of moderate severity. Increasingly, the intermediate or moderate categories are being incorporated by pediatric cardiologists into the severe group.

Severe stenosis can be assumed present in those patients where at least one of certain features is evident. These are cyanosis, congestive heart failure, a S wave in standard lead I of the electrocardiogram equal to or greater than 15 mm, a Q wave in V_1 or a negative T wave in aVf, and the sum of $RV_1 + SV_6$ equal to or greater than 35 mm. In such patients the pressure difference across the pulmonary valve averages 110 mm of mercury, higher gradients occurring if more than one criterion is present. This would still leave a large number of patients with simple pulmonary stenosis varying from mild to severe. Analysis of certain clinical features and simple accessory studies in relation to pressure gradient, found at cardiac catheterization, have long been used to seek predictions of pressure gradient that might be made for other patients without then resorting to

cardiac catheterization. These have included detailed consideration of the phonographic intervals, the murmur intensity and duration, and electrocardiographic and vectorcardiographic variables. No one clinical item permits reliable prediction of the pressure gradient or right ventricular pressure, and therefore multivariate analysis has been used more recently to arrive at prediction equations. Again, while many of these have reasonably good predictability, they do not cover all cases. Whether new additions to the available data pool in the future will improve the correlation remains to be seen, but for the present perhaps the most satisfactory solution is to settle for an ability to predict the presence of mild stenosis. In this way one can avoid cardiac catheterization for a sizable proportion of patients and confine that procedure to those who lie in the area of overlap, or intermediate, or occasionally even severe categories.

In the U.S. Joint Study of Congenital Heart Defects, prediction equations using universally available items were derived to this end (Ellison et al., 1977). The important final ingredients that emerged relate to auscultatory events and the electrocardiogram.

Pressure gradient RV − PA mm Hg

$$= 10.5(ISM) + 2.6(S_1)$$

$$+ S_2 \ SCORE + T \ SCORE.$$

ISM = Intensity of systolic murmur graded 1 − 6; S_1 = S in lead I in mm where 1 mm = 0.1 mv; S_2 SCORE = − 10 if P_2 is normal, + 2 if P_2 audible but diminished, and + 15 if P_2 is inaudible; T SCORE: + 15 if T is biphasic in V_1 when RV_1 is greater than 10 mm; otherwise the T SCORE is 0. If the estimated gradient is under 35 mm, from this equation one can predict that the cardiac catheterization would measure a gradient less than 65 mm of mercury. If the estimated gradient lies between 35 and 50 mm of mercury, a small proportion show a higher gradient, and if the estimation is greater than 50 mm of mercury, cardiac catheterization should probably be performed.

Complications

The patient with pulmonary stenosis and normal aortic root at the greatest risk for death is the infant with severe disease. In earlier editions of this book we showed that over half the deaths from pulmonary stenosis at The Hospital for Sick Children occurred during the course of the first year of life and similar experience was reported by Gibson and associates (1954). More recent data from the U.S. Joint Study has shown that almost all deaths today occur in newborn infants with severe disease (Nugent et al., 1977).

Congestive Heart Failure. In our earlier experience, heart failure was the immediate cause of death in one-third of the fatal cases seen at The

Hospital for Sick Children. It was recognized that this was a particularly ominous sign in the infant and that death often followed very quickly after presentation. Levine and Blumenthal (1965) reviewed 267 patients with pulmonary stenosis and intact ventricular septum in a pilot joint study of the natural history of this malformation and found 16 with congestive heart failure. All of these patients had right ventricular pressures in excess of 80 mm of mercury, and the proportion with congestive heart failure was much higher in those with pressures over 120 mm of mercury. Although congestive heart failure occasionally occurred in adults or younger children, by far the majority of patients with this complication were young infants. In the more recent U.S. Joint Study only 3 of 273 patients over the age of two years with right ventricular pulmonary artery pressure gradients in excess of 50 mm of mercury had this complication, whereas in 68 infants under the age of two years with a similar pressure gradient, 14 (or 1 in 5) had congestive heart failure. The complication was much more likely to arise when the pressure gradient exceeded 80 mm of mercury.

Hypoxic Spells. Cyanosis is very common in the severe form of pulmonary stenosis in infancy, and this sign is evident in as many as a third of those with gradients across the pulmonary valve of between 50 and 70 mm and almost a half of those who have gradients in excess of 80 mm of mercury. The occurrence of hypoxic episodes has, for many years, been recognized as a grave sign. Johnson and Johnson (1952) early pointed to the importance of episodes of paroxysmal dyspnea as a precursor of death, even before the development of frank congestive failure.

Infective Endocarditis. Abbott (1936) described two examples in 25 autopsies of pulmonary stenosis with normal aortic root, and Abrahams and Wood (1951) reported an incidence of almost 3 percent in their cases. In the U.S. Joint Study of Congenital Pulmonary Stenosis of 598 patients two gave a history of having had infective endocarditis and only one patient developed the disease during the study period. That patient survived. One interesting result of infective endocarditis in severe cases was the improvement in exercise tolerance that followed cure of the disease (Pollock et al., 1948; Abrahams and Wood, 1951). Nevertheless, the incidence of infective endocarditis is trivial in this condition, particularly when one compares the risk in other malformations such as aortic stenosis or ventricular septal defect.

Tuberculosis. Although tuberculosis was previously considered to be a common complication of the cyanotic form of pulmonary stenosis and normal aortic root, it has been found in recent times to be no more common than in the general population of the area (Aubertin, 1935; Abrahams and Wood, 1951).

Sudden Death. Discounting cardiac arrest at operation or death following cardiac catheterization, sudden death has been reported with no apparent relation to unusual effort. Blackford and Parker

(1941), Allanby and Campbell (1949), Marquis (1951), and Dimond and Lin (1954) have reported cases of this nature. The youngest was an infant with myocardial infarction at autopsy. Two others aged five years, one cyanosed, had extremely severe right ventricular hypertrophy in the electrocardiogram before death. These cases illustrate one more baneful effect of severe stenosis on cardiac function and presumably are due to myocardial ischemia from reduced systemic output.

Clinical Course

The worst immediate outlook, as always, lies in infants with gross cyanosis or congestive heart failure who are not offered immediate therapy. Unfortunately they often have complicating features such as small right ventricular cavity, or myocardial infarction, yet it is remarkable how high survival rates can be obtained, even in this high-risk group, today by prompt surgical intervention and first-rate preoperative and postoperative supportive care. The real questions lie in those who are asymptomatic and in little real distress.

Obviously some infants must have signs of mild stenosis that will be borne out by their subsequent course. The physician's task is to detect those infants who, having shown signs of mild or moderate stenosis, deviate from this picture by developing signs of very severe stenosis during the first few years of life. We have drawn attention to this particular problem in earlier editions and the matter has been highlighted recently by Mody (1975) and by Danilowicz and coworkers (1975). The latter workers found that the right ventricular systolic pressure rose by more than 20 mm of mercury in one-third in serial study of patients under five years old at the first investigation. Much smaller changes were encountered in patients first studied after the age of five years, findings earlier noted by others (Tinker et al., 1965; Moller et al., 1973; Johnson et al., 1972; Lueker et al., 1970). In the U.S. Joint Study of the Natural History of Congenital Heart Defects, among 261 patients treated medically it was shown that in patients with right ventricular to pulmonary artery gradients under 40 mm of mercury there is over a period of four to eight years either no change or a decrease in the gradient, whereas in those with severe obstruction with gradients in excess of 80 mm of mercury there is never improvement. The impressive rises in gradient occurred where the initial studies were performed in infancy. It is apparent from these studies that the truly mild pulmonary stenosis never increases in severity but that moderately severe stenosis commonly does so. Though the electrocardiogram often indicates this change, it may not do so, so that particular vigilance is needed for the follow-up of patients under the age of five years with mild-to-moderate stenosis, the probability of a need for recatheterization in selected cases being reasonably high. It seems likely that the majority of these potentially severe cases can be identified by careful

[handwritten margin note: critical gradient is 80 mm Hg]

analyses of auscultatory data and electrocardiograms in patients with initial right ventricular pressure levels at the borderline between the mild and severe stenosis.

Treatment

Medical Management. During early childhood mild cases do not require surgical treatment. Moderate cases should be operated upon only if they have symptoms or considerable cardiac enlargement from an associated arteriovenous shunt or if some detail in their investigation indicates that the obstruction is perhaps more severe than the clinical picture suggests. An assessment by complete heart catheterization with appropriate exercise studies and angiocardiography seems desirable eventually in borderline cases in view of recent suggestions that some such patients may ultimately develop significant disability that will not always be relieved by surgery. The main aim of the pediatrician should be to ensure, first, that the cases are, in fact, really mild in degree and, second, that the child is protected against infective endocarditis by penicillin prophylaxis at times of special risk.

antibiotic prophylaxis

Severe cases should be referred for confirmation and surgical treatment as soon as the diagnosis is made.

Surgical Management. Sellors (1948) and Brock (1948) reported the first successful attempts at relief of valvular pulmonary stenosis with normal aortic root. A significant experience of poor relief of stenosis from this technique in some hands led surgeons to attempt valvulotomy under hypothermia and direct vision by an approach through the pulmonary artery. In five cases operated in this way without a death (Blount et al., 1954) normal right ventricular and pulmonary artery pressures resulted. Larger numbers of patients have now been treated and the transarterial approach using cardiopulmonary bypass is now standard in most centers.

True isolated infundibular stenosis with a normal pulmonary valve was successfully treated by Glover and associates (1954) by infundibular resection based on the original method of Brock and Campbell (1950). This less common form of stenosis is not treated by open heart techniques (Slade, 1963).

The mortality from operation is relatively low in both adults and children. In 221 consecutive operations for pulmonary stenosis with intact ventricular septum at the Mayo Clinic between 1957 and 1967 the mortality rate was 4 percent (Danielson et al., 1971). Among 304 patients operated upon for pulmonary stenosis in the U.S. Joint Study nine died (3 percent) and all the deaths were patients operated upon in the first week of life. Among 109 patients from The Hospital for Sick Children, 84 of whom were less than ten years of age, there were six deaths when one includes the late complications (Mustard and Trusler, 1962). In 26 patients operated on in the first year of life, we had only one operative death (Mustard et al., 1968).

INDICATIONS FOR OPERATION. It is clear that the presence of cardiac enlargement is a late sign of severity in the malformation. One cannot rely on symptoms as an indication for operation, for many patients had none, and the first appearance of symptoms may be just prior to death (Johnson and Johnson, 1952). Marquis (1951) suggested that a right ventricular strain pattern in the electrocardiogram is an indication for urgent operation, and this is supported by Campbell (1954). A right ventricular pressure over 100 mm in systole was selected arbitrarily by Campbell and Brock (1955) by which level operation was recommended. Successes with direct-vision valvulotomy have led most groups to lower the right ventricular pressure level at which operative treatment is recommended to 70 mm or a gradient across the valve of more than 40 mm of mercury.

RV. → 70 40 mm

Tragic results may follow delay in surgery in severe cases in the first year. Many constitute surgical emergencies at this age.

RESULTS OF SUCCESSFUL VALVULOT-OMY. *Cyanosis.* In cyanotic cases the shunt is abolished except in patients in whom hypoplastic right ventricle is a feature, but in other infants the compliance of the right ventricle may be reduced from hypertrophy and/or ischemia but may be reversible over time. For these patients there is frequently a delay of several months before cyanosis completely clears. In a few cases the right-to-left atrial shunt may continue for a long time and eventually closure of an atrial defect may be required (DeCastro et al., 1970).

Exercise Tolerance. All patients claim they can exert themselves much more with fewer or no symptoms, but in many cases, especially children, the change is difficult to assess. This is particularly so when there was only equivocal reduction in exercise tolerance preoperatively.

Heart Size. When the heart was enlarged it becomes smaller. In Campbell and Brock's series (1955) the average reduction in cardiothoracic ratio was from 0.60 to 0.54. Only with cases complicated by major degrees of surgically induced pulmonary insufficiency is there any cardiac enlargement postoperatively.

Electrocardiogram. Evidence of severe right atrial hypertrophy and right ventricular hypertrophy becomes replaced by moderate hypertrophy or right bundle branch block. Particularly deep inversion T waves is greatly modified or abolished, and the height of R in V_1 is reduced. These changes begin immediately after operation but often take several months to be completed (Figure 40–9). Recent evidence indicates that a substantial number of children do not obtain a return to normal of their electrocardiogram (Dobell et al., 1971; Shams et al., 1973). The late consequences of this finding are at present uncertain.

Cardiac Catheterization. Postoperatively the right ventricular pressure falls considerably (Figure 40–9). Reduction rarely occurs to normal figures immediately, but in probably over three-quarters of

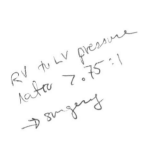
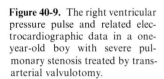

Bruce G.	mm Hg Right ventricular pressure	ECG V₁
Preoperative		
Two weeks postoperative		

Figure 40-9. The right ventricular pressure pulse and related electrocardiographic data in a one-year-old boy with severe pulmonary stenosis treated by transarterial valvulotomy.

those left with significant right ventricular hypertension, the pressure in the right ventricle returns to normal within a year or two (Engle et al., 1958; Brock, 1961). In a minority, reduction of the secondary infundibular stenosis responsible for these findings does not occur (Brock, 1961; McIntosh and Cohen, 1963). It does not seem at present that we are able to predict accurately which cases will fail to resolve their infundibular obstruction in the course of time. Our own results (Rowe et al., 1958) and those of McGoon and Kirklin (1958) suggested that age might be an important factor, secondary hypertrophy being more likely in the outflow tract of children more than five years of age. This has not always been true in the experience of others. The uncertainty of a favorable postoperative response of the outflow tract has led many surgeons to recommend resection of the infundibulum in any patient in whom adequate valvulotomy fails to reduce the right ventricular pressure to less than 100 mm of mercury (Johnson, 1959; Hosier et al., 1956). It is to be hoped that better evaluation of preoperative studies may soon lead to a clearer separation of those patients really requiring infundibular resections (Vogelpoel et al., 1964). Moulaert and associates (1976) believed that the response to a single small injection of propanolol given after valvotomy in the operating room can separate muscular from fixed causes of residual right ventricular hypertension.

One other important group of patients is that in which, after a long-standing moderate-to-severe pulmonary stenosis, adequate valvulotomy fails to improve the patient despite the abolition of pressure gradients across the pulmonary valve. It has been suggested that this complication is related to the

development of right ventricular fibrosis (Johnson, 1959, 1962, McIntosh and Cohen, 1963). Lewis and associates (1964) have confirmed the abnormal hemodynamic responses to exercise of all adult patients with resting right ventricular pressures exceeding 80 mm of mercury, while Ayres and Lukas (1960) found that approximately half their patients with even mild pulmonary stenosis had similar circulatory changes with exercise. These alterations are believed due to a reduction in right ventricular myocardial compliance, possibly due to fibrosis. This is seldom seen in children, suggesting that the present views on the severity required to recommend operation need changing. The U.S. Joint Study of Congenital Heart Defects demonstrated that of 294 operated patients only ten had a right ventricular to pulmonary artery gradient of more than 50 mm of mercury at recatheterization four to eight years after surgery and that only one of these had transarterial valvotomy on cardiopulmonary bypass. There is no evidence that restenosis occurs (Campbell and Brock, 1955). These data further strengthen the argument for surgical intervention in children when the resting right-ventricular-to-pulmonary-artery gradients exceed 50 mm of mercury.

A final problem concerns the production of pulmonary valve incompetence, which is obvious in about half the operative cases (Hanson et al., 1958; Rowe et al., 1958; Talbert et al., 1963). Although this does not seem to create immediate difficulties in most instances, the possibility of effects in later years from chronic diastolic overloading of the right ventricle is by no means excluded. This is the risk we are presently bound to take in severe cases. When the long-term consequences of this complication are ultimately

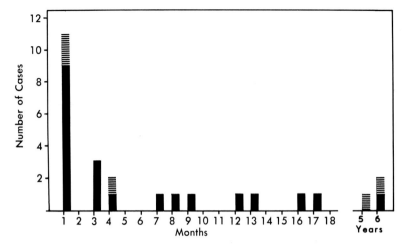

Figure 40-10. The age at death in 27 children with pulmonary stenosis and normal aortic root autopsied at The Hospital for Sick Children between 1946 and 1964. Surgical deaths are shown in shaded portion of the columns. Five patients (two operative deaths) had hypoplastic right ventricles, four dying in the neonatal period.

known, a decision regarding treatment for mild and moderate obstructions will clearly be influenced by the findings.

Prognosis

Up until very recently prognosis was based on the age at death reported in large autopsy series such as that of Abbott (1936) (see Figure 40–10). The average figure was close to 21 years. It is now apparent that the prognosis depends almost entirely on the severity of obstruction to pulmonary blood flow. Mild stenosis undoubtedly carries an excellent prognosis, and several cases have been reported surviving to 70 years. It is still uncertain how many cases of moderate stenosis develop eventual difficulty with increasing age because of right ventricular fibrosis.

Severe cases surviving the first year are likely to die from congestive failure in the second or third decade (Abrahams and Wood, 1951). The late results in survivors of pulmonary valvotomy are excellent (Reid et al., 1976; Nugent et al., 1977).

REFERENCES

Abbott, M. E.: *Atlas of Congenital Cardiac Disease.* American Heart Association, New York, 1936.

Abrahams, D. G., and Wood, P.: Pulmonary stenosis with normal aortic root. *Br. Heart J.,* **13**:519, 1951.

Adams, F. H.; Veasy, L. G.; Jorgens, J.; Diehl, A.; LaBree, J. W.; Shapiro, M. J.; and Dwan, P. F.; Congenital valvular pulmonary stenosis with or without an interatrial communication. *J. Pediat.,* **38**:431, 1951.

Allanby, K. D., and Campbell, M.: Congenital pulmonary stenosis with closed ventricular septum. *Guy Hosp. Rep.,* **98**:18, 1949.

Arcilla, R.; Tsai, P.; Thilenius, O.; and Ranniger, K.: Angiographic method for volume estimation of right and left ventricles. *Chest,* **60**:446, 1971.

Astley, R.; Oldham, J. S.; and Parsons, C.: Congenital tricuspid atresia. *Br. Heart J.,* **15**:287, 1953.

Aubertin, C.: Rétrécissement congénital de l'artere pulmonaire et tuberculose pulmonaire. *Paris Méd.,* 4 Mai, 413, 1935.

Ayres, S. M., and Lukas, D. S.: Mild pulmonic stenosis: a clinical and hemodynamic study of eleven cases. *Ann. Intern. Med.,* **52**:1076, 1960.

Bar-Or, O., and Shephard, R. J.: Cardiac output determination in exercising children—methodology and feasibility. In *Pediatric Work Physiology* Ed. Thorén, C. *Acta Paediatr. Scand.,* Suppl. **217**:49, 1971.

Barr, P. A.; Celermajer, J. M.; Bowdler, J. D.; and Cartmill, T. B.: Idiopathic hypertrophic obstructive cardiomyopathy causing severe right ventricular outflow tract obstruction in infancy. *Br. Heart J.,* **35**:1109, 1973.

Bassingthwaighte, J. B.; Parkin, T. W.; DuShane, J. W.; Wood, E. H.; and Burchell, H. B.: The electrocardiographic and hemodynamic findings in pulmonary stenosis with intact ventricular septum. *Circulation,* **28**:893, 1963.

Beard, E. F.; Cooley, D. A.; and Latson, J. R.: Combined congenital subaortic stenosis and infundibular subpulmonic stenosis. *Arch. Intern. Med.,* **100**:647, 1957.

Bécu, L.; Somerville, J.; and Gallo, A.: "Isolated" pulmonary valve stenosis as part of more widespread cardiovascular disease. *Br. Heart J.,* **38**:472, 1976.

Bentivoglio, L. G.; Maranhao, V.; and Downing, D. F.: The electrocardiogram in pulmonary stenosis with intact septa. *Am. Heart J.,* **59**:347, 1960.

Bing, R. J.; Reber, W.; Sparks, J. E.; Balboni, F. A.; Vitale, A. G.; and Hanlon, M.: Congenital pulmonary stenosis, *JAMA,* **154**:127, 1954.

Blackford, L. M., and Parker, F. P.: Pulmonary stenosis with bundle branch block: report of case with sound tracings and semi-serial studies of conduction bundle. *Arch. Intern. Med.,* **67**:1107, 1941.

Blount, S. G., Jr.; McCord, M. C.; Komesu, S.; and Lanier, R. R.; Roentgenological aspects of isolated valvular pulmonic stenosis. *Radiology,* **62**:337, 1954.

Bouchard, F., and Cornu, C.: Etude des courbes de pressions ventriculaire droite et arterielle pulmonaire dans les retrecissements pulmonaires. *Arch. Mal. Coeur,* **47**:417, 1954.

Boughner, D. R., and Roach, M. R.: Effect of low frequency vibration on the arterial wall. *Circ. Res.,* **29**:136, 1971.

Braunwald, E.; Goldblatt, A.; Aygon, M. M.; Rockoff, S. D.; and Morrow, A. G.: Congenital aortic stenosis. I. Clinical and hemodynamic findings in 100 patients. *Circulation,* **27**:426, 1963.

Broadbent, J. C.; Wood, E. H.; and Burchell, H. B.: Left to right intracardiac shunts in the presence of pulmonary stenosis. *Proc. Mayo Clin.,* **28**:101, 1953.

Brock, R. C.: Pulmonary valvulotomy for the relief of congenital stenosis: report of 3 cases. *Br. Med. J.,* **1**:1121, 1948.

Brock, Sir Russell: The surgical treatment of pulmonary stenosis. *B. Heart J.,* **23**:337, 1961.

Brock, R. C., and Campbell, M.: Infundibular resection or dilatation for infundibular stenosis. *Br. Heart J.,* **12**:403, 1950.

Brodsky, S. J.; Krovetz, L. J.; and Schiebler, G. L.: Assessment of severity of isolated valvar pulmonic stenosis using isoproterenol. *Am. Heart J.,* **80**:660, 1970.

Brown, J. W.; Health, D.; Morris, T. L.; and Whitaker, W.: Tricuspid atresia. *Br. Heart J.,* **18**:499, 1956.

Campbell, M.: Simple pulmonary stenosis. Pulmonary stenosis with closed ventricular septum. *Br. Heart J.*, **16**:273, 1954.

———: Relationship of pressure and valve area in pulmonary stenosis. *Br. Heart J.*, **22**:101, 1960.

———: Factors in the aetiology of pulmonary stenosis. *Br. Heart J.*, **24**:625, 1962.

Campbell, M., and Brock, R. C.: The results of valvotomy for simple pulmonary stenosis. *Br. Heart J.*, **17**:229, 1955.

Caralis, D. G.; Char, F.; Graber, J. D.; and Voigt, G. C.: Delineation of multiple cardiac anomalies associated with the Noonan syndrome in an adult and review of the literature. *Hopkins Med. J.*, **134**:346, 1974.

Case records of the Massachusetts General Hospital. *N. Engl. J. Med.*, **280**:714, 1969.

Catton, R. W.; Guntheroth, W. G.; and Reichenback, D. D.: A myxoma of the pulmonary valve causing severe stenosis in infancy. *Am. Heart J.*, **66**:248, 1963.

Cayler, C. G.; Ongley, P.; and Nadas, A. S.: Relation of systolic pressure in the right ventricle to the electrocardiogram. *N. Engl. J. Med.*, **258**:979, 1958.

Char, F.; Rodriquez-Fernandez, H. L.; Scott, C. I., Jr.; Borgaonkar, D. S.; Bell, B. B.; and Rowe, R. D.: The Noonan Syndrome—a clinical study of forty-five cases. *The Cardiovascular System. Birth Defects, Original Article Series*, **8**:110, 1972.

Chiche, P.: Etude anatomique et clinique des atrésies tri-cuspidiennes. *Arch. Mal. Coeur*, **45**:980, 1952.

Coblentz, B., and Mathivat, A.: Stenose pulmonaire congenital chez deux soeurs. *Arch. Mal. Coeur*, **45**:490, 1952.

Cournand, A.; Baldwin, J. S.; and Himmelstein, A.: *Cardiac Catheterization in Congenital Heart Disease*. The Commonwealth Fund, New York, 1949.

Currens, J. H.; Kinney, T. D.; and White, P. D.: Pulmonary stenosis with intact ventricular septum. Report of eleven cases. *Am. Heart J.*, **30**:491, 1945.

Danielson, G. K.; Exarhos, N. D.; Weidman, W. H.; and McGoon, D. C.: Pulmonic stenosis with intact ventricular septum. Surgical considerations and results of operation. *J. Thorac. Cardiovasc. Surg.*, **61**:228, 1971.

Danilowicz, D.; Hoffman, J. I. E.; and Rudolph, A. M.: Serial studies of pulmonary stenosis in infancy and childhood. *Br. Heart J.*, **37**:808, 1975.

Daty, K. K.; Deshmukh, M. M.; Engineer, J. D.; and Dalvi, C. P.: Straight back syndrome. *Br. Heart J.*, **26**:614, 1956.

D'Cruz, I. A.; Arcilla, R. A.; and Agustsson, M. H.: Dilatation of the pulmonary trunk in stenosis of the pulmonary valve and of the pulmonary arteries in children. *Am. Heart J.*, **68**:612, 1964.

deCastro, C. M.; Nelson, W. P.; Jones, R. C.; Hall, R. J.; Hopeman, A. R.; and Jahnke, E. J.: Pulmonary stenosis: Cyanosis, interatrial communication and inadequate right ventricular distensibility following pulmonary valvotomy. *Am. J. Cardiol.*, **26**:540, 1970.

DeLeon, A. C. Jr.; Perloff, J. K.; Twigg, H.; and Majd, M.: The straight back syndrome: Clinical cardiovascular manifestations. *Circulation*, **32**:193, 1965.

Deuchar, D. C., and Zak, G. A.: Cardiac catheterization in congenital heart disease. I. Four cases of pulmonary stenosis with increased pulmonary blood flow. *Guy Hosp. Rep.*, **101**:1, 1952.

Deverall, P. B.; Roberts, N. K.; and Stark, J.: Arrhythmias in children with pulmonary stenosis. *Br. Heart J.*, **32**:472, 1970.

Dimich, I.; Steinfeld, L.; Kahn, A.; and Rosenstock, N.: The use of glucagon and isoproterenol in the evaluation of isolated pulmonary stenosis. *J. Mt. Sinai Hosp. N.Y.*, **39**:598, 1972.

Dimond, E. G., and Lin, T. K.: The clinical picture of pulmonary stenosis (without ventricular septal defect). *Ann. Intern. Med.*, **40**:1108, 1954.

Dinsmore, R. E.; Sanders, C. A.; Harthome, J. W.; and Austen, W. G.: Congenital pulmonary stenosis with calcification. *Radiology*, **87**:429, 1966.

Disenhouse, R. B.; Anderson, R. C.; Adams, P., Jr.; Novick, R.; Jorgens, J.; and Levin, B.: Atrial septal defects in infants and children. *J. Pediat.*, **44**:369, 1954.

Dobell, A. R. C.; Fagan, J. E.; Sheverini, M.; Collins, G. F.; Murphy, D. R.; and Gibbons, J. E.: Results of pulmonary valvotomy—early and late. In Kidd, B. S. L., and Keith, J. D. (eds.): *The Natural History and Progress in Treatment of Congenital Heart Defects*. Charles C Thomas, Publisher, Springfield, Ill., 1971.

Donzelot, E., and D'Allaines, F.: *Traité des Cardiopathies Congenitales*. Masson & Cie, Paris, 1954.

Dow, J. W.; Levine, H. D.; Elkin, M.; Haynes, F. W.; Hellems, H. K.; Whittenberger, J. W.; Ferris, G. B.; Goodale, W. T.; Harvey, W. P.; Eppinger, E. C.; and Dexter, L.: Studies of congenital heart disease. IV. Uncomplicated pulmonic stenosis. *Circulation*, **1**:267, 1950.

Dubin, I. N., and Hollinshead, W. H.: Congenitally insufficient tricuspid valve accompanied by an anaomalous septum in the right atrium. *Arch. Pathol.*, **38**:225, 1944.

Edwards, J. E.: Congenital malformations of the heart and great vessels. In Gould, S. E. (ed.): *Pathology of the Heart*, Charles C Thomas, Publisher, Springfield, Ill., 1953.

Ehlers, K. H.; Hagstrom, J. W. C.; Lukas, D. S.; Redo, S. F.; and Engle, M. A.: Glycogen-storage disease of the myocardium with obstruction to left ventricular outflow. *Circulation*, **25**:96, 1962.

Ehlers, K. H.; Engle, M. A.; Levin, A. R.; Deely, W. J.; Levine, L. S.; and New, M. I.: Eccentric ventricular hypertrophy in familial and sporadic instances of 46 XX, XY Turner phenotype. *Circulation*, **45**:639, 1972.

Eldridge, F. L., and Hultgren, H. N.: Pulmonary stenosis with increased pulmonary blood flow. *Am. Heart J.*, **49**:838, 1955.

Ellison, R. C.; Freedom, R. M.; Keane, J. F.; Nugent, E. W.; Rowe, R. D.; and Miettinen, O. S.: Indirect assessment of severity in pulmonary stenosis. *Circulation*, **56**:(Suppl. 1) 1–14, 1977.

Ellison, R. C., and Miettinen, O. S.: Interpretation of RSR′ in pulmonic stenosis. *Am. Heart J.*, **88**:7, 1970.

Ellison, R. C., and Restieaux, N. J.: *Vectorcardiogram in Congenital Heart Disease. A method for Estimating Severity*. W. B. Saunders Co., Philadelphia, 1972, p. 60.

Engle, M. A.; Holswade, G. R.; Goldberg, H. P.; Lukas, D. S.; and Glenn, F.: Regression after open valvotomy of infundibular stenosis accompanying severe valvular pulmonic stenosis. *Circulation*, **17**:862, 1958.

Engle, M. A., and Taussig, H. B.: Valvular pulmonic stenosis with intact ventricular septum and patent foramen ovale: report of illustrative cases and analysis of clinical syndrome. *Circulation*, **2**:481, 1950.

Evans, J. R.; Rowe, R. D.; and Keith, J. D.: The clinical diagnosis of atrial septal defect in children. *Am. J. Med.*, **30**:345, 1961.

Findlay, D. W.: Malformation of the heart; stenosis of the pulmonary valve, with dilatation of the pulmonary artery and hypertrophy of the right ventricle; patency of the foramen ovale, with a cribriform opening in the septum of the auricles (ductus arteriosus closed). *Trans. Pathol. Soc. London*, **30**:262, 1879.

Folger, G. M.: Supravalvular tricuspid stenosis. *Am. J. Cardiol.*, **21**:81, 1968.

Fowler, R. S.: Terminal QRS conduction delay in pulmonary stenosis in children. *Am. J. Cardiol.*, **21**:669, 1968.

Fowler, R. S., and Keith, J. D.: The electrocardiogram in pulmonary stenosis—a reappraisal. *Can. Med. Assoc. J.*, **98**:433, 1968.

Franciosi, R. A., and Blanc, W. A.: Myocardial infarcts in infants and children. I. A necropsy study in congenital heart disease. *J. Pediatr.*, **73**:309, 1968.

Freed, M. D.; Rosenthal, A.; Bernhard, W. F.; Litwin, S. B.; and Nadas, A. S.: Critical pulmonary stenosis with a diminutive right ventricle in neonates. *Circulation*, **48**:875, 1973.

Freedom, R. M.: Unpublished observations.

Gabriele, O. F., and Scatliff, J. H.: Pulmonary valve calcification. *Am. Heart J.*, **80**:299, 1970.

Gamble, W. J., and Nadas, A. S.: Severe pulmonic stenosis with intact ventricular septum and right aortic arch. *Circulation*, **32**:114, 1965.

Gamboa, R.; Hugenholtz, P. G.; and Nadas, A. S.: Accuracy of the phonocardiogram in assessing severity of aortic and pulmonic stenosis. *Circulation*, **30**:35, 1964.

Gamboa, R.; Hugenholtz, P. G.; and Nadas, A. S.: Right ventricular forces in right ventricular hypertension. *Br. Heart J.*, **28**:62, 1966.

Gay, B. B., Jr., and Franch, R. H.: Pulsations in the pulmonary arteries as observed with roentgenoscopic image amplification. Observation in patients with isolated pulmonary valvular stenosis. *Am. J. Roentgenol.*, **83**:335, 1960.

Gibson, S.; White, H.; Johnson, F.; and Potts, W. J.: Congenital pulmonary stenosis with intact ventricular septum. *Am. J. Dis. Child.*, **87**:26, 1954.

Glancy, D. L.; Chang, M. Y.; Dorney, E. R.; and Roberts, W. C.: Parachute mitral valve. Further observations and associated lesions. *Am. J. Cardiol.*, **27**:309, 1971.

Glover, R. P.; O'Neill, J. E.; Gontigo, H.; McAuliffe, T. C.; and Wells, C. R. E.: The surgery of infundibular stenosis with intact ventricular septum (a type of "pure" pulmonic stenosis). *J. Thorac. Surg.*, **28**:481, 1954.

Godfrey, S., and Davies, C. T. M.: Estimates of arterial PCO_2 and their effect on the calculated values of cardiac output and dead space on exercise. *Clin. Sci.*, **39**:529, 1970.

Goldberg, S. J.; Allen, H. D.; and Sahn, D. J.: *Pediatric and Adolescent Echocardiography. A Handbook.* Year Book Medical Publishers, Inc., Chicago, 1975, p. 116.

Goldberg, S. J.; Mendes, F.; and Hurwitz, R.: Maximal exercise capability of children as a function of specific cardiac defects. *Am. J. Cardiol.*, **23**:349, 1969.

Gombert, H.: Beitrage zur pathologie der vorhofsscheidewand des herzens. *Beitr. Pathol., Anat.*, **91**:483, 1933.

Goodwin, J. F.: Cardiac function in primary myocardial disorders. *Br. Med. J.*, **1**:1527 and 1595, 1964.

Gorlin, R. J.; Anderson, R. C.; and Blaw, M.: Multiple lentigenes syndrome. *Am. J. Dis. Child.*, **117**:652, 1969.

Gorlin, R., and Gorlin, S. A.: Hydraulic formula for calculation of the area of the stenotic mitral valve, other cardiac valves and central circulatory shunts. *Am. Heart J.*, **41**:1, 1951.

Gottsegen, G.; Wessely, J.; Array, A.; and Temesvári, A.: Right ventricular myxoma simulating pneumonic stenosis. *Circulation*, **27**:95, 1963.

Graham, T. P., Jr.; Jarmakani, J. M.; Atwood, G. F.; and Canent, R. V., Jr.: Right ventricular volume determinations in children. Normal values and observations with volume or pressure overload. *Circulation*, **47**:144, 1973.

Gramiak, R.; Nanda, N. C.; and Shah, P. M.: Echocardiographic detection of the pulmonary valve. *Radiology*, **102**:153, 1972.

Greene, D. G.; Baldwin, E. de F.; Baldwin, J. S.; Himmelstein, A.; Roh, C. E.; and Cournand, A.: Pure congenital pulmonary stenosis and idiopathic congenital dilatation of the pulmonary artery. *Am. J. Med.*, **6**:24, 1949.

Greenwood, R. D.; Rosenthal, A.; Crocker, A. C.; and Nadas, A. S.: Syndrome of intrahepatic biliary dysgenesis and cardiovascular malformations. *Pediatrics*, **58**:243, 1976.

Grosse-Brockhoff, F., and Loogen, F.: Infundibular pulmonary stenosis in chronic left ventricular cardiopathy. *German Med. Monthly*, **7**:109, 1962.

Guller, B.; O'Brien, P. C.; Smith, R. E.; and Weidman, W. H.: Computer interpretation of right ventricular hypertrophy from Frank vectorcardiogram in children with congenital heart disease. *Mayo Clin. Proc.*, **49**:486, 1974.

Hansing, C. E.; Young, W. P.; and Rowe, G. G.: Cor triatriatum dexter. Persistent right sinus venosus valve. *Am. J. Cardiol.*, **30**:559, 1972.

Hanson, J. S.; Ikkos, D.; Crafoord, C.; and Ovenfors, C.-O.: Results of surgery for congenital pulmonary stenosis. Comparison of the transventricular and transarterial approaches. *Circulation*, **18**:588, 1958.

Harris, P.: Some variations in the shape of the pressure curve in the human right ventricle. *Br. Heart J.*, **17**:173, 1955.

Healey, R. F.; Dow, J. W.; Sosman, M. C.; and Dexter, J. L.: The relationship of the roentgenographic appearance of the pulmonary artery to pulmonary haemodynamics. *Am. J. Roentgenol.*, **62**:777, 1949.

Horlick, L., and Merriman, J. E.: Congenital valvular stenosis of pulmonary and aortic valves with atrial septal defect. *Am. Heart J.*, **54**:615, 1957.

Hosier, D. M.; Pitts, J. L.; and Taussig, H. B.: Results of valvulotomy for valvular pulmonary stenosis with intact ventricular septum. Analysis of 69 patients. *Circulation*, **14**:9, 1956.

Howitt, G.: Hemodynamic effects of exercise in pulmonary stenosis. *Br. Heart J.*, **28**:152, 1966.

Hubbard, T. F., and Koszewski, B. J.: Pulmonary stenosis with increased pulmonary blood flow. *Arch. Intern. Med.*, **97**:327, 1956.

Hugenholtz, P. G.; Hauck, A. J.; and Nadas, A. S.: Accuracy of valve area calculation in assessment of stenotic lesions. *Circulation*, **28**:740, 1963.

Hultgren, H. N.; Reeve, R.; Cohn, K.; and McLeod, R.: The ejection click of valvular pulmonic stenosis. *Circulation*, **40**:631, 1969.

Ito, T.; Engle, M. A.; and Holwade, G. R.: Congenital insufficiency of the pulmonic valve. A rare cause of neonatal heart failure. *Pediatrics*, **28**:712, 1961.

Izukawa, T., and Keith, J. D.: Unpublished observations.

Jeffrey, R. F.; Moller, J. H.; and Amplatz, K.: The dysplastic pulmonary valve: A new roentgenographic entity with a discussion of the anatomy and radiology of other types of valvular pulmonary stenosis. *Am. J. Roentgenol. Rad. Ther.*, **114**:322, 1972.

Johnson, A. M.: Hypertrophic infundibular stenosis complicating simple pulmonary valve stenosis. *Br. Heart J.*, **21**:429, 1959.

Johnson, R. P., and Johnson, E. E.: Congenital pulmonic stenosis with open foramen ovale in infancy. Report of five proved cases. *Am. Heart J.*, **44**:344, 1952.

Johnnson, L. W.; Grossman, W.; Dalen, J. E.; and Dexter, L.: Pulmonic stenosis in the adult. Long-term follow-up results. *N. Engl. J. Med.*, **287**:1159, 1972.

Kaufman, R. L.; Hartmann, A. F.; and McAlister, W. H.: Family studies in congenital heart disease. IV: Congenital heart disease associated with neurofibromatosis. *Birth Defects: Original Article Series*, **8**: #5, 1972.

Kjellberg, S. R.; Mannheimer, E.; Rudhe, U.; and Jönsson, B.: *Diagnosis of Congenital Heart Disease*, 2nd ed. Year Book Publishers, Inc., Chicago, 1959.

Klinge, T., and Laursen, H. B.: Familial pulmonary stenosis with underdeveloped or normal right ventricle. *Br. Heart J.*, **37**:60, 1975.

Koretzky, E. D.; Moller, J. H.; Korns, M. E.; Schwartz, C. J.; and Edwards, J. E.; Congenital pulmonary stenosis resulting from dysplasia of valve. *Circulation*, **40**:43, 1969.

Larsson, Y.; Mannheimer, E.; Moller, T.; Lagerlof, H.; and Werko, L. A.: Congenital pulmonary stenosis without overriding aorta. *Am. Heart J.*, **42**:70, 1951.

Lasser, R. P., and Genkins, G.: Chest pain in patients with isolated pulmonic stenosis. *Circulation*, **15**:258, 1957.

Leatham, A.: Phonocardiography. *Brit. Med. Bull.*, **8**:333, 1952.

————: Splitting of the first and second heart sounds. *Lancet*, **2**:607, 1954.

Leatham, A., and Weitzman, D.: Auscultatory and phonographic signs of pulmonary stenosis. *Br. Heart J.*, **19**:303, 1957.

Lev, M.: Pathology of congenital heart disease. In Luisada, A. A. (ed.): Cardiology, McGraw-Hill Book Co., New York, 1959, Vol. 3, pp. 6–28.

Levin, A. R.; Spach, M. S.; Canent, R. V.; and Boineau, J. P.: Dynamics of interatrial shunting in children with obstruction of the tricuspid and pulmonic valves. *Circulation*, **41**:503, 1970.

Levine, O. R., and Blumenthal, S.: Pulmonary stenosis. *Circulation*, **32**, Suppl. III:33, 1965.

Lewis, J. M.; Montero, A. C.; Kinard, S. A., Jr.; Dennis, E. W.; and Alexander, J. K.: Hemodynamic response to exercise in isolated pulmonic stenosis. *Circulation*, **29**:854, 1964.

Lucas, R. V., Jr., and Moller, H. J.: Pulmonary valvular stenosis. *Cardiovasc. Clin.*, **2**:155, 1970.

Lueker, R. D.; Vogel, J. H. K.; and Blount, S. G., Jr.: Regression of valvular pulmonary stenosis. *Br. Heart J.*, **32**:779, 1970.

McCarron, W. E., and Perloff, J. K.: Familial congenital valvular pulmonary stenosis. *Am. Heart J.*, **88**:397, 1974.

McGoon, D. C., and Kirklin, J. W.: Pulmonic stenosis with intact ventricular septum. Treatment utilizing extracorporeal circulation. *Circulation*, **17**:180, 1958.

McIntosh, H. D., and Cohen, A. I.: Pulmonary stenosis: the importance of the myocardial factor in determining the clinical course and surgical results. *Am. Heart J.*, **65**:715, 1963.

McKusick, V. A.: Carcinoid cardiovascular disease. *Bull. Hopkins Hosp.*, **98**:13, 1956.

Magidson, O.; Cosby, R. S.; Dimitroff, S. P.; Levinson, D. C.; and Griffith, G. C.: Pulmonary stenosis with left to right shunt. *Am. J. Med.*, **17**:311, 1954.

Mannheimer, E., and Jönsson, B.: Heart sounds and murmurs in congenital pulmonary stenosis with normal aortic root. *Acta Paediatr.*, **43** (suppl. 100): 167, 1954.

Maraist, F.; Daley, R.; Draper, A., Jr.; Heimbecker, R.; Dammann, F., Jr.; Keiffer, R., Jr.; King, J. T.; Ferencz, C.; and Bing, R. J.: Physiological studies in congenital heart disease. X. The physiological findings in 34 patients with isolated pulmonary valvular stenosis. *Bull. Hopkins Hosp.*, **88**:1, 1951.

Marquis, R. M.: Unipular electrocardiography in pulmonary stenosis. *Br. Heart J.*, **12**:265, 1951.

Miettinen, O. S., and Rees, J. K.: II. Methodology. Report from the Joint Study on the Natural History of Congenital Heart Disease. *Circulation*, 56: (Suppl. I), I–5, 1977.

Mody, M. R.: The natural history of uncomplicated valvular pulmonic stenosis. *Am. Heart. J.*, 90: 317, 1975.

Moffitt, G. R., Jr.; Zinsser, H. F., Jr.; Kuo, P. T.; Jönnson, J.; and Schnabel, T. G.: Pulmonary stenosis with left to right intracardiac shunts. *Am. J. Med.*, 16: 521, 1954.

Moller, J. H., and Adams, P., Jr.: A simplified method for calculating the pulmonary valvular area. *Am. Heart J.*, 72: 463, 1966.

Moller, J. H.; Rao, S.; and Lucas, R. V., Jr.: Exercise hemodynamics of pulmonary stenosis. Study of 64 children. *Circulation*, 46: 1018, 1972.

Møller, I.; Wennevold, A.; and Lyngberg, K. E.: The natural history of pulmonary stenosis: Long-term follow-up with serial heart catheterizations. *Cardiology*, 58: 193, 1973.

Moss, A. J., and Duffie, E. R., Jr.: The use of isoproterenol (isuprel) in the evaluation of cardiac defects. *Circulation*, 27: 51, 1963.

Moulaert, A. J.; Buis-Liem, T. N.; Geldof, W. Ch.; and Rohmer, J.: The postvalvulotomy propranolol test to determine reversibility of the residual gradient in pulmonary stenosis. *J. Thorac. Cardiovasc. Surg.*, 71: 865, 1976.

Mustard, W. T.; Jain, S. C.; and Trusler, G. A.: Pulmonary stenosis in the first year of life. *Br. Heart J.*, 30: 255, 1968.

Mustard, W. T.; Rowe, R. D.; and Firor, W. B., Jr.: Pulmonic stenosis in the first year of life. *Surgery*, 47: 678, 1960.

Mustard, W. T., and Trusler, G. A.: Pulmonic stenosis with normal aortic root. In Benson, C. D.; Mustard, W. T.; Ravitch, M. M.; Snyder, W. H., Jr.; and Welch, K. J. (eds.): *Pediatric Surgery*, Year Book Publishers, Inc., Chicago, 1962, Vol. 1.

Nadas, A. S., and Fyler, D. C.: *Pediatric Cardiology*, 3rd ed. W. B. Saunders Company, Philadelphia, 1972.

Nakazawa, M.; Marks, R. A.; Isabel-Jones, J.; and Jarmakani, J. M.: Right and left ventricular volume characteristics in children with pulmonary stenosis and intact ventricular septum. *Circulation*, 53: 884, 1976.

Neufeld, H. H.; Ongley, P. A.; and Edwards, J. E.: Combined congenital subaortic stenosis and infundibular pulmonary stenosis. *Br. Heart J.*, 22: 686, 1960.

Noonan, J. A., and Ehmke, D. A.: Associated non-cardiac malformations in children with congenital heart disease. *J. Pediatr.*, 63: 468, 1963.

Nora, J. J.; Lortscher, R. H.; and Spangler, R. D.: Echocardiographic studies of left ventricular disease in Ullrich-Noonan syndrome. *Am. J. Dis. Child.*, 129: 1417, 1975.

Nora, J. J.; Torres, F. G.; Sinha, A. K.; and McNamara, D. G.: Characteristic cardiovascular anomalies of XO Turner syndrome, XX and XY phenotype and XO/XX Turner mosaic. *Am. J. Cardiol.*, 25: 639, 1970.

Nugent, E. W.; Freedom, R. M.; Nora, J. J.; Ellison, R. C.; Rowe, R. D.; and Nadas, A. S.: Clinical course in pulmonary stenosis. *Circulation*, 56: (Suppl. 1) 1–38, 1977.

Okin, J. T.; Vogel, J. H. K.; Pryor, R.; and Blount, S. G., Jr.: Isolated right ventricular hypoplasia. *Am. J. Cardiol.*, 24: 135, 1969.

Phornphutkul, C.; Rosenthal, A.; and Nadas, A. S.: Cardio-myopathy in Noonan's syndrome. Report of three cases. *Br. Heart J.*, 35: 99, 1973.

Pickering, D.; Laski, B.; Macmillan, D. C.; and Rose, V.: The little Leopard syndrome—Description of 3 cases and review of 24 previously reported. *Arch. Dis. Child.*, 46: 84, 1971.

Pieroni, D. R.; Bell, B. B.; Krovetz, L. J.; Varghese, P. J.; and Rowe, R. D.: Auscultatory recognition of aneurysm of the membranous ventricular septum associated with small ventricular septal defect. *Circulation*, 44: 733, 1971.

Pollack, A. A.; Taylor, B. E.; Odel, H. M.; and Burchell, H. B.: Pulmonary stenosis without ventricular septal defect. *Proc. Mayo Clin.*, 23: 516, 1948.

Pung, S., and Hirsch, E. F.: Plexiform neurofibromatosis of the heart and neck. *Arch. Pathol.*, 59: 341, 1955.

Puyau, F. A.; Hastings, C. P.; and Collins, H. A.: Determination of orifice size in iolated pulmonary stenosis. Comparison of three methods. *Invest. Radiol.*, 3: 367, 1968.

Ramsay, H. W.; Torre, de la, A.; Linhart, J. W.; Krovetz, L. J.; Schiebler, G. L.; and Green, J. R., Jr.: Idiopathic dilatation of the pulmonary artery. *Am. J. Cardiol.*, 20: 324, 1967.

Rasmussen, K., and Sørland, S. J.: Electrocardiogram and vectorcardiogram in Turner phenotype with normal chromo-somes and pulmonary arteries. *Br. Heart J.*, 35: 937, 1973.

Rawlings, N. S.: The "straightback" syndrome: A new cause of pseudo-heart disease. *Am. J. Cardiol.*, 5: 333, 1960.

Reid, J. M.; Coleman, E. N.; Stevenson, J. G.; Inall, J. A.; and Doig, W. B.: Long-term results of surgical treatment for pulmonary valve stenosis. *Arch. Dis. Child.*, 51: 79, 1976.

Rodriguez-Fernandez, H. L.; Char, F.; Kelly, D. T.; and Rowe, R. D.: The dysplastic pulmonary valve and the Noonan syndrome. *Circulation*, 45–46 Suppl. II: 98, 1972.

Rose, V.; Hewitt, D.; and Milner, J.: Seasonal influences on the risk of cardiac malformations. Nature of the problem and some results from a study of 10,077 cases. *Int. J. Epidemiol.*, 1: 235, 1972.

Rosenquist, G. C.; Krovetz, L. J.; Haller, J. A., Jr.; Simon, A. L.; and Bannayan, G. A.: Acquired right ventricular outflow obstruction in a child with neurofibromatosis. *Am. Heart J.*, 79: 103, 1970.

Rowe, R. D.; Mitchell, S. C.; Keith, J. D.; Mustard, W. T.; and Barnes, W. T.: Severe valvular pulmonary stenosis with normal aortic root. Immediate results of transarterial valvotomy with notes on the clinical assessment of patients before and after operation. *Can. Med. Assoc. J.*, 78: 311, 1958.

Rowe, R. D.; Vlad, P.; and Keith, J. D.: Experiences in 180 cases of tetralogy of Fallot in infants and children. *Can. Med. Assoc. J.*, 73: 23, 1955.

Rudolph, A. M.; Nadas, A. S.; and Goodale, W. T.: Intracardiac left to right shunt with pulmonic stenosis. *Am. Heart J.*, 48: 808, 1954.

Rudolph, A. M.: *Congenital Disease of the Heart*. Year Book Medical Publishers, Inc., Chicago, 1974.

Rudhe, U.; Whitley, J. E.; and Herzenberg, H.: Mild pulmonary valvular stenosis studied functionally and anatomically. *Acta Radiol.*, 57: 161, 1962.

Scherlis, L.; Loenker, R. J.; and Lee, Y.-C.: Pulmonary stenosis. Electrocardiographic, vectorcardiographic and catheterization data. *Circulation*, 28: 288, 1963.

Schmidt, R. E., and Craige, E.: Recorded movements over the right ventricle in children with pulmonary stenosis. *Circulation*, 32: 241, 1965.

Schrire, V., and Vogelpoel, L.: The role of the dilated pulmonary artery in normal splitting of the second heart sound. *Am. Heart J.*, 63: 501, 1962.

Sellors, T.: Surgery of pulmonary stenosis: a case in which pulmonary valve was successfully divided. *Lancet*, 1: 988, 1948.

Selzer, A.; Carnes, W. H.; Noble, C. A.; Higgins, W. H.; and Holmes, R. C.: Syndrome of pulmonary stenosis with patent foramen ovale. *Am. J. Med.*, 6: 3, 1949.

Shams, A.; Keith, J. D.; Edibam, B.; Fukuda, H.; Rose, V.; and Fowler, R. S.: The rate of regression of ventricular hypertrophy in vectorcardiograms and electrocardiograms after surgery on congenital heart disease. *J. Electrocardiog.*, 6: 247, 1973.

Shephard, R. J.: Redistribution of systemic blood flow in pulmonary stenosis. *Br. Heart J.*, 17: 98, 1955.

Singh, S. P.: Unusual splitting of the second heart sound in pulmonary stenosis. *Am. J. Cardiol.*, 25: 28, 1970.

Sissman, N. J.; Neill, C. A.; Spencer, F. C.; and Taussig, H. B.: Congenital aortic stenosis. *Circulation*, 19: 458, 1959.

Slade, P. R.: Isolated infundibular stenosis. *J. Thorac. Cardiovasc. Surg.*, 45: 775, 1963.

Soulié, P.; Joly, F.; Carlotti, J.; Piton, A.; and Thuillez, B.: Sténoses valvulaires pulmonaires modérées. *Arch. Mal. Coeur*, 46: 695, 1953.

Soulie, P.; Joly, F.; Carlotti, J.; and Sicot, J.-R.: Etude comparee de l'hémodynamique dans les tétralogies et dans les trilogies de Fallot. *Arch. Mal. Coeur*, 44: 577, 1951.

Sternberg, C.: Cor triatriatum biventriculare. *Verh. Dtsch. Ges. Pathol.*, 16: 256, 1913.

Stoermer, J.; Beuren, A. J.; Gandjour, A.; and Grütte, E.: Überdreht Rinkstypische QRS-Acuse in EKg bei isolierter valvulärer pulmonal stenose. *Z. Kreislauff.*, 57: 1151, 1968.

Stone, F. M.; Bessinger, F. B., Jr.; Lucas, R. V., Jr.; and Moller, J. H.: Pre- and postoperative rest and exercise hemodynamics in children with pulmonary stenosis. *Circulation*, 49: 1102, 1974.

Swan, H. J. C.; Burchell, H. B.; and Wood, E. H.: The presence of venoarterial shunts in patients with interatrial communications. *Circulation*, 10: 705, 1954.

Swan, H. J. C.; Zapata-Diaz, J.; and Wood, E. H.: Dye dilution curves in cyanotic congenital heart disease. *Circulation*, 8: 70, 1953.

Talbert, J. L.; Morrow, A. G.; Collins, N. P.; and Gilbert, J. W.: The incidence and significance of pulmonic regurgitation after pulmonary valvulotomy. *Am. Heart J.*, **65**:591, 1963.

Tampas, J. P., and Lurie, P. R.: The roentgenographic appearance of the chest in children with functional murmurs. *Am. J. Roentgenol. Rad. Ther.*, **103**:78, 1968.

Taussig, H. B.: *Congenital Malformations of the Heart. II. Specific Malformations.* Harvard University Press, Cambridge, Mass., 1960, p. 119.

Taylor, B. E., and DuShane, J. W.: Patent ductus arteriosus associated with pulmonary stenosis. *Proc. Mayo Clin.*, **25**:60, 1950.

Thorson, A.; Bjorck, G.; Bjorkman, G.; and Walderstrom, J.: Malignant carcinoid of the small intestine with metastases to the liver, valvular disease of the heart (pulmonary stenosis and tricuspid regurgitation without septal defect), peripheral vasomotor symptoms, bronchoconstriction and an unusual type of cyanosis. A clinical and pathologic syndrome. *Am. Heart J.*, **47**:795, 1954.

Tinker, J.; Howitt, G.; Markman, P.; and Wade, E. G.: The natural history of isolated pulmonary stenosis. *Br. Heart J.*, **27**:151, 1965.

Truccone, N. J.; Steeg, C. N.; Dell, R.; and Gersony, W. M.: Comparison of the cardiocirculatory effects of exercise and isoproterenol in children with pulmonary or aortic valve stenosis. *Circulation*, **56**:79, 1977.

Van der Hauwaert, L., and Nadas, A. S.: Auscultatory findings in patients with a small ventricular septal defect. *Circulation*, **23**:886, 1961.

Vogelpoel, L., and Schrire, V.: Auscultatory and phonocardiographic assessment of pulmonary stenosis with intact septum. *Circulation*, **22**:55, 1960.

Vogelpoel, L.; Schrire, V.; Beck, W.; and Nellen, M.: The preoperative recognition of the "muscle bound" right ventricle in pulmonary stenosis with intact ventricular septum. *Br. Heart J.*, **26**:380, 1964.

Vogelpoel, L; Schrire, V.; Beck, W.; Nellen, M.; and Swanepoel, A.: The atypical systolic murmur of minute ventricular septal defect and its recognition by amyl nitrate and phenylephrine. *Am. Heart J.*, **62**:101, 1961.

Vogelpoel, L.; Schrire, V.; Nellen, M.; and Swanepoel, A.: The use of amyl nitrite in the differentiation of Fallot's tetralogy and pulmonary stenosis with intact ventricular septum. *Am. Heart J.*, **57**:803, 1959.

Watson, G. H.: Pulmonary stenosis, café au lait and dull intelligence. *Arch. Dis. Child.*, **42**:303, 1967.

Watson, H.; McArthur, P.; Somerville, J.; and Ross, D.: Spontaneous evolution of ventricular septal defect with isolated pulmonary stenosis. *Lancet*, **2**:1125, 1969.

Weyman, A. E.; Dillon, J. C.; Feigenbaum, H.; and Chang, S.: Echocardiographic patterns of pulmonary valve motion in valvular pulmonary stenosis. *Am. J. Cardiol.*, **34**:644, 1974.

Williams, J. C. P; Barratt-Boyes, B. G.; and Lowe, J. B.: Underdeveloped right ventricle and pulmonary stenosis. *Am. J. Cardiol.*, **11**:458, 1963.

Whitham, A. C.; Rainey, R. L.; and Edmonds, J. H.: Prediction of right ventricular pressure in pulmonic stenosis from sponge vectorcardiogram and electrocardiogram. *Am. Heart J.*, **75**:187, 1968.

Wood, P.: Congenital pulmonary stenosis with left ventricular enlargement associated with atrial septal defect. *Br. Heart J.*, **4**:11, 1942.

Zaret, B. L., and Conti, R. C.: Infundibular pulmonic stenosis with intact ventricular septum in the adult. *Hopkins Med. J.*, **132**:50, 1973.

41

Pulmonary Arterial Stenosis

Richard D. Rowe

UNDER the various terms of partial atresia of pulmonary arteries, supravalvular pulmonary stenoses, coarctation of the pulmonary arteries, and postvalvular, multiple, or peripheral stenoses of pulmonary arteries, a group of obstructions has been described in the pulmonary arterial tree at a number of points distal to the pulmonary valve but proximal to the small pulmonary arteries. A number of classifications of the disorder have been introduced into the literature, of which those of Smith (1958) and Franch and Gay (1963) are best known. In general, they identify the area of the pulmonary artery chiefly affected, e.g., proximal main pulmonary artery, bifurcation of the main pulmonary artery, distal pulmonary arteries, or various combinations. Our own preference is to use the following tabulation, which differs only in minor detail from existing ones. It places patients with complicated heart malformations in a separate group because, in our view, their clinical presentation and therapy are generally quite different from the others:

1. Simple Pulmonary Artery Stenoses. a. Isolated pulmonary artery stenosis. b. Pulmonary artery stenoses associated with basically simple intracardiac or extracardiac anomalies, e.g., pulmonary valve stenosis, patent ductus arteriosus, ventricular septal defect.

2. Complex Pulmonary Artery Stenoses. Part of a basically complex intracardiac anomaly, e.g., tetralogy of Fallot, transposition of great vessels, mitral atresia.

Each of these two groups may be further subdivided to indicate the position within the pulmonary arterial system of the major obstruction (Figure 41–1).

a. CENTRAL. Localized constriction within the main pulmonary artery usually at the origins of either right or left pulmonary arteries or both branches.

b. PERIPHERAL. Localized constriction at secondary branching of major pulmonary artery divisions.

c. INTERMEDIATE. A hypoplastic segment of the pulmonary artery usually commencing at either the distal end of the main pulmonary artery or at an origin of its major divisions extending for a significant distance into either or both branches.

Finally, the condition may be *unilateral or bilateral*.

Pathology

In 1938 Dr. Ella Oppenheimer described the findings in a 17-month-old baby born after a pregnancy complicated by pernicious vomiting. She presented in congestive heart failure, was grossly cyanosed and clubbed, and had a soft systolic murmur. Cardiomegaly was present in the chest x-ray and extreme right ventricular hypertrophy in the electrocardiogram. The infant died ten days after admission. At autopsy widespread obstruction of the elastic lobar arteries with medial calcification of these vessels was the main feature. An almost identical case, even with respect to sex, age, and heart rate, has been encountered in New Zealand (Lowe and Williams). This pregnancy was complicated by infectious hepatitis.

One further detailed autopsy has been reported in a 21-year-old Swedish woman dying in congestive failure (Orell et al., 1960). This showed gross obstruction of lobar pulmonary arteries without medial calcification. Although autopsy experience is at best sparse and, furthermore, in two or three cases was concerned with an exceedingly rare variant of the anomaly, it seems probable that, the primary disorder is an anomaly of medial elastic tissue with intimal proliferation at the bifurcation of the lobar arteries. Thrombotic changes may be a late cause of subsequent increase in the degree of obstruction to blood flow at these points. The vessel immediately beyond the point of obstruction has extremely thin walls rather like a vein (Franch and Gay, 1963). Since one sees occasional cases with both central and peripheral stenoses, it is not unreasonable to expect that a similar process may be involved in the more proximal variety. The solution to this problem awaits further autopsy reports but would probably be hastened if specially stained sections of lobar arteries were examined routinely at postmortem. There is no

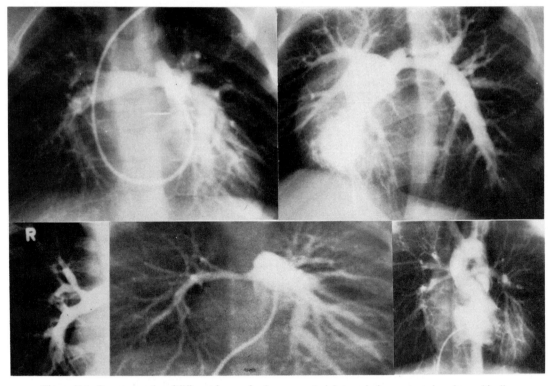

Figure 41-1. Some examples of different forms of pulmonary arterial stenosis demonstrated angiographically. *Top*: anteroposterior (*left*) and left anterior oblique (*right*) projections from a boy with mild pulmonary valve stenosis and the intermediate form of pulmonary arterial stenosis. *Bottom* (*left*): right upper lobe artery stenosis; (*center*): bilateral pulmonary arterial stenosis affecting the right branch to a greater degree than the left in a patient with secundum atrial septal defect; (*right*): extreme hypoplasia of the pulmonary artery divisions in a patient with tetralogy of Fallot and congenital rubella.

doubt that lobar arterial obstruction can be easily missed in gross autopsy specimens, and the same really applies to central and intermediate types. It is quite possible that relatively mild clinical cases exist not uncommonly and that they may survive to die of other diseases with perhaps no suspicion ever being aroused of there being an arterial anomaly present.

It has become appreciated recently that this arterial disorder is not necessarily confined to pulmonary arteries and that systemic conducting vessels may also be involved. The degree of involvement of each system varies considerably, even with the two major disorders in which this added dimension has been studied particularly—congenital rubella (Rowe, 1973) and idiopathic hypercalcemia (Beuren, 1972). The discovery of the combination in these disorders implies that there may be many more unsuspected examples in the population of patients with apparently isolated pulmonary arterial stenosis and that a more diligent search will uncover systemic arterial disease, even in them (Rowe et al., 1969).

Other secondary changes recognized in severe cases are a major degree of right ventricular hypertrophy and an increase in size of bronchial arteries. The disease may be isolated but is more commonly associated with other cardiovascular anomalies. Chief of these are patent ductus arteriosus,

pulmonary valve stenosis, coarctation of the aorta, aortic pulmonary septal defect, aortic stenosis, ventricular septal defect, atrial septal defect, tetralogy of Fallot, transposition of the great vessels, corrected transposition of the great vessels, total anomalous pulmonary venous drainage, and mitral atresia.

Etiology

In an early description Søndegaard (1954) invoked the Skodaic theory as causation since in a case of tetralogy of Fallot with bilateral central obstruction, he found fibers extending from the ligament of the ductus arteriosus around the origins of right and left pulmonary arteries in the form of a sling. A similar appearance was found in a case by Coles and Walker (1956). Though many cases appear to be of a strictly localized central type, the disorder occurs often where a patent duct exists in combination with peripheral stenoses, so that it is unlikely that this theory would explain the disease.

In our last edition we were impressed by the common presence of abnormal background features in the family or pregnancy history, or associations at the clinical examination that suggested that at least in the simple forms of the disease etiologic factors might frequently be identifiable. Since then, further evidence has been accumulated by others and ourselves, giving support to this view (see Table 41–1). In several situations so listed there are even more complex interrelationships, e.g., both metabolic and inherited. These data do not tell us the fundamental cause of the arterial disorder but they do indicate that somehow a wide variety of diseases ultimately affect the arterial wall in a similar way (Figure 41–2). The fascinating question of what factors determine the severity and distribution of the lesions in the vascular system within these different associations has so far given rise to more speculation than solution (Vince, 1970; Rowe, 1973; Rowe et al., 1974).

Hemodynamics

Obviously a difference in pressure between one site in the more proximal portion of the pulmonary artery and a more distal site indicates the presence of an obstructive element within the vessel. Absence of a pressure differential would argue against the presence of an obstruction, but such a view is not entirely valid.

To say that an obstruction is insignificant when it is demonstrated anatomically but not physiologically is to suggest that the obstruction is static—something that is not true even for the adult, let alone for the child in whom growth and development may create more rapid alterations in a dynamic situation. Since the consideration of pressure difference cannot be divorced from the question of quantitation of flow, it is clear that the determination of normal pressure difference across areas of bifurcation in the circulation must consider the nature, normal or otherwise, of the flow across the channel at the time of pressure measurements.

In normal individuals, even in the term infant, where variations in the pulmonary flow might normally be expected, the average pressure difference across the pulmonary bifurcation is not more than 5 to 5 mm of mercury. It has been noted in a number of adults with atrial septal defect and large pulmonary blood flow that a pressure difference exists across the bifurcation of the pulmonary artery of an order comparable to that which has been detected across the right ventricular outflow tract in similar circumstances. Repair of the atrial defect has been followed

---

Table 41–1.   CLINICAL ASSOCIATIONS IN SIMPLE PULMONARY ARTERIAL STENOSIS

FUNCTIONAL PULMONARY ARTERIAL STENOSIS

Infants of Low Birth Weight

  Prematurity (Danilowicz et al., 1972; Dunkle and Rowe, 1972)
  Racial*

Patients with High Pulmonary Blood Flow

  Atrial septal defect (Bouvrain et al., 1961; Perloff et al., 1967)
  Ventricular septal defect in infancy*

TRUE PULMONARY ARTERIAL STENOSIS

Familial

  (Van Epps, 1957; Arvidsson et al., 1955; 1961; Bouvrain et al., 1961; McCue et al., 1965)

Inherited

  The Noonan and related syndromes (Noonan and Ehmke, 1963; Linde et al., 1973; Roberts and Moes, 1973)
  Dolicho-ectasia (Beuren et al., 1969; Sacks and Lindenburg, 1968)
  Cutis laxa (Balboni, 1963; Hayden et al., 1968)
  Ehlers-Danlos (Lees et al., 1969)
  Keutel syndrome (Keutel et al., 1972)

Prenatal Infection

  Rubella (Arvidsson et al., 1955; Gyllensward et al., 1957; Williams et al, 1957; Rowe, 1963; Emmanouilides et al., 1964; and
    Chapter 53)
  Hepatitis (Rowe, 1963)
  Intrahepatic biliary dysgenesis (Greenwood et al., 1976)

Metabolic

  Idiopathic hypercalcemia syndrome (Beuren, 1972)
  Maternal diabetes (Fouron et al., 1967)
  Mucopolysaccharidoses*
  Hypothyroidism*

Hemodynamic

  Pulmonary arteriovenous fistula (Guller, 1972)

Uncertain

  Hypertension, mitral regurgitation (Loggie et al., 1968)

---

* Personal observations (R.D.R.).

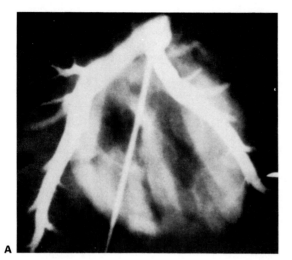 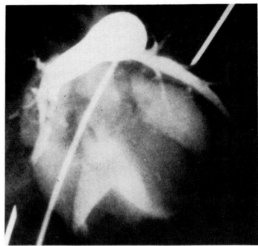

A   **B**

Figure 41-2. Postmortem pulmonary arteriogram in New Zealand white rabbit. *A.* A normal control. *B.* An animal infected in utero by rubella virus. Notice the left-branch hypoplasia.

by abolition of this pressure difference. Such arguments have been advanced to support the view that the pulmonary arteries of these patients are normal, and that any pressure differences are a consequence of physical factors related to the high flow through the pulmonary circuit. The point is not fully established. Many believe that even under these circumstances of large flow there is likely to be some anatomic abnormality in those patients who demonstrate the pressure difference. It is also not certain, given normal ranges of flow, that the absolute pressure difference between the main trunk and the distal pulmonary artery is in exact relationship to the severity of obstruction, or rather to the potential severity of the obstruction. It has long been known, however, that the diastolic pressure difference between the main trunk and a branch of the pulmonary artery is directly proportional to the severity of the obstruction.

The pressure pulse in the main trunk has been known since its description by Agustsson and colleagues (1962) to have a characteristic form in bilateral pulmonary artery stenosis (Figure 41-8, page 796). There is no guarantee that such a pressure pulse can differentiate between the obstruction that is revealed as truly anatomic and that in which no clear-cut stenosis can be seen angiographically. More recently, it has been suggested by Rios and associates (1969) that the rate of change of pressure rise in the pulse distal to the obstruction might provide an indication of real as opposed to spurious stenosis.

Clinically in unilateral disease there is usually no major change in cardiac dynamics unless there is atresia of the opposite pulmonary artery. Experimental studies in puppies (Falkenbach et al., 1959), however, showed progressive pulmonary hypertension after partial occlusion of the left pulmonary artery, but none where the left pulmonary artery was ligated, which suggests even in the apparently trivial

case that caution might be necessary in delivering a good prognosis. Where bilateral stenoses exist, right ventricular work increases to a degree apparently dependent upon the severity of the obstruction. In the isolated anomaly this is reflected in varying degrees of right ventricular and main pulmonary artery hypertension, which may be minimal where lesions are relatively limited, or even in extensive bilateral involvement in young patients before secondary thrombotic lesions have altered the degree of resistance to blood flow. In patients with associated anomalies the extent of the obstruction may not be easy to assess. In patients with intracardiac left-to-right shunt the pressure gradient across the obstruction may be considerable in mild disease. Conversely, in quite severe bilateral involvement where there is more proximal obstruction, as in cases of the simple group with pulmonary valve stenosis, but particularly in patients with tetralogy of Fallot, the arterial stenosis may appear relatively innocent before correction of the more proximal obstruction. In other types such as those associated with transposition of the great vessels or ventricular septal defect, the association may be really beneficial, at least for a time, in that the arterial stenosis is protective to the more distal pulmonary vascular bed.

Cyanosis, when present, is most often due to associated cardiac malformations and rarely is due to venoarterial interatrial shunting in the isolated types.

Clinical Features

The overall incidence of true pulmonary arterial stenosis has been reported in the order of 2 to 3 percent of all patients with congenital heart disease in a cardiac unit (Mudd et al., 1965; Fouron et al., 1967). Though these figures are our best approximation to date, they are very likely an underestimate of the situation.

The murmur caused by pulmonary artery stenosis is the most important diagnostic feature and is most often systolic in time and ejection in nature. Continuous murmurs are much less common, having been reported in about 10 percent of cases in the literature. It was pointed out by Eldridge and coworkers (1957) that a pressure gradient existed in these cases across a point of obstruction during diastole as well as in systole. Our own findings in three patients with continuous murmurs revealed diastolic gradients averaging 9 mm of mercury, whereas in those with systolic murmur, the diastolic gradient was less than 1 mm of mercury.

Though there is variation relating to severity, the murmur tends to peak in late systole, and while it is usually maximal in the pulmonary area, it is

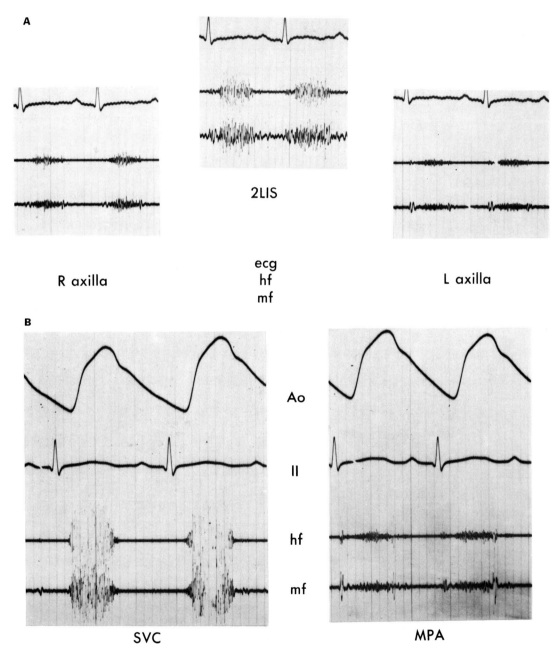

Figure 41-3. *A.* External phonocardiography in pulmonary artery stenoses. Records from the axillae and pulmonary area when using constant amplifier gain (*hf*, high-frequency banding: *mf*, medium-frequency banding). *B.* Internal phonocardiography in pulmonary arterial stenoses. Obtained by phonocatheter in a patient with bilateral obstructions. Note that with the same amplifier gain the intensity of the ejection murmur was maximal in the tracing recorded from the superior vena cava.

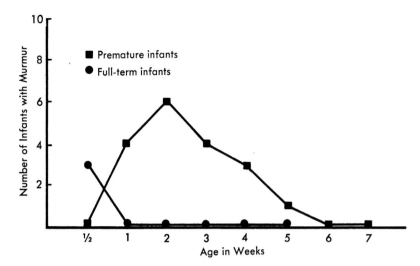

Figure 41-4. The transient murmur of functional pulmonary artery stenosis in a premature infant. The age at which the murmur is detected. Note that the murmur is commonly heard in the fourth week of life in the premature baby, whereas in the term infant, it is very uncommon and usually transient. (From Dunkle, Lisa M., and Rowe, Richard D.: Transient murmur simulating pulmonary artery stenosis in premature infants. *Am. J. Dis. Child.*, **124**:666, 1972. Copyright 1972, American Medical Association.)

transmitted widely, especially to the axillae and lower anterior and posterior aspects of the chest (Figure 41–3). The second heart sound is usually normal in intensity and in its width of splitting. The pulmonary closure sound may be delayed in the presence of associated pulmonary valve stenosis or an atrial septal defect (Rios et al., 1969; Perloff and Lebauer, 1969). With the isolated forms of the disease ejection clicks are absent.

A transient murmur resembling that of pulmonary arterial stenosis is heard frequently in healthy premature infants during the first six weeks of life. A similar observation has been made in other infants with low birth weight but of normal gestational age (Dunkle and Rowe, 1972). The presence of such a murmur shortly after birth in healthy, truly premature infants or in infants of some races who have low birth weight is not therefore a cause for alarm because it usually disappears within a few weeks (Figure 41–4). On the other hand, in an infant of low birth weight for gestational age, these signs

may imply the presence of true arterial stenosis. We have found that the association of these signs with an infant born between October and February in the northern hemisphere should raise the possibility of a rubella background (Rowe et al., 1966) (Figure 41–5). Similarly, the presence of the characteristic murmur in term infants should raise the possibility of some background factor. The family history should be assessed more closely for the presence of heart murmurs in relatives and the possibility of transmitted anomalies, such as the Noonan syndrome.

Associated lesions tend to distract the examiner from the usually important but less obvious arterial anomaly. Such is the case in both the simple and complex groups. It is the impressive cyanosis, clubbing, squatting, and single second heart sound of the patient with tetralogy of Fallot, or the pansystolic murmur, loud continuous murmur, or ejection systolic murmur of the acyanotic patient with ventricular septal defect, patent ductus arteriosus, or

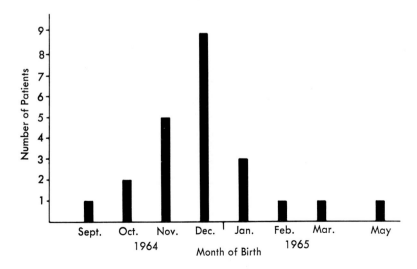

Figure 41-5. The month of birth in patients with rubella cardiovascular disease, mostly pulmonary arterial stenosis, seen during a major epidemic in the eastern seaboard of the United States. The majority of cases were born between October and January.

valvular pulmonary stenosis, which tends to limit further consideration and so lead to the pulmonary artery stenoses being missed. Nevertheless, in these examples, just as in the left common isolated pulmonary artery stenoses, it is possible to maintain a high index suspicion if due attention is paid to the distribution and character of the murmur. Of the two, distribution is the more important.

Other features, such as symptomatology, cyanosis, appearance of the jugular venous pulse, character of the apex beat, parasternal activity, and the second heart sound, are so dependent on associated cardiovascular anomalies as to be less valuable for consideration. Even in the isolated anomalies the symptoms may vary from being absent to gross congestive heart failure. It is usual for moderate fatigue and exertional dyspnea to develop during childhood. Progress from relatively slight to severe symptomatology occurred in one fatal case in a short space of two years (Orell et al., 1960). In severe cases of this group signs of right ventricular overwork are evident from the prominent "a" of the jugular venous pulse and the parasternal thrust, while accentuation of pulmonary valve closures is indicative of main pulmonary hypertension. Clubbing has been present in two fatal cases, and hemoptysis may occur as a terminal event.

Radiologic Examination

Conventional chest films in this disorder are not diagnostic. Usually the heart size is affected only minimally in isolated forms unless the obstructions are severe, when cardiomegaly and a prominence of the pulmonary artery segment on the left border can be expected (Figure 41–6). Associated anomalies more usually dictate the plain x-ray appearances. We have noticed that in most of the simple cases the main pulmonary artery segment is relatively inconspicuous rather than, as one might expect, more apparent than usual. In none of our cases was examination of the pulmonary vascularity rewarding, an experience shared by Delaney and Nadas (1964) but not by Baum and colleagues (1964).

Electrocardiography

In isolated forms with severe bilateral disease right-axis deviation and right atrial and right ventricular overloading are usually seen (Figure 41–7). Change from moderate right ventricular overload due to "strain pattern" has been reported (Orell et al., 1960). In the milder degrees of the anomaly, particularly in

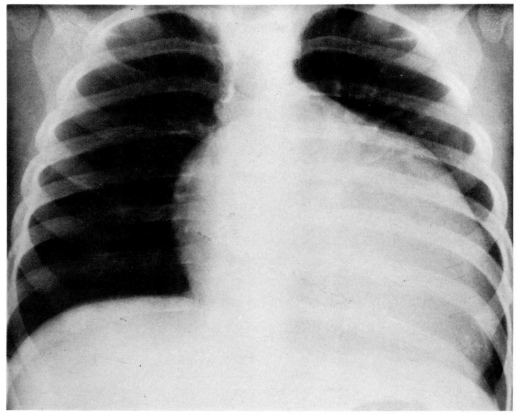

Figure 41-6. The radiologic picture in severe isolated pulmonary arterial stenosis. The chest film from a proved fatal case (Williams and Lowe) aged 17 months.

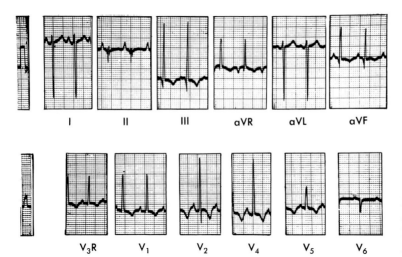

Figure 41-7. The electrocardiogram in severe isolated pulmonary artery stenosis. The tracing from the patient referred to in Figure 41-6.

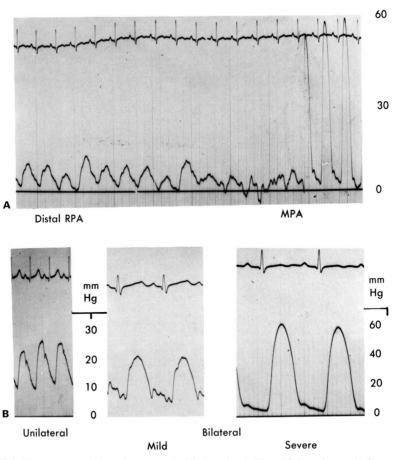

Figure 41-8. Pressure records in pulmonary arterial stenosis. *A.* The withdrawal record of a patient with bilateral central-type stenosis showing Venturi effect just before the entry of the catheter tip into the main pulmonary artery. *B.* The main pulmonary arterial pressure pulse in pulmonary arterial stenosis. The characteristic normal situation of the dicrotic notch in unilateral obstruction is contrasted with its low location on the pressure pulse of patients with bilateral stenosis, whether mild or severe.

very young patients, the electrocardiogram may be normal. In cases with associated anomalies the electrical picture varies greatly. In two of our cases with bilateral obstruction of moderate severity and a large patent ductus arteriosus we noted change from combined ventricular overloading to pure right ventricular overloading within a year of division of the ducts. In patients with the Noonan syndrome there may be left anterior hemiblock in the electrocardiogram (Roberts and Moes, 1973).

Cardiac Catheterization

Routine right heart catheterization is usually the first step in confirming the clinical diagnosis of pulmonary artery stenoses. The two principal means by which the arterial obstruction is demonstrated are the detection of the pressure gradient within the main pulmonary artery or its branches and an examination of the main pulmonary artery pressure pulse contour.

The pressure gradient is best revealed in severe disease of isolated simple type. In these cases pulmonary artery wedge pressure values are normal. Withdrawal to the free pulmonary artery main division still shows a low pressure, which is ultimately replaced by a higher pressure when the most proximal obstruction is passed. Sometimes there is evidence of the Venturi effect (Figure 41–8). The position at which this pressure change occurs varies and may sometimes be difficult to site accurately, particularly if the lesion is centrally placed. By virtue of the anteroposterior projection of the main pulmonary artery and the usual patient position screening at cardiac catheterization, it is almost impossible to tell in many cases whether the pressure gradient is occurring at the junction of a pulmonary artery branch origin.

The peculiar appearance of the main pulmonary artery pressure pulse and bilateral stenoses has recently been shown in an important paper by Agustsson and coworkers (1962). The features described by these authors are that the appearance of the systolic portion of the main pulmonary artery pulse is identical with that of the right ventricle, that while the diastolic level is usually normal the dicrotic notch is deep, and that the diastolic descent following pulmonary valve closure is flattened increasingly with increasing degrees of obstruction. Our own experience confirms the contention that on the basis of the main pulmonary artery pressure pulse alone, it should be possible to suspect the disorder if it is bilateral, even if occasionally a similar appearance is seen in patients without stenoses (Delaney and Nadas, 1964). In unilateral cases the pressure pulse is normal (Figure 41–8). Whereas the murmur in simple cases without pulmonary valve stenosis is loudest in the pulmonary area, the phonocatheter reveals only a relatively soft systolic murmur in the main pulmonary artery. There is a harsh systolic murmur in the pulmonary artery beyond the site of constriction (Deyrieux et al., 1961; Bouvain et al., 1961). A simple way to demonstrate this difference is to place the

catheter at the junction of superior vena cava and right atrium, a point which is close to the secondary divisions of the right pulmonary artery, or, better still, through a patent foramen ovale into a pulmonary vein. In either site in bilateral obstruction a loud murmur will be demonstrated (Figure 41–3).

Associated intra- or extracardiac defects may be revealed by usual methods.

When considering the changes in the degree of stenosis with time, it is important to remember that at birth the major branches of the pulmonary artery are small relative to the main pulmonary artery and that it takes several months for the size relationship between these segments characteristic of the older child and adult to develop. The individual with hypercalcemia does not necessarily have pulmonary arteries that are unusual in size in infancy. On the other hand, in patients with rubella syndrome, a more obvious degree of smallness or hypoplasia of the pulmonary artery branches is evident at birth. It has been shown that these branches enlarge distally with a more obvious bifurcation narrowing over the course of the next few months (Wasserman et al., 1968) (Figure 41–9). The speed with which this change develops seems likely related to the amount of pulmonary blood flow. The question arises as to whether a particular degree of smallness of the pulmonary arteries is critical in terms of future change. In premature infants at birth, a pressure differential across the bifurcation must be present that exists until the time when the infant would have been gestationally term. It is possible that a rubella infant with a lower degree of involvement or hypoplasia of the pulmonary artery branches, and who eventually loses the murmur characteristic of pulmonary artery stenosis in the first year of life, may be in a category comparable to the premature infant. In our hands and in those of others, systolic right ventricular pressure and right ventricular to pulmonary arterial systolic pressure differences tended not to increase over time (Rowe, 1963; Venables, 1965; Hastreiter et al., 1967; Hartman et al., 1968; Wasserman et al., 1968; Eldridge et al., 1972).

Only a limited amount of information is available about changes for those who demonstrate severe arterial stenosis at an early age. Such as exists indicates that the complication of the hemoptysis through rupture of the thin-walled distal vessels in the lung or thromboses in these dilated channels are the factors that lead to later demise. Also unsettled is the question of prognosis for the patient with milder degrees of stenosis. The problem is compounded by the fact that few instances of pulmonary arterial stenosis are of an isolated nature, so that there has been difficulty in sorting out the effects of arterial obstruction from those of other vascular or cardiac disease.

Angiocardiography

Pulmonary artery stenosis is a lesion par excellence where the combined studies of cardiac catheterization

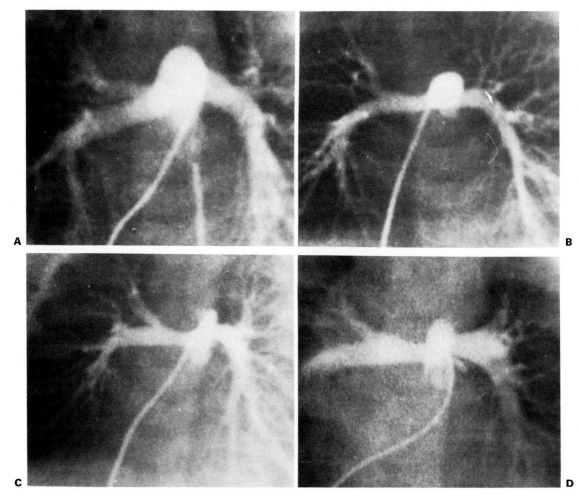

Figure 41-9. Angiography in pulmonary arterial stenosis. *A*. Pulmonary arteriogram in a two-month-old infant with patent ductus arteriosus for comparison. *B*. The pulmonary arteriogram of an infant with isolated pulmonary arterial stenosis at the age of five months. The pressure difference across the bifurcation of the pulmonary artery in this patient was 16 mm of mercury. *C*. A pulmonary arteriogram in an infant of one month with pulmonary arterial stenosis and patent ductus arteriosus. The pressure difference across the pulmonary artery bifurcation in this patient was 24 mm of mercury. *D*. The pulmonary arteriogram in an infant aged 11 months with isolated pulmonary arterial stenosis. The pressure difference across the bifurcation in this patient was 5 mm of mercury. These films show that from a hypoplastic appearance the more characteristic poststenotic dilatation appears over a period of time and that the presence of a left-to-right shunt accelerates this change.

and angiocardiography are essential to provide a complete picture of the malformation. The best demonstration follows injection of contrast material into the main pulmonary artery (Figures 41–1 and 41–9). A tilted patient position is preferable. Although it is an unusual finding, we have encountered the situation where a trivial pressure gradient at cardiac catheterization has been found in the presence of extensive bilateral disease shown by angiography. Rios and colleagues (1969) reported a similar situation in one patient who had a 7 mm systolic pressure gradient at the bifurcation of the main pulmonary artery. The implication is that in the appropriate circumstances of suspicion at cardiac catheterization, angiography should not be forgotten in patients where the hemodynamic support for

pulmonary arterial stenoses may be rather equivocal.

Angiocardiography has made it possible to classify the various types of obstruction, and in complex types it may be the only method of detecting unsuspected stenoses or confirming a clinical impression of the presence of the associated anomaly.

Increasing evidence of the association of systemic arterial disease with arterial disease of the pulmonary arteries emphasizes the need to consider exploration angiographically of the aorta and its branches in patients with pulmonary artery stenosis (Figure 41–10). More information from studies in such patients could define the probability of the association better than at present in order to reduce the need, if possible, for extensive mapping studies.

Diagnosis

The sign most helpful in the diagnosis of pulmonary artery stenosis is the wide transmission of the stenotic murmur into the anterolateral chest including the axillae. In any patient showing this sign the diagnosis must be seriously considered regardless of signs of other malformation that may be present. In fact the usual tendency is to accept the more obvious diagnosis presenting, such as patent ductus arteriosus, pulmonary stenosis with normal aortic group, coarctation of the aorta, tetralogy of Fallot, or transposition of the great arteries. Difficulty arises when very loud systolic murmurs due to other disorders, chiefly stenotic, exist and where wide transmission may be acceptable as originating from the more obvious lesions. Thus, often murmurs due to

pulmonary valve stenosis, coarctation of the aorta, or patent ductus arteriosus are well heard in the left axilla, left anterior chest, and back, while those due to aortic stenoses and less commonly ventricular septal defect may be propagated to the right chest. Accepting these possibilities, the fact remains that in bilateral disease, which after all is the only clinically important type, the diagnosis will seldom be missed if a careful auscultation is made over the whole of the right thorax. Because of the frequent association of other anomalies, symptoms and physical examination are quite variable and on the whole unhelpful. A history of maternal rubella in pregnancy, familial congenital heart disease, or the finding of facies or features suggestive of Noonan's syndrome or the idiopathic hypercalcemia syndrome should alert one to the possibility of the diagnosis.

The functional forms of pulmonary arterial

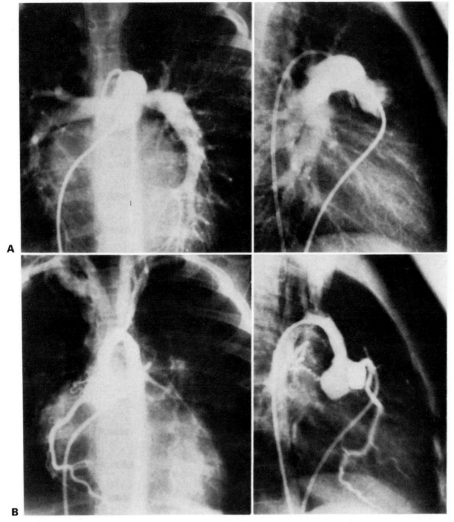

Figure 41-10. Anteroposterior and lateral projections of (A) the pulmonary arteriogram and (B) the aortogram of a boy with the vascular syndrome of idiopathic hypercalcemia. Note the bilateral bifurcation stenoses affecting the pulmonary artery and the unusually severe degree of narrowing of the aortic lumen as well as of the origins of the aortic branches and the left coronary artery.

stenosis that are encountered in the premature infant or in patients with septal defects are usually fairly easily distinguished from the true stenotic disorders.

In those patients with a continuous murmur from the pulmonary artery stenoses the diagnosis will revolve round other causes for continuous murmurs widely distributed over the chest. Seldom will this include simple patent ductus arteriosus, coronary arterial anomalies, or sinus or Valsalva rupture and more often will concern lesions with a diffuse collateral flow to the lung as in the various forms of pulmonary atresia or in truncus arteriosus.

In the relatively uncommon isolated anomaly, apart from murmur distribution, the degree of prominence of the jugular "a" wave, a parasternal right ventricular lift, and accentuation of the second sound will provide clinical indices of severity. Idiopathic pulmonary hypertension or pulmonary hypertension secondary to intracardiac lesions has been suggested as a differential diagnosis of importance, but seldom if ever should difficulty arise in practice because the murmur situation is so different.

Prognosis

A dearth of autopsy information on the disorder at present makes firm statements on prognosis impossible. What evidence there is available suggests that unilateral disease of the mild central type or mild stenosis immediately above the valve is associated with a good prognosis. Peripheral stenoses carry a poor prognosis, but the speed with which secondary thrombotic lesions accumulate probably varies a great deal. Progress may be quite rapid, as occurred over a two-year period in the 21-year-old fatal case of Orell and coworkers (1960). The relatively high incidence of thrombosis within the pulmonary arterial tree as the disease advances has led to the suggestion that anticoagulants might prove useful as a prophylactic measure (Baum et al., 1964).

It would seem that the majority will be asymptomatic or will have quite mild symptoms in the first decade and that only the rare exception with calcific changes will deteriorate in infancy.

More difficult to evaluate are the patients with intermediate-type stenosis since some of these have peripheral lesions as well, although perhaps visible only on a single branch in infants or children. One is suspicious that more widespread peripheral lesions in these subjects may be longer in appearing because of the protection given their lobar branches by the proximal obstruction.

In general, in isolated cases the disease is seldom severe in infancy so that congestive heart failure then is uncommon. There is a tendency for the disorder to appear static during childhood. The importance of elucidating the full extent of the disease at cardiac catheterization by exploring both sides of the circulation, and particularly by mapping the vascular circuits with appropriate angiography (Schlesinger and Meester, 1967; Rowe, 1972), cannot be overemphasized. All too often even now patients are subjected to study and, because relatively minor pressure gradients are found in the pulmonary circuit, are not further explored angiographically, or only one or the other side is examined in detail.

Surgical Treatment

Assistance can be offered in the case of supravalvular obstruction (Thrower et al., 1960). Other technically successful efforts have been made to relieve central obstructions at the pulmonary artery branch origins (Schumacker and Lurie, 1953; Sauvage et al., 1960; Baxter et al., 1961). It would seem likely that more attempts will soon be made to tackle the central types involving distal pulmonary artery or pulmonary artery branch origins and certain intermediate forms by means of extracorporeal circulation. The problem is more immediately important for patients with tetralogy of Fallot undergoing corrective surgery. Residual pulmonary and right ventricular hypertension will jeopardize the end result in such patients if the associated pulmonary arterial obstruction is not remedied simultaneously (Björk et al., 1963). There is no apparent prospect of surgical correction for the peripheral type of obstruction (Baum et al., 1964).

REFERENCES

Agustsson, M. H.; Arcilla, R. A.; Gasul, B. M.; Bicoff, J. P.; Nassif, S. I.; and Lendrum, B. L.: The diagnosis of bilateral stenosis of the primary pulmonary branches based on characteristic pulmonary trunk pressure curves. *Circulation*, **26**:421, 1962.

Arvidsson, H.; Carlsson, E.; Hartmann, A., Jr.; Argyrios, T.; and Crawford, C.: Supravalvular stenosis of the pulmonary arteries. Report of eleven cases. *Acta Radiol.*, **56**:466, 1961.

Arvidsson, H.; Karnell, J.; and Möller, T.: Multiple stenosis of the pulmonary arteries associated with pulmonary hypertension, diagnosed by selective angiocardiography. *Acta Radiol.*, **44**:209, 1955.

Balboni, F. A.: Cutis laxa and multiple vascular anomalies including coarctation of the aorta. *St. Francis Hosp. Bull.*, **19**:21, 1963.

Baum, D.; Khoury, G. H.; Ongley, P. A.; Susan, H. J. C.; and Kincaid, O. W.: Congenital stenosis of the pulmonary artery branches. *Circulation*, **29**:680, 1964.

Baxter, C. F.; Booth, R. W.; and Sirak, H. D.: Surgical correction of congenital stenosis of the right pulmonary artery accompanied by agenesis of the left pulmonary artery. *J. Thorac. Cardiovasc. Surg.*, **41**:796, 1961.

Beuren, A. J.: Supravalvular aortic stenosis: a complex syndrome with and without mental retardation. In *Birth Defects: Original Article Series*, **8**:No. 5, August, 1972, The National Foundation, Williams and Wilkins Co. Baltimore, p. 45.

Beuren, A. J.; Hort, W.; Kalbfleisch, H.; Muller, H.; and Stoermer, J.: Dysplasia of the systemic and pulmonary arterial system with tortuosity and lengthening of the arteries. A new entity, diagnosed during life, and leading to coronary death in early childhood. *Circulation*, **39**:109, 1969.

Björk, V. O.; Lodin, H.; and Michaelsson, M.: Fallot's anomaly with peripheral pulmonary artery malformations. *J. Thorac. Cardiovasc. Surg.*, **45**:764, 1963.

Bouvrain, Y.; Bourthoumieux, A.; and Nezry, R.: Souffles systoliques a irradiations axillaires et retrecissment des branches de l'artere pulmonaire. *Arch. Mal. Coeur*, **54**:999, 1961.

Coles, J. E., and Walker, W. J.; Coarctation of the pulmonary artery. *Am. Heart J.*, **52**:469, 1956.

Danilowicz, D. A.; Rudolph, A. M.; Hoffman, J. I. E.; and Heymann, M.: Physiologic pressure differences between main and branch pulmonary arteries in infants. *Circulation*, **45**:410, 1972.

Delaney, T. B., and Nadas, A. S.: Peripheral pulmonic stenosis. *Am. J. Cardiol.*, **13**:451, 1964.

Deyrieux, F.; Tartulier, M.; and Touriaire, A.: La stenose de l'artere pulmonaire droite phonocardiographe endocavitaire et etude hemodynamique de deux cas. *Arch. Mal. Coeur*, **54**:1004, 1961.

Dunkle, L. M., and Rowe, R. D.: Transient murmur simulating pulmonary artery stenosis in premature infants. *Am. J. Dis. Child.*, **124**:666, 1972.

Eldridge, W. J.; Tinglestad, J. B.; Robertson, L. W.; Mauck, H. P.; and McCue, C.: Observations on the natural history of pulmonary artery coarctations. *Circulation*, **45**:404, 1972.

Eldridge, F.; Selzer, A.; and Hultgren, H.: Stenosis of a branch of the pulmonary artery. An additional cause of continuous murmurs over the chest. *Circulation*, **15**:865, 1957.

Emmanouilides, G. C.; Linde, L. M.; and Crittenden, I. H.: Pulmonary artery stenosis associated with ductus arteriosus following maternal rubella. *Circulation*, **29**:514, 1964.

Falkenbach, K. H.; Zhentlin, N.; Dowdy, A. H.; and O'Loughlin, B. J.: Pulmonary hypertension due to pulmonary arterial coarctation. *Radiology*, **73**:575, 1959.

Fouron, J. C.; Favreau-Ethier, M.; Marion, P.; and Davignon, A.: Les stenoses pulmonaires peripheriques congenitales: Presentation de 16 observations et revue de la litterature. *Can. Med. Assoc. J.*, **96**:1084–94, 1967.

Franch, R. H., and Gay, B. B., Jr.: Congenital stenosis of the pulmonary artery branches. A classification, with post mortem findings in two cases. *Am. J. Cardiol.*, **35**:512–29, 1963.

Greenwood, R. D.; Rosenthal, A.; Crocker, A. C.; and Nadas, A. S.: Syndrome of intrahepatic biliary dysgenesis and cardiovascular malformations. *Pediatrics*, **58**:243, 1976.

Guller, B.: Stenosis of the pulmonary arteries: evolution and hemodynamic effects. *Chest*, **61**:70, 1972.

Gyllensward, A.; Lodin, H.; Lundberg, A.; and Moller, T.: Congenital multiple peripheral stenoses of the pulmonary artery. *Pediatrics*, **19**:399, 1957.

Hartmann, A. F. Jr.; Elliott, L. P.; and Goldring, D.: The course of peripheral pulmonary artery stenosis in children. *J. Pediatr.*, **73**:212, 1968.

Hastreiter, A. R.; Jarabchi, B.; Pujatti, G.; van der Herst, R. L.; Patacsil, G.; and Sever, J. L.: Cardiovascular lesions associated with congenital rubella. *J. Pediatr.*, **71**:59, 1967.

Hayden, J. G.; Taler, N. S.; and Klaus, S. M.: Cutis laxa associated with pulmonary artery stenosis. *J. Pediatr.*, **72**:506, 1968.

Keutel, J.; Jorgensen, G.; and Gabriel, P.: A new autosomal recessive syndrome peripheral stenoses, brachytelephalangism, neural hearing loss and abnormal cartilage calcifications/ossification. In *Birth Defects: Original Article Series*, **8**:No. 5, August, 1972.

Linde, L. M.; Turner, S. W.; and Sparkes, R. S.: Pulmonary valvular dysplasia. A cardiofacial syndrome. *Br. Heart J.*, **35**:301, 1973.

Loes, M. H.; Menashe, V. D.; Sunderland, C. O.; Morgan, C. L.; and Dawson, P. J.: Ehlers-Danlos syndrome associated with multiple pulmonary artery stenosis and tortuous systemic arteries. *J. Pediatr.*, **75**:1031, 1969.

Loggie, J. M. H.; Gaffney, T. E.; Kaplan, S.; and Hanenson, I. B.: Hypertension and mitral incompetence associated with multiple systemic and pulmonary artery stenosis in a Caucasian child. *J. Pediatr.*, **72**:101, 1968.

McCue, C. M.; Robertson, L. W.; Lester, R. G.; and Mauck, H. P., Jr.: Pulmonary artery coarctations. A report of 20 cases with review of 319 cases from the literature. *J. Pediatr.*, **67**:222, 1965.

Mudd, C. M.; Walter, K. E.; and Willman, V. L.: Pulmonary artery stenosis: Diagnostic and therapeutic considerations. *Am. J. Med. Sci.*, **249**:125, 1965.

Noonan, J. A., and Ehmke, D. A. Associated non-cardiac malformations in children with congenital heart disease. *J. Pediatr.*, **63**:468, 1963.

Oppenheimer, E. H.: Partial atresia of the main branches of the pulmonary artery occurring in infancy and accompanied by calcification of the pulmonary artery and aorta. *Bull. Hopkins Hosp.*, **63**:261, 1938.

Orell, S. R.; Karnell, J.; and Wahlgren, F.: Malformation and multiple stenoses of the pulmonary arteries with pulmonary hypertension. *Acta Radiol.*, **54**:449, 1960.

Perloff, J. K., and Lebauer, E. J.: Auscultatory and phonocardiographic manifestations of isolated stenosis of the pulmonary artery and its branches. *Br. Heart J.*, **31**:314, 1969.

Rios, J. C.; Walsh, B. J.; Massumi, R. A.; Sims, A. J.; and Ewy, G. A.: Congenital pulmonary artery branch stenosis. *Am. J. Cardiol.*, **24**:318, 1969.

Roberts, N., and Moes, C. A. F.: Supravalvular pulmonary stenosis. *J. Pediatr.*, **82**:838, 1973.

Rowe, R. D.: Maternal rubella and pulmonary artery stenoses. Report of eleven cases. *Pediatrics*, **32**:180, 1963.

Rowe, R. D.; Mehrizi, A.; Elliott, H. L.; and Neill, C. A.: Cardiovascular disease in the rubella syndrome. In Cassels, D. E. (ed.): *The Heart and Circulation in the Newborn and Infant.* Grune & Stratton, New York, 1966, p. 180.

Rowe, R. D.; Varghese, P. J.; and Simon, A. L.: Asymptomatic systemic arterial lesions in congenital rubella (abstr.). Amer. Ped. Soc., 79th Annual Meeting 1969, p. 40.

Rowe, R. D.: Stenosis of conducting arteries in infants and children. In *Birth Defects: Original Article Series*, **8**:No. 5, Aug. 1972, The National Foundation, Williams & Wilkins Co., Baltimore, p. 69.

Rowe, R. D.: Cardiovascular disease in the rubella syndrome. *Cardiovasc. Clin.*, **4**:5, 1973.

Rowe, R. D.; Kelly, D. T.; McCue, C.; and Ottesen, O.: Unusual distribution of vascular damage as sequelae of idiopathic hypercalcemia and congenital rubella syndrome. In *Birth Defects: Original Article Series*, **10**:No. 4, 1974. The National Foundation, Williams & Wilkins Co., Baltimore, p. 361.

Sacks, J. G.; and Lindenburg, R.: Dolicho-ectatic intracranial arteries: Symptomatology and pathogenesis of arterial elongation and distention. *J. Hopkins Hosp.*, **125**:95, 1969.

Sauvage, L. R.; Rudolph, A. M.; and Gross, R. E.: Replacement of the main pulmonary artery bifurcation by autogenous pericardium. *J. Thorac. Cardiovasc. Surg.*, **40**:567, 1960.

Schlesinger, F. G., and Meester, G. T.: Supravalvular stenosis of the pulmonary artery. *Br. Heart J.*, **29**:829, 1967.

Schumacker, H. B., Jr., and Lurie, P. R.: Pulmonary valvulotomy. *J. Thorac. Surg.*, **25**:173, 1953.

Smith, W. G.: Pulmonary hypertension and a continuous murmur due to multiple peripheral stenoses of the pulmonary arteries. *Thorax*, **13**:194, 1958.

Søndegaard, T.: Coarctation of the pulmonary artery. *Danish Med. Bull.*, **1**:46, 1954.

Thrower, W. B.; Abelmann, W. H. J.; and Harken, D. E.: Surgical correction of coarctation of the main pulmonary artery. *Circulation*, **21**:672, 1960.

Van Epps, E. F.: Primary pulmonary hypertension in brothers. *Am. J. Roentgenol.*, **78**:471, 1957.

Venables, A. W.: The syndrome of pulmonary stenosis complicating maternal rubella. *Br. Heart J.*, **27**:49, 1965.

Vince, D. J.: The role of rubella in the etiology of supravalvular aortic stenosis. *Can. Med. Assoc. J.*, **103**:1157, 1970.

Wasserman, M. P.; Varghese, P. J.; and Rowe, R. D.: The evolution of pulmonary arterial stenosis associated with congenital rubella. *Am. Heart J.*, **76**:638, 1968.

Williams, C. B.; Lange, R. L.; and Hecht, H. H.: Post valvular stenosis of the pulmonary artery. *Circulation*, **16**:195, 1957.

CHAPTER

42

Mitral Valve and Tricuspid Valve Stenosis

Kenneth R. Bloom

CONGENITAL stenosis of the atrioventricular (AV) valves may occur as isolated anomalies or may complicate other defects. A critical awareness of this latter possibility is of importance. Intended therapy may be modified as an otherwise-operable condition might be considered inoperable. Unrelieved AV valve stenosis following correction of intracardiac defects can compromise the outcome of surgery.

A number of structures are involved in the normal function of an AV valve (Roberts and Perloff, 1972). Abnormal development of any of these can result in hemodynamic stenosis.

MITRAL VALVE

Anatomy

There are four major components: leaflets, chordae tendineae, papillary muscles, and annulus.

Leaflets. Rusted and his coworkers (1952) showed that there is a continuous circumferential rim of leaflet tissue in the orifice of the mitral valve. The separation of this into anterior and posterior leaflets occurs at the posterolateral and anteromedial commissures. Ranganathan and coworkers (1970) confirmed that these commissures may be identified by the tips of the papillary muscles, and they also recognized chordae tendineae that inserted into these commissures.

The anterior leaflet extends much further into the orifice of the valve than does the posterior leaflet but is attached to only one-third of the annulus. It is continuous with the left and part of the noncoronary cusps of the aortic valve. Together with the adjacent portion of ventricular septum, it forms the borders of the left ventricular outflow tract. There is a rough zone into which the chordae tendineae insert and a clear zone.

The posterior leaflet has several clefts along its free margin and it is usually divided into three scallops (Ranganathan et al., 1970). Rough and clear zones are again identified here. There is also a basal zone into which chordae tendineae that originate directly from trabeculae carneae of the left ventricular myocardium insert (Ranganathan et al., 1970).

Chordae Tendineae. These arise from the two papillary muscles and insert into the ventricular surfaces of the rough areas of both leaflets, the basal area of the posterior leaflet, and the commissural areas (Lam et al., 1970). They branch several times from their origin, increasing in number from 25 to 120. Blood passes through the interchordal spaces, and fusion will narrow the effective mitral orifice.

Papillary Muscles. These are two in number and are related to the commissures on their ventricular surface. The anterolateral usually consists of a single muscle belly. Its arterial supply is from many branches of the left coronary system. The postero-medial papillary muscle is usually bifid. This arterial supply is from terminal branches of the right and left coronary arteries.

Annulus. This is part of the fibrous skeleton of the heart. The anteromedial leaflet attaches to its anterior third and the posterior leaflet to the posterior two-thirds. The cross-sectional area of the annulus is about 80 percent of the cross-sectional area of the leaflets, allowing for considerable overlap during closure (Du Plessis and Marchand, 1964).

Pathology

The unobstructed flow of blood across the mitral orifice is, therefore, dependent on the normal function of a number of structures. Essentially, there must be pliable valvular tissue; no restriction or fusion at the commissural junctions; proper position, function, and length of the chordae and papillary muscles; and an adequate annulus.

Leaflet Abnormalities. Thickened and fibrotic leaflets are usually combined with rudimentary and fused commissures. Anatomically, the valve is funnel-shaped and often resembles a classic "rheumatic" valve (Roberts et al., 1973). Davachi and coworkers (1971) have also described accessory mitral valvular tissue attached to the atrial aspect of the posterior leaflet. This tissue can obstruct the orifice of the mitral valve on the basis of its size.

Chordae Tendineae. Thickened and shortened chordae tendineae, often matted together, may obstruct the left ventricular inflow tract. Layman and Edwards (1967) described a bridge of fibrous tissue continuous with the free aspect of the anterior mitral leaflet resulting in direct continuity of the mitral valve leaflet with the papillary muscles.

Papillary Muscles. Shone and his coworkers (1963) described the developmental complex of "parachute" mitral valve, supravalvular ring of the left atrium, subaortic stenosis, and coarctation of the aorta. The mitral valve anatomy in this situation consists of the two mitral valve leaflets and commissures, but the chordae converge to insert into one major papillary muscle.

Compound Involvement of the Mitral Valve Mechanism. Daoud and coworkers (1963) describe cases in whom the leaflets are thickened as well as the chordae tendineae being shortened, thickened, and atrophic to variable degrees.

Mitral Stenosis Associated with Other Congenital Anomalies. At least 50 percent of congenital mitral stenosis coexists with other congenital anomalies (Kaplan, 1968). The recognition of this association is of critical importance in planning surgery. The clinical signs of mitral stenosis may be masked by the associated anatomic defects and may not be evident even on catheterization. Echocardiography has provided a useful additional diagnostic tool, but care in interpretation must be combined with a high index of suspicion. The more common associations will be mentioned.

COARCTATION OF THE AORTA. This association with parachute mitral valve (Shone et al., 1963) has been referred to. Rosenquist (1974) examined 53 specimens in whom coarctation of the aorta was the primary diagnosis. In only nine specimens was the mitral valve completely normal. Thirteen specimens had a basically normal valve mechanism, but the components were small compared to the normals. The remaining 31 cases showed abnormalities primarily of the papillary muscles or chordae tendineae.

TRANSPOSITION OF THE GREAT ARTERIES. Rosenquist and coworkers (1975) noted a spectrum of mitral valve anomalies associated with this defect. The majority of the anomalies are minor, such as minor chordal anomalies and slight reduction of the mitral annulus size. In some, fusion of papillary muscles and abnormal mitral valve leaflet attachments were noted.

DOUBLE-OUTLET RIGHT VENTRICLE. Sondheimer and coworkers (1976) found a high incidence (28 percent) of severe mitral valve anomalies in the group with subaortic ventricular septal defect without pulmonic stenosis. Fifteen percent of the group with subpulmonic ventricular septal defect without pulmonic stenosis also had significant mitral valve disease.

SINGLE OR PRIMITIVE VENTRICLES, VENTRICULAR SEPTAL DEFECT, AND DOUBLE-INLET LEFT VENTRICLE. Straddling AV valve orifices are frequently associated with hypoplastic valve orifices and abnormal valve tissue. This can result in mitral stenosis (Lieberthson et al., 1971). Double-inlet left ventricle (Mehrizi et al., 1966; de la Cruz and Miller, 1968) is also frequently associated with functional mitral stenosis.

ATRIAL SEPTAL DEFECT. The association of mitral stenosis with this defect (Lutembacher's syndrome) may result from rheumatic endocarditis (Espino-Vela, 1959; Steinbrunn et al., 1970). Congenital deformities of the mitral valve have also been described (Muller et al., 1965). The syndrome is rare, complicating about 4 to 6 percent of adults with atrial septal defects (Steinbrunn et al., 1970).

Pathophysiology

Isolated Mitral Stenosis. Transmission of the high left atrial pressure through to the bronchial veins results in edema of the bronchial mucosa and increased airway resistance. The elevated left atrial pressure is also transmitted freely through the pulmonary veins and pulmonary capillary bed. Pulmonary edema will occur when the hydrostatic pressure in the capillaries rises above the oncotic pressure of the blood and the lymphatics are unable to drain the increased amounts of tissue fluid formed. The vascular congestion results in decreased static and dynamic compliances of the lung (Wood et al., 1971). Tandon and Kasturi (1975) have described severe pulmonary vascular disease and marked interstitial fibrosis in young patients.

Compensatory mechanisms develop in the lung vascularity. These enable one to tolerate greater elevations of left atrial pressure than one could acutely. These mechanisms are:

1. An increased capacity of the lymphatic system (Rabin and Meyer, 1960).
2. The development of pulmonary bronchial collaterals.
3. Reflex pulmonary arteriolar constriction (Shoultz et al., 1971).
4. Possibly altered pulmonary capillary permeability.

Left ventricular function was assessed in adults with mitral stenosis by Heller and Carleton (1970). Significantly lower ejection fractions were found, suggesting some impairment of contraction presumably by the abnormal valve apparatus. This was confirmed in an echocardiographic study by McDonald (1976).

Mitral Stenosis with Other Defects. Here the hemodynamic effects of the associated defect must be considered. The finding of a larger left-to-right shunt at atrial level, or greater pulmonary hypertension than would otherwise be expected, may lead one to suspect the coexistence of an abnormal mitral valve. The hemodynamic diagnosis may be difficult with complicated associated defects.

Clinical Features

The hemodynamic features, combining both to reduce pulmonary compliance and to increase airway resistance, result in dyspnea in almost all cases. Effort intolerance is usually marked. This may be due to a disproportionate rise in the pulmonary vascular resistance on effort (Lasser and Amram, 1955). Paroxysmal nocturnal dyspnea and orthopnea are frequently seen. Right heart failure with peripheral edema may occur.

Cyanosis may occur in otherwise-uncomplicated mitral stenosis, presumably as a result of decreased oxygen saturation of the blood due to pulmonary edema. There may also be disturbance in the ventilation perfusion ratio of the lung secondary to abnormal capillary blood flow.

Examination of the Heart. There may be visual and palpable evidence of right ventricular hypertrophy.

Auscultation. A careful evaluation of the auscultatory findings can help in the final assessment of the nature of the pathology of the valve mechanism. The auscultatory features are (Figure 42–1):

1. MIDDIASTOLIC MURMUR. An apical rumble is often heard best when the patient lies in the left lateral position.

2. PRESYSTOLIC ACCENTUATION. This is due to the increased velocity of blood flow across the stenotic valve following atrial contraction. It is also noted in atrial fibrillation, particularly after short diastolic pauses (Lakier et al., 1972b).

3. LOUD AND DELAYED MITRAL COMPONENT OF THE FIRST HEART SOUND (van der Horst and Hastreiter, 1967). The presence of a loud mitral component of the first heart sound will normally indicate pliable valve leaflets and, in particular, mobile chordae (Lakier et al., 1972a). Therefore, a soft first heart sound—common in congenital mitral stenosis—suggests immobile leaflets with thickened short chordae.

4. OPENING SNAP. The presence of this sound indicates that the mitral leaflets are mobile. Again, this is frequently absent in congenital mitral stenosis (Daoud et al., 1963).

5. CAUSES OF A SYSTOLIC MURMUR. A systolic murmur may be due to either associated mitral regurgitation or, if pulmonary hypertension is present, tricuspid regurgitation.

6. OTHER CARDIAC DEFECTS. The presence of other cardiac defects will modify the clinical picture according to their hemodynamics.

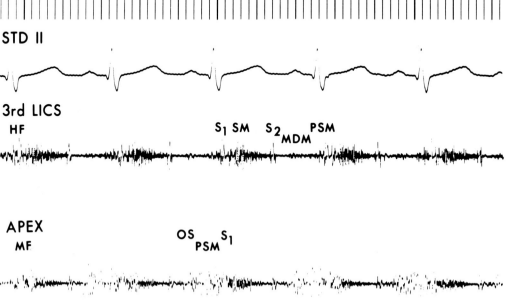

Figure 42-1. Phonocardiogram of a two-year-old child with moderate mitral stenosis associated with coarctation of the aorta. Leaflets appeared mobile at cardiac catheterization. *LICS* = left intercostal space; *HF* = high frequency; *MF* = midfrequency; *SM* = systolic murmur; *MDM* = middiastolic murmur; *PSM* = presystolic murmur; *OS* = opening snap.

Electrocardiography

Mean frontal plane QRS axis is normally between +90° and +150°. Right ventricular and biatrial hypertrophy is common (van der Horst and Hastreiter, 1967).

Radiologic Examination

Considerable cardiomegaly with left atrial and right ventricular enlargement is common. Severe stenosis may be indicated by the presence of Kerley's A and B lines (Chen et al., 1968).

Echocardiography

Echocardiography (Figure 42–2) gives the clinician the best chance of making an accurate diagnosis when mitral stenosis complicates other defects. The marked variations in the different types of mitral deformity that will result in functional stenosis make it important to evaluate all aspects of mitral valve motion. These must then be related to the functional hemodynamic state of the patient and the measured chamber size.

Cope and coworkers (1975) found a decreased E-F slope of the valve in all patients (average age 47 years). Forty-one percent of their patients had decreased amplitude of excursion (DE distance). These diseased mitral valves were predominantly rheumatic in etiology. There are many similarities between rheumatic involvement of the mitral valve mechanism and some congenital malformations.

Lundstrom (1972) evaluated seven patients with congenital mitral stenosis. Operative correlations were available. Patients in whom the chordae tendineae were fused had reduced amplitude of opening (DE). A reduced E-F slope was found in all cases. Posterior leaflet motion is usually abnormal in that the posterior leaflet echo usually moves anterior and parallel with the anterior leaflet echo, instead of away from it. Exceptions have been noted (Berman et al., 1975).

In our experience the E-F slope may be normal if the only valvar pathology is a small annulus. Henry and coworkers (1975) measured valvar orifice area successfully using real-time two-dimensional echocardiography.

An enlarged left atrium is seen in otherwise-uncomplicated cases. La Corte and coworkers (1976) described multiple diastolic echoes in one case.

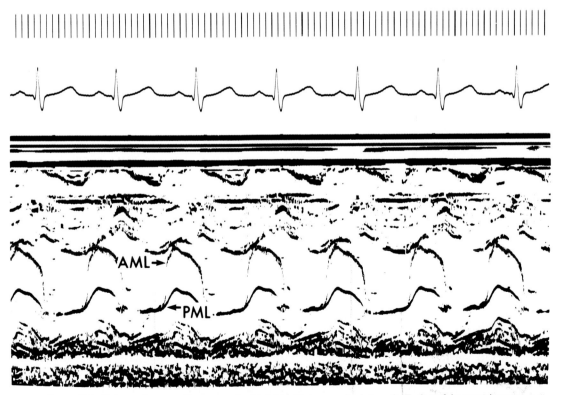

Figure 42-2. Echocardiogram of a ten-month-old child with severe mitral stenosis. Fusion of the commissures with pliable leaflets and somewhat thickened chordae was seen at open valvotomy. The annulus was nearly normal in diameter. Note slow E-F slope and small "a" wave of anterior mitral leaflet (*AML*). Posterior leaflet (*PML*) motion is abnormal. Amplitude of the AML excursion is normal.

Radionuclide Angiography

Kriss and coworkers (1971) have used 99 Mtc pertechnetate and shown enlargement of the left atrium with prolonged visualization and persistent dual visualization of the left atrium and ventricle in tight mitral stenosis.

Cardiac Catheterization

The left atrial pressure is elevated with a diastolic gradient across the mitral valve. There may be pulmonary hypertension.

Cineangiography may show a large left atrium with delayed emptying. Reduced mobility of the mitral valve mechanism and a "jet" of blood entering the left ventricle may be seen. The right anterior oblique view is best in children with otherwise-normal anatomy. Associated defects may modify this.

Differential Diagnosis

Other anomalies resulting in left ventricular inflow obstruction must be considered. These are: (1) pulmonary venous stenosis, (2) cor triatriatum, (3) anomalous pulmonary venous return, and (4) atrial tumors.

A careful examination utilizing the clinical and investigative parameters as outlined above can result in accurate localization of the site of obstruction. Obstruction may coexist at two different sites, as in the parachute mitral valve with supravalvar stenosing

ring (Shone et al., 1963a; Macartney et al., 1974) and also at pulmonary venous level (Shone et al., 1963a).

Management

Conservative management on comprehensive antifailure therapy may suffice in less severe obstruction. Digitalis preparations are indicated. Diuretics must be used cautiously as low-output states may be produced.

The need for anticoagulation can be assessed on an individual basis. Casella and coworkers (1964) found that systemic emboli occur more commonly with atrial fibrillation and increasing age, rather than with the degree of severity of the obstruction or the functional classification of the patient. Emboli occur only rarely in the pediatric age group. Surgery is the only effective method of treating severe obstruction. Relief of the obstruction will relieve or reduce pulmonary hypertension (Ward and Hancock, 1974). Closed or open valvotomy and prosthetic valve replacement have all been reported (Starkey, 1959; Young and Robinson, 1964; Trusler and Fowler, 1965). Children requiring surgery under one year of age have a high mortality. The improvement in design of low-profile prostheses makes replacement feasible if the annular size is adequate. Valvotomy or fenestration of the fused leaflets may give good palliation for years (Bernhard et al., 1972). The deformity of the valve usually dictates the surgical approach. Attempts to conserve the patient's own valve tissue should be made whenever possible.

An abnormal mitral valve affects the surgical approach to any associated defects. The possibility and feasibility of valve replacement must always be considered.

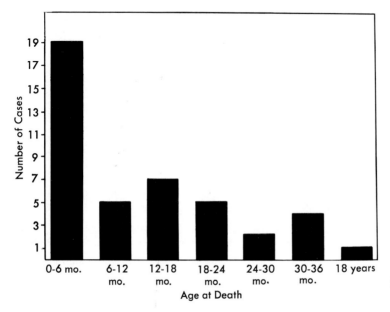

Figure 42-3. Age at death of 43 cases of congenital mitral stenosis.

Prognosis

Prognosis depends to a large extent on the severity of the obstruction and the nature of the associated lesions (Figure 42–3). Most children with severe disease die in the first year of life; the chances of survival, therefore, improve with age. The complications of endocarditis and emboli are rare in childhood but worsen prognosis when they occur.

All surgery is palliation. There are major long-term problems of prosthetic valve replacement in children. This malformation remains one of the challenges of pediatric cardiology.

TRICUSPID VALVE

ISOLATED tricuspid stenosis is a rare anomaly and usually forms the subject of individual case reports (Calleja et al., 1960; Henriques, 1963; Sapirstein and Baker, 1963; Keefe et al., 1970; Dimich et al., 1973).

This abnormality may complicate other congenital heart malformations, such as Uhl's anomaly and isolated hypoplasia of the right ventricle (Haworth et al., 1975). Persistence of tissue attributed to embryologic venous valves may result in supravalvar stenosis of the tricuspid valve with an associated hypoplastic valve orifice (Folger, 1968; Hausing et al., 1972). Straddling tricuspid valves may be functionally obstructive (Lieberthson et al., 1971).

Congenital polyvalvar disease, in which there is stenosis of the aortic, mitral, and tricuspid valves, is occasionally seen (Figure 42–4). The most common association is with the hypoplastic right heart syndrome, and this is considered in detail in Chapters 28 and 29.

Anatomy

Silver and coworkers (1971) describe the anatomy of this valve in detail. The annulus is triangular. Chordae tendineae are of five types. Free-edge and deep chordae—not seen in the mitral apparatus—are found, in addition to fan-shaped, rough-zone, and basal chordae. The leaflets have many indentations. They are divided by anteroseptal and anteroposterior commissures into anterior (largest), posterior, and septal leaflets.

Clinical Features

Women are more frequently affected. The jugular venous pressure may show a prominent "a" wave. Inspiration may result in an increase in the venous pressure.

A presystolic murmur that increases on inspiration is commonly heard. Opening snaps and middiastolic murmurs are rarely heard (Perloff and Harvey, 1960).

The electrocardiogram shows right atrial hypertrophy. Left axis has been reported (Keefe et al., 1970).

Cardiac catheterization shows a high right atrial pressure and "a" wave with a diastolic gradient across the valve.

Echocardiography will show limited amplitude of opening and a diminished diastolic slope much as in mitral stenosis (Joyner et al., 1967). This technique is of special value in the assessment of the tricuspid valve function in hypoplastic right heart syndromes.

Differential Diagnosis

Right atrial myxoma (Goldschlager et al., 1972), right atrial enlargement (Tenckhoff et al., 1969), and Ebstein's anomaly must be excluded.

Tricuspid Valve

Mitral Valve

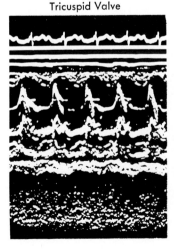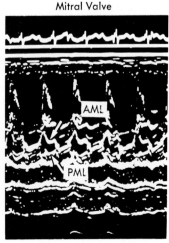

Figure 42-4. Congenital polyvalvar stenosis in a newborn infant. The tricuspid valve shows thick, coarse leaflet echoes. The mitral valve shows reduced amplitude of the anterior leaflet (*AML*). Posterior leaflet (*PML*) motion is near normal. At autopsy the tricuspid valve leaflets were gelatinous, the chordae were thickened. The mitral annulus was very small. There was a bicuspid (nonstenotic) aortic valve.

Treatment

Commissurotomy (Sapirstein and Baker, 1963) and valve replacement (Dimich et al., 1973) may be required if severe symptoms are present. Valves may be markedly dysplastic and, therefore, not amenable to conservative surgery.

Prognosis

A high percentage of reported cases have survived to adult life. Obviously, associated abnormalities and the severity of the lesion will influence survival.

REFERENCES

Mitral Valve Stenosis

Berman, N. D.; Gilbert, B. W.; McLaughlin, P. R.; and Morch, J. E.: Mitral stenosis with posterior diastolic movement of posterior leaflet. *Can. Med. Assoc. J.*, 112:976, 1975.

Bernhard, W. F., and Litwin, S. B.: The surgical treatment of unusual congenital mitral valve anomalies. *Circulation* (Suppl. II), 45:46, 135, 1972.

Casella, L.; Abelmann, W. H.; and Ellis, L. B.: Mitral stenosis and systemic emboli. *Arch. Intern. Med.*, 114:773, 1964.

Chen, J. T. T.; Behar, V. S.; Morris, J. J.; McIntosh, H. D.; and Lester, R. G.: Correlation of roentgen findings with hemodynamic data in pure mitral stenosis. *Am. J. Roentgenol.*, 102:280, 1968.

Cope, G. D.; Kisslo, J. A.; Johnson, M. L.; and Behar, V. S.: A Reassessment of the echocardiogram in mitral stenosis. *Circulation*, 52:664, 1975.

Daoud, G.; Kaplan, S.; Perrin, E. V.; Dorst, J. G.; and Edwards, F. K.: Congenital mitral stenosis. *Circulation*, 27:185, 1963.

Davichi, F.; Moller, J. H.; and Edwards, J. E.: Diseases of the mitral valve in infancy. An anatomical analysis of fifty-five cases. *Circulation*, 43:565, 1971.

De la Cruz, M. V.. and Miller, B. L.: Double inlet left ventricle. *Circulation*, 37:249, 1968.

Du Plessis, L. A., and Marchand, P.: The anatomy of the mitral valve and associated structures. *Thorax*, 19:221, 1964.

Espino-Vela, J.: Rheumatic heart disease associated with atrial septal defect: Clinical and pathological study of twelve cases of Lutembacher's syndrome. *Am. Heart J.*, 57:185, 1959.

Heller, S. J., and Carleton, R. A.: Abnormal left ventricular contraction in patients with mitral stenosis. *Circulation*, 42:1099, 1970.

Henry, W. C.; Griffith, J. M.; Michaelis, L. L.; McIntosh, C. L.; Morrow, A. G.; and Epstein, S. E.: Measurement of mitral orifice area in patients with mitral valve disease by real-time two-dimensional echocardiography. *Circulation*, 51:827, 1975.

Kaplan, S.: Congenital mitral stenosis. In Watson, E. H. (ed.): *Pediatric Cardiology*. Lloyd-Luke. London, 1968, p. 361.

La Corte, M.; Harada, K.; and Williams, R. G.: Echocardiographic features of congenital left ventricular inflow obstruction. *Circulation*, 54:562, 1976.

Lakier, J. B.; Fritz, V. N.; Pocock, W. A.; and Barlow, J. B.: Mitral components of the first heart sound. *Br. Heart J.*, 34:160, 1972a.

Lakier, J. B.; Pocock, W. A.; Grale, G. E.; and Barlow, J. B.: Hemodynamic and sound events preceding first heart sound in mitral stenosis. *Br. Heart J.*, 34:1152, 1972b.

Lam, J. H. C.; Ranganathan, N.; Wigle, E. D.; and Silver, M. D.: Morphology of the human mitral valve. Chordae tendinae: A new classification. *Circulation*, 41:449, 1970.

Lasser,, R. P., and Amram, S. S.: The effect of exercise upon the compression chamber function of the pulmonary artery in patients with mitral stenosis. *Clin. Res. Proc.*, 3:35, 1955.

Layman, T. E., and Edwards, J. E.: Anomalous mitral arcade. A type of congenital mitral insufficiency. *Circulation*, 35:389, 1967.

Lieberthson, R. R.; Paul, M. H.; Muster, A. J.; Arcilla, R. A.; Eckner, F. A. O.; and Lev, M.: Straddling and displaced atrioventricular orifices and valves with primitive ventricles. *Circulation*, 43:213, 1971.

Lundstrom, N. R.: Echocardiography in the diagnosis of congenital mitral stenosis and in evaluation of the results of mitral valvotomy. *Circulation*, 46:44, 1972.

Macartney, F. J.; Scott, O.; Ionescu, M. I.; and Deverall, P. B.: Diagnosis and management of parachute mitral valve and supravalvar mitral ring. *Br. Heart J.*, 36:641, 1974.

McDonald, I. G.: Echographic assessment of left ventricular function in mitral valve disease. *Circulation*, 53:865, 1976.

Mehrizi, A.; McMurphy, D. M.; Ottesen, O. E.; and Rowe, R. D.: Syndrome of double inlet left ventricle. Angiographic differentiation from single ventricle with rudimentary outflow chamber. *Bull. Johns Hopkins Hosp.*, 119:255, 1966.

Muller, W. H.; Littlefield, J. B.; and Beckwith, J. R.: Surgical treatment of Lutembacher's syndrome. *J. Thorac. Cardiovasc. Surg.*, 51:66, 1966.

Rabin, E. R., and Meyer, E. C.: Cardiopulmonary effects of pulmonary venous hypertension with special reference to pulmonary lymphatic flow. *Circ. Res.*, 8:324, 1960.

Ranganathan, N.; Lam, J. H. C.; Wigle, E. D.; and Silver, M. D.: Morphology of the human mitral valve. II The valve leaflets. *Circulation*, 41:459, 1970.

Roberts, W. C.; Dangel, J. C.; and Bulkley, B. H.: Nonrheumatic valvular cardiac disease: A clinico-pathological survey of twenty-seven different conditions causing valvular dysfunction. In Likoff, W. (ed.): *Cardiovascular Clinics*, Vol. 5, Number 2. F. A. Davis, Philadelphia, 1973, p. 346.

Roberts, W. C., and Perloff, J. K.: Mitral valvular disease. *Ann. Intern. Med.*, 77:939, 1972.

Rosenquist, G. C.: Congenital mitral valve disease associated with coarctation of the aorta. A spectrum that includes parachute deformity of the mitral valve. *Circulation*, 49:985, 1974.

Rosenquist, G. C.; Stark, J.; and Taylor, J. F. N.: Congenital mitral valve disease in transposition of the great arteries. *Circulation*, 51:731, 1975.

Rusted, I. E.; Schiefley, C. H.; and Edwards, J. E.: Studies of the mitral valve. 1. Anatomic features of the normal mitral valve and associated structures. *Circulation*, 6:825, 1952.

Shone, J. D.; Anderson, R. C.; Amplatz, K.; Varco, R. L.; Leonard, A. S.; and Edwards, J. E.: Pulmonary venous obstruction from two separate co-existent anomalies. *Am. J. Cardiol.*, 11:525, 1963.

Shone, J. D.; Sellers, R. D.; Anderson, R. C.; Adams, P.; Lillehei, C. W.; and Edwards, J. E.: The developmental complex of "parachute mitral valve", supravalvular ring of the left atrium, subaortic stenosis and coarctation of the aorta. *Am. J. Cardiol.*, 11:714, 1963b.

Shoultz, C. A.; Kelminson, L. L.; Vogel, J. H. K.; Pryor, R.; and Blount, S. G.: Hemodynamics in congenital mitral stenosis. *Chest*, 59:47, 1971.

Sondheimer, H. M.; Freedom, R. M.; and Olley, P. M.: Double outlet right ventricle: Clinical spectrum and prognosis. *Am. J. Cardiol.*, 39:709, 1977.

Starkey, G. W. B.: Surgical experiences in the treatment of congenital mitral stenosis and mitral insufficiency. *J. Thorac. Cardiovasc. Surg.*, 38:336, 1959.

Steinbrunn, W.; Chon, K. E.; and Selzer, A.: Atrial septal defect associated with mitral stenosis. The Lutembacher syndrome revisited. *Am. J. Med.*, 48:295, 1970.

Tandon, H. D.; and Kasturi, J.: Pulmonary vascular changes associated with isolated mitral stenosis in India. *Br. Heart J.*, 37:26, 1975.

Trusler, G. A.; and Fowler, R. S.: Congenital mitral stenosis in infancy: Report of a case with open correction. *Surgery*, 58:431, 1965.

van der Horst, R. L.; and Hastreiter, A. R.: Congenital mitral stenosis. *Am. J. Cardiol.*, 20:773, 1967.

Ward, C., and Hancock, B. W.: Extreme pulmonary hypertension caused by mitral valve disease. *Br. Heart J.*, 37:74, 1975.

Wood, T. E.; McLeod, P.; Anthonisen, N. R.; and Macklem, P. T.: Mechanics of breathing in mitral stenosis. *Am. Rev. Resp. Dis.*, 104:52, 1971.

Young, D., and Robinson, G.: Successful valve replacement in an infant with congenital mitral stenosis. *N. Engl. Med.*, 270:660, 1964.

Tricuspid Valve Stenosis

Calleja, H. B.; Hosier, D. M.; and Kissane, R. W.: Congenital tricuspid stenosis. *Am. J. Cardiol.*, **6**:821, 1960.

Dimich, I.; Goldfinger, P.; Steinfeld, L.; and Lukban, S. B.: Congenital tricuspid stenosis. *Am. J. Cardiol.*, **31**:89, 1973.

Folger, G. M.: Supravalvar tricuspid stenosis. *Am. J. Cardiol.*, **21**:81, 1968.

Goldschlager, A.; Popper, R.; Goldschlager, N.; Gerbode, F.; and Prozan, G.: Right atrial myxoma with right to left shunt and polycythemia presenting as congenital heart disease. *Am. J. Cardiol.*, **30**:82, 1972.

Hausing, C. E.; Young, W. P.; and Rowe, G. G.: Cor triatriatum dexter. *Am. J. Cardiol.*, **30**:559, 1972.

Haworth, S. G.; Shinebourne, E. A.; and Miller, G. A. H.: Right-to-left interatrial shunting with normal right ventricular pressure. *Br. Heart J.*, **37**:386, 1975.

Henriques, U.: Isolated tricuspid stenosis. *N. Engl. J. Med.*, **269**:1267, 1963.

Joyner, C. R.; Hey, E. B.; Johnson, J.; and Reid, J. M.: Reflected ultrasound in the diagosis of tricuspid stenosis. *Am. J. Cardiol.*, **19**:66, 1967.

Keefe, J. F.; Wolk, M. J.; and Levine, H. J.: Isolated tricuspid valvular stenosis. *Am. J. Cardiol.*, **25**:252, 1970.

Lieberthson, R. R.; Paul, M. H.; Muster, A. J.; Arcilla, R. A.; Eckner, F. A. O.; and Lev, M.: Straddling and displaced atrioventricular orifices and valves with primitive ventricles. *Circulation*, **43**:213, 1971.

Perloff, J., and Harvey, W. P.: Clinical recognition of tricuspid stenosis. *Circulation*, **22**:346, 1960.

Sapirstein, W., and Baker, C. B.: Isolated tricuspid valve stenosis. *N. Engl. J. Med.*, **269**:236, 1963.

Silver, M. D.; Lam, J. H. E.; Ranganathan, N.; and Wigle, E. D.: Morphology of the human tricuspid valve. *Circulation*, **43**:333, 1971.

Tenckhoff, L.; Stamm, S. J.; and Beckwith, J. B.: Sudden death in idiopathic (congenital) right atrial enlargement. *Circulation*, **40**:227, 1969.

CHAPTER

43

Mitral Valve Prolapse

Robert L. Gingell and *Peter Vlad*

A VARIETY of terms have come into common usage to describe this condition. Some are based on the angiographic appearance of the valve in systole (floppy mitral valve, ballooning mitral valve, billowing mitral valve, doughnut mitral valve); others reflect the clinical findings (systolic click–late systolic murmur syndrome); while still others are based on extrapolation from a limited number of pathologic observations (myxomatous mitral valve). Until more precise etiologic classification can be established, such descriptive terms will prevail. We feel that "mitral valve prolapse syndrome" is the most acceptable designation with the currently available information.

The modern history of this entity dates from 1963 when Barlow first demonstrated angiographically the association of the mitral regurgitation with the clinical syndrome of systolic click and late systolic murmur. Angiographic correlation with prolapse dates from the mid-1960s (Barlow and Bossman, 1966; Criley et al., 1966).

In retrospect, it seems clear that Osler (1880) and Cuffer and Barbillon (1887) described this clinical constellation characteristic of mitral valve prolapse. Although Griffith incriminated the mitral valve as early as 1892, such observations were largely held to be of extracardiac origin or of functional nature until these concepts were firmly dispelled by the advent of left ventricular angiography. In recent years, the noninvasive techniques of echocardiography have greatly enhanced the ability to establish the clinical diagnosis and detect unsuspected cases.

Subsequently, a large body of data has accumulated, indicating this malformation to be ubiquitous in the general population. Our experience indicates that a significant proportion of a pediatric population referred for cardiac evaluation is comprised of patients with the mitral valve prolapse syndrome.

Incidence

The available clinical data indicate that mitral valve prolapse is common in the general adult population. The studies of Brown and coworkers (1975), Markiewicz and associates (1975), and Procacci and colleagues (1976) emphasize the occult nature of this entity. Lachman and associates (1975) quoted data indicating an incidence of 1.4 percent detected on routine screening of a population of 12,050 South African schoolchildren, while Procacci and associates (1976) found evidence of mitral valve prolapse in 6.3 percent of a group of healthy women. Although the prevalence among the general childhood population remains undetermined, the observations of Chandramouli and coworkers (1969) and Alday and colleagues (1971) suggest this to be a common condition in the pediatric age group, as well. A review of a population referred for cardiac evaluation to the Children's Hospital of Buffalo over a period of ten years reveals about 10 percent had evidence of mitral valve prolapse, either isolated or in association with other forms of congenital heart disease.

The age and sex distribution at the time of referral of 159 proven cases (Figure 43–1) indicate that symptoms and/or auscultatory findings tend to become manifest in midchildhood and early adolescence. In addition, the female preponderance observed in adult populations (Jeresaty, 1974; Barlow et al., 1975) is preserved in the pediatric age group.

The potential for association of prolapsing mitral valve with various forms of congenital heart disease is important to the pediatric cardiologist, because a confusing auscultatory and electrocardiographic picture may be encountered. Our experience with 288 angiocardiographically documented cases is outlined in Table 43–1. Thirty-seven percent had associated congenital heart disease. The most frequently seen is the secundum atrial septal defect, accounting for 15 percent of all studied patients with mitral valve prolapse. This relationship has been observed by others (McDonald et al., 1971; Betriu et al., 1974; Jeresaty, 1974; Victorica et al., 1974; Keck et al., 1976). Keck and coworkers (1976) reviewed a series of documented secundum atrial septal defects and found concomitant prolapsing mitral valve in 41 percent.

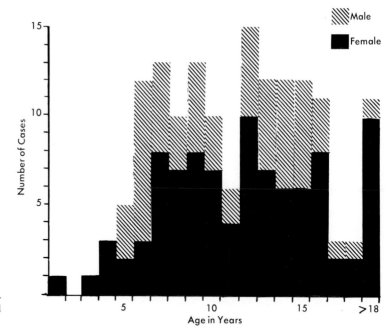

Figure 43-1. Age and sex distribution of 159 patients with isolated mitral valve prolapse.

As appreciation for the subtle and often evanescent physical findings is gained, a more substantial picture of the prevalence in childhood will be formed.

Table 43–1. ASSOCIATION WITH CONGENITAL HEART DISEASE, $N = 288$

Atrial septal defect (secundum type)	42
Ventricular septal defect	21
ASD plus VSD	3
Ebstein's anomaly	7
Membranous septum aneurysm	7*
Coarctation of aorta	3
Aortic regurgitation (Marfan's)	3
Pulmonic stenosis	13
Peripheral pulmonary stenosis	1
Transposition of great arteries	1
Tetralogy of Fallot	1
Aortic stenosis	1
Vascular ring	1
Myocardiopathy	1
	105

* 6 with VSD.

Etiology and Pathogenesis

The etiology of mitral valve prolapse remains obscure. This is in part due to the paucity of the pathologic material available for study, because of the favorable course enjoyed by the majority of patients. Further, any concept of the pathogenesis must encompass a broad spectrum of features, including incidence in the general population; female preponderance; sporadic and familial occurrence; clinical features and associations; electrocardio-

graphic changes, including the predisposition to arrhythmia, angiographic features, including left ventricular contraction patterns; and pathology.

Two major hypotheses have evolved through the reported observations (Jeresaty, 1976).

Valvular Theory.   This concept suggests that the myxomatous degeneration of the valve tissue itself is the primary event. As the degenerative changes advance, the valve area is increased, due to its redundancy. During systole, the increased surface area of the valve results in the transmission of increased tension to the chordae and papillary muscles. Such tension could produce local ischemia, account for the chest pain and ECG changes, and serve as an arrhythmogenic focus.

Myocardial Theory.   This theory indicates that a segmental or regional myocardiopathy is responsible for the prolapse by allowing the chordae to become slack during systole. Morphologic changes in the valve structure are then secondary to the abnormal stresses generated.

Although it is clear that many of these patients have abnormal left ventricular contraction patterns (Ehlers et al., 1970; Gooch et al., 1972; Scampardonis et al., 1973), evidence for the primacy of such findings is lacking. In 1973, Leidtke and associates reported detailed analyses of left ventricular angiographic studies in a series of adult patients with this syndrome. Their investigation indicated that there was a reduction in the circumferential fiber shortening of the proximal (inflow) portion of the left ventricle, reduced contraction of the inferior papillary muscle, and dilatation of the mitral ring. These observations were consistent, regardless of the degree of prolapse, suggesting that this may be an important initial condition for the prolapse to become manifest. We have reviewed a series of angiograms from a younger age group (mean age, 12.4 years) and found a significant reduction in the mean rate of shortening by the inferior papillary muscle, when compared with other forms of congenital and acquired heart disease. These data may imply a basic malfunction in the myocardium as a primary mechanism. Cobbs and coworkers (1974), however, have reported resolution of segmental contraction abnormalities after replacement of the mitral valve in such patients, challenging the validity of this concept.

The relative frequency of this lesion in the general population enhances chance associations and tends to confuse etiologic relationships. Prolapse of the mitral valve has thus been documented in patients with Turner's syndrome, homocystinuria, Ehlers-Danlos syndrome, muscular dystrophy, tuberous sclerosis, cardiomyopathy, acute rheumatic fever, and arteriosclerotic coronary artery disease.

The relationship of myxomatous degeneration of the mitral and aortic valves with Marfan's syndrome is more clear-cut. Phornphutkul and associates (1973) reviewed their experience with Marfan's syndrome in childhood. Mitral regurgitation was present in 47 percent and tended to be more frequent among girls. The electrocardiographic changes frequently associated with isolated prolapsing mitral valve were documented in about one-third of these patients. Indeed, some authors suggest that the isolated form of this condition may be a *forme fruste* of Marfan's syndrome (Read et al., 1965). Marfan's syndrome is known to occur sporadically or in families as a mendelian dominant trait. Familial occurrence with dominant inheritance is adequately documented in the isolated form (Hunt et al., 1969; Shell et al., 1969; Rizzon et al., 1972). These observations, together with the frequent occurrence of skeletal anomalies, particularly thoracic (Bon Tempo et al., 1975; Salomon et al., 1975), the demonstration of increased joint laxity (Evans et al., 1976), and the increased aortic root diameter demonstrated by echocardiography (Sahn et al., 1976), support the concept that idiopathic mitral valve prolapse represents a connective tissue disorder of subtle degree, the extreme of which constitutes the classic Marfan syndrome.

Clearly, more detailed pathologic, biochemical, genetic, and natural history studies are needed before these issues are resolved. At this time, because of the variance in prognosis, a distinction between the isolated idiopathic form and those patients with unequivocal Marfan's syndrome should be maintained.

Pathology

The pathologic features are based on a limited number of autopsy and surgical observations, which generally reflect more severe involvement. On gross examination, when viewed from the left atrial aspect (Figure 43–2*A*), the valve is seen to be thickened and

redundant, bulging into the annulus. The hemorrhoidal appearance of the posterior leaflet is the result of its normally triscalloped configuration. The deformity of the anterior leaflet is less obvious but equally severe (Figure 43–2*B* and *C*). When the valve ring is excised and opened, the involved scallops have a creamy soft appearance and are "hooded" over the free edge (Figure 43–2*C*).

The pathologic process may be limited to the posterior leaflet or isolated scallops (Ranganathan et al., 1973).

Advancing severity is characterized by involvement of the rough zone extending toward the base of the valve (Silver, 1976).

Carpentier and associates (1976), comparing rheumatic and nonrheumatic mitral insufficiency, were able to show distinct differences in mitral valve morphology. Both groups had significantly dilated annuli. The rheumatic group did not have increased leaflet height, and the chordae tendineae tended to be shortened. The nonrheumatic group had increased height of both the anterior and posterior leaflets, as well as significant elongation of the chordae. Rupture of the chordae is noted with regularity in pathologic specimens and most frequently involves the branches to the posterior leaflet (Ranganathan et al., 1973; Carpentier et al., 1976). The incidence of this complication in the pediatric age group is unknown. However, the rare occurrence of acute mitral regurgitation in childhood implies that spontaneous rupture is extremely infrequent.

The consistent microscopic findings are the myxomatous (mucinous) changes in the involved leaflet. This process is characterized by replacement of the collagen fibers of the fibrosa and spongiosa by loosely organized relatively acellular material. Marshall and Shappell (1974) reported detailed histochemical studies indicating the ground substance to be a protein acid-monopolysaccharide complex. These findings are not specific for the isolated form of mitral valve involvement. They are indistinguishable from those seen in Marfan's syndrome (Roberts et al., 1973). Since focal myxomatous changes can be seen associated with a variety of other conditions, Silver (1976) believes that diffuse involvement of the central plate must be demonstrated to support the diagnosis of prolapse.

Symptoms

The great majority of patients are asymptomatic and are referred for cardiac evaluation because of unusual physical findings detected during routine physical examination, frequently school-related. In rare instances, alarmed parents request urgent examination because of loud noises, beeps, or honks coming from the child's chest, which were heard by themselves in a quiet room, a distance from the patient—an occurrence first reported by Osler in 1879–1880. In our series, symptoms occurred in more than 10 percent of the group.

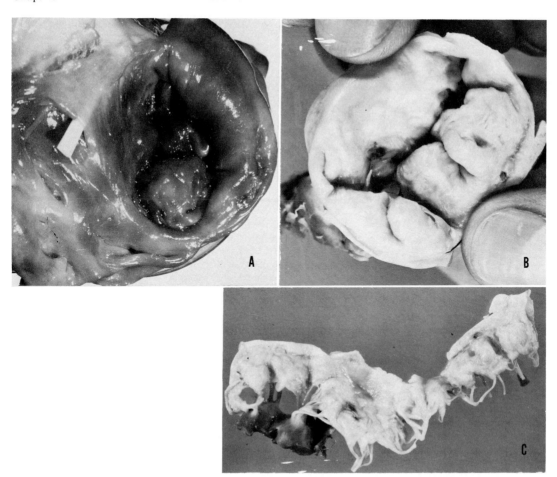

Figure 43-2. *A.* Mitral valve, viewed from the left atrial aspect, taken from a seven-week-old infant dying of uncontrolled massive mitral regurgitation. *B.* Excised valve ring from a 21-year-old female who died suddenly (ECG, Figure 43-5*A* and *B*) showing redundancy accentuated by the triscalloped structure of the posterior leaflet. The anterior leaflet is also involved. *C.* Opened valve ring demonstrating the thickened and "hooded" appearance of the individual scallops.

Nervousness, emotional instability, and tachycardia have been erroneously attributed to hyperthyroidism. Chronic fatigue, "shortness of breath," and palpitations were complaints in patients without any evidence of cardiac failure. Hypochondriac and hysterical manifestations were features of psychoneuroses leading to suicidal efforts in two girls. It appears probable, as intimated by Wooley (1976), that the clinical entities known in the past as neurocirculatory asthenia, soldier's heart, and DaCosta's syndrome represent cases of mitral valve prolapse.

Shortness of breath accompanied by cardiomegaly was a manifestation of congestive failure and invariably related to significant mitral regurgitation.

The acute development of cardiac failure suggests rupture of chordae tendineae. We have had none in our group and postulate that spontaneous rupture is age-related, occurring in adult life. Such an occurrence in childhood would suggest an infectious process and demands careful investigation for bacterial endocarditis.

Transient neurologic manifestations of cerebral embolization occurred once in a girl free of bacterial endocarditis.

Palpitations may be manifestations of arrhythmias (atrial or ventricular), but have also been documented to occur without any electrocardiographic changes. Syncopes and near syncopes occur with ventricular fibrillation (Wigle, 1976), although they were reported even without it (Winkle et al., 1975b).

Chest pains of the anginal type have been reported (Wigle, 1976). We have recognized no such case in our rather young population. On the other hand, in five girls, severe atypical chest pains occurred at rest, had no anginal transmission, and were prolonged and unrelenting. In one instance, such pains were disabling, persisted over a period of weeks, and were accompanied by electrocardiographic changes (flat-biphasic T waves), as well as a loud apical honk. Pain-free periods of 6 to 12 months separated recurrences and were free of both electrocardiographic changes and auscultatory findings. The pains were nonresponsive to coronary vasodilators, corticosteroids, or beta-blockade and required opiates for control. Sharp, stabbing precordial pains, often pleuritic in character, represent a rather common complaint of adolescence with or without associated prolapse. These symptoms therefore may not be causally related.

Auscultation

When *associated with other congenital heart disease*, the auscultatory findings of mitral valve prolapse are, in general, masked. Only rarely will the recognizable manifestations of the abnormal mitral valve surface. Atrial septal defect of the ostium secundum type offers a good and common example. An apical systolic click or a murmur of mitral regurgitation (late systolic of pansystolic) may become apparent only after surgical correction. On the other hand, in a rare case of the secundum-type defect, manifestations of mitral regurgitation may lead to the erroneous diagnosis of ostium primum defect, particularly when left-axis deviation by electrocardiogram is also present. Under these circumstances, the mitral

anomaly is detected by left ventricular angiocardiography or by echocardiography.

In the *uncomplicated prolapse*, the findings are preeminently variable within the same patient. The murmurs and clicks may differ from one examination to the next, in regard to their presence, their timing, or their combination. Patients with classic findings (apical midsystolic click followed by a late systolic murmur or honk) may go through short or prolonged silent periods. This intermittency, for which there is no ready explanation, is highly characteristic. Often the diagnostic findings will be absent when the patient is examined resting in the supine position, but will be uncovered with manipulations such as auscultation in held expiration, in left lateral supine, sitting and standing (Figure 43–3).

Variability also occurs in terms of natural history. A patient who starts with an isolated midsystolic click may be found to have a click and a late systolic murmur at a later date, and pansystolic murmur still later.

Further variations exist in relation to the degree of valvular deformity. With minor forms of prolapse there is a high incidence of atypical findings—namely, midsystolic murmurs of vibratory quality, resembling functional murmurs. Their suspicious nature is underscored by an apical location and by a frequent

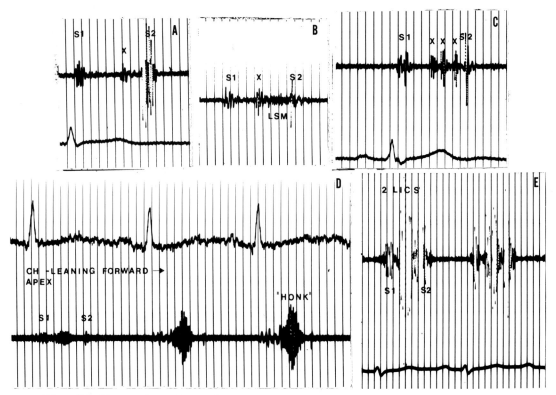

Figure 43-3. Phonocardiographic records. *A.* Isolated late systolic click (*X*). *B.* Midsystolic click and late systolic murmur (*LSM*). *C.* Multiple clicks in mid- to late systole. *D.* The evolution of a systolic honk as the patient leans forward in held expiration. *E.* Multiple clicks interrupting a long systolic murmur recorded at the base. Eight hours later, this or any other murmur was absent.

association with apical clicks. Angiographically, there is no mitral regurgitation; hence these murmurs are attributed to anomalies of the chordae tendineae.

The findings in 145 *uncomplicated*, angiocardiographically proven cases are tabulated in Table 43–2. An attempt was made to correlate physical findings with the degree of prolapse. The apical murmurs produced by mitral regurgitation are more frequent (78 percent) in the group with severe prolapse than in the group with slight prolapse (34 percent). However, the minor type of deformity does not preclude the occurrence of all classic findings.

In general, the auscultatory findings are located over the cardiac apex. Infrequently (10 percent in our series), the classic late systolic murmur, midsystolic click, or the late multiple systolic clicks are heard over the pulmonic area and not over the apex (Figure 43–3E).

It is postulated that the basal location of the auscultatory findings occurs when the mitral deformity of the anterolateral commissural region is dominant, and the clicks and murmurs are transmitted into an enlarged left atrial appendage.

The *systolic click* is usually single, is best heard over the cardiac apex, occurs during the middle third of the systole, and precedes a late systolic murmur. It marks the onset of prolapse and is attributed to sudden tensing of the chordae tendineae ("chordal snap," Read, 1961) or to the sudden billowing of the prolapsed valve ("sail sound," Criley, 1966). Clicks may be multiple, occurring in grating showers mimicking a friction rub (Figure 43–3C). An isolated click may become multiple with held expiration, in the left lateral supine position, or when sitting. It may disappear with inspiration. Clicks may occur in early systole or migrate toward the first sound with sitting, standing, head-up tilt position, the strain phase of the Valsalva maneuver, tachycardia, or administration or vasodilators (amyl nitrite) (Figure 43–4). With these maneuvers the valve prolapse occurs earlier in systole. This phenomenon was felt to be related to reduced left ventricular end-diastolic volume (Fontana et al., 1970). Mathey and associates (1976) have shown that the click occurs, in any individual patient, at a constant ventricular volume, and that migration

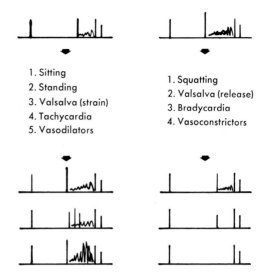

1. Sitting
2. Standing
3. Valsalva (strain)
4. Tachycardia
5. Vasodilators

1. Squatting
2. Valsalva (release)
3. Bradycardia
4. Vasoconstrictors

Figure 43-4. Effect of bedside maneuvers on clicks and murmurs of mitral valve prolapse.

of the click in systole is dependent on the combination of end-diastolic volume and the contractile state of the ventricle.

Squatting, vasoconstrictors, and bradycardia have the opposite effect. The click is delayed, diminished, or abolished. The murmur becomes shorter and fainter, and honks disappear. Pregnancy, known to expand the total blood volume, tends to diminish or abolish the auscultatory features. They return in the postpartum period (Haas, 1976). Differentiation of these clicks from the ejection clicks occurring in semilunar valve stenosis or with aneurysms of the membranous septum is established by producing migration with appropriate posturing or drugs (Mathey et al., 1976). The multiple clicks result from asynchronous tautening of individual chords or asynchronous prolapse of individual scallops (Wigle et al., 1975).

The late systolic murmur is typically initiated by a click, best heard over the apex, and of a crescendo or crescendo-decrescendo type. It may become audible only when provoked by held expiration, or posturing

Table 42–2. AUSCULTATORY FINDINGS AMONG UNCOMPLICATED CASES, $N = 145$

	SEVERE (95)	SLIGHT (50)
Apical murmurs:		
Late systolic	55 (26 clicks, 17 honks)	9 (3 clicks)
Pansystolic	19 (4 clicks)	8
Ejection systolic	8 (1 click)	12 (7 clicks)
Isolated mitral click	4	4
Other murmurs	9	17
Pulmonic (late, PAN, EJ)	9	10 (4 clicks)
Aortic, ejection	—	1 (click)
LLSB, ejection	—	6 (3 clicks)
Early diast. murmur	3 (AR)	3 (no AR)

in left lateral supine, sitting, or standing. The same maneuvers may increase its intensity or produce a "honk" or "whoop." On occasion, these may be so loud that they are heard by the child's parents across a quiet room, or by the patients, themselves. These "beeping hearts" are a source of parental alarm and may be the sole reason for referral to cardiologists.

The same maneuvers will make the already audible murmur longer and may change its acoustic quality into a grating, scratchy noise by superimposition of multiple clicks. Infrequently, a late systolic murmur becomes pansystolic.

Pansystolic murmurs occur less frequently (18 percent). The systolic click is commonly absent or obscured. It signifies a higher degree of regurgitation and may in time substitute a late systolic murmur. Under these circumstances, the click may be obscured or occur very early in systole, rendering it inaudible. The diagnosis of prolapse can be established only by echocardiography or left ventricular angiography.

Systolic ejection murmurs are atypical for the disease, but occur in some 18 percent of the patients. Commonly, they have the vibratory quality of Still's murmur and may be so classified. They may be recognized as suspicious for mitral valve deformities when they are heard over the cardiac apex (as occurred in 14 percent of the total group), and diagnostic when preceded or interrupted by clicks. It is postulated that, unlike the late systolic murmurs, they are not produced by mitral regurgitation; rather, that they are of chordal origin and produced by tautening of abnormal chordae tendineae.

Early diastolic murmurs are infrequent. They may be long and decrescendo when produced by aortic regurgitation in patients with Marfan's syndrome. Early diastolic scratches, on the other hand, are not related to aortic valve disease. They are similar to the diastolic scratch occurring in Ebstein's deformity of the tricuspid valve and may be attributed to sudden relaxation of abnormal chordae tendineae.

Radiologic Examination

The cardiac size and contour are normal, except in the patients with significant mitral regurgitation. In these, the left atrium may also be enlarged. It is not unusual, roentgenologically as well as angiographically, for the left atrial appendage to appear dilated. In the rare patient with progression of the mitral regurgitation, serial chest x-rays may demonstrate progressive cardiomegaly.

Calcification of the mitral valve was reported by Hancock and Cohn (1966), Goodman and Dorney (1969), Kittredge and associates (1970), and Jeresaty (1974).

When mitral valve prolapse is complicated by other congenital cardiac anomalies (e.g., atrial septal defect, Ebstein's anomaly), the roentgenologic features of these disorders will be dominant.

The frequent association with thoracic skeletal anomalies was noticed many years ago. The occurrence was documented by de Leon and Ronan (1971), Bon Tempo and coworkers (1975), and Salomon and colleagues (1975). Up to 75 percent of patients will be found to have some thoracic bony deformity. Pectus excavatum, an abnormally narrow anteroposterior diameter of the chest (straight back syndrome), and scoliosis are found in 62, 17, and 8 percent of cases, respectively. They occur in equal frequency in males and females and are frequently found in other members of their families. As pointed out by Salomon and associates (1975), the presence of these thoracic abnormalities on chest x-rays justifies a deliberate search for mitral valve prolapse. The "pseudoheart disease" traditionally associated with pectus excavatum and other deformities is likely to represent bona fide mitral valve prolapse.

Electrocardiography

The electrocardiographic disturbances reported to occur in association with prolapse of the mitral valve fall into three general categories: disorders of repolarization, disorders of conduction, and arrhythmias. The frequency of these findings is indicated by Barlow and Pocock (1975), who found abnormal electrocardiographic patterns in 53 percent of their cases. Unquestionably, the most common electrocardiographic abnormality observed consists of partial or complete reversal of T wave polarity in the inferior limb leads (II, III, AVF) (Jeresaty, 1974; Barlow and Pocock, 1975). These changes are less frequently seen in the lateral precordial leads as well (Figure 43–5A). Such repolarization disturbances are variable in degree (Figure 43–5B) and may resolve entirely. Accentuation of the T wave changes has been noted to occur spontaneously and may be precipitated by effort (Barlow and Pocock, 1975) with inhalation of amyl nitrite (Jeresaty, 1974) and on the simple assumption of the erect posture (Rizzon et al., 1973). Although the T wave pattern suggesting anterior myocardial ischemia has been reported, these changes are confined to the anterior precordial leads and are usually seen in combination with the inferior lead pattern. We have not seen a patient with isolated prolapse who had electrocardiographic evidence for anterolateral infarction, thus obviating confusion with the mitral regurgitation associated with anomalous origin of the left coronary artery. Alterations in the S-T segment are usually absent or show mild depression in the inferior limb leads (Figure 43–6A). Such changes may be induced by exercise (Sloman et al., 1972; Lobstein et al., 1973). Figure 43–6B was recorded from a seven-week-old infant with massive mitral regurgitation who subsequently died (see Figure 43–2A). The S-T segment elevation in II, III, and AVF probably represents true ischemic changes of the inferior subendocardium.

The electrophysiologic basis for these observations remains obscure. Abnormal tension on the papillary

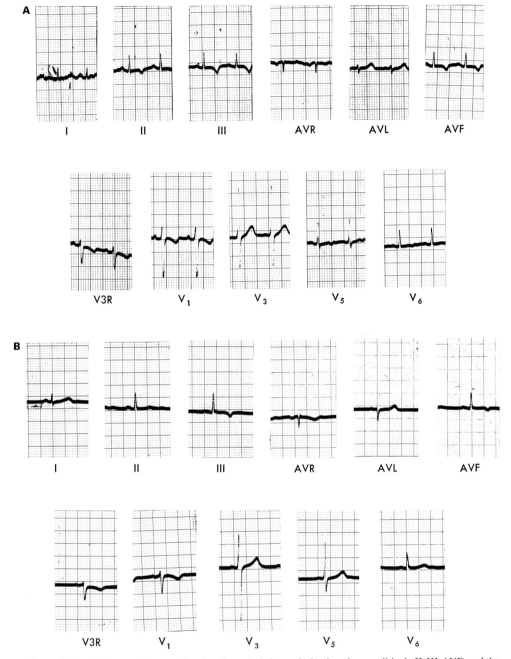

Figure 43-5. *A*. Electrocardiogram showing characteristic repolarization abnormalities in II, III, AVF, and the left precordial leads. *B*. A record from the same patient two years later shows resolution of abnormal T wave polarity in V_5 and V_6 (same case as in Figure 43-2*B* and *C*).

muscles creating local ischemia has been proposed by several authors (Lobstein et al., 1973; Cobbs, 1974; Jeresaty, 1974). Consideration must also be given to the possibility that tension may alter the myocardial membrane characteristics that become manifest as abnormalities or repolarization (Garello and Ribaldone, 1972, as quoted by Rizzon et al., 1973).

A review of the electrocardiographic features of 73

documented uncomplicated childhood cases is outlined in Table 43–3. Forty-nine percent had normal studies. Nearly half of those with abnormal ECGs (21 percent of the group, overall) showed the characteristic T wave aberrations described. The remaining 30 percent demonstrated a spectrum of electrophysiologic disturbances, including arrhythmias; conduction abnormalities, and selective

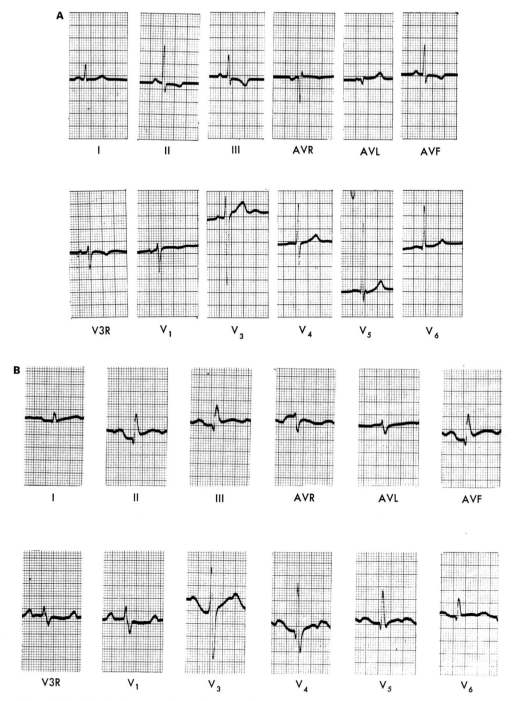

Figure 43-6. *A.* Resting electrocardiogram demonstrating S-T segment depression in the inferior limb leads (II, III, and AVF). *B.* Electrocardiographic record of a seven-week-old infant who died with uncontrollable massive mitral regurgitation (see Figure 43-2*A*). The S-T segment elevation in II, III, and AVF represents true ischemic changes.

chamber enlargement. Our experience with arrhythmias among these patients is limited. Two patients had recurrent supraventricular tachycardia, and two experienced ventricular tachycardia. Four patients consistently demonstrated premature ventri-

cular contractions, either occasional or persistent, and multifocal. When absent on the resting ECG, ectopic beats may be uncovered by exercise (Figure 43–7*A*, *B* and *C*). This incidence seems low in relation to that reported in adults (Jeresaty, 1974) and would most certainly be augmented by systematic ambulatory monitoring (Winkle et al., 1975b) (Figure 43–7D). Conduction disturbances were detected in about 10 percent. The frequency of first-degree AV block (3 percent) is consistent with that reported by others (Barlow and Pocock, 1975). Left-axis deviation occurred in four patients, and complete right bundle branch block was seen in one. One patient presented with 2:1 AV block and was observed to progress to complete heart block, which required pacemaker therapy. There was no instance of left bundle branch block, nor was there any evidence for associated accessory pathway conduction.

Ten patients were found to have patterns of right ventricular diastolic overload. That this finding may be a feature of individuals in the absence of atrial septal defect or Ebstein's anomaly is disconcerting, and cardiac catheterization may be required to exclude with certainty an associated anomaly. Evidence for left atrial hypertrophy was found in six patients. This observation would be expected in patients with significant mitral regurgitation; however, three of these were shown to have competent valves by angiography. Finally, left ventricular

Table 43–3. ELECTROCARDIOGRAPHIC ANALYSIS OF ANGIOGRAPHICALLY DOCUMENTED ISOLATED CASES, $N = 75$

Normal	37 (49%)
Repolarization disturbance	
Inferior ST-T wave changes	16 (21%)
Arrhythmias	
Ventricular tachycardia	2
Supraventricular tachycardia	2
Premature ventricular contractions	4
Conduction disturbances	
First-degree AV block	2
Complete heart block	1
CRBBB	1
Left-axis deviation	4
Selective chamber hypertrophy	
RVH	10
LAH	6
LVH	5

hypertrophy was noted in five patients. This finding could be justified hemodynamically in four instances. It can be appreciated that voltage criteria for left ventricular hypertrophy may coexist with the inferior T wave changes and produce a pattern of left

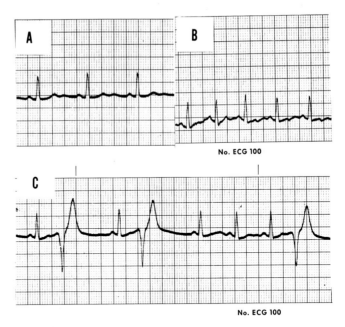

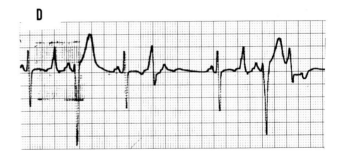

Figure 43-7. Samples of rhythm electrocardiograms taken before exercise, immediately after exercise, and later in recovery. The resting record shows normal sinus rhythm (*A*). No arrhythmia was induced by exercise (*B*). However, during recovery, multiple unifocal premature ventricular contractions emerged (*C*). *D*. A sample from a 24-hour ambulatory ECG showing multifocal and coupled ectopic beats.

ventricular "strain." Thus the severity of the hemodynamic status of the patient may be misjudged, and careful physiologic studies are indicated.

Echocardiography

Echocardiography plays an important role in the diagnosis of the syndrome, since it can frequently confirm the clinical impression. The common technique of single-beam scanning has limitations, however, since it may fail to demonstrate the abnormal systolic motion of the mitral valve leaflets. Popp (1976) estimates the incidence of negative echocardiograms to be 10 percent and points out that this will occur when the pathologic process is localized to single scallops. However, when used as a screening tool, echocardiography is capable of detecting the abnormal mitral valve motion when the auscultatory findings are absent—the so-called "silent prolapse" (DeMaria et al., 1974; Popp and Brown, 1974). In our institution, diagnostic confirmation by echocardiography was obtained in only 75 percent of cases proven to have mitral valve prolapse by left ventricular angiography. By using multiple-crystal scanning, Sahn and associates (1976, 1977) demonstrate that some pattern of prolapse is detectable in all patients. Until such time that real-time imaging by multibeam techniques becomes available, left ventricular angiography remains the absolute confirmatory method. There are no reports of documented prolapse by echocardiogram that could not be confirmed by adequate left ventricular angiography.

The echocardiographic patterns of mitral valve prolapse have been described by Shah and Gramiak (1970), Dillon and colleagues (1971), Kerber and associates (1971), and DeMaria and coworkers (1974). The two characteristic patterns (Figure 43–8) consist of:

1. Midsystolic posterior motion of the valve leaflets, with a discrete late systolic dip toward the left atrial wall, as described by Shah and Gramiak (1970) and Dillon and coworkers (1971).
2. Pansystolic posterior bowing (or hammocking), as described by DeMaria and colleagues (1974), consisting of gradual posterior motion during systole. This pattern occurs more frequently than the preceding.

Transition from one pattern to the other may occur. Multiple layering of the mitral valve during systole is frequent but not diagnostic and may represent technical artifacts.

Sahn and associates (1976) pointed out a high incidence of aortic root dilatation (85 percent of cases).

Angiography

At present, left ventricular angiography is the single definite diagnostic method for prolapse mitral

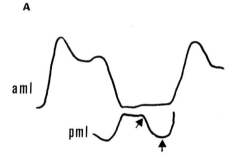

A

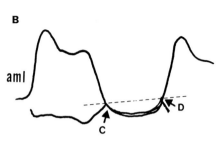

B

Figure 43-8. Schematic representation of the diagnostic echocardiographic patterns of mitral valve prolapse. *A.* The midsystolic posterior motion (arrows) of the posterior mitral leaflet (*pml*). *B.* The pansystolic prolapse of both anterior mitral leaflet (*aml*) and the posterior leaflet. Motion toward the left atrium begins at the point of mitral closure (*C* point) and extends through systole to the point of separation (*D* point). The *CD* line (dashed line) is used for reference.

valve, either isolated or in association with congenital heart disease. In a series of 180 left ventriculograms, two failed to document the prolapse for technical reasons. Conversely, overdiagnosis by misinterpretation of a persistent bulge of the inferior left ventricular wall adjacent to the mitral annulus in the right anterior oblique view or of an aneurysm of the membranous septum in the left anterior oblique projection must be guarded against.

The angiographic morphologic correlations have been investigated by Ranganathan and associates (1973). These studies were based on a detailed analysis of the normal mitral anatomy (Ranganathan et al., 1970). While different interpretations of similar data may be justified (Jeresaty et al., 1974), the right anterior oblique projection is traditionally considered the best analysis of the posterior leaflet (Figure 43–9*A*). In our view, the anteroposterior projection displays the anomaly in a more striking manner and best outlines the anterolateral commissural region (Figure 43–9*B*). Assessment of the degree of involvement of the anterior leaflet may be difficult in any view; however, the direct lateral view may prove to be superior (Figure 43–9*D*). It is our general plan that when possible angiograms in all four views

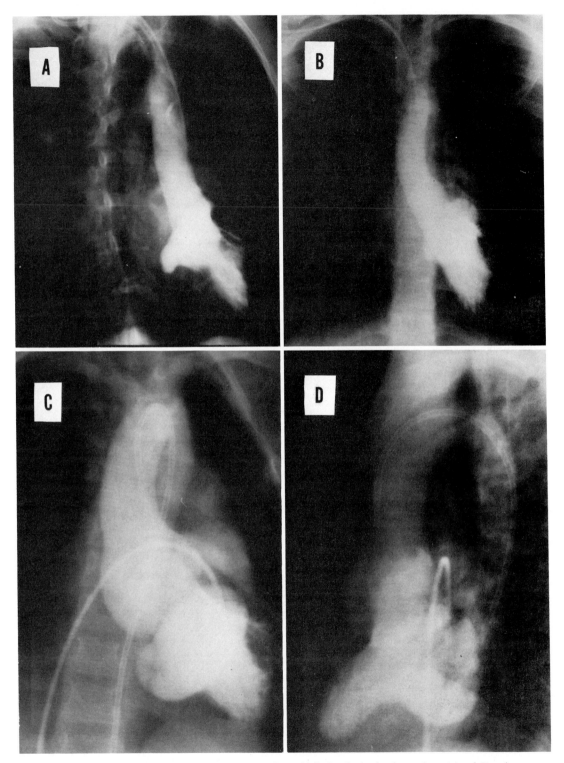

Figure 43-9. Left ventricular angiograms from a patient with isolated mitral valve prolapse (*A* and *B*) and a patient with Marfan's syndrome (*C* and *D*). *A.* Right anterior oblique projection showing the superior and inferior bulges at the poles of the mitral ring. The apparent midventricular contraction ring is actually the heads of the two papillary muscles. *B.* The anteroposterior projection is seen to allow the anterolateral commissural region to clear the aortic root, resulting in better definition. *C.* The anteroposterior projection showing massive mitral prolapse. The aortic valve is dilated. *D.* A direct lateral view of the same patient: "ballerina-foot" type of ventricular contraction pattern in addition to the mitral and aortic valve defects.

are obtained. In addition to the mitral valve, these provide the most complete information on the left ventricular morphology and function as well as the aortic root (Figure 43–9C and D). Each of these aspects has important bearing on the overall clinical behavior of the patient.

The frequent association of prolapsing mitral valve with secundum atrial septal defect warrants routine left ventricular angiography. Although the mitral deformity may not play a significant role in the hemodynamics, it has bearing on the long-term management (development of arrhythmia, need for infective endocarditis prophylaxis, frequency of follow-up visits) and may explain unexpected physical findings after surgical correction. Further, should significant mitral regurgitation be present, this may not be apparent by physiologic studies. Thus, left ventricular angiography should allow detection of the patient in whom mitral valve repair is indicated at the time of atrial septal defect closure.

Tricuspid valve prolapse has been shown as an associated defect (Gooch et al., 1972; Scarpandonis et al., 1973). The incidence in childhood is unknown. Right ventriculography is indicated for systematic review to determine the frequency of this association, as well as for diagnostic completeness.

Diagnosis

The presence of mitral valve prolapse may be suspected clinically in patients, particularly girls, who are tall, slender, have skeletal thoracic deformities, and who complain of palpitations, unjustified fatigue, or chest pains. With a family history, the index of suspicion is further increased.

The diagnosis is principally auscultatory. Care should be taken that examination is carried out in all body postures (recumbent, left lateral supine, sitting, standing), and with held expiration. The physician must be aware that abnormal physical findings may be entirely absent on any single examination.

Systolic clicks should be differentiated from the ejection click of semilunar valve stenosis, bicuspid aortic valve, and membranous septum aneurysm with small ventricular septal defect (see Auscultation). Midsystolic sounds may also occur with pericarditis, atrial myxoma, subvalvular ventricular aneurysms, and restrictive cardiomyopathy (Fontana et al., 1975). Late systolic honks have been heard with ventricular aneurysms. Blowing late systolic murmurs over the cardiac apex occur with coarctation of aorta. Their extension over the lateral chest (left and right) and over the back indicates the nature of the anomaly. Differentiation from Ebstein's anomaly becomes a problem in cases showing electro-cardiographic evidence of right bundle branch block or right ventricular overloading, loud systolic clicks, and early diastolic squeaks.

When patients present with an arrhythmia as the primary complaint, the search for a possible organic substrate should include the mitral valve prolapse, as well as myocardiopathies, idiopathic hypertrophic subaortic stenosis, Ebstein's anomaly of the tricuspid valve, myocardial tumors, catecholamine-producing tumors, or metabolic disturbances such as hypokalemia. With palpitations and tachycardia, hyperthyroidism needs to be excluded.

In presence of physical findings of mitral regurgitation (pansystolic murmur and no clicks) without a history of rheumatic fever, cardiac catheterization is required, inasmuch as mitral valve prolapse or other types of congenital regurgitation need to be differentiated.

Anginal or atypical anginal chest pains may require selective angiocardiographic studies, although the probability of detecting coronary anomalies in young patients is minimal.

Unlike adults, children are rarely referred for evaluation on the basis of an abnormal electrocardiogram in the absence of arrhythmia.

Prognosis

The natural history of the disease is not yet precisely established. Information regarding incidence, pathophysiology, diagnostic methods, and morbidity is still accumulating at a rapid pace. Long-term follow-up data are scarce (Allan et al., 1974; Appelblatt et al., 1975; Mills et al., 1977), limited to a small number of patients, and still confused by patient selection and classifications. Allan's study, for example, does not include the cases with manifestations of myocardiopathy or arrhythmias, who indeed represent the highest risk subgroups.

Estimates of mortality, incidence of sudden death, bacterial endocarditis, severe or progressive mitral regurgitation, rupture of chordae tendineae, or other morbid conditions are therefore at best provisional.

Undoubtedly the majority of patients are and remain symptom-free and have a good prognosis. Those without mitral regurgitation tend to preserve a good valvular function. Those with slight mitral regurgitation infrequently develop progression. Spontaneous rupture of chordae tendineae in childhood has not been reported, although it has occurred in association with infective endocarditis.

Bacterial Endocarditis. The theoretic possibility that bacterial endocarditis may complicate mitral valve prolapse was first raised by Barlow and associates (1963). Subsequent documentation was produced by Facquet and coworkers (1964), Read and Thal (1965), Linhart and Taylor (1966), LeBauer, Perloff and Harvey (1967), Shell and colleagues (1969), Cohn and associates (1972), Hill and colleagues (1973), Allan and coworkers (1974), and Lachman et al. (1975), and Mills et al. (1977).

LeBauer and colleagues (1967) demonstrated that this may occur even when the sole manifestation of the disorder is an isolated click. In our series, endocarditis

(*Staphylococcus aureus*) occurred in one case with click alone and excellent echocardiographic documentation. Our estimate is that the incidence of the infection should approximate 1 in 500 cases.

The association with ostium secundum atrial septal defect is most important in terms of infective complications, since the prolapsed mitral valve may be the site of such infections. In our view, the case reported by Danilowicz and coworkers (1971) represents such an example. The proof that uncomplicated secundum atrial defect carries any risk of bacterial endocarditis is still lacking. Prophylactic measures should, however, be taken when the two anomalies are combined.

The presence of endocarditis without apparent evidence of preexisting heart disease requires a systematic search for a prolapsed mitral valve (of the silent form), as well as for a bicuspid aortic valve.

Sudden Death. Sudden and unexpected deaths have been reported by Hancock and Cohn (1966), by Barlow and coworkers (1968), and by others (Shell et al., 1969; Trent et al., 1970; Jeresaty, 1973, Shappel et al., 1973; Gulotta et al., 1974), and appear to be more frequent as the awareness of this pathologic state has taken hold in both cardiology and pathology. In our 300-odd cases, we have had three such instances: a 21-year-old woman with intermittent slight ST-T abnormalities for the preceding 14 years, and single but early ventricular premature beats for four years; and a young man of the same age and with similar electrocardiographic findings, who was being treated with propranolol in an attempt to control the arrhythmia. In a 16-year-old girl, death was averted by six resuscitations for ventricular fibrillation, during the course of one night, and ventricular ectopy is being controlled with quinidine.

It is currently felt that these occurrences are produced by ventricular arrhythmias. It is yet uncertain if, in addition, repolarization defects (as manifested by ST-T wave changes) are required to produce ventricular fibrillation. It appears probable that the presence of ST-T abnormalities *in association* with ventricular premature beats has a predictive value. Hence an effort to detect arrhythmias at rest and with exertion in patients with repolarization defect is justified.

Cardiac Failure. Chronic uncontrolled *cardiac failure* occurred as the result of severe mitral regurgitation, the youngest patient being a baby who died at seven weeks of age. Acute and severe cardiac failure is a feature of ruptured chordae tendineae.

Cerebral Embolization. Cerebral embolization with transient neurologic manifestations and complete recovery was seen once in absence of bacterial endocarditis (Barnett et al., 1975). It is attributed to thrombosis not necessarily related to myocardiopathy. It could also occur with bacterial endocarditis as a result of septic embolization.

Table 43-4 lists complications that required some form of medical or surgical therapy in our group of 288 patients ranging in age from birth to 21 years. They were accumulated over an eight-year period. It

remains to be determined how many more will occur during a second decade of follow-up.

Table 43-4. MORTALITY AND SIGNIFICANT MORBIDITY, $N = 288$

Mitral regurgitation: severe (surgery)	3
progressive (no surgery)	3
Ventricular tachycardia or fibrillation	3
Ventricular ectopy (multifocal, exertional)	5
Supraventricular tachycardia	7
Cerebrovascular accident	1
Chest pain, disabling	5
Bacterial endocarditis	1
Complete heart block	1
Ruptured chordae tendineae	0
Deaths: cardiac failure, uncontrolled,	1
sudden, unexpected	3
	33 (11%)

Management

The asymptomatic patient needs no active treatment. Cardiac reevaluations at rare intervals are justified, in order to ascertain that no new and significant findings develop and that the electrocardiogram remains free of repolarization defects and of arrhythmias. The customary measures for prevention of bacterial endocarditis at appropriate times are indicated. In the case of secundum-type atrial septal defect, only the cases with proven absence of mitral valve prolapse may be absolved from prophylaxis.

Occasionally, mitral regurgitation (severe degree) will require treatment of cardiac failure and surgical therapy. The few patients surgically managed in our institution benefited from reconstructive procedures and required no replacement with prosthetic valves. In young patients, the abundance of mitral leaflet substance and the absence of ruptured chordae tendineae offer good opportunities for annuloplasty or suturing of pseudoclefts. The three patients so treated maintained a good result through the follow-up period (six to ten years). In patients with severe connective tissue disease (Marfan's syndrome), either surgical approach is fraught with uncertainties relating to dehiscence of sutures placed in tissues with myxomatous degeneration.

The presence of palpitations, syncopes, or chest pains requires electrocardiographic studies, including long-term monitoring, in order to clearly detect their possible presence and define the type of underlying arrhythmia. Occasional, benign, ventricular ectopic beats require no treatment. Ectopic activity of a significant nature, such as early premature ventricular beats (R on T type), bifocal or multifocal beats, repetitive firing (two to three premature ventricular contractions in succession), exercise-induced ectopy, or ventricular tachycardia, requires chemotherapy in an effort to suppress these potentially fatal disturbances, particularly in patients who also have repolarization abnormalities (ST-T wave depression or inversion).

Propranolol, quinidine, and procainamide, singly or in combination, have been used with varying degrees of success. Each of them may prove ineffective. Whether mitral valve replacement would provide a method of control of refractory ventricular arrhythmias in patients with syncopes, near-syncopes, or cardiac arrest remains to be established.

Supraventricular tachycardia tends to be responsive to quinidine or digitalis and is seldom a serious management problem.

The chest pains are not responsive to coronary dilators. Neither are they predictably responsive to beta-adrenergic blockade. Propranolol treatment needs, however, to be tried, and may be beneficial. Excision of the papillary muscles and replacement of the mitral valve for control of disabling chest pains has been considered but it is not recommended at the present. Justification for such a radical approach requires hitherto unavailable proof of effectiveness.

Emotional support of the symptomatic individual is most important and may occasionally be required in patients who have no objective findings.

REFERENCES

Abinader, E. G.: Adrenergic beta blockade and ECG changes in the systolic click murmur syndrome. *Am. Heart J.*, **91**:297, 1976.

Alday, L. E.; Moreyra, E.; and Vlad, P.: Click sistolico no eyectivo y soplo sistolico tardio. Revision. *Rev. Fac. Cienc. Med. Cardoba*, **29**:253, 1971.

Allan, H.; Harris, A.; and Leatham, A.: Significance and prognosis of an isolated late systolic murmur: A 9 to 22 year follow up. *Br. Heart J.*, **36**:525, 1974.

Appelblatt, N. H.; Willis, P. W.; Lenhart, J. A.; Shulman, J. I.; and Walton, J. A., Jr.: Ten to 40 year follow up of 69 patients with systolic click with or without late systolic murmur. *Am. J. Cardiol.*, **35**:119, 1975.

Barlow, J. B.; Pocock, W. A.; Marchand, P.; and Denny, M.: The significance of late systolic murmurs. *Am. Heart J.*, **66**:443, 1963.

Barlow, J. B.: Conjoint clinic on the clinical significance of late systolic murmurs and nonejection systolic clicks. *J. Chronic Dis.*, **18**:665, 1965.

Barlow, J. B., and Bosman, C. K.: Aneurysmal protrusion of the posterior leaflet of the mitral valve: An auscultatory-electrocardiographic syndrome. *Am. Heart J.*, **71**:166, 1966.

Barlow, J. B.; Bosman, C. K.; Pocock, W. A.; and Marchand, P.: Late systolic murmurs and non-ejection ("mid-late") systolic clicks. An analysis of 90 patients. *Br. Heart J.*, **30**:203, 1968.

Barlow, J. B., and Pocock, W. A.: The effort electrocardiogram in the billowing posterior mitral leaflet syndrome. *Circulation*, **40**:suppl. 3: 40, 1969.

Barlow, J. B., and Pocock, W. A.: The problem of non-ejection systolic clicks and associated mitral systolic murmurs: Emphasis on the billowing mitral leaflet syndrome. *Am. Heart J.*, **90**:636, 1975.

Barnett, H. J. M.; Jones, M. W.; and Boughner, D.: Cerebral ischemic events associated with prolapsing mitral valve. *Arch. Neurol.*, **32**:352, 1975.

Behar, V. S.; Whalen, R. E.; and McIntosh, H. D.: The ballooning mitral valve in patients with the "precordial honk" or "whoop." *Am. J. Cardiol.*, **20**:789, 1967.

Betriu, A.; Wigle, E. D.; Felderhof, C. H.; and McLoughlin, M. J.: Prolapse of the posterior leaflet of the mitral valve associated with secundum atrial septal defect. *Am. J. Cardiol.*, **35**:363, 1975.

Bittar, N., and Sosa, J. A.: The billowing mitral valve leaflet: Report on fourteen patients. *Circulation*, **38**:763, 1968.

Bon Tempo, C. P.; Ronan, J. A.; deLeon, A. C.; and Twigg, H. L.: Radiographic appearance of the thorax in systolic click-late systolic murmur syndrome. *Am. J. Cardiol.*, **36**:271, 1975.

Boughner, D. R.: Correlation of echocardiographic and angiographic abnormalities in mitral valve prolapse. *Ultrasound in Medicine*, **1**:55, 1975.

Bowden, D. H.; Favara, B. E.; and Donahoe, J. L.: Marfan's syndrome: accelerated course in childhood associated with lesions of mitral valve and pulmonary artery. *Am. Heart J.*, **69**:96, 1965.

Bowers, D.: An electrocardiographic pattern associated with mitral valve deformity in Marfan's syndrome. *Circulation*, **23**:30, 1961.

Bowers, D.: Pathogenesis of primary abnormalities of the mitral valve in Marfan's syndrome. *Br. Heart J.*, **31**:679, 1969.

Bowers, D.: Primary abnormalities of the mitral valve in Marfan's syndrome—electrocardiographic findings. *Br. Heart J.*, **31**:676, 1969.

Brown, O. R.; Kloster, F. E.; and DeMots, H.: Incidence of mitral valve prolapse in the asymptomatic normal. *Circulation*, **52**, suppl. 2:77, 1975.

Burch, G. E.; DePasquale, N. P.; and Phillips, J. H.: Clinical manifestations of papillary muscle dysfunction. *Arch. Intern. Med.*, **112**:112, 1963.

Burch, G. E.; DePasquale, N. P.; and Phillips, J. H.: The syndrome of papillary muscle dysfunction. *Am. Heart J.*, **75**:399, 1968.

Burgess, J.; Clark, R.; Kamigaki, M.; and Cohn, K.: Echocardiographic findings in different types of mitral regurgitation. *Circulation*, **48**:97, 1973.

Carpentier, A.; Guerinon, J.; DeLoche, A.; Fabiani, J.; and Rellaud, J.: Pathology of the mitral valve: Introduction to plastic and reconstructive surgery. In Kalmanson, D.: *The Mitral Valve*. Publishing Sciences Group, Inc., Publisher, Acton, Mass., 1976, p. 65.

Caves, P. K.; Sutton, G. C.; and Paneth, M.: Nonrheumatic subvalvar mitral regurgitation: Etiology and clinical aspects. *Circulation*, **47**:1242, 1973.

Chandramouli, B.; Alday, L. E.; Cornell, S. H.; Lambert, E. C.; and Vlad, P.: Myxomatous transformation of the mitral valve in children. *Circulation*, **39–40**. suppl 3:57, 1969.

Chandraratna, P. A. N.; Tolentino, A. O.; Mutucumarana, W.; and Lopez-Gomez, A.: Echocardiographic observations on the association between mitral valve prolapse and asymmetric septal hypertrophy. *Circulation*, **55**:622, 1977.

Cobbs, B. W., and King, S. B.: Mechanism of abnormal ventriculogram and ECG associated with prolapsed mitral valve. *Circulation*, **50**, suppl. 3:7, 1974.

Cohn, L. H.; Hultgren, H. N.; Angell, W. W.; Grehl, T. M.; and Kosek, J. C.: Prolapsing mitral valve with mucinous degeneration. *Calif. Med.*, **118**:43, 1972.

Criley, J. M.; Lewis, K. B.; Humphries, J. O.; and Ross, R. S.: Prolapse of the mitral valve: Clinical and cine-angiocardiographic findings. *Br. Heart J.*, **28**:482, 1966.

Crocker, D. W.: Marfan's syndrome confined to the mitral valve region: Two cases in siblings. *Am. Heart J.*, **76**:538, 1968.

Cuffer and Barbillon: Nouvelle recherches sur le bruit de galop. *Arch. Med. Gen. Trop.*, **1**:131–49, 301–20, 1887. Cited in Wigle et al., 1976.

Danilowicz, D. A.; Reed, S. E.; and Silver, W.: Ruptured mitral chordae after subacute bacterial endocarditis in a child with secundum atrial septal defect. *Johns Hopkins Med. J.*, **128**:45, 1971.

Davis, R. H.; Schuster, B.; Knoebel, S. B.; and Fisch, C.: Myxomatous degeneration of the mitral valve. *Am. J. Cardiol.*, **28**:449, 1971.

DeBush, R. F., and Harrison, D. C.: The clinical spectrum of papillary muscle disease. *N. Engl. J. Med.*, **281**:1458, 1969.

deLeon, A. C., and Ronan, J. A.: Thoracic bony abnormalities with the click and late systolic murmur syndrome. *Circulation*, **43**, suppl. 2:157, 1971.

DeMaria, A. N.; King, J. F.; Bogren, H. C.; Lies, J. E.; and Mason, D. T.: The variable spectrum of echocardiographic manifestations of the mitral valve prolapse syndrome. *Circulation*, **50**:33, 1974.

Devereux, R. B.; Perloff, J. K.; Reichek, N.; and Josephson, M. E.: Mitral valve prolapse. *Circulation*, **54**:3, 1976.

Dillon, J. C.; Haine, C. L.; Chang, S.; and Feigenbaum, H.: Use of echocardiography in patients with prolapsed mitral valve. *Circulation*, **43**:503, 1971.

Eckberg, D. L.; Gault, J. H.; Bouchard, R. L.; Karliner, J. S.; and

Ross, J.: Mechanics of left ventricular contraction in chronic severe mitral regurgitation. *Circulation,* 47:1252, 1973.

Edynak, G. M., and Rawson, A. J.: Ruptured aneurysm of the mitral valve in a Marfan-like syndrome. *Am. J. Cardiol.,* 11:674, 1963.

Ehlers, K. H.; Engle, M. A.; Levin, A. R.; Grossman, H.; and Fleming, R. J.: Left ventricular abnormality with late mitral insufficiency and abnormal electrocardiogram. *Am. J. Cardiol.,* 26:333, 1970.

Engle, M. A.: Editorial. The syndrome of apical systolic click, late systolic murmur, and abnormal T waves. *Circulation,* 39:1, 1969.

Epstein, E. J., and Coulshed, N.: Phonocardiogram and apex cardiogram in systolic click-late systolic murmur syndrome. *Br. Heart J.,* 35:260, 1973.

Facquet, J.; Alhomme, D.; and Raharison, S.: Sur la signification du souffle frequement associé au claquement télésystolique. *Acta Cardiol.,* 19:417, 1964.

Fisher, G. C.; Wessel, H. W.; and Sommers, H. W.: Mitral insufficiency following experimental papillary muscle infarction. *Am. Heart J.,* 83:382, 1972.

Fontana, M. E.; Pence, H. L.; Leighton, R. F.; and Wooley, C.: The varying clinical spectrum of the systolic click-late systolic murmur syndrome. A postural auscultatory phenomenon. *Circulation,* 41:807, 1970.

Fontana, M. E.; Kissel, G. L.; and Criley, J. M.: Function anatomy of mitral valve prolapse. In Leon, D. E., and Shaver, J. A. (eds.): *Physiologic Principles of Heart Sounds and Murmurs.* Monograph 46, American Heart Association, 1975, p. 126.

Frable, W. J.: Mucinous degeneration of the cardiac valves, the "floppy-valve" syndrome. *J. Thorac. Cardiovasc. Surg.,* 58:62, 1969.

Furbetta, D.; Bufalari, A.; Santucci, F.; and Solinas, P.: Abnormality of U wave and of the T-U segment of the electrocardiogram. The syndrome of the papillary muscle. *Circulation,* 14:1129, 1956.

Gentzler, R. D.; Gault, J. H.; Hunter, A. S.; and Liedtke, A. J.: Congenital absence of the left circumflex coronary artery in the systolic click syndrome. *Circulation,* 48, suppl. 4:65, 1973.

Gilbert, B. W.; Schatz, R. A.; Von Ramm, O. T.; Behar, V. S.; and Kisslo, J. A.: Mitral valve prolapse. Two-dimensional echocardiographic and angiographic correlation. *Circulation,* 54:716, 1976.

Giuliani, E. R.: Mitral valve incompetence due to flail anterior leaflet. A new physical sign. *Am. J. Cardiol.,* 20:784, 1967.

Gooch, A. S.; Vicencio, F.; Maranhao, V.; and Goldberg, H.: Arrhythmias and left ventricular asynergy in the prolapsing mitral leaflet syndrome. *Am. J. Cardiol.,* 29:611, 1972.

Gooch, A. S.; Maranhao, V.; Scampardonis, G.; Cha, S. D.; and Yang, S. S.: Prolapse of both mitral and tricuspid leaflets in systolic-murmur-click syndrome. *N. Engl. J. Med.,* 287:1218, 1972.

Goodman, H. B., and Dorney, E. R.: Marfan's syndrome with massive calcification of the mitral valve at age twenty-six. *Am. J. Cardiol.,* 24:426, 1969.

Gramiak, R., and Shah, P. M.: Cardiac ultrasonography. A review of current applications. *Radiol. Clin. North Am.,* 9:469, 1971.

Griffith, G. C.; Zinn, W. J.; and Stefanik, G.: The cardiovascular manifestations of Marfan's syndrome. *Cardiol. Digest,* 5:7, 1970.

Griffith, J. P. C.: Mid-systolic and late-systolic mitral murmurs. *Am. J. Med. Sci.,* 104:285, 1892.

Grossman, H.; Fleming, R. J.; Engle, M. A.; Levin, A. H.; and Ehlers, K. H.: Angiocardiography in the apical systolic click syndrome. Left ventricular abnormality, mitral insufficiency, late systolic murmur. *Radiology,* 91:898, 1968.

Gulotta, S. J.; Gulco, L.; Padmanabhan, V.; and Miller, S.: The syndrome of systolic click, murmur and mitral valve prolapse—a cardiomyopathy? *Circulation,* 49:717, 1974.

Haas, J. H.: The effect of pregnancy on the midsystolic click and murmur of the prolapsing posterior leaflet of the mitral valve. *Am. Heart J.,* 92:407, 1976.

Hall, J. N.: Late systolic mitral murmurs. *Am. J. Med. Sci.,* 125:663, 1903.

Hancock, E. W., and Cohn, K.: The syndrome associated with midsystolic click and late systolic murmur. *Am. J. Med.,* 41:183, 1966.

Hill, D. G.; Davies, M. J.; and Braimbridge, M. V.: The natural history and surgical management of the redundant cusp syndrome

(floppy mitral valve). *J. Thorac. Cardiovasc. Surg.,* 67:519, 1973.

Hunt, D., and Sloman, G.: Prolapse of posterior leaflet of mitral valve occurring in 11 family members. *Am. Heart J.,* 78:149, 1969.

Hutter, A. M.; Dinsmore, R. E.; Willerson, J. T.; and DeSanctis, R. W.: Early systolic clicks due to mitral valve prolapse. *Circulation,* 44:516, 1971.

Jamshidi, A., and Klein-Robbenhaar, J.: Myxomatous transformation of the aortic and mitral valve with subaortic "sail-like" membrane. *Am. J. Med.,* 49:114, 1970.

Jeresaty, R. M.: Mitral valve prolapse-click syndrome. *Prog. Cardiovasc. Dis.,* 15:623, 1973.

Jeresaty, R. M.: Ballooning of the mitral valve leaflet. *Radiology,* 100:45, 1971.

Jeresaty, R. M.: Etiology of the mitral valve prolapse-click syndrome. *Am. J. Cardiol.,* 36:110, 1975.

Jeresaty, R. M.: Mitral valve prolapse-click syndrome. In Sonnenblick, E. H., and Lesch, M. (eds.): *Valvular Heart Disease.* Grune & Stratton, Inc., New York, 1974, p. 203.

Jeresaty, R. M.: Sudden death in the mitral valve prolapse-click syndrome. *Am. J. Cardiol.,* 37:317, 1976.

Keck, E. W.; Henschel, W. G.; and Gruhl, L.: Mitral valve prolapse in children with secundum type atrial septal defect (ASDII). *Eur. J. Pediatr.,* 121:89, 1976.

Kerber, R. E.; Isaeff, D. M.; and Hancock, E. W.: Echocardiographic patterns in patients with the syndrome of systolic click and late systolic murmur. *N. Engl. J. Med.,* 284:691, 1971.

Kern, W. H., and Tucker, B. L.: Myxoid changes in cardiac valves: Pathologic, clinical and ultrastructural studies. *Am. Heart J.,* 84:294, 1972.

Kesteloot, H., and VanHoute, O.: On the origin of the telesystolic murmur preceded by a click. *Acta Cardiol.,* 20:197, 1965.

Khullar, S. C., and Leighton, R. F.: Mitral valve prolapse syndrome (MVPS). Left ventricular function and myocardial metabolism. *Am. J. Cardiol.,* 35:149, 1975.

Kittredge, R. D.; Shimomura, S.; Cameron, A.; et al.: Prolapsing mitral valve leaflets. Cineangiographic demonstration. *Am. J. Roentgenol.,* 109:84, 1970.

Kremrau, E. L.; Gilbertson, P. R.; and Bristow, J. D.: Acquired, nonrheumatic mitral regurgitation: clinical management with emphasis on evaluation of myocardial performance. *Prog. Cardiovasc. Dis.,* 15:403, 1973.

Lachman, A. S.; Bramwell-Jones, D. M.; Lakier, J. B.; Pocock, M. A.; and Barlow, J. B.: Infective endocarditis in the billowing mitral valve leaflet syndrome. *Br. Heart J.,* 37:326, 1975.

Lane, F. J.; Carroll, J. M.; Levine, D. H.; and Gorlin, R.: The apexcardiogram in myocardial asynergy. *Circulation,* 37:890, 1968.

Leachman, R. D.; Francheschi, A. D.; and Zamalloa, O.: Late systolic murmurs and clicks associated with abnormal mitral valve ring. *Am. J. Cardiol.,* 23:679, 1969.

LeBauer, E. J.; Perloff, J. K.; and Keliher, J.: The isolated systolic click with bacterial endocarditis. *Am. Heart J.,* 73:534, 1967.

Leighton, R. F.; Page, W. L.; Goodwin, R. S.; Molnar, W.; Wooley, C. F.; and Ryan, J. M.: Mild mitral regurgitation. Its characterization by intracardiac phonocardiography and pharmacologic responses. *Am. J. Med.,* 41:168, 1966.

Leon, D. F.; Leonard, J. J.; Kroetz, F. W.; Page, W. L.; Shaver, J. A.; and Lancaster, J. F.: Late systolic murmurs, clicks and whoops arising from the mitral valve. A transseptal intracardiac phonocardiographic analysis. *Am. Heart J.,* 72:325, 1966.

Lewis, H. P.: Midsystolic clicks and coronary heart disease. *Circulation,* 44:493, 1971.

Liedke, A. J.; Gault, J. H.; Lehman, D. M.; and Blumental, M. S.: Geometry of the left ventricular contraction in the systolic click syndrome: Characterization of a segmental myocardial abnormality. *Circulation,* 47:27, 1973.

Linhart, J. W., and Taylor, W. J.: The late apical systolic murmur. Clinical, hemodynamic and angiographic observations. *Am. J. Cardiol.,* 18:164, 1966.

Lobstein, H. P.; Horwitz, L. D.; Curry, G. C.; and Mullins, C. B.: Electrocardiographic abnormalities and coronary arteriograms in the mitral click-murmur syndrome. *N. Engl. J. Med.,* 289:127, 1973.

Markiewicz, W.; Stoner, J.; London, E.; Hunt, S. A.; and Popp, R. L.: Mitral valve prolapse in one hundred presumably healthy females. *Circulation,* 52:suppl. 2:77, 1975.

Marshall, D. E., and Shappell, S. D.: Sudden death and the

ballooning posterior leaflet syndrome. *Arch. Pathol.*, **98**:134, 1974.

Mathey, D. G.; DeCoodt, P. R.; Allen, H. N.; and Swan, H. J. C.: Determinants of the onset of the mitral valve prolapse in the systolic click-late systolic murmur syndrome. *Circulation*, **53**:872, 1976.

McDonald, A.; Harris, A.; Jefferson, K.; Marshall, J.; and McDonald, L.: Association of prolapse of posterior cusp of mitral valve and atrial septal defect. *Br. Heart J.*, **33**:383, 1971.

Mercer, E. N.; Frye, R. L.; and Giuliani, E. R.: Late systolic click in nonobstructive cardiomyopathy. *Br. Heart J.*, **32**:691, 1970.

Mills, P.; Rose, J.; Hollingsworth, J.; Amara, I.; and Craige, E.: Long-term prognosis of mitral valve prolapse. *New Engl. J. Med.*, **297**:13, 1977.

Moreyra, E.; Segal, B. L.; and Shimada, H.: The murmurs of mitral regurgitation. *Dis. Chest*, **55**:49, 1969.

O'Brien, K. P.; Hitchcock, G. C.; Barrat-Boyes, B. G.; and Lowe, J. B.: Spontaneous aortic cusp rupture associated with valvular myxomatous transformation. *Circulation*, **37**:273, 1968.

Oka, M.; Girerd, R. J.; Brodie, S. S., and Angrist, A.: Cardiac valve and aortic lesions in beta-amino-proprionitrite fed rats with and without high salt. *Am. J. Pathol.*, **48**:45, 1966.

Okada, R.; Glagov, S.; and Lev, M.: Relation of shunt flow and right ventricular pressure to heart valve structure in atrial septal defect. *Am. Heart J.*, **78**:781, 1969.

Osler, W.: On a remarkable heart murmur, heard at a distance from the chest wall. *Can. Med. Surg. J.*, **8**:518, 1879–1880.

Payvandi, M. N.; Kerber, R. E.; Phelps, C. D.; Judisch, G. F.; El-Khoury, G.; and Schrott, H. G.: Cardiac, skeletal and ophthalmologic abnormalities in relatives of patients with the Marfan syndrome. *Circulation*, **55**:797, 1977.

Perloff, J. K., and Roberts, W. C.: The mitral apparatus: functional anatomy of mitral regurgitation. *Circulation*, **46**:227, 1972.

Phillips, J. H.; Burch, G. E.; and DePasquale, N. P.: The syndrome of papillary muscle dysfunction: its clinical recognition. *Ann. Intern. Med.*, **59**:508, 1963.

Phornphutkul, C.; Rosenthal, A.; and Nadas, A. S.: Cardiac manifestations of Marfan's syndrome in infancy and childhood. *Circulation*, **47**:587, 1973.

Pocock, W. A., and Barlow, J. B.: An association between the billowing posterior mitral leaflet syndrome and congenital heart disease, particularly atrial septal defect. *Am. Heart J.*, **81**:720, 1971.

Pocock, W. A., and Barlow, J. B.: Etiology and electrocardiographic features of the billowing posterior mitral valve leaflet syndrome. Analysis of a further 130 patients with a late systolic murmur on nonejection systolic click. *Am. J. Med.*, **51**:731, 1971.

Pocock, W. A., and Barlow, J. B.: Post-exercise arrhythmias in the billowing posterior mitral leaflet syndrome. *Am. Heart J.*, **80**:740, 1970.

Pomerance, A.: Ballooning deformity (mucoid degeneration) of atrioventricular valves. *Br. Heart J.*, **31**:343, 1969.

Pomerance, A.: Pathology and valvular heart disease. *Br. Heart J.*, **34**:437, 1972.

Popp, R. L.: Echocardiographic assessment of cardiac disease. *Circulation*, **54**:538, 1976.

Popp, R. L.; Brown, O. R.; Silverman, J. F.; and Harrison, D. C.: Echocardiographic abnormalities in the mitral valve prolapse syndrome. *Circulation*, **49**:428, 1974.

Pridie, R. B.; Benham, R.; and Oakley, C. M.: Echocardiography of the mitral valve in aortic valve disease. *Br. Heart J.*, **33**:296, 1971.

Procacci, P. M.; Savran, S. V.; Schreiter, S. L.; and Bryson, A. L.: Prevalence of clinical mitral-valve prolapse in 1,169 young women. *N. Engl. J. Med.*, **294**:1086, 1976.

Rackley, C. E.; Whalen, R. D.; Floyd, W. L.; and McIntosh, H. D.: The precordial honk. *Am. J. Cardiol.*, **17**:509, 1966.

Raghib, G.; Jue, K. L.; Anderson, R. C.; and Edwards, J. E.: Marfan's syndrome with mitral insufficiency. *Am. J. Cardiol.*, **16**:127, 1965.

Ranganathan, N., and Burch, G. E.: Gross morphology and arterial supply of the papillary muscles of the left ventricle of a man. *Am. Heart J.*, **77**:506, 1969.

Ranganathan, N.; Lam, J. H. C.; Wigle, E. D.; and Silver, M. D.: Morphology of the human mitral valve. II. The valve leaflets. *Circulation*, **40**:459, 1970.

Ranganathan, N.; Silver, M. D.; Robinson, T. I.; Kostuk, W. J.; Felderhof, C. H.; Patt, N. L.; Wilson, J. K.; and Wigle, E. D.:

Angiographic-morphologic correlations in patients with severe mitral regurgitation due to prolapse of the posterior mitral valve leaflet. *Circulation*, **48**:514, 1973.

Ranganathan, N.; Silver, M. D.; Robinson, T. I.; and Wilson, J. K.: Idiopathic prolapse mitral leaflet syndrome. Angiographic-clinical correlations. *Circulation*, **54**:707, 1976.

Read, R. C.; Thal, A. P.; Wolf, P. L.; and Wendt, V. E.: Symptomatic valvular myxomatous degeneration: floppy valve syndrome. *Circulation*, **30**, suppl. 3:143, 1964.

Read, R. C.; Thal, A. P.; and Wendt, V. E.: Symptomatic valvular myxomatous transformation (the floppy valve syndrome). A possible forme fruste of the Marfan syndrome. *Circulation*, **32**:897, 1965.

Read, R. C., and Thal, A. P.: Surgical experience with symptomatic myxomatous valvular transformation (the floppy valve syndrome). *Surgery*, **59**:173, 1966.

Read, R. C.; White, H. J.; and Palacios, E.: The floppy valve syndrome: a possible expression of pituitary or mucopolysaccharide dysfunction. *Surg. Clin. North Am.*, **47**:1427, 1967.

Rizzon, P.; Biasco, G.; Brindici, G.; and Mauro, F.: Familial syndrome of midsystolic click and late systolic murmur. *Br. Heart J.*, **35**:245, 1973.

Roberts, W. C.; Dangel, J. C.; and Buckley, B. H.: Non-rheumatic valvular cardiac disease: a clinical pathologic survey of 27 different conditions causing valvular dysfunction. In Likoff, W. (ed.): *Cardiovasc. Clin.*, **5**:379, 1973.

Ronan, J. A.; Perloff, J. K.; and Harvey, W. P.: Systolic clicks and the late systolic murmur. Intracardiac phonocardiographic evidence of mitral valve origin. *Am. Heart J.*, **70**:319, 1965.

Sahn, D. J.; Allen, H. D.; Goldberg, S. J.; and Friedman, W. F.: Mitral valve prolapse in children. A problem defined by real-time cross-sectional echocardiography. *Circulation*, **53**:651, 1976.

Sahn, D. J.; Wood, J.; Allen, H. D.; Peoples, W.; and Goldberg, S. J.: Echocardiographic spectrum of mitral valve motion in children with and without mitral valve prolapse. Nature of false positive diagnosis. *Am. J. Cardiol.*, **39**:422, 1977.

Salomon, J.; Shah, P. M.; and Heinle, R. A.: Thoracic skeletal abnormalities in idiopathic mitral valve prolapse. *Am. J. Cardiol.*, **36**:32, 1975.

Scampardonis, G.; Yang, S. S.; Maranhao, V.; Goldberg, H.; and Gooch, A. S.: Left ventricular abnormalities in prolapsed mitral leaflet syndrome. Review of eighty-seven cases. *Circulation*, **48**:287, 1973.

Schwartz, D. C.; Kaplan, S.; and Meyer, R. A.: Mitral valve prolapse in children: clinical, echocardiographic and cineangiographic findings in 81 cases. *Am. J. Cardiol.*, **35**:169, 1975.

Schwartz, D. C.; Daoud, G.; and Kaplan, S.: Dysfunction of the mitral apparatus in children. *Am. J. Cardiol.*, **21**:114, 1968.

Segal, B. L., and Likoff, W.: Late systolic murmur of mitral regurgitation. *Am. Heart J.*, **67**:757, 1964.

Shah, P. M., and Gramiak, R.: Echocardiographic recognition of mitral valve prolapse. *Circulation*, **42**:45, 1970.

Shankar, K. R.; Hultgren, M. K.; Lauer, A. M.; and Diehl, A. M.: Lethal tricuspid and mitral regurgitation in Marfan's syndrome. *Am. J. Cardiol.*, **20**:122, 1967.

Shappell, S. D.; Marshall, C. E.; Brown, R. E.; and Bruce, T. A.: Sudden death and the familial occurrence of midsystolic click, late systolic murmur syndrome. *Circulation*, **48**:1128, 1973.

Shelburn, J. C.; Rubinstein, D.; and Gorlin, R.: A reappraisal of papillary muscle dysfunction. *Am. J. Med.*, **46**:862, 1969.

Shell, W. E.; Walton, J. A.; Clifford, M. E.; and Willis, P. W., III: The familial occurrence of the syndrome of mid-late systolic click and late systolic murmur. *Circulation*, **39**:327, 1969.

Sherman, E. B.; Char, F.; Dungah, W. T.; and Campbell, G. S.: Myxomatous transformation of the mitral valve producing mitral insufficiency. Floppy valve syndrome. *Am. J. Dis. Child.*, **119**:171, 1970.

Shrivastava, S.; Guthrie, R. B.; and Edwards, J. E.: Prolapse of the mitral valve. *Mod. Concepts Cardiovasc. Dis.*, **46**:57, 1977.

Silver, M. D.: Recent advances in the knowledge of pathology of natural and artificial valves. In Kalmanson, D.: *The Mitral Valve.* Publishing Sciences Group, Inc., Publisher, Acton, Mass., 1976, p. 5.

Silverman, M. E., and Hurst, J. W.: The mitral complex: Interaction of the anatomy, physiology, and pathology of the mitral annulus, mitral valve leaflets, chordae tendineae and papillary muscles. *Am. Heart J.*, **76**:399, 1968.

Simpson, J. W.; Nora, J. J.; and McNamara, D. G.: Marfan's syndrome and mitral valve disease: acute surgical emergencies. *Am. Heart J.*, **77**:96, 1969.

Sloman, G.; Stannard, M.; Hare, W. S. C., et al.: Prolapse of the posterior leaflet of the mitral valve. *Israel J. Med. Sci.*, **5/4**:727, 1969.

Sloman, G.; Wong, M.; and Walker, J.: Arrhythmias on exercise in patients with abnormalities of the posterior leaflet of the mitral valve. *Am. Heart J.*, **83**:312, 1972.

Spencer, W. H.; Behar, V. S.; and Orgain, E. S.: Apex cardiogram in patients with prolapsing mitral valve. *Am. J. Cardiol.*, **32**:276, 1973.

Sreenivasan, V. V.; Liebman, J.; Linton, D. S.; and Downs, T. D.: Posterior mitral regurgitation in girls possibly due to posterior papillary muscle dysfunction. *Pediatrics*, **42**:276, 1968.

Stannard, M., and Goble, A. J.: Endocarditis and the mitral valve. *Br. Med. J.*, **4**:683, 1967.

Stannard, M., and Rigo, S.: Prolapse of the posterior leaflet of the mitral valve. Chromosome studies in three sisters. *Am. Heart J.*, **75**:282, 1968.

Stannard, M.; Sloman, J. G.; Hare, W. S. C.; and Goble, A.: Prolapse of the posterior leaflet of the mitral valve: A clinical, familial and cineangiographic study. *Br. Med. J.*, **3**:71, 1967.

Steelman, R. B.; White, R. S.; Hill, J. C.; Nagle, J. P.; and Cheitlin, M. D.: Mid-systolic clicks in arterio-sclerotic heart disease. A new facet in the clinical syndrome of papillary muscle dysfunction. *Circulation*, **44**:503, 1971.

Tavel, M. E.; Campbell, R. W.; and Zimmer, J. F.: Late systolic murmurs and mitral regurgitation. *Am. J. Cardiol.*, **15**:719, 1965.

Taylor, D. E. M.; Wade, J. D.; and Hider, C. F.: Experimental study of mitral valve incompetence and mitral valve lesions following papillary muscle inactivation in the dog. *Cardiovasc. Res.*, **4**:319, 1970.

Tsakiris, A. G.; Rastelli, G. C.; Amorim, D.; Titus, J. L.; and Wood, E. H.: Effect of experimental papillary muscle damage on mitral valve closure in intact anesthetized dogs. *Mayo Clin. Proc.*, **285**:275, 1970.

Towne, W. D.; Rahimtoola, S. H.; Rosen, K. M.; Loeb, H. S.; and Gunnar, R.: The apex cardiogram in patients with systolic prolapse of the mitral valve. *Chest*, **63**:569, 1973.

Trent, J. K.; Adelman, A. G.; Wigle, E. D.; and Silver, M. D.: Morphology of a prolapsed posterior mitral valve leaflet. *Am. Heart J.*, **79**:539, 1970.

Vlad, P.: Editorial. Mitral valve anomalies in children. *Circulation*, **43**:465, 1971.

Victorica, B. E.; Elliot, L. P.; and Gessner, I. H.: Ostium secundum atrial septal defect associated with balloon mitral valve in children. *Am. J. Cardiol.*, **33**:669, 1974.

Weaver, A. L., and Spittell, J. A.: Lathyrism. *Mayo Clin. Proc.*, **39**:484, 1964.

Wigle, E. D.; Rakowski, H.; Ranganathan, N.; and Silver, M. D.: Mitral valve prolapse. *Ann. Rev. Med.*, **27**:165, 1976.

Willems, J.; Roelandt, J.; DeGeest, H.; Kesteloot, I.; and Joossens, J. V.: Late systolic murmurs and systolic nonejection clicks. *Acta Cardiol.*, **24**:456, 1969.

Winkle, R. A.; Goodman, D. J.; and Popp, R. L.: Simultaneous echocardiographic-phonocardiographic recordings at rest and during amyl nitrite administration in patients with mitral valve prolapse. *Circulation*, **51**:522, 1975a.

Winkle, R. A.; Lopes, M. G.; and Fitzgerald, J. W.: Arrhythmias in patients with mitral valve prolapse. *Circulation*, **52**:73, 1975b.

Winters, S. J. and Griggs, R. C.: Familial mitral valve prolapse and myotonic dystrophy. *Ann. Intern. Med.*, **85**:19, 1976.

Wooley, C. F.: Where are the diseases of yesteryear? DaCosta's syndrome, soldier's heart, the effort syndrome, neurocirculatory asthenia—and the mitral valve prolapse syndrome. Editorial. *Circulation*, **53**:749, 1976.

Young, D.: Noisy floppy mitral valve. *Am. Heart J.*, **93**:130, 1977.

44

Congenital Valvular Regurgitation

Robert M. Freedom

CONGENITAL MITRAL REGURGITATION

ALTHOUGH congenital mitral insufficiency is not uncommon in infancy and childhood, it is rarely dealt with as a distinct entity in pediatric cardiology, and there are few published reports in the literature under this heading alone. Most frequently it is associated with some other cardiac lesion and may be part of a well-known syndrome or combination of defects. Thus, we find it as part of the pathologic picture of atrioventricularis communis, ostium primum, corrected transposition of the great vessels, endocardial fibroelastosis, aneurysmal dilatation of the left atrium or left ventricle, and coarctation of the aorta. Mitral insufficiency can result from papillary muscle dysfunction resulting from ischemia or infarction and mitral valve dysfunction. This entity is dealt with in Chapter 47. Transient changes in myocardial perfusion in the neonate may lead to mitral valve incompetence (Rowe and Hoffman, 1972). In recent years, however, our interest has become focused on a group of cases of mitral insufficiency in which this is the chief or only defect. This group is characterized by such anomalies as cleft leaflet of the mitral valve, anomalous chordae, perforated valve, shortened or defective valve tissue, double-orifice thickenings and deformities, Ebstein's type of valve anomaly, and dilatation of the annulus. Prolapse may result in mitral incompetence.

Congenital mitral insufficiency is frequently associated with endocardial fibroelastosis of the left atrium and the left ventricle. This is not unexpected since the mitral valve is frequently involved when the endocardium is affected primarily. Shone and associates (1966) tested ten children with congenital mitral insufficiency with the mumps antigen skin test. This test proved to be definitely positive in seven of the ten cases, mildly positive in two, and negative in one. An interrelationship is suggested between congenital mitral insufficiency and endocardial fibroelastosis since this skin test is also positive in the majority of infants with fibroelastosis. However, subsequent studies did not confirm this apparent association.

The combined defects of mitral and tricuspid valves in atrioventricularis communis have been noted for many years (Abbott, 1932). Helmholz and associates emphasized the "mitral" insufficiency with corrected transposition in 1956, and Dorothy Anderson and many others have pointed out the effects on the mitral valve in certain cases of endocardial fibroelastosis. One of the earliest descriptions of the isolated defective mitral valve was that of Semans and Taussig in 1938. Prior, in 1953, reported two cases of mitral valve defects that survived into adult life. Linde and Adams (1959) reported three cases of mitral insufficiency associated with patent ductus arteriosus. Talner and associates (1961) have published an excellent review of the problem and presented their therapeutic results on six cases (Creech et al., 1962; Kay et al., 1961).

Renewed interest has been focused on this field by the recent reports of successful surgical therapy in many of the above-mentioned categories, and this has encouraged the pediatric cardiologist to search for cases that can be corrected.

Pathology

The character of the mitral valve offers opportunity for developmental defects in fetal life. Appreciation of the morphology of the normal mitral valve apparatus is necessary if one is to understand the wide variety of abnormalities that may affect this valve (Lam et al., 1970; Ranganatham et al., 1970). These authors have reviewed the morphology of the normal mitral valve with special attention to the chordae tendineae and valve leaflets. The posterior or lateral leaflet is attached to the annulus of the mitral valve at the junction of the left ventricle and left atrium, while the anterior or medial leaflet extends a good deal of its attachment up into the aortic root and is continuous with portions of the aortic valve above. The leaflets in the closed position are suspended by the chordae tendineae and papillary muscles, which insert into the ventricular wall just below the commissures. Davachi, Moller, and Edwards (1971) documented the pathologic findings of mitral valvular lesions in 29 infants with primary congenital anomalies of the mitral valve. Congenital anomalies were identified according to the components of the valve primarily involved: (1) leaflets; (2) commissures; (3) chordae tendineae; and (4) papillary muscles. The most common basis for primary congenital valvular disturbance in this study was an abnormality of the papillary muscle. Parachute mitral valve and abnormal position of the papillary muscles are representative of this group. Mitral insufficiency may also result from an anomalous mitral arcade (Layman and Edwards, 1967; Davachi et al., 1971). In this condition, there is connection of the left ventricular papillary muscles to the anterior mitral leaflet, either directly or through the interposition of unusually short chordae tendineae. Actis-Dato and Milocco (1966) reported a 21-year-old girl with anomalous attachment of the mitral valve to the ventricular wall. In this patient, the mitral valve leaflets were displaced downward into the ventricular wall and were not related to the fibrous ring surrounding the atrioventricular orifice, with shortening and fusion of the chordae tendineae. The findings in this patient suggest isolated Ebstein's anomaly of the mitral valve, without L-transposition.

In endocardial fibroelastosis thickening of the mitral valve occurs at times making it less mobile, and if the process involves the chordae tendineae, these structures become stiff, preventing full excursion of the leaflets. Shortened chordae tendineae and deformed valve leaflets frequently coexist and accentuate the insufficiency that either one may produce. Calcification of the valve is a rare phenomenon in childhood and, when it does occur, usually appears superimposed on a previously deformed or damaged mitral valve.

Dilation of the left atrium from any cause can proceed to a degree that enlarges the mitral ring and prevents the anterior and posterior cusps from approximating in systole, leading to a serious degree of insufficiency of the valve.

A cleft in the anterior leaflet is commonly associated with atrioventricular canal defects but may occur as an isolated phenomenon. In atrioventricularis communis, where both the mitral and tricuspid valves are cleft, the chordae tendineae may be inserted into unusual sites such as the margin of the ventricular septal defect. This is an important consideration since, when the cleft is closed surgically, unless the abnormal chordae are cut and the valve freed, insufficiency will persist.

Congenital mitral valve disease may be associated with coarctation of aorta. In Rosenquist's study of 53 specimens with aortic coarctation (1974), only nine had a mitral valve of normal size and configuration. Ten patients had a normally formed valve, which was small in comparison to both tricuspid valve and left ventricle. The majority of the remaining demonstrated various anomalies, including some forms of parachute mitral valve. Freed and his colleagues (1974) state that among 861 infants and children with coarctation of the aorta, examined between 1950 and 1973, 18 (2.1 percent) also had congenital mitral incompetence. The pathologic anatomy of the incompetent mitral valve associated with coarctation of the aorta includes leaflet abnormalities (clefts, perforation, and myxomatous change) and chordae abnormalities (short chordae, long chordae, ruptured chordae, and deficient chordae).

In corrected or L-transposition of the great vessels the mitral and tricuspid valves are transposed, and the resulting valve on the left side of the heart may be defective. Malers and associates (1960) reviewed 74 cases and found evidence of "mitral" regurgitation in 13. Five had an anomalous insertion of the chordae, four had an Ebstein's type of anomaly in the left atrioventricular valve, and four had some defect of the valve cusps. At times a major degree of insufficiency is found in the defective valve angiocardiographically when by other methods only a minor degree of regurgitation may be shown. It is probably safe to conclude that at least 20 percent of the children with corrected or L-transposition have a functional defect of the left-sided valve.

Accessory commissures may lead to a localized leak in the mitral valve. Edwards and Burchell (1958) demonstrated such anomalies and showed an associated jet lesion in the left atrium above the valve anomaly. A double orifice to the mitral valve may occur without functional impairment, but occasionally mitral insufficiency may be present and progressive in this anomaly.

Congenital regurgitation may be found in the patient with congenital polyvalvular disease. Bharati and Lev (1973) studied 36 hearts in which the valves were involved in a dysplastic process, characterized by an increase in valvular spongiosa, with vacuolar and lacunar degeneration. These cases were often, but not invariably, associated with trisomy 18 or 13–15. Usually, the dysplastic valve was stenotic, but in some patients studied at The Hospital for Sick Children, the valves were severely incompetent. Evans and his associates (1973) document, by angiography and necropsy examination, incomplete differentiation of cardiac valves.

With the enlargement and dilatation of the left ventricle that frequently characterize this lesion, the chordae tendineae spread out in a lateral fashion, until in some cases a situation may be reached where the valve leaflets cannot approximate each other and a further degree of insufficiency occurs. Thus Edwards and Burchell suggest that mitral insufficiency begets insufficiency.

Clinical Features

The history and clinical findings vary according to the underlying associated pathology as well as by the influence of the degree of mitral insufficiency. In the atrioventricular canal defects a distinctive picture is frequently presented, in corrected transposition another series of findings is characteristic, and when mitral insufficiency occurs as an isolated phenomenon, the clinical facets change again.

We are primarily concerned with the last group and with the history and clinical findings that mitral insufficiency produces when it is of congenital origin. There is almost invariably a history of fatigue and retarded growth and frequent respiratory infection. Although the cardiac findings may be suggestive of rheumatic heart disease, there will be no previous history of rheumatic fever, and the sedimentation rate and ASO titer will be within normal limits. The P-R interval may be normal or lengthened.

Heart failure is a common feature in congenital mitral insufficiency (Talner et al., 1961).

On physical examination there is usually an apical thrust due to the enlarged left ventricle, a mitral systolic murmur, a third heart sound, and, as a rule, an apical diastolic murmur of the inflow type. The systolic murmur is frequently accompanied by a thrill at the apex. The pulmonary second sound is likely to be accentuated since the pulmonary artery pressure is elevated in most instances. The defects of the atrioventricular canal form a special group. Those clinical findings have been set forth elsewhere and will

not be repeated in detail here, but it is worthwhile to refer to the apical systolic murmur. In ostium primum this murmur, indicative of mitral insufficiency, is present in 80 percent of cases (Evans et al., 1961). However, in most ostium primum cases with some central valve tissue, when mitral and tricuspid valves were both found to be cleft in the same patient, only one out of six cases had physical signs indicative of either mitral or tricuspid regurgitation. This one patient has a pansystolic murmur at apex but no left ventricular impulse.

Three cases proved to have a common atrium and a cleft mitral valve had no apical systolic murmur.

It is surprising to note that of 23 cases with atrioventricularis communis, ultimately proved to have a complete canal defect with cleft mitral and tricuspid valves, only one was thought to have mitral insufficiency on the basis of clinical signs. The others all had a harsh systolic murmur with thrill over the lower precordium near the sternum apparently related to the ventricular septal defect. Brockenbrough and associates (1962) have presented details of a case with cleft mitral valve and small atrial septal defect that behaved functionally like pure mitral insufficiency and had an enlarged left atrium. There

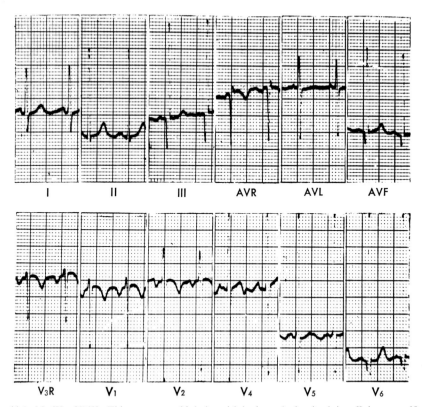

Figure 44-1. M. W., 5/1/62. This one-year-old baby girl had marked mitral insufficiency verified by cineangiogram and at operation. Section of left atrium and appearance of heart interior at time of surgical correction indicated underlying cause of insufficiency was endocardial fibroelastosis. Electrocardiogram shows marked left ventricular loading. (Reproduced from Keth, J. D.: Congenital mitral insufficiency. *Prog. Cardiovasc. Dis.,* **5**:264, 1962.)

was a pansystolic murmur at the apex transmitted to the axilla.

The apical systolic murmur is not a feature of corrected or L-transposition, since the physical signs of the associated anomalies such as ventricular septal defect usually predominate; however, a pansystolic murmur at the apex is recorded occasionally, apparently due to the mitral insufficiency (Malers et al., 1960).

Electrocardiography

In isolated mitral insufficiency the axis is usually in the quadrant from 0 to 90 degrees. Talner and associates report it to be occasionally over 90, up to 113 degrees. In a case reported by Braunwald and associates (1961) that had a small atrial septal defect and a cleft mitral valve, the axis was − 30 degrees. The anatomy was related to the group with AV canal defect, which, of course, characteristically has a negative axis. A broad, bifid P wave is almost invariably present in the cases of pure mitral insufficiency of a considerable degree. This group will also have evidence of left ventricular loading—most commonly characterized by a tall R wave in V_6 (see Figures 44–1 and 44–2).

A lengthened conduction time is associated with corrected transposition, as are the frequent presence of Q waves in the right precordium and their absence over the left.

Echocardiographic findings in mitral insufficiency have been described (Cosby et al., 1974; Burgess et al., 1973; Sweatman et al., 1972; Dillon et al., 1971; Kerber et al., 1971). Although mitral incompetence can be diagnosed by reflected ultrasound, the heterogeneity of anatomic types makes specific morphologic diagnosis difficult, but not impossible. Mitral valve prolapse is readily diagnosed by echo, and the salient echocardiographic findings of mitral incompetence secondary to ruptured chordae tendineae have also been described. The most characteristic echocardiographic findings in non-rheumatic mitral insufficiency are a marked increase in the diastolic slope and marked increase in both opening and closing heights of the mitral valve.

Radiologic Examination

The characteristic radiologic findings of this group of patients are left atrial and left ventricular enlargement. This is usually revealed by a somewhat diffuse cardiac enlargement in the anteroposterior view, and a double atrial contour may be recognized with the left atrium protruding through to the right margin. A barium swallow will confirm the left atrial enlargement, usually of noticeable degree (see Figure 44–2C). The large left atrium may at times elevate and spread the mainstem bronchi, as shown in the anteroposterior view of the chest. The aortic knuckle is not prominent in the conventional x-ray film, and angiocardiography usually reveals it to be small. The pulmonary vascular markings are increased, especially the shadows at the right apex, due to the back pressure in the pulmonary veins. The left anterior oblique view will most clearly outline the left ventricular enlargement. Kerley's lines may be present.

When corrected or L-transposition is present, the aorta can usually be seen coming up the left cardiac border, presenting the characteristic radiologic picture that has been described previously. In the group with common atrioventricular canal, since an atrial septal defect is present, the excessive left atrial flow due to mitral insufficiency is not forced into a confined left atrium but is allowed to escape through the atrial septal defect, thus enlarging the right side of the heart rather than the left. This produces a different radiologic picture from that of isolated mitral insufficiency. Occasionally, however, one may have a small atrial septal defect less than 1 cm in diameter in the atrioventricularis canal group. Then the left atrium may enlarge, and the clinical appearance is more like that in isolated mitral insufficiency (Ferencz et al., 1954; and Braunwald et al., 1961).

Angiocardiography

The clinical findings are usually sufficient to suggest the possibility of mitral insufficiency, thus permitting one to carry out angiocardiography in the most favorable site and position. This is best done with the tip of the catheter in the left ventricle (see Figure 44–3) either through a foramen ovale into the left atrium to the left ventricle or retrograde fashion through the aortic valve into the left ventricle. This will show the regurgitant flow of contrast material sweeping back with each systole into the left atrium; it will also show the immense dilatation of the left atrium with each systole. The left atrium may be aneurysmal in proportions and show up dramatically with angiocardiography. The contrast material is held up in the left atrium for a considerable period; the large left ventricle is revealed, as is also the somewhat small aorta. When the catheter is positioned across the mitral valve in the left ventricle, spurious mitral incompetence might result because the catheter itself mechanically interferes with the valve mechanism. Ideally, retrograde left ventricular cineangiographic techniques should be utilized to evaluate the presence (or absence) of mitral valve incompetence and the severity of the leak. The patient should be positioned in the right anterior oblique for best visualization of the mitral valve. Hopefully, the injection of contrast will not be complicated by ectopic beats, which may produce spurious mitral incompetence.

Selective aortic root angiography should be performed as part of the complete catheter assessment of the patient with isolated congenital mitral incompetence. One must be certain to exclude

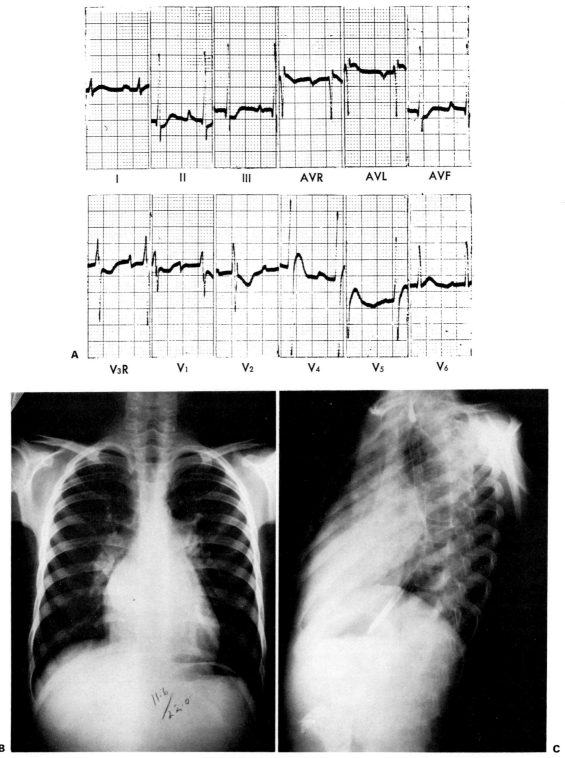

Figure 44-2. B. P., 2/3/62. Nine-year-old boy with congenital mitral insufficiency due to cleft in posterior cusp subsequently operated on successfully.

    A. Electrocardiogram—broad bifid P_1.

    B. AP view of heart—showing moderate cardiac enlargement and congested hilar shadows.

    C. Lateral view of heart—moderate left atrial enlargement. (Reproduced from Keith, J. D.: Congenital mitral insufficiency. *Prog. Cardiovasc. Dis.*, **5**: 264, 1962.)

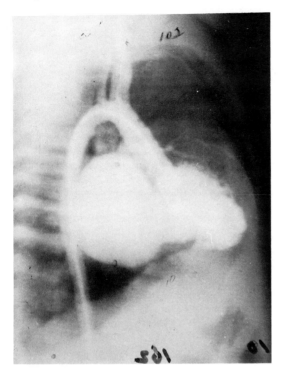

Figure 44-3. P. J.: female aged six weeks. Congenital mitral insufficiency showing reflux from left ventricle into left atrium. Greatly dilated left atrium is apparent.

an anomalous origin of the left coronary artery from the pulmonary artery as the etiology of the mitral incompetence.

Cardiac Catheterization

There have been many papers written on the hemodynamics of mitral regurgitation. These are associated with a high end-diastolic pressure in the left ventricle and a high mean-diastolic pressure in the left atrium. The left atrial pressure pulse is characterized by a tall peaked "v" wave followed by a rapid descent. A considerable "a" wave is also present in many cases. The left ventricular pressure pulse shows a rapid fall after the ejection peak. A withdrawal tracing from the left ventricle to the left atrium is helpful to rule out the associated presence of mitral stenosis. One may at times have difficulty in keeping the catheter in the left ventricle, since the regurgitant flow may carry the tip back into the left atrium (Musser et al., 1956). The pulmonary artery wedge pressure is always elevated when the mitral insufficiency is significant and is not accompanied by an atrial septal defect that decompresses the left atrium. The pulmonary artery wedge pressure tracing will also show the elevated "v" wave with its rapid descent. The right ventricular and pulmonary artery pressures are usually elevated to some degree.

Diagnosis

The obvious hemodynamic defect in mitral regurgitation is the flux of blood back into the atrium at the time the ventricle is attempting to empty its contents out into the aorta. This augments the volume of the left atrium during the next diastole and results in an abnormally large quantity of blood entering the left ventricle, producing diastolic overload. At the same time blood is forced backward from the atrium into the pulmonary veins. The left ventricle then gradually increases in size and dilates to a greater capacity in both systole and diastole.

Angiocardiography may clearly reveal the dilated left atrium, which bulges out in dramatic fashion with each ventricular systole and demonstrates the origin of the large venous pressure waves in the pulmonary veins. The enlarged left ventricle is also dilated. The heart increases its total stroke volume although the effective forward stroke volume is reduced.

These features can be especially well shown with cineangiocardiography, but they can also be shown by the pulse wave during cardiac catheterization. The characteristic left atrial pulse contour shows a high peaked "v" wave with little or no "c" wave, since the trough of the "x" wave between "c" and "v" is largely obliterated, and this wave is followed by rapid descent when ventricular systole is complete.

In infants, particularly in the first few weeks or months of life, it is usually not difficult to get across the foramen ovale into the left atrium and left ventricle and record the pressure contours. When this route is not possible, it may be necessary to do a left heart catheterization in retrograde fashion and maneuver the tip of the catheter into the left ventricle and, if possible, the left atrium.

Dye dilution curves will show a prolonged disappearance time that is suggestive of mitral regurgitation, but such methods may not be specific in the childhood age group because an atrial septal defect, ventricular septal defect, patent ductus, or other left-to-right shunts are frequently present, and one cannot be certain whether one is dealing with a shunt or valve regurgitation since the dye curves are similar. One might, however, employ this method successfully if the two-catheter double-dye dilution curve technique were used.

In the differential diagnosis of mitral insufficiency in infancy and childhood, there are seven main categories in which one may encounter this dynamic lesion:

1. Atrioventricularis communis and ostium primum are almost invariably associated with some degree of mitral regurgitation. Atrioventricularis communis is always associated with a cleft of the mitral valve, but in our experience approximately 6 percent of the children with ostium primum had no cleft in the mitral valve (Evans et al., 1961).

2. The second category is that of corrected or L-transposition, which may be associated with minor

degree of insufficiency of the left-sided valve but on occasion this may be severe.

3. The third category is that of rheumatic heart disease; such children may fail to give a history of rheumatic fever and the insufficiency may appear as an isolated finding.

4. The fourth category is that of congenital mitral insufficiency without any of the other associated anomalies listed above. In this group a patient may, of course, have an associated patent ductus or ventricular septal defect or a small atrial septal defect or other anomaly, but usually the hemodynamics are dominated by the mitral regurgitation.

5. Congenital mitral insufficiency may be associated with coarctation of the aorta as previously described. The coarctation will aggravate the severity of the regurgitation, and frequently, after coarctectomy, the mitral regurgitation will be improved.

6. The patient with anomalous left coronary artery originating from the pulmonary artery may have mitral regurgitation resulting from ischemic damage to the left ventricle and papillary muscle. Typically, the patient is an infant with cardiomegaly, mitral regurgitation, and characteristic electrocardiographic findings: abnormal Q waves in leads I, aVL, and evidence of left ventricular ischemia. Aortic root angiography will provide conclusive evidence for this anomaly.

7. Varying degrees of mitral regurgitation may accompany mitral valve prolapse. See Chapter 43.

The atrioventricularis communis and ostium primum group usually can be readily identified by the electrocardiogram and cardiac catheter findings. The negative axis in the electrocardiogram is a useful starting point. Ninety-five percent of our cases with either of these lesions had an axis between −50 and −150 degrees. Three cases had a figure-of-eight loop around the horizontal, but the major deviation was counterclockwise (Evans et al., 1961). Some of these cases have an apical systolic murmur, and at operation the surgeon will almost invariably find a cleft in the mitral valve. It is well to remember, however, that in patients with primum defects and clefts of both atrioventricular valves, clinical signs of mitral and tricuspid incompetence are often lacking, and one must depend on other signs in suspecting the presence of mitral valve insufficiency.

In corrected or L-transposition one usually finds an aorta that traverses the left cardiac border and can be recognized as such by x-ray, fluoroscopic, and electrocardiographic study. An angiogram, however, will confirm this anatomy with greater precision: preferably by a retrograde injection made into the outflow tract of the left ventricle. In this manner the diminutive outflow chamber, if present, can be shown as well as the body of the ventricle. This will help to identify whether one is dealing with a common ventricle or not and will also reveal mitral insufficiency if present. It is well to remember that approximately 20 percent of the cases of corrected transposition have "mitral" regurgitation (Malers et al., 1960). In the assessment of left AV valve

regurgitation in the patient with L- or corrected transposition of the great arteries, it is important to determine the morphologic state of the left AV (tricuspid) valve. Does the regurgitation through the left or systemic AV valve result from deformed but normally positioned and dilated valve ring, or from an Ebstein-type malformation? Jaffe (1976) suggests that the position of the left AV valve leaflets is best recognized in frontal angiocardiograms. The epicardial distribution of the coronary arteries will demonstrate the normal left AV groove. Displacement of valve tissue inferiorally with respect to the left AV groove should be interpreted as consistent with an Ebstein's malformation of the left-sided systemic AV valve.

In rheumatic heart disease and mitral insufficiency in the pediatric age group a patient may have a history of rheumatic fever, but, if this is lacking, the electrocardiogram rarely shows left ventricular loading of significant degree. The left atrium is usually not enlarged dramatically. The ASO titer may be elevated, or the sedimentation rate, making one suspect that the origin is rheumatic. Cardiac catheterization will reveal no shunt and usually shows a minimal degree of regurgitant flow. Such findings can be confirmed by angiocardiography. When mitral insufficiency due to rheumatic heart disease is severe, it may not be possible to differentiate it from that of congenital origin, and the signs and symptoms may be sufficient to warrant operation whatever the cause. In such instances the diagnosis can only be made with the valve exposed.

In congenital mitral insufficiency, apart from the atrial septal defect group, a history of cardiac failure is common and often associated with a failure to grow, a bifid P wave in the electrocardiogram, a large left atrium, and an apical systolic murmur transmitted to the axilla. There is an absence of cyanosis, and at cardiac catheterization a tall "v" wave is readily apparent in the left atrial pressure tracing. There is no gradient across the mitral valve on going from the left atrium to the left ventricle, and an angiocardiogram will clearly show the regurgitant flow when the injection is made into the left ventricle.

In aortic stenosis or aortic insufficiency one may have some enlargement of the left atrium and left ventricle, but the left atrial enlargement is usually not marked, the pressure curve in the left atrium will be different, and a left heart catheterization and angiogram will reveal the cause of the murmur.

Chronic myocarditis of a nonrheumatic origin may give one an apical systolic murmur with mitral insufficiency due to a dilated mitral ring. Such cases will usually have a history of onset with an acute illness, the electrocardiogram may be characteristic of acute myocarditis, and the disease is likely to be associated with progressive improvement if medically treated in the early stages. In the late stages, whether acute or chronic, the patient may run a progressive downhill course with further cardiac enlargement, failure, and demise. Acute myocarditis is not a common illness, but usually there is no difficulty in recognizing it as distinct from congenital mitral insufficiency. Chronic myocarditis with fibrosis and hypertrophy of the myocardium may be associated with cardiac enlargement and mitral regurgitation. Furthermore, the electrocardiogram may show left loading as in congenital mitral insufficiency. Electrocardiograms taken early in the course of myocarditis are characteristic of the acute phase of the disease and may thus reveal the true etiology, but if they are only available in the late recovery phase, it may be difficult to make an accurate differentiation at times. Fortunately the chronic type of myocarditis with such an electrocardiographic pattern is a very rare finding.

Acquired disturbances of the coronary arteries may result in coronary insufficiency and mitral incompetence. Infantile periarteritis nodosa may result in coronary arteritis, myocardial infarction, and papillary muscle dysfunction. The mucocutaneous lymph node syndrome may have significant coronary artery disturbances. Several reports have documented the coronary artery aneurysms typical of this syndrome. Although this disease has only rarely been reported in North America, several thousand cases have been documented in Japan.

There are unusual congenital defects of the mitral valve, such as that reported by Ferencz (1957), in which there was congenital mitral insufficiency and a defect in the membranous portion of the ventricular septum in such a fashion that the left ventricle injected blood through into the right atrium rather than the right ventricle. A similar case may be identified if a left heart catheterization with angiogram is done as well as right heart catheterization.

The case reported by Braunwald and associates (1961) was also an unusual exception to any of the above categories. There was congenital mitral insufficiency with a cleft of the anterior leaflet of the mitral valve and a very small atrial septal defect. Such a case apparently falls in the category of the atrioventricular canal anomalies but has not progressed to the full-blown stage. Atrial fibrillation occurred in both the case reported by Braunwald and associates (1961) and that reported by Semans and Taussig (1938), which latter case had mitral insufficiency with the mitral valve replaced by a perforated diaphragm.

In view of the bizarre associated findings in some cases of congenital mitral insufficiency, it would appear wise, when the diagnosis is suspected, to do both right and left heart catheterizations and to accompany the left heart catheterization with a pressure tracing in the left atrium and left ventricle and an angiogram with injection into the left ventricle.

Treatment

It is well known that patients with chronic severe mitral regurgitation can remain clinically asymptomatic for many years despite a significant regurgitant volume (Wilson and Lim, 1957; Ellis and Ramirez, 1969; Braunwald, 1969). These retrospective and longitudinal studies have been carried out in an adult patient with rheumatic heart disease. In the infant and child, the pathogenetic mechanism for the mitral incompetence (i.e., AV canal, anomalous left coronary artery, etc.) is a major determinant of the overall prognosis. Nonetheless, it is important to appreciate the myocardial mechanisms that allow mitral regurgitation to be tolerated. In the patient with chronic mitral incompetence, the cardiac index is usually nearly normal and the total left ventricular output (to left atrium and aorta) exceeds the normal (Eckberg et al., 1973). Mitral regurgitation reduces the radius of the ventricle more than normal during systole, resulting in a significant reduction of myocardial wall tension. The reduced tension of loading on the ventricle allows a larger proportion of the contractile energy of the myocardium to be expended in shortening than in tension development. The striking reduction in left ventricular tension that occurs in mitral regurgitation allows the left ventricle to increase its total output and accounts for the observation that patients with severe mitral regurgitation can sustain enormous regurgitant volumes for prolonged periods without clinical deterioration (Braunwald, 1969).

Because mitral insufficiency is not an uncommon lesion in adult life, a great deal of attention has been given over the past decade to its surgical correction. In the infant and child with mitral incompetence, the developmental bases for the regurgitation are quite varied, and treatment will, of course, vary considerably.

Considerable progress has been made in the past decade in the treatment of rheumatic mitral disease. Kirklin and Pacifico (1973) have reviewed their own experience and state that the hospital mortality rate for isolated mitral valve replacement for pure mitral incompetence is 20 percent. This significant mortality is possibly explained on the basis that the reserve of mitral incompetence is lost when the valve is made competent, and the resulting increased afterload may be an important determinant of the very low cardiac output seen in these patients. In recent years, attempts have been made to lower afterload (Harshaw et al., 1975). Kouchoukos (1973) has recently reviewed problems in mitral valve replacement.

Surgical correction of isolated congenital mitral regurgitation in childhood has been reported. Fortunately, the necessity for cardiac valve replacement in children is uncommon. Klint and associates in 1972 collected only 166 cases from the English literature and from their own experience. Van der Horst and colleagues (1973) reported the results of mitral valve replacement in 51 children, 39 having mitral incompetence.

One of the most useful procedures in the presence of a dilated ring or mitral annulus has been the placing of many through-and-through silk sutures in the region of one or both commissures in order to narrow the opening. This is probably the most acceptable method for children, but the suturing needs to be reinforced or it is likely to pull out. At best, it reduces the insufficiency rather than cures it. The immediate results are good. If the sutures hold and do not cut through the valve or annulus tissue, the long-term results should be good also. Although mitral valvuloplasty has been carried out in children with rheumatic mitral incompetence, there is little experience with the application of this technique to congenital mitral regurgitation (Kahn et al., 1967; Reed et al., 1974). The variety of anatomic defects that result in congenital mitral insufficiency will obviously necessitate individual therapy. Usually, only at the time of intraoperative intervention and observation can the decision be made whether valve plication will provide effective palliation.

When the mitral valve is deformed in the spectrum of endocardial cushion defect (Chapters 21, 22), it is almost impossible to routinely achieve complete functional integrity of valve using reconstructive operations. Pertinent anatomic observations on the complete form of common AV canal with special attention to the atrioventricular valves have been presented (Rastelli et al., 1966; Rastelli et al., 1968; McMullen et al., 1972; Rastelli et al., 1969). McGood (1973) has recently summarized the Mayo Clinic experience, using the Rastelli modifications of repair. The mortality was only 7 percent, indicating that the outlook for the patient with complete AV canal is no longer poor.

The cleft valve of the ostium primum type can usually be dealt with adequately. It is more difficult to adequately correct the defective valve of the atrioventricularis communis, partly because the cleft goes right through into the tricuspid valve and also because the tricuspid valve is usually deficient and defective to a degree that makes adequate repair almost impossible and thus prejudices the patient's chances of recovery in the postoperative period. Creech and associates (1962) reported the successful treatment of a two-year-old child with a posterior leaflet defect.

In the presence of ruptured chordae tendineae of the posterior leaflet, Ellis and associates (1959) fix the leaflet to the wall of the left ventricle in such a way that it acts as a baffle against which the anterior leaflet can meet during ventricular systole. They have usually found it necessary to narrow the mitral ring as well when using this technique. Another method, sponsored by McGoon (1960), consists of shortening the elongation portion of the leaflet whose chordae had been ruptured and tightening the leading edge by insertion of plicating sutures, thus prevent-ing eversion of the affected leaflet during systole.

Obviously each case will be a problem unto itself, and the surgeon will use one or more of the various techniques that may be required to make the valve function adequately.

Many authors have operated on mitral insufficiency in the adult age group by plicating or narrowing the mitral orifice. These techniques have been applied infrequently to the pediatric age group, but an excellent series has been reported by Talner, Stearn, and Sloan (1961), who operated on six cases of congenital mitral insufficiency with no death and good results in all of them. Mustard, at The Hospital for Sick Children, has recently operated on several children, with moderately satisfactory results. Each child continues to have some degree of mitral insufficiency.

The immediate mortality will depend on the severity of the lesion and the associated defects. Those who survive may show a varying degree of improvement. The apical systolic murmur may diminish, remain the same, or at times become intensified even when improvement occurs. X-ray films taken of the heart for size over a period of time may show gradual improvement for a period of several months. Left atrial pressure should decline considerably in the postoperative period but is likely to remain in the high-normal or slightly elevated area.

Dye dilution curves during right heart catheterization provide another method of evaluating the degree of mitral insufficiency persisting postoperatively, especially if one can compare the curve with that taken before operation was performed. Ellis and associates (1959) record a dramatic improvement in the contour of these curves when comparing them with the original tracings in all the cases restudied.

Cases for surgery in childhood should be selected with some care; a clear indication for operation is congestive heart failure. If the heart is enlarged, particularly the left ventricle and left atrium, and the patient has a reduced exercise tolerance (especially if progressive), one also has good reason for surgical intervention. Although it may be difficult to construct an entirely normal mitral valve in these children, the results appear to be satisfying in nearly every category that has been mentioned above. The recognition of this anomaly when it occurs, therefore, is imperative since the diagnostic techniques now make accurate assessment possible and the surgical techniques now offer several corrective procedures.

CONGENITAL TRICUSPID REGURGITATION

ISOLATED congenital tricuspid incompetence is most uncommon, and there have been only a few reports documenting this entity (Reisman et al., 1965; Shone et al., 1962; Talner and Campbell, 1973; Schiebler et al., 1968). Usually, tricuspid incompetence is associated with Ebstein's anomaly; right ventricular hypertension (pulmonary stenosis, atresia with intact ventricular septum); a cleft tricuspid valve as part of an endocardial cushion defect; and large ventricular defects with pulmonary hypertension and dilatation of the right ventricle and tricuspid annulus. Transient tricuspid regurgitation in the neonate may reflect a form of myocardial dysfunction in stressed babies (Brown and Pickering, 1974; Bucciarelli et al.,

1976, 1977; Riemenschneider et al., 1976). Tricuspid incompetence may also accompany Uhl's anomaly and congenitally unguarded tricuspid orifice. This latter entity has been associated with valve or subvalve pulmonary atresia in the reported cases (Kanjuh et al., 1964). The patient with incomplete differentiation of cardiac valves or congenital polyvalvular disease may have incompetence of the tricuspid valve. In this condition, the valve tissue is dysplastic, with an increase in valvular spongiosa and lacumar degeneration (Bharati and Lev, 1973; Evans et al., 1973). Infective endocarditis may distort the tricuspid valve and result in incompetence. This right-sided endocarditis is frequently seen in the drug abuser. The straddling or overriding tricuspid valve may occasionally be incompetent. Occasionally, the tricuspid valve will both participate in a complex malformation, as well as being congenitally dysplastic.

Pathology

Isolated congenital tricuspid valve insufficiency is usually due to maldevelopment of the septal leaflet. This cusp may be adherent to the interventricular septum and will have grossly deficient chordae tendineae. Occasionally, the most anterosuperior portion of the septal cusp has not developed. In some neonates with severe tricuspid regurgitation documented angiographically, there has been significant regression of the regurgitation. This would suggest a transient disturbance in hemodynamics or perhaps transient myocardial ischemia, with predominantly right-sided myocardial involvement (Rowe and Hoffman, 1972; Rowe, 1977). Significant dysplasia of the tricuspid valve resembling Ebstein's anomaly may result in tricuspid incompetence (Becker et al., 1971).

Clinical Features

Cyanosis has been conspicuous in the neonates with this disease.

The jugular venous pulse wave is distorted by tricuspid incompetence, although in the neonate this may be difficult to evaluate. The severity of the regurgitation will determine the extent of the alteration. With severe regurgitation, ventricularization of the jugular venous pulse may occur; this is best visualized during inspiration or abdominal compression.

Thrill.   With severe tricuspid regurgitation, there may be an associated thrill.

Heart Murmur.   The murmur of tricuspid incompetence is usually pansystolic and maximum along the lower sternal border. The murmur may be difficult to differentiate from that of ventricular septal defect or mitral insufficiency. A diastolic murmur of relative tricuspid stenosis is frequently heard with significant tricuspid regurgitation

Heart Sounds.   Frequently a third heart sound is heard, giving a triple rhythm. This occurs most commonly in those patients with a diastolic murmur. The heart sounds are usually of normal intensity.

Radiologic Examination

From the few patients from our institution with this disease, and from reports in the literature (Nielson et al., 1976), the symptomatic neonate has a very large heart, often massive, with diminished pulmonary vascularity (Figure 44–4).

Electrocardiography

The electrocardiogram would show right atrial and ventricular hypertrophy.

Diagnosis

A forward indicator-dye dilation curve performed by injection in the inferior vena cava with sampling in the femoral artery will demonstrate valve incompetence when compared to a normal curve performed with indicator distal to a competent tricuspid valve.

Cardiac catheterization findings will depend on the severity of the tricuspid regurgitation. When more than mild, the right atrial pressure is elevated, with the "ac" and "v" waves distorted or completely ventricularized. The right ventricular systolic pressure should be normal, but the end-diastolic pressure may be elevated.

Selective right ventricular angiocardiography should show regurgitation into the large right atrium, but this diagnosis must take into consideration the small amount of catheter-induced regurgitation and spurious regurgitation induced by ectopic beats. Barr and his associates (1974) recently reported the clinical and angiocardiographic features of two infants with tricuspid valvular dysplasia producing severe congenital tricuspid incompetence in the neonate. The patients were deeply cyanosed, and both had a loud heart murmur of tricuspid regurgitation. Angiocardiography in these patients suggested organic right ventricular outflow tract obstruction because very little contrast entered the pulmonary artery. In addition, the right ventricles were large, and there was retrograde flow of contrast material through the dilated tricuspid annulus into a large right atrium (Figure 44–5).

An electrode study should not show the pattern of discordance between atrial pressure and the ventricular electrogram.

Prognosis

The few number of reported cases makes it difficult to give an accurate prognosis. In the neonate with severe isolated tricuspid regurgitation, the fall of pulmonary vascular resistance may be accompanied by lessening of the tricuspid regurgitation. This is not always the case, and some infants have died in severe congenital heart failure. Severe tricuspid insufficiency in the neonate may be transient. This entity, considered a manifestation of myocardial dysfunction, is possibly precipitated by hypoxia and/or

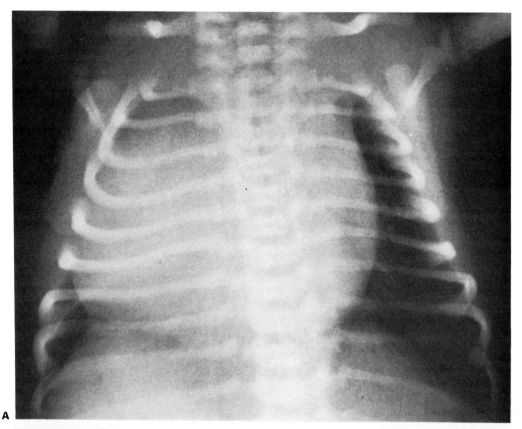

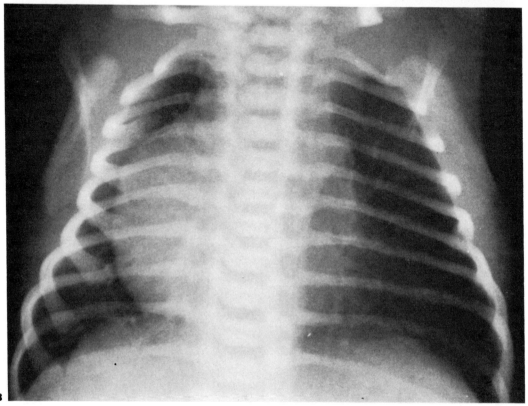

hypoglycemia. Bucciarelli and associates (1976, 1977) report 15 infants with transient tricuspid insufficiency. All infants were term, and the contrast features of perinatal stress, clinical findings of tricuspid regurgitation, ST-T wave abnormalities in the electrocardiogram, and spontaneous resolution of the tricuspid insufficiency suggested that this syndrome results from a reversible form of myocardial dysfunction.

Treatment

In the neonate, treatment is supportive, with judicious use of digoxin and diuretics. In the older patient with symptomatic isolated tricuspid valve incompetence, tricuspid annuloplasty, suture of the cleft, or tricuspid valve replacement may provide acceptable alternatives.

Right ventricular and atrial dilatation and hypertrophy would be expected in tricuspid regurgitation of long standing. During systole, the right ventricle ejects blood both into the pulmonary artery and also into the right atrium. The right ventricle has to increase its stroke volume in order to maintain a normal cardiac output. This necessitates volume overload and overwork of the right ventricle and right atrium. Thus, right ventricular and atrial dilatation and hypertrophy should be anticipated in tricuspid regurgitation of long standing.

CONGENITAL AORTIC INCOMPETENCE: AORTO-LEFT VENTRICULAR TUNNEL

AORTIC regurgitation may accompany a bicuspid aortic valve with stenosis; congenital aortic stenosis; prolapse of the aortic valve with ventricular septal defect; coronary AV fistula; dilatation of the aortic annulus as in Marfan's syndrome or relapsing polychondritis; rheumatic, syphilitic, and bacterial endocarditis; and a ruptured cusp. These disorders have been adequately covered in Chapters 13, 14, and 60.

Aorto–left ventricular tunnel is a most unusual form of congenital aortic runoff and must be considered in the differential diagnosis of congenital aortic incompetence (Levy et al., 1963; Bove and Schartz, 1967; Cooley et al., 1965; Fishbone et al., 1971; Roberts and Morrow, 1965; Perez–Martinez et al., 1973; Somerville et al., 1974). This tunnel represents an abnormal communication that begins in the ascending aorta above the origin of the coronary arteries, bypasses the aortic valve, and terminates in the left ventricle. Since Levy's description of this entity in 1963, less than 25 cases have been reported.

The pathologic anatomy has been quite similar in each of the reported cases. The tunnel originates from an aortic ostium high within the right sinus of Valsalva and about level with the ostium of the right coronary artery. Beyond the opening in the aorta is a true tunnel, with the supracardiac portion aneurysmally dilated. This tunnel passes as a wide ampullalike structure through the right ventricular infundibular portion of the ventricular septum, thus bypassing the aortic valve and entering the aortic vestibule beneath the intercoronary commissure. Associated aortic valve abnormalities have been contributed to the stretching of the aortic valve ring, with subsequent distortion of the aortic cusps.

The diagnosis of aorto–left ventricular tunnel should be considered in any infant or young child presenting with clinical findings suggesting severe aortic incompetence. Somerville (1974) suggested that the earlier the age at which these signs are found, the more likely the diagnosis of aorto–left ventricular tunnel, particularly so if the murmur is loud in the first months of life. Okoroma and associates reviewed 20 reported cases of aortico–left ventricular tunnel in 1976. In 15 patients, the characteristic to-and-fro murmur was heard during the first week of life. Nine patients developed congestive heart failure within the first year of life, and only two patients were described as asymptomatic. Fourteen of the twenty patients were male.

Chest radiography may show dilatation of the ascending aorta, left ventricular hypertrophy, and occasionally disproportionate dilatation of the right aortic sinus.

Ascending aortography will confirm the diagnosis of aorto–left ventricular tunnel. As pointed out by Somerville and associates (1974), the upper part of the right aortic sinus is almost always large, eccentric, and projects anteriorly. The intraventricular portion of the tunnel is frequently not clearly visualized. Central aortic valve regurgitation secondary to valve ring dilatation may occur.

Surgical intervention has been successful in some of the reported patients. In each case, the sole procedure was closure of the aortic ostium of the aorto–left ventricular tunnel. Early closure of the tunnel should prevent aortic valve deformity secondary to ring dilatation and should obviate the need for aortic valve replacement.

The differential diagnosis should include ventricular septal defect with aortic regurgitation, patent ductus arteriosus, aortic incompetence accompanying a bicuspid aortic valve, ruptured sinus of Valsalva, and coronary AV fistula. Congenital absence of the

Figure 44-4. [OPPOSITE] Although the initial chest radiograph suggested dextrocardia, the angiocardiograms revealed levocardia. The right atrium and ventricle are both huge, with severe atrial dilatation due to marked tricuspid regurgitation. *A.* Chest radiograph at 12 hours of age. *B.* At four days of age. There has been significant improvement during this interval.

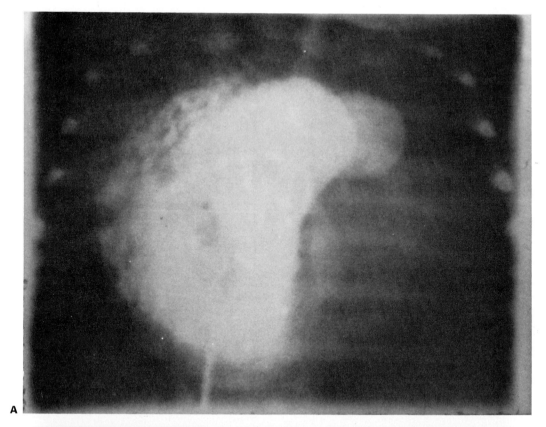

A

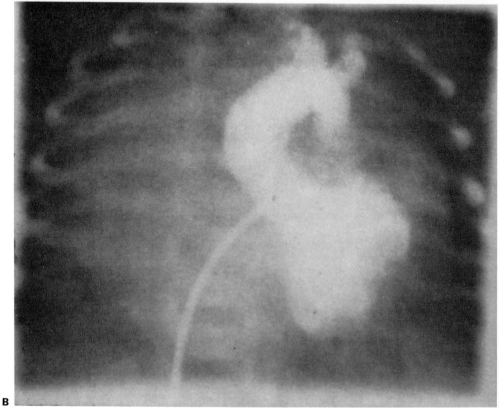

B

pulmonary valve may have a to-and-fro systolic and diastolic murmur, but the signs of aortic runoff will be lacking. Also, when present in the young infant,

bronchial compression secondary to the aneurysmally dilated pulmonary arteries may dominate the clinical picture

CONGENITAL PULMONARY REGURGITATION

PULMONARY valve regurgitation can occur in a variety of anatomic and hemodynamic situations. In general, these can be separated as to whether the pulmonary artery pressure is high or normal (Table 44–1). Isolated congenital pulmonary valve incompetence is uncommon, ranking twenty-first in incidence at the Boston Children's Hospital Medical Center, and accounting for about 0.94 percent of patients encountered there from 1950 to 1970 (Nadas and Fyler, 1972).

Table 44–1. PULMONARY REGURGITATION

I. LOW-PRESSURE PULMONARY ARTERY
A. Isolated congenital pulmonary regurgitation (idiopathic dilatation of the pulmonary artery)
B. Isolated pulmonary stenosis (Chapter 40)
C. Absence of the pulmonary valve
　1. Infantile presentation: associated with tetralogy of Fallot. Symptoms develop secondary to bronchial compression caused by aneurysmal dilatation of the pulmonary arteries (Chapter 27)
　2. Associated with VSD, or other intracardiac lesions
D. Postoperative pulmonary regurgitation
　1. After pulmonary valvotomy for pulmonary stenosis
　2. After outflow reconstruction in tetralogy of Fallot and other conotruncal anomalies
II. HIGH-PRESSURE PULMONARY ARTERY
A. Pulmonary vascular obstructive disease—Eisenmenger's syndrome
B. Primary pulmonary artery hypertension
C. Obstruction distal to pulmonary capillary bed
　1. Mitral stenosis
　2. Cor triatriatum
　3. Individual stenosis of pulmonary veins
　4. Pulmonary vein–occlusive disease
　5. Obstructed total anomalous pulmonary venous return
　6. Left ventricular outflow tract obstruction
　7. Miscellaneous lesions on left side of heart
D. Cor pulmonale

The symptomatic manifestations of congenital pulmonary regurgitation fall into three categories (Perloff, 1970). The largest group of patients are those asymptomatic children, adolescents, and adults with so-called idiopathic dilatation of the pulmonary artery. Although some cardiologists treat idiopathic dilatation of the pulmonary artery and congenital pulmonary valve regurgitation as separate entities (Brayshaw and Perloff, 1962; Perloff, 1970), there is certainly overlap between the two, and Nadas and Fyler, (1972) treat them as the same entity. Patients with idiopathic dilatation of the pulmonary artery are

asymptomatic, and death usually cannot be attributed to this anomaly.

The second category, although a distinct minority, are those patients who succumb in middle age from chronic right ventricular volume overload secondary to pulmonary regurgitation (Dickens et al., 1958; Fish et al., 1959; Fowler and Duchesne, 1958). Mild degrees of pulmonary regurgitation produce little hemodynamic distortion until the degree of regurgitation is worsened by pulmonary hypertension (Hambry and Gulotta, 1967). This rise in pulmonary artery pressure may result from pulmonary parenchymal disease or from left ventricular failure resulting from arteriosclerotic cardiovascular disease.

Finally, the least common type of isolated congenital pulmonary regurgitation consists of those cases of fetal or neonatal heart failure (Ito et al., 1961; Smith et al., 1959; Sanyal et al., 1964). As one might anticipate, the high resistance fetal state of the pulmonary vascular bed aggravates and augments the volume of regurgitation. Congenital absence or hypoplasia/dysplasia of the pulmonary valve can also be associated with ventricular septal defect, tetralogy of Fallot, endocardial cushion defect, and double-outlet right ventricle. Tetralogy of Fallot with absent pulmonary valve produces a unique clinical syndrome and is covered in Chapter 27. When congenital absence of the pulmonary valve occurs in concert with complex cardiac lesions, the clinical picture is often dominated by the intracardiac communication(s) or great artery anomalies, and by the bronchial compression that results secondary to the aneurysmally dilated pulmonary arteries.

Pathology

Complete absence of all three pulmonary cusps is exceedingly rare. Usually, small, nodular, verrucous, hypoplastic masses of primitive endocardium represent the undifferentiated valve tissue. In the symptomatic neonatal group, the valve ring is small and obstructive and is usually associated with a ventricular septal defect of the tetralogy of Fallot type. When associated with tetralogy of Fallot, the conal anatomy is characterized by conventricular malalignment, with deviation of the crista supraventricularis in an anterosuperior direction, producing right ventricular outflow tract obstruction. The pulmonary annulus is restrictive, and there is frequently massive dilatation of the main and branch

Figure 44-5. [OPPOSITE] *A.* Selective right ventriculogram in the AP projection of an infant with severe congenital tricuspid regurgitation, not due to Ebstein's anomaly. The right ventricle is huge and dilated and the pulmonary artery is well seen (studied at 14 hours of age). The left ventriculogram (*B*) of this infant shows a normal-sized left ventricle in levocardia.

pulmonary arteries. The ductus arteriosus is frequently absent. The bronchi are often compressed, and there are significant pulmonary parenchymal changes with obstructive emphysema and atelectasis. These infants are at one end of the clinical/pathologic spectrum of absent pulmonary valve. At the other end are the patients, usually asymptomatic, with isolated pulmonary insufficiency. In the asymptomatic patient with idiopathic dilatation of the pulmonary artery, the valve tissue is hypoplastic and dysplastic. The main and branch pulmonary arteries are dilated, and the right ventricle also shows signs of mild dilatation. The tricuspid valve is usually normal. In this situation, the left heart chambers and aorta are normal.

This chapter will concern itself primarily with the condition known as idiopathic dilatation of the pulmonary artery. This is an uncommon condition and was first described by Wessler and Jaches in 1923, in a patient with radiographic findings of an enlarged pulmonary artery, with no obvious etiology for this dilatation. This diagnosis can be made only after other organic causes are excluded. The etiology and pathogenesis of this anomaly are not known.

Clinical Features

The patient with idiopathic dilatation of the pulmonary artery is asymptomatic. In a physical examination, one not infrequently palpates a diastolic thrill along the left sternal border (Nadas and Fyler, 1972).

The most characteristic auscultatory finding is a moderately loud, low-frequency, decrescendo diastolic murmur at the second to fourth left interspace. A blowing systolic murmur, usually of lower intensity and frequency, may be heard in the pulmonic area. Rarely, there may be no murmur (Desmukh et al., 1960; Goetz and Nellen, 1953; Kjellberg et al., 1959). The second heart sound is often normal, but if the valve tissue is significantly deficient, then the pulmonic closure component may be inaudible. In addition, an early systolic ejection click (0.03 to 0.07 after the first heart sound) is audible at the left upper sternal border (Desmukh et al., 1960; Leatham and Vogelpoel, 1954; Minhas and Gasul, 1959). The arterial pulse pressure should be normal.

Electrocardiography

The electrovectorcardiogram is usually normal. Occasionally, findings of mild right ventricular hypertrophy will be evident.

Echocardiography

In our experience with trivial pulmonary regurgitation, the echocardiogram will be normal. With moderate pulmonary regurgitation, the right ventricular end-diastolic dimensions will be increased and the ventricular septal motion may be flattened or reversed.

Radiologic Examination

The chest radiograph will show a normal heart size, with a prominent main pulmonary artery (Wessler and Jaches, 1923; Lendrum and Shaffer, 1959). The peripheral pulmonary vascularity is normal. The aortic arch is left-sided. The chest radiography is indistinguishable from that of a patient with isolated valvar pulmonary stenosis.

Cardiac Catheterization

The catheterization findings in the patient with idiopathic dilatation of the pulmonary artery with mild pulmonary regurgitation will usually reveal normal hemodynamics (Deshmukh et al., 1960; Kjelberg et al., 1959; Greene et al., 1949). In those patients with pulmonary regurgitation, the pulmonary arterial pressure contour may appear ventriculoid, consistent with the low pulmonary diastolic pressure. A slight pressure gradient across the pulmonary orifice is commonly encountered, but the gradient is usually less than 10 mm of mercury. The pressure difference across the pulmonary valve annulus probably results from a fall in the pulmonary trunk pressure as blood is rapidly ejected into the compliant and dilated pulmonary artery.

Angiocardiography

Right ventricular biplane angiocardiography will show the dilatation of the main and branch pulmonary arteries. The levophase of this injection should opacify normal left heart chambers. Pulmonary angiography performed with the tip of the catheter quite distal from the pulmonary valve will also show the dilatation of the pulmonary trunk and should demonstrate any pulmonary regurgitation. With the venous catheter across the pulmonary valve, catheter recoil or inadequate positioning of the catheter may lead to spurious pulmonary regurgitation. Intracardiac phonocardiography can very easily detect the low-frequency murmur of pulmonary incompetence in equivocal cases. It is of importance to note that in these patients, the pulmonary annulus orifice is not obstructive, in contrast to the patient with tetralogy of Fallot and absent pulmonary valve. Also, in the group of patients with idiopathic dilatation of the pulmonary artery, there is no evidence of bronchial compression and these patients are symptom-free.

Differential Diagnosis

As mentioned earlier, pulmonary regurgitation can occur in a variety of clinical and anatomic situations. In the patient with idiopathic dilatation of the pulmonary artery, the heart is of normal size, and the electrocardiogram is normal. Cardiac catheterization will be normal, failing to demonstrate any significant hemodynamic abnormality. Deshmukh and associates (1960) suggested that the catheterization finding of a normal right ventricular pressure, with perhaps a trivial gradient across the pulmonary annulus, is essential before a diagnosis of idiopathic dilatation of the pulmonary artery can be made. Furthermore, this will enable differentiation from mild valvar pulmonary stenosis.

The differential diagnosis should include valvar pulmonary stenosis, pulmonary vascular obstruction, and aortic regurgitation. The auscultatory findings of mild aortic regurgitation are a high-frequency, decrescendo diastolic murmur beginning with aortic closure. Usually, there is no difficulty in distinguishing the low-frequency diastolic murmur of pulmonary regurgitation (with a low pulmonary artery pressure) from the murmur of aortic regurgitation. The patient with pulmonary regurgitation secondary to pulmonary vascular obstructive disease should have clinical findings of right ventricular and pulmonary artery hypertension. A sustained right ventricular lift should be palpated, and the pulmonary closure component of the second sound should be accentuated. The electrovectorcardiogram should document right ventricular hypertrophy. The echocardiogram will show increased right ventricular wall thickness and a long preejection period. Occasionally, the patient with very trivial valve pulmonary stenosis will have clinical findings similar to those observed in the patient with idiopathic dilatation of the pulmonary artery. In the patient with stenosis, the stenotic murmur should be more prominent than any diastolic murmur. The chest radiograph in both may be identical, and in very mild pulmonary stenosis, both the electrocardiogram and vectorcardiogram will be normal.

Prognosis

The prognosis of patients with idiopathic dilatation of the pulmonary artery is generally good, and yet some patients may experience difficulty in middle age. Yet it has been reported that major degrees of pulmonary regurgitation produced experimentally in animals may lead to chronic heart failure (Bender et al., 1963; Camp et al., 1964; Fowler and Duchesne, 1958). Indeed, right ventricular failure can result from congenital pulmonary regurgitation in the adult (Hambry and Gulotta, 1967). It must also be remembered that idiopathic dilatation of the pulmonary artery can be seen in patients with Marfan's syndrome (Van Buchem, 1958). Obviously, this genetically determined connective tissue disorder will add prognostic significance to this otherwise relatively benign disorder. Although rare, susceptibility to infectious endocarditis produces another hazard to those patients (Holmes et al., 1968; Ford et al., 1956).

The neonate with congenital pulmonary regurgitation and severe heart failure is most uncommon. Any one institution's experience with this small group of patients is far too small to make firm comments. Obviously, some of these infants will symptomatically improve with anticongestive therapy and with regression of the fetal pattern of pulmonary vasoconstrictions. Other infants may succumb to the effects of heart failure and hypoxia.

When congenital absence of the pulmonary valve is associated with tetralogy of Fallot, the clinical manifestations, course, therapy, and prognosis are vastly different. This clinical situation is covered in Chapter 27. The neonate with severe heart failure may improve with judicious use of digoxin and diuretics. This improvement may parallel the fall in pulmonary vascular resistance over the first few days of life. However, some infants with severe heart failure and hypoxia will die in this neonatal period.

REFERENCES

Congenital Mitral Regurgitation

Abbott, M. E.: *Nelson's Loose-Leaf Medicine.* Thomas Nelson & Sons, New York, 1932, Vol. 4, p. 223.

Actis-Dato, A., and Milocco, I.: Anomalous attachment of the mitral valve to the ventricular wall. *Am. J. Cardiol.,* **17**:278, 1966.

Anderson, D. H., and Kelly, J.: Endocardial fibroelastosis: I. Endocardial fibroelastosis associated with congenital malformations of the heart. II. A clinical and pathological investigation of those cases without associated cardiac malformations. *Pediatrics,* **18**:513, 1956.

Becker, A. E.; Becker, M. J.; and Edwards, J. E.: Anomalies associated with coarctation of aorta. Particular reference to infancy. *Circulation,* **41**:1067, 1970.

Bentivoglio, L. G.; Uricchil, J. F.; Waldow, A.; Likoff, W.; and Goldberg, H.: An electrocardiographic analysis of sixtyfive cases of mitral regurgitation. *Circulation,* **18**:572, 1958.

Bharati, S., and Lev, M.: Congenital poly-valvular disease. *Circulation,* **47**:575, 1973.

Bjork, V. O.; Lidin, H.; and Malers, E.: The evaluation of the degree of mitral insufficiency by selective left ventricular angiocardiography. *Am. Heart J.,* **60**:691, 1960.

Braunwald, E.: Mitral regurgitation: Physiologic, clinical and surgical considerations. *N. Engl. J. Med.,* **281**:425, 1969.

Braunwald, E.; Ross, E. S.; Morrow, A. G.; and Roberts, W. C.: Differential diagnosis of mitral regurgitation in childhood: clinical pathological conference at the National Institutes of Health. *Ann. Intern. Med.,* **54**:1223, 1961.

Braunwald, E., Welch, G. H., Jr.; and Morrow, A. G.: The effects of acutely increased systemic resistance on the left atrial pressure pulse: a method for the clinical detection of mitral insufficiency. *J. Clin. Invest.,* **37**:35, 1958.

Brockenbrough, E. C.; Braunwald, E.; Roberts, W. C.; and Morrow, A. G.: Partial persistent atrioventricular canal simulating pure mitral regurgitation. *Am. Heart J.,* **63**:9 1962.

Burgess, J.; Clark, R.; Kamigaki, M.; and Cohn, K.: Echocardiographic findings in different types of mitral regurgitation. *Circulation,* **48**:97, 1973.

Callaghan, J. C.: Mural leaflet advancement for free mitral valve regurgitation resulting from dilatation of the annulus. *Dis. Chest,* **43**:87, 1963.

Carney, E. K.; Braunwald, E.; Roberts, W. C.; Aygen, M.; and Morrow, A. G.: Congenital mitral regurgitation. *Am. J. Med.,* **33**:223, 1962.

Chiechi, M. A.; Lees, W. M.; and Thompson, R.: Functional anatomy of the normal mitral valve. *J. Thorac. Surg.,* **32**:378, 1956.

Cosby, R. S.; Giddings, J. A.; See, J. R.; Mayo, M.; and Boomershine, P.: The echocardiogram in non-rheumatic mitral insufficiency. *Chest,* **66**:642, 1974.

Creech, O., Jr.; Ledbetter, M. K.; and Reemtsma, K.: Congenital mitral insufficiency with cleft posterior leaflet. *Circulation,* **25**:390, 1962.

Dalith, F.: Systolic expansion or aortodiastolic displacement. *Acta Radiol.,* **45**:217, 1956.

Davila, J. C.: Hemodynamics of mitral insufficiency. *Am. J. Cardiol.,* **2**:135, 1958.

Davachi, F.; Moller, J. H.; and Edwards, J. E.: Diseases of the mitral valve in infancy. An anatomic analysis of 55 cases. *Circulation,* **43**:565, 1971.

Dillon, J.; Haine, C.; Chang, S.; and Felgenbaum, H.: Use of echocardiography in patients with prolapse mitral valve. *Circulation,* **43**:503, 1971.

Du Plessis, L. A.; Schnaid, E.; and Bloom, K. R.: Follow-up of Starr Edwards mitral valve replacements in children. *S. Afr. Med. J.*, **47**:1521, 1973.

Eckberg, D. L.; Gault, J. H.; Bouchard, R. L.; Karliner, J. S.; and Ross, J., Jr.: Mechanics of left ventricular contraction in chronic severe mitral regurgitation. *Circulation*, **47**:1252, 1973.

Edwards, J. E., and Burchell, H. B.: Pathologic anatomy of mitral insufficiency. *Proc. Mayo Clin.*, **33**:497, 1958.

Effler, D. B.; Groves, L. K.; Martinez, W. V.; and Kolff, W. J.: Open heart surgery for mitral insufficiency. *J. Thorac. Surg.*, **36**:665, 1958.

Ellis, F. H., Jr.; Brandenburg. R. O.; Callahan, I. A.; and Marshall, H. W.: Open heart surgery for acquired mitral insufficiency. *Arch. Surg.*, **79**:222, 1959.

Ellis, L. B., and Ramirez, A.: The clinical course of patients with severe "rheumatic" mitral insufficiency. *Am. Heart J.*, **78**:406, 1969.

Evans, J. R.; Rowe, R. D.; and Keith, J. D.: The clinical diagnosis of atrial septal defect in children. *Am. J. Med.*, **30**:345, 1961.

Evans, R. W.; Williams, T. H.; and Nelson, W. P.: Incomplete differentiation of cardiac valves. *Am. J. Cardiol.*, **31**:646, 1973.

Ferencz, C.: Atrio-ventricular defect of membranous septum: left ventricular-right atrial communication with malformed mitral valve simulating aortic stenosis. Report of a case, *Bull. Hopkins Hosp.*, **100**:209, 1957.

Ferencz, C.; Johnson, A. L.; and Wiglesworth, F. W.: Congenital mitral stenosis. *Circulation*, **9**:161, 1954.

Freed, M. R., Keave, J. F.; Van Praagh, R.; Castaneda, A. R.; Bernhard, W. F.; and Nadas, A. S.: Coarctation of the aorta with congenital mitral regurgitation. *Circulation*, **49**:1175, 1974.

Gilman, R. A.; Lehman, J. S.; Musser, B. G.; and Russell, R.: Mitral insufficiency—its quantitation by cardiac ventriculography. *JAMA*, **166**:2124, 1958.

Gott, V. L.; DeWall, R.; Gonzales, J. L.; Hodges, P. C.; Varco, R. L.; and Lillehei, C. W.: The direct vision surgical correction of pure mitral insufficiency by use of annuloplasty or a valvular prosthesis. *Univ. Minn. Med. Bull.*, **29**:69, 1957.

Harshaw, C. W.; Grossman, W.; Munro, A. B.; and McLaurin, L. P.: Reduced systemic vascular resistance as therapy for severe mitral regurgitation of valvular origin. *Ann. Intern. Med.*, **83**:312, 1975.

Helmholz, H. G., Jr.; Daugherty, G. W.; and Edwards, J. E.: Cardiac clinics: congenital "mitral" insufficiency in association with corrected transposition of the great vessels: report of probable clinical case and review of 6 cases studied pathologically. *Proc. Mayo Clin.*, **31**:82, 1956.

Jaffe, R. B.: Systemic atrioventricular valve regurgitation in corrected transposition of the great vessels. Angiographic differentiation of operable and nonoperable valve deformities. *Am. J. Cardiol.*, **37**:395, 1976.

Kahn, D. R.; Stern, A. M.; Sigmann, J. M.; Kirsh, M. M.; Lenox, S.; and Sloan, H.: Longterm results of valvuloplasty for mitral insufficiency in children. *J. Thorac. Cardiovasc. Surg.*, **53**:1, 1967.

Kay, E. B.; Mendelsohn, D.; and Zimmerman, H. A.: Evaluation of the surgical correction of mitral regurgitation. *Circulation*, **23**:813, 1961.

Kay, E. B.; Nogueira, C.; Heal, L. R.; Coenen, J. P.; and Zimmerman, H. A.: Surgical treatment of mitral insufficiency. *J. Thorac. Surg.*, **36**:677, 1958.

Kent, E. M.; Ford, W. B.; Neville, J. F., Jr.: and Fisher, D. L.: Experiences with the Davila-Glover purse-string suture in the correction of mitral insufficiency: a critical appraisal. *J. Thorac. Surg.*, **36**:421, 1958.

Kerber, R.; Isaeff, D.; and Haneolk, E.: Echocardiographic patterns in patients with the syndrome of systolic click and late systolic murmur. *N. Engl. J. Med.*, **284**:691, 1971.

King, H.; Su, C. S.; and Jontz, J. G.: Partial replacement of the mitral valve with synthetic fabric. *J. Thorac. Surg.*, **40**:12, 1960.

Kirklin, J. W. and Pacifico, A. D.: Surgery for acquired valvular heart disease. (second of two parts). *N. Engl. J. Med.*, **288**:194, 1975.

Klint, R.; Hernandez, A.; Weldon, C.; Hartmann, A. F., Jr.; and Goldring, D.: Replacement of cardiac valves in children. *J. Pediatr.*, **80**:980, 1972.

Kouchoukos, N. T.: Problems in mitral valve replacement. In Kirklin, J. W. (Ed.): *Advances in Cardiovascular Surgery*. Grune & Stratton, New York, 1973, p. 205.

Lam, J. H. C.; Ranganathan, N.; Wigle, E. D.; and Silver, M. D.:

Morphology of the human mitral valve. I. chordae tendineae: A new classification. *Circulation*, **41**:449, 1970.

LaMotta, E. P., and Gulotta, G. A.: Case report: analysis of left atrial curve and pulmonary capillary (wedge) curve in a patient with predominant mitral insufficiency. *Bull. St. Francis Hosp. (Roslyn)*, **16**:24, 1959.

Layman, T. E., and Edwards, J. E.: Anomalous mitral arcade. A type of congenital mitral insufficiency. *Circulation*, **35**:389, 1967.

Levinson, D. C.; Wilburne, M.; Meehan, J. P., Jr.; and Shubin, H.: Evidence for retrograde transpulmonary propagation of the V (or regurgitant) wave in mitral insufficiency. *Am. J. Cardiol.*, **2**:159, 1958.

Lind, J.; Rocha, M.; and Wegelius, M. D.: The value of fast angiocardiography in the early diagnosis of patent ductus arteriosus. *Am. J. Roentgenol.*, **77**:235, 1957.

Linde, L. M., and Adams, F. H.: Mitral insufficiency and pulmonary hypertension accompanying patent ductus arteriosus. *Am. J. Cardiol.*, **33**:713, 1959.

Long, D. M.; Gott, V. L.; Sterns, L. P.; Finsterbusch, W.; Meyne, N.; Varco, R. L.; and Lillehei, C. W.: Reconstruction and replacement of the mitral valve with plastic prosthesis. In *Prosthetic Valves for Cardiac Surgery*. Charles C Thomas, Publisher, Springfield, Ill., 1961, pp. 385–401.

Lowe, L.; and Bakst, A. A.: Basic criteria for effective surgical correction of mitral insufficiency. *Angiology*, **9**:112, 1958.

Luisada, A. A.; and Szatkowski, J.: Relative vs. organic mitral insufficiency. *Am. J. Cardiol.*, **5**:111, 1960.

McGoon, D. C.: Complex congenital malformations. Surgery for complete form of atrioventricular canal. In Kirklin, J. W. (ed.): *Advances in Cardiovascular Surgery*. Grune & Stratton, New York, 1973, p. 45.

McGoon, D. C.: Repair of mitral insufficiency due to ruptured chordae tendineae. *J. Thorac. Surg.*, **39**:357, 1960.

McMullen, M. H.; Wallace, R. B.; Weidman, W. H.; and McGovin, D. C.: Surgical treatment of complete atrioventricular canal. *Surgery*, **72**:905, 1972.

Malers, E.; Bjork, V. O.; Culhed, I.; and Lodin, H.: Transposition functionally totally corrected, associated with "mitral" insufficiency. *Am. Heart J.*, **59**:816, 1960.

Meredino, K. A., and Bruce, R. A.: One hundred seventeen surgically treated cases of valvular rheumatic heart disease with preliminary report of two cases of mitral regurgitation treated under direct vision with aid of a pump oxygenator. *JAMA*, **164**:749, 1957.

Morris, E. W. T.: Some features of the mitral valve. *Thorax*, **15**:70, 1960.

Musser, B. G.; Bongas, J. A.; and Goldberg, H.: Left heart catheterization; with particular reference to mitral and aortic valvular disease. *Am. Heart J.*, **52**:567, 1956.

Nichols, H. I.; Blanco, G.; Uricchio, J. F.; and Likoff, W.: Open heart surgery for mitral regurgitation and stenosis. *Arch. Surg.*, **72**:128, 1961.

Prior, J. T.: Congenital anomalies of the mitral valve—two cases associated with long survival. *Am. Heart J.*, **46**:649, 1953.

Ranganathan, N.; Lam, J. H. C.; Wigle, E. D.; and Silver, M. D.: Morphology of the human mitral valve. II. The valve leaflet. *Circulation*, **41**:459, 1970.

Rastelli, G. C.; Kirklin, J. W.; and Titus, J. L.: Anatomic observations on complete form of persistent common atrioventricular canal with special reference to atrioventricular valves. *Mayo Clin, Proc.*, **41**:296, 1966.

Rastelli, G. C.; Ongley, P. A.; Kirklin, J. W.; and McGoon, D. C.: Surgical repair of the complete form of persistent common atrioventricular canal. *J. Thorac, Cqrdiovasc. Surg.*, **55**:299, 1968.

Reed, G. E.; Kloth, H. H.; Kiely, B.; Danilowicz, D. A.; Rader, B.; and Doyle, E. F.: Longterm results of mitral annuloplasty in children with rheumatic mitral regurgitation. *Circulation*, **49** (suppl. II):II—189, 1974.

Rosenquist, G. C.: Congenital mitral valve disease associated with coarctation of aorta. A spectrum that includes parachute deformity of the mitral valve. *Circulation*, **49**:985, 1974.

Ross, J., Jr.; Braunwald, E.; and Morrow, A. G.: Clinical and hemodynamic observations in pure mitral insufficiency. *Am. J. Cardiol.*, **1**:11, 1958.

Ross, J., Jr.; Cooper, T.; and Lombardo, C. R.: Hemodynamic observations in experimental mitral regurgitation. *Surgery*, **47**:795, 1960.

Rowe, R. D., and Hoffman, T.: Transient myocardial ischemia of the newborn infant: A form of severe cardiorespiratory distress in fullterm infant. *J. Pediatr.*, **81**:243, 1972.

Scheiken, R. M.; Friedman, S.; Waldhausen, J.; and Johnson, J.: Isolated congenital mitral insufficiency. Pathologic and surgical variations in five children. *J. Pediatr. Surg.*, **6**:49, 1971.

Semans, J. H., and Taussig, H. B.: Congenital "aneurysmal" dilatation of the left auricle. *Bull. Hopkins Hosp.*, **63**:404, 1938.

Shone, J. D.; Armas, S. M.; Manning, J. A.; and Keith, J. D.: The mumps antigen skin test in endocardial fibroelastosis. *Pediatrics*, **37**:483, 1966.

Starkey, G. W. B.: Surgical experiences in the treatment of congenital mitral stenosis and mitral insufficiency. *J. Thorac. Surg.*, **38**:336, 1959.

Sweatman, T.; Selzer, A.; Kamagaki, M.; and Cohn, K.: Echocardiographic diagnosis of mitral regurgitation due to ruptured chordae tendinae. *Circulation*, **46**:580, 1972.

Tainer, N. S.; Stern, A. M.; and Sloan, H. E.; Jr.: Congenital mitral insufficiency. *Circulation*, **23**:339, 1961.

Tori, G., and Garusi, G. F.: Left cardiac ventriculography by means of percutaneous catheterization of a femoral artery in the diagnosis of mitral insufficiency. *Acta Radiol.*, **54**:170, 1960.

Trusler, G. A.; MacGregor, D. C.; and Keith, J. D.: Mitral valve replacement in a 14 month old child. *Can. Med. Assoc. J.*, **95**:1297, 1966.

Van der Horst, R. L.; le Roux, B. T.; Rogers, N. M. A.; and Gottsman, M. S.: Mitral valve replacement in childhood. A report of 51 patients. *Am. Heart J.*, **85**:624, 1973.

Vineberg, A.; Dobell, A. R. C.; and Gutelius, J.: Mitral insufficiency: report of an adult case treated by open heart surgery. *Can. Med. Assoc. J.*, **79**:273, 1958.

Wells, B. G.: The diagnosis of mitral incompetence from left atrial pressure curves. *Br. Heart J.*, **20**:321, 1958.

Wilson, M. G., and Lim, W. N.: Natural history of rheumatic heart disease in third, fourth and fifth decades of life. I. Prognosis with special reference to surroundings. *Circulation*, **16**:700, 1957.

Wilson, W. S.; Brandt, R. L.; Judge, R. D.; Morris, J. D.; and Clifford, M. E.: An appraisal of the double indicator-dilution method for the estimation of mitral regurgitation in human subjects. *Circulation*, **23**:64, 1961.

Congenital Tricuspid Regurgitation

Barr, P. A.; Celermajer, J. M.; Bowdler, J. D. and Cartmill, T. B.: Severe congenital tricuspid incompetence in the neonate. *Circulation*, **49**:962, 1974.

Becker, A. E.; Becker, M. J.; and Edwards, J. E. Pathologic spectrum of dysplasia of the tricuspid valve. Features in common with Ebstein's malformation. *Arch. Pathol.*, **91**:167, 1971.

Bharati, S. and Lev, M.: Congenital polyvalvular disease. *Circulation*, **47**:575, 1973.

Brown, R., and Pickering, D.: Persistent transitional circulation. *Arch. Dis. Child.*, **49**:883, 1974.

Bucciarelli, R. L.; Nelson, R. M., Jr.; Egan, E. A.; Eitzman, D. V.; and Gessner, I. H.: Transient tricuspid insufficiency: Manifestation of myocardial dysfunction in stressed newborns. *Am. J. Cardiol.*, **37**:124, 1976 (abstr.).

Bucciarelli, R. L.; Nelson, R. M.; Egan, E. A., II; Eitzman, D. V.; and Gessner, I. H.: Transient tricuspid insufficiency of the newborn: A form of myocardial dysfunction in stressed newborns. *Pediatrics*, **59**:330, 1977.

Evans, R. W.; Williams, T. H.; and Nelson, W. P.: Incomplete differentiation of cardiac valves. Angiographic diagnosis. *Am. J. Cardiol.*, **31**:646, 1973.

Kanjuh, V. I.; Stevenson, J. E.; Amplate, K.; and Edwards, J. E.: Congenitally unguarded tricuspid orifice with coexistent mitral atresia. *Circulation*, **30**:911, 1964.

Liberthson, R. R.; Paul, M. H.; Muster, A. J.; Arcilla, R. A.; Eckner, F. A. O.; and Lev, M.: Straddling and displaced atrioventricular orifices and valves with primitive ventricles. *Circulation*, **43**:213, 1971.

Nielson, H. C.; Riemenschneider, T. A.; and Jaffe, R. B.: Persistent transitional circulation. Roentgenographic findings in thirteen infants. *Radiology*, **120**:649, 1976.

Reisman, M.; Hipona, F. A.; Bloor, C. M.; and Talner, N. S.: Congenital tricuspid insufficiency. A cause of massive cardiomegaly and heart failure in the neonate. *J. Pediatri.*, **66**:869, 1965.

Riemenschneider, T. A.; Nielsen, H. C., Ruttenberg, H. D.; and Jaffe, R. B.: Disturbances of the transitional circulation. Spectrum of pulmonary hypertension and myocardial dysfunction. *J. Pediatri.*, **89**:622, 1976.

Rowe, R. D.: Abnormal pulmonary vasoconstriction in the newborn. *Pediatrics*, **59**:319, 1977.

Rowe, R. D., and Hoffman, T.: Transient myocardial ischemia of the newborn infant: A form of severe cardiorespiratory distress in full-term infants. *J. Pediatr.*, **81**:243, 1972.

Schiebler, G. L.; Van Mierop, L. HS.; and Krovetz, L. J.: Diseases of the tricuspid valve. In Moss, A. J., and Adams, F. M. (eds.): *Heart Disease in Infants and Children, and Adolescents.* Williams & Wilkins, Baltimore, 1968, Chap. 23.

Shone, J. D.; Anderson, R. C.; Elliott, L. P.; Amplate, K.; Lillehei, C. W.; and Edwards, J. E.: Clinical pathologic conference. *AmeAm. Heart J.*, **64**:547, 1962.

Talner, N. S., and Campbell, A. G. M.: Recognition and management of cardiologic problems in the newborn infant. In Friedman, W. F.; Leach, M.; and Sonnenblick, E. H. (eds.): *Neonatal Heart Disease.* Grune & Stratton, New York, 1972, pp. 100–101.

Congenital Aortic Incompetence: Aorto–Left Ventricular Tunnel

Bernhard, W. F.; Plauth, W.; and Fyler, D.: Unusual abnormalities of the aortic root or valve necessitating surgical correction in early childhood. *N. Engl. J. Med.*, **282**:68–71, 1970.

Bove, W. C., and Morrow, A. G.: Aorto-left ventricular tunnel. A cause of massive aortic regurgitation and of intra-cardiac aneurysm. *Am. J. Med.*, **39**:662, 1965.

Cooley, R. N.; Harris, L. C.; and Rodin, A. E.: Abnormal communication between the aorta and left ventricle. *Circulation*, **31**:564–571, 1965.

Fishbone, G.; DeLeuchtenberg, N.; and Stansel, H. C.: Aorto–left ventricular tunnel. *Radiology*, **98**:579, 1971.

Levy, M. J.; Lillehei, C. W.; Anderson, R. C.; Amplate, K.; and Edwards, J. E.: Aorto–left ventricular tunnel. *Circulation*, **27**:841–53, 1963.

Morgan, R. I., and Mazur, J. H.: Congenital aneurysm of aortic root with fistual to left ventricle. *Circulation*, **28**:589–94, 1963.

Roberts, W. C., and Morrow, A. G.: Aorto–left ventricular tunnel. A cause of massive aortic regurgitation and of intra-cardiac aneurysm. *Am. J. Med.*, **39**:662, 1965.

Somerville, J.; English, T.; and Ross, D. N.: Aorto-left ventricular tunnel. Clinical features and surgical management. *Br. Heart J.*, **36**:321–28, 1974.

Okoroma, E.; Perry, L. W.; Scott, L. P.; and McClenathan, J. E.: Aortico-left ventricular tunnel. Clinical profile, diagnostic features and surgical considerations. *J,. Thorac. Cardiovasc. Surg.*, **71**:238, 1976.

Perez-Martinez, V.; Quero, M.; Castro, C.; Moreno, F.; Brito, J. M.; and Merino, G.: Aortico–left ventricular tunnel. A clinical and pathologic review of this uncommon entity. *Am. Heart J.*, **85**:237, 1973.

Congenital Pulmonary Regurgitation

Bender, H. W.; Austin, W. G.; Ebert, P. A.; Greenfield, L. J.; Tsunakawa, T.; and Morrow, A. G.: Experimental pulmonary regurgitation. *J. Thorac. Cardiovasc. Surg.*, **45**:451, 1963.

Brayshaw, J. R., and Perloff, J. K.: Congenital pulmonary insufficiency complicating idiopathic dilatation of the pulmonary artery. *Am. J. Cardiol.*, **10**:282, 1962.

Camp, F. A.; McDonald, K. E.; and Schenk, W. G., Jr.: Hemodynamics of experimental pulmonic insufficiency. *J. Thorac, Cardiovasc. Surg.*, **47**:372, 1964.

Campeau, L. A.; Ruble, P. E.; and Cooksey, W. B.: Congenital absence of pulmonary valve. *Circulation*, **15**:397, 1957.

Desmukh, M.; Guvenc, S.: Bentivoglio, L.; and Goldberg, H.: Idiopathic dilatation of the pulmonary artery. *Circulation*, **21**:710, 1960.

Dickens, J.; Raber, G. T.; and Goldberg, H.: Dynamic pulmonary regurgitation associated with a bicuspid valve. *Ann. Intern. Med.*, **48**:851, 1958.

Fish. R. G.; Takaro, T.; and Cvymes, T.: Prognostic considerations in primary isolated insufficiency of the pulmonic valve. *N. Engl. J. Med.*, **261**:739, 1959.

Ford, A. B.; Hellerstein, H. K.; Wood, C.; and Kelly, H. B.: Isolated congenital bicuspid pulmonary valve. *Am. J. Med.*, **20**:474, 1956.

Fowler, N. O., and Duchesne, E. R.: Effect of experimental pulmonary valvular insufficiency on the circulation. *J. Thorac. Cardiovasc. Surg.*, **35**:643, 1958.

Fowler, N. O.; Mannix, E. P.; and Noble, W.: Some effects of partial pulmonary valvectomy. *Circ. Res.*, **4**:8, 1956.

Goetz, R. H., and Nellen, M. G.: Idiopathic dilatation of the pulmonary artery. *S. Afr. Med. J.*, **27**:360, 1953.

Greene, D. G.; Baldwin, E. deF.; Baldwin, J. S.; Himmelstein, A.; Roh, C. E.; and Cournand, A.: Pure congenital pulmonary stenosis and idiopathic congenital dilatation of the pulmonary artery. *Am. J. Med.*, **6**:24, 1949.

Hambry, R. I., and Gulotta, S. J.: Pulmonic valvular insufficiency: Etiology, recognition, and management. *Am. Heart J.*, **74**:110, 1967.

Holmes, J. C.; Fowler, N. O.; and Kaplan, S.: Pulmonary valvular insufficiency. *Am. J. Med.*, **44**:851, 1968.

Ito, T.; Engle, M. A.; and Holswade, G. R.: Congenital insufficiency of the pulmonic valve. A rare cause of neonatal heart failure. *Pediatrics*, **28**:712, 1961.

Kjellberg, S. R.; Mannheimer, E.; Ruohe, U.; and Jonsson, B.: "Idiopathic" dilatation of the pulmonary artery. In *Diagnosis of Congenital Heart Disease*, 2nd Year Book Publishers, Chicago, 1959, p. 831.

Leatham, A., and Vogelpoel, L.: The early systolic sound in dilatation of the pulmonary artery. *Br. Heart J.*, **16**:21, 1959.

Lendrum, B. L., and Shaffer, A. B.: Isolated congenital pulmonic valvular regurgitation. *Am. Heart J.*, **87**:298, 1959.

Minhas, K., and Gasul, B. M.: Systolic clicks: A clinical phonocardiographic and hemodynamic evaluation. *Am. Heart J.*, **57**:49, 1959.

Nadas, A. S., and Fyler, D. C.: *Pediatric Cardiology*. W. B. Saunders, Philadelphia, 1972.

Perloff, J. K.: *The Clinical Recognition of Congenital Heart Disease*. W. B. Saunders, Philadelphia, 1970.

Ratcliffe, J. W.; Hurt, R. L.; Belmonte, B.; and Gerbode, F.: The physiologic effects of experimental total pulmonary insufficiency. *Surgery*, **41**:43, 1957.

Sanyal, S. K.; Hipona, F. A.; Browne, M.; and Talner, N. S.: Congenital insufficiency of the pulmonary valve. *J. Pediatr.*, **64**:728, 1964.

Smith, R. D.; Dushane, J. W.; and Edwards, J. E.: Congenital insufficiency of the pulmonary valve, including a case of fetal cardiac failure. *Circulation*, **20**:554, 1959.

Van Buchem, F. S. P.: Cardiovascular disease in arachnodactyly. *Acta Med. Scand.*, **161**:197, 1958.

Wessler, H., and Jaches, L.: *Clinical Roentgenology of Diseases of the Chest*. Southworth, Troy, N. Y., 1923, p. 26.

CHAPTER

45

Ebstein's Disease

John D. Keith

Pathology

IN 1866 Wilhelm Ebstein, a German physician, reported the autopsy finding in a young man, aged 19, who had a malformation of the tricuspid valve and right ventricle. Since that date there have been close to 150 cases of this anomaly reported in the literature, approximately half of them postmortem studies. The clinical diagnosis has been made with relative frequency in the past 20 years. Prior to that the anomaly was recognized only at the autopsy table.

Pathology

In Figure 45–1 it will be noted that the right atrium is greatly enlarged and that the tricuspid valve, instead of being in its usual position, has prolapsed into the body of the right ventricle in such a manner

Ebstein's Disease   A286/54

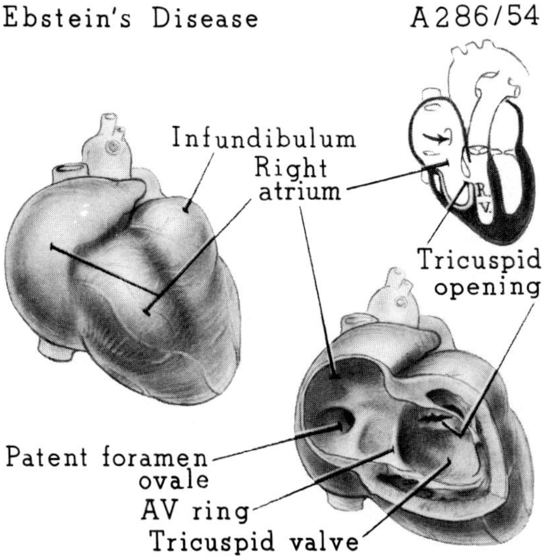

Figure 45-1. Drawing of specimen showing Ebstein's disease.

that the cavity is greatly reduced in size. The septal and posterior cusps of the tricuspid valve are grossly deformed and shortened, with their chordae tendineae appearing like small trabeculae in the reduced right ventricle. The attachment of these deformed valves and the trabeculae produces two chambers in the right ventricle, one toward the apex and the other toward the infundibulum, with a relatively small opening between. The wall of the right ventricle is unusually thin, while the pulmonary conus is slightly hypertrophied.

Figure 45–1 depicts a typical example of Ebstein's anomaly. All cases have deformities of some degree of the septal and posterior cusps. The anterior cusp of the tricuspid valve thus ballons out and guards the entrance of the right ventricle; it appears to be relatively adequate for this function, although tricuspid insufficiency may be demonstrated at times in the right atrial pressure tracing. The thin wall of the right ventricle shows a defective musculature and some fibrosis. This is also true of the wall of the right atrium, which in the younger cases shows hypertrophy and in the older cases fibrosis.

In three-fourths of the cases either the foramen ovale is patent or the fossa of the valve is fenestrated. The defective right ventricle cannot handle the returning blood adequately as a rule; hence a large proportion is shunted through the foramen ovale into the left ventricle and the systemic circulation. Thus this anomaly is commonly classified in the cyanotic group, although the onset of cyanosis is frequently delayed.

The conduction system is normally situated, but the AV node may be compressed and the right bundle branch fibrotic (Lev et al., 1970).

A number of associated lesions with Ebstein's anomaly have been reported. These include cases that had patent ductus arteriosus, pulmonary atresia, or ventricular septal defect (Mayer et al., 1957; Vacca et al., 1958; Caddell and Browne, 1963), and current opinion emphasizes a spectrum of involvement of the entire tricuspid apparatus and of the right ventricle (Lev et al., 1970; Becker et al. 1971).

Clinical Features

There is an equal number of males and females with Ebstein's disease. The majority of instances are sporadic in nature, but familial cases have been reported. There is division of opinion as to whether a hereditary basis for transmission exists (Emanuel et al., 1976; Rosenmann et al., 1976). Four of eight babies with congenital heart disease born to mothers exposed to lithium during pregnancy had Ebstein's anomaly (Nora et al., 1974). Variability of the clinical features has been well described in several major reports (Genton and Blount, 1967; Kumar et al., 1971; Bialostozky et al., 1972; Watson, 1974). In body build they are usually thinner than the average child. Dyspnea is commonly present, especially in those with cyanosis, but this symptom may precede the onset of cyanosis or failure.

Cyanosis.   Three-fourths of the cases reported in the literature have had evidence of cyanosis at some time. Such patients have a right-to-left shunt through a patent foramen ovale or a defect of the atrial septum. The opening may be a small one, but the raised pressure in the right atrium is sufficient to send blood through it into the left atrium. In two-thirds of the children the cyanosis has been present from birth or early infancy. In most of the others the cyanosis will appear insidiously between 3 and 12 years of age (Simca and Bonham-Carter, 1971).

It is thus a characteristic of this condition that cyanosis may at times be absent or minimal at birth but appear later in childhood; occasionally the onset may be delayed until adult life. At first there may simply be dyspnea and then dyspnea with cyanosis.

In Figure 45–2 is shown the arterial oxygen saturation at rest in 17 cases (15 cases reported in the literature; two cases from The Hospital for Sick Children, Toronto). It will be noted that this saturation varied from 64 to 97 percent and in many cases was at a level that did not show cyanosis except when the patient was exercised.

Pulse, Blood Pressure, Pulse Pressure.   The radial pulse is usually small and not brisk. The blood pressure is within normal limits or low normal levels. There is a relatively small pulse pressure.

Thrill.   If the heart is considerably enlarged, there may be a slight precordial bulge, occasionally a thrill may be palpable over the precordium.

Cardiac Impulse.   Over the lower precordium the cardiac impulse is likely to be quiet and subdued, whereas over the conus area, where the right ventricular muscle is sometimes a little thicker, a more powerful heartbeat may be felt. Thus, according to Blacket and associates (1952), a localized impulse over the conus may help to differentiate between this anomaly and pulmonary stenosis with patent foramen ovale where the cardiac impulse is felt over the whole precordium. The impulse is frequently associated with a coarse systolic thrill.

Heart Murmurs.   On auscultation a systolic and a short diastolic murmur are present in one-half of the cases. Most of the rest have only a systolic murmur. A few have no audible murmur. The murmur is best

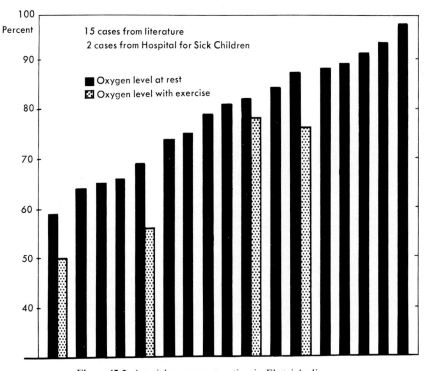

Figure 45-2. Arterial oxygen saturation in Ebstein's disease.

heard over the lower precordium and may be loud or faint. It was frequently described as scratching or crunching.

The majority have a diastolic murmur; this may be presystolic or middiastolic in time. Schiebler and associates (1959) point out it is usually accentuated in the inspiratory phase of respiration, suggesting a tricuspid valve origin.

To-and-fro murmurs have been noted by many authors. The effect may simulate a pericardial friction rub (Engle et al., 1950; Schiebler et al., 1959). The latter suggest the sound may be in fact due to pericardial friction at times.

Heart Sounds. Frequently a third heart sound is heard giving a triple rhythm. It occurs most commonly in those patients who have a diastolic murmur. As a rule, the heart sounds are of normal intensity, but at times they may be faint, as was emphasized by Engle and associates (1950) and Mayer and associates (1957). A consistent finding on phonocardiography is abnormally wide splitting of the first heart sound which has been shown to be caused by delayed closure of the large anterior tricuspid valve leaflet (Crews et al., 1972).

Radiologic Examination

In recent years the radiologic findings have been studied more intimately with the anatomic details and certain characteristic features delineated (Bialostozky et al., 1972; Deutsch et al., 1975). There is an impression of generalized enlargement in the majority of cases with prominence of both right and left heart borders. The convex left border is due primarily to the dilatation of the outflow tract to the right ventricle, but it is further displaced by the abnormal development of the right ventricle. A prominent right border is due to the enlarged right atrium, which is affected by the rise in internal pressure. These contours are shown in Figure 45–3 (Schiebler et al., 1959). The cardiac outline is highly suggestive of the underlying pathology and, when taken with the other clinical findings, permits an accurate diagnosis in the majority of cases.

Schiebler and associates (1959) pointed out that the newborn period presents particular problems because the heart is commonly within normal limits both for size and for shape. They found one case with a markedly enlarged heart at five hours of age, but in three others the measurements were within normal limits. In the first year of life it is helpful to take repeated x-rays of the heart even a few weeks apart to show the evolution of the typical contours.

The pulmonary vascular markings are either normal or decreased. Under the fluoroscope the cardiac borders are seen to be more quiet than usual. This is especially true of the right ventricle in the left anterior oblique view although there may be some movement of the pulmonary conus region in the right anterior oblique position. The lack of movement in the cardiac borders is more likely to be a feature of the

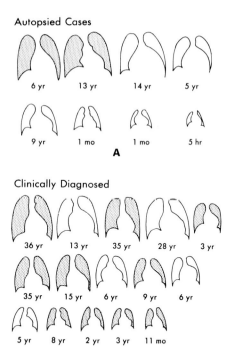

Figure 45-3. *A.* Tracings of chest roentgenograms of autopsied cases to show cardiac contour and pulmonary vasculature. *B.* Tracings of chest roentgenograms of living patients to show cardiac contour and pulmonary vasculature. (Reproduced from Schiebler, G. L.; Adams, P., Jr.; Anderson, R. C.; Amplatz, K.; and Lester, R. G.: Clinical study of twenty-three cases of Ebstein's anomaly of the tricuspid valve. *Circulation,* **19:** 170, 1959.)

older cases than of the very young ones. In a baby at The Hospital for Sick Children who died at three days the cardiac borders appeared to move normally. The hilar shadows did not pulsate. Schiebler and associates point out that there is a close correlation between the degree of cyanosis and the decrease in hilar markings. Furthermore, they found no increase in the hilar shadows in the presence of cardiac failure. Left atrial enlargement is not seen in children with this anomaly. Tourniaire and associates (1949) demonstrated calcification of the mitral valve and ring in Ebstein's disease.

Electrocardiography

Van Lingen and Bauerfeld (1953) and Bialostozky (1972) have summarized the electrocardiographic findings and have pointed out a pattern that is suggestively diagnostic.

The most striking feature of the electrocardiogram is the association of complete right bundle branch block with abnormally low R and S waves over the right precordium. This is an unusual combination in congenital heart disease and should immediately arouse one's suspicion. The QRS is long and usually multiphasic. The P waves are frequently abnormal, showing either increased amplitude or duration, or both. The P-R interval is usually lengthened to 0.16 second or more. The axis of the QRS is most frequently in the quadrant of 120 degrees, but the range varies widely from -30 to -170 degrees.

A summary of the electrocardiographic findings in 20 cases assembled from the literature of our own files is shown in Table 45–1; all of these were verified at postmortem or by cardiac catheterization or angiocardiography. In 19 of the 20 cases the R wave in V_1 was 7 mm or less. The exception was our case of two days of age, who had an R in V_1 of 9 mm. In only two cases was the S in V_1 over 7 mm. As Van Lingen and Bauerfeld (1953) have pointed out, these voltages are much less than the normal for adults, and in normal children the voltages are likely to be even higher than in adults.

The voltage in V_6 was within normal limits. Thus, these findings well fit the pathologic evidence since the right ventricular wall is thin and fibrotic and the left ventricular wall relatively normal. The electrocardiogram of one of our cases is shown in Figure 45–4.

Additional electrocardiographic studies in children have been reported by Mayer and associates (1957) and Schiebler and associates (1959). These findings were similar to those recorded above. The exceptional cases as far as electrocardiographic

changes are concerned are likely to appear in infancy.

Wolff-Parkinson-White syndrome was identified with Ebstein's disease by Sodi-Pallares (1956), who divided the cases with this association into two groups: those with right-axis deviation, and those with left. The latter simulated left bundle branch block. The right precordial leads show deep S waves and the left tall R waves. Tall, peaked P waves are also present as a reule. Many others have confirmed the association of Wolff-Parkinson-White syndrome and Ebstein's disease (Simca and Bonham-Carter, 1971; Bialostozky, 1972). Ventricular preexcitation was present in 10 percent of the international study patients (Watson, 1974). Although the conduction tissue is normally sited, electrophysiologic studies have revealed conduction delays at several levels of the system in patients with Ebstein's anomaly (Kastor et al., 1975). It is not too surprising that dysrhythmias of a paroxysmal nature occurred in more than a quarter of the 505 patients in Watson's survey (1974).

Echocardiography

An abnormally anterior position of the anterior leaflet during the entire period of diastole together with delayed closure of the tricuspid valve are the consistent features of the echocardiogram in Ebstein's anomaly (Lundstrom, 1973). Septal motion may also be abnormal (Yuste et al., 1974), but this

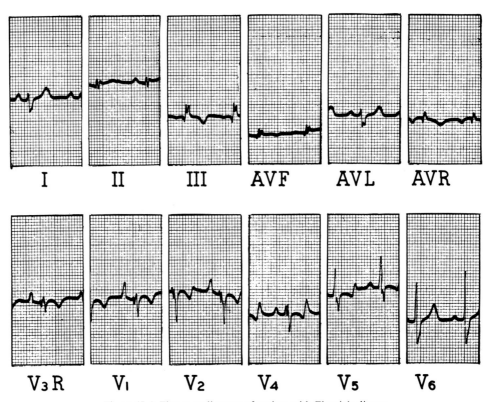

Figure 45-4. Electrocardiogram of patient with Ebstein's disease.

Table 45-1. EBSTEIN'S DISEASE—ELECTROCARDIOGRAM

Cases with Diagnosis Demonstrated by (1) Postmortem, (2) Catheterization, or (3) Angiocardiogram

AUTHORS	CASE	AGE	SEX	AXIS	P-R	QRS	P_2(MM)	RBBB	V_1	V_2	V_3	V_4	V_5	V^6
Blacket et al. (1952)	1	16 years	F	−30°	0.16	0.12	2	V_1	2/1	2/2	2/2	4/1	4/1	3/2
	2	2½ years	M	+120°	0.19	0.12	5	V_1	4/1	7/0		10/5		?/5
	3	18 years	F	+120°	0.20	0.11	2	V_1	2/3	1/5	1/13	5/5	6/3	7/1
	5	13 years	M	+120°	0.15	0.15	2	V_1	7/0	5/5	8/2	9/3	9/3	9/2
Medd et al. (1954)	1	7 years	F	+30°	0.24	0.12	3	V_1	2/2	2/7	2/6	8/6	16/6	18/5
Goodwin et al. (1953)	1	14 years	M	+120°	0.24	0.16	2	V_1	7/6	9/6		14/4		15/3
	2	13 years	M	+110°	0.22	0.12	2	V_1	1/6	4/8		17/6		16/4
Broadbent et al. (1953)	1	6 years	M	+120°	0.20	0.08	4		1/8		0/24			19/6
	2	35 years	M	+120°	0.24	0.12	3	V_1	3/5		10/2			8/0
	3	29 years	M	+150°	0.22	0.12	2	V_1	5/5	7/6	3/7	5/5	7/7	5/5
Van Lingen et al. (1952)	1	22 years	F	+140°	0.20	0.12	2	V_1	3/1	2/1	3/0.5	5/0	4/1	7/4
	2	20 years	F	+170°	0.21	0.12	3	V_1	3/2	1/8	1/8	4/6	10/4	15/7
Engle et al. (1950)	1	8 years	M	+118°	0.14	0.10	3.5		3.5/0					R + S in V_6/18.0
	2	4 years	M	+145°	0.18	0.12	2		3.0/0.5					
	3	10 years	F	+120°	0.16	0.13	8		1.5/0					R + S in V_6/16.0
Paul et al. (1951)	1	16 years	M	−170°	0.20	0.12	2.5	V_2		5/3		11/2	8/2	16/7
HSC * (1955)	1	7 years	F	+120°	0.21	0.11	1	V_1	2/4	2/7		2/6	15/3	20/8
	2	6 years	M	+60°	0.14	0.08	1	V_1	2/4	2/3		6/10	5/11	10/7
	3	2 days	M	+150°	0.17	0.08	3.5	V_1	9/8	5/14		23/20	24/15	9/2
Kerwin (1955)	1	18 years	M	+90°	0.17	0.16	1	V_1	6/4	16/7	21/4	16/1	7/1	
EBSTEIN'S DISEASE WITH PULMONARY VALVE ATRESIA AND MULTIPLE ATRIAL SEPTAL DEFECTS														
HSC * (1955)	1	6½ months	M	+60°	0.13	0.06	5		8/28	11/28		18/18	15/10	14/5
EBSTEIN'S DISEASE WITH VENTRICULAR SEPTAL DEFECT														
HSC *	1	7 months	F	−140°	0.14	0.11	5	V_1	21/0	7/9		16/20	17/25	15/18

* HSC = Hospital for Sick Children, Toronto.

feature is not normally encountered in newborns. The ability to record the anterior tricuspid leaflet farther to the left of the left sternal border than in controls has been regarded as a useful sign by Farooki and associates (1976).

Cardiac Catheterization

The information gathered by cardiac catheter may be pathognomonic of Ebstein's disease. First the catheter can be coiled up in the right atrium to reveal an abnormally large chamber. The pressure in the right atrium may be normal, but it is characteristically slightly raised, usually 10 to 25 mm of mercury. There may be difficulty in entering the right ventricle, and the pressure in the right ventricle is within normal range but not much higher than that of the right atrium. The pulmonary artery pressure is similar to that of the right ventricle or slightly lower.

The oxygen content of the right atrium is identical with that of the right ventricle and pulmonary artery. At the same time the blood in the systemic artery usually shows some degree of unsaturation, because at least three-fourths of the cases have a shunt from right atrium to left atrium. At times the catheter may pass through the atrial septal opening into the left atrium and left ventricle.

Cardiac irregularities are common in these patients and are especially likely to occur during cardiac catheterization. Extrasystoles, heart block, bundle branch block, and atrial fibrillation have been known to occur. Fatalities have been reported during the procedure; consequently, most cardiologists would prefer to avoid such investigation if it is not necessary. Now that the clinical picture is becoming increasingly clear, cardiac catheterization is less frequently required.

Hernandez and coworkers have demonstrated the value of the intracavity electrode catheter in recognizing Ebstein's disease. On the withdrawal of the catheter from the right ventricle to the right atrium, the QRS and P wave change, especially the latter. Fluoroscopic control will show this change when the catheter tip is an area one would expect to be in the body of the right ventricle, thus suggesting one of the diagnostic features of Ebstein's disease.

Angiocardiography

Selective angiocardiography has been considered to have danger, but in recent times this concern has proved less justified (Ellis et al., 1964; Fabian et al., 1966). The technique clearly defines the displaced tricuspid valve and its relation to the tricuspid annulus as two notches at the inferior cardiac border. Reciprocal volume changes occur between the atrialized right ventricle and the true right atrium (Dhanavaravibul et al., 1970). Fenestration of the anterior leaflet can rather commonly be identified (Deutsch et al., 1975).

In all reported cases there has been evidence of a large right atrium occupying over half of the cardiac shadow (see Figure 45–5). The trabeculae of the right atrium were well shown in one of our cases who died at a later date, and histologic sections confirmed the presence of marked hypertrophy of the atrial wall.

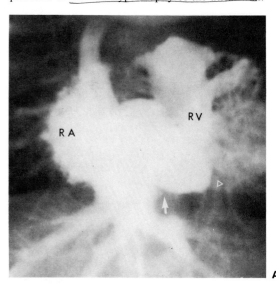

A

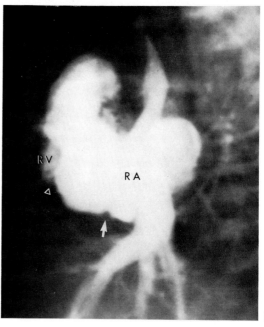

B

Figure 45-5. Angiocardiograms taken during ventricular diastole. Anteroposterior (*A*) and lateral (*B*) projections demonstrate the large atrialized portion of the right ventricle between the annulus of the tricuspid valve (↑) and the abnormally inserted tricuspid valve cusp(s) (△). *RA* = right atrium; *RV* = functioning right ventricle. (Courtesy of Dr. D. McNamara and the Department of Medical Photography, St. Luke's Episcopal Hospital and the Texas Children's Hospital, Houston, Texas.)

All observers have noted the late emptying time of the right atrium and right ventricle. The right-to-left shunt through the atrial opening can be demonstrated, and frequently the contrast medium penetrates the left atrium and the left ventricle before the pulmonary artery is filled (Kjellberg et al., 1955).

Prognosis

The prognosis is variable (see Figure 45–6). The oldest case on record lived to be 70 years of age, whereas one of our cases died at three days of age. However, the largest proportion of cases die in the second and fourth decades of life, the mean age at death being approximately 30 years. Twenty-five percent of the deaths occurred in the first ten years of life, 5 percent in the first year (Vacca et al., 1958). Our baby who died at three days of age appeared to have tricuspid insufficiency as well as a large cyanosis-producing shunt between the atria. It is not surprising that tricuspid insufficiency is an occasional accompaniment of this anomaly since the valve is so defective. Ebstein's original case appears to have had some insufficiency. Blount and coworkers (1957) also record it.

The degree of interference with the blood flow to the lung is one of the most important factors in prognosis. When it is marked, there will be progressive cardiac enlargement and early death. Thus, change in heart size is of prognostic significance. The defective wall of the right ventricle begins to weaken over the years, responding with distention and varying degrees of fibrosis and eventually leading to heart failure.

Watson (1974), reporting on the natural history of 505 cases, records that in the childhood years the majority were not significantly handicapped. Furthermore, 70 percent of the cases surviving 15 years remained in cardiac grades I or II during the follow-up period.

The pediatric mortality was highest in the first year of life. Few cases died between one and ten years. These later deaths occurred intermittently in the teen-age group.

Attempts at surgery carried a high mortality in childhood partly because the more severe cases were chosen for operation. The mortality from surgery at any age was more than 50 percent.

Two-thirds of the cases that die in childhood appear to die in congestive heart failure and most of the remaining third have the fatal event related to a cardiac arrhythmia. Vacca and associates (1958) noted that sudden death occurred 16 times out of 108 cases. This is usually related to some cardiac arrhythmia, but the arrhythmia may be initiated by a cardiac catheterization procedure or by heart failure.

The cyanosis is usually due to a shunt between the atria, from right to left, augmented by the tricuspid regurgitation or obstruction of the outflow tract of the diminished right ventricle. At times, these patients have an associated pulmonary stenosis.

Braunwald and Gorlin (1968) reported in the Cooperative Study on Cardiac Catheterization that while there were no fatalities among the 49 patients catheterized with Ebstein's anomaly, three developed complications. The risk is probably a little greater than in other forms of congenital heart disease, and the catheter operator should proceed with caution and be prepared to handle any arrhythmia that may develop. In the past, the risk has been over-emphasized.

The degree of interference with the blood flow to the lung is undoubtedly one of the important factors in prognosis. When it is marked, there will be progressive cardiac enlargement and early death. Thus, a change in heart size is of prognostic significance. The defective wall of the right ventricle begins to weaken over the years, responding with distention and varying degrees of fibrosis, eventually leading to cardiac failure.

Treatment

Since patients with this anomaly vary markedly in their exercise tolerance, no specific regimen can be advocated. However, it is important that they should live within their exercise tolerance and avoid dyspnea, excessive fatigue, and excessive cyanosis. This is especially so in the cases that show enlarged hearts or progressive cardiac enlargement. Suitable antibiotics should be given for respiratory illness since any infection may add to the burden of the heart. Antiarrhythmic therapy is frequently successful, but long-term prophylactic treatment with the objective of avoiding sudden death has not been attempted.

Surgical Treatment. A variety of forms of surgical approach have been attempted in recent years. In the presence of marked cyanosis some medical centers have used the Glenn anastomosis between the superior vena cava and the right pulmonary artery, thus allowing the systemic venous system to provide the slight pressure required to pass blood through the right lung. This may relieve the load on the abnormal right ventricle and right atrium to some degree. Several surgeons have reported some success with this procedure (Gasul et al., 1959; Weinberg and associates, 1960; Scott et al., 1963).

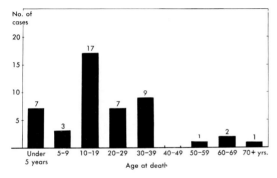

Figure 45-6. Age at death in Ebstein's disease.

854   OBSTRUCTIONS, REGURGITATIONS, AND OTHER MALFORMATIONS

The Blalock-Taussig type of shunt has been used occasionally, particularly in the presence of pulmonic stenosis. It is (not) recommended in the average type of Ebstein's anomaly. Several surgeons have reported success replacing the tricuspid valve with a prosthesis (Lillehei, 1967). Others have used a heterograft or homograft (Hardy, 1969; Senoo et al., 1976).

Trusler reserves the prosthesis for those who have a grossly defective valve that cannot be helped by annuloplasty. A circumferential annuloplasty is preferred, and currently a Carpentier ring would be the preferred method (Carpentier et al., 1971). In most cases this would be combined with the repair described by Hardy and associates (1964) in which the atrialized portion of the right ventricle is excluded by a plication suture which brings the false annulus and the true annulus together. Thus, regurgitation of the tricuspid valve is reduced or eliminated and the thin-walled expansion chamber of atrialized ventricle is also eliminated (Trusler, 1974).

▶The two major indications for heart surgery in this anomaly are (1) the presence of intractable congestive heart failure and (2) repeated arrhythmias, especially those that are difficult to control. However, as Watson (1974) has pointed out, the surgical approach should not be considered lightly since the mortality at operation is high.

REFERENCES

Baker, C.; Brinton, W. D.; and Channell, G. D.: Ebstein's disease. *Guy Hosp. Rep.*, 99:247, 1950.
Barger, J. D.; Henderson, C. E.; and Edwards, J. E.: Abscess of the brain in an adult with Ebstein's malformation of the tricuspid valve: report of a case. *Am. J. Clin. Pathol.*, 21:576, 1951.
Becker, A. E.; Becker, M. D.; and Edwards, J. E.: Pathologic spectrum of dysplasia of the tricuspid valve. *Arch. Pathol.*, 91:167, 1971.
Bialostozky, D.; Horwitz, S.; and Espino-Vela, J.: Ebstein's malformation of the tricuspid valve. *Am. J. Cardiol.*, 29:826, 1972.
Bialostozky, D.; Medrano, G. A.; Munoz, L.; and Contreras, R.: Vectorcardiographic study and anatomic observations in 21 cases of Ebstein's malformation of the tricuspid valve. *Am. J. Cardiol.*, 30:354, 1972.
Blacket, R. B.; Sinclair-Smith, B. C.; Palmer, A. J.; Halliday, J. H.; and Maddox, J. K.: Ebstein's disease: A report of five cases. *Aust. Ann. Med.*, 1:26, 1952.
Blount, S. G.; McCord, M. C.; and Gelb, I. J.: Ebstein's anomaly. *Circulation*, 15:120, 1957.
Braunwald, E., and Gorlin, R.: Total population studied, procedures employed and incidence of complications. *Circulation*, 37, 38:(Suppl. III) 8, 1968.
Broadbent, J. C.; Wood, E. H.; Burchell, H. B.; and Parker, R. L.: Ebstein's malformation of the tricuspid valve: report of 3 cases. *Proc. Mayo Clin.*, 28:79, 1953.
Caddell, J. L., and Browne, M. J.: Right ventricular hypertension and pulmonary stenosis in Ebstein's anomaly of the heart. *Am. J. Cardiol.*, 11:100, 1963.
Carpentier, A.; Deloche, A.; Dauptoin, J.; Soyer, R.; Blondeau, P.; Piwnica, A.; and Dubost, Ch.: A new reconstructive operation for correction of mitral and tricuspid insufficiency. *J. Thorac. Cardiovasc. Surg.*, 61:1, 1971.
Crews, T. L.; Pridie, R. B.; Benham, R.; and Leatham, A.: Auscultatory and phonocardiographic findings in Ebstein's anomaly. Correlation of first heart sound with ultrasonic records of tricuspid valve movement. *Br. Heart J.*, 34:681, 1972.
Deutsch, V.; Wexler, L.; Blieden, L. E.; Yahini, J. H.; and Neufeld, H. N.: Ebstein's anomaly of tricuspid valve: Critical review of roentgenological features and additional angiographic signs. *Am. J. Roentgenol. Radium Ther.*, 125:395, 1975.

Dhanavaravibul, S.; Nora, J. J.; and McNamara, D. G.: Angiocardiographic signs in Ebstein's anomaly. *Cardiovasc. Res. Cent. Bull.*, 9:50, 1970.
Ebstein, W.: Über einen sehr seltenen Fall von Insufficienz der Valvula tricuspidalis, bedingt durch eine tangeborene hochgradige Missbildung derselben. *Arch. Anat. Physiol. Wissensch. Med.*, 238, 1866.
Edwards, J. E.: Pathologic features of Ebstein's malformation of the tricuspid valve. *Proc. Mayo Clin.*, 28:89, 1953.
Ellis, K.; Griffiths, S. P.; Burris, J. O.; Ramsay, G. C.; and Fleming, R. J.: Ebstein's anomaly of the tricuspid valve: Angiocardiographic considerations. *Am. J. Roentgenol.*, 92:1338, 1964.
Emanuel, R.; O'Brien, K.; and Ng. R.: Ebstein's anomaly. Genetic study of 26 families. *Br. Heart J.*, 38:5, 1976.
Engle, M. A.; Payne, T. P. B.; Bruins, C.; and Taussig, H. B.: Ebstein's anomaly of the tricuspid valve. Report of three cases and analysis of clinical syndrome. *Circulation*, 1:1246, 1950.
Fabian, C. E.; Mundt, W. P.; and Abrams, H. L.: Ebstein's anomaly: the direct demonstration of contractile synchrony between the two parts of the right ventricle. *Invest. Radiol.*, 1:63, 1966.
Farooki, Z. Q.; Henry, T. G.; and Green, E. W.: Echocardiographic spectrum of Ebstein's anomaly of the tricuspid valve. *Circulation*, 53:63, 1976.
Genton, E., and Blount, S. G.: The spectrum of Ebstein's anomaly. *Am. Heart J.*, 73:395, 1967.
Goetzche, H., and Falholt, W.: Ebstein's anomaly of the tricuspid valve. *Am. Heart J.*, 47:587, 1954.
Goodwin, J. F.; Wynn, A.; and Steiner, R. E.: Ebstein's anomaly of the tricuspid valve. *Am. Heart J.*, 45:144, 1953.
Gulotta, G. A., and LaMotta, E. P.: Ebstein's anomaly associated with the Wolff-Parkinson-White syndrome. *Bull. St. Francis Hosp. (Roslyn)*, 16:14, 1959.
Hardy, K. L.; May, I. A.; Webster, C. A.; and Kimball, K. G.: Ebstein's anomaly: A functional concept and successful definitive repair. *J. Thorac Cardiovasc. Surg.*, 48:927, 1964.
Henderson, C. B.; Jackson, F.; and Swan, W. G. A.: Ebstein's anomaly diagnosed during life. *Br. Heart J.*, 15:360, 1953.
Hernandez, F. A.; Rochkind, R.; and Cooper, H. R.: The intracavitary electrocardiogram in the diagnosis of Ebstein's anomaly. *Am. J. Cardiol.*, 1:181, 1958.
Kastor, J. A.; Goldreyer, B. N.; Josephson, M. E.; Perloff, J. K.; Scharf, D. L.; Manchester, J. H.; Shelburne, J. C.; and Hirshfeld, J. W.: Electrophysiologic characteristics of Ebstein's anomaly of the tricuspid valve. *Circulation*, 52:987, 1975.
Kerwin, A. J.: Ebstein's anomaly: report of a case diagnosed during life. *Br. Heart J.*, 17:109, 1955.
Kjellberg, S. R.; Manheimer, E.; Rudhe, U.; and Jonsson, B.: *Diagnosis of Congenital Heart Disease.* Year Book Publishers, Inc., Chicago, 1955, p. 518.
Kumar, A. E.; Fyler, D. C.; Miettinen, O. S.; and Nadas, A. S.: Ebstein's anomaly. Clinical profile and natural history. *Am. J. Cardiol.*, 28:84, 1971.
Lambert, E. C.: Personal communication, 1956.
Lev, M.; Liberthson, R. R.; Joseph, R. H.; Seten, C. E.; Kunske, R. D.; Eckner, F. A. O.; and Miller, R. A.: The pathologic anatomy of Ebstein's disease. *Arch. Pathol.*, 90:334, 1970.
Lillehei, C. W., and Gannon, P. G.: Ebstein's malformation of the tricuspid valve. Method of surgical correction utilizing a ball-valve prosthesis and delayed closure of atrial septal defect. *Circulation*, 31:I-9, 1965.
Lillehei, C. W.; Kalke, B. R.; and Carlson, R. G.: Evolution of corrective surgery for Ebstein's anomaly. *Circulation*, 35:I-111, 1967.
Lundström, N-R.: Echocardiography in the diagnosis of Ebstein's anomaly of the tricuspid valve. *Circulation*, 47:597, 1973.
Matsumoto, M.; Matsuo, H.; Nagata, S.; Hamanaka, Y.; Fujita, T.; Kawashima, Y.; Nimura, Y.; and Abe, H.: Visualization of Ebstein's anomaly of the tricuspid valve by two-dimensional and standard echocardiography. *Circulation*, 53:1, 1976.
Mayer, F. E.; Nadas, A. S.; and Ongley, P. A.: Ebstein's anomaly: presentation of ten cases. *Circulation*, 16:1057, 1957.
McCredie, R. M.; Oakley, C.; Mahoney, E. B.; and Uy, P. N.: Ebstein's disease: diagnosis by electrode catheter and treatment by partial bypass of the right side of the heart. *N. Engl. J. Med.*, 267:174, 1962.

Medd, W. E.; Matthews, M. B.; and Thursfield, W. R.: Ebstein's disease. *Thorax*, **9**:14, 1954.

Najafi, H.; Hunter, J. A.; et al.: Ebstein's malformation of the tricuspid valve. *Ann. Thorac. Surg.*, **4**:334, 1967.

Nora, J. J.; Nora, A. H.; and Toews, W. H.: Lithium, Ebstein's anomaly and other congenital heart defects. *Lancet*, **2**:594, 1974.

Paul, O.; Myers, G. S.; and Campbell, J. A.: The electrocardiogram in congenital heart disease. *Circulation*, **3**:564, 1951.

Perez-Alvarez, J. J., et al.: Ebstein's anomaly with pulmonic stenosis. *Am. J. Cardiol.*, **20**:411, 1967.

Reynolds, G.: Ebstein's disease—a case diagnosed clinically. *Guy Hosp. Rep.*, **99**:276, 1950.

Rosenmann, A.; Arad, I.; Simcha, A.; and Schaap, T.: Familial Ebstein's anomaly. *J. Med. Genet.*, **13**:532, 1976.

Schiebler, G. L.; Adams, P., Jr.; Anderson, R. C.; Amplatz, K.; and Lester, R. G.: Clinical study of twenty-three cases of Ebstein's anomaly of the tricuspid valve, *Circulation*, **19**:165, 1959.

Scott, L. P.; Dempsey, J. J.; Timmis, H. H.; and McClenathan, J. E.: A surgical approach to Ebstein's disease. *Circulation*, **27**:574, 1963.

Senoo, Y.; Ohishi, K.; Nawa, S.; Teramoto, S.; and Sunada, T.: Total correction of Ebstein's anomaly by replacement with a biological aortic valve without plication of the atrialized ventricle. *J. Thorac. Cardiovasc. Surg.*, **72**:243, 1976.

Simcha, A., and Bonham-Carter, R. E.: Ebstein's anomaly. Clinical study of 32 patients in childhood. *Br. Heart J.*, **33**:46, 1971.

Sodi-Pallares, D.: *New Bases of Electrocardiography*. C. V. Mosby, St. Louis, 1956, p. 270.

Soloff, L. A.; Stauffer, H. M.; and Zatuchni, J.: Ebstein's disease: report of the first case diagnosed during life. *Am. J. Med. Sci.*, **222**:554, 1951.

Taussig, H. B.: *Congenital Malformations of the Heart*. The Commonwealth Fund, New York, 1947, p. 520.

Tourniaire, A.; Deyrieux, F.; Tartulier, M.: Maladie d'Ebstein: essai de diagnostic clinique. *Arch. Mal. Coeur*, **42**:1211, 1949.

Trusler, G.: Personal communication, 1974.

Uhl, H. S. M.: A previously undescribed congenital malformation of the heart: almost total absence of the myocardium of the right ventricle. *Bull. Hopkins Hosp.*, **91**:197, 1952.

Vacca, J. B.; Bussmann, D. W.; and Mudd, J. G.: Ebstein's anomaly: complete review of 108 cases. *Am. J. Cardiol.*, **2**:210, 1958.

Van Lingen, B., and Bauerfeld, S. R.: The electrocardiogram in Ebstein's anomaly of the tricuspid valve. *S. Afr. J. Med. Sci.*, **18**:88, 1953.

Van Lingen, B.; McGregor, M.; Kaye, J.; Meyer, M. J.; Jacobs, H. D.; Braudo, J. L.; Bothwell, T. H.; and Elliott, G. A.: Clinical and cardiac catheterization findings compatible with Ebstein's anomaly of the tricuspid valve: a report of two cases. *Am. Heart J.*, **43**:77, 1952.

Van Mierop, L. H. S.; Alley, R. D.; Kausel, H. W.: and Stranahan, A.: Ebstein's malformation of the left atrioventricular valve in corrected transposition, with subpulmonary stenosis and ventricular septal defect. *Am. J. Cardiol.*, **8**:270, 1961.

Walton, K., and Spencer, A. G.: Ebstein's anomaly of the tricuspid valve. *J. Pathol. Bact.*, **60**:387, 1948.

Watson, H.: Natural history of Ebstein's anomaly of tricuspid valve in childhood and adolescence. An international cooperative study of 505 cases. *Br. Heart J.*, **36**:417, 1974.

Weinberg, M., Jr.; Bicoff, J. P.; Agustsson, M. H.; Steiger, A.; Gasul, B. M.; Fell, E. H.; and Laun, L. L.: Surgical palliation in patients with Ebstein's anomaly and congenital hypoplasia of the right ventricle. *J. Thorac. Cardiovasc. Surg.*, **40**:310, 1960.

Wright, J. L.; Burchell, H. B.; Kirklin, J. W.; and Wood, E. H.: Congenital displacement of the tricuspid valve (Ebstein's anomaly). *Proc. Mayo Clin.*, **29**:278, 1954.

Yuste, P.; Minguez, I.; Aza, V.; Senor, J.; Asin, E.; and Martinez-Bordin, C.: Echocardiography in the diagnosis of Ebstein's anomaly. *Chest*, **66**:273, 1974.

CHAPTER

46

Vascular Rings and Anomalies of the Aortic Arch

C. A. F. Moës

CLASSIFICATIONS dealing with malformations of the aortic arch arrangement have been presented by Poynter (1916), Neuhauser (1946), Edwards (1948, 1953, 1960), Kirklin and Clagett (1950), Harley (1959), Stewart and coworkers (1964), Klinkhamer (1969), Shuford and Sybers (1974), and others.

The classification proposed by Stewart and coworkers (1964) is based on what has been termed the "hypothetic double aortic arch with bilateral ductus arteriosi" initially introduced by Edwards (1948, 1953). According to this plan, most aortic arch anomalies are the result either of persistent patency of a vascular segment that would normally regress or abnormal regression of a segment that would normally remain patent. This tends to take place at one or more specific locations. These are the right or left dorsal aortic roots or the right or left fourth aortic arch. The plan is completed by the presence or absence of the ductus arteriosus, which play a formidable role in formation of a vascular ring.

The diagram formulated in Figure 46–1 is based on the plan put forth by Edwards. In this schema an outline of most arch anomalies is depicted. The upper descending aorta may be left- or right-sided. The side on which the ductus arteriosus* persists may determine whether a vascular ring exists.

Double Aortic Arch. Both fourth arches and dorsal aortic roots remain patent. Rarely, however, atrophy of a segment on the left may occur. The upper descending aorta may be right- or left-sided, and the ductus arteriosus usually persists on the left, though it may be right-sided or bilateral. The anomaly results in the formation of a vascular ring.

Left Aortic Arch. The formation of a left aortic arch with a normal brachiocephalic artery branch pattern results from regression of the right dorsal aortic root (segment between the right subclavian artery and the descending aorta). The upper descending aorta is situated on the left. The left ductus

arteriosus persists, while the right disappears. Minor variations in the origin of the innominate or left common carotid artery can occur that may or may not cause tracheal compression, though there is no vascular ring formation. If the ductus arteriosus persists on the right rather than the left, it usually connects the right pulmonary artery to the base of the innominate artery with no vascular ring being formed. Rarely, in the presence of a persistent right ductus arteriosus, there is interruption of the right aortic arch between the right subclavian artery and right ductus arteriosus instead of between the right subclavian artery and descending aorta. In this instance, the ductus arteriosus connects the right pulmonary artery to a right-sided upper descending aorta via a partially persistent right dorsal aortic root, and a vascular ring is formed.

Formation of an aberrant right subclavian artery results from regression of the right aortic arch (segment between the right common carotid and right subclavian arteries). The subclavian artery, therefore, arises from the right dorsal aortic root. Usually the ductus arteriosus persists on the left and connects the left pulmonary artery to the left-sided upper descending aorta; thus no vascular ring exists. Persistence of a right ductus arteriosus with disappearance of the left will result in vascular encirclement of the trachea and esophagus. The ductus arteriosus in this instance extends between the right pulmonary artery and root of the aberrant right subclavian artery. The upper descending aorta may be right-sided.

Right Aortic Arch. The formation of a right aortic arch with mirror-image branching of the brachiocephalic arteries is the result of regression of the left dorsal aortic root (segment between the left ductus arteriosus and descending aorta). There is a disappearance of the right ductus arteriosus with persistence of the left ductus arteriosus, which connects the left pulmonary artery to the subclavian portion of the left innominate artery; thus no vascular ring exists. Rarely, when there is a persistent left ductus arteriosus there is regression of the left aortic arch between the left ductus arteriosus and left

---

* Throughout the text in this chapter, the term *ductus arteriosus* is used without any connotation as to whether the ductus is patent or ligamentous.

856

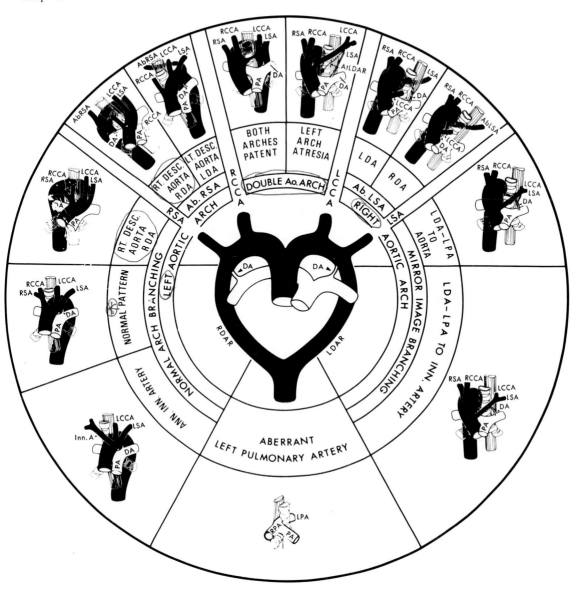

Figure 46-1. Schematic formulation of aortic arch anomalies.

subclavian artery. In this situation, a complete vascular ring is formed as the left ductus arteriosus connects the left pulmonary artery to the right-sided upper descending aorta via the remaining portion of the left dorsal aortic root. The presence of a right ductus arteriosus that passes between the right pulmonary artery and aorta is uncommon and is not associated with a vascular ring.

Formation of an aberrant left subclavian artery results from regression of the left aortic arch (segment between the left common carotid and left subclavian arteries). The subclavian artery thus arises from the left dorsal aortic root. When the left ductus arteriosus persists, it extends between the left pulmonary artery and the aberrant vessel and a ring is formed. Persistence of the ductus arteriosus on the right is

uncommon and will not be associated with a vascular ring.

▷**Aberrant Left Pulmonary Artery.** The vascular impingement on the trachea and esophagus depicted in the lower segment of the circle (Figure 46–1) is related to development of the pulmonary arteries rather than the aortic arches. The left pulmonary in this instance arises from the pulmonary artery on the right and passes to the left lung between the trachea and esophagus.

Diagnosis

A classification of aortic arch anomalies based on a knowledge of the embryologic features is essential in understanding the nature of the various complexes; however, it is of little value in arriving at a clinical diagnosis in a particular patient.

There are several aspects to diagnosis. First, the physician needs to determine whether a vascular ring is present or not. Second, if present, is it causing sufficient signs and symptoms to warrant surgery? Third, what is the nature of the vascular ring and what is the exact arrangement of anomalous vessels to guide the surgeon in his surgical approach?

Respiratory stridor in early life may occur from a variety of causes other than a vascular ring. Some of these include laryngomalacia, congenital webbing of the larynx, papilloma, tetany, foreign body, choanal atresia, etc. Thus, thorough examination of the nose and throat and a blood calcium study may be necessary to rule out these conditions. Part of the investigation of the above should include an esophagogram.

While a vascular ring may be asymptomatic, being discovered incidentally during chest radiography or a gastrointestinal series, nevertheless it may produce symptoms that are due to compression of either the trachea or esophagus or both. The severity of symptoms and age at which onset occurs tend to be proportional to the degree of compression and nature of the vascular ring. Thus the manifestations of a double aortic arch and anomalous left pulmonary artery tend to be severe and persistent and have their onset within the first six months of life. Compression due to a right aortic arch with vascular ring formation is often less severe as the ring is often relatively nonconstrictive. Thus, these patients tend to present beyond six months of age. The onset of symptoms referable to anomalous innominate artery compression of the trachea in patients seen at The Hospital for Sick Children, Toronto, ranged from birth to 30 months with a mean age of four months.

The simplest means of investigating a patient with a suspected mediastinal vascular anomaly is by means of a chest roentgenogram and esophagogram. The chest x-ray will show the laterality of the aortic arch and upper descending aorta in most instances, though in infancy difficulty is often encountered due to the presence of thymic tissue. The anteroposterior esophagogram in this instance can be very helpful as an indentation produced by the arch can frequently be visualized. The laterality of the aortic arch is appreciated on the plain film not only by the density produced by this structure, but by the indentation it produces on the lower lateral tracheal wall and the mild deviation of the trachea to the contralateral side. The position of the upper descending aorta can usually be recognized as an oblique density as it descends in the paraspinal region.

Attention to detail on the plain chest x-ray may help in arriving at a diagnosis as to the type of vascular malformation present. Thus in the presence of a right aortic arch, mirror-image brachiocephalic artery branching should be suspected if there is associated congenital heart disease, especially of the cyanotic variety such as tetralogy of Fallot, double-outlet right ventricle, or truncus arteriosus. On the other hand, a normal heart favors the existence of a right aortic arch with an aberrant left subclavian artery. The right aortic arch may be visibly enlarged if there is cyanotic heart disease with right-to-left shunting, such as tetralogy of Fallot. A visible right aortic arch that is of normal size suggests an associated aberrant left subclavian artery, while a right arch smaller than normal suggests a double aortic arch. In the last instance, the smaller size of the right arch is due to the fact that a portion of the blood from the left ventricle is directed through the left arch. Only occasionally are both arches visible on the plain chest film in the presence of a double aortic arch. An arch that extends into the cervical area, usually on the right, and causes superior mediastinal widening on the involved side with an upper descending aorta that lies on the same side and a lower descending aorta on the opposite side suggests a cervical aorta.

The site of the aortic arch in relationship to the upper descending aorta may be of further assistance in reaching a diagnosis. The arch and upper descending aorta are usually situated on the same side; however, when they are on opposite sides, one may suspect a double aortic arch, a left aortic arch with right descending aorta, or a right aortic arch with an aberrant left subclavian artery and left descending aorta.

The esophagogram is of immense value in differentiating the various types of malformation. Table 46–1 is a modified analysis of the vascular anomalies utilizing a lateral view of the trachea and barium-outlined esophagus as proposed by Berden and Baker (1972).

While the various anomalies in this classification are placed in specific groups, nevertheless the categorization is not absolute. Thus, a double aortic arch may exist and the ring produced may be relatively nonconstrictive so that anterior tracheal compression is not a prominent feature. The constriction produced by a right aortic arch, aberrant left subclavian artery, and left ductus arteriosus is modified by the site of attachment of the ductus arteriosus. Therefore, if the ductus arteriosus extends between the left pulmonary artery and the subclavian artery to the left of the esophagus, the ring tends to be relatively nonconstrictive so no tracheal compression is present. On the other hand, when the ductus passes behind the esophagus to join either the proximal bulbous portion of the subclavian artery or the adjacent right-sided upper descending aorta, the ring tends to be more constrictive with tracheal compression. Also, a left aortic arch with a right descending aorta, or a left arch with an aberrant right subclavian artery, may under some circumstances show some anterior tracheal compression.

The more common and some of the rarer types of vascular anomalies are discussed individually in the following pages.

Table 46–1.   ANALYSIS OF AORTIC VASCULAR ANOMALIES: LATERAL-VIEW TRACHEA AND ESOPHAGOGRAM

I. ANTERIOR TRACHEAL COMPRESSION/LARGE RETROESOPHAGEAL INDENTATION

A. Double aortic arch
     Both arches patent
     Atretic left arch
B. Right aortic arch
     * Aberrant left subclavian artery, left ductus arteriosus
     Mirror-image branching, left (retroesophageal) ductus arteriosus connecting left pulmonary artery to descending aorta

II. NO TRACHEAL COMPRESSION

(a) Large retroesophageal indentation
A. Left aortic arch, right descending aorta
B. Cervical aorta
(b) Shallow, oblique, retroesophageal indentation
A. Left aortic arch
     Aberrant right subclavian artery, left ductus arteriosus
B. Right aortic arch
     Aberrant left subclavian artery, right ductus arteriosus

III. ANTERIOR TRACHEAL COMPRESSION/NORMAL ESOPHAGUS

A. "Anomalous" innominate artery
B. "Anomalous" left carotid artery
C. "Brachiocephalic trunk" forming origin of innominate and left carotid arteries

IV. POSTERIOR TRACHEAL AND ANTERIOR ESOPHAGEAL INDENTATIONS

Aberrant left pulmonary artery

* Degree of tracheal compression is modified and may be absent depending on site of attachment and length of ductus arteriosus.

DOUBLE AORTIC ARCH

In 1737, Hommel was the first to describe a double aortic arch (Figure 46–2). Since then, reviews on the subject have been presented by Poynter (1916), Blincoe, Lowance, and Venable (1936), Wolman (1939), Griswold and Young (1949), Ekstrom and Sandblom (1951), Fearon and Shortreed (1963), Mahoney and Manning (1964), Lincoln and associates (1969), and Eklof and associates (1971).

More recently the excellent monographs by Stewart and associates (1964) and Klinkhamer (1969) on anomalies of the aortic arch system deal with double aortic arch anomalies extensively.

Arkin (1936) brought the condition out of the realm of pathology into the clinical field by describing the x-ray findings in patients with a double aortic arch. Gross (1945) was the first to perform successful surgery on a case and helped focus attention on the symptoms and signs and high mortality in the group that showed this defect in infancy.

Anatomy

A double aortic arch represents a persistence of both a right and left aortic arch. These arise from the ascending aorta anterior to the trachea, course dorsally on both sides of the trachea and esophagus,

and join posteriorly to form a descending aorta. If the descending aorta is on the left, there is a left anterior and right posterior arch. The left anterior arch lies against the anterior wall of the trachea, then arcs upward and posteriorly over the left main bronchus crossing the left side of the trachea and esophagus. The right posterior arch arcs upwards and to the right, curves posteriorly over the right main bronchus, and proceeds to the left behind the esophagus to join the left arch, forming a left descending aorta. If the descending aorta is right-sided, there is a left posterior and right anterior arch. The left posterior arch arcs upward and to the left, curves posteriorly over the left tracheobronchial angle, and proceeds to the right behind the esophagus. The right anterior arch arcs upward, then posteriorly crossing the right lateral wall of the trachea and esophagus to join the left branch forming a right descending aorta.

The relative size of the lumen of each arch in relationship to the other, the patency of each arch, the position of the upper descending aorta, and the side of the ductus arteriosus are all variables. While the size of each arch may be equal, or the left may be larger, nevertheless, a right arch that is larger than the left is most frequently encountered. Of 50 surgical or autopsy-confirmed cases at The Hospital for Sick Children, the right posterior was the major arch in 71

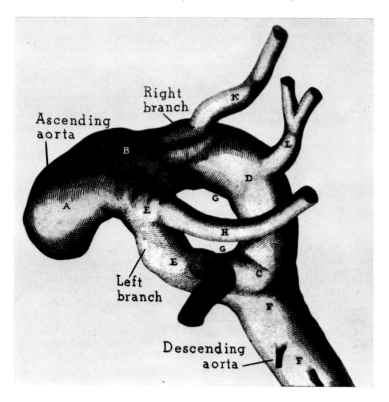

Right
branch

Ascending
aorta

Left
branch

Descending
aorta

Figure 46-2. First drawing of double aortic arch to appear in the literature. Drawing made by Hommel, 1737.

percent, in 25 percent it was the minor vessel, and in 4 percent the arches were of equal size when the upper descending aorta was left-sided. When the upper descending aorta was right-sided, the right anterior was the major arch in 86 percent, the arches were of equal size in 7 percent, while in the remaining 7 percent the left posterior arch was the larger. Klinkhamer, referring to 139 cases collected from the literature by Ekstrom and Sandblom (1951) and a thesis by Theodoridis (1960), reported that when the descending aorta was left-sided, the right arch was larger than the left in 72 percent, they were of equal size in 8 percent, while the left was the larger in 20 percent. With a right-sided descending aorta, the right was larger in 75 percent, they were of equal size in 11 percent, and in 14 percent the left was larger. The relative size of the arch is important since at operation the surgeon must divide the smaller arch. Atresia of one arch is uncommon. Stewart and associates (1964) in their monograph refer to ten cases in the literature but had none in their series of 14 cases. The atretic segment was distal to the origin of the left subclavian artery in eight and was between the left common carotid and left subclavian arteries in two. Symbas and associates (1971) have reported on three infants in whom atresia existed distal to the left subclavian artery. Shuford and colleagues (1972) have classified double aortic arch with atresia of the left arch into four subtypes according to the site of the atretic zone. In subtype 1 the atresia is between the left ductus arteriosus and descending aorta; in subtype 2 it is between the left ductus arteriosus and left subclavian artery; in subtype 3 the site is between the left

common carotid and left subclavian arteries; while in subtype 4 it is proximal to the left common carotid artery. In 8 of the 50 cases with double aortic arch encountered at The Hospital for Sick Children atresia of a segment of the left arch existed. The atretic zone in each was distal to the left subclavian artery. No case of an atretic right arch was found by Stewart and coworkers in the literature. In the reviews by Ekstrom and Sandblom (1951) and Theodoridis (1960) the upper descending aorta was left-sided in 77 percent and 71 percent, respectively. A right upper descending aorta was slightly more frequent in the cases studied at The Hospital for Sick Children, being encountered in 55 percent of the patients. Hypothetically, the ductus arteriosus may be left-sided, right-sided, or bilateral. All of the cases reported to date and all of the 50 patients reviewed at The Hospital for Sick Children, however, have had a left ductus arteriosus.

The ring formed by the arches encloses the trachea and esophagus. The left-sided ductus arteriosus connecting the aorta and pulmonary artery forms a very significant feature in determining the size of the ring. In the presence of a short ductus the pulmonary artery is pulled backward and compresses the trachea from in front while posteriorly the dorsal portion of the arch is pulled forward against the esophagus.

The origin of the brachiocephalic branches must be separate in this anomaly since an innominate artery is formed by disappearance of a dorsal aortic root. Existence of an innominate artery is reported by Gross (1945), Sweet and associates (1947), Potts and colleagues (1948), Dodrill (1952), Blumenthal and Ravitch (1957), and others. At operation, it is entirely possible not to visualize the vessels completely and thus assume that an innominate artery exists. Sweet and associates (1947) reported a case with an innominate artery at operation, though at autopsy four separate vessels existed.

Classification

Classifications dealing with types that are known to exist and hypothetical forms have been presented by Edwards (1948), Kirklin and Clagett (1950), Hartley (1959), Stewart and associates (1964), Shuford and colleagues (1972), and others. Utilizing the types that are known to exist, the following would seem to be a workable classification:

Double aortic arch, left or right upper descending aorta with:

a. Bilateral arch patency
b. Left arch segmental atresia

In the presence of bilateral arch patency the left arch may be smaller or larger than the right or they may be of equal size.

Associated Anomalies

A double aortic arch usually exists as an isolated anomaly, though the presence of associated congenital heart disease is reported. Eleven of fifty cases (22 percent) at The Hospital for Sick Children had defects. Three had a tetralogy of Fallot (two with a right-sided descending aorta), six had a ventricular septal defect (one also had a secundum atrial septal defect and another, a coarctation of the left arch), one had a preductal coarctation of the left arch, and one had a complete transposition of the great arteries. On review of the literature 12 cases had tetralogy of Fallot, eight with a right-sided descending aorta (Griswold and Young, 1949); Bahnson and Blalock, 1950; Jones and Walker, 1955; Blumenthal and Ravitch, 1957; Stewart et al., 1964; Binet et al., 1966; Klinkhamer, 1969). A coarctation of the aorta has been reported by Romanos and associates (1957) and Stewart and colleagues (1964). Lincoln and associates (1969) have reported the existence of a case with a ventricular septal defect and a left superior vena cava and a patient with a truncus arteriosus.

Clinical Features

Whether or not symptoms exist depends on the tightness of the vascular ring encircling the trachea and esophagus. If adequate space is available there will be no compression of the encircled structures and hence no symptoms. Of the cases reported in the literature, approximately 75 percent had symptoms. Griswold and Young (1949) noted that 89 percent of babies under age two years had symptoms referable to

the double arch, whereas, of those discovered over the age of two years, only 13 percent had symptoms. At The Hospital for Sick Children there are 61 cases of double aortic arch on record. Forty-one (67 percent) were operated on for relief of symptoms. The average age at the time of surgery was eight months with a range from three weeks to 24 months. In 11 patients the symptoms were not severe enough to warrant surgery. In three, the symptoms were referable to associated heart disease. The diagnosis in the remaining six was an incidental findings at autopsy in early infancy.

Symptoms in this type of vascular ring are usually present at birth or shortly after. They range from mild stridor with wheezing to attacks of dyspnea and cyanosis. In some, bouts of "reflex apnea" occur that usually last for a short period of time and no longer than three minutes. This term has been coined by Fearon and Shortreed (1963) to describe episodes of reflex respiratory arrest initiated by irritation of the area of tracheal compression. It may be initiated by a bolus of food passing through the esophagus or accumulation of secretions in the tracheobronchial tree. A wheezing type of respiration is noticeable whether the child is awake or asleep, but is made worse with crying or activity and especially with feeding or a respiratory infection. There is frequently a brassy cough. Feeding difficulties may be present though tend to become more apparent when solid foods are commenced. These children prefer to lie with the head extended, as flexion of the neck usually increases the respiratory difficulty.

There may be some increase in respiratory rate, occasionally to the point of intercostal indrawing, and on examination of the chest coarse rhonchi of a rattling type may be heard. Recurrent respiratory infections are frequent as it is difficult for these children to expel secretions past the tracheal narrowing. The heart sounds are normal without murmurs except in those cases with associated congenital heart disease.

Radiologic Examination

The radiographic patterns have been well documented by Arkin (1936), Neuhauser (1946), Stewart and associates (1964), Klinkhamer (1969), and others.

Recognition of a double aortic arch from the chest roentgenogram is difficult, and in young children with thymic tissue obscuring the superior mediastinum the diagnosis is virtually impossible. On the posteroanterior film the side of the larger of the two arches may be seen, especially if a high-kilovoltage technique is used. In a high proportion this is on the right, thus the appearance simulates a right aortic arch. An associated indentation of the adjacent lateral tracheal wall may be apparent. Only rarely is the smaller (usually the left) arch visible producing an indentation on the lateral tracheal wall at a slightly lower level. The lateral roentgenogram may demonstrate

[handwritten margin note: ® Arch is usually bigger]

narrowing of the trachea at the aortic arch level. The side of the descending aorta can usually be fairly readily identified from the posteroanterior film. The lungs may show areas of pneumonia, atelectasis, or emphysema.

⊕ Examination of the trachea and barium-outlined esophagus gives the most valuable diagnostic information. The degree of indentation of the esophagus and the size of the defect will of course vary with the size of each aortic arch. The arches indent the barium-outlined esophagus on both sides in the anteroposterior view. These indentations may be at the same level, though they are more commonly at different levels. Also, they may be of equal or, more frequently, unequal size depending on the size of each arch. If at the same level, bilateral indentations are present/If at different levels, the larger arch usually produces the larger indentation, which is often more cranially situated than the smaller arch (Figure 46–3A). The more cranial position of a large right arch indentation is not only due to the greater size of this arch, but is also due to the fact that it arcs over the right main bronchus, which is situated at a higher level than the left/The esophagus between the two arches appears kinked when the arches are at different levels. In the lateral projection, the union of the two arches with the upper descending aorta produces a large

indentation on the esophagus posteriorly. Anteriorly the esophagus is often flattened and may show a smaller indentation situated slightly cephaled to that which always exists posteriorly (Figure 46–3B). This represents pressure exerted on the trachea from the upper ascending aorta being transmi'ted to the esophagus. Klinkhamer (1969) describes the indentation as being due to a second ring produced by a short ductus arteriosus. The ductus pulls the pulmonary artery against the trachea so that the trachea and anterior aspect of the esophagus lie in close approximation and the anterior esophageal wall is notched by the trachea.

Additional diagnostic procedures, such as bronchoscopy, tracheography, esophagoscopy, and aortography may be performed. The possibility of trauma produced by bronchoscopy with resultant increase in respiratory difficulty must be considered, though this is probably slight in the hands of skilled bronchoscopists. The additional information gained in diagnosing double aortic arch variants is slight, however. Tracheography and esophagoscopy would not appear to be of value. Aortography gives the most precise details about the anatomy and will delineate the size of the arches, the sites of origin of the brachiocephalic branches (Figure 46–4), and the existence of associated anomalies, such as atresia of

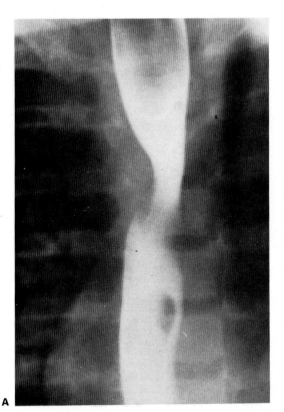 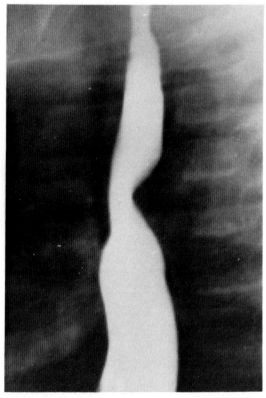

A **B**

Figure 46-3. Esophagogram in double aortic arch. *A.* Anteroposterior projection. The larger right arch produces a larger and slightly higher indentation than the smaller left. *B.* Lateral view. The large posterior concavity is produced by the union of both arches with the upper descending aorta. The anterior esophageal wall is flattened by pressure from the ascending aorta that is transmitted through the trachea.

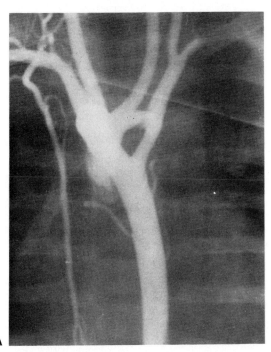
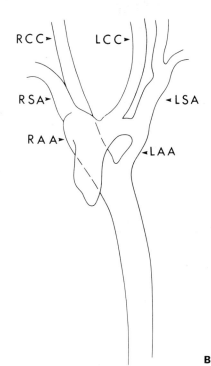

Figure 46-4. *A.* Aortogram (same case as Figure 46-3). Anteroposterior projection. *B.* The anatomy of the arches and the arrangement of the brachiocephalic branches are defined. Right aortic arch (*RAA*), left aortic arch (*LAA*), right and left subclavian arteries (*RSA* and *LSA*), right and left common carotid arteries (*RCC* and *LCC*).

one arch. As to whether this procedure should be performed must depend not only on the patient's condition, but also on the skill of the personnel carrying out the procedure and the availability of the proper specialized radiographic equipment.

Treatment

The type of treatment will be determined by the severity of symptoms. While it may be possible to carry some patients on a medical regime of liquid or semisolid foods with appropriate antibiotic therapy should the need arise, infants who exhibit stridor, wheezing, and recurrent chest infections will certainly require surgery. The presence of "reflex apneic" spells as described by Fearon and Shortreed (1963) is an absolute indication for immediate surgery.

Successful surgery was first performed by Gross (1945). Gross (1953) has pointed out that it is exceedingly important to identify the major aortic arch vessels in order to determine the proper site for ligation and section. Approximately 95 percent of cases can be dealt with by a left anterolateral approach as the left arch is usually the smaller of the two. In the presence of an atretic segment, division of this segment should be carried out so as not to sacrifice the blood supply of the left common carotid and left subclavian arteries. Division of the ligamentum arteriosum should also be carried out to complete the freeing of the vascular ring.

The operative mortality rate varies from 25 to 30 percent in the various reports in the literature. Forty-one of the sixty-one cases on record at The Hospital for Sick Children were operated on to relieve vascular compression with a mortality rate of 17 percent.

LEFT AORTIC ARCH

Embryology

The normal pattern of development of a left aortic arch with a left upper descending aorta and left ductus arteriosus as ascribed to the "hypothetical double aortic plan" of Edwards results from regression of the right dorsal root (segment between the right subclavian artery and descending aorta) and right ductus arteriosus. The innominate, left common carotid, and left subclavian arteries arise in sequence from the aortic arch. Anomalies in this arrangement may take place. The ductus arteriosus, while usually left-sided, may, nevertheless, persist on the right and regress on the left. Anatomically, these alterations may vary from no compression of the trachea or esophagus to the formation of a vascular ring.

Classification

1. Left aortic arch, left upper descending aorta, and left ductus arteriosus
   a. Anomalies of the brachiocephalic arteries with or without tracheal compression
   b. Aberrant origin of the right subclavian artery from the upper descending aorta
2. Left aortic arch, with right-sided upper descending aorta

ANOMALIES OF THE BRACHIOCEPHALIC ARTERIES WITH OR WITHOUT TRACHEAL COMPRESSION

While discussed under left aortic arch with left descending aorta, these variants may occur regardless of the side of the aortic arch or ductus.

Minor anomalies in this group include cases in which the innominate and left common carotid arteries have a common trunk arising from the aorta while the left subclavian artery arises separately. This variation was noted in approximately 10 percent of individuals by Edwards (1961) and 24 percent of 100 consecutive angiograms reported by Bosniak (1964). The term 'brachiocephalic" trunk or "bitruncus" has been coined to refer to this anomaly. While the anomaly usually causes no symptoms, one patient seen at The Hospital for Sick Children had a history of difficulty in breathing, stridor, and bouts of "reflex apnea" or respiratory arrest with unconsciousness. Death occurred during one of these attacks, and at necropsy there was tracheal compression by the innominate artery beyond the take-off of the left common carotid artery.

The separate origin of the left vertebral artery from the aorta between the left common carotid and left subclavian arteries is also reported to occur in 10 percent of individuals by Edwards (1961) and in 6 percent of the series presented by Bosniak (1964).

In the conditions often referred to as "anomalous" innominate artery or left carotid artery, tracheal compression may result.

Anomalous Innominate Artery. The innominate artery may compress the trachea anteriorly and give rise to respiratory difficulty. Cases have been reported by Gross and Neuhauser (1948), Fearon and Shortreed (1963), Maurseth (1966), Ericsson and Soderlung (1969), Berdon and associates (1969), Mustard and coworkers (1969), Eklof and associates (1971), and Moës and colleagues (1975).

A review of 60 operative cases at The Hospital for Sick Children revealed difficulty in breathing in every case, stridor in 49 patients, "reflex apnea" or respiratory arrest in 23, and recurrent respiratory infections in 20. The mean age at onset of symptoms was four months with a range from birth to 30 months. Bronchoscopy, according to Fearon and Shortreed (1963), shows anterior tracheal compression of varying degree running obliquely downward from right to left about 2 cm above the carina. The area pulsates synchronously with the heart rate, and when the bronchoscope tip is levered forward at the point of maximum pulsation, the right radial and temporal pulses either decrease or stop. The lateral chest x-ray may show a constant indentation on the anterior tracheal wall midway between the thoracic inlet and the carina. This was present in 59 percent of the 60 cases examined at The Hospital for Sick Children. Though a tracheogram may show the indentation to advantage, it is not considered that this examination is warranted. No abnormality is demonstrated on an esophagogram unless there is an associated anomaly, such as a tracheoesophageal fistula or stricture. Five of the reviewed cases had a previously repaired fistula and one a stricture.

Fearon and Shortreed (1963) have reported that there are cases in whom no tracheal compression was present in early infancy at bronchoscopy. Later symptoms developed and tracheal compression by the innominate artery was apparent.

The site of origin of the innominate artery may be of significance. While normally it almost always arises from the aorta to the left of the trachea at angiocardiography (Berdon et al., 1969), the origin may be further posterior in some patients. A posterior origin was noted in 7 of 15 patients who underwent angiography at The Hospital for Sick Children. Thus, it may be that the length of the artery is important. A congenitally short artery may give rise to tracheal compression and a posterior take-off of the artery may merely accentuate the degree of constriction.

At The Hospital for Sick Children 86 percent of the cases studied were treated conservatively (Mac-Donald and Fearon, 1971) with gradual improvement over a period of months or years due to increasing tracheal rigidity with growth and development of the cartilage rings. Surgical correction must be considered if "reflex apnea" occurs or if respiratory infections become chronic. Gross (1948) and Mustard (1969) have sutured the adventitia of the aorta or innominate artery to the sternum thus pulling the offending vessel forward. By this method, all of the patients treated at The Hospital for Sick Children without any additional abnormality obtained complete or moderate relief of symptoms. When subglottic stenosis, a tracheoesophageal fistula, or asthma was a complicating factor, the results were not as satisfactory.

Anomalous Left Carotid Artery. This anomaly is somewhat similar to the one described above. It occurs when the left common carotid artery arises farther to the right than usual. It then passes obliquely over the anterior surface of the trachea, and if it develops with sufficient tension, symptoms may be produced.

Gross (1951) has encountered two cases of this type. Neither had any difficulty in swallowing or any evidence of constriction of the esophagus on barium swallow, but both had moderate respiratory distress. Both were under one year of age when first seen.

Surgical correction is similar to that described for the anomalous innominate artery.

▶ABERRANT RIGHT SUBCLAVIAN ARTERY

In this anomaly the right subclavian artery arises as the last branch of the aortic arch and passes obliquely upward from left to right to reach the right arm. Hunault (1735) was the first to describe the condition. Bayford (1789) gave it the name of dysphagia lusoria. Klinkhamer (1966) reviewed the literature from 1763 to 1962 and collected 292 necropsy and surgical cases. Kommerell (1936) was the first to recognize the defect clinically and describe the radiologic findings.

Embryology and Anatomy

Embryologically using the "hypothetical double aortic arch plan" of Edwards, interruption of the right fourth arch occurs between the right common carotid and right subclavian arteries resulting in the origin of the right subclavian artery from the right dorsal aortic root, which remains patent. With growth, the subclavian artery migrates cephalad.

Anatomically, the right subclavian artery usually arises from the dorsal margin of the distal portion of the aortic arch beyond the origin of the left subclavian artery. In a small percentage the artery may arise from the descending aorta (Klinkhamer, 1964). The artery passes to the right side posterior to the esophagus and results in an incomplete vascular ring. Holzapfel (1899) and others have reported that in 15 percent of cases the vessel passes between the trachea and esophagus and in 5 percent anterior to the trachea. Neuhauser (1946) illustrates a case with the vessel anterior to the esophagus. Both Stewart and associates (1964) and Klinkhamer (1969) doubt the accuracy of many of these reports and suggest that cases in whom the artery passes other than posterior to the esophagus are few in number. The ductus arteriosus usually persists on the left and extends between the left pulmonary artery and left-sided upper descending aorta.

Incidence

A review of the literature indicates that the anomaly occurs in approximately 0.5 percent of cases seen at postmortem (Holzapfel, 1899; and Edwards, 1953). Maud Abbott (1932) noted it in 0.7 percent of 1000 cases. Usually it is found as an isolated defect, though it has been reported in association with congenital heart disease. A review of 53 proven cases

at The Hospital for Sick Children revealed the existence of an associated cardiac defect in 42. These consisted of 11 cases with a tetralogy of Fallot (two had pulmonary atresia), nine with a ventricular septal defect (four also had a patent ductus arteriosus), four with a patent ductus arteriosus, two with an endocardial cushion defect, and one case each of: tricuspid atresia, cor biloculare, aortic stenosis, and aortic atresia. A coarctation of the aorta existed in 12 patients (six with additional cardiac abnormalities). The aberrant right subclavian artery arose distal to the coarctation in ten, while in two both subclavian arteries originated beyond the coarctation. This rather high incidence of cardiovascular anomalies does not represent a true picture, as this is a selected group who underwent either surgery or necropsy because of an associated lesion.

When the site of coarctation is distal to the aberrant subclavian artery, the blood pressure in both arms is elevated. In this circumstance bilateral rib notching may be demonstrated radiologically. When the constriction is proximal to the aberrant vessel, the blood pressure in the left arm will be elevated and rib notching is confined to the left side. Similar unilateral rib notching may be present if the origin of the anomalous vessel is narrowed by the coarcted segment. In children it must be remembered, however, that rib notching is rare before the age of approximately seven years. Nine of forty-two proven cases of aberrant right subclavian artery reported by Stewart and associates (1964) were associated with coarctation. In three, the origin of the aberrant artery was proximal to the coarctation, though in one of these the artery was stenosed at its origin by the coarctation, while in six, the origin was distal to the coarctation. An excellent review of coarctation of the aorta in conjunction with an aberrant right subclavian artery is given in the monograph by Klinkhamer (1969).

A rather high incidence of aberrant right subclavian artery was found by Goldstein (1965) in Down's syndrome with congenital heart disease. The anomaly was noted in 37.5 percent of 28 children.

Clinical Features

Dysphagia may be present when the aberrant right subclavian artery passes posterior to the esophagus; however, the condition may exist and be asymptomatic, being discovered during a gastrointestinal series or at postmortem. It is possible, though uncommon, for the anomaly to present with respiratory distress, especially in children because the trachea is less rigid than in the adult. Mustard and associates (1962) reported a one-month-old infant with respiratory distress and regurgitation who required surgical division of the aberrant artery. Only temporary relief was obtained and the patient was subsequently found to have a hiatus hernia and reflux esophagitis. Of the 124 cases observed by Stewart and associates (1964) only eight had symptoms of a "lump in the throat" or some form of swallowing difficulty, while in the 120 cases reported by Klinkhamer (1969) only 12 were symptomatic. Two of these twelve were children with severe respiratory symptoms necessitating surgery, while ten were adults with a history of dysphagia. Eklof and coworkers (1971) encountered four children requiring surgical division of the subclavian artery with symptoms of dysphagia alone or in association with respiratory infections commencing at one week to one month of age. From these examples and a further review of the literature it would appear that the condition is usually asymptomatic. Klinkhamer is of the opinion that symptoms exist only when the right and left common carotid arteries have a common origin from the aorta (bicarotid trunk) or arise from the aorta closer to each other than normal thus forming a V anterior to the trachea. Under these circumstances, the esophagus is compressed by the right subclavian artery from behind and the trachea by the carotid arteries in front. On the other hand, when the right and left carotid arteries are normally separated the trachea and esophagus can bow forward and escape symptomatic compression by the retroesophageal vessel. This author found either a bicarotid trunk or a close origin carotid arteries in 39 percent of 292 necropsy or surgical cases collected from the literature. Only in these was there clinical evidence of tracheoesophageal compression.

Radiologic Examination

The esophagogram shows features that are diagnostic of the anomaly and are well described by Copleman (1945), Neuhauser (1946), Felson and associates (1950), Stewart and coworkers (1964), and Klinkhamer (1966). On the anterioposterior projection the artery produces an oblique linear defect in the esophagus. This commences on the left at the level of the third or fourth thoracic vertebral body and proceeds upward and to the right at an angle of about 70° from the horizontal to emerge on the right at the level of the second or third thoracic vertebra (Figure 46–5A). A somewhat similar appearance may be produced by the left main stem bronchus on the frontal projection; however, the defect in the esophageal indentation is caudal to that of an aberrant subclavian artery. Furthermore, differentiation between an aberrant subclavian artery and the more caudally situated bronchus is clearly seen on a left anterior oblique or lateral projection.

On the lateral projection, a wedge-shaped impression is seen on the posterior esophageal wall just at or below the aortic arch. The defect is fairly shallow and may appear to extend over a long segment of the esophagus due to the obliqueness of the artery (Figure 46–5B). The defect is smaller than that produced by a double aortic arch or other complete vascular rings. The anterior aspect of the esophagus is usually bowed forward opposite the retroesophageal indentation. A rather significant

feature is presented in the case of a two-year-old symptomatic child reported by Klinkhamer (1969). The esophagus and trachea at the level of the retroesophageal defect were straight and did not bow forward. The anterior tracheal wall at operation was compressed by the carotid arteries, which arose from a common stem vessel; thus tracheoesophageal constriction was produced by the aberrant right subclavian artery.

Confirmation of the vascular arrangement may be accurately defined by aortography (Figure 46–6). This procedure is rarely warranted unless symptoms exist.

Treatment

Since most cases are asymptomatic no treatment is necessary. If dysphagia is severe and not controlled by a soft diet or if respiratory obstruction is present, surgical division of the aberrant artery as suggested by Gross (1946) may be carried out.

LEFT AORTIC ARCH WITH RIGHT-SIDED UPPER DESCENDING AORTA

This anomaly is rare. The ascending aorta passes upward and arches over the left tracheobronchial angle to proceed backward, then crosses to the right, posterior to the esophagus. The descending aorta continues on the right. The ductus arteriosus may connect the right pulmonary artery to the upper right-sided descending aorta or root of an aberrant right subclavian artery. However, in one patient described by D'Cruz and associates (1966) a left ductus was found at operation. The brachiocephalic arteries may branch normally as in the cases presented by Paul (1948), Yang and colleagues (1965), D'Cruz and associates (1966), and Murthy and coworkers (1970), or there may be an aberrant right subclavian artery as in the cases of Edwards (1948), Schlamowitz and associates (1962), and Stewart and colleagues (1964). The arrangement of the brachiocephalic arteries was not ascertained in five further patients reported by Heinrich and Perez Tamayo (1956), Heim de Balsac (1960), Sterz (1961), and Gasul and coworkers (1966). These were diagnosed only by chest radiographs and esophagograms. One of the two cases noted by Gasul also had an angiocardiogram, though the position of these vessels is not mentioned.

The condition may exist as the only cardiovascular abnormality as in the cases reported by Edwards, Heinrich, and Perez Tamayo and an 11-month-old patient of D'Cruz and associates. On the other hand, associated defects were present in most patients. These consisted of a tetralogy of Fallot in one and probably tetralogy in the second case of Paul and the one of Stewart and colleagues; a ventricular septal defect and pulmonary stenosis in an eight-year-old girl of D'Cruz et al.; aortic insufficiency in the reports

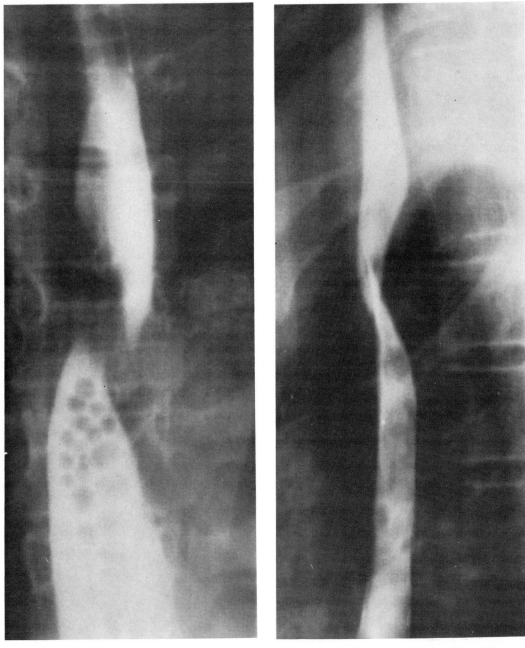

A

B

Figure 46-5. Esophagogram in aberrant right subclavian artery. *A.* Anteroposterior view. The oblique indentation produced by the subclavian artery commences on the left at the level of the fourth thoracic vertebra and proceeds upward and to the right to emerge at the third vertebra. *B.* Lateral projection. The aberrant vessel causes a relatively shallow, long retroesophageal impression.

by Heim de Balsac, Stirz, and Yang et al.; and aortic stenosis in one of the cases of Gasul et al. and D'Cruz et al. A preductal coarctation of the aorta and a persistent left superior vena cava was present in the cases described by Murthy et al. and Schlamowitz et al., respectively. Of the reported cases a true vascular ring due to a right ductus arteriosus was demonstrated only in three necropsied cases, one each of Edwards, Stewart et al., and Murthy et al., and probably in the patient described by Schlamowitz and coworkers.

A variant in this rare anomaly is one in which the aortic arch takes a pretracheal course rather than postesophageal. Two cases of this type have been described, one by Abrams (1951) and one by Klinkhamer (1969).

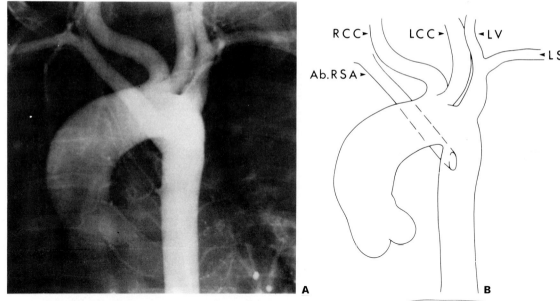

Figure 46-6. *A.* Aortogram. Anteroposterior projection. *B.* Schematic diagram. The aberrant subclavian artery arises from the aorta distal to the origin of the left subclavian artery. It passes upward and to the right. Aberrant right subclavian artery (*Ab. RSA*), left vertebral artery (*LV*).

Embryology

When the brachiocephalic arteries branch normally, the anomaly develops according to the "hypothetic double aortic arch plan" of Edwards if the right aortic arch is interrupted between the right subclavian artery and right ductus arteriosus. If the right ductus arteriosus persists and the left disappears, a vascular ring is formed. The ductus arteriosus connects the right pulmonary artery to the upper descending aorta by way of the partially persistent right dorsal aortic root.

When there is an aberrant right subclavian artery, regression of the right fourth arch between the right common carotid and right subclavian artery takes place. The subclavian artery is connected to the descending aorta by a persistent right dorsal aortic root. If the ductus arteriosus persists on the right, it passes from the root of the right subclavian artery to the right pulmonary artery. A vascular ring is thus formed consisting of the pulmonary artery anteriorly, the left-sided segment of the aortic arch on the left, the retroesophageal segment of the aorta posteriorly, and the ductus arteriosus on the right.

Clinical Features

Pressure symptoms resulting from the vascular anomaly would not appear to be common. Of the reported cases, dysphagia was present in the case reported by Edwards (1948) in whom there was an aberrant right subclavian artery and right ductus arteriosus forming a ring. Dysphagia was also a feature in the 69-year-old male presented by Stirz

(1961), though the exact vascular arrangement is not known as the diagnosis was made from an esophagogram only. Respiratory symptoms were noted in an 11-month-old patient of D'Cruz et al. (1966) in whom the ring was incomplete as the ductus arteriosus was found to be left-sided at operation.

Radiologic Examination

A high degree of suspicion as to the existence of this anomaly can be made from the chest x-ray and esophagogram as described by Paul (1948), Heinrich and Perez Tamayo (1956), Heim de Balsac (1960), Schlamowitz et al. (1962), and Gasul et al. (1966). On the posteroanterior chest film the aortic arch is left-sided and indents the left tracheobronchial angle, while the descending aorta is situated on the right. The descending aorta shadow below the knob on the left is absent. The esophagogram shows an indentation on the left, produced by the aorta; below this the esophagus is displaced to the left to a varying degree by the right-sided descending aorta. The lateral and oblique views show a retroesophageal indentation produced by the aortic arch as it passes from left to right. This defect will be nearly horizontal, though tends to slant downward slightly from left to right. The retroesophageal impression on the esophagus in the left anterior oblique view was more pronounced than in the right anterior oblique in the cases of Paul (1948) and Gasul et al. (1966). This, according to Paul, is explained on the basis of a transverse position of the aorta as it begins its retroesophageal course on the left and a somewhat diagonal position as it emerges on the right to form the descending aorta.

Aortography or angiocardiography as performed by Schlamowitz et al. (1962), Yang et al. (1965), Gasul et al. (1966), D'Cruz and coworkers (1966), and Murthy et al. (1970) will help establish the diagnosis and confirm the brachiocephalic artery arrangement.

Treatment

Surgery is warranted only if symptoms are severe. Ductus arteriosus division should be sufficient to loosen the ring in this event.

RIGHT AORTIC ARCH

The earliest report of a right aortic arch was by Fioratti and Aglietti in 1763. Since that time many excellent reviews have been published, which are listed in the monographs by Stewart et al. (1964, 1966) and Klinkhamer (1969). The first radiologically diagnosed cases were made on chest films by Mohr in 1913.

Classification

Classifications describing the various subgroups of right aortic arch have been proposed by Neuhauser (1946), Felson and Palayew (1963), Stewart et al. (1964, 1966), D'Cruz et al. (1966), Klinkhamer (1969), Shuford and coworkers (1970), and others.

The classification that is used is based on that proposed by Stewart and coworkers.

Right aortic arch:
1. With mirror-image brachiocephalic branching and
   a. Left ductus arteriosus connecting the left pulmonary artery to:
      i. Subclavian portion of left innominate artery
      ii. Upper descending aorta
   b. Right ductus arteriosus
2. With aberrant left subclavian artery and
   a. Left ductus arteriosus connecting the left pulmonary artery to:
      i. Aberrant subclavian artery
      ii. Upper descending aorta
   b. Right ductus arteriosus
3. Aberrant left innominate artery
4. With isolation of the left subclavian artery from the aorta.

Associated Anomalies

A significant difference exists regarding the presence of associated congenital heart disease in the types of right aortic arch. When there is mirror-image brachiocephalic artery branching, Stewart et al. (1966) found that there was a 98 percent chance that congenital heart disease exists. On the other hand, in the presence of a right aortic arch with an aberrant left subclavian artery and a left ductus arteriosus the existence of congenital heart disease was only 12 percent. In the series reported by Felson and Palayew (1963) 25 out of 26 patients with mirror-image branching had cyanotic heart disease, while only 4 out of 33 patients with an aberrant left subclavian had

cardiac defects (three with a patent ductus, one of whom also had a ventricular septal defect, and the fourth had a coarctation of the aorta). Twelve of the nineteen cases with an aberrant left subclavian artery at The Hospital for Sick Children had an intracardiac lesion. A ventricular septal defect was encountered in six, a tetralogy of Fallot in three (one had atresia of the pulmonary valve), a truncus arteriosus in two, and isolated pulmonary stenosis in one. This rather high incidence of associated defects is probably due to the fact that this represents a group who were primarily investigated for suspected congenital heart disease or were found to have the anomaly at necropsy performed in the neonatal period.

Incidence of Right Aortic Arch in Various Types of Congenital Heart Disease

The incidence of a right aortic arch in association with a tetralogy of Fallot varies in different reports from 13 percent by Lowe (1953) to 34 percent by Hastreiter et al. (1966). A review of 418 cases undergoing angiocardiography at The Hospital for Sick Children showed an incidence of 31 percent. In three cases, the left subclavian artery was aberrant, arising as the last branch from the arch. Four of fifteen patients with a right arch and aberrant left subclavian artery in the series reported by Stewart and coworkers (1964) had tetralogy of Fallot.

Double-outlet right ventricle demonstrates a moderately frequent occurrence of right aortic arch. This was found in twenty percent of 40 cases at The Hospital for Sick Children. Four of eighteen patients reported by Mehrizi (1965) had the arch on the right.

A right aortic arch in association with a truncus arteriosus was noted in 31 percent of 65 proven cases reviewed at The Hospital for Sick Children. In two of these there was an aberrant left subclavian artery. In the series reported by Collett and Edwards (1949) and Hastreiter et al. (1966) the incidence was 15 percent and 36 percent, respectively. Van Praagh (1965) has reported an incidence of 27 percent on review of 45 autopsied cases.

The incidence of a right aortic arch in patients with an isolated ventricular defect was encountered in 2.3 percent of 175 cases reported by Brotmacher and Campbell (1958) and 2.6 percent of 310 cases by Hastreiter et al. (1966). Becu et al. (1956) and Edwards et al. (1965) have quoted figures of 6 percent and 5 percent, respectively. Varghese et al. (1970)

state that the difference in incidence in various reports may be the result of the ages of the patients being studied. In infancy the incidence will be high. With age the defect will have closed spontaneously in a significant number, while others will have developed pulmonary stenosis. They found only two patients with a right aortic arch out of 100 children with a ventricular septal defect aged five years or over. At The Hospital for Sick Children an incidence of 2.3 percent was found out of 643 patients undergoing angiography.

Tricuspid atresia was associated with a right aortic arch in 3 of 65 (5 percent) proven cases at The Hospital for Sick Children. Hastreiter et al. (1966) has reported an incidence of 7.7 percent.

Complete transposition of the great arteries is less frequently associated with a right aortic arch. Elliott et al. (1963) reported an incidence of 4.9 percent, Hastreiter et al. (1966) an incidence of 6.7 percent. A review of 300 angiocardiograms carried out on patients with levocardia and situs solitus at The Hospital for Sick Children revealed seven cases (2.3 percent). A ventricular septal defect was present in all but one patient. One of those with a ventricular septal defect also had pulmonary valve and subvalve stenosis.

A right aortic arch in association with congenitally corrected (L) transposition of the great arteries is rare. A recent review of 100 cases at The Hospital for Sick Children revealed a right arch in one patient who had an associated ventricular septal defect and pulmonary stenosis.

RIGHT AORTIC ARCH WITH MIRROR IMAGE BRANCHING

Embryology and Anatomy

A right aortic arch with mirror-image branching of the brachiocephalic arteries results from regression of the left dorsal aortic root between the left ductus arteriosus and the descending aorta in the "hypothetic double aortic arch plan" of Edwards. The ascending aorta passes upward and to the right, anterior to the trachea. The arch then curves over the right main bronchus to proceed posteriorly, indenting the right margin of the trachea and esophagus. The upper portion of the descending aorta lies to the right of the mid line; then at or a short distance above the diaphragm it passes to the left through the normal left-sided diaphragmatic hiatus. The first branch to arise from the aortic arch is the left innominate artery followed by the right common carotid and right subclavian arteries. The ductus arteriosus may be left- or right-sided or bilateral. When left-sided, the ductus most commonly connects the left pulmonary to the subclavian portion of the left innominate artery; thus no vascular ring is formed. A rare exception is the situation in which the ductus arteriosus extends from the left pulmonary artery to the upper descending aorta. Embryologically, this is due to interruption of a segment of the left aortic arch between the left

subclavian artery and left ductus arteriosus. The remaining segment of the left dorsal aortic root between the ductus arteriosus and descending aorta persists, and it is by this that the ductus is connected to the descending aorta. The ductus, in this instance, passes behind the esophagus and a vascular ring is formed. Cases of this type have been described by Gruber (1912), Maude Abbott (1936), Neuhauser (1949), Klinkhamer (1969), Lincoln et al. (1969), Eklof et al. (1971), and Wychulis et al. (1971). When right-sided, the ductus arteriosus connects the right pulmonary artery and the aortic arch. Cases of this nature are relatively uncommon. Cases of bilateral ductus arteriosus have been described by Ghon (1908), Barger et al. (1956), and Stewart et al. (1964). In neither of these is a vascular ring formed.

Clinical Features

Symptoms of vascular compression are not a feature as no vascular ring exists. The clinical features, however, are determined by the intracardiac lesions that exist in a high proportion of these cases. An exception, however, is the situation in which the left ductus arteriosus extends from the left pulmonary artery to the upper right descending aorta. Symptoms of stridor, dysphagia, and recurrent respiratory infection usually exist due to the formation of a tight vascular ring.

Radiologic Examination

The radiologic features of a right aortic arch have been described by Fray (1936), Neuhauser (1946), Levene (1963), Felson and Palayew (1963), Stewart et al. (1964, 1966), Klinkhamer (1969), and others.

A right aortic arch with mirror-image branching of the brachiocephalic arteries and a left ductus connecting the subclavian portion of the left innominate and left pulmonary artery or a right-sided ductus arteriosus can usually be recognized on a posterior-anterior chest x-ray unless the aorta is obscured by the thymus. The aortic arch is visible where it indents the trachea slightly just above the right tracheobronchial angle and there is usually mild displacement of the trachea to the left. The arch is usually larger than normal because of the high incidence of cyanotic heart disease. On the left, in the expected position of the aortic knob, there is no vascular shadow. The upper descending aorta can usually be seen to the right of the spine. The cardiac shape is determined by the associated intracardiac abnormality. An esophagogram, which is often very helpful if the thymus is prominent, shows the aortic indentation on the right. There is no retroesophageal element except in the rare situation in which the left ductus arteriosus connects the upper descending aorta to pulmonary artery. The esophagogram in this instance as described by Neuhauser (1949), Klinkhamer (1969), and Lincoln et al. (1969) will show a nonpulsatile posterior indentation 0.5 to 1 cm in size at or just below the level of the aortic arch that is produced by the ductus arteriosus. The esophagus is not bowed forward at the site of the constriction, and the anterior oesophageal wall forms a straight line parallel to the lower tracheal airway. The pulmonary artery in this situation is pulled backward and causes the lower end of the trachea to impinge on the anterior esophageal wall. In addition to the aortic arch indentation on the right esophageal wall, a smaller and very shallow defect may be seen on the left produced by the ductus arteriosus. This appearance may simulate a double aortic arch with a small or partially atretic left arch or a right aortic arch with an aberrant left subclavian artery and left ductus arteriosus.

The arteriogram in this rare type of right aortic arch demonstrates the left innominate artery, right common carotid, and subclavian arteries arising in sequence from the aortic arch. An aortic diverticulum may be present projecting from the left lateral wall of the upper descending aorta (Wychulis et al., 1971).

RIGHT AORTIC ARCH WITH ABERRANT LEFT SUBCLAVIAN ARTERY

Embryology and Anatomy

A right aortic arch with an aberrant left subclavian artery results from regression of the left fourth arch between the left common carotid and left subclavian arteries in the "hypothetic double aortic arch plan" of Edwards. The arrangement of the brachiocephalic arteries is such that the left common carotid artery is the first branch to arise from the aortic arch. This is followed by the right common carotid and right subclavian arteries. The left subclavian artery arises as the last branch and passes to the left behind the esophagus. At this point of origin from the descending aorta the subclavian artery is frequently bulbous, as, embryologically, this portion is formed from the distal portion of the left dorsal aortic root. The position of the ductus arteriosus is more significant than in a right arch with mirror-image branching. Usually the ductus is left-sided and connects the aberrant left subclavian artery to the left pulmonary artery. The point of attachment of the left ductus to the subclavian artery is variable. Thus it may extend between the left pulmonary artery and the subclavian artery to the left of the esophagus and not run retroesophageally. This corresponds to the type lb$_2$ in the classification proposed by Klinkhamer (1969) and is the result of total persistence of the left dorsal aortic root. On the other hand, the ductus arteriosus may curve about the left esophageal margin and run retroesophageally to be connected to the bulbous origin of the aberrant subclavian artery (type lb$_3$ of Klinkhamer). This occurs when there is partial regression of the left dorsal aortic root. If total regression of the left dorsal aortic root occurs, the

subclavian artery arises from the aorta and the ductus arteriosus runs behind the esophagus to join the right aortic arch directly (type lb$_3$ of Klinkhamer). In this instance the ductus arteriosus does not join the origin of the subclavian artery. Therefore when there are a right aortic arch, aberrant left subclavian artery, and left ductus arteriosus, a vascular ring is formed encircling the trachea and esophagus. This consists of the ascending aorta and pulmonary artery anteriorly, the aortic arch on the right, and the ductus arteriosus and left subclavian artery on the left. Posteriorly the ring is completed by the proximal portion of the subclavian artery alone or the subclavian artery and the ductus arteriosus.

Two variations may exist regarding the position of the descending aorta. In one the ascending aorta is right-sided, the arch passes to the left, posterior to the esophagus, and the descending aorta is to the left of the spine. The retroesophageal vascular component is large and represents the retroesophageal position of the aortic arch principally (Baron, 1971). In the other the aorta descends to the right of the spine (Klinkhamer, 1969). In this type the retroesophageal component is smaller and represents the left subclavian artery.

Of 19 proven cases at The Hospital for Sick Children, the position of the upper descending aorta was on the right in 15 and on the left in four. The position of the upper descending aorta, when it could be determined, was left-sided in six and right-sided in 5 of 15 proven cases reported by Stewart et al. (1964).

If the ductus arteriosus is right-sided, it connects the right pulmonary artery and right-sided aortic arch; thus, the trachea and esophagus are not encircled. This anomaly is exceedingly rare, though cases have been reported by Lockwood (1884), Gross and Neuhauser (1951), and Sones and Effler (1951).

Clinical Features

The presence or absence of symptoms will depend on the degree of constriction of the trachea and esophagus by the ring. Six of the nineteen cases on record at The Hospital for Sick Children required surgical division of the aberrant left subclavian artery for respiratory difficulties alone in four and respiratory symptoms with dysphagia in two. Evidence of tracheoesophageal compression was noted in only 5 of 33 patients in the report by Felson and Palayew (1963), three of whom required surgical correction. Three of fifteen patients in the pediatric age group reported by Stewart et al. (1966) required surgery. On the other hand, Gross and Neuhauser (1951) reported on seven children with this type of anomaly requiring surgery. If the ductus arteriosus connects the right pulmonary artery and right-sided upper descending aorta, no vascular ring is formed and, thus, no compression symptoms are to be expected.

Radiologic Examination

The chest roentgenogram in the presence of an aberrant left subclavian artery and left ductus arteriosus usually reveals a normal cardiac configuration. The right-sided aortic arch is usually not enlarged, as intracardiac defects such as tetralogy of Fallot are uncommon in contradistinction to a right aortic arch with mirror-image branching. The right arch lies slightly more cephalad than a normal left arch as it arches over the right main bronchus. The bulbous origin of the left subclavian artery may form a soft tissue mass projecting to the left of the trachea in the position of a normal left aortic arch in the adult. The esophagogram is characterized by a shallow impression on the right produced by the aortic arch. On the left, no vascular indentation of the esophagus was noted by Stewart et al. (1964, 1966). Klinkhamer (1964) and Lincoln et al. (1969) have noted a small indentation produced by the subclavian artery or ductus arteriosus. The esophagogram in 6 of the 19 cases at The Hospital for Sick Children revealed a left-sided vascular impression in five (Figure 46–7A). When present this is less obvious than the defect that exists when there is a double aortic arch with a small

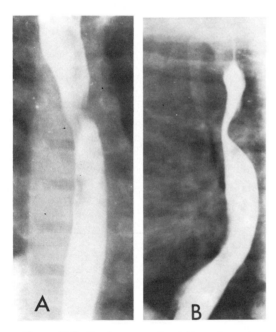

Figure 46-7. Esophagogram in right aortic arch, aberrant left subclavian artery, and left ductus arteriosus. *A.* Anteroposterior view. The aortic arch makes a shallow impression on the right, while the aberrant vessel and left ductus arteriosus produce a small indentation on the left. *B.* Lateral projection. The bulbous origin of the anomalous artery causes a large retroesophageal defect. The anterior esophageal wall in this patient is only slightly bowed forward as the ductus arteriosus pulls the pulmonary artery posteriorly against the trachea and the pressure is transmitted to the esophagus.

left arch. A large concave retroesophageal indentation, larger than that seen in most vascular rings, exists and is produced by the bulbous origin of the left subclavian artery (Figure 46–7B). When the ring is relatively nonconstrictive, there is often forward bowing of the trachea and esophagus. In the case of a constrictive ring, as tends to occur when the ductus arteriosus passes posterior to the esophagus to join either the bulbous origin of the subclavian artery or upper right-sided descending aorta, the anterior esophageal wall is not bowed anteriorly. The trachea is pulled backward in this situation and presses the trachea against the anterior esophageal wall. Confirmation of the vascular arrangement is well outlined by aortography, though the position of the ductus arteriosus cannot be defined unless it is patent (Figure 46–8).

If the ductus arteriosus is situated on the right, the radiologic features on the barium swallow are the mirror image of those seen when an aberrant right subclavian artery is present with a left aortic arch. The aberrant right subclavian artery passes behind the esophagus producing a shallow oblique defect that runs at about 70° to the horizontal plane. The trachea and esophagus are not compressed to any extent.

RIGHT AORTIC ARCH WITH ABERRANT LEFT INNOMINATE ARTERY

This is a rare type of anomaly. Grollman et al. (1968) have described a case and refer to five other reports in the literature. One such case is on record at The Hospital for Sick Children.

Embryology and Anatomy

This anomaly is the result of regression of the left arch between the ascending aorta and left common carotid artery in the "hypothetic double aortic arch" plan of Edwards. The right common carotid artery is the first branch to arise from the right aortic arch followed by the right subclavian artery and left innominate artery. The innominate artery is in effect connected to the aorta via a persistent left dorsal aortic root. The left ductus arteriosus persists. A vascular ring is thus formed by the right arch, retroesophageal left innominate artery, and left ductus arteriosus that passes from the innominate artery to the pulmonary artery in front.

Clinical Features

Symptoms of respiratory difficulties may be produced by the vascular ring.

Radiologic Examination

The aortic arch is right-sided on a chest x-ray. A barium esophageal study demonstrates a posterior

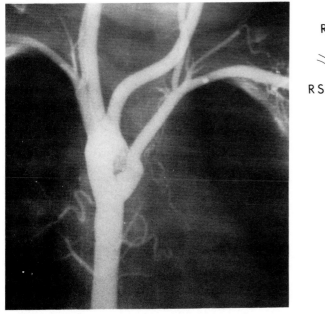
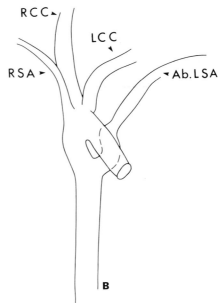

Figure 46-8. *A.* Aortogram (same case as Figure 46-7). Anteroposterior projection. *B.* Schematic diagram. The bulbous origin of the aberrant left subclavian artery is demonstrated arising from the right-sided descending aorta. The artery proceeds upward and to the left to reach the arm. Aberrant left subclavian artery (*Ab. LSA*).

compression at the aortic arch level. At angiography the brachiocephalic artery arrangement is as already described with the innominate artery arising as the third branch from the aortic arch (Grollman et al., 1968).

RIGHT AORTIC ARCH WITH ISOLATION OF THE LEFT SUBCLAVIAN ARTERY FROM THE AORTA

In this rare anomaly the left subclavian artery no longer arises from the aorta; instead it is connected to the left pulmonary artery by a left ductus arteriosus. The blood supply to the left subclavian artery is via mediastinal thoracic anastomosis or by the vertebral pathway (subclavian steal syndrome). Reports dealing with the abnormality have been presented by Stewart et al. (1964, 1966), Antia and Ottesen (1966), Levine and coworkers (1966), Gerber (1967), Maranhao et al. (1968), Shuford et al. (1970), Victoria et al. (1970), and Rodriguez et al. (1975).

Victoria et al. (1970) have divided the syndrome into three types. In the first type there is regression of the left aortic arch at two sites: one is between the left subclavian and left common carotid arteries, and the other involves the left dorsal aortic root distal to the attachment of the left ductus arteriosus. The left common carotid, right common carotid, and right subclavian arteries arise separately from the right aortic arch in that order. The left subclavian artery is connected by the ductus arteriosus to the left

pulmonary artery. No vascular ring is formed, as the aortic arch and brachiocephalic vessels are anterior to the trachea. The esophagogram shows no retroesophageal defect, and the radiographic appearance is thus similar to a right aortic arch with mirror-image brachiocephalic artery branching. Differentiation, however, can be made due to the fact that the pulse in the left arm is diminished. Angiography, preferably into the aorta, is necessary to substantiate the diagnosis. This reveals opacification of the left and right common carotid and right subclavian artery in that order directly from the aorta, while the left subclavian artery is only opacified later via the ipsilateral vertebral artery mediastinal pathways.

In the second type there is an aberrant left subclavian artery arising from a retroesophageal diverticulum with atresia or stenosis of the proximal portion of the subclavian artery. A vascular ring is completed by a left ductus arteriosus and an esophagogram shows a large posterior esophageal indentation. Again as in type I, the left arm pulse is diminished.

In the third type there is mirror-image branching of the brachiocephalic arteries. The left innominate artery is atretic and the left common carotid and left subclavian arteries may also be atretic. No vascular ring exists and there is no retroesophageal compression. Clinically, not only is the pulse in the left upper extremity diminished but the left carotid pulse is also decreased. This differentiates type III from types I and II.

Cases corresponding to type I have been reported by Gerber (1967), Maranhao et al. (1968), Shuford et al. (1970), Victoria et al. (1970), and Rodriguez et al. (1975); type II by Anita and Ottesen (1966) and Victoria et al. (1970); and type III by Levine et al. (1966).

The occurrence of this anomaly among patients with tetralogy of Fallot has been noted by Stewart et al. (1964) and Victoria and coworkers (1970). Knowledge of the situation is of importance if a left Blalock-Taussig anastomosis is contemplated.

DIFFERENTIAL DIAGNOSIS OF TYPES OF RIGHT AORTIC ARCH AND DOUBLE AORTIC ARCH

1. Differentiating a right aortic arch with mirror-image branching from a right aortic arch with an aberrant left subclavian artery may be made with a fair degree of certainty on the chest x-ray and esophagogram. In the former the ductus arteriosus connects the left subclavian artery to the left pulmonary artery; thus there is no vascular ring and hence no retroesophageal vessel is present on an esophagogram. The heart is frequently abnormal in shape and the aortic knob may be enlarged due to the high incidence of cyanotic congenital heart disease. In the latter, the ductus arteriosus connects the aberrant subclavian artery to the pulmonary artery and a vascular ring is formed. The esophagogram will confirm the existence of a posteriorly placed vessel. The heart is usually normal in configuration and the aortic knob is of normal size.

2. Differentiation of a right aortic arch with mirror-image branching and a left ductus arteriosus connecting the upper descending aorta to the left pulmonary artery (rare type) from a right aortic arch with an aberrant left subclavian artery and left ductus arteriosus cannot be made by the esophagogram. In both a retroesophageal vessel exists and the esophagus is usually indented bilaterally. Aortography, however, will depict the arrangement of the brachiocephalic arteries and differentiate these vascular rings.

3. Differentiating a right aortic arch with an aberrant left subclavian artery and left ductus arteriosus from a double aortic arch in which both arches are patent, though the left is the smaller of the two, may be difficult. In both, the feature of a right aortic arch are present on the x-ray. In the former, the aortic knob is of normal size, while in the latter, the

knob tends to be less prominent. Stewart et al. (1964) state that the smaller size of the right arch in the presence of a double aortic arch is due to the fact that this arch is supplying only a portion of the blood to the descending aorta. The esophagogram will show a prominent indentation on the left wall with a double aortic arch while this indentation is either small or absent when there is a right aortic arch, aberrant left subclavian artery, and left ductus arteriosus. Aortography will differentiate the type of abnormality that is present.

4. Differentiation of a right aortic arch with mirror-image branching from a double aortic arch with a left arch that is atretic between the left ductus arteriosus and descending aorta may be made by the esophagogram. In the former, the esophagus is indented only on the right and there is no retroesophageal indentation, while with a double aortic arch there is a bilateral indentation and there is also a retroesophageal vascular impression. Angiocardiograms in both conditions present a similar appearance. The innominate artery in the right aortic arch, however, tends to be directed cephalad and laterally. The combined left common and subclavian arteries, which present an appearance similar to a left innominate artery in a double aortic arch with atresia of the left arch, on the other hand, tend to pursue a more horizontal course as the arch is tethered by the left dorsal aortic root.

5. Differentiation of a right aortic arch with mirror-image branching and a left ductus arteriosus connecting the upper descending aorta to the left pulmonary artery (rare type) from a double aortic arch with atresia of a segment of the left arch between the left subclavian artery and left ductus arteriosus or distal to the ductus arteriosus cannot be made with certainty. In these a vascular ring is formed that encircles the trachea and esophagus. Aortography may be of help. Theoretically, the innominate artery in the former should be directed cephalad in a normal fashion, while in the latter the left arch giving rise to the left common carotid and subclavian arteries should lie in a more horizontal position as the arch is tethered by the left dorsal aortic arch.

6. Differentiation of a right aortic arch with an aberrant left subclavian artery and left ductus arteriosus from a double aortic arch with atresia of the left arch between the left common carotid and left subclavian arteries cannot be made by an esophagogram or by angiocardiography.

CERVICAL AORTA

A CERVICAL aorta is characterized by a malposition of the aortic arch so that it is situated in a position which is cephalad to the normal and is often in the neck. It often presents with a pulsatile mass in the supraclavicular region. In 16 of the 25 cases recorded to date the arch was situated on the right. This entity was first described by Reid in 1914. Since then isolated reports by Beavan and Fatti (1947), Lewis and Rogers

(1953), Harley (1959), Gravier et al. (1959), Massumi et al. (1963), Hastreiter et al. (1966), Shepherd and coworkers (1969), Chang and coworkers (1971), Shuford et al. (1972), Richie et al. (1972), Mullins et al. (1973), and Haughton and coworkers (1975) have occurred in the literature. Lewis and Rogers (1953) and Harley (1959) have described the same case. Less frequently, the arch is left-sided. Cases with a left arch have been presented by Mahoney and Manning (1964), Lipchik and Young (1967), Deffrenne and Verney (1968), Sissman (1968), Dejong and Klinkhamer (1969), Yigitbasi and Nalbantgil (1971), and McCue et al. (1973). In most of the reported cases the condition has been noted in childhood; however, the patient reported by Dejong and Klinkhamer (1969) was a 44-year-old female.

Three children with a right-sided cervical aorta have been observed at the Hospital for Sick Children.

Embryology and Anatomy

Various theories have been postulated to explain this anomaly. Persistence of the third brachial arch instead of the fourth has been suggested by Beavan and Fatti (1947), Shepherd et al. (1969), and Dejong and Klinkhamer (1969). Persistence of the second arch is suggested by Mahoney and Manning (1964). Massumi et al. (1963) are of the opinion that it is the result of failure of descent of the fourth aortic arch into the thorax along with the heart. Hastreiter et al. (1966) have postulated that confluence of the third and fourth arches when they are cervically located may be the explanation.

The aorta arises normally from the left ventricle and ascends into the neck on the right or left side. The apex of the arch has been described as being at the level of the hyoid bone or the fifth, sixth, or seventh cervical vertebra. In the patient seen by Sissman (1968) it ascended to the level of the second cervical vertebra.

Morphologic Types. Recently Haughton and coworkers (1975) have classified the cervical aorta into five morphologic types.

TYPE A. There is a contralateral descending aorta and absence of one common carotid artery. This type is usually associated with a right aortic arch. The first brachiocephalic branch to arise from the ascending aorta is the common carotid artery, usually the left. The internal and external carotid arteries, usually the right, arise as separate branches. The subclavian artery, usually the right, originates from the apex of the arch. The upper descending aorta lies on the same side as the arch and at about the level of the fourth thoracic vertebra crosses the midline to lie on the opposite side. After crossing the midline the last brachiocephalic artery arises as an aberrant subclavian artery, usually the left. Embryologically this type of cervical aorta is presumed to be due to a persistent third aortic arch on one side and involution of the fourth arches bilaterally. The aberrant subclavian is due to involution of the proximal contralateral dorsal aorta.

TYPE B. This is associated with a contralateral descending aorta and persistence of both common carotid arteries. In the reported cases the aortic arch is right-sided. The first branch to arise from the aorta is the left common carotid artery, followed by the right common carotid, right subclavian, and aberrant left subclavian in that order. This type can be explained by

the development of a right aortic arch from the fourth primitive arch with failure of migration of the arch from the cervical region into the thorax.

TYPE C. This demonstrates a contralateral descending aorta and bicarotid trunk. Deffrenne and Verney (1968) and McCue et al. (1973) have each reported a case of this type. In both, the arch was on the left and the descending aorta on the right. The common carotid arteries originate from a common stem vessel that arises from the aortic arch. The ductus arteriosus in this situation is right-sided and connects the pulmonary artery to the descending aorta.

TYPE D. There is an ipsilateral descending aorta and normal brachiocephalic artery branching. The aortic arch is situated on the left. Hypoplasia of the descending aorta is common. While development of this type of left aortic arch is normal in most respects, the segment between the left common carotid and left subclavian arteries is excessively long.

TYPE E. The aortic arch and descending aorta are situated on the right. The left common carotid, right common carotid, right subclavian, and left subclavian arteries arise from the aorta in that order. Embryologically this configuration may be explained by development of a right aortic arch with failure of migration of the arch from the cervical region into the thorax.

Clinical Features

Symptoms of tracheoesophageal compression were present in the cases reported by Beavan and Fatti (1947), Lewis and Rogers (1953), Massumi and coworkers (1963), Mahoney and Manning (1964), Lipchik and Young (1967), Deffrenne and Verney (1968), Chang et al. (1971), and Haughton et al. (1975). Physical signs of a pulsatile mass in the supraclavicular area, due to the apex of the aortic arch, are usually present, though may not be obvious unless looked for. There is a thrill and systolic murmur over the mass. Compression of the mass diminishes or obliterates the femoral pulse. The electrocardiogram is normal. Associated intracardiac lesions are rare though atrial and ventricular septal defects have been reported by Haughton et al. (1975). The three patients on record at The Hospital for Sick Children have had complicating lesions. In two there was a ventricular septal defect, while the third had a preductal coarctation of the aorta, ventricular septal defect, patent ductus arteriosus, and pulmonary stenosis.

Radiologic Examination

The chest x-ray shows widening of the superior mediastinum on the side of the aortic arch and the arch may be visualized in the apical area of the chest. The trachea may be displaced laterally by the mass and is compressed posteriorly by the descending aorta when it crosses the midline. The descending aorta, if it crosses the midline to the opposite side, indents the barium-filled esophagus posteriorly in a transverse or oblique fashion at the level of a normal aortic arch. Angiocardiography or aortography will define the nature of the anomaly and the arrangement of the brachiocephalic branches. Angiograms in the cases seen at The Hospital for Sick Children had a right aortic arch and would be classified according to Haughton et al. (1975) as type A; i.e., the left carotid artery was the first branch to arise from the aorta, followed by separate right internal and external carotid arteries, right subclavian, and aberrant left subclavian arteries.

Treatment

Treatment is required only in those cases that present with symptoms. If there is evidence of tracheoesophageal compression by a ring formed by the retroesophageal aorta, ductus arteriosus, and pulmonary artery, division of the ductus may relieve the symptoms, as in the cases of Massumi et al. (1963) and Lewis and Rogers (1964). Recognition of the nature of the cervical mass is essential. The case reported by Beavan and Fatti (1947) had ligation of the aorta carried out, mistaking the mass for an aneurysm of the right common carotid artery.

PERSISTENT LEFT FIFTH ARTERIAL ARCH

A persistent fifth left arterial arch is rare in man. Van Praagh and Van Praagh (1969) were the first to describe this anomaly in a patient with cor triatriatum. Three additional cases have been observed at The Hospital for Sick Children, two of which have been reported by Izukawa et al. (1973) and Moës and Izukawa (1974). In each instance there were associated cardiovascular anomalies. These consisted of a patent ductus arteriosus and small ventricular septal defect in one and a coarctation of the aorta, patent ductus, bicuspid aortic valve, and a single coronary artery in another. The third infant had an associated patent ductus arteriosus. No thymic tissue was present at autopsy in the first of these cases. In the reported cases the fifth arterial arch at autopsy has paralleled the left aortic arch from the level of the innominate to the left subclavian arteries with ostia at both ends that communicated with the aortic lumen. A band of tissue has been observed internally separating the two lumina.

Clinical Features

The persistence of a fifth left arterial arch in itself would not appear to give rise to symptoms. Those that are present are attributable to the associated anomalies.

Radiologic Examination

The abnormality cannot be diagnosed from the chest x-ray. Angiography, however, will demonstrate its existence. The left fifth arch may be seen as a vessel paralleling the inferior surface of the aortic arch between the levels of the origin of the innominate and left subclavian arteries (Moës and Izukawa).

ABERRANT LEFT PULMONARY ARTERY

THIS anomaly is characterized by an absence of a normal left pulmonary artery. The arterial supply to the left lung is derived from the right pulmonary artery with the anomalous vessel passing from right to left between the trachea and esophagus. The earliest report of the condition is attributed to Glaevecke and Doehle (1897). Scheid in 1938 described a similar necropsied case. Welsh and Munro (1954) were the first to recognize the condition during life. Potts et al. (1954) encountered a case at operation and carried out the first surgical correction. Wittenborg et al. (1954) and Heller and Maclean (1957) described the radiologic features. Contro and coworkers (1958) originated the term "vascular sling" to refer to the anomaly and so differentiate it from vascular rings produced by the aorta and its branches. Further reviews are presented by Stewart et al. (1964), Jue and coworkers (1965), Clarkson et al. (1967), Klinkhamer (1969), Lincoln et al. (1969), and Eklof and coworkers (1971).

Embryology and Anatomy

In this anomaly the pulmonary artery branch of the left sixth arch either fails to develop or, once formed, becomes obliterated at an early stage. As a result of the lack of arterial supply to a portion of the lung bud a collateral branch from the pulmonary segment of the right sixth arch extends into the primitive lung tissue, which is to become the future left lung. With maturation and separation of the pulmonary tissue into right and left lungs, the collateral vessel elongates and grows and assumes the function of the left pulmonary artery. The ductus arteriosus is found in a normal position indicating that the posterior portion of the left sixth arch is not involved in the malformation.

The main pulmonary artery is normally positioned and gives rise to the right pulmonary artery. The anomalous artery arises from the distal part of the main pulmonary artery or the right pulmonary artery to the right of the trachea. It passes over the right main bronchus and arches posteriorly about the tracheobronchial angle. It then pursues a course to the left between the trachea and esophagus to enter the hilus of the left lung. The sling that is formed compresses the proximal portion of the right main bronchus and distal end of the trachea. The pressure exerted may lead to defective development of the cartilage rings.

Clinical Features

Symptoms due to the "vascular sling" are solely respiratory in nature and are usually present at or shortly after birth. The case reported by Klinkhamer, however, did not exhibit signs until three months of age. The manifestations are stridor and wheezing, attacks of dyspnea and cyanosis, and recurrent respiratory infections. The stridor is likely to be expiratory, in contradistinction to the inspiratory stridor noted in aortic vascular rings. Symptoms are usually severe and are life-threatening within the first six months of life unless surgical intervention is carried out. Cases with only mild or no symptoms have been reported by Rudhe and Zetterqvist (1959), Murphy et al. (1964), Hiller (1965), and Klinkhamer (1969). Three cases are on record at The Hospital for Sick Children.

Cardiac findings are not a feature unless intracardiac anomalies exist. Cases with an atrial septal defect have been reported by Wittenborg et al. (1956), Jacobson et al. (1960), and Sissman (1968); a ventricular septal defect by Wittenborg et al. (1956), Jacobson and coworkers (1960), Jue et al. (1965), and Tan et al. (1968); a patent ductus by Jacobson et al. (1960); and a persistent left superior vena cava by Wittenborg et al. (1956), Jackson and coworkers (1960), and Jue et al. (1965). Aortic arch anomalies were present in two cases reported by Wittenborg et al. (1956). One patient had a coarctation of the aorta, while another had an aberrant right subclavian artery. A tetralogy of Fallot with a right aortic arch was present in one of the cases of Jacobson et al. (1960).

Radiologic Examination

The trachea and esophagus tend to be squeezed together radiologically in the vascular anomalies already described, while in the "vascular sling" they are displaced away from one another. The chest roentgenogram appearance will vary depending on the degree of obstruction of the right main stem bronchus and lower trachea. Thus, while the lungs may be equally inflated and clear, right-sided obstructive emphysema is most common. If the

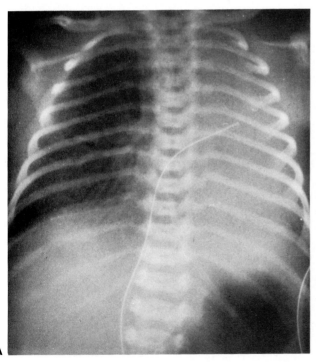
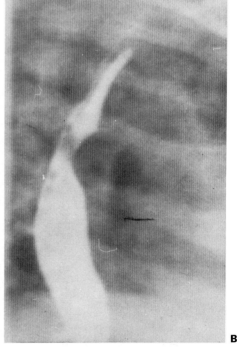

A   B

Figure 46-9. Aberrant left pulmonary artery. *A.* Anteroposterior chest x-ray showing hyperinflated right and atelectatic left lung with mediastinal shift to the left. *B.* Esophagogram, lateral projection. An anterior defect produced by the aberrant vessel passing between the esophagus and lower end of the trachea is present at the level of the tracheal bifurcation. At the same level the right main stem bronchus was bowed anteriorly on the lateral chest x-ray. (Reproduced from Martin, D. J.: Experiences with acute surgical conditions. *Radiol. Clin. North Am.,* **13:**324, 1975.)

obstruction is severe, however, atelectasis will occur. The obstructed segment of the right lung may present immediately after birth as an opaque area due to retained fetal lung fluid (Corbett, 1971). The presence of a right tracheal bronchus arising above the sling, as has been reported by Jacobson et al. (1960), Jue et al. (1965), Tan and coworkers (1968), and Capitanio et al. (1971), may result in compensatory hyperinflation of the upper lobe and atelectasis of the middle and lower lobes. Atelectasis or emphysema involving the left lung may also occur due to compression of the trachea by the anomalous pulmonary artery or there may be associated tracheal and/or bronchial hypoplasia or stenosis. In combination with either hyperinflation or atelectasis, pneumonia may be present.

The left hilus may be situated at a lower level than normal (Capitanio et al., 1971). Normally the left pulmonary artery is seen to branch at the level of the main pulmonary artery; however, in the presence of a "pulmonary sling," the branching may be noted at a lower level than the main pulmonary artery. On the lateral chest x-ray anterior bowing of the right main bronchus with an associated posterior indentation at the lower end of the trachea may be appreciated.

An esophagogram will frequently show an indentation of the anterior esophageal wall at the level of the tracheal bifurcation, first described by Wittenborg and coworkers (1956). Sprague and Kennedy (1976) state that when the right lung is hyperinflated the trachea is displaced from in front of the esophagus. This may result in an anterolateral or lateral esophageal indentation. It must be also stressed that the barium study may be normal.

Angiocardiography is the most accurate way of delineating the anatomy of the vascular anomaly. The left pulmonary artery is seen arising from the right and passing obliquely downward and to the left, posterior to the trachea, toward the hilus of the left lung.

The chest x-rays in two of the three patients seen at The Hospital for Sick Children showed a hyperinflated right lung with mediastinal shift to the left. In one patient there was also atelectasis of the left lung (Figure 46–9A). On the lateral chest film of this case there was anterior bowing of the right main stem bronchus. A barium swallow demonstrated an anterior indentation of the esophagus at the level of the tracheal bifurcation (Figure 46–9B). At bronchoscopy both main stem bronchi were slightly small but not occluded. Bronchoscopy in the other case, which has been reported by Mustard et al. (1962), revealed partial occlusion of the right bronchus by a nonpulsatile mass. A chest x-ray made at one day of age in the third patient demonstrated retained fluid in the right lung and hyperinflation of the left. An esophagogram was normal. Bronchoscopy revealed extrinsic stenosis of the distal trachea. At thoracotomy the true nature of the anomaly became apparent; however, death occurred after attempted correction. Angiocardiography was performed in only one patient. This outlined the left pulmonary

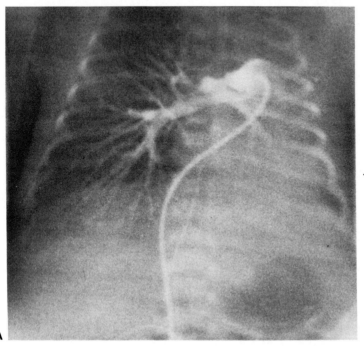
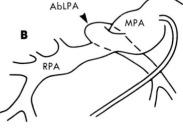

A

Figure 46-10. *A.* Pulmonary angiogram. Anteroposterior projection. A catheter is present in the main pulmonary artery. *B.* Schematic diagram. The aberrant left pulmonary artery arises from the proximal portion of the right pulmonary artery, then passes inferiorly and to the left to reach the left lung. Main pulmonary artery (*MPA*), right pulmonary artery (*RPA*), aberrant left pulmonary artery (*AbLPA*).

artery arising from the proximal segment of the right pulmonary artery and passing to the left, posterior to the trachea, to supply a hypoplastic left lung (Figure 46–10).

Treatment

Surgical division of the aberrant left pulmonary artery at its point of origin with redirection of its course anterior to the trachea and anastomosis to the main pulmonary artery as described by Potts and coworkers (1954), Contro et al. (1958), and Jacobson and associates (1960) would appear to be the procedure of choice. This procedure was attempted though unsuccessfully, on the second patient seen at The Hospital for Sick Children. The patient reported by Mustard et al. (1962) was treated by ligation and division of the ductus arteriosus with marked relief of symptoms.

REFERENCES

Abbott, M. E.: Congenital heart disease. *Nelson's Loose-leaf Medicine*, 4:155, 1932.

Abbott, M. E.: *Atlas of Congenital Cardiac Diseases*. American Heart Association, New York, 1936.

Abrams, H. L.: Left ascending aorta with right arch and right descending aorta. *Radiology*, 57:58, 1951.

Antia, A. U., and Ottesen, O. E.: Collateral circulation in subclavian stenosis or atresia: Angiographic demonstration of retrograde vertebral-subclavian flow in two cases with right aortic arch. *Am. J. Cardiol.*, 18:599, 1966.

Arkin, A.: Double aortic arch with total persistence of the right and isthmus stenosis of the left: A new clinical and x-ray picture: Report of six cases in adults. *Am. Heart J.*, 11:444, 1936.

Bahnson, H. E., and Blalock, A.: Aortic vascular rings encountered in surgical treatment of congenital pulmonic stenosis. *Ann. Surg.*, 131:356, 1950.

Barger, J. D.; Bregman, E. H.; and Edwards, J. E.: Bilateral ductus arteriosus with right aortic arch and right-sided aorta: Report of case. *Am. J. Roentgenol. Radium Ther. Nucl. Med.*, 76:758, 1956.

Baron, M. G.: Right aortic arch. *Circulation*, 44:1137, 1971.

Bayford, D.: An account of a singular case of obstructed deglutition. *Mem. Med. Soc.*, 2:271, 1789.

Beavan, T. E. D., and Fatti, L.: Ligature of aortic arch in the neck. *Br. J. Surg.*, 34:414, 1947.

Becu, L. M.; Fontana, R. S.; Du Shane, J. W.; Kirklin, J. W.; Burchell, H. B.; and Edwards, J. E.: Anatomic and pathologic studies in ventricular septal defect. *Circulation*, 14:349, 1956.

Berdon, W. E.; Baker, D. H.; Bordiuk, J.; and Mellins, R.: Innominate artery compression of the trachea in infants with stridor and apnea. *Radiology*, 92:272, 1969.

Berdon, W. E., and Baker, D. H.: Vascular anomalies and the infant lung: Rings, slings, and other things. *Semin. Roentgenol.*, 7:39, 1972.

Binet, J. P.; Carpentier, J.; Pottemain, M.; and Langlois, J.: Double aortic arch associated with tetralogy of Fallot in infants: Report of two cases. *J. Thorac. Cardiovasc. Surg.*, 51:116, 1966.

Blincoe, H.; Lowance, M. I.; and Venable, J.: A double aortic arch in man. *Anat. Rec.*, 66:505, 1936.

Blumenthal, S., and Ravitch, M. M.: Seminar on aortic vascular rings and other anomalies of the aortic arch. *Pediatrics*, 20:896, 1957.

Bosniak, M. A.: An analysis of some anatomic-roentgenologic aspects of the brachiocephalic vessels. *Am. J. Roentgenol. Radium Ther. Nucl. Med.*, 91:1222, 1964.

Brotmacher, L., and Campbell, M.: The natural history of ventricular septal defect. *Br. Heart J.*, 20:97, 1958.

Capitanio, M. A.; Ramos, R.; and Kirkpatrick, J. A.: Pulmonary sling, roentgen observations. *Am. J. Roentgenol. Radium. Ther. Nucl. Med.*, 112:28, 1971.

Chang, L. W. M.; Kaplan, E. L.; Baum, D.; and Figley, M. M.: Aortic arch in the neck: A case report. *J. Pediatr.*, 79:788, 1971.

Clarkson, P. M.; Ritter, D. G.; Rahimtoola, S. H.; Hallermann, F. J.; and McGoon, D. C.: Aberrant left pulmonary artery. *Am. J. Dis. Child.*, 113:373, 1967.

Collett, R. W., and Edwards, J. E.: Persistent truncus arteriosus: A classification according to anatomic types. *Surg. Clin. North Am.*, 29:1245, 1949.

Contro, S.; Miller, R. A.; White, H.; and Potts, W. J.: Bronchial obstruction due to pulmonary artery anomalies. I. Vascular sling. *Circulation*, 17:418, 1958.

Copleman, B.: Anomalous right subclavian artery. *Am. J. Roentgenol.*, 54:270, 1945.

Corbett, D. P., and Washington, J. E.: Respiratory obstruction in the newborn and excess pulmonary fluid. *Am. J. Roentgenol. Radium Ther. Nucl. Med.*, 18:112, 1971.

D'Cruz, I. A.; Cantiz, T.; Namin, E. P.; Licata, R.; and Hastreiter, A. R.: Right-sided aorta: Part II. Right aortic arch, right descending aorta, and associated anomalies. *Br. Heart J.*, 28:725, 1966.

Deffrenne, P., and Verney, R.: L'aorte cervicale. *Ann. Radiol.*, 11:525, 1968.

DeJong, I. H., and Klinkhamer, A. C.: Left-sided cervical aortic arch. *Am. J. Cardiol.*, 23:285, 1969.

Dodrill, F. D.: Double aortic arch. *Surgery*, 31:204, 1952.

Edwards, J. E.: Anomalies of the derivatives of the aortic arch system. *Med. Clin. North Am.*, 32:925, 1948.

Edwards, J. E.: Retro-esophageal segment of the left aortic arch, right ligamentum arteriosum and right descending aorta causing a congenital vascular ring about the trachea and esophagus. *Proc. Staff Meet. Mayo. Clin.*, 23:108, 1948.

Edwards, J. E.: Malformations of the aortic arch system manifested as "vascular rings." *Lab. Invest.*, 2:56, 1953.

Edwards, J. E.: Congenital malformations of the heart and great vessels. In Gould, S. E. (ed.): *Pathology of the Heart*, 2nd ed. Charles C Thomas, Publisher, Springfield, Ill., 1960.

Edwards, J. E.: *An Atlas of Acquired Diseases of the Heart and Great Vessels*. W. B. Saunders Co., Philadelphia, 1961.

Edwards, J. E.; Carey, L. S.; Neufeld, H. N.; and Lester, R. G.: Increased pulmonary arterial vasculature; cyanosis absent, intracardiac: Left to right shunts ventricular septal defect: Associated anomalies; mitral insufficiency. In: *Congenital Heart Disease: Correlation of Pathologic Anatomy and Angiocardiography*, Vol. I. W. B. Saunders Co., Philadelphia, 1965.

Eklöf, O.; Ekström, G.; Eriksson, B. O.; Michaëlsson, M.; Stephensen, O.; Söderlund, S.; Thorén, C.; and Wallgren, G.: Arterial anomalies causing compression of the trachea and/or the oesophagus: A report of 30 symptomatic cases. *Acta Paediatr. Scand.*, 60:81, 1971.

Ekström, G., and Sandblom, P.: Double aortic arch. *Acta Chir. Scand.*, 102:183, 1951.

Elliott, L. P.; Neufeld, H. N.; Anderson, R. C.; Adams, P., Jr.; and Edwards, J. E.: Complete transposition of the great vessels: I. An anatomic study of sixty cases. *Circulation*, 27:1105, 1963.

Ericsson, N. O., and Söderlund, S.: Compression of the trachea by an anomalous innominate artery. *J. Pediatr. Surg.*, 4:424, 1969.

Fearon, B., and Shortreed, R.: Tracheobronchial compression by congenital cardiovascular anomalies in children: Syndrome of apnea. *Ann. Otol. Rhinol. Laryngol.*, 72:949, 1963.

Felson, B.; Cohen, S.; Courter, S. R.; and McGuire, J.: Anomalous right subclavian artery. *Radiology*, 54:340, 1950.

Felson, B., and Palayew, M. J.: The two types of right aortic arch. *Radiology*, 81:745, 1963.

Fray, W. W.: Right aortic arch. *Radiology*, 26:27, 1936.

Gasul, B. M.; Arcilla, R. A.; and Lev, M.: *Heart Disease in Children, Diagnosis and Treatment*, 1st ed. J. B. Lippincott, Philadelphia, 1966.

Gerber, N.: Congenital atresia of the subclavia artery producing the "subclavian steal syndrome." *Am. J. Dis. Child.*, 113:709, 1967.

Ghon, A.: Ueber eine seltene Entwicklungsstörung des Getässystems. *Verh. Dtsch. Ges. Pathol.*, 12:242, 1908.

Glaeveche and Doehle: Ueber eine seltene angeborene Anomalie der Pulmonalarterie. *Munch. Med. Wochenschr.*, 44:950, 1897.

Goldstein, W. B.: Aberrant right subclavian artery in mongolism. *Am. J. Roentgenol.*, 95:131, 1965.

Gravier, J.; Vialtel, M.; and Pinet, F.: Apropos d'une Tumeur pulsatile du cou: Un cas d'aorte cervicale. *Pediatrie*, 14:437, 1959.

Griswold, H. E., and Young, M. D.: Double aortic arch and review of the literature. *Pediatrics*, 4:751, 1949.

Grollman, J. H.; Bedynek, J. L.; Henderson, H. S.; and Hall, R. J.: Right aortic arch with an aberrant retroesophageal innominate artery: angiographic diagnosis. *Radiology*, 90:782, 1968.

Gross, R. E.: Surgical relief for tracheal obstruction from a vascular ring. *N. Engl. J. Med.*, 233:586, 1945.

Gross, R. E.: Surgical treatment for dysphagia lusoria. *Ann. Surg.*, 124:532, 1946.

Gross, R. E., and Neuhauser, E. D. B.: Compression of the trachea by an anomalous innominate artery: An operation for its relief. *Am. J. Dis. Child.*, 75:570, 1948.

Gross, R. E., and Neuhauser, E. B. D.: Compression of the trachea or esophagus by vascular anomalies; surgical therapy in 40 cases. *Pediatrics*, 7:69, 1951.

Gross, R. E.: *The Surgery of Infancy and Childhood*. W. B. Saunders Co., Philadelphia, 1953.

Gruber, G. B.: Zwei Fälle von Dextropositio des Aortenbogens. *Frankfurt Z. Pathol.*, 10:375, 1912.

Harley, H. R. S.: The development and anomalies of the aortic arch and its branches: With the report of a case of right cervical aortic arch and intrathoracic vascular ring. *Br. J. Surg.*, 46:561, 1959.

Hastreiter, A. R.; D'Cruz, I. A.; and Cantez, T.: Right-sided aortic: Part I. Occurrence of right aortic arch in various types of congenital heart disease. *Br. Heart J.*, 28:722, 1966.

Haughton, V. M.; Fellows, K. E.; and Rosenbaum, A. E.: The cervical aortic arches. *Radiology*, 114:675, 1975.

Heim de Balsac, R.: Left aortic arch (posterior or circumflex type) with right descending aorta. *Am. J. Cardiol.*, 5:546, 1960.

Heinrich, W. D., and Perez Tamayo, R.: Left aortic arch and right descending aorta: Case report. *Am. J. Roentgenol.*, 76:762, 1956.

Hiller, H. G., and Maclean, A. D.: Pulmonary artery ring. *Acta Radiol.*, 48:434, 1957.

Hiller, H. G.: Vascular rings. *J. Coll. Radiol. Australasia*, 9:120, 1965.

Holzapfel, G.: Ungewöhnlicher Unsprung und Verlauf der arteria subclavia dextra. *Anat. Hefte.*, 12:369, 1899.

Izukawa, T.; Scott, M. E.; Durrani, F.; and Moës, C. A. F.: Persistent left fifth aortic arch in man. Report of two cases. *Br. Heart J.*, 35:1190, 1973.

Jacobson, J. H.; Morgan, B. C.; Anderson, D. H.; and Humphreys, G. H.: Aberrant left pulmonary artery: A correctable cause of respiratory obstruction. *J. Thorac. Cardiovasc. Surg.*, 39:602, 1960.

Jones, C. H., and Walker, J. K.: Double aortic arch with a report of a case. *J. Fac. Radiol.*, 6:281, 1955.

Jue, K. L.; Raghib, G.; Amplotz, K.; Adams, P., Jr.; and Edwards, J. E.: Anomalous origin of the left pulmonary artery from the right pulmonary artery. *Am. J. Roentgenol.*, 95:598, 1965.

Kirklin, J. W., and Clagett, O. T.: Symposium on respiratory obstruction in infancy and childhood: Vascular "rings" producing respiratory obstruction in infants. *Proc. Staff. Meet. Mayo Clin.*, 25:360, 1950.

Klinkhamer, A. C.: The significance of the oesophagogram for the demonstration of aberrant arteries in the superior mediastinum. *Medicamundi*, 10:28, 1964.

Klinkhamer, A. C.: Aberrant right subclavian artery: Clinical and roentgenologic aspects. *Am. J. Roentgenol. Radium. Ther. Nucl. Med.*, 97:438, 1966.

Klinkhamer, A. C.: Esophagography. In *Anomalies of the Aortic Arch System*. Excerpta Medica Foundation, Amsterdam, 1969.

Kommerell, B.: Verlagerung des ösophagus durch eine abnorm verlaufende arteria subclavia dextra (arteria-lusoria). *Fortschr. Geb. Roentgensfr. Nuklearmed.*, 54:590, 1936.

Levene, G.: A new roentgenologic sign of right aortic arch. *Radiology*, 80:434, 1963.

Levine, S.: Serfas, L. S.; and Rusinko, A.: Right aortic arch with subclavian steal syndrome (atresia of left common carotid and left subclavian arteries). *Am. J. Surg.*, 111:632, 1966.

Lewis, C., and Rogers, L.: The cervical aortic knuckle which resembles an aneurysm. *Lancet*, 1:825, 1953.

Lincoln, J. C. R.; Deverall, P. B.; Stark, J.; Aberdeen, E.; and Waterston, D. J.: Vascular anomalies compressing the oesophagus and trachea. *Thorax*, 24:295, 1969.

Lipchik, E. O., and Young, L. W.: Unusual symptomatic aortic arch anomalies. *Radiology*, 89:85, 1967.

Lockwood, C. B.: Right aortic arch. *Trans. Pathol. Soc. London*, 35:132, 1884.

Lowe, J. B.: The angiocardiogram in Fallot's tetralogy. *Br. Heart J.*, 15:319, 1953.

MacDonald, R. E., and Fearon, B.: Innominate artery compression syndrome in children. *Ann. Otol. Rhinol. Laryngol.*, 80:535, 1971.

Mahoney, E. B., and Manning, J. A.: Congenital abnormalities of the aortic arch. *Surgery*, 55:1, 1964.

Maranhao, V.; Gooch, A. S.; Ablaza, S. G. G.; Nakhjavan, F. K.; and Goldberg, H.: Congenital subclavian steal syndrome associated with right aortic arch. *Br. Heart J.*, 30:875, 1968.

Massumi, R.; Wiener, L.; and Charif, P.: The syndrome of cervical aorta: Report of a case and review of the previous cases. *Am. J. Cardiol.*, 11:678, 1963.

Maurseth, K.: Tracheal stenosis caused by compression from the innominate artery. *Ann. Radiol.*, 9:287, 1966.

McCue, C. M.; Mauck, H. P., Jr.; and Tingelstad et al.: Cervical aortic arch. *Am. J. Dis. Child.*, 125:738, 1973.

Mehrizi, A.: The origin of both great vessels from the right ventricle: I. With pulmonic stenosis: Clinico-pathological correlation in 18 autopsied cases. *Bull. Johns Hopkins Hosp.*, 117:75, 1965.

Moës, C. A. F., and Izukawa, T.: Persistent fifth arterial arch. Diagnosis during life, with post mortem confirmation. *Radiology*, 111:175, 1974.

Moës, C. A. F.; Izukawa, T.; and Trusler, G. A.: Innominate artery compression of the trachea. *Arch. Otolaryngol.*, 101:733, 1975.

Mohr, R.: Zur Diagnostik der Kongenitalen Herzfehler. *Dtsch. Z. Nervenheilkd.*, 47-48:371, 1913.

Mullins, C. E.; Gillette, P. C.; and McNamara, D. G.: The complex of cervical aortic arch. *Pediatrics*, 51:210, 1973.

Murphy, D. R.; Dunbar, F. S.; MacEwen, D. W.; Sanchez, F. R.; and Percy, D. Y. E.: Tracheobronchial compression due to a vascular sling. *Surg. Gynecol. Obstet.*, 118:572, 1964.

Murthy, K.; Mattioli, L.; Diehl, A. M.; and Holder, T. M.: Vascular ring due to left aortic arch, right descending aorta, and right patent ductus arteriosus. *J. Pediatr. Surg.*, 5:550, 1970.

Mustard, W. T.; Trimble, A. W.; and Trusler, G. A.: Mediastinal vascular anomalies causing tracheal and esophageal compression and obstruction in childhood. *Can. Med. Assoc. J.*, 87:1301, 1962.

Mustard, W. T.; Bayliss, C. E.; Fearon, B.; Pelton, D.; and Trusler, G. A.: Tracheal compression by the innominate artery in children. *Ann. Thorac. Surg.*, 8:312, 1969.

Neuhauser, E. B. D.: The roentgen diagnosis of double aortic arch and other anomalies of the great vessels. *Am. J. Roentgenol. Radium Ther. Nucl. Med.*, 56:1, 1946.

Neuhauser, E. B. D.: Tracheo-esophageal constriction produced by right aortic arch and left ligamentum arteriosum. *Am. J. Roentgenol. Radium Ther. Nucl. Med.*, 62:493, 1949.

Paul, R. N.: A new anomaly of the aorta: Left aortic arch with right descending aorta. *J. Pediatr.*, 32:19, 1948.

Potts, W. J.; Gibson, S.; and Rothwell, R.: Double aortic arch: Report of two cases. *Arch. Surg.*, 57:227, 1948.

Potts, W. J.; Hollinger, P. H.; and Rosenblum, A. H.: Anomalous left pulmonary artery causing obstruction to right main bronchus: Report of a case. *JAMA*, 155:1409, 1954.

Poynter, C. W. M.: Arterial anomalies pertaining to the aortic arches and the branches arising from them. *University Studies of the University of Nebraska*, Lincoln, Nebr., 1916, p. 129.

Reid, D. G.: Three examples of a right aortic arch. *J. Anat. Physiol.*, 48:174, 1913-1914.

Richie, R.; Del Rio, C.; Mullins, C. E.; et al.: Right-sided cervical aortic arch. *Am. Heart J.*, 84:531, 1972.

Rodriguez, L.; Izukawa, T.; Moës, C. A. F.; Trusler, G. A.; and Williams, W. G.: Surgical implications of right aortic arch with isolation of left subclavian artery. *Br. Heart J.*, 37:931, 1975.

Romanos, A. N.; Bruins, C. L.; and Brom, A. D.: Rare anomaly of the aortic arch combined with coarctation of the aorta. *Dis. Chest*, 31:540, 1957.

Rudhe, U., and Zetterqvist, P.: Aberrant left pulmonary artery. *Acta Chir. Scand.*, 245:331, 1959.

Scheid, P.: Missbildung des Trachealskelettes und der linken: Arteria pulmonalis mit Erstickungstod bei 7 monate altem Kind. *Frankfurt Z. Pathol.*, 52:114, 1938.

Schlamowitz, S. T.; Di Giorgi, S.; and Gensini, G. G.: Left aortic arch and right descending aorta. *Am. J. Cardiol.*, 10:132, 1962.

Shepherd, R. M.; Kerth, W. J.; and Rosenthal, J. H.: Right cervical aortic arch with left descending aorta. *Am. J. Dis. Child.*, **118**:642, 1969.

Shuford, W. H.; Sybers, R. G.; and Schlant, R. C.: Right aortic arch with isolation of the left subclavian artery. *Am. J. Roentgenol. Radium Ther. Nucl. Med.*, **109**:75, 1970.

Shuford, W. H.; Sybers, R. G.; and Edwards, F. K.: The three types of right aortic arch. *Am. J. Roentgenol. Radium Ther. Nucl. Med.*, **109**:67, 1970.

Shuford, W. H.; Sybers, R. G.; and Weens, H. S.: The angiographic features of double aortic arch. *Am. J. Roentgenol. Radium Ther. Nucl. Med.*, **116**:125, 1972.

Shuford, W. H.; Sybers, R. G.; Milledge, R. D.; et al.: The cervical aortic arch. *Am. J. Roentgenol. Radium Ther. Nucl. Med.*, **116**:519, 1972.

Shuford, W. H., and Sybers, R. G.: *The Aortic Arch and Its Malformations.* Charles C Thomas, Publisher, Springfield, Ill., 1974, 110.

Sissman, N. J.: Anomalies of the aortic arch complex. In Moss, A. J., and Adams, F. H. (eds.): *Heart Disease in Infants, Children and Adolescents.* Williams & Wilkins Co., Baltimore, 1968.

Sones, F. M., Jr., and Effler, D. B.: Diagnosis and treatment of aortic rings. *Cleveland Clin. Quart.*, **18**:310, 1951.

Sprague, P. L., and Kennedy, J. C.: Anomalous left pulmonary artery with an unusual barium swallow. *Pediatr. Radiol.*, **4**:188, 1976.

Sterz, H.: Dysphagie durch eine seltene Anomalie der Aorta thoracalis: Arcus aortae sinistir circumflexus und Dextroposition dir Aorta discendins. *Wien Z. Inn. Med.*, **42**:420, 1961.

Stewart, J. R.; Kincaid, O. W.; and Edwards, J. E.: *An Atlas of Vascular Rings and Related Malformations of the Aortic Arch System.* Charles C Thomas, Publisher, Springfield, Ill., 1964.

Stewart, J. R.; Kincaid, O. W.; and Titus, J. L.: Right aortic arch: Plain film diagnosis and significance. *Am. J. Roentgenol. Radium Ther. Nucl. Med.*, **97**:377, 1966.

Sweet, R. H.; Findlay, C. W., Jr.; and Reyersbach, G. C.: The diagnosis and treatment of tracheal and esophageal obstruction due to congenital vascular ring. *J. Pediatr.*, **30**:1, 1947.

Symbas, P. N.; Shuford, W. H.; Edwards, F. K.; and Sehdena, J. S.: Vascular ring: Persistent right aortic arch, patent proximal left arch, obliterated distal left arch, and left ligamentum arteriosum. *J. Thorac. Cardiovasc. Surg.*, **61**:149, 1971.

Tan, P. M.; Loh, T. F.; Yong, N. K.; and Sugai, K.: Aberrant left pulmonary artery. *Br. Heart J.*, **30**:110, 1968.

Van Praagh, R., and Van Praagh, S.: The anatomy of common aorticopulmonary trunk (truncus arteriosus communis) and its embryologic implications. *Am. J. Cardiol.*, **16**:406, 1965.

Van Praagh, R., and Van Praagh, S.: Persistent fifth arterial arch in man. *Am. J. Cardiol.*, **24**:279, 1969.

Varghese, P. J.; Allen, J. R.; Rosenquist, G. C.; and Rowe, R. D.: Natural history of ventricular septal defect with right-sided aortic arch. *Br. Heart J.*, **32**:537, 1970.

Victoria, B. E.; Van Mireop, L. H. S.; and Elliott, L. P.: Right aortic arch associated with contralateral congenital subclavian steal syndrome. *Am. J. Roentgenol. Radium Ther. Nucl. Med.*, **108**:582, 1970.

Welsh, T. M., and Munro, I. B.: Congenital stridor caused by an aberrant pulmonary artery. *Arch. Dis. Child.*, **29**:101, 1954.

Wittenborg, M. H.; Tantiwongse, T.; and Rosenberg, B. F.: Anomalous course of left pulmonary artery with respiratory obstruction. *Radiology*, **67**:339, 1956.

Wolman, I. J.: Syndrome of constricting double aortic arch in infancy. Report of a case. *J. Pediatr.*, **14**:527, 1939.

Wychulis, A. R.; Kincaid, O. W.; and Danielson, G. K.: Congenital vascular ring: Surgical considerations and results of operation. *Mayo Clin. Proc.*, **46**:182, 1971.

Yang, S. S.; Maranhao, V.; and Goldberg, H.: Left aortic arch and right descending aorta. *Lancet*, **85**:133, 1965.

Yigitbasi, O., and Nalbantgil, I.: Murmur over an abnormal left apical mass. *Chest*, **59**:561, 1971.

47

Congenital Anomalies of the Coronary Arteries

J. A. Gordon Culham

CONGENITAL anomalies of the coronary arteries are important not only because of primary hemodynamic disturbances that they may cause, but also in the diagnosis and surgical management of congenital cardiac disease. Furthermore they may play a significant role in the performance and interpretation of selective coronary angiograms.

Classification

1. Major coronary anomalies
2. Minor coronary anomalies
3. Coronary anomalies associated with specific congenital heart lesions

Major Coronary Anomalies. These abnormalities include congenital fistulae, aneurysms, and aberrant origin of one, both, or an accessory coronary artery from the pulmonary artery (see Chapter 61).

An anomaly, in which both coronary arteries arise from the right aortic sinus, is often considered minor; however, as it may result in myocardial infarction or even sudden death it deserves special mention at this time. The left coronary artery arises from the right aortic sinus and courses abruptly leftward between the aorta and pulmonary artery (Figure 47–1*A* and *B*). Kinking of the artery at its origin, or compression between the great arteries during exercise, may cause acute left ventricular ischemia and infarction (Benson, 1970; Cohen and Shaw, 1967; Liberthson et al., 1974; Cheitlin et al., 1974).

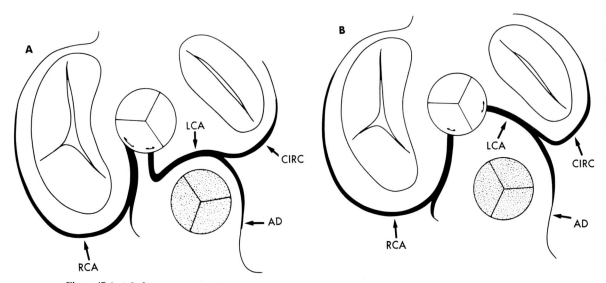

Figure 47-1. *A.* Left coronary artery from the right aortic sinus. This schematic drawing illustrates the coronary artery distribution in relationship to the heart valves as viewed from above. The left coronary artery arises from the right aortic sinus and passes leftward between the aorta and pulmonary artery. *RCA, LCA, AD,* and *CIRC* indicate the right coronary artery, left coronary artery, anterior descending coronary artery, and circumflex coronary artery. *B.* Normal coronary distribution.

Minor Coronary Anomalies. In this group the coronary arteries arise from the aorta, but are abnormal in number, position, or origin and course. Their significance largely concerns the performance and interpretation of coronary angiograms.

NUMBER. The number of coronary arteries may vary from one to four. A single coronary artery is rare and usually a benign anomaly; however, myocardial ischemia, infarction, and sudden death have been reported. A single coronary artery is frequently associated with congenital heart disease, most commonly transposition of the great arteries, coronary artery fistula, bicuspid aortic valve, and tetralogy of Fallot (Ogden and Goodyear, 1970). Ogden and Goodyear (1970) proposed a classification of five types based upon the number of initial major divisions and their subsequent course. A single coronary artery should not be considered as complete absence of a coronary artery but as an interruption of the proximal portion of one coronary artery at the aortic root. The distal portion of the artery has a normal epicardial distribution and is supplied by the single artery. In approximately 10 percent of cases a blind pouch is found in the aortic sinus of the "absent" coronary artery (Ogden, 1970). In these cases the proximal coronary artery failed to connect with the more distal epicardial vessels or the communication either failed to canalize or became atretic. In two reported cases a fibrous cord connected the blind pouch with the distal segment of the "absent" coronary artery (Ogden and Goodyear, 1970). A single coronary artery may be mimicked by two or more coronary ostia arising from one aortic sinus or by hypoplasia of the proximal portion of one artery with its distal circulation arising from the other artery (Gooding, 1974).

Surgery must be carefully planned in patients with a single coronary artery. Coronary perfusion should be done cautiously to prevent occlusion of a major branch. Right ventriculotomy also must be carefully planned as in 25 percent of patients with a single coronary artery a major branch crosses the right ventricular outflow tract.

A third coronary artery is reported to occur in 50 percent of individuals (Schlesinger et al., 1949). This third artery, the conus coronary artery, arises just anterior to the right coronary artery and perfuses the anterior portion of the right ventricular outflow tract. Rarely two conus coronary arteries are present, resulting in four coronary arteries (Vlodaver et al., 1972). Three coronary arteries may also exist when the left circumflex and left anterior descending coronary arteries have separate origins from the left aortic sinus (Adams et al., 1972). The latter variation when combined with a conus coronary artery also results in four coronary arteries.

POSITION. The coronary ostia are normally within the sinuses of Valsalva; however, one, both, or all ostia may arise from the tubular portion of the ascending aorta (Vlodaver et al., 1972). This variation is of significance to the physician performing selective coronary angiograms and the surgeon at aortotomy.

ORIGIN AND COURSE. The coronary arteries are subject to numerous variations. Vlodaver and associates (1972) describe six types. In type I both coronary arteries arise from the left aortic sinus, while in type II they both arise from the right aortic sinus. As previously discussed, the type II anomaly may be associated with myocardial infarction or death when the left coronary artery passes between the aorta and pulmonary artery (Figure 47–1A). In type III, the left circumflex coronary artery arises from the right aortic sinus or from the right coronary artery. This occurs in 1:300 otherwise normal hearts. The anterior descending coronary artery arises from the right coronary artery in type IV. This anomaly occurs in tetralogy of Fallot and will be subsequently discussed. The right coronary artery in type V arises from the posterior aortic sinus. This configuration is rare in the normal heart, but common in D-(complete) transposition of the great arteries. This will be discussed below. In type VI the anterior descending coronary artery and circumflex coronary arteries arise from separate ostia in the left aortic sinus. This occurs in 1 percent of normal hearts.

Coronary Anomalies Associated with Specific Congenital Heart Lesions. Coronary anomalies are important in the surgical management of children with congenital heart disease. The correction of intracardiac lesions is complicated by anomalously positioned major coronary branches. The preoperative or intraoperative recognition of these anomalies is of vital importance. The origin and proximal course of the coronary arteries may aid in the diagnosis of the underlying cardiac disorder. Van Praagh (1975) points out that the epicardial distribution of the coronaries is the most reliable indication of the underlying ventricular relationships.

PULMONARY ATRESIA. Patients with pulmonary atresia and an intact ventricular septum often have communications between the right ventricle and the coronary arteries via myocardial sinusoids. Bidirectional coronary flow has been observed in these patients angiographically (Ogden and Stansel, 1971). All coronary flow was via these communications, in a patient reported by Lenox and Briner (1972).

HYPOPLASTIC LEFT HEART SYNDROME. Anomalies of the coronary arteries may exist in patients with the hypoplastic left heart syndrome. At The Hospital for Sick Children, Toronto, we have encountered cases where coronary artery fistulae were present between the left coronary artery and the cavity of the left ventricle. Similar communications have been reported in a variety of left-sided obstructive lesions (Edmunds et al., 1975).

TETRALOGY OF FALLOT. With modern surgical techniques an anomalous coronary artery can be of vital importance. Many authors have reported fatalities due to a major coronary artery being severed during surgical repair (Kirklin et al., 1959; Senning, 1959; Friedman et al., 1960; Gadboys et al., 1961; Meng et al., 1965; Fellows et al., 1975).

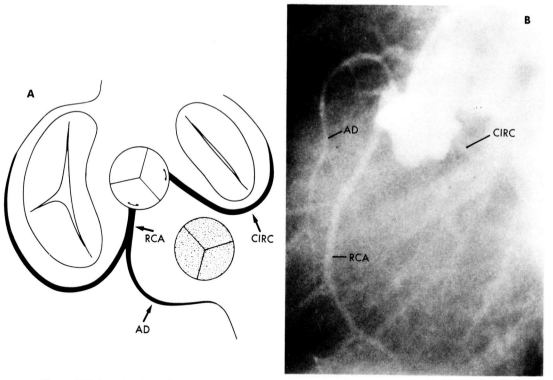

Figure 47-2. Anterior descending coronary artery arising from the right coronary artery. A drawing (*A*) and selective aortogram in lateral view (*B*) illustrate the anterior descending coronary artery arising from the right coronary artery and crossing the right ventricular outflow tract to reach the anterior interventricular groove.

Enlarged coronary arteries supplying the hypertrophied right ventricular myocardium may make ventriculotomy difficult (Longenecker et al., 1961). White and associates (1972) found a 40 percent incidence of long and large conus coronary arteries in these patients. Ectasia of the coronary arteries has been described in three cases (Bjork, 1966).

Two important coronary artery anomalies occur. These are aberrant origin of the anterior descending coronary artery from the right coronary artery or right aortic sinus and single coronary artery. The former results in a major artery crossing the right ventricular outflow tract (Figure 47–2*A* and *B*). If this artery is severed during ventriculotomy, morbidity or mortality may result. Even when recognized, this vessel may compromise the surgical procedure. The anterior descending coronary artery arises from the right coronary artery in 2 to 9 percent of cases. In the cumulative data of Fellows and associates (1975) the incidence as assessed by angiography, autopsy, or surgery was approximately 2.5 percent. At angiography these authors found an incidence approaching 5 percent. A single coronary artery may pose similar problems as a major branch crosses the right ventricular outflow tract in 25 percent of cases. A single coronary artery occurs in approximately 1.5 percent of patients with tetralogy of Fallot (Fellows et al., 1975).

The assessment of coronary artery anatomy may be

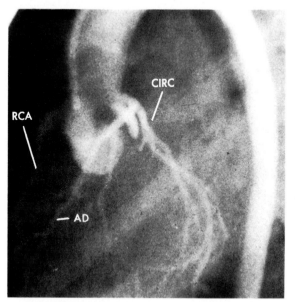

Figure 47-3. Normal coronary arteries. A selective aortic root angiogram reveals a normal coronary distribution.

possible from ventriculograms; however, selective injections in the proximal ascending aorta are often required (Figure 47–3). In tetralogy of Fallot this may be accomplished by passing a catheter from the right heart through the ventricular septal defect into the aorta. Selective coronary arteriography is not usually necessary.

Anomalies of the coronary arteries are often obvious to the surgeon; however, the anomalous artery may pursue an intramyocardial course or be obscured by adhesions if previous surgery has been performed. Thus, angiographic assessment is mandatory. Infants being considered for complete repair should have their coronary arteries evaluated. Many of these patients require an outflow patch at surgery, and thus the presence of an anomalous artery may make the repair difficult. The preoperative recognition of a coronary anomaly may influence the surgeon to perform palliative rather than corrective surgery.

An anomalous coronary artery encountered at surgery may be circumvented by performing the ventriculotomy below the anomalous artery or by incising the ventricle both above and below the artery. If these measures should fail to relieve the infundibular stenosis, a conduit may be inserted from the right ventricle to the pulmonary artery (Berry and McGoon, 1973).

TRANSPOSITION OF THE GREAT ARTERIES. The origin and course of coronary arteries in D-(complete) transposition of the great arteries are variable. Shaher and Puddu (1966) examined 149 specimens. They describe nine types of coronary pattern and cite two additional patterns from the literature not seen in their review. The commonest pattern, type I (Figure 47–4), occurs in approximately two-thirds of patients. The left coronary artery arises from the left sinus and the right coronary artery from the posterior aortic sinus. The next commonest pattern, type II (Figure 47–5), is found in approximately one-quarter of patients. The anterior descending coronary artery arises from the left aortic

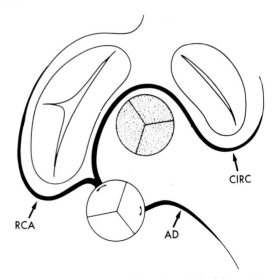

Figure 47-5. D-Transposition (complete) of the great arteries, type II.

sinus while the right coronary artery and circumflex coronary arteries originate from the posterior aortic sinus either together or separately. These two patterns account for 80 to 90 percent of cases of D-transposition of the great arteries (Elliot et al., 1966; Shaher and Puddu, 1966; Van Praagh et al., 1967). In the majority of cases, the circumflex coronary artery passes in front of the left ventricle and may be a complicating factor if left ventriculotomy is required to relieve associated pulmonary stenosis. A major vessel may cross the right ventricular outflow tract, complicating right ventriculotomy.

The coronary pattern in D-transposition of the great arteries has been noted to bear a relationship to the orientation of the great arteries (Elliot et al., 1966). When the great arteries were obliquely related, the coronaries in 34 of 39 cases had a type I coronary distribution, whereas when the great arteries were side-by-side, only 4 of 19 were type I.

In L-(congenitally corrected) transposition of the great arteries the anterior sinus is usually non-coronary and the anterior descending branch arises from the coronary artery that originates from the right sinus (Figure 47–6). This artery has been called the right coronary artery in spite of the fact that it supplies the left ventricle.

SINGLE VENTRICLE. In single ventricle (double-inlet left ventricle, outlet chamber) with D-, AP-, or L-transposition* related great arteries the coronary pattern is similar to Shaher's type I (Figure 47–4). The anterior descending artery arises from the left-sided coronary artery. This differs from patients with L-transposition of the great arteries with two ventricles in whom the anterior descending coronary artery arises from the right-sided coronary artery

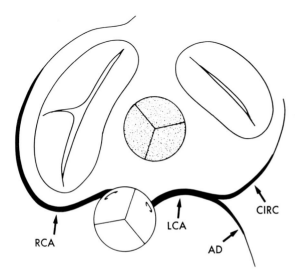

Figure 47-4. D = Transposition (complete) of the great arteries, type I.

---

* D-, AP-, or L-transposition related great arteries means that the aorta is situated anterior to the pulmonary artery and to the right (D), to the left (L), or directly in front (AP) of the pulmonary artery.

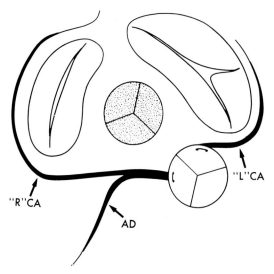

Figure 47-6. L-Transposition (congenitally corrected) of the great arteries.

(Figure 47–6). Thus in a patient with L-transposition related great arteries and the anterior descending coronary arising from the left-sided coronary artery one should suspect single ventricle.

DOUBLE-OUTLET RIGHT VENTRICLE. This anomaly may be difficult to differentiate from normally related great arteries and from D-(complete) transposition of the great arteries. The coronary pattern can be helpful. With double-outlet right ventricle the coronary pattern is usually normal, while in transposition of the great arteries a normal coronary distribution is rare.

REFERENCES

Adams, D. F.; Abrams, H. L.; and Ruttley, M.: The roentgen pathology of coronary artery disease. *Semin. Roentgenol.*, 7:344, 1972.

Benson, P. A.: Anomalous aortic origin of coronary artery with sudden death: Case report and review. *Am. Heart J.*, 79:254, 1970.

Berry, B. E., and McGoon, D. C.: Total correction for tetralogy of Fallot with anomalous coronary artery. *Surgery*, 74:894, 1973.

Bjork, Lars: Ectasia of the coronary arteries. *Radiology*, 87:33, 1966.

Cheitlin, M. D.; DeCastro, C. M.; and McAllister, H. A.: Sudden death as a complication of anomalous left coronary origin from the anterior sinuses of Valsalva: A not-so-minor congenital anomaly. *Circulation*, 50:780, 1974.

Cohen, L. S., and Shaw, L. D.: Fatal myocardial infarction in an 11 year old boy associated with a unique coronary artery anomaly. *Am. J. Cardiol.*, 19:420, 1967.

Edmunds, H. L., Jr.; Friedman, S.; Rashkind, W. J.; Dodd, P. F.; and Saxena, N. C.: Transatrial resection of right ventricular infundibulum for infundibular pulmonary stenosis and tetralogy of Fallot. *Circulation*, 51 and 52: Suppl. 699, 1975.

Elliot, L. P.; Amplatz, K.; and Edwards, J. E.: Coronary arterial patterns in transposition complexes: anatomic and angio-cardiographic studies. *Am. J. Cardiol.*, 17:362, 1966.

Fellows, K. E.; Freed, M. D.; Keane, J. F.; Van Praagh, R.; Bernhard, W. F.; and Castaneda, A. C.: Results of routine preoperative coronary angiography in tetralogy of Fallot. *Circulation*, 51:561, 1975.

Friedman, S.; Ash, R.; Klein, D.; and Johnson, J.: Anomalous single coronary artery complicating ventriculotomy in a child with cyanotic congenital heart disease. *Am. Heart J.*, 59:140, 1960.

Gadboys, H. L.; Slomin, R.; and Litwak, R. S.: Treacherous anomalous coronary artery. *Am. J. Cardiol.*, 8:854, 1961.

Gooding, C. A.: Angiography of the thoracic aorta and its branches. In Gyepes, M. T. (ed.): *Angiography in Infants and Children.* Grune & Stratton, Inc., New York, 1974, p. 49.

Kirklin, J. W.; Ellis, F. H., Jr.; McGoon, D. C.; DuShane, J. W.; and Swan, H. J. C.: Surgical treatment for tetralogy of Fallot by open intracardiac repair. *J. Thorac. Surg.*, 37:22, 1959.

Lenox, C. C., and Briner, J.: Absent proximal coronary arteries associated with pulmonary atresia. *Am. J. Cardiol.*, 30:666, 1972.

Liberthson, R. R.; Dinsmore, R. E.; Bharati, S.; Rubenstein, J. J.; Caulfield, J.; Wheeler, E. O.; Harthorne, J. W.; and Lev, M.: Aberrant coronary artery origin from the aorta: Diagnosis and Significance. *Circulation*, 50:774, 1974.

Longenecker, C. G.; Reemtsma, K.; and Creech, O., Jr.: Anomalous coronary artery distribution associated with tetralogy of Fallot: A hazard of open cardiac repair. *J. Thorac. Surg.*, 42:258, 1961.

Meng, C. C. L.; Ecker, F. A. O.; and Lev, M.: Coronary artery distribution in tetralogy of Fallot. *Arch. Surg.*, 90:363, 1965.

Ogden, J. A.: Congenital anomalies of the coronary arteries. *Am. J. Cardiol.*, 25:474, 1970.

Ogden, J. A., and Goodyear, A. V.: Patterns of distribution of the single coronary artery. *Yale J. Biol. Med.*, 43:11, 1970.

Ogden, J. A., and Stansel, H. C., Jr.: Roentgenographic manifestations of congenital coronary artery disease. *Am. J. Roentgenol. Radium Ther. Nucl. Med.*, 113:538, 1971.

Schlesinger, M. J.; Zoll, P. A.; and Wessler, S.: The conus artery: a third coronary artery. *Am. Heart J.*, 38:823, 1949.

Senning, A.: Surgical treatment of right ventricular outflow tract stenosis combined with ventricular septal defect and right-left shunt (Fallot's tetralogy). *Acta Chir. Scand.*, 117:73, 1959.

Shaher, R. M., and Puddu, G. C.: Coronary arterial anatomy in complete transposition of the great arteries. *Am. J. Cardiol.*, 17:355, 1966.

Van Praagh, R.; Durnin, R. E.; Jockin, H.; Wagner, H. R.; Korns, M.; Garabedian, H.; Ando, M.; and Calder, L.: Anatomically corrected malposition of the great arteries (S.D.L.). *Circulation*, 51:20, 1975.

Van Praagh, R.; Vlad, P.; and Keith, J. D.: Complete transposition of the great arteries. In Keith, Rowe, and Vlad (eds.): *Heart Disease in Infancy and Childhood*, 2nd ed. Macmillan Publishing Co., Inc., New York, 1967.

Vlodaver, Z.; Neufeld, H. N.; and Edwards, J. E.: Pathology of coronary disease. *Semin. Roentgenol.*, 7:376, 1972.

White, R. I., Jr.; Frech, R. S.; Castaneda, A.; and Amplatz, K.: The nature and significance of anomalous coronary arteries in tetralogy of Fallot. *Am. J. Roentgenol. Radium Ther. Nucl. Med.*, 114:350, 1972.

48

Congenital Pulmonary Arteriovenous Aneurysm

John D. Keith

Congenital arteriovenous aneurysm of the lung is primarily a pediatric problem since 80 percent of cases present signs and symptoms in infancy and childhood. Although it had been seen at postmortem for some time (Churton, 1897), it was not until 1939 that it was recognized clinically (Smith and Horton, 1939). The first successful treatment of a case was reported in 1942 by Hepburn and Dauphinee. The subject is reviewed by Bosher and colleagues (1958), Moyer and associates (1962), Hodgson and Kaye (1963), Jerasaty and associates (1966), Utzon and Brandrup (1973), and Zavanella and associates (1975).

Prevalence

This is not a common lesion, but several hundred cases have been described in the literature (Stringer et al., 1955). Sloan and Cooley (1953) report that out of 15,000 consecutive postmortems at Johns Hopkins Hospital only three such defects were found. At The Hospital for Sick Children, Toronto, in data collected on 15,104 cases of congenital heart disease, six cases of congenital pulmonary arteriovenous aneurysm were recognized.

Many of the cases described in the past were not identified until adult life. Since the majority have signs or symptoms in infancy and childhood, it is now more common for cases to be recognized early in life and treated promptly before serious complications occur.

Pathology

At postmortem the aneurysm is seen incorporated into the lung tissue, with an enlarged pulmonary artery entering it and an equal-size vein emerging. The vascular channels of the aneurysm are tortuous, lined with endothelium, and supported by a connective tissue stroma. The wall is likely to be thin, an explanation of why rupture may occur either into the parenchyma of the lung or into a bronchus.

Such aneurysms are commonly fairly large and vary in size from a pinpoint up to that of a small orange (Standefer et al., 1964). Nearly half of the patients have two or more. A widespread telangiectatic form occurs in about 10 percent of the reported cases (Utzon and Bandrup, 1973).

In most instances the shunt is from the pulmonary artery to the pulmonary vein, but on occasion the communicating artery may arise from the aorta directly or as a branch of the bronchial artery (Watson, 1947).

Hemodynamics

A dilated branch of the pulmonary artery carries venous blood into the aneurysm and quickly recirculates it through tortuous channels, permitting it to return to the pulmonary vein without being oxygenated. There is a shunt of venous blood into the systemic circulation, producing cyanosis and a secondary rise in the red blood cell count and hemoglobin (a red blood cell count of 11 million has been reported). It has been estimated that from 18 to 89 percent of the right ventricular output may pass through the aneurysm (Sloan and Cooley, 1953). It is of interest that Gray and associates (1952) found no relationship between the size of the arteriovenous aneurysm and the size of the shunt.

Usually the cardiac output is not increased significantly in pulmonary arteriovenous aneurysm. This is a feature that is characteristic of this type of lesion only when it is in the lung, since the systemic arteriovenous aneurysms usually produce a marked increase in cardiac output.

Because the cardiac output is not large, increased size of the heart is uncommon and is found in approximately 10 percent of cases. The blood pressure, heart rate, and circulation time are usually within normal limits, but exceptional cases may show changes. In a few cases the aneurysms or the channels through the aneurysm are so small that no significant shunt exists and no abnormal signs or symptoms result.

Clinical Features

Approximately 10 percent of cases of arteriovenous aneurysm of the lung have no symptoms whatever. In the vast majority, however, some of the characteristic clinical features occur, and these include a history of dyspnea, nosebleeds, cerebral manifestations, hemoptysis, and chest pain. On physical examination there may be cyanosis, clubbing, or a murmur over the involved lung. Hemangiomas of the skin or mucous membranes occur in between one third and one half of these patients and the association with Rendu–Osler–Weber disease is now well established (Hodgson et al., 1959). The heart is usually within the normal limits of size.

Dyspnea is present in the majority of cases and is of a mild degree noticeable with exercise. The associated finding of cyanosis is present in approximately 80 percent of recorded cases (Muri, 1955; Sloan and Cooley, 1953). Nosebleeds are frequent (32 percent) and are an indication of the associated telangiectasis in the nasal mucosa.

Numbness, dizziness, convulsive seizures, or other related neurologic manifestations occur in at least 25 percent of the total group and appear to have their basis in cerebral anoxemia or localized thrombosis.

Hemoptysis occurs occasionally and is an expected complication since the wall of the aneurysm may become very thin and rupture into the bronchus, yielding either blood-stained sputum or varying quantities of blood up to a massive fatal hemorrhage.

On physical examination one is first impressed with the presence of cyanosis and clubbing (80 percent of cases), occurring without other obvious cardiac signs such as one expects in congenital heart disease. Murmurs of varying types are frequently heard over the chest at the site of the aneurysm, sometimes limited to systole and in others audible continuously. They have been noted to increase in intensity with deep inspiration.

Children with this condition usually look well nourished and are not underdeveloped. There is no difference in frequency between the sexes.

Electrocardiography

Since the heart is not significantly enlarged and in most cases the cardiac output is within normal limits, it is understandable that the electrocardiogram should show little or no change. It may occasionally show slight evidence of right ventricular hypertrophy.

Radiologic Examination

Nearly every case shows some radiologic evidence of the aneurysm in the lung fields, and because of this an x-ray of the chest should be examined with care in all suspected patients (see Figure 48–1B).

A rounded or slightly nodular opacity may be seen in either lung field, but occurs most frequently in the lower lobes. The borders of the aneurysm are usually well defined, and with careful inspection two cordlike strands may be seen proceeding from the shadow to the hilum of the lung. These consist of the dilated arteries and veins supplying the lesion.

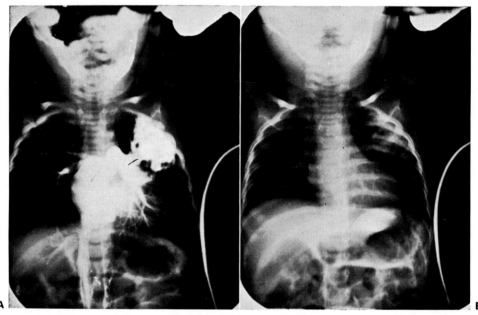

Figure 48-1. D. B., aged nine months. *A* shows the arteriovenous aneurysm of the left lung connected to the hilum with a narrow stalk of artery and vein demonstrated by venous angiocardiogram. *B* is the conventional chest x-ray of the same patient showing a similar but less clearly defined shadow in the left lung.

Fluoroscopy reveals pulsation of the aneurysmal shadow in the majority of patients. It is also reported that the mass increases in size with the Valsalva experiment (which diminishes the pulmonary pressure) and decreases in size with the Müller maneuver (which increases the pulmonary pressure).

In the dispersed, telangiectatic type the chest x-ray may be normal (Utzon and Brandrup, 1973).

Other

Contrast echocardiography has been shown to be a useful screening method in patients with suspicion of having pulmonary arteriovenous fistulas. Appearance of echoes in the left ventricle, very prompt in patients with intracardiac right to left shunts, are delayed for several cardiac cycles in individuals with a lung fistula (Shub et al., 1976). Application of nuclide techniques to this malformation has also proved useful (Weiss et al., 1975).

Angiocardiography

Angiocardiography helps greatly to clarify the diagnosis by revealing the anatomic details of the lesion. The mass is then well delineated, and the dilated communicating vessels are clearly visible (see Figure 48–1*A*). The tortuous vascular channels show up as nodular prominences in, and at the margin of, the lesion. Small aneurysms, which are ill-defined in the conventional chest plate, may be distinctly delineated by this method, but again in the less common dispersed telangiectatic form, the pulmonary arteriogram can be normal (Utzon and Brandrup, 1973)

Treatment

Since 1942 when Hepburn and Dauphinee reported the first case successfully treated by surgery, excision has been the method of choice. This is carried out by lobectomy or segmental resection, removing the minimal amount of pulmonary tissue required to extract the aneurysm safely and completely.

The patients most suitably selected for surgery are those with dyspnea, cyanosis, hemoptysis, or neurologic disturbances such as convulsions. When the lesion is not producing signs or symptoms and the patient is well and active, it is probably safer to recommend a period of observation before contemplating surgery.

Prognosis

With surgical excision the operative mortality has been approximately 10 percent (Sloan and Cooley, 1953). The majority of operative survivors are completely cured and are able to lead a normal life. When additional aneurysms remain in the lung or when pulmonary insufficiency is present as a complication, complete return to normal may not be achieved.

Without surgery, many of these patients have died of rupture of the aneurysm, massive hemoptysis, brain abscess, or convulsions. In the series reported by Sloan and Cooley (1953) outlining the natural history of pulmonary arteriovenous aneurysms, 27 percent had died in childhood or adult life, 12 percent were alive but continued to have symptoms, and 37 percent were alive and well and apparently leading a normal existence. Twenty-four percent had died from other causes.

REFERENCES

Bosher L. H.; Blake, A.; Byrd, B. R.; and Richmond, V.: An analysis of the pathologic anatomy of pulmonary arteriovenous aneurysms with particular reference to the applicability of local excision. *Surgery*, **45**:91, 1958.

Churton, T.: Multiple aneurysm of pulmonary artery. *Br. Med. J.*, **1**:1223, 1897.

Gray, F. D.; Lurie, P. R.; and Whittemore, R.: Circulatory changes in pulmonary arteriovenous fistula. *Yale J. Biol. Med.*, **25**:107, 1952.

Hepburn, J., and Dauphinee, J. A.: Successful removal of hemangioma of the lung followed by the disappearance of polycythemia. *Am. J. Med. Sci.*, **204**:681, 1942.

Hodgson, C. H.; Burchell, H. B.; Good, A.; and Claggett, O. T.: Hereditary hemorrhagic telangiectasis and pulmonary arteriovenous fistula. Survey of a large family. *N. Engl. J. Med.*, **261**:625, 1959.

Hodgson, C. H., and Kage, R. L.: Pulmonary arteriovenous fistula and hereditary hemorrhagic telangiectasia. *Dis. Chest*, **43**:449, 1963.

Husson, G. S.: Pulmonary arteriovenous aneurysm in childhood. *Pediatrics*, **18**:871, 1956.

Jerasaty, R. M.; Knight, H. F.; and Hart, W. E.: Pulmonary arteriovenous fistulas in children. Report of two cases and review of literature. *Am. J. Dis. Child.*, **111**:256, 1966.

Moyer, J. H.; Glantz, S.; and Brest, A. N.: Pulmonary arteriovenous fistulas. *Am. J. Med.*, **32**:417, 1962.

Muri, J. W.: Arteriovenous aneurysm of the lung. *Am. J. Surg.*, **89**:265, 1955.

Shub, C.; Tajik, A. J.; Seward, J. B.; and Dines, D. E.: Detecting intrapulmonary right-to-left shunt with contrast echocardiography. Observations in a patient with diffuse pulmonary arteriovenous fistulas. *Mayo Clin. Proc.*, **51**:81, 1976.

Sloan, R. D., and Cooley, R. N.: Congenital pulmonary arteriovenous aneurysm. *Am. J. Roentgenol.*, **70**:183, 1953.

Sluiter-Eringa, H.; Orie, N. G. M.; and Sluiter, H. J.: Pulmonary arteriovenous fistula. Diagnosis and prognosis in noncomplainant patients. *Am. Rev. Resp. Dis.*, **100**:177, 1969.

Smith, H. L., and Horton, B. T.: Arteriovenous fistula of the lung associated with polycythemia vera; report of a case in which the diagnosis was made clinically. *Am. Heart J.*, **18**:589, 1939.

Standefer, J. E.; Tabakin, R. S.; and Hanson, J. S.: Pulmonary arteriovenous fistulas. *Am. Rev. Resp. Dis.*, **89**:95, 1964.

Steinberg, I.: Diagnosis and surgical treatment of pulmonary arteriovenous fistula. *Surg. Clin. North Am.*, **41**:523, 1961.

Stringer, C. J.; Stanley, A. L.; Bates, R. C.; and Summers, J. E.: Pulmonary arteriovenous fistula. *Am. J. Surg.*, **89**:1054, 1955.

Utzon, F., and Brandrup, F.: Pulmonary arteriovenous fistulas in children. A review with special reference to the telangiectatic type, illustrated by report of a case. *Acta Paediatr. Scand.*, **62**:422, 1973.

Watson, W. L.: Pulmonary arteriovenous aneurysm. *Surgery*, **22**:919, 1947.

Weiss, M. A.; Koenigeberg, M.; and Freeman, L.: Pulmonary arteriovenous malformation: Scintigraphic demonstration and analysis. *J. Nucl. Med.*, **16**:180, 1975.

Zavanella, C.; Jaffe, A.; Tellez, J. G.; Rufilanchas, J. J.; Agosti, J.; and Figuera, D.: Pulmonary arteriovenous fistula. A review. *Vasc. Surg.*, **9**:244, 1975.

49

Ectopia Cordis and Diverticulum of the Left Ventricle

John D. Keith

ECTOPIA CORDIS

THE TERM "ectopia cordis" has been used to include all abnormally placed hearts not within the thoracic cavity. The first recorded case is attributed to Haller (1706), and many examples have been published since then. Byron (1948) was able to refer to a total of 142 cases that have appeared in the literature.

Table 49–1. DISTRIBUTION BY SITE OF DEFECT

SITE	NUMBER
Thoracic	81
Abdominal	38
Combined thoracoabdominal	10
Cervical	4
Unclassified	9
Total	142

There are four groups described: The most common is the thoracic type, in which the sternum is split and the heart protrudes out of the thoracic cage. The second most common is the abdominal type, in which the heart extrudes through the diaphragm into the abdomen and may appear through a hernia in the abdominal wall. The third group is a combination of the thoracic and the abdominal types. The fourth is the cervical type, which is very rare, with the heart protruding in the neck.

The incidence recorded by Byron (1948) is shown in Table 49–1.

There have been debates and confusion over what constitutes ectopia cordis. Many reported cases have been examples of either simple cleft sternum or Cantrell's pentalogy, an association of defects of the lower sternum, ventral diaphragm, abdominal wall, and the heart (Cantrell et al., 1958). Ravitch (1977) in a critical review of the world literature concluded that

an extrathoracic presentation was the only situation where the heart could certainly be regarded as ectopic.

Clinical Features

In ectopia cordis the heart is displaced out of the thorax so that it comes to lie on the outer surface of the neck or thorax or within the abdominal cavity. One is usually presented with a newborn baby with a pulsating mass protruding out of the midline of the thorax or epigastrium (see Figure 49–1). The skin overlying the mass is usually thinner than normal skin and may appear stretched and contain small blood vessels. At times the complete outline of the heart is apparent, with ventricles and atria showing, but more often the ectopic heart simply takes the outline of a herniated, pulsating mass and anatomic details are not apparent. A loud systolic murmur may be heard occasionally, as in the case reported by Holt (1897), but frequently no murmur is audible. Several electrocardiograms have been reported in the past, and these have been found to be normal.

An x-ray in the anteroposterior and lateral views will confirm the abnormal position of the heart. This may be especially useful in differentiating ectopia cordis from diverticulum of the left ventricle.

Prognosis

Survival depends on the site of the anomalous heart, the presence or absence of associated defects, and the general condition of the baby. Approximately one-third of infants with ectopia cordis are prematures and frequently do not survive the passage of the birth canal. If they do survive, it is only for a few hours or a few days. Many of the full-term babies with this anomaly are also stillborn.

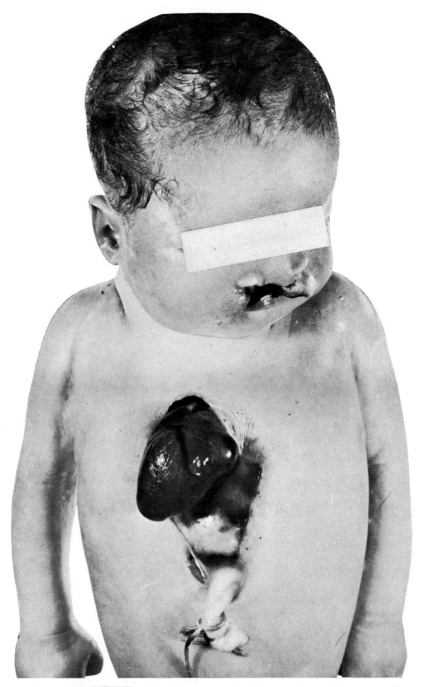

Figure 49-1. Thoracic ectopia cordis with split sternum, left diaphragmatic hernia, tricuspid and pulmonary atresia, and other congenital anomalies. Male infant who lived 67 minutes. (Courtesy of Drs. H. G. Pritzker and J. Steiner, Department of Pathology, New Mount Sinai Hospital, Toronto.)

A number of cases have other defective anatomy within the heart, such as tricuspid atresia, single ventricle with or without atrial septal defect and anomalies of the aorta, pulmonary artery, or great veins (Greig, 1926).

In general, the prognosis is related to the type of ectopia cordis. In the thoracic type only one case has survived longer than 16 days (this is Greig's case [1926], who lived 13 months). The abdominal type has the best outlook. A number of these cases have survived infancy, a few even reaching adult life; two were in good health in the fourth decade (Bouchard, 1888; Foy, 1909). One unusual instance was that of an old soldier (reported by Deschamps, 1826), whose heart was found to have replaced the position normally occupied by the left kidney in the abdominal cavity and whose great vessels entered the thorax through a small opening in the diaphragm.

Treatment

Surgical correction has been attempted in 20 cases, and only one survived (Ravitch, 1977). When the heart is manipulated into a new position, its action becomes embarrassed and it is necessary to allow it to return to the original ectopic situation. Additionally most patients have severe intracardiac anomalies for which repair as newborns or young infants poses considerable difficulty. One is forced to the conclusion that this anomaly is better managed without surgical intervention.

DIVERTICULUM OF THE LEFT VENTRICLE

DIVERTICULUM of the left ventricle is of interest to pediatricians because it can be readily recognized on physical examination in infancy and because it can be treated surgically with success. It is a rare anomaly, only about 30 cases having been reported. We have encountered two patients among 15,104 cases of congenital heart disease at The Hospital for Sick Children.

Pathology

The anomaly consists of a diverticulum of the left ventricle that projects downward and forward to protrude into the epigastrium. It is contained in a serous sac that is continuous with the pericardium and involves a defect in the diaphragm as well as in the anterior abdominal wall. The pouch of the diverticulum is continuous with the left ventricular cavity and therefore contains the usual components of the heart wall, including endocardium, myocardium, and pericardium. The diverticulum is therefore part of the cardiac abnormality of many patients with degrees of the Cantrell syndrome and may exist in hearts that are otherwise normal or with other intracardiac anomalies (Ravitch, 1977).

The developmental origin of the diverticulum is not entirely clear, but it seems likely that it is a congenital defect that has its origin in the early stages of fetal development.

Duckworth (1958) considers that the diverticulum of the left ventricle is most likely to be due to a simple herniation of the heart wall at its thinnest part (which normally occurs at the apex) due to a developmental upset in the arrangement of the muscle forming the apical whorl, and that once the diverticulum is formed it presses on the diaphragm causing it to thin out or perforate so that protrusion into the anterior abdominal wall occurs.

Clinical Features

Babies with the diverticulum of the left ventricle present symptoms in infancy, and three-fourths of the cases do not survive the first six months of life. The cardinal diagnostic feature is a pulsating hernia in the upper epigastrium. Usually this takes the form of a pulsating mass protruding out into the abdominal wall just below the xiphisternum. As a rule there are no murmurs present and no other evidence of congenital heart disease, but occasionally a systolic murmur and thrill may be recognized just above the pulsating mass (Potts et al., 1953). Incomplete left bundle branch block has been reported in the electrocardiogram.

Angiocardiography

Cardiac catheterization and angiocardiography are reasonable preoperative studies to exclude associated anomalies and clearly define the ventricular anatomy. Contrast injection usually identifies the diverticulum well. Although selective injection into the left ventricle has been safely performed (Skapinker, 1951; Potts et al., 1953), because one of the known risks of the disorder is rupture, it is probably wiser to rely on contrast visualization from injections made upstream to the left ventricle.

Diagnosis

The diagnosis is readily made by finding a pulsating mass protruding through the upper epigastrium. As Potts and associates (1953) point out, it must be differentiated from ectopia cordis. Byron (1948) has reviewed 142 cases of this latter condition—81 of the thoracic type and 38 of the abdominal type. The thoracic type can be readily recognized by the defect in the chest wall and the cleft sternum. The abdominal type, although not as common, is compatible with life and has been reported in patients who survived into the fourth decade. In ectopia cordis abdominalis the entire heart lies outside the thoracic cage, whereas the diverticulum of the left ventricle has the heart lying within the thoracic cage and the diverticulum protrudes from it. The two may be readily differentiated by x-rays in lateral and anteroposterior views and, if necessary, by angiocardiography.

Treatment

The treatment of choice is a resection of the diverticulum and a repair of the defect in the abdominal wall and diaphragm. The earliest successful surgery for this type has been reported by Roessler (1944), Skapinker (1951), and Potts and associates (1953). One of our two cases was reported earlier (Mustard et al., 1958), and the other was treated, also successfully, in 1974.

It is quite feasible to expose the diverticulum, put a clamp on it where it joins the normal left ventricle, and excise the abnormal portion. The heart tolerates the procedure very well.

Since three-fourths of the cases die in the first six months of life and many of them die suddenly, it is imperative to treat these babies when they are first seen in infancy. Once corrected they should be able to lead normal lives.

REFERENCES

Blatt, M. L., and Zellas, M.: Ectopia cordis—report of a case and review of the literature. *Am. J. Dis. Child.*, **63**:515, 1942.

Byron, F.: Ectopia cordis—case with attempted operative correction. *J. Thorac. Surg.*, **7**:717, 1948.

Cantrell, J. R.; Haller, J. A.; and Ravitch, M. M.: A syndrome of congenital defects involving the abdominal wall, sternum, diaphragm, pericardium and heart. *Surg. Gynecol. Obstet.*, **197**:602, 1958.

Deschamps: Cited by Breschet, G.: Memoire sur un vice de conformation congénitale des enveloppes du coeur. *Rep. Gén. Anat. Physiol. Pathol.*, **1**:67, 1826.

Duckworth, J. W. A.: See Mustard et al. (1958).

Foy, G.: Ectopie cardiaque par malformation sternale. *Bull. Mém. Soc. Anat. Paris*, **11**:446, 1909.

Greig, D. M.: Cleft sternum and ectopia cordis. *Edinburgh Med. J.*, **33**:480, 1926.

Holt, E. L.: A remarkable case of ectocardia with displacement, the heart beating in the abdominal cavity. *Med. News N.Y.*, **71**:769, 1897.

Mustard, W. T.; Duckworth, J. W. A.; Rowe, R. D.; and Dolan, F. G.: Congenital diverticulum of the left ventricle of the heart (case report). *Can. J. Surg.*, **1** (Jan.):149, 1958.

Potts, W. J.; DeBoer, A.; and Johnson, F. R.: Congenital diverticulum of the left ventricle. *Surgery*, **33**:301, 1953.

Ravitch, M. M.: *Congenital Deformities of the Chest Wall and Their Operative Correction.* W. B. Saunders Co., Philadelphia 1977.

Roessler, W.: Erfolgreiche operative Enternung eines ektopischen herzdivertikles an einem neugeborenen. *Deutsch. Z. Chir.*, **258**:561, 1944.

Skapinker, S.: Diverticulum of the left ventricle of the heart. *Arch. Surg.*, **63**:629, 1951.

Swyer, A. J.; Mans, H. I.; and Rosenblatt, P.: Congenital diverticulosis of the left ventricle. *Am. J. Dis. Child.*, **79**:111, 1950.

Von Sydow: Ruptur des Herzens bei einem Kinder. *Jahrb. Kinderh.*, **47**:427, 1866.

50

Heart Disease Associated with
Chromosomal Abnormalities

Richard D. Rowe, Irene A. Uchida, and *Florence Char*

A DISCUSSION of congenital heart disease would be incomplete without examining the role of chromosomes in its etiology since cardiac defects are among the most frequently occurring malformations in chromosome syndromes.

BASIC PRINCIPLES OF CYTOGENETICS

THE 23 pairs of chromosomes in man have been classified into seven groups from A to G according to similarity in size and shape and numbered in descending order of size (Chicago Conf., 1966). The shape is determined by the position of the centromere seen as a constricted region at or near the center (metacentric), closer to one end (submetacentric), or at one end (acrocentric). Because of similarity in shape, only a few chromosomes could be identified with certainty when karyotypes were prepared with conventional stains. A few more chromosomes could be identified and paired by a laborious process involving radioactive thymidine labeling based on the principle that pairs of chromosomes (with the exception of the X chromosomes) replicate synchronously. Newer staining techniques now permit accurate identification of every chromosome in the human karyotype by characteristic banding patterns produced by fluorescent quinacrine stains referred to as Q-bands (Figure 50–1) or by modified Giemsa staining called G-bands (Paris Conf., 1972).

Descriptions of karyotypes follow standard formulations. First the total number of chromosomes is given, then the sex chromosome complement followed by a description of any aberrations. The presence or absence of a chromosome is designated by + or − placed immediately before the chromosome in question, e.g., 47,XY,+21 for a male with 21 trisomy syndrome. The − or + sign follows the chromosome number when there is partial loss of or addition to a chromosome; e.g., a female cri du chat is 46,XX,5p− (p = short arm, q = long arm).

Any variation from the normal diploid number of chromosomes is termed aneuploidy. Trisomy refers to the presence of three homologous chromosomes and monosomy when only one is present. Aneuploidy results from abnormal segregation or nondisjunction during formation of the gamete. Among the autosomal abnormalities the most familiar is the 21 trisomy or Down's syndrome. Best-known sex chromosome aneuploids are Turner's and Klinefelter's syndromes. Mosaicism, the presence of two or more different cell lines in a subject, has been found for almost all chromosome aberrations but most frequently involves the sex chromosomes. Although trisomies are not usually inherited, a familial tendency to nondisjunction is sometimes apparent. This may be caused by a gene or a chromosomal variant (see inversion below). In most instances, however, chromosome segregation is influenced by environmental factors, among which late maternal age is the best documented. Evidence for radiation and viruses as causative agents is also mounting.

The most common structural aberration is translocation (Figure 50–4, page 900). A reciprocal translocation is formed when two nonhomologous chromosomes break and exchange segments. Since no chromatin material is lost, carriers of reciprocal translocations are phenotypically normal. A carrier can, theoretically, produce several different types of gametes, but most combinations will be inviable and lost. Three viable combinations, i.e., normal, carrier, and abnormal, should be found in equal frequencies among the offspring, but the actual proportion of abnormal children varies with the chromosomes involved and is usually less than the expected frequency. Most unbalanced translocations are not

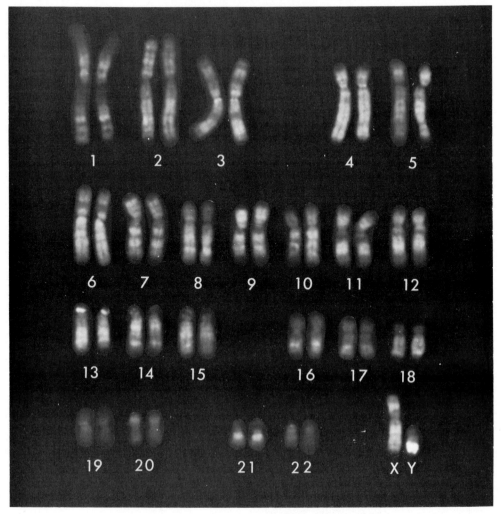

Figure 50-1. Normal karyotype stained with quinacrine.

inherited but arise de novo in a gamete. They are caused by chromosome-breaking agents such as ionizing, radiation, viruses, drugs, and chemicals.

Deletions are another form of fairly common aberration. They were thought at first to be nonviable but some patients have been noted to be less severely affected than trisomics. When both ends of a chromosome are deleted, the broken ends may fuse to form a ring (Figure 50–2A). Deletions, including rings, are probably lethal for most chromosomes in the absence of mosaicism. Y chromosomes may vary in length and shape, this variation being caused mainly by loss or duplication of the brilliantly fluorescent distal portion of the long arm (Figure 50–2B). This region appears to be genetically inert since Y variants affect neither the phenotype nor the reproductive capacity. A special type of deficiency and duplication is the isochromosome (Figure 50–2C) formed by misdivision of the centromere: it may divide across the transverse rather than the

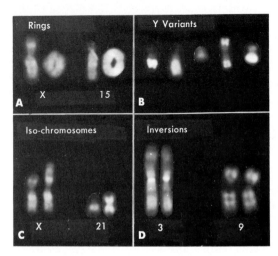

Figure 50-2. Some structural aberrations seen in chromosomal disorders. *A*. Ring forms. *B*. Length variations. *C*. Isochromosomes. *D*. Inversions.

longitudinal plane. The result will be one chromosome with two long arms carrying identical genes and no short arm and the other chromosome with two short arms. Isochromosomes for the long arm, i(Xq), are found most frequently in patients with atypical Turner's syndrome. Some apparent translocations between two D or two G chromosomes could be isochromosomes.

Inversions arise when two breaks occur in a single chromosome and the segment between is inverted (Figure 50–2D). The order of the genes is disarranged, but since none are lost or duplicated the carrier of an inversion is usually phenotypically normal. The change in order may cause difficulties when chromosomes synapse during meiosis and induce abnormal segregation and nondisjunction. Inversions have been frequently observed in chromosome no. 9.

The simplest cell to use for cytogenetic analysis is the small lymphocyte of the peripheral blood. Bone marrow cells are examined in blood dyscrasias and fibroblasts are cultured from abortuses. Techniques have recently been developed to culture amniotic fluid cells for prenatal diagnosis. The chromosomes of male and female meiotic cells can be examined to look for the cause of reduced fertility or sterility. These newer techniques are invaluable for obtaining more accurate data for genetic counseling and for the prevention of births of abnormal children.

Additional aids for chromosome diagnosis are sex chromatin and dermatoglyphic analyses. A simple technique, long in use, to screen for sex chromosome aberrations has been the examination of interphase nuclei for the presence of the S chromatin or Barr body (Figure 50–3C). The principle underlying the formation of the X chromatin body is the inactivation of all X chromosomes in excess of one, i.e., the Lyon hypothesis. The number of Barr bodies in a cell is thus one less than the total number of X chromosomes present. This test is not always reliable for detecting mosaicism nor can a structurally abnormal X be predicted. In a comparable test for the presence of Y chromatin the brilliantly fluorescent region of the Y chromosome can be seen in the interphase nucleus as a brilliant spot (Figure 50–3A, B, D). Occasionally a false positive or negative may result from normal variants in fluorescent karyotypes. Consequently, when a diagnosis of sex is crucial, such as in the prenatal diagnosis of amniotic fluid cells for X-linked abnormalities, complete karyotyping is essential.

The correlation between dermatoglyphics and

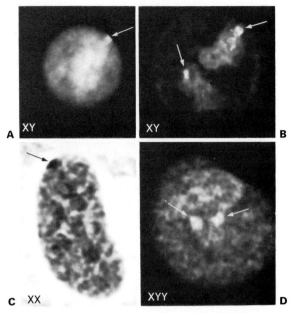

Figure 50-3. Sex chromatin. *A.* Normal male with one fluorescent body. *B.* Normal male with two fluorescent bodies, one of which is a bright variant found on chromosome no. 22. *C.* Normal female with Barr body. *D.* True YY.

abnormal karyotypes is clear. The important diagnostic criteria are the type and size of the patterns on the distal phalanges of the fingers, the position of the axial triradius on the palm, the type of pattern in the hallucal area of the sole, and the type and number of flexion creases on the palm and little finger (see Figure 50–4; also Figures 50–6, 50–7, and 50–16, pages 907, 909, and 919). This technique has been most valuable in the diagnosis of autosomal trisomies and has less value in the deficiency disorders and sex chromosome aberrations. Although identification by chromosome banding patterns has limited the use of dermatoglyphics as a diagnostic tool, it still remains useful in places where there is no convenient access to a cytogenetics service.

Patients who are the most likely candidates for chromosomal aberrations have an array of physical and mental defects of unknown origin. They frequently have an unusual facies, abnormal ears, malformations of the heart and kidneys, abnormalities of the hands and feet, and disturbances in dermal configurations and flexion creases.

HEART DEFECTS AND CHROMOSOMES

It has been estimated that 3.5 percent of all pregnancies contain a recognizable chromosomal abnormality. By the time abortions take their toll the number with abnormal chromosomes has been reduced to 0.5 percent of live births (Polani, 1968; Walzer et al., 1969; Sergovich et al., 1969). Of the survivors, the heart is involved in a variable proportion ranging from a few to 100 percent in specific syndromes; the most striking are trisomies 13 and 18 with 90 to 100 percent. Intermediate in frequency (40 to 50 percent) are trisomy 21, partial short arm deletion of chromosome no. 4 (4p−), and partial long arm deletion of no. 18 (18q−), while less common frequencies (20 percent) are reported in

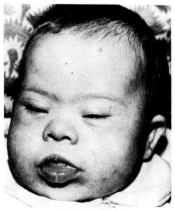

A

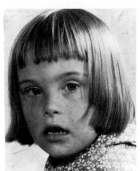

B

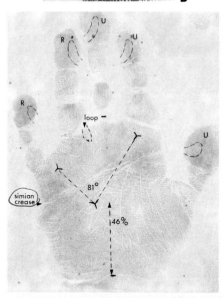

C

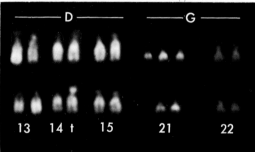

D

INCIDENCE

1:600 to 1:700

GENERAL

Mean maternal age at birth: 33 years

HEAD

Brachycephaly

Short neck

Straight fine hair

FACE

Tongue protrudes

Delayed dentition

Epicanthic folds

Brushfield spots

HEART

Heart malformation 45 per cent

Atrioventricular canal and ventricular
septal defects 75 per cent

Atrial septal defect, tetralogy of Fallot,
and patent ductus arteriosus

ABDOMEN

Prominent

Duodenal atresia increased frequency;
cryptorchidism

EXTREMITIES

Short broad hands

Clinodactyly 5th finger

Gap between 1st and 2nd toe

OTHER

Decreased acetabular angle

Psychomotor retardation

High incidence leukemia

DERMATOGLYPHICS

Distal axial triradius;
radial loop on 4th and 5th fingers;
simian crease

CHROMOSOMES

Partial karyotypes

Top: regular 21 trisomy: 47,+21

Bottom: translocation t(14q21q)

Figure 50-4. A composite of the major clinical
features, the specific karyotypic abnormality, and the
physical appearance of patients with trisomy 21
(Down's syndrome).

partial short arm deletion of no. 5 (5p−) and 45,X Turner's syndrome. In syndromes involving additional sex chromosomes the proportion with congenital heart disease is uncertain but probably much lower than the above. In other miscellaneous syndromes there is insufficient documentation to estimate the frequency of congenital heart disease. Hence the frequency in chromosomally abnormal births is about 1 in 700 (roughly 30 percent of those with a chromosomal abnormality). Since the incidence of cardiac malformations in the general population is about 1 percent, the contribution of chromosomal abnormalities to the total population of congenital heart disease can be seen to be appreciable (Polani, 1968).

The chromosomes of patients with inherited or sporadic heart defects have been examined in an effort to explain the production of congenital heart disease in chromosomal abnormalities (Sasaki et al., 1963; Anders et al., 1965; German et al., 1966; Rohde, 1966; Polani, 1968; Emerit et al., 1973; Dahl, 1970). What emerges is that, except in known syndromes, there is no clear evidence of major chromosomal abnormality to account for the heart defect. In most studies minor structural chromosomal changes were encountered in rather fewer than 10 percent of the populations sampled. Although the findings could be fortuitous, they have led to the hypothesis that the transmission of these variations in phenotypically normal individuals constituted a chromosomal structural load that might produce maldevelopment of the heart (Rohde, 1966; German et al., 1966). It remains to be seen whether reexamination of these variants utilizing the newer staining techniques could refine this problem to some solution.

The unusual distribution of the anatomic type of congenital heart disease encountered within the chromosomal syndromes has tempted consideration of possible modes by which chromosomal abnormality could cause a cardiac malformation such as excess, loss, or rearrangement of genetic material (Polani, 1968; German et al., 1972), but there is not presently an entirely satisfactory theory, let alone proof, of the mechanism involved. The possibility that a specific locus for congenital heart disease will prove to be the answer to these questions seems unlikely. The almost overwhelming evidence to date would support a polygenic cause for heart malformation (Nora, 1968; Patterson et al., 1972).

The association between dermatoglyphics and chromosomes has stimulated the cardiologist to ask if a particular dermal ridge or crease pattern has any specificity for the presence of congenital heart disease itself. This area was explored briefly in some of our earlier work on Down's syndrome (Rowe and Uchida, 1961). It was found that 21 trisomics with heart disease tended to have axial triradii more distally located on the palm. This was given some support by Reed and associates (1973). The same tendency has been noted in nonmongoloid patients with congenital heart disease (Hale et al., 1961; Burguet and Collard, 1968). Speculation as to the role that dermatoglyphics may play in identifying a subgroup of genetically determined congenital heart disease has been made (Sanchez Cascos, 1968; Alter and Schulenberg, 1970). However, these conclusions were not borne out by Preus and associates (1970) who reported that dermatoglyphics were not diagnostically useful because the differences found were so small.

AUTOSOMAL ABNORMALITIES

THE TRISOMIES

Trisomy 21 (47, +21 Mongolism; Down's Syndrome)

Mongolism (Down, 1866) is a well-known syndrome characterized by gross mental retardation, muscle hypotonia, multiple congenital malformations, and a characteristic facies (Figure 50–4). Most reports have concerned white populations, but Down's syndrome has also been found in other races. Because of this widespread occurrence and on the assumption that the use of the term "mongolism" offends persons of other races, the alternative titles of Down's syndrome (Allen et al., 1961) and trisomy 21 (Lennox, 1961) have been suggested.

Other features of this disorder include typical dermatoglyphics (Cummins et al., 1950; Walker, 1957; Holt, 1961; Reed et al., 1970), reduced acetabular angle (Caffey and Ross, 1956; Kaufmann and Taillard, 1961), disturbance of tryptophan metabolism, and failure of polymorphonuclear leukocytes to mature fully. More variable traits include brachycephaly, a third fontanelle, deformed middle phalanx of the little finger, Brushfield spots, and congenital malformations of the heart, alimentary canal, and lungs. The monographs of Penrose and Smith (1966), the Ciba Foundation Study Group (Wolstenholme and Porter, 1967), and Smith and Berg (1976) provide complete descriptions of the disorder.

Genetics. The disorder is characteristically associated with an extra chromosome (Lejeune et al., 1959), identified by its banding pattern as the smallest in the human karyotype (Caspersson et al., 1970). Since mongolism has long been associated with chromosome no. 21 it was decided to retain this classification (rather than the correct no. 22) in order to avoid confusion (Paris Conf., 1971). Regular trisomics form 95 percent of patients with Down's syndrome, 4 percent are translocations involving mostly nos. 14 and 21, i.e., t(14q21q), or two no. 21 chromosomes, t(21q21q), and 1 percent exhibit mosaicism. The latter patients are usually less severely affected, but there is considerable variation. The mentality in one case appears normal and heart malformation is unusual (Nichols et al., 1962; Clarke et al., 1961; Smith et al., 1962; Medenis et al., 1962; Kohn et al., 1970).

Nondisjunction is responsible for most cases of 21 trisomy. The majority are born to older mothers (Carter and McCarthy, 1951; Oster, 1953) and paternal age is irrelevant. Recent data from several countries show a decrease in the mean age of mothers giving birth to infants with trisomy 21 (Uchida, 1970; Gardner et al., 1973; Lowry et al., 1976; Kuroki et al., 1977). Translocation mongolism is not associated with parental age. The relation between age and nondisjunction is as yet uncertain, but suggestions as to causation have included X-irradiation (Uchida and Curtis, 1961; Sigler et al., 1965; Uchida et al., 1968; Alberman et al., 1972), hormone imbalance (Rundle et al., 1961), and infection (Collman and Stoller, 1962; Robinson and Puck, 1966). Proof of the maternal origin of nondisjunction in older women has become available with examination of chromosome banding patterns (Robinson, 1973; Licnerski and Lindsten, 1972). On the other hand paternal nondisjunction in young parents has been observed (Sasaki and Hara, 1973; Uchida, 1973).

It has been estimated that one-tenth of the children of translocation carrier mothers will be affected rather than the expected one-third (Hamerton, 1968), while half the offspring of a trisomic female will also be trisomic (Penrose, 1961). It requires emphasis that translocation is not the responsible mechanism for most cases of repetitive mongolism or mongoloids born to young mothers (Penrose, 1961); the majority are regular trisomics. In twins monozygous pairs are concordant except for the rare event when nondisjunction occurs after zygote formation to give rise to monozygous twins with different chromosome complements. Double nondisjunction with 21 trisomy and XXY Klinefelter's syndrome has been noted by several groups.

Frequency. It is generally accepted that one in every 600 to 700 births in Europeans will be a mongoloid infant (Carter and McCarthy, 1951; Collman and Stoller, 1962). Heart defect as an associated anomaly in mongolism was not reported until the end of the nineteenth century (Garrod, 1894, 1899; Thomson, 1898), and although a large literature on this aspect has accumulated since, there has been considerable disagreement over the proportion of mongoloids affected in this manner. In a series of autopsy studies (Table 50–1) totaling 300 mongoloids, over half had heart disease. Clinical estimates in most reports have shown smaller proportions with heart malformation. In a comprehensive review of the literature conducted by Berg and associates (1960) almost 2500 cases of mongolism in series not exclusively autopsy were examined. Heart disease was detected in 424 cases, an incidence of 19 percent. The median value for the 27 studies was 17 percent. About 5 percent of all congenital heart disease deaths are associated with Down's syndrome (Cullum and Liebman, 1969).

This wide variation in the frequency of congenital heart disease found in postmortem and clinical surveys is mainly due to factors of selection but is also due to differences in criteria for diagnosis. A prospective study of a large group of Down's patients was achieved over a two-year period (Rowe and Uchida, 1961) through the availability for several years prior to the cardiac investigation of a widely used outpatient confirmatory diagnostic service for interpretation of dermal ridge configurations by the Department of Genetics, Hospital for Sick Children, Toronto. Mongoloids referred for confirmation of the diagnosis by this service or for counseling were examined specifically for congenital heart disease. It is believed that practically all mongoloids born in the city of Toronto in this period were seen. Apart from clinical examination by a pediatric cardiologist, chest x-rays, electrocardiogram, and, in the majority, fluoroscopy with barium swallow were performed. Cardiac catheterization, requested in all cases irrespective of the clinical state, was performed in about one-third. Specially stringent criteria were used for newborn infants, and wherever possible, follow-up was obtained. A total of 184 mongoloids was seen, and in 174 where a decision on the cardiovascular status could be reached, 70 (40 percent) had heart defect. Although even this approach has flaws, it seems likely that the real frequency of heart malformation is high and lies close to this figure.

The Nature of the Cardiac Defect. Abbot (1936) referred to the frequent combination of mongolian idiocy and persistent ostium atrioventriculare commune and ostium primum. Nadas (1957), Lev and Kaveggia (1960), and Potter (1961) have also considered persistent atrioventricular canal to be the

Table 50–1. THE PROPORTION OF SUBJECTS
WITH DOWN'S SYNDROME HAVING HEART
DISEASE AT AUTOPSY

AUTHOR	NUMBER IN SERIES	NUMBER WITH HEART DEFECT	PERCENT
Evans, 1950	63	28	44
Strauss, 1953	12	6	50
Hambach, 1956	24	17	71
Esen, 1957	31	12	39
Berg et al., 1960	141	79	56
Rowe and Uchida, 1961	29	17	59

Table 50–2.　A COMPARISON OF TYPE AND FREQUENCY OF HEART DEFECT IN DOWN'S SYNDROME FROM AUTOPSY AND FROM PROSPECTIVE CLINICAL STUDIES

AUTOPSY SERIES DEFECT	CULLUM AND LIEBMAN, 1969		PROSPECTIVE SERIES (ROWE AND UCHIDA, 1961)		CLINICAL SYNDROME WITH HEART DEFECT HSC 1950–1972	
	Number	*Percent*	*Number*	*Percent*	*Number*	*Percent*
Atrioventricular canal defect						
Complete	34	25	23 } 25	36	174 } 211	36
Incomplete	?	?	3		37	
Atrial septal defect	14	10	6	9	42	7
Ventricular septal defect	54	39	23	33	180	30
Patent ductus arteriosus	7	5	7	10	45	8
Isolated aberrant right subclavian artery	0	0	5	7	NK	—
Tetralogy of Fallot	15	10	1	1	37	6
Bicuspid aortic valve	0	0	?	?	?	
Pulmonary stenosis	1	—	1	1	5	1
Endocardial fibroelastosis	2	—	—	—	0	—
Miscellaneous	9	7	—	—	24	4
Coarctation of aorta	2	—	—	—	5	1
Aortic stenosis	1	—	—	—	5	1
Equivocal classification	—	—	2	3	36	6
Total	139	100	70	100	590	100

common cardiac anomaly in mongoloids. Recent studies have confirmed that defects of the cardiac septa account for over three-quarters of the heart malformations found in mongoloids (Table 50–2). It may be seen from this table that the total proportion with atrioventricular canal defects, ventricular septal defects, and secundum atrial defects is about the same in the three series. In the clinical study isolated patent ductus arteriosus and aberrant right subclavian artery accounted for almost one-sixth of the number with heart disease, while they were not seen once in the postmortem group. Though not a major defect, aberrant right subclavian artery has been noted in relatively high frequency in mongolism by Evans (1950), Strauss (1953), and Liu and Corlett (1959). In the study at The Hospital for Sick Children the anomaly was present in 5.6 percent of mongoloids, compared with the 1.3 percent noted in 1000 autopsies by Anson (1960).

Frankly cyanotic lesions are less common, although the very first report of congenital heart disease in mongolism concerned a cyanotic infant (Garrod, 1894).

Tetralogy of Fallot has been reported 42 times from 14 series (including six patients with atrioventricular canal defect (Lev et al., 1961; Tandon and Edwards, 1973) and transposition of the great vessels in 15 patients from eight series. Six of the latter anomaly came from one series of 17 mongoloids with congenital heart disease (Hambach, 1956). Aortic coarctation, aortic stenosis, truncus arteriosus, mitral atresia, aortic atresia, pulmonary stenosis, endocardial fibroelastosis, and single ventricle while not unknown in Down's syndrome are rare.

The morphologic study of specific defects of Tandon and Edwards (1973) makes some important observations. In addition to confirming that atrial septal defect, ventricular septal defect, and patent ductus arteriosus were present, in one form or another in 76 percent, 87 percent, and 47 percent, respectively, of cases associated with Down's syndrome and congenital heart disease, these authors examined the detailed anatomy of additional anomalies of the common, mitral, and tricuspid valve in the different forms of the atrioventricular canal malformation in the disorder. The fact that a third of the complete form of the canal have a variety of added disturbances (parachute deformity, plastered valve, double orifice, free floating leaflet, etc.) provides good reason for the enormously different clinical courses in that malformation. These authors also draw attention to the fact that the ventricular septal defect is in the membranous and atrioventricular canal position in roughly equal proportions, that spontaneous closure of the ventricular septal defect by tricuspid valve adhesion can occur in mongolism, and that the tetralogy of Fallot may be associated with complete atrioventricular canal defect or not in a possibly equal division.

A variety of left- and right-sided obstructions was identified in their series. While the left-sided obstructions are a relatively new emphasis, this adds to other questions about the importance of left-sided disease seen in older patients with this trisomy (Gerstmann et al., 1972).

Recently, Rosenquist and colleagues (1974) have demonstrated that the proportion of the ventricular septum that is membranous is increased from the normal 2 percent to 9 percent in individuals with Down's syndrome.

The important points that may be taken from these facts are that septal defects account for most heart malformations in mongolism, that atrioventricular canal defects form a higher proportion of heart disease in mongoloids than in the nonmongoloid population, and that the relatively uncommon purely cyanotic lesion in a mongoloid will more often prove to be tetralogy of Fallot than complete transposition of great vessels.

Clinical Features. GENERAL. The diagnosis of mongolism by inspection at birth is possible in all but about 1 percent of cases. The characteristic facies provides the initial and principal clue, although other signs previously described are helpful to the physician making the important clinical decision. The more features of the syndrome that can be detected, the more certain will be the diagnosis. In our experience the situation is more readily accepted by parents when confirmatory studies such as dermatoglyphic or cytogenetic analyses are carried out. Such objective studies, although desirable in obvious Down's patients, are essential in doubtful cases because of the serious prognosis carried by the disorder. It is especially important to analyze the chromosomes of the affected offspring of a young mother and the young mother herself in case a translocation may be present. If an inherited translocation is found, a search for carriers in all close relatives is indicated.

CARDIOVASCULAR. Mongoloid infants are reputed to exhibit more cyanosis and coldness of the extremities than normal infants, and it is believed that their peripheral vasculature has some differences from the normal (Benda, 1949). There is some evidence to show that the postnatal transitional circulation may be delayed in these subjects in the sense that higher pulmonary arterial pressures and functional left-to-right shunts through the ductus arteriosus may occur for a longer-than-usual period after birth (Rowe and James, 1957). The suggestion that pulmonary vascular obstructive disease may develop in patients having large interventricular communications or aorticopulmonary defects and Down's syndrome earlier than would be found in phenotypically normal patients with defects of similar size (Shaher et al., 1972) has recently been confirmed by Chi and Krovetz (1975). One possible explanation for these differences could lie in the low-grade, mildly hypoxic state present most of the time in many patients with the trisomy as a result of airways obstruction, weak thoracic musculature, or a combination.

The detection of associated congenital heart disease is not always simple. Since frankly cyanotic lesions are rare, one useful pointer toward congenital

heart disease is absent in the majority of cases. The principal feature on examination is the presence of a heart murmur, especially after the second week of life. Prior to this time, owing among other things to the presence of the transitional circulation, murmurs may be absent. We have found it virtually impossible to declare the heart of a mongoloid infant normal in this period without the aid of cardiac catheterization. Three such infants who showed no cardiac murmur, no cardiac enlargement, and lung vascularity within normal limits at x-ray when first seen at two, five, and six days, respectively, underwent cardiac catheterization at the age of three, four, and three months, and the presence of a secundum atrial septal defect, atrioventricularis communis, and ventricular septal defect, respectively, was detected. Similar experiences were encountered in several infants catheterized in the first two weeks of life. The decision regarding the cardiac status becomes easier after one month of age, and with very few exceptions the correct diagnosis of heart disease is possible after that age. The clinical diagnosis of a normal heart may likewise be made then and has been confirmed by cardiac catheterization or autopsy in our series.

The anatomic diagnosis is reached in affected mongoloid infants from a combination of physical findings, electrocardiographic changes, and radiologic and other accessory investigations, in a manner outlined in chapters relevant to the particular malformation.

It needs emphasis that although the usual clinical diagnostic criteria can be applied, exceptions will be found just as they are in the clinical picture of cardiac malformations in patients with normal phenotype. For example, where it might be assumed particularly in a mongoloid with signs of an atrial septal defect that a frontal plane axis of $+150°$ might imply a secundum type or one of $+270°$ an endocardial cushion–type defect, the reverse may be found in about 10 percent of patients. The great majority with confirmed atrial defects of either variety have quite appropriate and expected frontal plane axes for the defect site. Likewise the presence of ventricular septal defect with a frontal plane axis QRS in the range of $+270°$ to $+330°$ does not necessarily imply the presence of an atrioventricular canal–type of ventricular communication. If the data of Tandon and Edwards (1973) indicating equal proportions of atrioventricular canal–type and membranous ventricular defects are representative, then this is not reflected in the electrocardiogram, which in our experience shows that the great majority of mongoloids with ventricular defect have A QRS ranging from $+50°$ to $+150°$ (Park et al., 1977). Again, spontaneous closure of ventricular defects can occur in Down's syndrome (Berg et al., 1960; Tandon and Edwards, 1973), and one suspects from the high frequency of cushion anomalies that a favorable climate for spontaneous closure or reduction in size of ventricular defects could be predicted. We know of no data about the incidence of spontaneous closure, however, and it is not our impression that such an event is at all common by contrast with our experience in nonmongoloids with ventricular septal defect.

Prognosis. From an average age at death of about nine years in the late 1920s (Brousseau, 1928; Penrose, 1932), there has been a steady improvement to almost double that figure (Polani, 1968). Studies of mortality on large numbers of patients with Down's syndrome in England, Australia, and Sweden have been made during the past decade (Carter, 1958; Collman and Stoller, 1963; Forssman and Åkesson, 1965). These newer life tables indicate still a high though lessened mortality in the first six months of life. In Forssman and Akesson's study (1965) the group had an overall mortality 6 percent higher than the general population through the 5-to-40-year age group. After 50 years the excess over general population mortality was 30 percent. For the Australian patients the expectation of life at birth is 16.2 years; at one year, 22.4 years; at five to nine years, 26.7 years; and at 50, 2.5 years (Collman and Stoller, 1963). It has long been accepted that those infants with congenital heart disease or other serious associated malformations die in infancy, whereas premature death after that age is due to infections, particularly respiratory, which are poorly tolerated by the mongoloid child. According to Benda (1949), the heart is abnormal in 75 percent of mongoloid infants dying in the first two years of life. Of 14 mongoloids in the Toronto study dying in the first month after birth, only five had congenital heart defect. Those with a normal heart died from severe anomalies of the gastrointestinal tract (such as duodenal atresia, imperforate anus, or tracheo-esophageal fistula), respiratory distress syndrome, or infection. After the newborn period deaths due directly or indirectly to congenital heart malformation become relatively more prominent. In our series the likelihood of congenital heart disease being present in mongoloids dying after the first month of life was more than 70 percent. Similarly, other workers have found that about two-thirds of the deaths in mongolism in the first year of life are associated with heart malformation (Benda, 1949; Lunn, 1959; Berg et al., 1960). These observations have been amply confirmed in a large population of mongols (Fabia and Drolette, 1970) where additionally it was shown that females with congenital heart disease were less likely to survive the early years (Figure 50–5). These figures emphasize the importance to the family of knowing whether heart disease is present or absent in a particular mongoloid infant. Although it should not be expected that there might be any difference in the incidence of congenital heart malformation in the various chromosomal types of true mongolism both from theoretic grounds and indirect evidence, this matter awaits confirmation.

It has been suggested that 21 trisomics, being frail members of the species, do not tolerate insults such as angiocardiography (Abrams and Kaplan, 1956). Disturbances were not noted during either lengthy cardiac catheterization or angiographic examination of such patients in our unit. Leukemia is 20 times more

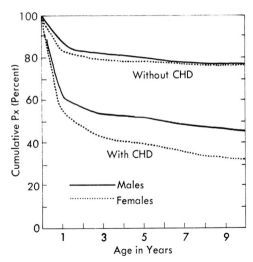

Figure 50-5. Cumulative survival rates for the first ten years of life by sex. Mongols with and without congenital heart disease. *CHD* = congenital heart defect. (Reproduced from Fabia, J., and Drolette, M. J.: Life tables up to age ten for mongols with and without congenital heart disease. *Ment. Defic. Res.,* **14**:235, 1970.)

frequent in Down's patients than in the general population (Penrose, 1961). This observation led to the assumption that the Philadelphia (Ph') chromosome, found in chronic myelogenous leukemia, probably represented a deletion of part of the long arm of chromosome no. 21 and was accepted as the connecting link between mongolism and leukemia. This reasoning, however, broke down when chromosome banding identified the Ph' chromosome as no. 22 (Caspersson et al., 1970) and, rather than being deleted, the broken end was translocated to chromosome no. 9 (Rowley, 1973). With the exception of leukemia, it may be said that once the dangers of infancy are successfully passed, the patient with a normal heart appears capable of survival to a much older age than formerly if provided with modern therapy at times of illness.

A joint analysis of patients with trisomy 21 and congenital heart disease seen in children over the past 15 years was made by the pediatric cardiology divisions at the Children's Hospital, Pittsburgh, and at the Johns Hopkins Hospital (Park et al., 1977). From a total of 251 patients it was concluded that palliative surgery carried a distinct but not prohibitive mortality during the first six months of life. Thereafter there was no mortality from this form of treatment while open heart surgery was feasible at moderate risk. The limiting factor in surgical intervention is not therefore a technical one but is quite obviously a matter where decisions are most often being rendered against surgical intervention by pediatricians and parents on the basis of the underlying Down's syndrome.

Treatment. There is no cure for mongolism. Despite many claims to the contrary, no pharmacologic agent has yet produced significant lasting improvement in the general or intellectual development of children with Down's syndrome. For many, in addition to attention to providing a favorable climate for the best intellectual development possible, the only acceptable program is one that includes all therapeutic measures available to any child for any illness. This includes cardiac surgery (Park et al., 1977). The very difficult ethical problems surrounding therapy that affect pediatricians daily (Veeder, 1961; Gustafson, 1973) are now being examined in the public forum to an increasing degree (Shaw, 1972).

Aside from the important issues about the actual patient and his management, a number of preventive measures may be taken. Parents want to know what factors determine high risk for the production of Down's syndrome and how they can avoid these risks. Affected families want to know the chances for recurrence. The answers to these questions are now known in large measure. Following the observation that the incidence of mongolism rises as maternal age approaches 40 years, Oster (1953) claimed that the incidence could be reduced about 30 percent by the avoidance of pregnancies after the fourth decade.

The factors determining the recurrence risk for pregnancies subsequent to an affected birth have been discussed by Polani (1963). Table 50–3, in addition to showing the importance of increasing maternal age on the risk of occurrence, gives the recurrence risks for trisomics, which are the same for all age groups and are similar to the occurrence risk for women over the age of 45 years. Translocation carriers are at particular risk, being in the order of 1:10. In the rare case where a mother is a t(21q21q) carrier, 100 percent of her offspring will be affected. Amniocentesis for prenatal diagnosis is indicated for mothers who have balanced translocation, a previous trisomic infant, or who are over the age of 40 years. In a broader view, since there is some evidence suggesting that cumulative x-ray exposure can influence nondisjunction, efforts directed at reducing such exposure in females need continuing emphasis.

Trisomy 18 (47, +18; E Syndrome; Edwards' Syndrome)

A syndrome of multiple congenital anomalies caused by an extra chromosome in the E group was described independently by two groups of investigators (Smith et al., 1960; Edwards et al., 1960). Subsequent reports confirmed their observations (German et al., 1962; Smith, 1962; Uchida et al., 1962a; Warkany et al., 1966). The clinical features are now almost as familiar to pediatricians as those of mongolism. The small delicate facial features distinguish these patients from other trisomics. The chief signs are a low birth weight for gestational age, scaphocephaly, low-set malformed ears, micrognathia, a nonfixed flexion deformity of the fingers, deformed feet, spasticity, and mental retardation. A number of anomalies, including renal, gastrointestinal, and skeletal, occur less uniformly (Figure 50–6). Failure to thrive and heart malformation are almost invariable (Taylor, 1967), 1968).

Genetics. The incidence of the disorder is about 1:4,000 births. Late maternal age is etiologically important. Females preponderate, the sex ratio being 4:1. The chromosome involved has been certainly identified as no. 18 (Smith et al., 1960). Identification by amniotic fluid cell culture at $16\frac{1}{2}$ weeks, subsequently confirmed at 20 weeks after induced abortion, has been reported. The fetus had atrial and ventricular septal defects and a bicuspid aortic valve (Hsu et al., 1973). Mosaics and doble trisomics have been recorded (Weiss et al., 1962; Uchida et al., 1962b). Translocations are rare and give rise to partial trisomy syndromes; i.e., only part of the no. 18 chromosome is in triplicate.

A single crease on the fifth finger (sometimes on all fingers) is common while a high frequency of arches on the fingers and toes is the characteristic dermatoglyphic pattern (Uchida et al., 1962c). Less than six arches or more than two whorls argues strongly against the diagnosis (Preus and Fraser, 1972).

Heart Malformation. Cardiac defect is present in almost all cases (Kurien and Duke, 1968). A ventricular septal defect was present in the first three cases reported and has continued to be the most frequent of the heart malformations. There is, however, frequently associated patent ductus arteriosus and atrial septal defect. There is some contention over whether many patients or few within this large group have double-outlet right ventricle (Rogers et al., 1965). Aneurysmal transformation

Table 50–3. RISK OF RECURRENCE OF TRISOMY 21 ACCORDING TO MATERNAL AGE AT BIRTH OF PROBAND (MOSAICS AND TRANSLOCATIONS EXCLUDED)

| MATERNAL AGE | TRISOMY BIRTH RATE MANITOBA 1960–1968 | CHILDREN BORN AFTER PROBAND | | RECURRENCE RISK |
		Total Sibs	Trisomy 21	
<25	1/2000	181	2	1/90
25–34	1/1300	254	5	1/50
35–44	1/250	94	1	1/90
45+	1/80	0	0	—
Totals	1/900	529	8	1/65

Combined data from Manitoba study (Uchida, 1970) and Carter and Evans (Lancet, **2**:785, 1961).

INCIDENCE

1:6700 to 1:3500 live births

GENERAL

Hydramnios, small placenta
Mean birth weight 2200 G
More females affected
Most die by one 1 year
Hypertonia
Failure to thrive
Mental retardation

HEAD

Scaphocephaly with prominent occiput

FACE

Low set, malformed ears

HEART

Congenital heart disease: almost 100 per cent

Ventricular septal defect: 96 per cent

Atrial septal defect: 22 per cent

Patent ductus arteriosus: 69 per cent

ABDOMEN

Single umbilical artery
Renal anomalies - horseshoe, cystic double ureters
Diaphragm eventration
Meckel's diverticulum

EXTREMITIES

Clinodactyly
Rocker bottom feet
Short dorsiflexed hallux

OTHER

Shield chest
Short sternum

DERMATOGLYPHICS

Arch pattern: high frequency of simple arches on most fingers
Single crease fifth finger

CHROMOSOMES

Partial fluorescence karyotype showing three #18 chromosomes

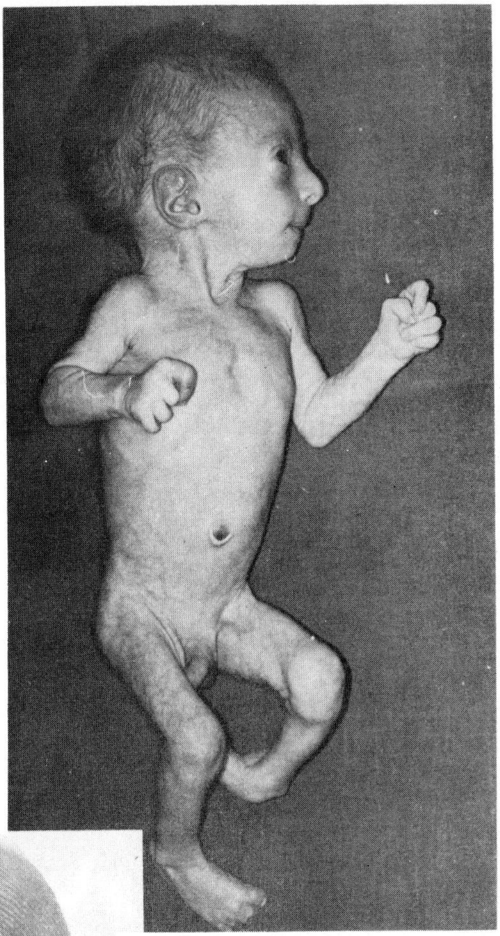

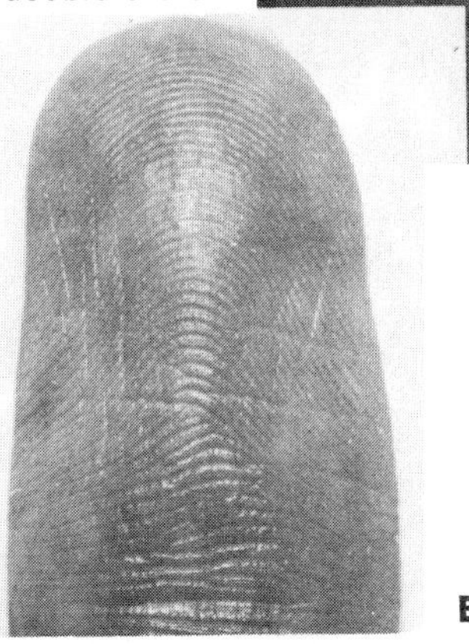

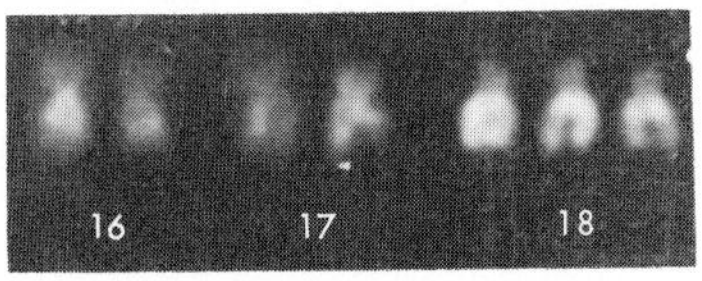

Figure 50-6. A composite of the major clinical features, the specific karyotypic abnormality, and the physical appearance in a patient with trisomy 18 (Edwards' syndrome).

around a ventricular septal defect has been observed in partial trisomy (Chesler et al., 1970). A high incidence of bicuspid semilunar valves is evident in the literature, and moderate degrees of aortic and pulmonary stenosis have been described (Townes et al., 1963; Holman et al., 1963; Kurien and Duke. 1968). Only occasionally does ventricular defect occur as part of a more complex situation such as coarctation of the aorta, atrial septal defect, transposition of the great vessels, atrioventricular canal defect, or mitral atresia (Rohde et al., 1964; Scarpa and Borgaonkar, 1966). Myocardial disease (fibrosis of uncertain origin or endocardial fibroelastosis) has been the subject of several reports (Townes et al., 1963; Lewis, 1964; Kurien and Duke, 1968). There is little doubt that the cardiac anomaly contributes significantly to the early death of these patients. Long-term survivors may have relatively mild cardiac disease (Weiss et al., 1962; Surana et al., 1972; Chesler et al., 1970).

Prognosis. The outlook is bad, death during early infancy being usual. The mean survival time for males is appreciably shorter than that for females (Conen and Erkman, 1966). Survival to the second or third decade is exceptional (Weiss et al., 1962; Surana et al., 1972). Although most trisomy 18 cases are sporadic and second recurrence is rare, parental mosaicism in trisomy 18 has been reported (Beratis et al., 1972). Parents of children with trisomy 18 should be investigated for their chromosome constitution. The indications for amniocentesis have been outlined on page 906.

Trisomy 13 (47, +13; D Syndrome; Patau's Syndrome)

A syndrome of multiple congenital anomalies associated with an extra chromosome of the D group was first reported by Patau and associates (1960). Since then several groups have confirmed these observations (Atkins and Rosenthal, 1961; Ellis and Marwood, 1961; Lubs et al., 1961; Northcutt, 1962; Smith et al., 1963; Conen et al., 1966; Warkany et al., 1966; Taylor, 1968). A review of 120 published cases has appeared recently (Taylor et al., 1970).

The average birth weight is 2500 gm. Mental retardation, seizures, deafness, and failure to thrive are usual. Cleft lip and palate and polydactyly are the most striking external anomalies, occurring in 75 percent of the patients. Ocular deformities are common and include colobomata, cataract, and anophthalmia. Flexion deformities of the hands, ear deformities, and renal tract anomalies have all been reported, and a capillary hemangioma over the forehead is common. Males have inguinal or abdominal cryptorchidism with anomalous scrotal development (Smith et al., 1963). Bicornuate uterus is common in females. There is characteristically abnormal elevation of fetal Hgb F, and polymorphonuclear leucocytes have nuclear projections about 12 times more frequently than normal (Taylor et al., 1970). Although most cases show a remarkably similar pattern of congenital anomalies (Figure 50–7), there have been exceptions. Patients with trisomy 13 have been reported where the clinical features were classic for trisomy 18 (Goodman and Kaufman, 1962; Rhode et al., 1965). We have a proved trisomy 13 in a five-and-a-half-year-old boy

with a repaired cleft palate and harelip who is blind and yet has an otherwise normal physical and mental status (Conen, personal communication) (Figure 50–8).

Genetics. The incidence of trisomy 13 is in the order of 1:7000 to 1:14,500. Increased maternal age is noted in patients with nondisjunction but not in those with translocation. The sex ratio is equal. Trisomy of chromosome 13 was first distinguished from other D-group chromosomes by autoradiography. Fluorescent and Giemsa staining are the methods of choice for identification today. Trisomies for the other two pairs of the D group have not been found and are probably lethal. Mosaics are not infrequent—about 5 to 10 percent (Green et al., 1968; Polani, 1969). Translocation occurs in about 20 percent of cases by contrast with about 5 percent for mongolism (Taylor et al., 1970; Erkman et al., 1965). This is most often of the t(13qDq) constitution.

Simian creases are characteristic and about twice as commonly observed as in either trisomy 18 or 21. There is a marked increase in bilateral distal axial triradii (Uchida et al., 1962; Preus and Fraser, 1972).

Heart Malformation. Over 80 percent of patients with trisomy 13 have had heart defect. Transposition of great vessels, truncus arteriosus, atrial septal defect, dextroposition, and ventricular septal defect have presented as single defects in approximately that order of frequency. This demonstrates real differences in the types of congenital heart disease in trisomy 13 from those encountered in both trisomy 18 and 21 syndromes (Polani, 1968). Rarely hypoplastic left ventricle, atrioventricularis communis (Nusbacher and Hirschhorn, 1968), and Ebstein's disorder (Murphyn et al., 1967) have been associated with trisomy 13. Ventricular septal defect, patent ductus arteriosus, and atrial septal defect of course have been commonly encountered (Patau et al., 1960; Townes et al., 1962; Smith et al., 1963) and in one combination or another make up the majority of defects seen.

Prognosis. The outlook for these patients is poor. The average time for survival is 100 days, about half dying during the first month. There is no survival difference between the sexes (Conen and Erkman, 1966). Many observers feel the cardiac lesion is usually responsible for death. While it may be that the cardiac contribution may be very important to the demise of some, in our experience and that of Polani (1968) apnea and aspiration from the cerebral abnormality seem more often to be the major cause of early death. Renal agenesis and other renal anomalies, e.g., polycystic kidneys and hypoplastic kidneys, are an additional factor in early demise.

Parents of trisomy D children should be studied for their chromosome constitution. Amniocentesis should be available for mothers with a previously affected infant as outlined for Down's syndrome (see page 906).

Figure 50-7. A composite of the major clinical features, the specific karyotypic abnormality, and the physical appearance of a patient with trisomy 13 (Patau's syndrome).

INCIDENCE

1:9000 to 1:7600 live births

GENERAL

Low normal birth weight

3/4 die by 6 months

Mental retardation

HEAD

Arhinencephaly

Microcephaly

Scalp defects

FACE

Micropthalmia or anopthalmia

Colobomata

Cleft lip/palate

Micrognathia

HEART

Congenital heart disease 88 per cent

Ventricular septal defect 60 per cent

Atrial septal defect 44 per cent

Patent ductus arteriosus 48 per cent

Dextrocardia 65 per cent

Transposition great arteries 11 per cent

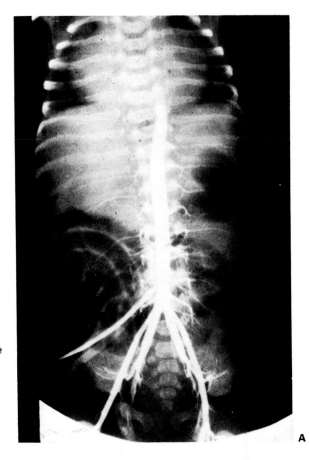

A

ABDOMEN

Midline wall defect

Malrotation of gut

Polycystic kidneys

Hydronephrosis

Renal agenesis (see aortogram: absent renal arteries,
autopsy confirmed)

EXTREMITIES

Polydactyly

Hyperconvex nails

OTHER

Hemangiomata

Persistence of fetal hemoglobin

Nuclear polymorphonuclear projections

Abnormal external genitalia

B

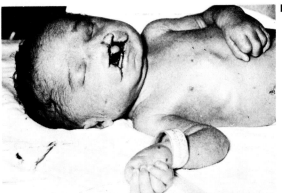

DERMATOGLYPHICS

1. Simian crease

2. Distal axial triradius

3. Arch fibular pattern hallucal area

C

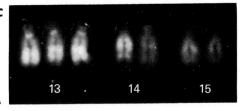

CHROMOSOMES

Partial karyotype showing three #13 chromosomes

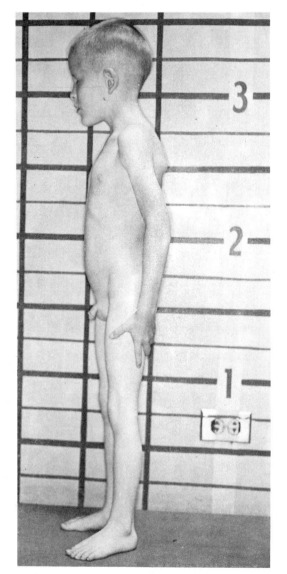

Figure 50-8. A five-and-one-half-year-old boy with trisomy 13. He is blind and had a repair of harelip and cleft palate at an earlier age. Mentality is normal, and he has no other obvious physical defects.

Trisomy 22 (47, +22)

This is a recently confirmed syndrome in patients with mental and growth retardation, microcephaly, micrognathia, preauricular skin tags, low-set or malformed ears, mild neck webbing, deformed lower extremities, and congenital heart disease (Crawfurd, 1961; Gustavson et al., 1962; Uchida et al., 1968; Hsu et al., 1971.) Birth weight has been normal (Figure 50-9).

Karyotypes have shown an extra small acrocentric chromosome, which marker chromosomes, autoradiography, and fluorescent techniques have identified in some cases as one of three no. 22

chromosomes. Advanced maternal age favors the probability that meiotic nondisjunction is responsible for the event.

Dermatoglyphics have been unremarkable (Uchida et al., 1968; Hsu et al., 1971).

Heart malformation has been reported in approximately half the cases. Atrial septal defect of the secundum type, ventricular septal defect (including a two-month-old autopsy with dextrocardia and double-outlet right ventricle) (Crawfurd, 1961)), and patent ductus arteriosus have been reported.

Other Trisomies

Trisomies of other autosomes have been reported but for most of these real documentation is lacking. That would include the case of trisomy 19–20 with secundum atrial septal defect noted in earlier editions of this chapter (Böök et al., 1961). More recent examples have involved mainly the C group and the majority have been mosaics. As a result of improved identification of individual chromosomes it may soon be possible to delineate new syndromes, but it would appear that full trisomy of this group is probably lethal. Cardiac malformation noted to date has been relatively simple and quite compatible with life (atrial or ventricular septal defect). We have encountered one patient with the chromosomal mosaicism 46/47,9 +. His mother was 32 years old when he was born. He had multiple anomalies at birth including dextrocardia. At nine years he was severely retarded and short of stature. The previously confirmed ventricular septal defect of large size was now associated with signs of high pulmonary vascular resistance. His congestive failure responded to anticongestive measures but he died at home a month after discharge. An autopsy showed communicating hydrocephalus, ventricular septal defect, and pulmonary vascular obstruction.

"Cat Eye" Syndrome

The "cat eye" syndrome is an uncommon syndrome with anal atresia, choroidal and iridal colobomata, and an additional small abnormal acrocentric chromosome (47,XX or XY, +mar). The choroidal and iridal colobomata are usually vertical, thus giving the appearance of cat eyes. Renal and cardiac malformations are common (35 percent). The cardiovascular lesions found most frequently include total anomalous pulmonary venous return, tetralogy of Fallot, tricuspid atresia, and atrial and ventricular septal defect (Freedom and Gerald, 1973).

THE DELETION SYNDROMES

Originally thought to be lethal in man, chromosomal deletions have now been documented as causing a number of clinical syndromes. The more common involve chromosomes no. 4, 5, 13, and 18 but a variety of chromosomal deficiencies in the F and G

GENERAL

Hypotonia

Mental retardation

Growth retardation

More common in females

HEAD

Microcephaly

FACE

Characteristic facies

Micrognathia

Low-set ears

Preauricular skin tags

Cleft palate

Epicanthic folds

HEART

Congenital heart disease 50 per cent

EXTREMITIES

Deformed lower extremities

Malopposed thumbs

Cubitus valgus

Slender fingers

Dislocation of hips

DERMATOGLYPHICS

No distinctive pattern

CHROMOSOMES

Partial karyotype from a girl with trisomy 22 identified by autoradiography

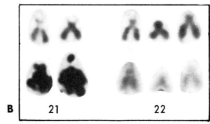

Figure 50-9. A composite of the major clinical features, the specific karyotypic abnormality, and the physical appearance in a patient with trisomy 22.

group, particularly the latter, are being reported. So far it has been established that congenital heart malformation is a common accompaniment only in short-arm deletions of chromosomes 4 and 5 (4p − and 5p −) and in long-arm deletions of chromosomes no. 13 and 18 (13q − and 18q −). It is possible that the spectrum could enlarge with further refinements of techniques of identification.

Short-Arm Deletion of Chromosome No. 5 (5p − ; Cri du Chat Syndrome)

Lejeune and coworkers reported the first three cases of this disorder in 1963. The catlike cry present

only during the early year of life accompanies a collection of anomalies in a physically and mentally retarded infant (Figure 50–10).

Congenital cardiac malformation is present in about 20 percent of patients (Taylor, 1967; Polani, 1968), and although the detailed information on the type and degree of cardiac defect is at present rather vague, there seems little question that complex or severe malformations of the heart are rare. In the report of Breg and associates (1970) some 13 older subjects with the syndrome had no true malformation of the heart. One patient had an aberrant right subclavian artery. It would seem reasonable to assume that heart defect when present has trivial influence on mortality.

INCIDENCE

Rare

GENERAL

Cat cry in infancy, disappears with age

Hypotonia

Mental and motor retardation

Survival beyond infancy common

HEAD

Microcephaly

FACE

Hypertelorism

High forehead

Micrognathia

Low-set ears, preauricular tags

Downward slant to palpebral fissures

HEART

Congenital heart disease in approximately
20 per cent

DERMATOGLYPHICS

Simian line 80 per cent

CHROMOSOMES

B group chromosomes in a patient with partial deletion
of the short arm of chromosome #5

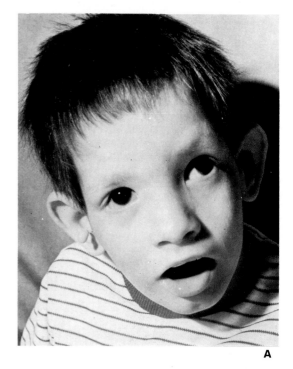

A

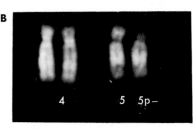

B

4   5 5p−

Figure 50-10. A composite of the major clinical features, the specific karyotypic abnormality, and the physical appearance in a patient with 5p − (cri du chat syndrome).

Since in about 13 percent of patients so far reported one parent had a balanced translocation, the increased inheritance risk should be investigated by chromosomal analysis of sibs and parents of affected infants.

Short-Arm Deletion of Chromosome No. 4 (4p − ; Wolf Syndrome)

The 4p − syndrome (Wolf et al., 1965) was initially grouped with 5p− because these patients were considered as having short-arm deletion of the B chromosome. In this way the features became mixed in clinical descriptions, when, in fact, the stigmata are largely different. In the 4p − syndrome the associated malformations are complex and the degree of mental retardation is severe (Figure 50–11). The facies are distinctive with disturbance of midline fusion. Prominence of the glabella and cleft palate are common. Deformity of the iris, hypertelorism, misshapen nose, preauricular skin tags, hypospadias,

and hypoplastic dermal ridges are commonly found. There is no catlike cry.

Congenital heart malformation has been found in a higher proportion of patients than with 5p − (Polani, 1968) and possibly is present in as high as 50 percent (Guthrie et al., 1971). Atrial septal defects of secundum type (Passarge et al., 1970; Guthrie et al., 1971) or of the endocardial cushion variety (Arias et al., 1970), ventricular septal defect, and patent ductus arteriosus (Miller et al., 1970) are probably the most frequently encountered cardiac abnormalities in the syndrome. Cases with dextrocardia (Taylor et al., 1970) and hypoplastic left ventricle have been noted, and single cases of such relatively mild anomalies as pulmonary stenosis, bicuspid aortic valve, and persistent left superior vena cava are on record (Guthrie et al., 1971). A study of fatalities indicates that deaths in early infancy are most often associated with frank congestive heart failure.

Because of the profound total deficiency present in many patients, Guthrie and associates (1971) recommend supportive management alone, along the lines usually adopted for trisomy 13 and 18.

Partial Long-Arm Deletion of Chromosome No. 18 (18q − ; Carp Mouth Syndrome)

First described by de Grouchy and associates (1964) over a score of patients with this syndrome have now been described. The disorder is characterized by growth failure, mental retardation, midface dysplasia, and a carp mouth. The digital patterns are mainly whorls with a high ridge count (Figure 50–12).

Although 13/29 patients in the literature have had congenital heart disease (Wertelecki and Gerald, 1971), individual detail on the nature of the cardiac disorder is scanty. Atrial septal defect with or without mild pulmonary valve stenosis is documented for affected patients in the only complete reports on this aspect of the syndrome (Curran et al., 1970; Kushnick and Matsushita, 1968). At least two patients have suggestive signs for ventricular defect—one large and one small—but the evidence is far from conclusive (Lejeune et al., 1966; Borkowf et al., 1969). Yet it is apparent that heart defect when present is usually simple in form and does not influence the prognosis to any major degree.

Short-Arm Deletion of Chromosome No 18 (18p −)

This chromosomal abnormality produces an extremely variable phenotype, some patients having

INCIDENCE

Rare

GENERAL

Severe mental and motor retardation

Absence of cat cry

Hypotonia

HEAD

Microcephaly

Midline scalp defects

FACE

Fish-shape mouth

Hypertelorism

Flat beaked nose

Colobomata

HEART

Congenital heart disease about <u>50 per cent</u>

Atrial septal defect most common

EXTREMITIES

Deformed fingers

Clubbed feet

OTHER

Seizures

CHROMOSOMES

B group chromosomes showing partial deletion of the short arm of chromosome #4

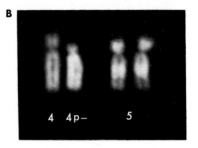

A

B

4   4p−   5

Figure 50-11. A composite of the major clinical features, the specific karyotypic abnormality, and the physical appearance in a patient with 4p− (<u>Wolf syndrome</u>).

INCIDENCE

?

GENERAL

Prognosis for life not impaired
Mental retardation
Hypotonia

HEAD

Microcephaly

FACE

Carp mouth
Smooth upper lip with no columella
Characteristic ear with prominent antihelix and antitragus; small canal

HEART

Congenital heart disease 40 per cent

EXTREMITIES

Long tapering fingers, elongated palm
Dimpled knees and elbows
Club feet

OTHER

Rudimentary external genitalia
Seizures
Hearing defect
Eye defects

DERMATOGLYPHICS

Excess finger whorls

CHROMOSOMES

E group chromosomes showing partial short arm deletion of chromosome #18

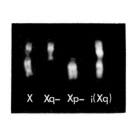
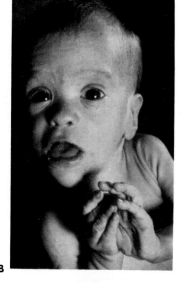
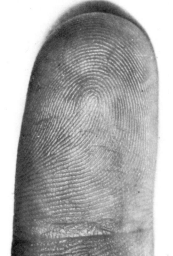

Figure 50-12. A composite of the major clinical features, the specific karyotypic abnormality, and the physical appearance in a patient with 18q– (carp mouth syndrome).

severe and others mild anomalies (Uchida et al., 1965) (Figure 50–13). Heart malformation has not been a cause for comment in case reports of this subgroup but the numbers are few and the point may need reexamination. One reason is that the so-called Turner phenotype occurs in many patients. The high incidence (50 percent) of cardiac malformation and the known propensity for heart malformation to appear trivial on physical examination in the Noonan syndrome (Char et al., 1972) argue for this approach.

Ring Chromosome No. 18; r(18)

Since both ends of the chromosome are lost during ring formation, the clinical consequence might be expected to resemble the effect seen in both 18p – and 18q – or in one more than the other to varying degrees. As far as the cardiac consequences are concerned, there may be differences from those seen in patients with either of the single-arm deletions in this chromosome.

In an early report (Gropp et al., 1964) a cardiac malformation was described. From the murmur description the defect might have been due to a persistent ductus arteriosus or a ventricular septal defect. In two other reports major venous anomalies were encountered. In one (Wald et al., 1969) a persistent left superior vena cava drained into the left atrium (there was associated hypertrophic subaortic stenosis). In the other there was total anomalous pulmonary venous return to the coronary sinus (Palmer et al., 1967).

Long-Arm Deletion of Chromosome No. 13 (13q −)

A few instances with loss of part of the long arm of a D chromosome have been found (Bain and Gauld, 1963; Adams, 1965; Sparkes et al., 1967; Laurent et

al., 1967; Opitz et al., 1969). Autoradiography has identified this chromosome as no. 13. The phenotypic abnormality is uniform (Figure 50–14).

It is difficult to define the cardiac side with so few data, but so far there have been two patients with cyanotic congenital heart disease, probably tetralogy of Fallot, and two patients with ventricular septal defect of which one was stillborn. One other patient had no intracardiac abnormality but a vascular ring formed by a right aortic arch, retroesophageal left subclavian artery, and a closed ductus arteriosus arising from it.

G-Deletion Syndromes (Ring 21; Ring 22)

G-deletion syndromes are caused by loss of all or part of chromosome no. 21 or 22. The karyotype may

GENERAL

Low birth weight

Short stature

Variable mental retardation

Turner -like stigmata

HEAD

Low set large ears

FACE

Hypertelorism

Flat nasal bridge

Micrognathia

HEART

Congenital heart disease incidence ? low

EXTREMITIES

Stubby hands

High-set thumbs

Partial syndactyly toes

DERMATOGLYPHICS

Large digital patterns

High total ridge count

CHROMOSOMES

Partial karyotype showing 18 short arm deletion

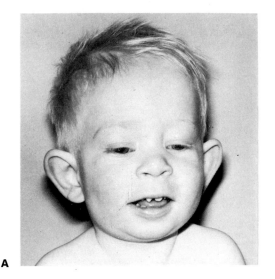

A

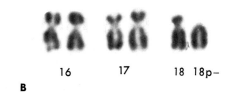

16　　　　17　　　　18 18p−

B

Figure 50-13. A composite of the major clinical features, the specific karyotypic abnormality, and the physical appearance in a patient with 18p− .

GENERAL

Low birth weight

Severe mental retardation

Failure to thrive

HEAD

Microcephaly

Trigonocephaly

FACE

Flat nasal bridge

Hypertelorism

Ptosis

Microphthalmia

Micrognathia   **A**

Retinoblastoma

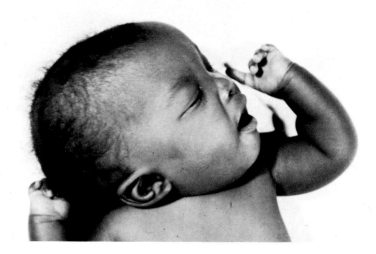

HEART

Congenital heart disease uncertain frequency ?   50 per cent

EXTREMITIES

B

Hip dysplasia

Cryptorchidism

Hypoplasia or absent thumbs

Short 5th finger

CHROMOSOMES

Affected infant and partial karyotype. There it is partial

deletion of the long arm of chromosome #13

(Courtesy of Dr. F. Sergovich, University of Western Ontario)

Figure 50-14. A composite of the major clinical features, the specific karyotypic abnormality, and the physical appearance in a patient with 13q–.

show monosomy, partial loss of the long arm, or ring formation of a G chromosome. The majority have been associated with a ring chromosome. Lejeune and coworkers (1964) first described the clinical features of 21 deletion as the antithesis of Down's syndrome and introduced the concept or hypothesis that chromosome 21 if present in triplicate causes mongolism and if deleted causes "antimongolism." Before cytogenetic techniques were available to distinguish chromosomes 21 and 22, it was noted that G-deletion individuals present different clinical features. Warren and Rimoin (1970) described two distinct G-deletion syndromes and suggested the terms G-deletion syndrome I (antimongolism) and G-deletion syndrome II. With the use of chromosome banding techniques, two syndromes have been identified and shown to be associated with a deletion of chromosome 21 or chromosome 22 (Crandall et al., 1972; Warren et al., 1973).

The clinical features of ring 21 include microcephaly, hypertonicity, hypotelorism, antimongoloid slant, prominent ears and nasal bridge, micrognathia, and mental retardation. Variably present are cleft palate, pyloric stenosis, inguinal hernias, and skeletal abnormalities. Heart murmurs and unspecified congenital heart disease have been reported (Lejeune et al., 1964; Reisman et al., 1966). (See Figure 50–15.)

Patients with ring 22 have less distinctive clinical features. Mental retardation, hypotonia, epicanthal folds, and prominent ears are constant features. Ptosis, bifid uvula, clinodactyly, and syndactyly are sometimes present. Congenital heart disease is not usually associated (Warren and Rimoin, 1970).

The two types of G-deletion syndromes can be differentiated by differences in their dermato-glyphics (Schindeler and Warren, 1973). Ring 21 is characterized by a marked increase in radial loops on the

GENERAL

Hypertonia

Mental retardation

Growth retardation

HEAD

Microcephaly

FACE

Antimongoloid slant

Prominent nasal bridge

Large ears

HEART

Congenital heart disease <u>uncommon</u> and non-specific

(This patient had mild isolated pulmonary stenosis)

ABDOMEN

Inguinal hernia

Pyloric stenosis

EXTREMITIES

Nail dysplasia

DERMATOGLYPHICS

Distinctive for the two types

CHROMOSOMES

G group showing deletion in ring form of chromosome # 21

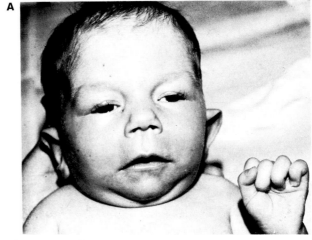

Figure 50-15. A composite of the clinical features, specific karyotypic abnormality, and physical appearance in a patient with G-deletion syndrome (antimongolism; r[21]).

digits. The axial triradius is usually found in a proximal position. Ring 22, on the other hand, differs from 21 deletion by an increased frequency of whorls on the digits and a distally placed axial triradius.

SEX CHROMOSOME ABNORMALITIES

ABNORMALITIES involving either too few or (more frequently) too many sex chromosomes are actually the most common of all chromosomal disorders. Patients with the sex chromosome trisomies XXY, XXX, and XYY together occur once in every 526 live births (Polani, 1968). Only those varieties where there is undisputed presence of or some debate about their association with congenital cardiac malformation will be considered here.

XXY Abnormality (Klinefelter's Syndrome)

This term has been used to describe the syndrome of male phenotype with small or atrophic male genital organs, mental retardation, and frequently gynecomastia and eunuchoid appearance with increased urinary excretion of gonadotropin (Klinefelter et al., 1942). Broader interpretations of the disorder, in keeping with advances in the cytogenetics. have been reviewed by Ferguson-Smith and associates (1960) and Harnden and Jacobs (1961).

Eighty percent of the subjects are chromatin-positive and have 47 chromosomes with mainly XXY constitution or variants involving more sex chromosomes or mosaicism. There are some differences between the dermatoglyphics of patients with Klinefelter's syndrome and normal males, such as small digital patterns with many arches and distal displacement of the axial triradius, but they are not distinct enough to be of diagnostic value (Preus and Fraser, 1972).

An earlier view that the incidence of congenital heart malformation was possibly not greater than that in the population at large (Polani, 1968) has given way to one that indicates that heart defects are probably four to five times more frequent (5/233 cases of XXY constitution) than the general incidence of heart malformation (Ferguson-Smith, 1966; Rosenthal, 1972). A wide variety of malformations has been reported, but tetralogy of Fallot may be one of the more common (Gautier and Nouaille, 1964; Gautier, 1966). Among others, Ebstein's anomaly of the tricuspid valve, atrial septal defect, ventricular septal defect, aortic stenosis, and arteriovenous fistula have been reported (Rao and Mooring, 1970; Rosenthal, 1972). Double-outlet right ventricle confirmed by autopsy has been diagnosed in the newborn (Edlow et al., 1969).

While individually the cardiac malformation can affect life expectancy in some patients, the larger clinical problem in Klinefelter's syndrome is infertility frequently accompanied by personality difficulties and mental deficiency.

XYY Abnormality

This sex chromosome complement, present in 1:700 males, is sometimes characterized by hypogonadism, webbing of the neck, vascular, bone, and joint abnormalities, varicose ulceration, and skin disorders although the majority of subjects appear normal physically. Their height is greater than normal but the risk for sociopathic behavior is questionable.

Heart malformation is not a feature. The observation that conduction abnormalities in the electrocardiogram (prolonged P-R interval; notching of R in V_1) were abnormally frequent (Price, 1968) has not been supported by others (Steiness and Nielsen, 1970; Char and Borgaonkar, 1971).

XXX Abnormality

The triple X subject, recurring once in every 1000 females, is usually physically normal and has normal gonads. A relatively high incidence of older XXX women in schizophrenic populations is not certainly related to congenital abnormality. Three patients with this constitution and atrial septal defect (two) or pulmonary atresia (one) were found among 500 infants with severe congenital heart malformation (Gautier, 1966).

XXXX Abnormality

Among 21 reported cases of this rare condition is one confirmed instance of multiple atrial septal defects in a patient dying at age 50 years (Keane et al., 1974). The incidence of congenital heart disease appears to be less than 10 percent.

X Monosomy (Turner's Syndrome)

The original report of this disorder described six women with short stature, absence of breast development, small amounts of pubic and axillary hair, webbing of the neck, and cubitus valgus (Turner, 1938). It is now known that in addition to a fairly extensive number of anatomic abnormalities and failure to achieve secondary sex characteristics at puberty, these phenotype females have raised urinary gonadotropin excretion and replacement of ovaries by streaks of connective tissue. Short stature is a uniform finding even at birth, while broad chest, congenital lymphedema or its sequelae, low posterior hairline, prominent ears, narrow high-arched palate, abnormal nails, and a small mandible were found in 80 percent of 25 patients studied by Lemli and Smith (1963) (Figure 50–16). Lymphedema of the feet occurs in about one-quarter of affected infants (Bishop et al., 1960). It is not surprising that this valuable clue to diagnosis is sometimes mistaken for evidence of congestive heart failure in those subjects with congenital heart disease.

Genetics. There has been considerable debate over which patients should be labeled as having Turner's syndrome and where, within a group of phenotypically similar patients, one withdraws from the classic definition and assigns another name to the disorder.

English workers have, for years, considered Turner's syndrome to be very strictly only those patients having the clinical features described by Turner himself, i.e., infantilism (short stature, absence of secondary sex characteristics after expected puberty) and webbing of the neck. Ninety-four percent of such subjects have the 45,X constitution and 6 percent are mosaic 45,X/46,XX (Polani, 1968).

A second group of patients with the same phenotype but without webbing of the neck have been labeled "ovarian dysgenesis." Half of these patients have 45,X, one-quarter are mosaic, and another quarter have structural chromosome anomalies, such as deletions or isochromosomes (Polani, 1969). Phenotypic variation in Turner's syndrome thus appears to be the result of sex chromosome mosaicism, deletion, or a combination of both (Ferguson-Smith, 1965, 1969). Detailed chromosomal analysis with chromosome banding could conceivably assist in clarifying matters even further.

Other patients with short or normal stature, with or without neck webbing and other somatic abnormalities, but with normal ovarian function and 46,XX constitution without mosaicism (Bishop et al., 1960; Polani, 1969) have been labeled Bonnevie-Ullrich syndrome (Ullrich, 1949). A group of males with a similar phenotype has been termed Turner syndrome in the male (if the patient had abnormal sexual development such as undescended testis) or Bonnevie-Ullrich syndrome in the male (if there was no sexual abnormality). Although attitudes toward

GENERAL

Low birth weight
Short stature
Sexual infantilism
Webbed neck
Normal intelligence

HEART

Congenital heart disease
(about 20 per cent)
Coarctation of the aorta
Aortic stenosis
Ventricular septal defect

EXTREMITIES

Short 4th metacarpal
Hypoplasia nails

OTHER

Cubitus valgus
Shield chest
Multiple pigmented nevi
Lymphedema

DERMATOGLYPHICS

Large whorls and loops
Otherwise non-specific

CHROMOSOMES

Variants of the X chromosome found in Turner's syndrome
(Partial fluorescence karyotypes)

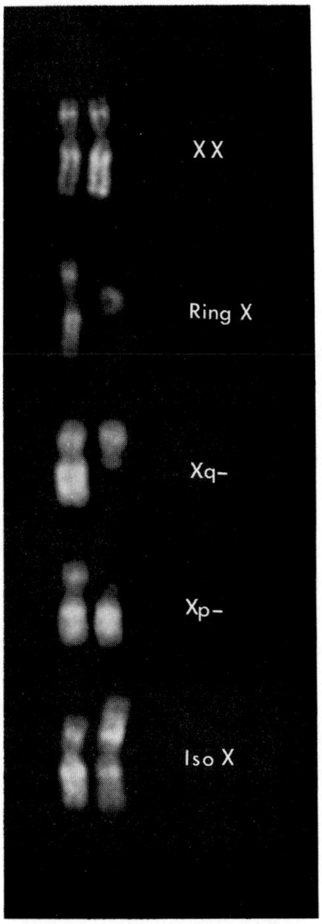

Figure 50-16. A composite of the major clinical features and the X chromosome variants in X monosomy.

the nosology of these disorders have varied within all medical communities, American investigators have recently preferred to make the separation of Turner's syndrome from Turner-simulating conditions by the karyotypic approach (McKusick, 1972) and have replaced the Bonnevie-Ullrich and the male Turner's syndromes for the moment with another inclusive eponym, the Noonan syndrome (Noonan and Ehmke, 1963; Char, 1971; Char et al., 1972; McKusick, 1972) (Figure 50–17). While the total digital ridge count is significantly higher than normal in classic and mosaic Turner's syndrome, in the Noonan syndrome ridge counts are normal.

Heart Disorder. Although cases of coarctation of the aorta were not mentioned by Turner, they were reported by other authors discussing ovarian insufficiency (Pich, 1937; Albright et al., 1942). Much later the frequent association of heart defect was emphasized (Haddard and Wilkins, 1959). In a review of 55 cases of Turner's syndrome these authors noted eight cases of adult-type coarctation of the aorta. In

two of these, subaortic stenosis was an additional feature. In a series of 24 patients Bishop and associates (1960) found seven with coarctation of the aorta. The latter authors did not find other types of heart malformation in their group, but the review of Haddard and Wilkins (1959) included examples of isolated subaortic stenosis, ventricular septal defect, and dextrocardia. We have encountered two autopsy-proved cases with aortic atresia (Conen and Glass, 1963). The confusion that subsequently developed over other types of cardiac malformation was mainly due to the inclusion of patients with what is now generally referred to as the Noonan syndrome (Rainier-Pope et al., 1964), an error to which most of us contributed. Of 46 patients with 45,X Turner's syndrome Polani (1968) found ten with congenital cardiac defect: nine with coarctation of the aorta and one with aortic stenosis. In a further 25 patients with 45,X karyotype but no neck webbing there were no instances of heart disease. Nora and associates (1970) examined the question by looking specifically at the

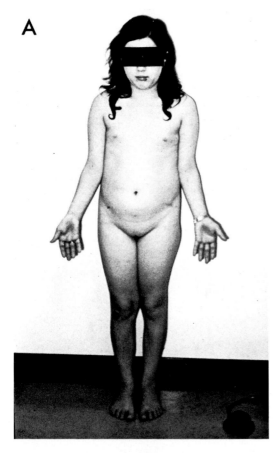

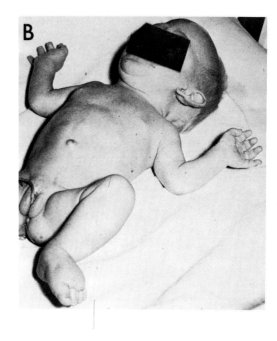

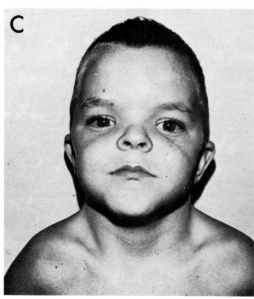

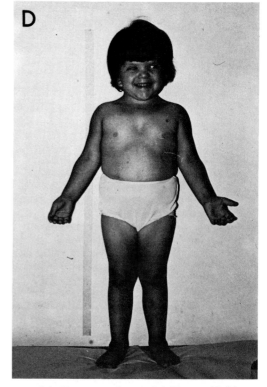

Figure 50-17. The appearance of children with X monosomy and the Noonan syndrome. *A.* A 15-year-old girl with X monosomy. *B.* A two-week-old infant with X monosomy and coarctation of the aorta. Neck webbing and lymphedema are present. *C.* A boy with Noonan syndrome and pulmonary arterial stenosis. *D.* A 5½-year-old XX girl with the Noonan syndrome.

precise type of heart malformation. They studied 40 patients with unequivocal "Turner" stigmata and heart disease all of whom had been examined not only by buccal smear and full chromosomal analysis but also by complete cardiac catheterization studies:

16 were 45,X and of these 11 had coarctation of the aorta.

4 were 45,X/46,XX mosaics and all had pulmonary stenosis.

16 were 46,XX; 14 of these had pulmonary stenosis and two had ventricular septal defect.

4 were 46,XY, 3 having pulmonary stenosis and 1 aortic stenosis.

There were thus two main groupings of the cardiovascular lesion. Coarctation of the aorta was present in 70 percent of patients with heart disease and 45,X constitution but not in mosaics or in the Noonan syndrome. Pulmonary stenosis with or without atrial septal defect was present in 90 percent of patients with the Noonan syndrome or with mosaic Turner's syndrome but never in the true 45,X Turner's syndrome (with heart disorder) (Nora et al., 1974).

The clinical consequence is that if a patient with apparent Turner phenotype is found to have pulmonary stenosis, one can confidently assume that the chromosomal arrangement will *not* be 45,X. On the other hand, if the patient has coarctation of the aorta, she cannot have pure 46,XX, and there is an extremely high probability that she will have 45,X constitution. Heart disease of any other variety, e.g., ventricular septal defect, isolated atrial septal defect, or aortic stenosis, present in such patients does not of itself permit prediction of the chromosomal constitution.

Systemic hypertension was noted in about one-quarter of the subjects studied by Haddard and Wilkins (1959). It was usually mild and apparently unrelated to frank renal disease or vascular anomaly. The high frequency of renal anomalies in Turner's syndrome—12 of 30 studied by Bishop and associates (1960)—suggests that the explanation for hypertension in an individual patient should be accepted as idiopathic with caution. The point is even further emphasized through observations that by 40 years of age the proportion with significant systemic hypertension has risen to 80 percent (Engel and Forbes, 1965). For these authors the high incidence of hypertension, diabetes mellitus, and "old-for-age" appearance in these subjects suggests that precocious aging may be a part of the syndrome.

REFERENCES

General

Alter, M., and Schulenberg, R.: Dermatoglyphics in congenital heart disease. *Circulation*, 41:49, 1970.

Anders, J. M.; Moores, E. C.; and Emanuel, R.: Chromosome studies in 156 patients with congenital heart disease. *Br. Heart J.*, 27:756, 1965.

Burguet, W., and Collard, P.: Dermatoglyphics in congenital heart-disease. *Lancet*, 2:106, 1968.

Chicago Conference: *Standardization in Human Genetics*. Birth Defects: Original Article Series II, 2. National Foundation, New York, 1966.

Dahl, G.: Chromosomal conditions in congenital heart disease. *Acta Paediatr. Scand.*, 59:65, 1970.

Emerit, I.; de Grouchy, J.; Vernant, P.; and Corone, P.; Chromosomal abnormalities and congenital heart disease. *Circulation*, 36:886, 1967.

German, J.; Ehlers, K. H.; and Engle, M. A.: Familial congenital heart disease. II. Chromosomal studies. *Circulation*, 34:517, 1966.

German, J.; Ehlers, K. H.; Crippa, L. P.; and Engle, M. A.: The chromosomes in congenital heart disease. Birth Defects: Original Article Series VIII, 5. National Foundation, New York, 1972, p. 285.

Hale, A. R.; Phillips, J. H.; and Burch, G. E.: Features of palmar dermatoglyphics in congenital heart disease. *JAMA*, 176:41, 1961.

Nora, J. J.: Multifactorial inheritance hypothesis for the etiology of congenital heart diseases. *Circulation*, 38:604, 1968.

Paris Conference (1971): *Standardization in Human Cytogenetics*. Birth Defects: Original Article Series VIII, 7. National Foundation, New York, 1972.

Patterson, D. F.; Pyle, R. L.; and Buchanan, J. W.: Hereditary cardiovascular malformations of the dog. Birth Defects: Original Article Series VIII, 5. National Foundation, New York, 1972, p. 160.

Polani, P. E.: Chromosomal abnormalities and congenital heart disease. *Guy's Hosp. Rep.*, 117:323, 1968.

Preus, M.; Fraser, F. C.; and Levy, E. P.: Dermatoglyphics in congenital heart malformations. *Hum. Hered.*, 20:388, 1970.

Reed, T.; Shields, L.; and Nance, W. E.: Dermatoglyphic heterogeneity in mongols with congenital heart disease. *Am. J. Hum. Genet.*, 25:109, 1973.

Rohde, R. A.: The chromosomes in heart disease. *Circulation*, 34:484, 1966.

Rowe, R. D., and Uchida, I. A.: Cardiac malformation in mongolism. A prospective study of 184 mongoloid children. *Am. J. Med.*, 31:726, 1961.

Sanchez Cascos, A.: Dermatoglyphs in congenital heart disease. *Acta Paediatr. Scand.*, 57:9, 1968.

Sasaki, M.; Makino, S.; and Kajii, T.: Chromosomal aberrations in congenital cardiovascular disorders in man. *Proc. Japan. Acad.*, 39:388, 1963.

Sergovich, R.; Valentine, G. H.; Chen, A. T. L.; Kinch, R. A. H.; and Smout, M. S.: Chromosome aberrations in 2159 consecutive newborn babies. *N. Engl. J. Med.*, 280:851, 1969.

Walzer, S.; Breau, G.; and Gerald, P. S.: A chromosome survey of 2,400 normal newborn infants. *J. Pediatr.*, 74:438, 1969.

Autosome Abnormalities

Trisomy 21: (Mongolism)

Abbot, M.: *Atlas of Congenital Cardiac Disease*. The American Heart Association, New York, 1936.

Abrams, H. L., and Kaplan, H. S.: *Angiocardiographic Interpretation in Congenital Heart Disease*. Charles C Thomas, Publisher, Springfield, Ill., 1956.

Alberman, E.; Polani, P. E.; Fraser Roberts, J. A.; Spicer, C. C.; Elliott, M.; and Armstrong, E.: Parental exposure to X-irradiation and Down's syndrome. *Ann. Hum. Genet., Lond.*, 36:195, 1972.

Allen, G., et al.: Mongolism. *Lancet*, 1:775, 1961.

Anson, B. J.: The aortic arch and its branches. In Luisada, A. A. (ed.): *Cardiology*. McGraw-Hill Book Co., New York, 1960, Vol. 1, p. 123.

Benda, C. E.: *Mongolism and Cretinism*. Grune & Stratton, Inc., New York, 1949.

Berg, J. M.; Crome, L.; and France, N. E.: Congenital cardiac malformation in mongolism. *Br. Heart J.*, 22:331, 1960.

Brousseau, K.: *Mongolism*. Williams & Wilkins Co., Baltimore, 1928.

Caffey, J., and Ross, S.: Mongolism (mongoloid deficiency) during early infancy—some newly recognized diagnostic changes in the pelvic bones. *Pediatrics*, 17:642, 1956.

Carter, C. D., and McCarthy, D.: Incidence of mongolism and its diagnosis in the newborn. *Br. J. Soc. Med.*, 5:83, 1951.

Carter, C. O.: A life-table for mongols. *J. Ment. Defic. Res.* 2:64, 1958.

Caspersson, T.; Gahrton, G.; Lindsten, J.; and Zech, L.: Identification of the Philadelphia chromosome as a number 22 by quinacrine mustard fluorescence analysis. *Exp. Cell Res.*, **63**:238, 1970a.

Caspersson, T.; Hultén, M.; Lindsten, J.; and Zech, L.: Distinction between extra G-like chromosomes by quinacrine mustard fluorescence analysis. *Exp. Cell Res.*, **63**:240, 1970b.

Chi, T. L., and Krovetz, L. J. The pulmonary vascular bed in children with Down syndrome. *J. Pediatr.*, **86**:533, 1975.

Clarke, C.; Edwards, J. H.; and Smallpiece, V.: 21-Trisomy/normal mosaicism. *Lancet*, **1**:1028, 1961.

Collman, R. D., and Stoller, A.: A survey of mongolism and congenital anomalies of the central nervous system in Victoria. *N.Z. Med. J.*, **61**:24, 1962.

Collman, R. D., and Stoller, A.: Data on mongolism in Victoria, Australia. Prevalence and life expectation. *J. Ment. Defic. Res.*, **7**:60, 1963.

Cullum, L., and Liebman, J.: The association of congenital heart disease with Down's syndrome (mongolism). *Am. J. Cardiol.*, **24**:354, 1969.

Cummins, H.; Talley, G.; and Platou, R. V.: Palmar dermato-glyphics in mongolism. *Pediatrics*, **5**:241, 1950.

Down, J. L.: Observations on an ethnic classification of idiots. *Clin. Lect. Rep. Lond. Hosp.*, **3**:259, 1866.

Evans, P. R.: Cardiac anomalies in mongolism. *Br. Heart J.*, **12**:258, 1950.

Fabia, J., and Drolette, M.: Life tables up to age 10 for mongols with and without congenital heart disease. *J. Ment. Defic. Res.*, **14**:235, 1970.

Forssman, H., and Akesson, H. O.: Mortality in patients with Down's syndrome. *J. Ment. Defic. Res.*, **9**:146, 1965.

Gardner, R. J. M.; Veale, A. M. O.; Parslow, M. I.; Becroft, D. M. O.; Shaw, R. L.; Fitzgerald, P. H.; Hutchings, H. E.; McCreanor, H. R.; Wong, J.; Eiby, J. R.; Howart, D. A.; and Shyte, S. E.: A survey of 972 cytogenetically examined cases of Down syndrome. *N.Z. Med. J.*, **78**:403, 1973.

Garrod, A. E.: On the association of cardiac malformations with other congenital defects. *St. Bart. Hosp. Rep.*, **30**:53, 1894.

———: Cases illustrating the association of congenital heart disease with the 'mongolian' form of idiocy. *Trans. Clin. Soc. Lond.*, **32**:6, 1899.

Gerstmann, P. E.; Baum, D.; and Guntheroth, W. G.: Prevalence of cardiovascular disease in the retarded. *JAMA*, **219**:1171, 1972.

Gustafson, J. M.: Mongolism, parental desires, and the right to life. *Perspect. Biol. Med.*, **16**:529, 1973.

Hambach, R., and Prispevek, K.: Otazce kombinace vrozenych srdecnich vad s mongolismem. *Cas. Lek. Cesk.*, **95**:317, 1956.

Hamerton, J. L.: Robertsonian translocations in man: evidence for prezygotic selection. *Cytogenetics*, **7**:260, 1968.

Holt, S. B.: Quantitative genetics of finger-print patterns. *Br. Med. Bull.*, **17**:247, 1961.

Kaufmann, H. J., and Taillard, W. F.: Pelvic abnormalities in mongols. *Br. Med. J.*, **1**:948, 1961.

Kohn, G.; Taysi, K.; Atkins, T. C.; and Mellman, W. J.: Mosaic mongolism. I. Clinical correlations. *J. Pediatr.*, **76**:874, 1970.

Kuroki, Y.; Yamamoto, Y.; Matsui, I.; and Kurita, T.: Down syndrome and maternal age in Japan, 1950–1973. *Clin. Genet.*, **12**:43, 1977.

Lejeune, J.; Turpin, R.; and Gautier, M.: Les chromosomes humaines en culture de tissues. *C.R. Acad. Sci. (Paris)*, **248**:602, 1959.

Lennox, B.: Down's syndrome (mongolism). *Lancet*, **2**:1093, 1961.

Lev, M.; Agustsson, M. H.; and Arcilla, R.: The pathologic anatomy of common atrioventricular orifice associated with tetralogy of Fallot. *Am. J. Clin. Pathol.*, **36**:408, 1961.

Lev, M., and Kaveggia, E.: Etiology and pathogenesis of congenital cardiac disease. In Luisada, A. A. (ed.): *Cardiology*. McGraw-Hill Book Co., New York, 1960, Vol. 3.

Licznerski, G., and Lindsten, J.: Trisomy 21 in man due to maternal non-disjunction during the first meiotic division. *Hereditas*, **70**:153, 1972.

Liu, M. C., and Corlett, K.: A study of congenital heart defects in mongolism. *Arch. Dis. Child.*, **34**:410, 1959.

Lowry, R. B.; Jones, D. C.; Renwick, D. H. G.; and Trimble, B. K.: Down syndrome in British Columbia. 1952–1973: Incidence and mean maternal age. *Teratology*, **14**:29, 1976.

Lunn, J. E.: A survey of mongol children in Glasgow. *Scot. Med. J.*, **4**:368, 1959.

Medenis, R.; Forbes, A.; and Rosenthal, I. M.: Mosaicism associated with mongolism. *Proc. Soc. Pediatr. Res.*, p. 75, 1962.

Nadas, A. S.: *Pediatric Cardiology*. W. B. Saunders Co., Philadelphia, 1957, p. 268.

Nichols, W. W.; Coriell, L. L.; Fabrigio, D. P.; Bishop, H. C.; and Boggo, T. R., Jr.; Mongolism with mosaic chromosome pattern. *J. Pediatr.*, **60**:69, 1962.

Øster, J.: *Mongolism*. Danish Science Press, Copenhagen, 1953.

Paris conference: Standardization in human cytogenetics. Birth Defects: Original Article Series VIII, 7, 1972. National Foundation, New York, 1971.

Park, S. C.; Mathews, R. A.; Zuberbuhler, J. R.; Rowe, R. D.; Neches, W. H.; and Lennox, C. C.: Down syndrome with congenital heart malformation. *Am. J. Dis. Child.*, **131**:29, 1977.

Penrose, L. S.: On the interaction of heredity and environment in the study of human genetics with special reference to mongolism imbecility. *J. Genet.*, **25**:407, 1932.

Penrose, L. S., and Smith, G. F.: *Down's Anomaly*. Little, Brown and Co., Boston, 1966.

Penrose, L. S.: Mongolism. *Br. Med. Bull.*, **17**:184, 1961.

———: Paternal age in mongolism. *Lancet*, **1**:1101, 1962.

Polani, P. E.: Cytogenetics of Down's syndrome (mongolism). *Pediatr. Clin. North Am.*, **10**:423, 1963.

Polani, P. E.: Chromosomal abnormalities and congenital heart disease. *Guy's Hosp. Rep.*, **117**:323, 1968.

Potter, E. L.: *Pathology of the Fetus and Infant*, 2nd ed. Year Book, Publishers Inc., Chicago, 1961, p. 262.

Reed, T. E.; Borgaonkar, D. S.; Conneally, P. M.; Yu, P.-L.; Nance, W. E.; and Christian, J. C.: Dermatoglyphic nomogram for the diagnosis of Down's syndrome. *J. Pediatr.*, **77**:1024, 1970.

Robinson, A., and Puck, T. T.: The epidemiology of non-disjunction. *Proc. Am. Pediatr. Soc.*, p. 18, 1966.

Robinson, J. A.: Origin of extra chromosome in trisomy 21. *Lancet*, **1**:131, 1973.

Rosenquist, G. C.; Sweeney, L. J.; Amsel, J.; and McAllister, H. A.: Enlargement of the membranous ventricular septum: an internal stigma of Down's syndrome. *J. Pediatrics*, **85**:4890, 1974.

Rowe, R. D., and James, L. S.: The normal pulmonary arterial pressure during the first year of life. *J. Pediatr.*, **51**:1, 1957.

Rowe, R. D., and Uchida, I. A.: Cardiac malformation in mongolism. A prospective study of 184 mongoloid children. *Am. J. Med.*, **31**:726, 1961.

Rowley, J. D.: A new consistent chromosomal abnormality in chronic myelogenous leukemia identified by quinacrine fluore-scence and Giemsa staining. *Nature (London)*, **243**:290, 1973.

Rundle, A.; Coppen, A.; and Cowie, V.: Steroid excretion in mothers of mongols. *Lancet*, **2**:846, 1961.

Sasaki, M., and Hara, Y.: Paternal origin of the extra chromosome in Down's syndrome. *Lancet*, **2**:1257, 1973.

Shaher, R. M.; Farina, M. A.; Porter, I. H.; and Bishop, M.: Clinical aspects of congenital heart disease in mongolism. *Am. J. Cardiol.*, **29**:497, 1972.

Shaw, A.: A 47th chromosome. The life and death decision for mongoloid baby with fatal defect. *Globe and Mail*, Toronto 3, Feb., 1972, p. W5.

Sigler, A. T.; Lilienfeld, A. M.; Cohen, B. H.; and Westlake, J. E.: Radiation exposure in parents of children with mongolism. *Bull. Hopkins Hosp.*, **117**:374, 1965.

Smith, D. W.: Therman, E.; Patau, K.; and Inhorn, S. L.: Mosaicism in mother of two mongoloids. *Proc. Soc. Pediatr. Res.*, p. 20, 1962.

Smith, G. F., and Berg, J. M.: *Down's Anomaly*. 2nd ed. Churchill Livingstone, Edinburgh, 1976.

Strauss, L.: Congenital cardiac anomalies associated with mongolism. *Trans. Am. Coll. Cardiol.*, **2**:214, 1953.

Tandon, R., and Edwards, J. E.: Cardiac malformations associated with Down's syndrome. *Circulation*, **47**:1349, 1973.

Thomson, J.: On the diagnosis and prognosis of certain forms of imbecility in infancy. *Scot. Med. Surg. J.*, **2**:203, 1898.

Uchida, I. A., and Curtis, E. J. A possible association between maternal radiation and mongolism. *Lancet*, **2**:848, 1961.

Uchida, I. A.; Holunga, R.; and Lawler, C.: Maternal radiation and chromosomal aberrations. *Lancet*, **2**:1045, 1968.

Uchida, I. A.: Epidemiology of mongolism: The Manitoba study. *Ann. N.Y. Acad. Sci.*, **171**:361, 1970.

Uchida, I. A.: Paternal origin of the extra chromosome in Down's syndrome. *Lancet*, **2**:1258, 1973.

Veeder, B. S.: A pediatric ethical question. *J. Pediatr.*, **58**:604, 1961.

Walker, N. F.: The use of dermal configurations in the diagnosis of mongolism. *J. Pediatr.*, **50**:19, 1957.

Wolstenholme, G. E. W., and Porter, R. (eds.): *Mongolism.* Ciba Foundation Study Group No. 25, London, 1967.

Trisomy 18: (Edwards' Syndrome)

Beratis, N. G.; Kardon, N. B.; Hsu, L. Y. F.; Grossman, D.; and Hirschhorn, K. Parental mosaicism in trisomy 18, *Pediatrics*, **50**:908, 1972.

Chesler, E.; Freiman, I.; Rosen, E.; and Wilton, E.: Congenital aneurysm of the membranous septum associated with partial trisomy E syndrome. *Am. Heart J.*, **79**:805, 1970.

Conen, P. E., and Erkman, B.: Frequency and occurrence of chromosomal syndromes II. E-trisomy. *Am. J. Hum. Genet.*, **18**:387, 1966.

Edwards, J. H.; Harden, D. G.; Cameron, A. H.; Crosse, V. M.; and Wolff, O. H.: A new trisomic syndrome. *Lancet*, **1**:787, 1960.

German, J. L., III; Rankin, J. K.; Harrison, P. A.; Donovan, D. J.; Hogan, W. J.; and Bearn, A. G.: Autosomal trisomy of a group 16–18 chromosome. *J. Pediatr.*, **60**:503, 1962.

Holman, G. H.; Erkman, B.; Zacharias, D. L.; and Koch, H. F.: The 18-trisomy syndrome—two new clinical variants. One with associated tracheoesophageal fistula and the other with probable familial occurrence. *N. Engl. J. Med.*, **268**:982, 1963.

Hsu, L. Y. F.; Strauss, L.; Dubin, E.; and Hirschhorn, K.: Prenatal diagnosis of trisomy 18. Pathologic findings in a 20-week conceptus. *Am. J. Dis. Child.*, **125**:290, 1973.

Kurien, V. A., and Duke, M.: Trisomy 17-18 syndrome. Report of a case with diffuse myocardial fibrosis and review of cardiovascular abnormalities. *Am. J. Cardiol.*, **21**:431, 1968.

Lewis, A. J.: The pathology of trisomy 18. *J. Pediatr.*, **65**:92, 1964.

Preus, M., and Fraser, F. C.: Dermatoglyphics and syndromes. *Am. J. Dis. Child.*, **124**:933, 1972.

Rogers, T. R.; Hagstrom, J. W. C.; and Engle, M. A.: Origin of both great vessels from the right ventricle associated with the trisomy-18 syndrome. *Circulation*, **32**:802, 1965.

Rohde, R. A.; Hodgman, J. E.; and Cleland, R. S.: Multiple congenital anomalies in the E₁-trisomy (group 16–18) syndrome. *Pediatrics*, **33**:258, 1964.

Scarpa, F. J., and Borgaonkar, D. S.: A-V communis defect in trisomy E₁ (17–18): report of a case. *Bull. Hopkins Hosp.*, **118**:395, 1966.

Smith, D. W.; Patau, K.; Therdman, E.; and Inhorn, S. L.: A new autosomal trisomy syndrome: multiple congenital anomalies caused by an extra chromosome. *J. Pediatr.*, **57**:338, 1960.

———: The no. 18 trisomy syndrome. *J. Pediatr.*, **60**:513, 1962.

Surana, R. B.; Bain, H. W.; and Conen, P. E.: 18-Trisomy in a 15 year old girl. *Am. J. Dis. Child.*, **123**:75, 1972.

Taylor, A. I.: Patau's, Edwards' and Cri du chat syndromes: a tabulated summary of current findings. *Develop. Med. Child. Neurol.*, **9**:78, 1967.

Taylor, A. I.: Autosomal trisomy syndromes: A detailed study of 27 cases of Edwards' syndrome and 27 cases of Patau's syndrome. *J. Med. Genet.*, **5**:227, 1968.

Townes, P. L.; Kreutner, K. A.; Kreutner, A.; and Manning, J.: Observations on the pathology of the trisomy 17–18 syndrome. *J. Pediatr.*, **62**:703, 1963.

Uchida, I. A.; Bowman, J. M.; and Wang, H. C.: The 18-trisomy syndrome. *N. Engl. J. Med.*, **26**:1198, 1962a.

Uchida, I. A.; Lewis, A. J.; Bowman, J. A.; and Wang, H. C.: A case of double trisomy: trisomy no. 18 and tripolo-X. *J. Pediatr.*, **60**:498, 1962.

Uchida, I. A.; Patau, K.; and Smith, D. W.: Dermal patterns of 18 and D₁ trisomics. *Am. J. Hum. Genet.*, **14**:345, 1962c.

Warkany, J.; Passarge, E.; and Smith, L. B.: Congenital malformations in autosomal trisomy syndromes. *Am. J. Dis. Child.*, **112**:502, 1966.

Weiss, L.; Di George, A. M.; and Baird, H. W.: 111.: Four infants with the trisomy 18 syndrome and one with trisomy mosaicism. *Proc. Soc. Pediatr. Res.*, p. 20, 1962.

Trisomy 13 (Patau's Syndrome)

Atkins, L., and Rosenthal, M. K.: Multiple congenital anomalies

associated with chromosomal trisomy. *N. Engl. J. Med.*, **265**:314, 1961.

Conen, P. E.; Erkman, B.; and Metaxotou, C.: The "D" syndrome. *Am. J. Dis. Child.*, **111**:236, 1966.

Conen, P. E., and Erkman, B.: Frequency and occurrence of chromosomal syndromes I. D-trisomy. *Am. J. Hum. Genet.*, **18**:374, 1966.

Ellis, J. R., and Marwood, J. C.: Autosomal trisomy syndromes. *Lancet*, **2**:263, 1961.

Erkman, B.; Basrur, V. R.; and Conen, P. E.: D/D translocation "D" syndrome. *J. Pediatr.*, **67**:270, 1965.

Goodman, R. M., and Kaufman, B. N.: A 13–15 trisomy with clinical features of the 16–18 trisomy. *Proc. Soc. Pediatr. Res.*, p. 73, 1962.

Green, J. R., Jr.; Krovetz, L. J.; and Taylor, W. J.: Two generations of 13–15 chromosomal mosaicism: Possible evidence for a genetic defect in the control of chromosomal replications. *Cytogenetics*, **7**:286, 1968.

Lubs, H. A., Jr.; Koenig, E. U.; and Brandt, I. K.: Trisomy 13–15: a clinical syndrome. *Lancet*, **2**:1001, 1961.

Murphy, J. W.; Sing, S.; and Reisnan, L. E.: Ebstein's anomaly in an infant with D. Trisomy. *J. Kentucky Med. Assoc.*, **65165**:585, 1967.

Northcutt, R. C.: Multiple congenital anomalies in a negro infant with 13–15 trisomy. *South Med. J.*, **55**:385, 1962.

Nusbacher, J., and Hirschhorn, K.: Autosomal anomalies in man. *Adv. Tetratology*, **3**:1–63, 1968.

Patau, K.; Smith, D. W.; Therman, E. Z.; Inhorn, S. L.; and Wagner, H. P.: Multiple congenital anomaly caused by an extra chromosome. *Lancet*, **1**:790, 1960.

Polani, P. E.: Autosomal imbalance and its syndromes, excluding Down's. *Br. Med. Bull.*, **25**:81, 1969.

Preus, M., and Fraser, F. C.: Dermatoglyphics and syndromes. *Am. J. Dis. Child.*, **124**:933, 1972.

Rohde, R. A.; Bowles, A.; and Hodgman, J.: Mimicry in the chromosomal syndromes: two cases of the E syndrome. *Human Chromosome Newsletter*, **15**:18, 1965.

Smith, D. W.; Patau, K.; Therman, E.; Inhorn, S. L.; and DeMars, R. I.: The D₁ trisomy syndrome. *J. Pediatr.*, **62**:326, 1963.

Taylor, M. B.; Juberg, R. C.; Jones, B.; and Johnson, W. A.: Chromosomal variability in the D, trisomy syndrome. Three cases and review of the literature. *Am. J. Dis. Child.*, **120**:374, 1970.

Townes, P. L.; Dettart, G. K., Jr.; Hect, F.; and Manning, J. A.: Trisomy 13–15 in a male infant. *J. Pediatr.*, **60**:528, 1962.

Uchida, I. A.; Patau, K.; and Smith, D. W.: Dermal patterns of 18 and D₁ trisomics. *Am. J. Hum. Genet.*, **14**:345, 1962.

Warkany, J.; Passarge, E.; and Smith, L. B.: Congenital malformations in autosomal trisomy syndromes. *Am. J. Dis. Child.*, **112**:502, 1966.

Trisomy 22

Crawfurd, M. d'A.: Multiple congenital anomaly associated with an extra autosome. *Lancet*, **2**:22, 1961.

Gustavson, K.-H.; Hagberg, B.; Finley, S. C.; and Finley, W. H.: An apparently identical extra autosome in two severely retarded sisters with multiple malformations. *Cytogenetics*, **1**:32, 1962.

Hsu, L. Y. F.; Shapiro, L. R.; Gertner, M.; Lieber, E.; and Hirschhorn, K.: Trisomy 22: A clinical entity. *J. Pediatr.*, **79**:12, 1971.

Uchida, I. A.; Ray, M.; McRae, K. N.; and Besant, D. F.: Familial occurrence of trisomy 22. *Am. J. Hum. Genet.*, **20**:107, 1968.

Other Trisomies

Böök, J. A.; Santesson, B.; and Zetterqvist, P.: Association between congenital heart malformation and chromosomal variations. *Acta Paediatr.*, **50**:217, 1961.

Freedom, R. M., and Gerald, P. S.: Congenital cardiac disease and the "cat eye" syndrome. *Am. J. Dis. Child.*, **126**:16, 1973.

Deletion Syndromes

5p−

Breg, W. R.; Steel, M. W.; Miller, O. J.; Warburton, D.; de Capoa, A.; and Alderdice, P. W.: The cri du chat syndrome in adolescents and adults. Clinical findings in 13 older patients with partial deletion of the short arm of chromosome no. 5 (tp-). *J. Pediatr.*, **77**:782, 1970.

Lejeune, J.; Lafourcade, J.; Berger, R.; Vialatte, J.; Boeswillwald, M.; Seringe, P.; and Turpin, R.: Trois cas de deletion partieppe du bras court d'un chromosome 5. *Compt. Rend. Acad. Sci. (Paris)*, **257**:3098, 1963.

Polani, P. E.: Chromosomal abnormalities and congenital heart disease. *Guy's Hosp. Rep.*, **117**:323, 1968.

Taylor, A. J.: Patau's, Edwards' and cri du chat syndrome: A tabulated summary of current findings. *Develop Med. Child. Neurol.*, **9**:78, 1967.

4p −

Arias, D.; Passarge, E.; Engle, M. A.; and German, J.: Human chromosomal deletion: Two patients with the 4p- syndrome. *J. Pediatr.*, **76**:82, 1970.

Guthrie, R. D.; Aase, J. M.; Asper, A. C.; and Suritt, D. W.: The 4p-syndrome. A clinically recognizeable chromosomal deletion syndrome. *Am. J. Dis. Child.*, **122**:421, 1971.

Miller, O. J.; Breg, W. R.; Warburton, D.; Miller, D. A.; de Capoa, A.; Allerdice, P. W.; Davis, J.; Klinger, H. P.; McGilvray, E.; and Allen, F. H., Jr.; Clinical studies in five unrelated cases. *J. Pediatr.*, **77**:792, 1970.

Passarge, E.; Altrogge, H. C.; and Rudiger, R. A.: Human chromosomal deficiency: The 4p- syndrome. *Humangenetik.*, **10**:51, 1970.

Polani, P. E.: Chromosomal abnormalities and congenital heart disease. *Guy's Hosp. Rep.*, **117**:323, 1968.

Taylor, A. I.; Challacombe, D. N.; and Howlett, R. M.: Short-arm deletion, chromosome 4, (4p −), a syndrome? *Ann. Hum. Genet.*, **34**:137, 1970.

Wolf, U.; Porsch, R.; Baitsch, H.; and Reinwein, H.: Deletion of short arms of B-chromosome without "cri du chat" syndrome. *Lancet*, **1**:769, 1965.

18q −

Borkowf, S. P.; Wadia, R. P.; Borgaonkar, D. S.; and Bias, W. B.: Partial deletion of the long arm of a chromosome 18. Birth Defects: Original Article Series V, 5. National Foundation, New York, 1969, p. 155.

Curran, J. P.; Al-Salihi, F. L.; and Allderdice, P. W.: Partial deletion of the long of chromosome E-18. *Pediatrics*, **46**:721, 1970.

de Grouchy, J.; Royer, P.; Salmon, C.; and Lang, M.: Deletion partielle des bras longs du chromosome 18. *Pathol. Biol.*, **12**:579, 1964.

Kushnick, T., and Matsushita, G.: Partial deletions of long arms of chromosome 18. *Pediatrics*, **42**:194, 1968.

Lejeune, J.; Berger, R.; Lafourcade, J.; and Rethore, M.: La deletion partielle du bras long du chromosome 18. Individualisation d'un novel etat morbide. *Ann. Genet.*, **9**:32, 1966.

Wertelecki, W., and Gerald, P. S.: Clinical and chromosomal studies of 18—syndrome. *J. Pediatr.*, **78**:44, 1971.

18p −

Char, F.; Rodriguez-Fernandez, H. L.; Scott, C. I., Jr.; Borgaonkar, D. S.; Bell, B. B.; and Rowe, R. D.: The Noonan syndrome—a clinical study of forty-five cases. Birth Defects: Original Article Series VIII, 5. National Foundation, New York, 1972, p. 110.

Uchida, I. A.; McRae, K. N.; Wang, H. C.; and Ray, M.: Familial short arm deficiency of chromosome 18 concomitant with arhinencephaly and alopecia congenita. *Am. J. Hum. Genet.*, **17**:410, 1965.

18r

Gropp, A.; Jussen, A.; and Offeringer, K.: Multiple congenital anomalies associated with a partially mug-shaped chromosome probably derived from chromosome no. 18 in man. *Nature (Lond.)*, **202**:829, 1964.

Palmer, C. G.; Fareed, N.; and Merritt, A. D.: Ring chromosome 18 in a patient with multiple anomalies. *J. Med. Genet.*, **4**:117, 1967.

Wald, S.; Engel, E.; Nance, W. E.; Davies, J.; Puyau, F. A.; and Sinclair-Smith, B. C.: E ring chromosome with persistent left superior vena cava and hypertrophic subaortic stenosis. *J. Med. Genet.*, **6**:328, 1969.

13q −

Adams, M. S.: Palm prints and a ring-D chromosome. *Lancet*, **2**:494, 1965.

Bain, A. D., and Gauld, I. K.: Multiple congenital abnormalities associated with ring chromosome. *Lancet*, **2**:304, 1963.

Laurent, C.; Cotton, J. B.; Nivelon, A.; and Freycon, M.: Deletion partielle du bras long d'un chromosome du groupe D (13–15): Dq-. *Ann. Genet.*, **10**:25, 1967.

Opitz, J. M.; Slungaard, R.; Edwards, R. H.; Inhorn, S. L.; Muller, J.; and de Venecia, G.: Report of a patient with a presumed dq-syndrome. Birth Defects: Original Article Series V, 5. National Foundation, New York, 1969, p. 93.

Sparkes, R. S.; Carrel, R. E.; and Wright, S. W.: Absent thumbs with a ring D2 chromosome: a new deletion syndrome. *Am. J. Hum. Genet*, **19**:644, 1967.

G-Deletion Syndromes

Crandall; B. F., Weber, F.; Muller, H. M.; and Burwell, J. K.: Identification of 21r and 22r chromosomes by quinacrine fluorescence. *Clin. Genet.*, **3**:264, 1972.

Lejeune, J.; Berger, R.; Rethore, M. O.; Archambault, L.; Jerome, H.; Thieffry, S.; Aicardi, J.; Brayer, M.; Lafourcade, J.; Cruveiller, J.; and Turpin, R.: Monosomie partielle pour un petit acrocentrique. *C.R. Acad. Sci. (D) (Paris)*, **259**:4187, 1964.

Reisman, L. E.; Kasahara, S.; Chung, C.-Y.; Darnell, A.; and Hall, B.; Antimongolism. Studies in an infant with partial monosomy of the 21 chromosome. *Lancet*, **1**:394, 1966.

Schindeler, J., and Warren, R. J.: Dermatoglyphics in the G deletion syndromes. *J. Ment. Defic. Res.*, **17**:149, 1973.

Warren, R. J., and Rimoin, D. L.: The G-deletion syndromes. *J. Pediatr.*, **77**:658, 1970.

Warren, R. J.; Rimoin, D. L.; and Summitt, R. L.: Identification by fluorescent microscopy of the abnormal chromosomes associated with G-deletion syndromes. *Am. J. Hum. Genet.*, **25**:77, 1973.

Sex Chromosome Abnormalities

XXY (Klinefelter's Syndrome)

Edlow, J. B.; Shapiro, L. R.; Hsu, L. Y. F.; and Hirschhorn, K.: Neonatal Klinefelter's syndrome. *Am. J. Dis. Child.*, **118**:788, 1969.

Ferguson-Smith, M. A.; Lennox, B.; Stewart, J. S. S.; and Mack, W. S.: Klinefelter's syndrome. *Mem. Soc. Endocr.*, **7**:173, 1960.

Ferguson-Smith, M. A.: In Moore, K. L. (ed.): *The Sex Chromatin.* W. B. Saunders Co., Philadelphia, 1966, p. 277.

Gautier, M.: Chromosomes in congenital heart disease. *Lancet*, **2**:641, 1966.

Gautier, M., and Nouaille, J.: Deux cas de syndrome de Klinefelter's associé a une tetralogie de Fallot (étude systematique du corpuscule de Barr chez 210 nourrissons atteints de cardiopathies congenitales). *Arch. Fr. Pediatr.*, **21**:761, 1964.

Harden, D. G., and Jacobs, P. A.: Cytogenetics of abnormal sexual development in man. *Br. Med. Bull.*, **17**:206, 1961.

Klinefelter, H. F., Jr.: Reifenstein, E. C., Jr.; and Albright, F.: Syndrome characterized by gynecomastia, aspermatogenesis without A-leydigism, and increased excretion of follicle-stimulating hormone. *J. Clin. Endocrinol.*, **3**:615, 1942.

Polani, P. E.: Chromosomal abnormalities and congenital heart disease. *Guy's Hosp. Rep.*, **117**:323, 1968.

Preus, M., and Fraser, F. C.: Dermatoglyphics and syndromes. *Am. J. Dis. Child.*, **124**:933, 1972.

Rao, V. S., and Mooring, P.: Ebstein's anomaly in XXY syndrome Klinefelter. *Am. J. Dis. Child.*, **120**:164, 1970.

Rosenthal, A.: Cardiovascular malformations in Klinefelter's syndrome: Report of three cases. *J. Pediatr.*, **80**:471, 1972.

XYY

Char, F., and Borgaonkar, D. S.: Electrocardiogram in males with 47,XXY karyotype. *Lancet*, **1**:1242, 1971.

Price, W. H.: The electrocardiogram in males with an extra Y chromosome. *Lancet*, **1**:1106, 1968.

Steiness, E., and Nielson, J.: The electrocardiogram in males with the 47,XYY karyotype. *Lancet*. **1**:140, 1970.

XXX

Gautier, M.: Chromosomes in congenital heart disease. *Lancet*, **2**:641, 1966.

XXXX

Keane, J. F.; McLennan, J. E.; Chi, Je G.; Monedjikova, V.; Vawter,

G. F.; Hilles, F. H.; and Van Praagh, R.: Congenital heart disease in a tetra-X woman. *Chest*, **66**:726, 1974.

X Monosomy (Turner's Syndrome)

Albright, F.; Smith, P. H.; and Fraser, R.: A syndrome characterized by primary ovarian insufficiency and decreased stature. *Am. J. Med. Sci.*, **204**:625, 1942.

Bishop, P. M. F.; Lessof, M. H.; and Pollani, P. E.: Turner's syndrome and allied conditions. *Mem. Soc. Endocrinol.*, **7**:162, 1960.

Char, F.: "Turner phenotypes" vs Noonan's syndrome. *JAMA*, **216**:679, 1971.

Char, F.; Rodriguez-Fernandez, H. L.; Scott, C. I., Jr.; Borgaonkar, D. S.; Bell, B. B.; and Rowe, R. D.: The Noonan syndrome—a clinical study of forty-five cases. Birth Defects. Original Article Series VIII, 5. National Foundation, New York, 1972, p. 110.

Conen, P. E., and Glass, I. H., 45/XO Turner's syndrome in the newborn: report of two cases. *J. Clin. Endocrinol.*, **23**:1, 1963.

Engel, E., and Forbes, A. P.: Cytogenetic and clinical findings in 48 patients with congenitally defective or absent ovaries. *Medicine*, **44**:135, 1965.

Ferguson-Smith, M. A.: Karyotype-phenotype correlations in gonadal dysgenesis and their bearing on the pathogenesis of malformations. *J. Med. Genet.*, **2**:142, 1965.

Ferguson-Smith, M. A.: Phenotypic aspects of sex chromosome aberrations. Birth Defects: Original Article Series V, 5. National Foundation, New York, 1969, p. 3.

Haddard, H. M., and Wilkins, L.: Congenital anomalies associated with gonadal dysplasia. Review of 55 cases. *Pediatrics*, **23**:885, 1959.

Lemli, L., and Smith, D. W.: The XO syndrome: A study of the differentiated phenotype in 25 patients. *J. Pediatr.*, **63**:577, 1963.

McKusick, V. A.: Clinical delineation in hereditary and congenital disorders of the cardiovascular system. Birth Defects: Original Article Series VIII, 5. National Foundation, New York, 1972, p. 2.

Noonan, J. A., and Ehmke, D. A.: Associate noncardiac malformations in children with congenital heart disease. *J. Pediatr.*, **63**:468, 1963.

Nora, J. J.; Torres, F. G.; Sinha, A. K.; and McNamara, D. G.: Characteristic cardiovascular anomalies of XO Turner syndrome, XX and XY phenotype and XO/XX Turner mosaic. *Am. J. Cardiol.*, **25**:639, 1970.

Nora, J. J.; Nora, A. H.; Sinha, A. K.; Spangler, R. D.; and Lubs, H. A.: The Ullrich–Noonan syndrome (Turner phenotype). *Am. J. Dis. Child.*, **127**:48, 1974.

Pich, G.: Uber den angeborenen, eierstockmangel. *Beitr. Pathol. Anat.*, **98**:218, 1937.

Polani, P. E.: Chromosomal abnormalities and congenital heart disease. *Guy's Hosp. Rep.*, **117**:323, 1968.

Polani, P. E.: Autosomal imbalance and its syndromes, excluding Down's. *Br. Med. Bull.*, **25**:81, 1969.

Rainier-Pope, C. R.; Cunningham, R. D.; Nadas, A. S.; and Crigler, J. F., Jr.: Cardiovascular malformations in Turner's syndrome. *Pediatrics*, **33**:919, 1964.

Turner, H. H.: Syndrome of infantilism, congenital webbed neck and cubitus valgus. *Endocrinology*, **25**:566, 1938.

Ullrich, O.: Turner's syndrome and Stalus Bonnevie-Ullrich; a synthesis of animal phenogenetics and chemical observations on a typical complex of developmental anomalies. *Am. J. Hum. Genet.*, **1**:179, 1949.

51

Myocarditis

John D. Keith

INFECTIVE MYOCARDITIS

YOCARDITIS in the pediatric age group related in the past chiefly to rheumatic fever. Gradually other forms have attracted increasing attention. The problem was brought to the fore in an excellent pathologic study by Saphir and coworkers in 1944. The investigations of Williams and coworkers (1953), of Rosenbaum and coworkers (1953), and of Kreutzer and coworkers (1959) have indicated the clinical importance of certain forms of myocarditis and reemphasized the value of digitalis therapy. Important review articles on the subject have been published by Rosenberg and McNamara (1964), Harris and Nghiem (1972), and Wenger (1972).

In infancy and childhood the cases of myocarditis can be readily divided into two main groups: (1) those with myocarditis secondary to a specific infection and (2) those with myocarditis of unknown etiology. Among those with myocarditis due to a specific infection, the largest number over the years has had rheumatic fever. This is a special problem and will not be dealt with here. The object of this study is to analyze the findings in the other groups of myocarditis referred to above with a view to discussing diagnosis, treatment, and prognosis.

Prevalence

At Bellevue Hospital, New York, where patients of all ages are accepted, there were 1250 autopsies over a period of two years, with the majority over ten years of age. De La Chapelle and Kossmann (1954) found that 3.3 percent of this adult group had myocarditis. Saphir and associates have drawn attention to the prevalence of myocarditis in children. In their review of 1944 they presented information on 97 instances of myocarditis, which comprised 6.8 percent of 1420 autopsies in the pediatric age group. These cases were divided as follows: rheumatic carditis, 32 percent; abscesses in the myocardium, 16 percent; broncho-pneumonia or lobar pneumonia, 15 percent; polio-

myelitis, 7 percent; subacute bacterial endocarditis, 7 percent; bacterial endocarditis; 5 percent; meningitis, 4 percent; tuberculosis, 4 percent; nephritis, 3 percent; nonspecific myocarditis, 3 percent; and scattered information on cases of measles, mumps, chickenpox, and diphtheria was also reported. More recently Saphir and Field (1954) have reported on 15 cases of isolated myocarditis seen over an eight-year period. De La Chapelle and Kossmann (1954) reviewed 1000 autopsies at the Willard Parker Infectious Diseases Hospital in New York, covering a period from 1932 to 1952. In this hospital the overall incidence of myocarditis in postmortem studies was 7 percent. These investigators found that of 78 such cases, 18 were associated with diphtheria, 14 had poliomyelitis, 14 had various forms of tuberculosis, nine had measles, seven had scarlet fever, six had meningococcal infections, two had whooping cough, and six had miscellaneous conditions such as pneumonia, otitis media, influenza, meningitis, anemia, croup, and erythema multiforme bullosum. There were two instances of isolated myocarditis.

Myocarditis in infancy has received increasing attention in recent years, partly because of the interest of such students of myocarditis as Kreutzer and associates (1959), but also because of the recognition of Coxsackie virus infection in the newborn period (Javett et al., 1956; Suckling and Vogelpoel, 1958). Other infectious diseases that have been associated with myocarditis in recent years are infectious mononucleosis, encephalomyocarditis, influenza, Asian flu, silicosis, infectious hepatitis, Chagas' disease, Rocky Mountain spotted fever, scrub typhus, epidemic typhus, and echoviruses.

At The Hospital for Sick Children, Toronto, during the past 25 years the cases of myocarditis that have been identified apart from the rheumatic fever group have been assembled. In a number not included, the diagnosis has been suspected but clear-cut evidence has been lacking. Besides these available for review are 11 autopsy-proved cases of Becu each of which has a full electrocardiographic tracing with precordial leads.

Lind and Hulquist reported five cases in 1949. This was followed by a series of 14 cases by Williams and coworkers in 1953. In the same year Rosenbaum and associates presented ten more. Saphir and Field in 1954 added 15 to the total, and Van Crevold and associates in 1954, 11 cases. Kreutzer, Berrie, and Becu (1959) reported one of the largest series up to the present, consisting of 70 cases. Kilbrick has assembled data on 45 cases of myocarditis reported in the literature, all of Coxsackie origin.

Epidemiology

Epidemics of myocarditis have been described by several authors. One hundred and forty cases were reported by Stoeber (1952) between 1937 and 1944, between the ages of one month and two years, and all had died. No etiologic agent was identified. In the epidemics recorded in Johannesburg (1952), Southern Rhodesia (1954), and Amsterdam (1955), Coxsackie virus was obtained from the stool and from autopsy material. Since then an epidemic has been described by Freundlich and associates in Israel (1958). Fifty-seven cases were recognized. Eighty-seven percent of them died, with death occurring in the majority less than 24 hours after a prodromal stage of a mild respiratory infection. No organism or virus was identified.

There is a slight tendency for cases of myocarditis of unrecognized etiology to occur in the summer or in the winter months. This was also noted by Hosier and Newton in 1958, whose maximum incidence was in July and August.

The most commonly identified etiologic agent in myocarditis today in the pediatric age group is Coxsackie virus. This is especially true of the newborn period, but it also applies to a lesser degree to the cases seen from one to three years of age. Of our 45 cases past the neonatal period, 32 were of unknown etiology, eight had antibody evidence of Coxsackie infection, two were due to diphtheria, one to chickenpox, one to mumps, and one to infectious mononucleosis. During epidemics rubella myocarditis may be recognized (Ainger et al., 1966).

Pathology

The heart usually appears flabby, pale, and dilated with enlarged ventricular chambers and a wall that, in comparison, appears thin, but by weight is found to be hypertrophied. Occasionally, however, gross inspection of the heart may show it to be normal, and it may be of normal weight in the event of a sudden overwhelming infection.

Histologically, myocarditis is characterized by an interstitial infiltration of lymphocytes, polymorphs, and plasma cells. The muscle fibers may show focal necrotic lesions at times and a diffuse degeneration at others. When septicemia has preceded death, leukocytes clumped in abscess formation may appear throughout the myocardium. Interstitial edema is common. In those in whom the disease has lasted for several weeks or more, patchy fibrosis appears.

A virus infection such as poliomyelitis, infectious hepatitis, or measles may show lesions with collections of lymphocytes in the interstitial tissues accompanied by occasional monocytes and polymorphs. The pathologic picture under the microscope is not constant, but in isolated myocarditis, one is more likely to see an interstitial type of lesion. This histologic pattern Saphir distinguishes from the one he considers to be associated with a known virus infection. The latter, he points out, may also have an interstitial cellular reaction, but it is characterized by patchy muscle fragmentation and necrosis, which, he says, are less likely to occur in the isolated myocarditis. He says, however, that this does not rule out the possibility that isolated myocarditis may be due to some unrecognized virus.

Rickettsial lesions are primarily associated with vasculitis. In such cases the virus multiples within the cell and produces muscle fragmentation and necrosis. Diphtheria and other bacterial toxins are protoplasmic poisons that alter cellular respiration (Woodward et al., 1960). Experimentally, endotoxins and gram-negative bacteria produce fibrinoid in the walls of coronary vessels and myocardial destruction. The changes seen resemble the overwhelming intoxication due to epinephrine or the syndrome of traumatic shock. Becu (1963) has recognized children with leptospirosis infection and enlarged hearts at postmortem with no evidence of degeneration or infection in the heart muscle in spite of hypertrophy.

It has been our finding, and also that of Sayers (1958), that the chronic cases have a good deal of fibrosis when they are examined at the autopsy table. An occasional case may have fibrosis of the heart tissues as a permanent complication and lead to myocardial insufficiency only after many years. Sayers (1958) reports such a case 12 years after an attack of diphtheritic myocarditis.

Clinical Features

In infants and children one should suspect the presence of myocarditis if any of the following are present in an acute or chronically ill patient: gallop rhythm, persistent tachycardia, enlargement of the heart, cardiovascular collapse, congestive heart failure, dyspnea, enlarged liver, a characteristic electrocardiographic pattern, or the new appearance of a significant apical systolic murmur.

In isolated myocarditis there may be no preceding illness whatever; the child may suddenly become dyspneic in a few minutes or a few hours. The larger proportion, however, have a somewhat more gradual onset, and many cases follow a preceding upper respiratory infection or pneumonia. Some begin with a history of vomiting, either once, twice, or repeatedly, while in others the first sign of illness is a cough associated with a mild degree of irritability, and in some babies there is simply a failure to gain weight.

The most common history in young infants is a mild respiratory infection associated with a red throat and followed by dyspnea over a period of two or three days; then it is suddenly realized by the parents that the baby is looking significantly ill and medical attention is sought. In the first few weeks of life such a history may be followed by dyspnea, cyanosis, and later death; in older cases survival is more likely.

The infant with myocarditis is usually acutely or severely ill with a respiratory rate between 60 and 120 per minute. At times there is a somewhat ashen type of cyanosis, which deepens with the severity of the illness. Peripheral edema may occur in a few cases, but this is the exception rather than the rule in infants and children. In a group of adults described by De La Chapelle and Kossman in 1954, edema occurred in 14 percent.

In children over one year of age the illness is usually less acute than in infancy, although they too may at times show the same cyanosis and peripheral collapse that is seen in the severely involved babies with Coxsackie virus infection and myocarditis. There is a tachycardia of 120 or higher, and the heart rate is frequently out of proportion to the temperature. In most cases there is no heart murmur to be heard. Occasionally there may be a soft systolic murmur at the apex, particularly in the chronic cases; in others an apical systolic murmur may appear after many weeks or months. The heart sounds may be normal or weak; a gallop rhythm is heard in the majority; the pressure of a gallop rhythm and no murmur are highly suggestive of myocarditis.

The apex beat is weak and diffuse and may be palpated in the fifth space beyond the nipple line. An x-ray of the heart shows it to be enlarged to a fairly marked degree in the majority of cases. In a few instances the enlargement may be minimal by x-ray and the weight not abnormally increased at postmortem, yet a gallop rhythm may be present associated with electrocardiographic changes. The sedimentation rate is usually elevated but has been reported as normal in several instances (De La Chapelle and Kossmann, 1954). The white blood cell count is also variable, being slightly elevated as a rule, but may be normal or occasionally in the twenty thousands.

Electrocardiography

The electrocardiogram is an integral part of the diagnostic picture. Tachycardia is the rule; con-

duction defects are not uncommon with varying degrees of heart block up to complete atrioventricular dissociation, which is a rare finding but may occur, particularly in the severe cases in the terminal state.

The two most important electrocardiographic features are:

1. A lowering of the voltages of the QRS in the standard leads, or the precordial leads, or both together. (See Figure 51–1.)
2. A flattening or inversion of the T waves, of the standard leads, or the left precordial leads. These features are illustrated in the accompanying electrocardiograms. (See Figure 51–1.)

In evaluation of the diagnostic significance of the electrocardiogram, the voltage of the QRS is considered depressed when less than 5 mm in each of the standard leads. The R wave in V_1 in the right precordium is frequently less than 4 mm and often less than 2 mm. In the left precordium the R wave is considered depressed if less than 6 mm in V_6. Minor degrees of lowered voltage become apparent as the child improves and the voltage increases toward the normal. Many children with myocarditis have a precordial electrocardiogram that is rather characteristic; in addition to low R waves across the whole chest the S waves are larger in comparison (see Figures 51–2).

The normal T wave in V_6 usually approximates 3 mm in height and may be as high as 5 or 6 mm and is rarely under 2 mm after six months of age. In the first six months of life it may be between 1 and 2 mm, but only under exceptional circumstances is it less than 1 mm in height (Ziegler, 1951).

In 45 cases of myocarditis the abnormalities of the T wave may be listed as follows (see Tables 51–1 and 51–2).

The T wave in myocarditis is most commonly flat but when inverted is usually inverted only to a minor degree, less than 1 mm of negativity as a general rule. This type of T wave may be positive but still lower than normal. As is indicated above, this occurred in 18

Table 51–1. MYOCARDITIS, 45 CASES—T WAVE IN V_5 OR V_6

	PERCENT
Flat or inverted T V_5 or V_6	68
Low T V_5 or V_6	18
Normal T V_5 or V_6	4
Markedly deviated ST (myocardial infarction pattern)	10
	100

Table 51–2. MYOCARDITIS, 45 CASES—T WAVE IN V_5 OR V_6

Myocarditis (no. of cases)			1	3	4	1	15	8		3	1		
T wave (mm)	+5	+4	+3	+2	+1	+.5	0	−.5	−1	−2	−3	−4	−5

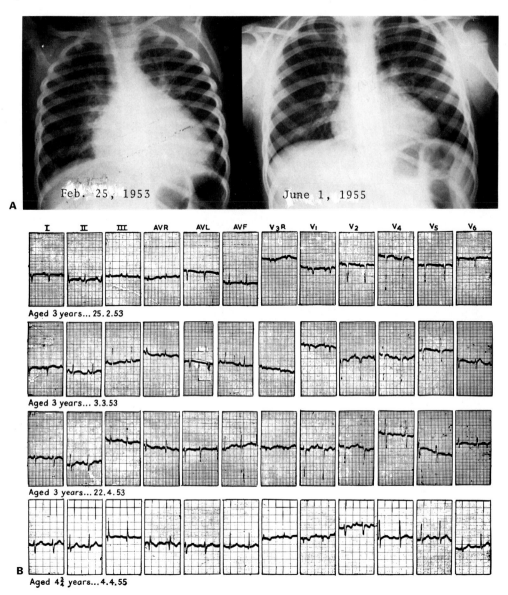

Figure 51–1. Patient developed acute isolated myocarditis at three years of age with enlargement of the heart and electrocardiographic change. The second x-ray, taken two and one-fourth years after the first, indicates a marked reduction in heart size; the final electrocardiogram shows a return to normal.

percent of our cases and a normal T wave in V_5 or V_6 in 4 percent. It should be pointed out that if repeated electrocardiograms are performed, eventually the minimal effects will revert to normal, and one may then decide whether or not they are due to myocarditis.

A marked elevation of the S-T portion of the electrocardiogram was present in one case reported by Weber and associates in 1949, in two cases reported by Dominguez, Lendrum, and Pick in 1959, and in three of the cases examined at The Hospital for Sick Children (see Figure 51–3). It is difficult to determine the exact frequency of this abnormality in the

electrocardiogram in myocarditis because certain cases are reported in the literature simply because they have this finding present. It is our impression that it occurs in approximately 5 percent of the patients with acute myocarditis and occasionally among the chronic cases. In one of our children with this electrocardiographic finding, the free wall of the left ventricle had fibrosis of the myocardium through its entire thickness. None of these cases mentioned had any evidence of coronary disease at postmortem, and the electrocardiographic abnormality appears to be due either to a diffuse fibrotic process in the ventricular wall or to acute localized necrosis of the

R.G.

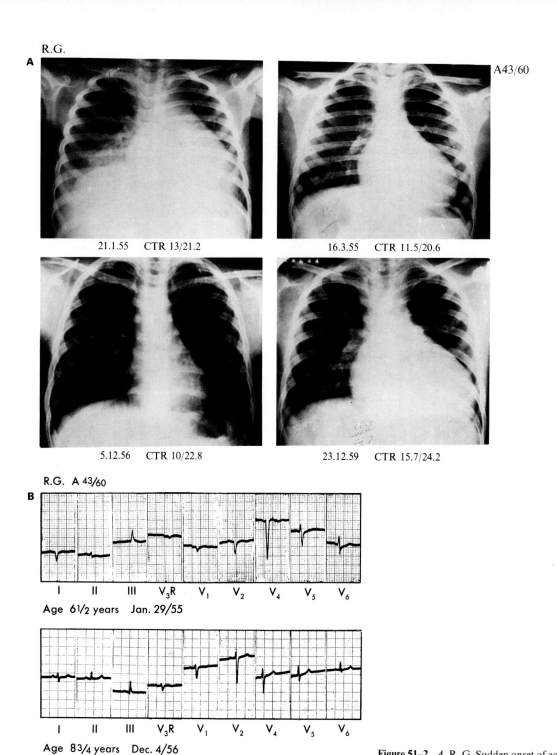

A43/60

21.1.55   CTR 13/21.2

16.3.55   CTR 11.5/20.6

5.12.56   CTR 10/22.8

23.12.59   CTR 15.7/24.2

R.G. A 43/60

B

I   II   III   V₃R   V₁   V₂   V₄   V₅   V₆
Age 6½ years   Jan. 29/55

I   II   III   V₃R   V₁   V₂   V₄   V₅   V₆
Age 8¾ years   Dec. 4/56

I   II   III   V₃R   V₁   V₂   V₄   V₅   V₆
Age 11¾ years   Nov. 11/59

Figure 51–2. *A.* R. G. Sudden onset of acute myocarditis with severe failure in January, 1955. Gradual improvement with bed rest and digitalis over many months. Recurrence of failure in 1959, followed by death early in 1960. The electrocardiogram did not regain normal voltage between 1955 and 1959. Autopsy showed some replacement of damaged cardiac muscle fibers with fibrous tissue. *B.* Electrocardiogram of R. G. shown in *A.* Tracing showed improvement in 1956 but deterioration in 1959.

C.B. #489422

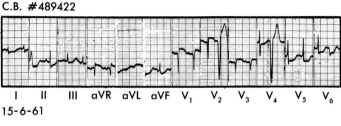

| I | II | III | aVR | aVL | aVF | V₁ | V₂ | V₃ | V₄ | V₅ | V₆ |

15-6-61

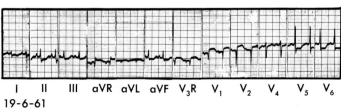

Figure 51–3. C. B., aged eight years, with acute myocarditis, showing elevation of the S-T portion of the electrocardiogram in leads V_1 and V_2 and depression of the S-T in V_5 and V_6. Low voltage of the QRS and T is shown in the standard leads.

| I | II | III | aVR | aVL | aVF | V₃R | V₁ | V₂ | V₄ | V₅ | V₆ |

19-6-61

myocardium. It is not necessarily a sign of fatal myocarditis, because one of our cases who presented with this abnormality recovered completely and is now active and well.

Another feature of the electrocardiographic pattern in myocarditis relates to the Q wave in precordial lead V_6. In 25 cases studied there was no Q wave in V_6 in 74 percent, a Q wave of 0.5 to 1 mm in 12 percent, and a Q wave of over 1 mm in 14 percent. This 14 percent represents five cases, and three of the five had a myocardial infarctation pattern, and associated marked necrosis or fibrosis of the ventricular wall and the Q wave was obviously due to this pathology. There were two cases in which the Q wave was between 1 and 3 mm in depth and did not appear to be associated either with left ventricular hypertrophy or with myocardial necrosis with fibrosis of a significant degree.

Some 85 percent of normal infants and children have a Q wave in precordial lead of V_6 of 1 mm or more; a finding of a Q wave of less than 1 mm in 86 percent of our cases of myocarditis is of some significance and may be of some help in the differential diagnosis.

If the low voltage of the QRS or the T wave abnormalities persist after the patient has apparently recovered, it is quite probably that some degree of myocardial fibrosis is present. As a rule, this does not interfere with a normal active life but occasionally may lead to heart failure, an event that has occurred in one of our cases and has also been reported by Sayers (1958).

Diagnosis

The diagnosis of myocarditis is based chiefly on two things:

1. Evidence of clinical or laboratory signs of myocarditis and
2. The exclusion of other forms of heart disease.

Myocarditis is usually indicated by a gallop rhythm, enlarged heart, tachycardia, congestive heart failure, circulatory collapse, absence of murmurs, appearance of certain electrocardiographic abnormalities, and identification of etiologic factors that precipitate myocarditis. In patients with frank failure the echocardiogram will show a large, poorly contracting left ventricle with a reduced ejection fraction, and velocity of circumferential fiber shortening is seen. The left atrium is usually also enlarged (Sahn et al., 1976). Rarely in early stages of the disorder and especially in newborn infants, the echocardiogram may be normal.

Differential Diagnosis. In excluding various forms of heart disease, rheumatic fever must be considered as well as the infectious diseases, toxic drugs, and congenital heart disease: (1) pericarditis, (2) endocardial fibroelastosis, (3) Coxsackie virus infection, (4) glycogen-storage disease of the heart, (5) anomalous left coronary, (6) coronary calcinosis, and (7) medial necrosis of coronary arteries.

PERICARDITIS. Pericarditis can enlarge the heart shadow, produce tachycardia, and cause T wave abnormalities in the electrocardiogram similar to those described. The first point of diagnostic import is the presence or absence of a friction rub. The second point is the change in size of the heart shadow. In pericarditis the heart shadow is usually large and a change of size occurs more rapidly than with myocarditis. One may see a return to normal size over a period of one to four weeks, a feature that is unusual in myocarditis. Paracentesis with a withdrawal of a quantity of pericardial fluid will settle the problem, of course, but such a procedure is rarely indicated. The electrocardiographic changes are sufficiently similar in the two conditions so that they are of little help in making the differentiation. Today echocardiography is a sensitive method of confirming the diagnosis. Finally, it should be remembered that pericarditis and myocarditis may occur together. When there is continued doubt, digitalis should be administered.

ENDOCARDIAL FIBROELASTOSIS. The most difficult problem is to differentiate clearly between endocardial fibroelastosis and myocarditis. Both conditions are likely to be associated with heart failure, and frequently murmurs are absent or insignificant. Gallop rhythm is common to both, and both diseases respond to digitalis in a high percentage of cases. However, a review of 79 cases of myocarditis and 45 cases of endocardial fibroelastosis has helped to clarify the differences between these two pathologic states.

First, a specific etiologic agent may be identified that is commonly associated with myocarditis, Coxsackie virus, diphtheria, and many of the childhood infectious diseases, encephalomyocarditis virus, pneumonia, and influenza. A Coxsackie virus infection, particularly in the first week or two of life, is likely to cause myocarditis. Later it is much less likely to do so. A history of pleurodynia or pyrexial illness in the mother a week or so before delivery suggests the possibly of such an infection.

Second, apart from the newborn period, myocarditis is much more likely to have its onset after the first year of life. In endocardial fibroelastosis the onset occurs in the first eight months of life in 90 percent of cases. Excluding the Coxsackie myocarditis of the newborn, only 30 percent of cases of myocarditis have their onset during the first eight months.

Perhaps the most useful differential point of all is the information recorded by the electrocardiogram. The majority of cases with endocardial fibroelastosis have an increase in voltage with certain precordial leads indicating a left ventricular loading pattern. On the other hand, 93 percent of the cases with acute myocarditis have decreased or normal voltage of the same precordial leads (see Table 51–3).

Table 51–3. MYOCARDITIS,
45 CASES—QRS VOLTAGE

	PER CENT	
Low voltage	58	93% normal or
Normal voltage	35	decreased voltage
Increased voltage	7	

Both endocardial fibroelastosis and myocarditis characteristically have a flat or inverted T wave in V_5 or V_6 and both frequently produce congestive heart failure, gallop rhythm, large heart, etc. In endocardial fibroelastosis over half the cases will have some evidence of a significant Q wave in V_5 or V_6. Such a finding is rare in cases of myocarditis unless a myocardial infarction pattern is present.

Furthermore, the T wave in V_5 or V_6 in endocardial fibroelastosis is more likely to be inverted to a greater degree than the T wave in myocarditis. Characteristically, the T wave in V_5 or V_6 in myocarditis is flat. At times it may be very slightly inverted, usually not more than a millimeter. In endocardial fibroelastosis, on the other hand, it may be inverted to a depth of 4 or 5 mm, and in a relatively high percentage of cases it is inverted to more than 1 mm.

The mumps antigen skin test is usually positive in endocardial fibroelastosis and unlikely in myocarditis, especially under four or five years of age.

GLYCOGEN-STORAGE DISEASE OF THE HEART. In glycogen-storage disease of the heart one finds a cardiac enlargement of a marked degree, usually involving right and left ventricles with increased thickness of the myocardium, the left predominating over the right. At times the thickening of the septum may take the form of infundibular obstruction with the characteristic findings of infundibular stenosis of the left ventricle.

These pathologic findings may be reflected in the electrocardiogram (Ehlers et al., 1962). There is characteristically a short P-R interval, a high voltage of the QRS, and in some instances upright T waves over the right precordium and inverted T waves over the left. The T waves characteristically show considerable voltage whether they are upright or inverted—a point that helps in differentiating this condition from myocarditis. Congestive heart failure usually occurs as a terminal event. If there is a family history of this condition, it is helpful in making the diagnosis. Perhaps the most useful differentiating point is the fact that when the heart is involved in glycogen-storage disease, there is likely to be involvement of the muscles throughout the other parts of the body. The biopsy and histochemical analysis will reveal excess glycogen deposition. The buffy coat of the centrifugal blood may also contain an unusual amount of glycogen. In this condition as many as 76 percent die in the first six months, 18 percent between 6 and 12 months, and only 6 percent survive for a short time after one year of age; thus the mortality distribution varies from that of myocarditis.

ABERRANT LEFT CORONARY ARTERY. Another congenital defect that may give somewhat similar findings is the aberrant left coronary arising from the pulmonary. Here there are left ventricular loading in the electrocardiographic pattern and inverted T waves over the left precordium as a rule. The heart is also enlarged and there may be no murmur present. These children have tachycardia and eventually develop congestive heart failure. The echocardiogram will show a large dilated left ventricle with poor function as in any congestive cardiomyopathy. Angiocardiography reveals a huge left ventricle and a small right ventricle compressed by a deviated septum, and the aortogram will demonstrate a right coronary coming off the aorta in normal fashion but present no evidence of a left coronary from that vessel. The electrocardiogram, however, will permit an accurate differentiation from other conditions in most instances, since babies with an aberrant left coronary off the pulmonary show an anterior myocardial infarction pattern affirming the underlying pathology. The age of the baby, the course of the illness, the operative findings, or ultimate death with subsequent postmortem reveals the correct diagnosis and allows time to distinguish the anomaly from endocardial fibroelastosis and myocarditis. The typical electrocardiographic pattern of myocardial infarction may now show up on the first examination, but if repeated electrocardiograms are taken, the classic tracing will eventually appear. Occasionally a somewhat similar pattern is seen in a patient with myocarditis (Dominguez et al., 1959). Myocardial perfusion scanning using thallium is a reliable new method of demonstrating the ischemic zone and differentiating other forms of cardiomyopathy.

MEDIAL NECROSIS OF THE CORONARY ARTERIES. Another rare condition that should be considered in the differential diagnosis is that of medial necrosis of the coronary arteries. This was first described completely by Bryant and White in 1901. The pulmonary and renal arteries are often involved, and there may be signs of renal disease that may help in making the diagnosis. The age of onset in this group is usually in the first three months of life. Although a tachycardia may be present, it is usually not associated with heart failure.

Specific Diseases Causing Myocarditis

Coxsackie Virus Myocarditis. Although myocarditis is considered an uncommon illness in the first year of life, in the past 25 years an increasing number of reports have been appearing in literature of Coxsackie infections in the neonatal period. Javett and associates (1956) and Suckling and Vogelpoel (1958) drew attention to small groups of cases that appeared in epidemic fashion. Kilbrick (1961) has summarized the literature in this category and has recorded 45 cases of Coxsackie myocarditis with a 73 percent mortality. They have all been in the neonatal period. In many instances the mother had a Coxsackie infection with fever, or pleurodynia, or both, in the last week of pregnancy. A week or two after birth the infant developed the same infection but with damaging effect on the heart muscle. It was pointed out that this transmission of the infection appears to be serious only during the neonatal period since no ill effects have been noticed earlier in pregnancy and are usually not fatal after the first month or two of life. While the disease is a diffuse one and produces generalized effects including encephalitis, it is only the myocarditis that leads to the high mortality. The reason for this is not clear, but it may be related to the extra burden the heart is called upon to bear in the circulatory adjustments of the newborn.

Since Coxsackie infection in the newborn frequently involves the other systems besides, the symptoms may be widely distributed throughout the body. Loss of appetite, feeding difficulties, breathlessness, and severe degree of dyspnea are present in the vast majority. Fever and red throat are commonly seen initially; hepatomegaly occurs if heart failure supervenes. Encephalitic signs may be evident but are less common features.

Tachycardia, dyspnea, hepatomegaly, and radiologic evidence of an enlarged heart are all indications of cardiac involvement. The electrocardiogram will reveal confirming evidence of myocarditis in nearly all cases. In the acute myocarditis with failure electrocardiographic changes will usually appear as shown in Figure 51–1. In the milder cases it may be necessary to do several electrocardiograms and demonstrate changes for better or for worse before incriminating evidence is elicited.

Saphir reports a pathologic appearance of a virus type of myocardial infection at postmortem that leads him to suspect that such cases have been damaged in a somewhat specific manner. This is characterized by a patchy necrosis of muscle tissue and is somewhat different from the diffuse reaction that he associates with other types of myocarditis.

The newborn babies with Coxsackie infection are usually acutely ill for a few days or a week, but the majority die after a relatively short course of illness. If they are going to recover, recovery takes place fairly rapidly over the next week or two, with the electrocardiographic changes persisting for one or two months but rarely longer. Digitalis, antibiotics, oxygen, and other supportive measures are indicated and may be lifesaving.

The outlook in such infants is usually good if they recover, and there are no reports in literature so far of cases developing the chronic picture that one sometimes sees in older children with myocarditis.

COXSACKIE MYOPERICARDITIS IN CHILDREN AND ADULTS. It is now recognized that this type of infection occurs at all ages (Smith, 1970; Burch, 1969; Koontz et al., 1971; Hirschman and Hammer, 1974). Arthalgia and myalgia are common symptoms occurring more frequently where there is evidence of Coxsackie B infection. Due to the ubiquitous presence of Coxsackie infections in many communities around the world, elevated neutralizing antibodies cannot be trusted as diagnostic of an acute infection. Koontz and Gray (1971) suggest, however, that a fourfold increase in the titer is good supporting evidence of relationship between such an infection and the current illness.

It should be pointed out that recurrences have been recorded in approximately a third of Coxsackie B infections and about 50 percent of other Coxsackie infections when the patients are followed for several months. Such recurrences may be associated with return of abnormalities in the electrocardiogram. Koontz describes relapses occurring when corticosteroids were stopped or reduced.

Abscesses of the Myocardium. In the past these cases were due to a septicemia from an associated infection, such as osteomyelitis, cellulitis, local abscess, otitis media, and mastoid. They were undoubtedly due to a septicemia, with a localization of the pyemic infection in the heart muscle. Saphir's study covered a period of years leading up to 1944, a period before antibiotics were available. A similar study today would show few instances of myocardial abscesses. The decline would probably parallel that of septic pericarditis. Obviously, treatment consists of determining the causative agent and prescribing the adequate amount of suitable antibiotic to eliminate the organism. The drugs and their dosage are the same as those used in treating subacute bacterial endocarditis due to similar organisms.

Pneumonia. In 1922, Stone reported that 2.7 percent of patients dying with bronchopneumonia had interstitial myocarditis. Today, deaths from bronchopneumonia are much less common in infancy and childhood. These cases are less likely to have myocarditis than they would have been 30 years ago, especially if they are adequately treated with a suitable antibiotic. Deaths now rarely occur from lobar pneumonia in childhood, and, when they do, the heart is unlikely to be involved. However, myocarditis may simulate pneumonia or the two infections may involve both heart and lungs. Unusual dyspnea associated with enlargement of the liver suggests a complicating myocarditis in pneumonia or the presence of gallop rhythm. The electrocardiogram will often be of decisive diagnostic help. A trial of digitalis is indicated in the doubtful cases as well as in those in which diagnosis is confirmed. Occasionally, the response to digitalis is dramatic.

Diphtheria. Myocarditis in diphtheria is due to the toxin liberated by the diphtheria bacillus. It occurs in approximately 10 percent of patients with this disease. Since the infection has been eliminated almost totally by immunization, an opportunity to study a diphtheritic heart is rarely presented. In the past 25 years three children suffering from this form of myocarditis have been seen at The Hospital for Sick Children: one died in heart failure and the two others recovered.

In the past, rhythm abnormalities, such as extrasystoles, gallop rhythm, lengthened conduction time, heart block, ventricular tachycardia, and atrial fibrillation, have been noted. In severe cases heart failure and death may occur. An electrocardiogram may show changes indicative of myocarditis, such as flattened and inverted T waves or low voltage. Usually children with diphtheria, when adequately treated with antitoxin, make a complete recovery with no residual signs of heart disease. When they do show signs of heart failure, digitalis may be lifesaving.

An occasional case may have fibrosis of the heart as a permanent complication that will eventually lead to myocardial insufficiency (Sayers, 1958).

Nihoyannopoulos (1963) records a reservoir of diphtheria cases in children in Greece averaging 400 to 500 cases a year. Electrocardiographic abnormalities were noted in approximately 25 percent, but the mortality, which was largely due to myocarditis, was in the neighborhood of only 2 to 3 percent. The youngest patient was three months and the oldest 14 years. The majority of cases occurred in the preschool age group. In few patients between four and seven years a fatal outcome after progressive damage to the conduction system was described (Nihoyannopoulos and Agoroyannis, 1972).

Measles. In the city of Toronto there is approximately one death a year due to measles, and it is usually associated with an overwhelming infection in a young child. Pneumonia or complicating infections may be a responsible factor. Rarely is there any associated heart disease. Saphir and coworkers (1944) record only two cases with postmortem evidence of myocarditis following measles.

Electrocardiographic abnormalities may occur in measles but are not related to the severity of the disease. One study cited by Goldfield and associates (1955) reported electrocardiographic changes in 19 percent of the cases, including abnormalities of the T waves and a prolonged P-R interval. Another study by Ross (1952) revealed the conduction time to be 0.18 second or over in 30 percent of 71 children with measles. These electrocardiographic changes are of minor importance and do not affect the prognosis in a child with measles. None of these cases had gallop rhythm or murmurs of significance. One can conclude that significant myocarditis in measles is an exceedingly rare phenomenon.

Mumps. One case of a patient dying suddenly during an attack of mumps, with myocarditis demonstrated at postmortem, is recorded in the literature (Bengtsson and Orndahl, 1954). Although occasions of irregularity of rate and rhythm have been noted in children with mumps, myocarditis is a rarity.

Chickenpox. Approximately one case a year dies with chickenpox in the city of Toronto. It is usually associated with secondary infection or encephalitis. Myocardial involvement with interstitial inflammatory lesions has been described in this condition, but as in mumps and measles it is a rare event. One of our cases had transient heart failure with electrocardiographic changes following an attack of chickenpox, and then made a complete recovery.

Poliomyelitis. In 1941, Larson first described poliomyelitis with myocarditis. Since that time there have been numerous reports of pathologic and electrocardiographic studies. Jurow and Dolgopol (1953) examined the hearts of 73 patients who died with poliomyelitis at the Willard Parker Infectious Disease Hospital, New York. Thirty-two percent had evidence of focal myocarditis. The lesion usually consisted of histiocytes, polymorphs, and a few lymphocytes.

Gefter and associates (1947) reported electrocardiographic findings in 226 patients with poliomyelitis. Significant abnormalities were found in 14 percent of these patients: tachycardia in 4 percent; extrasystoles in 0.9 percent; abnormally high P waves in 2.7 percent; a long P-R interval in 3.1 percent; a slurring of the QRS in 0.04 percent; left-axis deviation in 3.5 percent; right-axis deviation in 2.2 percent; and flat, diphasic, or inverted T waves in 3.5 percent. At The Hospital for Sick Children the study of electrocardiograms in 226 cases of poliomyelitis revealed only minor abnormalities, similar to those recorded by Gefter and associates. Abnormal T wave inversion was found in only one case.

Hypertension has been recorded frequently in poliomyelitis. In 226 cases we found that the majority of patients (two-thirds) showed elevation in blood pressure from the third to the seventh day. After that the blood pressure subsided steadily until, at the end of two weeks, it was within normal limits in all but an occasional case. Hypertension was more common in the paralytic group: It occurred in 65 percent of the 186 cases in the paralytic group, whereas it was found in only 12 percent of the 40 cases of the nonparalytic group.

The cause of hypertension is not entirely clear. A renal origin has been suggested, but this seems unlikely. Hypoxia has been mentioned as the cause in some cases since with the use of oxygen the blood pressure at times has come down. Weinstein and Shelokov (1951) related the hypertension to involvement of the hypothalamus, which may occur in the bulbar type. The hypertension may appear suddenly or progressively. It may reach very high levels and persist long after the acute phase of the infection is over. The eyegrounds in such cases may show spasm of the arterioles.

In the fatal bulbar poliomyelitis, peripheral vascular collapse with hypotension may occur. Such collapse appears to be irreversible and does not respond to supportive therapy.

When the signs of myocarditis, either clinically or in the electrocardiogram, are associated with hypertension, especially in poliomyelitis, it would seem reasonable to digitalize the patient as one does in acute nephritis.

Heart failure has been reported rarely in poliomyelitis; however, pulmonary edema may occur as a terminal event.

Treatment

Whenever the diagnosis of isolated myocarditis is made, digitalis should be administered. In infants and children who are desperately ill, this should be given intravenously, starting with one-fourth of the digitalizing dose, giving another fourth an hour later, and giving the rest of the digitalizing dose intravenously or by mouth as indicated by the severity of the condition. In the less severely ill patients, digitalization may be carried out over a 24-hour period, as described in the discussion of congestive heart failure (Chapter 10). Oxygen, a low-sodium diet, diuretics, and antibiotics should be used when indicated, as in other cases of congestive heart failure.

One of the most important aspects of treatment is the length of time the digitalis is administered. It should be continued until all signs of heart disease have completely disappeared and the patient is entirely recovered—three months should be a minimum. Relapses are common; consequently, if treatment is stopped early, the patient's condition may become worse than it was at the initial admission. Before digitalis therapy is stopped, the electrocardiogram should be normal, the heart should be normal or close to normal in size, there should be no signs of heart failure, and the health should be good. This may entail giving digitalis for one to two years or more in some instances. When it is finally decided to discontinue digitalis, the drug should be reduced gradually in step doses and the patient watched for returning signs of myocarditis or heart failure.

The use of ACTH in the treatment of myocarditis has been reported by Garrison and Swisher (1953). The authors have also used this hormone in several instances. However, since ACTH has usually been given as an adjunct to digitalis, it is difficult to draw conclusions as to its value. Kreutzer and associates (1959) report the use of steroids before the administration of digitalis with beneficial effects.

Prognosis

There are two main clinical types of myocarditis: (1) the acute form and (2) the subacute or chronic form. The acute form is characteristic of the newborn period but may occur at any time, particularly in the presence of Coxsackie infection, during childhood (see Figure 51-4). The onset of symptoms is rapid, and in many cases death comes within a few days after the first signs of illness. Cardiac arrhythmias are a common complication (Abelmann, 1973). Digitalis is usually inadequate to control this fulminating process. The age and the rapidity of onset of severe signs and symptoms are a useful guide to prognosis. Early therapy with rest, digitalis, and, when necessary, oxygen will decrease the mortality. One of our severest cases survived, as did two of those reported by Williams and associates (1953).

In our recent experience, fewer cases have been appearing in the first year of life, whereas more have been seen between 2 and 12 years. In this age group the condition is more frequently of the subacute or chronic variety, which permits supportive therapy with bed rest and digitalis to control the signs of heart failure, thus leading ultimately to a successful cure. The majority of the milder cases will recover completely. A few of the more severely involved may have some residual myocardial fibrosis (Sayers, 1958). One of our cases exhibited this finding when he died three years after the original attack.

In certain parts of the world a particularly severe form of myocarditis may appear in epidemic proportions with a high mortality. This was true of the Israeli epidemic reported by Freundlich and associates (1958). In adults death may be due to other causes, the myocarditis being contributory (Smith, 1970; Koontz and Ray, 1971).

CHAGAS' DISEASE

CHAGAS' disease (Carlos Chagas, 1909) is the result of infection with *Trypanosoma cruzi*. This is usually transmitted to man in the feces of the triatomid bug. The *T. cruzi* enters the cells of the reticuloendothelial

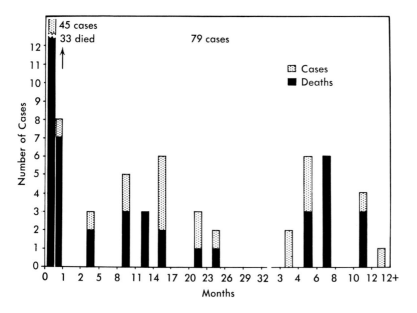

Figure 51–4. The age of onset of myocarditis in infancy and childhood is recorded in 79 cases reported in the literature and from our own files. Epidemics of myocarditis such as that reported by Freundlich and associates (1958) with a large number of cases concentrated in a short period of time were not included, since they appear to be isolated phenomena and do not present any problem in the differential diagnosis with endocardial fibroelastosis. Furthermore, all the cases reported by Freundlich were six months old or more at the time of onset.

system and muscles and is transformed in the leishmanial form. This disease is found particularly in South America, especially Brazil, and is confined to the American continents. It tends to occur in the lower economic group, particularly those living in houses in the country that have cracks in the walls harboring the infecting bug. An excellent review of the subject has been published recently (Prata et al., 1974).

The disease is characterized by an acute phase that occurs in the first week or two following the initial infection. In the endemic areas this occurs usually in the first decade of life. The invasion is characteristically via a lesion on the skin or through inoculation in the mucous membranes. It is characterized by fever, malaise, anorexia, generalized nontender lymphoadenopathy, moderate hepatosplenomegaly, and, in some instances, peripheral edema. Very often the local signs of the portal of entry can be recognized. Frequently there is unilateral periorbital edema with mild conjunctivitis and hypertrophy of the preauricular lymph node (Romaña's sign). These manifestations subside in two or three months, and it is said that 5 to 10 percent of the cases die at this stage of acute meningoencephalitis or acute myocarditis.

The majority of cases of Chagas' disease are seen in the chronic phase of the illness. Initially these patients are asymptomatic (latent phase), and the diagnosis can be made only on a positive complement fixation test or, occasionally, identifying the organism in the peripheral blood. Much later signs develop of cardiomyopathy and disturbances of the digestive tract or of the nervous system.

The cardiomyopathy may become evident in the first ten years of life but is more likely to be identified when the individual is between 10 and 50 years of age, with the peak reached between 30 and 40. The cardiovascular signs are characterized by tachycardia unrelated to fever and arterial hypotension with low pulse pressure. The cardiac sounds may be decreased in intensity; there may be a gallop rhythm; cardiac enlargement of varying degrees is present, which may go on to heart failure. The electrocardiogram usually shows a prolongation of the P-R interval and of the Q-T interval, disturbance of the T wave and S-T segment, and at times low voltage of the QRS complex. Such findings are characteristic of the early acute stages of the disease. In the final stages there is marked cardiac enlargement, congestive heart failure leading to death in two or three years, mitral or tricuspid insufficiency, and arrhythmias that may lead to complete heart block and at times sudden death.

The diagnosis is based on the history and the finding of positive complement fixation test or detection of the parasite in the peripheral blood through direct examination (acute phase) or through the xenodiagnosis. One may look for evidence of myocardial involvement excluding other recognized causes of cardiac disease such as congenital heart disease, hypertensive heart disease, or ischemic heart disease. Circulating immunoglobulins in patients with Chagas' heart disease react consistently with endocardium, blood vessel, and interstitium. Use of this fact to improve diagnosis of the chronic cardiopathy seems promising (Cossio et al., 1974).

A congenital form of Chagas' disease has been described in the endemic areas with a transmission rate as high as 10 percent (Bittencourt et al, 1972) and associated with spontaneous abortion and low-birth-weight infants. The clinical manifestations (Rocha, 1971) are those of an intrauterine infection, and characteristically there are jaundice, hepatosplenomegaly, petechiae, generalized edema, and signs of meningoencephalitis. The diagnosis is made by finding the *Trypanosoma* in the blood or in the placenta. The differential diagnosis should include other causes of intrauterine infection, particularly syphilis, rubella, toxoplasmosis, and cytomegalic inclusion disease.

In spite of the availability of many drugs in modern therapy there is little that can be done specifically for Chagas' disease. Symptomatic treatment is directed toward correction of the heart failure or the arrhythmias or at times thromboembolic accidents.

The chief form of control is prophylaxis, providing adequate housing and public health measures, and the use of insecticides, particularly in the country or farm dwellings.

THE HEART AND KWASHIORKOR

THIS condition occurs in the tropics and is a form of malnutrition that is a protein deficiency with relatively adequate caloric intake. The child becomes thin, wasted, and weak, the hair changes color to a slightly reddish sheen, and activity is minimized.

Among the children suffering from kwashiorkor there is very little evidence of cardiac involvement on examination of the heart. Heart sounds may be diminished but murmurs are not usually heard and there is no enlargement of the heart. In fact, on x-ray the heart appears unusually small and atrophic and is associated with a diminished cardiac output. The electrocardiogram shows changes in the S-T segment with low voltage or inversion of the T wave.

Such clinical findings are supported by histologic examination at autopsy for interstitial edema, and vacuolation of the muscle fibers occurs proceeding to necrosis in some cases. The heart, as one would expect, is markedly reduced in weight. These signs gradually regress under therapy.

MYOCARDIAL FIBROSIS AND CYSTIC FIBROSIS OF THE PANCREAS

MYOCARDIAL fibrosis and cystic fibrosis of the pancreas has been reported by McGiven (1962), Powell and associates (1957), and Barnes and coworkers (1970). In the recent report by Barnes (1970) there are six cases that died between the age of five months and two and one-half years. Some of them were treated with pancreatic enzymes. At autopsy there was cardiac involvement of a similar fashion in all. The muscle of the left ventricle was pallid, and there was focal scarring that histologically showed replacement of the muscle fibers by simple fibrous connective tissue of varying degrees of maturity and vascularity. Inflammatory cells were not frequently seen. An electrocardiogram was performed on two, which showed changes in the S-T segment. X-ray showed cardiac enlargement. Since the pathologic changes were not those of inflammation, primary muscle degeneration, or ischemia, they appear to be possibly metabolic or nutritional and might arise from the malabsorption of fat or fat-soluble vitamins such as one might expect to occur in this condition.

The above pathology should not be confused with the response of the heart to emphysema, which is often associated with increased pulmonary artery pressure and may occur in cystic fibrosis of the pancreas leading to changes in heart size and in the electrocardiogram, particularly right ventricular hypertrophy.

CARDIOMYOPATHY

GOODWIN (1972) quite rightly points out that the term *cardiomyopathy* means no more than disease of the heart muscle and in current use is a definition implying ignorance of etiology. He excludes from the definition those diseases of the heart muscle that are due to a known cause or due to disease elsewhere in the body. And he reserves the term *primary cardiomyopthy* for those heart muscle diseases in which the heart alone is affected. He suggests the classification of three main types: (1) hypertrophic, with or without obstruction, characterized by impaired ventricular distensibility and compliance; (2) congestive, notable for poor systolic ejection function; and (3) obliterative, characterized by obliteration of the ventricular cavities.

The hypertrophic or obstructive type is exemplified by ventricular hypertrophy, increased ventricular power, but reduced compliance. Under the heading "congestive" are listed infective, toxic, allergic, alcohol, cobalt, drugs, etc., in which there is minimal ventricular hypertrophy, maximum dilatation of the heart, reduced power, and possibly normal compliance. In the obliterative category are grouped endomyocardial fibrosis and Loeffler's eosinophilic disorder in which there is little or no ventricular hypertrophy or dilatation but there is reduced power and reduced compliance.

Such cardiomyopathies as are included in the above definition are uncommon in childhood. The one that does appear in childhood, although it is not common, is hypertrophic obstructive cardiomyopathy or idiopathic hypertrophic subaortic stenosis characterized by massive hypertrophy of the outflow tract to the left ventricle producing significant pressure gradients. This is described elsewhere in this book in Chapter 37 on aortic stenosis.

We have not included the endocardial fibroelastosis of infancy under cardiomyopathies because it appears more likely to be a congenital defect. It is present apparently at birth, or shortly after, is associated with a bicuspid aortic valve in 20 percent of the cases, and is present along with other congenital heart anomalies not infrequently such as coarctation of the aorta and aortic atresia. Furthermore a family history of a similar defect occurs in a modest proportion of cases (10 percent).

Congestive cardiomyopathy occurs occasionally in childhood. We have one boy who developed heart failure and a dilated and enlarged heart at two years of age who is now 18 and has been in the state of chronic failure all his life, who has dilated, flabby ventricles and does not fit into any other category in the pediatric group.

The current approach to cardiomyopathies is well described by Perloff (1971), Goodwin (1972), and Harris and Nghiem (1972).

Goodwin's group of obliterative cardiomyopathy is typified by endomyocardial fibrosis (EMF).

Endomyocardial fibrosis is a disease that was first described in Africans but has been seen in many other countries: in South America, India, Ceylon, Brazil, Sudan, and the Middle East. It is characterized by a fibrosis of the endocardium, the myocardium, and the ventricular cavities, particularly the apex and subvalvular areas.

Like many other diseases, it tends to occur in a lower economic group, but it does occur from time to time in well-nourished Europeans, which suggests that malnutrition is not a primary factor. Its etiology is unknown although it has been suggested that it may be a hypersensitivity disorder similar to rheumatic fever, but there is no direct evidence that the *Streptococcus* is an etiologic factor.

At autopsy the heart may be normal in size, but frequently it is increased in weight. The lesion consists of dense fibrous thickening of the endocardium. This may occur only in the right ventricle, or only in the left, or in a combined form in about 50 percent of cases.

The lesion is clinically recognizable only when the disease has progressed for some time with common presenting features such as cardiac failure. It is a disease that occurs in younger people, and about a third of the patients are under 15 years of age when first recognized. Fatigue and weakness are common features; dyspnea, palpitations, and ascites may be present by the time the patient seeks medical advice. There may be a systolic murmur of tricuspid incompetence with or without a gallop rhythm, but an absence of murmurs is not uncommon.

When endomyocardial fibrosis affects the left ventricle alone, a form of pulmonary hypertension usually develops, giving rise to right ventricular hypertrophy associated with a prominent left parasternal lift. When the fibrosis involves the right ventricle, the tricuspid valve is usually rendered incompetent producing a murmur and raising the venous pressure. The only unrestricted part of the right ventricle is the infundibulum, and this hypertrophies and dilates giving rise to visible and palpable pulsation in the second, third, and fourth left interspaces and is a physical sign unique to right ventricular endomyocardial fibrosis. The right atrium enlarges; gross hepatomegaly and ascites are common and atrial fibrillation may occur. In the advanced stages pericardial effusion may occur and persist for some time.

The electrocardiogram usually shows low voltage in the QRS complex with increased potential of the P wave. S-T segment depression and T wave inversion in the right precordial leads may be present, but generalized flattening of the T waves across the whole precordium is not unusual.

A cardiac catheterization is helpful as it rules out mitral stenosis, constrictive pericarditis, and lesions that might simulate endomyocardial fibrosis. Whether there is left ventricular involvement, right ventricular involvement, or combined, treatment is usually disappointing; digitalis and diuretics are of limited value.

Infantile Xanthomatosus Cardiomyopathy

MacMahon (1971) has suggested the term "infantile xanthomatosus cardiomyopathy" to describe a group of cases in infancy and childhood who have large and small islands of xanthomatous cells throughout the myocardium. Similar cases were reported by Hudson (1965) and Reid and associates (1968). The clinical picture may be accompanied by disturbances of rate and rhythm, and finally by heart failure. The diagnosis is made at autopsy and comprises areas of compact xanthomatous cells scattered throughout the heart, causing a displacement of myocardial fibers. The prime pathologic process appears to be confined to the heart. Other changes in the body are secondary.

REFERENCES

Abelmann, W. H.: Viral myocarditis and its sequelae. *Annu. Rev. Med.*, **24**:145, 1973.

Abt, A. F., and Vinnecour, M. I.: Electrocardiographic studies during pneumonia in infants and children. *Am. J. Dis. Child.*, **47**:737, 1934.

Ainger, L. E.; Lawyer, N. G.; and Fitch, C. W.: Neonatal rubella myocarditis. *Br. Heart J.*, **28**:691, 1966.

Alleyne, G. A. O.: Cardiac function in severely malnourished Jamaican children. *Clin. Sci.*, **30**:553, 1966.

Baker, P. S.; Johnston, F. D.; and Wilson, F. N.: The duration of systole in hypocalcemia. *Am. Heart J.*, **14**:82, 1937.

Baker, P. S.; Shrader, E. L.; and Ronzoni, E.: The effects of alkalosis and acidosis upon the human electrocardiogram. *Am. Heart J.*, **17**:169, 1939.

Barnes, G. L.; Gwynne, J. F.; and Watt, J. M.: Myocardial fibrosis in cystic fibrosis of the pancreas. *Aust. Paediatr. J.*, **6**:81, 1970.

Beasley, O. C., Jr.: Familial myocardial disease, a report of three siblings, and a review of the literature. *Am. J. Med.*, **29**:476, 1960.

Becu, Louis: Personal communication, 1963.

Bell, E. J., and Grist, N. R.: Echoviruses, carditis and acute pleurodynia. *Lancet*, **1**:326, 1970.

Bengtsson, E., and Orndahl, G.: Complications of mumps with special reference to the incidence of myocarditis. *Acta Med. Scand.*, **144**:381, 1954.

Bittencourt, A. L.; Barbosa, H. S.; Rocha, T.; Sodré, I.: Sodré, A.:

Incidência da transmissão congênita da doenca de Chagas em partos prematuros na Maternidade Tsylla Balbino (Salvador, Bahia). *Rev. Inst. Med. Trop. São Paulo*, **14**:131, 1972.

Brockington, I. F.; Olsen, E. G. J.; and Goodwin, J. F.: Endomyocardial fibrosis in Europeans resident in tropical Africa. *Lancet*, **1**:583, 1967.

Bryant, J. H., and White, W. H.: A case of calcification of the arteries and obliterative endarteritis, associated with hydronephrosis, in a child aged 6 months. *Guy. Hosp. Rep.*, **55**:17, 1901.

Burch, G. E., and Colcolough, H. L.: Progressive Coxsackie viral pancarditis and nephritis. *Ann. Intern. Med.*, **71**:963, 1969.

Campbell, S.; and Macafee, C. A. J.: A case of idiopathic pulmonary heamosiderosis with myocarditis. *Arch. Dis. Child.*, **34**:218, 1959.

Churg, J., and Sender, B.: Precipitation of sulfadiazine in the heart. *Arch. Pathol.*, **62**:174, 1956.

Clagett, A. H.: The electrocardiographic changes following artificial hyperpyrexia. *Am. J. Med. Sci.*, **208**:81, 1944.

Clinical features and diagnosis of primary myocardial disease (II). *Mod. Conc. Cardiovasc. Dis.*, **30**:683, 1961.

Connor, D. H.; Somers, K.; Hutt, M. S. R.; Manion, W. C.; and D'Arbela, P. G.: Endomyocardial fibrosis in Uganda (Davies' disease). *Am. Heart J.*, I, **74**:687, 1967; II, **75**:107, 1968.

Cook, G. C., and Hutt, M. S. R.: The liver after kwashiokor. *Lancet*, **3**:454, 1967.

Cossio, P. M.; Diez, C.; Szarfman, A.; Kreutzer, E.; Candiola, B.; and Arana, R. M.: Chagasic cardiomyopathy. Demonstration of a serum gamma globulin factor which reacts with endocardium and vascular structures. *Circulation*, **49**:13, 1974.

Crawford, S. E.; Crook, W. G.; Harrison, W. W.; and Somervill, B.: Histoplasmosis as a cause of acute myocarditis and pericarditis. Report of occurrence in siblings and a review of the literature. *Pediatrics*, **28**:92, 1961.

Crevald, S. van; Groot, J. W. de; Hartog, H. A. P.; and Lie, Sing Kiem: Diagnosis and treatment of acute interstitial myocarditis in infancy. *Ann. Paediatr.*, **183**:193, 1954.

Dalgaard, J. B.: Fatal myocarditis following smallpox vaccination. *Am. Heart J.*, **54**:156, 1957.

De La Chapelle, C. E., and Graef, I.: Acute isolate myocarditis with report of a case. *Arch. Intern. Med.*, **47**:942, 1931.

De La Chapelle, C. E., and Kossman, C. E.: Myocarditis. *Circulation*, **10**:747, 1954.

Di Sant'Agnese, P.; Anderson, D. H.; and Mason, H. H.: Glycogen storage disease of heart. *Pediatrics*, **6**:607, 1950.

Dolgopol, V. B., and Cragan, M. D.: Myocardial changes in poliomyelitis. *Arch. Pathol.*, **46**:202, 1948.

Dominguez, P.; Leindrum, B. L.; and Pick, A.: False "coronary patterns" in the infant electrocardiogram. *Circulation*, **19**:409, 1959.

Drennan, J. M.: Acute isolated myocarditis in newborn infants. *Arch. Dis. Child.*, **28**:288, 1953.

Ehlers, K. H.; Hagstrom, J. W. C.; Lukas, D. S.; Redo, S. F.; and Engle, M. A.: Glycogen-storage disease of the myocardium with obstruction to left ventricular outflow. *Circulation*, **25**:96, 1962.

Farber, R.: Personal communication, 1955.

Fejfar, Z.: Cardiomyopathies—An international problem. *Cardiologia*, **52**:9, 1968.

Fiedler, A.: *Festschrit zur Feier des 50 jahringen Bestehens des Stadtkrankenhauses zu Dresden*. Friedrichstadt, Dresden, 1899.

Fine, I.; Brainerd, H.; and Sokolow, M.: Myocarditis in acute infectious diseases. A clinical and electrocardiographic study. *Circulation*, **2**:859, 1950.

Friedman, I.; Laufer, A.; Ron, N.; and Davies, A. M.: Experimental myocarditis. In vitro and in vivo studies of lymphocytes sensitized to heart extracts and group A streptococci. *Immunology*, **20**:225, 1971.

French, A. J., and Weller, C. V.: Interstitial myocarditis following the clinical and experimental use of sulfonamide drugs. *Am. J. Pathol.*, **18**:109, 1942.

Freundlich, E.; Berkowitz, M.; Elkon, A.; and Wilder, A.: Primary interstitial myocarditis. *Am. J. Dis. Child.*, **96**:43, 1958.

Garrison, R. F., and Swisher, R. C.: Myocarditis of unknown etiology (Fiedler's) treated with ACTH; report of a case in a 7 year old boy with improvement. *J. Pediatr.*, **42**:591, 1953.

Garrow, J. S., and Pike, M. C.: The long-term prognosis of severe infantile malnutrition. *Lancet*, **1**:1, 1967.

Gefter, W. I.; Leaman, W. G., Jr.; Lucchesi, P. F.; Mager, I. E.; and

Dworin, M.: The heart in acute anterior poliomyelitis. *Am. Heart J.*, **33**:228, 1947.

Goldberg, G. M.: Myocarditis of giant-cell type in an infant. *Am. J. Clin. Pathol.*, **25**:510, 1955.

Goldfield, M.; Boyer, N. H.; and Weinstein, L.: Electrocardiographic changes during the course of measles. *J. Pediatr.*, **46**:30, 1955.

Goodwin, J. F.: Clarification of the cardiomyopathies. *Mod. Conc. Cardiovasc. Dis.*, **41**:41, 1972.

Gore, I.: Myocardial changes in fatal diphtheria. A summary of observations in 221 cases. *Am. J. Med. Sci.*, **215**:257, 1948.

Gore, I., and Saphir, O.: Myocarditis. A classification of 1402 cases. *Am. Heart J.*, **34**:827, 1947.

Harris, L. E., and Nghiem, Q. X.: Cardiomyopathies in infants and children. *Prog. Cardiovasc. Dis.*, **15**:255, 1972.

Hirschman, S. Z., and Hammer, G. S.: Coxsackie virus myopericarditis—A microbiological and clinical review. *Am. J. Cardiol.*, **34**:1974.

Hodge, P. R.; and Lawrence, J. R.: Two cases of myocarditis associated with phenylbutazone therapy. *Med. J. Aust.*, **1**:640, 1957.

Horton, G. E.: Mumps myocarditis: case report with review of the literature. *Ann. Intern. Med.*, **49**:1228, 1958.

Hosier, D. M., and Newton, W. A.: Serious coxsackie infection in infants and children. *Am. J. Dis. Child.*, **96**:251, 1958.

Hudson, G.: Bone-marrow volume in the human foetus and newborn. *Br. J. Haematol.*, **11**:446, 1965.

Iams, A. M., and Keith, H. M.: Histoplasmosis in infancy. *J. Pediatr.*, **30**:123, 1947.

Javett, S. W.; Heymann, S.; Mundel, B.; Pepler, W. J.; Lurie, H. I.; Gear, J.; Measroch, V.; and Kirsch, Z.: Myocarditis in the newborn infant. *J. Paediatr.*, **48**:1, 1956.

Joos, H. A., and Yu, P. N. G.: Electrocardiographic observations in poliomyelitis. Changes of the Q-T interval in twenty-three cases. *Am. J. Dis. Child.*, **80**:22, 1950.

Jurow, S. S., and Dolgopol, V. B.: Interstitial pneumonia and focal mycarditis in poliomyelitis. *Am. J. Med. Sci.*, **226**:393, 1953.

Karni, H.: Sudden death due to myocarditis, A clinical and pathological study. *Acta Med. Scand.*, **149**:243, 1954.

Kavelman, D. A.: Myocarditis. *Can. Med. Assoc. J.*, **79**:33, 1958.

Keith, J. D.: Unpublished findings, 1955.

Kilbrick, S.: Viral infections of the fetus and newborn. In *Perspectives in Virology*. Burgess, Minneapolis, 1961, Vol. II, p. 140.

Kilbrick, S.; and Benirschke, K.: Acute aseptic myocarditis and meningoencephalitis in the newborn child infected with coxsackie virus group B type 3. *N. Engl. J. Med.*, **225**:883, 1956.

Kipkie, G. F., and McAuley, J. S. M.: Acute myocarditis occurring in bulbar poliomyelitis. *Can. Med. Assoc. J.*, **70**:315, 1954.

Koontz, C. H., and Ray, C. G.: The role of Coxsackie group B virus infections in sporadic myopericarditis. *Am. Heart J.*, **82**:750, 1971.

Lambert, E. C.: Personal communication, 1955.

Lambert, E. C.; Shumway, C. N.; and Terplan, K.: Clinical diagnosis of endocardial fibrosis. Analysis of literature with report of four new cases. *Pediatrics*, **11**:255, 1953.

Laranja, F. S.; Dias, E.; Nobrega, G.; and Miranda, A.: Chagas' disease. A clinical epidemiologic and pathologic study. *Circulation*, **14**:1035, 1956.

Larson, C. P.: Pathology of poliomyelitis. *Northwest Med.*, **40**:448, 1941.

Lerner, A. M.; Klein, J. O.; and Finland, M.: A laboratory outbreak of infections with coxsackie virus group A, type 9. *N. Engl. J. Med.*, **263**:1302, 1960.

Lind, J., and Hulquist, G. T.: Isolated myocarditis in newborn and young infants. *Am. Heart J.*, **38**:123, 1949.

Lipman, W. H.: Idiopathic myocarditis in infants and children. *Wisconsin Med. J.*, **53**:578, 1954.

Lustok, M. J.; Chase, J.; and Lubitz, J. M.: Myocarditis: a clinical and pathologic study of forty-five cases. *Dis. Chest*, **28**:243, 1955.

MacMahon, H. E.: Infantile xanthomatous cardiomyopathy. *Pediatrics*, **48**:312, 1971.

McCue, C. M.: Three cases of myocarditis in children less than one year of age. *Pediatrics*, **21**:710, 1958.

McGiven, A. R.: Myocardial fibrosis in fibrocystic disease of the pancreas. *Arch. Dis. Child.*, **37**:656, 1962.

Mainzer, F.: Electrocardiographic study of typhoid myocarditis. *Br. Heart J.*, **9**:145, 1947.

Miall, W. E., and Bras, G.: Heart disease in the tropics. *Br. Med. Bull.*, **28**:79, 1972.

Mogabgab, W. J.: Virus myocarditis. *Am. Heart J.*, **53**:485, 1957.

Moritz, A. R., and Zamcheck, N.: Sudden and unexpected deaths of young soldiers. *Arch. Pathol.*, **42**:459, 1946.

Neustadt, D. H.: Transient electrocardiographic changes simulating an acute myocarditis in serum sickness. *Ann. Intern. Med.*, **39**:126, 1953.

Nihoyannopoulos, J.: Personal communication, 1963.

Nihoyannopoulos, J., and Agoroyannis, S.: Disorders of cardiac rhythm in diphtheria. Fascicular blocks and their prognostic value. *Proc. Ass. Eur. Pediatr. Cardiol.*, **8**:61, 1972.

Perloff, J. K.: The cardiomyopathies—Current perspectives. *Circulation*, **44**:942, 1971.

Powell, L. W.; Newman, S.; and Hooker, J. W.: Cystic fibrosis of the pancreas complicated by myocardial fibrosis. *V. Med. Mon.*, **87**:187, 1957.

Prata, A.; Andrade, Z.; and Guimaraes, A.: Chagas' heart disease. In Shaper, A. G.; Hutt, M. S. R.; and Fejfar, Z. (eds.): *Cardiovascular Disease in the Tropics.* International Society of Cardiology, British Medical Association, London, 1974, p. 264.

Puigbo, J. J.; Nava-Rhode, J. R.; Garcia, Barrios, H.; Suarez, J. A.; and Til Yepex, C.: Clinical and epidemiological study of Chagas' chronic heart involvement. *Bull. WHO*, **34**:655, 1966.

Reid, J. D.; Hajdun, S. I.; and Attah, E.: Infantile cardiomyopathy; previously unrecognized type with histiocytoid reaction. *J. Pediatr.*, **73**:335, 1968.

Rocha, H.: Chagas' disease. In Beeson, Paul B.: *Cecil-Loeb Textbook of Medicine*, 13th ed. Philadelphia, W. B. Saunders, 1971, p. 717.

Rosenbaum, H. D.; Nadas, A. S.; and Neuhauser, E. B. D.: Primary myocardial disease in infancy and childhood. *Am. J. Dis. Child.*, **86**:28, 1953.

Rosenberg, H. S., and McNamara, D. G.: Acute myocarditis in infancy and childhood. *Prog. Cardiovasc. Dis.*, **7**:179, 1964.

Ross, L. J.: Electrocardiographic findings in measles. *Am. J. Dis. Child.*, **83**:282, 1952.

Sahn, D. J.; Vaucher, Y.; Williams, D. E.; Allen, H. E.; Goldberg, S. J.; and Friedman, W. F.: Echocardiographic detection of large left-to-right shunts and cardiomyopathies in infants and children. *Am. J. Cardiol.*, **38**:73, 1976.

Saphir, O.: Encephalomyocarditis. *Circulation*, **6**:843, 1952.

———: Nonrheumatic inflammatory diseases of the heart. C. Myocarditis. In Gould, S. E. (ed.): *Pathology of the Heart.* Charles C Thomas, Publisher, Springfield, Ill., 1953, pp. 784–835.

———: Myocarditis. *Am. Heart J.*, **57**:639, 1959.

Saphir, O., and Field, M.: Complications of myocarditis in children. *J. Pediatr.*, **45**:457, 1954.

Saphir, O.; Wile, S. A.; and Reingold, I. M.: Myocarditis in children. *Am. J. Dis. Child.*, **67**:294, 1944.

Sayers, E. G.: Diphtheric myocarditis with permanent heart damage. *Ann. Intern. Med.*, **48**:146, 1958.

Schnitzer, R.: Myocardial tuberculosis with paroxysmal ventricular tachycardia. *Br. Heart J.*, **9**:213, 1947.

Segar, L. F.; Kashtan, H. A.; and Miller, Captain, P. B.: Trichinosis with myocarditis, report of a case treated with ACTH. *N. Engl. J. Med.*, **252**:397, 1955.

Shaper, A. G.: Endomyocardial fibrosis and rheumatic heart disease. *Lancet*, **1**:639, 1966.

Shaper, A. G.; Hutt, M. S. R.; and Coles, R. M.: Necropsy study of endomyocardial fibrosis and rheumatic heart disease in Uganda 1950–65. *Br. Heart J.*, **30**:391, 1968.

Sims, B. A.: Conducting tissue of the heart in kwashiorkor. *Br. Heart J.*, **34**:828, 1972.

Smith, W. G.: Coxsackie B myopericarditis in adults. *Am. Heart J.*, **80**:34, 1970.

Smythe, P. M.; Swanepoel, A.; and Campbell, J. A. J.: The heart in kwashiorkor. *Br. Med. J.*, **1**:67, 1962.

Somers, K.; Brenton, D. P.; and Sood, N. K.: The clinical features of endomyocardial fibrosis of the right ventricle. *Br. Heart J.*, **30**:309, 1968.

Stoeber, E.: Weitere untersuchungen uber epidemische myocarditis (Schwielenherz) des Sauglings. *Ztschr. Kinderheilk.*, **71**:319, 1952.

———: Weitere untersuchungen uber epidemische myocarditis (Schwielenherz) des Sauglings. *Ztschr. Kinderheilk.*, **71**:592, 1952.

Stone, W. J.: The heart muscle changes in pneumonia with remarks on digitalis therapy. *Am. J. Med. Sci.*, **163**:659, 1922.

Suckling, P. V., and Vogelpoel, L.: Viral myocarditis. *Med. Proc.*, **4**:372, 1958.

Surawicz, B.; and Lepeschkin, E.: The electrocardiographic pattern of hypopotassemia with and without hypocalcemia. *Circulation*, **8**:801, 1953.

Swanepoel, A.; Smythe, P. M.; and Campbell, J. A. H.: The heart in kwashiorkor. *Am. Heart J.*, **67**:1, 1964.

Tedeschi, C. G., and Stevenson, T. D., Jr.: Interstitial myocarditis in children. *N. Engl. J. Med.*, **244**:352, 1951.

Van Creveld, S.; De Groot, J. W.; Hartof, H. A. PH.; and Kiem, L. S.: Diagnosis and treatment of acute interstitial myocarditis in infancy. *Ann. Paediatr.*, **183**:193, 1954.

Van Der Spuy, J. C.: Mitral valve pericardioplasty—A long-term follow-up study. *Thorax*, **27**:207, 1972.

Weber, M. W.; Baldwin, J. S.; and Hall, J. W.: Acute isolated myocarditis: review of the literature and a report of a case in a 10 year old child. *Pediatrics*, **3**:829, 1949.

Weinstein, L., and Shelokov, A.: Cardiovascular manifestations in acute poliomyelitis. *N. Engl. J. Med.*, **244**:281, 1951.

Wells, A. H., and Sax, S. G.: Isolated myocarditis probably of sulfonamide origin. *Am. Heart J.*, **30**:522, 1945.

Wenger, N. K.: Infectious myocarditis. *Cardiovasc. Clin.*, **4**:167, 1972.

Williams, H.; O'Reilly, R. N.; and Williams, A.: Fourteen cases of idiopathic myocarditis in infants and children. *Arch. Dis. Child.*, **28**:271, 1953.

Woodward, T. E.; McCrumb, F. R., Jr.; Carey, T. N.; and Togo, Y.: Viral and rickettsial causes of cardiac disease, including the coxsackie virus etiology of pericarditis and myocarditis. *Ann. Intern. Med.*, **53**:1130, 1960.

Woody, N. C., and Woody, H. B.: American trypanosomiasis. I. Clinical and epidemiologic background of Chagas' disease in the United States. *J. Pediatr.*, **58**:568, 1961.

World Health Organization: Study group on Chagas' disease. Techn. Rep. Ser. 202, 1960.

Yarom, R.; Laufer, A.; and Davies, A. M.: Effect of repeated isoproterenol administration in young rats—a histological and serological study. *Pathol. Microbiol.*, **36**:65, 1970.

Ziegler, R.: Characteristics of the unipolar precordial electrocardiogram in normal infants. *Circulation*, **3**:438, 1951.

Zuppinger, H.: Zur Kenntniss der diffusen chronischen Myocarditis bei Kindern. *Arch. Kinderh.*, **35**:381, 1902–3.

52

Endocardial Fibroelastosis

John D. Keith, Vera Rose, and *James A. Manning*

ENDOCARDIAL fibroelastosis is a disease entity that has been described under a variety of terms in past years. "Fetal endocarditis," "endocardial sclerosis," and "endomyocardial fibroelastosis" are the chief ones. Undoubtedly many cases were listed over the years under the term "idiopathic hypertrophy of the heart." From the reports of Rauchfuss (1878), it seems likely that Kreysig was the first to describe this lesion in 1816, and at that time he applied to it the term "fetal endocarditis." A thorough pathologic review of the subject by Gross (1941) has helped to clarify the abnormal findings.

Classification

Several classifications of endocardial fibroelastosis have appeared in the literature (Anderson and Kelly, 1956; Hastreiter, 1969; Forfar et al., 1964).

The international classification published recently is as follows:

1. Endocardial fibroelastosis of left ventricle, left atrium, right ventricle, right atrium.
2. Involvement of the valves may be specified—aortic, mitral, pulmonary, or tricuspid.
3. Associated congenital heart defect, such as coarctation of the aorta, patent ductus arteriosus, complete heart block, Wolff–Parkinson–White syndrome, anomalous coronary artery arising from the pulmonary artery, aortic atresia, mitral stenosis, etc.

In most cases the left ventricle is involved and the chamber enlarged and dilated. However, in a few cases, it may be contracted, and in such instances, it is more likely to be associated with aortic or mitral valve stenosis and occasionally is contracted as an isolated lesion.

Endocardial fibroelastosis occurs characteristically in the left ventricle, but when it is involved, the left atrium is also affected to some degree in approximately 60 percent of cases. If the endocardium is inspected carefully in the right ventricle,

some endocardial fibroelastosis may also be present in 20 percent of cases. Rarely is the right atrium involved.

Incidence

The prevalence of endocardial fibroelastosis has been reported in the past as an autopsy diagnosis and related to the total number of congenital heart defects seen at postmortem in any particular institution. Such prevalence may vary, depending on how diligently one looks for minor degrees of endocardial fibroelastosis found at autopsy. Table 52–1 shows figures from four reviews appearing in the literature.

Table 52–1. INCIDENCE OF ALL TYPES (COMPLICATED, UNCOMPLICATED) OF ENDOCARDIAL FIBROELASTOSIS FOUND AT AUTOPSY

Lambert and Vlad, 1958	7% of children with congenital heart disease seen at postmortem
Fontana and Edwards, 1962	5% of children seen with congenital heart disease
Forfar et al., 1964	17% of children seen with congenital heart disease
Gasul et al., 1967	7.7% of children seen with congenital heart disease

It is generally recognized that approximately 75 percent of children who exhibit endocardial fibroelastosis when the heart is opened have a complicated form associated with other heart defects. In twenty-five percent it appears as an isolated or uncomplicated lesion (Forfar et al., 1964, 22 percent; Halliday, 1954, 23 percent; Fontana and Edwards, 1962, 33 percent).

It is most essential to realize that the above figures relate to an autopsy diagnosis. Another approach to the problem of incidence relates to the numbers found in the total clinical population of congenital heart disease. In 15,104 cases of congenital heart disease from The Hospital for Sick Children 0.94 percent had endocardial fibroelastosis. Mitchell and associates

(1971) reported seven cases out of 350 cases of congenital heart disease, giving an incidence of 2.4 percent.

Forfar and associates (1964) pointed out the interesting fact that the longer these affected babies survive in the first year of life, the more likely they are to have a more extensive form of endocardial fibroelastosis and more chambers involved. Thus, those that have one chamber involved live an average of 120 days; when two chambers were affected it was 260 days, and with three chambers it was 300 days. They found no cases of endocardial fibroelastosis among their 50 stillbirths, although it has occasionally been reported in the past by other authors.

Pathology

Almost invariably there is considerable cardiac enlargement present, the heart being two to four times the normal weight for the age group concerned (Prior and Wyatt, 1950). Dennis and coworkers (1953) report that 94 percent of 119 cases reviewed in the literature had cardiac enlargement. The endocardium of the left side of the heart was involved in 98 percent of the cases: as well as right and left sides in 16 percent and the left side alone in 82 percent. Thus, only occasionally does the right side of the heart show either hypertrophy or endocardial change.

The characteristic lesion is a thickened layer of pearly whiteness covering the inner wall of the left ventricle and left atrium. It feels stiff and rubbery in consistency and is spread diffusely over the endocardium of both ventricle and atrium, although at times its distribution may be patchy (see Figure 52–1).

Valvular deformities are present in 34 to 51 percent of cases (Lambert et al., 1953; Dennis et al., 1953). The aortic and mitral valves are most commonly involved, although the tricuspid and pulmonary valves may occasionally show a similar pathologic structure. Some involvement of the valve is present in many cases with or without physical signs.

Microscopically, there is seen a hyperplasia of the fibrous and elastic tissue of the endocardium. The subendocardial-myocardial junction usually shows a few degenerating muscle fibers; diffuse round-cell infiltration of a minor degree and vacuolation may occasionally be seen in the same area. The mass of the myocardium is not involved except by hypertrophy in the vast majority of cases, but occasionally an associated myocarditis may be present and exhibit a cellular infiltration.

Blumberg and Lyon (1952) and Halliday (1954) found that 28 to 53 percent of cases of endocardial fibroelastosis have associated congenital heart defects. The most common of these are coarctation of the aorta, patent ductus arteriosus, and aortic atresia, but other types may be found in combination with endocardial fibroelastosis.

The hypoplastic left ventricle stands as a special group between primary endocardial fibroelastosis without valvular lesion, on the one hand, and aortic atresia, on the other. In such cases the aortic valve ring is hypoplastic and the aortic valve may appear small but normal. Frequently, however, the aortic valve with hypoplastic left ventricle presents a gnarled, abnormal edge with a narrowed aperture. These children have a left ventricular cavity that is reduced in size and is characteristically surrounded by a massively hypertrophied ventricular wall. This hypertrophy may not be related to an excessive work load during fetal life any more than it is in aortic atresia where the cavity of the left ventricle usually does not function at all. However, after birth this contracted and somewhat hypoplastic left ventricle is responsible for maintaining the systemic circulation. This type of case is almost invariably associated with endocardial fibroelastosis. In spite of the gross muscular hypertrophy of the ventricular wall, the heart is unable to maintain the circulation, and the infant dies early as a rule. It seems unlikely that any of these cases survive since one never finds this type of pathologic picture in infants dying after one to two years of age.

History During Pregnancy

There is rarely any evidence in the pregnancy history of an etiologic factor that might be related to endocardial fibroelastosis. Two mothers in our series had difficulty at the later stages of pregnancy: one had toxemia and the baby had respiratory distress for a short time after delivery, and the other gave birth to a baby who appeared well initially but soon developed congestive heart failure. Kelly and Anderson (1956) and Chen and associates (1971) also found no significant history of maternal illness in 17 pregnancy cases. Noren and associates (1963) recorded two instances of mumps during early pregnancy.

Birth Rank

Data regarding birth order were reported by Sellers, Keith, and Manning (1964) in 51 families and by Chen and associates (1971) in 119 families. There was evidence of increased probability of endocardial fibroelastosis with increase in birth rank.

Birth Weight

The average birth weight of male and female infants in our series was 3246 and 3133 gm, respectively. Eighty percent of both groups of cases had birth weights within the 10 to 90 percentile range. Approximately 8 percent were premature by weight, that is, weighed 2180 to 2450 gm. Chen and associates (1971) showed that the mean birth weight was not significantly different for affected patients when compared with normal infants.

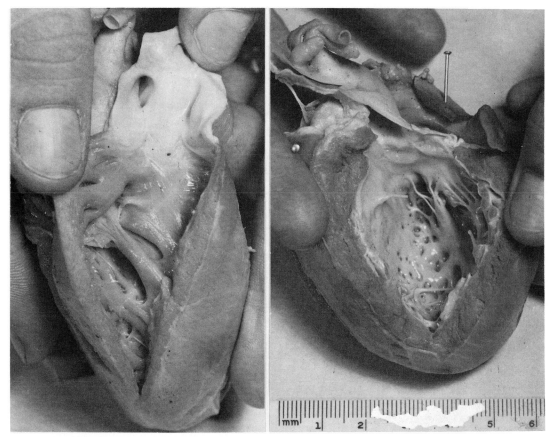

Figure 52-1. Right and left ventricles of M. W., aged five and one-half months. Right ventricle has normal endocardium; left ventricle shows typical endocardial fibroelastosis, pearly-white thickness.

Sex Ratio

The females predominated slightly over the males in the experience at The Hospital for Sick Children. However, this was only true in the absence of associated valvular disease. When the latter complication was present, males predominated.

Maternal Age

Infants with endocardial fibroelastosis were born most frequently to mothers in the age group 25 to 29 years. This corresponds to the peak incidence of childbirth in the general population. Analysis of the data, however, suggests that endocardial fibroelastosis does not occur as frequently in older mothers as in the younger ones despite the higher frequency of primary endocardial fibroelastosis with progressive birth rank. This observation could have resulted from deliberate restriction of pregnancies following the birth of an affected child.

Familial Incidence

In several studies reported elsewhere multiple cases have occurred. This is the situation in nine of the families investigated at The Hospital for Sick Children. The presence of one known case of endocardial fibroelastosis in the family increases the recurrence risk to over 17 percent. After a second affected child the figure jumps to 33 percent (Chen et al., 1971).

Etiology

The etiology is unknown. Several concepts of pathogenesis have been suggested: (1) inflammation, (2) congenital developmental defect, (3) anoxia, (4) deposition of fibrin, and (5) hereditary defect.

Inflammation. In the time of Kreysig in 1816, intrauterine infection was considered the prime etiologic factor. However, both Gross (1941) and Campbell (1949) presented evidence against this hypothesis. No maternal rubella was found in the history of these infants, and it was pointed out that pathologic material was not indicative of infection but, rather, suggested a hyperplastic or degenerative process. Leary and associates (1949), however, reported one case of endocardial fibroelastosis following infectious mononucleosis. Frühling and associates (1962) and Hastreiter and Miller (1964) have assembled evidence suggesting that Coxsackie virus may be an etiologic factor. Studies of animal models by Noren and associates (1970) indicated that endocardial fibroelastosis comes by the end stage of an inflammatory process in the myocardium secondary to viral infection.

Congenital Developmental Defect.   Weinberg and Himmelfarb (1943) advanced the hypothesis that a congenital developmental defect of the endocardium was responsible. This was supported by the fact that a high percentage of the cases are associated with other congenital heart defects, with the lesions obviously existing before birth in many instances, and also because elastic tissue is known to be influenced by a variety of factors during embryologic development. There have been reports of ten sets of twins, and only one set had both children affected. Monozygosity did not appear to be a factor.

Data regarding siblings were available in 45 cases reported by Sellers, Keith, and Manning (1964) and 119 patient families studied by Chen et al. (1971). In nine families multiple cases occurred. Thus the presence of a known case of endocardial fibroelastosis in the family increased slightly the possibility of another case occurring in a later pregnancy.

Hypoxia.   Many authors have mentioned the possible relation of the endocardial lesion to hypoxia (Paul and Robbins, 1955). Johnson (1952) suggested that premature closure of the foramen ovale before birth might lead to left atrium and ventricular vascular stasis and anoxia.

This theory is largely invalidated by the fact that endocardial fibroelastosis has been demonstrated in a number of cases with an open foramen ovale (Halliday, 1954). Furthermore, the evidence is rather in the opposite direction and suggests that oxygen itself might be the noxious agent. The noxious effects of hyperoxia on developing vascular tissue are now established as the cause of retrolental fibroplasia, a similar lesion in premature infants. The fact that the left side of the heart is involved in endocardial fibroelastosis is also significant, since the lesion appears to develop in most cases after birth when the oxygen content of the arterial blood of the left side of the heart is raised. When it occurs in aortic atresia, it is only found in those cases with open mitral valves. Thus, when there is a closed mitral valve and stasis in the small left ventricle, no endocardial fibroelastosis occurs. When endocardial fibroelastosis appears in conjunction with other congenital heart defects, it is usually found in the noncyanotic lesions, such as coarctation of the aorta and patent ductus arteriosus. It has not been reported in tricuspid atresia, in which defect the blood in the left ventricle is always cyanotic.

Anderson and Kelly have pointed out endocardial fibroelastosis of a mild degree may occur with anomalous left coronary from the pulmonary artery. This form of fibroelastosis may well be related to the inadequate circulation to the left ventricle.

Deposition of Fibrin.   Still and Boult (1956) have studied the endocardial tissue of six cases of endocardial fibroelastosis by electron microscopy and report that the surface layers are composed almost solely of fibers morphologically indistinguishable from fibrin. This hypothesis of the deposition on the endocardium of fine layers of fibrin from the blood appears to be supported by the finding of endocardial fibroelastosis in the left ventricle only in those cases of aortic atresia that have an open mitral valve during development. When the left ventricle is sealed off with an atretic mitral valve, no endocardial lesion occurs.

Hereditary Defect.   Until recently the possible role of heredity in the etiology of endocardial fibroelastosis was not considered to be of importance. However, in 1955 Rosahn presented evidence in support of a recessive gene hypothesis by reporting similar endocardial involvement in two sibs and by citing two comparable cases from the literature (Weinberg and Himelfarb, 1943; Dordick, 1951). For further evidence he referred to Ullrich (1938), who reported that in a set of triplets the anomaly was found in two members who were identical whereas their fraternal triplet was unaffected. Sprague and associates (1931) also reported a case of endocardial fibroelastosis whose sib had remarkably similar symptoms, but no autopsy was obtained for proof. Hunter and Keay (1973) described four families each with more than one child affected, and autopsy-proven diagnosis in eight of nine cases. They suggested that the condition may be an autosomal dominant rather than a recessive trait. Lindenbaum et al. (1973), on the basis of one kindred examined, suggested that a proportion may be determined by X-linked genes. In nine pairs of twins reported in the literature only one member of each set was affected (Dissman, 1932; Wesson and Beaver, 1935; Roberts, 1936; Craig, 1949; Morison, 1949; Prior and Wyatt, 1950; and Kempton, 1953). The twin pairs reported by Morison and Kempton are known to be identical. In 119 patient families of endocardial fibroelastosis seen at The Hospital for Sick Children there have been nine families with more than one affected sib: seven with two affected sibs and two with three affected sibs. No single pattern of inheritance fitted the family data, but empiric risk figures were derived for family counseling. The hereditary factor present in some families, must play a role in patients with the disease.

Nonspecific Reaction Secondary to Ventricular Dilatation.   The concept that idiopathic endocardial fibroelastosis may be a nonspecific response to a number of causes of an increased mural tension was originally advanced by Black-Schaffer (1957) and has recently been attractively supported by Hutchins and Vie (1972). The basic idea is that any number of causes, such as interstitial myocarditis, obstructive lesions, etc., cause a marked ventricular dilatation and that this increase in endocardial tension in some physical way causes the development of fibroelastosis. This is an interesting hypothesis but it does not explain the remarkably similar clinical presentation that so many of these infants show, nor does it encompass the familial aspects of the process.

Clinical Features

It is necessary, first, to refer to the cases that have endocardial fibroelastosis associated with other congenital heart anomalies. The diagnosis of the endocardial lesion is difficult in these instances since there is usually no evidence to suggest its presence. One may suspect endocardial fibroelastosis when the diagnosis of aortic atresia is made since in our experience 60 percent of such cases also have the endocardial lesion. The association occurs in approximately 4 percent of cases of coarctation of the aorta and 1 percent of cases of patent ductus arteriosus and in 50 percent of children with evidence of aortic stenosis who develop heart failure in the first year of life.

The group that requires special attention is that of endocardial fibroelastosis without other anomalies. The age at death is shown in Figure 52–2. Death may occur at any age from birth to adult life. However, the greatest mortality is in the first six months of life; 75 percent have died by the end of the first year.

Many of these babies develop normally and appear healthy and well nourished until there is a sudden onset of signs and symptoms. In the more chronic cases, anorexia and failure to gain are common features, and approximately a third of the cases fall into this category (Dennis et al., 1953). Irritability is also a common finding; vomiting is less frequent.

The chief signs and symptoms are related to various stages of heart failure. When the infant is brought to the hospital, the liver is usually enlarged three to five finger-breadths below the costal margin.

Dyspnea. Dyspnea is one of the most common clinical manifestations, occurring in 91 percent (Lambert et al., 1953) and 89 percent (Dennis et al., 1953) of the cases. The dyspnea is usually characterized by a single increase in the respiratory rate, which varies from 40 to 100 per minute. There may be associated signs of distress, such as a grunt or crowlike sound, and frequently in the chronic cases there is a respiratory wheeze. A cough has been reported in approximately 40 percent, and it is most commonly due to the congestive heart failure but may be brought on by associated respiratory infection.

Cyanosis. As a general rule these babies do not appear significantly cyanotic, and in the cases in our group on whom oximetry was performed the arterial oxygen saturation was always above 85 percent and usually in the ninetieth percentile. Lambert and associates (1953), in their review of the literature, found that cyanosis was absent or intermittent in three-fourths of the cases. Except for the infants who

died in the first week of life, there was only one case where persistent cyanosis was reported. When present, the cyanosis was associated with severe heart failure or occurred as a terminal event. Oximetry findings suggest that it is peripheral in origin in some cases although in others it may be due to the marked pulmonary congestion.

Gallop Rhythm. Gallop rhythm is a common finding, occurring in 80 percent of our cases with congestive heart failure.

Valvular Involvement and Heart Murmurs. Lambert and associates (1953) noted that 34 percent of their cases had evidence of valvular involvement, and this coincided fairly well with their figure on the incidence of heart murmurs since 21 percent had significant murmurs audible. In order of frequency, mitral valvular involvement was first, aortic second.

In the series reported by Sellers, Keith, and Manning (1964), among 25 cases whose lesions were proved at autopsy to have no valvular disease, 15 had no murmur whatever, and ten had functional murmurs that could be differentiated from those due to valvular disease, but at times repeated examinations were necessary before a definitive opinion was established. Similarly, several examinations were also required in the 33 cases in the clinically diagnosed group. Eighteen percent of primary endocardial fibroelastosis patients have bicuspid aortic valve (see Chapter 38).

Radiologic Examination

Radiologic evidence of cardiac enlargement is found in all cases. The average cardiothoracic ratio is 69 percent, with a range of 56 to 80 percent in those who come to autopsy. Although the average heart size is similar in these two groups, only 14 percent of the clinical (surviving) group have a ratio greater than 70 percent, whereas 64 percent of the postmortem group have larger ratios (Sellers, Keith, and Manning, 1964) (see Figure 52–3).

On fluoroscopy left atrial enlargement, left ventricular enlargement, and low cardiac action are seen commonly. Except during congestive heart failure, the lung fields appear normal. Left atrial enlargement may at times be simulated by the hypertrophied and expanded left ventricle pressing back against the esophagus. This sign may also be present in the case of an aberrant left coronary arising from the pulmonary artery.

Electrocardiography

The electrocardiographic findings have been reviewed by Vlad and coworkers (1955) and Sellers, Keith, and Manning (1964). The material in both these papers was based primarily on complete electrocardiographic tracings on cases whose diagnosis was confirmed later at postmortem. The second study also included a group for comparison whose

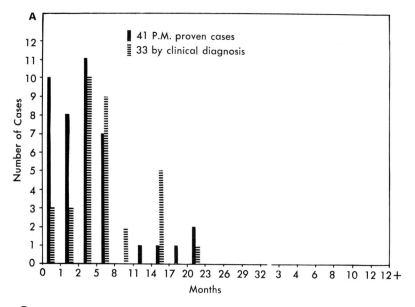

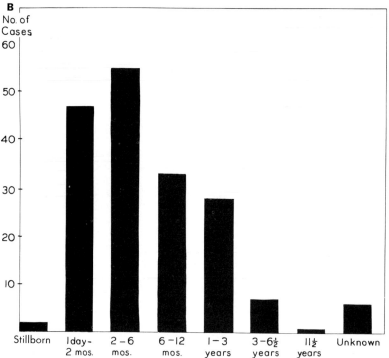

Figure 52-2. *A.* Clinical and postmortem cases of endocardial fibroelastosis at The Hospital for Sick Children, Toronto. *B.* Age at death of 179 cases of endocardial fibroelastosis.

diagnosis was made by clinical findings. Sinus rhythm is the rule, but heart block, complete or intermittent, may occasionally occur, particularly in the terminal stages.

The P-R interval is usually within normal limits (range 0.08 to 0.16 second, mean 0.12 second). The duration of the P wave averages 0.05 second, and only in rare occasions is it prolonged to 0.10 second.

The amplitude of the P wave averaged 2 mm, but in 35 percent of the autopsy cases it was 3 mm or more in height, whereas it was of this level in only 14 percent of

the clinically demonstrable cases. The QRS interval is rarely beyond the normal limits except in the terminal stages of the illness.

The T wave deflection in V_5 and/or V_6 was characteristically flattened or inverted both in the autopsy-proved group and in the clinical cases prior to the administration of digoxin. In the postmortem group reported by Sellers, Keith, and Manning, the average depth of the T wave in V_6 was -1.5 mm, and in 75 percent it was clearly inverted. The clinical cases had T waves that were a little deeper. The average depth was 2.5 mm, and in 95 percent they were clearly inverted. (See Figure 52–3.)

The mean electrical axis ranges from − 10 to + 110 and in 77 percent of the cases lies between + 20 and + 80 degrees. The frontal loop is almost invariably clockwise, although a counterclockwise loop was found in 5 to 10 percent of the cases.

The most significant part of the electrocardiographic tracing is the presence or absence of left loading patterns usually associated with increased voltage in the left ventricular precordial leads. Eighty-six percent of the cases proved at autopsy have left ventricular hypertrophy patterns as an isolated phenomenon. The remaining 14 percent have right ventricular loading alone or combined right and left patterns. Thus, the characteristic tracing may show a tall R wave in precordial lead V_6, or a tall R wave in RV_6 coupled with a deep S in precordial lead V_1, or a deep S wave in V_1 may be the only evidence of left ventricular hypertrophy. Thus, the overwhelming majority have evidence of left ventricular loading on voltage alone, and only occasionally does one need to depend on the R/S ratio in precordial lead V_1 for evidence of left ventricular dominance. Only with rare exceptions does one have difficulty in differentiating the electrocardiographic curves of endocardial fibroelastosis from myocarditis. The latter characteristically have low-voltage patterns (Sellers, Keith, and Manning, 1964).

These figures agree closely with the incidence of chamber hypertrophy reported by Lambert and coworkers (1953) and Dennis and associates (1953) on autopsy studies. Only occasionally was right ventricular hypertrophy noticed, and then it was usually associated with a tall R or a QR pattern in V and a deep S in V_6. There are several circumstances in which right ventricular hypertrophy may occur in endocardial fibroelastosis: (1) in the early weeks of life when the right ventricular pattern is likely to predominate; (2) in certain types such as the

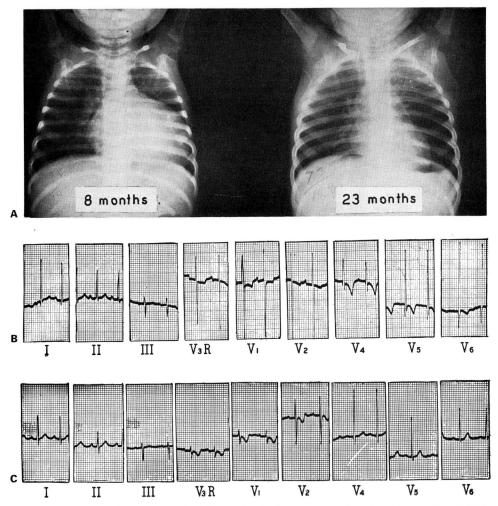

Figure 52-3. Endocardial fibroelastosis. *A.* X-rays showing heart grossly enlarged at eight months and within normal limits at 23 months. *B.* Electrocardiogram showing a left ventricular hypertrophy pattern at eight months of age. *C.* Normal electrocardiogram at three years.

contracted left ventricle with dilated right ventricle as described by Edwards (1953) and in the four-chamber involvement reported by Metianu and associates (1954); (3) with associated presence of other forms of congenital heart disease such as preductal coarctation in the aorta; and (4) in acute failure associated with a deep S in V_6 suggesting right ventricular hypertrophy probably due to a dilated heart; this S wave is likely to disappear with the administration of digitalis, and as clinical improvement takes place, the high voltage pattern of left ventricular dominance appears once more (see Figure 52–3).

Diagnosis

There has been some controversy over the years as to whether one can make a clinical diagnosis of endocardial fibroelastosis. We have been successful in doing so during life in 85 percent of those who later died, and we believe those who survived, since they had identical clinical findings, must have had the same pathology. However, leaving such discussions aside, it is generally agreed there is a syndrome in babies and young children with congestive heart failure and electrocardiographic signs that include left ventricular loading and flattening or inversion of the T waves in V_5 and V_6. We have excluded the cases with organic murmurs or with myocardial cellular infiltrate at autopsy.

This syndrome can be recognized and treated but requires a systematic review of the differential diagnosis.

There are two primary groups of endocardial fibroelastosis relating to diagnosis. The first is the group with associated congenital heart anomalies. The second group includes those cases without other defects.

In the first group the diagnosis of endocardial fibroelastosis is usually impossible or very difficult before necropsy. One may suspect it in the presence of aortic atresia since 60 percent have the endocardial lesion. An occasional case of coarctation of the aorta with endocardial fibroelastosis may reveal a greater degree of left ventricular hypertrophy in the electrocardiogram than one would expect (Vlad et al., 1955) and thus suggest the diagnosis, but in most instances the congenital heart anomaly dominates the clinical picture. The recognition of the endocardial lesion in this group is not important since the associated defect is dominant and usually controls the prognosis.

Over the past 25 years we have been impressed with the clinical findings in babies of congestive heart failure, a large heart, no murmurs, and a distinctive electrocardiographic pattern. In such cases we have made a diagnosis of endocardial fibroelastosis, and in many instances the baby has died in the next few days and the diagnosis has been confirmed.

During the course of this study we observed a group of cases that responded initially to therapy. They were followed for several years. Five of them died during the course of the follow-up, one to three years after the original clinical diagnosis had been made. All five were found to have the typical endocardial lesion at autopsy.

One case not included in this series had been diagnosed as endocardial fibroelastosis in 1953 and responded well to therapy, with return of the heart size and electrocardiogram to normal. At the age of seven years this child developed an unrelated attack of nephritis and died. At autopsy pearly-white thickening of the endocardium of the left ventricle was readily seen and appeared similar to that seen in infants dying in the first year of life.

The problem in diagnosis involves differentiation of conditions in which congestive heart failure occurs in infancy unaccompanied by a significant heart murmur and in which the electrocardiogram indicates a left ventricular overload. Idiopathic myocarditis and an anomalous left coronary artery arising from the pulmonary artery, calcification of the coronary arteries, glycogen-storage disease of the heart, medial necrosis of the coronary arteries, coarctation of the aorta, aortic stenosis, and mitral insufficiency are the chief defects that must be considered. Many of these lesions may be associated with a mild secondary endocardial fibrotic reaction that is, however, relatively insignificant when compared with the endocardium in the classic picture of primary endocardial fibroelastosis. The problem of differential diagnosis has been greatly helped by the noninvasive technique of echocardiography and radionuclear investigations.

Recently ultrasound echocardiography has been used in the definition of endocardial fibroelastosis from hypertrophic cardiomyopathies. Studies by Chung, Manning, and Gramiak (1973) in patients with endocardial fibroelastosis have shown a left ventricular diameter and left ventricular outflow width twice as large as control; septal thickness and mitral valve systolic motion were normal. In hypertrophic cardiomyopathy, there was a marked narrowing of the left ventricular outflow tract, left ventricular diameter was diminished slightly, and there was an abnormal systolic movement of the anterior leaflet of the mitral valve. Nuclear medicine is valuable in the noninvasive assessment of cardiac function and performance in endocardial fibroelastosis. Radionuclide angiography and gated blood pool studies are used for this purpose. Myocardial perfusion and viability are assessed using radionuclides which accumulate maximally in normal myocardium as is the case with thallium 201.

Coarctation of the aorta is readily ruled out by determination of the blood pressure in arm and leg. When both coarctation and endocardial fibroelastosis exist together, the electrocardiogram usually shows a left ventricular strain pattern that is unusual in coarctation of the aorta alone. Thus, the correct diagnosis of the double lesion is usually possible and may be confirmed at operation by a biopsy of the left atrium. We have done this in one of our cases. Patent ductus arteriosus usually has the characteristic continuous murmur. When such murmur is not present, the more marked left ventricular hypertrophy pattern in the electrocardiogram plus enlargement of the left atrium may distinguish endocardial fibroelastosis. Babies with tricuspid atresia have much more cyanosis as a rule than those with endocardial fibroelastosis and, furthermore, the cyanosis shows a significant increase with crying. The heart shape is often characteristic in tricuspid atresia, whereas in endocardial fibroelastosis the heart shows generalized enlargement. Furthermore, the electrocardiogram shows a horizontal heart in tricuspid atresia and most frequently the T waves in the left precordium are upright. Doubtful cases may have the diagnosis clarified by echocardiography and angiography. In aortic pulmonary septal defect there is usually less evidence of left ventricular hypertrophy; the hilar shadows are more engorged as a rule and may be pulsating. However, it may require an angiocardiogram and cardiac catheterization to fully differentiate the two.

Aortic stenosis may show a similar electrocardiographic picture, but a loud murmur is usually heard in the aortic area accompanied by a thrill. Occasionally the murmur of aortic stenosis may be absent or heard down the left sternal border. In such cases, if the differential diagnosis becomes of crucial importance, one may be justified in obtaining a left ventricular pressure curve either by the Björk needle through the left atrium or via the trachea into the left atrium. Finally, it should be remembered that aortic stenosis and endocardial fibroelastosis may coexist.

Differential Diagnosis

Anomalous Left Coronary Artery. Many reports have appeared in the literature of an anomalous left coronary artery arising from the pulmonary artery. A few cases survived into adult life, but such individuals did not present signs or symptoms during infancy. Infants with this anomaly usually have a distinctive picture, the vast majority show signs and symptoms in the first four months of life, rarely before two months of age. The onset is heart failure, dyspnea, large liver, and, in a few cases, screaming or crying as if the infant were in pain.

The electrocardiogram is very helpful in making the differential diagnosis. All the cases of anomalous coronary from the pulmonary artery that develop congestive failure in infancy eventually show the ischemic pattern of myocardial infarction. This change is associated with a left ventricular loading pattern usually of the type that produces a deep S in V_1 rather than a tall R in V_6. Characteristically, there is a deep Q wave in leads I, aV_L, and V_5 and V_6. The S-T segment in V_5 and V_6 is elevated distinctly in the majority of cases, although it may be depressed. The pattern is that of an anterolateral myocardial infarction. While the electrocardiogram is almost invariably diagnostic, confirmatory evidence can be obtained noninvasively from myocardial imaging

using thallium 201 which will show defective uptake of the radionuclide in the infarcted myocardium. An aortogram with the tip of the catheter in the region of the coronary arteries will reveal a large, completely filled right coronary artery arising from the aorta and will show an absence of left coronary arising from the aorta, indicating its anomalous presence elsewhere. The cases of anomalous left coronary artery arising from the pulmonary artery that develop heart failure in infancy, almost without exception, are dead by the end of the first year of life.

It should be noted that the number of cases of anomalous coronary arising from the pulmonary artery have a mild, pallid degree of endocardial fibroelastosis of the left ventricle at postmortem examination, which is obviously a secondary phenomenon and does not rival the dense lesion of primary endocardial fibroelastosis.

Calcification of Coronary Arteries. Calcification of the coronary arteries in infancy is associated with widespread calcification of the arteries throughout the body and may involve the renal and thyroid vessels and the arteries of numerous other vital organs (Cochrane and Bowden, 1954). In the majority of cases these infants die because of the general arterial involvement rather than the specific effect on the heart, but occasionally congestive heart failure may occur and produce an electrocardiographic pattern similar to that found in endocardial fibroelastosis. Thus, the clinical picture, the electrocardiographic findings, and the calcification of the coronary arteries may at times be indistinguishable from primary endocardial fibroelastosis. Although this condition must be considered in the differential diagnosis, it apparently does not represent a real problem, since it is so rare. It is uniformly fatal and does not respond to digitalis. X-ray of the various portions of the body may reveal calcification of the arteries and thus lead to the correct diagnosis.

Glycogen-Storage Disease of the Heart. Glycogen-storage disease of the heart is a uniformly fatal disease in infancy, and death usually occurs during the first eight months of life. The electrocardiogram may show left ventricular loading with T wave inversion in V_6, and usually has a short PR interval. The echocardiogram usually confirms the presence of an infective myocardial lesion.

The majority of these children have a history of generalized muscular weakness from birth and characteristically have macroglossia. A histologic section from an involved muscle may reveal the true diagnosis.

Myocarditis. A review of the clinical findings and especially the electrocardiogram indicates that the differentiation between endocardial fibroelastosis and myocarditis can usually be made during life.

The pattern of age of onset in myocarditis differs somewhat from that of endocardial fibroelastosis. Recent literature demonstrates that Coxsackie myocarditis, when it occurs in the mother at the end of pregnancy, is likely to produce the same infection in the newborn baby and will almost invariably be associated with myocarditis with a mortality of approximately 70 percent. After the first month of life the incidence of myocarditis with Coxsackie infection falls precipitously and the mortality becomes very low. After the neonatal period myocarditis appears to be scattered irregularly through the pediatric age group and is not concentrated in any particular year. On the other hand, in endocardial fibroelastosis the age of onset is in the first eight months of life in 85 per cent of cases (see Figure 52–2). In myocarditis, on the other hand, if one rules out the Coxsackie virus infections in the neonatal period, only 30 percent have their onset in the first eight months of life.

The electrocardiogram in myocarditis and endocardial fibroelastosis show differences of diagnostic significance. The voltage of the R wave in V_6 or the voltage of the S wave in V_1 is abnormally high in most cases of endocardial fibroelastosis; it is rarely increased in myocarditis. The R wave in V_6 is abnormally high in most cases of endocardial fibroelastosis; it is rarely increased in myocarditis. The T wave in V_6 is more deeply inverted in endocardial fibroelastosis than in myocarditis in most cases, and it tends to be flat or slightly inverted in the myocarditis group. A pattern of myocardial infarction may be seen in 10 percent of children with myocarditis but is very rare in endocardial fibroelastosis. A Q wave in V_6 of 1 mm or greater is seen in 60 to 70 percent of the cases of endocardial fibroelastosis, but a Q wave in V_6 is uncommon in myocarditis unless a pattern of myocardial infarction is present (Sellers, Keith, and Manning, 1964).

Eighty-five percent of the cases of endocardial fibroelastosis have a left loading pattern, and 93 percent of these also have an increase in voltage in the leads pertaining to the left ventricle. On the other hand, in myocarditis only 7 percent of cases show an increase in voltage in the same leads, and any left loading present is associated with a simple lowering of the R/S ratio in V_1. This striking difference provides security of diagnosis in cases showing the characteristic clinical and electrocardiographic picture. As a result, all the autopsy-proved cases (20) showed this pattern and were diagnosed correctly during life, and myocarditis was correctly ruled out.

One may not always reach the correct diagnosis, since an occasional case of myocarditis may have a left loading pattern with increased voltage of S in V_1 or R in V_6. This is not an uncommon finding, and we have not been misled in this manner to date. An occasional case of endocardial fibroelastosis may show a low-voltage pattern similar to that seen in myocarditis. This occurrence does not, however, invalidate the statement that all cases that satisfied the criteria and came to autopsy had endocardial fibroelastosis.

In the majority of cases with myocarditis the diagnosis was correctly identified from the clinical findings and the electrocardiogram. Confirmation was subsequently obtained at autopsy. None of our cases of myocarditis was considered to be endocardial fibroelastosis during life. We have encountered one case with endocardial fibroelastosis that was considered to be myocarditis because of the low voltage in the electrocardiogram. An autopsy revealed the correct diagnosis.

Decourt and coworkers (1962) reported on a punch-biopsy study of the heart. Five patients had clinical evidence of endocardial fibroelastosis, and the presence of this lesion was confirmed in each case by biopsy of the endocardium. These children are doing well.

Endocardial Fibroelastosis Associated with Valvular Involvement. The cases with valvular involvement were excluded from the main body of this study because it is difficult to be certain about the type and origin of the valvular pathology. There may well be an intimate relationship between the mural endocardial fibroelastic reaction and the pearly-white thickening of the mitral valve. This combination was regarded as primary endocardial fibroelastosis by Kelly and Anderson (1956). At The Hospital for Sick Children 11 such cases have been encountered at autopsy: ten had mitral valve involvement as well as the typical endocardial lesion, and six of these also had a similar process imposed on the aortic valve. The eleventh case had aortic valve involvement without the mitral lesion.

Seven of the eleven cases showed a left ventricular overload pattern in the electrocardiogram. Of those cases that did not show left loading, three had evidence of right ventricular overload, and one electrocardiogram recorded in a moribund child was difficult to assess. One of the cases showing right ventricular overload had aortic stenosis, mitral stenosis, and endocardial fibroelastosis with a nondilated left ventricle. The remaining two cases showed right ventricular overloading and were found to have mitral valve involvement at autopsy.

One may suspect the presence of endocardial fibroelastosis in a baby with congestive heart failure and a systolic murmur in the first year of life with inverted T waves over the left precordium, with or without increased voltage of the R in V_6 or the S in V_1. In the face of the murmurs that go with these valvular lesions, one cannot make the diagnosis with accuracy, since isolated aortic stenosis or large intracardiac left-to-right shunts may at times give similar electrocardiographic findings.

We did not encounter any infants who had evidence of involvement of the pulmonary or tricuspid valve associated with the endocardial lesion. Kelly and Anderson (1956) had two cases with an involvement of the tricuspid valve; some degree of involvement of all four chambers was noted in 15 of their 17 cases. At the same time they indicated that the left ventricular or the left atrial lesions were usually more marked and obvious.

Kelly and Anderson demonstrated that all but 2 of their 17 cases had dilated hearts, an observation that was confirmed in our autopsy-proved material. They referred to these two cases as having an absence of dilatation, whereas Edwards used the term "contracted left ventricle." It would seem more suitable to designate them as nondilated, as the former authors do, since such hearts are hypertrophied and somewhat enlarged.

The contracted left ventricle of aortic or mitral atresia is an entirely different entity.

Noren and associates (1963) and Ainger (quoted by Noren) have presented studies on the use of a mumps antigen skin test in primary endocardial fibroelastosis. They have found a high incidence of positive reactions in their clinicaly diagnosed cases and a very low incidence in the normal infant. While their emphasis was on etiology, to us this appeared to offer a test of some diagnostic significance, and as a result 50 cases of clinically diagnosed endocardial fibroelastosis at The Hospital for Sick Children have been skin-tested with the mumps antigen. Ninety-one percent of the infants under the age of two years had a positive test, while only 9 percent of the control group in the same category were positive (Shone et al., 1966). Over the age of two the test was less useful because of the increased number of positives in the controls. Our conclusion was that the test did not appear to be specific.

Treatment

Manning, Sellers, Bynum, and Keith (1964) presented well-documented evidence that clinically diagnosed endocardial fibroelastosis can be treated and, in the majority of cases, may lead to a healthy, active, surviving child.

Whenever a diagnosis of endocardial fibroelastosis is made or suspected, digitalis should be administered promptly. In infants who are desperately ill, this should be given intravenously, starting with a quarter of the digitalizing dose and giving another quarter an hour later; the rest of the digitalizing dose may be given intravenously or by mouth as the severity of the condition indicates in the next few hours. In the less severely ill cases digitalization may be carried out in the usual way over a period of 24 hours.

Oxygen, antibiotics, and diuretics may be used when indicated. Oxygen is needed only when cyanosis is present. Antibiotics are useful since it is frequently difficult to tell whether the pulmonary signs are due to infection or failure. Sedatives should be given for restlessness.

Another important aspect of treatment is the length of time digitalis should be administered. This has not been finally settled. However, there is no doubt that digitalis should be kept up until all signs and symptoms of the disease have disappeared and the electrocardiogram shows a normal tracing. In the light of our present knowledge, digitalis should be administered for two to three years at least, preferably until both heart size and electrocardiogram are normal (see Figure 52–4).

Results of Therapy and Prognosis

In the past, since the diagnosis was based on necropsy findings, it was thought that in all probability the mortality was 100 percent. The recent reporting of occasional older cases between 5 and 11, or 22 and 70 years of age, who have led active lives over many years, has suggested that there may be individuals who do survive without special therapy for a long time (Panke and Rottino, 1955, 22 years; White and Fennell, 1954, 71 years), although those cases occurring in adult life may have had their origin after childhood. However, the autopsy files indicate that endocardial fibroelastosis is mainly a disease of the first year of life. Linde and Adams (1963) have reported a favorable result with early and adequate therapy.

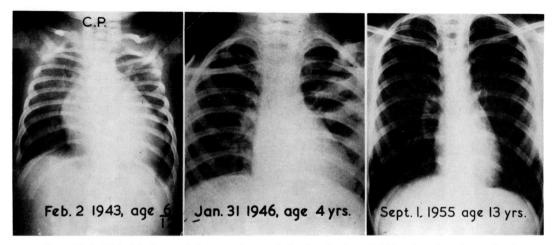

Figure 52-4. Clinical findings and electrocardiogram indicative of endocardial fibroelastosis at six months of age. At 13 years of age this child had a normal heart and normal exercise tolerance.

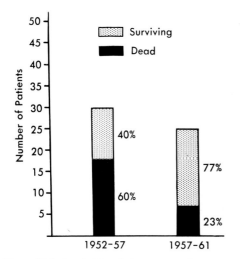

Figure 52-5. Survival in relation to year of treatment and age of patient.

Manning and associates (1964) evaluated the therapy in 56 patients. With more vigorous therapy the mortality fell from 60 percent to 23 percent (see Figure 52–5). The length of time digitalis therapy was administered in those who died is indicated in Figure 52–6. Thus, in the overwhelming majority death occurred in the first few days of treatment before the congestive heart failure could be brought adequately under control. The infants who received therapy early in the course of their illness were much more likely to survive. Prompt use of digitalis helps to elicit a favorable response, and this is reflected in Figure 52–5, which reveals a lowering in mortality in the years 1957–1970 as compared with 1950–1956.

The experience at The Hospital for Sick Children

and the Strong Memorial Hospital (1964) is shown in Figure 33–6. It is obvious that early therapy is important before the heart has reached excessive proportions. The vast majority of children who died had a cardiothoracic ratio over 70 percent, whereas only 40 percent of the survivors had hearts enlarged to this degree. After several years of therapy 80 percent had cardiothoracic rates 55 percent or less (Figure 52–7).

Evidence of left ventricular overload was present in nearly every case. The few exceptions were referred to previously. When digitalis was started and improvement began, one of the first salutary signs was a return of the T waves in the left precordium to a positive position. This was usually accompanied by a decrease in amplitude of the R wave in the same leads. Among the long-term survivors the electrocardiogram was normal in one-third after two years. Close to three-quarters were normal after five years.

The mortality is shown in Figure 52–5. With increasing experience and early therapy the mortality has fallen from 66 percent to 44 percent. In the past such a pessimistic view was taken of the outcome of the disease that therapy was frequently neglected. Now that there is clear evidence for optimism in the ultimate outcome, the future should see a lower mortality and a return to normal activity of the majority of these infants and children.

Late deaths in children under apparently adequate therapy may occur. Manning and associates report five such cases, three between one month and two years, one at two and one-half years, and one at three years, after beginning of treatment. Of the three who died between one month and two years, two had an excellent response symptomatically. Their heart sizes had decreased, but the electrocardiograms were still abnormal. In both cases digitalis therapy was stopped

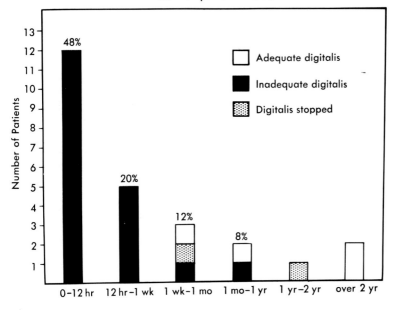

Figure 52-6. Duration of survival in relation to digitalization in patients who died.

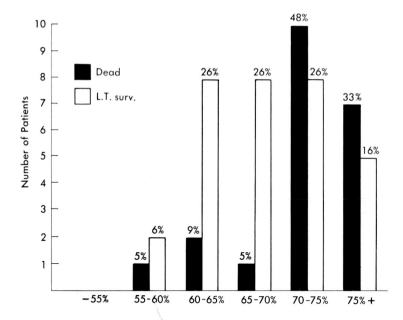

Figure 52-7. Initial cardiothoracic ratios in relation to survival.

by the parents. This led to a recurring and fatal episode of congestive heart failure—one died at home, the other shortly after rehospitalization (two hours), with clinical evidence of severe congestive heart failure. The third patient who died between one month and two years never did have a good response to therapy. There have been no late-deaths associated with arrhythmias.

A comparative experience at The Hospital for Sick Children in Toronto and the Strong Memorial Hospital at Rochester, using similar diagnostic and therapeutic criteria, throws light on the long-term prognosis in those who have survived. It also helps to clarify the age at which death may occur.

In 155 patients followed from 1 to 20 years, there have been 72 deaths and 83 survivors with an overall mortality rate of 47 percent. The age at death is shown in Figure 52–8. The overwhelming majority of those who died did so in the first year of life, two died in the second year, only six died after the age of two, and only three after the age of four. Thus, if a child survives to his fifth birthday it is likely that he will live on with little or no handicap.

The electrocardiogram became normal in 47 out of the 83 in an average time of 4.3 years with a range of six months to 12 years. Those that have remained abnormal show some increased voltage of the R and V_6 or the S and V_1 with or without some changes in the T wave and V_6.

A review of the x-rays at the time of the last visit in the follow-up of survivors indicates that after an average follow-up of ten years, 67 percent had a cardiothoracic ratio of 55 percent or less (see Figure 52–9).

In those who survived, when digitalis was started, improvement was noted early on in the return of the T wave and the left precordium to a positive position. This was usually accompanied by a decrease in the R

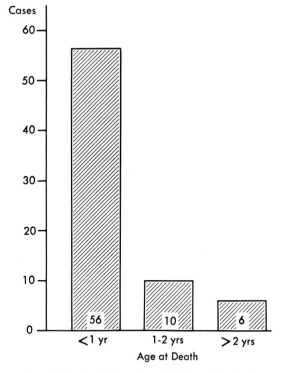

Figure 52-8. Deaths in endocardial fibroelastosis, 72 patients (47 percent mortality).

wave in the same lead. A third of the electrocardiograms of the survivors were normal in two years and three-quarters in five years.

When one compares a mortality between 1950 and 1956 with that of 1957–1970, it is seen that in the early years the mortality was 69 percent and in more recent years, 40 percent (see Figure 52–10). This coincides

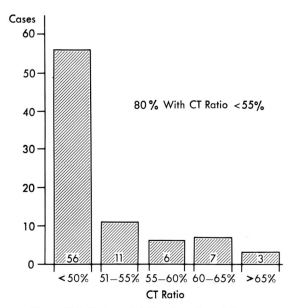

Figure 52-9. Endocardial fibroelastosis in follow-up study. Most recent cardiothoracic ratio, 83 survivors.

follow-up series who had normal hearts. electrocardiograms, x-rays, etc., had a longer follow-up than that those with residual signs, and it may be that if one follows those with residual signs for another five or ten years, their abnormalities will disappear also (see Figure 52–11).

Bicycle ergometry was performed in six patients, five of them with maximum endurance; the maximum endurance index was within normal range suggesting a normal left ventricular performance. In one patient the test was terminated following the development of a supraventricular tachycardia. The resting electrocardiogram was entirely normal in this case and was not known to have had any previous arrhythmia.

Complete cardiac catheterization studies on patients with well-documented endocardial fibroelastosis have been reported by a number of workers (McLoughlin and Schiebler, 1968; Davignon, 1972).

In a group of 13 cases studied by Davignon, meeting all of the diagnostic criteria we have set forth, left and right heart catheterization defined diminished left ventricular dp/dt, diminished ejection fraction, increased left ventricular end diastolic pressure, and cardiac output within normal limits. Lambert (1974) has identified distinctly abnormal responses to workload in a follow-up of ten patients clinically meeting the diagnostic criteria for endocardial fibroelastosis.

Somerville, studying 55 children who presented under the age of 18 months with left heart failure, concluded that primary endocardial fibroelastosis was a pathologic end-point of many different diseases of the myocardium in the fetus, neonate, or infant and had a variable and not necessarily predictable prognosis.

with persistent long-term therapy with digitalis and careful observation and control of respiratory infections.

In those patients in whom more clinical parameters are presently normal, the height and weight measurements follow a normal distribution, whereas in those patients with one or more residual abnormalities, both height and weight tended to be below normal standard for the age. The children in the

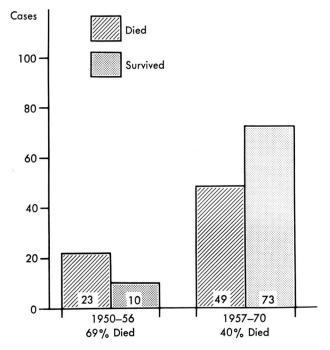

Figure 52-10. Early and late mortality in endocardial fibroelastosis, 155 cases.

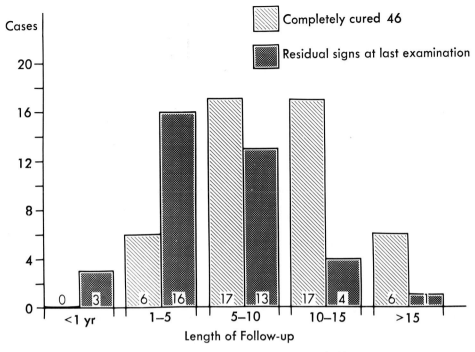

Figure 52-11. Endocardial fibroelastosis prognosis, 83 cases.

It would appear that she is reporting on a group of patients who do not meet the specific criteria necessary for the clinical diagnosis of primary endocardial fibroelastosis, indeed representing a potpourri of all types of undefined left heart disease in infants and young children. Reviewing her data and method of management, we would expect to find many different disease processes and a definitely unpredictable prognosis.

A long-term prognosis of primary endocardial fibroelastosis, therefore, appears to be good in those patients whose heart size and electrocardiogram become normal. What happens to the thickened endocardium is unknown. Meager data at present would indicate that endocardial thickening is maintained, and echocardiographic studies in some of these cases suggest that diminished left ventricular function persists. It remains to be seen whether these hearts will effectively handle the degenerative diseases of later life. There also remains to be seen whether those with persistent changes in electrocardiograms or some increase in heart size may show gradual improvement in the next five or ten years or may take a progressively downhill course.

REFERENCES

Adams, F. H., and Katz, B. L.: Endocardial fibroelastosis. Case reports with special emphasis on the clinical findings. *J. Pediatr.*, **41**:141, 1952.

Ainger, L. E.: Mitral and aortic valve incompetence in endocardial fibroelastosis. *Am. J. Cardiol.*, **28**:309, 1971.

Ainger, L. E.: Quoted by Noren.

Anderson, D. H., and Kelly, J.: Endocardial fibroelastosis associated with congenital malformations of the heart. *Pediatrics*, **18**:513, 1956.

Black-Schaffer, B.: Infantile endocardial fibroelastosis. *Arch. Pathol.*, **63**:281, 1957.

Blankenship, B. E.: Endocardial fibroelastosis: pathology and proposed pathogenesis. *Bull. Tulane Med. Fac.*, **13**:99, 1954.

Blumberg, R. W., and Lyon, R. A.: Endocardial sclerosis. *Am. J. Dis. Child.*, **84**:291, 1952.

Campbell, M.: Genetic and environmental factors in congenital heart disease. *Q. J. Med.*, **18**:379, 1949.

Chen, S.; Thompson, M. W.; and Rose, V.: Endocardial fibroelastosis: Family studies with special reference to counseling. *J. Pediatr.*, **79**:385, 1971.

Chung, K. J.; Manning, J. A.; and Gramiak, R.: Presentation—Association of European Pediatric Cardiologists, May, 1973.

Cochrane, W. A., and Bowden, D. H.: Calcification of the arteries in infancy and childhood. *Pediatrics*, **14**:222, 1954.

Craig, J. M.: Congenital endocardial sclerosis. *Bull. Intern. A. M. Museums*, **30**:15, 1949.

Crome, L.: Epiloia and endocardial fibroelastosis. *Arch. Dis. Child.*, **29**:136, 1954.

————: The structural features of epiloia, with special reference to endocardial fibroelastosis. *J. Clin. Pathol.*, **7**:137, 1954.

Davignon, A.: Presentation, Canadian Heart Association, October, 1972.

Decourt, L. V.; Macruz, R.; Garcia, D. P.; and Torloni, H.: Endocardial fibroelastosis, its study by punch-biopsy of the heart. Fourth World Congress of Cardiology, Mexico City, 1962.

Dennis, J. L.; Hansen, A. E.; and Corpening, T. N.: Endocardial fibroelastosis. *Pediatrics*, **12**:130, 1953.

Di Sant'Agnese, P. A.; Andersen, D. H.; and Mason, H. H.: Glycogen, storage disease of the heart. *Pediatrics*, **6**:607, 1950.

Dissman, E.: Ein Fall von kongenitaler Aortenstenose und Endokardhyperplasie bei einem Neugeborenen. *Frankfurt Z. Pathol.*, **43**:476, 1932.

Dordick, J. R.: Diffuse endocardial fibrosis and cardiac hypertrophy in infancy. *Am. J. Clin. Pathol.*, **21**:743, 1951.

Edwards, J. E.: In Gould, S. E. (ed.): *Pathology of the Heart.* Charles C Thomas, Publisher, Springfield, Ill., 1953, p. 420.

Ferencz, C.; Johnson, A. L.; and Wiglesworth, F. W.: Congenital mitral stenosis. *Circulation,* 9:161, 1954.

Folger, G. M., Jr.: Endocardial Fibroelastosis. A continuing and unsolved dilemma. *Clin. Pediatr.,* 10:246, 1971.

Fontana, R. S., and Edwards, J. E.: *Congenital Cardiac Disease. A Review of 357 Cases Studied Pathologically.* W. B. Saunders Co., Philadelphia, 1962, p. 141.

Forfar, J. O.; Miller, R. A.; Bain, A. D.; et al.: Endocardial fibroelastosis. *Br. Med. J.,* 2:7, 1964.

Freer, J. L., and Matheson, W. J.: Left auricular enlargement in endocardial fibroelastosis. *Arch. Dis. Child.,* 28:284, 1953.

Frieundlich, E.; Berkowitz, M.; Elkon, A.; and Wilder, A.: Primary interstitial myocarditis. *Am. J. Dis. Child.,* 96:43, 1958.

Frühling, L.; Korn, R.; Lavillaureix, J.; Surjus, A.; and Foussereau, S.: La myoendocardite chronique fibro-elasticue du nouveau-ne et du nourrisson (fibroelastose). *Ann. Anat. Pathol.,* 7:227, 1962.

Gasul, B. M.; Arcilla, R. A.; and Lev, M.: *Heart Disease in Children.* J. B. Lippincott, Philadelphia, 1966, p. 365.

Golper, M. N.: Endocardial fibroelastosis. *Radiology,* 61:865, 1953.

Greaves, J. L.; Wilkins, P. S. W.; and Pearson, S.: Endocardial fibroelastosis in identical twins. *Arch. Dis. Child.,* 29:447, 1954.

Gross, P.: Concept of fetal endocarditis. General review with report of illustrative case. *Arch. Pathol.,* 31:163, 1941.

Haldane, J. B. S., and Smith, C. A.: A simple exact test for birth order effect. *Ann. Eugenics,* 14:114, 1947.

Halliday, W. R.: Endomyocardial fibroelastosis. *Dis. Chest,* 26:27, 1954.

Hastreiter, A. R., and Miller, R. A.: Management of primary endomyocardial disease, the myocarditis-endocardial fibroelastosis syndrome. *Pediatr. Clin. North Am.,* 11:401, 1964.

Hill, W. T., and Reilly, W. A.: Endocardial fibroelastosis. *Am. J. Dis. Child.,* 82:579, 1951.

Hunter, A. S., and Keay, A. J.: Primary endocardial fibroelastosis. An inherited condition. *Arch. Dis. Child.,* 48:66, 1973.

Hutchins, G. M., and Vie, S. A.: The progression of interstitial myocarditis to idiopathic endocardial fibroelastosis. *Am. J. Pathol.,* 66:483, 1972.

Johnson, F. R.: Anoxia as a cause of endocardial fibroelastosis in infancy. *Arch. Pathol.,* 54:237, 1952.

Katz, B. E., and Adams, F. H.: Endocardial fibroelastosis. *Am. J. Dis. Child.,* 86:186, 1953.

Kelly, J., and Anderson, D. H.: Congenital endocardial fibroelastosis. II. A clinical and pathologic investigation of those cases without associated cardiac malformation, including report of two familial instances. *Pediatrics,* 18:539, 1956.

Kempton, J. J.: Endocardial fibroelastosis in one of 3-year-old twins. *Proc. Roy. Soc. Med.,* 46:271, 1953.

Kibrich, D.: Viral infections of fetus and newborn. In Polland, M. (ed.): *Perspectives in Virology.* Burgess Publishing Company, Minneapolis, 1961, p. 140.

Lambert, E. C.; Shumway, C. N. and Terplan, K.: Clinical diagnosis of endocardial fibrosis. Analysis of literature with report of four new cases. *Pediatrics,* 11:255, 1953.

Lambert, E. D., and Vlad, P.: Primary endomyocardial disease. *Pediatr. Clin. North Am.,* 5:1057, 1958.

Lambert, E. D.: Personal communication, 1974.

Leary, D. C.; Welt, L. G.; and Beckett, R. S.: Infectious mononucleosis complicating pregnancy with fatal congenital anomaly of infant. *Am. J. Obstet. Gynecol.,* 57:381, 1949.

Linde, L. M.; Adams, F. H.; and O'Loughlin, B. J.: Endocardial fibroelastosis angiocardiographic studies. *Circulation,* 17:40, 1958.

Linde, L. M., and Adams, F.: Prognosis in endocardial fibroelastosis. *Am. J. Dis. Child.,* 105:329, 1963.

Lindenbaum, R. H.; Andrews, P. S.; and Khan, A. S. S. I.: Two cases of endocardial fibroelastosis—possibly X-linked determination. *Br. Heart J.,* 35:38, 1973.

Lowenburg, H., Jr., and Meyer, H.: Endocardial fibroelastosis. *J. Einstein Med. Cent.,* 2:127, 1954.

Lunfield, J.; Gasul, B. M.; Luan, L. L.; and Dillon, R. F.: Right and left heart catheterization and angiocardiographic findings in idiopathic cardiac hypertrophy with endocardial fibroelastosis. *Circulation,* 21:386, 1960.

Manning, J. A.; Sellers, F. J.; Bynum, R.; and Keith, J. D.: Medical

management of clinical endocardial fibroelastosis. *Circulation,* 29:60, 1964.

Maxwell, G. M., and Young, W. P.: Isolated mitral stenosis in an infant of three months: report of a case treated surgically. *Am. Heart J.,* 48:787, 1954.

McLoughlin, T. G.; Schiebler, G. L.; and Krovetz, L. J.: Hemodynamic findings in children with endocardial fibroelastosis. *Am. Heart J.,* 75:162, 1968.

Metianu, C.; Guillemot, R.; Durand, M.; and Bardin, P.; Un nouveau cas de fibroelastose cardiaque du nourrisson. *Sem. Hôp. Paris,* 30:434, 1954.

Mitchell, S. C.; Sellmann, A. H.; et al.: Etiologic correlates in a study of congenital heart disease in 56,109 births. *Am. J. Cardiol.,* 28:653, 1971.

Morgan, A. D.; McLoughlin, T. G.; et al.: Endocardial fibroelastosis of the right ventricle in the newborn. *Am. J. Cardiol.,* 18:933, 1966.

Morison, J. E.: Congenital malformations in one of monozygotic twins. *Arch. Dis. Child.,* 24:214, 1949.

Mortensen, O.; Kissmeyer-Nielsen, F.; and Jorgensen, P. K.: Endocardial fibroelastosis in infancy. *Acta Paediatr.,* 43:87, 1954.

Nadas, A. S.: *Pediatric Cardiology.* W. B. Saunders Company, Philadelphia, 1957.

Noren, G. R.; Adams, P., Jr.; and Anderson, R. C.: Positive skin reactivity to mumps virus antigen in endocardial fibroelastosis. *J. Pediatr.,* 62:604, 1963.

Noren, G. R.; Jenkins, E. F.; Staley, N. A.; and Stevenson, J. E.: A new experimental model of myocarditis. (Abstr.) *Pediatr. Res.,* 4:377, 1970.

Oppenheimer, E. H.: The association of adult-type coarctation of the aorta with endocardial fibroelastosis in infancy. *Bull. Hopkins Hosp.,* 93:319, 1953.

Panke, W., and Rottino, A.: Endocardial fibroelastosis occurring in the adult. *Am. Heart J.,* 49:89, 1955.

Paul, R. N., and Robbins, S. G.: A surgical treatment proposed for either endocardial fibroelastosis or anomalous left coronary artery. *Pediatrics,* 16:147, 1955.

Prior, J. T., and Wyatt, T. C.: Endocardial fibroelastosis: A study of eight cases. *Am. J. Pathol.,* 26:969, 1950.

Rauchfuss, C.: Cited in Gerhardt, C.: *Handbuch der Kinderkrankheiten.* H. Laupp, Tubingen, 1878, Vol. 4, p. 12.

Roberts, J. T.: A case of congenital aortic atresia. *Am. Heart J.,* 12:448, 1936.

Rosahn, P. D.: Endocardial fibroelastosis: old and new concepts. *Bull. N.Y. Acad. Med.,* 31:453, 1955.

Rose, V.; O'Connor, J. R.; Keith, J. D.; et al.: Computer-based data storage and retrieval in pediatric cardiology. *Can. Med. Assoc. J.,* 107:305, 1972.

Rosenbaum, H. D.; Nadas, A. S.; and Neuhauser, E. B.: Primary myocardial disease in infancy and childhood. *Am. J. Dis. Child.,* 86:28, 1953.

Sellers, F. J.; Keith, J. D.; and Manning, J. A.: Diagnosis of primary endocardial fibroelastosis. *Circulation,* 29:49, 1964.

Shah, C. V.; Patel, M. K.; and Hastreiter, A. R.: Hemodynamics of complete atrioventricular canal and its evolution with age. *Am. J. Cardiol.,* 24:326, 1969.

Shone, J.; Munoz, Armas; Manning, J. A.; and Keith, J. D.; The mumps antigen skin test in endocardial fibroelastosis. *Pediatrics,* 37:483, 1966.

Snyder, C. H.; Bost, R. B.; and Platou, R. V.: Hypertension in infancy with anomalous, renal artery; diagnosis by renal arteriography, apparent cure after nephrectomy. *Pediatrics,* 15:88, 1955.

Somerville, J.: Primary myocardial disease in children or the myth of fibroelastosis. Proceedings of the Assoc. Europe. Paed. Cadriologists 11th Annual General Meeting, May 1973.

Sprague, H. B.; Bland, E. F.; and White, P. D.: Congenital idiopathic hypertrophy of the heart. *Am. J. Dis. Child.,* 41:877, 1931.

Still, W. J. S.: Endocardial fibrosis. *Lancet,* 2:1261, 1954.

Still, W. J. S., and Boult, E. N.: Pathogenesis of endocardial fibroelastosis. *Lancet,* 2:117, 1956.

Tingelstad, J. B.; Shiel, F. O.; and McCue, C. M.: The electrocardiogram in the contracted type of primary endocardial fibroelastosis. *Am. J. Cardiol.,* 27:304, 1971.

Ullrich, O.: Angeborene Herzhypertrophie mit Endokardfibrose bei zwei eineiigen Partnern von männlichen Drillingen. *Z. Menschl. Vererb.*, **21**:585, 1938.

Vlad, P.; Rowe, R. D.; and Keith, J. D.: The electrocardiogram in primary endocardial fibroelastosis. *Br. Heart J.*, **17**:189, 1955.

Weinberg, T., and Himelfarb, A. J.: Endocardial fibroelastosis. *Bull. Hopkins Hosp.*, **72**:299, 1943.

Wesson, H. R., and Beaver, D. C.: Congenital atresia of aortic orifice. *J. Tech. Methods*, **14**:86, 1935.

White, P. D., and Fennell, R. H.: Endocardial fibro-elastosis with marked cardiac enlargement and failure in a man who died at the age of 71 after 15 years of angina pectoris and two years of congestive heart failure. *Ann. Intern. Med.*, **41**:333, 1954.

Williams, H.; O'Reilly, R. N.; and Williams, A.: Fourteen cases of idiopathic myocarditis in infants and children. *Arch. Dis. Child.*, **28**:271, 1953.

Zeigler, R. F.: *Electrocardiographic Studies in Normal Infants and Children.* Charles C Thomas, Publisher, Springfield, Ill., 1951.

53

Cardiovascular Disease in the Rubella Syndrome

Richard D. Rowe

T HE INFECTIOUS disease we now know as rubella was first described in 1752 in the German literature when it was felt to be a variety of measles, scarlet fever, or a hybrid form of the two. It was subsequently identified in 1815 as a separate disease by an Englishman and eventually named rubella by a Scot. Not before 140 years had passed did anybody notice that the infection during the first trimester of the pregnancy could result in malformation in the fetus. Even then it was an ophthalmologist who in 1941 recognized that a bunching of cases in congenital cataract could be explained by an epidemic of rubella that had occurred in eastern Australia in the spring of 1940 (Gregg, 1941). In all but 1 of the 13 patients in this original report there was heart disease, and in four autopsies patent ductus arteriosus was the lesion identified. This association was confirmed elsewhere with minor differences, and for a number of reasons patent ductus arteriosus became fixed as the principal cardiovascular malformation of rubella infants in experiences recorded from widely separated parts of the world.

Pathology

Only the cardiovascular aspects of rubella at this stage of pathology will be described here. The apparently high incidence of extensive involvement of the fetus found in pregnancy rubella has led in the past to a considerable number of therapeutic abortions for first-trimester infection. Examination of this material has shown patchy changes of necrotic nature in the endothelium of blood vessels in the chorion, the brain, and the subendocardial myocardium of the atria. There is some evidence that there is delay in the development of the cardiac septa but there is no evidence of inflammation (Tondury and Smith, 1966; Driscoll, 1969).

A wide variety of intracardiac malformations has been encountered in live births including such early

malformations as transposition of the great arteries, truncus arteriosus, atresia of atrioventricular valves, atrioventricular communis, and tetralogy of Fallot. Of these the tetralogy appears to be the most frequently encountered malformation, but altogether these complex defects are responsible for not more than 5 to 10 percent of all rubella cardiovascular disease.

Simpler defects such as secundum atrial defects or ventricular defects may possibly account for 5 percent of the total proportion of cases affected if one takes a generous view. It is our feeling that the incidence of ventricular septal defect has been overreported. It is quite impossible to tell from the literature whether the size of the ventricular defect under these circumstances follows the usual distribution or whether there are more larger or smaller defects than occur in patients without rubella background. The distribution in our own material is similar to that usually encountered for ventricular defects, but atrial defects where present are most always small. Problems regarding the presence or absence of atrial communication are compounded by the frequent association of left-to-right shunts at atrial level through stretching of the foramen ovale flap in very young infants. We have encountered one patient with cardiac catheterization evidence of a small left-to-right shunt at atrial level in association with mild pulmonary arterial stenosis who subsequently died from the effects of the rubella infection and who had small but true defects on an apparently thinned foramen ovale flap (Rowe, 1972). It is thus possible that small atrial defects of this nature are more common after gestational rubella than had been previously thought although they would be impossible to detect in all likelihood on a clinical basis.

Valvular lesions have been noted in the rubella syndrome from autopsy information. The lesion is nodular and distributed on the leaflets of all four valves. There seems to be no predilection for one or other side of the heart. Whether these lesions found in infant autopsies would in older individuals create obstructive problems is uncertain. Amongst autopsy material in infancy there have been no examples of severe valvular pulmonary stenosis although this has been encountered in clinical situations in older subjects (Campbell, 1961; Rowe, 1972).

Changes in the myocardium have been reported in both fetal and postnatal material by several groups of investigators (Korones et al., 1965; Singer et al., 1967; Esterly and Oppenheimer, 1969; Way, 1967). At autopsy the affected myocardium forms gray or brown patches over the ventricle. The microscopic appearance is that of swelling of myocardial fibers that have loss of cross-striation and pleomorphic nuclei (Figure 53–1). There is no evidence of inflammation.

Frank myocarditis with inflammatory cells has not been encountered except probably as a separate situation postnatally (Esterly and Oppenheimer, 1969). The same question surrounds the detection of two cases of primary endocardial fibroelastosis in patients with serologic evidence of gestational rubella (Hardy, 1968).

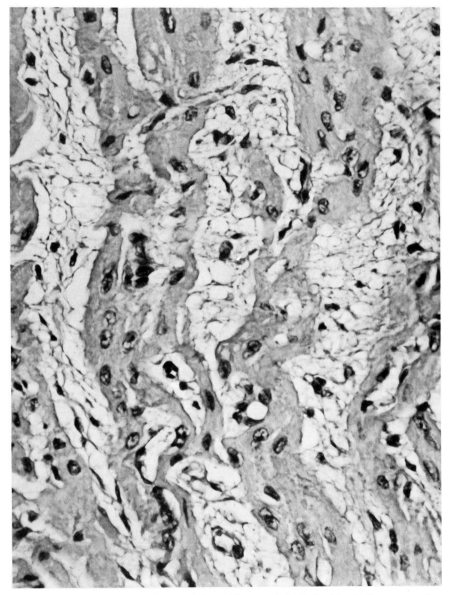

Figure 53-1. Section of myocardium from an infant with congenital rubella. Muscle fibers are swollen and extensively vacuolated. Nuclei are pleomorphic. There is no inflammatory reaction. × 250. (Reproduced from Korones, S. B.; Ainger, L. E.; Monif, G. R. G.; Roane, J.; Sever, J. L.; and Fuste, F.: Congenital rubella syndrome: new clinical aspects with recovery of virus from affected infants. *J. Pediatr.*, **67**:166, 1965.)

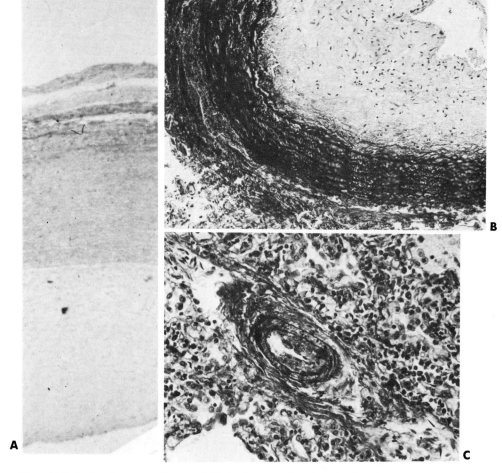

Figure 53-2. Sections from ascending aorta (*A*, intima lower portion), from a major pulmonary artery branch (*B*), and from the lung (*C*) illustrating the changes in severe rubella vascular disease. The patient, JHH #1146265, died at age six months (autopsy #33848). (Reproduced from Rowe, R. D.: Cardiovascular disease in the rubella syndrome. *Cardiovasc. Clin.,* **5**:61, 1973.)

The most important recent observation in relation to rubella disease of the cardiovascular system is the damage that has been found in blood vessels. A patchy distribution of such changes has been noted in large conducting arteries, in muscular arteries, and in smaller vessels of both circuits (Figures 53–2 to 53–4).

In the pulmonary circulation the main pulmonary artery divisions in the newborn infant affected by the disease may be quite small in size though there may be little histologic evidence of morphologic change (Rowe et al., 1966; Esterly and Oppenheimer, 1967). In older infants and children more obvious thickening of the vessel wall is evident in the gross and commonly there is narrowing at the bifurcation of the main pulmonary artery.

The changes originally reported by Campbell (1965) include an intimal thickening with irregular arrangement of elastic fibers in the media of such subjects. Where the elastic tissue is particularly

distorted and fragmented, intimal proliferation appears to be maximal. Poststenotic dilatation of the vessel may occur with thinning of vessel wall. Such changes may occasionally be present in small muscular vessels of the lung and occlusive changes in arterioles have also been noted.

In the aorta there may be considerable thickening of the entire vessel. Most of the change has been reported in the descending aorta, but the area immediately above the aortic valve has also been a site for change in many infants seen at autopsy. Again the lesion appears to be a fibromuscular proliferation from below the endothelium.

The ductus arteriosus, which normally has a well-developed muscular layer and a prominent elastic lamina with breakage near the intimal mounding, forms a striking contrast to the abnormal duct in some patients with rubella syndrome where elastic tissue tends to be absent and where there is no myointimal heaping. The muscular wall has been noted to be defective with an increased amount of collagen between smooth muscle cells (Campbell, 1965).

Focal changes have been reported in many of the major systemic arteries including those to abdominal organs, to the lung, to the heart, and to the brain. The intimal thickening present is similar to that seen in the pulmonary circuit and is localized within areas of the wall that are deficient in elastic tissue. There is considerable interest in the probability that endothelial swelling produces obstruction to flow of blood to critical areas in the brain and abdomen, which may be responsible on the one hand for the mental retardation so characteristic of this syndrome and the occasional incidence of atretic malformations of the gut.

Etiology

The pathogenesis of the disorder has been greatly advanced by the isolation of the rubella virus (Weller and Neva, 1962; Parkman et al., 1962). It is believed that viremia occurs in the mother before the rash appears and that the placenta is infected in that process. The fetus becomes involved through endothelial shedding from the placenta or through the passage of infected white cells. A curious immunologic situation follows in which antibodies

are formed but the virus remains alive. Breaks in the chromosome structure have been reported but there is no convincing evidence that there is any increase in the incidence of the better known syndromes of chromosomal addition or deletion. The evidence is very strong, however, that cell replication is slowed. From a number of sources it has been determined that the total cell number in liveborn infants is considerably reduced (Naeye and Blanc, 1965; Hill et al., 1970). Some cytopathic damage is believed to occur as well as the reduction in cell number. The evidence suggests that growth may be sufficiently disturbed from very early infection to induce teratogenetic effects in growing organs while later infection produces damage to the fetus of a much more subtle variety.

Although the proportion of susceptible adult females varies from one community to another, in the United States in urban communities it is probably no more than 15 percent. Even during epidemics not all exposed susceptible gravida become infected. In addition, the risk of damage to the fetus declines with progressive fetal age at the time of maternal illness (Katz et al., 1968). Furthermore, recent evaluation of the impact of rubella immunization gives encouragement to the view that the program can result in a decline in incidence of congenital rubella and prevent viremia in the event of reinfection (Krugman and Katz, 1974; Welch, 1977).

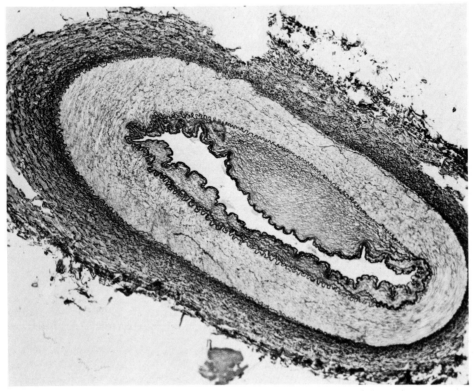

Figure 53-3. The renal artery of a seven-year-old boy with congenital rubella and systemic hypertension showing intimal proliferation. × 60. (Reproduced from Fortuin, N. J.; Morrow, A. G.; and Roberts, W. C.: Late vascular manifestations of the rubella syndrome. *Am. J. Med.,* **51**:134, 1971.)

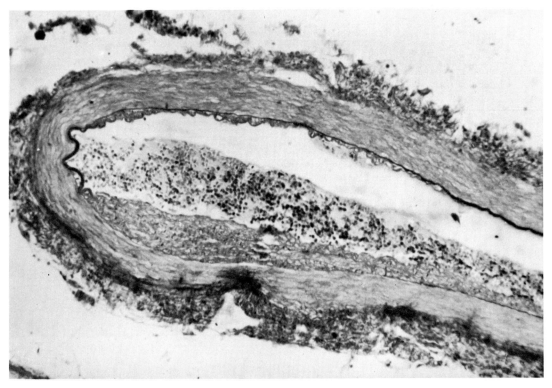

Figure 53-4. A cerebral artery from a four-month-old infant with congenital rubella showing patchy deficiency of the internal elastic lamina and overlying intimal proliferation. × 203. (Reproduced from Campbell, P. E.: Vascular abnormalities following maternal rubella. *Br. Heart J.*, **27**:134, 1965.)

Hemodynamics

In most individuals with complex cardiac anomalies (Ainger, 1966) changes in hemodynamics will be appropriate for the individual malformation and readily elucidated by cardiac catheterization and angiocardiography.

Of more interest is the detection of valvular lesions, of pulmonary arterial stenoses, and of lesions in a systemic circulation. Obviously those elements of the disease that involve very small vessels are unlikely to be clarified by the usual procedures in the hemodynamic laboratory, but a great deal of knowledge has ensued following routine study of these patients.

Subjects with pulmonary arterial stenosis have now been studied in considerable numbers, and the observations in terms of both the degree of abnormality in pressure difference across the obstruction and the anatomic appearance through angiography have been clarified. There is evidence of little change of the dynamics with age during childhood, but a striking alteration in the anatomic appearances occurs during the same interval (Figure 53–5) (Rowe, 1963; Emmanouilides et al., 1964; Venables, 1965; Hastreiter et al., 1967; Wasserman et al., 1968). Pulmonary valvular stenosis in both mild and severe forms has been noted (Heiner and Nadas,

1958; Rowe, 1963, 1972) but little attention has been paid to tricuspid or mitral valve involvement in the disorder. Angiographic observations have produced most information in dealing with the systemic arterial lesions. Supravalvar aortic stenosis, which was initially suggested with studies in sick infants (Figure 53–6) (Rowe et al., 1966), was detected in older patients (Varghese et al., 1969), and there has been evidence angiographically of stenoses of other aortic branches (Rowe et al., 1969; Fortuin et al., 1971; Siassi et al., 1970).

Clinical Features

Postnatal rubella is a mild and self-limiting disease of children and young adults but fetal infection produces a series of clinical manifestations that are known together as the rubella syndrome (Dudgeon, 1975). There is abundant evidence that in susceptible women the risk to the fetus is greatest in the first trimester of the pregnancy with a stepwise reduction in the frequency of affliction from the first month. This does not mean that there cannot be manifestations from late infection but they seem to be considerably fewer and exhibit less florid features. Most epidemics show a high proportion of infected infants, but the data are weighted toward infants with congenital disease of various types because the

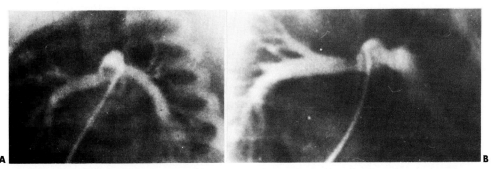

Figure 53-5. Serial pulmonary cinearteriograms from an infant with congenital rubella and isolated pulmonary arterial stenosis at age two months (*A*) and 15 months (*B*). The systolic pressure difference across the bifurcation of the main pulmonary artery at each study was 26 mm of mercury. Note the more obvious distal poststenotic dilatation of both major pulmonary arteries at the second study. (Modified from Wasserman, M. P.; Varghese, P. J.; and Rowe, R. D.: The evolution of pulmonary arterial stenosis associated with congenital rubella. *Am. Heart J.*, **76**:638, 1968.)

history and other information are obtained retrospectively. In prospective studies the proportions are lower. The most severe abnormalities include congenital cardiovascular disease, hearing loss, cataracts or glaucoma, psychomotor retardation, and neonatal purpura.

In the newborn severely affected group there is often difficulty in making an unequivocal diagnosis of heart failure because of the high frequency of pneumonitis, hepatosplenomegaly, and tachycardia. Despite this, profound heart failure has been noted in babies with myocardial necrosis and in infants with large patent ductus arteriosus. As with prematurely born infants, the heart failure in those with a large

ductus is likely to occur earlier in patients with lower rather than high birth weights (Rowe and Neill, 1971; Lynfield et al., 1966).

On other occasions congestive failure encountered in the sick newborn on further investigation may be proved to be the result of a combination of problems rather than a single entity. Included in this list would be patients with moderate ductal shunts, with some myocardial necrosis, and with pulmonary arterial stenosis.

In other infants and in older children the manifestations will not be so florid but the cardiovascular disorder may be revealed in a variety of ways. Patients may be referred to a cardiologist

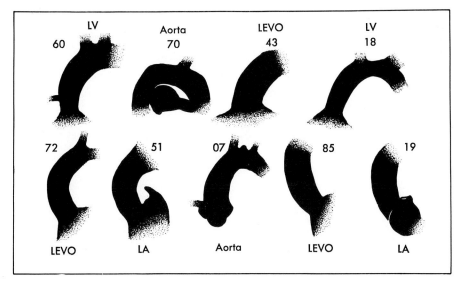

Figure 53-6. Tracings of contrast visualization of the ascending aorta in the left anterior oblique position in nine patients with the rubella syndrome. The numbers are patient identification. *Aorta* = aortogram. *LV* = left ventricular contrast injection. *LA* = left atrial injection of contrast. *LEVO* = pulmonary arterial injection of contrast. Despite less than optimal visualization the possibility of supravalvular stenosis is suggested in at least two patients. (Reproduced from Rowe, R. D.; Mehrizi, A.; Elliott, H. L.; and Neill, C. A.: Cardiovascular disease in the rubella syndrome. In Cassels, D. E. [ed.]: *The Heart and Circulation in the Newborn and Infant.* Grune & Stratton, Inc., New York, 1966, p. 180.)

because of the detection of a murmur. In some cases this may be the murmur of a ductus arteriosus but more often it is a murmur of pulmonary arterial stenosis with characteristic transmission from the precordium to the axilla and the back. We have also encountered children with aortic stenosis, pulmonary valvar stenosis, and tetralogy of Fallot referred because of the detection of the murmur and for whom the evidence was conclusive eventually that the background was congenital rubella. The clues to that background may frequently be suggested by the presence of a low birth weight for gestational age, the birth of the patient between October and March in North America, or by testing for minor abnormalities of vision or hearing.

Occasionally a child may present with systemic hypertension that is found to be due to renal artery stenosis. Under those circumstances there is a high probability of a rubella background. One might expect also that case-finding mechanisms for cardiovascular disease in the rubella system would be found in individuals detected in screening programs for hearing and speech defects, for eye dysfunction, and for diabetes (Karmody, 1968; Weinberger et al., 1970).

Radiologic Examination

In young infants with congenital rubella syndrome, particularly those severely ill in the newborn period, the appearance of the chest film may be extremely variable. It may not truly reflect the state of affairs hemodynamically. In older infants and in those with large left-to-right shunts, cardiomegaly with plethora is usually an indication of substantial left-to-right shunt through the ductus arteriosus. Because in the very small baby a combination of lesions in the cardiovascular system may produce a very similar picture it becomes necessary to perform further studies in order to arrive at accurate diagnosis. In those with isolated pulmonary arterial stenosis especially in older age groups the heart size is usually within normal range. Changes in the lung vascular markings due to poststenotic dilatation of the arterial lesion in the lung are uncommon in infancy and not particularly obvious for some years thereafter unless the lesion is particularly severe. Fortunately, the majority of pulmonary arterial stenotic problems in the young child are relatively mild.

In patients with tetralogy of Fallot, especially in very young, ill infants, the radiologic appearance may be quite misleading in that cardiomegaly and plethora may be present due to the presence of an associated ductus arteriosus. Later the appearance may be more consistent with the presence of the classic tetralogy.

Electrocardiography

In complex anomalies the electrocardiogram is usually helpful in directing attention to chamber enlargement. In older children with relatively simple defects such as ductus arteriosus or pulmonary arterial stenosis the electrical changes are not striking though they are in the expected directions. In the very young infant, particularly in the newborn period, one must be alerted toward the possible detection at any time in a sick infant of myocardial ischemia by the appearance in electrocardiograms of frank infarction patterns (Figure 53–7) (Korones et al., 1965). We have seen relatively minor changes strongly suggestive of infarction of lesser degree with abnormal T and S-T segments in patients who have survived, but a major infarcted zone that persists is rather more ominous.

A high incidence of an unusually oriented frontal plan QRS axis has been reported by one group of observers (Halloran et al., 1966). Although we have not ourselves encountered such a high incidence as in their study, the presence of that finding in the tracings of a baby with congenital rubella syndrome would be suspicious of some degree of involvement of the left bundle. The changes are apparently not necessarily permanent but frequently are.

Diagnosis

The diagnosis of congenital rubella syndrome in epidemic form is not difficult because of the characteristic manifestations nor should it be even in the sporadic disease. The ability to separate patients with rubella from those with other types of severe intrauterine infection is now available through culture of the virus and the demonstration of appropriate antibodies. It is to be remembered that virus shedding can continue for many months even in infants who appear normal (Katz et al., 1968). Most infants with congenital rubella cease excreting virus and have normal immunoglobin levels at age one year (Cooper and Krugman, 1967). The diagnosis of myocardial necrosis of extensive nature, ductus arteriosus, and pulmonary arterial stenosis or combinations, as well as of more complicated intracardiac malformations, follows a fairly standard approach. What is more difficult is to map the extent of the arterial damage in both circulations with certainty particularly on the systemic side. It is unlikely that much will accrue from extensive studies in the very small infant, for most changes in the vascular system appear more obvious with the passage of time. Until more evidence one way or the other is produced about the incidence of vascular lesions in children who are otherwise well, all that might properly be done is for the clinician to remember the possibility of involvement throughout the body and consider this at periodic follow-up examinations.

Prognosis

There seems to be a fairly high mortality in the florid form of the disease. For example, the mortality rate in a group of 58 infants with neonatal

Baby 3 (12-8-64)

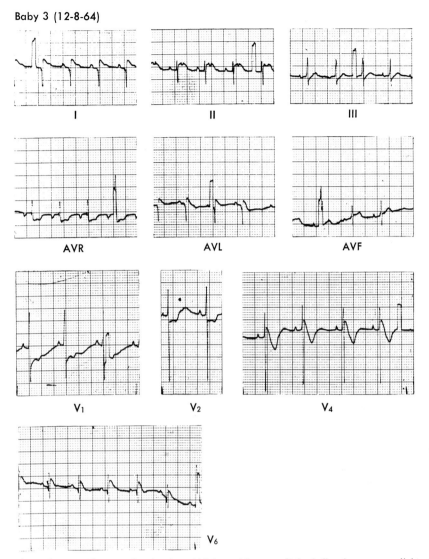

Figure 53-7. Electrocardiogram of a nine-day-old infant with congenital rubella whose myocardial section is shown in Figure 53-1. A pathologic Q wave is present in lead I. S-T segments are elevated in leads I, II, aVL, V$_4$, and V$_6$, and depressed in aVR, V$_1$, and V$_2$. T waves are blended into the S-T segments. (Reproduced from Korones, S. B.; Ainger, L. E.; Monif, G. R. G.; Roane, J.; Sever, J. L.; and Fuste, F.: Congenital rubella syndrome: new clinical aspects with recovery of virus from affected infants. *J. Pediatr.*, **67**:166, 1965.)

thrombocytic purpura and other manifestations of rubella described in 1965 had by 1967 exceeded 65 percent (Cooper and Krugman, 1967). The cardiac contribution to death has usually been in those with massive ductal shunts or with extensive myocardial necrosis. Other lesions are hemodynamically reasonably well tolerated, and provided the general systemic upset is not major, the prognosis for the immediate future for them seems good. Some uncertainty exists over what the contribution of vascular disease will be for the future of these patients. Slightly less than 30 percent of 50 survivors followed for 25 years had cardiovascular abnormalities (Menser et al., 1969). One is concerned that the demonstration of arterial disease in vessels of such

critical importance as the coronary, cerebral, adrenal, pancreatic, and mesenteric regions may have implications for occlusive disease of these organs at a later age. The question has not been answered for any but the renal arteries so far, and it may be that more time will be necessary to elucidate the bowel and myocardial infarctions together with strokes and subarachnoid hemorrhages that may be implicated from this source. Too few of the more complex malformations have been studied in regard to prognosis to make useful comment. From our experience atrial defects in general are small; one would not expect great difficulties in later life because of such malformation. On the other hand, patients with tetralogy of Fallot have often had severe obstruction to right ventricular outflow together with marked stenosis of the pulmonary arteries so that the outlook for this group has been bad. Where pulmonary arterial stenosis is the principal cardiovascular manifestation there has been little published attempt to move to surgical therapy. The reason for this may be that the majority of patients in the childhood range have not had very severe obstruction. Some surgical experiences have been apparently successful but others with more peripheral lesions have not produced great benefit (Schumacker and Lurie, 1953; Sauvage et al., 1960; Baum et al., 1964).

REFERENCES

Ainger, L. E.: Cardiovascular lesions in rubella. Letter to Editor. *J. Pediatr.*, **68**:829, 1966.

Baum, D.; Khoury, G. H.; Ongley, P. A.; Swan, H. J. C.; and Kincaid, O. W.: Congenital stenosis of the pulmonary artery branches. *Circulation*, **29**:680, 1964.

Campbell, J.: Place of maternal rubella in the aetiology of congenital heart disease. *Br. Med. J.*, **1**:691, 1961.

Campbell, P. E.: Vascular abnormalities following maternal rubella. *Br. Heart J.*, **27**:134, 1965.

Cooper, L. Z., and Krugman, S.: Clinical manifestations of postnatal and congenital rubella. *Arch. Ophthalmol.*, **77**:434, 1967.

Driscoll, S. G.: Histopathology of gestational rubella. *Am. J. Dis. Child.*, **118**:49, 1969.

Dudgeon, J. A.: Congenital rubella. *J. Pediatr.*, **87**:1978, 1975.

Emmanouilides, G. C.; Linde, L. M.; and Crittenden, I. H.: Pulmonary artery stenosis associated with ductus arteriosus following maternal rubella. *Circulation*, **29**:514, 1964.

Esterly, J. R., and Oppenheimer, E. H.: Vascular lesions in infants with congenital rubella. *Circulation*, **36**:544, 1967.

Esterly, J. R., and Oppenheimer, E. H.: Pathological lesions due to congenital rubella. *Arch. Pathol.*, **87**:380, 1969.

Fortuin, N. J.; Morrow, A. G.; and Roberts, W. C.: Late vascular manifestations of the rubella syndrome. *Am. J. Med.*, **51**:134, 1971.

Gregg, N. McA.: Congenital cataract following German measles in the mother. *Trans. Ophthal. Soc. Aust.*, **3**:35, 1941.

Halloran, K. H.; Sanyal, S. K.; and Gardner, T. H.: Superiorly oriented electrocardiographic axis in infants with the rubella syndrome. *Am. Heart J.*, **72**:600, 1966.

Hardy, J. B.: Viruses and the fetus. *Postgrad. Med.*, **43**:156, 1968.

Hastreiter, A. R.; Joorabchi, B.; Pujatti, G.; Van der Horst, R. L.; Patacsil, G.; and Sever, J. L.: Cardiovascular lesions associated with congenital rubella. *J. Pediatr.*, **71**:59, 1967.

Heiner, D. C., and Nadas, A. S.: Patent ductus arteriosus in association with pulmonic stenoses. A report of six cases with additional noncardiac congenital anomalies. *Circulation*, **17**:232, 1958.

Hill, D. E.; Arellano, C. P.; Izukawa, T.; Holt, A. B.; and Cheek, D. B.: Studies in infants and children with congenital rubella: oxygen consumption, body water, cell mass, muscle and adipose tissue composition. *Johns Hopkins Med. J.*, **127**:309, 1970.

Karmody, C. S.: Subclinical maternal rubella and congenital deafness. *N. Engl. J. Med.*, **278**:809, 1968.

Katz, R. G.; White, L. R.; and Sever, J. L.: Maternal and congenital rubella. *Clin. Pediatr.*, **7** (No. 6):323, 1968.

Korones, S. B.; Ainger, L. E.; Monif, G. R. C.; Roane, J.; Sever, J. L.; and Fuste, F.: Congenital rubella syndrome: New clinical aspects with recovery of virus from affected infants. *J. Pediatr.*, **67**:166, 1965.

Krugman, S., and Katz, S. L.: Rubella immunization: a five-year progress report. *N. Engl. J. Med.*, **290**:1375, 1974.

Lynfield, J.; Vichitbandha, P.; Yao, A. C.; Rodriguez-Torres, R.; Karlson, K. E.; and Kauffman, S.: Neonatal heart failure following rubella in utero. *Am. J. Cardiol.*, **17**:130, 1966.

Menser, M. A.; Dods, L.; and Harley, J. D.: A twenty-five-year follow-up of congenital rubella. *Lancet*, **2**:1347, 1967.

Naeye, R. L., and Blanc, W.: Pathogenesis of congenital rubella. *JAMA*, **194**:1277, 1965.

Parkman, P. D.; Buescher, E. L.; and Artenstein, M. S.: Recovery of rubella virus from Army recruits. *Proc. Soc. Exp. Biol. Med.*, **3**:225, 1962.

Rowe, R. D.: Maternal rubella and pulmonary artery stenoses. Report of eleven cases. *Pediatrics*, **32**:180, 1963.

Rowe, R. D.; Mehrizi, A.; Elliott, H. L.; and Neill, C. A.: Cardiovascular disease in the rubella syndrome. In Cassels, D. E. (ed.): *The Heart and Circulation in the Newborn and Infant.* Grune & Stratton, New York, 1966, p. 180.

Rowe, R. D.; Varghese, P. J.; and Simon, A. L.: Asymptomatic systemic arterial lesions in congenital rubella (abstr.). American Pediatric Society, 79th Annual Meeting, 1969, p. 40.

Rowe, R. D., and Neill, C. A.: Patent ductus arteriosus in the first year of life: Factors influencing spontaneous closure. In Kidd, B. S. L., and Keith, J. D. (eds.): *The Natural History and Progress in Treatment of Congenital Heart Defects.* Charles C Thomas, Publisher, Springfield, Ill., 1971, p. 33.

Rowe, R. D.: Cardiovascular disease in the rubella syndrome. *Cardiovasc. Clin.*, **5**:62, 1972.

Sauvage, L. R.; Rudolph, A. M.; and Gross, R. E.: Replacement of the main pulmonary artery bifurcation by autogenous pericardium. *J. Thorac. Cardiovasc. Surg.*, **40**:567, 1960.

Schumacker, H. B., Jr., and Lurie, P. R.: Pulmonary valvulotomy. *J. Thorac. Surg.*, **25**:173, 1953.

Siassi, B.; Klyman, G.; and Emmanouilides, G. C.: Hypoplasia of the abdominal aorta associated with the rubella syndrome. *Am. J. Dis. Child.*, **120**:476, 1970.

Singer, D. B.; Rudolph, A. J.; Rosenberg, H. S.; Rawls, W. E.; and Boniuk, M.: Pathology of the congenital rubella syndrome. *J. Pediatr.*, **71**:665, 1967.

Tondury, G., and Smith, D. W.: Fetal rubella pathology. *J. Pediatr.*, **68**:867, 1966.

Varghese, P. J.; Izukawa, T.; and Rowe, R. D.: Supravalvular aortic stenosis as part of rubella syndrome, with discussion of pathogenesis. *Br. Heart J.*, **31**:59, 1969.

Venables, A. W.: The syndrome of pulmonary stenosis complicating maternal rubella. *Br. Heart J.*, **27**:49, 1965.

Wasserman, M. P.; Varghese, P. J.; and Rowe, R. D.: The evolution of pulmonary arterial stenosis associated with congenital rubella. *Am. Heart J.*, **76**:638, 1968.

Way, R. C.: Cardiovascular defects and the rubella syndrome. *Can. Med. Assoc. J.*, **97**:1329, 1967.

Weinberger, M. M.; Masland, M. W.; Asbed, R. A.; and Sever, J. L.: Congenital rubella presenting as retarded language development. *Am. J. Dis. Child.*, **120**:125, 1970.

Welch, J. P.: Prevention of congenital rubella. *Can. Med. Assoc. J.*, **117**:151, 1977.

Weller, T. H., and Neva, F. A.: Propagation in tissue culture of cytopathic agents from patients with rubella-like illness. *Proc. Soc. Exp. Biol. Med.*, **3**:215, 1962.

54

Cardiac Involvement in Acute Glomerulonephritis

John D. Keith

THERE is an increasing body of evidence to indicate that acute nephritis occurs as the result of a hemolytic streptococcal infection, types 4 and 12 of the bacteria having been implicated especially. Goodhart (1879) recognized that heart failure could develop as a complication of this disease, but neither the clinical nor pathologic picture is one that would be anticipated in a streptococcal infection. At postmortem, when death has occurred with cardiovascular signs associated with acute nephritis, there is usually very little to show in the myocardium (Whitehill et al., 1939)—no toxic myocarditis and no valvular disease. Gore and Saphir (1948) did find a few patchy areas of myocardial change in 10 percent of 160 cases studied.

Clinically the evidence of myocardial involvement has been remarked on by several authors. Master and associates (1937) reported the heart affected in 33 percent of cases. Marcolongo (1935) found it in 40 percent; Ellis (1942), in 20 percent; Murphy (1949), in 17 percent; Rubin and Rapoport (1938), in 25 percent; and Whitehill and associates (1939), in 71 percent. Thus some evidence of cardiac involvement is not uncommon in acute nephritis. If the above authors were believed, it would precede hypertensive encephalopathy (9 percent) and uremia (4 percent) (Rubin and Rapoport, 1938). However, true myocardial damage may be less common than thought in the past (Fleischer et al., 1966; Strauss and Welt, 1971).

Clinical Features

In the past the myocardium has been considered to be affected in acute nephritis when enlargement of the heart, electrocardiographic abnormalities, or congestive heart failure has been noted. These signs present difficulty in interpretation, especially heart size and electrocardiographic change.

Heart Size. Moderate degrees of cardiac enlargement are difficult to assess since the normal varies considerably. Furthermore, it is possible that in some cases slight increase in heart size may be related to increased blood volume or retention of fluid in the myocardium rather than myocardial disease itself. Such an explanation has also been suggested in studies with hormone therapy in rheumatic fever (Cooperative Rheumatic Fever Study, 1955). Cardiac enlargement was noted by Murphy and Murphy (1954) to occur in 58 percent of acute nephritis cases. At The Hospital for Sick Children, enlargement was noted in 20 percent (whereas evidence of heart failure occurred in only 4 percent).

Electrocardiographic Changes. In the past, electrocardiographic abnormalities have been reported as a frequent occurrence (Langendorf and Pick; 1937; LaDue and Ashman, 1946; Ash et al., 1944; Ashman and Hull, 1949; Murphy and Murphy, 1954). Master and coworkers (1937) found a higher incidence of electrocardiographic abnormalties such as a low, flat, or inverted T_1 and T_2 in the standard leads or similar changes in the T waves of the left precordium; alteration of the S-T segment and lengthening of the QRS interval were also noted. Tachycardia, bradycardia, minor alterations in the Q-T interval, and arrhythmias were occasionally seen but could not be linked as definitely to myocardial damage.

In our series of electrocardiographic studies in children, Disenhouse (1954) reviewed the electrocardiograms of 30 children with acute nephritis. Two-thirds of the electrocardiograms were made with precordial leads, and over half of the children had serial electrocardiograms. Only 5 percent were noted to have evidence suggestive of myocardial damage. The electrocardiographic changes usually disappeared quickly after improvement began, but occasionally the negative T waves persisted for several weeks.

Congestive Heart Failure. In the past the presence or absence of heart failure has been considered to be a guide in indicating the degree of myocardial involvement. Twenty-five percent of Murphy and

Murphy's group (1954) were considered to have congestive heart failure. We question this since it occurred in only 4 percent of our series. It is interesting to note the differing incidence of failure with age. In Murphy and Murphy's study only 18 percent of those under 20 years of age developed congestive heart failure, whereas among those over 20 years the incidence was 45 percent.

Peters (1953) has suggested that the edema of nephritis is due to cardiac failure. In our series edema was found much more frequently than failure, periorbital edema being present in half the cases and pitting edema of the legs in a fifth. It seems likely, therefore, that edema is usually not cardiac in origin.

Clinical signs suggestive of heart failure in acute nephritis are dyspnea associated with enlargement of the liver and pulmonary congestion. Moist rales are often heard at the lung bases, and on rare occasions in children pulmonary edema with copious sputum may develop.

Heart failure should be suspected or looked for in the presence of such indirect signs as tachycardia, gallop rhythm, apical systolic murmur, cardiac enlargement, and electrocardiographic abnormalities. Evidence may be found among the cases that have hypertensive encephalopathy with convulsions. It should be remembered that failure does not occur in the absence of cardiac enlargement.

The heart failure is usually accompanied by hypertension (90 to 95 percent). An occasional case has been reported in which the blood pressure was normal (Levy, 1930; Murphy et al., 1934). A number of children have only a slight elevation of blood pressure and yet develop some evidence suggestive of congestive heart failure. In the vast majority the pressure is considerably raised and there is, therefore, a good correlation between the presence of hypertension and heart failure. Thus the failure may be related to, but not wholly dependent on, the hypertension. It appears likely that the mechanism, possibly a toxic factor, that affects cellular membranes throughout the body causes edema in acute nephritis and may also alter the response of the myocardium. Other factors may be increased blood volume, hydremia (suggested by Addis, 1948), and salt retention (Fishberg, 1954).

The recent studies of Fleisher (1966) and Strauss and Welt (1971) question whether true heart failure ever occurs in acute glomerulonephritis. Thus the clinical signs should be evaluated carefully before such conclusion is reached.

Treatment

Treatment of acute nephritis involves a variety of therapeutic approaches.

Since acute nephritis is commonly precipitated by a streptococcal infection, it is logical as in acute rheumatic fever to eradicate the organism from the body. Adequate penicillin therapy maintaining a suitable blood level for ten days will usually achieve this. Three injections a day apart of an all-purpose-type penicillin, 1,200,000 units, which will include aqueous, procaine, and benzathine penicillin, will also produce this effect successfully.

After the investigations of a case are complete and there is evidence of some circulatory congestion, we can decide the therapy. If the circulatory congestion is mild, one can simply wait out the natural course of the disease, which will involve a diuresis, and this usually occurs within a few days. If the congestion is more severe, one should carry out a careful fluid balance, restrict fluid intake, and use a diuretic such as furosemide. At the same time one should carefully monitor the serum potassium, which might be elevated as the result of oliguria or lowered because of the use of the diuretic.

When there is evidence of circulatory involvement in acute glomerulonephritis, there is frequently evidence of hypertension. If this is mild no therapy is required, but at times the intramuscular use of reserpine and hydralazine may be necessary. In a severe crisis where there is a headache, vomiting, or convulsions it is recommended that Diazoxide, 5 mg/kg, be given intravenously over a ten-second period to relieve the crisis.

In recent years, it has been recognized that heart failure is a rare occurrence in acute glomerular-nephritis (Fleischer et al., 1966; Strauss and Welt, 1971). Slight cardiac enlargement and pulmonary congestion may be explained on the basis of peripheral venoconstruction and hypervolemia. Systemic hypertension does not appear essential for the occurrence of cardiac or pulmonary vascular changes, which are seen at times in glomerular nephritis, although they usually go together.

The value of digoxin is therefore in question when vascular changes are present in heart or lungs. They are usually relieved when diuresis occurs and blood pressure falls. If, however, both heart and liver are enlarged, with suggestive evidence of true heart failure, digitalis may reasonably be given. Fortunately such need appears rarely in this condition. If oliguria or anuria is present, the digitalis dose must be scaled down accordingly.

The incidence of various types of cardiac involvement in acute glomerulonephritis has been studied by Disenhouse and Keith at The Hospital for Sick Children, Toronto. The results are shown in Table 54–1. Our findings indicate how infrequently congestive heart failure is identified in this condition.

Salt restriction and adequate hydration are now recognized as an integral part of modern therapy. Since intravenous fluids or transfusions are not commonly given to children suffering from acute nephritis, it should be remembered that overrapid administration of fluid especially in the anuric or oliguric patient, may precipitate heart failure. Such has been noted to occur with transfusions. If this should happen, venesection and rapid withdrawal of 2 to 3 oz. of blood may be required.

Table 54–1. CARDIAC INVOLVEMENT IN ACUTE GLOMERULONEPHRITIS*

Number of cases of acute nephritis with or without cardiac involvement (1950–1955)	167
Cardiac failure	4%
Cardiac enlargement	20%
Electrocardiographic abnormalities (30 cases reviewed)	5%
Bradycardia	2%
Hypertension	54%
Hypertensive encephalopathy	9%
Age range of total group	
0–23 months	4
2– 5 years	68
6–10 years	75
11–15 years	20

* Disenhouse, R. B.: Hospital for Sick Children, Toronto.

Prognosis

A current view of the problem suggests that evidence of myocardial damage in nephritis is decreasing. Heart failure is less common, enlargement of the heart is less frequently noted, and electrocardiographic abnormalities are now relatively rare. It is possible that this improvement is related to therapy. The widespread use of penicillin, the more adequate use of fluids by mouth, the dietary restriction of salt, the administration of blood pressure–lowering drugs, and the occasional use of digitalis may all be playing a part in this improved prognosis.

REFERENCES

Addis, T.: *Glomerular Nephritis: Diagnosis and Treatment.* The Macmillan Co., New York, 1948.

Ash, R.; Rubin, M. I.; and Rapoport, M.: Electrocardiographic variations in acute glomerulonephritis. *Am. J. Dis. Child.,* **67**: 106, 1944.

Ashman, R., and Hull, E.: *A Primer of Electrocardiography,* 2nd ed. Lea & Febiger, Philadelphia, 1949.

Disenhouse, R. B.: Personal communication, 1956.

Ellis, A.: Natural history of Bright's disease: Clinical, histological, and experimental observations. Croonian lectures. *Lancet,* **1**: 1, 34, 72, 1942.

Fishberg, A. M.: Symposium on differential diagnosis of internal disease: differential diagnosis of high blood pressure. *Med. Clin. North Am.,* **38**: 753, 1954.

Fleisher, D. S., et al.: Hemodynamic findings in acute glomerulonephritis. *J. Pediatr.,* **69**: 1054–62, 1966.

Goodhart, J. F.: On acute dilatation of the heart as a cause of death in scarlatinal dropsy. *Guy Hosp. Rep.,* **24**: 152, 1879.

Gore, I., and Saphir, O.: Myocarditis associated with acute and subacute glomerulonephritis. *Am. Heart J.,* **36**: 390, 1948.

LaDue, J. S., and Ashman, R.: Electrocardiographic changes in acute glomerulonephritis. *Am. Heart J.,* **31**: 685, 1946. ·

Langendorf, R., and Pick, A.: Elektrokardiogramm bei akuter Nephritis. *Med. Klin.,* **33**: 126, 1937.

Levy, I. J.: The cardiac response in acute diffuse glomerulonephritis. *Am. Heart J.,* **5**: 277, 1930.

Marcolongo, F.: Il cuore nella glomerulonefrite acta diffusa. *Arch. Med. Scand.,* **59**: 975, 1025, 1935.

Master, A. M.; Jaffe, H. L.; and Dack, S.: Electrocardiographic changes in acute nephritis. *J. Mt. Sinai Hosp. N.Y.,* **4**: 98, 1937.

Murphy, F. D.: *Acute Medical Disorders,* 3rd ed. F. A. Davis Co., Philadelphia, 1949.

Murphy, F. D.; Grill, J.; and Moxon, G. F.: Acute diffuse glomerular nephritis: study of 94 cases with special consideration of stage of transition into chronic form. *Arch. Intern. Med.,* **54**: 483, 1934.

Murphy, T. R., and Murphy, F. D.: The heart in acute glomerulonephritis. *Ann. Intern. Med.,* **41**: 510, 1954.

Peters, J. P.: Edema of acute nephritis. *Am. J. Med.,* **14**: 448, 1953.

Rubin, M. I., and Rapoport, M.: Cardiac complications of acute hemorrhagic nephritis. *Am. J. Dis. Child.,* **55**: 244, 1938.

Strauss, M. B., and Welt, L. G.: *Diseases of the Kidney,* 2nd ed. Little, Brown and Co., Boston, 1971.

Whitehill, R.; Longcope, W. T.; and Williams, R.: The occurrence and significance of myocardial failure in acute hemorrhagic nephritis. *Bull. Hopkins Hosp.,* **64**: 83, 1939.

55

Cardiac Involvement in the Collagen Diseases

Robert M. Freedom and *John D. Keith*

DURING recent years, several well-known disease entities, such as rheumatic fever, rheumatoid arthritis, disseminated lupus erythematosus, periarteritis nodosa, scleroderma, dermatomyositis, and serum sickness, have been grouped under the heading of "diffuse collagen disease." This grouping is based on the concept that all have as their common denominator some alteration in the connective tissue elements (collagen tissue) of the body. They have also been called autoimmune diseases.

Klinge in 1930 noted that the changes in rheumatic fever had their basis in alteration of the connective tissue and emphasized the similarity to periarteritis nodosa and serum sickness.

The term "collagen diseases" was first suggested in 1941 by Klemperer and coworkers, who showed that the lesions of disseminated lupus erythematosus and diffuse scleroderma were the result of changes in the collagenous tissue. The term met with immediate popularity; however, to prevent it from being used as a wastebasket for puzzling syndromes, Klemperer (1955) later stressed that, although many of these diseases had a basic anatomic site and similar histopathologic change, this did not mean that they were identical or even related.

The connective tissue of the body is composed of cells and intercellular substance, and its structure differs according to local requirements. The cells are fibroblasts, and the intercellular substance consists of fibers (collagen, elastic, reticulum) and a homogeneous ground substance, the nature of which has not yet been elucidated but which is probably composed of complicated mucoproteins.

Fibrinoid degeneration of the connective tissue of the body is the most characteristic pathologic change in these conditions, but proliferation and inflammation may also occur in varying degrees. Thus in rheumatic fever, proliferation (heart valves) and inflammation (joints) predominate, although necrosis does occur in the center of the Aschoff nodule. In periarteritis nodosa, the lesions are limited to the small- and medium-sized arteries, with proliferation and inflammation standing out. In disseminated lupus erythematosus, fibrinoid de-

generation of connective tissue dominates the scene with involvement of skin, joint capsules, serous membranes, blood vessels, endocardium, lymph nodes, etc., while proliferation and inflammation are at a minimum. In diffuse scleroderma, the lesions are essentially proliferative with thickening and sclerosing of the collagen tissue of the blood vessels, alimentary tract, lungs, and skeletal muscles, but fibrinoid changes have also been noted. As Duff states: "These differences, together with the differences in the anatomical distribution of the lesions, permit the recognition of distinct disease entities.... The same theme runs through all of them, but the variations on the theme are distinct for each disease."*

As to the etiology of these conditions, much has been written. Since fibrinoid degeneration is present to some degree in most of them, and since fibrinoid changes are characteristic of allergic tissue reactions, it has been postulated that many of the collagen diseases have an allergic origin. Observations of Klinge (1930), Rich (1945), and Rich and Gregory (1943) strongly support this view; nevertheless, as has been pointed out by Klemperer and coworkers (1941), fibrinoid collagen alteration must not be interpreted solely and invariably as an expression of an allergic reaction. Thus simple squeezing of the skin results in fibrinoid degeneration; it may occur in acute bacterial infections, in the base of a chronic peptic ulcer, and in the vicinity of acute pancreatic necrosis. It is superfluous to state that the nature of these maladies has yet to be clarified.

The cardiovascular system is involved in all of these diseases, but there is considerable variation in the extent and degree, partly dependent on the underlying disease process and partly on the individual response of the patient concerned. This subject is well reviewed by Taubenhaus and associates (1955) and Sokoloff (1964).

---

* Duff, G. L.: The collagen diseases. In Ashford, M. (ed.): *The Musuloskeletal System* (symposium presented at Twenty-third Graduate Fortnight of the New York Academy of Medicine). Macmillan Publishing Co., Inc., New York, 1952, p. 251.

PERIARTERITIS NODOSA

PERIARTERITIS nodosa was first described as a clinical entity in 1866 by Kussmaul and Maier. It may be defined as a form of necrotizing inflammatory panarteritis affecting small- and medium-sized arteries throughout the body, characterized by the signs of a systemic infection and by focal signs and symptoms due to scattered arterial lesions with local circulatory disturbances varying from relative ischemia to gross infarction.

Etiology

Clinical and experimental data strongly support the theory that periarteritis is caused by an allergic response to a variety of antigens. These may be bacterial or nonbacterial (e.g., sulfonamides, arsenicals, desoxycorticosterone acetate). Rich (1945) and Rich and Gregory (1943) produced acute necrotizing arteritis, accompanied by acute carditis and glomerulonephritis, by repeated injections of foreign serum in rabbits.

Pathology

Pathologically the lesions are limited to small- and medium-sized arteries of muscular type, which are affected segmentally. The adventitia and media are involved in a proliferative reaction that is accompanied by edema and infiltration of inflammatory cells, polymorphonuclear cells, and eosinophils. There is extensive necrosis of the media with resultant aneurysms. The inflammation extends to the intima with destruction of endothelium and thrombosis. (Fibrinoid degeneration is found in the ground substance of the media and/or intima, followed by fibroblastic proliferation and narrowing of the vessels.) The vessels of the kidneys appear to be the most susceptible followed by the coronary, adrenal, pancreatic, mesenteric, hepatic, splenic, and cerebral vessels.

Clinical Features

Periarteritis may present a multiplicity of manifestations. The onset is usually insidious. Several systems or organs may be involved. Frequently there is a protracted fever with pronounced tachycardia but no obvious cause. A very high sedimentation rate and anemia are relatively constant. Other vague symptoms may include arthralgia, abdominal distress, weight loss, lethargy, general malaise, weakness, and headache.

The kidneys are involved (pathologically) in 90 percent of the cases, and urinary changes, such as albuminuria, casts, and microscopic hematuria, are found in two-thirds. Hypertension eventually develops in two-thirds of the cases. There may be evidence of renal failure and associated changes in the ocular fundi.

Pain may be a prominent feature due to such things as mesenteric vessel involvement, arthritis, polyneuritis (in 50 percent), polymyositis, peripheral ischemia of the Raynaud type, or visceral infarction. There may be painful subcutaneous nodules.

Edema may occur in as many as 50 percent of the cases due to nephropathy, congestive failure, or polymyositis. A high polymorphonuclear leukocytosis (count often more than 20,000) is common, but a significant eosinophilia occurs in only 20 percent of the cases. Peripheral neuritis may be manifested by wasting, weakness, paresthesias, and reflex changes. Central nervous system involvement may lead to convulsions, coma, and death. Involvement of mesenteric arteries may lead to abdominal pain, nausea, vomiting, diarrhea, or gastrointestinal hemorrhage. Perforation of bowel with peritonitis may occur.

Myocardial Involvement

Myocardial involvement is usually secondary to coronary disease augmented by hypertension, if such is present. Occasionally a myocardial infarction occurs. Failure may develop and is not uncommonly a terminal event. Enlargement of the heart may be visible by fluoroscopy, and the electrocardiogram at times shows T wave and S-T segment changes indicative of myocardial infarction, pericarditis, or myocarditis. Left ventricular hypertrophy may be exhibited in the presence of severe hypertension.

Systolic murmurs may appear at times, and are related to pathologic change in the valve margins.

Pericarditis is not as common as in lupus erythematosus, but it does occur occasionally and may be accompanied by a friction rub or suggestive electrocardiographic or x-ray changes.

Diagnosis

The diagnosis is made partly by exclusion, partly by the diffuse nature of the disease coupled with leukocytosis and at times an eosinophilia. Urinary findings and a reverse of the albumin-globulin ratio may be of help. For complete confirmation a biopsy is required, showing the characteristic invasion of the arterial wall.

Recently, a new infantile acute febrile mucocutaneous lymph node syndrome has been described in Japan (Kawasaki, 1967). This disease, affecting infants and children, is an acute febrile mucocutaneous condition, accompanied by swelling of cervical lymph nodes. The principal symptoms include: (1) fever of one to two weeks, not responsive to antibiotics; (2) congestion of ocular conjunctivae; (3) changes of lips and oral cavity, including dryness, redness, and fissuring of lips, protuberance of tongue papillae, and reddening of oral and pharyngeal mucosa; (4) changes of peripheral extremities, characterized initially by reddening of palms and soles, with an indurative edema, and followed by membranous desquamation from the fingertips; (5) polymorphous exanthema of trunk; and (6) acute nonsuppurative cervical lymphadenopathy (Kawasaki et al., 1974). Kawasaki of Tokyo in 1967 initially described 50 cases of this seemingly self-limited disease. Subsequently, more than 6000 cases have been reported in Japan. One to two percent of these patients have died suddenly of cardiac failure (Yanagisawa et al., 1974). The autopsies have showed periarteritis nodosa-like arteritis, accompanied by coronary thrombosis and aneurysm, and in some surviving patients coronary artery aneurysms have been demonstrated by aortography (Kato et al., 1975; Radford et al., 1975). Serial coronary arteriography has shown resolution of the coronary aneurysms in some patients.

There are obvious similarities between infantile periarteritis and the mucocutaneous lymph node syndrome. Laboratory tests will show similar abnormalities. There is a view that infantile polyarteritis nodosa and mucocutaneous lymph node syndrome are diseases of a common basic process. However, infantile polyarteritis nodosa has been a rare disease, with a very poor prognosis. In Japan, the mucocutaneous lymph node syndrome has occurred in great numbers, and the prognosis has been excellent in the majority of cases.

The etiology of the mucocutaneous lymph node syndrome is unknown. Hamashima has recently demonstrated Rickettsia-like bodies by electron microscopy in biopsy specimens obtained from the skin or lymph nodes in 12 of 23 patients with mucocutaneous lymph node syndrome. These bodies were located in the cytoplasm of macrophages, in arteriolar endothelial cells, and inside the vascular lumen. The bodies were isolated by yolk sac culture, but their pathogenicity has not as yet been proven.

Prognosis and Treatment

The disease is usually fatal. The average length of life as reported by Harris and associates (1939) is 8.6 months. However, a few cases have survived up to 5 years from the time of onset, and a number followed for a shorter time have shown apparent recovery.

The treatment in the past has been palliative and supportive with the use of transfusion, digitalis, and antibiotics. Cortisone has proved valuable in controlling signs and symptoms in children and is much more effective in some cases than in others. In some children the disease proceeds to its termination in spite of the use of such hormonal therapy. In others, varying degrees of relief up to apparent cure have resulted.

DISSEMINATED LUPUS ERYTHEMATOSUS

THIS disease was first described by Kapozi in 1872 and is characterized by an erythematous skin rash, involving the face particularly, with a butterfly type of malar flush. It is associated with varying signs of arthritis, arthralgia, polyserositis, large lymph nodes, splenomegaly, leukopenia and anemia, and central nervous system manifestations. It usually has its onset in the second decade of life but has been found a number of times in children between the ages of five and ten years. The diagnosis is now usually made by the appearance of LE cells in the bloodstream. These have been found to occur in 75 percent of cases at some time.

Pathology

Pathologic studies show evidence of fibrinoid degeneration of the connective tissue, and the cardiovascular system is always involved to some degree. There is endothelial fibrinoid degeneration appearing indiscriminately in the arteries of various organs. Such lesions may extend throughout the entire thickness of the vessel wall. The epicardium and pericardium of the heart are frequently involved; the myocardium may show degeneration and fibrosis; and verrucae are frequently seen on some or all of the valves, particularly the tricuspid (Gross, 1940). Renal vascular disease is a common finding and is associated with evidence of kidney damage in two-thirds of the cases. Hypertension secondary to the renal pathology is frequently noted.

Clinical Evidence of Involvement of the Cardiovascular System

A pericardial friction rub and x-ray evidence of pericardial effusion are common findings since pericardial involvement has been reported at postmortem in nearly half of the cases (Dubois, 1953). Heart murmurs may be heard in any area of the precordium, depending on the valves affected. One or more heart valves are involved in approximately 40 percent of the cases (Taubenhaus et al., 1955). It should be remembered, however, that endocarditis has been found at postmortem without murmurs having been present during life. Furthermore, heart murmurs may occur without the presence of valve damage. The electrocardiogram may reveal evidence of myocarditis with flattened or inverted T waves over the precordium. Enlargement of the heart is common, and congestive heart failure has been reported as occurring in approximately one-fourth of these patients (Shearn and Pirofsky, 1952).

Severe valvular dysfunction is an unusual clinical occurrence in the patient with disseminated lupus erythematosus, despite the frequent finding on noninfective Libman-Sacks endocardial lesions at necropsy. Recently, however, Paget and his associates (1975) described severe mitral regurgitation in an 18-year-old woman with lupus erythematosus. Because of severe congestive heart failure and a catheter study that demonstrated a mean pulmonary wedge pressure of 28 mm Hg, with "a" waves of 32 and "v" waves of 40 mm Hg, mitral valve replacement was performed, using a 29-mm porcine xenograft. Examination of the excised valve demonstrated healed and calcified Libman-Sacks lesions. Hemotoxylin bodies, Aschoff bodies, and stainable organisms were not observed.

Significant aortic valve regurgitation has also been associated with lupus erythematosus, and aortic valve replacement has been performed (Oh et al., 1974; Shulman and Christian, 1969).

Raynaud's phenomenon, due to interference in the circulation of the fingers and toes, has been reported in nearly one-fourth of the patients (Dubois, 1953). Central nervous system involvement secondary to cardiovascular change is not uncommon, and when it does occur it is frequently associated with convulsions. Pancreatitis secondary to vascular change has also been reported. Arteritis may be found in any organ system of the body, and thus bizarre signs and symptoms are to be expected in diffuse, irregular patterns (Brigden et al., 1960).

Treatment

The skin and joint manifestations are usually controlled by cortisone, ACTH, or newer steroids.

Myocardial function may also improve. The renal involvement, if present, may be improved by the use of steroids and immunosuppressive agents.

The natural history of the cardiovascular manifestations of disseminated lupus erythematosus has been substantially altered by the use of corticosteroids, which exert their own cardiovascular effects. Bulkley and Roberts (1975) described clinical and necropsy observations in 36 corticosteroid-treated patients with lupus and compared them to necropsy observations in patients with disseminated lupus reported before the use of corticosteroid therapy. Hypertension was five times more common in the steroid-treated group, and congestive heart failure was eight times more frequent than that reported in the nonsteroid-treated patients. Subepicardial and myocardial fat was increased in all 36 patients.

The frequency of lupus carditis was similar between the two groups, but differed morphologically. Libman-Sacks endocardial lesions were smaller and fewer in number in the steroid-treated patients and tended to be left-sided and univalvular, rather than multivalvular. The majority of the verrucae were partially or totally healed, and some were calcified. Pericarditis was predominantly fibrous and myocarditis was found in only three patients. In 42 percent of the 50 patients who had received corticosteroids for more than one year, the lumen of at least one of the three major coronary arteries was narrowed more than 50 percent by atherosclerotic plaques. In none of 17 patients treated for less than a year was this narrowing found.

These authors conclude that corticosteroids, while vital to the management of lupus erythematosus, have an overall deleterious effect on the heart: Systemic hypertension and left ventricular hypertrophy either appear or worsen; congestive heart failure increases; epicardial and myocardial fat increases; and coronary atherosclerosis seems accelerated.

DERMATOMYOSITIS

DERMATOMYOSITIS was first described by Wagner, Hepp, and Unervicht independently in 1887. There have been a number of reviews on the subject since. In 1939, Schuermann analyzed 263 cases collected from the literature and noted that 47 of them were in children under the age of 15 years. Since then Selander (1950) has reported 20 new cases in children under seven years of age; Roberts and Brunsting (1954), 40 cases under 15 years; Wedgwood and associates (1953), 26 cases in childhood.

Clinical Features

The chief clinical features are muscular weakness and involvement of skin and subcutaneous tissues. The muscles of the trunk and extremities, the muscles of respiration, and those of swallowing are

characteristically affected. Pain and tenderness are associated with a progressive weakness that eventually makes the patient bedridden. Death is frequently due to failure of respiratory or swallowing muscles, and in advanced cases calcinosis of muscles or other tissues is found.

Involvement of the skin and subcutaneous tissues shown in a dermatitis with indurated tissues of the trunk and extremities. There may be facial skin lesions and periorbital swelling or generalized edema. Involvement of the skin over the joints may lead to contractures.

Pathology

Pathologically, the skeletal muscle and skin are predominantly affected. The earliest lesions show

Table 55-1. CARDIAC INVOLVEMENT IN THE COLLAGEN DISEASES

DISEASE	ARTERITIS	ENDOCARDIAL	MYOCARDIAL	PERICARDIAL	RAYNAUD'S PHENOMENON	ECG CHANGES	LABORATORY	CLINICAL
Disseminated lupus erythematosus	Many organs of body Kidney Cerebral Gastrointestinal Coronary	+++ All 4 valves may be involved 40 percent (Libman-Sacks)	Cardiac enlargement Heart failure—24 percent	++ Up to 45 percent of cases	25 percent	T and S-T changes of myocarditis or pericarditis	LE cells in 75 percent of cases	Sex incidence: M:F, 1:3.5 Common age of onset: 15–40 years Erythematous skin changes: face ++ Heart murmurs Heart failure Pericardial friction rub or ECG changes Raynaud's phenomenon
Periarteritis nodosa	Renal Coronary Mesenteric Muscular Splenic Cerebral	Occasionally	Cardiac enlargement Left heart strain with hypertension Heart failure is common	+ Occurs occasionally	Rare	Changes of pericarditis or myocarditis	Leukocytosis Eosinophilia Reversal of albumin-globulin ratio	Sex incidence: M:F, 4:1 Common age of onset: 20–40 years Muscle tenderness Signs of renal involvement, hematuria, nocturia Heart failure Abdominal pain, G.I. hemorrhage Convulsions Weakness Peripheral neuritis, paresthesia, pain Erythema
Dermatomyositis	+	±	++ 10 percent of children have heart murmurs May have terminal heart failure	±	++	+		Sex incidence: M:F, 1:1 Common age of onset: 10–50 years Muscle weakness: shoulder, pelvis, swallowing, respiratory Skin: dermatitis, edema Pneumonia

974

Disease	Pathology						Clinical features
Scleroderma	+ Perivascular fibrosis Intimal proliferation Skin Extremities Lungs Heart	±	+ Fibrosis Hypertrophy in 50 percent	0	±	+	Sex incidence: M:F, 1:2.7 Common age of onset: 30–50 years Swollen, thickened, leathery skin Heart failure Dyspnea Pulmonary hypertension ECG changes of myocardium Cardiac enlargement Right ventricular hypertrophy
Serum sickness	– Fibrinoid: degree of vessel walls	±	±	0	±	± T wave inversion, S-T alteration occasionally	Urticaria Joint swelling Fever
Rheumatic fever	±	+++	+++	+15 percent	0	+	Arthritis, 50 percent Nodules, 10 percent Chorea, 15 percent Carditis, 70 percent Erythema marginatum, 5 percent Heart failure, 15 percent
Rheumatoid arthritis in children	0	Children—1 percent	0	Children—5 percent	Changes of pericarditis may be seen in 5 percent	0	Arthritis Rash, 25 percent Nodules, 5–15 percent No heart failure Pericarditis, 5 percent

RHEUMATOID ARTHRITIS IN ADULTS.* TYPES OF CARDIAC INVOLVEMENT

Idiopathic pericarditis—40 percent adults, 5 percent—children
Interstitial myocarditis—occasional
Rheumatic heart disease—6–10 percent
Rheumatoid heart disease
granulomatous process—5–20 percent
Coronary arteritis—2 percent

* Sokoloff L.: Cardiac involvement in rheumatoid arthritis and allied disorders: current concepts. *Mod. Concepts Cardiovasc. Dis.*, **33**:847, 1964.

edema of the subendothelial connective tissues with collections of inflammatory cells in both skin and muscle. Vascular changes are found with a hyalinized material in the media of the arterioles and slight inflammatory reaction in and around the vessels. The myocardium may show pathologic change with loss of striation, fragmentation, and vascularization of muscle fibers. Interstitial tissues of the heart may show swelling and edema, and the disease process may at times involve the epicardium, but the pericardium is usually spared.

Clinical Evidence of Involvement of the Cardiovascular System

Clinically the most common finding of the cardiovascular system is tachycardia of a greater degree than one would expect from the age of the child. The electrocardiogram may be normal but at times may show a lowering, flattening, or inversion of the T wave due to myocardial involvement. Arrhythmias have been reported. Enlargement of the heart is uncommon, but if myocardial disease is present heart murmurs may be heard. Roberts and Brunsting (1954) report that 10 percent of children have a murmur. The edema referred to is part of the disease process involving the skin and tissues, and only under exceptional circumstances is it due to heart failure. Dyspnea may be present, but this again is associated with respiratory failure in most instances and is not myocardial in origin. The blood pressure is usually within normal limits. Raynaud's phenomenon in the fingers or toes is not uncommon.

Treatment

The majority of children with this condition are clinically improved by cortisone or ACTH. A few are not improved.

Prognosis

Wedgewood and associates (1953) record a follow-up of 26 cases in childhood. Ten died four months to two years from the onset of the disease. Of the 16 that survived, four were still active, four were severely crippled, and eight were leading normal lives but had some muscle weakness.

SCLERODERMA

In common with most other collagen diseases scleroderma is found more frequently in adult life. It has been reported occasionally in childhood (Leinwand et al., 1954).

Pathology

Scleroderma is characterized by a widespread replacement of cutaneous and subcutaneous fibrous tissue by collagen, which results in a generalized thickening of the skin. The onset may be associated with an erythema, but this soon gives way to swelling and eventually to a leathery, stiff dermoid layer that is unpliable. It may at times have a shiny appearance.

The face and extremities are affected first. Joint movement may be limited because of the overlying skin involvement. Atrophy of muscles occurs; pulmonary involvement is common since a fibrosis develops in the interstitial tissues of the lung with obliteration of alveoli and capillaries and eventual formation of cysts.

Vascular changes occur with intimal proliferation and perivascular fibrosis. Such vessel alterations may be found in skin, kidney, extremities, and pulmonary arteries. Interstitial fibrosis is common in the heart and may lead to heart failure. The heart weight has been found to be moderately increased in approximately one-half of the cases.

Clinical Evidence of Involvement of the Cardiovascular System

Heart failure may occur from the myocardial involvement or because of pulmonary hypertension secondary to pulmonary vascular and interstitial change. Occasionally it is the presenting symptom (Weiss et al., 1943). Enlargement of the heart may be demonstrated by x-ray, in many cases with or without failure.

Pericardial disease, has been extensively studied in patients with scleroderma (McWhorter and LeRoy, 1974; D'Angelo et al., 1969). Basically there are two clinical patterns of pericardial disease: (1) chronic pericardial effusion and (2) acute pericarditis (with associated dyspnea, chest pain, friction rub, fever, and cardiomegaly). Clinical evidence of pericardial involvement occurred in 15 of 210 patients with scleroderma studied by McWhorter and LeRoy. In the same study, the incidence of pericardial involvement at autopsy was twice as frequent as the incidence of significant myocardial fibrosis. These authors suggest that pericardial scleroderma represents a fairly common form of cardiac involvement in this connective tissue disorder.

Prognosis

The prognosis shows marked variability, some

cases rapidly reaching a fatal termination in less than a year and others showing arrest of the disease process and surviving 16 years or more (Biegelman et al., 1953; Leinwand et al., 1954). Leinwand describes a case three years of age at onset of the disease who died at 35 years. The localized or circumscribed cases do better than those with a more generalized involvement. ACTH and cortisone are usually of transient benefit only, but may occasionally contribute to the arrest of the disease.

For discussion of rheumatoid arthritis, see Chapter 15.

For rheumatic fever, see Chapter 13.

REFERENCES

Barrett, N. W., and O'Brien, W.: Heart disease in scleroderma. *Br. Heart J.*, **14**:421, 1952.

Biegelman, P. M.; Goldner, F., Jr.; and Bayles, T. B.: Progressive systemic sclerosis (scleroderma). *N. Engl. J. Med.*, **249**:45, 1953.

Brigden, W.; Bywaters, E.; Lessof, M.; and Ross, I.: The heart in systemic lupus erythematosus. *Br. Heart J.*, **22**:1, 1960.

Bulkley, B. H., and Roberts, W. C.: The heart in systemic lupus erythematosus and the changes induced in it by corticosteroid therapy. A study of 36 necropsy patients. *Am. J. Med.*, **58**:243, 1975.

Dorfman, A.: Metabolism of the mucopolysaccharides of connective tissue. *Pharmacol. Rev.*, **7**:1, 1955.

Dubois, E. L.: The effect of the LE cell test on the clinical picture of systemic lupus erythematosus. *Ann. Intern. Med.*, **38**:1265, 1953.

Duff, G. L.: The collagen diseases. In Ashford, M. (ed.): *The Musculoskeletal System* (symposium presented at twenty-third Graduate Fortnight of the New York Academy of Medicine). The Macmillan Co., New York, 1952, p. 243.

Ehrich, W. E.: Nature of collagen diseases. *Am. Heart J.*, **43**:121, 1952.

Friedberg, C. K., and Gross, L.: Periarteritis nodosa (necrotizing arteritis) associated with rheumatic heart disease, with a note on abdominal rheumatism. *Arch. Intern. Med.*, **54**:170, 1934.

Goetz, R. H.: The heart in generalized scleroderma (progressive systemic sclerosis). *Angiology*, **2**:555, 1951.

Goldman, M. J., and Lau, F. J. K.: Acute pericarditis associated with serum sickness. *N. Engl. J. Med.*, **250**:278, 1954.

Gross, L.: The cardiac lesions in Libman-Sacks disease with a consideration of its relationship to acute diffuse lupus erythematosus. *Am. J. Pathol.*, **16**:375, 1940.

Hamashima, Y.; Kishi, K.; and Tasaka, K.: Rickettsia-like bodies in infantile acute febrile mucocutaneous lymph node syndrome. *Lancet*, **1**:42, 1973.

Harris, A. W.; Lynch, G. W.; and O'Hare, J. P.: Periarteritis nodosa. *Arch Intern. Med.*, **63**:1163, 1939.

Jessar, R. A.; Lamont-Havers, W.; and Ragan, C.: Natural-history of lupus erythematosus disseminatus. *Ann. Intern. Med.*, **38**:717, 1953.

Kato, H.; Koike, S.; Yamamoto, M.; Ito, Y.; and Yano, E.: Coronary aneurysms in infants and young children with acute febrile mucocutaneous lymph node syndrome. *J. Paediatr.*, **86**:892, 1975.

Kawasaki, T.: Clinical observations of 50 cases (in Japan). *Jap. J. Allerg.*, **16**:178, 1967.

Kawasaki, T.; Kosaki, F.; Okawa, S.; Shigematsu, I.; and Yanagawa, H.: A new infantile acute febrile mucocutaneous lymph node syndrome (M.L.N.S.) prevailing in Japan. *Paediatrics*, **54**:271, 1974.

Kinney, T. D., and Maher, M. M.: Dermatomyositis: a study of 5 cases. *Am. J. Pathol.*, **16**:561, 1940.

Klemperer, P.: Pathology of systemic lupus erythematosus. In McManus, J. F. A. (ed.): *Progress in Fundamental Medicine*, Lea & Febiger, Philadelphia, 1952, p. 51.

———: The significance of the intermediate substance of the connective tissues. *The Harvey Lectures, 1953–1954*. Charles C Thomas, Publisher, Springfield, Ill., 1955, p. 100.

Klemperer, P.; Pollack, A. D.; and Baehr, G.: Pathology of disseminated lupus erythematosus. *Arch. Pathol.*, **32**:569, 1941.

Klinge, F.: Das Gewebsbild des fieberhaften Rheumatismus; das rheumatische Frühinfiltrat. (Akutes degenerativ-exsudatives Stadium.) *Virchows Arch. Pathol. Anat.*, **278**:438, 1930.

Oh, W. M. C.; Taylor, R. T.; and Olsen, E. G. J.: Aortic regurgitation in systemic lupus erythematosus requiring aortic valve replacement. *Br. Heart J.*, **36**:413, 1974.

Paget, S. A.; Bulkley, B. H.; Grauer, L. F.; and Seningen, R.: Mitral valve disease of systemic lupus erythematosus. A cause of severe congestive heart failure reversed by valve replacement. *Am. J. Med.*, **59**:134, 1975.

Radford, D. J.; Sondheimer, H. M.; Williams, G. J.; and Fowler, R. S.: A case of mucocutaneous lymph node syndrome with coronary artery aneurysm. *Am. J. Dis. Child.*, **130**:596, 1976.

Shulman, H. J., and Christian, C. L.: Aortic insufficiency in systemic lupus erythematosus. *Arthritis Rheum.*, **12**:138, 1969.

Sokoloff, L.: Cardiac involvement in rheumatoid arthritis and allied disorders: current concepts. *Mod. Concepts Cardiovasc. Dis.*, **33**:847, 1964.

Yanagisawa, M.; Kobayashi, N.; Matsuya, S.: Myocardial infarction due to coronary thromboarteritis, following acute febrile mucocutaneous lymph node syndrome (M.L.N.S.) in an infant. *Paediatrics*, **54**:277, 1974.

56

The Heart in Neuromuscular Disorders

Richard D. Rowe and *Robert M. Freedom*

THE HEART IN FRIEDREICH'S ATAXIA

RIEDREICH'S ataxia is a hereditary neurologic disorder characterized pathologically by a degeneration of the optic nerves, cerebellum, olive, and lateral and posterior columns of the spinal cord. It is usually caused by a recessive gene. Less commonly, a dominant form of inheritance from father to daughter has been observed (Boyer et al., 1962). Microscopically the neurologic changes are those of parenchymal atrophy and gliosis. Similar histologic changes have been seen in the hearts of patients dying with the disease. Marked eccentric hypertrophy of both ventricles is present, but usually there is no grossly visible fibrosis or infarction. Histologic examination shows extensive fibrosis separating hypertrophied muscle fibers in all cardiac chambers. Focal degenerative changes within the cardiac muscle can also be identified, but there have been no changes found in bulbar nuclei or in the cardiac conducting system. Round cell infiltration has been reported as present (Russell, 1946; Manning, 1950) and absent (Ivemark and Thorén, 1964; Hewer, 1969). Minor degrees of left atrial fibroelastosis and occasional thrombi have been found, but no generalized vascular or muscular abnormalities have been observed in other parts of the body (Ivemark and Thorén, 1969). There has been a recent difference of opinion over the importance to be attached to subintimal fibrosis of large coronary arteries or to the patchy luminal narrowing of smaller coronary arteries. These changes are not infrequently seen in large coronary vessels but particular interest has arisen over involvement of the smaller vessels (Nadas et al., 1951; Ivemark and Thorén, 1964; James and Fisch, 1963; Hewer, 1969; Krongrad and Joos, 1972).

Five of the six cases reviewed by Friedreich (1863) had cardiac abnormalities. Pitt (1887) reported a case dying in congestive failure whose autopsy showed diffuse myocardial fibrosis. Reports of cardiac involvement in Friedreich's ataxia later appeared in the French literature (Debre et al., 1936; van Bogaert and van Bogaert, 1936; Laubry and Heim de Balsac,

1936), and subsequently a number of papers on this aspect have been published (Evans and Wright, 1942; Russell, 1946; Piron, 1946; Hejtmancik et al., 1949; Manning, 1950; Flipse et al., 1950; Schilero et al., 1952; Gach et al., 1971; Perloff, 1971). The publications of Lorenz and associates (1950), Nadas and associates (1951), Novick and associates (1955), Thilenius and Grossman (1961), Thorén (1964), Boehm and colleagues (1970) Ruschhaupt and associates (1972), and Krongrad and Joos (1972), in particular, have drawn attention to the fact that heart involvement in Friedreich's ataxia may be pronounced in childhood.

Etiology

The basic cause of the neurologic degeneration in Friedreich's ataxia is unknown. It seems very likely that there is a close etiologic relationship between the neurologic and cardiac aspects of the disorder. Theories on this relationship have been many and varied. Certainly heart involvement is not directly related to the time of onset of the neurologic disorder or to the age of the patient, and its presence is not dependent on the severity of neurologic involvement. Nevertheless, heart disease, more often than not, is associated with severe and diffuse neurologic disease (Evans and Wright, 1942; Manning, 1950). In most series the cases with a positive family history have had heart disease more often and in greater severity than those without a family history of neurologic disease (Evans and Wright, 1942; Lorenz et al., 1950; Schilero et al., 1952), but the reverse was found in the patients studied by Boyer and coworkers (1962).

The histologic picture in the myocardium and the abnormal appearance of the coronary arteries have led to several views on the pathogenesis of the cardiac involvement. These have included an ischemic cause secondary to small-vessel disease (James and Fisch, 1963), neurologic dysfunction (Russell, 1946), and the suggestion that there is a common genetic basis for both the neurologic and the cardiac disorder (Evans, 1949; Manning, 1950; Thorén, 1964). Support for the vascular concept has been most strongly provided by the detailed pathologic studies of James and Fisch (1963), by the frequently encountered electrocardiographic (Thorén, 1964) and vectorcardiographic (Gregorini et al., 1974) signs of myocardial damage, and by a detailed clinical case report suggesting myocardial infarction (Krongrad and Joos, 1970). Against these views are other histologic studies that show that less than 10 percent of small coronary arteries to be affected, that active myocardial necrosis can occur without nearby arterial alterations, and that involved arteries tend to be close to areas of fibrous replacement (Hewer, 1969). Clearly the mechanism of cardiac involvement is far from settled.

Clinical Features

The onset of neurologic symptoms, usually during childhood, is gradual, disturbance of gait always being the first feature. Upper-limb involvement and dysarthria then appear. In the fully developed case the tendon reflexes and position and vibration sense are lost and nystagmus is present. The plantar response is extensor early in the disease. Secondary skeletal changes such as scoliosis and pescavus are found in the majority of patients. The disease is progressive, with an average duration of about 30 years.

There may be no symptoms referable to the cardiovascular system in patients with Friedreich's ataxia, even when there is extensive heart disease present in childhood (Novick et al., 1955). On the other hand, both Thilenius and Grossman (1961) and Thorén (1964) found about 10 percent of their series had heart disease before clinical signs of the neurologic disorder became manifest. No correlation has been found between the degree of neurologic disorder and the severity of heart disease. In cases having only incidental electrocardiographic findings, symptoms are invariably absent. In older patients exertional dyspnea or palpitations may be the presenting symptom of cardiac involvement. Sudden death has been reported.

Clinically the heart may be of normal size or moderately enlarged. The heart sounds are frequently normal, but gallop rhythm, paroxysmal atrial tachycardia, atrial fibrillation, or frequent extrasystoles may be found. A soft systolic murmur is not uncommonly heard in the pulmonary or mitral area and may occasionally be harsh and organic in quality and have a regurgitant basis. Diastolic murmurs, including presystolic apical murmurs, audible after exercise, are uncommon. Their origin is probably the result of dilatation of the heart. Congestive failure is most often a terminal manifestation and occurred in over two-thirds of 82 fatal cases of Friedeich's ataxia reported by Hewer (1969).

Radiologic Examination

In many cases the heart size is normal. Gross enlargement is rare (see Figure 56–1). In the majority

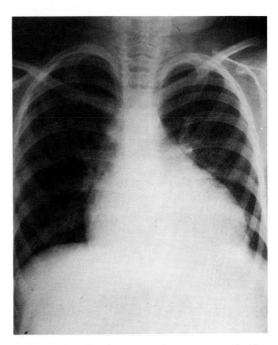

Figure 56-1. The chest x-ray of a seven-year-old girl with Friedreich's ataxia of about three years' duration. Congestive failure appeared at six and one-half years but was controlled with bed rest and diuretics. The electrocardiogram showed T inversion in leads II, III, aVF, and V_6, and moderate left ventricular hypertrophy was present.

with lesser degrees of cardiac enlargement, the apex is downpointing and suggestive of left ventricular hypertrophy.

Electrocardiography

The electrocardiogram was abnormal in about one-third of the cases with Friedreich's ataxia of Evans and Wright (1942), in 55 percent of seven cases under 16 years of Boyer and associates (1962), and in 90 percent of the large series of Thorén (1964) and Hewer (1969). The principal pattern appears to be of T inversion in the standard leads (I + II; II + III; or I + II + III), in aVF, and in the precordial leads over the left ventricle—V_5 and V_6. Furthermore, normalization of the T wave occurs after exercise in almost 80 percent of patients who have resting T wave abnormalities (Thorén, 1964), and in follow-up studies reversion to normality occurs in almost one-third of those showing initial T wave inversion (see Figure 56–1).

Sinus tachycardia is common, and dysrrhythmias with exercise have been observed in advanced cases of the disease (Thorén 1964). The axis QRS is only rarely deviated to the left in the frontal plane, usually being normal or toward the right. The voltage of QRS is not uncommonly reduced in the standard leads, whereas in the precordial leads it is usually within normal range. As many as half the cases may have evidence of ventricular hypertrophy of one or other side. The relatively consistent T wave pattern raises the suggestion of myocardial infarction, but few cases of frank infarction have been seen at autopsy. Gregorini and associates (1974) have recently shown that while the electrocardiogram may be normal, the vectorcardiogram is abnormal in all cases, showing by notches in horizontal or sagittal loops evidence of diffuse myocardial damage.

Cardiac Catheterization

Seventeen patients studied by cardiac catheterization in the series of Thorén (1964) showed normal values for those patients who had heart disease of mild or moderate severity. In the very severely affected patients the right atrial pressure was elevated, as was the end-diastolic pressure in the right ventricle. The cardiac output was usually reduced in this group. Angiocardiograms from earlier studies showed a thick left ventricular wall but no evidence of obstruction or hypercontractility (Thorén, 1964), but more recently hypertrophic disease of left ventricular muscle with or without obstructive features has been described (Soulie et al., 1966; Boehm et al., 1970; Gach et al., 1971; Elias et al., 1972; Ruschaupt et al., 1972). This association lends itself to evaluation by echocardiography. Of six patients so studied by Flemington and associates (1974) all were shown to have septal/posterior left ventricular wall thickness ratios of 1.43 to 1.89. One of these in addition had systolic anterior movement of the anterior mitral leaflet. The obstructive element in the disorder has not seemed severe to date, and because there have been no histologic studies of the precise architectural arrangement of cardiac muscle, it cannot yet be said what relation the findings have to true hypertrophic obstructive cardiomyopathy.

It seems rather unlikely that coronary arteriography could detect lesions in the major coronary artery branches since these sites in the coronary system are seldom effected by appreciable intimal thickening.

Diagnosis

A positive family history is naturally an extremely helpful pointer in any particular case. In the early stages of Friedreich's ataxia, neurologic signs not infrequently are incorrectly interpreted. Apart from a suspicion of cerebellar tumor, the label of chorea may be applied to these patients until the elicitation of other signs, such as nystagmus, extensor plantar responses, and vibration sense impairment, permits a correct diagnosis (Nadas et al., 1951). Where an affected child with ataxia and an intercurrent infection is found to have a cardiac murmur or cardiac enlargement, protracted bed rest because of suspected rheumatic heart disease may be ordered (Novick et al., 1955). Congenital heart disease has also been the initial diagnosis in a number of cases (Boyer et al., 1962). The clinical picture from the cardiac standpoint may at times resemble myocarditis or myoendocardial disease of other types, and in a small proportion the presentation may be entirely cardiac.

The pattern of the electrocardiogram is so consistent as to be an important confirmatory aid in the diagnosis when present. A normal tracing does not, of course, exclude Friedreich's ataxia. Significant murmurs may suggest congenital or acquired heart disease. In these instances the heart is seriously affected and the neurologic signs should be very obvious. Errors in diagnosis are extremely unlikely if the possibility of Friedreich's ataxia is kept in mind and particularly if the significant neurologic signs are sought for diligently.

Prognosis

Patients with Friedreich's ataxia may survive 30 or 40 years after the onset of symptoms before dying of intercurrent infection. At least half have evidence of cardiac involvement, and it is not yet established whether all these invariably die a cardiac death or whether the proportion with cardiac disease increases in later years. The majority of cases survive childhood. The youngest autopsies with heart involvement reported were two girls dying suddenly at 10 and 13 years (Russell, 1946). Of those dying from cardiac reasons, congestive heart failure is the chief cause. Reported cases of sudden death may be due to gross coronary insufficiency, either from the disease process or as a result of the development of arrhythmias. Manning (1950) believes that an abnormal electrocardiogram indicates eventual death from congestive heart failure, and that a normal electrocardiogram in a case of Friedreich's ataxia probably indicates that the patient will not develop heart disease later. We have some evidence that this is not invariably so (Figure 56–2), suggesting that in some cases, at least, cardiac involvement may be progressive in the same way as the neurologic features.

A long-term clinical study of a large group of cases with Friedreich's ataxia would go far in settling these debatable points relevant to the prognosis.

Treatment

In those with gross congestive heart failure or arrhythmias, the usual therapeutic measures are

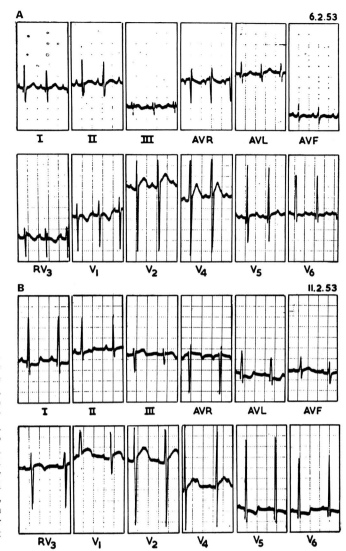

Figure 56-2. The electrocardiograms· in an 11-year-old girl with moderately severe Friedreich's ataxia of one year's duration. The initial (*A*) tracing is equivocally abnormal, while the tracing recorded five days later (*B*) reveals definite left ventricular hypertrophy and signs of anterior myocardial infarction. In the interval between tracings there were no signs or symptoms to suggest cardiac disease. Serial tracings over the next nine days showed gradual return to the initial record. Yearly tracings for the next two years showed moderate left ventricular hypertrophy only, but ischemic changes reappeared in an electrocardiogram taken at 14 years. Neither cardiac symptoms nor cardiac enlargement has resulted.

indicated. In such instances improvement may be noted (Thorén, 1964), but this is usually temporary and the prognosis is more often poor once this complication has appeared (Manning, 1950). Where electrocardiographic signs only are evident, there seems little point in physical restriction since other features of the disorder usually limit the patient's activity. We have not noticed any deterioration in the cardiac status from exertion in those able to move about.

PROGRESSIVE MUSCULAR DYSTROPHY

PROGRESSIVE muscular dystrophy is a hereditary disease of unknown etiology, characterized by weakness and wasting of striated muscle groups (Meryon, 1852). It has been usual to recognize three main types of clinical representation. The Duchenne (pseudohypertrophic) form starts in early childhood almost exclusively in boys. The condition is rapidly progressive, death occurring from respiratory tract infection or congestive heart failure before the age of 20. The disorder is usually transmitted as a sex-linked recessive, but in about 10 percent of the cases the transmission is by an autosomal recessive trait. In such patients the deterioration is considerably slower.

The limb girdle form starts in the second decade of life, affecting both sexes and leading to severe disability only by middle life. Death occurs before the normal span. The condition is usually inherited as an autosomal recessive trait, and according to most observers, cardiac involvement is uncommon.

The facio-scapular-humeral form (Landouzy-Déjerine) may begin at any age and affects both sexes. The facial and shoulder girdle muscles are affected first, and the condition later extends to other muscle groups. The condition is the most benign of the three forms and allows a normal life duration, but with increasing later disability transmission is an autosomal dominant. The heart is rarely abnormal in this form.

Pathologically there is atrophy of muscle cells with fatty and fibrous tissue replacement. These findings may be encountered in the heart muscle as well as in the skeletal muscle (Ross, 1883; Globus, 1923; Bevans, 1945; Nothacker and Netsky, 1950; Weisenfeld and Messinger, 1952; Moore, 1954; Storstein and Austarheim, 1955; Schott et al., 1955). At autopsy, the heart usually shows pale left ventricular muscle, which is thicker than that of the right ventricle. The large coronary arteries are normal. In two individuals the histologic changes were maximal in sections taken from the posterior portion of the left ventricle (Schott et al., 1955). Bowden (1956) has described a streaky fibrosis visible in the posterolateral wall of the left ventricle, which, on section, was shown to have a perivascular distribution. Recent detailed study of the smaller vessels of the coronary system by James (1962) has shown that degenerative alteration may be present, particularly in the size of vessels supplying nodal tissue. This may have relationship to the possibility of sudden death (Zatuchni et al., 1951) and arrhythmias that exists with the malformation.

Clinical Features

The common form in childhood begins insidiously. Although the first case in the family may not be recognized until the age of four or five years, subsequent affected members may be detected in the first year of life by the delay in the usual physical milestones. Easy fatigue and difficulty in climbing stairs are early symptoms after infancy. Dyspnea is a late manifestation seen in adults and has not been encountered in patients under the age of 12 years (Moore, 1954). Sudden death is likewise uncommon and confined to adults.

In examining child patients with the disease, a waddling gait and difficulty in rising from the lying position are classic signs. Although weakness and wasting of shoulder, girdle, and thigh muscles develop, the calves are disproportionately large. The knee jerks are diminished or absent. Most often, physical examination reveals no abnormal cardiac findings. Tachycardia is the only consistent and early sign of cardiac involvement. Arrhythmias have been reported. The heart sounds are frequently normal, but a soft, first mitral sound has been noted (Boas and Lowenberg, (1931). The usual murmur is a soft ejection type in the pulmonary area. Occasionally harsher murmurs in that region (Weisenfeld and Messinger 1952) or at the apex (Perloff et al., 1966)

have been noted. Third and fourth heart sounds are quite commonly encountered. The development of congestive heart failure is ominous, and, though amenable to the usual therapy, lengthy survival after its first appearance is unusual. The blood pressure is normal.

Radiologic Examination

Cardiac enlargement is uncommon but is always present when congestive heart failure exists. A few patients without symptoms will show slight enlargement and the radiologic appearance of left ventricular hypertrophy (Moore, 1954). Decreased cardiac excursion at fluoroscopy is reputedly common (Sandberg et al., 1952). Scoliosis, a common sequel of the disease, may influence the cardiac position and contour so that the heart may appear abnormal when in fact it is not.

Electrocardiography

A number of electrocardiographic studies have been made in patients with progressive muscular dystrophy. Puddu and Mussafia (1939) found abnormal tracings in 10 percent; Rubin and Buchberg (1952), in 50 percent; Weisenfeld and Messinger (1952), in 80 percent; Walton and Nattrass (1954), in 25 percent; and Schott and associates (1955) and Lowenstein and coworkers (1962), in 44 percent of their patients. Figures between 70 and 80 percent were noted by Skyring and McKusick (1961), Wahi (1963), Gilroy and associates (1963), and Perloff and colleagues (1966). The changes most frequently reported have been tachycardia, right ventricular hypertrophy, relatively short P-R interval, flat or negative T waves in limb or left chest leads, and abnormalities of the Q in left chest leads and aVL. The enumerated changes have been sufficiently frequent to lead Wahi (1963) to discuss a myopathic pattern in the electrocardiogram of such patients. There appears to be some distinct relationship between the electrocardiographic changes and the age of the patient in the Duchenne type. In the series described by Gilroy and associates (1963), 50 percent of their younger patients had normal tracings, but after the age of ten years normal tracings were encountered in only one quarter. Diffuse myocardial damage patterns with S-T segment changes and abnormal T waves, together with Q waves suggestive of myocardial infarction, were not observed in patients under the age of 12 years.

The findings in 17 consecutive patients with muscular dystrophy examined by electrocardiography at The Hospital for Sick Children are shown in Table 56–1. The importance of a rapid heart rate may be questioned in children of the age studied, although none of these patients seemed at all upset during the examination. The majority had evidence of mild degrees of abnormal right ventricular dominance,

Table 56-1.   AN ANALYSIS OF THE ELECTROCARDIOGRAMS OF 17 CONSECUTIVE PATIENTS WITH PROGRESSIVE MUSCULAR DYSTROPHY SEEN IN THE SPECIAL CLINIC OF THE HOSPITAL FOR SICK CHILDREN, TORONTO

Age	2 to 12 years (80 percent between 5 and 10 years)	
Heart rate	80 to 150 per minute (only four cases under 100 per minute)	
Electrical position	Vertical	11
	Intermediate	3
	Horizontal	3
ÂQRS	Normal	14
	Left	1
	Right	1
	Indeterminate	1
P-R interval	0.10 to 0.14 second	
P wave	No abnormalities	
Q-T$_c$ interval	Range, 0.350 to 0.380 second (except for two cases: 0.400 and 0.410 second)	
Ventricular activation times	Normal in all cases	
Right ventricular hypertrophy	10	
Abnormal R/S ratio in V$_1$	10	
Abnormal voltage R in V$_1$	5	
Left ventricular hypertrophy	3	
Abnormal voltage R in V$_6$	1	
Abnormal voltage Q or S in aVR	2	
Incomplete right bundle branch block	10 (all minimal)	

and the minority showed the features of minimal left ventricular hypertrophy. It would seem unwise to attach too great a significance to such minor changes, yet on this basis over 75 percent of this unselected group showed electrocardiographic abnormalities.

The high proportion with changes in the electrocardiogram is confined to the Duchenne type, and the electrocardiographic alterations have not been a feature in the facio-scapular-humeral form (Schott et al., 1955; Murphy, 1964). Most reports have also indicated that the electrocardiogram is normal in the limb girdle group (Murphy, 1964). This conclusion has been questioned by Welsh and coworkers (1963), whose series contained only 7 of 26 patients of this form with a normal electrocardiogram and by Perloff and associates (1966).

Cardiac Catheterization

Relatively few hemodynamic studies have been done in patients with these disorders. In 12 patients showing no murmur or cardiomegaly Gailani and associates (1958) discovered normal right heart pressures at rest and on exercise in all except two patients in whom abnormalities were detected with exercise. Similarly normal findings were noted by Perloff and associates (1966).

In the examination of a 32-year-old man in congestive heart failure by Rubeiz and Saab (1962) low cardiac output, elevated end-diastolic and right ventricular systolic pressures, and a high wedge pressure suggested the presence of left ventricular failure. There have been no reports of coronary arteriography in this condition, although from the nature of the abnormality so far described in the coronary arteries it would seem unlikely that this type of study will be very fruitful during life.

Diagnosis

The classic procedures for confirmation of the diagnosis have included electromyography, muscle biopsy, and serum enzyme estimations, especially creatine kinase. The latter enzyme activity is increased markedly in the important period of infancy prior to the onset of muscle weakness. Most carriers have moderate elevation of creatine kinase when they are young (Pearce et al., 1964), and they may also show other minimal features of the disease (Monckton and Ludvigsen, 1968). The value of combining histochemical techniques with electron microscopy as a means of establishing better markers for the different myopathies is becoming increasingly apparent (Dubowitz, 1975). An assessment combining family history and evidence of slight myopathy (from enzyme, electromyogram, electrocardiogram, and biopsy) offers the best chance of detection of carriers (Walton and Gardner-Medwin, 1974).

Since symptoms due to cardiac disease are never the presenting symptoms in progressive muscular dystrophy, the problem for the cardiologist in assessing the cardiac status in such patients is relatively straightforward. Apart from a persistent tachycardia, the electrocardiogram provides the earliest and most frequent indication of cardiac involvement in the Duchenne type. X-rays of the chest are of secondary assistance. Systolic time indices appear to be sensitive means of detecting cardiac involvement in patients with muscular dystrophy (Bonanno et al., 1973). Cardiac catheterization seems to be unhelpful (Sandberg et al., 1952; Gailani et al., 1958).

Prognosis

The disorder is a progressive one, death occurring approximately 10 to 15 years after the onset of symptoms in the Duchenne type. The mode of exit is most commonly intercurrent infection. Death as the result of cardiac involvement is rare. It seems fairly clear that significant heart disease is a late manifestation correlating with a widespread and advanced skeletal muscle change.

Treatment

No specific treatment is available for progressive muscular dystrophy at the present time (Zundel and Tyler, 1965). The uncommon appearance of congestive heart failure requires the usual therapy. Physical restriction because of lesser degrees of cardiac involvement is obviously unnecessary. Carrier detection programs look to be a promising means of reducing the incidence of the disease (Hutton and Thompson, 1976).

OTHER NEUROMUSCULAR DISORDERS

AMONGST a rather large number of rare chronic diseases falling into this general heading are a few where cardiac abnormalities have been reported. Exceptionally these have produced major symptoms and signs related to the heart. It is beyond the scope of this section to examine the matter in great detail but a few warrant mention.

Refsum's Syndrome

This is a slowly progressive disorder inherited as a recessive trait. The symptoms, which start in childhood, include nerve deafness, cerebellar ataxia, mental retardation, pes cavus, and retinitis pigmentosa. The cardiac involvement usually concerns conducting elements of the heart, and the Q-T interval may be prolonged. Other rather nonspecific changes in the T-wave and the S-T segments may occur. At autopsy subendocardial fibrosis and increase in size of conducting tissue have been found (Gordon and Hudson, 1959).

Peroneal-Muscular Atrophy

This is a hereditary disease associated with distal muscular wasting and weakness with loss of reflexes. Symptoms tend to develop in childhood or adolescence, but the disease is compatible with long life. Whether or not there is change in the myocardium of such patients is not known, but abnormalities of heart rhythm and heart failure have been reported in an adult (Leak, 1961).

Myotonic Dystrophy

This is a chronic disorder transmitted as an autosomal dominant that affects both sexes.

The disease may start in infancy with hypotonia, poor sucking, and delay in developmental milestones. In a study of 70 patients in Britain (Harper, 1975) it was shown that about half had respiratory problems in the newborn period. Diagnosis then was often difficult and sometimes was confused with congenital heart disease. Associated findings helpful in diagnosis at this age were talipes equinovarus and a history of hydramnios. Mental retardation was fairly common while cataracts were rare.

Presentation more often occurs later in childhood with weakness and atrophy of facial muscles. Testicular atrophy, cataracts, and baldness are well-known features in the established adult case. While it is very unusual for patients to present with significant heart disease other than in the form of arrhythmia, electrocardiographic changes are extremely common, being detected in 200 of 300 cases reviewed by Church (1967). The most common abnormality is prolongation of the P-R interval, while next is frequency in the presence of left-axis deviation. Nonspecific T wave and S-T segment changes have been noted. The presence of left-axis deviation may occur early, and in one two-year-old child with borderline features of the disease its presence greatly assisted in diagnosis (Payne and Greenfield, 1963). Few patients coming to autopsy have had detailed consideration given the cardiovascular system, and no consistent or striking abnormalities have been noted. The coronary vessels and conducting system have been reported normal (Hudson, 1965).

Progressive External Ophthalmoplegia

This is a slowly progressive external ophthalmoplegia usually of a heredofamilial type. The onset is usually in infancy or childhood and often occurs before the sixth year. Rarely symptoms have been noted in the first few days of life. Bilateral ptosis of the eyelids is usually the first evidence of disease, and later the weakness extends to the superior recti and other muscles that rotate the eyeballs, resulting in a complete external ophthalmoplegia. The course of the disease is very slow and the paralysis may not be complete until the fourth or fifth decade of life. As a rule, the process is confined to the extraocular muscles, but in some cases skeletal muscles are involved, giving a picture of progressive muscular dystrophy (Ford, 1960).

In recent years, complete heart block and other cardiac dysrhythmias have been recognized in patients with progressive external ophthalmoplegia (Kearns, 1958; Ross et al., 1969; Morriss et al., 1972). Conduction disturbances with electrocardiographic evidence of right bundle branch block and left anterior hemiblock have preceded the development of complete heart block in some instances. Morriss and her associates (1972) have performed His bundle recordings in a 16-year-old white girl with progressive external ophthalmoplegia and retinitis pigmentosa ophthalmoplegia; in addition, her cardiac rhythm was irregular. An initial electrocardiogram was interpreted as showing sinus rhythm interrupted by periods of second-degree heart block and occasional premature ventricular contractions. In addition, there was left anterior fascicular block. A later ECG showed the development of complete right bundle branch block, with persistence of left-axis deviation and second-degree heart block. His bundle electrogram revealed prolongation of the H-V conduction time interval. A permanent demand cardiac pacemaker was implanted and paced the patient during episodes of complete heart block that subsequently developed.

The myopathy is progressive, and if skeletal muscle becomes involved, respiratory failure may result. Additionally, progressive heart block may result in complete heart block, with Stokes-Adams attacks. These can be treated with a demand pacemaker.

Idiopathic Dystonia Musculorum Deformans

This is an extrapyramidal degenerative disease resulting in involuntary movements and postures. Early, juvenile, and late forms of the disorder occur. Heart disease at autopsy has not been reported but arrhythmias and sudden death can occur. A patient who first exhibited involuntary movements at the age of 12 years developed paroxysmal nodal tachycardia, which proved to be extremely difficult to control by the age of 19 years (Waal-Manning et al., 1971). The source of the dysrhythmia may be the hypothalamic disease that exists in these patients.

REFERENCES

Friedreich's Ataxia

Boyer, S. H., Iv.; Chisholm, A. W.; and McKusick, V. A.: Cardiac aspects of Friedreich's ataxia. *Circulation*, **25**:493, 1962.

Boehm, T. M.; Dickerson, R. B.; and Glasser, S. P.: Hypertrophic subaortic stenosis occurring in a patient with Friedreich's ataxia. *Am. J. Med. Sci.*, **260**:279, 1970.

Debre, R.; Marie, J.; Soulié, P.; and de Font-Reaulx, P.: Coronary type of electrocardiogram in child with Friedreich's disease. *Bull. Mém. Soc. Med. Hôp. Paris*, **52**:749, 1936.

Dubowitz, V.: Neuromuscular disorders in childhood: Old dogmas, new concepts. *Arch. Dis. Child.*, **50**:335, 1975.

Elias, G.; Guerin, R.; Spitaels, S.; Fouron, J.; and Davignon, A.: Muscular sub-aortic stenosis and Friedreich's ataxia. *Union Med. Can.*, **101**:474, 1974.

Evans, W.: Familial cardiomegaly. *Br. Heart J.*, **11**:68, 1949.

Evans, W., and Wright, G.: The electrocardiogram in Friedreich disease. *Br. Heart J.*, **4**:91, 1942.

Fleming, C. S.; Smith, E. R.; and Heffernan, L. P.: The cardiomyopathy of Friedreich's ataxia: echocardiographic study of six patients and their families. *27th Annual Meeting*, Canadian Cardiovascular Society, 1974, p. 46.

Flipse, F. D.; Dry, T. J.; and Woltman, W. H.: Heart in Friedreich's ataxia. *Minnesota Med.*, **33**:1000, 1950.

Freidreich, N.: Über degenerative atrophie der spinal en Hinterstrange. *N. Arch. Pathol. Anat.*, **26**:391, 433, 1863.

Gach, J. V.; Andriange, M.; and Franck, G.: Hypertrophic obstructive cardiomyopathy and Friedreich's ataxia. Report of a case and review of literature. *Am. J. Cardiol.*, **27**:36, 1971.

Gregorini, L.; Valentini, R.; and Libretti, A.: The vectorcardiogram in Friedreich's ataxia. *Am. Heart J.*, **87**:158, 1974.

Harper, P. S.: Congenital myotonic dystrophy in Britain. I. Clinical aspects. *Arch. Dis. Child.*, **50**:505, 1975.

Hejtmancik, M. R.; Bradfield, J. Y., Jr.; and Miller, G. V.: Myocarditis and Friedreich's ataxia: report of two cases. *Am. Heart J.*, **38**:757, 1949.

Hewer, R. L.: The heart in Friedreich's ataxia. *Br. Heart J.*, **31**:5, 1969.

Ivemark, B., and Thorén, C.: The pathology of the heart in Friedreich's ataxia. *Acta Med. Scand.*, **175**:227, 1964.

Thilenius, O. G., and Grossman, B. J.: Friedreich's ataxia with heart disease in children. *Pediatrics*, **27**:246, 1961.

Thorén, C.: Cardiomyopathy in Friedreich's ataxia. *Acta Paediatr.*, **53**:Suppl. 153, 1964.

van Bogaert, A., and van Bogaert, L.: Concerning the electrocardiographic alterations in Friedreich's disease. *Arch. Mal. Coeur*, **29**:630, 1936.

Progressive Muscular Dystrophy

Bevans, M.: Changes in musculature of gastro-intestinal tract and in myocardium in progressive muscular dystrophy. *Arch. Pathol.*, **40**:225, 1945.

Boas, E. P., and Lowenberg, H.: The heart rate in progressive muscular dystrophy. *Arch. Intern. Med.*, **47**:376, 1931.

Bonanno, J. A.; Lies, T.; Taylor, R. G.; Kraus, J. F.; Amsterdam, E. A.; and Mason, D. T. Early detection of cardiomyopathy in muscular dystrophies. *Am. J. Cardiol.*, **31**:121, 1973 (abstr.).

Bowden, D. H.: Unpublished data, 1956.

Gailani, S.; Danowski, T. S.; and Fisher, D. S.: Muscular dystrophy. Catheterization studies indicating latent congestive heart failure. *Circulation*, **27**:583, 1958.

Gilroy, J.; Cahalan, J. L.; Berman, R.; and Newman, M.: Cardiac and pulmonary complications in Duchenne's progressive muscular dystrophy. *Circulation*, **27**:484, 1963.

Globus, J. H.: The pathologic findings in the heart muscle in progressive muscular dystrophy. *Arch. Neurol. Psychiat.*, **9**:59, 1923.

Hutton, E. M., and Thompson, M. W.: Carrier detection and genetic counselling in Duchenne muscular dystrophy: a follow-up study. *Can. Med. Assoc J.*, **115**:749, 1976.

James, T. N.: Observations on the cardiovascular involvement, including the cardiac conduction system, in progressive muscular dystrophy. *Am. Heart J.*, **63**:48, 1962.

James, T. N.: Observations on the cardiovascular involvement, including the cardiac conduction system, in progressive muscular dystrophy. *Am. Heart J.*, **63**:48, 1962.

James, T. N., and Fisch, C.: Observations on the cardiovascular involvement in Friedreich's ataxia. *Am. Heart J.*, **66**:164, 1963.

Krongrad, E., and Joos, H. A.: Friedreich's ataxia in childhood. Case report with possible myocardial infarction, cerebrovascular thrombembolization and persistent elevation of cardiac specific LDH. *Chest*, **61**:644, 1972.

Laubry, C., and Heim de Balsac, R.: A propos de troubles cardiaques de la maladie de Friedreich. *Bull. Mêm. Soc. Méd. Hôp. Paris*, **52**:756, 1936.

Lorenz, T. H.; Kurtz, C. M.; and Shapiro, H. H.: Cardiopathy in Friedreich's ataxia. *Arch. Intern. Med.*, **86**:412, 1950.

Lowenstein, A. S.; Arbeit, S. R.; and Rubin, I. L.: Cardiac involvement in progressive muscular dystrophy. An electrocardiographic and ballistocardiographic study. *Am. J. Cardiol.*, **9**:528, 1962.

Manning, G. W.: Cardiac manifestations in Friedreich's ataxia. *Am. Heart J.*, **39**:799, 1950.

Meryon, E.: On granular and fatty degeneration of the voluntary muscles. *Med. Clin. Trans. Lond.*, **35**:73, 1852. Cited by Rubin and Buchberg (1952).

Monckton, G., and Ludvigsen, B.: The identification of carriers in Duchenne muscular dystrophy. *Can. Med. Assoc. J.*, **89**:333, 1963.

Moore, W. F., Jr.: Cardiac involvement in progressive muscular dystrophy. *J. Pediatr.*, **44**:683, 1954.

Murphy, E. G.: *The Chemistry and Therapy of Disorders of Voluntary Muscles.* Charles C Thomas, Publisher, Springfield, Ill., 1964.

Nadas, A. S.; Alimururing, M. M.; and Sieracki, L. A.: Cardiac manifestations of Friedreich's ataxia. *N. Engl. J. Med.*, **244**:239, 1951.

Nothacker, W. G., and Netsky, M. G.: Myocardial lesions in progressive muscular dystrophy. *Arch. Pathol.*, **50**:578, 1950.

Novick, R.; Adams, P., Jr.; and Anderson, R. C.: Cardiac manifestations of Friedreich's ataxia in children. *J. Lancet*, **75**:62, 1955.

Pearce, J. M. S.; Pennington, R. J.; and Walton, J. N.: Serum enzyme studies in muscle disease. I. Variations in serum creatine kinase activity in normal individuals. *J. Neurol. Neurosurg. Psychiat.*, **27**:1, 1964.

Perloff, J. K.: Cardiomyopathy associated with heredofamilial neuromyopathic diseases. *Mod. Concepts Cardiovasc. Dis.*, **40**:23, 1971.

Perloff, J. K.; De Leon, A. C., Jr.; and O'Doherty, D.: Cardiomyopathy of progressive muscular dystrophy. *Circulation*, **33**:625, 1966.

Piron, A.: La cardiopathie de la maladie de Friedreich. *Acta Cardiol.*, **1**:305, 1946.

Pitt, G. N.: On a case of Friedreich's disease. Its clinical history and postmortem appearance. *Guy Hosp. Rep.*, **44**:369, 1887.

Puddu, V., and Mussafia, A.: L'electrocardiogramme dans la dystrophie musculaire progressive. *Arch. Mal. Coeur*, **32**:958, 1939.

Ross, J.: On a case of pseudo-hypertrophic paralysis. *Br. Med. J.*, **1**:200, 1883.

Rubeiz, G. A., and Saab, N. G.: Hemodynamic study in a case of progressive muscular dystrophy involving the heart. *Am. J. Cardiol.*, **10**:890, 1962.

Rubin, I. L., and Buchberg, A. S.: The heart in progressive muscular dystrophy. *Am. Heart J.*, **43**:161, 1952.

Ruschhaupt, D. G.; Thilenius, D. G.; and Cassels, D. E.: Friedreich's ataxia associated with hypertrophic subaortic stenosis. *Am. Heart J.*, **84**:95, 1972.

Russell, D. S.: Myocarditis in Friedreich's ataxia. *J. Pathol. Bact.*, **58**:739, 1946.

Sandberg, A. A.; Hecht, H. H.; and Tyler, F. H.: The heart in muscular dystrophy. *Am. J. Med.*, **13**:495, 1952.

Schilero, A. J.; Antzis, E.; and Dunn, J.: Friedreich's ataxia and its cardiac manifestations. *Am. Heart J.*, **44**:805, 1952.

Schott, J.; Jacobi, M.; and Wald, M. A.: Electrocardiographic patterns in the differential diagnosis of progressive muscular dystrophy. *Am. J. Med. Sci.*, **229**:517, 1955.

Skyring, A. P., and McKusick, V. A.: Clinical, genetic and electrocardiographic studies of childhood muscular dystrophy. *Am. J. Med. Sci.*, **242**:534, 1961.

Soulie, P.; Vernant, P.; Gaudeau, S.; Calisti, G.; Joly, F.; Bouchard, F.; and Forman, J.: Le Coeur dans la maladie de Freidreich; etude hemodynamque droite et gauche. *Mal. Cardiovasc.*, **7**:369, 1966.

Storstein, O., and Austarheim, K.: Progressive muscular dystrophy of the heart. *Acta Med. Scand.*, **150**:431, 1955.

Wahi, P. L.: Cardiac changes in myopathy. *Am. Heart J.*, **66**:748, 1963.

Walton, J. N., and Nattrass, F. J.: On classication, natural history and treatment of myopathies. *Brain*, **77**:169, 1954.

Walton, J. N., and Gardner-Medwin, D.: Progressive muscular dystrophy and the myotonic disorders. In Walton, J. N. (ed.): *Disorders of Voluntary Muscle.* 3rd ed. Churchill and Livingstone, Edinburgh and London, 1974, p. 561.

Weisenfeld, S., and Messinger, W. J.: Cardiac involvement in progressive muscular dystrophy. *Am. Heart J.*, **43**:170, 1952.

Zatuchni, J.; Aegerter, E. E.; Melthan, L.; and Shuman, C. R.: The heart in progressive muscular dystrophy. *Circulation*, **3**:846, 1951.

Zundel, W. S., and Tyler, F. H.: The muscular dystrophies. *N. Engl. J. Med.*, **273**:537, 1965.

Other Neuromuscular Disorders

Church, S. C.: The heart in myotonia atrophica. *Arch. Intern. Med.*, **119**:176, 1967.

Ford, F. R.: *Diseases of the Nervous System in Infancy, Childhood, and Adolescence*, 4th ed. Charles C Thomas, Publisher, Springfield, Ill., 1960, pp. 1274–76.

Gordon, N., and Hudson, R. E. B.: Refsum's syndrome— heredopathia atactica polyneuritiformis. *Brain*. **82**:41, 1959.

Hudson, R. E. B.: *Cardiovascular Pathology.* Edward Arnold (Publishers), London, 1965, Vol. 1, p. 743.

Kearns, T. P., and Sayre, G. P.: Retinitis pigmentosa, external ophthalmoplegia and complete heart block. *Arch. Ophthalmol.*, **60**:280, 1958.

Leak, D.: Paroxysmal atrial flutter in peroneal muscular dystrophy. *Br. Heart J.*, **23**:326, 1961.

Morriss, J. H.; Eugsten, G. S.; Nora, J. J.; and Pryor, R.; His bundle recording in progressive external ophthalmoplegia. *J. Pediatr.*, **81**:1167, 1972.

Payne, C. A., and Greenfield, J. C., Jr.: Electrocardiographic abnormalities associated with myotonic dystrophy. *Am. Heart J.*, **65**:436, 1963.

Ross, A.; Lipschultz, D.; Austin, J.; and Smith, J., Jr.: External ophthalmoplegia and complete heart block. *N. Engl. J. Med.*, **280**:313, 1969.

Waal-Manning, H. J.; Ng, J.; Holst, P. E.; and Kilpatrick, J. A.: Idiopathic dystonia musculorum deformans and paroxysmal nodal tachycardia. *N.Z. Med. J.*, **73**:204, 1971.

57

The Heart in Hyperthyroidism
and Hypothyroidism

John D. Keith

THE HEART IN HYPERTHYROIDISM

HYPERTHYROIDISM, or thyrotoxicosis, is a disease that occurs occasionally in childhood, but it is very rare before the age of six years. Twenty-eight cases under one year have been reported (White, 1951; Margett, 1950; Farrehi and associates, 1966). Two-thirds of cases in childhood occur after ten years of age (McClintock et al., 1956). Lyons (1949) found that it occurred approximately once in 10,000 admissions to the Children's Hospital, Washington. Girls are more frequently affected than boys. It has become less frequent over the years, and as a cause of heart disease is steadily diminishing. White (1951) found that he had only one-eighth as many cases of thyroid heart disease in the 1940s as he had in the 1920s.

At The Hospital for Sick Children, Toronto, during the period 1930 to 1940, there was an average admission of 18 cases a year. Presently the Endocrine Service of The Hospital for Sick Children sees 15 to 20 per year.

Farrehi and associates record 22 cases of infants born to mothers with thyrotoxicosis. Seven of the infants had evidence of heart failure.

Clinical Features

The onset is characterized by tachycardia, restlessness, irritability, sweating, and tremor. These are accompanied by a flushed, moist skin; exophthalmos; and enlargement of the thyroid gland.

Examination of the cardiovascular system reveals a tachycardia, raised systolic blood pressure, and lowered diastolic pressure, giving a high pulse pressure. With the increased heart rate go an increased blood flow, increased blood volume, and, in the cases with heart involvement, cardiac enlargement. A systolic murmur may be present.

Atrial fibrillation occurs in approximately 20 percent of adults but is rarely encountered in children. McClintock and associates (1956) record its presence in one case out of 50 children with hyperthyroidism. If the involvement of the heart is severe enough, heart failure will occur. Atrial fibrillation increases the likelihood of heart failure.

Diagnosis

The diagnosis of hyperthyroidism is made on the clinical findings, to which reference has been made, coupled with a serum thyroxine level higher than 13 μg/100 ml. Twenty-four hour radioactive iodine uptake by the thyroid gland should normally not exceed 50 percent, but in thyrotoxicosis it is greatly increased. Another diagnostic feature is the response to therapy.

Treatment

Medical Treatment. The medical treatment of hyperthyroidism with cardiac involvement, or where there are sympathomimetic effects, consists of propranolol. Bed rest and propylthiouracil are the first choice of therapy in infants and children.

If heart failure is present this must be treated in the usual way with digitalis. In the case of thyroid storm, oral iodine and parenteral corticosteroids are usually added. If the response to medical treatment is inadequate, subtotal thyroidectomy or radioactive iodine ablative therapy may be recommended. Fifty percent of these children eventually need such alternative therapy. After successful therapy signs of cardiac involvement rapidly recede.

THE HEART IN HYPOTHYROIDISM AND CRETINISM

BOTH cretinism in infants and hypothyroidism in older children are relatively uncommon clinical events now. Endemic cretinism used to be more common in areas where mothers were suffering from iodine deficiency goiters. With the iodinization of salt, this type of cretinism has become distinctly uncommon. Sporadic cretinism of unknown etiology still occurs occasionally. Juvenile myxedema is rarely found now but may occur spontaneously or following an infection; in the pediatric age group it occurs approximately one-tenth as frequently as cretinism.

HYPOTHYROIDISM (JUVENILE MYXEDEMA)

In juvenile myxedema the child has a dull, apathetic appearance, exhibiting little evidence of normal childhood energy. Growth is likely to be retarded. The skin and hair are dry, and there may be increased subcutaneous fat. There may be enlargement of the heart, bradycardia, and evidence of low voltage in the electrocardiogram. X-rays of the bones reveal delay in centers of ossification. The blood cholesterol is raised.

Among adults with myxedema the heart is considered to be involved in three-fourths of the cases (White, 1951). Enlargement of the heart, pericardial effusion, and electrocardiographic changes are common. Hypothyroidism with evidence of heart involvement is distinctly rare in childhood. The following is an example taken from the files of The Hospital for Sick Children.

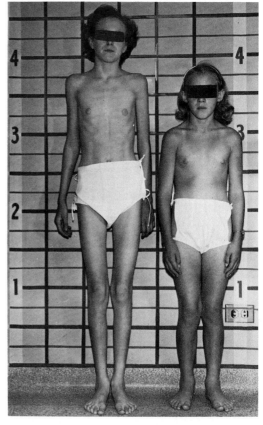

Figure 57-1. B. C., aged 11 years. Hypothyroidism patient (*right*) compared with a girl her own age (*left*).

Case Report

An 11-year-old girl was admitted to The Hospital for Sick Children on December 1, 1951, with a history of failure to grow normally, anemia that did not respond to iron therapy, and the finding of an enlarged heart (see Figure 57–1).

Examination revealed that she was small for her age and had coarse, dry hair; dry, rough skin that was thickened; some increase in fat pads; and an enlarged heart. There were a soft, blowing systolic murmur in the aortic and pulmonary areas and a short diastolic murmur down the left sternal border. The cardio-thoracic ratio was 13.3/18.7. The electrocardiogram showed low or inverted T waves in the standard leads and over the left precordium (see Figure 57–2). The x-ray of the heart showed generalized enlargement.

Laboratory Findings. Laboratory findings were as follows: basal metabolic rate, −40 and −47 on two occasions; protein-bound iodine, 1.74 mg percent; cholesterol, 263 mg percent. Cardiac catheterization revealed a small atrial septal defect.

Diagnosis. A diagnosis of juvenile myxedema with an atrial septal defect of the ostium secundum type was made.

Treatment. She was started on thyroid extract, 60 mg a day, and this was gradually increased to 120 mg a day. On this regimen her heart findings gradually improved, the heart size decreasing slightly in relation to the body growth. The diastolic murmur disappeared, and the systolic murmur became very faint. Four years after being started on thyroid, she was fully active and getting along well at home and at school. The electrocardiogram improved dramatically (see Figure 57–2).

Clinical Features Relating to the Heart

Usually there are no symptoms referable to the heart, but on physical examination the heart is quiet in action and the x-ray shows it to be enlarged. The electrocardiogram shows a slow pulse, low or absent P waves and T waves, and, at times, left-axis deviation

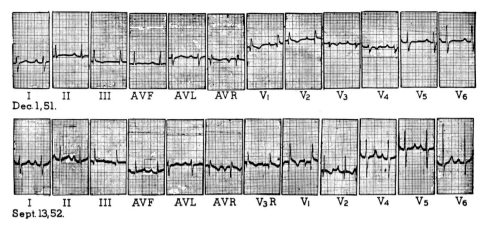

I   II   III   AVF   AVL   AVR   V₁   V₂   V₃   V₄   V₅   V₆
Dec. 1, 51.

I   II   III   AVF   AVL   AVR   V₃R   V₁   V₂   V₄   V₅   V₆
Sept. 13, 52.

Figure 57-2. B. C., aged 11 years. First electrocardiogram taken during hypothyroid state. Second electrocardiogram taken after nine months of thyroid therapy.

which disappears with treatment. The response to thyroid is usually excellent in these children.

CRETINISM

Cretins appear normal at birth. Signs and symptoms may begin to appear in about two to four weeks, and cases are characterized by inactivity, slowness or refusal of feeding, constipation, and apathy. Typical facies, with prominent eyelids, wrinkled skin, large tongue, and dry, scanty hair, may develop within the next few weeks or months.

Diagnosis

The diagnosis is usually possible on the basis of clinical findings and a low serum thyroxine level. An x-ray of the bones may show a delay in ossification centers. The blood cholesterol is over 200 to 250 mg percent as a rule.

Heart Involvement

Frank signs of heart disease are rarely found in cretins, but the electrocardiographic changes are common, having been noted in all cases in a series of ten studied before therapy by Schlesinger and Landtman (1949).

The heart is normal in size and shape, but it may appear in transverse position owing to the relatively high diaphragm, since the growth in cretinism is usually delayed and leads to a squat-shaped chest.

The electrocardiogram shows a rate that is slightly below average, but sinus arrhythmia is less frequently found before treatment than after. Left-axis deviation is uncommon but may occur. It disappears when thyroid therapy is begun. Low or flat T waves and P waves are found in most cases; these more than double their size with treatment. The Q-T interval is

prolonged slightly on the average and decreases with thyroid extract. The QRS-T angle is widened in a third.

Schlesinger and Landtman (1949) found that the electrocardiogram may be helpful in making the diagnosis in doubtful cases of cretinism since the basal metabolic rate is not obtainable at this early age; the cholesterol level may be equivocal and the clinical findings inadequate. A normal electrocardiogram is very suggestive evidence that one is not dealing with cretinism.

The electrocardiogram is also of use in evaluating the adequacy of treatment. Tracings should appear normal within a month of starting treatment if sufficient thyroid is administered. If the electrocardiogram still shows flat T or P waves, one should consider the possibility of instituting a higher dosage schedule.

Treatment

The therapy of choice is 1-thyroxine in doses of between 5 and 10 µg/kg/day. In those with cardiomegaly or frank heart failure this dosage is usually halved for the first week of treatment.

REFERENCES

Hyperthyroidism

Boas, N. F., and Ober, W. B.: Hereditary exophthalmic goitre—report of eleven cases in one family. *J. Clin. Endocrinol.,* **6**:575, 1946.

Dinsmore, R. S.: Hyperthyroidism in children. *Surg. Gynec. Obstet.,* **42**:172, 1926; *JAMA,* **99**:636, 1932.

Drake, M. E.; Howard, A.; Heldrick, F.; Joslin, B. S.; and Imburg, J.: Treatment of juvenile thyrotoxicosis with propylthiouracil. *Am. J. Dis. Child.,* **82**:43, 1951.

Farrehi, C.; Mitchell, M.; and Fawcett, D. M.: Heart failure in congenital thyrotoxicosis. *Pediatrics,* **37**:460, 1966.

Helmolz, H. F.: Exophthalmic goiter in childhood. *JAMA,* **87**:157, 1926.

Kunstadter, R. H., and Stein, A. F.: Treatment of thyrotoxicosis in children with thiouracil derivatives. *Pediatrics,* **6**:244, 1950.

Lyons, J. H.: Treatment of hyperthyroidism in children. *Ann. Surg.*, **129**:631, 1949.

McClintock, J. C.; Frawley, T. F.; and Holden, J. H. P.: Hyperthyroidism in children: observations in 50 treated cases, including an evaluation of endocrine factors. *J. Clin. Endocrinol.*, **16**:62, 1956.

Margett, B. M.: Thyrotoxicosis in a new born infant. *Proc. Roy. Med.*, **43**:615, 1950.

Van Wyk, J. J.; Grumbach, M. M.; Shepard, T. H.; and Wilkins, L.: The treatment of hyperthyroidism in childhood with thiouracil drugs. *Pediatrics*, **17**:221, 1956.

White, P. D.: *Heart Disease*, 4th ed. The Macmillan Co., New York, 1951.

Hypothyroidism and Cretinism

Burgess, A. M.: Myxedema controlled by thyroid extract for 52 years. *Ann. Intern. Med.*, **25**:146, 1946.

Lerman, J.; Clark, R. J.; and Means, J. H.: The heart in myxedema: electrocardiograms and roentgen-ray measurements before and after therapy. *Ann. Intern. Med.*, **6**:1251, 1933.

Schlesinger, B., and Landtman, B.: Electrocardiographic studies in cretins. *Br. Heart J.*, **11**:237, 1949.

Van Wyk, J. J.: Hypothyroidism in childhood. *Pediatrics*, **17**:427, 1956.

White, P. D.: *Heart Disease*, 4th ed. The Macmillan Co., New York, 1951, p. 453.

58

Glycogen-Storage Disease of the Heart

John D. Keith and *Andrew Sass-Kortsak*

GLYCOGEN-STORAGE disease involving the heart is part of a generalized entity that is now biochemically well defined. It is clinically characterized by enlargement of the heart, muscular weakness, and at times macroglossia. A few cases have minimal cardiac involvement and survive for some years. In the overwhelming majority, however, the heart is seriously affected and death usually occurs in the first year of life.

This condition was first described in 1932 by Pompe and Bischoff and independently by Putschar. They noted infants dying with marked cardiac enlargement due to excessive deposition of glycogen. Over the years further cases were reported, and in 1950 Di Sant'Agnese and coworkers reviewed the literature on the subject and presented data on 14 cases. They integrated the clinical and pathologic material more thoroughly than had been done before, further establishing glycogen-storage disease of the heart as a separate entity and outlining the features that might make diagnosis possible during life.

The hepatic type of glycogen-storage disease had previously been described by van Creveld (1928) and von Gierke (1929). It was soon recognized that the cardiac type was a separate entity distinct from the hepatic type. This separation was further delineated when Clement and Godman (1950) pointed out the association of skeletal muscle weakness occurring in a case of glycogen-storage disease.

In 1964 Hers demonstrated that the tissues from normal individuals contain an acid alpha 1,4-glucosidase (acid martase). This enzyme activity is absent in type II glycogen-storage disease and leads to the signs and symptoms described below. Since this enzyme lack occurs throughout the body it is not specific for the heart, but the cardiac involvement plays a major part in the early onset of symptoms.

Classification

A variety of classifications of glycogen disease have appeared in the literature and change with the addition of new knowledge on the subject. The classification listed in Table 58–1 is that of Van Hoof and colleagues (1972).

Prevalence

This is a relatively rare condition. However, Hers (1970) has identified 47 cases. At The Hospital for

Table 58–1.   CLASSIFICATION OF GLYCOGENOSES *

TYPE	ENZYMATIC LESION	PRINCIPAL SITE OF GLYCOGEN STORAGE	PREVALENCE %
I	Glucose 6-phosphatase	Liver, kidney	26.0
II	Acid α-glucosidase	Generalized disease	15.9
III	Amylo-1, 6-glucosidase	Liver, muscle (erythrocytes)	20.0
IV	Branching enzyme	Liver	0.3
V	Phosphorylase	Muscle	—
VI	Either no detectable lesion or low hepatic phosphorylase	Liver	39.0
VII	Phosphofructokinase	Muscle	—
			100.0

* Van Hoof, F.; Hue, I.; et al.: Glycogen storage disease. *Biochimie*, **54**:745, 1972.

Sick Children, Toronto, eight cases have been seen in 25 years.

A review of the literature by Muller and associates (1961) and Ehlers and colleagues (1962) coupled with the data of Hers (1968) and Van Hoof (1973) indicated that reports on over 100 such cases are available. The distribution among the sexes is equal.

Etiology

The etiology now appears to be clarified. It is recognized as an enzyme deficiency disease involving a lack of acid alpha 1,4-glucosidase (acid martase). This leads to an accumulation of glycogen in many organs throughout the body, particularly in heart, liver, and skeletal muscle. Glycogen increase has also been found in the leukocytes, kidney, mucous-secreting glands of the gastrointestinal tract, muscle fibers of the bladder, blood vessels, and pyramidal cells of the cerebral cortex. Glucose, lactose, and adrenaline tolerance tests are within normal limits. There are no hypoglycemia and no ketone bodies in the urine.

Clinical Features

The clinical signs and symptoms usually appear between two and six months of age. In a few cases evidence of the disease was noted in the first month of life, and in one case symptoms did not appear until the second year. Most commonly there are a lack of appetite and a failure to gain. This starts insidiously but may become more marked over a period of weeks or months. In several cases the failure to gain was evident shortly after birth.

Rapid or labored respirations may be evident to the parents before they seek medical advice since, as the disease progresses, most of these cases develop congestive heart failure. Muscular weakness has been noted a number of times by the parents but is more likely to be found on physical examination by the examining physician.

Not uncommonly, infection may be a precipitating event that brings the baby to the doctor's office. Vomiting may occur, and in those with failure there may be intermittent attacks of a mild degree of cyanosis.

Physical Findings. The baby is poorly nourished as a rule and is acutely ill in approximately half of the cases. The liver is usually enlarged due to either heart failure or increased glycogen deposition. Macroglossia has been reported in approximately 25 percent of cases and, if looked for, would probably be found more frequently. If reflex and muscle power are studied with care, particularly in the babies who have survived the neonatal period, weakness may be demonstrated.

Heart. The heart is usually enlarged and reveals a shape that is suggestive (see Figure 58-1). Generalized enlargement is characteristic, involving the

ventricles chiefly. The atria are likely to be enlarged if failure is present. A murmur has been reported in over half of the cases in which a record of the heart sounds was made. When present, the murmur is usually at the apex and not widely propagated. Gallop rhythm is likely to be noted. Ehlers and coworkers (1962) have recorded details of a case with obstruction of the outflow tract of the left ventricle.

Radiologic Examination

Enlargement of the heart has always been found in the cases where radiologic examination was made (see Figure 58-1). There is evidence of generalized enlargement of the heart with a smooth, convex border and an apex that is pointing down and out close to the left costal margin. The right atrium may be enlarged if a considerable degree of failure is present. A barium swallow will usually show a pushing back of the left atrium due to generalized enlargement of the heart. In one of the cases reported by Martin and Bonte (1951) some specific degree of enlargement of

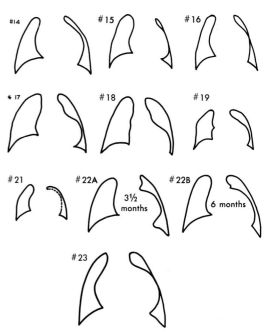

Figure 58-1. Glycogen-storage disease of the heart. Cardiac outlines, all showing some degree of generalized enlargement. #14, Age at death, four months (Di Sant'Agnese et al., 1950, case two). #15, Age at death, six months (Martin and Bonte, 1951, case one). #16, Age at death, nine weeks (Martin and Bonte, 1951, case two). #17, Age at death, 14 months (Childs et al., 1952, case one). #18, Age at death, 17½ months (Childs et al., 1952, case two). #19, Age at x-ray, six months (Levine and Taubenhaus, 1954). #21, Age at death, four and one-half months (Langewisch and Bigler, 1952). #22, Age at x-ray, three and one-half months; age at death, six months (Clement and Godman, 1950). #23, Age at death, four months (Landing and Bangle, 1950, case one).

the left atrium appeared to be present. In one case an x-ray of the chest taken at birth showed a normal heart size and shape; when this was repeated at 16 months of age, gross enlargement was evident (case 18). The hilar shadows and lung fields may be congested. The angiocardiographic and hemodynamic features have been presented in two thoroughly studied cases by Ruttenberg and associates (1964).

Electrocardiography

Electrocardiographic data have been summarized on at least 21 cases (Ehlers et al., 1962). The heart rate is increased usually over 140 beats per minute. The conduction time is characteristically short, less than 0.12 second in 85 percent (range, 0.05 to 0.12 second). This is shorter than is usually seen in the first year of life and shorter than one would expect with the tachycardia. The QRS interval is wide in the majority. The T wave is inverted in 70 percent in standard leads I and II. A normal axis is present in a similar percentage and a left axis in the remainder. Right atrial enlargement occurs in a third. The precordial leads showed evidence of left ventricular hypertrophy in 80 percent. Right ventricular hypertrophy of some degree is present in one-third.

The characteristic tracing, therefore, is one with a short P-R interval, wide QRS, left ventricular hypertrophy with or without the strain pattern. A normal QRS is usually present in the frontal plane, but it may be slightly to the left.

Diagnosis

For the cardiologist the diagnosis depends on recognition of cardiac enlargement early in life, usually in the first six months. Because of the hereditary tendency of this disease, one is much more likely to suspect its occurrence when it has appeared in another member of the family. Two or more members affected in one family have been reported in ten definitive instances and seven possible.

Since the term "idiopathic hypertrophy of the heart" has been used often in the literature of the past, it seems likely that a good many cases have occurred without being recognized or reported.

In the presence of an enlarged heart in a baby in the first year of life, one should suspect glycogen-storage disease if there is a history of poor appetite and a lack of weight gain associated with a large tongue and muscular weakness. Supporting evidence is provided by the absence of a specific type of heart murmur occurring in a noncyanotic baby who has evidence of left ventricular hypertrophy or combined ventricular hypertrophy in the electrocardiogram with a normal axis and a short P-R interval. The short conduction time is highly suggestive if the Wolff-Parkinson-White syndrome is eliminated.

A muscle biopsy may suggest the diagnosis if it shows an increased glycogen content (over 1 percent of net weight). The histologic picture of the muscle fibers is also distinctive, revealing evidence of increased glycogen storage. A definitive diagnosis depends on demonstrating the absence of acid martase in the tissues coupled with an increase in glycogen. The presence of increased amounts of glycogen in the white blood cells is a simple approach to the diagnosis.

Since glycogenosis type II appears to be inherited as an autosomal recession, when one child with this defect has occurred in a family, a second pregnancy creates the need for early diagnosis. This can be achieved by amniocentesis. The cultured amniocytes reveal a deficiency of the critical enzyme.

Differential Diagnosis. The differential diagnosis includes those conditions in early life that have left ventricular hypertrophy in the electrocardiogram, such as endocardial fibroelastosis, coronary calcinosis, aberrant left coronary artery arising from the pulmonary artery, aortic stenosis, and coarctation of the aorta. Coarctation of the aorta does not present much difficulty when blood pressures are taken. Left coronary artery arising from the pulmonary artery usually has a suggestive electrocardiographic picture. Aortic stenosis may be separated by its murmur or by angiocardiogram, although it should be remembered that subaortic stenosis may occur in glycogen-storage disease of the heart. Coronary calcinosis runs a brief course after the onset of symptoms, and, on occasion, calcification of certain vessels throughout the body may be shown by means of x-ray. Endocardial fibroelastosis is the most common cause of heart failure combined with left ventricular hypertrophy in the first year of life. It will show a more marked picture of left ventricular hypertrophy usually, with a normal P-R interval and QRS interval, whereas the P-R interval is likely to be shortened in glycogen-storage disease. A most important differential point is the muscle-biopsy revelation of excess glycogen.

Any baby who presents flaccid musculature suggesting amyotonia congenita or Werdnig-Hoffmann's disease must be considered as possibly suffering from glycogen-storage disease of the heart.

Prognosis

The age at death is shown in Figure 58–2. It will be seen that all but two cases died in the first year of life; most of them died between four and eight months. As far as is known, the condition is uniformly fatal. One of the cases is alive at the time of being reported (Levine and Taubenhaus, 1954) and is receiving digitalis.

The increasing deposition of glycogen in the heart muscle interferes with its function, causing progressive weakness and enlargement of that organ, eventually leading to congestive heart failure. Failure is either precipitated or hurried when the baby contracts an infection. Another debilitating feature is the presence of muscle weakness through the body,

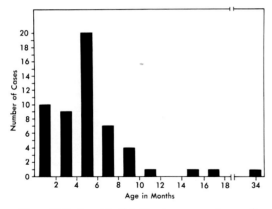

Figure 58-2. Age at death in 54 autopsy-proved cases of glycogen-storage disease involving the heart.

which may eventually lead to difficulty in swallowing and respiration.

Treatment

These babies should be given a trial on digitalis: first, until the diagnosis is established; second, to see whether life can be prolonged significantly by that means. Specific enzyme replacement has been tried but so far without success (Van Hoof, 1972).

REFERENCES

Andersen, D. H.: Familial cirrhosis of the liver with storage of abnormal glycogen. *Lab. Invest.*, 5:11, 1956.

Bischoff, G.: Zum klinischen Bild der Glykogen-Speicherungs-krankheit-(Glykogenose). *Z. Kinderh.*, 52:722, 1931–32.

Childs, A. W.; Crose, R. F.; and Henderson, P. H.: Glycogen disease of heart; report of 2 cases occurring in siblings. *Pediatrics*, 10:208, 1952.

Clement, D. H., and Godman, G. C.: Glycogen disease resembling mongolism, cretinism and amyotonia congenita. *J. Pediatr.*, 36:11, 1950.

Cori, G. T., and Larner, J.: Action of amylo-1, 6-glucosidase and phosphorylase on glycogen and amylopectin. *J. Biol. Chem.*, 188:17, 1951.

Creveld, S. van: Peculiar disturbance of carbohydrate metabolism in childhood. *Nederl. Maandschr. Geneesk.*, 15:349, 1928.

Di Sant'Agnese, P. A.: Diseases of glycogen storage with special reference to cardiac type of generalized glycogenosis. *Ann. N.Y. Acad. Sci.*, 72:439, 1959.

Di Sant'Agnese, P.; Andersen, D. H.; and Mason, H. H.: Glycogen storage disease of heart. *Pediatrics*, 6:607, 1950.

Ehlers, K. H., Hagstrom, J. W. C.; Lukas, D. A.; Redo, S. F.; and Engle, M. A.: Glycogen storage disease of the myocardium with obstruction to left ventricular outflow. *Circulation*, 25:96, 1962.

Gierke, E. von: Hepato-Nephromegalia glykogenica. (Glykogen-speicherkrankheit der Leber und Neiren.) *Betr. Pathol. Anat.*, 82:497, 1929.

Hers, H. G.: Etudes enzymatique sur fragments hepatiques. Application a la classification des glycogenoses. *Rev. Internat. Hepatol.*, 9:35, 1959.

Hers, H. G.: In Levine, R., and Luft, R. (eds.): *Advances in Metabolic Disorders*. Academic Press, N.Y., 1964, vol. 1, p. 1.

Hers, H. G., and Van Hoof, F.: In Dickens, F.; Randie, P. J., and Whelan, W. J. (eds.): *Carbohydrate Metabolism and Its Disorders*. Academic Press, N.Y., 1968, vol. 2, p. 151.

Hers, H. G.; De Wulf, H.; and Stalmans, W.: *FEBS Letters*, 12:73, 1970.

Illingworth, B., and Cori, G. T.: Structure of glycogens and amylopectins. III. Normal and abnormal human glycogen. *J. Biol. Chem.*, 199:653, 1952.

Krivit, W.; Polglase, W. J.; Gunn, F. D.; and Tyler, F. H.: Studies in disorders of muscle; glycogen storage disease primarily affecting skeletal muscle and clinically resembling amyotonia congenita. *Pediatrics*, 12:165, 1953.

Lambert, E. C., and Vlad, P.: Primary endomyocardial disease. *Pediatr. Clin. North Am.*, 5:1057, 1958.

Landing, B. H., and Bangle, R., Jr.: Glycogen storage disease. Histochemical studies of glycogenolysis in human hearts obtained postmortem, with special reference to glycogen storage disease. *Bull. Internat. A. M. Museums*, 31:110, 1950.

Langewisch, W. H., and Bigler, J. A.: Disorders of glycogen metabolism with special reference to glycogen storage disease and galactosemia. *Pediatrics*, 9:263, 1952.

Levine, R., and Taubenhaus, M.: Clinical conference on metabolic problems—glycogen storage disease. *Metabolism*, 3:173, 1954.

Martin, J. F., and Bonte, F. J.: Glycogen disease: report of two cases with cardiomegaly. *Am. J. Roentgenol.*, 66:922, 1951.

Mehrizi, A., and Oppenheimer, E. H.: Heart failure associated with unusual deposition of glycogen in the myocardium. *Bull Hopkins Hosp.*, 107:329, 1960.

Miller, R. A.: Symposium on cardiovascular diseases: the electrocardiogram in congenital malformations of the heart. *Pediatr. Clin. North Am.*, 1:51, 1954.

Mommaerts, W. F. H. M.; Illingworth, B.; Pearson, C. M.; Guillory, R. J.; and Seray-Darian, K.: A functional disorder of muscle associated with absence of phosphorylase. *Proc. Nat. Acad. Sci. U.S.A.*, 45:791, 1959.

Muller, O. F.; Bellet, S.; and Ertrugrul, A.: Glycogen-storage disease. Report of a case with generalized glycogenosis and review of the literature. *Circulation*, 23:261, 1961.

Nadas, A. S.: *Pediatric Cardiology*. W. B. Saunders Co., Philadelphia, 1957, p. 212.

Pompe, J. D.: Over idiopatische hypertrophy van het hart. *Nederl. Tijdschr. Geneesk.*, 76:304, 1932.

———: Hypertrophie idiopathique du coeur. *Ann. Anat. Pathol.*, 10:23, 1933.

Putschar, W.: Ueber engevorene Glykogen-speicherkrankheit des Herzens—"Thesaurismosis glykogenika" (von Gierke). *Beitr. Pathol. Anat.*, 90:222, 1932.

Ruttenberg, H. D.; Steidl, R. M.; and Carey, L. S.: Glycogen-storage disease of the heart. Hemodynamic and angiocardiographic features in 2 cases. *Am. Heart J.*, 67:469, 1964.

Schmid, R.; Robbins, P. W.; and Traut, R. R.: Glycogen synthesis in muscle lacking phosphorylase. *Proc. Nat. Acad. Sci. U.S.A.*, 45:1236, 1959.

Von Gierke, E.: Hepato-nephromegalia glykogenica (Glykogen-speichkrankheit der Leben und Nieren). *Beitr. Pathol. Anat.*, 82:497, 1929.

Van Hoof, F.; Hue, I.; et al.: Glycogen storage disease. *Biochimie*, 54:745, 1972.

Cardiac Involvement in the Mucopolysaccharidoses

J. Alexander Lowden, Richard G. Pearse, and *Richard D. Rowe*

THE MUCOPOLYSACCHARIDOSES (MPS) are a group of inherited metabolic disorders in which there is impaired degradation of various glycosaminoglycans due to defective or absent activity of specific lysosomal enzymes (Frattatoni et al., 1968; Neufeld, 1973; McKusick, 1972). The disorders are characterized by deposits of mucopolysaccharides in various tissues and by mucopolysacchariduria. Lowry and Renwick (1971) have assessed the relative frequency of live births of MPS in British Columbia as 1:100,000 (Hurler), 0.66:100,000 (Hunter), and 0.33:100,000 (Morquio).

The first examples of what are now known as the MPS were noted by John Thompson of the Royal Hospital for Sick Children, Edinburgh, between 1900 and 1913 (Henderson and Ellis, 1940). It was not until later that the first case reports appeared in the literature (Hunter, 1917; Hurler, 1919).

Ellis and associates (1936) introduced the term "gargoylism" to describe the ugly facies and dwarfism characteristic of some types of mucopolysaccharidosis. At that time the disorder was thought to lie in the metabolic pathway of lipid storage. However, evidence was steadily mounting in favor of its being an abnormality of mucopolysaccharide metabolism, and when in 1952 Brante isolated dermatan sulfate (chondroitin sulfate B) from the liver of the two patients with Hurler syndrome, the term "MPS" was suggested.

One of the first two cases described by Charles Hunter of Winnipeg in 1917 had cardiac involvement, and since that time there has been frequent mention of cardiovascular symptoms during life and of death from congestive cardiac failure. Detailed autopsy reports and the clinical findings in the cardiovascular system were much less commonly documented. Lindsay (1950) reviewed these disorders with special regard to the effects on the cardiovascular system and this aspect has since been covered by Berensen and Geer (1963) and Krovetz and associates (1963, 1965, 1972).

Clinical Features

The mucopolysaccharidoses are characterized by the abnormal storage and excretion in the urine of excess quantities of mucopolysaccharides. The various syndromes are differentiated by the clinical signs, the substance or substances in the urine, and by the measurement of the activity of specific mucopolysaccharide-catabolizing enzymes. Classification originally proved difficult, but in 1972 on the basis of specific enzymology and the use of "corrective factors" (see Biochemistry) McKusick published a revised classification that will be used in the ensuing discussion.

All the MPS except Hunter syndrome (type II) are transmitted as autosomal recessives. Hunter syndrome is an X-linked disorder. There are no clinical signs of the disease in the heterozygotes.

MPS Type I H (Hurler Syndrome). Early signs may be variable in appearance. Some children are recognized in the first few months while others may be 8 to 12 months old before the diagnosis is made. The infants have a chronic nasal discharge, frequent upper respiratory infections, and occasional episodes of pneumonia. Often the diagnosis is suspected on examination of radiographs of the chest. The classic "gargoyle" facies develops slowly during the first year and continues to progress throughout life. Hepatosplenomegaly, inguinal and umbilical hernias, deafness, clouding of the cornea, a lumbar gibbus, claw hands, and deformities of the chest are seen. Growth slows in the second year and usually ceases before four years of age. Mental deterioration is severe to moderate, although most children learn to walk and may say a few words. Mitral and aortic valve regurgitation are the most common clinical expressions of cardiac involvement. Death occurs at seven to ten years from cardiopulmonary complications.

MPS Type I S (Scheie Syndrome) (Previously Type V). Intelligence is normal in this condition.

However, the other features of type I H are present but to a minor degree. Impaired vision due to clouding of the cornea is the major problem, but aortic valve disease (regurgitation, stenosis, or both) is seen in most cases. Many patients have lived to the fifth decade.

MPS Type I HS Compound. There are some children who present with features of both the type I H and S disorders. They have severe bony changes, short stature, gargoyle facies, hernias, and hepatospleno- megaly but only mild retardation if any. They are probably the offspring of a Hurler carrier and a Scheie carrier. Both disorders involve defects in α- iduronidase activity (Table 59–1) but are presumably isoenzymically different (McKusick, 1972).

MPS Type II (Hunter Syndrome). Clouding of the cornea is not seen clinically and development of a lumbar gibbus is rarer. Otherwise the clinical signs resemble type I H closely, although they are much less marked. Deafness is prominent. Patients usually survive boyhood to die in early adult life but mild and severe forms within this type have recently been described (Lichtenstein et al., 1972). The cardiovas- cular involvement in these patients is similar to that encountered in MPS type I H.

MPS Type III (Sanfilippo Syndrome). These children present with mild-to-moderate retardation at two to four years. They have few somatic changes but growth usually slows by seven to eight years and they become severe aggressive behavior problems. They may survive to early adulthood. Heart disease has recently been described (Herd et al., 1973). Two types of Sanfilippo syndrome (A and B) can be distinguished biochemically (Table 59–1) but they are clinically identical.

MPS Type IV (Morquio Syndrome). Spondylo- epiphyseal dysplasia is the hallmark of this condition with clouding of the cornea and deformities of the teeth. Intelligence is normal but odontoid hypoplasia and other spinal deformities may cause spastic paraplegia or other neurologic symptoms. Death often occurs before the age of 20 from acute atlantoaxial subluxation, but cardiorespiratory deaths are also common. Aortic regurgitation often appears during adolescence.

MPS Type VI (Maroteaux-Lamy Syndrome). Dwarfism is the primary feature of this disease. Intelligence is normal, although most other features of MPS I H are present to a greater or lesser degree. Skeletal changes are so marked as to cause death from cardiorespiratory complications at an early age. Specific descriptions of cardiac abnormalities have recently been made (Krovetz and Schiebler, 1972; Di Ferranti et al., 1974).

MPS Type VII (β-Glucuronidase Deficiency). Two cases only described with differing clinical symptoms and signs, neither including heart disease (Glasser and Sly, 1973).

Mucolipidoses. Several conditions have clinical features that resemble those of the MPS. Spranger and Wiedeman (1970) have classified some of these as "mucolipidoses." Affected children do not excrete increased quantities of mucopolysaccharides in their urine but have similar radiologic findings and usually have cardiac involvement. The commonest cardiac defects are mitral or aortic regurgitation. The mucolipidoses include: *Type I*—(GM$_1$- gangliosidosis) a multisystem disorder due to a defect in β-galactosidase activity (O'Brien, 1969). These children fail to thrive, have hepatosplenomegaly, cloudy corneas, cherry red spots, and abnormal facies. Chest x-rays show infiltration of lungs. Histologically the alveoli are filled with foamy histiocytes, which are also found in the bone marrow. Mitral insufficiency is often severe, causing congestive failure in the first six months of life. *Type II*—(I-cell disease) a remarkable syndrome with growth failure, bony changes, mental retardation, and "gargoyle" features but with little hepatosplenomegaly and usually clear corneas (Leroy et al., 1971). Cardiac involvement in these children develops at the end of the first or the second year of life. *Type III*—(pseudo- Hurler polydystrophy) a milder form of mucolip- idosis. The first symptom usually begins in the second year of life with restricted joint movement. The children are short, have scoliosis, hip dysplasia, and mild mental retardation. Fine corneal opacities are found on slit-lamp examination (Spranger and Weidemann, 1970). Cardiac involvement is rare or absent.

Table 59–1. BIOCHEMICAL FINDINGS IN THE MUCOPOLYSACCHARIDOSES

TYPE	COMMON NAME	URINARY MUCOPOLYSAC- CHARIDES	ENZYME DEFECT	REFERENCE
I H	Hurler	Dermatan sulfate 60–80% heparan sulfate	α-Iduronidase	Bach et al., 1972
I S	Scheie	Dermatan sulfate 60–80% heparan sulfate	α-Iduronidase	Bach et al., 1972
II	Hunter	Dermatan sulfate ~50%	Sulfo-iduronate sulfatase	Bach et al., 1973
III A	Sanfilippo	Heparan sulfate	Heparan sulfate sulfatase	Kresse and Neufeld, 1972
B	Sanfilippo	Heparan sulfate	N-Acetyl-α-D-glucosaminidase	O'Brien, 1972
IV	Morquio	Keratan sulfate	N-Acetylhexosamine sulfate sulfatase	Mataton et al., 1974
VI	Maroteaux- Lamy	Dermatan sulfate	Arylsulfatase B	DiFerrante et al., 1974
VII	"Atypical"	?	β-Glucouronidase	Glasser and Sly, 1973

Cardiovascular Features

Over half the cases of MPS show evidence of heart disease, and the proportion may be higher if serial examinations are made on known cases (Berenson and Geer, 1963; Krovetz and Schiebler, 1972). Heart disease is often recognized by the development of an organic murmur. Clinically, aortic regurgitation is probably the most frequently diagnosed lesion (Krovetz and Schiebler, 1972) (Figure 59–1), although at autopsy the mitral valve is found to be the most commonly affected. In many of the patients studied by Krovetz, a grade I–II/VI typically descrescendo systolic murmur, which started after the first sound and lasted for about half systole, was heard. Our own experience would support the view that most of these shorter softer systolic murmurs are regurgitant and have a mitral or tricuspid origin. Occasionally we have heard heart murmurs strongly suggesting mild pulmonary arterial stenosis. Murmurs detected early in infancy and childhood tend to increase in amplitude with the passage of time as the disease process causes ever-increasing damage to the heart valves. A number have a decrease in precordial activity with a first heart sound of diminished intensity (Krovetz and Schiebler, 1972). In the adults studied by Emanuel (1954), the second heart sound in the pulmonary area was greatly accentuated. A third heart sound at the apex is frequently heard.

Cardiac enlargement and/or congestive heart failure may be the presenting feature of cardiac involvement. In others, sudden death is the first and only sign of heart disease. The blood pressure is often normal; however, 29 percent of the cases studied by Krovetz and associates (1963) had systemic hypertension. Occasionally, heart disease may be the presenting feature in an infant (Strauss and Platt, 1957).

It seems probable that heart disease may occur in all types of MPS, but the number of cases of each type so far described is insufficient to show the full cardiovascular extent of the disease.

In summary, cardiovascular disease has to date been found associated with every form of MPS, except type VII. Its clinical expression has been evident as aortic valvular disease (almost all regurgitation) and terminal heart failure. Krovetz and Schiebler (1972) believe it unlikely that the involvement of coronary or other arteries is individually the cause of death. They believe that hypoxia from respiratory obstruction, together with compromise of left ventricular function from a combination of the accumulation of mucopolysaccharide in the myocardium, presence of systemic hypertension, valvular regurgitation, and coronary artery disease, accounts for cardiorespiratory demise.

The presence of a heart murmur in MPS has led in the past to a diagnosis of congenital heart malformations, particularly ventricular septal defect (Lindsay, 1950) but also pulmonary and aortic stenosis. Mitral regurgitation, cor pulmonale, and anemic heart disease are other diagnoses that have been entertained. On rare occasions, sudden death in

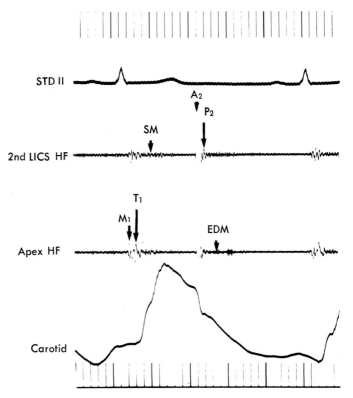

Figure 59-1. Phonocardiogram of a nine-year-old boy with MPS type III showing an early systolic murmur and an early diastolic murmur. *HF* = high frequency. There was clinical and other evidence of aortic regurgitation.

infancy, first thought to be due to other causes even after necropsy, has been found, following detailed histologic examination, to be due to cardiac involvement by the mucopolysaccharidoses. It seems probable that echocardiography will be useful in diagnosis by identifying abnormal left heart dimensions and by showing mitral and aortic valvular abnormalities (Di Ferrante et al., 1974) (Figure 59–2).

Electrocardiography

Most cases show prolongation of the Q-T interval (Krovetz and Schiebler, 1972). Right-axis deviation

was reported in patients with clinical heart disease at four years and six years, by Craig (1954) and Jelke (1951). Emanuel (1954) analyzed the electrocardiograms with standard and unipolar leads in two adult cases, both of which showed some evidence of right ventricular hypertrophy. Our records include several patients with normal electrocardiograms who had no clinical evidence of heart involvement. Others have shown abnormal tracings (Figure 59–3). Krovetz and Schiebler (1972) studied the electrocardiograms of 32 patients with MPS and found ten with left ventricular hypertrophy and nine with evidence for left atrial enlargement. Six patients had combined ventricular hypertrophy and four patients

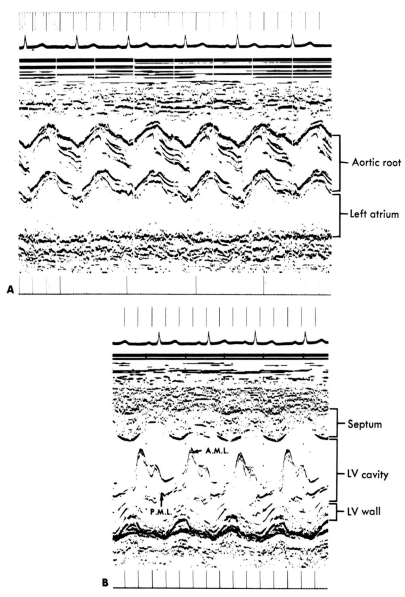

Figure 59-2. The echocardiogram of a nine-year-old boy with MPS type III. *A.* The aortic root echo showing multilayered diastolic echoes consistent with an abnormal aortic valve. *B.* Flutter of the anterior mitral leaflet is consistent with aortic regurgitation.

right ventricular hypertrophy alone. Arrhythmias were not seen, apart from some cases of first-degree heart block.

Cardiac Catheterization

There is only one major report on cardiac catheterization in this disorder. In 15 individuals, Krovetz and associates (1965) found only three patients with pulmonary hypertension, and this was mild. Nine of their fifteen cases had normal cardiac indices, although both systemic and pulmonary vascular resistance was slightly increased. There was some abnormality in the appearance of the upstroke of the pressure pulse in both right ventricle and pulmonary artery in this series, and two cases had aortic regurgitation, one mitral and one pulmonary regurgitation. Coronary artery disease was not observed angiographically. Indices of left ventricular function obtained by measurements of left ventricular and diastolic pressure and the response to angiotensin infusion by these authors were frequently abnormal. Cardiac catheterization in one 26-year-old patient with physical signs suggesting pulmonary hypertension was confirmed by revealing a pressure of 88/50 (mean 61) mm of mercury in the main pulmonary artery (Emanuel, 1954).

Pathology

Dawson (1954) demonstrated abnormal storage of mucopolysaccharides in the parenchymal cells and fibroelastic tissue throughout the body. Following observations of Dorfman and Lorincz (1957) and Meyer and associates (1958) that patients with "gargoylism" excreted two chemically unrelated mucopolysaccharides, chondroitin sulfate B (der-

matan sulfate) and heparitin sulfate (heparan sulfate), Meyer and associates (1959) reported the unequal accumulation of these two substances in various organs of patients with this group of diseases. Dermatan sulfate is mainly stored in the spleen, bone, brain, and kidney, whereas heparan sulfate is the major mucopolysaccharide in the liver. Because of its widespread distribution, the mucopolysaccharide that is stored produces a diffuse disease that varies in both its clinical and pathologic picture, depending on the speed, degree, and site of accumulation of the abnormal substance as well as on the nature of the material itself. Symptoms are produced by the effect on the organ structure and function and by interference with growth. No region escapes involvement, and although bones, skin, eyes, brain, liver, and spleen are affected, attention here will be confined to the cardiovascular system.

In 80 percent of reported autopsies hypertrophy of the heart has been noted. The left ventricle is more affected than the right. The myocardium is normal in most cases, but a grayish-red color in the fresh state has also been reported (Lindsay, 1950). The endocardium of either ventricle may be thickened. Most striking of the gross findings is the appearance of the heart valves, which are affected in over 60 percent of cases. The valve is usually thickened and has a fibrous or gelatinous nodular appearance at its free edge (Jelke, 1955; Dawson, 1954; Bishton et al., 1956; Emanuel, 1954). Regurgitation is the commonest clinical sequela, but if the process is extreme, then stenosis may occur. The order of frequency of involvement of the heart valves reported by Krovetz and associates (1965) in 58 autopsied cases was mitral 29, tricuspid 19, aortic 16, and pulmonary 8. The chordae tendineae may also be thickened and shortened in severe cases. Occasionally the coronary arteries appear as thickened white cords (Emanuel, 1954).

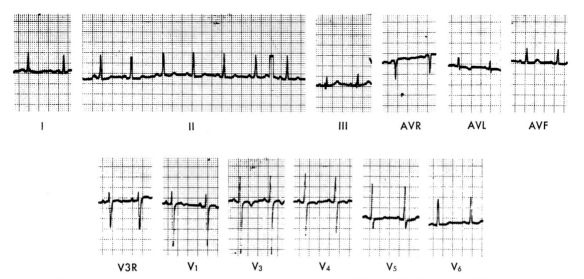

Figure 59-3. The electrocardiogram of a nine-year-old boy with MPS type III. There is no QRS voltage abnormality, but T waves are abnormal in I and aVL, and the S-T segment is depressed in I, II, V$_5$ and V$_6$.

A normal microscopic examination of the heart is a rarity (Dawson, 1954). Characteristic is the swollen and vacuolated appearance of cells in the connective tissue of all layers of the heart, particularly of the valves and intima of the main vessels and coronary arteries. Electron microscopy has revealed two types of abnormal cells in the mitral valve of a three-year-old female patient with MPS I H, one a glycolipid cell and the other containing acid mucopolysaccharide (Lagunoff et al., 1962). Over 30 percent of all detailed autopsies have shown marked narrowing of the coronary arteries. It is important to emphasize that this change has been found in children (Lindsay et al., 1948; Strauss, 1948; Lindsay, 1950; Magee, 1950; Henderson et al., 1952; Dawson, 1954; Emanuel, 1954; Krovetz and Schiebler, 1972). Alterations in other vessels have been noted infrequently, possibly because they have not been looked for. The pancreatic arteries have shown minimal intimal involvement (Lindsay et al., 1948) as have other regional arteries, including those in the brain, spleen, and kidney (Henderson et al., 1952). The narrowing of these arteries is due in part to plaque formation, and it is probable that these contain mucopolysaccharide and thus are different from true atheromatous plaques (Krovetz and Schiebler, 1972). Gross changes in myocardial fibers are less common, although the appearance of chronic myocarditis has been described (Morris and Waldman, 1953).

Biochemistry

The mucopolysaccharides are macromolecules composed of disaccharide units of a hexosamine and either a hexuronic acid or hexose. They are O-sulfated in either sugar and may be N-sulfated (heparan sulfate). They are covalently bound to a peptide or small protein. The chemical composition of the various glycosaminoglycans has been reviewed in detail by Neufeld (1973).

Children with mucopolysaccharidoses excrete 3 to 20 times the normal quantity of mucopolysaccharides in their urine. There are some differences in the types of mucopolysaccharides excreted by the different genotypes (Table 59–1).

In 1964 van Hoof and Hers noted the similarity of the storage organelles in the liver of a child with Hurler syndrome to the lysosomes of rats treated with dextran or WR 1339. Their work led to the concept that mucopolysaccharidoses were "lysosomal defects" probably due to an inactive lysosomal hydolase. Danes and Bearn (1965) showed that the storage could be replicated in cultured fibroblasts. They showed that cells from a child with Hurler syndrome accumulated metachromatic material in culture. Fratatoni, Hall, and Neufeld (1968) added $^{35}SO_4$ to these cell cultures and found the label was accumulated more extensively in MPS cells than normal. They concluded the increased incorporation was due to a block in degradation of mucopolysaccharides that these cells formed at normal rates.

Subsequently Fratatoni, Hall, and Neufeld (1969) demonstrated that the cell secretions in culture medium from fibroblasts of a different genotype could correct the storage in MPS cells. For example, the radiosulfate accumulation in Hurler cells could be corrected not only with culture medium from normal cells, but also with medium from Hunter or Sanfilippo cells. The mucopolysaccharide storage resulted from a defect in a factor that was present in genotypically different cells.

Different "corrective factors" were found for Hurler, Hunter, Morquio, Morateaux-Lamy, and two varieties of Sanfilippo syndromes. The corrective factor in Scheie syndrome was similar to the Hurler corrective factor. This latter observation was of interest because the syndromes were clinically quite distinct.

The catabolism of complex oligosaccharides of other types (glycogen and the carbohydrate portion of gangliosides) proceeds in a stepwise fashion. Each individual hexose is hydrolyzed from the nonreducing end of the macromolecule. Sulfated glycolipid cannot be catabolized until the sulfate has been removed from the terminal sugar (Brady, 1973). In the catabolism of mucopolysaccharides the same general rules apply. For complete degradation of the macromolecule, each of the specific glycosidases and sulfatases must be active. A defect in the activity of any one results in failure of catabolism and storage. The first enzyme defect to be described in the MPS was the absence of α-iduronidase activity in Hurler syndrome (Matalon, Cifonelli, and Dorfman, 1971). The Hurler corrective factor was then identified as α-iduronidase (Bach et al., 1972). Subsequently each of the enzyme defects in the different MPS have been identified (Table 59–1).

Radiologic Examination

The striking range of skeletal abnormalities in the MPS has been well described (McKusick, 1972). Briefly, they center on an abnormality of bony texture with loss of trabeculation and thinning of the cortex. The long bones, including ribs and metacarpals, become wider and misshapen. The lumbar vertebrae are often notched, the skull has prominent frontal bones and a shallow sella turcica, and there is a decrease in mastoid and ethmoid air spaces. In those chest radiographs published by Emanuel (1954) of two adults, aged 20 and 29 years, and of two children (Costello, 1954; Lyon and Kaplan, 1954) the cardiothoracic ratio exceeded 0.60. The cardiac enlargement was generalized and the pulmonary artery segment prominent. Similar findings were noted in an infant recently seen at The Hospital for Sick Children (Figure 59–4).

Diagnosis

The mucopolysaccharidoses may be diagnosed by the specific clinical appearance, the genetic history,

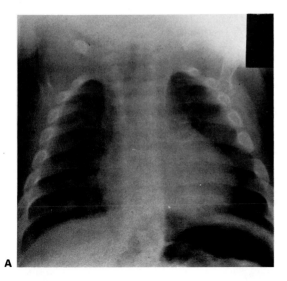

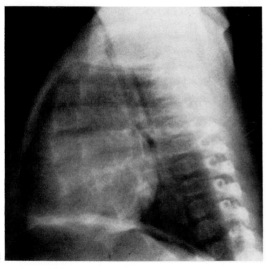

Figure 59-4. The anteroposterior (*A*) and lateral (*B*) chest x-rays showing cardiomegaly in an infant aged three months with MPS type I.

Using $^{35}SO_4$ incorporation (Fratatoni, Hall, and Neufeld, 1968) mucopolysaccharide storage can be demonstrated with cultured fibroblasts. Differentiation of genotypes can then be accomplished by cross-correction studies with known genotypes. Enzymologic diagnosis is not generally available for all the mucopolysaccharidoses because of the substrates that must be synthesized in the laboratory. Supplies of phenyl-α-iduronide are small (Freidman and Weissman, 1972). The sulfatase defects can only be demonstrated with ^{35}S-labeled substrates, which have a limited shelf-life because of radioactive decay. However, N-acetyl-α-D-glucosaminide as the 4-methylumbilliferyl derivative is commercially available for the diagnosis of Sanfilippo B syndrome, as is $^{35}SO_4$ heparin sulfate for the diagnosis of Sanfilippo A.

In families with a previously affected infant, antenatal diagnosis of MPS can be considered. We have monitored three such pregnancies at The Hospital for Sick Children and have aborted an affected Hurler fetus (Lowden et al., 1975).

Treatment

Supportive therapy for orthopedic problems, respiratory infections, and congestive cardiac failure may postpone the end and is indicated, especially in those with normal mental development. Valve replacement for severe mitral regurgitation has been successfully performed (Herd et al., 1973). Corneal grafting, particularly lamellar grafting, has been tried with success in some cases (Lahdensuu, 1964; King, 1943; Rosen et al., 1968; Scheie et al., 1962). The major problem in each disease, however, is the inactivity of a specific enzyme.

Many attempts have been made at generalized therapy for children with MPS. Hurler (1919) and Ernould (1949) tried thyroid and pituitary extracts without effect. Vitamin A, prednisone, and diets low in vitamin C have all been used because they stimulate synthesis and release of lysomal hydrolases. None of these methods have proved successful.

Neufeld's demonstration of a corrective factor in serum, urine, and culture medium prompted Di Ferrante and associates (1971) to attempt treatment with infusions of normal plasma and leukocytes. They claimed a clinical improvement in patients with MPS I H. The same group (Knudson et al., 1971) found even more marked improvement after infusing leukocytes into a six-year old with MPS II. However, Dekaban et al. (1972) and Erikson et al. (1972) could not repeat this work. Probably the infused plasma or leukocytes contained so little enzyme that it had no sustained effect.

Reports by Brady's group (1973, 1974) indicate that infusion of purified enzyme is feasible in other diseases due to inactive lysosomal hydrolyses. Perhaps it may be a reasonable form of therapy at some future date when the mucopolysaccharide-degrading enzymes have been purified.

x-rays of the spine, ribs, long bones, and hands, and by a combination of laboratory tests. At The Hospital for Sick Children, we measure mucopolysaccharide excretion in 24-hour urines (Whiteman, 1973) and quantitate the results as milligrams of hexuronic acid excreted per 24 hr. Normals excrete less than 20 mg/24 hr. Patients with types I, II, and VI excrete from 5 to 10 times the normal. Those with type III excrete 2 to 4 times the normal. Patients with type IV excrete keratan sulfate, which contains no hexuronic acid. For quantitation of the different species, we isolate the mucopolysaccharides on DEAE cellulose columns (modified from Di Ferrante, 1967) and separate the individual species by cellulose acetate electrophoresis (Breen et al., 1970). The electrophoretograms can be quantitated by densitometry.

REFERENCES

Bach, G.; Friedman, R.; Weissmann, B.; and Neufeld, E. F.: The defect in the Hurler and Scheie syndromes: Deficiency of α-L-iduronidase. *Proc. Natl. Acad. Sci. U.S.A.*, **69**:2048, 1972.

Bach, G.; Eisenberg, F., Jr.; Crantz, M.; and Neufeld, E. F.: The defect in Hunter syndrome: Deficiency of sulfoiduronate sulfatase. *Proc. Natl. Acad. Sci. U.S.A.*, **70**:2134, 1973.

Berenson, G. S., and Geer, J. C.: Heart disease in Hurler and Marfan syndromes. *Arch. Intern. Med.*, **111**:58, 1963.

Bishton, R. L.; Norman, R. M.; and Tingey, A.: Pathology and chemistry of a case of gargoylism. *J. Clin. Pathol.*, **9**:305, 1956.

Brady, R. O.: The sphingolipodystrophies. In *Duncan's Diseases of Metabolism*, Vol. 1. W. B. Saunders, Philadelphia, 1973.

Brady, R. O.; Tallman, J. F.; Johnson, W. G.; Gal, A. E.; Leahy, W. R.; Quirk, J. M.; and Dekaban, A. S.: Replacement therapy for inherited enzyme deficiency in Fabry's disease. *N. Engl. J. Med.*, **289**:9, 1973.

Brady, R. O.; Pentchev, P. G.; Gal, A. E.; Hibbert, S. R.; and Dekaban, A. S.: Replacement therapy with purified glucocerebrosidase in Gaucher's disease. *N. Engl. J. Med.*, **291**:989, 1974.

Brante, G.: Gargoylism: a mucopolysaccharidosis. *Scand. J. Clin. Lab. Invest.*, **4**:43, 1952.

Breen, M.; Weinstein, H. G.; Anderson, M.; and Veis, A.: Microanalysis and characterization of acidic glycosaminoglycans in human tissues. *Anal. Biochem.*, **35**:146, 1970.

Costello, P.: Gargoylism: clinical case. *Bull. Child. Mem. Hosp. (Chicago)*, **12**:3428, 1954.

Craig, W. S.: Gargoylism in a twin brother and sister. *Arch. Dis. Child.*, **29**:293, 1954.

Danes, B. S., and Bearn, A. G.: Hurler's syndrome: demonstration of an inherited disorder of connective tissue in cell culture. *Science*, **149**:987, 1965.

Dawson, J. M.: The histology and histochemistry of gargoylism. *J. Pathol. Bact.*, **67**:587, 1954.

Dekaban, A. S.; Holden, K. R.; and Constantapoulos, G.: Effects of fresh plasma or whole blood transfusions on patients with various types of mucopolysaccharidosis. *Pediatrics*, **50**:688, 1972.

Di Ferrante, N.; Nichols, B. L.; Donnelly, P. V.; Neri, G.; Hrgovcic, R.; and Berglund, R. K.: Induced degradation of glycosaminoglycans in Hurler's and Hunter's syndromes by plasma infusion. *Proc. Natl. Acad. Sci.*, **68**:303, 1971.

Di Ferrante, N.; Hyman, B. H.; Klish, W.; Donnelly, P. V.; Nichols, B. L.; Dutton, E. V.; and Gniot-Szulzycka, J.: Mucopolysaccharidosis VI (Maroteaux-Lamy disease): Clinical and biochemical study of a mild variant case. *Johns Hopkins Med. J.*, **135**:42, 1974.

Dorfman, A.; and Lorincz, A. E.: Occurrence of urinary mucopolysaccharides in the Hurler syndrome. *Proc. Natl. Acad. Sci. U.S.A.*, **43**:443, 1957.

Ellis, R. W. B.; Sheldon, W.; and Capon, N. B.: Gargoylism (chondo-osteodystrophy, corneal opacities, hepatosplenomegaly and mental deficiency). *Q. J. Med.*, **5**:119, 1936.

Emanuel, R. W.: Gargoylism with cardiovascular involvement in two brothers. *Br. Heart J.*, **16**:417, 1954.

Erickson, R. P.; Sandman, R.; Robertson, W. van B., and Epstein, C. J.: Inefficiency of fresh frozen plasma therapy of mucopolysaccharidosis II. *Pediatrics*, **50**:693, 1972.

Ernould, H. J.: *Arch. Pediatr.*, **6**:238, 1949. Quoted by Jelke, 1951.

Fratatoni, J. C.; Hall, C. W.; and Neufeld, E. F.: The defect in Hurler and Hunter syndromes: II Deficiency of specific factors involved in mucopolysaccharide degeneration. *Proc. Natl. Acad. Sci. U.S.A.*, **64**:360, 1969.

Fratatoni, J. C.; Hall, C. W.; and Neufeld, E. F.: The defect in Hurler's and Hunter's syndromes: Faulty degeneration of mucopolysaccharidosis. *Proc. Natl. Acad. Sci. U.S.A.*, **60**:699, 1968.

Friedman, R. B., and Weissman, B., The phenyl α and β-L-idopyranosiduronic acids and some other aryl-glycopyranosiduronic acids. *Carbohydr. Res.*, **24**:123, 1972.

Glaser, J. H., and Sly, W. S.: β-Glucuronidase deficiency mucopolysaccharidosis: Methods for enzymatic diagnosis. *J. Lab. Clin. Med.*, **82**:969, 1973.

Henderson, J. L.; MacGregor, A. R.; Thannhauser, S. J.; and Holden, R.: The pathology and biochemistry of gargoylism. A report of three cases with a review of the literature. *Arch. Dis. Child.*, **27**:230, 1952.

Henderson, J. L., and Ellis, R. W. B.: Gargoylism. A review of the principal features with a report of five cases. *Arch. Dis. Child.*, **15**:201, 1940.

Herd, J. K.; Subramanian, S.; and Robinson, H.: Type III mucopolysaccharidosis: Report of a case with severe mitral involvement. *J. Pediatr.*, **82**:101, 1973.

Hunter, C. H.: A rare disease in two brothers. *Proc. Roy. Soc. Med.*, **10**:104, 1917.

Hurler, G.: Uber einen Typ multiplier Abartungen, vorwiegend am Skeletsystem. *Z. Kinderheilk.*, **24**:220, 1919.

Jelke, H.: Gargoylism. Report of a case. *Ann. Pediatr.*, **177**:355, 1951.

Jelke, H.: Gargoylism II. Postmortem findings in an earlier published case. *Ann. Pediatr.*, **184**:101, 1955.

King, J. H., Jr.: Personal communication to V. A. McKusick, 1964; quoted in *Heritable Disorders of Connective Tissue*, 4th ed., 1972.

Knudson, A.; Di Ferrante, N.; and Curtis, J. E.: The effects of leukocyte transfusion in a child with mucopolysaccharidosis II. *Proc. Natl. Acad. Sci. U.S.A.*, **68**:1738, 1971.

Kresse, H., and Neufeld, E. F.: The Sanfilippo A corrective factor. Purification and mode of action. *J. Biol. Chem.*, **247**:2164, 1972.

Krovetz, L. J.; Lorincz, A. E.; and Schiebler, G. L.: Hemodynamic studies in the Hunter-Hurler syndrome (gargoylism). *Circulation*, **82**:753, 1963.

Krovetz, L. J.; Lorincz, A. E.; and Schiebler, G. L.: Cardiovascular manifestations of the Hurler syndrome: Hemodynamic and angiocardiographic observations in 15 patients. *Circulation*, **31**:132, 1965.

Krovetz, L. J., and Shiebler, G. L.: Cardiovascular manifestations of the genetic mucopolysaccaridoses. *Birth Defects: Original Article Series*, **8**:August, 1972.

Lagunoff, D.; Ross, R.; and Benditt, E. P.: Histochemical and electron microscopic study in a case of Hurler's disease. *Am. J. Pathol.*, **41**:273, 1962.

Lahdensuu, S.: Falle der sogenannten Pfaundler-Hurlersche Krankheit. (Dysostosis multiplex). *Mschr. Kinderheilk.*, **92**:340, 1943.

Leroy, J. G.; Spranger, J. W.; Feingold, M.; Optiz, J.; and Crocker, A.: I-cell disease: A clinical picture. *J. Pediatr.*, **79**:360, 1971.

Lichtenstein, J. R.; Bilbrey, G. L.; and McKusick, V. A.: Clinical and probable genetic heterogeneity within mucopolysaccharidosis II. Report of a family with a mild form. *Johns Hopkins Med. J.*, **131**:425, 1972.

Lindsay, S.: The cardiovascular system in gargoylism. *Br. Heart J.*, **12**:17, 1950.

Lindsay, S.; Reilly, W. A.; Gotham, T. J.; and Skahen, R.: Gargoylism II. Study of pathologic lesions and clinical review of 12 cases. *Am. J. Dis. Child.*, **76**:239, 1948.

Lowden, J. A.; Rudd, N.; Cutz, E.; and Doran, T. A.: Antenatal diagnosis of sphingolipid and mucopolysaccharide storage disease. *Can. Med. Assoc. J.*, **113**:507, 1975.

Lowry, R. B., and Renwick, D. H.: Relative frequency of the Hurler and Hunter syndromes. *N. Engl. J. Med.*, **284**:221, 1971.

Lyon, R. A., and Kaplan, S.: Disease of the myocardium. In Nelson, W. E. (ed.): *Textbook of Pediatrics*, 6th ed. W. B. Saunders Co., Philadelphia, 1954.

Mages, K. R.: Leptomeningeal changes associated with lipochondrodystrophy (gargoylism). *Arch. Neurol. Psychiat.*, **63**:282, 1950.

Matalon, R.; Cifonelli, J. A.; and Dorfman, A.: α-L-iduronidase in cultured human fibroblasts and liver. *Biochem. Biophys. Res. Comm.*, **42**:340, 1971.

Matalon, R.; Arbogast, B.; Parvin, J.; Brandt, I. K.; and Dorfman, A.: Morquio's syndrome: Deficiency of chondroitin sulfate N-acetylhexosamine sulfate sufatase. *Biochem. Biophys. Res. Comm.*, **61**:709, 1974.

McKusick, V. A.: *Heritable Disorders of the Connective Tissue*, 4th ed. C. V. Mosby Co., St. Louis, 1972, Chap. 11.

Meyer, K.; Grumbach, M. M.; Linker, A.; and Hoffman, P.: Excretion of sulphated mucopolysaccharides in gargoylism (Hurler's syndrome). *Proc. Soc. Exp. Biol. Med.*, **97**:275, 1958.

Meyer, J.; Hoffman, P.; Linker, A.; Grumbach, M. M.; and Sampson, P.: Sulphated mucopolysaccharides of urine and organs in gargoylism (Hurler's syndrome) II. Additional studies (25327). *Proc. Soc. Exp. Biol. Med.*, **102**:587, 1959.

Morris, P., and Waldman, S.: Gargoylism. *J. Einstein Med. Cent.*, **2**:12, 1953.

Neufeld, E.: F.: Genertic disorders of mucopolysaccharide metabolism. In Gaull, G. E. (ed.): *Biology of Brain Dysfunction*, Vol. 1. Plenum Press, New York, 1973.

O'Brien, J. S.: Generalized gangliosidosis. *J. Pediatr.*, **75**:167, 1969.

O'Brien, J. S.: Sanfilippo syndrome: Profound deficiency of α-acetylglucosaminidase activity in organs and skin fibroblasts from type B patients. *Proc. Natl. Acad. Sci. U.S.A.*, **69**:1720, 1972.

Rosen, D. A.; Haust, M. D.; Yamashite, T.; and Bryans, A. M.: Keratoplasty and electron microscopy of the cornea in systemic mucopolysaccharidosis (Hurler's syndrome). *Can. J. Ophthalmol.*, **3**:218, 1968.

Scheie, H. G.; Hambrick, G. W., Jr.; and Barness, L. A.: A newly recognized forme fruste of Hurler's disease (gargoylism). *Am. J. Ophthalmol.*, **53**:753, 1962.

Spranger, J. W., and Wiedeman, H. R.: The genetic mucolipidoses. *Humangenetik*, **9**, 113, 1970.

Strauss, L., and Platt, R. L.: Endocardial sclerosis in infancy associated with abnormal storage (gargoylism). *J. Mt. Sinai Hosp. N.Y.*, **24**:1258, 1957.

Strauss, L.: The pathology of gargoylism: Report of a case and review of the literature. *Am. J. Pathol.*, **24**:855, 1948.

Van Hoof, F., and Hers, H. G.: L'ultrastructure des celles hepatiques dans la maladie de Hurler. *Compt. Rend. Acad. Sci. (Paris)*, **259**:1281, 1964.

Whiteman, P.: The quantitative determination of glycosaminoglycans in urine with Alcian blue 8GX. *Biochem. J.*, **131**:351, 1973.

CHAPTER

60

Marfan's Syndrome—Arachnodactyly

Beat Friedli and *Richard D. Rowe*

I N 1896, Marfan described a 5½-year-old girl who had long limbs, hyperextensible joints, atrophied musculature, and an abnormally long head (dolichocephaly) (see Figure 60–1). Her feet and hands were particularly slender ("spider legs"). This collection of abnormalities had been recognized at birth by the midwife. The eyes and heart were apparently normal. Marfan labeled the condition "dolichostenomelie," while Achard (1902) in reporting an 18-year-old girl with the disorder, used the term "arachnodactyly." This latter title focuses attention

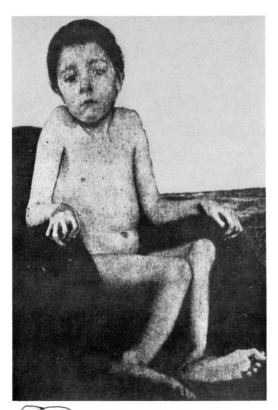

Figure 60-1. Gabrielle P., aged five and one-half years. The original case reported by Marfan (1896).

on the skeletal changes. Since the disorder has been shown to have other important aspects, such as ocular and cardiac lesions, "Marfan's syndrome" has been preferred as a more embracing term for the disorder. Some doubt has been cast recently on the diagnosis of Gabrielle P. (Figure 60–1), the patient originally described by Marfan, because she had joint contractures and probable mental retardation. This led Bianchine (1971) to consider the true diagnosis in that child to have been homocystinuria. Hecht and Beals (1972) described two families with an autosomal dominant phenotype without heart disease or mental retardation that they named congenital contractural arachnodactyly. They found a dozen descriptions in the earlier literature of arachnodactyly and judged Gabrielle P. to be an example of the disorder. Their view was supported by McKusick (1972a). Sixteen years after Marfan's original description, the first association of heart disease was reported by Salle (1912) in a 2½-month-old infant with obvious features of the syndrome at birth and evidence of aortic and tricuspid disease at autopsy. Borger (1914), having recognized a loud, mitral systolic murmur during life in an infant who died in the second year, found only a patency of the foramen ovale at autopsy. This case had ocular abnormality. By 1924, numerous reports of the syndrome had appeared, and in that year Ormond and Williams reviewed the literature and described the features in a 12-year-old boy, with particular emphasis on the ocular manifestations. It was not, however, until 1942 that diffuse aortic dilatation was reported in detail by Baer and associates. The following year dissecting aneurysm was described in association with the syndrome by Etter and Glover (1943).

Subsequently other reports and reviews of the cardiac aspects of Marfan's syndrome have appeared in the literature (Rados, 1942; Ross, 1949; Reynolds, 1950; Marvel and Genovese, 1951; Goyette and Palmer, 1953; McKusick, 1955, 1972b; Van Buchem, 1958; Sinclair et al., 1960; Breton et al., 1961; Hirst and Gore, 1973). The cardiovascular features of the syndrome in infants and children have been

1004

emphasized in the papers of Papaioannou and associates (1961) and Phornphutkul and associates (1973).

Etiology

Marfan's syndrome is a heritable disorder of connective tissue. It appears to be transmitted as a simple, dominant autosomal gene, about 50 percent of the offspring being affected. There is a relatively high grade of penetrance (Lutman and Neel, 1949). De novo mutation has been considered to occur in not more than 15 percent of cases, and there seems to be a relationship between the presentation of this unusual type and advanced paternal age (McKusick, 1972b).

The finding by Bacchus (1958) of abnormal serum seromucoid levels could not be confirmed by Leeming and McKusick (1962). Increased urinary excretion of hydroxyproline has been demonstrated in patients below 20 years of age (Sjoerdsma et al., 1958) but this may merely be a reflection of their increased growth (McKusick, 1972b).

The fact that disruption of elastic fibers in the aorta is a striking histologic finding in Marfan's syndrome suggests that the primary defect may be in the elastic tissue. However, the absence of any change in elastic tissue of the trachea, spinal ligaments, and intervertebral disks argues against this theory (Roark, 1959). Also, Bolande (1963) has demonstrated by histochemical and histologic techniques that deposition of metachromatic material in the aorta may precede elastic tissue changes; on the basis of his histochemical studies, he believes that the fundamental lesion may be overaccumulation of chondroitin sulfate C. More recently, Priest and colleagues (1973) found that collagen produced by fibroblasts from patients with Marfan's syndrome is abnormally soluble. This finding however is not specific of arachnodactyly since it was found in Ehlers Danlos syndrome as well (Francis et al., 1976).

Pathology

Only details of the pathology in relation to the cardiovascular system will be discussed here. Less than 10 percent of cases of Marfan's syndrome have a normal heart at autopsy (Reynolds, 1950; Goyette and Palmer, 1953). In an earlier analysis at The Hospital for Sick Children, Toronto, one heart in an infant aged only $2\frac{1}{2}$ months was normal in a total of six postmortems of the condition. The principal lesions found consist of aortic and pulmonary arterial aneurysms, aortic and pulmonary wall dissection, valvular incompetence, particularly of aortic and mitral valves, and true congenital malformations of the heart (Wagenvoort et al., 1962).

Aorta. *A fusiform aneurysm* of the ascending aorta is the most common cardiovascular lesion in Marfan's syndrome and accounts for the majority of cardiovascular problems in the adult age group (Goyette and Palmer, 1953; Murdoch et al., 1972). The dilatation usually extends from the aortic valve to the innominate artery, the portion of the aorta that normally undergoes the maximal hemodynamic stress. This particular change in its fully established form creates the typical "waterflask appearance" of the ascending aorta in the aortogram as well as on gross inspection. Aneurysm of the sinuses of Valsalva is often described. McKusick (1955) has emphasized that the process starts at the aortic ring and may cause so much sacculation of the aortic cusps and dilatation of the ring that aortic incompetence may be present in an individual who shows no true aneurysmal formation of the ascending portion of the vessel. This particular point has been well appreciated by pediatricians who see patients at an early stage (Papaiannou et al., 1961). *Dissection of the aorta* may occur with or, less commonly, without previous dilatation. It is often a terminal event and may cause death by cardiac tamponade. Although dissecting aneurysm is a threat mainly to adult patients, being responsible for 29 to 43 percent of deaths in this age group (Hirst and Gore, 1973), it has been described in children down to the age of four years (Traisman and Johnson, 1954; Coleman, 1955; Wong et al., 1964).

Involvement of other parts of the arterial system has been infrequently reported, mainly dissection of the innominate and carotid arteries (Austin and Schaefer, 1957; Traisman and Johnson, 1954) and fusiform aneurysm of the descending aorta (McKusick, 1972b).

The *microscopic picture* is one of total disruption of normal aortic architecture; elastic fibers are interrupted and scarce. Smooth muscle tissue is hyperplastic and irregular, and vasa vasorum invade the media. Cystic spaces are filled with metachromatically staining material. The picture is indistinguishable from Erdheim's cystic medial necrosis (Baer et al., 1943; Wagenvoort et al., 1962; Bolande, 1963; McKusick, 1972b). MacLeod and Williams (1956), however, preferred not to use this term for the reason that there are neither true cysts nor notable necrosis in sections of the vessels.

Pulmonary Artery. A similar aneurysmal dilatation of the pulmonary artery may occur (Bowden et al., 1965). It is more common to find only microscopic changes in this vessel, however. Baer and associates (1942) described pulmonary arterial lesions of this sort in association with aortic aneurysms in their two patients. Subsequent reports of pulmonary arterial involvement were provided by Lillian (1949), and more striking changes in the pulmonary artery contributing to death were noted by Gardner and associates (1939), Anderson and Pratt-Thomas (1953), Tung and Liebow (1952), and McKusick (1955). Again the dilatation of the vessel commences at the artery root in a manner similar to that seen in the aorta. Dissection of the aneurysm may likewise occur.

Valves.   Lesions of the *mitral valve* were described as early as 1912 by Salle, but were given little attention until it became clear, much later, that significant mitral regurgitation often ensues and is, in fact, the most frequent cardiovascular problem in children with Marfan's syndrome (Phornphutkul, 1973; Papaionnou et al., 1961; Perrin et al., 1966; Raghib et al., 1965; and Hohn and Webb, 1971). Severe heart failure and death from mitral regurgitation has been reported in patients as young as four months (Bowden et al., 1965; Shankar et al., 1967). The mitral valve in Marfan's syndrome is described as redundant, folded, and thickened, with an almost cartilaginous translucency (Tung and Liebow, 1952; Raghib et al., 1965; Grondin et al., 1969; Hohn and Webb, 1971). The chordae are thickened and elongated. The valve bulges into the left atrium. Rupture of chordae and avulsion of the posterior leaflet have been reported (Sirak and Ressallat, 1973). The *microscopic picture* is one of myxomatous degeneration: the material accumulated has the same staining characteristics as that contained in the aortic cysts (Bolande, 1963). The *tricuspid valve* and the *aortic valve* may rarely be affected by the same process (Shankar et al., 1967; McKusick, 1972b). Apart from any hemodynamic upset such lesions may cause, they may predispose to subacute bacterial endocarditis (Vivas-Salas and Sanson, 1948; Olcott, 1940; McKusick, 1955; Bowers and Lim, 1962; Wunsch et al., 1965; Soman et al., 1974; Mehl et al., 1976).

Congenital Malformations of the Heart.   Many of the original reports claiming the presence of an atrial septal defect on closer examination were shown to exhibit only a probe patency of the foramen ovale. There are several autopsy-proved cases of atrial septal defect in the literature—a case of ostium primum reported by Piper and Irvine-Jones (1926), two infants with large secundum atrial septal defects (Bolande and Tucker, 1964; Bowden et al., 1965). Relatively few ventricular septal defects have been reported in the literature (Tolbert and Birchall, 1956; Ross and Gerbode, 1960; Bolande and Tucker, 1964; McKusick, 1972), and there are two such examples in our own autopsy group. McKusick also reported two instances of tetralogy of Fallot in association with the syndrome. Patent ductus arteriosus and coarctation of the aorta are also rarely seen (Goyette and Palmer, 1953; Uyeyama et al., 1947; Bingle, 1957; Eldridge, 1964; Fischl and Ruthberg, 1951). Pulmonary artery stenosis and partial anomalous pulmonary venous drainage have also been encountered (Papaioannou et al., 1961). Some believe the chance of associated congenital heart defect to be greater than for the population at large (Headley et al., 1963).

Much confusion exists in the earlier literature regarding the association of rheumatic heart disease with Marfan's syndrome. There is very little pathologic evidence to support the combination, and, with the wider recognition of valvular lesions of nonrheumatic type in association with Marfan's syndrome, the diagnosis of rheumatic valvular disease has become less frequent.

Clinical Features

Severely affected cases of Marfan's syndrome will be recognized at birth. Many are noted at least to be thin during the first year, and it is only occasionally that a history of "thinning out" in the second or third year is given. Where relatives have been tall and thin, the physical picture in an affected infant is usually accepted without question by the parents. Sporadic cases are more likely to seek medical treatment for failure to thrive.

As the child grows older, the excessive height, wasted appearance, deformed chest, or scoliosis may make the family consult a doctor. Visual difficulties may be emphasized on entry to school. Symptoms of easy fatigue and limb pains with failure to gain weight not infrequently appear. Add to this a heart murmur and minor electrocardiographic abnormalities and it is not surprising that a diagnosis of rheumatic fever may be made. In adolescence, psychologic difficulties become prominent, especially in girls.

In childhood, some cases will present the complaint of dyspnea from congestive heart failure. One of our patients (whose angiogram is shown in Figure 60–5, page 1009) developed sudden congestive heart failure at two years and was found at open operation at five years to have a flail mitral valve due to a ruptured cord. More often this picture, as well as sudden death from aortic rupture, is delayed until adult life.

The physical appearance of the severe case is characteristic (see Figure 60–1). The wasted look is due to a combination of excessive length of bones of the extremities, poor musculature, and lack of subcutaneous fat. The inadequate musculature results in scoliosis and kyphosis. Excessive over-growth in length of the ribs results in pectus excavatum or pigeon-breast deformity. The nose, ears, and teeth are frequently misshapen. The skull is dolichocephalic, and the palate is narrow and high-arched. Ocular abnormalities, which are often progressive, occur in up to 75 percent of the cases and include dislocated lenses, tremulous irides, deformed anterior chambers or corneae, and myopia. Re-spiratory symptoms may be related to infection in abnormal lungs or to spontaneous pneumothorax (Hudson, 1965).

Symptoms from cardiovascular lesions may appear in childhood, although they are more often delayed into adulthood. In Phornphutkul and associates' (1973) series only 6 of 36 children with Marfan's syndrome developed symptoms of heart failure, although 22 (61 percent) had cardiac involvement. Symptoms are usually related to mitral and aortic regurgitation. Two children under 13 years died in our institution from congestive heart failure due to aortic insufficiency. One child died at ten years with underlying mitral regurgitation (Figure 60–3, page 1008). Chest pain or sudden death from aortic dissection is rarely seen in children. *Auscultatory signs* help define the site and severity of cardiac lesions. *Mitral regurgitation* is the most common finding in childhood. A classic pansystolic apical murmur may be heard, but often the murmur is mid- to late systolic (Papaioannou et al., 1961; Perrin et al., 1966; Phornphutkul et al., 1973). Midsystolic clicks or multiple nonejection clicks near the apex are commonly a clue to the presence of a prolapsed posterior mitral valve leaflet (Criley et al., 1966; Barlow et al., 1968; Ronan et al., 1965) for which Marfan's syndrome is but one cause. The mitral murmur varies with the position of the patient and is usually maximal with the patient upright, so that from being late systolic in the recumbent position, it may become pansystolic when the patient sits up (Barlow et al., 1968). One of our patients, a five-year-old-girl with Marfan's syndrome, had no murmur at all when lying down, but a late systolic click and murmur appeared in the sitting position (Figure 60-2). *Aortic or pulmonary regurgitation* will be suspected when an early diastolic decrescendo murmur is heard along the left sternal border. Ejection clicks may also be audible in patients who have dilatation of one or another great vessel. Severe aortic regurgitation can occur in both sexes (Glaser et al., 1973), although it appears more common in males (Phornphutkul et al., 1973).

In a study of 35 patients Brown and associates (1975) noted that aortic regurgitation was present in 23 percent, occurred only in males, and was more common in adults than children with the disorder. By contrast, in this series the mitral valve abnormalities encountered in almost half the patients did not suggest a sex or age predilection.

McKusick (1972b) describes a musical, vibratory, or buzzing systolic murmur in the aortic area as indicating dissection of the aorta. The murmur is believed to be generated on fibrous cords in the lumen of the aorta or on the "lips" of an endothelial tear.

Radiologic Examination

At x-ray the heart may be of normal appearance. The two characteristic radiologic pointers to vessel involvement in childhood are dilatation of the ascending aorta and a peculiar bulge in the usual position of the outflow tract of the right ventricle (best seen in anteroposterior and right anterior oblique views) due to sacculated descent of the pulmonary valve cusps. The latter is often mistaken for left atrial enlargement. These features may be associated with moderate to gross cardiac enlargement in the more severe cases (see Figure 60-3).

Electrocardiography

Cases with aortic or mitral incompetence develop progressive left ventricular hypertrophy. The tracings of 5 out of 55 patients with Marfan's syndrome showed S-T depression and T wave inversion in standard leads II and III and unipolar lead aVF in association with autopsy-proved deformity of the mitral valve (Bowers, 1961). These signs are not specific to Marfan's syndrome and may be seen with a variety of causes of mitral regurgitation.

Changes suggesting subendocardial ischemia are present in the electrocardiograms of some reports, e.g., that of Shankar and associates (1967).

Conduction abnormalities and arrhythmias have been described even in the absence of major associated hemodynamic disturbance. They include right and left bundle branch block, junctional rhythm, atrial flutter, atrial fibrillation, Wolff-Parkinson-White syndrome, and complete heart block (McKusick, 1972b).

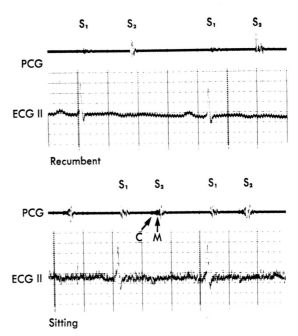

Figure 60-2. Phonocardiogram (*PCG*) of a five-year-old girl with Marfan's syndrome. Normal heart sounds (S_1, S_2) and no murmurs are recorded in the recumbent position. A late systolic click (*C*) and murmur (*M*) appear in the sitting position.

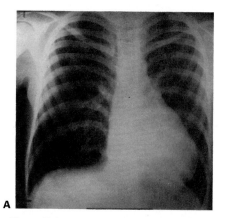 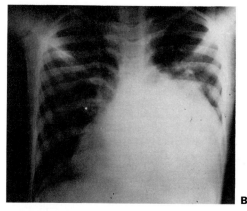

Figure 60-3. M. McG. A girl with classic physical features of Marfan's syndrome who died at ten years in atrial fibrillation and congestive heart failure secondary to gross mitral regurgitation. Chest films at eight years (*A*) and ten years (*B*) showing progressive cardiomegaly and the development of a giant left atrium.

We have seen a small number of children with Marfan's syndrome who, although free of symptoms and signs of cardiac involvement, have shown minor electrocardiographic abnormalities, particularly marked incomplete right bundle branch block and P-R and Q-T interval prolongation. Such abnormalities may be due to as yet undetermined pathologic changes or to changes in small coronary arteries, both generally (Berenson and Geer, 1963) or from a specific cystic degeneration of nodal arteries (James et al., 1964).

Echocardiography

As might be expected in a disorder where proximal areas of the great arteries become dilated and mitral valve function is frequently abnormal, echocardiography offers considerable and precise information both at initial diagnosis and for long-term follow-up.

In the studies of Brown and associates (1975) 91 percent of 35 subjects had evidence of mitral valve prolapse. Both sexes were clearly affected, the females 100 percent. Sixty percent showed an increased aortic root dimension. Although males have more frequent aortic abnormality, one-third of the females also showed these changes and the changes did not appear to be age-related. These observations indicate a very high incidence of vascular and valve involvement in the syndrome in either sex and strongly point to echocardiography as being a very important part of the full assessment of such patients. Support for this view is provided from the report of Spangler and associates (1976) who found an abnormal aortic root or mitral valve in the echocardiograms of 85 percent of 26 patients with Marfan's syndrome.

Cardiac Catheterization

Right and left heart catheterization will confirm hemodynamically significant valvular lesions and congenital malformations. More information will be obtained, however, from selective angiocardiography.

Angiocardiography

Angiocardiographic evidence of aneurysmal dilatation of the aortic sinuses was first demonstrated in three cases of Marfan's syndrome by Steinberg and Geller (1955). It has been shown that this is a very early sign and may be observed in infants without frank cardiovascular disease (Papaioannou et al., 1961). A similar change in the pulmonary artery was demonstrated in an asymptomatic male patient aged 12 years at The Hospital for Sick Children. This boy had no murmurs, but his second heart sound was greatly accentuated and closely split. At x-ray there were slight cardiac enlargement, a huge bulge below the left middle arc in the anteroposterior view, slight increase in lung vascularity, and a normal barium swallow. Cardiac catheterization revealed normal pressures and no shunts and indicated the bulge to be the root of the main pulmonary artery. This was better demonstrated by selective angiocardiography from the right ventricle (see Figure 60–4).

Mitral regurgitation, with or without aortic root alterations, can be demonstrated following left ventricular contrast injection (Figure 60–5).

Diagnosis

The classic case of a tall, thin child with long fingers and toes, chest deformity, and poor eyesight is unlikely to be missed. If dislocated lenses are present and if the accompanying parent is also tall and thin or describes a similar build in the partner or siblings, the diagnosis is certain. With a positive family history, the diagnosis of Marfan's syndrome can often be made

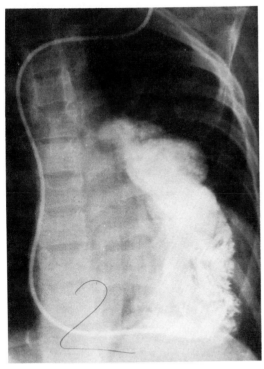

Figure 60-4. The angiocardiogram in a twelve-year-old boy, G. B., with Marfan's syndrome and pulmonary arterial lesions. Gross dilatation of the pulmonary sinuses, producing a bulge on the left cardiac border and descent of the valve within the outflow tract of the right ventricle, is evident.

with confidence in the neonate (Heldrich and Wright, 1967; McKusick, 1972b). In patients with negative family history, late paternal age can provide supportive evidence for mutation.

The most important condition requiring differentiation from the Marfan syndrome is *homocystinuria*. This metabolic disorder (Carson and Neill, 1962) results from one of several possible enzyme deficiencies inherited as autosomal recessive traits. The physical appearance in patients with homocystinuria closely resembles that of the Marfan syndrome. Affected individuals are tall and thin. Scoliosis and pectus deformities are common. Joint action is "tight" when compared with the Marfan group (McKusick, 1972b). Osteoporosis and bone fractures are common. Lens dislocation is common after the age of ten years, occurs downward, and usually is of more marked degree than in the Marfan disorder. Mental retardation is present in at least half the reported patients and psychiatric or seizure disturbances are also common. Light-colored and prematurely gray hair is usual (McKusick, 1972a) though variable (Bianchine, 1972). The cardiovascular abnormalities in the two conditions are totally dissimilar. In homocystinuria there is malar flushing after exertion or exercise and an increasing incidence of thrombosis in medium-sized arteries and in veins after adolescence. A patient aged 11 years has

died from coronary thrombosis (Carey et al., 1968), and major infarction of brain, heart, lung, or kidney eventually occurs by early adult life (Sensenbrenner, 1972). Such patients are at risk from angiographic study or from use of contraceptive pills. Valvular dysfunction and vessel rupture do not occur in homocystinuria. A positive cyanide-nitroprusside test on the urine is suggestive of homocystinuria and urine chromatography establishes the diagnosis. Tests for metabolic abnormalities have proved unrewarding in the Marfan syndrome. Patients with homocystinuria may be helped by dietary restriction or specific vitamin therapy (McKusick, 1972b).

It has become clear that incomplete forms of Marfan's syndrome, sometimes spoken of as *formes frustes*, may occur since families with unequivocal examples of the disorder may contain some members with only one manifestation. In this way a tall, slender physique, or dislocated lenses, or heart involvement may be the solitary evidence of Marfan's syndrome. Formes frustes pose a problem when the family history is negative. Attention to ocular and radiologic manifestations is often rewarding in equivocal cases but cannot resolve all such diagnostic problems (Bear and Tung, 1971; Hirst and Gore, 1973). Certain physiques may resemble the disorder. McKusick (1955) has drawn attention to the normal, lanky variant seen in the Negro and similar physique of eunuchoidism. Severe wasting from a variety of disorders may superficially resemble Marfan's syndrome. There have been a number of reports of a possible "cardiovascular forme fruste" involving the mitral valve only or, less commonly, the aortic valve (Emanuel et al., 1977). Familial cases of prolapsed

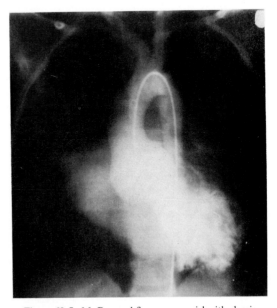

Figure 60-5. M. B., aged five years, a girl with classic physical features of Marfan's syndrome and mitral regurgitation. The anteroposterior projection after contrast injection into the left ventricle. Note the massive mitral regurgitation and aortic root dilatation.

mitral leaflet have been described (Read et al., 1965; Crocker, 1968; Shahin et al., 1969; Sherman et al., 1970; Davis et al., 1971), but none of the patients has a typical example of Marfan's syndrome in the family, and none has ocular abnormalities. Some of these cases could be a forme fruste of Marfan's syndrome, although the evidence suggests the great majority are not. Similarly, "idiopathic" pulmonary artery dilatation, aortic aneurysm, and aortic and mitral insufficiency (with no previous history or with equivocal history of rheumatic fever), as isolated findings, warrant a closer inspection for other manifestations of Marfan's syndrome, but we agree with the statement by McKusick (1972b) that "the diagnosis of Marfan's syndrome can usually not be made with complete confidence when ectopia lentis or a positive family history are not found."

In childhood the main differential diagnosis of the cardiovascular manifestations of arachnodactyly is from rheumatic or congenital heart disease. The latter may be associated, but nonrheumatic valvular lesions should always be suspected first.

Prognosis

Life expectancy is greatly reduced in Marfan's syndrome. Cumulative probability of survival has been calculated by Murdoch and associates (1972) on the basis of 257 patients (Figure 60–6). Mean age at death is 32 years for males and 29.5 years for females. Women between 24 and 45 years have a somewhat better life expectancy than males; the cumulative death curve reaches 50 percent at the age of 48 for women but at the age of 40 for men. Only about 10 percent died in the first two decades in Murdoch's report. A figure approximately similar is found by

Phornphutkul and associates (1973), who report five deaths in their series of 36 children with Marfan's syndrome (14 percent).

The cause of death is almost always cardiovascular (93 percent in Murdoch's series), the aortic lesions taking the highest toll (rupture of aortic aneurysm and aortic dissection). Mitral regurgitation may cause death from heart failure or at cardiac surgery (valve replacement) in children (Phornphutkul et al., 1973; Shankar et al., 1967; Bowden et al., 1965) and even in infants (Hohn and Webb, 1971). Subacute bacterial endocarditis, usually on the mitral valve, has also been a cause of death (Wunsch et al., 1965; Murdoch et al., 1972).

Treatment

There is no treatment for the underlying disorder. Assistance for ocular defects is necessary. There are few contraindications to correction of associated malformations such as cleft palate, sternal deformities, and scoliosis. Attempts to curb excessive growth by inducing precocious puberty have been made (McKusick, 1972b).

Cardiovascular lesions remain the major therapeutic problem. Halpern and associates (1971) are conducting a trial of medical treatment with propranolol (120 to 160 mg/day) to prevent aortic dissection. Since aortic dissection and rupture are the result of medial degeneration plus hemodynamic stress, reducing this stress may delay rupture. Propranolol reduces myocardial contractility and decreases the pulsatile force in the aorta, but a controlled long-term follow-up study will be necessary to determine whether this treatment is effective.

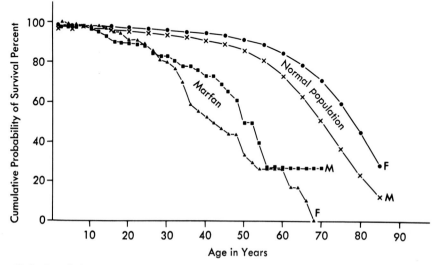

Figure 60-6. Cumulative probability of survival for patients with Marfan's syndrome, compared to the normal population. M = males; F = females. (Reproduced from Murdoch, J. L.; Walker, B. A.; Halpern, B. L.; Kuzma, J. W.; and McKusick, V. A.: Life expectancy and causes of death in the Marfan syndrome. *N. Engl. J. Med.,* **286**:804, 1972.)

Numerous reports on cardiac surgical procedures have appeared in the literature. These include excision of aortic aneurysm with bicuspidation of the aortic valve (excision of the noncoronary aortic leaflet to decrease valve surface), (Muller et al., 1960; Merendino et al., 1967; Durnin et al., 1965); graft replacement of the ascending aorta and prosthesis (Chapman et al., 1965; Symbas et al., 1970; Caves and Paneth, 1972; Ross et al., 1972); and replacement of the mitral valve (Raghib et al., 1965; Simpson et al., 1969; Shahin et al., 1969; Caves and Paneth, 1972). Plication of the redundant mitral valve has been tried but mitral regurgitation is likely to recur (Sirak and Ressallat, 1968). There has been one report of successful reimplantation of a ruptured mitral chorda (Barratt-Boyes, 1963). One of the difficulties in replacement of myxomatous valves and dilated aortas is the fact that tissues hold the stitches poorly and dehiscence of the prosthesis may occur (Read et al., 1966; Caves and Paneth, 1972). Here again, long-term follow-up is required to assess whether these procedures prolong the life of patients with Marfan's syndrome significantly.

REFERENCES

Achard, M. C.: Arachnodactylie. *Bull. Mem. Soc. Med. Hop. Paris*, **19**:834, 1902.
Anderson, M., and Pratt-Thomas, H. R.: Marfan's syndrome. *Am. Heart J.*, **46**:911, 1953.
Austin, M. G., and Schaefer, R. F.: Marfan's syndrome, with unusual blood vessel manifestations; primary medionecrosis dissection of right innominate, right carotid and left carotid arteries. *Arch. Pathol.*, **64**:205, 1957.
Bacchus, H.: A quantitative abnormality in serum mucoproteins in the Marfan syndrome. *Am. J. Med.*, **25**:744, 1958.
Baer, R. W.; Taussig, H. B.; and Oppenheimer, E. H.: Congenital aneurysmal dilatation of the aorta associated with arachnodactyly. *Bull. Hopkins Hosp.*, **72**:309, 1942.
Barlow, J. B.; Bosman, C. K.; Pocock, W. A.; and Marchand, P.: Late systolic murmurs and non-ejection ("mid-late") systolic clicks; an analysis of 90 patients. *Br. Heart J.*, **30**:203, 1968.
Barratt-Boyes, B. G.: Surgical correction of mitral incompetence resulting from bacterial endocarditis. *Br. Heart J.*, **25**:415, 1963.
Bear, E. S., and Tung, M. Y.: Marfan's syndrome. Letter to Editor. *JAMA* **218**:597, 1971.
Berenson, G. S., and Geer, J. C.: Heart disease in the Hurler and Marfan syndromes. *Arch. Intern. Med.*, **111**:58, 1963.
Bianchine, J. W.: The Marfan syndrome revisited. *J. Pediatr.*, **79**:717, 1971.
Bianchine, J. W.: Reply (letter). *J. Pediatr.*, **80**:530, 1972.
Bingle, J.: Marfan's syndrome. *Br. Med. J.*, **1**:629, 1957.
Bolande, R. P.: The nature of the connective tissue abiotrophy in the Marfan syndrome. *Lab. Invest.*, **12**:1087, 1963.
Bolande, R. P., and Tucker, Z. S.: Pulmonary emphysema and other cardiorespiratory lesions as part of the Marfan abiotrophy. *Pediatrics*, **33**:356, 1964.
Borger, F.: Ueber zwei Faelle von Arachnodaktylie. *Z. Kinderh.*, **12**:161, 1914.
Bowden, D. H.; Favara, B. E.; and Donahoe, J. L.: Marfan's syndrome. Accelerated course in childhood associated with lesions of mitral valve and pulmonary artery. *Am. Heart J.*, **69**:96, 1965.
Bowers, D.: An electrocardiographic pattern associated with mitral valve devormity in Marfan's syndrome. *Circulation*, **23**:30, 1961.
Bowers, D., and Lim, D. W.: Subacute bacterial endocarditis and Marfan's syndrome. *Can. Med. Assoc. J.*, **86**:455, 1962.
Breton, A.; Francois, P.; Lekieffre, M.; Dupuis, C.; and Lekieffre, J.: Cardiopathies et syndrome de Marfan. *Arch. Mal. Coeur*, **54**:900, 1961.
Brown, O. R.; DeMots, H.; Kloster, F. E.; Robats, A.; Menashe, V.

D.; and Beals, R. K.: Aortic root dilatation and mitral valve prolapse in Marfan's syndrome. An echocardiography study. *Circulation*, **52**:651, 1975.
Carey, M. C.; Donovan, D. E.; Fitzgerald, O.; and McAuley, F. D.: Homocystinuria, I. A clinical and pathological study of nine subjects in six families. *Am. J. Med.*, **45**:7, 1968.
Carson, N. A. J., and Neill, D. W.: Metabolic abnormalities detected in a survey of mentally backward individuals in northern Ireland. *Arch. Dis. Child.*, **37**:505, 1962.
Caves, P. K., and Paneth, M.: Replacement of the mitral valve, aortic valve, and ascending aorta with coronary transplantation in a child with the Marfan syndrome. *Thorax*, **27**:58, 1972.
Chapman, D. W.; Beazley, H. L.; Peterson, P. K.; and Cooley, D. A.: Annulo-aortic ectasia with cystic medial necrosis; diagnosis and surgical treatment. *Am. J. Cardiol.*, **16**:679, 1965.
Coleman, P. N.: A case of dissecting aneurysm in a child. *J. Clin. Pathol.*, **8**:313, 1955.
Criley, J. M.; Lewis, K. B.; Humphries, J. O'N.; and Ross, R. S.: Prolapse of the mitral valve: clinical and cine-angiocardiographic findings. *Br. Heart J.*, **28**:488, 1966.
Crocker, D. W.: Marfan's syndrome confined to the mitral valve region; two cases in siblings. *Am. Heart J.*, **76**:538, 1968.
Davis, R. H.; Schuster, B.; Knoebel, S. B.; and Fisch, G.: Myxomatous degeneration of the mitral valve. *Am. J. Cardiol.*, **28**:449, 1971.
Durnin, R. E.; Lindesmith, G.; and Meyer, B.: Aorta surgery in a child with Marfan's syndrome. *Am. J. Dis. Child.*, **110**:547, 1965.
Eldridge, R.: Coarctation in the Marfan syndrome. *Arch. Intern. Med.*, **113**:342, 1964.
Emanuel, R.; Ng, R. A. L., Marcomichelakis, J., Moores, E. C.; Jefferson, K. E., Macfaul, P. A.; and Withers, R.: Formes frustes of Marfan's syndrome presenting with severe aortic regurgitation. *Br. Heart J.*, **39**:190, 1977.
Etter, L. E., and Glover, L. P.: Arachnodactyly complicated by dislocated lens and death from rupture of dissecting aneurysm of aorta. *JAMA*, **123**:88, 1943.
Fischl, A. A., and Ruthberg, J.: Clinical implications of Marfan's syndrome. *JAMA*, **146**:704, 1951.
Francis, G.; Donnelly, P. V.; and DiFerrante, N.: Abnormally soluble collagen produced in fibroblast cultures. *Experientia*, **32**:691, 1976.
Gardner, E.; Galbraith, A. J.; and Hardwick, J. W.: A huge dissecting aneurysm. *Lancet*, **2**:1019, 1939.
Glaser, J.; Whitman, V.; and Liebman, J.: Aortic regurgitation in a young girl with severe form of Marfan syndrome. *J. Pediatr.*, **83**:685, 1973.
Goyette, E. M., and Palmer, P. W.: Cardiovascular lesions in arachnodactyly. *Circulation*, **7**:373, 1953.
Grondin, C. M.; Steinberg, C. L.; and Edwards, J. E.: Dissecting aneurysm complicating Marfan's syndrome (arachnodactyly) in a mother and son. *Am. Heart J.*, **77**:301, 1969.
Halpern, B. L.; Char, F.; Murdoch, J. L.; and Horton, V. A.: A prospectus on the prevention of aortic rupture in the Marfan syndrome with data on survivorship without treatment. *Johns Hopkins Med. J.*, **129**:123, 1971.
Headley, R. N.; Carpenter, H. M.; and Sawyer, C. G.: Unusual features of Marfan's syndrome including two postmortem studies. *Am. J. Cardiol.*, **11**:259, 1963.
Hecht, F., and Beals, R. K.: "New" syndrome of congenital contractural arachnodactyly originally described by Marfan in 1896. *Pediatrics*, **49**:574, 1972.
Heldrich, F. J., Jr., and Wright, C. E.: Marfan's syndrome; diagnosis in the neonate. *Am. J. Dis. Child.*, **114**:419, 1967.
Hirst, A. E., Jr., and Gore, I.: Marfan's syndrome: A review. *Progr. Cardiovasc. Dis.*, **16**:187, 1973.
Hohn, A. R., and Webb, H. M.: Cardiac studies of infant twins with Marfan's syndrome. *Am. J. Dis. Child.*, **122**:526, 1971.
Hudson, R. E. B.: *Cardiovascular Pathology*, Vol. 1. Edward Arnold (Publishers) Ltd., London, 1965.
James, T. N.; Frame, B.; and Schatz, I. J.: Pathology of cardiac conduction system in Marfan's syndrome. *Arch. Intern. Med.*, **114**:339, 1964.
Leeming, J. T., and McKusick, V. A.: Serum seromucoid levels in the Marfan syndrome. *Bull. Hopkins Hosp.*, **110**:38, 1962.
Lillian, M.: Multiple pulmonary artery aneurysms. *Am. J. Med.*, **7**:280, 1949.
Lutman, F. C., and Neel, J. V.: Inheritance of arachnodactyly,

ectopia lentis and other congenital anomalies (Marfan's syndrome) in the E. family. *Arch. Ophthalmol.*, **41**:276, 1949.

MacLeod, M., and Williams, A. W.: The cardiovascular lesions in Marfan's syndrome. *Arch. Pathol.*, **61**:143, 1956.

McKusick, V. A.: The cardiovascular aspects of Marfan's syndrome: a heritable disorder of connective tissue. *Circulation*, **11**:321, 1955.

——: *Heritable Disorders of Connective Tissue*, 4th ed. C. V. Mosby Co., St. Louis, 1972a.

——: More speculation on Marfan syndrome (letter). *J. Pediatr.*, **80**:530, 1972b.

Marfan, A. B.: Un cas de déformation congenitale des quatre membres, plus prononcée aux extremités, characterisée par l'allongement des os avec un certain degré d'amincissement. *Bull. Mém. Soc. Méd. Hôp. Paris*, **13**:220, 1896.

Marvel, R. J., and Genovese, P. D.: Cardiovascular disease in Marfan's syndrome. *Am. Heart J.*, **42**:814, 1951.

Mehl, S. J.; Kronton, I.; and Zimmerman, D.: Bacterial endocarditis in a patient with Marfan's syndrome. *Chest*, **70**:784, 1976.

Merendino, K. A.; Winterscheid, L. C.; and Dillard, D. H.: Cystic medial necrosis with and without Marfan's syndrome; surgical experience with 20 patients and a note about the modified bicuspidization operation. *Surg. Clin. North Am.*, **47**:1403, 1967.

Muller, W. H., Jr.; Dammann, J. F., Jr.; and Warren, W. D.: Surgical correction of cardiovascular deformities in Marfan's syndrome. *Ann. Surg.* **152**:506, 1960.

Murdoch, J. L.; Walker, B. A.; Halpern, B. L.; Kuzma, J. W.; and McKusick, V. A.; Life expectancy and causes of death in the Marfan syndrome. *N. Engl. J. Med.*, **286**:804, 1972.

Olcott, C. T.: Arachnodactyly (Marfan's syndrome) with severe anemia. *Am. J. Dis. Child.*, **60**:660, 1940.

Ormond, A. W., and Williams, R. G.: A case of arachnodactyly with special reference to ocular symptoms. *Guy Hosp. Rep.*, **74**:385, 1924.

Papaioannou, A. C.; Agustsson, M. H.; and Gasul, B. M.: Early manifestations of the cardiovascular disorders in Marfan's syndrome. *Pediatrics*, **27**:255, 1961.

Perrin, A.; Gravier, J.; Verney, R. N.; Pasternac, A.; and Froment, R.: L'insufficisance mitrale au cours du syndrome de Marfan. *Actual. Cardiol. Angeiol. Int.*, **15**:229, 1966.

Phornphutkul, C. H.; Rosenthal, A.; and Nadas, A. S.: Cardiac manifestations of Marfan syndrome in infancy and childhood. *Circulation*, **47**:587, 1973.

Piper, R. K., and Ivrine-Jones, E.: Arachnodactylia and its association with congenital heart disease; report of case and review of literature. *Am. J. Dis. Child.*, **31**:832, 1926.

Priest, R. E.; Moinuddin, J. F.; and Priest, J. H.: Collagen of Marfan syndrome is abnormally soluble. *Nature*, **245**:264, 1973.

Rados, A.: Marfan's syndrome (arachnodactyly coupled with dislocation of the lens). *Arch. Ophthalmol.*, **27**:477, 1942.

Raghib, G.; Jeu, K. L.; Anderson, R. C.; and Edwards, J. E.: Marfan's syndrome with mitral insufficiency. *Am. J. Cardiol.*, **16**:127, 1965.

Read, R. C.; Thal, A. P.; and Wendt, V. E.: Symptomatic valvular myxomatous transformation (the floppy valve syndrome): a possible forme fruste of Marfan's disease. *Circulation*, **32**:897, 1965.

Reynolds, G.: The heart in arachnodactyly, *Guy's Hosp. Rep.*, **99**:178, 1950.

Roark, J. W.: Marfan's syndrome; report of one case with autopsy, special histological study and review of the literature. *Arch. Intern. Med.*, **103**:123, 1959.

Ronan, J. A.; Perloff, J. K.; and Harvey, W. P.: Systolic clicks and the late systolic murmur. *Am. Heart J.*, **70**:319, 1965.

Ross, L. J.: Arachnodactyly. Review of recent literature and report of a case with cleft palate. *Am. J. Dis. Child.*, **78**:417, 1949.

Ross, J. K., and Gerbode, F.: The Marfan syndrome associated with an unusual interventricular septal defect. *J. Thorac. Cardiovasc. Surg.*, **39**:746, 1960.

Ross, D. N.: Frazier, T. G.; and Gonzalez-Lavin, L.: Surgery of Marfan's syndrome and related conditions of the aortic root. (annulo-aortic ecstasia). *Thorax*, **27**:52, 1972.

Salle, V.: Ueber einen Fall von angeborener abnormer Groese der Extremiteten mit eineman Akromegalia erinnenden Symptomen komplex. *Jahrb. Kinderh.* **75**:540, 1912.

Sensenbrenner, J. A.: Homocystinuria with vascular complications. In *Birth Defects: Original Article Series* **8**:No. 5, 1972, p. 286.

Shahin, W.; Eskhol, D.; and Levy, M. J.: Valve replacement for mitral insufficiency in an infant with Marfan's syndrome. *J. Pediatr. Surg.*, **4**:350, 1969.

Shankar, K. R.; Hultgren, M. K.; and Lauer, R. M.; and Diehl, A. M.: Lethal tricuspid and mitral regurgitation in Marfan's syndrome. *Am. J. Cardiol.*, **20**:122, 1967.

Sherman, E. B.; Char, F.; Duncan, W. T.; and Campbell, G. S.: Myxomatous transformation of the mitral valve producing mitral insufficiency. *Am. J. Dis. Child.*, **119**:171, 1970.

Simpson, J. W.; Nora, J. J.; and McNamara, D. G.: Marfan's syndrome and mitral valve disease—acute surgical emergencies. *Am. Heart J.*, **77**:96, 1969.

Sinclair, R. J. G.; Kitchin, A. H.; and Turner, R. W. D.: The Marfan syndrome. *Q. J. Med.*, **29**:19, 1960.

Sirak, H. D., and Ressallat, M. M.: Surgical correction of mitral insufficiency in Marfan's syndrome: Late follow-up results in two cases. *J. Thorac. Cardiovasc. Surg.*, **55**:493, 1968.

Sjoerdsma, A.; Davidson, J. D.: Udenfriend, S.; and Mitoma, C.: Increased excretion of hydroxyproline in Marfan's syndrome. *Lancet*, **2**:994, 1958.

Soman, V. R.; Breton, G.; Hershkowitz, M.; and Mark, H.: Bacterial endocarditis of mitral valve in Marfan syndrome. *Br. Heart J.*, **36**:1247, 1974.

Spangler, R. D.; Nora, J. J.; Lortscher, R. H.; Wolfe, R. R.; and Okin, J. T.: Echocardiography in Marfan's syndrome. *Chest*, **69**:72, 1976.

Steinberg, I., and Geller, W.: Aneurysmal dilatation of aortic sinuses in arachnodactyly: Diagnosis during life in three cases. *Ann. Intern. Med.*, **43**:120, 1955.

Symbas, P. N.; Baldwin, B. J.; Silverman, M. E.; and Galambos, J. T.: Marfan's syndrome with aneurysm of ascending aorta and aortic regurgitation, surgical treatment and new histochemical observations. *Am. J. Cardiol.*, **25**:483, 1970.

Tolbert, L. E., Jr., and Birchall, R. B.: Marfan's syndrome with interventricular defect found at autopsy. *Ochsner Clin. Rep.*, **2**:48, 1956.

Traisman, H. S., and Johnson, F. R.: Arachnodactyly associated with aneurysm of the aorta. *Am. J. Dis. Child.*, **87**:156, 1954.

Tung, H. L., and Liebow, A. A.: Marfan's syndrome. Observations at necropsy with special reference to medionecrosis of the great vessels. *Lab. Invest.*, **1**:382, 1952.

Uyeyama, H.; Kondo, B.; and Kamins, M.: Arachnodactylia and cardiovascular disease. Report of an autopsied case with a summary of previously autopsied cases. *Am. Heart J.*, **34**:580, 1947.

Van Buchem, F. S. P.: Cardiovascular disease in arachnodactyly. *Acta Med. Scand.*, **161**:197, 1958.

Vivas-Salas, E., and Sanson, R. E.: Sindrome de Marfan, con cardiopatia congenita y con endocarditis lenta conformada par la autopsia. *Arch. Inst. Cardiol. Mexico*, **18**:217, 1948.

Wagenvoort, C. A.; Neufeld, H. N.; and Edwards, J. E.: Cardiovascular system in Marfan's syndrome and in idiopathic dilatation of the ascending aorta. *Am. J. Cardiol.*, **9**:496, 1962.

Wong, F. L.; Friedman, S.; and Yakovac, W.: Cardiac complications of Marfan's syndrome in a child; report of a case with rapidly progressive course terminating with rupture of dissecting aneurysm. *Am. J. Dis. Child.*, **107**:404, 1964.

Wunsch, M. C.; Steinmetz, E. F.; and Fisch, C.: Marfan's syndrome and subacute bacterial endocarditis. *Am. J. Cardiol.*, **15**:102, 1965.

61

Diseases of Coronary Arteries and Aorta

John D. Keith

VARIOUS forms of involvement of the coronary arteries have been noted in infants and children. These include specific infection, hyperplastic changes, sclerosis, coronary calcification, arteritis, thrombosis, aneurysms, fistuli, congenital defects of the coronary arterial system, various syndromes, hypertension, and atherosclerosis.

The rubella syndrome may involve the coronary arteries with intimal proliferation and at times changes in the internal elastic lamina and the media. Such changes occur in rubella at the time of birth or in the few weeks following it, but may also lead to changes that have become apparent if death occurs at a later date (Fortuin et al., 1971).

Meyer and Lind (1972) noted evidence of early calcific deposits in carotid arteries of 28 children coming to autopsy, between the ages of 1 and 16 years.

Lev and coworkers (1967) believe calcification may occur in infants and children who have widespread necrosis of an artery. This is supported by Gruenwald (1949) who has demonstrated that newborn infants may have necrosis of the media in septic states and suggests that such may be the site of development of subsequent coronary calcific deposits. Menten and Fetterman (1948) report siblings, with infantile coronary sclerosis. This is also reported by Moran and Becker (1959). Pesonen (1974) noted a relationship between histologic changes in the coronary arteries in various infections in childhood. Meyer and Lind (1972) described small calcium deposits in the internal elastic lamina of iliac arteries of infants and young children. In the latter there were also gross lipid deposits. They related their findings to the hemodynamic load on the iliacs early in life.

Coronary Calcinosis

This is a rare disease in infancy characterized by deposition of calcium in the walls of a variety of vessels throughout the body. The coronary arteries are affected as part of this pathologic picture (Baggenstoss and Keith, 1941).

Approximately 50 cases have been reported in the literature (Cochrane and Bowden, 1954; Stryker, 1946). These have been chiefly in the first six months of life. A few instances have been reported in older children between two and five years of age, but a study of such case reports suggests that the arterial calcification may be of a different origin.

Pathology

The coronary vessels are usually involved, especially in the infants, and present a characteristic appearance in the gross specimen. They are raised, tortuous, calcareous vessels showing prominently on the surface of the heart as soon as the pericardium is opened. The muscle is hypertrophied, the left ventricle more than the right. The hearts of these infants weigh approximately twice the normal for the age concerned.

Myocardial infarction may occur occasionally as a complicating feature in infants with calcified coronary arteries (Traisman et al., 1956).

The earliest change is seen in the internal elastic lamina of the various-sized arteries throughout the body. Slight or moderate staining alterations are seen initially in these areas, and later calcium is deposited. The latter may assume the appearance of a ring or a segment of a circle on either side of the internal elastic lamina, extending at times into the media, although frequently this portion of the artery is spared. Intimal proliferation and thickening occur at all cases, and the lumen of some vessels is almost occluded. The disease may then be distinguished from Monckeberg's sclerosis, which characteristically involves the media rather than the intima. Since the lesions are widespread, many organs of the body are affected.

Clinical Features

Characteristically, these babies are affected in the first two to eight months of life (one case was reported of an infant ten hours old). The infants appear well in

1013

the neonatal period and later (Rich and Gregory, 1947) present a sudden onset of the signs and symptoms, which last from one to five days. Death occurs rapidly after the onset of symptoms.

Dyspnea is noted first, usually coupled with an ashen-gray color of the face that suggests shock. The respiratory rate increases. Signs of heart failure appear, with enlargement of the liver and rales in the chest. Gallop rhythm may be heard with the stethoscope, but no murmurs were reported in three cases (Cochrane and Bowden, 1954; Nestor et al., 1953). A normal axis and left ventricular hypertrophy with strain are shown in pericordial leads.

Usually these babies die before the diagnosis can be made, but the rapid onset of dyspnea, coupled with heart failure and the appearance of shock, as well as evidence of the left ventricular hypertrophy in the electrocardiogram may lead one to suspect the diagnosis during life.

In the differential diagnosis one should consider aortic stenosis and coarctation of the aorta. These can usually be differentiated by further study with angiocardiogram, catheterization, or phonocardiogram. Biochemical or adrenal insufficiency may lead to a similar cardiovascular collapse.

In endocardial fibroelastosis the electrocardiogram will frequently show more left hypertrophy than in coronary calcinosis. The course in some cases is longer and less severe. When an aberrant left coronary arising from the pulmonary artery is present, a characteristic electrocardiographic pattern is found. Glycogen-storage disease may be associated with a family history. However, at times it may be impossible to differentiate between endocardial fibroelastosis, glycogen-storage disease of the heart, and coronary calcinosis unless evidence of calcified vessels over the surface of the heart can be demonstrated radiographically.

Prognosis and Treatment

Death occurs in the first year of life and usually in the first six months.

These babies should receive oxygen and digitalis since it may not be immediately possible to exclude endocardial fibroelastosis or coarctation of the aorta, conditions that will respond to therapy.

ANOMALOUS ORIGIN OF THE LEFT CORONARY ARTERY FROM THE PULMONARY ARTERY

THE anomalous origin of the left coronary artery from the pulmonary artery in a heart without other defects was originally described by Abrikosoff in 1911, but clinical interest was not aroused until Bland, White, and Garland (1932) integrated clinical and pathologic data and recorded an electrocardiogram in an infant with this condition. Since then sporadic cases have been reported intermittently, and in the past ten years interest has been further stimulated by the possibilities of surgical correction. Many suggestions have been advanced in this regard. It is clear from a review of the literature that while this is a rare anomaly, an increasing number are being reported in the literature (approximately 200). It is present in approximately 0.24 percent of our total group of congenital heart disease and occurs once in 300,000 children.

Most instances of this defect have been found in babies who have died in the first year of life. In some instances survival is possible into adult life. Kaunitz (1947) has presented data on seven such cases. The oldest was 64 years of age and was first reported by Abbott (1927). These adults were discovered at autopsy to have an abnormally large right coronary artery, which yielded a relatively copious blood supply to the left ventricle via collaterals and thus compensated for the defective circulation of the aberrant left coronary.

Pathology. At the autopsy table the dissection of the root of the aorta and pulmonary artery will show

the right coronary artery arising in its usual position, while the left coronary originates from the base of the pulmonary artery, often somewhat posteriorly.

Examination of the heart at postmortem reveals a grossly enlarged left ventricle of aneurysmal proportions with a greatly dilated chamber. The left ventricle is hypertrophied but not markedly so, the wall at times being relatively thin. The right ventricle, by comparison, is small and compressed. Patchy fibrosis is apparent in the left ventricle but is especially prominent at the apex and over the anterior portion of the myocardium. It appears with decreasing frequency as one approaches the collateral branches of the right coronary on either side. Besides the increase in fibrous tissue there is an increase in elastic tissue and a patchy disintegration of muscle fiber. In the more advanced cases, calcareous infiltration may be apparent in the anterior portion of the left ventricle. Kaunitz (1947) reported this finding in slightly over half of his cases.

Many infants with the left coronary arising from the pulmonary artery also have evidence of endocardial fibroelastosis. The sex incidence is approximately equal, being slightly more common in females than males (Kaunitz, 1947).

A focal atelectasis may be apparent in the lung tissue adjacent to the enlarged heart, and the alveoli may show evidence of the chronic passive congestion of heart failure.

Hemodynamics

Before birth the oxygen content of the blood in the right and left ventricles is essentially the same. Furthermore, the pressures are similar. Thus the presence of a left coronary taking its origin from the pulmonary artery had no deleterious effect on the heart prior to birth.

Among the cardiovascular adjustments that take place at, or shortly after, birth is a fall in pressure in the right ventricle and pulmonary artery, as compared to that in the left side of the heart. A coronary artery arising from the pulmonary artery will thus be receiving venous blood under low pressure; or the flow may be reversed, the collaterals from the right coronary supplying the left ventricle and the left coronary merely acting as a vein. This is most likely to be the situation in the few adult cases, who have been shown at postmortem to have huge right coronary arteries with abundant collaterals. In early infancy the pulmonary artery pressure may be high enough to provide a moderate blood flow to the left ventricle. This will soon fall, however, to an insignificant trickle or reverse flow. An angiocardiogram at three to six months usually shows no flow into the left coronary from the pulmonary artery. Whatever the source, some of the coronary blood supply to the left ventricle must come during diastole, and, since in infants diastole may be shorter than systole, a further inadequacy of blood flow to the left ventricle results. Pathologic changes occur over a period of several weeks or months and lead to failure of the left ventricle. Tachycardia and the circulatory inadequacies of congestive heart failure further increase the ischemia of the left ventricle, thus producing rapid deterioration and death.

In the past the division of anomalous coronary arising from the pulmonary artery into two types, adult and infantile, has been rather sharp. This was so because those that presented with signs and symptoms in infancy appeared to succumb in the first year or two of life with no obvious survivals, except those that turned up unexpectedly in adult life without evidence of the anomaly during childhood. More recently, however, the condition has been recognized throughout the childhood years and with varying degrees of severity (Agustsson et al., 1962; Rudolph et al., 1963; Nadas et al., 1964). It is now clear that death may occur at any age up to 64 years or more, but the overwhelming majority do not survive the first year of life. Survivals appear to be related primarily to the amount of direct or indirect circulation reaching the left ventricle.

Edwards (1954) raised the question of the direction of the flow of blood through the pulmonary artery, but it has now been shown, in numerous angiocardiographic studies as well as at surgery, that the flow is frequently from the right coronary artery through collaterals to the left and thus into the pulmonary artery. The left coronary then acts as vein with the flow reversed (Sabiston, 1963; Goldberger, 1960;

Agustsson et al., 1962; Nadas, 1963; Rudolph et al., 1963; Nadas et al., 1964).

It is obvious that a period of postnatal adjustment of the circulation must occur before the flow is reversed. The earliest this has been demonstrated angiocardiographically is two months (Friedenberg et al., 1963). In an infant approximately the same age, Jameson and associates have recorded a case in which the flow was still from the pulmonary artery to the left ventricle. Armer and associates found this latter type of circulation at four months of age. On the other hand, of infants who survive four months, the majority will have the left coronary artery acting as a vein.

Clinical Features

History. Infants with this anomaly appear normal at birth and, as a rule, continue to react as normal babies for the first month. They may even appear in good health until the second, third, or fourth month of life, but most frequently symptoms begin to appear in the second or third month of life. These symptoms may be grouped under three headings: (1) discomfort, (2) heart failure, and (3) respiratory infections.

In some instances there are no signs or symptoms until the onset of congestive heart failure, but in a large portion of babies with this anomaly there is a history of irritability and discomfort for several weeks, occurring intermittently during the day. A look of anxiety or pain may be suggested on the baby's face. Episodes of pain and distress during and after feeding have been recorded in many published reports and have been considered to be anginal in origin. Paroxysms of distress with pallor, sweating, and dyspnea have also been noted, and are probably related to the same cause.

The chief symptoms, however, are intimately associated with the onset of heart failure, and include dyspnea, tachycardia, wheezing respirations, cough, and, occasionally, secondary cyanosis.

In the past the heart failure has frequently been precipitated by a respiratory infection as either nasopharyngitis, bronchitis, or pneumonia. Such evidence should not mislead the diagnostician away from the underlying cardiac origin of the pathology.

The few cases that survive until adult life have not had signs or symptoms present during infancy or childhood.

Physical Examination. On examination (1) the baby is usually fairly well developed but may at times appear slightly underweight; (2) an increased respiratory rate is the rule, and the baby appears uncomfortable and irritable; (3) a minor degree of pallor is common, intermittent cyanosis may be noted with crying if failure is present, but the appearance of the baby does not suggest that one is dealing with congenital heart disease in the cyanotic group.

Most of these babies are uncomfortable, and thus cry intermittently. Their faces show irritability and, at times, pain. The legs may be drawn up. Crying is likely to occur in paroxysms and may be associated with pallor, profuse sweating, and even shock. Such paroxysms may occur at any time but are most likely to be seen during or after feedings.

The respiratory rate, as a rule, is between 50 and 100 per minute and usually is associated with dyspnea, wheezing respirations, retraction of the costal margin, and dilatation of the alae nasi. There may be a grunt and a cough, and, on examination of the chest, fine rales may be heard. The liver is frequently more than 3 cm below the costal margin. Slight puffiness of the tissues may be evident, but definite edema is uncommon.

Evidence of a respiratory infection is commonly present, with fever, cough, nasal discharge, or rales in the chest.

There is generalized cardiac enlargement visible under the fluoroscope, but this is mainly on the left due to the greatly dilated left ventricle. In spite of the signs pointing to cardiac involvement, murmurs are usually not heard. They have been reported to occur occasionally in such cases, but they are short, unimpressive, and usually heard at the apex.

Radiologic Examination

The heart size and shape may vary. Generally there is marked enlargement with a blunt apex protruding out and down into the left axilla. The left cardiac border is usually full and convex. The right atrial shadow, whether normal or slightly enlarged, appears small in comparison with the left cardiac enlargement. The lung fields are congested. In the left anterior oblique view the left ventricle protrudes back, overlapping the vertebral column markedly.

Under the fluoroscope the cardiac borders appear quiet. The left ventricle is greatly enlarged, particularly when considered in the lateral or left anterior oblique view. Hilar shadows are congested but not pulsating. Barium swallow shows a normal left aortic arch. The left atrium may be within normal limits or show enlargement due to increased pressure from the failing left ventricle. The right ventricle is not enlarged, but its border in the left anterior oblique view may appear more active than that of the left ventricle.

Angiocardiography

Angiocardiography dramatically demonstrates the small right ventricle, compressed into a small portion of the cardiac shadow, giving rise to a normal pulmonary artery and branches. The most striking feature is the greatly enlarged left ventricle, which occupies nearly two-thirds of the cardiac outline. It has a round, symmetric shape and may be seen so clearly that one can determine the thickness of the left ventricular wall. There is not as much hypertrophy as one would expect with large chamber size.

The anomalous coronary may occasionally be demonstrated arising from the pulmonary artery, but usually the flow is from the coronary into the pulmonary vessel and under such circumstances is not visible by venous angiogram. An arteriogram from the base of the aorta shows the absence of a left coronary at that site and reveals the right coronary clearly (see Figure 61–1A). If one follows the circulation through the collaterals, it may then fill the left coronary branches and eventually make visible the main left coronary and its attachment to the pulmonary artery.

Electrocardiography

The electrocardiograms in 24 proved cases, 19 of them with precordial leads, have been analyzed. They have revealed the following characteristics:

Rate: varied from 135 to 260.
Conduction time: 0.09 to 0.14 second.
Axis: −60 to +90 degrees.
Electrical position: usually horizontal.

STANDARD LEADS

T_1 inverted (22 of 24 cases) (1 upright, 1 diphasic)
T_2 inverted (12 of 24 cases).
T_3 inverted (2 of 24 cases).

S-T SEGMENT IN STANDARD LEAD I

Slightly raised (10 of 24 cases).
Slightly depressed (7 of 24 cases).

QR PATTERN IN STANDARD LEAD I

Occurred in 21 of 24 cases.
In 2 of the remaining 3, the qR portion of the ECG was slurred (see Figure 61–1B).

QR PATTERN IN UNIPOLAR LIMB LEAD AVL

A qR pattern was present in all cases in which aVL was recorded (14 cases). The q wave was almost invariably more than 50 percent of the R wave, but in 1 case it was 20 percent.
The T wave was inverted in aVL in 12 of 14 cases: flat in 1; upright in 1.

PRECORDIAL LEADS (15 CASES)

Evidence of left ventricular hypertrophy present in all cases (usually indicated by a low ratio in R/S in V_1 [less than 1]).

T WAVES

Inverted T waves in V_5 or V_6 in 12 of 19 cases. (T_1 was inverted in only 1 case.)

S-T SEGMENT

Raised S-T segment over the left precordium in 13 of 19 cases. Usually evident in V_5.
S-T depressed slightly in 2 of 15 cases. No deviation of S-T in 2 of 15 cases.
S-T segment usually cove-shaped when elevated.

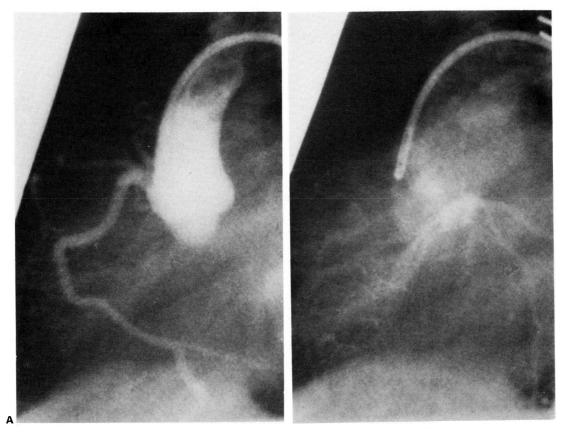

Figure 61-1A. C. L., aged 2½. Aortogram in lateral projection shows filling of the right coronary artery from the aorta (*left*). Subsequently (*right*) the left coronary artery is opacified and contrast material flows retrograde into the pulmonary artery.

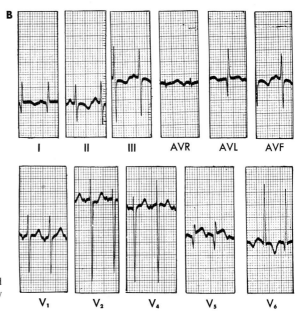

Figure 61-1B. Electrocardiogram of a three-month-old girl with anomalous origin of the left coronary artery from the pulmonary artery.

In the majority of cases the electrocardiogram reveals a pattern that is associated with anterior myocardial infarction in adults. Almost invariably there is a QR pattern and inverted T wave in standard lead I and unipolar lead aVL. This is accompanied by deep Q waves in V_5 and V_6. In 60 percent there are also inverted T waves in these leads. The majority of cases have evidence of a raised S-T segment over the left precordium followed by a T wave that is cove-shaped and symmetric in outline. A characteristic tracing is shown in Figure 61–1*B*.

Diagnosis

A diagnosis should be possible in all the cases that appear in infancy. It may be based on the following criteria.

The appearance of signs and symptoms related to the heart occurs in the first year of life. There may be irritability or even pain during or after feeding. Congestive heart failure usually appears between the second and fifth month of life. Signs suggesting pneumonia are common.

The physical examination reveals a baby who has little or no cyanosis. An x-ray of the chest will show a moderate or grossly enlarged heart, generalized fullness of the left cardiac border, and an especially large left ventricle. The most useful diagnostic tool is the electrocardiogram, which shows evidence of a pattern consistent with anterior myocardial infarction and is characterized by a QR pattern and inverted T in standard lead I and a similar pattern in aVL. This is coupled with evidence of left ventricular hypertrophy in the precordial leads, deep Q wave in V_5 or V_6, often with a cove-shaped S-T in the same lead. This pattern found in a baby with congestive heart failure in the first year of life is pathognomonic of the condition and should permit a firm diagnosis. Thallium-201 myocardial perfusion scans give direct confirmation of the infarction in this condition by showing a wedge-shaped defect in the image of the left ventricular wall (Finley et al., 1977) and may prove useful in following changes in the extent of the infarct. If doubt exists, a selective angiogram, with the tip of the catheter in the base of the aorta, will demonstrate the right coronary only and show no evidence of a left coronary arising in its usual place. It may show collaterals filling the left coronary from the right.

Differential Diagnosis. The differential diagnosis includes those congenital heart defects that are associated with left ventricular hypertrophy, such as endocardial fibroelastosis, tricuspid atresia, aortic stenosis, patent ductus arteriosus, coarctation of the aorta, ventricular septal defect, myocarditis, or coronary calcinosis. The diagnostic problem that arises most frequently is to differentiate between endocardial fibroelastosis and an aberrant left coronary arising from the pulmonary. Since both defects are most likely to be found in the first year of life, age is not of much value in differentiation. However, when the onset of symptoms occurs at the end of the first year or in the second year of life, it is much more likely that one is dealing with endocardial fibroelastosis than an aberrant left coronary. The electrocardiogram will usually permit a definitive diagnosis since the aberrant coronary gives a pattern of anterior myocardial infarction associated with left ventricular hypertrophy, whereas endocardial fibroelastosis simply presents evidence of left ventricular hypertrophy. A QR pattern in the standard lead I occurs in 80 percent of aberrant coronary cases, whereas the Q wave in standard lead I in endocardial fibroelastosis occurs only rarely, and then it is a positional effect. Elevation of the S-T segment in left precordial leads is rare in endocardial fibroelastosis but common in aberrant coronary. The T wave inversion in the left precordial leads frequently involves all of the complexes of the left precordium in endocardial fibroelastosis, whereas it is found in V_6 alone in the majority of aberrant coronary cases.

A marked Q wave followed by an inverted T wave is almost invariably present in aVL in the aberrant coronary cases, whereas this pattern is rarely found in endocardial fibroelastosis.

Tricuspid atresia rarely constitutes a problem since it is associated with more obvious cyanosis. The murmur usually differentiates aortic stenosis, although, on rare occasions in early life, aortic stenosis may show deeply inverted T waves over the left precordium associated with heart failure. However, the infarct pattern is lacking. Patent ductus arteriosus and ventricular septal defect can be readily differentiated. Blood pressures will rule out coarctation of the aorta. Myocarditis may present inverted T waves on the left precordium, but the anterior infarct pattern is lacking. Coronary calcinosis may lead to left ventricular hypertrophy, but, in spite of the coronary disease, gross myocardial infarction has not yet been reported in this group although slight apical necrosis was recorded in one of Cochrane and Bowden's cases (1954).

Prognosis

Among the cases in the pediatric age group that present signs and symptoms, the prognosis is uniformly poor. The largest number die in the first six months of life, usually between the third and fifth month. A few babies have survived into the second year. Deaths have not been reported in childhood after the second year of life.

A few cases have reached adult life, but in all instances examined at postmortem there has been a large right coronary artery with an unusually copious collateral supply to the left side of the heart. Many of these cases have not been recognized in infancy or childhood but develop symptoms in adult life and die either of heart failure or suddenly and unexpectedly. Several had a history of anginal attacks over a period of several years.

The infants who die early are apparently those with little or no communication between the right and left coronary branches. Reiner and associates (1961) found 22 percent of neonates had no visible collaterals connecting the two circulations. A similar percentage may occur in the group with anomalous coronaries. In any case, the stimulus to the opening up of such channels must come following birth after the pulmonary artery pressure falls. As Edwards (1964) suggests, it is the intermediate phase that is crucial and survival may depend on a number of factors including the coronary artery anatomy, the growth and size of the baby, the response of the infant to medical therapy, and the ability of the left ventricular muscle to carry on with minimal nourishment. (See also Coates and associates, 1966.)

Treatment

From the natural history of the anomalous left coronary arising from the pulmonary artery there are two groups of cases that require different surgical management and treatment.

Group I. Group I consists of those who have survived infancy because of sufficient collateral circulation from the right coronary to the left coronary, thus nourishing the left ventricle and permitting survival for several years. Such cases in the past have been identified in childhood or the teen-age group or occasionally in adult life for the first time. These cases may be helped by a saphenous vein bypass graft between the aorta and the anomalous coronary. This has been carried out successfully at The Hospital for Sick Children in Toronto. Successful results have also been reported by Chaitman et al. (1975), Thomas et al. (1973), and Akhtar and associates (1973). In 1975 Chiariello and associates reported their long-term results with the above procedure and indicated that the graft did not always remain patent or, if it did remain patent, it might become narrowed or stenotic.

The above technique depends on the survival of the child beyond the first year or two of life and it is dependent on an adequate left coronary flow and pressure through the collateral circulation. This occurs in relatively few cases. Furthermore, the aorticocoronary bypass graft technique requires a sufficient size of the coronary artery to permit the surgeons to ensure an adequate flow. Thus this approach is limited to children over the age of two or three although Ben Venugopal and associates (1975) reported a successful result in a 17-month-old child.

Group II. This group consists of those cases who present in infancy with an anomalous left coronary off the pulmonary and thus constitutes the majority of cases (85 percent). Every case whose diagnosis is made and confirmed in the first year of life fits into this category since one cannot be certain of survival even if one demonstrates good collaterals to the left ventricle; sudden death may occur or unexpected

heart failure. Thus, the diagnosis having been made in infancy, surgical management becomes of paramount importance. It is usually required without much delay. Medical treatment with digitalis, diuretics, and oxygen should be initiated early and may postpone the fatal outcome for a short time while surgical management is being considered. Several surgical techniques are in current use. One consists of ligation of the anomalous coronary at its origin. The surgeons have in the past replaced the left coronary artery region and noted the effect on the heart of temporary clamping. If the effect on the heart of coronary circulation was satisfactory, ligation of the coronary was proceeded with. This approach has proved successful in some cases. However, the mortality is high and usually runs to the order of 50 percent (Sabiston, 1963; Mustard 1964; Nadas et al., 1964). Several instances of sudden death or heart failure have been reported after ligation of the anomalous left coronary (Keith, 1959; Wesselhoeft, 1968).

The use of a systemic artery to anastomose to the anomalous coronary was first suggested by Mustard (1967), and some success with this technique has been reported by several groups (Meyer et al., 1968; Neches and associates, 1974; Pinsky et al., 1973; Senderoff and associates, 1975). However, the success of this technique depends on an adequate flow from the systemic artery to the coronary system, and this in turn depends on the size of the coronary artery and the resistance of subsequent branches.

Doty, Lauer, and Eberhoft (1975) have recently reported a patient with an anomalous left coronary and a congenital aorticopulmonary window in whom the window was tunneled to the anomalous coronary artery. This technique was used recently at The Hospital for Sick Children and has been reported by Lee and colleagues. An orifice of 5 mm in diameter was made in the adjacent wall of the aorta and pulmonary artery at the same level as the anomalous coronary orifice. The vessels were then anastomosed in a side-to-side fashion from within the pulmonary artery, producing an aorticopulmonary window. A strip of pericardium was used to form a tunnel leading from the aorta across the posterior wall of the pulmonary artery into the anomalous left coronary orifice. The aortic blood was thereby pumped into the left coronary portion of the circulation. The aortocoronary tunnel remained patent, but the patient developed an arrhythmia a day or two following surgery and did not survive.

This latter technique appears to have several advantages in that it is technically easier to perform than a bypass graft. The size of the coronary artery is not a limiting factor. There is no need to mobilize the left coronary artery, which may damage some of the proximal branches. In an AP window of sufficient size full coronary flow is permitted, and since the pulmonary artery forms part of the tunnel, it may grow along with the child. In any event the tunnel can be made large enough to accommodate the flow for a normal adult.

ORIGIN OF BOTH CORONARY ARTERIES FROM THE PULMONARY ARTERY

THE presence of both coronary arteries having their origin from the pulmonary artery is a very rare anomaly, having been reported only five times in the literature (Tedeschi and Helpern, 1954). The age at death was within the first two weeks of life in four of the five cases, and in the other case the child survived to five months. Survival in the latter case was due to the fact that there was an associated truncus arteriosus delivering blood at systemic pressure to both coronaries.

Three of the five cases were associated with serious congenital heart disease, such as truncus arteriosus, atresia of the tricuspid valve, and tetralogy of Fallot. In the other two cases there was simply an associated patent ductus arteriosus.

In the two cases with no serious associated anomalies, the short life was apparently due to a relatively low pressure in the pulmonary artery and, therefore, a diminished blood flow to both ventricles. Both these cases had cyanosis on crying and cardiac enlargement. One died on the tenth day and the other on the thirteenth day of life. An electrocardiogram was available in one case and showed right-axis deviation with right ventricular hypertrophy. There was nothing in this clinical picture of any diagnostic value; therefore, it is unlikely that any of these cases will be recognized before death.

It should perhaps be pointed out that, unless a careful search is made for the origin of the coronary arteries in all cases of congenital heart disease, many instances of coronary artery anomalies will remain identified.

ORIGIN OF THE RIGHT CORONARY ARTERY FROM THE PULMONARY ARTERY

AN aberrant right coronary artery arising from the pulmonary artery is an exceedingly rare anomaly: three cases have been reported in the literature (Cronk et al., 1951). One, reported by Monckeberg in 1914, occurred in a 30-year-old man who died of an epileptic fit and cerebral hemorrhage. The second, reported by Schley in 1925, occurred in a 60-year-old man with syphilis. The third case, reported by Cronk and associates, occurred in a Negro who died at 90 years of age of hypertension and arteriosclerosis and was found to have the right coronary arising from the pulmonary. After its abnormal origin from the pulmonary artery, the right coronary was distributed in a normal fashion over the right ventricle. The wall of the artery was thin, resembling that of a vein, and showed no evidence of atherosclerosis. On the other hand, the left coronary artery was dilated and tortuous, showing signs of atherosclerosis throughout its entire length. Operative repair has been successfully performed (Tingelstad et al., 1972).

The prognosis appears to be excellent. There is no evidence in any of these three cases that the presence of this aberrant coronary interfered with normal life. No electrocardiograms were recorded.

There is nothing to suggest that this anomaly can be, or need be, recognized during life.

POLYARTERITIS NODOSA IN INFANCY

THIS subject was well reviewed by Munro-Faure as a necrotizing arteritis of the coronary arteries in infancy and published in 1959 (see also Roberts and Fetterman, 1963). The clinical manifestations are usually indicated by a prolonged intermittent fever, often accompanied by an erythematous rash, which comes and goes. There may be conjunctivitis and/or a cough. Half the cases have congestive heart failure. Heart murmurs are usually absent, although they have been described in two or three cases. Myocardial infarction of some degree may be present ultimately in many cases and, therefore, electrocardiogram changes may indicate such pathology by the time the child is admitted to hospital. Thus, the electrocardiogram may show left hypertrophy, evidence of myocardial damage, and occasionally right ventricular hypertrophy with strain. Urinary findings may show leukocytes and an occasional erythrocyte.

The pathologic features include cardiomegaly, myocardial infarction, pericardial infusion, or occasionally pericarditis or hemopericardium. In two-thirds of the cases, there is aneurysmal dilatation of the coronary artery. The adventitia is frequently infiltrated with polymorphonuclear leukocytes and lymphocytes, the muscle fibers may show evidence of degeneration, edema may be present, the elastic lamina may be undergoing degeneration, and there may be marked endarterial fibroelastic proliferation. Such lesions commonly present in the coronaries, but may extend through other vessels throughout the body, and focal calcification may develop in some arteries.

In summary, one finds severe arteritis involving the coronaries, intercostals, common iliacs, left lumbar arteries, and smaller arteries of the spleen, kidney, heart, bladder, and adrenal. This diagnosis should be suspected in the presence of prolonged intermittent fever with muscular exanthem, conjunctivitis, cardiomegaly, heart failure, electrocardiographic changes, and abdominal urinary sediment.

Older children may develop the clinical picture of periarteritis nodosa as found in adults with resulting coronary arteritis and at times occlusion and infarction. This complication is less commonly associated with rheumatoid arthritis. Its occurrence with occlusive coronary arteritis in systemic lupus erythematosus is unusual. Keat and Shore in 1958 reported a case of a 14-year-old girl who had systemic lupus erythematosus and occlusion of the popliteal artery. Bonfiglio and coworkers (1972) report four women who had lupus erythematosus and coronary artery disease. One, aged 16, had severe coronary arteritis and thrombosis and acute myocardial infarction.

MUCOCUTANEOUS LYMPH NODE SYNDROME (MLNS)

ACUTE febrile mucocutaneous lymph node syndrome (MLNS) in infancy may produce autopsy findings that are similar to infantile polyarteritis nodosa. MLNS was reported by Kawasaki in 1967 in the Japanese literature. Since then more than 6000 cases have been collected by the research committee from all over Japan and this has resulted in a well-defined syndrome. It is characterized by fever, usually persisting for five to seven days or longer and not responding to antibiotics, hyperemia of the conjunctiva, edema of hands and feet, and an erythematous appearance of the palms and soles, which may eventually lead to membraneous desquamation; the mouth and lips are dry and red, sometimes associated with fissures, and the pharyngeal mucosa is reddened. There is usually a rash over the trunk. The cervical lymph nodes are enlarged and hard and occasionally there is diarrhea, arthralgia, and mild jaundice.

The above clinical picture may be associated with leukocytosis, raised sedimentation rate, a positive CRP, and proteinuria.

The majority of cases have run their course and survived and been returned to what appears to be normal health. However, a few have died and these have usually shown coronary thromboarteritis involving one or more branches of the coronary arterial system. There may be focal aneurysmal dilatation of part of the coronary artery with destruction of the media, mural thrombi, dilatation and hypertrophy of the left ventricle, and at times fibroelastosis of the endocardium. Such cases will show electrocardiographic patterns characteristic of myocardial infarction.

While MLNS at autopsy is somewhat similar to infantile polyarteritis as is seen in North America, a large number of cases in Japan suggest almost epidemic proportions, whereas infantile polyarteritis occurs only occasionally in other parts of the world. Polyarteritis nodosa has been considered to be a serious and usually fatal condition whereas MLNS is usually accompanied by a good prognosis and only an occasional case dies with the pathologic picture described above. Examples are now appearing in the North American literature (Russell et al., 1975; Radford et al., 1976).

CORONARY ARTERIOVENOUS FISTULA

Anatomy

The communication between the arterial and venous systems in coronary arteriovenous fistula may consist of a single dilated coronary artery or numerous tortuous loops of artery on the surface or embedded in the myocardium. The entrance of the coronary artery is enlarged and thin and dilated. Either the right or the left coronary may be involved or both, the right more commonly than the left. Thus the communication is noted more frequently with the right heart chambers.

Coronary arteriovenous fistula is a rare anomaly. Upstraw summarized the literature up to 1962 with reports on 73 cases.

Physical Examination

These lesions do not usually lead to major symptoms and usually present with a continuous murmur over the precordium similar to the patent ductus arteriosus but more often over the myocardium rather than in the pulmonary area. In our experience, failure is not a common occurrence, although it has been noted by Nora and MacNamara (1968).

Gasul (1960) points out that if the point of entry is into either right or left atrium, the systolic component is the dominant one with midsystolic accentuation. If the fistula communicates with the left ventricle, the diastolic murmur is loud, and with right ventricular entry the two phases of the murmur are approximately equal in intensity.

Radiologic Examination

X-ray usually shows little or no enlargement of the heart, although occasionally right or left ventricular enlargement or atrial enlargement has been noted. The electrocardiogram may show either right or left ventricular involvement, depending on the site of the AV fistula and its anatomic direction.

Cardiac Catheterization

Catheterization characteristically shows evidence of a step-up in either of the atria or ventricles depending on the site of entry. Angiography is usually the best way of demonstrating the lesion and its anatomic details, preferably by combining anteroposterior and lateral views.

Treatment

The majority of these cases can be operated on without difficulty. Cooley (1962) records a 7 percent mortality. Our course has usually been to follow these cases for a period of time. If there is no enlargement, the electrocardiogram is normal, and the patient has a normal exercise tolerance, we frequently recommend a delay in surgical correction. However, if there is any evidence of progression of the lesion or enlargement of the heart, etc., an exploratory operation can be performed and the vessel ligated. As a rule this is readily feasible.

ARTERIOVENOUS ANEURYSM OF THE BRAIN

FORD in 1968 described arteriovenous aneurysm of the brain as circoid aneurysm, which he indicates is a twisted mass of dilated vessels in which the arteries and veins are in direct communication. This cerebral type may give rise to epilepsy, hemorrhage, or migraine.

Physical sounds may include a systolic murmur in the region of the eyeball on the affected side or sometimes over the throat. The region can be confirmed by angiocardiography. Such findings are rarely seen in childhood and are much more likely to occur in adult life as the patient grows older.

In the pediatric age group, signs and symptoms are more likely to occur in the neonate, although in later infancy progressive hydrocephalus or convulsions or both may occur.

We should be on the lookout for an unusual type of congestive heart failure occurring in the first few weeks of life characterized by dyspnea, cyanosis, and signs of elevated blood pressure, and enlargement of the liver. Examination of the heart and circulation should not reveal any obvious cause of such signs or symptoms, although bruits may occur over the head and neck. If an arteriovenous fistula is suspected, an angiogram should be done to clarify the diagnosis in a newborn, or cardiac catheterization can be advanced across the foramen ovale into the left heart and the contrast material delivered to the left ventricle, which will outline the aorta and the cerebral fistula's communications. Retrograde brachial arteriography may also be used (Keith and Forsyth, 1950).

PRIMARY ARTERITIS

PRIMARY arteritis is a term suggested to relate to Takayasu's disease, or the aortic arch syndrome, which affects segments of the aorta and its major branches. It is commonly found among young females.

In 1908, Takayasu reported that at a meeting of Japanese ophthalmologists, a patient with diminished pulses and changes in eye-grounds was discovered. Since then sporadic cases have been reported. In 1926, Harbitz and Raeder presented a similar case. In 1944, Martorell and Fabre published the first complete description of the clinical picture of obliteration of portions of the aortic arch. In 1965, Ueda and associates reviewed 321 cases. It is now recognized that the majority of instances have occurred in Japan (approximately two-thirds); a few cases have been reported in Sweden, the U.S.A., Great Britain, Norway, Hungary, and other countries.

The disease is characterized by a diffuse chronic arteritis involving the aorta, proximal segments of its largest branches, the descending aorta, and the renal arteries, each in varying degrees. There is an inflammatory process affecting all layers of the artery, and it is characterized by a marked thickening of the intima. The latter appears a pearly-gray white on its inner surface, and the intimal lesions are found to consist of a mucopolysaccharide and do not resemble atheroma. The media may show evidence of necrosis and granuloma formation and elastic tissue degeneration. The adventitia is thickened and may show lymphocytic infiltration.

The carotid arteries may be involved, producing cerebral symptoms. The subclavian artery involvement may produce changes in the upper extremities. A narrowed thoracic aorta may give rise to hypertension in the upper extremities and diminished pressure in the lower extremities. Involvement of the abdominal aorta also produces hypertension above the constricted area. According to Ueda (1965), in 321 cases in Japan the order of frequency was the left subclavian and carotid artery, next the right subclavian, followed by the abdominal and thoracic aorta.

The chief symptoms in children involve hypertension, dyspnea, cardiomegaly, diminution or absence of pulses, murmurs over the abdomen, electrocardiographic changes in the left ventricular hypertrophy or left-axis deviation, edema, palpitations, and headache. The disease may begin as early as four or five years of age, but the majority develop signs and symptoms in their early 20s. Survival may occur for many years and ranges from 1 to 20 years from the time of onset.

The diagnosis is most readily made by a careful physical examination of the various arteries, including aortography, which will reveal more accurately the location and degree of involvement.

The electrocardiogram and x-ray of the heart are also helpful.

The prognosis depends on the degree and the extent of involvement of any particular artery, and death may result from acute cerebrovascular insufficiency, cerebrovascular accident, cardiac failure, or pulmonary edema.

No medical therapy has been able to alter the ultimate course of the disease, although digitalis and diuretics can be helpful if heart failure is present. Steroids and anticoagulants have been tried with questionable success, and the steroids are probably contraindicated in the presence of hypertension.

When surgical procedures have been carried out to relieve segmental obstructions, modern cardiovascular surgical techniques can be quite successful in a temporary way, if the obstruction in the aorta or great vessels is eliminated. However, these corrections are of limited value and the disease ultimately runs its full course. The etiology is still unidentified and it is still not understood why there should be a majority of cases appearing in Japan and Korea, rather than other countries. The current hypothesis is that this syndrome is part of the autoimmune group of diseases. Ito (1966) and Ikeda (1966) demonstrated the presence of antibodies against the aorta, and Asherson and associates (1968) found a raised level of IgG, IgM, and IgA in patients with arteritis.

DISSECTING ANEURYSM OF THE AORTA

THIS is rare in children. In a review of 580 cases, Schnitker and Boyer (1944) pointed out its presence as a relatively common complication of Marfan's disease. It may also occur at times in coarctation of the aorta or independently of either of these underlying defects. An aortic aneurysm due to arteriosclerosis is a rare finding in the pediatric age group, but has been reported by MacKay (1964) in a 15-year-old boy.

MYOCARDIAL INFARCTION

MYOCARDIAL infarction is occasionally noted in infants and children and has been reported by Seganti (1968) and Bor (1969) and Talner (1973). Each of these authors collected data from various European countries. Seganti, for example, was able to collect 44 cases, proved by postmortem examination, and he presented data on an additional four cases suspected of having myocardial infarction from clinical and electrocardiographic evidence. Bor records 29 cases of myocardial infarction in infants and children, from a few days of age to 13 years. He lists underlying causes such as embolism, inflammatory disease, lupus erythematosus, syphilis, polyarteritis nodosa, interstitial myocarditis and degeneration disease, hypertension, and a variety of miscellaneous causes such as thrombocytosis, trauma, aneurysm, fibroelastosis, tumors, and congenital anomalies, such as abnormalities of the coronary arteries. He also reports a case of congenital aortic stenosis with heart failure, which, at autopsy, had evidence of posterior myocardial infarction. Becu (1974) reports the finding of some evidence of myocardial infarction in 4 percent of autopsies in the pediatric age groups. He has not noted any evidence of healed myocardial infarction in older children who might have survived such pathology in early life.

One cannot escape the conclusion that while areas of infarction are found in the heart from time to time at autopsy in infants and in the first year or two of life, it appears to be an uncommon cause of death or of subsequent pathology if they survive.

Myocardial infarction from atherosclerosis may also occur in childhood, in diabetes, progeria, and homozygous type II hyperlipoproteinemia. Thus it is apparent that the etiologic factors of myocardial infarction commonly found among adults are also operating occasionally among children.

While congenital anomalies of the coronary circulation have been associated with the development of myocardial infarction in infancy (anomalous origin of the left coronary artery from the pulmonary artery), occlusive disease of the coronary circulation producing characteristic electrocardiographic and serum enzyme changes consistent with acute myocardial infarction has been rarely encountered in the newborn period. Talner (1973) reported two such newborn infants who presented with clinical signs of low systemic perfusion, i.e., diminished arterial pulsations, metabolic acidemia, and pulmonary venous congestion, following difficult deliveries. In each infant, the scalar electrocardiogram showed pathologic Q waves in leads I, AVL, and precordial leads V_5 and V_6 compatible with anterolateral myocardial infarction. Serum lactic dehydrogenase was over 1500 units in each infant along with significant elevation of transaminase and creatinine phosphokinase levels. Cardiac catheterization was performed in one infant and demonstrated a left-to-right shunt at the atrial level and right-to-left ductal shunting. There was striking elevation of the left-sided filling pressures (LA mean = 15 mm of mercury) and diminished ventricular contractility. The infant expired and postmortem findings consisted of massive hemorrhagic necrosis of the left ventricle with a thrombus occluding the left anterior descending coronary artery. The second infant improved on cardiac glycoside and diuretic therapy, and serum enzyme levels returned to normal values. The electrocardiogram showed persistent T wave abnormalities.

While apparently rare, occlusion of a major coronary vessel can take place during delivery or at birth, usually leading to a fatal outcome. However, survival can occur as indicated by the second patient.

Talner (1973) points out, "It would appear that acute myocardial infarction in the newborn infant constitutes a distinct entity producing characteristic electrocardiographic and serum enzyme changes permitting antemortem clinical diagnosis. The

association of asphyxial problems encountered during delivery and the development of myocardial infarction in these cases confirm the experience reported by others. This condition must be included in the differential diagnosis of low cardiac output states encountered in the newborn period."

ATHEROSCLEROSIS IN CHILDHOOD

MITCHELL and Schwartz (1965) attribute the term *arteriosclerosis* to Lobstein (1829) and point out that from the outset it has been a generic term not a specific word. It is simply intended to describe any disease of the arteries in which there are thickening of the wall and induration. In childhood, there may be a variety of factors operating that make it difficult to choose a title word that covers the various facets in this age group. Atherosclerosis suggests a closer relationship to atheroma.

A variety of forms of involvement of the coronary arteries may occur in the pediatric age group, some leading to early death, others to the slowly progressive changes in the arterial wall that ultimately result in adult atherosclerosis and the complications that occur in the latter half of human life.

Atherosclerosis in the aorta and coronary, cerebral, and other peripheral arteries is now entrenched as a major cause of morbidity and mortality in most countries around the world, particularly the more affluent ones. Although death usually occurs in middle age or in the elderly, recently concern has been directed to the vessels in childhood or early adult life. An increasing number of studies in this age group are being reported (Enos et al., 1953; Rigal et al., 1960; Mason, 1963; McNamara et al., 1971). These authors found early atherosclerosis in approximately half the young men examined whose average age was in the midtwenties.

Atherosclerosis of Coronary Arteries and Aorta

It has now become obvious that vascular changes take place over many years, leading to significant pathology and coronary events after the age of 40. It is not yet clear when the original pathologic alterations begin to evolve, but histologic investigations of arteries from infants and children and adolescents accidentally dying in the first two decades of life suggest that a significant number are developing early atherosclerotic lesions that make this a pediatric problem initially.

Many investigators have studied the histologic and structural changes in the coronary arteries in infants and children. Fangman (1947), Minkowski (1947), Moon (1957), Neufeld and colleagues (1962), and Oppenheimer (1967) have all added to our knowledge

in this field. Moon (1957) found changes that he considered to be early atherosclerotic lesions present from time to time in infants and also noted some degree of intimal fibrosis in infants only a few months old. He associated the degeneration and regeneration and depositions of mucopolysaccharides and of intimal fibrosis as characteristic of the early nonlipid phase of atherosclerosis that is seen in adults. Vladover and Neufeld (1967) pointed out that the smooth muscle cells of the coronary arteries in infancy are of a primitive structure and it is possible that they retain their embryologic properties for some time after birth. This explains their capacity to change and adapt to hemodynamic conditions in the growing infant and child. The same authors (1968) studied the coronary arteries in infants of different tribal origins in the Middle East, between birth and ten years of age. The three groups were Ashkenazim, Yemenites, and Bedouins. The prevalence of coronary atherosclerosis in young Yemenite Jews and among Bedouins is low, both as an absolute rate and in comparison with other ethnic groups in Israel. It is higher in the Ashkenazim. The authors found that soon after birth the intima in the Ashkenazy males became thicker than that of the other groups studied. The difference increased from birth to ten years. (See Figure 61–1C.) In a parallel study they investigated those that had coarctation in the same tribal goups and noted that changes were present in both the media and intima. However, these changes, which first appeared in the media and later in the intima, were thought to be accelerated by the higher pressure in the systemic arteries in coarctation of the aorta.

There is some difference in opinion regarding the significance of fatty streaks that may appear in the endothelium of the aorta of infants in the first year of life. They occur in populations of all countries studied and at all ages. While they may develop into atherosclerotic plaques, they may at times remain unchanged or regress. When such streaks are associated with disintegrating cells of lipid debris, they appear more likely to develop into atherosclerotic plaques.

The progression of events in atherosclerosis is easier to identify in later life than in the pediatric age group. However, many pathologists associate the first decade of life with some degree of musculoelastic intimal thickening and minimal fatty streaking. The second decade of life is associated with more diffuse fatty streaking of the aorta and coronaries; the third

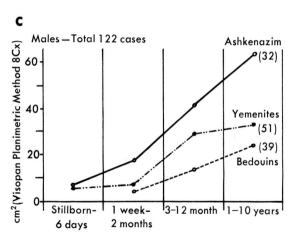

Figure 61-1C. Mean values of measurement of intima and musculoelastic layer in coronary arteries of males in three ethnic groups. (Reproduced from Vlodaver, Z.; Kahn, H. A.; and Neufeld, H. N.: The coronary arteries in early life in three different ethnic groups. *Circulation,* **39**:541, 1969. By permission of the American Heart Association, Inc.)

decade of life is characterized by a gradual increase in the incidence of fibrous plaques; the fourth decade of life is associated with the evolution of more complicated lesions such as early necrosis, ulceration, minimal hemorrhage, or thrombosis, with or without calcification. In the fifth decade of life one begins to see more commonly clinical manifestations of these underlying pathologic processes.

All children have some evidence of aortic fatty streaking by five years of age, but such streaking occurs later in the coronary arteries and is usually not present in the majority of cases until age 20. Raised atherosclerotic plaques may begin to appear in both the aorta and coronary arteries before 20, but they are more characteristic of the 20s and 30s. Some investigators question the relationship of coronary artery fatty streaks to raised lesions and the clinical disease, but the association appears closer and more significant in the coronaries than in the aorta. A number believe that fatty streaking in the aorta may at times be reversible in the human, particularly in the first two or three decades of life. This is based chiefly on animal investigations, and such studies on primates may well be applicable to the human. Strong and McGill (1969) conclude that populations with extensive coronary artery fatty streaks in childhood tend to have more extensive raised atherosclerotic lesions in middle age. This parallel relationship did not hold as consistently for aortic fatty streaks. From such studies they concluded that the data were consistent with the hypothesis that advanced atherosclerotic lesions develop by progression and transformation appears to vary from one artery to another and among racial groups. Holman (1961) discussed the problem under the heading, "Atherosclerosis, a Pediatric Nutrition Problem."

It may be important to prevent excessive fatty streaking or prevent the progression of fatty streaks to more advanced lesions if one is attempting to control atherosclerosis in later life. A key to the problem may well reside in the pediatric years, and there is now increasing evidence from both human and experimental animals that a program to control dietary habits, blood lipid levels, hypertension, atherosclerosis, and

coronary progression of events in the arteries should be directed toward the first two or three decades of life.

As indicated above, several studies have demonstrated that at birth the aorta is clear of fatty streaks. During the first few years of life all infants gradually deposit a little lipid in some portion of the aorta until by age five it is present in all aortas even though it may be only to a minor degree. Schwartz and associates (1968) have investigated this in detail and reported that between the ages of one and ten an average of 5 percent of the aorta is involved with lipid streaks; between 10 and 20 it increases to 10 percent.

Table 61-1. PERCENTAGE OF AORTA WITH LIPID STREAKS*

AGE	CASES	% OF AORTA INVOLVED
Stillbirth	9	0
1 mo	11	0
1–12 wk	16	5
1–5 yr	13	5
6–10 yr	10	5
11–15 yr	7	10
16–20 yr	12	10

* Data of Schwartz et al., 1967.

A striking feature of the above study was the early and characteristic localization of lipid deposits in the aortic valve ring, in the region of the ductus scar, and just below the orifices of the intercostal arteries.

The above findings fit in with those of the international study reported by McGill (1968), which covered the age groups from 10 to 39 as shown in Figure 61-2. The latter study demonstrated that the lipid-streaking process proceeds at a slower pace in the coronary arteries than in the aorta, and it is also of interest that the development of raised plaques parallels the fatty streaking much more closely in the coronaries than in the aorta (see Figure 61-3).

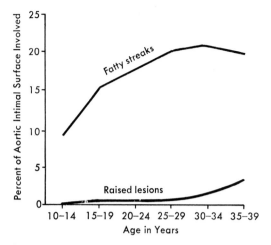

Figure 61-2. Fatty streaks in the aorta. (Reproduced from McGill, H. C., Jr.: Fatty streaks in the coronary arteries and aorta. *Lab. Invest.*, **18**:100, 1968.)

Asymptomatic atherosclerosis has been identified at autopsy in persons in their twenties, dying of accidental or war deaths (Enos, 1953; Rigal, 1960; Mason, 1963; MacNamara, 1971). Each had a somewhat different answer.

Enos, examining battle casualties in the Korean War in 1953, found that 77 percent had some degree of atherosclerosis. On the other hand, in the Vietnam War in 1971, MacNamara demonstrated some degree of atherosclerosis in only 45 percent, again healthy American males. He points out this is a reduction from the figure obtained by Enos (1953) and he suggests that the two series were similar in many respects and, therefore, the reduction might be significant.

Yater and associates (1948) recorded that the amount of atherosclerosis of the aorta was slight or

moderate in comparison with the degree of sclerosis in the coronary arteries. Rigal and associates (1960) are in agreement with Yater and conclude that in younger persons the process in the coronary arteries may proceed independently and is not necessarily part of generalized atherosclerosis.

Strong and McGill (1968) concluded from their studies on the coronary arteries in accidental death that it is impossible to divide American males into those having and not having coronary atherosclerosis, since after the age of 20 years the only distinction lies in the severity of the disease process, rather than its presence.

Oppenheimer and Esterle (1967) evaluated the coronary arteries in 140 hypertensive infants and children; 53 of the children had hypertension of renal origin, and of these 36 had an elevated serum cholesterol. Coronary atherosclerosis was much more common in those who had hypertension than in those in whom the blood pressure was normal, even though the latter did have elevated serum lipids. Their conclusion was that the elevated serum lipids appear to be less significant than the hypertension in the pathogenesis of vascular lesions in childhood.

French and Dock (1944) reviewed the findings of 80 cases of fatal coronary atherosclerosis among soldiers. Nine of them occurred between the ages of 23 and 25, five between the ages of 20 and 22. Sprague and Orgain (1935) recorded the case of a boy 15 years of age who had substernal distress on exertion for three years before his death and who, at autopsy, was found to have had atheroma with thrombus of the left circumflex artery. Benda (1925) reported sudden death in a 13-year-old girl who had atherosclerosis of the aorta and coronary arteries with coronary occlusion, myocardial infarction, and rupture of the left ventricle. Jokl and Greenstein (1944) presented the details of a ten-year-old boy who died three minutes after participating in a boxing match. At postmortem, atheromatous changes were found in the coronary arteries and thrombosis had apparently occurred in the left descending branch.

Somer and Schwartz (1970) demonstrated the focal nature of aortic uptake of 3H cholesterol in vivo in young pigs and also showed that there is a similar focal accumulation of Evans blue. Because of the consistent location and focal nature of the patterns of dye uptake, it was suggested that they might be determined by regional patterns of aortic blood flow. Supporting this latter possibility is the work of Somer and associates (1972) who studied the influence of aortic coarctation on the pattern of Evans blue uptake in the pig in vivo. This type of anomaly resulted in an increased area of dye uptake proximal to the coarctation and a decreased uptake distal to the coarctation, and some small areas related to jet lesions. The potential importance of hemodynamic factors in endothelial permeability is also emphasized by Fry (1969) who has shown that the flux of Evans blue into the arterial intima is greater with increased pressure of wall strain, increased by stress, and increased by turbulence.

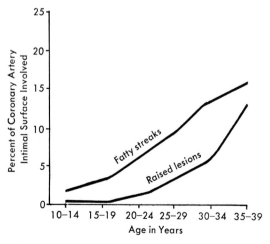

Figure 61-3. Fatty streaks in coronary arteries. (Reproduced from McGill, H. C., Jr.: Fatty streaks in the coronary arteries and aorta. *Lab. Invest.*, **18**:100, 1968.)

The factors of stress and turbulence may be related to the pathophysiology of the bicuspid aortic valve. The bicuspid aortic valve has long been recognized as an apparently minor abnormality that may ultimately be associated with a gradual thickening of the cuspid distortion and deposition of calcium. These changes may lead to a modest systolic murmur and later full-blown aortic stenosis or at times the alternative pathway of aortic regurgitation. This process may begin insidiously in the first two decades of life without significantly altering valve function. However, in the 30s, 40s, and 50s calcific deposits begin to appear, producing an increasing rigidity and malfunction of the cuspids.

Lipid stains on the bicuspid valve and base of the aorta in the second decade of life suggest that the evident lipid streaking in such cases is related to the altered hemodynamics. This may be brought about by the fact that initially a bicuspid aortic valve may not open as fully as a tricuspid one, or because one cuspid is frequently larger than the others, thus further distorting the blood flow. Whatever the basis of the resulting malfunction, it frequently leads to a series of histologic and pathologic changes that might then be included under the term *arteriosclerosis*. It seems likely that part of this is accompanied by some degree of slowly progressive atherosclerosis or arteriosclerosis involving both the valve and the base of the aorta. Whatever the origin, a superimposed pathology is present in the overwhelming majority of bicuspid aortic valves examined in the latter half of life. The full significance of the congenital bicuspid aortic valve is seen when it is recognized that it occurs in 1 percent of the normal population (Osler, 1890; Silver 1973; Izukawa and Keith, 1973). Furthermore, it occurs in approximately 7 percent of children with congenital heart defects, particularly coarctation of the aorta (37 percent), ventricular septal defect (19 percent), and endocardial fibroelastosis (20 percent).

Jaffe at The Hospital for Sick Children in Toronto (1971), in an attempt to elucidate the natural history of coronary atherosclerosis, studied 750 pairs of coronary arteries in infants and children who had medicolegal or hospital autopsies. The arteries were dissected free and embedded in gelatin to permit the study of lipids and sectioned at close intervals, mostly longitudinally, which gives one a broader view of the histology of the coronary vessels.

Bloch and associates (1976) carried out coronary arteriography in patients with type II and type IV hyperlipoproteinemia, most of whom had angina. Type II was characterized by distal disease of the coronary circulation (92 percent) and involvement of the left main coronary artery (42 percent). In type IV the lesions were characteristically localized to the proximal part of the coronary arteries (65 percent) with infrequent occurrences of stenosis of the left main coronary artery (15 percent).

James, Glueck, Fallat, Millett, and Kaplan (1976) carried out exercise electrocardiograms in normal and hypercholesterolemic children. The latter were 73 children heterozygous for familial hyper-cholesterolemia. These authors also performed similar tests on 97 normal children. The mean age of each group was 13 years. All of the children had normal resting electrocardiograms. An S-T depression of 1 mm or greater in V_5 was considered significant. Eighteen percent of the hypercholesterolemic group showed a significant S-T depression on exercise compared with only 7 percent in the normal group. They concluded that there is latent ischemic heart disease in many children with familial hypercholesterolemia.

Newborn

In the newborn period, musculoelastic intimal thickenings were regularly found, forming pads at the branch sites and also involving additional surface areas. The quantity of intimal tissue varied greatly from infant to infant. Scanty superficial intimal lipid was frequently present, either extracellular or intracellular in smooth muscle cells. Edema was noted in about a fifth of the cases. Such thickenings of the intima were similar in both sexes. As the study progressed from infancy through to 12 months, intimal thickenings increased in extent and bulk and were more frequently edematous, and fatty streaks were found to increase gradually.

Age 2 to 9 Years

Intimal thickenings continued to increase in extent.

Age 15 to 19 Years

The most significant finding in this age group was probably the presence of focal deposits of debris from disintegrating lipid cells, a finding that was present in practically all the children from 15 to 19 and was seldom noted in the younger age groups. These changes were especially common at the branch pads and opposite branch orifices. Surface encrustation of blood constituents forming intimal layers, seen in the older age groups when coronary artery disease is obvious, was not present in these children, and, as has been noted before, foci or lipid necrosis tended to occur where there was thickening of the intima near the bifurcation of the vessels. Jaffe thus considered thickening of the intima to be a possible precursor of the disintegrating foci. (See Figures 61–4 and 61–5.) The mean intimal depth in the proximal portion of the coronary arteries increases in the second and third decades of life. A significant incidence of focal intimal fibrosis appears in the third decade (Jaffe and Manning, Hospital for Sick Children, Toronto, 1974). Grossly visible intracellular lipid is scanty during the first decade. It becomes a common finding in the 10-to-20-year age group but is present in the majority between 20 and 30 years.

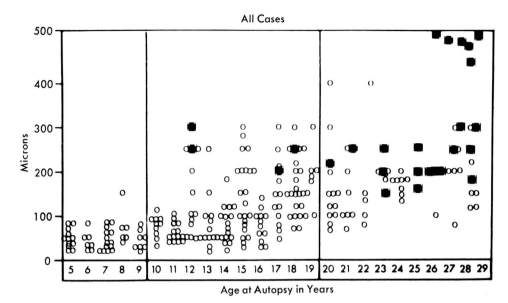

Figure 61-4. Mean intimal depth ("diffuse intimal thickening") in proximal portions of coronary arteries. ○ Focal increase in intimal fibrosis absent or questionable. ▣ Focal increase in intimal fibrosis present. (Jaffe and Manning, 1973.)

Progeria

A condition that is characteristically associated with generalized atherosclerosis and coronary thrombosis in childhood is progeria. Thirty-two cases had been reported up to 1962 (Makous et al., 1962). In eight of these autopsy details were published and all showed evidence of widespread and advanced atherosclerosis. In six of the eight, occlusion of the coronary arteries and myocardial infarcts were

demonstrated. Six had had angina on effort. The youngest patient with progeria, for whom postmortem details were available, was that reported by Talbot and associates (1945). This was a seven-year-old boy who had angina with effort and died at seven years of age with myocardial infarction and generalized atheroma.

Keay and associates (1955) also presented the details of a three-year-old child with progeria who, although he did not have demonstrable evidence of atherosclerosis clinically, had abnormal levels of

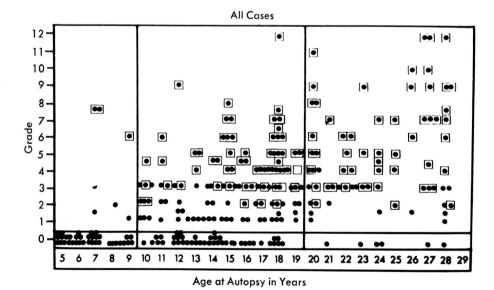

Figure 61-5. Amount of intracellular lipid in intima of coronary arteries (HSC series). • Intimal lipid, if present, visible microscopically only. ▣ Intimal lipid in grossly visible "fatty streaks". (Jaffe and Manning, 1973.)

cholesterol and total circulating phospholipids reflected in moderately raised beta lipid fractions, a finding that is commonly associated with atherosclerosis. There was no evidence of pituitary or other glandular dysfunction in the child. Consequently, Keay and associates suggested that the premature development of atherosclerosis and progeria might be similar in character to the development in adults, except that the metabolic error may be inborn in the former and acquired in the latter. Certainly, it would be useful to study such cases carefully in an effort to discover errors in metabolism that might prove reversible. In this regard MacNamara and associates (1970) reported a case of progeria that was followed for several years and was treated with a diet in which the fat was predominantly unsaturated. This did not appear to alter the course significantly, although it did lower the serum cholesterol. The child died at ten years of age and postmortem showed atheromatous ulceration of the aorta, narrowed coronary arteries, and multiple myocardial infarcts. (See Figure 61–6.)

The lipid levels in progeria are only moderately raised and are not comparable to those seen in most cases of type II hyperlipoproteinemia. Chance (1970) examined the conjunctival vessels in progeria and found they had an unusual palisaded appearance quite different from normal children. Most vessels appeared to be placed at right angles to each other, which in turn may have affected the blood supply to the vessel wall.

Risk Factors

The main risk factors leading to atherosclerosis in adults include a family history of atherosclerotic pathology; hyperlipidemia; hypertension; diabetes mellitus; obesity; a diet intake rich in saturated fats, cholesterol, and sucrose; cigarette smoking; and habitual physical inactivity. Males also appear more susceptible than females. All of these factors are relevant, to some degree, in the pediatric age group.

In childhood diabetes may be controlled; obesity may be obviated or minimized; hypertension may now be alleviated or controlled; and physical inactivity is uncommon in the first two decades. Cigarette smoking may be a problem in certain age groups in some countries.

Other possible contributing factors that may accelerate or produce atherosclerosis, but less likely to be active in childhood, are as follows: genetic traits of the arterial wall; of structure, metabolism, permeability and nutrition, or deterioration of the vessel wall with age; the effect of testosterone; hypothyroidism; obstructive liver disease; specific drugs, psychic stress; occupation; culture; and trauma.

Hyperlipidemia

Hyperlipidemia, as a possible cause of atherosclerosis, may be acting early in life. Primary hyper-pre-beta-lipoproteinemia is a frequent finding in young adults with occlusive vascular disease (Allbrink et al., 1961; Hatch et al., 1966; Blankenhorn et al., 1968). Recent evidence from the Framingham study suggests that, at least in young and middle-aged adults, the risk of coronary heart disease is reflected equally as well by the degree of elevation of cholesterol as by the presence or degree of hyper-pre-beta-lipoproteinemia, or perhaps even better (Kannel et al., 1971). Proof that its control through primary prevention diets will improve the prognosis in later decades is still lacking or is incomplete, but there is sufficient evidence to suggest that studies should be begun in the pediatric age group to help clarify this problem.

Numerous investigations are in progress in the adult field to determine whether, after a coronary episode, life may be prolonged, or further episodes prevented, by the use of a low-fat or polyunsaturated fat diet (secondary prevention). Such diets appear to be effective in some studies but not in all (Nelson, 1956; Leren, 1966; Hood, 1965; Bierenbaum and Green, 1967; Morris, 1968; Mietliven et al., 1972; Turpeinen, 1968; Stamler, 1969; Dayton et al., 1969; Christakis et al., 1969).

Tamir et al. (1971) studied the lipid profiles of the families of 64 men who were hospitalized for acute myocardial infarction under the age of 41. Thirty-eight of the sixty-four men were noted to have abnormal serum lipid patterns. Among the progeny of these 38, slightly over one-third (36.4 percent) also had abnormally elevated lipid levels. The picture was further clarified when it was found that there was no significant deviation from the normal in the 55 children born to the fathers who had normal serum lipids.

It is difficult, or impossible, to control or change the eating habits of the whole population of the country, especially when the evidence is not clarified that such changes will be universally beneficial. However, the familial hyperlipoproteinemias, especially type II, which can be identified in childhood and are associated with premature coronary artery disease, might well be helped by a suitable diet.

Types of Hyperlipoproteinemia

Familial hyperlipoproteinemias have been divided by Frederickson and Lees (1965) into five groups by ultracentrifuge and electrophoretic methods. Type I (hyperchlomicronemias, hypertriglyceridemia) is characterized by eruptive skin xanthomata, abdominal pain, lipemia rationalis, and marked increase in triglycerides and is associated with a typical electrophoretic pattern. It is brought about by delayed clearance of exogenous lipid use to a lipoprotein lipase enzyme deficiency and, if necessary, may be treated by a low-fat diet. It is a rare condition and considered an autosomal recessive. Goodman et al. (1940) described an example in a 20-month-old

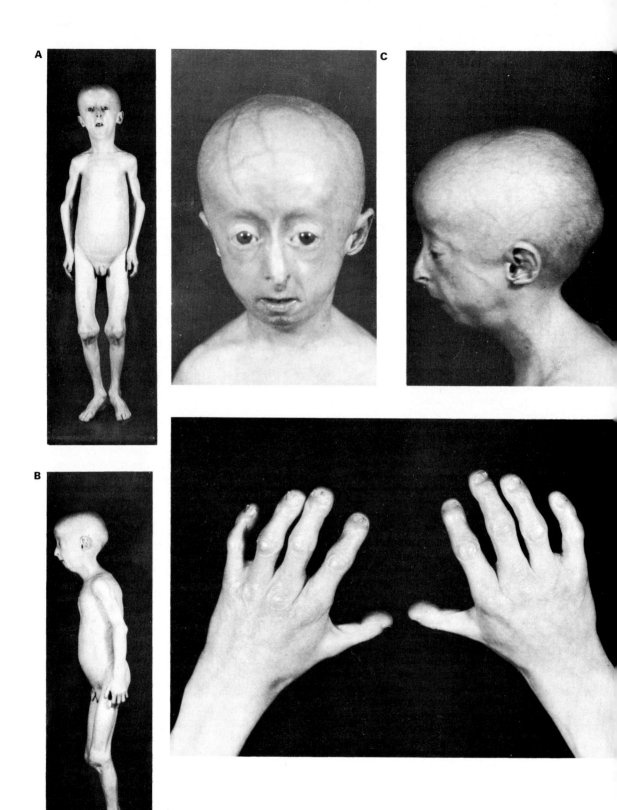

Figure 61-6. Ten-year-old boy who died at the age of 11 years with myocardial infarction. Diffuse atherosclerosis found at postmortem examination. (Courtesy of Dr. Clifford Parsons, Children's Hospital, Birmingham, England.)

boy. Bruton and Kanter (1951) reported a two-year-old child also with type I. It does not appear to be associated with premature atherosclerosis.

Type II (hyper-beta-lipoproteinemia) is apparently associated with excess production, or inadequate clearance, of low-density lipoprotein (Frederickson, 1972). It may at times have its onset in childhood with arcus cornea, tendon and tuberous xanthomata, accelerated atherosclerosis, and an increase in serum cholesterol. Triglycerides are normal, or only slightly increased; the plasma is clear; the electrophoretic pattern is characteristic. Such cases can be treated with a reduced cholesterol diet, coupled with the use of polyunsaturated fats and, if necessary, suitable drug therapy. This group appears as an autosomal dominant with incomplete penetrance. In childhood, heterozygotes usually show no signs or symptoms with the occasional exception of arcus senilis.

At The Hospital for Sick Children, Toronto, we have had a homozygotic case in recent years with a family history of similar defect in both parents. The child was first seen at four years of age and had a total cholesterol varying between 755 and 914 mg percent. He developed angina at six years of age with characteristic transient changes in his electrocardiogram. He died suddenly before his seventh birthday. His electrocardiograms under various circumstances are shown in Figure 61–7. He exhibited typical xanthomatosis as shown in Figure 61–8.

Type III has its onset in adult life with atherosclerosis of coronary and peripheral vessels and tuberous eruptive lesions. Cholesterol and triglycerides are increased. There is an abnormal glucose tolerance and a characteristic "broad beta" electrophoretic pattern. It can be treated with drugs, low-carbohydrate diet, and weight control. Type III is much less common than type II or type IV and is considered to be a recessive mendelian relationship.

Type IV usually has its onset in adult life with obesity, abdominal pain, and/or cardiovascular disease. The cholesterol is either normal or slightly increased and the triglycerides are moderately to markedly increased. The glucose tolerance is abnormal. There is a characteristic prebeta band in the electrophoretic pattern and there may be eruptive tuberosities in the skin. It also can be treated with weight control, restriction of carbohydrates, and drug therapy. Type IV may be seen at times in children.

Type V has an eruptive lesion seen early in adult life, with hepatosplenomegaly, obesity, abdominal pain, and lipemia retinalis. Cholesterol is normal, or slightly increased, and the triglycerides increased. Glucose tolerance is abnormal. There is a characteristic combined chylomicron and "prebeta" electrophoretic pattern. It is described as an excess of very low-density lipoprotein combined with poor chylomicron removal. It can be treated with weight control, a diet low in fat and carbohydrates, and the addition of drugs or hormones.

Since some hyperlipoproteinemias may lead to early coronary atherosclerosis and coronary epi-sodes, it would seem reasonable to attempt dietary prophylaxis in childhood. This is particularly true of type II, which can usually be identified at birth, in infancy, or in early childhood and is well recognized as a cause of premature coronary episodes. Since in type II more than one member of the family may be at risk, the family group may all cooperate and significant reduction of cholesterol levels may be achieved.

Frederickson suggests the following table for categorizing the types of hyperlipoproteinemia using cholesterol and triglyceride levels:

Cholesterol high, triglycerides normal, type II(a)
Cholesterol high, triglycerides 150–400, type II(b), III, or IV
Cholesterol high, triglycerides 400–1000, type III, IV, or V
Cholesterol high, triglycerides over 1000, type I or V
Cholesterol normal, triglycerides high, type IV

In children we are dealing chiefly with type II(a) with cholesterol above the 94 percentile level. Borderline cases may be due to dietary excess. More severe forms are usually related to genetic abnormalities and are referred to as familial type II. The inheritance is via a single mutant allelic gene causing elevation of serum cholesterol and an increase of the low-density lipoprotein. Carriers of this gene are not uncommon and usually one of the parents and about half of the other relatives are affected.

When the cholesterol is high and triglycerides are between 150 and 400, patients usually fall into the category of type II(b) or type IV. The nomogram of Frederickson (1972) is helpful in differentiating between these two. He points out that as the low-density lipoprotein levels move progressively above 170 to 200, the need for type II diets and drugs that are designed to enhance excretion of cholesterol and its breakdown products becomes increasingly important. When the low-density lipoprotein levels are lower, greater emphasis is placed on type IV diet and drugs that are aimed at curbing the excess of very low-density lipoprotein production associated with high triglyceride level.

Serum Cholesterol Levels in Infants and Children

In the human at birth, the total serum cholesterol levels are low, varying from 55 to 120 mg/100 ml according to different authors. At two weeks of age infants fed either breast milk, or evaporated milk formula, show levels usually between 96 and 99 mg/ml. By four to six weeks of age, the levels have risen to between 120 and 190 mg/ml. Fomon and Bartels (1960), however, found levels of approximately 172 mg in breast-fed babies from one to six months of age, often a little higher than the bottle-fed babies of the same age. Goalwin and Pomeranze (1962) compared the total cholesterol levels in three groups of infants: one group breast-fed, the second

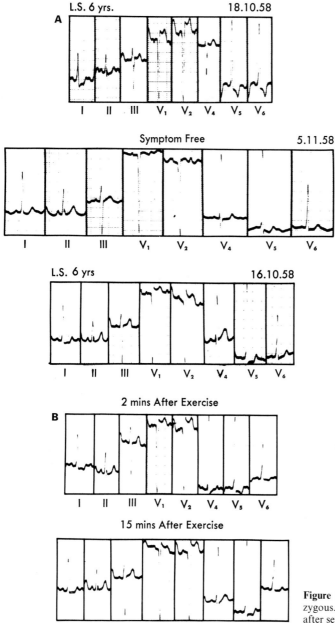

Figure 61-7. Familial hypercholesterolemia, homozygous. *A*. Electrocardiographic changes 15 minutes after severe spontaneous angina. *B*. Effect of exercise testing on the electrocardiogram.

group fed evaporated milk formula, and the third group fed a similar formula but with milk fat replaced by corn oil. All babies were given fruit. By 12 weeks of age the cholesterol levels in the first two groups had reached 188 mg/ml. The level in the babies fed corn oil formula, on the other hand, had reached only 127 mg/ml. At that time cereals, meats, vegetables, and other "dairy products" were added to the diets of the babies fed the usual evaporated milk feedings and to the diets of a number of those receiving the special corn oil feedings. Four weeks later the levels in the babies on the usual evaporated milk feedings were unchanged whereas levels in those on the special corn

oil feedings had risen to 173 mg/ml. (The control babies who were continued on the corn oil feeding alone did not show this rise and their average level at 16 weeks was 132 mg/ml.) Apparently, therefore, the cholesterol-depressing effect of corn oil feedings is practically nullified by the addition of other foods.

The effect of nutrition early in life on the ultimate blood cholesterol levels in adult life has yet to be determined in the human. Nevertheless, there are some laboratory experiments that should be considered in this context. In 1966 Hahn and Kolkovsky reported interesting results in an experiment performed on animals. Newborn female

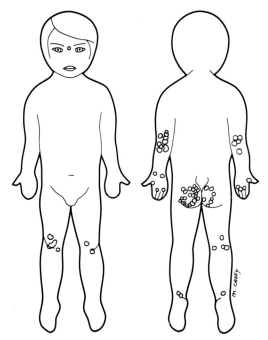

Figure 61-8. Distribution of xanthomatosis in the child with homozygous familial hypercholesterolemia referred to in Figure 61–7.

rats were divided into two groups: one group weaned on day 18 and the other on day 30 after birth. Both groups were then fed the same laboratory diet for nine months. There was no difference between the two groups when aged ten months. After that they were fed an atherogenic diet with high fat and 5 percent cholesterol for two and one-half months and their blood cholesterol levels were determined. The cholesterol level of the prematurely weaned rats (day 18) had risen to 1400 mg percent while the level in the normally weaned group was 900 mg percent. These authors concluded that early exclusion of fat from the diet (since weaning on day 18 means eliminating milk and feeding a high-carbohydrate laboratory diet) may lead to hypercholesteremia in adult life of the rat.

In 1972 Reiser and Sidelman showed that in male

rats there was an inverse relationship between the cholesterol content in the dam's milk and the blood cholesterol levels in the animals at 24 weeks. Thus, if the cholesterol content in the milk was 35 mg percent, then the blood cholesterol was 145 mg percent at 24 weeks, whereas a milk cholesterol of 24 mg percent resulted in a blood cholesterol of 252 mg percent.

Scrimshaw et al. (1957) reported total cholesterol levels in groups of Guatemalan children from 7 to 12 years inclusive attending a city private school (group A), a public school in a poor city area (group B), and a public school in a poor rural area (group C). The serum cholesterol in the children referred to in these three groups is shown in Table 61–2 as well as the calories as fat and protein in the parents' diet. It will be noted that the serum cholesterol in the children in the well-to-do urban district had levels much the same as those in Canada and the United States whereas in the poor urban and poor rural districts the levels were distinctly lower.

Familial hypercholesterolemia or familial type II hyperlipoproteinemia is associated with tendon and subcutaneous xanthomas and a risk of premature ischemic heart disease and is characterized by a marked elevation in beta lipoprotein fraction. This lipid abnormality appears to be inherited as an autosomal dominant trait. Kwiterovitch and associates (1973) have analyzed data from 238 children, aged 1 to 19 years, born of 90 type II individuals who are mated with normal individuals. Forty-five percent of the offspring had hyper-beta-lipoproteinemia.

Darmondy et al. (1972) reported a longitudinal study of serum cholesterol in 302 children. They determined the cord blood total cholesterol and found it difficult to predict precisely which children might have familial hypercholesterolemia at age one on the basis of the cord blood cholesterol. They concluded that a diagnosis of this condition should be deferred until one year of age.

Kwiterovitch and associates (1973) studied the cord bloods of 29 infants where one parent had familial type II hyperlipoproteinemia. Using cord blood plasma concentration of low-density lipoprotein (LDL) cholesterol, they found that this exceeded a cut-off limit of 41 mg/100 ml, representing

Table 61-2.   DIET AND SERUM CHOLESTEROL IN GUATEMALAN CHILDREN*

	SOCIOECONOMIC GROUP		
	A. WELL-TO-DO URBAN	B. POOR URBAN	C. POOR RURAL
Parents' diet			
Calories as fat (%)	37	15	8
Total protein (gm/day)	69	47	67
Animal protein (gm/day)	39	10	6
Calories/day (adult)	2500	1600	2300
Serum cholesterol (mg/100 ml) in children			
Boys (7–12 years)	187	143	121
Girls (7–12 years)	188	156	128

* Scrimshaw, N. S.; Balsam, A.; and Arroyave, G.: The nutrition of children and adolescents. *Am. J. Clin. Nutr.*, **5**:629, 1957.

the upper 5 percentile for LDL cholesterol in a control population. The children with normal low-density lipoprotein cholesterol at birth remained in the normal range at follow-up a year or two later. Eleven of the twelve who had an elevated low-density lipoprotein cholesterol at birth later had obvious hyper-beta-lipoproteinemia. The exception was one infant who had been put on a strict low-cholesterol diet from birth.

These results indicate that the concentration of low-density lipoprotein in the cord blood permits the identification of affected children of a parent with type II hyperlipoproteinemia. Thus, when the low-density lipoproteinemia measured in cord blood exceeds 41 mg/100 ml, one can reliably conclude that the infant has this lipid abnormality.

Levels of serum cholesterol in 587 children of various age groups at The Hospital for Sick Children in Toronto are shown in Figure 61–9; secondary cases of hypercholesterolemia are excluded. Ninety-five percent of those from birth to five years were under 200 mg percent; from 5 to 15 years, 95 percent are under 220. There is minimal overlap of serum cholesterol levels when normal children are compared with those with familial hypercholesterolemia. However, the upper 5 percent and the nonfamilial hypercholesterolemic children may also be at risk in this regard. Further investigation is needed to clarify the various subgroups.

Preventive Measures

Although adequate control of diabetes is an accepted approach in preventing atherosclerosis at an early age in children with this disease, the direct evidence that this is effective is lacking. However, there is evidence that lack of control of blood sugar in the known diabetic may be associated with elevation of serum lipids, which, in turn, may accelerate arterial change (Schrade et al., 1963). Careful control of diabetes in childhood and adolescence results in normal serum lipoprotein patterns in the majority of patients. Vigorous attempts at superimposition of polyunsaturated fat diets already restricted in carbohydrates may lead to patient noncooperation with resultant increased consumption of carbohydrate, worsening control, and a high incidence of pre-beta-lipoproteinemia (Chance et al., 1969). Use of a carbohydrate-regulated diet in which moderate reductions of cholesterol and saturated fat intake are achieved within the limits of palatability and adolescent social acceptability could conceivably produce better results. Indeed, it may be appropriate to translate this to all of childhood since the evidence from several sources suggests that a suitable diet for optimum health in this age group should not include an excessive use of sucrose.

Control of obesity is often difficult for the adolescent, but if it is significant for future arterial health as well as for appearance, children may be persuaded to maintain dietary control of their weight.

The evidence that smoking contributes to atherosclerosis is recorded in numerous investigations in the age groups over 30 years. This information is being widely disseminated now.

While the serum cholesterol in type II hyperlipoproteinemia can usually be reduced to some degree by diet at all ages in childhood, it appears easier to achieve a significant decrease relatively early in life than later (Glueck, 1972). At the present time, it seems reasonable to use the dietary approach in such cases, even though it will be years before it can be demonstrated whether or not this decrease diminishes the progression of atherosclerosis in such individuals.

Friedman et al. (1973) are attempting to evaluate a program of diminishing the risk factors in pediatrics. Beginning in infancy, they interest the parents in preventing obesity in their children. They attempt to keep the total fat intake to 25 percent of the total calories and to have no more than 10 percent of the total calories as saturated fat. They are also recommending that the children's diet should keep the total cholesterol intake in 24 hours to 150 mg. Carrying out these recommendations, they are attempting to follow the guidelines of the American Heart Association in emphasizing to each family how they may maintain an optimum nutrition among their children. Such advice includes comment regarding adequate protein, iron, and vitamin intake.

So far they have followed a group of 21,777 infants and children on the above regime for a period of 18 months. The following parameters have been evaluated: percentile height; weight; head circumference; hemoglobin; total serum protein; serum cholesterol; number of sick visits per year; and skinfold thickness. Their conclusion is that the group that adhered to the diet, as evidenced by a decreased cholesterol, were found to have no significant interference with the measured parameters in any one age group.

Physical Activity and Cardiovascular Health

In 1970 the Inter-society Commission on Heart Disease Resources supported the view that regular exercise, particularly those forms of endurance exercise that enhance cardiovascular fitness, may have a role to play in the prevention of atherosclerotic disease.

Fox, Naughton, and Gorman (1972) have summarized the mechanisms by which physical activity may reduce the occurrence, or severity, of coronary heart disease. They suggest that physical exercise may increase coronary collateral vascularization, vessel size, myocardial efficiency, efficiency of peripheral blood distribution and return, electron transport capacity, fibrinolytic capability, arterial oxygen content, red blood cell mass and blood volume, thyroid function, growth hormone production, tolerance to stress, prudent living habits, and

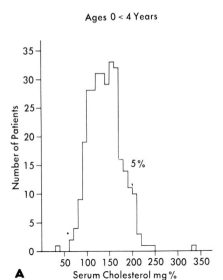

Ages 0 < 4 Years

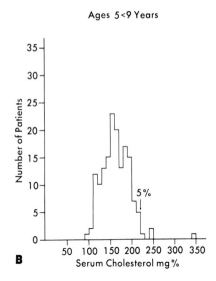

Ages 5 <9 Years

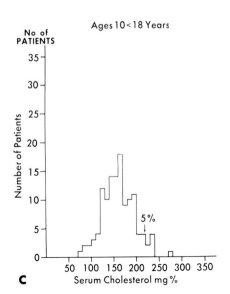

Ages 10 < 18 Years

Figure 61-9. Levels of serum cholesterol in 587 children of various age groups at The Hospital for Sick Children, Toronto. Secondary cases of hypercholesterolemia are excluded.

joie de vivre. At the same time it may decrease to some degree serum lipid levels, triglycerides, cholesterol glucose intolerance, obesity-adiposity, platelet stickiness, arterial blood pressure, heart rate, vulnerability to dysrhythmias, neurohormonal overreaction, and the strain associated with psychic stress.

Improved myocardial efficiency is suggested by the work of Detry et al. (1971). Improved peripheral blood distribution has been confirmed by the work of Larsen and Malmberg (1971). The same authors indicated that a greater arterial oxygen content may be acquired by exercise and fibrinolytic activity may be significantly decreased temporarily.

The work of Ikkala et al. (1966) showed a decreased tendency for platelet aggregation with moderate exertion. Psychologic factors have been recognized

for some time as playing a significant role in determining cardiac health and the presence, or absence, of coronary heart disease. Useful information is available in the publication by Heinzelmann and Bagley (1970).

Exercise has minimal effect on serum cholesterol unless it is associated with weight loss in the activity and physical training process. However, Larsen and Malmberg (1971) demonstrated a significant decrease in serum triglycerides lasting a day or two. It has long been recognized that a training bradycardia occurs with physical activity and this improves the efficiency of the heart. Such physical activity may reduce the blood pressure during activity compared with the untrained person, but controlled studies have reported only a modest reduction in resting pressures.

The possible benefits listed above do not persist indefinitely, and it appears important for an individual to keep up some form of regular and pleasurable exercise.

Dietary Management of Hyperlipoproteinemia in Children

Opinion is not yet fully crystallized in regard to efforts to control serum cholesterol and triglycerides when this occurs as a primary abnormality in childhood. However, since there are many children who may require some form of dietary therapy, particularly those with type II(a) and (b), the following material is presented to guide the physician in the management of his patient.

The diet can be prescribed in two ways: either a very strictly controlled diet specifying the exact quantities of foods to be taken, or a less rigid one arrived at by listing foods allowed and foods to avoid, which permits the patient to select the suitable quantities from the list of foods allowed.

Diet no. 1 is a controlled type of diet that involves more work in menu planning on the part of the mother, but is more likely to achieve a greater reduction in blood lipids. Since the calorie level is usually specified, the diet would also be suitable for those requiring weight reduction. Diet no. 2 is a less rigid form of diet that would be more suitable for children with mildly raised lipids, or in cases where there is an aversion to strict dietary treatment or a lack of clear understanding of it. The chances of successful dieting are greatly enhanced by the whole family being on, and sharing, the same diet.

REFERENCES

Abbott, M. E.; Congenital heart disease. In Osler, W., and McCrae, T. (eds.): *Modern Medicine: Its Theory and Practice*. Lea and Febiger, Philadelphia, 1927, Vol. 4, p. 794.

Abrikosoff, A.: Aneurysma des linken Harzventrikels mit abnormer Abgangsstelle der linken Koronararterie von de pulmonalis bei einem Funfmonatlichen Kinde. *Arch. Pathol. Anat.*, **203**:413, 1911.

Akhtar, N.; Hyland, J. W.; and Adam, M.: Anomalous origin of left coronary artery from the pulmonary artery in an adult. *J. Thorac. Cardiovasc. Surg.*, **66**:112, 1973.

Albrink, M. J.; Meigs, J. W.; and Mann, E. B.: Serum lipids, hypertension and coronary artery disease. *Am. J. Med.*, **31**:4, 1961.

American Heart Association: *Planning Fat-Controlled Meals for 1200 and 1800 Calories*, New York, 1962, 1966.

American Heart Association: *Planning Fat-Controlled Meals for Approximately 2000–2600 Calories*. New York, 1962, 1967.

American Heart Association: *Recipes for Fat-Controlled, Low Cholesterol Meals*, New York, 1968, 1972.

American Heart Association: *Reduce Your Risk of Heart Attack*. New York, 1969.

American Heart Association: *The Way to a Man's Heart*. New York, 1972.

American Heart Association: *You and Your Heart*. New York, 1970.

Andersen, G. E., and Friis-Hansen, B.: Neonatal diagnosis of familial type II hyperlipoproteinemia. *Pediatrics*, **52**:2, 1976.

Annand, J. C.: Further evidence in the case against heated milk protein. *Atherosclerosis*, **15**:129, 1972.

Askenazi, J., and Nadas, A. S.: Anomalous left coronary artery originating from the pulmonary artery. Report on 15 cases. *Circulation*, **51**:976, 1975.

Atherosclerosis. *Physician's Bull.*, **22**:17, 1955.

Becu, L.; Personal communication, 1974, Buenos Aires, Argentina.

Bell, F. P.; Somer, J. B.; Craig, I. H.; and Schwartz, C. J.: Patterns of aortic Evans blue uptake in vivo and in vitro. *Atherosclerosis*, **15**:369, 1972.

Benda, C.: Quoted in Stryker, 1946.

Benda, C.: Uber einen Fall von schwerer infantiler Koronararteriensklerose als Todesurasache. *Virchows Arch. Pathol. Anat.*, **254**:600, 1925.

Bennett, M. J., and Medwadowski, B. V.: Vitamin A, vitamin E, and lipids in serum of children with cystic fibrosis or congenital heart defects compared with normal children. *Am. J. Clin. Nutr.*, **20**:415, 1967.

Bialostozky, D.; Iuengo, M.; Magos, C.; and Zorrilla, E.: Coronary insufficiency in children. *Am. J. Cardiol.*, **36**:509–13, 1975.

Bierenbaum, M. L.; Green, D. P.; Florin, A.; Fleischman, A. I.; and Caldwell, A. B.: Modified-fat dietary management of the young male with coronary disease. *JAMA*, **202**:1119–23, 1967.

Bland, E. F.; White, P. D.; and Garland, J.: Congenital anomalies of coronary arteries: report of unusual case associated with cardiac hypertrophy. *Am. Heart J.*, **8**:787, 1932.

Blankenhorn, D. H.; Chin, H. P.; and Lau, F. Y. K.: Ischemic heart disease in young adults. Metabolic and angiographic diagnosis and the prevalence of type IV hyperlipoproteinemia. *Ann. Intern. Med.*, **69**:21, 1968.

Bloch, A.; Dinsmore, R. E.; and Lees, R. S.: Coronary arteriographic findings in type-II and type-IV hyperlipoproteinemia. *Lancet*, May **1**:928, 1976.

Blumgart, H. L.; Freedberg, A. S.; and Kurland, G. S.: Hypercholesterolemia, myxedema and atherosclerosis. *Am. J. Med.*, **14**:665, 1953.

Bor, I.: Myocardial infarctation and ischaemic heart disease in infants and children. *Arch. Dis. Child.*, **44**:268, 1969.

Bruton, O. C., and Kanter, A. J.: Idiopathic familial hyperlipemia. *Am. J. Dis. Child.*, **82**:153, 1951.

Buchwald, H.; Lee, G. B.; Amplatz, K.; Moore, R. B.; Frantz, I. D., Jr.; and Varco, R. L.: Severe atherosclerotic cardiovascular disease. *Minnesota Med.*, **51**:477, 1968.

Chaitman, B. R.; Bourassa, M. G.; Lesperance, J.; and Grondin, P.: Anomalous left coronary artery from pulmonary artery. *Circulation*, **51**:552, 1975.

Chance, G. W., and Albutt, E. C.: The relative effects of diabetic control and corn oil diet on serum lipids in childhood diabetes (abstr.). *Diabetologia*, **5**:206, 1968.

Chance, G. W.; Albutt, E. C.; and Edkins, S. M.: Control of hyperlipidamin in juvenile diabetes. Standard and corn-oil diets compared over a period of 10 years. *Br. Med. J.*, **3**:616, 1969.

Chance, G. W.: Personal communication, 1970.

Chapman, J. M., and Massey, F. J., Jr: Interrelationship of serum cholesterol, hypertension, body weight and risk of coronary disease: results of the first 10 years' follow-up in the Los Angeles Heart Study. *J. Chronic Dis.*, **17**:933, 1964.

Chiariello, L.; Meyer, J.; Reul, G. J.; Hallman, G. L.; and Cooley, D. A.: Surgical treatment for anomalous origin of left coronary artery from pulmonary artery. *Ann. Thorac. Surg.*, **19**:443, 1975.

Christakis, G., and Rinzler, S. H.: Diet in atherosclerosis. Schettler, F. G., and Boyd, G. S., eds. Elsevier Publ. Co., New York, **10C**:823–54, 1969.

Cochrane, W. A., and Bowden, D. H.: Calcification of the arteries in infancy and childhood. *Pediatrics*, **14**:222, 1954.

Committee on Exercise, American Heart Assn.: *Exercise Testing and Training of Apparently Healthy Individuals*. American Heart Association, New York, 1972.

Conn, J. H.; Chavez, C. M.; and Fain, W. R.: The short bowel syndrome. *Ann. Surg.*, **175**:803, 1972.

Cooley, D. A., and Ellis, P. R.: Surgical considerations of coronary arterio fistula. *Am. J. Cardiol.*, **10**:467, 1962.

Creed, D. L.; Baird, W. F.; and Fisher, E. R.: The severity of arteriosclerosis in certain diseases: a necropsy study. *Am. J. Med. Sci.*, **230**:385, 1955.

Darmondy, J. M.; Fosbrooke, A. S.; and Lloyd, J. K.: Prospective study of serum cholesterol levels during first year of life. *Br. Med. J.*, **2**:685, 1972.

Day, A. J.; Schwartz, C. J.; and Peters, J. A.: Serum lipid responses to heparin and to protamine in rabbits. *Aust. J. Exp. Biol. Med. Sci.*, **35**:457, 1957.

Day, A. J.; Wilkinson, G. K.; and Schwartz, C. J.: The effect of toluidine blue on serum lipids and lipoproteins in rabbits. *Aust. J. Exp. Biol. Med. Sci.*, **34**:415, 1956.

Day, A. J.; Wilkinson, G. K.; Schwartz, C. J.; and Peters, J. A.: Changes in serum lipids and in aortic atherosclerosis following toluidine blue and heparin administration to cholesterol fed rabbits. *Aust. J. Exp. Biol. Med. Sci.*, **35**:277, 1957.

Day, A. J.; Schwartz, D. J.; Wilkinson, G. K.; and Peters, J. A.: The effect of uranium acetate on serum lipids and on atherosclerosis in cholesterol fed rabbits. *Aust. J. Exp. Biol. Med. Sci.*, **35**:1, 1957.

Dayton, S.; Pearce, M. L.; Hashimoto, S.; Dixon, W. J.; and Tomiyasu, U.: *A Controlled Clinical Trial of a Diet High in Unsaturated Fat.* American Heart Association Mono. 23, New York, 1969.

Detry, J. M.; Rousseau, M.; Vandenbrouche, G.; et al.: Increased arteriovenous oxygen difference after physical training and coronary heart disease. *Circulation*, **44**:109, 1971.

Doty, D. B.; Lauer, R. M.; and Eberhoft, J. L.: Congenital cardiac anomalies. *Am. J. Thorac. Surg.*, **20**:316–25, 1975.

Duff, G. L., and McMillan, G. C.: Pathology of atherosclerosis. *Am. J. Med.*, **11**:92, 1951.

Duguid, J. B.: The etiology of atherosclerosis. *Practitioner*, **175**:241, 1955.

Duguid, J. B., and Robertson, W. B.: Effects of atherosclerosis on the coronary circulation. *Lancet*, **1**, 525, 1955.

Eisalo, A.; Ahrenberg, P.; and Nikkila, E. A.: Treatment of hyperlipidemia with D-thyroxine. *Acta Med. Scand.*, **173**:639, 1963.

Enos, W. F.; Holmes, R. H.; and Beyer, J.: Coronary disease among United States soldiers killed in action in Korea. *JAMA*, **152**:1090, 1953.

Epstein, S. E.; Redwood, D. R.; Goldstein, R. E.; Beiser, G. D.; Rosing, D. R.; Glancy, D. L.; Reis, R. L.; and Stinson, E. B.: Angina pectoris: Pathophysiology, evaluation and treatment (NIH conference). *Ann. Intern. Med.*, **75**:263, 1971.

Fangman, R. S., and Hellwig, C. A.: Histology of the coronary arteries in newborn infants. *Am. J. Pathol.*, **23**:901, 1947.

Fetterman, G. H., and Hashida, Y.: Mucocutaneous lymph node syndrome (MLNS): A disease widespread in Japan which demands our attention. *Pediatrics*, **54**:268, 1974.

Finley, J.; Howman-Giles, R.; Gilday, D.; Olley, P.; and Rowe, R. D.: Normal thallium scan following surgery of anomalous left coronary arising from pulmonary artery. Programme and Abstracts, Canadian Cardiovascular Society, page 86, 1977.

Fomon, S. J., and Bartels, D. J.: Concentration of cholesterol in serum of infants in relation to diet. *Am. J. Dis. Child.*, **99**:27, 1960.

Fomon, S. J.: A pediatrician looks at early nutrition. *Bull. N. Y. Acad. Med.*, **47**:569, 1971.

Fortuin, N. J.; Morrow, A. G.; and Roberts, W. C.: Late vascular manifestations of the rubella syndrome. A roentgenographic-pathologic study. *Am. J. Med.*, **51**:134, 1971.

Fox, S. M.; Naughton, J. P.; and Gorman, P. A.: Physical activity and cardiovascular health. *Mod. Concepts Cardiovasc. Dis.*, **41**:25, 1972.

Frederikson, D. S., and Lees, R. S.: A system for pheno-typing hyperlipoproteinemia. *Circulation*, **31**:321, 1965.

Frederikson, D. S.: A physician's guide to hyperlipidemia. *Mod. Concepts Cardiovasc. Dis.*, **41**:31, 1972.

French, A. J., and Dock, W.: Fatal coronary arteriosclerosis in young soldiers. *JAMA*, **124**:1233, 1944.

Fry, D. L.: Certain chemorheologic considerations regarding the blood vascular interface with particular reference to coronary artery disease. *Circulation*, **39** and **40**:38, 1969.

Geer, J. C.; McGill, H. C., Jr.; Robertson, W. B.; and Strong, J. P.: Histologic characteristics of coronary artery fatty streaks. *Lab. Invest.*, **18**:105, 1968.

Glueck, C. J.; Heckman, F.; Schoenfeld, M.; Steiner, P.; and Pearce, W.: Neonatal familial type II hyperlipoproteinemia; cord blood colesterol in 1800 births. *Metabolism*, **20**:597, 1971.

Goalwin, A., and Pomeranze, J.: Serum cholesterol studies in infants. *Arch. Pediatr.*, **79**:58, 1962.

Gofman, J., et al.: Blood lipids and human atherosclerosis. *Circulation*, **5**:119, 1952.

Goldsmith, R.; Gribetz, D.; and Strauss, L.: Mucocutaneous Lymph node syndrome (MLNS) in the continental United States. *Pediatrics*, **57**:431, 1976.

Goodman, M.; Schuman, H.; and Goodman, S.: Idiopathic lipemia

with secondary zanthomatosis hepatosplenomegaly and lipemic retinalis. *J. Pediatr.*, **16**:596, 1940.

Gruenwald, P.: Necrosis in coronary arteries of newborn infants. *Am. Heart J.*, **38**:889, 1949.

Gubner, R., and Ungerleider, H. E.: Arteriosclerosis. A statement of the problem. *Am. J. Med.*, **6**:60, 1949.

Hahn, P., and Koldovsky, O.: *Utilization of Nutrients During Postnatal Development.* Pergamon Press, Oxford, 1966.

Hamashinma, Y.; Kishi, K.; and Tasaka, K.: Rickettsia-like bodies in infantile acute febrile mucocutaneous lymph node syndrome. *Lancet*, **2**:819, 1973.

Harbitz, F., and Raeder, J. G.: Atrophy of face and eyes (presenile cataract and "glaucoma") caused by symmetrical carotid affection. *Norsk. Mag. f. Laegevidensk*, **87**:529, 1926.

Hartroft, W. S.: Natural history of athermatous lesions. Unpublished data.

Hatch, F. T.; Reissell, P. K.; Poon-King, T. M. W.; Canellos, G. P.; Lees, R. S.; and Hagopian, L. M.: A study of coronary heart disease in young men. *Circulation*, **33**:679, 1966.

Heinzelmann, F., and Bagley, R. W.: Response to physical activity programs and their effects on health behavior. *Public Health Rep.*, **85**:905, 1970.

Hellerstein, H. K., et al.: Effects of physical activity: Patients and normal coronary prone subjects. *Minnesota Med.*, **52**:1335, 1969.

Holman, R. L.: Atherosclerosis—A pediatric nutrition problem? *Am. J. Clin. Nutr.*, **9**:565, 1961.

Holman, R. L., and Strong, J. P.: Analysis of juvenile atherosclerosis. *Circulation*, **8**:442, 1953.

Hood, B.; Sanne, H., Orndahl, G., Ahlstrom, M.; and Welin, G.: Long-term prognosis in essential hypercholesterolemia. The effect of strict diet. *Acta Med. Scand.*, **178**:161–73, 1965.

Hueper, W. C.: Arteriosclerosis. *Arch. Pathol.*, **39**:51, 117, 187, 1945.

Ikeda, M.: Immunologic studies on Takayasu's arteritis. *Jap. Circ. J.*, **30**:87, 1966.

Ito, I.: Aortitis syndrome, with reference to detection of antiaorta antibody from patient's sera. *Jap. Circ. J.*, **39**:75, 1966.

Jaffe, D.; Hartroft, W. S.; Manning, M.; and Eleta, G.: Coronary arteries in newborn children. *Acta Paediatr. Scand. Suppl.*, 219, 1971.

Jaffe, D., and Manning, M.: Unpublished observations, 1974.

James, F.; Glueck, C. J.; Fallat, R. W.; Millett, F.; and Kaplan, S.: Exercise electrocardiograms in normal and hypercholesterolemic children. Presented at Pediatric Research and American Pediatric Society Meeting, 1975.

Jokl, E., and Greenstein, J.: Fatal coronary sclerosis in a boy of 10 years. *Lancet*, **2**:659, 1944.

Kannel, W. B.; Castelli, W. P.; Gordon, T.; and McNamara, P. M.: Serum cholesterol, lipoproteins and the risk of coronary heart disease. *Ann. Intern. Med.*, **74**:1, 1971.

Katz, L. N.: Experimental atherosclerosis. *Circulation*, **5**:101, 1952.

Katz, L. N., and Stamler, J.: *Experimental Atherosclerosis.* Charles C Thomas, Publisher, Springfield, Ill., 1953.

Kaunitz, P. E.: Origin of the left coronary artery from pulmonary artery. *Am. Heart J.*, **33**:182, 1947.

Kawasaki, T.: Acute febrile mucocutaneous lymph node syndrome and sudden death (in Japanese). *Acta Paediatr. Jap.*, **75**:433, 1971.

Kawasaki, T.: Acute febrile mucocutaneous syndrome with lymph node involvement with specific desquamation of the fingers and toes in children (in Japanese). *Jap. J. Allerg.*, **16**:178, 1967.

Kawasaki, T., and Kousaki, F.: Febrile aculo-aculo-orocutaneoacrodesquamatous syndrome with or without acute nonsuppurative cervical lymphadenitis in infancy and childhood: Clinical observations of 50 cases (English abstr.). *Jap. J. Allerg.*, **16**:225, 1967.

Keay, A. J.; Oliver, M. F.; and Boyd, G. S.: Progeria and atherosclerosis. *Arch. Dis. Child.*, **30**:410, 1955.

Keith, J. D.; The anomalous origin of the left coronary artery from the pulmonary artery. *Am. J. Cardiol.*, **27**:149, 1959.

Keys, A.: Cholesterol, "giant molecules," and atherosclerosis. *JAMA*, **147**:1514, 1951.

Keys, A.: Human atherosclerosis and the diet. *Circulation*, **5**:115, 1952.

Keys, A.: Physical activity and the epidemiology of coronary heart disease. In Brunner, D., and Jokl, E. (eds.): *Medicine and Sport*, vol. 4: *Physical Activity and Aging.* University Park Press, Baltimore, 1970.

Kotz, O., and Manning, M. F.: Fatty streaks in the intima of arteries. *J. Pathol. Bact.* **16**:211, 1911.

Krikler, D. M., and Lewis, B.: Coronary artery disease in a young man with normal serum lipids. *Br. Heart J.*, **34**:1186, 1972.

Kuo, P. T.; Huang, N. N.; and Bassett, D. R.: The fatty acid composition of the serum chylomicrons and adipose tissue of children with cystic fibrosis of the pancreas. *J. Pediatr.*, **60**:394, 1962.

Kwiterovich, P. O., Jr.; Levy, R. I.; and Frederickson, D. S.: Neonatal diagnosis of familial type II hyperlipoproteinemia. *Lancet*, **1**:118, 1973.

Larsen, O. A., and Malmberg, R. O.: *Coronary Heart Disease and Physical Fitness.* University Press, Baltimore, 1971.

Leach, E. B.: Calcific arteriosclerosis of infancy. *Can. Med. Assoc. J.*, **73**:733, 1955.

Lee, J.; Freedom, R. M.; Williams, W. G.; Trusler, G. A.; and Mustard, W. T.: Anomalous origin of left coronary artery from the left pulmonary artery—Review of 11 cases and presentation of a new surgical technique (unpublished observations).

Leren, P.: The effect of plasma cholesterol lowering diet in male survivors of myocardial infarction. A controlled clinical trial. *Acta Med. Scand.*, Suppl. **466**:1, 1966.

Lev, M.; Craenen, J.; Lambert, E. C.: Infantile coronary sclerosis with atrioventricular block. *J. Pediatr.*, **70**:87, 1967.

Levy, R. I., et al.: Dietary and drug treatment of primary hyperlipoproteineumia. *Ann. Intern. Med.*, **77**:267, 1972.

McGill, H. C., Jr.: Fatty streaks in the coronary arteries and aorta. *Lab. Invest.*, **18**:100, 1968.

McGill, H. C., Jr.: The geographic pathology of atherosclerosis. *Lab. Invest.*, **18**:463, 1968.

McKenzie, A. D., and Robertson, H. R.: Arterial reconstruction (thromboendarterectomy) in arteriosclerotic vascular disease. *Surgery*, **36**:808, 1954.

McMillan, G. C.; Horlick, L.; and Duff, G. L.: Cholesterol content of aorta in relation to severity of atherosclerosis. *Arch. Pathol.*, **59**:285, 1955.

McNamara, J. J.; Molot, M. A.; Stremple, J. F.; and Cutting, R. T.: Coronary artery disease in combat casualties in Vietnam. *JAMA*, **216**:1185, 1971.

Macnamara, B. G. P.; Farr, K. T.; Mitra, A. K.; Lloyd, J. K.; and Fosbrooke, A. S.: Progeria case report with long-term studies of serum lipids. *Arch. Dis. Child.*, **45**:553, 1970.

Makous, N.; Freidman, S.; Yakovac, W.; and Maris, E. P.: Cardiovascular manifestations in progeria. Report of clinical and pathologic findings in a patient with severe arteriosclerotic heart disease and aortic stenosis. *Am. Heart J.*, **64**:334, 1962.

March, Z.; Jaegermann, K.; and Ciba, T.: Atherosclerosis and levels of serum cholesterol in postmortem investigations. *Am. Heart J.*, **63**:768, 1962.

Martorell-otzet, F., and Fabre, T.: El sindrome de obliteración de los troncos supraaórticos. *Med. Clin. Barcelona*, **2**:26, 1944.

Mason, J. K.: Asymptomatic disease of coronary arteries in young men. *Br. Med. J.*, **2**:1234, 1963.

Mawatari, S.; Iwashita, H.; and Kuroiwa, Y.: Familial hypo-3-lipoproteinemia. *J. Neurol. Sci.*, **16**:93, 1972.

Menten, M. L., and Fetterman, G. H.: Coronary sclerosis in infancy: report of three autopsied cases, two in siblings. *Am. J. Clin. Pathol.*, **18**:805, 1948.

Meyer, B. W.; Stefanski, G.; Stiles, O. R.; Hindsmith, G. G.; and Jones, J. P.: A method of defective surgical Rx of AOLCA. *J. Thorac. Cardiovasc. Surg.*, **56**:104, 1968.

Meyer, W. W., and Lind, J.: Calcifications of the carotid siphon—a common finding in infancy and childhood. *Arch. Dis. Child.*, **47**:355, 1972.

Miettinen, M.; Karvonen, M. J.; Turpeinen, O.; Elosuo, R.; and Paavilainen, E.: Effect of cholesterol-lowering diet on mortality from coronary heart disease and other causes. *Lancet*, **2**:835, 1972.

Miller, H.; Hirschman, A.; and Kraemer, D. M.: Calcium and magnesium content of albuminoid fraction of human aortae. *Arch. Pathol.*, **56**:607, 1953.

Minkowski, W. L.: Coronary arteries of infants. *Am. J. Med. Sci.*, **214**:623, 1947.

Mitchell, J. R., and Schwartz, C. J.: *Aortic Disease.* Blackwell Scientific Publications Ltd., Oxford, 1965, vol. 5, p. 87.

Mitchell, J. R., and Schwartz, C. J.: *The Localization of Arterial Plaques.* Blackwell Scientific Publications Ltd., Oxford, 1965, vol. 3, p. 50.

Mitchell, J. R., and Schwartz, C. J.: *Intramural Haemorrhage in the Aetiology and Pathogenesis of the Raised Arterial Plaque.* Blackwell Scientific Publications Ltd., Oxford, 1965, vol. 5, p. 313.

Montenegro, M. R., and Eggen, D. A.: Topography of atherosclerosis in the coronary arteries. *Lab. Invest.*, **18**:126, 1968.

Moon, H. D.: Coronary arteries in fetuses, infants and juveniles. *Circulation*, **16**:263, 1957.

Moran, J. J., and Becker, S. M.: Idiopathic arterial calcification of infancy. *Am. J. Clin. Pathol.*, **31**:517, 1959.

Morris, J. N.: Controlled trial of soya-bean oil in myocardial infarction. *Lancet*, **2**:693, 1968.

Morris, J. N., and Crawford, M. D.: Coronary heart disease and physical activity of work: Evidence of a national necropsy survey. *Br. Med. J.*, **2**:1485, 1968.

Morris, J. N.; Heady, J. A.; Raffle, P. A. B.; Roberts, C. G.; and Parks, J. W.: Coronary heart-disease and physical activity of work. *Lancet*, **2**:1053, 1953.

Morris, J. N.; Heady, J. A.; and Raffle, P. A. B.: Physique of London busmen: Epidemiology of uniforms. *Lancet*, **2**:569, 1956.

Morris, J. N.; Kagan, A.; Pattison, D. C.; Gardner, M. J.; and Raffle, P. A. B.: Incidence and prediction of ischaemic heart-disease in London busmen. *Lancet*, **2**:553, 1966.

Mustard, W. T.: *Pediatric Surgery*, ed. by Mustard, W. T.; Ravitch, M. M.; Snyder, W. H.; Welch, K. J.; Benson, C. D. Yearbook Medical Publishers, Chicago, 1964, vol. 1, p. 539.

Neches, W. H.; Mathews, R. A.; Park, S. C.; Lenox, C. C.; Zuberbuhler, J. R.; Siewers, R. D.; and Bahnson, H. T.: Anomalous origin of left coronary artery from the pulmonary artery—a new method of surgical repair. *Circulation*, **50**:582, 1974.

Nelson, A. M.: The effect of fat controlled diet on patients with coronary disease. *Med. Welt.*, 2063:8, 1965 and *Northwest. Med.*, **55**:643:9, 792:5, 874:8, 1956.

Nestor, J. A. O.; Folston, J. M.; and Howard, W. A.: Arteriosclerotic heart disease in infants. *Proc. Child. Hosp. Washington*, **9**:10, 1953.

Neufeld, H. N., and Vlodaver, Z.: Structural changes in the coronary arteries of infants. *Proc. Assoc. Eur. Paediatr. Cardiol.*, **4**:35, 1968.

Neufeld, H. N.; Wagenvoort, C. A.; and Edwards, J. E.: Coronary arteries in fetuses, infants, juveniles and young adults. *Lab. Invest.*, **11**:837, 1962.

Nikkila, E. A., et al.: Modulation of triglyceride kinetics by fructose versus glucose in the rat. *Scand. J. Clin. Lab. Invest.*, **18**:76, 1966.

Nora, J. J., and MacNamara, D. G.: Anomalies of the coronary arteries and coronary artery fistula. In Watson, H.: *Pediatric Cardiology.* C. V. Mosby Co., St. Louis, 1968.

Onouchi, Z.; Tanaka, K.; Shinkawa, M.; et al.: A study of acute febrile mucocutaneous lymph node syndrome: (1) Cardiac involvement (in Japanese). *Acta Pediatr. Jap.*, **77**:320, 1973.

Oppenheimer, E. H., and Esterly, J. R.: Cardiac lesions in hypertensive infants and children. *Arch. Pathol.*, **84**:318, 1967.

Page, I. H.: Atherosclerosis. An introduction. *Circulation*, **10**:1, 1954.

Parmley, L. F., Jr.: Introduction to supplement. National Workshop on Exercise in the Prevention, in the Evaluation, in the Treatment of Heart Disease. *J. S. C. Med. Assoc.*, **65**:Suppl. 1:i–ii, 1969.

Paterson, J. C.; Dyer, L.; and Armstrong, E. C.: Serum cholesterol levels in human atherosclerosis. *Can. Med. Assoc. J.*, **82**:6, 1960.

Pesonen, E.; Martimo, P.; and Rapola, J.: Histometry of the arterial wall. A new technique with the aid of automatic data processing. *Lab. Invest.*, **30**:550, 1974.

Pinsky, W. W.; Fagan, L. R.; Kraeger, R. R.; Mudd, J. F. G.; and Willman, V. L.: Anomalous left coronary artery—a report of 2 cases. *J. Thorac. Cardiovasc. Surg.*, **65**:810, 1973.

Radford, D. J.; Sondheimer, H. M.; Williams, G. J.; and Fowler, R. S.: Mucocutaneous lymph node syndrome with coronary artery aneurysm. *Am. J. Dis. Child.*, **130**:596, 1976.

Reiser, R., and Sidelman, Z.: Control of serum cholesterol homeostasis by cholesterol in the milk of the suckling rat. *J. Nutr.*, **102**:1009, 1972.

Report of Inter-Society Commission for Heart Disease Resources: Primary Prevention of the Atherosclerotic Diseases. *Circulation*, **42**:55, 1970.

Rich, A. R., and Gregory, J. E.: Experimental anaphylactic lesions of coronary arteries of "sclerotic" type, commonly associated with rheumatic fever and disseminated lupus erythematosus. *Bull. Johns Hopkins Hosp.*, **81**:312, 1947.

Rigal, R. D.; Lovell, F. W.; and Townsend, F. M.: Pathologic findings in the cardiovascular systems of military flying personnel. *Am. J. Cardiol.*, 6:19, 1960.

Robbin, S. R., and Dack, S.: Atherosclerosis: A review of the predisposing factors and the problems of treatment. *J. Mt. Sinai Hosp. N.Y.*, 22:34, 1955.

Roberts, F. B., and Fetterman, G. H.: Polyarteritis nodosa in infancy. *J. Pediatr.*, 63:519, 1963.

Robertson, E. D.: The nutrition of children and adolescents. *Nutrition*, 3:43, 1966.

Rota, A.: Surface studies on the arterial intima. M.S. thesis, in pathology, McGill University, 1953.

Rudel, L. L.; Morris, M. D.; and Felts, J. M.: The transport of exogenous cholesterol in the rabbit. *J. Clin. Invest.*, 51:2686, 1972.

Russell, A. S.; Zaragoza, A. J.; and Shea, R.: Mucocutaneous lymph node syndrome in Canada. *Can. Med. Assoc. J.*, 112:1210, 1975.

Sabiston, D. C.; Ross, R. S.; Oriley, J. M.; Gaertner, R. A.; Neill, C.; and Taussig, H. B.: Surgical management of congenital lesions of the coronary circulation. *Ann. Surg.*, 157:908, 1963.

Schornagel, H. E.: Internal thickening in the coronary arteries of infants. *Arch. Pathol.*, 62:427, 1956.

Schrade, W.; Boehle, E.; Biegler, R.; and Harmuth, E.: Fatty-acid composition of lipid fractions in diabetic serum. *Lancet*, 1:285, 1963.

Schreuder, O. B., and Constantino, J. G.: Cardiovascular system of the aging pilot. *Am. J. Cardiol.*, 6:26, 1960.

Scrimshaw, N. S.; Balsam, A.; and Arroyave, G.: The nutrition of children and adolescents. *Am. J. Clin. Nutr.*, 5:629, 1957.

Segal, M. M.: Treatment of familial hypercholesterolaemia in childhood. *Arch. Dis. Child.*, 43:748, 1968.

Seganti, A.: Myocardial infarction in children. *Proc. Assoc. Eur. Paediatr. Cardiol.*, 4:43, 1968.

Seltzer, C. C.: Overweight and obesity. Minnesota Symposium on Prevention in Cardiology, 1968.

Senderoff, E.; Slovis, A. J.; Moallem, A.; and Kahn, R. E.: Subclavian-coronary artery anastomosis. *J. Thorac. Cardiovasc. Surg.*, 71:142, 1975.

Slack, J., and Nevin, N. C.: Hyperlipidaemic zanthomatosis. *J. Med. Genet.*, 5:4, 1968.

Sladden, R. A.: Coronary arteriosclerosis and calcification in infancy. *J. Clin. Pathol.*, 5:175, 1952.

Somer, J. B.; Evans, G.; and Schwartz, C. J.: Influence of experimental aortic coarctation on the pattern of aortic Evans blue uptake in vivo. *Atherosclerosis*, 16:127, 1972.

Somer, J. B., and Schwartz, C. J.: Focal ^{3}H-cholesterol uptake in the pig aorta. *Atherosclerosis*, 13:293, 1971.

Somer, J. B., and Schwartz, C. J.: Focal ^{3}H-cholesterol uptake in the pig aorta. *Atherosclerosis*, 16:377, 1972.

Sprague, H. B., and Orgain, E. S.: Electrocardiographic study of cases of coronary occlusion proved at autopsy at Massachusetts General Hospital, 1914–1934. *N. Engl. J. Med.*, 212:903, 1935.

Stambul, J.: Atherosclerosis: interpretation of its mechanisms and new approach to prevention and treatment. *J. Einstein Med. Cent.*, 3:149, 1955.

Stamler, J.: Prevention of atherosclerotic coronary heart disease. In

Morgan Jones, A. (ed.): *Modern Trends in Cardiology—2.* Butterworths, Glasgow, 1969, vol. 6, pp. 88, 132.

Strong, J. P., and McGill, H. C., Jr.: The pediatric aspects of atherosclerosis. *J. Atheroscl. Res.*, 9:251, 1969.

Stryker, W. A.: Coronary occlusive disease in infants and in children. *Am. J. Dis. Child.*, 71:280, 1946.

Takayasu, M.: A case with peculiar changes of central retinal vessels. *Trans. Soc. Ophthal. Jap.*, 12:554, 1908.

Talbot, N. B., et al.: Progeria; clinical metabolic and pathologic studies on patient. *Am. J. Dis. Child.*, 69:267, 1945.

Talner, N. S.: Myocardial infarction in the newborn infant, European Pediatric Cardiology meeting, Rhodes, Greece, 1973.

Tamir, I.; Bojanower, Y.; Levtow, O.; Heldenberg, D.; Dickerman, Z.; and Werbin, B.: Serum lipids and lipoproteins in children from families with early coronary heart disease. *Arch. Dis. Child.*, 47:808, 1972.

Tamir, I.; Levtow, O.; Dickerman, Z.; and Werbin, B.: Serum lipids in children of families with a history of early coronary heart disease. *Arch. Dis. Child.*, 47:808, 1972.

Thomas, C. S.; Campbell, W. B.; Alford, W. C.; Burrus, G. R.; and Stoney, W. S.: Complete repair of anomalous origin of left coronary artery in the adult. *J. Thorac. Cardiovasc. Surg.*, 66:439, 1973.

Tingelstad, J. B.; Lower, R. R.; and Eldredge, W. J.: Anomalous origin of the right coronary artery from the main pulmonary artery. *Am. J. Cardiol.*, 39:670, 1972.

Traisman, H. S.; Limperis, N. M.; and Traisman, A. S.: Myocardial infarction due to calcification of arteries in infants. *A.M.A.J. Dis. Child.*, 91:34, 1956.

Turpeinen, O.; Miettinen, M.; Karvonen, M. J.: Roine, P.; Pekkarinen, M.; Lehtosuo, E. J.; and Alivirta, P.: Dietary prevention of coronary heart disease. A long-term experiment. *Am. J. Clin. Nutr.*, 21:255–76, 1968.

U.S. Department of Health, Education and Welfare: *Arteriosclerosis.* Report by National Heart and Lung Institute, June, 1971.

Venugopal, P., and Subramanian, S.: Anomalous origin of left coronary artery from the pulmonary artery. *Ann. Thorac. Surg.*, 19:451, 1975.

Vlodaver, Z.; Kahn, H. A.; and Neufeld, H. N.: The coronary arteries in early life in three different ethnic groups. *Circulation*, 39:541, 1969.

Wesselhoeft, H.; Fawcett, J. S.; and Johnston, A.: Anomalous origin of the left coronary artery from the pulmonary artery. *Circulation*, 38:403, 1968.

Williams, C. N., and Dickson, R. C.: Cholestyramine and medium-chain triglyceride in prolonged management of patients subjected to ileal resection or bypass. *Can. Med. Assoc. J.*, 107:626, 1972.

Wilmore, J. H., and Haskell, W. L.: Use of the heart rate-energy expenditure relationship in the individualized prescription of exercise. *Am. J. Clin. Nutr.*, 24:1186, 1971.

Wiese, H. F.; Bennet, M. J.; Braun, I. H. G.; Yamanaka, W.; and Coon, E.: Blood serum lipid patterns during infancy and childhood. *Am. J. Clin. Nutr.*, 18:155, 1966.

Yater, W. M., et al.: Coronary artery disease in men 18 to 39 years of age. Report of 866 cases, 450 with necropsy examinations. *Am. Heart J.*, 36:334, 1948.

62

Cardiac Tumors

Rodney S. Fowler and *John D. Keith*

CARDIAC tumors are uncommon in adults and extremely rare in infants and children. At The Hospital for Sick Children, Toronto, 22 children have been seen in the last 30 years with heart tumors, and during the same interval there were 11,500 necropsies and 683,300 hospital admissions. There were 12 primary heart tumors and ten secondary heart tumors excluding cases with leukemia.

PRIMARY TUMORS IN CHILDREN

Pathology

Pathologic Classification. Classification is as follows: (1) clinically unimportant, (2) rhabdomyomas, (3) intramural fibromas, (4) myxomas, (5) sarcomas, (6) pericardial tumors, and (7) miscellaneous tumors.

CLINICALLY UNIMPORTANT TUMORS OF THE HEART. These tumors cause no symptoms and are not clinically significant.

Congenital Blood Cysts. These are small red nodules that are often found on the heart valves of infants. They rarely exceed 1 mm in diameter and are usually multiple. They are most commonly seen on the atrial surfaces of the mitral and tricuspid valves, but are rarely found there or on other heart valves after six months of age. Congenital blood cysts have no clinical significance and presumably disappear after a few weeks or months of life.

Focal Myxomas. These are small lesions on the valves of stillborn and newborn infants, which are composed of loose myxomatous tissue. They are not found in older children and have no clinical significance.

Lambe's Excrescences. These are small villous projections on the free borders of the valves. They consist of subendocardial fibrous and elastic tissue covered with endocardium. Unlike the congenital blood cysts their incidence increases with age. They do not change in size and have no clinical significance.

RHABDOMYOMA. This is the most common primary heart tumor in children comprising 62 percent of the collected series of Bigelow (1954), Nadas (1968), Van der Hauwaert (1970), and Williams (1972) (89 of 144).

The youngest case reported occurred in a six-month fetus, and the oldest case was found in a 45-year-old female. Forty percent died in the first six months of life, 60 percent by the age of one year, and 80 percent by five years.

The nodules protrude through the epicardium in a gross heart specimen. On cut section there are circumscribed tumor masses, commonly 0.3 to 1 cm in diameter, in the myocardium. Histologically, the tumors are composed of swollen cardiac muscle fibers with protoplasmic strands extending from the nucleus to the periphery of the cells in a spiderlike pattern. Between these fibers are large vacuoles containing glycogen.

Half of the cases are associated with tuberous sclerosis. Of the 12 cases of primary heart tumor seen at The Hospital for Sick Children, Toronto, there were six examples of rhabdomyoma and three of these accompanied tuberous sclerosis (Williams, 1972).

INTRAMURAL FIBROMA. This tumor comprises 11 percent (16 of 144) of the combined experience of Bigelow (1954), Nadas (1968), Van der Hauwaert (1970), and Williams (1972). At The Hospital for Sick Children, Toronto, of the 12 primary tumors seen, four were ventricular fibromas. It has a predilection for infants and children, and in Geha's review (1967) of 36 reported cases in the literature 14 are under one year, 17 are from 1 to 15 years, and only five are over 15 years.

Usually, the lesion consists of a single large tumor in the myocardium of the left ventricle or interventricular septum. The cut surface presents a whorled appearance, which microscopically is composed of coarse bands of collagen-containing fibroblasts with strands of cardiac muscle between them. (See Figures 62–1, 62–2, and 62–3.)

MYXOMA. Among adults, the myxoma is the most common tumor of the heart and comprises 50 percent of all primary cardiac tumors. It has been reported in patients from the age of three months to the age of 68 years, the majority of cases occurring between 30 and 60 years. It usually arises by a pedicle from the atrial wall in the region of the fossa ovalis. Three-fourths of these tumors develop in the left atrium, and most of the rest appear in the right atrium.

This is a rare type of cardiac tumor in childhood comprising about 5 percent of primary cardiac tumors. Bigelow and associates (1954) could find in the literature only five instances of myxoma of the heart in children. Van der Hauwaert (1970) discussed three cases of atrial myxoma in their 22 pediatric primary heart tumors and Steinke and associates (1972) reported the successful removal of a left atrial myxoma from a nine-year-old child.

SARCOMA. Approximately 125 cases of primary sarcoma of the heart have been reported in the literature. In a review of the subject, Prichard in 1951 found that the age varied from three days to 79 years. Eighty percent of these cases were mural and only 20 percent polypoid. Nearly a third had metastasized to the lung, lymph nodes, liver, kidney, etc.

Very few of the reported cases have occurred in childhood. Engle and Glenn (1955) report the case of a rhabdomyosarcoma of the right ventricle with secondaries in the lung, mediastinum, and thymus. It occurred in a four-month-old boy who presented sudden onset of signs of congestive heart failure. The electrocardiogram showed elevation of the S-T segment in the left precordium and inversion of the T waves. At postmortem the tumor was found to have partly obstructed the lumen of the anterior descending branch of the left coronary artery. This case was diagnosed before death.

PERICARDIAL TUMORS. These account for up to 20 percent of cardiac tumors in children collected by Reynolds (1969) and Pernot (1968) and include teratomas, fibromas, lipomas, angiomas, and leiomyofibromas. Longino and Meeker (1953) have reported a malignant tumor of the pericardial sac of a three-month-old baby.

MISCELLANEOUS TUMORS. These include lipoma, hemangioma, lymphangioma, and congenital cyst.

Clinical Features

The clinical findings depend on the position of the tumor in the heart. It may be intramural, pericardial, or intracavitary.

Intramural Tumors. These heart tumors often grow slowly and cause no symptoms. The most recent patient with an intramural heart tumor seen at The Hospital for Sick Children, Toronto, had a

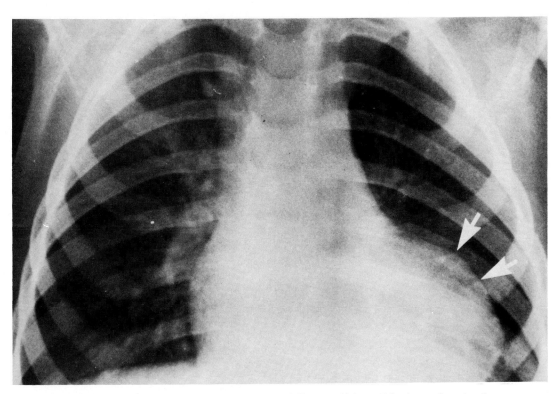

Figure 62-1. X-ray of the heart of two-year-old child with fibroma of left ventricle. *Arrows* show site of tumor.

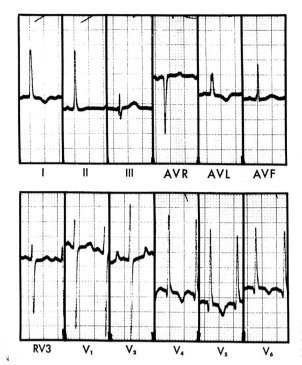

Figure 62-2. Electrocardiogram of two-year-old child with fibroma of left ventricle showing left ventricular hypertrophy with T wave inversion over the left side.

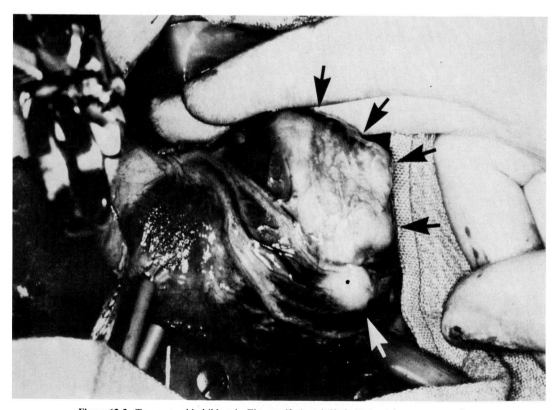

Figure 62-3. Two-year-old child as in Figures 62–1 and 62–2. Tumor shown at operation.

roentgenogram of his chest done because of a respiratory infection at one year of age and a mass projecting from his left ventricle was found. The discovery of an unusual cardiac shape on a routine chest roentgenogram is a common presenting complaint in patients with intramural cardiac tumors. In some adult patients calcification of the tumor can be seen on the "roentgen."

A significant heart murmur is heard if the tumor encroaches on the cardiac cavities. In Van der Hauwaert's (1970) review there were 14 intramural tumors and nine had a significant heart murmur. Shaher and associates (1971, 1972) reported four patients with tuberous sclerosis and cardiac rhabdomyoma and two had harsh murmurs, one typical of discrete subvalvular aortic stenosis. Rhabdomyoma is often multiple and 50 percent of cases occur with tuberous sclerosis. The neurologic findings of convulsions and mental retardation are more striking than the cardiac findings, but heart tumor should always be suspected in such patients.

Intramural tumors sometimes cause severe heart failure, particularly in infants. Of the 12 primary heart tumors seen at The Hospital for Sick Children, Toronto, all were intramural and five presented with severe heart failure at ten hours, two days, ten days, three months, and ten months.

The case reported from The Hospital for Sick Children by Williams and associates (1972) was originally seen for the assessment of a heart murmur. It was an innocent vibratory murmur, but in the routine investigation of the patient a mass in the left ventricle was seen in the roentgenogram (Figure 62–1) and the electrocardiogram revealed left ventricular hypertrophy and inverted T waves over the left ventricle (Figure 62–2). A left ventricular angiocardiogram revealed a mass in the free wall of the ventricle. At surgery, a fibroma measuring 5 by 3.5 cm was excised (Figure 62–3). The patient was seen two years afterward and he was well and the T waves over his left chest had become upright.

The electrocardiogram is often helpful in diagnosing intramural tumors. In the combined series of Williams et al. (1972) and Van der Hauwaert (1970) were 18 intramural tumors in patients who had had an electrocardiogram and all showed some abnormality. A hypertrophy pattern was common, occurring in 61 percent of cases (6 LVH, 3 RVH, 2 CVH, 1 LAH). Arrhythmias occurred in 39 percent including paroxysmal supraventricular tachycardia leading eventually to atrial fibrillation, ventricular extrasystoles (three cases), intermittent Wolff-Parkinson-White syndrome, intermittent ventricular tachycardia, one case of 2:1 atrioventricular block, and one case of complete atrioventricular block. There was one case of complete right bundle branch block in a child with a rhabdomyoma of the ventricular septum. Four cases had electrocardiograms that suggest myocardial infarction with wide, deep abnormal Q waves and S-T and T changes.

Pericardial Cysts and Tumors. These tumors cause an abnormal contour of the heart on the roentgenogram or a rapid pericardial effusion. Particularly in infants where 46 percent of intrapericardial teratomas occur (Reynolds et al., 1969), heart failure and tamponade are common. The effusion is profuse, recurrent, and is sometimes bloodstained. In Van der Hauwaert's series (1971) there were five pericardial teratomas of whom four had electrocardiograms. One was normal and the other three had low voltages consistent with pericardial effusion. Only two of Reynolds' series (1969) of 37 intrapericardial teratomas (all ages) were malignant. A persistent pericardial effusion in an infant should suggest a pericardial tumor.

Intracavity Tumors. The clinical picture in this group is often bizarre and includes such characteristics as sudden onset of dyspnea, loss of consciousness, congestive heart failure, cyanosis, shock, or death. In some cases these clinical features are precipitated by change of position. The murmur of mitral stenosis may be found without any preceding history of rheumatic fever, and such a murmur may change or disappear with change in body position. Embolic phenomena are found due to fragmentation either of the tumor itself or of a thrombus formed on the surface of the tumor. Intractable congestive heart failure not relieved by digitalis has been described.

An interesting example of myxoma of the left atrium in childhood is reported by Goldberg and associates (1952) in a three-year-old boy whose first symptom was transient right-sided hemiparesis. Subsequently he had two similar episodes, and on examination after his third attack mitral presystolic and apical systolic murmurs were heard for the first time. Van der Hauwaert (1971) reports two left atrial myxomas and one left ventricular myxoma.

Steinke et al. (1972) described a nine-year-old girl with mitral regurgitation, heart failure, and an elevated sedimentation rate. Left atrial myxoma was eventually diagnosed and successfully removed. These authors reviewed 23 cases reported in the literature of left atrial myxoma in children. They may present with embolic or constitutional symptoms and often have signs of mitral regurgitation.

When any of the signs suggestive of an intracavity tumor is found, a useful initial examination is echocardiography, particularly when the two-dimensional mode is used. Angiocardiography, however, remains a widely used and reliable diagnostic method.

An accurate diagnosis preoperatively is important because successful surgery depends on the proper approach for excision of the tumor.

Treatment

Successful removal of cardiac tumors in childhood is being reported more frequently than in the past. Van der Hauwaert (1971) notes eight survivals in his collected series of 22 cases. Two surgical successes are reported by Reynolds (1969), Geha (1967), and Simcha (1971), and one each by Williams (1972),

Thomson (1971), Shaher (1972), Longmire (1962), Beck (1942), Goldberg (1955), and Steinke (1972).

Recently at The Hospital for Sick Children, Toronto, another child of five years was investigated and found to have a heart tumor since the report of Williams (1972). At surgery, two fibromas of the free wall of the left ventricle were excised successfully and the child is now well.

Successful surgery depends on early diagnosis usually involving angiocardiography.

SECONDARY TUMORS IN CHILDREN

SECONDARY tumors are much more common in adults than primary tumors and are of academic interest rather than of clinical importance. In the pediatric age group, secondary tumors of the heart are rare. At The Hospital for Sick Children, Toronto, *ten* children with secondary tumors of the heart were seen, excluding cases of acute leukemia. The majority were sarcomas with three lymphosarcomas, one botryoid sarcoma from the cervix, one Ewing's sarcoma, and three nonspecific types. In addition, there were one nephroblastoma and one hepatoblastoma. One boy presented with signs of constrictive pericarditis due to a widespread thoracic sarcoma. Another boy had his hepatoblastoma removed at two years and then was well until four years later when he developed atrial fibrillation and heart failure and died with secondary tumor in his lungs and left atrium. The only other child with secondary heart tumor with cardiac symptoms had a Ewing's sarcoma discovered at seven months and treated with radiation and antitumor drugs. At one and one-half years a heart murmur was heard and an angiocardiogram revealed two pedunculated tumors, one in the right atrium and one in the right ventricle. The heart was radiated and an angiocardiogram was repeated two months later revealing no evidence of the tumors.

Acute leukemia often affects the heart. Roberts (1968) studied necropsies of 420 cases of leukemia of all ages and 69 percent of the patients had either focal myocardial hemorrhages or leukemic infiltrates in the heart. Despite these abnormalities few of the patients had any cardiac signs or symptoms. A few had chest pain due to pericarditis with thickening of the visceral and parietal pericardium due to leukemic infiltrates.

CONCLUSIONS

A CARDIAC tumor should be suspected if any of the following are present:

1. An unusual heart shape, particularly with a protrusion from the left ventricle.
2. An electrocardiogram in a child with abnormal wide deep Q waves and S-T deviations or abnormal T waves (infarct pattern).
3. Underlying disease such as leukemia, tuberous sclerosis, or a primary malignant tumor in some other organ.
4. An organic murmur that varies with body position.
5. Persistent pericardial effusion in an infant.

Angiocardiography is helpful in making the diagnosis. Spontaneous resolution can occur (Khattar et al., 1975).

REFERENCES

Beck, C. S.: An intrapericardial teratoma and a tumor of the heart: both removed operatively. *Ann. Surg.*, **116**:161, 1942.

Bigelow, N. H.; Klinger, S.; and Wright, A. W.: Primary tumours of the heart in infancy and childhood. *Cancer*, **7**:549, 1954.

Boyd, T. A. B.: Blood cysts on the heart valves of infants. *Am. J. Pathol.*, **25**:757, 1949.

Craig, J. M.: Congenital endocardial sclerosis. *Bull. Internat. A. M. Museums*, **30**:15, 1949.

Edlund, S., and Holradable, K. A.: Primary tumor of the heart. *Acta Paediatr.*, **46**:59, 1957.

Engle, M. A., and Glenn, F.: Primary malignant tumor of the heart in infancy. Case report and review of the subject. *Pediatrics*, **15**:562, 1955.

Geha, A. S.; Weidman, W. H.; Soule, E. H.; and McGoon, D. C.: Intramural ventricular cardiac fibroma. *Circulation*, **36**:427, 1967.

Goldberg, H. P.; Glenn, F.; Dotter, C. T.; and Steinberg, I.: Myxoma of the left atrium: diagnosis made during life with operative and postmortem findings. *Circulation*, **6**:762, 1952.

Goldberg, H. P., and Steinberg, I.: Primary tumours of the heart. *Circulation*, **11**:963, 1955.

Gross, P.: Concept of fetal endocarditis: a general review with a report of an illustrative case. *Arch. Pathol.*, **31**:163, 1941.

Gunzel, W.: Über Entstehung und Maufigkeit der Lambl'schen Exkeszenzen an den Herzklappen. *Beitr. Pathol. Anat.*, **91**:305, 1933.

James, V., and Stanfield, M.: A case of fibroma of the left ventricle in a child of four years. *Arch. Dis. Child.*, **30**:187, 1955.

Khattar, H.; Guerin, R.; Fouron, J-C.; Stanley, P.; Kratz, C.; and Davignon, A.: Les tumeurs cardiaques chez l'enfant. Rapport de 3 observations avec evolution spontanee favorable. *Arch. Mal. Coeur*, **68**:419, 1975.

Kidder, L. A.: Congenital glycogenic tumours of the heart. *Arch. Pathol.*, **49**:55, 1950.

Longino, L. A., and Meeker, I. A.: Primary cardiac tumours in infancy. *J. Pediatr.*, **43**:724, 1953.

Mago, P.: Intrathoracic neuroblastoma in a newborn infant. *J. Thorac. Cardiovasc. Surg.*, **45**:720, 1963.

Nadas, A. S., and Ellison, R. C.: Cardiac tumors in infancy. *Am. J. Cardiol.*, **21**:363, 1968.

Parks, F. R.; Adams, F.; and Longmire, W. P.: Successful excision of a left ventricular hamartoma. *Circulation*, **26**:1316, 1962.

Patterson, E. L., and Spink, M. S.: Congenital epicardial cyst. *J. Pathol. Bact.*, **76**:601, 1958.

Pernot, P. C.: Frisch, R.; Mathieu, P.; Olive, D.; and Vidailhet, M.: Les teratomes intrapericardiques du nourrissou. *Arch. Mal. Coeur*, **61**:546, 1968.

Prichard, R. W.: Tumours of the heart: review of the subject and report on one hundred and fifty cases. *Arch. Pathol.*, **51**:98, 1951.

Reynolds, J. R.; Donahue, J. K.; and Pearce, C. W.: Intrapericardial teratoma. *Pediatrics*, **43**:71, 1969.

Roberts, W. C.; Bodey, G. P.; and Wertlake, P. T.: The heart in acute leukemia: A study of 420 autopsy cases. *Am. J. Cardiol.*, **21**:388, 1968.

Shaher, R. M.; Farina, M.; Alley, R.; Hansen, P.; and Bishop, M.: Congenital subaortic stenosis in infancy caused by rhabdomyoma of the left ventricle. *J. Thorac. Cardiol. Surg.*, **62**:157, 1972.

Simcha, A.; Well, B. G.; Tynan, M. J.; and Waterston, D. J.: Primary cardiac tumors in childhood. *Arch. Dis. Child.*, **46**:508, 1971.

Steinberg, I.; Dotter, C. T.; and Glenn, F.: Myxoma of the heart: roentgen diagnosis during life in three cases. *Dis. Chest*, **24**:509, 1953.

Steinke, W. C.; Perry, L. W.; Gold, H. R.; McClenathan, J. E.; and Scott, L. P.: Left atrial myxoma in a child. *Pediatrics*, **49**:580, 1972.

Thomson, J. H.; Corliss, R. J.; Sellers, R. D.; Mooring, P. K.; and Wilson, W. J.: Left ventricular intramural fibroma. *Am. J. Cardiol.*, **28**:726, 1971.

Van der Hauwaert, L.: Cardiac tumors in infancy and childhood. *Proc. Assoc. Eur. Paediatr. Cardiol.*, **6**:31, 1970.

Von Recklinghausen: Ein Herz von einem Neugeborenen, welches mehrere theils noch aussen, theils noch den Höhlen prominierende Tumoren (Myomen) Trug. *Monatsschr. Geburtsch. Frauenkr.*, **20**:1, 1862.

Williams, W. G.; Trusler, G. A.; Fowler, R. S.; Scott, M. R.; and Mustard, W. T.: Left ventricular myocardial fibroma: A case report and review of cardiac tumors in children. *J. Pediatr. Surg.*, **7**:324, 1972.

Drugs and Dosages Useful in Heart Disease in Infancy and Childhood

Every effort has been made to ensure that the drug dosage schedules herein are accurate and in accord with the standards accepted at the time of publication. However the reader is cautioned to check the product information sheet included in the package of each drug and verify indications, contraindications and recommended dosages.

Acetylsalicylic Acid (Aspirin)	60 mg/kg of body weight total daily dose; given in 5 divided doses.
Adrenaline (Epinephrine)	1:1000 solution subcut. For infants: 0.1 ml For children: 0.1–0.5 ml.
Alcohol	For acute pulmonary edema, bubble O_2 through 50% ethyl alcohol to a mask; give for 5–10 min and repeat as necessary, with pauses of 10–15 min between each administration.
Aldomet	*See* Methyldopa.
Aminophylline	IM or IV: 3 mg/kg q.6h. Rectally: 6 mg/kg q.6h.

Antibiotics–Prophylactic Use

*Infective Endocarditis Prevention**

I. Dental procedures, oropharyngeal surgery, instrumentation of the respiratory tract.

Patients Tolerant of Penicillin

A. Children
1. Aqueous penicillin G 30,000 units/kg IM *mixed* with procaine penicillin G 600,000 units. Give 30 minutes to 1 hour prior to procedure. Follow with penicillin V 250 mg q. 6h. for 8 doses

or

2. Pencillin V 2.0 gm PO 30 min to 1 h. prior to procedure, then 500 mg q. 6h. for 8 doses. For children less than 30 kg use 1 gm and 250 mg.

B. Adults
1. Aqueous penicillin G 1 million units IM *mixed* with procaine penicillin G 600,000 units 30 minutes to 1 h. prior to procedure. Follow with penicillin V 500 mg PO q. 6h. for 8 doses

or

2. Penicillin V 2.0 gm PO 30 min to 1 h. prior to procedure. Follow with 250 mg q. 6h. for 8 doses.

Patients Sensitive to Penicillin

1. Erythromycin 20 mg/kg PO 1 to 2 h. prior to procedure, then 10 mg/kg q.6h. for 8 doses.

or

2. Vancomycin 20 mg/kg by IV infusion 30 min to 1 h. prior to procedure, then erythromycin 10 mg/kg PO q. 6h. for 8 doses.

1. Erythromycin 1.0 gm PO 1 to 2 h. prior to procedure, then 500 mg q. 6h. for 8 doses

or

2. Vancomycin 1.0 gm by IV infusion 30 min to 1 h. prior to procedure, then erythromycin 500 mg PO q. 6h. for 8 doses.

*Data from American Heart Association Committee Report. *Circulation*, **56**:139A, 1977.

II. Gastrointestinal and Genitourinary Procedures or Instrumentation

Patients Tolerant of Penicillin   *Patients Sensitive to Penicillin*

A. Children

Ampicillin 50 mg/kg IM or IV 30 min to 1 h.   Replace ampicillin with single dose of
prior to procedure *and* q. 8h. × 2.   vancomycin 20 mg/kg by IV infusion

                          plus   plus

Gentamicin 2.0 mg/kg IM or IV at same   Streptomycin 20 mg/kg IM.
time and q. 8h. × 2.

                           or

Streptomycin 20 mg/kg IM and q. 8h. × 2.

B. Adults

Ampicillin 1.0 gm IM or IV 30 min to 1 h.   Replace ampicillin with single dose of
prior to procedure *and* q. 8h. × 2.   vancomycin 1.0 gm by IV infusion

                          plus   plus

Gentamicin 1.5 mg/kg (maximum 80 mg)   Streptomycin 1.0 gm IM.
IM or IV at same time *and* q. 8h. × 2

                           or

Streptomycin 1.0 gm IM *and* q. 8h. × 2.

III. Patients with prosthetic valves

Should receive streptomycin (as above) in addition to penicillin or vancomycin (in patients sensitive to penicillin).

Rheumatic Fever (Prevention of Recurrences) *

Sulfadiazine	By mouth:	0.5 gm daily for patients less than 30 kg. 1.0 gm daily for patients over 30 kg.
Penicillin G	By mouth:	200,000 to 250,000 units b.i.d.
Benzathine penicillin G		Intramuscular injections: 1,200,000 units, monthly.
Erythromycin	By mouth:	for patients *sensitive to both penicillin and sulfonamides*: 250 mg b.i.d.
Tetracycline	Not indicated.	

Apresoline	*See* Hydralazine.
Atropine	0.01 mg/kg/day; may repeat q.4–6h.
Benadryl	*See* Diphenhydramine KCl.
Calcium Gluconate	PO: 5–10 gm/day. IV: 0.5–1.0 gm in 2–5 % solution. Must be given very slowly, preferably with a stethoscope on the heart to watch for possible cardiac arrest. May be repeated q.4h., if indicated. Small doses may be given IV during cardiac surgery to stimulate cardiac contraction: 30 mg at a time to small babies; 0.1–0.2 gm to older children. During exchange transfusion, 10 ml of 2 % calcium gluconate is given IV for each 100 ml of citrated blood to maintain an adequate ionized calcium content of the blood.

* Data from American Heart Association Committee Report. *Circulation*, **55**; 223, 1977.

Chloral Hydrate	Capsule: 250 and 500 mg. Elixir: 300 mg/5 ml. Suppository: 300 mg. Dose: 20–40 mg/kg (max. 1 gm) q.6–8h. PO or rectal.
Chlorothiazide (Diuril)	Tab.: 250–500 mg. 10 mg/kg b.i.d.
Chloropromazine Mixture (Largactil Mixture, Thorazine Mixture, CM₃)	1 ml contains 6.25 mg of promethazine (Phenergan), 6.25 mg of chlorpromazine (Largactil), and 25 mg of meperidine (Demerol).

Chloropromazine Mixture — Sedation for cardiac catheterization:

{ 1 ml/10 kg given deeply IM 1 h. before procedure, to a maximum of 2 ml. In cyanosed children or infants weighing less than 5 kg, give one half the calculated dose. Not to be given to neonates. }

Corticosteroids

Type	Relative Dose Anti-inflammatory Effects	Preparations
Cortisone	25.0 mg	Tab: 5, 10, 25 mg IM: susp. 25 or 50 mg/ml
Hydrocortisone	20.0 mg	Tab: 5, 10, 20 mg IM or IV: vial 100 mg Topical: 0.5, 1.0, 2.5% Intra-articular: 25 mg/ml
Prednisone	5.0 mg	Tab.: 1, 2.5, 5 mg
Prednisolone	4.0 mg	Tab.: 1, 2.5, 5 mg IM or IV: 10, 20 mg/ml Intra-articular: 10–25 mg Topical: 0.1–0.5%
Methylprednisolone	4.0 mg	Tab.: 4 mg
Triamcinolone	4.0 mg	Tab.: 1, 2, 4 mg
Dexamethasone	0.75 mg	Tab.: 0.75 mg
Betamethasone	0.5 mg	Tab.: 0.5 mg

Cortisone dosage varies with patient and disease. Average dose for active treatment is 10 mg/kg/day up to 300 mg daily in 4 or more divided doses. IM dose is the same, given b.i.d. or daily. Maintenance therapy may range 5–75 mg or more daily. Replacement therapy in adrenal hyperplasia or Addison's disease is usually 25–75 mg daily. The dose of other corticosteroids can be calculated from the table. Hydrocortisone Na succinate (Solu-Cortef)—IV in emergencies 15–100 mg stat. The daily dose is then added to the intravenous solutions or given q.4–6h. IV until oral therapy can be started.

Coumadin	*See* Warfarin Sodium.
Demerol	*See* Meperidine.
Diazepam (Valium)	IV: 0.1 mg/kg.
Diazoxide (Hyperstat)	IV rapid push: 5–10 mg/kg.

Digitalis Preparations   *See also* Chapter 10.

	DIGITALIZATION			MAINTENANCE THERAPY		
DRUG	*Route*	*Age*	*Total Dose in 24 Hours*	*Route*	*Age*	*Total Dose in 24 Hours*
Digoxin	Oral	Under 2 yr	0.05 mg/kg	Oral*	Under 2 yr	0.01 mg/kg
		Over 2 yr	0.04 mg/kg		Over 2 yr	0.008 mg/kg
	Intravenous or intramuscular	Under 2 yr	0.04 mg/kg			
		Over 2 yr	0.03 mg/kg			
Digitoxin	Oral	Under 2 yr	0.035 mg/kg	Oral	Under 2 yr	0.0035–0.007 mg/kg
		Over 2 yr	0.02 mg/kg	Over	Over 2 yr	0.002–0.004 mg/kg
	Intravenous or intramuscular	Under 2 yr	} 0.02 mg/kg			
		Over 2 yr				
Lanatoside C		Under 2 yr	0.03 mg/kg			
		Over 2 yr	0.01–0.02 mg/kg			

The digitalizing dose should be given in divided doses over 24 hours unless an emergency arises. The lower
 dose is less likely to produce toxicity than the larger dose.
* Digoxin is best administered by dividing the maintenance dose into two and giving one-half in the morning
 and one-half in the evening.

Dilantin   *See* Phenytoin Sodium.

**Dimenhydrinate
(Dramamine,
  Gravol)**
PO: 50-mg tablets.
     12.5 mg/4 ml elixir.
IM: 50 mg/ml.
IV: 10 mg/ml.
Rectal: 100-mg suppository.
Dose: 1 mg/kg q.6h.
Rectal: twice oral dose.

**Diphenhydramine HCl
(Benadryl)**
PO: 25- and 50-mg capsules.
Elixir: 10 mg/4 ml
Dose: 1–3 mg/kg/q.6h.
Adult: 25–50 mg q.6h.

Diuril   *See* Chlorothiazide.

Dopamine   IV drip: 2–3 mcg/kg/min to a maximum of 10 mcg/kg/min.

Dramamine   *See* Dimenhydrinate.

**Edrophonium Chloride
(Tensilon)**   0.2 mg/kg IV, give $\frac{1}{5}$ of dose slowly in 1 min; if tolerated, give remainder.

Epinephrine   *See* Adrenaline.

Ethacrynic Acid
Infants' single PO dose: 1–2.5 mg/kg.
IV: 0.5–1.0 mg/kg.

**Furosemide
(Lasix)**
PO: 1–2 mg/kg/day.
IV: 1–2 mg/kg/dose.

Gravol   *See* Dimenhydrinate.

Guanethedine	PO: 0.2 mg/kg/day in 3–4 doses; may increase weekly to 3–4 times dose until desired effect is achieved.
Heparin	10-ml vial, 1000 IU/ml. 100 units = 1 mg. *Initial dose:* 0.5 mg/kg/dose q.1h. IV drip: heparin diluted 10 IU/ml; clotting time then checked, and further heparin given to maintain clotting time at 15–20 min.
Hydralazine	Initial PO dose: 0.75 mg/kg/day, divided q.6h.; may increase to 7.5 mg/kg/day over 3 weeks if necessary. If given above IM or IV: 1.7–3.5 mg/kg/day, divided q.6h.
Hyperstat	*See* Diazoxide.
Inderal	*See* Propranolol.
Indomethacin (Indocin)	0.1 mg/kg orally.
Iron	
Ferric and Ammonium Citrate	0.2 gm (2 ml of 10% solution)/kg of body weight/day; may be added to the full day's formula for infants, or given in divided doses in fruit juice.
Ferrous Sulfate	Up to 2 yr: 0.25–0.4 gm/day in divided doses. 2–6 yr: 0.4–0.5 gm/day. Over 6 yr: 0.6–0.8 gm/day.
Isoproterenol (Isuprel)	Sublingually: 5–10 mg 3 or 4 times a day. Subcut.: 0.5–1.0 mg. IV: 1–4 mcg/min as constant infusion.
Kayexalate	Rectal: 1.0 gm/kg.
Lanoxin	*See* Digitalis Preparations.
Largactil Mixture	*See* Chlorpromazine Mixture.
Lasix	*See* Furosemide.
Levophed	*See* Norepinephrine.
Lidocaine	2% solution Slow IV: stat. 0.5–1.0 mg/kg. Continuous infusion: 20–40 mcg/kg/min (maximum total dose = 5 mg/kg).
Meperidine (Demerol)	Subcut. or PO: 1 mg/kg q.4–6h. Supplied: tablets, 50 mg solution, 60 mg/ml
Methyldopa (Aldomet)	PO: 10–60 mg/kg/day, divided q.8–q.12h. IV: 20 mg/kg/day, divided q.6h. PO: 250 mg/day in 3 doses; increase to 750 mg/day. IV: 20–40 mg/kg/day in 3–4 doses.
Methylene Blue	1–2 mg/kg or 0.1–0.2 ml/kg or 1% solution.
Morphine	0.2 mg/kg (maximum dose, 15 mg).
Nallorphine (Nalline)	IV or IM: 0.1–0.2 mg/kg/dose.

Narloxone (Narcan)	For children: 5 mcg, single dose. For adolescents: 0.4 mg/dose, IV q.3 min until effective.
Nitroprusside	*See* Sodium Nitroprusside.
Norepinephrine (Levophed)	By IV infusion only: use 1.0 ml of 0.2% solution in 250 ml; infuse at 0.5 ml/min; titrate dose with blood pressure. Slough results if interstitial.
Paraldehyde	PO, IM, and rectal: 0.2 ml/kg up to 10 ml. IV: 0.1 ml/kg diluted to 5% with IV solution.
Phenytoin Sodium (Dilantin)	IV: slow push: 1–5 mg/kg.
Procainamide HCl (Pronestyl)	PO: 30–50 mg/kg/24 h.; divide into 4–6 doses/24 h. IV: Emergency only, 3–8 mg/kg at rate not over 0.5–1.0 mg/kg/min, continuous ECG and BP q.1 min. 2.0 mg/kg/dose in D5W IV slowly over 5 min.
Propranolol (Inderal)	IV: 0.05–0.15 mg/kg. PO (infants): 1.0 mg/kg/day in three doses.
Prostaglandin E$_1$ (under investigational use only)	0.1 mcg/kg/min infused intra-arterially proximal to the patent ductus arteriosus.
Protamine Sulfate	1.0 mg for each 1.0 mg of heparin given in previous 4 hours, up to 50 mg q.4–6h.
Quinidine Sulfate	4 mg/kg q.2h. for 4 or 5 doses.
Reserpine (Serpasil)	PO: 0.02 mg/kg/day. IM: 0.07 mg/kg/dose q.4–6h.
Sodium Nitroprusside	5–10 mcg/kg/min; titrate dose with blood pressure.
Tensilon	*See* Edrophonium Chloride.
Thorazine	*See* Chlorpromazine Mixture.
Valium	*See* Diazepam.
Vitamin K$_1$ (Phylloquinone, Mephytone)	5–10 mg IV as single dose for a child.
Warfarin Sodium (Coumadin)	Titrate according to prothrombin time to twice the control value.

INDEX